KU-740-123

Neurology in
Clinical Practice

www.nicp.com

is the Internet companion to *Neurology in Clinical Practice*, Third Edition.
Inside the back cover of Volume I, you will find your unique user name
and password, which will allow you to access all of the online features:

- continuous updates by contributors and editors
- powerful search capabilities
- full-color photos
- reference linking to Medline abstracts
- audio and video clips

Library
Stepping Hill Hospital
Poplar Grove
Stockport SK2 7JE

This book is to be returned
the last date

- 3 APR 2006

616.8 BRA

Volume II

Neurology in Clinical Practice

The Neurological Disorders

Third Edition

Edited by Walter G. Bradley, D.M., F.R.C.P.
Professor and Chairman, Department of Neurology,
University of Miami School of Medicine;
Chief, Neurology Service,
University of Miami–Jackson Memorial Medical Center

Robert B. Daroff, M.D.
Chief of Staff and Senior Vice President for Academic Affairs,
University Hospitals of Cleveland;
Professor of Neurology and Associate Dean,
Case Western Reserve University School of Medicine, Cleveland

Gerald M. Fenichel, M.D.
Professor of Neurology and Pediatrics and Chairman, Department of
Neurology, Vanderbilt University School of Medicine, Nashville, Tennessee;
Neurologist-in-Chief, Vanderbilt University Hospital and
Vanderbilt Children's Hospital, Nashville

C. David Marsden, D.Sc., F.R.C.P., F.R.S.
Professor of Neurology, University Department of Neurology,
The National Hospital for Neurology and Neurosurgery, London

With 152 contributing authors

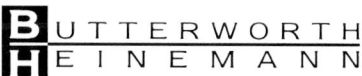

Boston   Oxford   Singapore   Auckland   Johannesburg   Melbourne   New Delhi

Copyright © 2000 by Butterworth–Heinemann

 A member of the Reed Elsevier group

All rights reserved.

No part of this publication may be reproduced, stored in a retrieval system, or transmitted in any form or by any means, electronic, mechanical, photocopying, recording, or otherwise, without the prior written permission of the publisher.

Every effort has been made to ensure that the drug dosage schedules within this text are accurate and conform to standards accepted at time of publication. However, as treatment recommendations vary in the light of continuing research and clinical experience, the reader is advised to verify drug dosage schedules herein with information found on product information sheets. This is especially true in cases of new or infrequently used drugs.

 Recognizing the importance of preserving what has been written, Butterworth–Heinemann prints its books on acid-free paper whenever possible.

 Butterworth–Heinemann supports the efforts of American Forests and Global ReLeaf program in its campaign for the betterment of trees, forests, and our environment.

Library of Congress Cataloging-in-Publication Data

Neurology in clinical practice / edited by Walter G. Bradley ... [et al.] ; with 152 contributing authors. --3rd ed.

    p.   cm.

    Includes bibliographical references and index.

    Contents: v. 1. Principles of diagnosis and management -- v. 2. The neurological disorders.

        ISBN 0-7506-9973-6 (set). -- ISBN 0-7506-7205-6 (v. 1). -- ISBN 0-7506-7212-9 (v. 2)

    1. Neurology.   2. Nervous system--Diseases.   I. Bradley, W. G. (Walter George)

    [DNLM: 1. Nervous System Diseases. 2. Diagnostic Techniques, Neurological. WL 140 N493 2000]

    RC346.N4535   2000

    616.8--dc21

    DNLM/DLC

    for Library of Congress   99-31264

                                     CIP

British Library Cataloguing-in-Publication Data

A catalog record for this book is available from the British Library.

The publisher offers discounts on bulk orders of this book. For information, please write:

Manager of Special Sales
Butterworth–Heinemann
225 Wildwood Avenue
Woburn, MA 01801–2041
Tel: 781-904-2500
Fax: 781-904-2620

For information on all Butterworth–Heinemann medical publications available, contact our World Wide Web home page at: http://www.bh.com

10 9 8 7 6 5 4

Printed in the United States of America

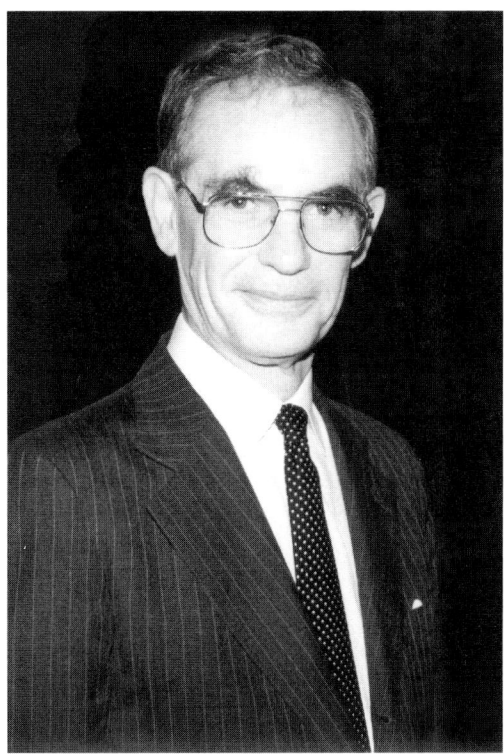

C. David Marsden (1938–1998)

We were in the final stages of receiving the manuscripts for the third edition of *Neurology in Clinical Practice* when we learned of the tragic death of David Marsden on 29 September 1998. For us, as editors and publisher of *Neurology in Clinical Practice*, David's death is a very personal loss, and for that reason, we dedicate this book to his memory.

David was with us from the very inception of *Neurology in Clinical Practice*. We first asked him to join us because of his prodigious knowledge of movement disorders, but we came to rely on him for his broad understanding of the whole of neurology.

From the beginning, we all had the same burning desire to write a textbook of neurology for those in training that would be more than just a description of the neurological diseases, their causes, and treatments. Neurology is a discipline in which clinical skills and experience are more important than a deep understanding of the basic neurosciences. That is not to minimize the importance of neuroscience research, for all the editors based our careers on combining neuroscience research with clinical practice. For no one was this more true than for David. Nevertheless, the clinical skills of lesion localization and disease recognition are of crucial importance to being a good neurologist. These skills come from having outstanding mentors, a keen power of observation, an inquiring mind, and experience. Again, for no one was this more true than for David. He wanted to pass on the wisdom he had derived from many years dedicated to the care of patients. The first section of *Neurology in Clinical Practice* embodies much of the flair that David brought to this work.

We had too little time with David, even though we produced three editions of a large two-volume textbook over a 10-year period. We spent more time communing by letter and later by e-mail. However, it was our editorial board meetings that provided a rare insight into David's genius. He was a man of relatively few spoken words, even though he was so prolific in his writings. He would often sit back and listen to the discussion in silence and would then make the incisive and definitive comment for which we had all been searching.

This third edition of *Neurology in Clinical Practice* was developed and produced almost entirely using electronic technology and the Internet. The development of the Internet companion to the textbook (www.nicp.com) expands our ability to teach clinical neurology by allowing us to provide clips of audiotapes and videotapes that users can download, as well as ongoing updates of the text and references and interaction with readers. David was at the forefront of teaching with audiovisual aids. For his many accomplishments, we and our patients owe David an undying debt.

Walter G. Bradley
Robert B. Daroff
Gerald M. Fenichel
Susan F. Pioli, Director of Medical Publishing

Contents

Volume II   The Neurological Disorders

CONTENTS xi

Contributing Authors

Michael J. Aminoff, M.D., F.R.C.P.
Professor of Neurology, University of California, San Francisco, School of Medicine; Attending Physician, Department of Neurology, Medical Center at the University of California, San Francisco
55A. Neurological Complications of Systemic Disease: In Adults; 64A. Effects of Toxins and Physical Agents on the Nervous System: Effects of Occupational Toxins on the Nervous System; 64E. Effects of Toxins and Physical Agents on the Nervous System: Effect of Physical Agents on the Nervous System

Lisa C. Arguello, M.Ed., C.C.C.-A.
Clinical Audiologist, Wake Forest University Baptist Medical Center, Winston-Salem, North Carolina
19. Hearing Loss and Tinnitus without Dizziness or Vertigo; 42. Neuro-Otology

Mario F. Mendez Ashla, M.D., Ph.D.
Associate Professor of Neurology and Psychiatry, University of California, Los Angeles, UCLA School of Medicine; Director, Neurobehavior Unit, The Veterans Administration Greater Los Angeles Healthcare System
4. Delirium

Viken L. Babikian, M.D.
Professor of Neurology, Boston University School of Medicine
38D. Neuroimaging: Ultrasound Imaging of the Cerebral Vasculature

Alberto O. Barroso, M.D.
Clinical Associate Professor of Internal Medicine, Baylor College of Medicine, Houston; Associate Medical Director, Digestive Disease Department, The Methodist Hospital, Houston
13. Difficulties with Speech and Swallowing

Roy W. Beck, M.D., Ph.D.
Director, Jaeb Center for Health Research, Tampa, Florida
15. Abnormalities of the Optic Nerve and Retina

Joseph R. Berger, M.D.
Professor and Chairman of Neurology and Professor of Internal Medicine, University of Kentucky College of Medicine, and Kentucky Clinic, Lexington
5. Clinical Approach to Stupor and Coma

José Biller, M.D.
Professor and Chairman, Department of Neurology, Indiana University School of Medicine; Chief, Neurology Services, Department of Neurology, Indiana University Medical Center, Indianapolis
57A. Vascular Diseases of the Nervous System: Ischemic Cerebrovascular Disease

Thomas D. Bird, M.D.
Professor of Neurology and Medicine, University of Washington School of Medicine, Seattle; Neurologist, Geriatrics Research Education and Clinical Center, Veterans Administration Medical Center, Seattle
45. Clinical Neurogenetics

Thomas P. Bleck, M.D., F.C.C.M.
The Louise Nerancy Professor of Neurology and Professor of Neurological Surgery and Internal Medicine, University of Virginia School of Medicine, Charlottesville; Director, Neuroscience Intensive Care Unit, University of Virginia Health Sciences Center, Charlottesville
52. Principles of Neurointensive Care

Hans-Georg O. Bock, M.D., Ph.D., F.A.C.M.
Associate Professor, University of Mississippi School of Medicine, Jackson; Division Chief of Preventive Medicine, University of Mississippi Medical Center, Jackson
68. Inborn Errors of Metabolism of the Nervous System

E. Peter Bosch, M.D.
Professor of Neurology, Mayo Medical School, Rochester, Minnesota; Consultant in Neurology, Mayo Clinic Scottsdale, Scottsdale, Arizona
80. Disorders of Peripheral Nerves

Brian C. Bowen, Ph.D., M.D.
Associate Professor of Radiology, University of Miami School of Medicine; Attending Radiologist, University of Miami–Jackson Memorial Medical Center
38B. Neuroimaging: Computed Tomographic and Magnetic Resonance Vascular Imaging

Walter G. Bradley, D.M., F.R.C.P.
Professor and Chairman, Department of Neurology, University of Miami School of Medicine; Chief, Neurology Service, University of Miami–Jackson Memorial Medical Center
1. Diagnosis of Neurological Disease; 36. Laboratory Investigations in Diagnosis and Management of Neurological Disease; 49. Management of Neurological Disease

Michael H. Brooke, M.B., B.Ch., F.R.C.P.C.
Professor of Neurology, University of Alberta Faculty of

Medicine, Edmonton, Alberta, Canada; Neurologist, University of Alberta Hospitals, Edmonton

29. Proximal, Distal, and Generalized Weakness; 83. Disorders of the Skeletal Muscle

Paul Brown, M.D.
Senior Research Scientist, Laboratory of Central Nervous System Studies, National Institute of Neurological Disorders and Stroke, National Institutes of Health, Bethesda, Maryland

59F. Infections of the Nervous System: Transmissible Spongiform Encephalopathies

Joseph Bruni, M.D., F.R.C.P.C.
Associate Professor of Medicine, University of Toronto Faculty of Medicine; Consultant Neurologist, St. Michael's Hospital, Toronto

2. Episodic Impairment of Consciousness

Thomas N. Byrne, M.D.
Clinical Professor of Neurology and Internal Medicine, Yale University School of Medicine, New Haven, Connecticut; Assistant Chief of Neurology, Yale–New Haven Medical Center

28. Paraplegia and Spinal Cord Syndromes

David J. Capobianco, M.D.
Assistant Professor of Neurology, Mayo Medical School, Rochester, Minnesota; Consultant in Neurology, Mayo Clinic Jacksonville, Jacksonville, Florida

73. Headache and Other Craniofacial Pain

David A. Chad, M.D.
Professor of Neurology and Pathology, University of Massachusetts Medical School, Worcester; Attending Neurologist, University of Massachusetts Medical Center, Worcester

79. Disorders of Nerve Roots and Plexuses

Tanuja Chitnis, M.D.
Fellow in Neurology, Harvard Medical School and Brigham and Women's Hospital, Boston

46. Neuroimmunology

Sudhansu Chokroverty, M.D.
Professor of Neurology, New York Medical College, Valhalla, New York; Associate Chairman of Neurology, Chairman, Division of Neurophysiology, and Director, Center of Sleep Medicine, Saint Vincents Hospital and Medical Center, New York

6. Excessive Daytime Somnolence; 72. Sleep Disorders

Michael E. Cohen, M.D.
Chairman of Neurology and Professor of Neurology and Pediatrics, State University of New York at Buffalo School of Medicine and Biomedical Sciences, Buffalo

58. Primary and Secondary Tumors of the Central Nervous System: Introduction; 58B. Primary and Secondary Tumors of the Central Nervous System: Molecular Biology of Nervous System Tumors; 58C. Primary and Secondary

Tumors of the Central Nervous System: Clinical Presentation and Therapy of Nervous System Tumors; 58D. Primary and Secondary Tumors of the Central Nervous System: Clinical Presentation and Therapy for Spinal Tumors; 58E. Primary and Secondary Tumors of the Central Nervous System: Clinical Presentation and Therapy of Peripheral Nerve Tumors; 58G. Primary and Secondary Tumors of the Central Nervous System: Quality of Life and Late Effects of Treatment

Paul E. Cooper, M.D., F.R.C.P.C.
Associate Professor of Neurology, University of Western Ontario Faculty of Medicine, London, Ontario, Canada; Chief of Clinical Neurological Sciences, St. Joseph's Health Centre, London

48. Neuroendocrinology

John R. Corboy, M.D.
Assistant Professor of Neurology, University of Colorado School of Medicine, Denver; Staff Neurologist, University of Colorado Health Sciences Center, Denver

47. Neurovirology

Jody Corey-Bloom, M.D., Ph.D.
Associate Professor of Neurosciences, University of California, San Diego, School of Medicine and University of California Medical Center, La Jolla

59C. Infections of the Nervous System: Fungal Infections

Terry A. Cox, M.D.
Assistant Consulting Professor of Ophthalmology, Duke University Medical Center, Durham, North Carolina

17. Pupillary and Eyelid Abnormalities

Thomas O. Crawford, M.D.
Associate Professor of Neurology and Pediatrics, Johns Hopkins University School of Medicine, Baltimore; Child Neurologist, John Hopkins Hospital, Baltimore

31. The Floppy Infant

Robert B. Daroff, M.D.
Chief of Staff and Senior Vice President for Academic Affairs, University Hospitals of Cleveland; Professor of Neurology and Associate Dean, Case Western Reserve University School of Medicine, Cleveland

1. Diagnosis of Neurological Disease; 3. Falls and Drop Attacks; 17. Pupillary and Eyelid Abnormalities; 36. Laboratory Investigations in Diagnosis and Management of Neurological Disease; 49. Management of Neurological Disease; 61. Anoxic and Ischemic Encephalopathies

David M. Dawson, M.D.
Professor of Neurology, Harvard Medical School and Brigham and Women's Hospital, Boston

60. Multiple Sclerosis and Other Inflammatory Demyelinating Diseases of the Central Nervous System

W. Dalton Dietrich, Ph.D.
Kinetic Concepts Distinguished Chair in Neurosurgery and
Professor of Neurological Surgery, Neurology, and Cell Biology and Anatomy, University of Miami School of Medicine; Scientific Director, The Miami Project to Cure
Paralysis, University of Miami School of Medicine
*56A. Trauma of the Nervous System: Basic Neuroscience
of Neurotrauma*

Bruce H. Dobkin, M.D.
Professor of Neurology, University of California, Los Angeles, UCLA School of Medicine
54. Principles of Neurological Rehabilitation

David W. Dodick, M.D.
Assistant Professor of Neurology, Mayo Medical School,
Rochester, Minnesota; Consultant in Neurology, Mayo
Clinic, Rochester
73. Headache and Other Craniofacial Pain

Sean P. Donahue, M.D., Ph.D.
Assistant Professor of Ophthalmology, Neurology, and Pediatrics, Vanderbilt University School of Medicine, Nashville,
Tennessee
40. Neuro-Ophthalmology: Ocular Motor System

Patricia K. Duffner, M.D.
Professor of Neurology and Pediatrics, State University of
New York at Buffalo School of Medicine and Biomedical
Sciences, Buffalo; Attending Physician in Child Neurology,
Children's Hospital of Buffalo
*58C. Primary and Secondary Tumors of the Central Ner-
vous System: Clinical Presentation and Therapy of Nervous
System Tumors; 58G. Primary and Secondary Tumors of
the Central Nervous System: Quality of Life and Late Ef-
fects of Treatment*

Ronald G. Emerson, M.D.
Associate Professor of Neurology, Columbia University
College of Physicians and Surgeons, New York; Associate
Attending Neurologist, Columbia Presbyterian Medical
Center, New York
*37A. Clinical Neurophysiology: Electroencephalography
and Evoked Potentials*

Owen B. Evans, M.D.
Professor and Chairman of Pediatrics, University of Mississippi School of Medicine, Jackson
68. Inborn Errors of Metabolism of the Nervous System

Martha J. Farah, Ph.D.
Professor of Psychology, University of Pennsylvania,
Philadelphia
*11B. Cognitive-Motor Disorders, Apraxias, and Ag-
nosias: Agnosias*

Todd E. Feinberg, M.D.
Associate Professor of Neurology and Psychiatry, Albert
Einstein College of Medicine of Yeshiva University, Bronx,
New York; Chief, Yarmon Division of Neurobehavior and
Alzheimer's Disease, Beth Israel Medical Center, New York
*11B. Cognitive-Motor Disorders, Apraxias, and Ag-
nosias: Agnosias*

Gerald M. Fenichel, M.D.
Professor of Neurology and Pediatrics and Chairman, Department of Neurology, Vanderbilt University School of
Medicine, Nashville, Tennessee; Neurologist-in-Chief, Vanderbilt University Hospital and Vanderbilt Children's Hospital, Nashville
*1. Diagnosis of Neurological Disease; 8. Developmental
Delay and Regression in Infants; 36. Laboratory Investigations in Diagnosis and Management of Neurological Disease; 49. Management of Neurological Disease*

Pasquale F. Finelli, M.D.
Professor of Neurology, University of Connecticut School
of Medicine, Farmington; Associate Director of Neurology,
Hartford Hospital, Hartford, Connecticut
20. Disturbances of Taste and Smell

Laura Flores, M.D.
Professor of Pediatric Neurology, Universidad Nacional
Autónoma Mexico School of Medicine, Mexico City; Head
of Pediatric Neurology, Instituto Nacional de Pediatría,
Mexico City
66. Developmental Disorders of the Nervous System

Clare J. Fowler, M.Sc., F.R.C.P.
Reader in Clinical Neurology, Institute of Neurology, Uni-
versity College London; Consultant in Uro-Neurology,
The National Hospital for Neurology and Neurosurgery,
London
*33. Neurological Causes of Bladder, Bowel, and Sexual
Dysfunction; 43. Neurourology*

Richard S. J. Frackowiak, M.A., M.D., B.Sc., F.R.C.P.
Professor and Chairman, Wellcome Department of Cogni-
tive Neurology; Dean, Institute of Neurology, University
College London; Consultant Neurologist, The National
Hospital for Neurology and Neurosurgery, London
38E. Neuroimaging: Functional Neuroimaging

David G. Gadian, D.Phil.
Professor of Biophysics, Institute of Child Health and Great
Ormond Street Hospital, London
38E. Neuroimaging: Functional Neuroimaging

David S. Geldmacher, M.D.
Assistant Professor of Neurology, Case Western Reserve University School of Medicine, Cleveland; Clinical Director, Uni-

versity Alzheimer Center, University Hospitals of Cleveland
  57F. Vascular Diseases of the Nervous System: Spinal Cord Vascular Disease

Steven J. Greenberg, M.D.
Associate Professor of Neurology, State University of New York at Buffalo School of Medicine and Biomedical Sciences, Buffalo; Chairman, Department of Neurology, Roswell Park Cancer Institute, Buffalo
  58B. Primary and Secondary Tumors of the Central Nervous System: Molecular Biology of Nervous System Tumors

Richard H. Haas, M.A., M.B., B.Chir., M.R.C.P.
Professor of Neurosciences and Pediatrics, University of California, San Diego, School of Medicine; Director, Mitochondrial Laboratory, University of California Medical Center, La Jolla
  68. Inborn Errors of Metabolism of the Nervous System

Robert W. Hamill, M.D.
Professor and Chair of Neurology, University of Vermont College of Medicine, Burlington; Physician Leader, Neurology Health Care Service, Fletcher Allen Health Care, Burlington
  86. Geriatric Neurology

Maurice R. Hanson, M.D.
Physician, Clinical Neurology and Neurophysiology, Cleveland Clinic Florida, Ft. Lauderdale, Florida
  21. Disturbances of Lower Cranial Nerves; 74. Cranial Neuropathies

Anita E. Harding, M.D., F.R.C.P.
Professor of Clinical Neurology, Institue of Neurology, London; Consultant Neurologist, National Hospital for Neurology and Neurosurgery, London
  24. Ataxic Disorders; 76. Cerebellar and Spinocerebellar Disorders

John F. Healy, M.D.
Clinical Professor of Radiology, University of California, San Diego, School of Medicine; Chief of Radiology, San Diego Veterans Administration Medical Center
  59A. Infections of the Nervous System: Bacterial Infections

Reid R. Heffner, Jr., M.D.
Professor and Chair, Department of Pathology, State University of New York at Buffalo School of Medicine and Biomedical Sciences, Buffalo; Chair, University at Buffalo Pathologists, Buffalo General Hospital, Buffalo
  58A. Primary and Secondary Tumors of the Central Nervous System: Pathology of Nervous System Tumors

Kenneth M. Heilman, M.D.
The James E. Rooks, Jr., Distinguished Professor of Neurology, University of Florida College of Medicine,

Gainesville; Chief of Neurology, Veterans Administration Medical Center, Gainesville
  11A. Cognitive-Motor Disorders, Apraxias, and Agnosias: Cognitive-Motor Disorders and Apraxias

Deborah O. Heros, M.D.
Director of Neuro-Oncology, Mt. Sinai Comprehensive Cancer Center, Miami Beach, Florida
  53. Principles of Neurosurgery

Roberto C. Heros, M.D.
Professor, Co-Chairman, and Program Director, Department of Neurological Surgery, University of Miami School of Medicine
  53. Principles of Neurosurgery

Albert Hijdra, M.D.
Staff Neurologist, Academisch Medisch Centrum, University of Amsterdam, Amsterdam, The Netherlands
  70C. The Dementias: Vascular Dementia

Alan Hill, M.D., Ph.D.
Professor and Head of Neurology, University of British Columbia Faculty of Medicine, Vancouver, British Columbia, Canada; Head of Neurology, British Columbia Children's Hospital, Vancouver
  84. Neurological Problems of the Newborn

James F. Howard, Jr., M.D.
Chief, Neuromuscular Disorders Section, Department of Neurology, University of North Carolina at Chapel Hill School of Medicine and University of North Carolina Hospitals, Chapel Hill
  82. Disorders of Neuromuscular Transmission

Kurt A. Jaeckle, M.D.
Associate Professor of Neuro-Oncology and Medicine, University of Texas Houston Medical School, M. D. Anderson Cancer Center, Houston
  58C. Primary and Secondary Tumors of the Central Nervous System: Clinical Presentation and Therapy of Nervous System Tumors

Jack I. Jallo, M.D.
Assistant Professor of Neurosurgery, Temple University School of Medicine, Philadelphia
  56B. Trauma of the Nervous System: Craniocerebral Trauma

Cheryl A. Jay, M.D.
Assistant Clinical Professor of Neurology, University of California, San Francisco, School of Medicine; Attending Neurologist, San Francisco General Hospital
  59A. Infections of the Nervous System: Bacterial Infections; 59E. Infections of the Nervous System: Neurological Manifestations of Human Immunodeficiency Virus Infection

Luke D. Kartsounis, M.Sc., Ph.D.
Consultant Neuropsychologist, Regional Neurosciences Centre, Oldchurch Hospital, Romford, Essex, United Kingdom
39. Neuropsychology

Carlos S. Kase, M.D.
Professor of Neurology, Boston University School of Medicine; Attending Neurologist, Boston University Medical Center
57B. Vascular Diseases of the Nervous System: Intracerebral Hemorrhage

Samia J. Khoury, M.D.
Associate Professor of Neurology, Harvard Medical School, Boston; Associate Physician, Department of Neurology, Brigham and Women's Hospital, Boston
46. Neuroimmunology

Jun Kimura, M.D.
Professor Emeritus, Kyoto University Graduate School of Medicine, Kyoto, Japan; Professor of Neurology, University of Iowa College of Medicine, Iowa City
37B. Clinical Neurophysiology: Electrodiagnosis of Neuromuscular Disorders

Howard S. Kirshner, M.D.
Professor of Neurology, Psychiatry, and Hearing and Speech Sciences, and Vice Chairman of Neurology, Vanderbilt University School of Medicine, Nashville, Tennessee; Director, Adult Neurology Service and Director, Vanderbilt Stroke Center, Vanderbilt University Medical Center, Nashville; Associate Medical Director, Vanderbilt Stallworth Rehabilitation Hospital, Nashville
7. Approaches to Intellectual and Memory Impairments; 12A. Language Disorders: Aphasia

David G. Kline, M.D.
Boyd Professor and Head of Neurosurgery, Louisiana State University School of Medicine in New Orleans; Active Staff Member, Department of Neurosurgery, Ochsner Foundation Hospital, New Orleans
56D. Trauma of the Nervous System: Peripheral Nerve Trauma

Nobuo Kohara, M.D.
Assistant Professor of Neurology, Kyoto University Graduate School of Medicine, Kyoto, Japan
37B. Clinical Neurophysiology: Electrodiagnosis of Neuromuscular Disorders

John F. Kurtzke, M.D.
Professor of Neurology, Georgetown University School of Medicine, Washington, D.C.; Chief, Neuroepidemiology Section, Neurology Service, Veterans Administration Medical Center, Washington, D.C.
44. Neuroepidemiology

Anthony E. Lang, M.D., F.R.C.P.C.
Professor of Neurology, University of Toronto Faculty of Medicine; Director of Movement Disorders, The Toronto Western Hospital, Division of the University Health Network
25. Movement Disorders: Symptoms; 75. Movement Disorders

Donald W. Larsen, M.D.
Associate Professor of Neurological Surgery, University of Southern California School of Medicine, Los Angeles, and University of Southern California University Hospital, Los Angeles
38C. Neuroimaging: Radiological Angiography

Patrick J. M. Lavin, M.B., B.Ch., B.A.O., M.R.C.P.I.
Associate Professor of Neurology, Vanderbilt University School of Medicine, Nashville, Tennessee
16. Eye Movement Disorders: Diplopia, Nystagmus, and Other Ocular Oscillations; 40. Neuro-Ophthalmology: Ocular Motor System

Ronald P. Lesser, M.D.
Professor of Neurology, Johns Hopkins University School of Medicine, Baltimore; Staff Physician, Department of Neurology, Johns Hopkins Hospital, Baltimore
71. The Epilepsies

Alan H. Lockwood, M.D.
Professor of Neurology and Nuclear Medicine, State University of New York at Buffalo School of Medicine and Biomedical Sciences, Buffalo; Director of Operations, Center for Positron Emission Tomography, Veterans Administration Western New York Health Care System, Buffalo
62. Toxic and Metabolic Encephalopathies

Betsy B. Love, M.D.
Clinical Assistant Professor of Neurology, Indiana University School of Medicine, Indianapolis
57A. Vascular Diseases of the Nervous System: Ischemic Cerebrovascular Disease

Mícheál P. Macken, M.B., B.Ch., B.A.O., M.R.C.P.I.
Fellow in Clinical Neurophysiology, Cleveland Clinic Foundation
74. Cranial Neuropathies

Robert G. Mair, Ph.D.
Professor of Psychology, University of New Hampshire, Durham
20. Disturbances of Taste and Smell

C. David Marsden, D.Sc., F.R.C.P., F.R.S.
Professor of Neurology, University Department of Neurology, The National Hospital for Neurology and Neuro-

surgery, London
1. Diagnosis of Neurological Disease; 26. Walking Disorders; 36. Laboratory Investigations in Diagnosis and Management of Neurological Disease; 49. Management of Neurological Disease

Alberto Martinez-Arizala, M.D.
Associate Professor of Neurology, University of Miami School of Medicine; Staff Neurologist, University of Miami–Jackson Memorial Medical Center
35. Low Back and Lower Limb Pain

Christopher J. Mathias, D.Phil., D.Sc., F.R.C.P.
Professor of Neurovascular Medicine, Imperial College School of Medicine and University Department of Clinical Neurology, Institute of Neurology, University College London; Consultant Physician, Neurovascular Medicine Unit, St. Mary's Hospital, London; Consultant Physician, Autonomic Unit, The National Hospital for Neurology and Neurosurgery, London
81. Disorders of the Autonomic Nervous System

John C. Mazziotta, M.D., Ph.D.
Professor of Neurology, Radiological Sciences, and Molecular Pharmacology, and Director, Brain Mapping Center, University of California, Los Angeles, UCLA School of Medicine
38E. Neuroimaging: Functional Neuroimaging

Rosaleen A. McCarthy, M.D.
University Lecturer in Experimental Psychology, University of Cambridge, Cambridge, United Kingdom; Honorary Clinical Research Associate, Addenbrooke's Hospital, Cambridge
39. Neuropsychology

Michael J. McLean, M.D., Ph.D.
Associate Professor of Neurology and Pharmacology, Vanderbilt University School of Medicine, Nashville, Tennessee
50. Principles of Neuropharmacology and Therapeutics

Laszlo L. Mechtler, M.D.
Associate Professor of Neurology, State University of New York at Buffalo School of Medicine and Biomedical Sciences, Koleida Health Care, Roswell Park Cancer Institute, and Catholic Health System, Buffalo
58D. Primary and Secondary Tumors of the Central Nervous System: Clinical Presentation and Therapy for Spinal Tumors; 58E. Primary and Secondary Tumors of the Central Nervous System: Clinical Presentation and Therapy of Peripheral Nerve Tumors

Van S. Miller, Ph.D., M.D.
Associate Professor of Neurology, University of Texas Southwestern Medical Center at Dallas Southwestern Medical School
69. Neurocutaneous Syndromes

Karl E. Misulis, M.D., Ph.D.
Clinical Professor of Neurology, Vanderbilt University School of Medicine, Nashville, Tennessee; Neurologist, Semmes-Murphy Clinic, Jackson, Tennessee
27. Hemiplegia and Monoplegia

Hiroshi Mitsumoto, M.D., D.M.Sc.
Professor of Neurology and Attending Neurologist, Columbia University College of Physicians and Surgeons, New York; Director, Amyotrophic Lateral Sclerosis/Muscle Center, and Head of Division, Amotrophic Lateral Sclerosis and Muscle Disease, The Neurological Institute, New York
78. Disorders of Upper and Lower Motor Neurons

Paul L. Moots, M.D.
Associate Professor of Neurology and Assistant Professor of Medicine, Vanderbilt University School of Medicine, Nashville, Tennessee; Neurologist, Vanderbilt University Medical Center and Veterans Administration Medical Center, Nashville
51. Principles of Pain Management

Hugo W. Moser, M.D.
Professor of Neurology and Pediatrics, Johns Hopkins University School of Medicine, Baltimore; Director of Neurogenetics Research, Kennedy Krieger Institute, Baltimore
68. Inborn Errors of Metabolism of the Nervous System

Sakkubai Naidu, M.D.
Associate Professor of Neurology, Johns Hopkins University School of Medicine, Baltimore; Pediatric Neurologist, Kennedy Krieger Institute, Baltimore
68. Inborn Errors of Metabolism of the Nervous System

Raj K. Narayan, M.D.
Professor and Chairman of Neurosurgery, Temple University School of Medicine, Philadelphia; Chairman of Neurosurgery, Temple University Hospital, Philadelphia
56B. Trauma of the Nervous System: Craniocerebral Trauma

Ruth Nass, M.D.
Professor of Clinical Neurology, New York University Medical Center
12B. Language Disorders: Developmental Speech and Language Disorders; 67. Developmental Disabilities

David Neary, M.D.
Professor of Neurology, University of Manchester, Manchester, United Kingdom; Consultant Neurologist, Manchester Royal Infirmary
70D. The Dementias: Progressive Focal Cortical Syndromes

Michael J. Olek, D.O.
Instructor in Neurology, Harvard Medical School, Boston;

Attending Physician, Department of Neurology, Brigham and Women's Hospital and Massachusetts General Hospital, Boston
60. Multiple Sclerosis and Other Inflammatory Demyelinating Diseases of the Central Nervous System

Colette C. Parker, M.D.
Associate Professor of Pediatric Neurology, University of Mississippi School of Medicine, Jackson
68. Inborn Errors of Metabolism of the Nervous System

Timothy A. Pedley, M.D.
Henry and Lucy Moses Professor of Neurology and Chairman, Department of Neurology, Columbia University College of Physicians and Surgeons, New York; Neurologist-in-Chief, Columbia-Presbyterian Medical Center, New York
37A. Clinical Neurophysiology: Electroencephalography and Evoked Potentials

Alan Pestronk, M.D.
Professor of Neurology and Pathology, and Director, Neuromuscular Clinical Laboratory, Washington University School of Medicine, St. Louis
30. Muscle Pain and Cramps

David M. Pilgrim, M.D.
Clinical Instructor in Neurology, Harvard Medical School, Boston; Chief of Neurology, Harvard Vanguard Medical Associates, Boston; Associate Neurologist, Brigham and Women's Hospital, Boston
86. Geriatric Neurology

Jerome B. Posner, M.D.
Professor of Neurology and Neuroscience, Cornell University Medical College, New York; Attending Neurologist, Memorial Sloan-Kettering Cancer Center, New York
58F. Primary and Secondary Tumors of the Central Nervous System: Paraneoplastic Syndromes

J. Ned Pruitt II, M.D.
Assistant Professor of Neurology, Medical College of Georgia School of Medicine, Augusta
34. Arm and Neck Pain

Robert M. Quencer, M.D.
Chairman and Professor of Radiology, University of Miami School of Medicine; Chief of Radiology Service, University of Miami–Jackson Memorial Hospital
38A. Neuroimaging: Structural Neuroimaging

Robert A. Ratcheson, M.D.
Harvey Huntington Brown, Jr., Professor and Chairman of Neurological Surgery, Case Western Reserve University School of Medicine, Cleveland; Director of Neurological Surgery, University Hospitals of Cleveland
57C. Vascular Diseases of the Nervous System: Intracranial

Aneurysms and Subarachnoid Hemorrhage; 57D. Vascular Diseases of the Nervous System: Arteriovenous Malformations

Bernd F. Remler, M.D.
Associate Professor of Neurology, Medical College of Wisconsin, Milwaukee; Staff Physician, Department of Neurology, Froedtert Memorial Lutheran Hospital, Milwaukee
3. Falls and Drop Attacks

David E. Riley, M.D.
Associate Professor of Neurology, Case Western Reserve University School of Medicine, Cleveland; Director, Movement Disorders Center, University Hospitals of Cleveland
75. Movement Disorders

Marco A. Rizzo, M.D., Ph.D.
Assistant Professor of Neurology, Yale University School of Medicine, New Haven, Connecticut; Attending Staff, Department of Neurology, Yale–New Haven Hospital
32. Sensory Abnormalities of the Limbs, Trunk, and Face

E. Steve Roach, M.D.
Helen and Robert S. Strauss Professor of Neurology, University of Texas Southwestern Medical Center at Dallas Southwestern Medical School; Director, Division of Child Neurology, Children's Medical Center of Dallas
69. Neurocutaneous Syndromes

Richard B. Rosenbaum, M.D.
Clinical Professor of Neurology, Oregon Health Sciences University, Portland; Neurology Division, The Oregon Clinic, Portland
77. Disorders of Bones, Joints, Ligaments, and Meninges

Gary A. Rosenberg, M.D.
Professor and Chairman of Neurology, University of New Mexico School of Medicine, Albuquerque
65. Brain Edema and Disorders of Cerebrospinal Fluid Circulation

David B. Rosenfield, M.D.
Professor of Neurology and of Otorhinolaryngology, and Communication Sciences, Baylor College of Medicine, Houston; Professor of Neurology, The Methodist Hospital, Houston; Director, Stuttering Center–Speech Motor Control Laboratory, Baylor College of Medicine, Houston
13. Difficulties with Speech and Swallowing

Martin N. Rossor, M.A., M.D., F.R.C.P.
Professor of Clinical Neurology, Institute of Neurology, University College London; Consultant Neurologist, The National Hospital for Neurology and Neurosurgery and St. Mary's Hospital, London
70. The Dementias; 70A. The Dementias: Primary Degenerative Dementia; 70B. The Dementias: Dementia as Part of Other Degenerative Diseases; 70E. The Dementias: Other Causes of Dementias

Leslie J. Gonzalez Rothi, Ph.D.
Associate Professor of Neurology, University of Florida
College of Medicine, Gainesville; Staff Speech Pathologist,
Neurology Service, Gainesville Veterans Administration
Medical Center
  11A. *Cognitive-Motor Disorders, Apraxias, and Agnosias: Cognitive-Motor Disorders and Apraxias*

Armando Ruiz, M.D.
Assistant Professor of Radiology and Neurological Surgery,
University of Miami School of Medicine and University of
Miami–Jackson Memorial Medical Center
  38A. *Neuroimaging: Structural Neuroimaging; 38B. Neuroimaging: Computed Tomographic and Magnetic Resonance Vascular Imaging*

Donald B. Sanders, M.D.
Professor of Medicine (Neurology), Duke University School
of Medicine, Durham, North Carolina
  82. *Disorders of Neuromuscular Transmission*

Harvey B. Sarnat, M.D., F.R.C.P.C.
Professor of Neurology, Pediatrics, and Pathology (Neuropathology), University of Washington School of Medicine, Seattle; Active Staff, Departments of Neurology,
Pediatrics, and Pathology, Children's Hospital and Regional
Medical Center, Seattle
  66. *Developmental Disorders of the Nervous System*

James W. Schmidley, M.D.
Professor of Neurology, University of Arkansas College of
Medicine, Little Rock; Neurologist, University Hospital,
Little Rock
  57G. *Vascular Diseases of the Nervous System: Central Nervous System Vasculitis*

Warren R. Selman, M.D.
Professor of Neurological Surgery, Case Western Reserve University School of Medicine, Cleveland; Vice
Chairman, Department of Neurological Surgery, University Hospitals of Cleveland
  57C. *Vascular Diseases of the Nervous System: Intracranial Aneurysms and Subarachnoid Hemorrhage; 57D. Vascular Diseases of the Nervous System: Arteriovenous Malformations*

D. Malcolm Shaner, M.D.
Assistant Clinical Professor of Neurology, University of
California, Los Angeles, UCLA School of Medicine; Consultant in Neurology, Southern California Permanente
Medical Group, Los Angeles
  85. *Neurological Problems of Pregnancy*

Roger P. Simon, M.D.
Professor of Neurology, University of Pittsburgh School of
Medicine
  63. *Deficiency Diseases of the Nervous System*

Ghassan S. Skaf, M.D., F.R.C.S.C.
Assistant Professor of Surgery, Division of Neurosurgery,
American University of Beirut, Beirut, Lebanon; Head, Spinal
Program, American University of Beirut Medical Center
  56C. *Trauma of the Nervous System: Spinal Cord Trauma*

Evelyn M. L. Sklar, M.D.
Professor of Clinical Radiology, University of Miami School
of Medicine; Attending Neuroradiologist, University of
Miami–Jackson Memorial Hospital
  38A. *Neuroimaging: Structural Neuroimaging*

Benn E. Smith, M.D.
Assistant Professor of Neurology, Mayo Medical School,
Rochester, Minnesota; Consultant in Neurology, Mayo
Clinic Arizona, Scottsdale
  80. *Disorders of Peripheral Nerves*

Julie S. Snowden, Ph.D.
Clinical Scientist (Neuropsychologist), Manchester Royal
Infirmary, Manchester, United Kingdom
  70D. *The Dementias: Progressive Focal Cortical Syndromes*

Bruce D. Snyder, M.D.
Clinical Professor of Neurology, University of Minnesota
Medical School, Minneapolis
  61. *Anoxic and Ischemic Encephalopathies*

Yuen T. So, M.D., Ph.D.
Associate Professor of Neurology, Stanford University
School of Medicine, Stanford, California
  63. *Deficiency Diseases of the Nervous System; 64B. Effects of Toxins and Physical Agents on the Nervous System: Effects of Drug Abuse on the Nervous System; 64C. Effects of Toxins and Physical Agents on the Nervous System: Neurotoxins of Animals and Plants; 64D. Effects of Toxins and Physical Agents on the Nervous System: Marine Toxins*

Marylou V. Solbrig, M.D.
Assistant Adjunct Professor of Neurology, University of
California, Irvine, School of Medicine; Attending Neurologist, University of California, Irvine, Medical Center
  59. *Infections of the Nervous System: Introduction; 59A. Infections of the Nervous System: Bacterial Infections; 59B. Infections of the Nervous System: Viral Infections; 59C. Infections of the Nervous System: Fungal Infections; 59D. Infections of the Nervous System: Parasitic Infections*

Jerry W. Swanson, M.D.
Associate Professor of Neurology, Mayo Medical School,
Rochester, Minnesota; Consultant in Neurology, Mayo
Clinic, Rochester
  22. *Cranial and Facial Pain; 73. Headache and Other Craniofacial Pain*

Patrick J. Sweeney, M.D., F.A.C.P.
Department of Neurology, Case Western Reserve University School of Medicine, Cleveland; Director, Neurology Residency Program, The Cleveland Clinic Foundation
21. Disturbances of Lower Cranial Nerves; 74. Cranial Neuropathies

Thomas R. Swift, M.D.
Professor and Chair of Neurology, Medical College of Georgia School of Medicine, Augusta
34. Arm and Neck Pain

Stephen J. Tapscott, M.D., Ph.D.
Associate Professor of Neurology, University of Washington School of Medicine, Seattle; Associate Member, Division of Molecular Medicine, Fred Hutchinson Cancer Research Center, Seattle
45. Clinical Neurogenetics

Robert W. Tarr, M.D.
Associate Professor of Radiology and Neurosurgery, Case Western Reserve University School of Medicine, Cleveland; Director of Interventional Neuroradiology, University Hospitals of Cleveland
57C. Vascular Diseases of the Nervous System: Intracranial Aneurysms and Subarachnoid Hemorrhage 57D. Vascular Diseases of the Nervous System: Arteriovenous Malformations

Charles H. Tator, M.D., M.A., Ph.D., F.R.C.S.C.
Professor of Neurosurgery, University of Toronto Faculty of Medicine
56C. Trauma of the Nervous System: Spinal Cord Trauma

Charles H. Tegeler, M.D.
Associate Professor of Neurology, Head, Section of Stroke and Cerebrovascular Disease, and Director, Neurosonology Laboratory, Wake Forest University School of Medicine, Winston-Salem, North Carolina
38D. Neuroimaging: Ultrasound Imaging of the Cerebral Vasculature

George P. Teitelbaum, M.D.
Associate Professor of Neurological Surgery, University of Southern California School of Medicine and University of Southern California Hospital, Los Angeles
38C. Neuroimaging: Radiological Angiography

Alan J. Thompson, M.D., F.R.C.P., F.R.C.P.I.
Garfield Weston Professor of Clinical Neurology and Neurorehabilitation, Institute of Neurology, University College London; Consultant Neurologist, The National Hospital for Neurology and Neurosurgery, London
54. Principles of Neurological Rehabilitation

Philip D. Thompson, M.B.B.S., Ph.D., F.R.A.C.P.
Professor of Neurology, Royal Adelaide Hospital, Adelaide, South Australia
26. Walking Disorders

Robert L. Tiel, M.D.
Associate Professor of Neurosurgery, Louisiana State University Medical Center, New Orleans; Department of Neurosurgery, University Hospital, New Orleans
56D. Trauma of the Nervous System: Peripheral Nerve Trauma

Robert L. Tomsak, M.D., Ph.D.
Clinical Associate Professor of Ophthalmology and Neurology, Case Western Reserve University School of Medicine, Cleveland
14. Vision Loss; 41. Neuro-Opthalmology: Afferent Visual System

William H. Trescher, M.D.
Assistant Professor of Neurology, Johns Hopkins University School of Medicine, Baltimore; Department of Neurology and Developmental Medicine, Kennedy Krieger Institute, Baltimore
71. The Epilepsies

Michael R. Trimble, M.D., F.R.C.P., F.R.C.Psych.
Professor of Behavioural Neurology, Institute of Neurology, University College London; Consultant Physician in Psychological Medicine, The National Hospital for Neurology and Neurosurgery, London
9. Behavior and Personality Disturbances; 10. Depression and Psychosis in Neurological Practice

B. Todd Troost, M.D.
Professor and Chairman of Neurology, Wake Forest University School of Medicine, Winston-Salem, North Carolina
18. Dizziness and Vertigo; 19. Hearing Loss and Tinnitus without Dizziness or Vertigo; 42. Neuro-Otology

Kenneth L. Tyler, M.D.
Vice-Chairman and Professor of Neurology and Professor of Medicine, Microbiology and Immunology, University of Colorado Health Sciences Center, Denver; Chief, Neurology Service, Denver Veterans Administration Medical Center
47. Neurovirology

Edward Valenstein, M.D.
Professor of Neurology, University of Florida College of Medicine, Gainesville; Attending Neurologist, Shands Hospital at the University of Florida, Gainesville
11A. Cognitive-Motor Disorders, Apraxias, and Agnosias: Cognitive-Motor Disorders and Apraxias

Paul M. Vespa, M.D.
Assistant Professor of Neurosurgery and Neurology, Univer-

sity of California, Los Angeles, UCLA School of Medicine
52. Principles of Neurointensive Care

Joseph J. Volpe, M.D.
Bronson Crothers Professor of Neurology, Harvard Medical School, Boston; Neurologist-in-Chief, Children's Hospital, Boston
84. Neurological Problems of the Newborn

Michael Wall, M.D.
Professor of Neurology and Ophthalmology, University of Iowa College of Medicine, Iowa City; Staff Physician, University of Iowa Hospitals and Clinics and Veterans Administration Medical Center, Iowa City
23. Brainstem Syndromes

Mitchell Taylor Wallin, M.D., M.P.H.
Clinical Instructor in Neurology, Georgetown University Medical School, Washington, D.C.; Assistant Chief of Neuroepidemiology, Veterans Administration Medical Center, Washington, D.C.
44. Neuroepidemiology

Robert T. Watson, M.D.
Professor of Neurology and Senior Associate Dean for Educational Affairs, University of Florida College of Medicine, Gainesville; Neurologist, Shands Hospital at the University of Florida, Gainesville
11A. Cognitive-Motor Disorders, Apraxias, and Agnosias: Cognitive-Motor Disorders and Apraxias

Stephen G. Waxman, M.D., Ph.D.
Professor and Chairman of Neurology, Yale University

School of Medicine, New Haven, Connecticut; Director, Paralyzed Veterans of America/Eastern Paralyzed Veterans of America Neuroscience Research Center, Veterans Administration Healthcare System, West Haven, Connecticut; Visiting Professor of Neurology, Anatomy, and Biology, University College London; Neurologist-in-Chief, Yale–New Haven Hospital
28. Paraplegia and Spinal Cord Syndromes; 32. Sensory Abnormalities of the Limbs, Trunk, and Face

Nicholas W. Wood, M.B., Ch.B., M.R.C.P., Ph.D.
Reader in Clinical Neurology, Institute of Neurology, University College London; Honorary Consultant Neurologist, The National Hospital for Neurology and Neurosurgery, London
24. Ataxic Disorders; 76. Cerebellar and Spinocerebellar Disorders

Richard S. K. Young, M.D, M.P.H.
Associate Clinical Professor of Pediatrics and Neurology, Yale University School of Medicine, New Haven, Connecticut; Chair of Pediatrics, Hospital of Saint Raphael, New Haven
57E. Vascular Diseases of the Nervous System: Stroke in Childhood

Donald P. Younkin, M.D.
Associate Professor of Neurology and Pediatrics, University of Pennsylvania School of Medicine, Philadelphia; Senior Physician, Department of Neurology, Children's Hospital of Philadelphia
55B. Neurological Complications of Systemic Disease: In Children

Preface to the Third Edition

Our original concept in developing *Neurology in Clinical Practice* (NICP) was to produce a complete, but concise, textbook of neurology that would meet the needs of clinicians both in practice and in training. We thought it best to have three parts: the first describing how an experienced neurologist approaches the most common neurological problems; the second covering the neurological subspecialties, related disciplines, and relevant laboratory investigations as well as general principles of management of patients with neurological problems; and the third, which is the second volume of the book, covering the individual neurological diseases, emphasizing clinical diagnosis and treatment and including sufficient basic science to facilitate understanding of the diseases.

The first edition was awarded the Most Outstanding Book Published in 1991 by the Professional and Scholarly Publishing Division of the Association of American Publishers and received critical acclaim in scholarly reviews.

For the second edition, published in 1996, we rewrote much of the text, and almost one-third of the authors were new contributors. For many neurologists, this edition became the standard clinical textbook. The Resident In-Service Training Examination of the American Academy of Neurology used it as the reference for more than half of the questions.

With this third edition, almost half of the authors are new contributors, but we have maintained the successful format of the first two editions. We also added considerable material, including a chapter on neurointensive care.

We entered the electronic era with this new edition. The writing of manuscripts, their editorial review, and their production into the final published book relied on heavy use of both the Internet and an *NICP* intranet. For facilitating these procedures, we thank Electronic Press of Cambridge, Massachusetts. Despite problems with the electronic medium, it has expedited the handling of the manuscript and its publication.

The publication of these two volumes is accompanied by the launch of a companion Web site, www.nicp.com, which expands the educational capacity of the text. This electronic version of the textbook provides audiotapes and videotapes to download, continuous updating of information, a sophisticated search engine, links to relevant Internet sites, and cross-references to related texts for further reading. In addition, a question-and-answer book, based on the material in the text, will be published, to assist candidates for neurological board and certification examinations. We will also publish the second edition of *Pocket Companion to Neurology in Clinical Practice*.

Many people contributed to the success of this third edition. First and foremost are the authors who responded to our call for manuscripts and who have been patient with our demands. Susan Pioli, Director of Medical Publishing at Butterworth–Heinemann, played a crucial part in completing the text version and achieving the transition into the electronic age. Rita Kessel was the Managing Editor, and her steady guiding hand brought this book to fruition. Our loyal administrative assistants and secretaries, Janice Setney, Beth Howell-Hughes, Vicki Fields, and Nelda Tilley were essential throughout the production of the third edition. Kim Langford and the staff of Silverchair Science + Communications, Charlottesville, Virginia, did an excellent job of converting the final manuscripts to the finished product, both for the printed book and for the Internet companion.

Walter G. Bradley
Robert B. Daroff
Gerald M. Fenichel

Part III

Neurological Diseases

Chapter 55
Neurological Complications of Systemic Disease

A. IN ADULTS
Michael J. Aminoff

This chapter discusses neurological complications of systemic disease in adults. A separate chapter discusses the same subject in children (see Chapter 55B). Some disorders are discussed in both chapters but with a different emphasis.

CARDIAC DISORDERS AND THE NERVOUS SYSTEM

Neurological complications are an important cause of morbidity in patients with cardiac disease. Cardiogenic emboli may result from cardiac disease or its surgical treatment, and cardiac dysfunction can cause global cerebral hypoperfusion leading to syncope, stroke, or death, depending on the severity and duration of cerebral ischemia.

Cardiogenic Embolism

Cardiogenic emboli are most prevalent in patients with mitral stenosis and atrial fibrillation, intramural thrombi, prosthetic cardiac valves, atrial myxoma, infective endocarditis, sick sinus syndrome, and atrial fibrillation. Other causes include recent myocardial infarct, left atrial thrombus or turbulence, mitral valve prolapse, mitral annulus calcification, atrial flutter, hypokinetic left ventricular segments, and congestive cardiac failure. Emboli from congenital heart disease are discussed in Chapter 55B. The possibility of cardiac emboli must be considered in young people with either valvular heart disease or mitral valve prolapse.

Echocardiography is an important investigative procedure when cardiogenic emboli are suspected. Transesophageal echocardiography is preferable to the transthoracic approach in the evaluation of suspected atrial disease, such as myxoma or thrombus, and to demonstrate a patent foramen ovale (Manning 1997), but transthoracic echocardiography is an important method of visualizing the ventricular apex, mitral or aortic valvular disease, and left ventricular thrombus.

Transesophageal echocardiography is an appropriate method to investigate people younger than 45 years with suspected cardiogenic emboli who may need anticoagulation or surgery and older people without signs of cardiac disease, but transthoracic echocardiography is generally adequate when clinical evidence of cardiac disease is present.

Emboli are more likely when atrial fibrillation is associated with valvular heart disease. The incidence of stroke is increased 17-fold or fivefold, respectively, among patients with atrial fibrillation, depending on the presence or absence of rheumatic heart disease. Atrial fibrillation, in the absence of cardiovascular disease or other predisposing illness, has a considerably lower risk of neurological complications. The neurological prognosis of paroxysmal atrial fibrillation is not established, but the risk of embolism is probably less than with chronic atrial fibrillation.

The benefit of anticoagulation in reducing the risk of stroke in people with atrial fibrillation is established. A consensus conference recommended long-term oral warfarin therapy for atrial fibrillation unless there were specific contraindications or the atrial fibrillation was an isolated finding in people younger than 60 years without other evidence of cardiovascular disease. Aspirin (325 mg/day) is recommended when warfarin is contraindicated. In 1992 Laupacis and colleagues recommended that warfarin be started 3 weeks before elective cardioversion in people with atrial fibrillation of more than 2 days' duration and continued until normal rhythm has been maintained for 4 weeks.

Myocardial infarcts, especially apical, anterolateral, or large infarcts, have a risk of embolic stroke. Most occur within a week, but the risk persists for approximately 2 months. Therefore, patients not on thrombolytic therapy are heparinized after myocardial infarction and then treated for 3 months with warfarin if they have an increased risk of embolism. The groups with increased risk are those with congestive heart failure, previous emboli, evidence of a mural thrombus, left ventricular dysfunction, or atrial fibrillation.

Emboli are an important cause of death in people with rheumatic valvular disease. The risk of embolism is increased in the presence of atrial fibrillation, intra-atrial thrombus, or a past history of emboli, and long-term warfarin treatment is recommended. Aspirin (160–325 mg/day) is added for recurrent systemic emboli despite adequate warfarin therapy.

Mitral valve prolapse is a common anomaly, especially among young women, and its relationship to cerebral emboli is now recognized. The risk of emboli is relatively small, and long-term warfarin is only recommended for people who have had previous embolic phenomena or are in atrial fibrillation. Long-term aspirin therapy (325–975 mg/day) is recommended for people with mitral valve prolapse and transient cerebral ischemic attacks of uncertain nature.

Among patients with a history of cardiogenic emboli, recurrent stroke is more likely in those with cardiac valve disease and congestive heart failure. Nevertheless, the main cause of death in such patients is from the heart disease rather than neurological complications. The conversion of a cerebral infarct into a hemorrhage is a concern when patients with stroke from cardiogenic emboli are anticoagulated. The concern is especially justified in patients with large infarcts or when imaging studies suggest pre-existing hemorrhagic transformation. It is good practice to delay anticoagulation therapy after a small infarct for at least 24 hours, and then to initiate it only if computed tomography shows no evidence of major hemorrhagic transformation. Anticoagulation is best delayed for 7 days after large infarcts. Atrial fibrillation is associated with an increased mortality during the acute phase of a stroke and in the subsequent year (Kaarisalo et al. 1997).

Syncope

Transitory global cerebral ischemia secondary to cardiac arrhythmia causes syncope, sometimes preceded by nonspecific premonitory symptoms such as visual disturbances, paresthesias, and lightheadedness. Syncope is associated usually with loss of muscle tone, but prolonged ischemia causes tonic posturing and irregular jerking movements that are easily mistaken for seizures (Stokes-Adams attacks). The syncopal patient is pale, and postictal confusion is either absent or short-lived, usually lasting for less than 30 seconds. Obstructed outflow from aortic stenosis or left atrial tumor or thrombus is one cardiac cause of syncope; other causes are arrhythmias, especially from ventricular tachycardia or fibrillation, chronic sinoatrial disorder or sick sinus syndrome, and paroxysmal tachycardia. Additional causes of syncope are central and peripheral dysautonomias, postural hypotension, and endocrine and metabolic disorders. Vasovagal syncope, the most common variety, and the prolonged QT interval syndrome are discussed in Chapter 55B.

Cardiac Arrest

Brain function is critically dependent on the cerebral circulation. The brain receives approximately 15% of the total cardiac output. Ventricular fibrillation or asystole causes circulatory failure that, depending on its duration, can cause irreversible anoxic-ischemic brain damage. The prognosis generally depends on age, the duration of the arrest before cardiopulmonary resuscitation is started, and the interval before starting defibrillating procedures. The prognosis is better when circulatory arrest is caused by ventricular fibrillation rather than asystole.

The pathophysiology of neurological damage caused by transitory interruption of cerebral blood flow is unclear. Suspected mechanisms are the accumulation of intracellular calcium, increased extracellular concentrations of glutamate and aspartate, and increased concentrations of free radicals.

In the mature brain, gray matter is generally more sensitive to ischemia than white matter, and the cerebral cortex is more sensitive than the brainstem. The premature brain has the reverse pattern of sensitivity (see Chapter 84). Cerebral or spinal regions lying between the territories supplied by the major arteries (watershed areas) are especially vulnerable to ischemic injury.

The severity of neurological complications of circulatory arrest correlates with the duration of the arrest. Brief (<5 minute) arrests cause temporary loss of consciousness and impaired cognitive function. Recovery may be followed by a demyelinating encephalopathy 7–10 days later, characterized by increasing cerebral dysfunction with cognitive disturbances and pyramidal or extrapyramidal abnormalities that may lead to a fatal outcome. Thus, some patients regain consciousness after several hours and then develop progressive neurological deficits affecting cognitive and cortical function: intellectual decline, seizures, visual agnosia, cortical blindness, amnestic syndromes, and personality changes. Less common residua are the locked-in syndrome, parkinsonism or other extrapyramidal syndromes, abnormal ocular movements, bilateral brachial paresis, or action myoclonus. Spinal cord dysfunction is unusual and usually involves the watershed region at T5: Flaccid paraplegia with sensory loss, areflexia, and sphincter dysfunction are the immediate findings.

Prolonged cardiac arrest causes widespread and irreversible brain damage characterized by prolonged coma or a persistent vegetative state. Prolonged coma and loss of brainstem reflexes indicate a poor prognosis for survival or useful recovery. Absence of the pupillary response to light is perhaps the most useful clinical guide to prognosis; its absence even on initial examination indicates a poor prognosis for useful recovery. See Chapter 5 for further discussion.

Complications of Cardiac Catheterization and Surgery

Comments pertinent to children are provided in Chapter 55B. Cardiac catheterization causes cerebral emboli in less than 1% of cases; for unexplained reasons, these more often involve the posterior than the anterior circulation. The frequency of cerebral emboli following percutaneous transluminal coronary angioplasty is generally also less than 1% and may involve either the carotid or vertebral circulation. However, in a study of 1,184 patients with acute myocardial infarction treated by angioplasty, 6% died of a stroke and 7% of anoxic encephalopathy (Brodie et al. 1997).

Encephalopathy, seizures, and cerebral infarction after cardiac surgery are usually caused by hypoxia or emboli. Postoperative psychoses or encephalopathies may be caused by metabolic disturbances, medication, infection, or multiorgan failure. Intracranial infection should be suspected when behavioral disturbances develop several weeks postoperatively in patients receiving immunosuppressive agents. Postoperative seizures are usually caused by focal or generalized cerebral ischemia, electrolyte or metabolic disturbances, or multiorgan failure. Intracranial hemorrhage is a rare complication of cardiopulmonary bypass. It is usually attributed to diminished platelet adhesiveness and reduced coagulation factors.

Compression or traction injuries to the brachial plexus, especially the lower trunk, and phrenic and recurrent laryngeal nerves may occur during cardiac surgery.

Other common early complications of cardiac transplantation are organ rejection with consequent cardiac failure and side effects of immunosuppressive drugs. Infections (meningitis, meningoencephalitis, or cerebral abscess) secondary to immunosuppressive therapy are the most important late complications. The infecting organisms include *Aspergillus*, *Toxoplasma*, *Cryptococcus*, *Candida*, *Nocardia*, and viruses. The risk of lymphoma and reticulum cell sarcoma is increased also in patients on long-term immunosuppressive agents. Primary central nervous system (CNS) lymphoma may be impossible to distinguish clinically or radiologically from infection (see Chapter 58).

Stroke occurs in approximately 5% of patients undergoing coronary artery bypass surgery. The risk is increasing because of the tendency to operate on older patients with more severe vascular disease (Nussmeier 1996). The mechanism is either embolic or, less commonly, a watershed infarction from hypoperfusion. A history of previous stroke increases the risk, but a carotid bruit or radiological evidence of atherosclerotic disease of the carotid artery does

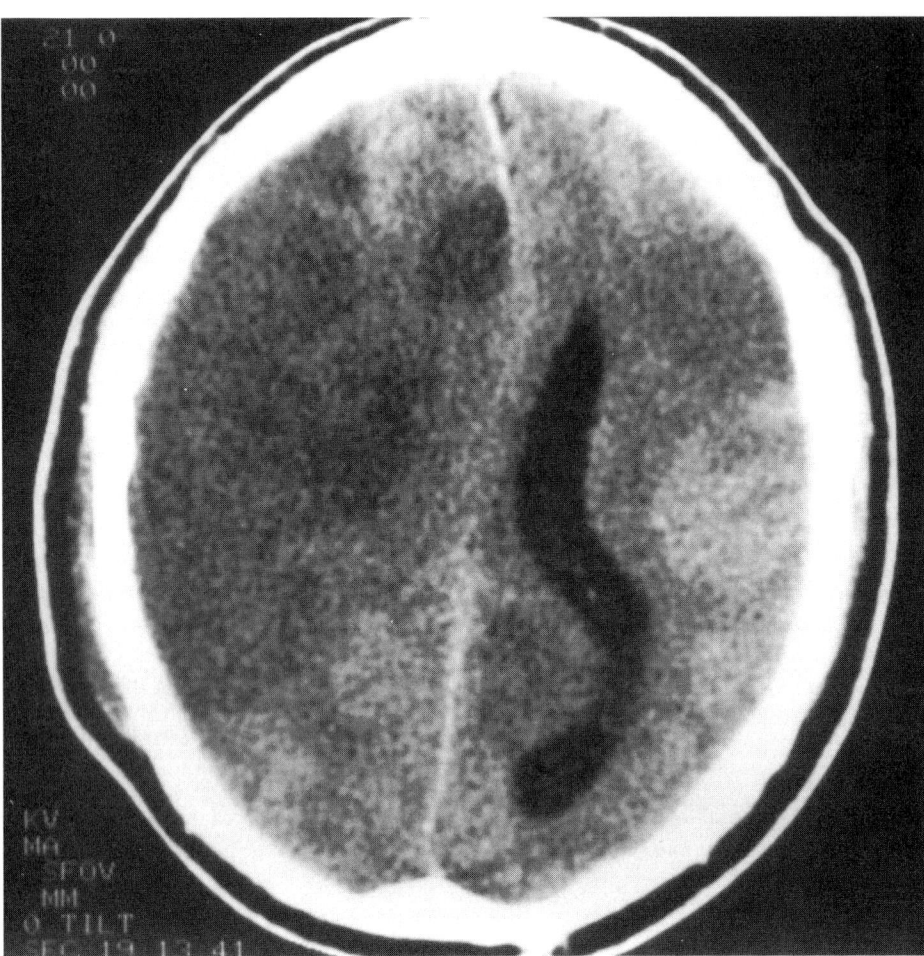

FIGURE 55A.1   A noncontrast computed tomographic scan performed to evaluate persistent coma 2 days after coronary artery bypass graft. Multiple bilateral ischemic lesions can be seen.

not, and carotid endarterectomy prior to the cardiac surgery is not justified.

Rare patients who fail to recover consciousness after surgery despite the absence of any identified metabolic cause have probably suffered diffuse cerebral ischemia or hypoxia. Hemispheric or multifocal infarction (Figure 55A.1) is responsible in some cases.

Neurological Complications of Medication

The infectious and neoplastic complications of immunosuppressive agents are discussed in the previous section. The other adverse events associated with corticosteroids are behavioral disturbances, psychoses, proximal weakness with type II muscle fiber atrophy, postural tremor, cataracts, and osteoporotic fractures. Benign intracranial hypertension may occur during treatment with or on withdrawal of corticosteroids. Neurological complications of cyclosporine include tremor, seizures, focal deficits, paresthesias, encephalopathy, and ataxia.

Among antiarrhythmic agents, amiodarone causes tremor, sensorimotor peripheral neuropathy, myopathy, ataxia, optic neuropathy, and pseudotumor cerebri. Pro-

cainamide may unmask latent myasthenia gravis or precipitate a lupuslike syndrome with secondary vascular occlusive complications that are probably associated with lupus anticoagulant and antiphospholipid antibodies. Quinidine has neurological side effects similar to those of procainamide and also causes headache, tinnitus, and syncope.

Lidocaine and related agents may cause seizures, tremor, paresthesias, and confusional states. Calcium channel–blocking agents occasionally cause encephalopathy. Beta blockers are associated with mental changes, paresthesias, and disturbances of neuromuscular transmission, and digoxin and thiazide diuretics with an encephalopathy and disturbances of color vision.

Infective Endocarditis

The incidence of infective endocarditis has been increasing because of intravenous substance abuse and the increasing use of prosthetic cardiac valves. The overall incidence of neurological complications of infective endocarditis is approximately 35% but varies with the infecting organism. Neurological manifestations are especially common in patients with mitral valve abnormalities and consist of

FIGURE 55A.2 Carotid angiogram, lateral view with subtraction, in a 48-year-old man with multiple peripheral mycotic aneurysms (*arrows*) verified at autopsy.

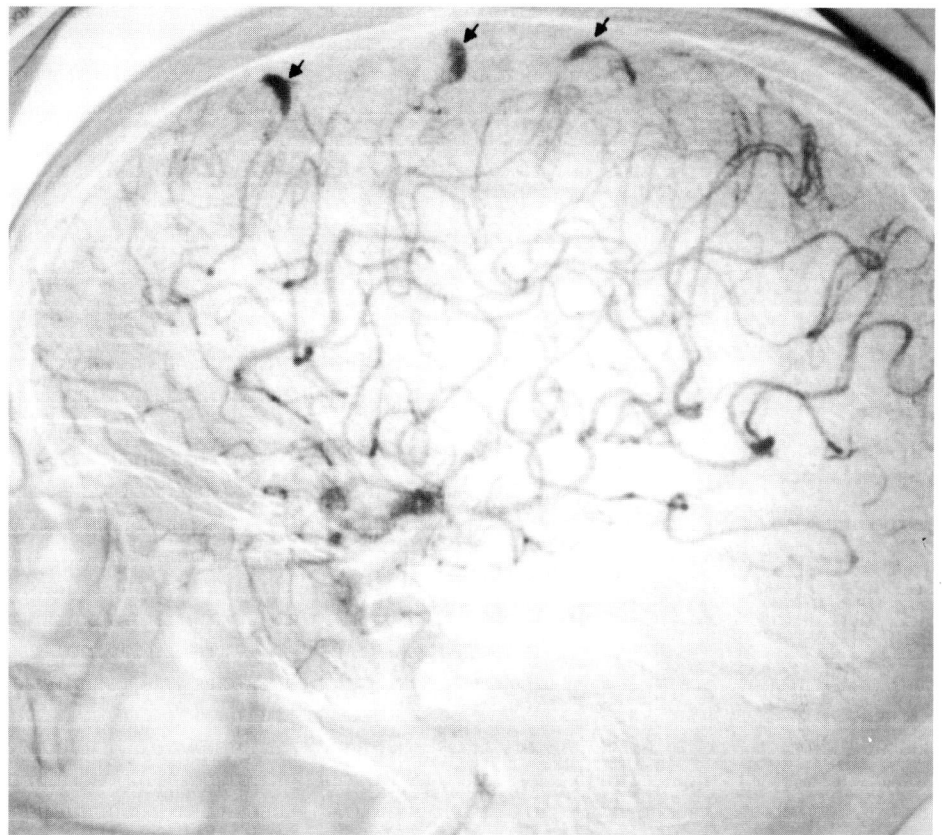

embolic or hemorrhagic stroke and infections such as meningitis or brain abscess (Bitsch et al. 1996).

Cerebral mycotic aneurysms (Figure 55A.2) are recognized complications of infective endocarditis and may result in intracranial hemorrhage. They generally develop at the point of bifurcation of peripheral arteries and have a more distal location than congenital berry aneurysms. The pathogenesis of mycotic aneurysms is unclear. The most likely cause is impaction of infected material in the vasa vasorum, with resulting destruction of the wall of an artery. Intraluminal occlusion of the vessel by infected material, with subsequent aneurysmal formation, is less likely but has been documented in some cases. Mycotic aneurysms may be clinically silent and sometimes resolve with antibiotic therapy. They are less common, but occur earlier, in acute than in subacute bacterial endocarditis. Their natural history is poorly defined.

Intracranial hemorrhage is caused also by septic arteritis that destroys the vessel wall without causing aneurysm, and by hemorrhagic transformation of cerebral infarcts. Arteriography is needed, therefore, in patients with intracranial hemorrhage to distinguish mycotic aneurysm from septic arteritis.

Intracranial bleeding from a ruptured mycotic aneurysm can be the initial feature of an underlying cardiac disorder or may occur during the management of previously recognized infective endocarditis. Four-vessel arteriography is indicated in every patient with infective endocarditis who

develops focal neurological deficits or has a subarachnoid hemorrhage. Arteriography should be performed before starting anticoagulation therapy in infective endocarditis unless an appropriate course of antibiotics has been completed without the development of neurological symptoms.

Embolization of infected material causes cerebral microabscesses and meningitis. Multiple septic emboli may cause meningoencephalitis or a diffuse encephalopathy that is characterized by a confusional state, headache, meningismus, and a cerebrospinal fluid (CSF) profile suggesting an aseptic process. The basis of these symptoms is probably multifactorial: infection, vascular occlusion, metabolic abnormalities, and mycotic aneurysms.

Antibiotic therapy to resolve the cardiac infection is the mainstay of treatment. Neurological abnormalities usually resolve. Imaging studies are indicated in patients with progressive or persistent neurological deficits or an abnormal CSF. Arteriography is needed when magnetic resonance imaging (MRI) suggests mycotic aneurysm. It is not clear whether mycotic aneurysms require surgical resection or should be treated with antibiotics alone. Resection is recommended when cardiac valve replacement is planned in order to reduce the risk of rupture from anticoagulants used during cardiopulmonary bypass. Anticoagulants are usually withheld from patients with infective endocarditis and cerebral embolism because of the risk of rupture of an unrecognized mycotic aneurysm. Moreover, control of the underlying infection with antibiotics reduces the risk of further embolism sufficiently to make anticoagulation unnecessary. Anticoagulation also may increase the risk of hemorrhagic transformation of embolic infarcts.

DISEASES OF THE AORTA

The aorta supplies blood to the CNS and peripheral nervous system (PNS). Several neurological syndromes result from aortic disease, depending on the site and severity of obstruction.

Spinal cord ischemia may result from congenital aortic abnormalities such as coarctation, acquired disorders such as aortic aneurysm or occlusive atherosclerotic disease, and aortic surgery or aortography. The level of myelopathy depends to some extent on the site of aortic disease. In general, aortic pathology that causes cord ischemia is above the origin of the renal arteries; obstruction more distally is less likely to affect the segmental vessels that feed the spinal cord. Risk factors for cord ischemia during aortic surgery include the presence of dissection or extensive thoracoabdominal disease, and a long cross-clamp time (Mauney et al. 1995). The thoracic cord is more susceptible to ischemia than the cervical or lumbosacral regions.

Spinal cord ischemia from aortic disease usually causes a complete transverse myelopathy or an anterior spinal artery syndrome. Weakness, loss of sphincter control, and impaired pain and temperature appreciation occur below the level of myelopathy. Initial flaccidity and areflexia are eventually replaced by spasticity, hyperreflexia, and bilateral extensor plantar responses. The existence of a true posterior spinal artery syndrome is doubtful, because the posterior spinal arteries have multiple feeding vessels along their length. Occasional reports of a clinical disorder resembling progressive spinal muscular atrophy have been attributed to cord ischemia from aortic disease affecting the anterior horn cells especially.

Neurogenic claudication may be caused by ischemia of the nerve roots or cauda equina (as by a protruded lumbar disk in spinal stenosis), by intermittent cord ischemia from spinal vascular malformations, or by aortic disease. Pain, weakness, or a sensory disturbance develops in one or both legs while walking or in relation to certain postures. Symptoms are relieved by rest or change of posture. Neurogenic claudication must be distinguished from the intermittent claudication of peripheral vascular disease, because their treatments are different.

Disease of the aortic arch or its main branches also may lead to transient cerebral ischemic attacks or strokes. The risk of embolization from the aortic arch has been grossly underestimated until recently, especially in patients older than 60 years. Transesophageal echocardiography is an important means of evaluating the aortic arch (Heinzlef et al. 1997).

Aortic Aneurysms

In Marfan's syndrome, there is an unusually high incidence of dissecting aneurysm of the ascending aorta that is associated with a dilated aortic root, but dissecting aortic aneurysms also occur in the absence of connective tissue disease. The neurological features usually consist of acute cerebral or cord deficits from ischemia. Acute chest pain often is associated with it.

Thoracic aortic aneurysms suggest a syphilitic etiology. Left recurrent laryngeal nerve palsy may result from compression or traction of the nerve, especially when the aneurysm involves the aortic arch. Horner's syndrome is a rare finding caused by pressure on the sympathetic trunk and superior cervical ganglion. Cerebral emboli are a complication of thoracic aortic aneurysms.

Abdominal aortic aneurysms are caused usually by atherosclerosis. The femoral or obturator nerve may be compressed, usually by hematoma and rarely from the aneurysm itself, or injured at surgery. Occlusive disease of the terminal aorta sometimes leads to an ischemic monomelic neuropathy, characterized by pain and loss of all sensation in the distal portion of the leg. Disturbances of micturition and sexual function also may result from aortic aneurysms.

Aortitis

The causes of aortitis include syphilis, Takayasu's disease, irradiation, transient emboligenic aortoarteritis, rheumatic fever, various connective tissue diseases (giant cell arteritis, rheumatoid arthritis, systemic lupus erythematosus [SLE], scleroderma), ankylosing spondylitis, and Reiter's syndrome. Neurological complications occur when arteries are involved that perfuse neural tissues or in relation to secondary aortic pathology such as an aneurysm.

Takayasu's disease is primarily a disease of young women. Nonspecific symptoms are fever, weight loss, myalgias, and arthralgia. Obstruction of major vessels of the aortic arch causes loss of pulses in the neck and arms, hypertension, and aortic regurgitation. Less common symptoms are headache, seizures, transient cerebral ischemic attacks, and stroke. Corticosteroids are the treatment of choice.

Transient emboligenic aortoarteritis is an inflammatory process affecting the aorta and other central elastic arteries, but not the more peripheral vessels. It is a cause of stroke or transient ischemic attacks in young people.

Coarctation of the Aorta

Congenital coarctation of the aorta is a narrowing of the thoracic aorta just after the origin of the left subclavian artery. Acquired coarctation may follow irradiation during infancy; the narrowing is in the irradiated region. A narrowed segment that is atypically located for congenital coarctation and unrelated to prior irradiation should suggest Takayasu's disease.

Headache occurs in more than 25% of patients with coarctation. Subarachnoid hemorrhage may occur when an associated cerebral aneurysm ruptures, and episodic loss of consciousness of uncertain basis is reported also. Spinal cord dysfunction occurs when the lower part of the cord, supplied by vessels arising from the aorta beyond the narrowed segment, becomes ischemic. Neurogenic intermittent claudication may result from the stealing of blood from the cord by retrograde flow through the anterior spinal artery, a part of the collateral circulation bypassing the narrowed segment. Marked enlargement of collateral vessels within the spinal canal may compress the cervicothoracic cord and cause myelopathy. Enlargement of the anterior spinal artery or one of its feeders may lead to aneurysmal distention and rupture, resulting in spinal subarachnoid hemorrhage. Treatment is by correction of the underlying coarctation.

Subclavian Steal Syndrome

Occlusion of either the innominate or left subclavian artery before the origin of the vertebral artery reverses the direction of blood flow in the vertebral artery on the affected side. This often causes no symptoms, but may cause ischemia in the posterior cerebral circulation. Neurological features are weakness, vertigo, visual complaints, and syncope. The pulse is typically diminished or absent in the affected arm, and systolic pressure is reduced usually by at least 20 mm Hg compared with the opposite arm. Reconstructive surgery is sometimes helpful but is unnecessary in most patients.

Complications of Aortic Surgery

Spinal cord infarction remains the most serious neurological complication of aortic surgery. Others are neuropathy, radiculopathy, postsympathectomy neuralgia when the sympathetic chain is surgically divided, and disturbances of penile erection or ejaculation when the superior hypogastric plexus is divided surgically (Goodin 1995).

CONNECTIVE TISSUE DISEASES AND VASCULITIDES

Neurological complications may be direct consequences of connective tissue diseases, secondary to other organ involvement, or secondary to treatment. The adverse effects of corticosteroids and immunosuppressive agents were discussed earlier. Connective tissue disorders are characterized by an autoimmune inflammatory response, especially necrotizing vasculitis. The mechanism of vasculitis is uncertain but may involve the deposition of immune complexes in vessel walls or cell-mediated immunity and release of lymphokines; autoantibodies also may be important in some instances (Moore 1995). The common direct CNS manifestations of connective tissue diseases are cognitive or behavioral changes and focal neurological deficits. Peripheral neuropathies also occur and may take the form of a vasculitic neuropathy, distal axonal polyneuropathy, compression neuropathy, sensory neuronopathy, trigeminal sensory neuropathy, acute or chronic demyelinating polyneuropathy, or plexopathy.

Vasculitic neuropathy is caused by nerve infarction from occlusion of the vasa nervorum. It is a mononeuropathy multiplex that becomes increasingly confluent as more nerves are affected until it resembles a distal symmetric polyneuropathy. Nerves tend to be affected in watershed regions that lie between different vascular territories, such as the mid thigh or mid upper arm.

Polyarteritis Nodosa, Churg-Strauss Syndrome, and Overlap Syndrome

Peripheral neuropathy occurs in up to 60% of patients with polyarteritis nodosa, Churg-Strauss syndrome, or overlap syndrome. It is usually a painful mononeuropathy multiplex that, at least in polyarteritis, often develops during the first year. As more nerves are affected, the deficits become more confluent and come to resemble a polyneuropathy. Occasional patients exhibit only patchy hypesthetic areas; others develop a secondary polyneuropathy, for instance, from renal failure, a plexopathy, radiculopathy, or cauda equina syndrome. Electrophysiological studies and nerve histology are frequently abnormal even when there is no clinical evidence of peripheral nerve involvement.

CNS involvement usually occurs later in the course than peripheral involvement. Common features are headache, which sometimes indicates aseptic meningitis, and behavioral disturbances such as cognitive decline, acute confusion, and affective or psychotic disorders. The electroencephalogram (EEG) is sometimes diffusely slow, but neuroimaging studies are generally normal. Focal CNS deficits are uncommon, are typically sudden in onset, and may be caused by infarction (Figure 55A.3) or hemorrhage. Angiography may not show the underlying vasculitis. Ischemic or compressive myelopathies from extradural hematomas are rare complications.

The 6-month survival rate of patients with untreated polyarteritis nodosa is only 35%. Prompt diagnosis and treatment are critical. Weight loss, fever, cutaneous abnormalities, and arthralgias are common, and there may be hypertension and renal, cardiac, pulmonary, or gastrointestinal involvement. Laboratory studies show multiorgan involvement and immunological abnormalities. Common abnormalities are an increased erythrocyte sedimentation rate (ESR), anemia, and a peripheral leukocytosis. Hepati-

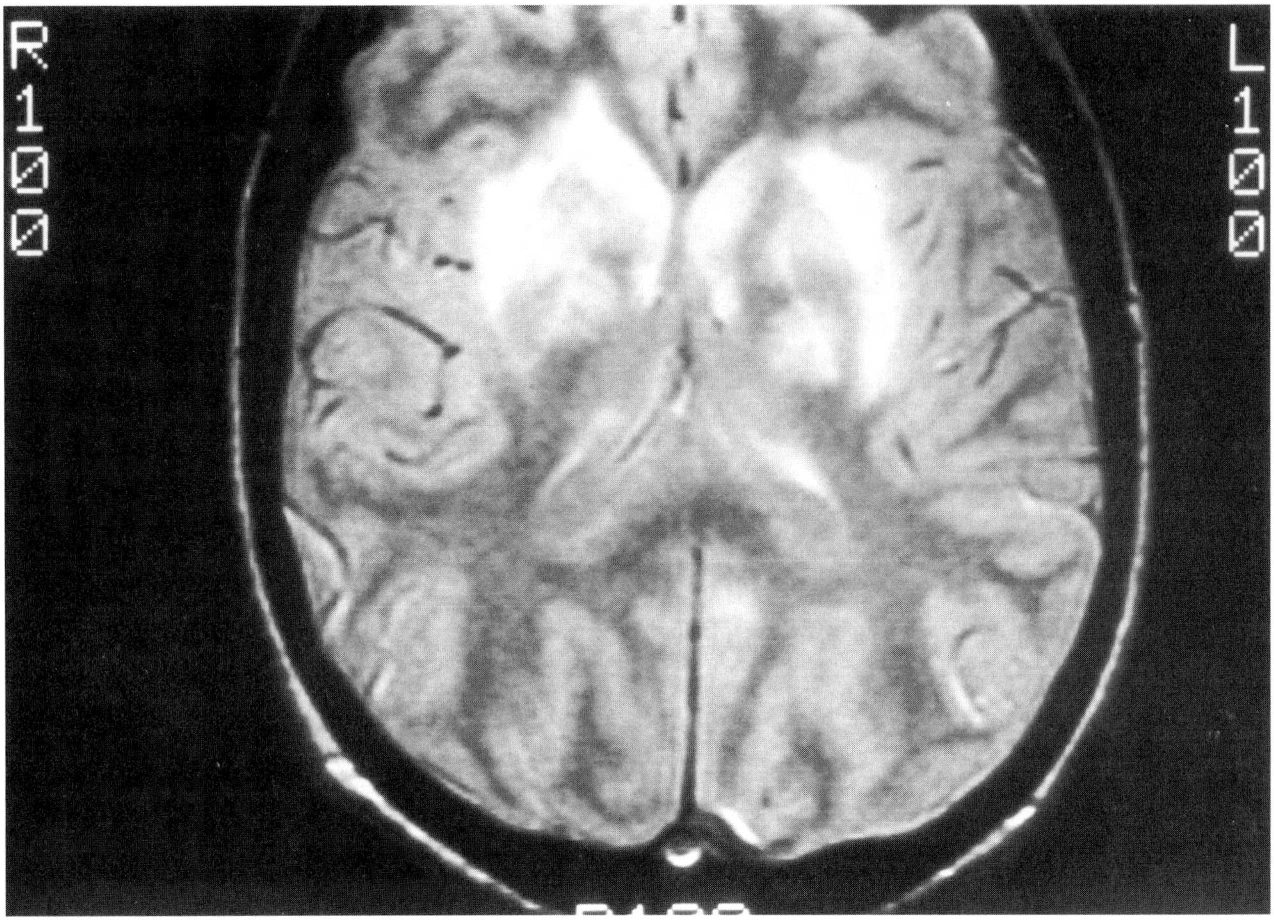

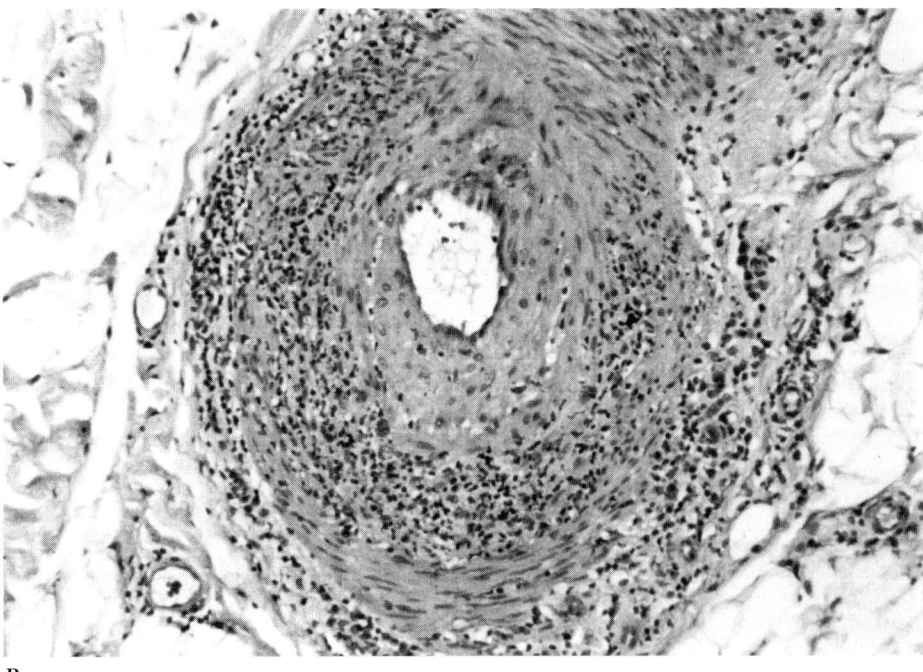

A

B

FIGURE 55A.3   (A) Proton density–weighted magnetic resonance imaging showing patchy high signal in the basal ganglia bilaterally. (B) Microscopical section of a biopsied blood vessel showing marked thickening and inflammatory infiltrates indicative of a vasculitis in this patient with polyarteritis nodosa (hematoxylin and eosin, 120×).

tis B surface antigen, hypocomplementemia, and uremia each occur in at least 20% of cases. Nerve or muscle biopsy often shows the necrotizing vasculitis, and angiography shows segmental narrowing or aneurysmal distention, especially in the renal, mesenteric, or hepatic vessels. Treatment is with corticosteroids, sometimes combined with cyclophosphamide.

Giant Cell Arteritis

Headache is the most common initial complaint of patients with giant cell arteritis, some of whom also complain of masticatory claudication. The temporal and other scalp arteries are often erythematous, tender, and nodular. A more serious initial symptom is acute transitory or permanent blindness, affecting one or both eyes, caused by ischemic optic neuropathy. Other CNS complications are rare, but neuropsychiatric disturbances, strokes, diplopia, or seizures are occasionally the presenting feature. Peripheral neuropathies occur in up to 15% of cases and are generalized peripheral neuropathies in approximately one-half of cases.

One-half of all patients have an elevated ESR, and polymyalgia rheumatica is often associated. High-dose corticosteroid treatment should be started once the diagnosis is suspected, without waiting to perform a temporal artery biopsy; any delay increases the risk of vision loss. Treatment is monitored by the clinical response and the ESR. The dose of corticosteroids is gradually tapered with time, but treatment is usually required for 18–24 months.

Wegener's Granulomatosis

Neurological involvement occurs in up to 50% of patients with Wegener's granulomatosis. Peripheral involvement is manifest usually by a mononeuropathy multiplex or, less often, a symmetrical polyneuropathy. The brain may be affected directly by vasculitis or by extension of granulomas from the upper respiratory tract; the associated clinical syndromes are basal meningitis, temporal lobe dysfunction, cranial neuropathies, cerebral infarction, or venous sinus obstruction.

In one study of 109 patients with neurological complications, 53 had a peripheral neuropathy, consisting of mononeuropathy multiplex in 42, symmetrical polyneuropathy in 6, and unclassified involvement in 5 (Nishino et al. 1993). Cranial neuropathy was found in 21 patients (usually second, sixth, and seventh nerve involvement); 8 had multiple cranial neuropathies. Other neurological features were external ophthalmoplegia from orbital pseudotumor in 16, cerebrovascular events in 13, seizures (from metabolic, septic, or other complications, or from vasculitis) in 10, cerebritis in 5, and miscellaneous abnormalities in 25.

Isolated Angiitis of the Nervous System

Isolated angiitis (granulomatous angiitis) of the CNS is discussed in Chapter 57G, and of the PNS in Chapter 80.

Rheumatoid Arthritis

Rheumatoid arthritis is the most common of the connective tissue diseases. Juvenile rheumatoid arthritis is discussed in Chapter 55B. Systemic vasculitis occurs in up to 25% of adult patients, but the CNS is rarely affected. Pathological involvement of the cervical spine (Figure 55A.4), or atlantoaxial dislocation, may cause a myelopathy, headaches, or hydrocephalus, or lead to brainstem deficits from direct medullary compression or vertebral artery involvement. Special care is needed when hyperextending the neck, as during endotracheal intubation, in patients with rheumatoid arthritis. Surgical fixation of subluxation (Coyne et al. 1995) is usually unnecessary unless displacement is marked or an associated myelopathy is severe or progressive.

Peripheral nerve involvement is frequent in rheumatoid arthritis. A distal sensory or sensorimotor polyneuropathy is common; clinical or electrophysiological evidence of sensory dysfunction is found in up to 75% of patients. Mononeuropathy multiplex and entrapment or compression neuropathies are also common. Compression injuries occur to the median nerve in the carpal tunnel, medial plantar nerve in the tarsal tunnel, ulnar nerve in the cubital tunnel or canal of Guyon, and peroneal nerve at the fibular head.

Several antirheumatic agents have adverse effects on the neuromuscular system. Gold treatment causes peripheral neuropathy in up to 1% of cases. Its onset is rapid and the evolution of weakness and the CSF profile may suggest Guillain-Barré syndrome. Chloroquine can cause neuropathy, myopathy, or both, and D-penicillamine causes disturbances of taste, an inflammatory myopathy, and a reversible form of myasthenia gravis.

Systemic Lupus Erythematosus

As many as 75% of patients with SLE have neurological involvement at some point during their course, often during the first year. Neurological complications may lead to a fatal outcome. The mechanism of CNS involvement is unknown. Neither the presence of antineuronal and antiastrocyte antibodies nor the deposition of antibody in the choroid plexus correlates with CNS involvement.

The most common neurological manifestations are episodic affective or psychotic disorders that may be difficult to distinguish from corticosteroid-induced mental changes. Cognitive dysfunction is often temporary. Treatment is empirical, depending on presentation and the prob-

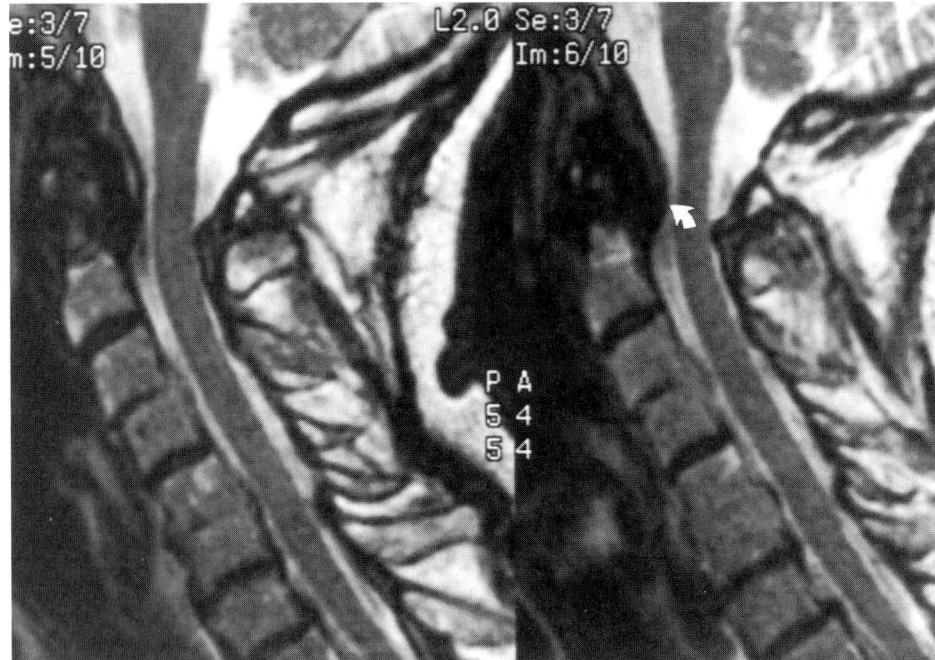

A

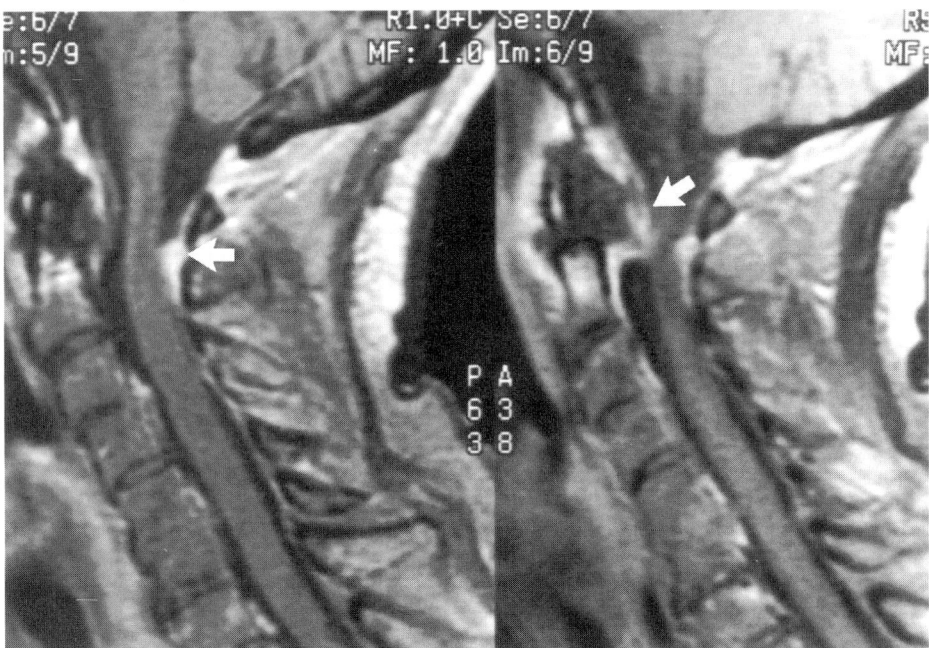

B

FIGURE 55A.4   Two contiguous sagittal magnetic resonance images of the craniocervical region in a patient with rheumatoid arthritis. (A) T2-weighted and (B) T1-weighted gadolinium-enhanced images. Arrows show pannus formation at C1, causing narrowing of the subarachnoid space and a suggestion of posterior displacement of the upper cervical cord.

able underlying pathophysiology. Disturbances of consciousness sometimes occur, especially in patients with systemic infections. Focal neurological deficits may result from strokes, the pathogenesis of which in SLE includes cardiac valvular disease, thrombosis associated with antiphospholipid antibodies, and cerebral vasculitis. Anticoagulant or fibrinolytic therapy may prevent stroke recurrence. Dyskinesias, especially chorea, occur in some patients with SLE, but underlying structural pathology of the basal ganglia cannot be detected usually; chorea is associated with the presence of antiphospholipid antibodies. The occurrence of generalized or partial seizures is probably caused by microinfarcts, metabolic disturbances, and systemic infections (see Chapter 55B for additional information on the pediatric aspects of SLE).

PNS involvement occurs less often and is characterized usually by a distal sensory or sensorimotor polyneuropathy. Other forms of neuropathy include an acute or chronic demyelinating polyneuropathy that resembles Guillain-Barré syndrome, single or multiple mononeuropathies, and optic neuropathy. Corticosteroids, immunosuppressive agents, and plasmapheresis are beneficial when neuropathy is caused by necrotizing vasculitis but are of less certain value in other circumstances.

Sjögren's Syndrome

Sjögren's syndrome may be a primary disorder or secondary to other connective tissue diseases. The main features are xerostomia and xerophthalmia. Women are more often affected than men. Definite diagnosis requires a positive result of the rose bengal dye test for keratoconjunctivitis, evidence of diminished salivary gland flow, abnormalities on biopsy of a minor salivary gland, and an abnormal test result for rheumatoid factor or antinuclear antibody. Neurological complications are not common but include psychiatric disturbances, late-onset migrainous episodes, aseptic meningitis, meningoencephalitis, focal neurological deficits, and in rare instances, an acute or chronic myelopathy. Cranial MRI may show hyperintense, small subcortical lesions (Escudero et al. 1995). Polyneuropathy is the most frequent peripheral manifestation, but mononeuropathy multiplex may occur also. Sensory neuronopathy is unusual but is more characteristic of Sjögren's syndrome than other connective tissue diseases.

Progressive Systemic Sclerosis

Progressive systemic sclerosis (scleroderma) was believed to affect the nervous system only rarely, but Averbuch-Heller and coworkers in 1992 suggested there is neurological involvement in as many as 40% of patients. The PNS is usually affected: Distal sensorimotor polyneuropathy, entrapment mononeuropathy, trigeminal neuropathy, myopathy, or myositis may occur.

Behçet's Disease

Behçet's disease, of unknown etiology, is defined by the combination of uveitis and oral and genital ulcers. Aseptic meningitis or meningoencephalitis occurs in 20% of cases. Focal or multifocal deficits also may occur and are caused by ischemic disease of the brain or spinal cord. The CSF commonly shows a mild pleocytosis, and the protein concentration may be increased. Peripheral nerve involvement is rare and takes the form of polyneuropathy or mononeuropathy multiplex.

Relapsing Polychondritis

Relapsing polychondritis is an infrequently diagnosed inflammatory condition of cartilage such as that of the nose, ears, trachea, and joints. Episodes of ear or nose inflamma-

tion typically last 1–4 weeks, then either resolve completely or leave deformities because of cartilage destruction. Both genders are affected equally, with peak age incidence between 30 and 60 years. Eye inflammation, especially episcleritis or conjunctivitis, may be associated with the attacks. Systemic vasculitis or features of other connective tissue disorders may develop. The diagnosis requires a typical clinical picture of chondritis. The ESR is elevated usually. Although autoimmunity against type II collagen may play a role in pathogenesis, only one-half of patients have serological evidence of anti–type II collagen antibodies.

Auditory or vestibular dysfunction occurs in nearly one-half of patients. The mechanism is usually otic rather than eighth nerve inflammation. Other cranial neuropathies, such as optic or facial neuropathy, may be associated. Headache, when it occurs, is more often caused by extracranial chondritis than intracranial inflammation. Aseptic meningitis, which may be recurrent, and vasculitic meningoencephalitis are sometimes associated.

Corticosteroids are the traditional treatment, and other inflammatory or immunosuppressive drugs have been tried in some cases. The efficacy of treatment is difficult to assess because of the remitting and relapsing pattern of the disease.

RESPIRATORY DISEASES

Ventilation requires the integrity of the CNS and PNS to support its coordinated motor activity. Diseases of the forebrain, brainstem, and spinal cord cause abnormal ventilatory patterns or ventilatory arrest, and diseases of the motor unit cause hypoventilation and ventilatory failure. This section is concerned with the neurological consequences of respiratory abnormalities rather than the neurological causes of ventilatory disturbances.

Hypoxia

The neurological manifestations of hypoxia depend on its rate of onset, duration, and severity. Hypoxia may be complicated by acid–base imbalance and leads to other hematological and biochemical changes that affect cerebral function. The precise mechanisms responsible for the neurological abnormalities discussed here are therefore complex.

Encephalopathies caused by chronic pulmonary insufficiency are characterized by headache, disorientation, confusion, and depressed cognitive function. Postural tremor, myoclonus, asterixis, and brisk tendon reflexes are found commonly on examination, and papilledema is present sometimes. These features are caused not only by cerebral hypoxia but also by hypercapnia, which leads to cerebral vasodilatation, increased CSF pressure, and altered pH of the CSF.

Sleep apnea syndromes cause chronic nocturnal hypoxia and become symptomatic as excessive daytime sleepiness.

Many affected patients are obese, plethoric, and snore heavily. The treatment is summarized in Chapter 72.

High-altitude sickness is characterized by headache, lassitude, anorexia, nausea, difficulty in concentration, and disturbances of sleep. Symptoms begin within hours or days of ascending higher than 10,000 feet. At even higher altitudes, consciousness may be disturbed; coma occurs in severe cases and may lead to a fatal outcome. Cerebral edema of uncertain cause is the major underlying feature that causes papilledema, retinal hemorrhages, cranial neuropathies, focal or multifocal motor and sensory deficits, and behavioral disturbances. Corticosteroids avert or relieve the syndrome.

Hypercapnia

Ventilatory impairment causes hypercapnia as well as hypoxemia, and the neurological manifestations of each are difficult to distinguish.

Hypocapnia

The hypocapnia that results from hyperventilation causes cerebral vasoconstriction, a shift of the oxyhemoglobin dissociation curve so that peripheral availability of oxygen is reduced, and an alteration in the ionic balance of calcium. The clinical features are lightheadedness, paresthesias, visual disturbances, headache, unsteadiness, tremor, nausea, palpitations, muscle cramps, carpopedal spasms, and loss of consciousness.

Hyperventilation occurs in hepatic and diabetic coma, with certain brainstem lesions, with various cardiopulmonary diseases, with certain drugs causing acidosis, and on an iatrogenic basis. Episodic hyperventilation often occurs without any identifiable systemic disease.

SYSTEMIC INFLAMMATORY RESPONSE SYNDROME

Neurological complications may occur when infection and trauma have induced a systemic inflammatory response affecting the microcirculation to multiple organs. For example, patients with sepsis and multiorgan (including respiratory) failure sometimes develop an axonal neuropathy that only comes to attention when attempts are made to withdraw ventilatory support. The neuropathy, which is called *critical illness neuropathy* (Bolton 1996), improves only slowly as the critical illness subsides.

Corticosteroids and neuromuscular blocking drugs may induce a myopathy, especially in patients with obstructive airway diseases. Its highest prevalence is among asthmatics who require ventilatory support in addition to corticosteroids and who have also received the neuromuscular blocking agent vecuronium. It sometimes occurs in patients who have received corticosteroids or neuromuscular blockers, but not both (Hanson et al. 1997). Muscle biopsy may show muscle fibers with specific loss of myosin (thick filaments).

A diffuse encephalopathy is a complication of sepsis and is most likely in patients with respiratory distress syndrome. Its pathogenesis is probably multifactorial and may relate to direct cerebral infection or to toxins produced by infecting organisms. Other contributing factors include alterations in the cerebral microcirculation, metabolic abnormalities, and the effects of medication (Bolton et al. 1993). The encephalopathy tends to fluctuate in severity, is often worse at night, and is associated with marked abnormalities of the EEG.

SARCOIDOSIS

Sarcoidosis is a disorder of unknown cause with multiorgan involvement and many different clinical presentations. It is more frequent in blacks than in whites and in women than in men. The disease is often discovered incidentally on routine chest roentgenography. The prevalence of neurological involvement in any series varies with case selection and diagnostic criteria but may be as high as 5%. The nervous system may be involved directly by the disease or secondary to opportunistic infections associated with abnormalities of the immune system. Only direct involvement (Figure 55A.5) is considered in this section.

Cranial neuropathies from chronic basal meningitis are the most common neurological manifestations of sarcoidosis. The facial nerve is affected most often, sometimes bilaterally. The optic nerve may be swollen or atrophied. Increased intracranial pressure from a space-occupying lesion, meningeal involvement, or obstructive hydrocephalus may cause papilledema. Visual changes are caused also by direct involvement of the optic nerves or their meningeal covering, or by uveitis. Unilateral or bilateral recurrent laryngeal, trigeminal, or auditory nerve involvement is also frequent, and multiple cranial neuropathies may occur.

Disturbances of the hypothalamic region are associated with diabetes insipidus, abnormalities in thermoregulation, amenorrhea, impotence, hypoglycemia, disturbances of sleep, obesity, personality changes, and evidence of hypopituitarism.

Other neurological features depend on intracranial or intraspinal meningeal or parenchymal involvement. Diffuse meningoencephalitis causes cognitive abnormalities or affective disorders. An enlarging granuloma may mimic a cerebral tumor and lead to seizures and focal neurological deficits.

Peripheral nerve involvement may take the form of a symmetrical polyneuropathy or an asymmetrical mononeuropathy multiplex. This may result from polyradicular involvement by extension of meningeal sarcoidosis or from direct involvement of the nerves by sarcoid granulomas. Muscle granulomas may cause clinical features of a

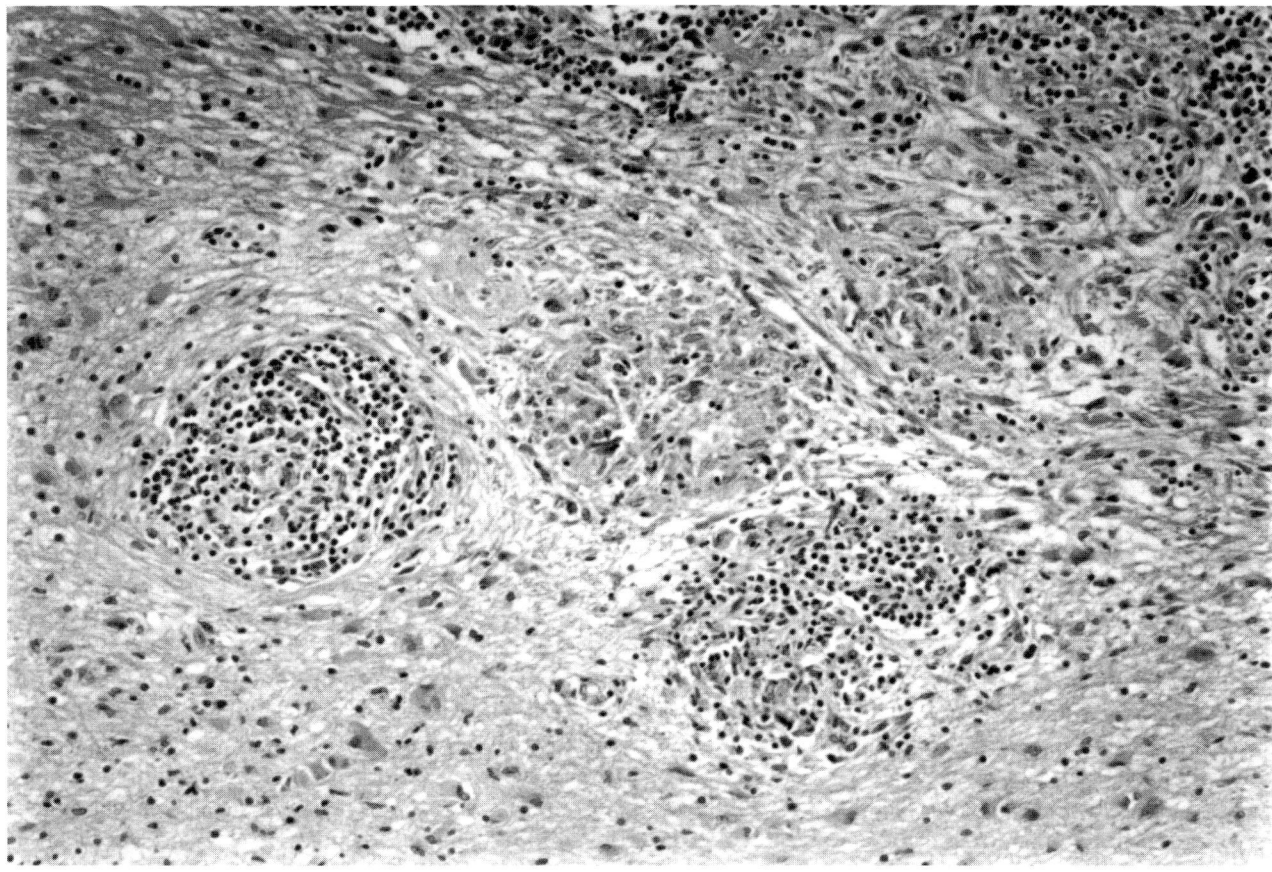

FIGURE 55A.5   Photomicrograph showing sharply delimited granulomas without necrosis in hypothalamus of a patient with sarcoidosis (hematoxylin and eosin, 40×).

myopathy and also are found commonly in clinically unaffected muscles.

Neurosarcoidosis often remits spontaneously but progressive neurological disease occurs in approximately 30% of cases. The diagnosis of neurosarcoidosis is difficult in the absence of systemic disease, especially cutaneous or pulmonary involvement. Histological confirmation often requires biopsy of seemingly unaffected tissue (e.g., muscle or conjunctiva) if other lesions are not accessible. Neither the tuberculin skin test nor the blood concentration of angiotensin-converting enzyme is definitive in establishing the diagnosis. Corticosteroid treatment is recommended generally, but its long-term value is not established. The initial dose of prednisone is 60 mg per day, and the dose is adjusted depending on clinical response. Irradiation of a focal lesion or cyclosporine is beneficial in some cases. Useful surgical measures are the excision of focal, enlarging granulomas and the placement of a shunt to relieve hydrocephalus.

HEMATOLOGICAL DISORDERS WITH ANEMIA

Anemia often causes nonspecific behavioral symptoms such as lassitude, lightheadedness, inattentiveness, irritability, headache, and unsteadiness. Iron-deficiency anemia is associated with pica, restless legs syndrome, and benign intracranial hypertension, and with an increased risk of stroke or transient cerebral ischemic attacks because of thrombocytosis. Severe anemia may rarely cause focal neurological deficits in patients with pre-existing cerebral atherosclerotic disease. Pancytopenia may cause hemorrhagic CNS complications.

Megaloblastic Anemia

Vitamin B_{12} deficiency causes myelopathy, encephalopathy, optic neuropathy, peripheral neuropathy, or some combination of these disorders. The neurological complications do not necessarily correlate with the presence or severity of associated megaloblastic anemia. Folic acid masks the anemia without preventing the neurological complications. The food supply in the United States was fortified with folic acid beginning in 1994 to prevent spina bifida and hence anemia is no longer a marker of vitamin B_{12} deficiency.

The Schilling test is an important means of diagnosing the most common cause of vitamin B_{12} deficiency, impaired absorption from deficiency of intrinsic factor. Vitamin B_{12} is absorbed exclusively by the terminal ileum, and deficiency may occur also in patients with urinary intestinal diversion (Terai et al. 1997). Treatment with intramuscular injections of vitamin B$_{12}$ reverses the neurological disorder. The extent of residua correlates with the severity and duration of symptoms before treatment.

Sickle Cell Disease

Sickle cell disease causes vascular occlusion of both large and small vessels. Sickling is aggravated by hypoxia, infection, dehydration, and acidosis.

The most frequent neurological complication of sickle cell disease is stroke, which occurs more often in children than in adults. Other complications are convulsions, intracranial (usually subarachnoid) hemorrhage, behavioral disturbances, and alteration in consciousness. The cause of intracranial hemorrhage cannot always be determined despite detailed investigation, but some cases are caused by rupture of an aneurysm that may be surgically accessible. Blindness sometimes results from proliferative retinopathy; retinal detachment or infarction also occurs. Spinal cord infarction is rare.

Thalassemias

Extramedullary hematopoiesis occurs in the liver, spleen, and lymph nodes of patients with severe forms of beta-thalassemia, but it may also occur in the spinal epidural space and cause a compressive myelopathy. Treatment includes local irradiation, surgical decompression, corticosteroids, and repeat blood transfusions. Bone marrow hypertrophy also causes facial deformity, nerve root compression, and auditory impairment. Surgical decompression or radiation therapy is beneficial in some cases.

ACANTHOCYTIC SYNDROMES

Acanthocytes, or spiny red cells, are associated with abetalipoproteinemia (see Chapter 68), neuroacanthocytosis (see Chapter 75), and McLeod's syndrome (see Chapter 83).

PROLIFERATIVE HEMATOLOGICAL DISORDERS

Leukemias

The neurological complications of leukemia are caused by leukemic infiltration of the nervous system, hemorrhage, infection, electrolyte disturbances, hyperviscosity, and complications of treatment. Localized leukemic deposits are more likely to affect the brain than the spinal cord; peripheral nerve involvement is rare.

The clinical features of meningeal leukemia are headache, nausea and vomiting, somnolence, irritability, convulsions, and coma. Obstructive or communicating hydrocephalus,

papilledema, and meningismus may be associated. Cranial neuropathies and spinal radiculopathies are common, and their multifocal distribution should always suggest meningeal leukemia. Examination of the CSF shows abnormal leukemic cells, especially if cytospin techniques are used, but a normal CSF result does not exclude the diagnosis of meningeal leukemia. Treatment is with intrathecal chemotherapy.

Intracerebral hemorrhage is more common than subarachnoid or subdural hemorrhage. It is associated with platelet counts less than 20,000/μl. The hemorrhage is often multifocal and varies in severity from microscopic to fatal. Spinal subdural or subarachnoid hemorrhage is less common than intracranial bleeding but is a potentially serious complication of lumbar puncture, sometimes requiring surgical decompression.

The hyperviscosity syndrome occurs when resistance to blood flow is increased markedly, so that transit through the microcirculatory system is impaired in consequence. It is characterized by headache, somnolence, impaired consciousness, stroke or transient cerebral ischemia, and visual disturbances. Venous sinus thrombosis, nonbacterial thrombotic endocarditis, and disseminated intravascular coagulation (DIC), discussed later in this chapter, may occur also. The most common cause of this syndrome is an increase in the concentration of circulating gamma globulins, which is discussed in the following section.

Infection is a common complication of chemotherapy or corticosteroid therapy. The use of broad-spectrum antibiotics often encourages infection by unusual organisms. Progressive multifocal leukoencephalopathy is an uncommon complication of leukemia (see Chapter 60).

Plasma Cell Dyscrasias

Plasma cell dyscrasias are classified on the basis of the protein synthesized. They may be complicated by paraneoplastic syndromes (see Chapter 58) and by an increased susceptibility to infections that may involve the CNS.

Myelomatosis

Multiple myeloma, the most common plasma cell dyscrasia, is associated with a monoclonal IgG or IgA paraprotein in the serum or urine. The clinical features are pain, fracture, and destruction of bone. Tumor infiltration of the vertebrae causes compression of the spinal cord or nerve roots. Back pain is conspicuous, radicular pain is common, and cord or root dysfunction may be present. Treatment by local irradiation and high-dose corticosteroids prevents or minimizes residual neurological deficits, but urgent decompressive surgery is required if the diagnosis is uncertain. Cranial involvement is less common than spinal involvement. Cranial neuropathies, especially of nerves II, V, VI, VII, and VIII, may occur. A reversible optic neuropathy of uncertain etiology, but probably not caused by infiltration, has been described.

Increased intracranial pressure does not necessarily indicate intracranial infiltration: Pseudotumor cerebri sometimes occurs without evidence of intracranial myeloma or hyperviscosity syndromes.

Peripheral neuropathy is a well-recognized complication of myeloma. A symmetrical axonal sensory or sensorimotor polyneuropathy occurs as a complication of the circulating immunoglobulin, and a predominantly motor neuropathy resembling chronic inflammatory demyelinating polyradiculoneuropathy may occur with osteosclerotic myeloma. Treatment with cytotoxic agents and plasmapheresis sometimes slows or reverses the neuropathy, as may irradiation of bony lesions. Tumor infiltration of nerves leads to an asymmetrical neuropathy that has the features of mononeuropathy multiplex. Amyloidosis is sometimes associated with myeloma and causes a neuropathy characterized by dysautonomia, marked loss of pain and temperature appreciation, and weakness.

The POEMS syndrome consists of *p*olyneuropathy, *o*rganomegaly, *e*ndocrinopathy, *M* protein, and *s*kin changes in patients with plasma cell dyscrasia. It is most often associated with osteosclerotic myeloma, but also occurs with osteolytic myeloma accompanied by only minor sclerotic changes and in patients without myeloma. Osteosclerotic myeloma usually is considered a variant of solitary or early multiple myeloma but may be a distinct entity. The neuropathy is a distal, sensorimotor polyneuropathy with both axonal degeneration and segmental demyelination. Other clinical features are papilledema; lymphadenopathy; hepatosplenomegaly; impotence; gynecomastia; amenorrhea; glucose intolerance; peripheral edema; ascites; pleural effusions; and cutaneous pigmentation, thickening, and hypertrichosis. Corticosteroids, cyclophosphamide, and irradiation of solitary osteosclerotic lesions may be beneficial.

Other neurological manifestations are caused by infections related to immunodeficiency, hypercalcemia, uremia, and hyperviscosity. The hyperviscosity syndrome is characterized by headache, visual disturbances, and encephalopathy. Hemorrhages, exudates, and venous engorgement are seen on funduscopic examination.

Waldenström's Macroglobulinemia

Waldenström's macroglobulinemia is a plasma cell dyscrasia associated with IgM gammopathy. Neurological complications are common. A progressive sensorimotor polyneuropathy is attributed to binding of monoclonal IgM to peripheral nerves or results from lymphocytic infiltration of the nerves. Other neurological complications relate to hyperviscosity or a bleeding tendency resulting from platelet abnormalities. Presentation is with a diffuse encephalopathy or focal neurological deficits. Common manifestations are fatigue, lassitude, lethargy, confusion, altered consciousness, and seizures. Visual, auditory, and vestibular disturbances also occur.

Neurological examination shows pyramidal, cerebellar, or brainstem abnormalities, and funduscopical examination may reveal papillitis, venous engorgement, hemorrhages, and exudates. Plasmapheresis relieves symptoms caused by hyperviscosity and helps the peripheral neuropathy in some cases.

Monoclonal Gammopathy of Undetermined Significance

Many patients with a monoclonal gammopathy have no evidence of serious underlying pathology, but some eventually develop a malignant plasma cell dyscrasia. Chronic inflammatory demyelinating polyradiculoneuropathy is the characteristic polyneuropathy associated with monoclonal gammopathy of undetermined significance. IgM autoantibodies that react with myelin-associated glycoproteins or with other target antigens may be present in the blood. Short-term treatment with intermittent cyclophosphamide and prednisone may provide long-term benefit (Notermans et al. 1996).

Amyloidosis

Amyloidosis may occur as a familial disorder with dominant inheritance. Portuguese, Japanese, Swedish, and other varieties are described. The main neurological complication is a small-fiber sensory neuropathy, with marked impairment of pain and temperature appreciation and lesser involvement of other sensory modalities (see Chapter 80). An associated dysautonomia is conspicuous. Weakness develops later.

Nonfamilial amyloidosis is divided into primary and secondary varieties. Primary amyloidosis occurs in the absence of other disorders (except multiple myeloma), whereas secondary amyloidosis occurs in association with such disorders as chronic infection. Peripheral neuropathy is a common feature of primary but not secondary amyloidosis. It is characterized by a progressive sensory or sensorimotor polyneuropathy with autonomic involvement or by carpal tunnel syndrome. Cranial neuropathy is uncommon; cranial nerves III, V, and VII are most often affected. Cardiovascular and renal dysfunction are common, and other organ systems also may be involved. The diagnosis is suggested by the clinical findings and the presence, in most cases, of a monoclonal protein in the serum. There is no effective treatment. Death usually results from systemic complications.

Accumulation of β_2-microglobulin–associated amyloid in patients undergoing long-term hemodialysis may cause carpal tunnel syndrome, a cervical myelopathy, or a cauda equina syndrome (Marcelli et al. 1996). Surgical decompression may be helpful in such circumstances.

Cryoglobulinemia

Cryoglobulins are proteins that precipitate in the cold and dissolve when heated. They are classified as monoclonal IgM, IgG, IgA, or light chains (type 1), mixed but with one monoclonal immunoglobulin (type 2), and polyclonal, without any monoclonal protein (type 3).

Primary cryoglobulinemia occurs in the absence of other disease. Secondary cryoglobulinemia occurs in association with disorders such as myelomatosis or macroglobulinemia with monoclonal protein production, or disorders with polyclonal protein production, such as vasculitis or chronic inflammatory disease. Cryoglobulinemia is associated with transient cerebral ischemic attacks, strokes, and a peripheral neuropathy that is probably ischemic in origin. The extent to which neurological complications are caused by the cryoglobulinemia, as opposed to the accompanying vasculitis, is unclear. Treatment with corticosteroids, plasmapheresis, or both, may be beneficial.

Lymphoma

Neurological complications of lymphoma can be caused by direct spread of tumor, compression of the nervous system by extrinsic tumor, or paraneoplastic syndromes (see Chapter 58). They may also result from irradiation or chemotherapy, thrombocytopenic hemorrhage, or opportunistic infections. Primary CNS lymphoma is a known complication of immunosuppression and occurs most frequently in patients with acquired immunodeficiency syndrome (see Chapter 58) and less frequently in transplant recipients.

Polycythemia

The thrombotic and hemorrhagic complications of polycythemia frequently affect the nervous system. Occlusion of small or large arteries or venous channels may cause cerebral infarcts that are sometimes recurrent and fatal. This thrombotic tendency has been attributed to increased blood viscosity, thrombocytosis, and possibly chronic disseminated intravascular clotting. Intracranial hemorrhage is caused by abnormalities of clot retraction, thromboplastin generation, and platelet function. Spinal cord infarction is rare. Patients with polycythemia often complain of headache, poor concentration, unsteadiness, tinnitus, blurred vision, dysesthesias, and other nonspecific symptoms. The basis of such symptoms is unclear, but disturbances in the retinal circulation may account for the visual complaints. Pseudotumor cerebri and chorea may occur with polycythemia. Chorea reverses when the underlying hematological disorder is treated.

HEMORRHAGIC DISEASES

Hemophilia

Intracranial hemorrhage is a major cause of death in patients with hemophilia. Hemorrhages may be epidural, subdural, subarachnoid, or intracerebral and may occur spontaneously or following trivial head injury. Neurological symptoms may

not develop for several days after injury. The severity of bleeding generally correlates with the severity of coagulopathy. Spinal subdural or epidural hemorrhage may occur but is uncommon; the clinical features are back or neck pain and a progressive painful paraparesis or quadriparesis. Surgical decompression is necessary to preserve neurological function, and the deficient factor VIII must be provided as well.

Peripheral neuropathies secondary to compression of individual nerves by intramuscular or retroperitoneal hematomas are a common complication. Urgent operative decompression may be needed to preserve function.

Seizures may result from brain injury caused by previous intracranial hemorrhage. Their control with anticonvulsant agents helps prevent further bleeding.

Other Congenital Hemorrhagic Disorders

Other congenital coagulopathies have a lower frequency of neurological complications than hemophilia, but these are similar to those already described.

Disseminated Intravascular Coagulation

DIC is characterized by thrombotic occlusion of small vessels and concomitant hemorrhagic complications because clotting factors (including fibrinogen and factors V and VIII) and platelets are consumed in the thrombotic process. DIC occurs in association with primary brain disease, diseases of other organs, septicemia, immune-mediated disorders, diabetic ketoacidosis, neoplastic disease, and obstetrical complications. Several different organs may be affected, but the brain is commonly involved. The underlying cause, rate of onset, and severity of DIC influence the clinical features, as do the organs affected and the predominance of thrombosis or hemorrhage.

Neurological features fluctuate in severity. Encephalopathy is common and varies in severity from a mild confusional state to coma. Comatose patients may recover completely, and continuing support is therefore indicated. The prothrombin time is usually prolonged, the serum level of fibrin degradation products increased, and thrombocytopenia may be present. The serum fibrinogen concentration is sometimes normal. Neuroimaging shows multifocal cerebral hematomas and infarctions. Treatment is directed at the underlying cause of DIC. Heparin may limit thrombotic complications but can worsen hemorrhagic complications; its value is uncertain. The same can be said of antiplatelet agents and antithrombin concentrates.

Thrombocytopenia

Thrombocytopenia, which is caused by reduced production or increased breakdown of platelets, may lead to hemorrhage. Intracerebral hemorrhage is usually from capillaries

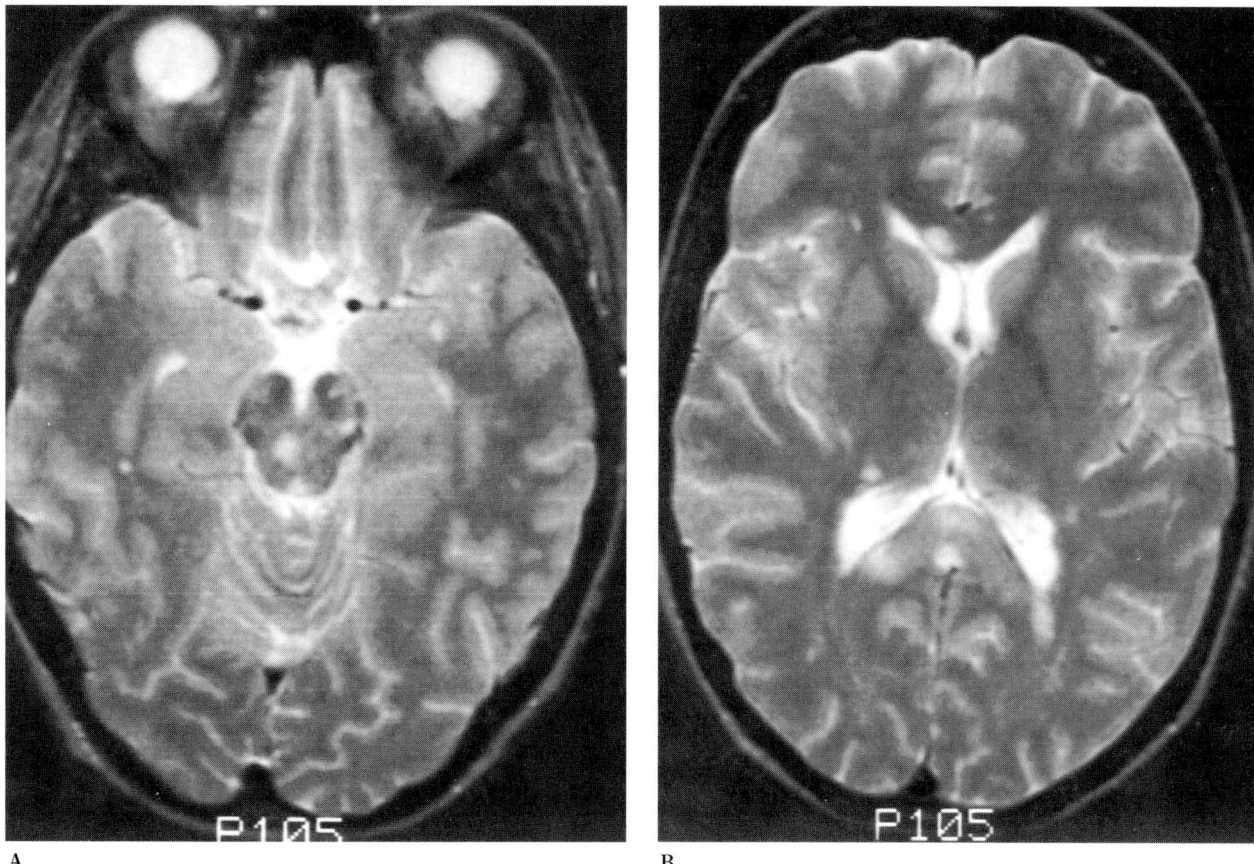

A   B

FIGURE 55A.6   A 27-year-old woman with Sneddon's syndrome (livedo reticularis and cerebrovascular disease). T2-weighted magnetic resonance imaging showing multiple foci of high signal intensity in the mesencephalon (**A**) and in the corpus callosum and periventricular white matter (**B**).

and is characterized first by clinically silent petechial hemorrhages and later by symptomatic hematomas. Spinal or peripheral nerve involvement by hemorrhage is uncommon. Platelet transfusions arrest further bleeding. Corticosteroids may be beneficial when platelet function is abnormal; splenectomy is sometimes indicated.

Thrombotic Thrombocytopenic Purpura

Thrombotic thrombocytopenic purpura is a disorder of uncertain cause, possibly immune-mediated, that often has a fatal outcome. The clinical features are thrombocytopenic purpura, hemolytic anemia, fever, neurological abnormalities, and renal disease. The neurological features may include headache, mental changes, altered states of consciousness, seizures, and focal deficits. Treatment options are plasma exchange or infusion, splenectomy, and administration of corticosteroids or antiplatelet agents.

Iatrogenic Hemorrhagic Disorders

Patients treated with heparin or warfarin may develop intracranial or spinal hemorrhage. The bleeding may be

parenchymal, subarachnoid, subdural, or extradural in location. It can occur spontaneously or after injury and cause the acute or subacute onset of a neurological deficit. Treatment includes reversal of the coagulopathy, definition of the pathology by neuroimaging studies, and urgent decompressive surgery if necessary. Intramuscular hemorrhage may cause a plexopathy or peripheral neuropathy that requires urgent decompression.

ANTIPHOSPHOLIPID ANTIBODY SYNDROMES

Antiphospholipid antibodies (the lupus anticoagulant and anticardiolipin antibodies) are detectable in several disorders, but especially in SLE, Sneddon's syndrome (Figure 55A.6), and other connective tissue disorders. They are found also in patients taking certain medications, with some infections and obstetrical complications, and as an incidental finding in healthy people. The presence of antiphospholipid antibodies increases the risk of thrombotic disease. Cerebral ischemia is caused by either arterial or venous occlusion. Visual abnormalities include amaurosis fugax and ischemic optic neuropathy or retinopathy. The occurrence of migrainelike headaches may be fortuitous. An acute ischemic encephalopathy, characterized by confusion,

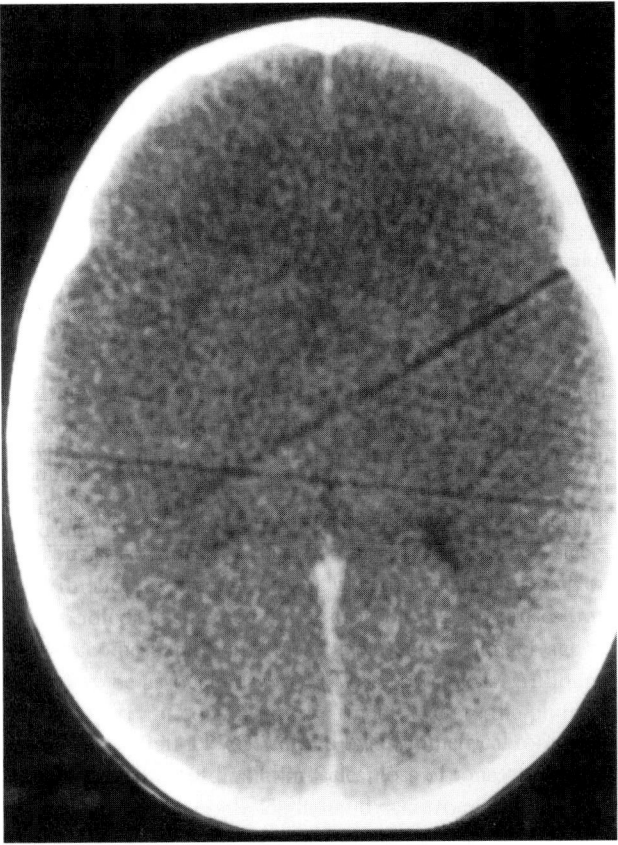

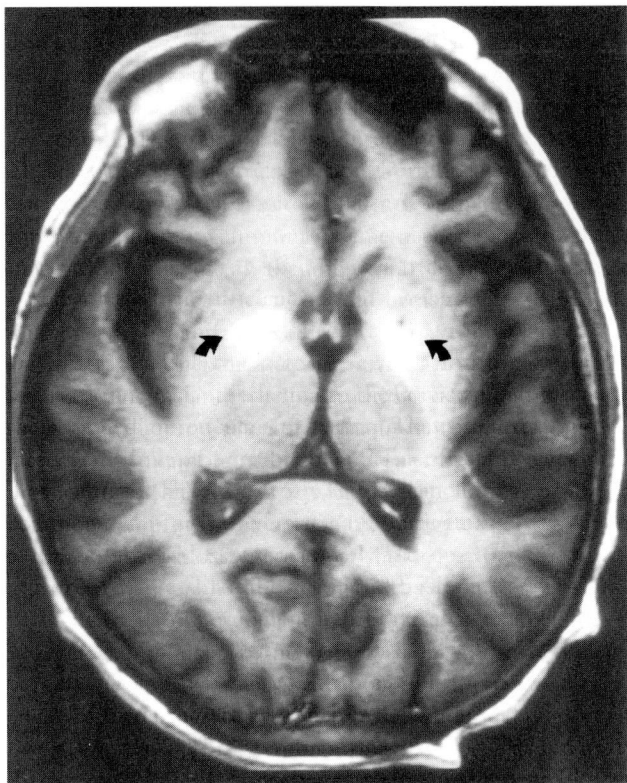

FIGURE 55A.8 Patient with chronic liver disease related to ethanol abuse. T1-weighted magnetic resonance imaging, without contrast, shows bright signal in the region of the globus pallidus bilaterally (*arrows*). T2-weighted images (not shown) were normal.

FIGURE 55A.7 A 15-year-old girl with fulminant viral hepatitis. Computed tomographic scan without contrast shows severe diffuse cerebral edema. (The two diagonal dark bands represent artifact from an intracranial pressure monitor.)

obtundation, quadriparesis, and bilateral pyramidal signs, may occur. Dementia, chorea, transient global amnesia, transverse myelopathy, Guillain-Barré syndrome, and seizures have been described also (Brey et al. 1993).

The pathogenesis of the thrombotic tendency is not established. The presence of antiphospholipid antibodies does not require immunosuppression. Cerebral thrombosis is managed in the same way as that from other causes.

LIVER DISEASE

Patients with acute hepatic failure often develop severe cerebral edema (Figure 55A.7). A variety of other neurological manifestations occur with chronic hepatic disorders.

Portal Systemic Encephalopathy

Chronic liver disease causes a portal systemic encephalopathy, characterized by an abnormal mental status (see Chapter 62). Points to emphasize here are that the encephalopathy may have an insidious onset, delaying its clinical recognition and treatment; a flapping tremor (asterixis) may be the only other neurological sign; and liver function test results, other than the fasting arterial ammonia concentration, do not always correlate with the severity of the clinical disturbance. EEG abnormalities also correlate with the severity of encephalopathy. MRI may show abnormal signal intensities in the basal ganglia on T1-weighted images (Figure 55A.8). The mechanism of the encephalopathy is unknown. Treatment is discussed in Chapter 62.

Chronic Nonwilsonian Hepatocerebral Degeneration

Some patients with chronic liver disease develop a permanent neurological deficit, even in the absence of prior portal systemic encephalopathy. The neurological features are similar to those of Wilson's disease (see Chapter 68): Intention tremor, ataxia, dysarthria, and choreoathetosis are common. As with portal systemic encephalopathy, the severity of the neurological disorder correlates best with the fasting arterial ammonia level. Neuroimaging studies may be abnormal. Specific treatment is not available.

Liver Transplantation

The neurological consequences of liver transplantation are similar to those of other organ transplants. The earliest postoperative disturbances are caused by organ rejection (with worsening hepatic encephalopathy), cerebral anoxia, cerebrovascular disease, or the side effects of immunosuppressant drugs, especially cyclosporine. Seizures are common. They result from metabolic disturbances, cerebrovascular disease, CNS infections, or adverse effects of treatment. Coagulopathies are also a complication and may cause fatal cerebral hemorrhage.

Late complications are usually caused by infections or malignancies affecting the nervous system.

PANCREATIC ENCEPHALOPATHY

It is not established whether acute pancreatitis is associated with a transient encephalopathy. The symptoms are nonspecific and similar to those of other metabolic encephalopathies, which must be excluded.

GASTROINTESTINAL DISEASES

Nutritional deficiency is the usual cause of neurological complications from gastrointestinal disorders (see Chapter 63). Several different dietary components are simultaneously deficient, and a single responsible nutrient is rarely defined.

Gastric Surgery

Neurological complications occur in 10–15% of patients after gastric resection. Impaired vitamin B_{12} absorption because of the loss of gastric intrinsic factor may be responsible in part for neuropathy or myelopathy. However, postgastrectomy neuropathy does not usually respond to vitamin B_{12} replacement alone. The myopathy that sometimes occurs is probably caused by vitamin D deficiency.

Gastric plication has been associated with encephalopathy, myelopathy, polyneuropathy, Wernicke's syndrome, and a nutritional amblyopia, but the precise nutritional deficiencies responsible remain to be established.

Small Bowel Disease

Neuropathy and myelopathy are associated with the malabsorption syndromes caused by small bowel disease, biliary atresia, or blind loop syndrome, or with previous extensive gastrointestinal resection. The findings may include pigmentary retinal degeneration, external ophthalmoplegia, dysarthria, peripheral neuropathy, and pyramidal and cerebral signs in the limbs. Ataxia may be an especially conspicuous feature, so that the neurological disorder resembles a spinocerebellar degeneration with an associated polyneuropathy. The syndrome is caused by vitamin E deficiency and responds to supplementation.

Chronic gluten enteropathy may cause a progressive and sometimes fatal CNS disorder in which there is some combination of encephalopathy, myelopathy, and cerebellar disturbance. Peripheral neuropathy is sometimes associated. An axonal neuropathy also occurs alone and without a measurable vitamin deficiency; restriction of dietary gluten leads to gradual resolution of neuropathic symptoms.

WHIPPLE'S DISEASE

Whipple's disease is a multisystem disorder that is believed to be caused by infection with the bacillus *Trophermyma whippleii*. It is characterized clinically by steatorrhea, abdominal pain, weight loss, arthritis, lymphadenopathy, and a variety of systemic complaints. Neurological involvement is rare but may occur in the absence of gastrointestinal symptoms. The most common neurological feature is dementia. Less common are seizures, myoclonus, cerebellar ataxia, clouding of consciousness, visual disturbances, papilledema, supranuclear ophthalmoplegia, myelopathy, and hypothalamic dysfunction. A characteristic movement disorder, oculomasticatory myorhythmia, is peculiar to Whipple's disease; pendular vergence oscillations of the eyes occur with concurrent contractions of the masticatory muscles and persist during sleep. Oculo-facial-skeletal myorhythmia is also pathognomonic when present; it resembles oculomasticatory myorhythmia but also involves nonfacial muscles (Louis et al. 1996). Postmortem examination shows abnormalities of the gray matter of the hypothalamus, cingulate gyrus, basal ganglia, insular cortex, and cerebellum.

The diagnosis is usually made by jejunal biopsy. Patients with neurological involvement also show cells that stain positively with periodic acid–Schiff stain in the CSF and brain parenchyma (Figure 55A.9). Polymerase chain reaction analysis of intestinal tissue is sometimes helpful (Louis et al. 1996). Treatment is with antibiotic drugs such as trimethoprim-sulfamethoxazole, penicillin, tetracycline, or erythromycin, which should be prescribed in patients with a compatible clinical syndrome even when the jejunal biopsy result is negative.

RENAL FAILURE

Renal failure is associated with several neurological manifestations. Uremic encephalopathy is discussed in Chapter 62. Its clinical features resemble other metabolic encephalopathies, and its severity does not correlate well with any single laboratory abnormality. The mechanism of encepha-

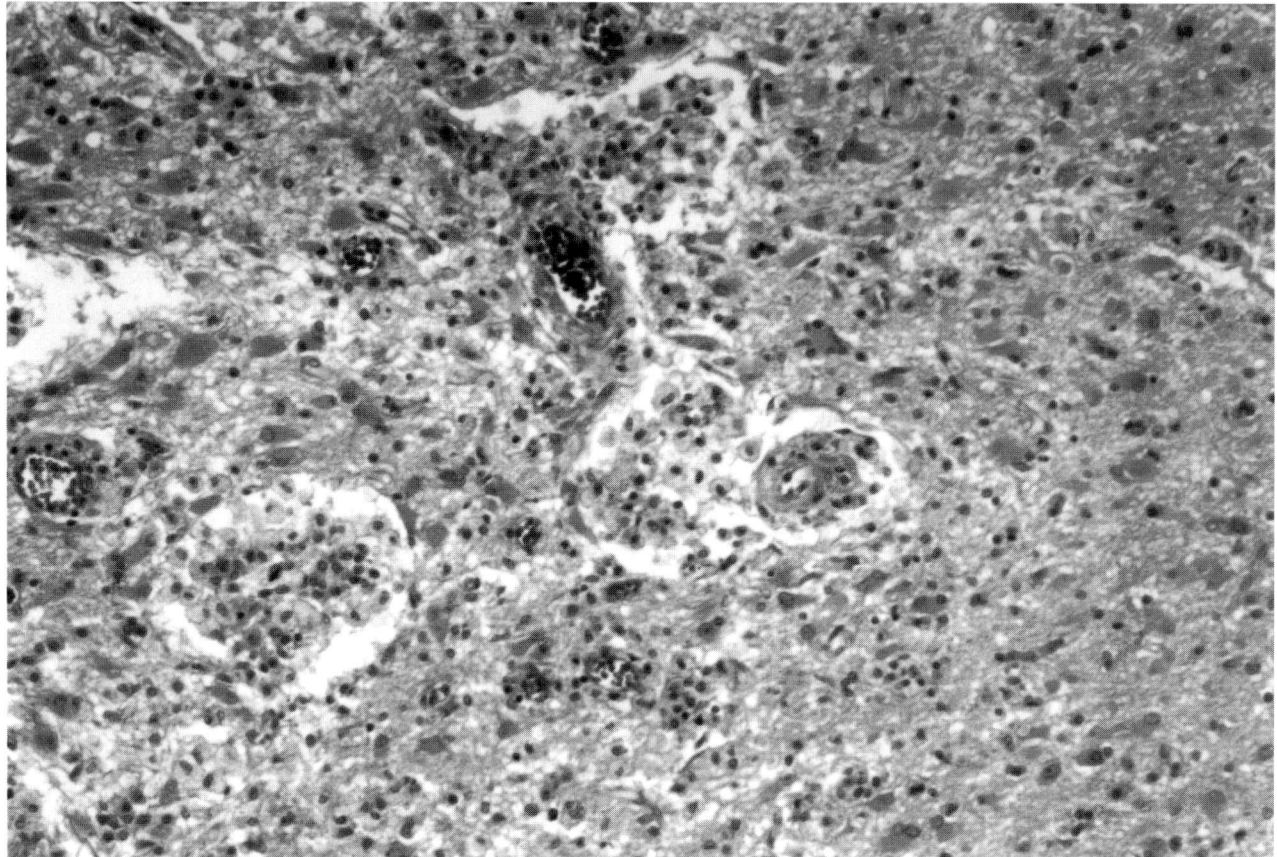

FIGURE 55A.9   Photomicrograph showing macrophages in brain tissue and around blood vessels, with prominent astrogliosis in involved brain, in a patient with Whipple's disease (hematoxylin and eosin, 40×).

lopathy is not established but has been attributed to the accumulation of toxic organic acids in the CNS or to direct toxic effects on the CNS of parathyroid hormone.

A length-dependent, symmetrical, sensorimotor polyneuropathy is a common complication of uremia. It usually worsens over several months but may progress more rapidly until the patient is profoundly disabled. Dysesthesias, muscle cramps, and restless legs are common early features. The neuropathy may stabilize or improve with long-term dialysis. Renal transplantation produces progressive improvement over the following year or longer, and complete recovery is possible. The neuropathy has been attributed to the accumulation of metabolites that have a molecular weight of 500–2,000 d, but its precise pathogenesis is not established.

Autonomic dysfunction leads to postural hypotension, sudomotor abnormalities, impotence, and gastrointestinal disturbances. Dysautonomia may be important in the development of hypotension during hemodialysis, but other factors, such as volume depletion, are undoubtedly involved as well.

Uremic optic neuropathy causes a rapidly progressive vision loss that responds to hemodialysis and corticosteroid treatment. Isolated peripheral mononeuropathies occur in uremic patients from compression or entrapment, or from intramuscular hemorrhage. Hyperkalemia is sometimes responsible for a flaccid quadriparesis that responds to electrolyte correction. Treatment of uremic patients with aminoglycoside antibiotics can lead to cochlear, vestibular, or neuromuscular junction disturbances, and a myopathy sometimes results from electrolyte disturbances or corticosteroid treatment.

Neurological Complications of Dialysis

Hemodialysis requires an arteriovenous shunt in the forearm that sometimes causes a carpal tunnel syndrome attributed to ischemia and venous congestion, or to β_2-microglobulin amyloidosis.

The dialysis disequilibrium syndrome is probably caused by shifts of water into the brain. It is characterized by headache, irritability, agitation, somnolence, seizures, muscle cramps, and nausea during or after hemodialysis or peritoneal dialysis. Less common features are exophthalmos, increased intraocular pressure, increased intracranial pressure, and papilledema.

Patients undergoing dialysis for longer than 1 year may develop a fatal encephalopathy called *dialysis dementia*.

Hesitancy of speech, leading to speech arrest, is a characteristic early feature. Intellectual function declines with time, and delusions, hallucinations, seizures, myoclonic jerking, asterixis, gait disturbances, and other neurological abnormalities ultimately develop. Death usually occurs within 6–12 months of onset of symptoms. The cause of dialysis dementia is uncertain, but aluminum intoxication was suggested by increased cerebral concentrations of aluminum at postmortem examination. Dialysis dementia has become less common since aluminum was removed from dialysates. Treatment with deferoxamine, a chelating agent that binds aluminum, is usually prescribed for patients with dialysis dementia but the optimal duration of treatment is unclear. Deferoxamine may actually exacerbate or precipitate encephalopathy in patients with very high serum aluminum concentrations, and it also causes visual and auditory disturbances.

Another cause of encephalopathy in patients undergoing dialysis is Wernicke's disease. Thiamine, a water-soluble vitamin, is removed by dialysis and must be replaced by thiamine supplementation.

Neurological Complications of Renal Transplantation

The placement of the transplanted kidney close to the inguinal ligament increases the risk of retraction injury or hematoma formation around the femoral nerve. The result can be a postoperative femoral neuropathy that often resolves completely. Dysfunction of the ipsilateral lateral femoral cutaneous nerve also may be caused by retraction or hematoma. The neurological complications associated with long-term immunosuppressive treatment are the same as for other organ transplants.

ELECTROLYTE DISTURBANCES

Sodium

Serum osmolarity is primarily determined by the serum sodium concentration. Rapid changes in serum sodium concentration cause CNS dysfunction by altering the osmotic equilibrium between the brain and body fluids. The typical clinical features are disturbances of cognition and arousal that can progress to coma. Myoclonus, asterixis, and tremulousness are common. Seizures, when they occur, are often refractory to anticonvulsant medications until the underlying metabolic disturbance is corrected. Focal symptoms (such as a hemiparesis) may occur during hyponatremia without any demonstrable structural basis but may indicate a prior or subclinical focal abnormality that is aggravated by the metabolic disturbance.

Focal abnormalities associated with hypernatremia often reflect intracerebral or subdural hemorrhage. The hemorrhage is caused by brain shrinkage from osmotic forces, with secondary tearing of blood vessels. Hypernatremia, a common consequence of dehydration, may occur in patients receiving inadequate parenteral fluid replacement. It also occurs with diabetes insipidus, pathological involvement of the hypothalamic thirst center by tumor, and excessive salt intake.

Hyponatremia, defined as a serum sodium concentration less than 132 mEq/liter, is associated with hypo-osmolarity, except in patients with hyperlipidemia or hyperglycemia. It occurs in several pathological states: excessive salt loss from the kidney or gastrointestinal tract, impaired water excretion, the syndrome of inappropriate secretion of antidiuretic hormone (SIADH), adrenocortical insufficiency, and iatrogenic water intoxication.

Hyponatremia in patients with acute brain syndromes, such as subarachnoid hemorrhage, is often attributed to SIADH. In fact, hyponatremia in this circumstance is more likely to be caused by salt wasting than SIADH, and patients have a reduced plasma volume, rather than a normal or increased plasma volume as expected with SIADH. In such cases, fluid restriction further exacerbates the hypovolemia and may cause cerebral ischemia.

The rapid correction of hyponatremia may cause central pontine myelinolysis, a disorder initially associated with alcoholism or malnutrition but now more often iatrogenic in origin. Neurological deterioration from central pontine myelinolysis may obscure or follow the resolution of hyponatremic encephalopathy. Severe cases are characterized by a spastic or flaccid quadriparesis, pseudobulbar palsy, and decreased states of consciousness. In some patients, the clinical features are minimal compared with the abnormalities seen on MRI. Central pontine myelinolysis is prevented when hyponatremia is corrected at a rate of less than 12 mEq/liter per day.

Potassium

The difference in the concentration of intracellular and extracellular potassium creates the resting membrane potential of nerve and muscle cells. Disturbances of serum potassium concentrations adversely affect cardiac and neuromuscular function. The hereditary periodic paralyses are discussed in Chapter 83.

Hyperkalemia usually causes cardiac arrhythmia before disturbing neurological function. The arrhythmia is sometimes associated with rapidly progressive flaccid paralysis and depressed tendon reflexes. Weakness may last for several hours, may be preceded by burning paresthesias, and is sometimes accompanied by mental changes. Treatment is determined by the underlying cause, severity of the hyperkalemia, and electrocardiographic findings.

Hypokalemia usually causes neuromuscular disturbances rather than encephalopathy. Mild hypokalemia causes myalgia, fatigability, and proximal weakness that spares the bulbar muscles. Severe hypokalemia causes rhabdomyolysis and myoglobinuria, and hypokalemic alkalosis causes tetany. All symptoms remit when normokalemia is re-established.

Calcium

Hypercalcemia is associated with metastatic disease, myeloma, paraneoplastic syndromes, primary or secondary hyperparathyroidism, vitamin D intoxication, and milk-alkali syndrome. Its main CNS complication is an encephalopathy, characterized by altered state of consciousness, apathy or agitation, depression or mania, headache, and, in rare instances, seizures that may be a result of vascular occlusive complications. In the PNS, there is muscle weakness and fatigability, especially in patients with hyperparathyroidism, who may develop myopathy.

Hypocalcemia may follow thyroid or parathyroid surgery and is a well-recognized feature of hypoparathyroidism, malabsorption syndromes, vitamin D deficiency, and acute pancreatitis. Tetany is the main symptom of hypocalcemia. Perioral and distal limb paresthesias are the initial feature and are followed by muscle cramps, a feeling of muscle spasms, and then actual spasm of the hands and feet.

CNS complications of hypocalcemia are focal or generalized seizures and an encephalopathy characterized by hallucinations, delusions, psychosis, altered states of consciousness, and cognitive impairment. The seizures respond poorly to anticonvulsant drugs but stop when hypocalcemia is corrected. Other CNS complications of hypocalcemia are parkinsonism or chorea that responds to correction of the calcium abnormality, increased intracranial pressure (in patients with hypoparathyroidism), and myelopathy.

Magnesium

Intracellular magnesium is involved in the activation of several enzymatic reactions, and extracellular magnesium is important in synaptic transmission.

Hypomagnesemia is caused by reduced intake or absorption of magnesium or by excessive loss from diuretics, kidney disorders such as renal tubular acidosis, and diabetic acidosis. Serum concentrations do not reflect accurately the severity of magnesium depletion, because magnesium is predominantly an intracellular ion.

The neurological complications of hypomagnesemia are similar to those of hypocalcemia, and the two often coexist. The possibility of concurrent hypomagnesemia must be considered when managing hypocalcemia, especially when parenteral calcium supplementation fails to provide the expected response. Complaints of weakness in patients with hypomagnesemia may be caused by magnesium deficiency alone or with other electrolyte abnormalities. Hypomagnesemia is treated with magnesium sulfate given orally, unless there is an absorptive defect, when it is given intramuscularly or intravenously.

Hypermagnesemia is caused by excessive intake or impaired excretion of magnesium. The usual cause is renal failure. Clinical features are drowsiness and diminished responsiveness, confusion, and depressed or absent tendon reflexes. Other features are hypotension, respiratory depression, and weakness from impaired neuromuscular transmission. Severe hypermagnesemia causes coma and may be fatal.

PITUITARY DISEASE

Pituitary Adenomas

The initial features of prolactin-secreting pituitary adenomas are amenorrhea and galactorrhea in women and impotence in men. However, the diagnosis of prolactinoma is often not considered until the patients develop symptoms of increased intracranial pressure originating in the sellar region. The treatment choices are transsphenoidal surgery or dopaminergic agonists such as bromocriptine. Radiation therapy is used when these choices are either unhelpful or not feasible.

Growth hormone–secreting pituitary tumors cause acromegaly; gigantism occurs in children, and enlargement of the jaw, extremities, and skull in adults. Approximately 50% of patients have a myopathy, which improves over many months when the underlying hormonal disorder is treated. Carpal tunnel syndrome in patients with acromegaly is from hypertrophy of the transverse carpal ligament. Symptoms usually resolve 2–3 months after surgical excision of the pituitary tumor, but electrophysiological abnormalities may persist for longer. Patients with acromegaly also may develop a mild, usually subclinical, polyneuropathy.

Cushing's Disease and Syndrome

Cushing's disease is caused by excessive secretion of adrenocorticotropic hormone from the pituitary gland. The clinical features are truncal obesity, hypertension, acne, hirsutism, osteoporosis, diabetes mellitus, and menstrual irregularities. Mental changes are common and include anxiety, agitation, insomnia, depression, euphoria, mania, and psychoses. Proximal muscle weakness and wasting are common, especially in the legs. Muscle biopsy shows type II fiber atrophy, a characteristic feature of muscle in patients treated with corticosteroids (see Chapter 83); electromyography is generally normal. The constellation of clinical features that constitutes Cushing's syndrome is seen also as a paraneoplastic syndrome, in association with adrenal adenomas, and after long-term corticosteroid treatment.

An enlarging pituitary adenoma may cause a visual field defect (Figure 55A.10). Treatment of Cushing's disease by bilateral adrenalectomy sometimes leads to rapid expansion

FIGURE 55A.10 T1-weighted gadolinium-enhanced magnetic resonance imaging. (**A**) Sagittal view. (**B**) Coronal view. A heterogeneously enhancing mass arises out of the sella turcica and extends up to involve the region of the optic chiasm. Surgery confirmed a pituitary adenoma.

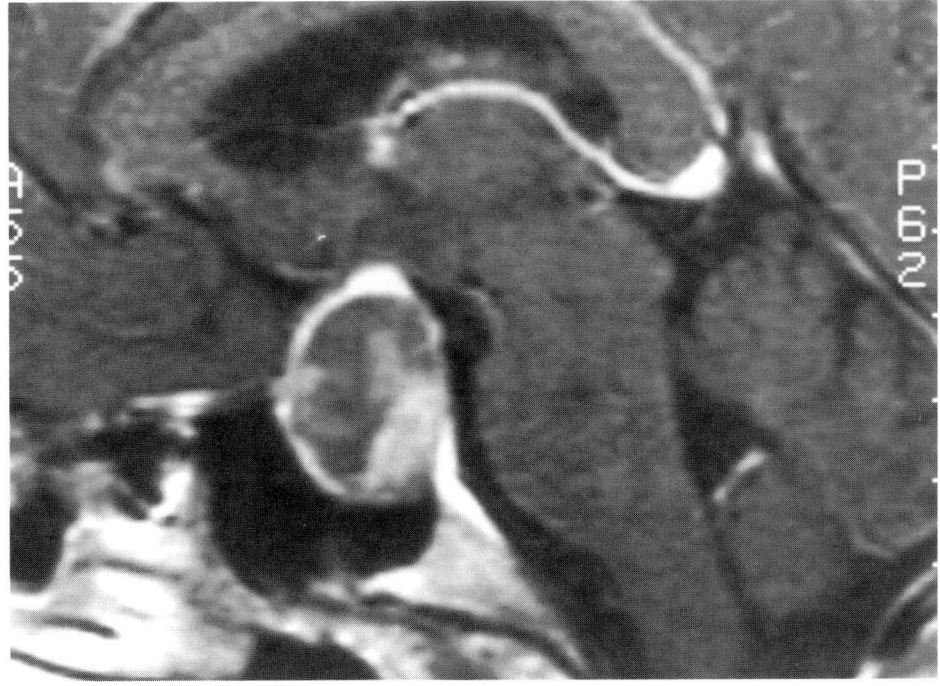

A

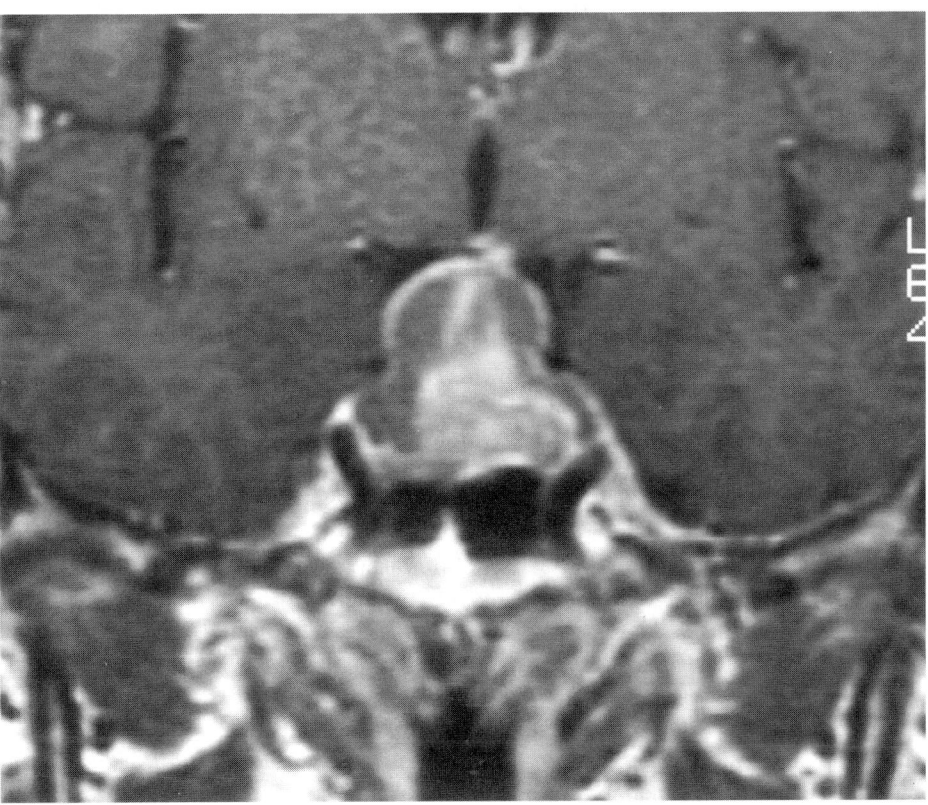

B

of the underlying pituitary adenoma (Nelson's syndrome), with compression of other cranial nerves, especially III. Intracranial hypertension is a well-recognized complication of Cushing's syndrome and occurs particularly after the pituitary adenoma is resected.

Hypopituitarism

Hypopituitarism results from diseases of the pituitary gland or hypothalamus. The neurological features depend on the severity of secretory impairment and on the hormones affected. Common features are apathy and intellectual decline, which are often difficult to attribute to a single hormone deficiency because several are affected concurrently.

Diabetes Insipidus

Diabetes insipidus, the inability to conserve water, results from disorders of the hypothalamus or pituitary gland or from interruption of the neurohypophyseal tract. Transitory diabetes insipidus is often a complication of head injury or intracranial surgery and may occur without explanation in previously well patients. Nephrogenic diabetes insipidus is caused by impaired renal responsiveness to vasopressin, which is synthesized in the hypothalamus and transported to the posterior pituitary gland. The main neurological feature is an encephalopathy that varies in severity from irritability to somnolence and ultimately to coma. Hypotension and hyperthermia also occur. Treatment is with vasopressin or a long-acting vasopressin analogue.

THYROID DISEASE

Hyperthyroidism

The features of hyperthyroidism are anxiety, restlessness, irritability, emotional lability, impaired concentration, headaches, and insomnia. Elderly patients may become depressed and lethargic, a condition designated *apathetic hyperthyroidism*. An enhanced physiological tremor and generalized hyperreflexia are common. Hyperthyroidism itself may cause seizures or may trigger a pre-existing seizure disorder. Chorea and paroxysmal choreoathetosis also have been described.

Thyrotoxic crisis is characterized by confusion and agitation leading to coma. Fever, cardiac arrhythmias, diarrhea and vomiting, and other systemic disturbances are associated. Treatment consists of hydration and cooling, beta-blocking drugs, corticosteroids, and, in some cases, plasmapheresis.

Dysthyroid orbitopathy (ophthalmic Graves' disease), characterized by exophthalmos and ophthalmoplegia, is common. Orbital edema and infiltration by inflammatory cells lead to orbital fullness, conjunctival edema and hyperemia, proptosis, and some limitation of ocular movements. Eyelid retraction may be caused by sympathetic overactivity affecting Müller's muscle in the upper lids and fibrosis of the levator muscle. The occasional occurrence of optic neuropathy is related to infiltration of the optic nerve, crowding of the orbital apex, and enlargement of the extraocular muscles. Dysthyroid orbitopathy may occur in patients without a history of thyroid disease or clinical signs of hyperthyroidism. Treatment options include corticosteroids, radiation therapy, and orbital decompression.

Compression of the recurrent laryngeal nerve or cervical sympathetic fibers by an enlarged thyroid gland, commonly neoplastic, may lead to vocal cord paralysis or Horner's syndrome, respectively.

Several neuromuscular disorders are associated with hyperthyroidism. Most common is a proximal myopathy accompanied by fasciculations. Its mechanism is unknown, but the severity of myopathy does not correlate with the severity of thyroid abnormality. Serum creatine kinase levels are generally normal. Improvement occurs with treatment of the underlying thyroid disorder. Hyperthyroidism and myasthenia gravis often coexist. Both are immune-mediated disorders (see Chapter 82). Treatment of one disorder, however, does not have any predictable effect on the other.

Thyrotoxic periodic paralysis is similar to familial hypokalemic period paralysis (see Chapter 83). It is particularly seen in Asians, and the hyperthyroidism may be clinically silent. Episodes of weakness occur after activity or after meals with high carbohydrate content. Potassium administration treats the acute attacks, and correction of the thyroid disorder cures the periodic paralysis as well.

A sensorimotor polyneuropathy has been reported in hyperthyroidism, but the association may be fortuitous.

Hypothyroidism

Mental changes are common in hypothyroidism. Apathy, somnolence, and impaired concentration are typical and are often attributed to depression. Confusion, delirium, and psychosis (myxedema madness) may occur also and improve with treatment of the underlying thyroid disorder. In severe hypothyroidism, decreased states of consciousness are associated with hypotension, hypothermia, respiratory failure, hypoglycemia, and other metabolic derangements; untreated, the disorder progresses to coma and sometimes death.

Other features of hypothyroidism are an increased incidence of seizures, truncal ataxia caused by a cerebellar degeneration, hearing loss, and cranial neuropathies. Hoarseness of the voice is caused by structural changes in the vocal cords rather than neurological disease. The neurological complications of hypothyroidism usually recover with thyroid replacement, especially if the deficiency is not long-standing.

The PNS is often involved in hypothyroidism. Most common is a proximal myopathy accompanied by myalgia and muscle stiffness. The affected muscles may be enlarged (Hoffmann's syndrome) and have myoedema (transient local mounding when a muscle is percussed).

Carpal tunnel syndrome occurs in as many as 30% of patients and usually responds to correction of the thyroid disorder. Less common is a sensory or sensorimotor neuropathy; both segmental demyelination and axonal degeneration have been implicated. There may be slow relaxation of tendon reflexes. Myasthenia gravis is associated also but occurs less commonly than in hyperthyroidism.

Hashimoto's Thyroiditis

Hashimoto's thyroiditis has been associated with myasthenia gravis and less clearly with giant cell arteritis and vasculitic peripheral neuropathy. In addition, a relapsing encephalopathy may occur in association with Hashimoto's thyroiditis and high titers of antithyroid antibodies. Clinical presentation is with confusion, altered conscious level, and seizures. Tremulousness and myoclonus may be conspicuous, and strokelike episodes of deterioration are frequent. The EEG is diffusely abnormal, the CSF protein concentration is increased without any associated pleocytosis, and neuroimaging studies are normal except for patchy abnormal uptake on isotope brain scan. Treatment is with corticosteroids. The long-term prognosis is good (Ghika-Schmid et al. 1996).

PARATHYROID DISEASE

Hyperparathyroidism

Neurological manifestations of hyperparathyroidism are common. They are essentially those of hypercalcemia (discussed previously under Calcium). A mild proximal myopathy may occur also and improves with surgical treatment of the parathyroid disorder. A picture like that of amyotrophic lateral sclerosis has also been described.

Hypoparathyroidism

Hypoparathyroidism commonly follows thyroidectomy or has an idiopathic basis. Pseudohypoparathyroidism is caused by peripheral resistance to the effects of parathyroid hormone rather than to any deficiency of hormone secretion. The neurological manifestations of these disorders relate primarily to the effects of hypocalcemia on the nervous system. Intracranial calcification is common in patients with hypoparathyroidism and occurs especially in the basal ganglia; it is usually asymptomatic. Benign intracranial hypertension also may be associated with hypoparathyroidism and is reversed by correction of the underlying metabolic disorder.

ADRENAL GLANDS

Pheochromocytoma

Pheochromocytoma is associated with neurofibromatosis and von Hippel–Lindau disease (see Chapter 69). The initial features of pheochromocytoma are paroxysmal symptoms of excessive catecholamine secretion: headache, hyperhidrosis, palpitations, tremulousness, and anxiety. Most patients have hypertension and seizures occur in approximately 5%.

Addison's Disease

Adrenal failure results from diseases of the pituitary or adrenal gland, or from adrenal suppression by long-term use of exogenous corticosteroids. The major features are generalized weakness, fatigability, lassitude, depression, headache, weight loss, anorexia, and hyperpigmentation of the skin. Increased intracranial pressure may be present. Adrenal failure is a feature of X-linked adrenomyeloleukodystrophy.

DIABETES MELLITUS

Peripheral Nervous System

In developed countries, diabetes is the most common cause of polyneuropathy (see Chapter 80). The mechanism of neuropathy is not established but may be either metabolic or vascular.

Diabetic polyneuropathy has both axonal degeneration and demyelination. It may be asymptomatic; the diagnosis is suggested by depressed tendon reflexes and impaired vibratory sense in the legs. When the neuropathy becomes symptomatic, the feet are affected more than the hands. The initial symptoms are pain, paresthesias, or numbness. Profound weight loss sometimes precedes the development of an acute painful neuropathy. Progressive neuropathy is characterized by distal sensory loss and weakness in the limbs and areflexia. Severe impairment of pain and temperature appreciation occurs occasionally and results in distal ulceration and arthropathy (acrodystrophic neuropathy).

Autonomic neuropathy is an important feature of diabetes mellitus. The clinical features range from lack of symptoms to a syndrome that includes postural hypotension, abnormal cardiovascular and thermoregulatory control, and impotence. Pupillary abnormalities, gastroparesis, and diarrhea from intestinal dysmotility may occur also, and responses to hypoglycemia may be blunted.

Diabetic polyradiculoneuropathy is characterized by pain and asymmetrical limb weakness, usually involving the thighs and often accompanied by weight loss. A diabetic plexopathy or polyradiculopathy, rather than a femoral neuropathy, probably accounts for most cases of diabetic amyotrophy. Symptoms are rapidly progressive but stabilize after a few weeks; gradual but often incomplete recovery occurs over the following months or years.

The typical syndrome of diabetic thoracoabdominal polyradiculopathy consists of nonradicular truncal pain that may initially suggest intra-abdominal or intrathoracic pathology requiring surgical exploration. Sensory loss and weakness are mild.

Diabetic mononeuropathy multiplex has a vascular basis. Simple mononeuropathies are also common in diabetics. Entrapment neuropathies, especially carpal tunnel syndrome, occur with an increased incidence. Cranial neuropathies, usually isolated involvement of nerves III, IV, and VI, cause a painful extraocular palsy. Diabetes-induced palsies of cranial nerve III are generally distinguished from compressive lesions by sparing of the pupillary reflex. Cranial nerve VII may also be affected, causing unilateral facial weakness. Specific treatment for diabetic neuropathy is not available, but it is important to ensure that the diabetes itself is well controlled.

Central Nervous System

Stroke is more common in diabetics than in the general population, because of an increased incidence of hypertension and atherosclerosis. Diabetes increases stroke severity and mortality, and predisposes to deep subcortical infarcts (Caplan 1996).

Diabetic ketoacidosis, an important cause of morbidity and mortality, may be the presenting feature of previously unrecognized diabetes. Severe hyperglycemia and a metabolic acidosis cause an osmotic diuresis that dehydrates the patient. Clinical presentation is with an altered state of consciousness that progresses to coma. Focal or lateralizing signs are absent usually unless the patient has underlying brain disease. The pathogenesis of diabetic coma is poorly understood and probably multifactorial. Serum hyperosmolality and acidosis are probably important contributing factors. Postmortem examination in some patients with severe diabetic ketoacidosis shows evidence of DIC, which may contribute to the altered level of consciousness. Potential contributory factors are other metabolic derangements, infection, vascular occlusive phenomena, and cerebral edema.

Nonketotic hyperosmolar coma may be precipitated in diabetic patients by an acute medical complication, such as a myocardial infarction. Affected patients are typically elderly with mild disease. Hyperglycemia and hyperosmolality occur without significant ketosis. Progressive obtundation is the principal feature, but seizures and focal deficits may develop. Treatment includes fluid, potassium, and phosphate replacement as necessary and correction of hyperglycemia.

HYPOGLYCEMIA

Hypoglycemia can cause an acute metabolic encephalopathy, with initial features of tremulousness, anxiety, confusion, stupor, or coma, depending on the level of hypoglycemia. Later features are brainstem dysfunction and transitory focal neurological deficits that resemble strokes but either resolve or alternate from side to side. Seizures are sometimes the only manifestation of hypoglycemia. Administration of glucose reverses the symptoms. Severe hypoglycemic cerebral injury causes MRI abnormalities localized to the basal ganglia, cerebral cortex, substantia nigra, and hippocampus, suggesting a particular vulnerability of these areas (Fujioka et al. 1997). Neuromuscular syndromes resembling a peripheral sensorimotor polyneuropathy or lower motor neuron degeneration have been described in patients with insulinomas or who receive excessive insulin for therapeutic purposes.

REFERENCES

Bitsch A, Nau R, Hilgers RA, et al. Focal neurologic deficits in infective endocarditis and other septic diseases. Acta Neurol Scand 1996;94:279–286.

Bolton CF. Sepsis and the systemic inflammatory response: neuromuscular manifestations. Crit Care Med 1996;24:1408–1416.

Bolton CF, Young GB, Zochodne DW. The neurological complications of sepsis. Ann Neurol 1993;33:94–100.

Brey RL, Gharavi AE, Lockshin MD. Neurologic complications of antiphospholipid antibodies. Rheum Dis Clin North Am 1993;19:833–850.

Brodie BR, Stuckey TD, Hansen CJ, et al. Timing and mechanism of death determined clinically after primary angioplasty for acute myocardial infarction. Am J Cardiol 1997;79:1586–1591.

Caplan LR. Diabetes and brain ischemia. Diabetes 1996;45(Suppl. 3):S95–S97.

Coyne TJ, Fehlings MG, Wallace MC, et al. C1-C2 posterior cervical fusion: long-term evaluation of results and efficacy. Neurosurgery 1995;37:688–692.

Escudero D, Latorre P, Codina M, et al. Central nervous system disease in Sjögren's syndrome. Ann Med Intern 1995;146:239–242.

Fujioka M, Okuchi K, Hiramatsu KI, et al. Specific changes in human brain after hypoglycemic injury. Stroke 1997;28:584–587.

Ghika-Schmid F, Ghika J, Regli F, et al. Hashimoto's myoclonic encephalopathy: an underdiagnosed treatable condition? Mov Disord 1996;11:555–562.

Goodin DS. Neurological Sequelae of Aortic Disease and Surgery. In MJ Aminoff (ed), Neurology and General Medicine. New York: Churchill Livingstone, 1995;27–52.

Hanson P, Dive A, Brucher J-M, et al. Acute corticosteroid myopathy in intensive care patients. Muscle Nerve 1997;20:1371–1380.

Heinzlef O, Cohen A, Amarenco P. An update on aortic causes of ischemic stroke. Curr Opin Neurol 1997;10:64–72.

Kaarisalo MM, Immonen-Raiha P, Marttila RJ, et al. Atrial fibrillation and stroke. Stroke 1997;28:311–315.

Louis ED, Lynch T, Kaufmann P, et al. Diagnostic guidelines in central nervous system Whipple's disease. Ann Neurol 1996;40:561–568.

Manning WJ. Role of transesophageal echocardiography in the management of thromboembolic stroke. Am J Cardiol 1997;80:19D–28D.

Marcelli C, Perennou D, Cyteval C, et al. Amyloidosis-related cauda equina compression in long-term hemodialysis patients. Spine 1996;21:381–385.

Mauney MC, Blackbourne LH, Langenburg SE, et al. Prevention of spinal cord injury after repair of the thoracic or thoracoabdominal aorta. Ann Thorac Surg 1995;59:245–252.

Moore PM. Neurological manifestations of vasculitis: update on immunopathogenic mechanisms and clinical features. Ann Neurol 1995;37:S131–S141.

Nishino H, Rubino FA, DeRemee RA, et al. Neurological involvement in Wegener's granulomatosis: an analysis of 324 consecutive patients at the Mayo Clinic. Ann Neurol 1993;33:4–9.

Notermans NC, Lokhorst HM, Franssen H, et al. Intermittent cyclophosphamide and prednisone treatment of polyneuropathy associated with monoclonal gammopathy of undetermined significance. Neurology 1996;47:1227–1233.

Nussmeier NA. Adverse neurologic events: risks of intracardiac versus extracardiac surgery. J Cardiothorac Vasc Anesth 1996;10:31–37.

Terai A, Okada Y, Shichiri Y, et al. Vitamin B_{12} deficiency in patients with urinary intestinal diversion. Int J Urol 1997;4:21–25.

Zeuner M, Straub RH, Rauh G, et al. Relapsing polychondritis: clinical and immunogenetic analysis of 62 patients. J Rheumatol 1997;24:96–101.

Chapter 55
Neurological Complications of Systemic Disease

B. IN CHILDREN
Donald P. Younkin

Many of the systemic diseases that affect the nervous system of children are similar to those of adults (see Chapter 55A). This chapter is limited to disorders that are unique to or common in children.

CARDIAC DISEASE

Congenital Heart Disease

Congenital heart disease (CHD) occurs in 1% of newborns. It is probably caused by an interaction of genetic and environmental factors. CHD is divided into cyanotic and noncyanotic types. Cyanotic CHD includes tetralogy of Fallot, transposition of the great arteries, truncus arteriosus, hypoplastic left-sided heart syndrome, and pulmonary atresia. Noncyanotic CHD includes ventricular septal defect, atrial septal defect, patent ductus arteriosus, endocardial cushion defect, coarctation of the aorta, and aortic stenosis. Although cyanotic CHD represents less than 20% of CHD, it accounts for most of the neurological complications of CHD (duPlessis 1997b).

Children with CHD usually have normal cognitive development, but those with cyanotic CHD have an increased incidence of delayed psychomotor development, especially when surgical repair is delayed until late childhood. Proposed mechanisms of developmental delay in children with CHD are associated congenital brain malformations, chronic hypoxia, multiple cerebral infarctions, and recurrent seizures. The current practice of early surgical repair or palliation during infancy has reduced the incidence of developmental delay by preventing chronic hypoxia (Samango-Sprouse and Suddaby 1997).

CHD is often associated with cerebral dysgenesis. Several chromosomal abnormalities (trisomy 13, trisomy 18, trisomy 21, 4p-) cause major anomalies of the brain and heart. Other syndromes in which both organs are involved are the CHARGE association (coloboma; heart disease; atresia choanae; retarded growth, development, and central nervous system [CNS] anomalies; genital anomalies; and ear anomalies), Dandy-Walker syndrome, Kallmann's syndrome, de Lange's syndrome, velocardiofacial syndrome, and Williams syndrome. Fetal toxins (alcohol, phenytoin) and infections (rubella) also may affect both the heart and brain.

Some forms of CHD have a higher frequency of cerebral dysgenesis than others: tetralogy of Fallot, 2–5%; transposition of the great vessels, 2–5%; truncus arteriosus, 4–10%; and hypoplasia of the left side of the heart, 2–10%. In postmortem series, the overall incidence of cerebral anomalies is 68% among children with different types of CHD, and 29% in children with hypoplastic left-sided heart syndrome.

Cyanotic attacks are an important cause of neurological disturbances in children with cyanotic CHD. The event is precipitated usually by activity or feeding and is characterized by tachypnea and increased cyanosis. Prolonged events cause loss of consciousness and generalized tonic-clonic seizures. These seizures are anoxic in origin and do not respond to anticonvulsant drugs. Cyanotic attacks may herald cerebral infarction.

Stroke is a major complication of cyanotic CHD, especially tetralogy of Fallot and transposition of the great vessels. Venous thrombosis occurs more frequently than arterial obstruction or embolic stroke. Children younger than 2 years with polycythemia and dehydration are at greatest risk. The typical initial features are sudden hemiparesis, increased intracranial pressure, seizures, and depressed consciousness.

In 1992, Tekkok found that brain abscess occurs in 2% of patients with CHD, particularly with the cyanotic variety, and 19% of patients with brain abscess have an underlying CHD. In contrast to stroke, which usually occurs during infancy, the peak age for brain abscess is between 4 and 7 years. Most abscesses are solitary and supratentorial in location. The most common pathogens are *Streptococcus*, *Staphylococcus*, and *Haemophilus*. The pathogenesis of brain abscess formation is multifactorial: right-to-left shunting of blood that bypasses lung filtration, chronic hypoxic-ischemic cerebral injury, multiple systemic microemboli, and septic embolization from infective endocarditis.

Cardiac Catheterization and Surgery

Cardiac catheterization is used in pediatrics for diagnosis and therapy. The current incidence of neurological complications is probably far less than the 1% reported in 1985. The most common complication is a hypoxia-induced seizure. Precatheterization sedation, usually a mixture of meperidine, promethazine, and chlorpromazine, can cause irritability and dystonic reactions. Embolic cerebral infarction from air introduced during catheter exchange or dislodged thrombi is a rare complication.

The frequency of neurological complications following open heart surgery using extracorporeal circulatory support is 10–40%. Complications include seizures, ischemic and hemorrhagic stroke, movement disorders, mental retardation, and learning disorders (duPlessis 1997b). Cardiac surgery does not have a deleterious effect on developmental outcome or IQ. However, infants operated on with hypothermic (12° to 24°C) total circulatory arrest longer than 45–50 minutes often show a significant decline in their developmental outcome. In addition, infants with seizures in the perioperative period have an even greater incidence of developmental delay at 1 year of age.

Abnormal magnetic resonance imaging (MRI) scan results of the brain are found in up to 75% of children following open heart surgery for CHD. Findings include diffuse changes consistent with hypoxic-ischemic encephalopathy, cortical infarction, and developmental defects (agenesis of the corpus callosum, abnormalities of neuronal migration). Focal injury is more likely after open heart surgery without total circulatory arrest; and diffuse injury is associated usually with prolonged periods of total circulatory arrest. Children with normal MRIs or focal infarction usually have normal IQ scores.

Syncope, Prolonged QT Interval, and Breath-Holding Spells

Syncope occurs in 15% of children, causes 3% of all emergency room visits, and may be the most common transitory neurological problem of childhood. Benign syncope is probably a familial trait. The causes of syncope are cardiac (arrhythmia, obstruction), neurological (breath-holding spells, vasovagal, vasodepressor), and metabolic (hypoglycemia, hypocalcemia, hyponatremia, hypokalemia, anemia). Most syncopal episodes are harmless, and the diagnosis can be established by history and physical examination. Some syncopal events are associated with apparent convulsive activity, stiffening of the body, and trembling of the limbs, and electroencephalography (EEG) may be requested to exclude epilepsy. Pallor at the time of loss of consciousness is the single best indicator of syncope. Studies of underlying disease, including tilt-table testing, are indicated in selected cases, but an underlying etiology is rarely established in children.

The prolonged QT interval syndrome, an autosomal-dominant trait, may cause syncope between the ages of 2 and 6 years (Ackerman and Clapham 1997). Exertion or fright is a rare cause of sudden death in affected children. The diagnosis is easily confirmed by measuring the QT interval on a standard electrocardiogram or on the electrocardiogram rhythm strip obtained during an EEG. The diagnosis should be considered in children with seizures preceded by lifelessness or syncope. It usually responds well to beta blockers.

Breath-holding spells are a benign, hereditary disorder with onset between 6 months and 2 years (Breningstall 1996). The spells stop by 6–8 years. They are either cyanotic or pallid. In cyanotic breath-holding spells, the child is frightened, hurt, or angered; cries for a few breaths; and has a prolonged expiratory apnea, becomes cyanotic and limp, and falls to the ground. There is no actual breath holding. Infants and young children cannot voluntarily hold their breath. Cyanotic spells may be associated with clonic activity, and it is important to determine if cyanosis precedes or follows the onset of clonic movements. Pallid syncope is associated with sudden, vagal-mediated asystole that can be induced with ocular compression and treated with atropine. Both cyanotic and pallid syncope may induce an opisthotonic posture, but neither form is associated with neurological sequelae. It is important to distinguish breath-holding spells from epilepsy. Breath-holding spells usually decrease in frequency and duration after the age of 2 years.

ENDOCRINE DISORDERS

Growth Hormone

Growth hormone deficiency is relatively common in children. Most cases are caused by decreased hypothalamic growth hormone–releasing factor. Growth hormone is not required for intrauterine growth; therefore, birth weight and length are normal. Weight gain and linear growth are abnormally slow during infancy, but head circumference increases normally. Bone age (assessed by radiography of the hand and wrist) is delayed, but the upper-to-lower-segment ratio (distance from symphysis pubis to top of head divided by distance from symphysis pubis to floor) is normal. Neurological development is usually normal. The exception is when hypoglycemia and adrenocorticotropic hormone deficiency are associated and cause hypoglycemic neonatal seizures. Growth hormone deficiency should be considered in any newborn with hypoglycemic neonatal seizures and should prompt a search for micropenis, optic nerve hypoplasia, and midline cerebral defects (see Chapter 66).

Growth hormone–secreting pituitary adenomas occur in childhood and increase linear growth as long as the epiphyses are open. The complete syndrome consists of the typical coarse features of acromegaly, macrocephaly, organomegaly, glucose intolerance, and diabetes mellitus. Neurological complications include proximal muscle weakness, paresthesias in the legs, enlarged peripheral nerves, and carpal tunnel syndrome. Transsphenoidal microadenomectomy is the treatment of choice. Children with persistent growth hormone secretion after surgery may respond to octreotide, a long-acting somatostatin analogue.

Growth hormone secretion may be increased or decreased in the diencephalic syndrome. This syndrome is caused by a glioma in the floor of the third ventricle or optic chiasm that involves the hypothalamus. The typical initial features are progressive emaciation despite normal caloric intake during the first year. Affected infants are usually alert and cheerful despite the failure to thrive. Associated features are emesis, nystagmus, optic atrophy, poor temperature regulation, increased intracranial pressure, and an increased concentration of protein in the cerebrospinal fluid (CSF).

Growth hormone therapy is a rare cause of benign intracranial hypertension in children (Koller et al. 1997). Many cases of Creutzfeldt-Jakob disease occurred in children treated with human cadaveric growth hormone contaminated with prion protein.

Puberty

Precocious puberty is defined as the appearance of secondary sexual characteristics in a boy before the age of 9 years and in a girl before the age of 8 (Merke and Cutler 1996). Girls are more frequently affected. Precocious puberty may be complete when caused by premature maturation of the hypothalamic-pituitary axis, but is usually incomplete when caused by autonomous secretion of sex steroids or human chorionic gonadotropin. If unrecognized and untreated, precocious puberty causes rapid growth and skeletal maturation; it results in a tall child who stops growing early and becomes a short adult.

Precocious puberty is a feature of hamartomas of the tuber cinereum, hypothalamic and optic nerve gliomas, human chorionic gonadotropin–secreting germinomas, teratomas, ependymomas, neurofibromatosis 1 with or without optic glioma (Cnossen et al. 1997), increased intracranial pressure, hydrocephalus, meningomyelocele, and head trauma. MRIs are abnormal in one-third of children with central precocious puberty.

Delayed puberty is defined as the absence of secondary sexual development in a boy by age 14 years or a girl by age 13. It is rare, but like precocious puberty, may be caused by neurological disorders. The differential diagnosis of delayed puberty is not limited to tumors of the hypothalamic-pituitary axis but includes craniopharyngiomas, pineal germinomas, tuberculosis, sarcoidosis, vasculitis, head trauma, and increased intracranial pressure. Almost any intracranial mass can exert pressure on the hypothalamus and cause endocrine dysfunction in children.

Diabetes Mellitus

Insulin-dependent diabetes mellitus (IDDM) is the most common endocrine disorder of childhood. It is characterized by inadequate insulin production, a tendency to ketosis and ketoacidosis, circulating antibodies to pancreatic cell components, and an association with other autoimmune diseases.

In contrast to adults (see Chapter 55A), most neurological complications of IDDM in children are acute. Intractable cerebral edema is a rare but potentially fatal complication of diabetic ketoacidosis (Hale et al. 1997). It should be considered in any child whose mental status fails to improve or deteriorates after successful treatment of ketoacidosis. Subclinical cerebral edema may be an expected part of the treatment of diabetic ketoacidosis in children.

Transitory hemiparesis associated with headache and respiratory infections are reported in normoglycemic children with IDDM. All have had normal computed tomographic (CT) scans of the brain; recovery is always complete.

Symptomatic peripheral neuropathy is unusual in childhood diabetes, but 11% of adolescents with diabetes have slowed peroneal nerve conduction velocities. Abnormal somatosensory evoked potentials are reported also.

Hyperglycemia caused by undiagnosed IDDM may cause intractable seizures in children with epilepsy. Acute hyperglycemia causes impaired cognitive function in diabetic children.

Thyroid

The frequency of congenital hypothyroidism is 1 in 4,000 (Dussault 1997). Affected newborns are often large and "postdated." Common features are delayed stooling, prolonged jaundice, unstable temperature, and decreased activity. Within a few months, the infants develop coarse facial features, thick tongue, protruding abdomen, irritability, and hoarse cry. Untreated congenital hypothyroidism always causes mental retardation and may also cause spasticity and cerebellar ataxia. The severity of retardation is proportional to the delay in treatment. Histopathological examination of the brain shows immature, disordered synaptic connections. The United States, Great Britain, and most developed countries screen newborns for hypothyroidism, provide early treatment, and have almost eliminated congenital hypothyroidism as a cause of mental retardation. However, newborn screening may be missed as maternity stays are progressively shortened and more babies are born at home. The diagnosis should be considered in any infant with severe developmental delay and coarse features.

Iodine deficiency is the most common preventable cause of mental retardation in the world (Pharoah and Connolly 1996). In 1990, the World Health Organization estimated that 20 million people had preventable brain damage caused by iodine deficiency. Cretinism is still endemic in Asia, Africa, and Latin America where the incidence may be up to 10%. Involvement of the neocortex, cochlea, and basal ganglia results in the characteristic neurological signs of mental retardation, deaf-mutism, and motor rigidity. Correction of iodine deficiency before pregnancy prevents cretinism, but treatment during the pregnancy does not.

Children with Down syndrome (trisomy 21) have an increased incidence of hypothyroidism, which may be overlooked because the Down phenotype is similar to congenital hypothyroidism. For this reason, most Down syndrome clinics check thyroid function annually.

Neurological complications of hyperthyroidism are similar in children and adults (see Chapter 56A). However, children have a lower incidence of neuromuscular abnormalities, though these are more common in girls than in boys.

RENAL DISORDERS

Acute Renal Failure

Acute renal failure in children is caused usually by prerenal factors (hypovolemia, hypotension, renal artery thrombosis) that decrease renal blood flow and may overlap with renal parenchymal injury (glomerulonephritis, interstitial nephritis, vasculitis, acute tubular necrosis). Acute renal failure is better tolerated when it develops slowly; however, it usually occurs rapidly in children. Neurological symptoms occur more frequently when acute renal failure is associated with anuria or oliguria. Symptoms are usually secondary to acute water intoxication or hyperkalemia. Water intoxication occurs within hours to days of the onset of renal failure and is characterized by altered mental status, headache, emesis, and fasciculations or coarse fibrillations. In addition to causing cardiac arrhythmia, hyperkalemia also slows nerve conduction velocity and causes skeletal muscle weakness. Treatment is directed at correcting fluid and electrolyte balance.

Hemolytic-uremic syndrome is a leading cause of acute renal failure in children younger than 5 years. It is defined by the combination of thrombocytopenia, uremia, and Coombs-negative hemolytic anemia. There is considerable overlap between hemolytic-uremic syndrome in infants and young children and thrombotic thrombocytopenic purpura in older children and adults. The pathogenesis of the two syndromes may be the same, but clinical involvement in hemolytic-uremic syndrome is more restricted. Thirty percent to 50% of patients have neurological symptoms, including seizures, altered mental status (stupor, hallucinations, coma), and focal neurological deficits. CT scan may demonstrate ischemic or hemorrhagic infarction. Most children recover, but may have chronic hypertension. Survivors have normal cognitive function, but may have hyperactivity and inattentiveness (Qamar et al. 1996).

Chronic Renal Failure

The neurological complications and treatment of end-stage renal disease, uremia, and dialysis are the same in children and adults (see Chapter 55A). A congenital uremic encephalopathy can develop in infants with the onset of severe chronic uremia before the age of 1 year. This is a slowly progressive encephalopathy that may be caused by chronic aluminum toxicity. The initial features are a delay in the acquisition of new skills, followed by a plateau in development. Coordination and motor skills are affected early, and children develop tremor, ataxia, dysmetria, hyperreflexia, and extensor plantar responses. As the encephalopathy progresses, children lose previously acquired skills and become severely dysarthric and hypotonic; most develop myoclonus and seizures. The end result is a chronic vegetative state. Serial EEGs show progressive slowing of the background rhythm with bursts of 2- to 4-Hz polyspike wave discharges. Head CT scan and MRI show progressive cerebral atrophy. Dialysis and renal transplantation do not reverse the encephalopathy.

RESPIRATORY DISORDERS

Congenital Anomalies of the Respiratory Tract

Malformations of the outer ear are often associated with malformations of the middle ear and conductive hearing loss, but are associated rarely with inner ear anomalies. Commonly encountered external malformations include pits, tags, anomalies of the pinna, protruding ears, low-set ears, and small ears. Most of these anomalies are not associated with CNS problems, but some indicate chromosomal aberrations (trisomy 18), recognizable genetic syndromes (Treacher Collins syndrome), or a constellation of malformations (CHARGE syndrome). Small ears are part of the Down phenotype and large ears of the fragile X syndrome. Cholesteatomas, acquired or congenital rests of epithelial tissue in the external auditory canal, can enlarge, cause bony destruction, spread to the intracranial cavity, and cause facial palsy.

The normal anterior migration of the forebrain is partially responsible for anterior midline facial development. Therefore, the nose, sinuses, and oropharynx are important external markers of CNS malformations (see Chapter 66). Congenital anomalies of the lower respiratory tract, including tracheoesophageal fistulas, are rarely associated with CNS malformations. The CNS is secondarily affected by hypoxia from respiratory compromise.

Infections of the Respiratory Tract

Otitis media is common in childhood. Neurological complications are rare but can include hearing loss, facial nerve palsy, and the contiguous spread of infection, resulting in mastoiditis, venous sinus thrombosis, meningitis, subdural empyema, cerebritis, and cerebral abscess.

Rhinitis and sinusitis are common in children but rarely cause neurological complications. The major concern with chronic sinusitis is extension of infection to the skull, CSF, and venous sinuses. Fractures in the cribriform plate, paranasal sinuses, and temporal bone can result in meningitis and brain abscess. Such fractures may cause CSF to leak as a clear nasal discharge. The glucose content of CSF is sufficient to cause a positive dipstick test result, whereas mucus has a negative dipstick result. Chronic or persistent sinusitis, particularly if associated with recurrent pneumonia, may be the first sign of ataxia-telangiectasia (see Chapter 76).

Postinfectious demyelinating syndromes are often late effects of upper respiratory infections (see Chapter 60). These are monophasic demyelinating illnesses that may affect all parts of the CNS. The mechanism is believed to be immune-mediated. Acute hemorrhagic leukoencephalitis is a rare disorder that develops days to weeks after a mild viral respiratory tract illness, frequently varicella or measles. Neurological signs develop over a few days. The initial features are headache, lethargy, confusion, and nuchal rigidity. These are followed by seizures, long tract signs, and increased intracranial pressure. Most children become comatose, and some die. Postmortem examination reveals parenchymal edema, diffuse involvement of the white matter with perivascular hemorrhage, inflammation and demyelination, and necrotizing angiitis of the capillaries and venules in the white matter.

Apnea and Periodic Breathing

Apnea and periodic breathing are common problems in premature and full-term neonates (see Chapter 84). *Apnea* is defined as cessation of respiration for more than 10–20 seconds; periodic breathing is a regular pattern lasting more than 2 minutes, with cycles of regular respirations lasting 18–20 seconds, followed by respiratory cessation lasting 2–3 seconds. Most infants have central apnea, presumably secondary to immaturity of respiratory control mechanisms. Most apneic episodes occur during rapid eye movement or transitional sleep when respiratory patterns are irregular in timing and amplitude. The incidence of intraventricular hemorrhage, hydrocephalus, and developmental delay is increased in newborns with apnea, especially those with obstructive apnea. Apnea can be part of the clinical expression of seizures in the newborn but is rarely the only expression. Bradycardia does not complicate convulsive apnea, unless it lasts longer than 60 seconds.

Bronchopulmonary dysplasia (BPD) is a chronic progressive lung disease that occurs in infants after mechanical ventilation for severe respiratory distress syndrome. Infants with BPD have an increased frequency of intraventricular hemorrhage and hydrocephalus. Long-term neurological sequelae are more common in infants with BPD than in comparable low-birth-weight newborns without BPD. Two neurological syndromes are reported. Most common is cerebral palsy, mental retardation, and blindness. A few have progressive motor disability, developmental delay and regression, visual impairment, and intractable seizures. The syndrome culminates in death from continued and progressive respiratory compromise.

Asthma

Asthma is a complex syndrome of recurrent, reversible airway obstruction caused by airway hyperreactivity and characterized by wheezing, coryza, breathlessness, and increased sputum production. Most neurological complications are from medication or hypoxia. Headaches are common in asthmatic children and they occur independent of bronchodilators. A poliomyelitislike syndrome with flaccid monoplegia, hemiplegia, or diplegia has been described in a few asthmatic children. It usually occurs within 1 week of an asthmatic attack. The most likely explanation is infection with a neurotropic virus that coincidentally triggered an asthmatic attack. Frequent corticosteroid use may make asthmatic children more susceptible to viral invasion of the anterior horn cells.

Aminophylline is used commonly in the management of childhood asthma. Seizures may occur when theophylline levels are above 25 μg/ml, but usually do not occur until the level is above 50 μg/ml. In children with epilepsy, therapeutic levels of aminophylline may lower the seizure threshold and increase seizures. In addition, aminophylline may alter seizure control by affecting the metabolism of antiepileptic drugs such as phenobarbital, phenytoin, and carbamazepine.

Cystic Fibrosis

Cystic fibrosis is a multisystem disorder that affects all exocrine glands, with the eccrine sweat glands producing increased concentrations of sodium and chloride. Exocrine gland dysfunction leads to obstructive pulmonary disease, pancreatic insufficiency, intestinal obstruction, gallstones, biliary cirrhosis, and electrolyte imbalance. Abnormalities of the autonomic nervous system can occur, including increased sensitivity to adrenergically stimulated pupillary constriction, parotid saliva secretion, and eccrine sweat secretion. Other ocular features are retinal hemorrhages, papilledema, preganglionic oculosympathetic paresis, and decreased light contrast sensitivity.

Pancreatic insufficiency may cause malabsorption of vitamins E and D, leading to neuromuscular abnormalities. Children with cystic fibrosis can develop a sensory ataxia with diminished joint position sense and vibratory perception, and a spinocerebellar degeneration. A proximal myopathy and rickets were reported in one child with vitamin D deficiency that resolved after vitamin replacement.

GASTROINTESTINAL DISORDERS

The most common gastrointestinal disorders associated with serious neurological complications are chronic liver failure with hepatic encephalopathy, hepatitis, inflammatory bowel disease, and liver transplantation. These conditions are the same in children and adults and are reviewed in Chapter 55A.

Reye's syndrome is unique to children, but it has been virtually eliminated as a clinical entity. It is an acute encephalopathy with brain edema and elevated intracranial pressure associated with microvesicular fatty degeneration of the liver (Hardie et al. 1996). It is usually associated with a concurrent viral illness, frequently varicella. The incidence of Reye's syndrome decreased dramatically in the 1980s, coincident with a decreased use of aspirin products in children (Smith 1996).

Gastroesophageal Reflux

The prevalence of gastroesophageal reflux (GER) in normal infants is estimated at 1 in 300, but is considerably higher in infants with cerebral palsy or severe mental retar- dation (Roberts 1996). The high acidity of gastric contents irritates and inflames the esophagus and causes apnea. The main neurological features of children with GER are episodes of dystonia and torticollis that occur during or immediately after feeding. Other features are episodes of apnea, cyanosis, and stiffening that may be misdiagnosed as seizures. GER-induced apnea is rarely a cause of hypoxic seizures, but must be considered in the differential diagnosis of seizures that occur shortly after feeding (Tirosh and Jaffe 1996). Neurological symptoms resolve when GER is treated successfully.

Cyclic Vomiting

Children with cyclic vomiting have recurrent episodes of unexplained emesis lasting hours to days (Withers et al. 1998). Between events, the child enjoys good health and does not have metabolic, gastrointestinal, or neurological problems. The condition usually occurs in children between the ages of 2 and 4 years but has been described in older children. Vomiting can begin at any time of the day or night and can last more than a week. It frequently leads to dehydration requiring hospitalization and intravenous fluids. Many infants with cyclic vomiting develop classic migraine headaches during childhood, and it is assumed that the vomiting is a migraine attack without a headache. Cyclic vomiting is easily diagnosed after recurrent episodes but often necessitates a thorough evaluation of underlying causes during the initial episode. Inderal, amitriptyline, and cyproheptadine are helpful in preventing recurrent attacks (Andersen et al. 1997). Sumatriptan may abort individual episodes, but is contraindicated if focal neurological signs accompany the emesis.

Nausea, but not vomiting, is a common feature of complex partial epilepsy in children. Most children with complex partial epilepsy have other symptoms of epilepsy and an abnormal EEG.

Valproate-Induced Hepatic Failure

The incidence of valproate-induced acute hepatic failure is estimated at 1 in 500 treated children younger than age 2 years. This is much higher than the incidence in adults. It usually occurs within 6 months of starting valproate. The highest incidence is in children receiving multiple antiepileptic drugs or with other neurological problems. Valproate-induced hepatic failure may be related to inborn errors of metabolism. The incidence of fatal valproate hepatic toxicity is declining, possibly because of increased awareness of the problem. Hepatic failure cannot be predicted by monitoring serum transaminase or ammonia concentrations; these are usually normal or mildly elevated until the onset of hepatic failure, which is usually abrupt. The major features are altered mental status (apathy, lethargy, coma), nausea, vomiting, and increased seizures. Other, less frequent features are asterixis, hyperventilation, and alkalosis. Treatment is symptomatic with protein restriction and sodium benzoate to reduce serum ammonia. Outcome is variable; some children regain liver function, and others have irreversible liver failure. The role of carnitine in preventing and treating hepatic failure is controversial. Most experts recommend carnitine supplementation in high-risk patients and when there are signs of hepatic toxicity or failure.

Moderate, two- to threefold increases in serum transaminases are common in children treated with valproate. These children have normal liver function and are asymptomatic. Mildly elevated transaminases do not predict later hepatotoxicity and may be dose related.

HEMATOLOGICAL DISORDERS

The neurological complications of most hematological disorders are comparable in children and adults (see Chapter 55A). Two hematological conditions, bilirubin toxicity and sickle cell anemia, are unique to childhood and are discussed in this section. Factor V Leiden deficiency is associated with neurological problems in newborn infants and children but is not a risk factor for ischemic stroke or transient ischemic attacks in adults.

Bilirubin Toxicity

Bilirubin is the end product of heme catabolism. The normal destruction of senescent red blood cells in newborns accounts for 75% of bilirubin production. Bilirubin is produced in the reticuloendothelium, bound to serum albumin, and transported to the liver, where it is conjugated and excreted in bile. Physiological jaundice (hyperbilirubinemia) occurs in most babies during the first postnatal week, and mean bilirubin concentrations peak at 6 mg/dl by 48–72 hours.

Factors that may cause excessive bilirubin concentrations are blood group incompatibility, hemorrhage, polycythemia, defects of liver conjugation, increased enterohepatic circulation, and hypothyroidism (Gourley 1997). Bilirubin levels below 20 mg/dl are rarely associated with neurotoxicity; however, 33% of babies with concentrations between 25 and 29 mg/dl and 73% of infants with bilirubin concentrations greater than 30 mg/dl develop kernicterus. Other factors in the pathogenesis of bilirubin neurotoxicity are low serum albumin concentrations, low albumin bilirubin binding affinity, high concentrations of endogenous organic acids and exogenous anions that compete with bilirubin for albumin-binding sites, and disruption of the blood-brain barrier.

Neurons are more susceptible than glial cells to bilirubin neurotoxicity. Neurons with specific susceptibility are those in the globus pallidus, subthalamic nucleus, hypothalamus, Sommer's sector H2-3 of the hippocampus, substantia nigra, cranial nerve nuclei, brainstem reticular formation, dentate nuclei, and anterior horn.

Kernicterus produces an identifiable neurological syndrome. During the first few days, newborns are stuporous and hypotonic and suck poorly. Seizures are not a prominent feature of bilirubin neurotoxicity, and their occurrence suggests concurrent hypoxic-ischemic encephalopathy (see Chapter 84). Three to 5 days later, hypertonia with prominent retrocollis, opisthotonos, or both develops. The initial hypertonia is followed, after the first week, by hypotonia, brisk tendon reflexes, obligate tonic neck reflexes, and delayed motor development. Extrapyramidal and oculomotor signs develop after the age of 1 year. Athetosis is more prominent in the arms than in the legs and usually increases during voluntary activity. Many children have difficulty with facial movements, swallowing, and phonation. Less common movement disorders are dystonia, ballismus, tremor, and chorea. Supranuclear gaze palsies with absent voluntary upward gaze are an almost constant feature.

The auditory system is uniquely sensitive to bilirubin neurotoxicity. Cochlear nuclei and auditory nerve injury resulting in moderate to severe hearing loss are the most consistent abnormalities of bilirubin neurotoxicity. Brainstem auditory responses should be measured and language development monitored in all newborns with significantly elevated bilirubin levels. Mental retardation is not a prominent feature of kernicterus, although hearing loss and profound motor impairment may suggest retardation and interfere with adequate intelligence testing.

Sickle Cell Anemia

Sickle cell disease (SCD) is the most common hemoglobinopathy and a frequent cause of stroke in children. SCD is caused by a homozygous substitution of valine for glutamate at position 6 in the β chain. Approximately 0.16% of the black population in the United States are homozygous for hemoglobin S. Most children with SCD become symptomatic before 5 years of age. Approximately 17% of homozygotes have cerebrovascular disorders, and stroke can be the first clinical manifestation of disease. Preliminary data from the Cooperative Study of Sickle Cell Disease show an incidence of 0.5% per year of first stroke in SCD, with a slight increase in children between 5 and 10 years (Ohene-Frempong et al. 1998). This risk is 500 times greater than in normal children of similar age.

Cerebral infarction accounts for 75% of stroke in SCD and 77% of infarctions are in children (Moser et al. 1996). Two-thirds of untreated children have recurrent stroke within 3 years. Factors associated with an increased risk of cerebral infarction are family history of stroke, frequent sickle cell crises, cardiomegaly, and low hemoglobin concentration. Children with persistent hemoglobin F beyond the neonatal period or with thalassemia have relatively few strokes.

Symptomatic cerebral infarction usually occurs during a sickle cell crisis. Crises are often precipitated by intercurrent infection; the usual features are fever, diffuse pain, and dehydration. Altered mental status is probably caused by cerebral hypoperfusion but may be difficult to distinguish from general malaise and narcotic effects. Focal or generalized seizures during a crisis are common, and postictal weakness must be distinguished from cerebral infarction. Either large or small vessels may be occluded, and the resulting infarctions vary in location and size. Neurological findings depend on the site of infarction. Most are in the cerebral hemispheres; the brainstem and spinal cord are rarely involved. Most children recover from their first infarction, but unusually large or recurrent infarctions result in residual neurological morbidity. Periodic transfusions to keep the level of hemoglobin S below 30% reduce the rate of recurrent infarction by 90%. Asymptomatic or *silent* infarction occurs in up to 13% of children with SCD. Silent infarctions are usually confined to the white matter. Children with silent infarction have a greater risk for symptomatic infarction.

Children with SCD between the ages of 2 and 16 years should be screened with transcranial Doppler (Adams et al. 1997). Children with flow rates greater than 200 cm per second have a significantly increased risk for stroke and should be imaged and treated with periodic blood transfusions (Adams et al. 1998).

Intraparenchymal and subarachnoid hemorrhage account for the other 25% of strokes in children with SCD. Intracranial hemorrhage is usually an isolated event in children. In contrast to older adolescents and adults, it is unusual to identify an aneurysm or arteriovenous malformation as the source of bleeding in children.

The clinical presentation of intracranial hemorrhage in SCD is not unique. The diagnosis should be considered in any child with sudden onset of neurological symptoms, markedly altered mental status, signs of meningeal irritation, and evidence of increased intracranial pressure. Infection and cerebral infarction also must be considered when a child with SCD presents with these symptoms. Intracranial hemorrhage usually occurs during a sickle cell crisis. Diagnosis and appropriate therapy may be delayed if treating physicians attribute symptoms of intracranial hemorrhage to sickle cell crisis. Recurrent hemorrhages have been reported.

If an arteriovenous malformation or arterial aneurysm is not identified with angiography or another neuroimaging modality, then intracranial hemorrhage is usually attributed to hemorrhagic infarction. Some authorities suggest chronic arterial changes with increased vascular fragility as a possible mechanism. A syndrome of acute hypertension, seizures, and intracranial hemorrhage has been reported during transfusion therapy in SCD.

The prognosis after intracranial hemorrhage in SCD is variable. The mortality from hemorrhage is greater than 50%. Children who survive subarachnoid hemorrhage usually recover completely, but recovery after intraparenchymal hemorrhage depends on its size and location.

Factor V Leiden Mutation

Activated protein C resistance caused by factor V Leiden mutation is the most common cause of familial thrombosis. It is found in 2–7% of people and is 10 times as common as protein C, protein S, and antithrombin III deficiencies. In one study, 38% of neonates and children with arterial thromboembolic disease had factor V Leiden mutation. The fetus and newborn may be predisposed to infarction from this and other prothrombotic conditions. Factor V Leiden mutation has been reported in children with hemiplegic cerebral palsy (Thorarensen et al. 1997). This and other coagulation factors may prove to be an important cause of undiagnosed cerebral palsy.

VASCULITIC DISORDERS

Juvenile Rheumatoid Arthritis

Juvenile rheumatoid arthritis (JRA) is a chronic inflammatory disease that always involves the joints but may cause extensive systemic disease. JRA is defined as an onset before age 16, but the peak incidence is between 1 and 3 years. Approximately 30% of the children have pauciarticular JRA, 50% have polyarticular JRA, and 20% have systemic JRA. Systemic JRA, also referred to as *Still's disease*, is characterized by fever, rash, arthritis, lymphadenopathy, splenomegaly, and variable degrees of cardiac, liver, and gastrointestinal involvement. Neurological symptoms occur in 5% of children with systemic JRA. Iridocyclitis may occur as an isolated finding in pauciarticular JRA, but neurological involvement in pauciarticular and polyarticular JRA is uncommon. Adolescent boys with JRA may develop ankylosing spondylitis and atlantoaxial subluxation with cervical myelopathy.

An acute encephalopathy characterized by altered mental status and seizures may occur in children with systemic JRA. CSF protein concentration is increased and leukocytosis is present. The encephalopathy responds to high doses of intravenous corticosteroids.

A Reye's-like syndrome characterized by abnormal liver function, hyperammonemia, hyponatremia, and increased intracranial pressure is another potential complication of children with JRA. Intracranial hemorrhage and disseminated intravascular coagulopathy may be associated. The CSF may show an increased protein concentration and pleocytosis. The syndrome may be caused by chronic salicylate therapy.

A child with JRA may develop bilateral basal ganglia lesions and hypotonia, dystonia, and dysphasia during an exacerbation of systemic JRA. The neurological symptoms resolve and the basal ganglia lesions improve after corticosteroid treatment. Two different neurological syndromes occur in infants with JRA. One is developmental motor delay caused by painful joints. The other occurs only during the first year and includes chronic meningitis, seizures, hydrocephalus, papilledema, developmental delay, and hearing loss. The mechanism of the second syndrome is not established.

Several neuromuscular disorders are associated with JRA. Motor and sensory neuropathies occur in children with protracted JRA. The frequency of myasthenia gravis is increased (see Chapter 82). Treatment of the myasthenia has no affect on arthritis. Finally, the serum concentration of creatine kinase may be slightly increased, but symptomatic muscle disease is rare.

Nonspecific EEG changes occur in more than 50% of children with JRA. Focal or generalized slowing is typical, but paroxysmal activity can occur. These abnormalities may reflect CNS vasculitis, but this has not been confirmed by angiography.

Acute Rheumatic Fever

Acute rheumatic fever (ARF) is an inflammatory disease that follows infection with group A hemolytic streptococci. ARF affects the skin, heart, joints, subcutaneous tissue, and CNS. Diagnosis is based on the Jones criteria: The major manifestations are carditis, polyarthritis, chorea, erythema marginatum, migratory polyarthritis, and subcutaneous nodules. The incidence of ARF has increased considerably in the past several years after decades of decline. Pediatric autoimmune neuropsychiatric diseases associated with streptococcal infections (PANDAS) include tics, explosive obsessive-compulsive symptoms, and psychosis (Swedo et al. 1998).

Sydenham's chorea is the only feature of ARF in up to 30% of children. During adolescence, it occurs almost exclusively in girls. The clinical features and treatment are reviewed in Chapter 75. Carditis may develop as chorea resolves. It is unusual for children with ARF to have chorea and arthritis. Sydenham's chorea is a relatively benign neurological problem, and neuropathological findings are rarely reported. There are limited reports of a proliferative endarteritis in smaller cortical vessels with patches of gray matter degeneration. Anticardiolipin antibodies may be positive, but cerebral infarction has not been reported in ARF. CSF is normal. MRI and CT studies are normal. The EEG may have nonspecific abnormalities with slowing and paroxysmal activity.

Systemic Lupus Erythematosus

Systemic lupus erythematosus (SLE) is an autoimmune disorder with multisystem involvement (see Chapter 55A).

Approximately 25% of SLE begins during childhood, even during infancy. The female-to-male ratio is 8 to 1. The systemic features are a characteristic butterfly rash, arthralgia, and arthritis. Hematological, renal, and cardiac abnormalities are common; however, discoid lupus and severe arthritis are uncommon in childhood SLE. Diagnosis is made on a clinical basis with laboratory confirmation of positive antinuclear antibody, anti-DNA or anti-RNA, and low serum complement (C3, C4, CH50) levels. Neurological complications may be the first sign of SLE in children. Generalized or multifocal seizures occur in 10% of children with SLE. Although seizures can occur at any stage of the disease, they are associated usually with active systemic disease, including uremia, electrolyte abnormalities, metabolic encephalopathy, or severe hypertension. Treatment is directed at correcting systemic problems. Antiepileptic drugs may be helpful, but chronic anticonvulsant therapy is rarely necessary.

Psychiatric symptoms are a prominent feature of childhood SLE. Some combination of depression, mood swings, anxiety, personality change, acute psychosis, confusion, and progressive dementia occurs in 25% of children. In 20–30% of children, psychiatric problems are the initial symptom of SLE. It can be difficult to distinguish SLE-induced psychiatric symptoms from complications of corticosteroid therapy.

Chorea can precede systemic symptoms of SLE by up to 1 year and can resolve before other symptoms appear. Differentiation from Sydenham's chorea can be difficult, because serum antistreptococcal antibody titers may be falsely positive in SLE. The presence of antinuclear antibodies or low CSF complement titers is suggestive of SLE. Chorea usually improves with chlorpromazine, haloperidol, or corticosteroid therapy.

Occlusive cerebrovascular disease occurs in children but is rarely the initial manifestation of SLE. It is caused usually by a small vessel vasculitis and may respond to high doses of intravenous corticosteroids.

Visual complaints are common in children and include retinal artery occlusion, retinal hemorrhages, cotton-wool exudates, optic neuritis, and papilledema. Either SLE or corticosteroids can cause pseudotumor cerebri and papilledema.

Other neurological complications of lupus in children are hypertensive encephalopathy, cerebral vein thrombosis, cranial neuropathies, brainstem dysfunction, transverse myelopathy, bacterial and fungal meningitis, brain abscess, chronic aseptic meningitis, peripheral neuropathies, and myalgia but rarely myositis.

REFERENCES

Ackerman MJ, Clapham DE. Ion channels—basic science and clinical disease. N Engl J Med 1997;336:1575–1586.
Adams RJ, McKie VC, Carl EM, et al. Long-term stroke risk in children with sickle cell disease screened with transcranial Doppler. Ann Neurol 1997;42:699–704.

Adams RJ, McKie VC, Hsu L, et al. Prevention of a first stroke by transfusions in children with sickle cell anemia and abnormal results on transcranial Doppler ultrasonography. N Engl J Med 1998;339:5–11.

Andersen JM, Sugerman KS, Lockhart JR, Weinberg WA. Effective prophylactic therapy for cyclic vomiting syndrome in children using amitriptyline or cyproheptadine. Pediatrics 1997;100:977–981.

Breningstall GN. Breath-holding spells. Pediatr Neurol 1996;14:91–97.

Cnossen MH, Stam EN, Cooiman LC, et al. Endocrinologic disorders and optic pathway gliomas in children with neurofibromatosis type 1. Pediatrics 1997;100:667–670.

duPlessis AJ. Cerebral hemodynamics and metabolism during infant cardiac surgery. Mechanisms of injury and strategies for protection. J Child Neurol 1997a;12:285–300.

duPlessis AJ. Neurologic complications of cardiac disease in the newborn. Clin Perinatol 1997b;24:807–826.

Dussault JH. Childhood primary hypothyroidism and endemic cretinism. Curr Ther Endocrinol Metab 1997;6:107–109.

Gourley GR. Bilirubin metabolism and kernicterus. Adv Pediatr 1997;44:173–229.

Hale PM, Rezvani I, Braunstein AW, et al. Factors predicting cerebral edema in young children with diabetic ketoacidosis and new onset type I diabetes. Acta Paediatr 1997;86:626–631.

Hardie RM, Newton LH, Bruce JC, et al. The changing pattern of Reye's syndrome 1982–1990. Arch Dis Child 1996;74:400–405.

Koller EA, Stadel BV, Malozowski SN. Papilledema in 15 renally compromised patients treated with growth hormone. Pediatr Nephrol 1997;11:451–454.

Merke DP, Cutler GB. Evaluation and management of precocious puberty. Arch Dis Child 1996;75:269–271.

Moser FG, Miller ST, Bello JA, et al. The spectrum of brain MR abnormalities in sickle-cell disease: a report from the Cooperative Study of Sickle Cell Disease. Am J Neuroradiol 1996;17:965–972.

Ohene-Frempong K, Weiner SJ, Sleeper LA, et al. Cerebrovascular accidents in sickle cell disease: rates and risk factors. Blood 1998;91:288–294.

Pharoah PO, Connolly KJ. Iodine and brain development. Dev Med Child Neurol 1996;37:744–748.

Qamar IU, Ohali M, MacGregor DL, et al. Long-term neurologic sequelae of hemolytic uremic syndrome: a preliminary report. Pediatr Nephrol 1996;10:504–506.

Roberts KB. Gastroesophageal reflux in infants and children who have neurodevelopmental disabilities. Pediatr Rev 1996;17:211–212.

Samango-Sprouse C, Suddaby EC. Developmental concerns in children with congenital heart disease. Curr Opin Cardiol 1997;12:91–98.

Smith TC. Reye's syndrome and the use of aspirin. Scott Med J 1996;41:4–9.

Swedo SE, Leonard HL, Garvey M, et al. Pediatric autoimmune neuropsychiatric disorders associated with streptococcal infections: clinical description of the first 50 cases. Am J Psychiatry 1998;155:264–271.

Thorarensen O, Ryan S, Hunter J, Younkin DP. Factor V Leiden mutation: an unrecognized cause of hemiplegic cerebral palsy, neonatal stroke, and placental thrombosis. Ann Neurol 1997;42:372–375.

Tirosh E, Jaffe M. Apnea of infancy, seizures, and gastroesophageal reflux: an important but infrequent association. J Child Neurol 1996;11:98–100.

Withers GD, Silburn SR, Forbes DA. Precipitants and aetiology of cyclic vomiting syndrome. Acta Paediatr 1998;87:272–277.

Chapter 56
Trauma of the Nervous System

A. BASIC NEUROSCIENCE OF NEUROTRAUMA
W. Dalton Dietrich

The mortality and morbidity associated with traumatic brain injury (TBI) is considered one of the major public health problems in Western industrialized countries. To investigate the pathophysiology of brain injury and to develop novel therapeutic strategies to treat this condition, experimental models of TBI have been established. Although no experimental model completely mimics the human condition, individual models produce many features of human brain injury. Based on these models, therapeutic strategies directed at specific pathomechanisms have been initiated. This chapter reviews the basic neuroscience of neurotrauma and summarizes the various experimental strategies used to investigate and treat TBI.

EXPERIMENTAL MODELS OF TRAUMATIC BRAIN INJURY

Severe closed head injury produces a range of cerebral lesions that may be divided into four general categories: (1) diffuse axonal injury; (2) vascular lesions, including subdural hematoma; (3) contusion; and (4) neuronal degeneration within selectively vulnerable regions. In a review of animal models of head injury, Gennarelli (1994) classified models of head injury according to the method of producing injury. Fluid-percussion (F-P) and rigid indentation models are characterized as percussion concussion, whereas inertial injury models and impact acceleration models are included under acceleration concussion. In an attempt to investigate the effects of mechanical deformation on specific cell types, in vitro models of stretch-induced injury have also been developed.

Percussion Concussion

The central and parasagittal F-P models are characterized by brief behavioral responsiveness (e.g., coma), metabolic alterations, changes in local cerebral blood flow (lCBF) and blood-brain barrier (BBB) permeability, and behavioral deficits. The central F-P model tends to have variable and relatively small contusions in the vicinity of the fluid pulse and scattered axonal damage, mostly restricted to the brainstem. In contrast, parasagittal F-P is characterized by a lateral cortical contusion that is remote from the impact site. Evidence for axonal damage is seen throughout the white matter tracts within the ipsilateral cerebral hemisphere as well as tissue tears at gray-white matter interfaces. Hippocampal damage is pronounced in the parasagittal F-P injury model with little brainstem damage. The parasagittal F-P injury model therefore produces a range of pathologies, including contusion, widespread axonal injury, and selective neuronal necrosis. In addition, varying injury severity, including mild (1.1–1.3 atm), moderate (2.0–2.3 atm), and severe (2.4–2.6 atm), can be studied in a reproducible fashion. This is an important model characteristic because of the heterogeneous nature of human TBI and the possibility that treatment strategies may vary with injury severity.

Acceleration Concussion

Inertial acceleration models can produce relatively pure acute subdural hematomas and diffuse axonal injury. Tissue-tear

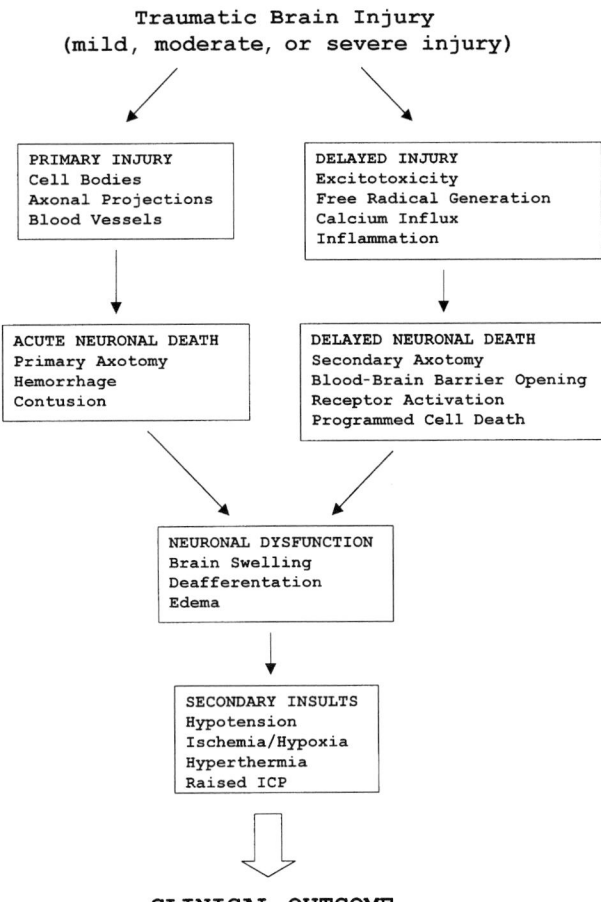

**Traumatic Brain Injury
(mild, moderate, or severe injury)**

PRIMARY INJURY
Cell Bodies
Axonal Projections
Blood Vessels

DELAYED INJURY
Excitotoxicity
Free Radical Generation
Calcium Influx
Inflammation

ACUTE NEURONAL DEATH
Primary Axotomy
Hemorrhage
Contusion

DELAYED NEURONAL DEATH
Secondary Axotomy
Blood-Brain Barrier Opening
Receptor Activation
Programmed Cell Death

NEURONAL DYSFUNCTION
Brain Swelling
Deafferentation
Edema

SECONDARY INSULTS
Hypotension
Ischemia/Hypoxia
Hyperthermia
Raised ICP

CLINICAL OUTCOME

FIGURE 56A.1   Schematic diagram of key primary and secondary pathological events important to traumatic outcome. (ICP = intracranial pressure.)

hemorrhages occur in the central white matter, and gliding contusions occur in the parasagittal gray-white matter junctions. These models are characterized by a variable period of coma and widespread axonal damage within the upper brainstem and cerebellum. Impact acceleration models produce prolonged coma and widespread axonal damage. These models are characterized by variable and somewhat uncontrolled skull fractures.

Cerebral contusion is the most common head injury. In this regard, both acceleration and concussion models reproduce this histopathological outcome. Diffuse brain injury is an important phenomenon with regard to patients who die or remain in persistent vegetative state. The parasagittal F-P model produces widespread axonal perturbations (Bramlett et al. 1997b). Human head injury is never as pure as an experimental model, and the total human injury condition may not be addressed adequately with a single animal model. However, once a particular feature of human brain injury is produced in an experimental model, the pathogenesis of the injury can be critically investigated.

In Vitro Models

A shortcoming of animal models is that they preclude a critical assessment of individual cell responses to trauma. In animal experiments, for example, the initial cellular response to injury may be a consequence of both primary and secondary events initiated by a complex cascade of cellular interactions (Figure 56A.1). Thus, to critically investigate the consequences of injury on a specific cell type in the absence of confounding cellular and systemic factors, several in vitro cell culture models have been developed (Ellis et al. 1995). Models range from "scratching" the culture with a pipette tip to inducing cellular deformation by stretching cultured cells.

Using these approaches, investigators have found that trauma induces a wide range of primary cellular alterations. Astrocytic responses include hyperplasia, hypertrophy, and increased glial fibrillary acidic protein content. Increases in intracellular calcium occur, which are blocked by specific receptor antagonists. Traumatized astrocytes also produce interleukins and neurotropic factors. Neonatal cortical neurons that are stretched undergo delayed depolarization that depends on the activation of specific receptor populations. In vitro experimental approaches provide novel data concerning mechanisms underlying cellular responses to trauma and the role of specific cell types in the pathophysiology of brain trauma.

NEURONAL DAMAGE AFTER TRAUMATIC BRAIN INJURY

Temporal Patterns of Neuronal Death

The neuropathological sequelae of human TBI has been well described (Graham 1996). In experimental TBI, temporal patterns of neuronal damage have also been characterized (Figure 56A.2). As early as 6 hours after cortical contusion injury, the contused tissue appears edematous, and pyknotic neurons are apparent at the injury site. By 8 days, a cortical cavity has developed that is surrounded by a border containing necrotic tissue or a glial scar, or both. The temporal profile of neuronal damage after parasagittal F-P brain injury has also been assessed with light and electron microscopy. As early as 1 hour after impact, dark shrunken neurons indicative of irreversible damage are seen in cortical layers overlying the gliding contusion that displays BBB breakdown to protein tracers (Figure 56A.3). Ultrastructural studies demonstrate that early BBB dysfunction results from mechanical damage of small venules within vulnerable regions, including the external capsule. In some brain regions, focal sites of acute neuronal damage are associated with extravasated protein, whereas neuronal damage within other regions appears to occur without overt BBB breakdown. Astrocytic swelling is observed early after injury with increased glial fibrillary acidic protein

FIGURE 56A.2 The temporal profile of neuronal death after brain injury is highly variable. Factors that influence the maturation of irreversible damage include injury severity, intrinsic neuronal properties, and whether secondary insults take place.

I.   Acute Neuronal Injury

   Brain Trauma ➡️ Neuronal Death

II. Delayed Neuronal Death

   Brain Trauma ➡️ ➡️ Neuronal Death

III. Slowly Progressive Neuronal Death

   Brain Trauma ➡️ ➡️ ➡️ ➡️ ➡️ Neuronal Death

IV. Secondary Injury Mechanisms

   Brain Trauma ➡️ Secondary Insult ➡️ Neuronal Death

immunoreactivity apparent at later times in areas demonstrating histopathological damage (Figure 56A.4). In terms of neuroprotection, the acuteness of this pathology limits the potential for therapeutic interventions directed against the neuronal and glial response to TBI.

More subacute patterns of neuronal injury have been documented in various TBI models. At 3 days after moderate parasagittal F-P brain injury, scattered necrotic neurons are present throughout the frontoparietal cerebral cortex remote from the impact site (Figure 56A.5). In addition, selective neuronal necrosis is seen in the CA3 and CA4 hippocampal subsectors, the dentate hilus, and lateral thalamus ipsilateral to the trauma. These patterns of selective neuronal damage are associated with a well-demarcated contusion overlying the lateral external capsule. Molecular events leading to apoptosis have been described after TBI (Rink et al. 1995). Therefore, delayed patterns of neuronal cell death may involve necrotic as well as programmed cell death processes.

Only relatively recently has the progressive nature of the histopathological consequences of TBI been appreciated (Bramlett et al. 1997a). At 2 months after moderate parasagittal F-P injury, significant atrophy of the cerebral cortex, hippocampus, and thalamus is apparent in histological sections (Figure 56A.6). Atrophy of gray matter structures is associated with a significant enlargement of the lateral ventricle. Ventricular expansion not associated with hydrocephalus or increased intracranial pressure is felt to be a sensitive indicator of structural damage and an indirect measurement of white matter atrophy. Ventricular size has been correlated with memory disturbances, when patients with the highest ventricular volumes demonstrated significantly lower memory scores (Anderson and Bigler 1995).

The importance of a progressive injury cascade after TBI in terms of other neurological conditions merits consideration. For example, if mild head trauma leads to "reduced neuronal reserve," would the individual who sustained such trauma be more susceptible than others to neurodegenera-

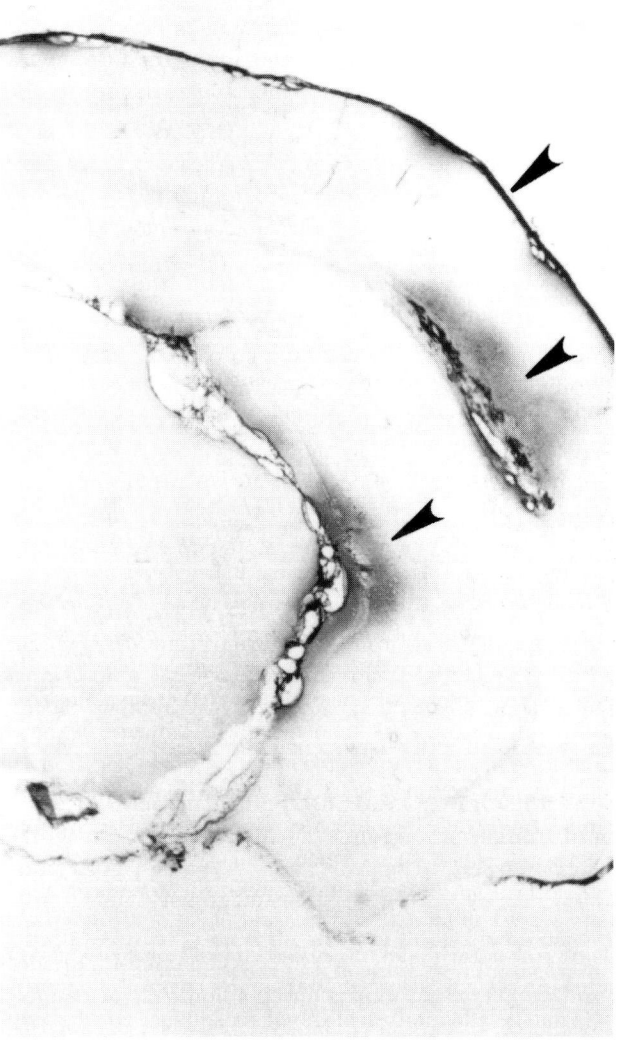

FIGURE 56A.3 This cross section of rat brain demonstrates focal sites of blood-brain barrier breakdown to the protein tracer horseradish peroxidase (*arrowheads*) 1 hour after fluid-percussion brain injury.

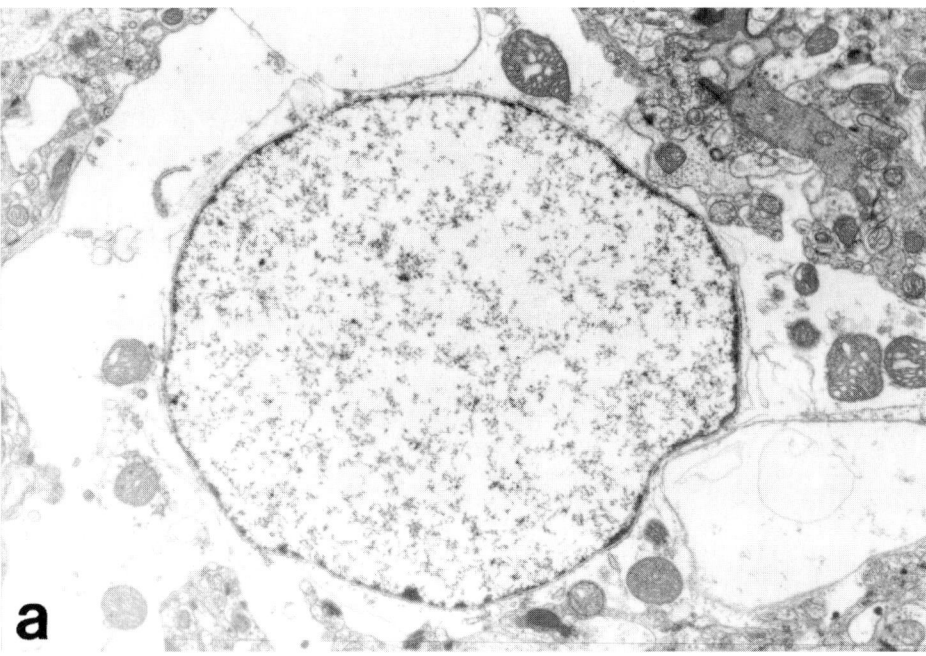

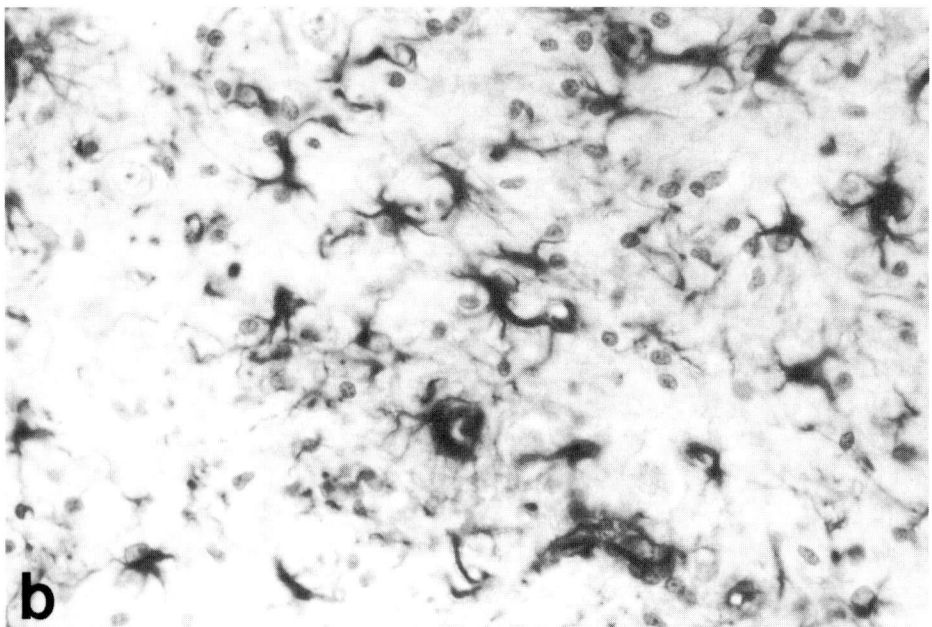

FIGURE 56A.4 (A) Astrocytic swelling 1 hour after fluid-percussion injury (×15,000). (B) At 3 days after trauma, reactive astrocytes express glial fibrillary acidic protein.

tive processes associated with aging? Indeed, some epidemiologic studies have indicated that a history of brain trauma is a risk factor for Alzheimer's disease.

Selective Neuronal Vulnerability

Damage to the hippocampus is commonly reported in autopsy studies of head-injured patients. Clinical and experimental studies describe cognitive abnormalities thought to be associated with hippocampal dysfunction. In an acceleration model of brain injury in nonhuman primates, CA1

hippocampal histopathological damage was reported in the majority of animals. CA1 damage was not produced by secondary global ischemia, raised intracranial pressure, or seizure activity. Significantly, CA1 hippocampal damage is not routinely reported in other TBI models, including cortical contusion and moderate F-P injury. However, midline F-P injury followed by a delayed sublethal global ischemic insult leads to CA1 neuronal damage. In contrast to moderate parasagittal F-P injury, severe trauma causes hemodynamic reductions that reach ischemic levels and CA1 neuronal damage. Taken together, these findings indicate an increased sensitivity of the post-traumatic brain to sec-

FIGURE 56A.5 (A) Well-demarcated contusion (*) overlying the external capsule is shown at 3 days after traumatic brain injury. (B) Perivascular inflammation is a prominent feature within the contusion (*arrowheads*).

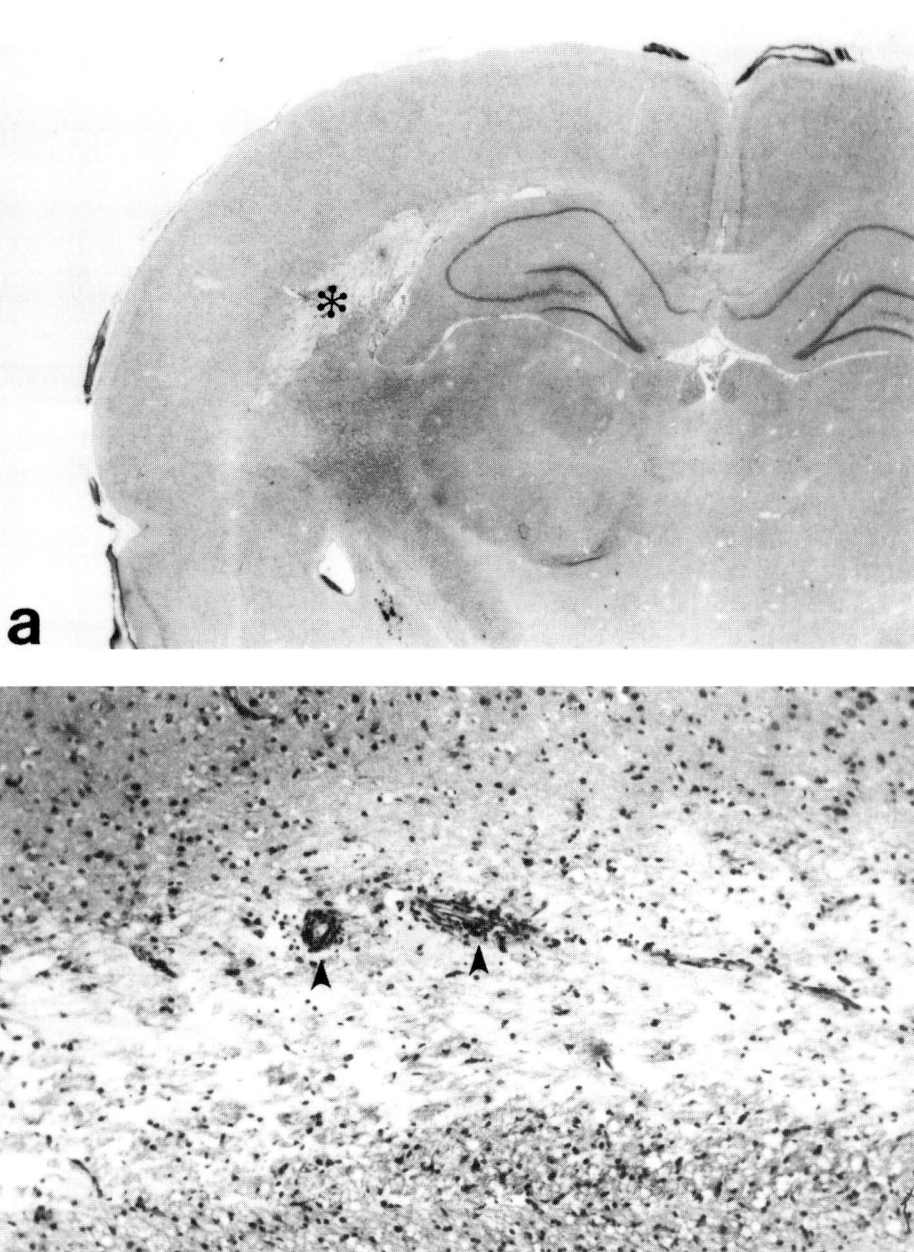

ondary insults. Finally, the dentate gyrus and CA3 hippocampus have also been reported to be selectively damaged in F-P models, with bilateral damage to dentate hilus reported after F-P injury.

Thalamic damage after brain injury is described in clinical and experimental studies. In human brain injury, the loss of inhibitory thalamic reticular neurons is proposed to underlie some forms of attention deficits. In radiographic studies of TBI patients using magnetic resonance imaging, relationships between injury severity, lesion volume, ventricle-to-brain ratio, and thalamic volume have been reported. Patients with moderate-to-severe injuries had smaller thalamic volumes and greater ventricle-to-brain ratios than did patients with mild-to-moderate injuries. Decreased thalamic volumes suggest that subcortical brain structures may be susceptible to transneuronal degeneration after cortical damage. Focal damage to thalamic nuclei seen after long-term F-P injury may result from progressive circuit degeneration after axonal damage, from neuronal cell death, or from the lack of neurotrophic delivery.

Axonal and Dendritic Injury

In 1992, Povlishock wrote that axonal injury exists as a spectrum involving widespread areas of the brain in exper-

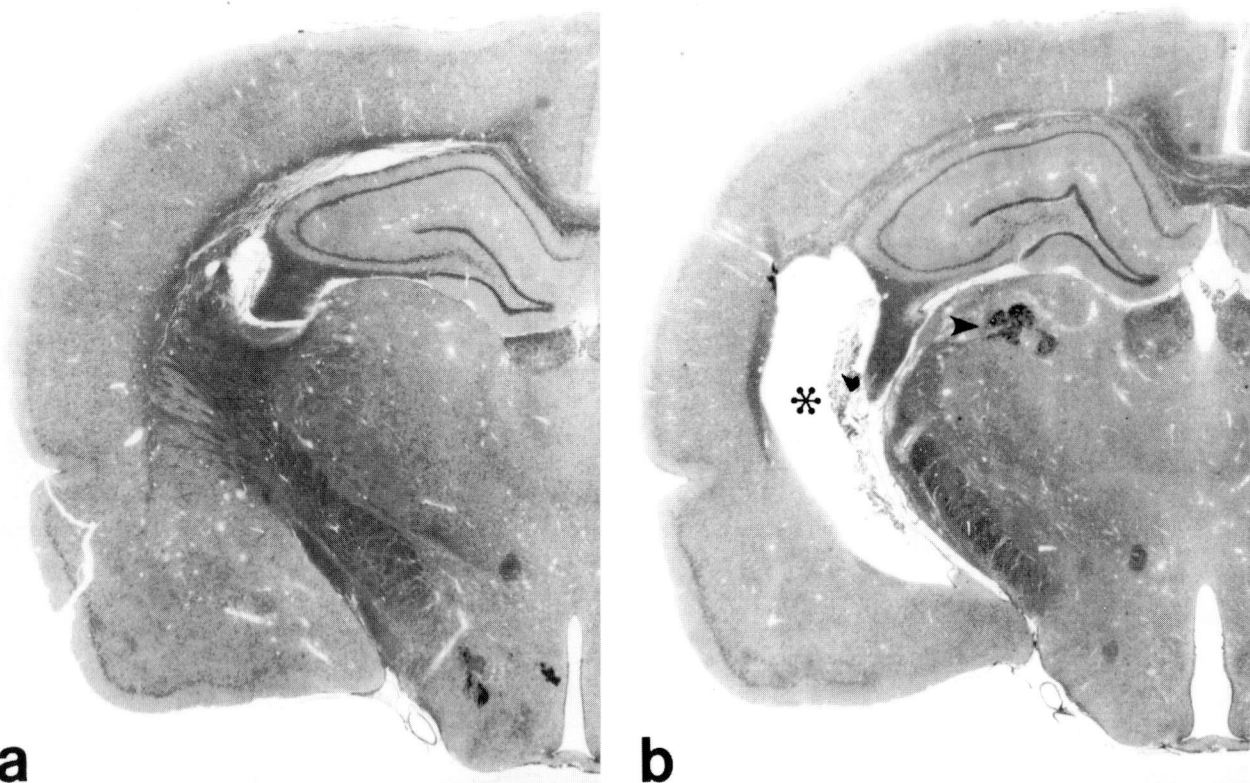

FIGURE 56A.6   Comparison between (**A**) noninjured rat and (**B**) rat 2 months after moderate fluid-percussion injury. Note cortical atrophy, enlarged lateral ventricle (*), and thalamic lesion (*arrowhead*) in traumatized rat.

imental models of TBI. Patterns of reactive axonal change using monoclonal antibodies targeted at neurofilament subunits or β-amyloid precursor protein have been characterized after F-P brain injury and controlled cortical impact injury. Within 1–2 hours of injury, reactive axonal change is most conspicuous in brainstem regions, including the pontomedullary junction. This pattern of axonal damage seen in experimental models is in contrast to the human condition, in which callosal and subcortical white matter axonal damage predominates. Significantly, moderate parasagittal F-P brain injury leads to widespread axonal damage in forebrain regions that represent reversible, irreversible, and delayed axonal perturbations (Bramlett et al. 1997b). These findings may explain some of the transient and delayed functional consequences of TBI.

In addition to axonal damage, studies indicate that TBI also leads to significant changes in neuronal dendrites (Posmantur et al. 1996). A common feature of damage of injured neurons is loss of microtubule-associated protein 2 (MAP2) antigenicity. MAP2 is an important microtubule cross-linking protein that is found predominantly in somatodendritic environments. Changes in MAP2 may therefore reflect damage to dendrites. Using this strategy, evidence for dendritic damage has been reported within and beyond areas of overt histopathological damage. Thus, den-

dritic damage not necessarily associated with neuronal death may participate in some of the functional consequences associated with TBI.

BASIC MECHANISMS OF INJURY

Primary Injury Mechanisms

Two major types of forces are responsible for brain injury, one localized at the impact site and a second characterized by rotational forces. Depending on the force and location of the primary impact, head trauma can produce acute damage to blood vessels and axonal projections. Contact phenomena generate superficial or contusional hemorrhages through coup and contrecoup mechanisms. Direct injury is commonly superficial, and the coup-contrecoup hemorrhages may be adjacent or central.

Axonal shearing is a common lesion of the cerebral white matter and occurs particularly in acceleration-deceleration injury. Only recently has morphological evidence for axonal shearing (primary axotomy) become available. Ultrastructural evidence demonstrates the tearing or shearing of axons in nonhuman primates exposed to lateral acceleration of the head. Axonal separation can occur without prior formation of axonal swelling. Perturbations of the axolemma leading to the accumulation of cytoskeletal components and organelles may represent a secondary injury process that can be treated.

Shearing strains may also damage blood vessels and cause petechial hemorrhages, deep intracerebral hematomas, and brain swelling. Mechanical damage to small venules resulting in focal BBB breakdown is reported immediately after F-P injury. Vascular damage leads to the formation of hemorrhagic contusions. Early vascular damage may increase neuronal vulnerability by causing post-traumatic perfusion deficits and the extravasation of potentially neurotoxic blood-borne substances.

Secondary Injury Mechanisms

In many head-injured patients, the extent of neurological recovery depends on the contribution of post-traumatic secondary insults (DeWitt et al. 1995). In the clinical setting, secondary insults include hypotension, hypoxia, hyperglycemia, anemia, sepsis, and hyperthermia. Experimental evidence indicates an increased susceptibility of the post-traumatic brain to secondary insults. For example, after mild F-P brain injury, CA1 hippocampal vulnerability is enhanced with superimposed secondary ischemia. An important area of research regarding the treatment of brain injury involves the characterization of secondary injury processes, which may be targeted for intensive care management or for pharmacotherapy.

A high frequency of hypoxic or ischemic brain damage occurs in patients who die as a result of nonmissile head injury (Graham 1996). Hypoxic damage in the form of hemorrhagic infarction and diffuse neuronal necrosis is most frequent in arterial boundary zones between the major cerebral arteries. Hypoxic damage is also common in patients who have experienced an episode of intracranial hypertension. A significant correlation between hypoxic brain damage and arterial spasm in nonmissile TBI patients has been reported. Post-traumatic hypoxia aggravates the BBB consequences of F-P brain injury.

Post-traumatic hemodynamic impairments represent another injury mechanism. Clinical and experimental investigations report moderate reductions in lCBF after TBI. After moderate parasagittal F-P brain injury, widespread reductions in lCBF range from 40% to 80% of control. In contrast, severe F-P injury leads to lCBF reductions that reach ischemic levels. Focal reductions in lCBF are associated with subarachnoid and intracerebral hemorrhage and local platelet accumulation. Reductions in lCBF result from the mechanical occlusion of cerebral vessels, the release of vasoactive substances, or possibly as a secondary consequence of reductions in neuronal activity or metabolism. Injury severity is a critical factor in determining the hemodynamic and pathological consequences of experimental TBI.

Hypotension is present in a significant number of patients with TBI. In severely injured patients, outcome is correlated with reduced mean arterial blood pressure. Hemorrhagic hypotension after F-P injury results in more severe depletion of high-energy phosphates compared with TBI alone. The increased sensitivity of the post-traumatic brain to moderate levels of hypotension may result from deficits in autoregulation, which have been reported in patient and experimental studies. Hypotensive periods that may occur during surgical procedures and anesthesia may produce secondary insults and be hazardous to the head-injured patient.

In experimental brain injury, organ reperfusion has been shown to exacerbate tissue injury (i.e., reperfusion injury). In models of cerebral ischemia, for example, evidence for inflammatory processes influencing pathological outcome has been reported. In models of TBI, the temporal profile of polymorphonuclear leukocyte accumulation has been examined. In the cortical impact model, myeloperoxidase activity, an indicator of neutrophil accumulation, increased within the traumatized hemisphere at 1 day. In the lateral F-P model, neutrophils are present as early as 4 hours after injury. Future studies are required to determine whether attenuating neutrophil infiltration or general inflammatory processes (or both) improves structural and functional improvement after TBI.

Many patients experience fever after head injury, and clinical data indicate that brain temperature after TBI may be higher than core or bladder temperature. Experimentally, post-traumatic brain hyperthermia induced artificially 24 hours after trauma increases mortality rate and aggravates histopathological outcome (Dietrich et al. 1996a). Post-traumatic hyperthermia also increases the frequency of swollen myelinated axons (Figure 56A.7). Thus, in the clinical setting, post-traumatic hyperthermia may represent a secondary injury mechanism that might negate the beneficial effects of a therapeutic agent. Because delayed post-traumatic hyperthermia has been shown to have detrimental effects on outcome, aggressive attempts should be made to reduce brain temperature.

THERAPEUTIC INTERVENTIONS DIRECTED AGAINST PATHOPHYSIOLOGICAL PROCESSES

The pathophysiology of TBI has been investigated using a variety of animal models. Based on experimental data, new therapies have been initiated. Several reviews have summarized the agents that have been investigated in TBI (Faden 1996). The problem of TBI involves injury pathways that are common to other brain injuries, including cerebral ischemia. However, the pathogenesis of TBI is unique in other ways and requires therapeutic approaches specifically targeted at brain trauma. The present discussion is limited to several of the major therapeutic strategies currently being assessed experimentally and clinically.

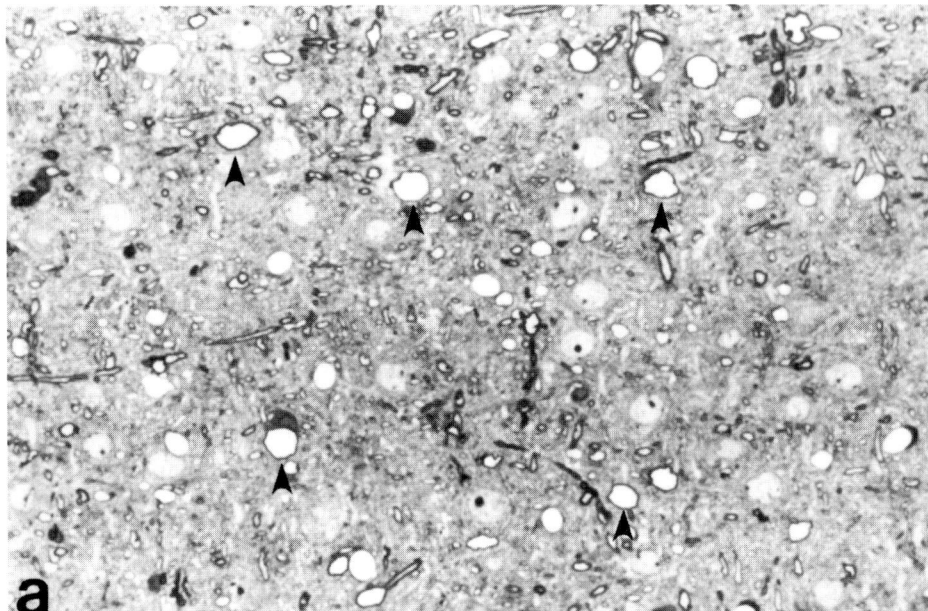

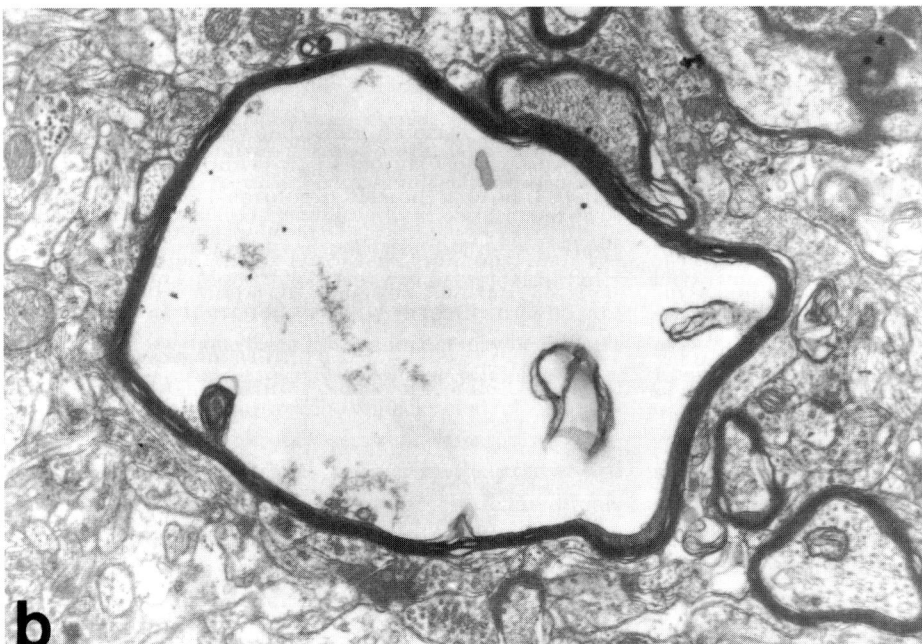

FIGURE 56A.7   (A) Three hours of hyperthermia induced 24 hours after fluid-percussion injury increases the frequency of swollen axons (*arrowheads*). (B) Ultrastructural features of severely swollen and damaged myelinated axon (×14,000).

Glutamate Antagonists

Excitatory amino acid neurotransmitters have been implicated in the pathophysiology of TBI (Baker et al. 1993). Microdialysis techniques have documented elevated levels of extracellular amino acids, whereas N-methyl-D-aspartate (NMDA) receptor antagonists, including MK-801 (dizocilpine), provide behavioral and histopathological protection against brain trauma. The role of glutamate antagonists for the treatment of central nervous system injury has been reviewed, and clinical stroke trials of the competitive NMDA antagonists are in progress. The noncompetitive

NMDA antagonist MK-801 was withdrawn due to harmful side effects. Clinical data are still required to determine whether NMDA receptor blockage will provide a significant benefit in clinical head trauma.

Free Radical Scavengers

The genesis of oxygen free radicals has also been implicated in the pathophysiology of TBI. Experimental F-P injury increases the production of oxygen radicals, and free radical scavenger inhibitors have been reported to be protective in brain injury models. Using sensitive indicators of hydroxy radical production and microdialysis, elevations in extracellular hydroxy radical production after F-P injury have been reported. The free radical scavenger superoxide dismutase (SOD) reduces BBB opening and the genesis of brain edema after TBI. Transgenic mice who overexpress human copper-zinc SOD are protected against brain trauma (Chan et al. 1996). Clinical trials using polyethylene glycol SOD have been initiated in brain trauma.

Neurotrophic Factors

A unique problem of brain trauma is diffuse axonal injury. Axonal injury leading to circuit disruption may not only produce immediate functional consequences but may also affect trophic signaling between neuronal populations. The addition of trophic factors after TBI may help maintain neuronal survival as well as promote circuit reorganization and functional recovery (Mattson and Scheff 1994). Neurotrophins have been shown to be neuroprotective by in vitro and in vivo models of neuronal injury. One neurotrophic factor, basic fibroblast growth factor (bFGF) or FGF type 2 (FGF2), has been reported to protect neuronal cell cultures from a variety of lethal injuries, including hypoxia and ischemia. bFGF has been shown to be neuroprotective in the F-P model, in which intravenous bFGF infusion initiated 30 minutes after trauma significantly reduced histopathology damage (Dietrich et al. 1996b). If experimental studies continue to show a benefit of bFGF on neuronal injury and behavioral outcome in TBI models, this may be an important direction for future clinical trials in brain trauma.

Protection by Nitric Oxide–Related Species

Within the nervous system, nitric oxide (NO) may serve as a neurotransmitter and as a signal between cells, as well as an autocrine signal within a given cell. After brain injury, an increase of neuronal Ca^{2+} triggers constitutive NO synthase (cNOS) activity, leading to the release of NO that may enhance excitotoxicity (Dawson et al. 1994). Studies of mutant mice deficient in neuronal (nNOS) or endothelial NOS (eNOS) activity have demonstrated that, whereas nNOS exacerbates ischemic injury, eNOS protects.

Therapeutic strategies directed at the NO pathway have been reported in models of brain injury. The selective inhibition of nNOS by 3-bromo-7-nitroindazole improves histopathological outcome after cerebral ischemia. Data indicate that F-P injury leads to the acute activation of cNOS and that treatment with 7-nitroindazole protects histopathologically and behaviorally. In addition, the inhibition of inducible NOS with aminoguanidine also led to improved histopathological outcome. Future studies using mutant mice deficient in nNOS or eNOS activity will be important to advance this area of investigation.

Antiapoptotic Agents

Apoptosis is a mode of cell death in both physiological and pathological processes. Apoptosis has also been observed after TBI (Rink et al. 1995). After F-P injury, apoptotic cells have been identified in the ipsilateral cortex, hippocampus, and thalamus as soon as 4 hours after injury. The effects of F-P injury on the expression of the bcl-2 protein, which regulates developmental programmed cell death, has also been investigated. Evidence for apoptosis of oligodendroglia in long tracts undergoing wallerian degeneration has been reported after spinal cord injury. Thus, demyelination of tracts after brain or spinal cord trauma may result from apoptotic death of oligodendrocytes.

Although the molecular events leading to apoptosis are not fully understood, the family of cysteine proteases (caspases) play an active role in its pathogenesis. In addition, in vitro studies have demonstrated that protease inhibitors specific to caspase 3 inhibit apoptosis. In vivo data also indicate that specific inhibitors of the caspase family improve histological and behavioral outcome after TBI. The role of apoptosis in the pathophysiology of brain trauma is important because therapeutic strategies directed at this injury mechanism may be initiated to prevent delayed degeneration. Using agents specific to apoptosis or in combination with agents that target necrosis is a potential research direction.

Therapeutic Hypothermia

Numerous studies have demonstrated that, although mild-to-moderate hypothermia is neuroprotective in models of TBI, mild hyperthermia worsens outcome. After brain trauma, hypothermia has been shown to improve histopathological and behavioral outcomes in a variety of injury models. Therapeutic hypothermia has been shown to influence a wide range of injury processes (Dietrich et al. 1996c). Microdialysis studies report that post-traumatic hypothermia reduces the acute surge in levels of extracellular glutamate and hydroxyl radicals after injury (Globus et al. 1995). Post-traumatic hypothermia protects against BBB dysfunction. In terms of long-term outcome measures, hypothermia inhibits progressive cortical atrophy and subsequent ventricular enlargement. The ability of any therapeutic intervention to provide long-term protection is an important requirement for the advancement of any therapeutic strategy to the clinical setting.

The use of moderate levels of hypothermia (>32°C) also improves outcome in patient studies. Systemic hypothermia (32–33°C) begun within 6 hours of injury (Glasgow Coma Scale 4–7; see Chapter 5, Table 5.4) resulted in no cardiac or coagulopathy-related complications, a lower seizure frequency, and more patients in the good recovery–to–moderate disability category (Marion et al. 1997). In other studies, therapeutic hypothermia attenuated intracranial hypertension but did not affect the frequency of delayed intracerebral hemorrhage. The duration of cooling is an important variable in determining the extent of neuroprotection. In TBI studies, prolonged periods of hypothermia may therefore be necessary to protect the brain from primary and secondary injury processes.

Continued experimental studies directed at the pathogenesis of TBI will enhance our understanding of the neuroscience of brain trauma. The clarification of what injury processes dominate the injury cascade will improve our strategies directed at brain protection. The continued communication between basic scientists involved in brain injury research and clinicians responsible for treating this patient population will enhance our efforts toward these goals.

REFERENCES

Anderson CV, Bigler ED. Ventricular dilation, cortical atrophy, and neuropsychological outcome following traumatic brain injury. J Neuropsychiatry Clin Neurosci 1995;7:42–48.

Baker A, Moulton RJ, MacMillian VH, Shedden PM. Excitatory amino acids in cerebrospinal fluid following traumatic brain injury in humans. J Neurosurg 1993;79:369–372.

Bramlett HM, Dietrich WD, Green EJ, Busto R. Chronic histopathological consequences of fluid-percussion brain injury in rats: effects of posttraumatic hypothermia. Acta Neuropathol 1997a;93:190–199.

Bramlett HM, Kraydieh S, Green EJ, Dietrich WD. Temporal and regional patterns of axonal damage following traumatic brain injury: a beta-amyloid precursor protein immunocytochemical study in rats. J Neuropathol Exp Neurol 1997b;56:1132–1141.

Chan PH, Epstein CJ, Kinouchi H, et al. Neuroprotective Role of CuZn-Superoxide Dismutase in Ischemic Brain Damage. In BK Siesjo, T Wieloch (eds), Cellular and Molecular Mechanisms of Ischemic Brain Damage. Philadelphia: Lippincott–Raven, 1996; 271–280.

Dawson TM, Snyder SH. Gases as biological messengers: nitric oxide and carbon monoxide in the brain. J Neurosci 1994;14:5147–5159.

DeWitt DS, Jenkins LW, Prough DS. Enhanced vulnerability to secondary ischemic insults after experimental traumatic brain injury. New Horizons 1995;3:376–383.

Dietrich WD, Alonso O, Busto R, et al. Post-traumatic brain hypothermia reduces histopathological damage following concussive brain injury in the rat. Acta Neuropathol 1994;87:250–258.

Dietrich WD, Alonso O, Busto R, Finklestein SP. Posttreatment with intravenous basic fibroblast growth factor reduces histopathological damage following fluid-percussion brain injury in rats. J Neurotrauma 1996b;13:309–316.

Dietrich WD, Alonso O, Halley M, Busto R. Delayed posttraumatic brain hyperthermia worsens outcome after fluid percussion brain injury: a light and electron microscopic study in rats. Neurosurgery 1996a;38:533–541.

Dietrich WD, Busto R, Globus MY-T, Ginsberg, MD. Brain damage and termperature: cellular and molecular mechanisms. Adv Neurol 1996c;71:177–197.

Ellis EF, McKinney JS, Willoughby KA, et al. A new model for rapid stretch-induced injury in culture: characterization of the model using astrocytes. J Neurotrauma 1995;12:325–339.

Faden AI. Pharmacological Treatment Approaches for Brain and Spinal Cord Trauma. In RK Narayan, JE Wilberger, JT Povlishock (eds), Neurotrauma. New York: McGraw-Hill, 1996;1479–1490.

Gennarelli TA. Animate models of human head injury. J Neurotrauma 1994;11:357–368.

Globus MY-T, Alonso O, Dietrich WD, et al. Glutamate release and free radical production following brain injury: effects of posttraumatic hypothermia. J Neurochem 1995;65:1704–1711.

Graham DI. Neuropathology of Head Injury. In RK Narayan, JE Wilberger, JT Povlishock (eds), Neurotrauma. New York: McGraw-Hill, 1996;43–59.

Marion DW, Penrod LE, Kelsey SF, et al. Treatment of traumatic brain injury with moderate hypothermia. N Engl J Med 1997;336:540–546.

Mattson MP, Scheff SW. Endogenous neuroprotection factors and traumatic brain injury: mechanisms of action and implications for therapy. J Neurotrauma 1994;11:3–33.

Posmantur RM, Kampfl A, Taft WC, et al. Diminished microtubule-associated protein 2 (MAP2) immunoreactivity following impact brain injury. J Neurotrauma 1996;13:125–137.

Rink A, Fung KM, Trojanowski JQ, et al. Evidence of apoptotic cell death after experimental traumatic brain injury in the rat. Am J Pathol 1995;147:1575–1583.

Chapter 56
Trauma of the Nervous System

B. CRANIOCEREBRAL TRAUMA
Jack I. Jallo and Raj K. Narayan

Trauma is a major cause of death and disability in developed and developing countries around the world. In the United States, traumatic injury is the leading cause of death and disability for people aged 1–44 years and is the third most common cause of death overall. In more than one-half of trauma-related deaths, head injury contributes significantly to mortality (Kraus et al. 1996). Perhaps even more important, for each death, there are at least two survivors with some degree of permanent disability, usually secondary to head injury.

In the United States, accurate data relating to the incidence of head injury are difficult to obtain because there is no nationwide registry. Furthermore, the incidence and cause of head injury can vary dramatically from one locale to the next, even within the same city (Table 56B.1). Keeping these limitations in mind, the average incidence of traumatic brain injury (TBI) in the United States is conservatively estimated at 180–220 per 100,000 population per year (Kraus et al. 1996). With an approximate population of 250 million, this translates into 500,000 new cases per year in the United States. Of these, 50,000 patients die before reaching the hospital; the remaining 450,000 are admitted. These figures do not include an indeterminate number of persons who do not come to medical attention. Of those that do get to the hospital, 80% are categorized as mild

head injuries and 10% each as moderate and severe. Much of the research and attention to date has focused on the severe head injury population.

If the frequency of permanent disability is 10%, 66%, and 100% in the mild, moderate, and severe head injury groups, respectively, then 82,814 new patients with varying degrees of impairment are being added to the population each year in the United States. This figure includes approximately 2,000 who remain in a permanent vegetative state. The total direct and indirect cost to the nation from TBI, including acute care and rehabilitation, support services, and lost income is estimated to be around $25 billion. Thus, TBI is a major public health problem. Any organizational, social, or therapeutic measure that reduces the incidence, mortality, or morbidity from this condition even slightly can be very significant in both human and economic terms.

The mortality associated with severe head injury has dropped from approximately 50% in the 1970s to the 30% range in the 1990s. This dramatic improvement can be ascribed to several factors, including improved rescue systems, the widespread introduction of computed tomographic (CT) scanners, the establishment of designated trauma centers with better-trained personnel, prompt surgery, and aggressive neurocritical care. Apart from reducing mortality, these developments have also improved

Table 56B.1: Distribution of head injury by location

Cause of injury	Inner-city Chicago (%)	Suburban Chicago (%)	Aquitaine, France (%)
Motor vehicle accident	31	39	60
Fall	20	31	33
Assault	40	10	9 (includes recreation or other)
Recreation or other	9	20	—

the neurological condition of the survivors. However, it is hard to statistically document these trends, except by comparison with historical data. Furthermore, trying to tease out the impact of any single intervention on the ultimate outcome is even more difficult.

It was originally believed that most of the damage resulting from TBI occurred at the moment of impact, and thereafter the outcome was a *fait accompli*. We now know that only part of the injury occurs *ab initio*. The initial impact sets into motion a series of biochemical processes having ultrastructural concomitants. In the future, modification of these processes by pharmacological or other means might significantly protect the injured brain and improve the ultimate neurological outcomes.

The impact of secondary insults on the injured brain is well documented. Common post-traumatic events, such as raised intracranial pressure (ICP), hypotension, hypoxia, hyperthermia, hyperglycemia, and infection, among others, can markedly affect outcome. Compulsory attention to preventing, or promptly treating, these secondary insults is responsible for improved outcomes.

Although we largely focus on treating patients with head injury, clearly it is better to have prevented the injury in the first place. Seat belts, air bags, and helmets seem to be making a substantial impact on the incidence of vehicular head injury. Think First, an educational program aimed at school-age children, was developed by American neurosurgeons to help prevent risk-taking behavior by this vulnerable group. Limiting the availability of firearms could reduce the incidence of gunshot wounds to the head, but this is constrained by legal and socioeconomic issues in the United States.

This chapter reviews the key issues relating to TBI and its clinical management. The pathophysiology of head injury has been detailed in Chapter 56A. For a comprehensive treatise on TBI, the interested reader is referred to Narayan et al. (1996).

CLASSIFICATION

Head injuries may be classified by mechanism, severity, and morphology (Table 56B.2).

Classification by Mechanism

Based on mechanism, head injury may be classified as *blunt* or *penetrating*, or as *open* or *closed*. Penetrating injuries are by definition open, whereas blunt head injuries may be open or closed. Open head injuries have an elevated risk of cerebrospinal fluid (CSF) leak and infection. Penetrating injuries are usually due to gunshot wounds (Figure 56B.1) or stab wounds, whereas closed injuries usually result from motor vehicle accidents, falls, or assault.

Penetrating injuries in a civilian environment most commonly result from handgun use. Missile size and velocity are important because these factors determine the amount of energy that is transmitted to the brain. The energy deposited is determined by the formula $KE = \frac{1}{2} MV^2$ (where *KE* is kinetic energy, *M* is mass, and *V* is the velocity of the missile). Hence, the extent of injury caused by a bullet depends on velocity and bullet type. Deformable, hollow-point bullets produce more severe damage by expanding on impact and producing a larger-diameter cavity.

Classification by Severity

A number of scales are available to measure injury severity, such as the Abbreviated Injury Scale, the Reaction Level Scale, and the Injury Severity Scale, but the most commonly used brain injury severity scale is the Glasgow Coma Scale (GCS) (see Chapter 5, Table 5.4). This scale was introduced by Teasdale and Jennett in 1974 and has three components:

Table 56B.2: Classification of head injury

A. By mechanism
  1. Closed
  2. Penetrating
B. By severity
  1. Glasgow Coma Scale score
  2. Mild, moderate, severe
C. By morphology
  1. Skull fractures
    a. Vault
      (1) Linear or stellate
      (2) Depressed or nondepressed
    b. Basilar
  2. Intracranial lesions
    a. Focal
      (1) Epidural
      (2) Subdural
      (3) Intracerebral
    b. Diffuse
      (1) Mild concussion
      (2) Classic concussion
      (3) Diffuse axonal injury

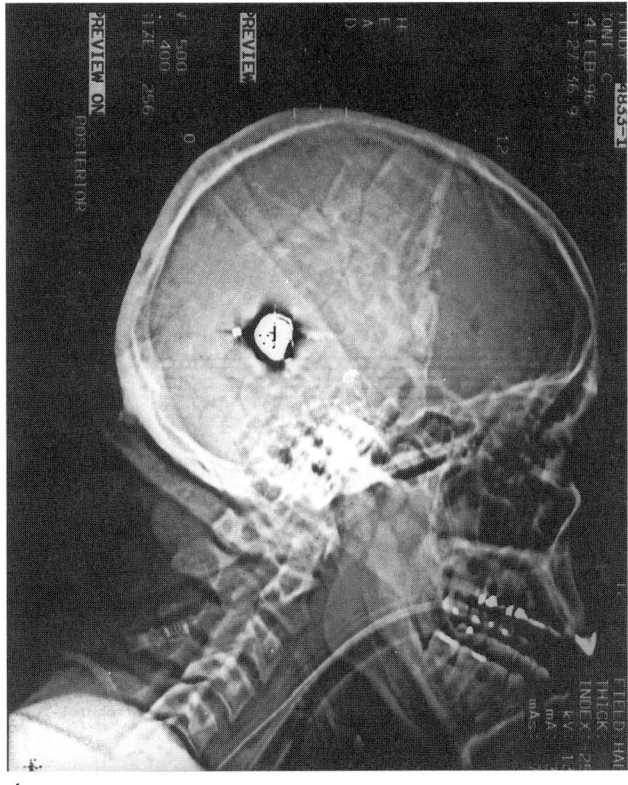

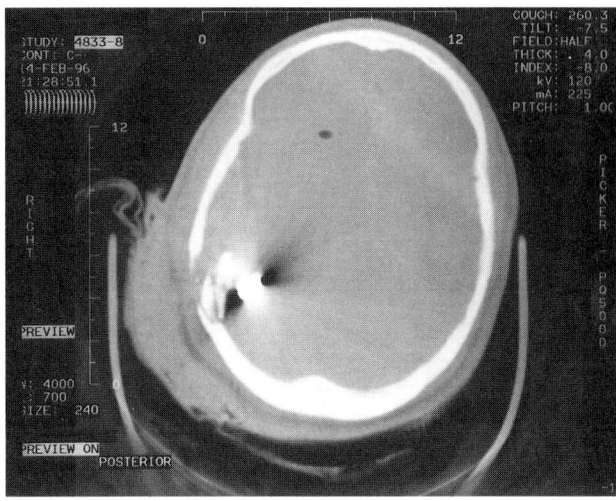

B

FIGURE 56B.1   (A) Scout view of bullet penetrating right parietal skull. (B) Axial computed tomographic view of same bullet.

eye opening, best verbal response, and best motor response. The score should be ascertained after resuscitation because hypotension or hypoxia can markedly alter the neurological examination. The GCS score is a sum of the three scores (eye opening, best motor response, and best verbal response). The patient who follows commands, is oriented, and has spontaneous eye opening achieves the maximum score of 15. At the other extreme of the GCS, the patient without a motor and verbal response or eye opening to a noxious stimulus is assigned a score of 3. Coma, according to the GCS, is generally defined as a score of 8 or less and represents patients who do not follow commands, speak, or open their eyes.

Head injury is further classified as mild, moderate, or severe according to the GCS. Mild head injury is defined by a score of 14–15, moderate head injury by a score of 9–13, and severe head injury by a score of 3–8. The patient who is intubated receives a letter score of "T" to replace the verbal score. In a comatose patient, the motor response is clearly the most important prognostic feature (Table 56B.3).

Classification by Morphology

Classifying head injury based on morphology broadly divides injuries into intracranial lesions and skull lesions (see Table 56B.2). Skull fractures may further be catalogued as skull base or cranial vault. Fractures of the cranial vault may be linear or stellate, depressed or nondepressed, and open or closed. In general, fractures that are open and have evidence of dural laceration and those that are depressed beyond the inner table of the skull require surgical repair. Patients with a skull fracture are also much more likely to harbor an intracranial hematoma. Fractures of the skull base are associated with an increased risk of CSF leak and cranial nerve injury. The facial nerve is particularly vulnerable because it passes through the petrous temporal bone, but olfactory nerve injury with loss of smell and vestibulocochlear injuries with abnormalities of balance are more common.

Table 56B.3:   Comparison of outcome after head injury with different motor responses

		Outcome (%)		
Motor response	No. of cases	G/MD	SD/V	Dead
Not posturing or flaccid	83	74	7	19
Uni- or bilaterally decorticate	20	60	5	35
Uni- or bilaterally decerebrate	19	21	16	63
Bilaterally flaccid	11	27	9	64
Total	133	60	8	32

G = good outcome; MD = moderately disabled; SD = severely disabled; V = vegetative.
Source: Reprinted with permission from RK Narayan, RP Greenberg, JD Miller, et al. Improved confidence of outcome prediction in severe head injury: a comparative analysis of the clinical examination, multimodality evoked potentials, CT scanning, and intracranial pressure. J Neurosurg 1981;54:756.

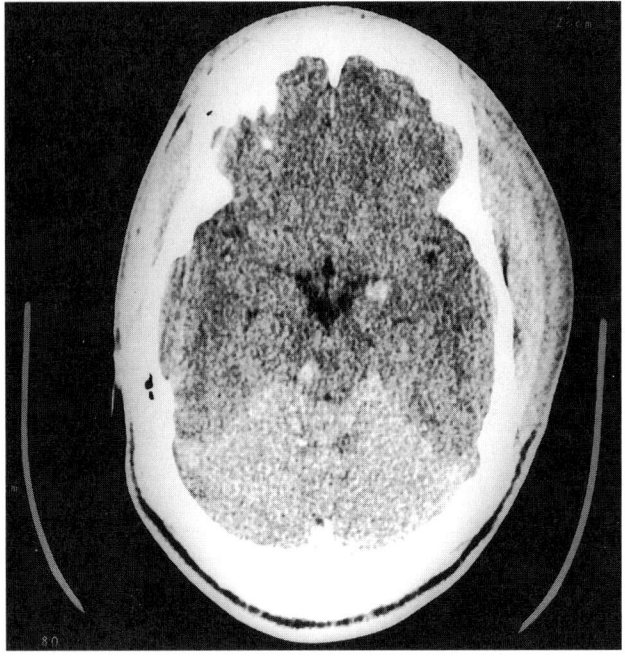

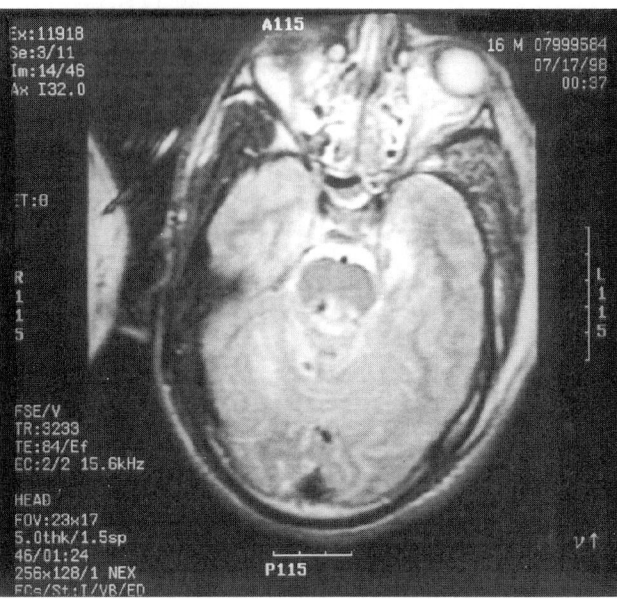

A   B

FIGURE 56B.2   (A) Axial computed tomographic view demonstrating punctate hemorrhagic lesions suggestive of diffuse axonal injury. (B) Axial T2-weighted magnetic resonance image illustrating punctate hemorrhagic lesions suggestive of diffuse axonal injury.

Intracranial lesions may be broadly categorized as focal or diffuse, although it is not uncommon to find both in the same patient. Focal lesions may be epidural, subdural, or intracerebral hematomas and frequently represent surgical emergencies. Diffuse lesions are concussions or diffuse axonal injury (DAI) (Figure 56B.2).

Axonal Injury

DAI may be one of the most important factors determining outcome in blunt head injury. It is also the most common cause of coma in the absence of an intracranial mass lesion. DAI is seen most frequently in patients who have been injured in vehicular accidents, but it may also occur after injuries that occur at much lower velocity, such as falls. DAI is characterized by distinct gross and microscopic features, including axonal swellings that are widely distributed in the cerebral white matter, corpus callosum, and upper brainstem; gross hemorrhagic lesions of the corpus callosum; and gross hemorrhagic lesions involving one or both dorsolateral quadrants of the rostral brainstem.

To make a diagnosis of DAI, evidence of axonal injury must be found independent of other lesions, such as infarcts and hematomas. A pathological grading system for DAI is based on the distribution of injury. Grade 1 DAI demonstrates histologic evidence of axonal damage in the white matter of the cerebral hemispheres, corpus callosum, brainstem, and less commonly, the cerebellum. In grade 2 DAI, in addition to evidence of axonal injury, there are also focal lesions of the corpus callosum. In grade 3 DAI, in addition to the axonal injury found in grade 1 and the focal lesion of

the corpus callosum found in grade 2, there are lesions of the dorsolateral quadrant of the rostral brainstem.

Acute Subdural Hematoma

Acute subdural hematoma (SDH; Figure 56B.3) is the most common focal intracerebral lesion and occurs in approximately 30% of patients with severe head injury. They have the highest morbidity and mortality of all traumatic focal lesions because of underlying parenchymal injury and intracranial hypertension. They are frequently associated with cerebral contusions, intracerebral hematomas, and brain lacerations. Classically, chronic SDH arises from torn bridging veins between the cerebral cortex and the major venous sinuses, but acute SDH may also arise from laceration of cortical vessels.

Epidural Hematoma

Epidural hematoma (Figure 56B.4) is less common than SDH but has a better overall outcome, provided it is detected and evacuated quickly. The better outcome results from the fact that less underlying parenchymal brain injury is associated with these lesions. Outcome after evacuation of an epidural hematoma is directly related to the level of consciousness before surgery. With epidural hematomas, blood accumulates between the skull and dura, resulting in a lens-shaped or biconvex collection. These hematomas typically arise from a laceration of the middle meningeal artery caused by a skull fracture. They may also develop more slowly from diploic bleeding from skull fractures.

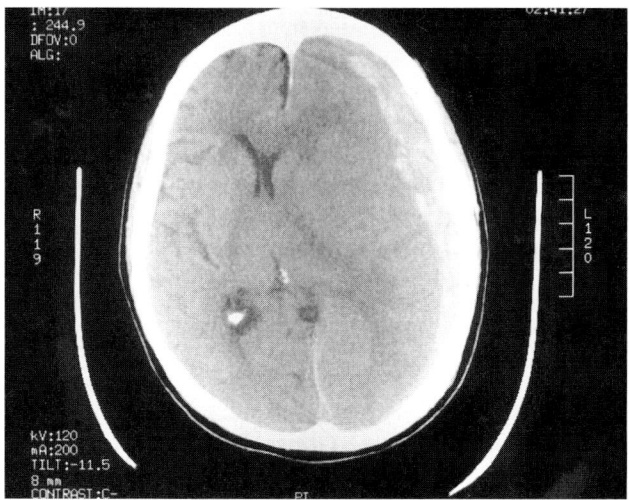

FIGURE 56B.3   Axial computed tomographic scan showing an acute subdural hematoma.

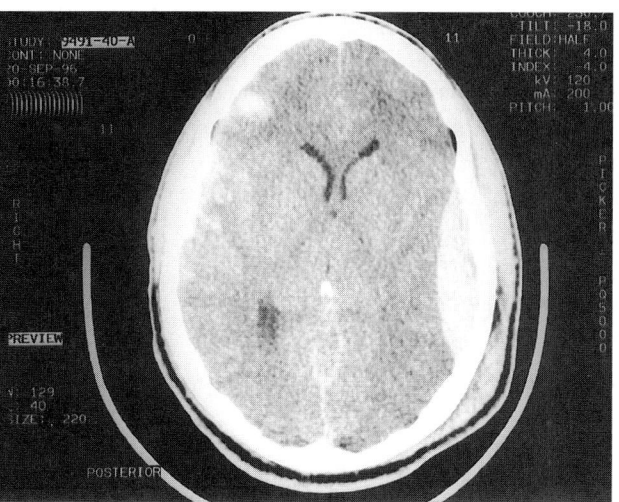

FIGURE 56B.4   Axial computed tomographic scan demonstrating a left epidural hematoma, a right frontal contusion, and right frontal and temporal subarachnoid hemorrhage.

Contusion and Intracerebral Hematoma

Contusions and intracerebral hematomas (Figure 56B.5; see also Figure 56B.4) may be found in isolation or associated with other lesions, such as SDH, epidural hematomas, subarachnoid hemorrhage (SAH), or skull fractures. Contusions and intracerebral hematomas represent a continuum. Contusions are bruises of the brain characterized by extravasation of blood from small, lacerated vessels, whereas intracerebral hemorrhages are large blood clots in the brain parenchyma. Contusions are sometimes described as *coup* (abnormalities seen directly below the site of impact) and *countercoup* (abnormalities located on the diametrically opposite side of the brain). The majority of contusions are in the inferior frontal or temporal lobes, and most of these do not require evacuation. Careful clinical observation and follow-up CT scans are helpful in assessing the evolution of these lesions and determining the need for surgery, based primarily on the degree of mass effect.

Subarachnoid Hemorrhage

SAH, or bleeding into the subarachnoid space, is common in TBI. SAH may be the only manifestation of head injury, although it is frequently found in association with other lesions, such as contusions or hematomas. When it is found in isolation, surgical intervention is not indicated, although one must be alert for cerebral vasospasm, raised ICP, and hydrocephalus.

INITIAL EXAMINATION

Meagher and Narayan (1999) reviewed some of the key issues relating to the role of the neurosurgeon in the initial management and triage of the TBI patient.

Primary Survey

On presentation, a primary survey is performed and resuscitation initiated. Hypotension and hypoxia adversely affect outcome from brain injury. Hypotension on admission, defined as a systolic blood pressure of less than 90 mm Hg, is associated with a doubling of mortality in patients with severe head injury (Chesnut et al. 1993a). When both hypotension and hypoxia are present, the mortality is as high as 75%. Rapid cardiopulmonary resuscitation and maintenance of an adequate blood pressure is therefore crucial.

Airway

Securing an airway begins with clearing the oropharynx and supplying supplemental oxygen. Patients with severe

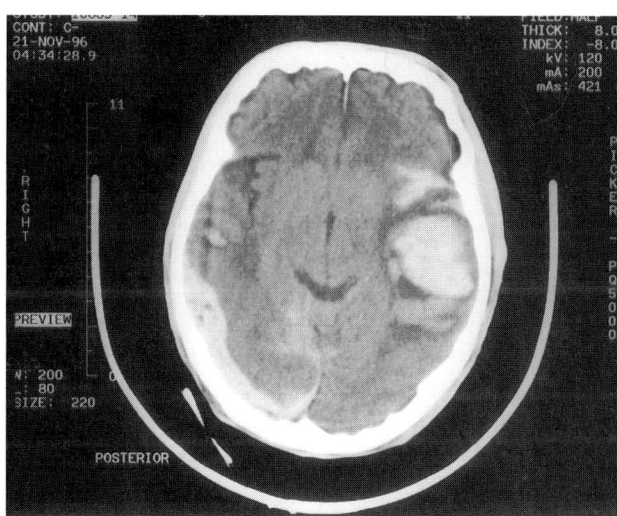

FIGURE 56B.5   Axial computed tomographic scan illustrating a large left intracerebral hematoma and a right occipital subdural hematoma.

head injury, those unable to maintain adequate ventilation, and those with impending airway loss from neck or pharyngeal injury should undergo early oral endotracheal intubation with in-line stabilization of the cervical spine. Nasotracheal intubation is contraindicated in patients with anterior cranial base or midface fractures and is generally not needed in this setting. In patients with major facial or upper airway trauma, a surgical airway may be required.

Breathing

Patients are ventilated with 100% oxygen until blood gases can be obtained to guide adjustments. Care must be taken to avoid persistent and excessive hyperventilation in patients who are neurologically stable because this may promote cerebral ischemia. However, moderate hyperventilation (PCO_2 of 25–30 mm Hg) is appropriate along with mannitol in patients with a deteriorating neurological examination or pupillary dilatation.

Circulation

Once adequate ventilation is established, attention is directed toward circulatory support. Hypotension is present in almost 35% of patients with severe head injury and is associated with increased mortality. In the trauma patient, hypotension is generally due to hypovolemia from hemorrhage and not from the head injury *per se*. Hypotension resulting from primary brain injury only results from brainstem failure and represents a terminal event. Physiologically, the initial response to hypovolemia is tachycardia in an attempt to maintain cardiac output when stroke volume is reduced. Tachycardia is followed by a narrowing of the pulse pressure as peripheral vasoconstriction attempts to maintain blood flow to vital organs. Hypotension ensues when these compensatory mechanisms are exhausted and represents approximately a 30% loss of blood volume. The ideal resuscitation fluid has been a source of controversy for three decades. Available fluids include isotonic crystalloid, hypertonic crystalloid, colloid solution, and blood. Normal saline is most commonly used for resuscitation and is an appropriate resuscitation fluid for volume losses of up to 30%. For patients who lose more than 30% of blood volume, blood transfusion must be provided. Hypertonic saline has some theoretical advantages because, in addition to providing volume expansion, it may reduce intracranial hypertension by reducing brain edema and improving cerebral perfusion. However, clinical studies are in their infancy, and normal saline remains the standard of care. Despite many studies, colloid resuscitation is not superior to crystalloid resuscitation and is more expensive.

Secondary Survey

Once the patient has airway and circulation stabilized, attention is directed to a secondary survey of individual body regions. Patients with severe head injury often have multiple injuries. Throughout the secondary survey, attention to the patient's respiratory and circulatory status is essential. The secondary survey should be completed quickly and efficiently to correctly prioritize further evaluation and treatment of the multiply injured patient.

As part of the assessment of the brain-injured patient, the head and neck should be evaluated for external signs of trauma; these include contusions, soft tissue swelling, lacerations, or hemorrhage. The scalp may be palpated for lacerations or fractures. Signs of a basilar skull fracture should be sought, such as raccoon eyes (periorbital ecchymosis), Battle's sign (ecchymosis over the mastoid region), and CSF otorrhea or rhinorrhea. The neck and thoracolumbar spine is palpated for tenderness, with care taken not to manipulate the cervical spine until stability can be evaluated.

Neurological Examination

It is during the secondary survey that a directed neurological examination is performed, which is focused on level of consciousness as measured by the GCS, pupillary light reflexes, and, if necessary, extraocular movements (oculocephalic reflexes, such as doll's eye and caloric responses).

As soon as the patient's cardiopulmonary status is stable, a rapid and directed neurological examination is performed. Although various factors can prevent an accurate evaluation of the patient's neurological state at this point (e.g., hypotension, hypoxia, or intoxication), valuable data can nevertheless be obtained. Between the fully alert and the deeply comatose patient lies a continuum of altered consciousness that is difficult to quantify objectively, and the GCS is widely used for this purpose.

If a patient demonstrates variable responses to stimulation, or if the response on each side is different, the best response appears to serve as a more accurate prognostic indicator than does the worst response. To follow trends in an individual patient's progress, however, it is better to report both the best and the worst responses. The right- and left-sided motor responses should be recorded separately. Deep nail-bed pressure should be used as the standard painful stimulus.

The physician should not, however, limit the examination to the factors of unconsciousness used in the GCS (i.e., eye opening, motor response, and verbal response). Of equal importance in the initial assessment are the patient's age, vital signs, pupillary response, and eye movements (Table 56B.4). The GCS provides a simple grading of the arousal and functional capacity of the cerebral cortex, whereas the pupillary responses and eye movements serve as measures of brainstem function. Advanced age, hypotension, and hypoxia all adversely affect outcome. Indeed, there is considerable interplay among all these factors in determining the ultimate prognosis in the severely head-injured patient.

Pupils

Notation of pupil size and response to light is of utmost importance during the initial examination. A well-known early sign of temporal lobe herniation is mild dilatation of the ipsilateral pupil and a sluggish pupillary light response (Table 56B.5). Compression or distortion of the oculomotor nerve during tentorial-uncal herniation impairs the function of the parasympathetic axons that transmit efferent signals for pupillary constriction, resulting in mild pupillary dilatation. Although bilateral miotic pupils (1–3 mm) are usually associated with narcotics, this finding may be seen in the early stages of central cephalic herniation. This is due to bilateral compromise of the pupillomotor sympathetic pathways originating in the hypothalamus, permitting a predominance of parasympathetic tone and pupillary constriction. Continued herniation causes increasing dilatation of the pupil and paralysis of its light response. With full mydriasis (8- to 9-mm pupil), ptosis and paresis of the medial rectus and other ocular muscles innervated by the oculomotor nerve appear. A bright light is always necessary to determine pupillary light responses. A magnifying lens, such as the plus-20-diopter lens on a standard ophthalmoscope, is helpful in distinguishing between a weak pupillary light reaction and absence of a reaction, especially if the pupil is small.

Bilateral small pupils, in addition to drug effect and central herniation, may be due to a destructive lesion of the pons. In these conditions, pupillary light responses usually can be seen if examined with a magnifying lens. Unilateral Horner's pupil is seen occasionally with brainstem lesions, but in the trauma patient, attention should be given to the possibility of a disrupted efferent sympathetic pathway at the apex of the lung, base of the neck, or ipsilateral carotid sheath. Midposition pupils with variable light responses are observed in all stages of coma (see Chapters 5 and 17).

Traumatic oculomotor nerve injury is the diagnosis in patients with a history of a dilated pupil from the onset of injury, an improving level of consciousness, and appropriate ocular muscle weakness. A mydriatic pupil (6 mm or more) occurs occasionally with direct trauma to the globe of the eye. This traumatic mydriasis is usually unilateral and is not accompanied by ocular muscle paresis.

Finally, bilaterally dilated and fixed pupils in patients with head injury may be the result of inadequate cerebral vascular perfusion. This situation can be due to hypotension secondary to blood loss or to elevation of ICP to a degree that impairs cerebral blood flow (CBF). Return of the pupillary response may occur promptly after the

Table 56B.4: Outcomes associated with different clinical features noted soon after admission in severe head injury

Clinical features	No. of cases	Outcome (%)		
		G/MD	SD/V	Dead
1. Age (yrs)[a]				
0–20	46	72	11	17
21–40	50	66	6	28
41–60	28	43	11	46
61+	9	22	0	78
2. GCS admission score[b]				
3–5	39	23	15	62
6–8	74	74	6	20
9–11	17	76	6	18
12–14	3	100	0	0
3. Pupillary reaction[b]				
Normal	87	76	8	16
Bilaterally impaired	46	30	9	61
4. Eye movements[b]				
Normal	74	76	7	17
Uni- or bilaterally impaired	57	39	10	51
5. Surgical decompression[b]				
None	74	76	7	17
Once	47	47	11	42
Two or three times	12	17	8	75
6. Motor posturing[a]				
None (includes flaccidity)	94	68	7	25
Unilateral or bilateral	39	41	10	49

G = good recovery; GCS = Glasgow Coma Scale; MD = moderately disabled; SD = severely disabled; V = vegetative.
[a]$P <0.02$.
[b]$P <0.0002$.
Source: Reprinted with permission from RK Narayan, RP Greenberg, JD Miller, et al. Improved confidence of outcome prediction in severe head injury: a comparative analysis of the clinical examination, multimodality evoked potentials, CT scanning, and intracranial pressure. J Neurosurg 1981;54:756.

restoration of blood flow if the period of inadequate perfusion has not been too long.

Eye Movements

Ocular movements are an important index of the functional activity that is present within the brainstem reticular formation. If the patient is sufficiently alert to follow simple

Table 56B.5: Interpretation of pupillary findings in head-injured patients

Pupil size	Light response	Interpretation
Unilaterally dilated	Sluggish or fixed	Cranial nerve III compression secondary to tentorial herniation
Bilaterally dilated	Sluggish or fixed	Inadequate brain perfusion
		Bilateral cranial nerve III palsy
Unilaterally dilated or equal	Cross-reactive (Marcus Gunn)	Optic nerve injury
Bilaterally constricted	May be difficult to determine	Drugs (opiates)
		Metabolic encephalopathy
		Pontine lesions
Unilaterally constricted	Preserved	Injured sympathetic pathway (e.g., carotid sheath injury)

Table 56B.6:   Medical Research Council scale

Normal power	5
Moderate weakness	4
Severe weakness (just antigravity)	3
Severe weakness (not antigravity)	2
Trace movement	1
No movement	0

commands, a full range of eye movements is easily obtained and the integrity of the entire ocular motor system within the brainstem can be affirmed. In states of depressed consciousness, voluntary eye movement is lost and there may be dysfunction of the neural structures activating eye movements. In these instances, doll's eye or caloric responses are used to determine the presence or absence of an eye movement disorder. For a discussion of these tests and the anatomical connections involved in the normal response, readers are referred to Chapters 16, 18, 40, and 42.

Motor Function

The basic examination is completed by a gross test of motor strength (severely head-injured patients are not sufficiently responsive for a detailed determination of muscle strength). Each extremity is examined and graded on the Medical Research Council scale (Table 56B.6).

Herniation Syndromes

Rising ICP or the presence of a mass lesion can result in distortion and displacement of the brain, which can cause compression of critical brain structures. There are a number of herniation syndromes, the most common being uncal herniation, central herniation, cingulate herniation, and tonsillar herniation (Figure 56B.6).

Uncal herniation occurs with lesions of the middle cranial fossa, such as epidural hematoma, SDH, and intracerebral contusion. With this herniation syndrome, the uncus herniates between the rostral brainstem and the ten-

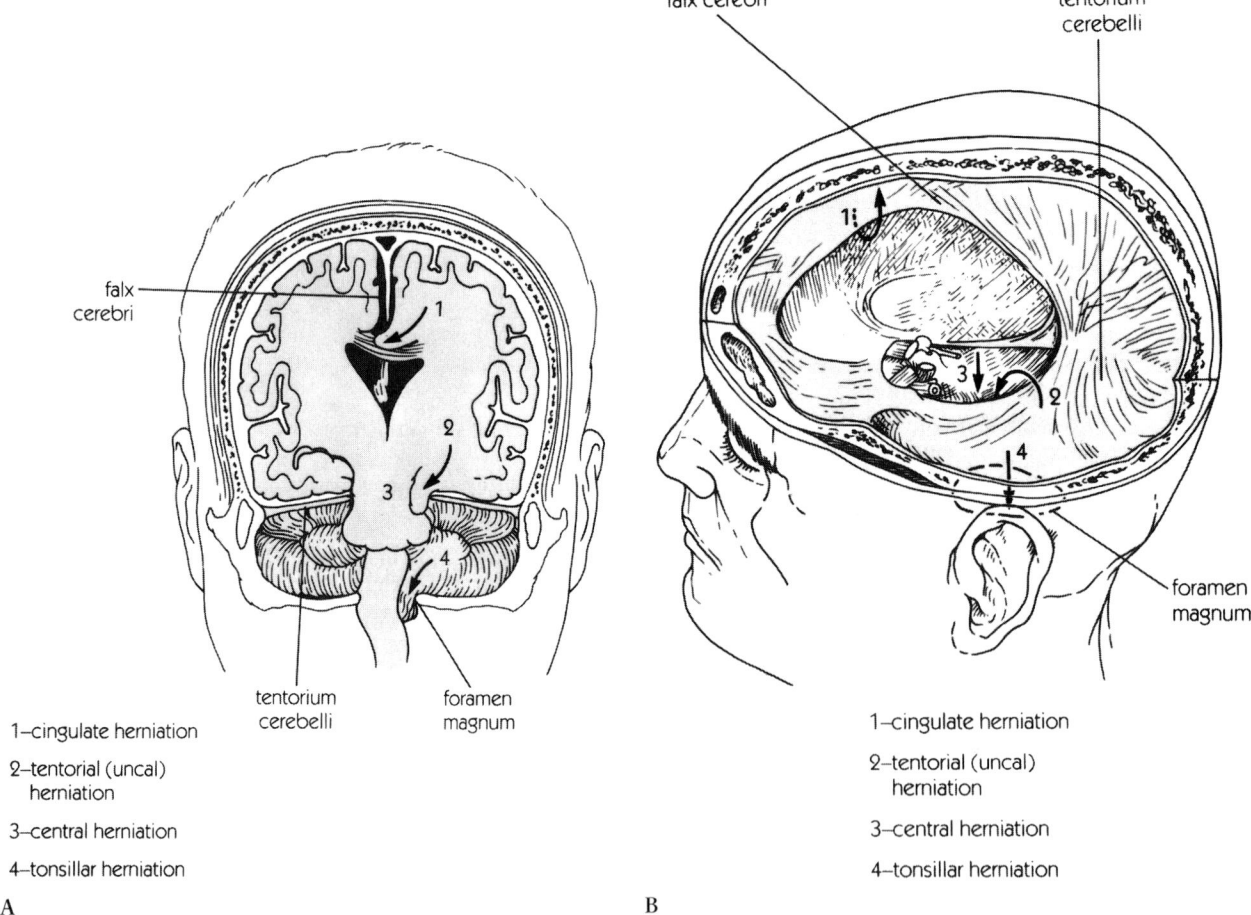

falx cerebri

tentorium cerebelli

falx cerebri

tentorium cerebelli

foramen magnum

foramen magnum

1–cingulate herniation

2–tentorial (uncal) herniation

3–central herniation

4–tonsillar herniation

A

1–cingulate herniation

2–tentorial (uncal) herniation

3–central herniation

4–tonsillar herniation

B

FIGURE 56B.6   **(A)** Types of brain herniation. **(B)** Dural folds within the cranial cavity and associated herniation sites. (Reprinted with permission from SS Rengachary, DE Duke. Increased Intracranial Pressure, Cerebral Edema, and Brain Herniation. In SS Rengachary, RH Wilkens (eds), Principles of Neurosurgery. New York: McGraw-Hill, 1994.)

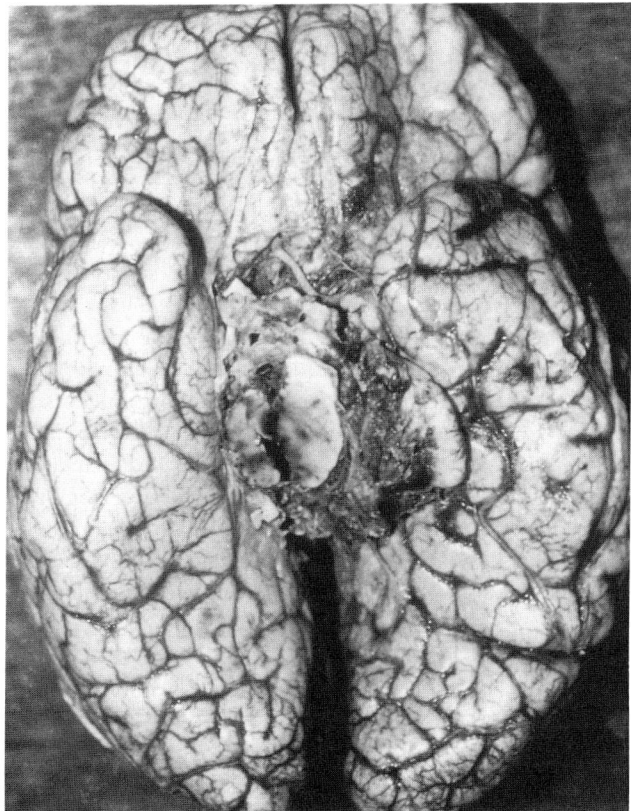

FIGURE 56B.7   Inferior view of the brain of patient with left cerebral hemisphere injury and swelling, showing the result of tentorial herniation, including the damage to the uncus and the hippocampus. Brainstem distortion and secondary hemorrhage (Duret's) have also taken place. (Reprinted with permission from the American Association of Neurologic Surgeons, Joint Section on Neurotrauma and Critical Care. Guidelines for the Management of Severe Head Injury. New York: Brain Trauma Foundation, 1995.)

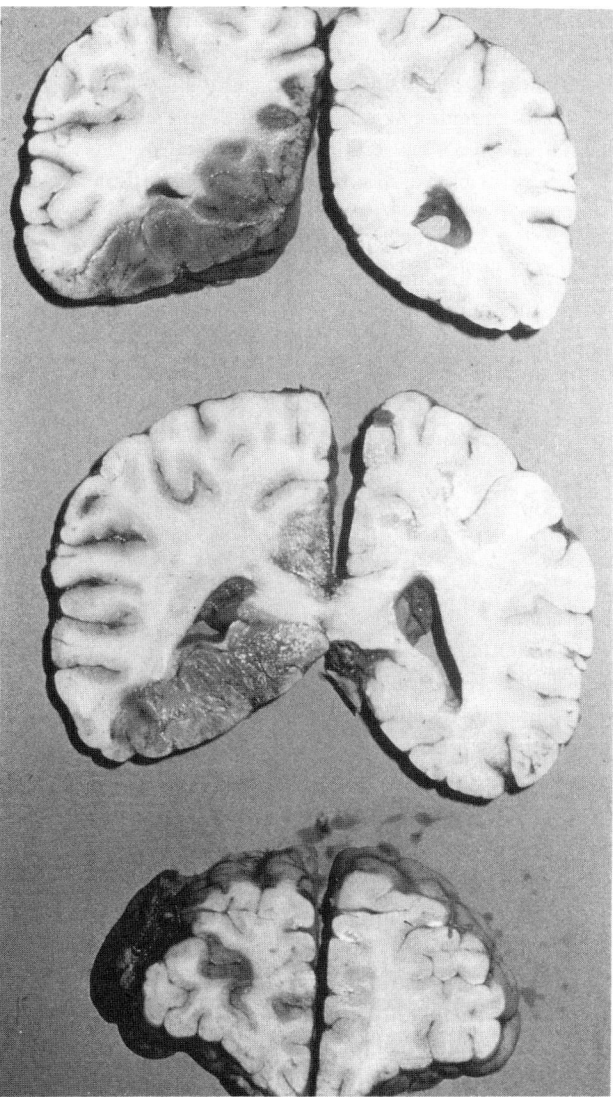

FIGURE 56B.8   Infarction of the occipital lobe as a result of tentorial herniation compressing the posterior cerebral artery.

torial edge into the posterior fossa (Figure 56B.7). This is usually recognized by pupillary dilatation due to compression of the third cranial nerve, which lies near the tentorial edge. Compression of the posterior cerebral artery against the tentorium cerebelli in transtentorial herniation can cause infarction of the occipital and inferior temporal lobes (Figure 56B.8).

Cingulate herniation is seen when there is a mass lesion in the supratentorial compartment causing displacement of the cingulate gyrus across the free edge of the falx cerebri. This can frequently be seen on CT scan, although there are no specific signs or symptoms of this herniation.

Central herniation occurs when a large supratentorial mass causes downward displacement of the diencephalon and midbrain through the tentorial incisura. The clinical findings with this syndrome include a lowered state of consciousness, bilaterally small reactive pupils, and Cheyne-Stokes respirations.

Tonsillar herniation results from an expanding posterior fossa mass causing herniation of the cerebellar tonsils through the foramen magnum into the upper cervical spinal canal. The clinical manifestations include hypertension, Cheyne-Stokes respirations, neurogenic hyperventilation, cardiorespiratory impairment, and impaired consciousness. Decorticate or decerebrate posturing may also be present. Mass lesions in the posterior fossa can cause progressive deterioration in consciousness and, eventually, death due to brainstem compression without any increase in supratentorial ICP.

EMERGENCY ROOM MANAGEMENT

Over the past three decades, there has been a widening implementation of emergency medical services and the formation of regional trauma systems in the United States and other developed countries. This has resulted in an overall improved survival from head injury and a reduction in the frequency of preventable deaths. Key factors contributing to better outcome include establishing an airway, adequate oxygenation, fluid resuscitation, spinal stabilization, tamponade of external hemorrhage, and rapid transportation to an appropriate trauma facility.

Standardization of care for the head-injured patient has been advanced by evidence-based *Guidelines for the Management of Severe Head Injury*, published by the American Association of Neurological Surgeons with the support of the Brain Trauma Foundation. These guidelines are well integrated into the consensus-based Advanced Trauma Life Support course of the American College of Surgeons Committee on Trauma (Figure 56B.9). Care is optimal when there is a designated trauma team, a readily available neurosurgeon, and a continuously staffed and available operating room, intensive care unit (ICU), and laboratory for treating neurotrauma patients.

Mild Head Injury

The evaluation of patients with mild head injury must identify those at risk for developing potentially lethal complications. The magnitude of the importance of mild head injury is evident from the fact that approximately 80% of all head injuries may be classified as mild. Of patients with mild head injury, 1–2% deteriorate into coma or require neurosurgical intervention. The sequelae that result from mild brain injuries may include cognitive dysfunctions of memory, attention, problem solving, speech, affect, and personality.

The initial management of mild head injury is similar to that of severe injuries in the need for identifying and treating associated injuries. We advocate the routine use of CT scanning in this patient group because missing a developing mass may have disastrous consequences. A patient with a normal examination and a normal CT scan of the head may be sent home under the care of a suitable caregiver. Although it is more sensitive to the changes in brain injury than CT, magnetic resonance imaging (MRI) is not routinely performed in the acute setting.

A commonly accepted method of managing these patients involves emergency CT scanning of all patients with a GCS score less than 15. Patients with a GCS score of 15 who have a focal neurological deficit, an altered mental status, an open injury, a history of significant loss of consciousness, or intoxication are also routinely scanned (Figure 56B.10).

Much debate has centered on the use of skull radiographs for patients with mild head injury. Skull radiographs are important as a diagnostic aid when CT scanning is unavailable. Fortunately, this is not a problem at most institutions in the United States. The likelihood of intracranial pathology increases 400-fold in the presence of a skull fracture. As a result, admission for observation and CT scanning is suggested when plain films reveal a skull fracture.

Moderate and Severe Head Injury

Along the continuum of head injury, patients classified as having a moderate or severe injury are more likely to have an intracranial hematoma. An important early consideration in these patients is determining when surgery is indicated; the neurosurgical consultant makes this determination. Defining the indications for surgical evacuation of intracranial hematomas is not a simple exercise. A brief summary of general principles is included here, but it is by no means comprehensive (Figures 56B.11 and 56B.12). Furthermore, there are many exceptions to any rules in this context. Subdural and epidural hematomas are grouped together as extra-axial hematomas.

RADIOGRAPHIC STUDIES

A number of imaging studies are possible to supplement the initial neurological evaluation. These include plain skull films, CT scanning, MRI, transcranial Doppler ultrasonography, positron emission tomography (PET) or single-photon emission computed tomography (SPECT) imaging, near-infrared spectroscopy (NIRS), and xenon-CT. Despite the variety of imaging modalities available, CT scanning is the cornerstone of diagnostic imaging of the trauma patient. Since its clinical introduction in the 1970s, CT has revolutionized the evaluation and management of the brain injured patient. Advantages of CT include its rapid, safe, and non-invasive nature. CT has made possible accurate anatomic localization of space-occupying lesions, skull fractures, metallic foreign bodies, and hydrocephalus. This allows for rapid diagnosis, triage, and surgical evacuation of mass lesions. Shortcomings of CT imaging include poor visualization of vascular lesions, such as arterial dissections and traumatic aneurysms, fractures at the vertex, and the posterior fossa. Although uncommon, traumatic aneurysms have a tendency to rupture. They tend to be pseudo-aneurysms, meaning that the vascular adventitia is not intact. These aneurysms also tend to be more peripheral and less likely to occur at branch points. Traumatic aneurysms are probably less frequently diagnosed now that CT has replaced cerebral angiography in the routine evaluation of the severely head-injured patient. As a result, clinical suspicion should be raised when there is a delayed intracranial hemorrhage or an unexpected deterioration after head injury. Cerebral angiography may be undertaken when the neurological examination cannot be explained by the CT picture.

MRI has a number of advantages in evaluating brain injury. It is more sensitive than CT in detecting acute abnormalities and delayed effects of head trauma. Advantages of MRI include visualization of shearing injuries and non-hemorrhagic contusions, improved localization due to multiplanar imaging, and improved imaging of posterior fossa injury. MRI also allows the evolution of a hemorrhage to

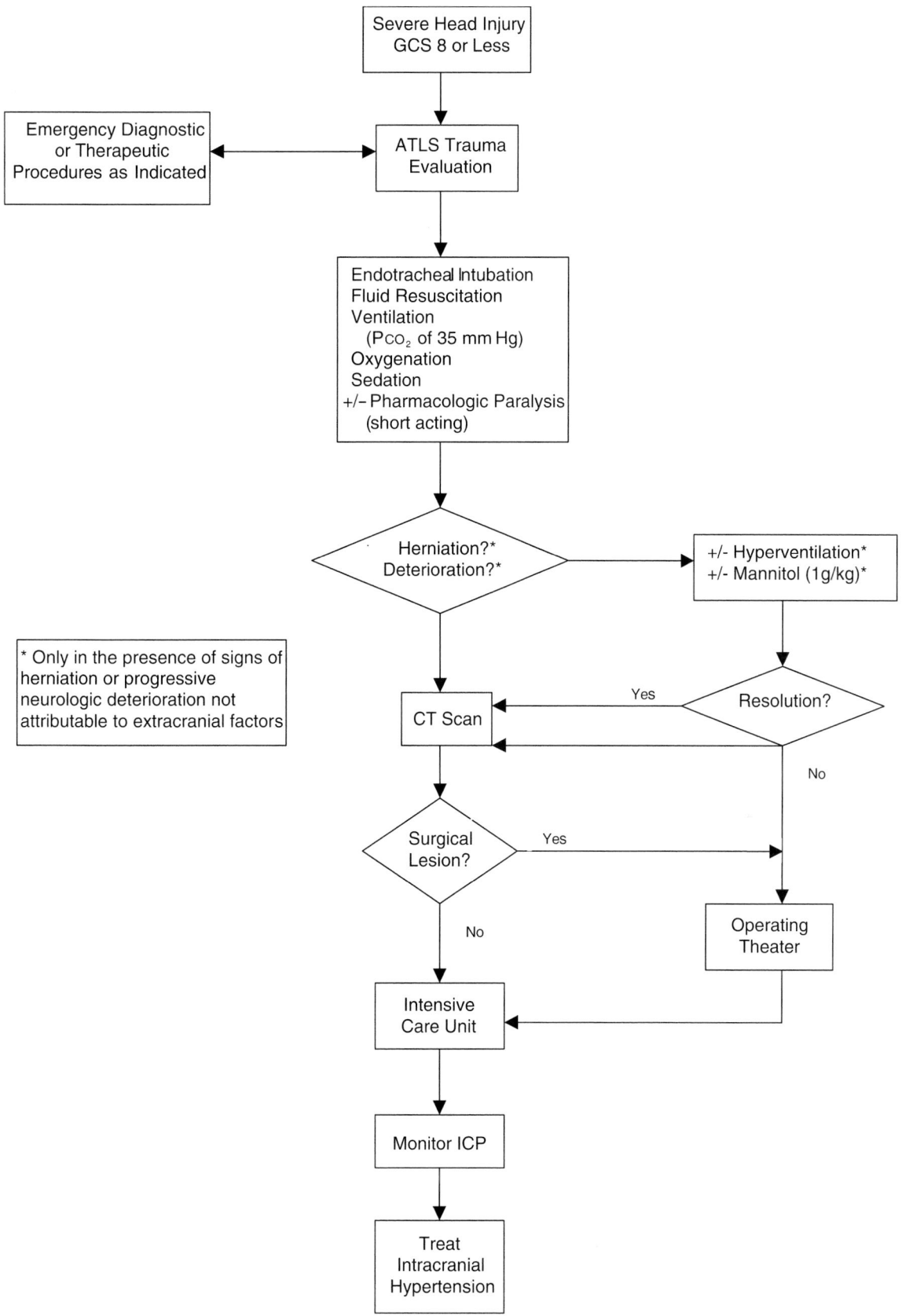

FIGURE 56B.9   Initial resuscitation of the patient with severe head injury. (ATLS = Advanced Trauma Life Support; CT = computed tomography; GCS = Glasgow Coma Scale; ICP = intracranial pressure.) (Reprinted with permission from the American Association of Neurologic Surgeons, Joint Section on Neurotrauma and Critical Care. Guidelines for the Management of Severe Head Injury. New York: Brain Trauma Foundation, 1995.)

Definition: Patient is awake and may be oriented (GCS 14 or 15)

History

- Name, age, sex, race, occupation
- Mechanism of injury
- Time of injury
- Loss of consciousness immediately after injury
- Subsequent level of alertness
- Amnesia: retrograde, anterograde
- Headache: mild, moderate, severe
- Seizures

General examination to exclude systemic injuries

Limited neurological examination

Cervical spine and other radiographs as indicated

Blood alcohol level and urine toxic screen

CT scan of the head in all patients except completely asymptomatic and neurologically normal patients is ideal

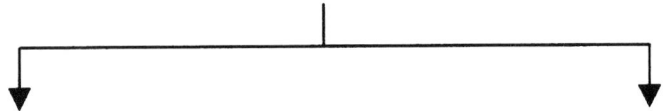

Observe in/admit to hospital

- No CT scanner available
- Abnormal CT scan
- All penetrating head injuries
- History of loss of consciousness
- Deteriorating level of consciousness
- Moderate to severe headache
- Significant alcoholic/drug intoxication
- Skull fracture
- CSF leak rhinorrhea or otorrhea
- Significant associated injuries
- No reliable companion at home
- Unable to return promptly
- Amnesia

Discharge from hospital

- Patient does not meet any of the criteria for admission
- Discuss need to return if any problems develop and issue a "warning sheet"
- Schedule follow-up clinic visit, usually within 1 week

FIGURE 56B.10   Algorithm for the management of mild head injury. (CSF = cerebrospinal fluid; CT = computed tomography; GCS = Glasgow Coma Scale.) (Adapted with permission from AB Valadka, RJ Narayan. Emergency Room Management of the Head-Injured Patient. In RK Narayan, J Wilberger, J Povlishock, eds. Neurotrauma. New York: McGraw-Hill, 1996.)

be followed. Disadvantages of MRI include longer imaging times of potentially critically ill patients, requirement for MRI-compatible monitoring and ventilator equipment, and poor visualization of bone and SAH.

Other imaging modalities, such as transcranial Doppler TCD ultrasonography, and PET or SPECT imaging, cur-rently play no role in the routine evaluation of the brain-injured patient but do help to elucidate the pathophysiol-ogy of brain injury. TCD provides information on blood flow velocity, is a useful way to monitor for the develop-ment of vasospasm, and can help direct therapy for vasospasm. NIRS may develop as a bedside technique for

Definition: Patient may be confused or somnolent but is still able to follow simple commands (GCS 9 to 13)

Initial workup
- Same as for mild head injury, plus baseline blood work
- CT scan of the head obtained in all cases
- Admission for observation

After admission
- Frequent neurological checks
- Follow-up CT scan if condition deteriorates or preferably before discharge

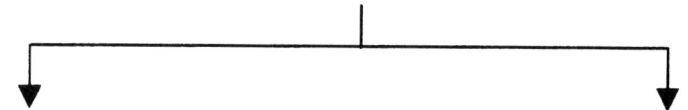

If patient improves (90%)

- Discharge when appropriate
- Follow-up in clinic

If patient deteriorates (10%)

- If the patient stops following simple commands, repeat CT scan and manage per severe head injury protocol.

FIGURE 56B.11   Algorithm for the management of moderate head injury. (CT = computed tomography; GCS = Glasgow Coma Scale.) (Adapted with permission from AB Valadka, RJ Narayan. Emergency Room Management of the Head-Injured Patient. In RK Narayan, J Wilberger, J Povlishock, eds. Neurotrauma. New York: McGraw-Hill, 1996.)

determining brain tissue oxygenation and detecting intracranial hematomas. PET and SPECT studies provide information about CBF and metabolism.

INDICATIONS FOR SURGERY

It is difficult to lay down hard-and-fast rules on managing a disease as diverse as head injury, but we have arrived at certain guidelines that have proved to be useful. Some of these practices are based on hard data, some on clinical prejudice, and some on our desire to simplify a complicated problem.

In its simplest form, our criterion for considering a mass lesion operable is a midline shift of 5 mm or more. Such a shift is usually demonstrated by CT scan. Virtually all acute epidural, subdural, or intracerebral hematomas associated with a midline shift of 5 mm or more should be surgically evacuated unless the patient is brain-dead. This policy is based on evidence that a few patients with bilaterally nonreactive pupils, impaired oculocephalic responses, and decerebrate posturing can nevertheless make a good recovery. In one series, 3 of 19 such patients who were treated maximally ended up in the "good" or "moderately disabled" category, despite their initially forbidding constellation of signs.

A conservative approach is certainly justified in a patient with a small hematoma with minimal shift who is alert and neurologically intact. The patient may deteriorate, however, and very close observation is critical. Should there be a significant change in mental status, a repeat CT scan should be obtained immediately.

The management of brain contusions is somewhat less clear-cut. In one series of 26 patients with acute traumatic intracranial hematomas who were managed without surgery, all patients with an ICP greater than 30 mm Hg eventually deteriorated and required surgery. In contrast, only one patient with ICP levels of less than 20 mm Hg deteriorated. Patients in the 20- to 30-mm Hg range were about evenly divided between surgical and nonsurgical groups.

We analyzed our experience with 130 head-injured patients with pure contusions who were managed with CT scanning and, as needed, ICP monitoring in a neurosurgical ICU setting. This study showed that patients with brain contusions who could follow commands at admission did not require ICP monitoring and, as a rule, did well with simple observation. However, those who could not follow commands (in the absence of a focal lesion in the speech area) often had intracranial hypertension and deserved to have their ICP monitored. The majority of these patients, who had a shift of 5 mm or more, required surgery.

Definition: Patient is unable to follow even simple commands because of impaired consciousness (GCS 3 to 8)

Assessment and management
- ABC
- Primary survey and AMPLE history

Neurological reevaluation
- Eye opening
- Motor response
- Verbal response
- Pupillary light reaction
- Oculocephalics (doll's eyes)
- Oculovestibulars (caloric)

Therapeutic agents
- Mannitol
- Moderate hyperventilation
- Anticonvulsant

Diagnostic tests (in descending order of preference)
- CT scan, all patients
- Air ventriculogram
- Angiogram

Consider only if CT is not available

FIGURE 56B.12   Algorithm for the management of severe head injury. (ABC = mnemonic for *a*irway, *b*reathing, and *c*irculation; AMPLE = mnemonic for *a*llergies, *m*edications currently taken, *p*ast illnesses, *l*ast meal, and *e*vents/environment related to the injury; CT = computed tomography; GCS = Glasgow Coma Scale.) (Adapted with permission from AB Valadka, RJ Narayan. Emergency Room Management of the Head-Injured Patient. In RK Narayan, J Wilberger, J Povlishock, eds. Neurotrauma. New York: McGraw-Hill, 1996.)

Patients with a large (>30 ml) temporal lobe hematoma have a much greater risk of developing tentorial herniation than do those with similar frontal or parieto-occipital lesions. The bias should tilt toward early surgery in such cases. The same holds true for posterior fossa hematomas.

When CT scanning is not available, decisions regarding surgery may be based on air ventriculography and ICP measurements. Here again, a midline shift of 5 mm or more indicates a need for immediate surgical decompression. If there is no midline shift, but the ICP is elevated above 20 mm Hg, angiography should be performed promptly to rule out bilateral balancing lesions, such as SDH.

When angiography is undertaken in patients with severe head injury, the following findings should be considered indications for an operation:

1. An intra- or extra-axial mass lesion, causing a shift of the anterior cerebral vessels across the midline to an extent of 5 mm or more.
2. An extra-axial mass lesion more than 5 mm from the inner table, if it is associated with any degree of anterior or middle cerebral artery displacement.
3. Bilateral extra-axial mass lesions more than 5 mm from the inner table; except for patients who have marked brain atrophy, such intracranial masses usually cause major elevations of ICP.
4. A temporal lobe intra-axial mass lesion causing a major elevation of the middle cerebral artery or any degree of midline shift. These patients are in a most precarious position because only slight swelling can cause a tentorial herniation syndrome that progresses very rapidly.

Once a decision has been made that the patient is a surgical candidate, he or she is promptly moved to the operating room. Mannitol (1–2 g/kg) should be administered en route to the operating room. In addition, the patient should be moderately hyperventilated to achieve an arterial P_{CO_2} of 25–30 mm Hg. As in all the maneuvers undertaken thus far, time is of the essence. The sooner the mass lesion is evacuated, the better the possibility of a good recovery. If, on the other hand, no surgical lesion is found, the patient is carefully monitored in the neurosurgical ICU, both clinically and with various physiological parameters, notably ICP and cerebral perfusion pressure (CPP) recordings and serial CT scans. Any persistent rise in ICP above 20 mm Hg that cannot be readily explained and reversed, or any deterioration in neurological status, warrants prompt repetition of the CT scan followed by the appropriate corrective measures.

CRITICAL CARE

Secondary Insults

As with the initial management of head injury, management in the ICU consists primarily of ensuring adequate ventilation and cerebral perfusion. A central aim of the management of the head-injured patient is the prevention of secondary injury, of which cerebral ischemia is perhaps the most important. Others include hyponatremia, meningitis or ventriculitis, pneumonia, acute respiratory distress syndrome, urinary tract infection, sepsis, and anemia. Factors that contribute to cerebral ischemia include hypotension, hypoxemia, and elevated ICP. Although little can be done in the hospital setting to correct or prevent the primary injury, the clinician can take steps to prevent secondary injury. There are a number of agents under investigation that hold promise for interrupting the cascade of events involved in the progression of brain swelling and ischemia.

Intracranial Pressure

Several pathological processes that affect the brain can cause elevation of ICP. In turn, intracranial hypertension can have consequences that adversely affect outcome. Thus, not only does elevated ICP indicate the presence of a problem, it often contributes to the problem. Continuous monitoring of ICP is now selectively applied to severely head-injured patients in virtually all major neurosurgical centers in the United States.

Basic Physiology

Normal ICP in the resting state is approximately 10 mm Hg (136 mm H_2O). As a broad generalization, pressures greater than 20 mm Hg are considered abnormal, and pressures greater than 40 mm Hg can be categorized as severe elevations. Higher ICP after head injury is associated with a poorer outcome.

The Monro-Kellie Doctrine

The Monro-Kellie doctrine is a simple yet vitally important concept relating to the understanding of ICP dynamics. It states that the total volume of intracranial contents must remain constant. This is fairly obvious because the cranium is essentially a non-expansile box. Thus, if V denotes volume:

$$V_{brain} + V_{CSF} + V_{blood} + V_{mass\ lesion} = constant$$

As the size of an intracranial mass lesion, such as a hematoma, increases, there is a compensatory squeezing out of CSF and of venous blood. The ICP initially remains normal. However, eventually no more CSF or venous blood can be eliminated and the compensatory mechanisms are no longer effective. At this point, an exponential increase in ICP begins, associated with even a small increase in the size of the intracranial mass. The pressure-volume curve illustrates this phenomenon. The ICP is generally within normal limits until a patient reaches a point of decompensation and enters the exponential phase of the pressure-volume curve. The ICP number *per se* does not initially give any indication of where a patient is along this curve.

Brain Elastance

To better understand ICP dynamics, the concept of brain elastance was introduced. This is defined as the change in ICP resulting from a unit change in intracranial CSF volume. It is usually quantified in terms of the volume-pressure response (VPR), which is defined as the immediate rise in ICP resulting from an injection of 1 ml of fluid over 1 second. In a normal subject, the VPR is 0–2 mm Hg/ml. Values of 3–4 mm Hg/ml are often seen after surgery for head trauma, and values of 10–20 mm Hg/ml usually indicate the presence of a mass lesion.

Pressure-Volume Index

Another measure of intracranial compliance is the pressure-volume index (PVI). PVI is defined as the volume of fluid that would theoretically have to be injected into the craniospinal axis to produce a 10-fold increase in ICP. Clinically, this is a calculated figure based on the following formula:

$$PVI = change\ in\ volume/(\log P_1/P_2)$$

where P_1 is the initial ICP and P_2 is the final ICP after an injection of, for example, 1 ml of fluid. Normal PVI is 26 ± 4 ml; values of 13 ml or less are considered clearly indicative of markedly compromised intracranial compliance. Although VPR and PVI are not widely used in the management of neurosurgical patients, it is helpful to understand their basis and significance.

Cerebral Perfusion Pressure

The single most important secondary occurrence that affects outcome after severe traumatic closed head injury is cerebral ischemia. CPP, or the mean arterial blood pressure (MAP) minus ICP, is closely related to ischemia because it is the pressure gradient driving CBF and metabolic delivery. Brain trauma can produce a significant frequency of post-traumatic vasospasm plus changes in pressure and metabolic autoregulation; hence, cerebral vascular resistance is often increased by trauma. Thus, a region of the brain with pre-existing ischemia may be further injured by a low CPP or, conversely, improved by increasing CPP. Often, with clinical manipulation, the CPP can be increased to aid in avoiding both global and regional ischemia. Although the optimal CPP is unknown, several clinical studies suggest that 70–80 mm Hg may be the critical threshold. In McGraw's 1989 model relating outcome to CPP, mortality was 35–40% when CPP was 80 mm Hg versus approximately 95% for CPP less than 60. Some institutions use CPP rather than ICP alone for the routine monitoring of patients. Rosner and co-workers (1995) advocated a method of management of head injury based on maintenance of CPP. Too great a perfusion pressure after head injury may be deleterious. *Guidelines for the Management of Severe Head Injury* recommends maintenance of CPP at a minimum of 70 mm Hg to substantially reduce mortality, improve quality of survival, and enhance perfusion to areas of cerebral ischemia after severe closed head injury.

Autoregulation

The phenomenon of autoregulation tends to maintain fairly constant CBF between mean blood pressures of 50–160 mm Hg. Below 50 mm Hg, the CBF declines steeply, and above 160 mm Hg, there is a passive dilatation of the cerebral vessels and an increase in CBF. Autoregulation is often severely disturbed in the head-injured patient. Because increases in cerebral blood volume can contribute significantly to intracranial hypertension, it is as important to avoid systemic arterial hypertension as it is to avoid shock in the severely head-injured patient. Although the optimal level at which blood pressure should be maintained is not known, an overly aggressive correction of moderate hypertension or less than prompt correction of hypotension can be disastrous, especially in elderly patients.

Technical Aspects of Intracranial Pressure Monitoring

ICP can be monitored in several locations. These are listed below along with commonly available monitoring devices:

- Lateral ventricle: ventricular catheter, fiberoptic device
- Intraparenchymal: fiberoptic device, strain gauge
- Subdural or subarachnoid: Richmond bolt, catheter, fiberoptic device
- Epidural: Gaeltec, Ladd, Philips
- Anterior fontanelle (in neonates)

Three major types of devices are used for ICP monitoring. The intraventricular catheter remains the gold standard, but other devices are available and demonstrate varying degrees of accuracy. The commonly available devices include (1) catheters (intraventricular or subdural); (2) hollow adapters (screws, bolts), such as the Richmond, Philadelphia, Leeds, and Philips devices; and (3) pressure-sensitive devices, such as the Camino fiberoptic, Codman Microsensor, and Ladd devices.

We use ventricular catheters in almost all cases. In the few instances in which the ventricles cannot be successfully cannulated, we use the Camino fiberoptic device or Codman Microsensor. Nevertheless, the vast majority of our patients are still monitored through a ventriculostomy. The advantages and disadvantages of these devices are shown in Table 56B.7.

Value of Intracranial Pressure Monitoring

ICP data can be used in three ways:

1. As a diagnostic adjunct:
   - Elevated ICP and midline shift on an air ventriculogram serve as useful indicators of a mass lesion if a CT scanner is not immediately available.
   - ICP data facilitate early diagnosis of a developing mass lesion.
   - Data allow therapy to be initiated before irreversible neurological damage occurs, especially in sedated or paralyzed patients in whom the clinical examination is difficult to follow.
2. As a therapeutic adjunct:
   - Ventriculostomies are useful for CSF drainage, which can lower ICP, at least temporarily.
   - Knowledge of the ICP takes the guesswork out of therapy. ICP fluctuates greatly, and the response of different patients to different maneuvers to lower ICP is very unpredictable. Empirical therapy with agents such as mannitol, without a means of monitoring response, is therefore not optimal.
3. As a prognostic tool: In general terms, ICP trends can be used together with clinical signs in judging prognosis.

Whether ICP monitoring *per se* improves outcome from head injury is a rather controversial issue that has been debated in neurosurgical conferences and in courts of law. There has been no randomized study of the effect of ICP monitoring *per se*, but certain large, well-documented, nonrandomized studies have indicated that, as part of an intensive care package, the monitoring and control of ICP may be associated with improved outcome in patients with severe head injury. There is no doubt that ICP monitoring has greatly added to our understanding of intracranial dynamics and helped to make the basis on which we manage patients more scientific. We monitor ICP in all head-injury patients who have a significantly altered level of consciousness and find the data to be very valuable in patient management. However, facilities for ICP monitoring are not universally available, and it is certainly feasible to use alternative management strategies.

Indications for Intracranial Pressure Monitoring

Head injury is the most common indication for ICP monitoring. As a general rule, patients who are able to follow

Table 56B.7:   Features of certain intracranial pressure monitoring devices

Device	Advantages	Disadvantages
Ventricular catheter	Gold standard of accuracy Allows drainage of CSF for intracranial pressure control, CSF sampling, monitoring infection	Sometimes difficult to cannulate ventricle Requires fluid-filled column, which can get blocked by air bubbles and debris Artifact from tube movement Needs repositioning of transducer level with change in head position
Subarachnoid bolt	Does not invade brain May have a lower infection rate No need to cannulate ventricle	Blocking of port by swollen brain may cause artificially low readings Requires fluid-filled column, which can get blocked by air bubbles and debris Artifact from tube movement Needs repositioning of transducer level with change in head position
Fiberoptic device	Can be placed subdurally, intraparenchymally, or intraventricularly Minimal artifact and drift High resolution of waveform No need to reposition transducer with change in head position	Inability to check calibration once intraparenchymally or inserted, unless a ventriculostomy is used simultaneously Fiber breakage

CSF = cerebrospinal fluid.

simple commands do not need to be monitored. They may satisfactorily be followed clinically. In patients who are unable to follow commands and have an abnormal CT scan, the frequency of intracranial hypertension is high (53–63%), and monitoring is warranted. Severely head-injured patients with normal CT scans generally have a low frequency of intracranial hypertension (13%), unless they have two or more of the following adverse features at the time of admission.

1. Systolic blood pressure less than 90 mm Hg
2. Unilateral or bilateral motor posturing
3. Age older than 40 years

ICP should be monitored in patients with cerebral contusions who are unable to follow simple commands. If the ICP rises and persists over 25–30 mm Hg, surgical débridement is usually indicated. Clinicians should be aware that ICP is not always elevated in the presence of an intracranial process. This is particularly true of temporal lobe lesions, which can cause tentorial herniation in the absence of ICP elevation, and in posterior fossa lesions, in which brainstem compression often precedes any significant elevation of the supratentorial ICP.

Treating Raised Intracranial Pressure

There has been some debate as to what constitutes elevated ICP. Initially, it was decided somewhat arbitrarily to treat ICP greater than 25 mm Hg in patients with severe head injury. Since then, this figure has been moved down by other groups to 20 mm Hg and then to 15 mm Hg. Transient elevations of ICP associated with patient manipulation, such as suctioning, turning, or coughing, do not constitute adequate reason for treatment. The following stepwise approach to ICP elevation is suggested:

1. Ensure optimal body and neck position. The neck should be in a neutral position to facilitate venous drainage. Turning the neck to an extreme position can result in reduced venous outflow and elevation of ICP. The optimal degree of head elevation remains somewhat controversial. Although most believe that raising the head of the bed is a uniformly useful maneuver, Rosner and co-workers (1995) argued that this should be individualized and head elevation may adversely affect cerebral perfusion in certain cases.

2. Check calibration. Before more involved steps are taken to treat raised ICP, one must calibrate the monitoring system and make sure that the readings are not artifactual.

3. Check serum Na^+ and arterial blood gases. Hyponatremia is a common problem in neurosurgical patients, often as a result of the syndrome of inappropriate secretion of antidiuretic hormone (SIADH) or cerebral salt wasting. Hyponatremia should be treated aggressively in these patients because it contributes dramatically to brain swelling. Hypercapnia can also result in brain swelling secondary to vasodilatation. We used to use hyperventilation (down to a P_{CO_2} of 25 mm Hg) as a routine measure to treat patients with potential brain swelling. Hyperventilation over a period of time may contribute to cerebral ischemia due to vasoconstriction, and we therefore use this modality aggressively only when necessary, and then for as short a time as needed to keep ICP within normal limits.

4. Rule out seizures. Although they are not a common occurrence, subclinical seizures may result in unexplained increases in ICP.

5. Rule out mass lesions with a CT scan. Elevated ICP is a sign of some other problem and should not be considered a diagnosis in and of itself. Hence, if the previous measures do not resolve the ICP problem, a CT scan of the brain should be obtained to make sure there is no developing mass lesion. This cannot be emphasized enough.

6. Hyperventilate to a P_{CO_2} of 25–30 mm Hg (see no. 3 in this list).

7. CSF drainage via ventriculostomy. Intermittent drainage of CSF via the ventriculostomy is a very useful method of controlling ICP. For this reason, a ventricular catheter is much more useful than the other monitoring devices.

8. Administer mannitol (0.25–2.0 g/kg). This remains our drug of choice for treating ICP elevations. Although urea and glycerol have been used, mannitol is clearly the most widely useful agent. Its ability to be used intravenously, its rapidity of action, and its relative safety have contributed to its popularity.

9. Induce barbiturate coma. When all these measures have failed to control ICP, barbiturate coma may be considered. As a general guideline, one should consider this when the ICP has remained elevated above 25 mm Hg for 30 minutes or above 30 mm Hg for 15 minutes, in spite of all the therapies mentioned in steps 1–8. The commonly used agent is pentobarbital (Nembutal) in a dose of 10 mg/kg as a loading dose over 30 minutes, 5mg/kg every hour for 3 hours, followed by a maintenance dose of 1mg/kg per hour adjusted to obtain a serum level of 3–4 dl.

Mannitol

Mannitol administration is routinely used in the treatment of head injury and has replaced other osmotic diuretics over the last 20 years. Although the exact mechanism by which mannitol functions is debated, its beneficial effects on ICP, CPP, CBF, and brain metabolism are well accepted. There are two distinct mechanisms by which mannitol exerts its beneficial effects:

1. As a plasma expander, it improves CBF and cerebral oxygen delivery while reducing hematocrit and blood viscosity. These rheologic effects are thought to explain the rapid response seen in ICP reduction with mannitol administration, especially in patients with low CPP.

2. As an osmotic diuretic, mannitol extracts water from the brain by increasing the osmotic pressure of plasma. This effect on ICP is delayed because osmotic exchange can take 15–20 minutes.

Mannitol is entirely excreted by the kidneys, and there is significant risk of renal failure when it is administered in large doses. This is a matter of concern especially when other nephrotoxic drugs are administered or in the presence of pre-existing renal failure. Serum osmolarity is generally kept below 320 mosm because of concern about potential renal toxicity. Concurrent with mannitol administration, it is important to maintain adequate intravascular volume because hypotension increases the risk of ischemic brain injury. Mannitol, along with other osmotic agents, is known to cause an opening of the blood-brain barrier, resulting in accumulation of mannitol and other small molecules in the brain. This process may result in a reverse osmotic shift that *raises* brain osmolarity and theoretically *increases* brain edema.

Hyperventilation

Hyperventilation rapidly reduces ICP by causing cerebral vasoconstriction and thus a reduction of intracranial blood volume in a tight craniospinal compartment. Given that elevated ICP occurs in a significant number of patients with severe head injury and is associated with death and neurological disability, most clinicians have assumed that hyperventilation is beneficial in this setting. Unfortunately, hyperventilation also reduces ICP by causing cerebral vasoconstriction. Cerebral vasoconstriction is mediated by a reduction of CSF pH, not by hypocapnia. Therefore, hyperventilation, which reduces CBF, may be harmful. A prospective randomized trial comparing prophylactic hyperventilation (P_{CO_2} 25 ± 2 mm Hg) with ventilation aiming for normocapnia (P_{CO_2} 35 ± 2 mm Hg) found that patients who were hyperventilated had a significantly worse outcome at 3 and 6 months after injury.

In conclusion, prophylactic hyperventilation (P_{CO_2} <30 mm Hg) should be avoided in patients with head trauma. However, hyperventilation (P_{CO_2} = 25 mm Hg) may be necessary for *short periods* when there is an acute neurological deterioration or for longer periods if intracranial hypertension is refractory to other measures.

Barbiturates

Barbiturates are cerebroprotective and lower ICP. Barbiturates decrease cerebral metabolism and inhibit free radical–mediated lipid peroxidation. Suppressing cerebral metabolism results in a reduction of CSF and cerebral blood volume, which causes a lowering of ICP. Barbiturate use is based on the fact that pentobarbital can control ICP when other treatments have failed and that ICP control in general is associated with better outcomes.

Unfortunately, barbiturate use is also associated with a number of complications, the most important of which is hypotension. Hypotension is detrimental to outcome in head injury and contributes to secondary injury. Other possible difficulties associated with the use of barbiturates include hypothermia, cardiac suppression, and pneumonia. Although barbiturate use has been found to control ICP, no significant difference in outcome has been clearly demonstrated because of constraints in study design due to ethical concerns. Because of potential complications, the prophylactic use of barbiturates for the treatment of raised ICP is not recommended. High-dose barbiturate use is an option in hemodynamically stable patients with severe head injury and refractory intracranial hypertension.

A multicenter, randomized, blinded pilot study has shown propofol to be a promising alternative to pentobarbital in the treatment of severe head injury.

Glucocorticoids

One of the few standards (i.e., an accepted principle of patient management that reflects a high degree of clinical certainty) from Guidelines for the Management of Severe Head Injury is the role of glucocorticoids. These were first used in the early 1960s for the treatment of brain edema. The proposed mechanisms of action of corticosteroids included a reduction of CSF production, decrease in free radical production, and restoration of vascular permeability, to name a few. The significant clinical benefit of glucocorticoids in patients with primary and metastatic brain tumors was well documented, but several prospective double-blinded studies have failed to demonstrate any benefit of high-dose corticosteroids in the treatment of severe head injury. Thus, the use of glucocorticoids is not recommended for improving outcome or reducing ICP in patients with severe head injury, as stated in later guidelines for the management of severe head injury (Bullock et al. 1996).

Hypothermia

There has been a resurgence of interest in the use of moderate hypothermia (30–32°C for 48 hours) in the treatment of patients with severe head injury (Clifton et al. 1993; Marion et al. 1997). Hypothermia offers cerebral protection from ischemia. Its mechanisms of action are multifactorial. Hypothermia has been shown to reduce cerebral metabolism, decrease intracellular acidosis, diminish blood-brain barrier alterations, and inhibit excessive release of excitatory neurotransmitters. Clinical concerns with the use of hypothermia include an intracellular shift of potassium, a prolongation of the prothrombin time and partial thromboplastin time, and suppression of cardiac function with reduced heart rate and MAP.

Complications of Intracranial Pressure Monitoring

The main risk of ICP monitoring is infection. With optimal care, this incidence should be 5% or less. If monitoring is conducted for less than 3 days, the infection rate should be virtually zero. Beyond 5 days, the incidence of infection begins to increase significantly. It is therefore our practice to monitor for as short a period as possible. If monitoring must be continued beyond 5 days, the catheter is removed, and a new catheter is inserted at a different site. The incidence of hemorrhage relating to the placement of an ICP monitoring device is approximately 1%. The need for evacuation of a catheter-related bleed is very uncommon. Furthermore, because these devices are usually placed in the frontal region, it is rare to have a neurological deficit relating to catheter placement.

COMPLICATIONS

Infection

Severely injured patients are particularly susceptible to infectious complications, especially those with severe neurotrauma. Depressed respiratory function, prolonged mechanical ventilation, multiple invasive procedures and monitoring devices, prolonged immobilization, and post-traumatic immunosuppression all conspire to make infection a significant cause of delayed mortality and morbidity. Penetrating brain injury constitutes the greatest infection risk.

Meningitis

The development of a CSF fistula, secondary to a skull fracture and an associated dural tear, is the most common cause of post-traumatic meningitis. Fractures that predispose to meningitis involve the cribriform plate, frontal and ethmoidal sinuses, and temporal bone. Post-traumatic meningitis can occur even in the absence of an immediate CSF leak. This can be due to entrapment of a meningeal sleeve within a fracture and the subsequent development of a dural breach. Delayed post-traumatic meningitis can occur months and even years after head injury.

The microbiology of post-traumatic meningitis varies with the nature of the injury. More than 80% of cases of early post-traumatic meningitis, less than 5 days after injury, are pneumococcal meningitis, which can be associated with a closed head injury, skull fracture, or CSF leak. After the first 5 days post injury, there is an increasing incidence of meningitis due to other microbes. Gram-positive cocci, such as Staphylococcus aureus, aerobic gram-negative bacilli, Escherichia coli, and enteric gram-negative bacilli, Klebsiella pneumonia, Pseudomonas aeruginosa, Haemophilus influenzae, and Neisseria meningitides, are the most common pathogens after open and penetrating head injuries.

The clinical and laboratory features of post-traumatic meningitis differ significantly from spontaneously acquired cases of meningitis because of the severity of the systemic and neurological injury. Diagnosis of post-traumatic meningitis can therefore be difficult. The common symptoms and signs of lethargy, headache, fever, chills, photophobia, nuchal rigidity, and seizures may all be masked by the underlying brain injury. Traumatic SAH causes chemical meningitis and alters the CSF examination, which further confuses the diagnosis of post-traumatic meningitis. A significant traumatic SAH causes an inflammatory response, creating an increase in CSF protein and CSF polymor-phonuclear leukocytes, with a decrease in CSF glucose. The diagnosis and treatment of post-traumatic meningitis should be made from a high degree of clinical suspicion and laboratory and microbiological investigations.

For the eradication of post-traumatic meningitis, the CSF concentration of antibiotics must exceed the minimum bactericidal concentration of the isolated species by 10–20 times. Therefore, the choice of agent and its CSF penetration is crucial. The initial antibiotic regimen should be based on the results of Gram's stain and the type of head injury. Empirical coverage should be based on the most likely infecting organisms. An important part of infection treatment and prevention includes early meticulous wound débridement and closure. Cultures obtained during closure can be useful in guiding the initial choice of antibiotics.

Bacteremia and Sepsis

Patients sustaining major neurotrauma and requiring prolonged specialized care are at significant risk for the development of systemic infection. Prolonged mechanical ventilation and indwelling monitoring devices and catheters all serve as potential routes for the introduction of life-threatening systemic infections. After as few as 3 days in the ICU, patients with severe traumatic injuries have as high as a 50% risk of colonization by exogenous bacteria and a 20–25% risk of infection. By day 10, these risks jump to 90% and 75%, respectively. Most gram-negative pathogens are normal gastrointestinal (GI) tract flora. The overall mortality from gram-negative septicemia varies between 25% and 55%.

A significant body of evidence suggests that transmigration of GI flora secondary to impaired mucosal integrity plays a large role in increased infection rates after injury. Enteral feeding appears to maintain mucosal integrity. Most gram-positive infections arise from skin and respiratory tract commensals. Frequent hand washing, unit hygiene, and the meticulous maintenance of all catheters and all indwelling equipment are vital elements in the prevention of ICU sepsis. Fungal infections commonly occur after the prolonged use of broad-spectrum antibacterial drugs.

The pathophysiology of septic shock involves both host and microbial elements. The host elements involved include the complement system, the coagulation cascade and kinin systems, and their activated derivatives. The bradykinins are potent vasodilators that increase vascular permeability, decrease systemic vascular resistance, and increase GI motility. The complement system has similar effects and serves to activate macrophages and polymorphonuclear lymphocytes.

The lipopolysaccharide coating of certain bacteria permit them to resist opsonization, phagocytosis, and complement lysis. The lipopolysaccharide and other bacterial products induce the synthesis of interleukin-1 and tumor necrosis factor by macrophages and endothelial cells. These inflammatory mediators have profound effects on a multitude of organ systems. The inflammatory cascade of septic shock appears to be mediated by tumor necrosis factor.

Endothelial cells and organ microcirculation are the principal targets of the inflammatory cascade in sepsis. Precapillary shunting, clotting within postcapillary venules, fibrin deposition, platelet activation, and cytotoxicity are the direct effects of the inflammatory response on the microcirculation. A disseminated capillary leak ensues, with tissue hypoxia and cell death resulting from microcirculatory changes.

The clinical manifestations of sepsis commonly include fever, rigors, myalgia, tachycardia, tachypnea, cyanosis, lethargy, and confusion. Less frequently, hyperglycemia, hypothermia, respiratory distress, lactic acidosis, oliguria, thrombocytopenia, anemia, and disseminated intravascular coagulation (DIC) are part of the clinical presentation.

Septic shock occurs when hypotension and signs of organ hypoperfusion develop. The sepsis syndrome therefore includes infection, fever or hypothermia, tachypnea, tachycardia, and evidence of impaired organ system function. A high index of suspicion is required for the diagnosis because many of these presenting features can be masked by severe neurotrauma.

A rigorous investigation for the origin of the infection should be instituted. Intravenous lines should be changed and cultured. Urinary and other catheters should be replaced. Tissue oxygenation must be maximized by respiratory support, blood pressure support, and the correction of anemia. Volume resuscitation is crucial. The successful management of sepsis requires early recognition and rapid resuscitation. Aggressive treatment includes antibiotics and respiratory and hemodynamic support guided to optimize organ perfusion by central venous or pulmonary artery catheters. Arterial catheters also prove useful for continuous blood pressure monitoring and blood sampling. Persistent hypotension should be treated with vasopressors, after adequate volume resuscitation.

The cause and diagnosis of sepsis is confirmed by finding organisms in blood and other cultures. Bacteremia is intermittent; therefore, multiple cultures of sufficient quantity obtained during febrile spikes are of the greatest diagnostic use. Yield is improved by obtaining large volumes of blood (30 ml). The administration of antibiotics should not be delayed. Gram's stain and the buffy coat can speed the identification of pathogenic bacteria.

For the initial management of sepsis, a third-generation cephalosporin combined with an aminoglycoside is of greatest use for broad-spectrum coverage. For suspected anaerobic infection, clindamycin or metronidazole should be added. Antibiotic therapy is then tailored once definitive culture results are available.

Although there are a multitude of newer and more powerful antibiotics, the frequency and outcome of septic shock has not changed significantly over the past two decades. Nosocomial gram-negative bacilli are becoming increasingly resistant to third-generation cephalosporins. In this setting, aztreonam and imipenem are of significant usefulness. Amikacin and ciprofloxacin are helpful in the management of gentamicin-resistant *Pseudomonas aeruginosa*. Naloxone, glucocorticoids, and immunotherapy have been investigated in this setting as adjunctive agents, but there is no evidence to support their use.

Unit personnel remain the greatest vector for the transmission of microbes. Therefore, strict antisepsis and hygiene are paramount in the prevention of infection. Prophylactic antibiotics are of no benefit. Improper and injudicious use of antibiotics has led to the emergence of resistant bacterial strains and increases the risk of fungal infections and superinfections.

Pneumonia

Pneumonia is an extremely common complication of severe neurotrauma. In patients with a GCS score of less than 8, the frequency of pneumonia is approximately 40–45%. In severe brain injury, pneumonia is a powerful predictor of an unfavorable outcome. The peak time when a patient is at risk for pneumonia is between days 5 and 10 after injury.

The diagnosis of pneumonia requires a positive sputum culture combined with an infiltrate on the chest radiograph. The loss or alteration of airway reflexes, immunocompromise, mechanical ventilation, and prophylaxis against peptic ulcers all increase the risk of pneumonia. Aspiration pneumonia is a common sequel of severe neurotrauma. Clinically occult regurgitation, nasogastric tubes, tracheostomies, emergent surgical procedures on patients with full stomachs, and decreased swallowing and protective mechanisms are just some of the predisposing risk factors.

There are two patterns of infection in aspiration pneumonia. With the aspiration of a small volume of heavily contaminated particles, patients are prone to develop nonspecific lung abscesses, empyemas, or necrotizing bacterial pneumonia. Oropharyngeal flora is the usual isolate. With large volumes of acidic aspiration, gram-negative aerobic infections predominate, with *Pseudomonas* being commonly grown in cultures.

The clinical features of aspiration pneumonia include hypoxemia, fever, leukocytosis, increased sputum production, increased pulmonary adventitial sounds, dyspneic episodes, and infiltrates on chest radiographs. Hypotension is not uncommon; it may represent a reflex action or the result of intravascular volume depletion secondary to the aggregation of fluid within the lung. A ventilation-perfusion mismatch, manifested by a Po_2 of 35–50 mm Hg with a low or normal Pco_2, is commonly encountered. Lung compliance may be reduced secondary to pulmonary edema, hemorrhage, or atelectasis. Acute respiratory distress syndrome may develop.

An uncomplicated chemical pneumonitis includes increased sputum production, fever, leukocytosis, and radiographic pulmonary infiltrates. Therefore, it is extremely difficult initially to clinically differentiate chemical pneumonitis from aspiration pneumonia. Carefully obtained sputum cultures should be sought. The exclusion of oropharyngeal contamination is paramount. Transtracheal aspiration or bronchoscopic collection of sputum cultures is helpful. Before the initiation of antibiotics, aerobic and anaerobic cultures must be obtained. Colonization must be separated from clinical infection when positive sputum cultures are obtained.

The management of community-acquired aspiration pneumonia differs significantly from that of hospital-acquired pneumonia. The use of penicillin G is an inexpensive and efficacious choice for the treatment of community-acquired aspiration pneumonia. Clindamycin or metronidazole can be added in cases of relapse or poor response to initial therapy. There is some data to suggest that clindamycin is more efficacious than penicillin G. In critically ill patients with a hospital-acquired aspiration pneumonia, agents such as vancomycin for antistaphylococcal coverage plus a third-generation cephalosporin for gram-negative coverage, may be employed.

Fluid management is critical in severely brain-injured patients, especially those with serious medical complications. Head-injured patients with aspiration pneumonia therefore should be closely monitored with invasive hemodynamic monitors. Endotracheal suctioning should be used immediately if aspiration is observed, but this is inadequate to completely evacuate the aspirate. Bronchoscopy should be performed, but the use of large fluid volumes for lavage should be avoided. To improve ventilation-perfusion mismatch and survival, positive pressure ventilation with positive end expiratory pressure (PEEP) is of proved benefit.

Coagulopathies

Coagulopathies and platelet abnormalities are commonly encountered in the ICU. Coagulopathy is an early complication of severe brain injury and multisystem trauma, occurring in up to 20% of patients. Its peak incidence is within the first 3 days of injury. If present, a coagulopathy is an independent predictor for a poor outcome in head-injured patients.

Disorders involving the coagulation cascade and platelets may have intracranial and extracranial causes. DIC due to massive blood product transfusion, destruction of brain substance, and gram-negative septicemia are the most common causes in this scenario. The acute DIC that is commonly associated with severe brain injury is related to the systemic release of tissue thromboplastin, which in turn induces a consumptive coagulopathy. A positive correlation between degree of brain injury and DIC has been demonstrated.

Thrombocytopenia or platelet dysfunction may also be secondary to many of the medications employed in severe head injury. Antibiotics, dextran, calcium-channel blockers, beta blockers, and theophylline all can alter platelet function.

DIC is characterized by increased prothrombin and partial thromboplastin times, the clinical signs of an increased tendency to bleeding with intravascular coagulation, and a decrease in clotting factors, fibrinogen, and platelets. Only a small percentage of brain-injured patients go on to develop full-blown DIC. Most DIC is associated with an increase in fibrin split products. Consequently, therapy is directed at controlling the primary process and restoring adequate clotting factors, usually via the administration of fresh frozen plasma. Antithrombin levels drop rapidly in sepsis and shock. Low antithrombin levels increase the tendency toward subclinical DIC and multiple organ failure.

Seizures

Post-traumatic epilepsy is a public health concern with profound economic and social impact. Between 5,000 and 30,000 new cases of post-traumatic epilepsy are encountered each year in the United States. Approximately 20–25% of moderately to severely brain-injured patients experience at least one post-traumatic seizure. Post-traumatic epilepsy is divided into two types: early and late.

Early post-traumatic seizures are those that occur within the first week of injury. They occur in about 5% of people admitted to the hospital with the diagnosis of head injury. Children appear to have an increased susceptibility toward early post-traumatic seizures. Early post-traumatic seizures can be life threatening because they may develop into status epilepticus. Thirty percent of early seizures occur within the first hour of injury.

Approximately 50% of early seizures are focal in onset. Even when associated with mild brain injury, early seizures are associated with late seizures in up to 25% of cases. Therefore, early seizures are an important predictor for the development of late post-traumatic epilepsy. The subsequent development of late post-traumatic epilepsy is not affected by the frequency or type of early seizures. Twenty-five to 30% of adults with early seizures will develop late seizures. Less than 10% of children who have early seizures develop late post-traumatic seizures.

Seizures that occur after the first week post injury are considered late post-traumatic epilepsy. Injury severity is a major predictor. Nearly 50% of patients with SDH, intracerebral hematomas, or penetrating brain injury develop late post-traumatic epilepsy, whereas 20% of patients with epidural hematomas develop late post-traumatic seizures. The highest incidence of late post-traumatic epilepsy occurs in relation to combat missile injuries to the brain. More than 50% of patients experiencing these injuries develop late post-traumatic epilepsy. Patients with depressed skull fractures in association with other injuries, including post-traumatic amnesia (PTA) greater than 24 hours, early post-traumatic seizures, focal brain injuries, and dural lacerations, have a 40–50% chance of developing late post-traumatic epilepsy. Most seizures occur within the first 2 years of injury; approximately 50% occur within 1 year, and 70% of late seizures will have occurred by 2 years.

Prophylaxis

A double-blinded, placebo-controlled trial in severely head-injured patients at high risk for post-traumatic seizures evaluated the long- and short-term use and efficacy of phenytoin administration in the prevention of post-traumatic seizures. The initial loading dose of phenytoin was given within the first 24 hours after injury. Phenytoin reduced the incidence of early seizures by 73%. It must be remembered that anticonvulsants, particularly phenytoin, are associated with a multitude of serious and potentially lethal adverse reactions. Therefore at this time, based on the evidence available, the prophylactic administration of anticonvulsants, phenytoin specifically, cannot be recommended to prevent early or late seizures. Should an early seizure occur, however, phenytoin should be administered in the effort to prevent subsequent seizures. Phenytoin should be given for 10 days and then discontinued. No prophylaxis should be instituted for the prevention of late seizures. If a late seizure does occur, an anticonvulsant (e.g., phenytoin, carbamazepine, or valproate) should be administered. Late post-traumatic seizures are most commonly multiple; therefore, maintenance anticonvulsant treatment should be instituted after the first seizure.

Deep Venous Thrombosis and Pulmonary Embolism

Deep venous thrombosis (DVT) occurs in 15–20% of people with severe central nervous system (CNS) trauma. Accompanying pulmonary embolism (PE) occurs in 5–10% of these patients. DVT and PE prophylaxis should therefore be instituted as soon as possible. Intermittent pneumatic compression stockings should be employed early after injury, barring contraindications. Low-dose heparin should be prescribed when the patient has been stabilized from the multisystem trauma and after any operative procedures. In patients for whom the use of anticoagulants is contraindicated, strong consideration must be given to the placement of an inferior vena cava filter.

The development of any change in cardiopulmonary status should be considered a possible PE. Chest radiograph, electrocardiogram, and even blood gas analyses are not themselves individually or in concert reliable for the diagnosis of PE. A ventilation-perfusion study is the first diagnostic step. Patients with severe CNS trauma have altered pulmonary mechanics, which therefore almost eliminates the possibility of a normal ventilation-perfusion scan. The common occurrence of false-positive, false-negative, and intermediate-probability reports leads to pulmonary angiography as part of the diagnostic algorithm. Complete anticoagulation or thrombolysis is often undesirable or absolutely contraindicated in the acute setting of CNS trauma. The placement of an inferior vena cava filter is often the mode of treatment, but it presents serious short- and long-term implications.

Stress Ulcers

Stress ulcers occur often with patients in the ICU, particularly those with CNS trauma. Endoscopic evidence of gastric erosions has been observed within 24 hours of severe CNS injury. GI hemorrhage has been associated with mortality rates as high as 50%. The pathophysiology for the development of stress ulceration is multifactorial. Hypersecretion of gastric acid and pepsin peak secondary to intracranial disease occurs within 3–5 days of injury. Pepsin contains several proteolytic enzymes that compound the destruction of gastric mucosa. Bile salts, which are known to reflux in the severely injured, also disrupt gastric mucosa and thereby increase mucosal injury. Injury to the parasympathetic centers in the hypothalamus and their connections to vagal nuclei in the medulla interrupts gastric acid secretion inhibitory pathways. This leads to elevated gastric acid production and consequent gastric erosions.

A frequency of hemorrhagic ulcers of 12.5% has been reported in brain-injured patients. Severe head injury with a GCS score of less than 8 is associated with acid hypersecretion and gastric ulceration rates as high as 17%. Bleeding from gastric ulceration occurs most frequently within the first 2 weeks of hospitalization. Hypotension, age greater than 60, CNS infection, gastric pH less than 4, respiratory failure, and the development of SIADH are all significant risk factors for the development of bleeding gastric ulceration in head injury.

The ideal method of preventing GI ulceration in the neurotraumatized patient is widely debated. The standard treatments include antacids, histamine-receptor antagonists, and sucralfate. All these therapeutic ministrations have their own associated risks and benefits. Antacids historically have been the mainstay of stress ulcer prophylaxis. Raising gastric pH above 3.5 has been demonstrated to decrease the incidence of gastric hemorrhage. Attaining a pH of greater than 5 inactivates pepsin and neutralizes 99% of stomach acid. Magnesium hydroxide is the most efficacious antacid compound for elevating stomach pH for a sustained period. Some common side effects resulting from antacids include diarrhea, hypophosphatemia, and metabolic alkalosis.

A number of studies document the efficacy of histamine antagonists in the prevention of GI ulceration and bleeding (Lu et al. 1997), but there is controversy about whether these drugs are better in GI ulcer prophylaxis than antacids. Histamine-receptor antagonists reduce gastric acid secretion by the reversible inhibition of gastric parietal cells. The stimulation of gastric acid production by pentagastrin, food, and pepsin are all suppressed by H_2 blockade in a dose-related manner. From the data available, H_2 blockers are at least as good as antacids. Continuous infusion of H_2-receptor antagonists abolishes the peaks and troughs of pH that are associated with intermittent-dose regimens and appears to provide better prophylaxis than antacids do.

Sucralfate is a mixture of sucrose, aluminum hydroxide, and sulfates. It exerts a protective effect against stress ulceration by strengthening the gastric mucosa. By binding to both normal and damaged gastric mucosa, sucralfate increases the mucin content of the stomach lining, increases the viscosity of gastric mucus, and increases the hydrophobic character of the gastric mucosa. Other beneficial effects of sucralfate include stimulation of gastric prostaglandin production, improvement of mucosal blood flow, inhibition of peptic digestion, and facilitation of mucosal repair and regeneration. No major adverse reactions to sucralfate have been reported.

PROGNOSIS

Many factors have been evaluated for their prognostic abilities after TBI. We review the available data briefly, but certain caveats must be emphasized. The clinician must remain aware that numbers derived from groups of patients give only a general sense of the prognostic correlations. Moreover, when these various prognostic factors are subjected to a logistic regression analysis, most factors are found to be insignificant. In daily practice, each patient must be considered as an individual, with unique characteristics that affect outcome. Prognostic factors are merely associations between a clinical finding and outcome; they do not provide a definitive answer in each case. In addition, head injury initiates a dynamic process in brain tissues, with changes that occur over variable time spans. Thus, ongoing assessments are required to reflect a patient's current status. Decisions about the level of medical care must be based on firm clinical and diagnostic data, especially when considering the withdrawal of support. Finally, the field of neuroscience is in a state of rapid growth, and advances in knowledge may have implications for the TBI patient.

Preinjury Factors

Several preinjury factors have been shown to have an impact on recovery from TBI: age, gender, genetics, race, and substance abuse.

Age

Age is a strong independent predictor of mortality. Higher mortality rates are seen in children younger than 5 years and

Table 56B.8:   Glasgow Outcome Scale

Unfavorable outcomes			Favorable outcomes	
1	2	3	4	5
Death	Persistent vegetative state	Severe disability	Moderate disability	Good recovery
Loss of life due to head injury	Unresponsive, + sleep cycles, + eye opening	Conscious but disabled, dependent for daily care	Disabled but independent, able to care for self	Resumes normal life, minor residual deficits

in individuals older than 65 years. Age also has an impact on the level of residual disability, with effects reported on both functional and cognitive outcomes. A study of 40 elderly patients with severe TBI found no functional improvement after 3 years (Kilaru et al. 1996). Another study found that functional change did occur in patients older than age 55, but they required longer rehabilitation programs and had a lower rate of change compared with those younger than 55 (Cifu et al. 1996). Goldstein and co-workers (1994) found that patients older than age 50 with only mild-to-moderate injuries had marked problems with memory and executive function tasks on neurobehavioral studies. Brain injuries before the age of 8 years result in a greater likelihood of severe disability on the Glasgow Outcome Scale (GOS) (Table 56B.8) as well as evidence of impaired motor and visuomotor development (Asikainen et al. 1996).

Gender

A significant difference between genders is seen in TBI data on frequency and mortality. TBI occurs much more frequently in males, with a 3 to 1 male-to-female mortality ratio that may simply represent differences in severity of injury. The effect of gender on recovery after TBI remains unclear. Animal studies imply that gonadal hormones can influence outcome from brain injury, but only a few human studies have suggested a gender effect. One study of penetrating brain injury in children and adolescents found that gender did correlate with outcome (Levy et al. 1993). Gender was also found to be a predictor of the length of rehabilitation stay in a recent study.

Genetics

The influence of genetics on recovery from brain injury has received recent attention. The increased risk of Alzheimer's disease with the presence of an apolipoprotein ε-4 (apo E-4) genotype is well known. Recent studies suggest that TBI patients with this same genotype may have a greater risk of persistent deficits due to the possibility of histopathological changes in response to the injury. Boxers with the apo E-4 genotype and more than 12 professional bouts have significantly higher impairments on a scale specifically designed to test for the traumatic encephalopathy associated with boxing (Jordan et al. 1997). Teasdale and co-

workers (1997) reported on the results of a prospective study assessing the apo E genotype in 93 TBI patients. A higher proportion of the patients with the apo E-4 genotype had a GCS less than 13. In addition, the 6-month GOS determination found that 57% of the patients with apo E-4 had a poor outcome compared with 27% of the patients without apo E-4 ($P = 0.006$). Further studies are needed on the long-term predictive value provided by this information.

Race

Race and socioeconomic factors correlate with the frequency of TBI by placing people in an environment with higher risks for head injury. Sosin and co-workers (1995) reported that the TBI mortality rates for black males have risen since 1984, whereas the rates have fallen for white males. This was attributed to a significant increase in black male firearm-related deaths, with an associated decrease in motor vehicle-related deaths in white males. Median family income has shown an inverse relationship to both the incidence and the mortality rate of TBI. Patients with a higher premorbid level of education and intelligence carry a better prognosis for recovery from TBI. Neuropsychological testing of intelligence in the acute phase after TBI has a positive correlation with outcome. This may relate in some way to the neural reserve available to a person after TBI. Recurrent head injuries have been shown to result in cumulative damage over time, and even mild trauma may result in significant deficits if there is a prior history of TBI.

Substance Abuse

Corrigan (1995) found that alcohol intoxication was present in one-third to one-half of all TBI hospitalizations. A history of some form of substance abuse is present in approximately two-thirds of TBI patients going on to rehabilitation. Higher mortality rates, increased acute complications with longer hospitalizations, worse discharge status, and a greater likelihood of repeat injuries were all associated with a history of substance abuse. A history of substance abuse also has a negative influence on cognitive performance after TBI. This association was confirmed by Kelly et al. (1997), who found lower scores on multiple neuropsychological tests in TBI patients with a positive toxicology screen on admission.

Nature of the Injury

Type of Injury

The pathology of TBI has a bearing on the outcome. Brain injury can be described in terms of the mechanism and morphology of injury. *Mechanism of injury* refers to blunt versus penetrating trauma, whereas *morphology* describes the presence of focal or diffuse intracranial injury. The mechanism of injury carries implications about outcome. Penetrating trauma occurs less frequently than blunt trauma in most series, but the mortality rate is significantly higher. Outcome after penetrating head injury follows a strongly bimodal pattern (i.e., either patients do quite well or they die). In closed head injury, the intermediate outcomes are much better represented. An overall mortality rate of 55% was seen at 1 week after penetrating brain injury in a retrospective study of 62 patients with severe TBI. A prospective study found that patients with penetrating head injuries with a GCS of 6–8 had a 70% mortality rate; the rate jumped to 94% when the initial GCS was 3–5. The presence of a traumatic SAH is a poor prognostic sign after penetrating head injury. Although there is greater likelihood of death after a penetrating head injury, survival does not necessarily imply a poor long-term outcome. A study comparing the functional outcome of 25 cases of penetrating TBI survivors with the same number of blunt TBI survivors found no significant differences in the outcome variables 1 year after injury (Zafonte et al. 1997b).

DAI is a diffuse effect of trauma and may occur either in isolation or with coexisting focal hematomas. Neuroimaging studies are generally not diagnostic, and DAI remains a histological diagnosis. Clinically, the syndrome of DAI has three separate stages: (1) immediate unconsciousness, (2) a longer period of confusion and associated PTA, and (3) a prolonged recovery period. The amount and density of DAI determine the clinical course. The factors that are most predictive of outcome include the length of PTA, duration of coma, and GCS. Secondary injuries, most notably due to hypotension and hypoxia, are often associated with brain injury. Furthermore, metabolic and neurochemical disturbances can contribute to the cellular injury and influence the clinical course.

SAH is another form of diffuse injury seen in TBI. Greene and co-workers (1997) compared the clinical course of TBI patients with SAH to patients of similar GCS scores without SAH. The traumatic SAH patients were found to have more medical complications as well as an increased number of days in both the ICU and the hospital. The clinical outcome for traumatic SAH was also worse; these patients had higher mortality rates and lower GOS scores on discharge, and a smaller number were discharged to home. However, all these studies are based on relatively few patients, thus precluding valid statistical analyses.

Cortical contusions and subdural, extradural, and intracranial hematomas comprise the majority of focal pathologies. The recovery from these types of injuries is variable and depends on the location, size, and depth of the lesion. At one time, it was suggested that lesions in the left hemisphere were associated with an increased duration of unresponsiveness. Further studies found that the length of time to develop localized pain responses was similar regardless of the hemispheric localization of injury. The interpretation of this result was that impaired language skills provided the explanation for any delayed responsiveness seen with left hemisphere lesions.

The presence of SDH and epidural hematoma can affect outcome, and they often require neurosurgical intervention. Outcome from SDH is related to the length of time between injury and surgical decompression. In one study, patients had a 30% mortality rate if decompression was accomplished within 4 hours, whereas delays of more than 4 hours increased the mortality rate to 90%. The presence of a greater than 15-mm midline shift on CT due to an SDH has also been associated with late deterioration and death. An outcome study focusing on patients with epidural hematoma suggests that 23% have a poor outcome and 77% have good recovery or moderate disability by GOS. These results were found to have an association with GCS scores, other intracerebral injuries, and ICP management (Heinzelmann et al. 1996). The depth of a lesion on brain MRI done 3 months after TBI has been found to be predictive of the 6-month GOS.

Severity of Injury

TBI is the single largest contributor to trauma center deaths, with a higher mortality rate than other forms of trauma. In 1989, a review by Gennarelli and co-workers of 95 trauma centers found an overall trauma mortality rate of 6.1%, but this rate increased to 18.2% in the TBI patients. One of the strongest predictors of mortality is severity of injury, and this is usually determined by assessing the level of consciousness. This information can also provide some guidance regarding the possibility and amount of any residual disability. The most widely used scale to assess the level of consciousness is the GCS. As a measure of injury severity, the GCS has shown a strong relationship to outcome in numerous studies. Another scale to assess the severity of injuries frequently used in trauma centers is the Revised Trauma Score (RTS) (developed by Boyd in 1987); this is arrived at by adding the GCS, systolic blood pressure, and respiratory rate. Although it has good predictive value regarding mortality, it has limited usefulness in predicting disability.

The GCS can change rapidly in response to medical interventions in the early stages after TBI. For this reason, the developers of the GCS have recommended that a standardized postresuscitation time be identified for assessment of the GCS. Other researchers have found that both the first GCS obtained and the worst postresuscitation GCS can be highly predictive of neurobehavioral functioning 1 year after injury. An isolated GCS may actually have a somewhat lim-

Table 56B.9:   Multidimensional assessments for outcome prediction after traumatic brain injury

Author, year	Variables affecting outcome	Outcome measurement
Braakman et al. 1980	Age, GCS, pupil reactivity, spontaneous and reflex eye movements, length of coma	6-month GOS
Narayan et al. 1981	GCS, pupillary response, intracranial pressure, evoked potentials, age	2-category GOS (D + VS + SD; MD + GR)
Choi et al. 1988	Best motor response by GCS, admission pupillary response, age	4-category GOS (D + VS; SD; MD; GR)
Levin et al. 1990	Lowest post-resuscitation GCS, pupil reactivity	1-year GOS
Michaud 1992 (pediatric)	Brain and extracranial injury severity, pupil response	Survival
	72-hour GCS motor response, early oxygenation status	Disability

D = death; GCS = Glasgow Coma Scale; GOS = Glasgow Outcome Scale; GR = good recovery; MD = moderate disability; SD = severe disability; VS = vegetative state.

Source: R Braakman, G Gelpke, J Habbema, et al. Systemic selection of prognostic features in patients with severe head injury. Neurosurgery 1980;6:362–370; R Narayan, R Greenberg, J Miller, et al. Improved confidence of outcome prediction in severe head injury. A comparative analysis of the clinical examination, multimodality evoked potentials, CT scanning and intracranial pressure. J Neurosurg 1981;54:751–762; SC Choi, RK Narayan, RL Anderson, et al. Enhanced specificity of prognosis in severe head injury. J Neurosurg 1988;69:381–385; H Levin, H Gary, H Eisenberg, et al. Neurobehavioral outcome 1 year after severe head injury: experience of the Traumatic Coma Data Bank. J Neurosurg 1990;73:699–709; L Michaud, F Rivara, M Grady, et al. Predictors of survival and severity of disability after severe brain injury in children. Neurosurgery 1992;31:254–264.

ited value as a predictor of functional outcome. Alternative scales have been proposed, but although these other scales may provide more specific information, the GCS remains the most widely used and has reasonably good interobserver reliability. However, significant variations have been noted, depending on who is assessing the GCS.

Although recent advances in emergent and acute care have resulted in improved outcomes, severe TBI (GCS <8) continues to have a significant mortality and disability rate. The National Institutes of Health Traumatic Coma Data Bank was a cooperative effort of six clinical head-injury centers to collect data regarding acute and long-term prognosis after severe TBI. This study reported a decrease in TBI mortality from 50% in the 1970s to approximately 30% in a 1991 review. It also found that moderate disability or good recovery occurred in only 16% of patients with a GCS less than 6. Poor or substantially limited reintegration in the community has been found in 76% of severe TBI patients for up to 6 years after injury. The subgroup of patients with good recovery or moderate disability by the GOS showed only a 50% rate of good community reintegration. Moderate TBI carries a much better prognosis, with one study finding that patients with a GCS of 9–13 had a mortality rate of 0.9%. The 6-month outcome analysis found 86% with moderate disability or good recovery, 7% with severe disability, and only 7% in the vegetative or dead category.

Overall mild head injury (GCS = 14) has a good prognosis, although some recommend classifying it into uncomplicated or complicated (or high-risk) categories. Complicated mild TBI patients are those with a GCS of 13–14, or 15 with radiographic abnormalities. This group demonstrates worse outcomes compared to patients with a GCS of 15 without radiographic findings (Hsiang et al. 1997).

Postconcussion syndrome (PCS) can follow a mild head injury. The symptoms are diverse but commonly include headache, irritability, dizziness, and cognitive impairments. Levin (1996) reports that there is consistent evidence for the recovery of the cognitive deficits within 1–3 months of injury. The majority of patients experience substantial or complete recovery of symptoms by 3 months after injury, but 1 year after injury, residual symptoms are still reported in 7% of mild TBI patients. The persistence of PCS 6 months after injury raises concerns that psychological factors may contribute to the symptoms. Researchers have reported on the high prevalence of PCS-like symptoms in the general population and in patients with medical or psychiatric problems. TBI patients may underestimate the prevalence of these symptoms in the general population, thus causing them to associate the symptoms directly to their injury.

Prognosis from TBI may be better determined by looking at more than one variable, especially in the severely head-injured patient. Many researchers have proposed the need for multidimensional analysis tools (Table 56B.9). The combination of patient's age, best GCS motor response, and pupillary response at admission provided the most accurate prediction of outcome; it has been proposed to use these variables in a decision-tree algorithm (Figure 56B.13).Clinical use of this tool found it to have an accuracy rate of 77.7%. The prediction accuracy was highest for patients at the GOS extremes (i.e., death or good recovery) compared with those in the intermediate categories. Outcome can be predicted by using the lowest postresuscitation GCS, pupil reactivity, age, and spontaneous and reflex eye movements; ICP data and multimodal evoked potentials may add to the confidence of the prediction. In the pediatric population, brain injury severity, extracranial injury severity, and intermediate pupillary response have been shown to be predictive of mortality. The most prognostic factors for disability in the same

FIGURE 56B.13 Traumatic brain injury outcome prediction tree based on pupillary response, motor response, and age. The predicted 12-month outcomes (defined by the Glasgow Outcome Scale) are: good recovery (GR); moderately disabled (MD); severely disabled (SD); vegetative state (VS); and dead (D). (Adapted with permission from S Choi, J Muizelaar, T Barnes, et al. Prediction tree for severely head-injured patients. J Neurosurg 1991;75:251–255.)

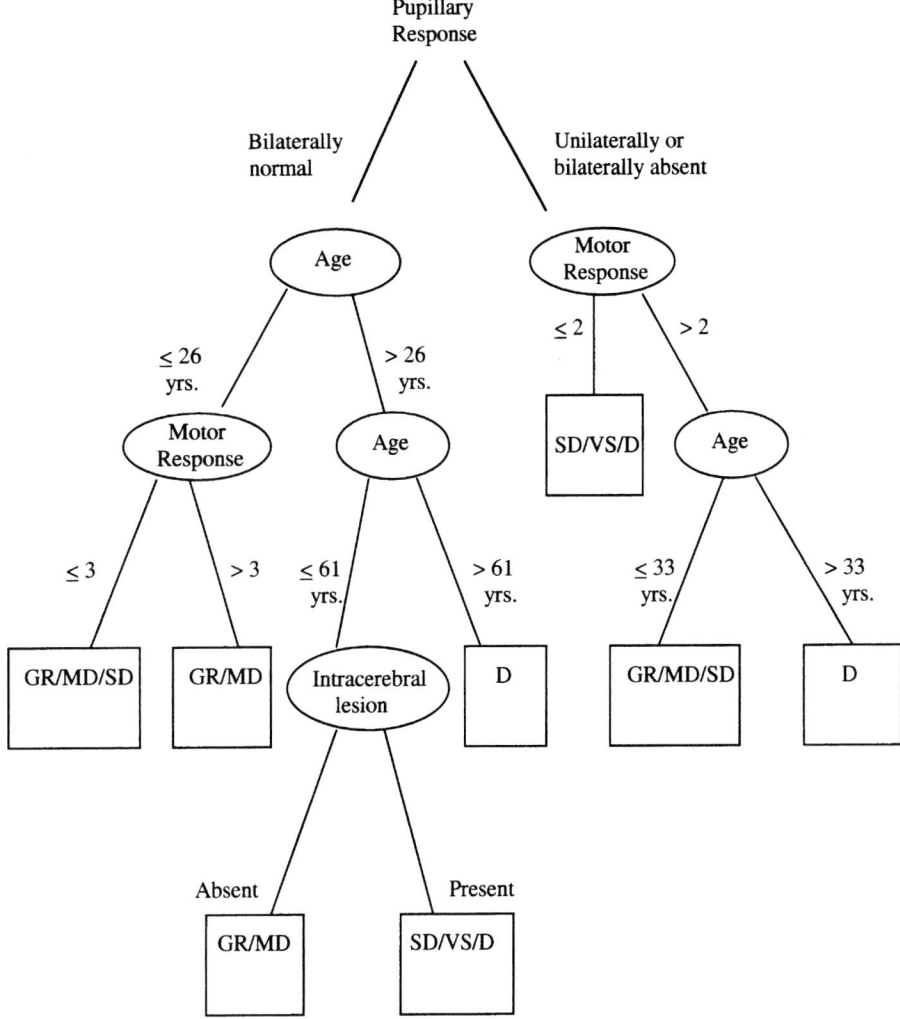

cohort were 72-hour postinjury GCS motor response and early oxygenation status.

Present information supports efforts to make mortality predictions by using a limited number of variables in the acute phase after injury, with the primary focus on age, injury severity (especially the GCS motor component), and pupillary reactions. Although this is the trend, it must be emphasized that life is inherently unpredictable. Inaccurate predictions can have serious and devastating implications. Quigley et al. (1997) reported a "3-4-5" rule after evaluating the use of age and admission GCS for predicting survival. They found only nonfunctional survival (death or vegetative state) in patients whose age was beyond the 30s with a GCS of 3, beyond the 40s with a GCS of 4, or beyond the 50s with a GCS of 5. In their discussion, they stressed that any rule has exceptions. Thus, prognostic factors should not be used for definitive decisions to treat or not to treat but instead should act as guides for treatment decisions and expectations. The prediction of long-term dis-

ability poses even greater challenges and requires a broader base of information gathered over a longer period.

Associated Injuries

The presence of extracranial traumatic injuries can have a significant effect on recovery after TBI. In one review of 1,709 patients with TBI, 60% had associated systemic injuries and 40% had an isolated TBI. The patients with systemic injuries had a mortality rate of 21.8% compared with an 11% rate in the isolated TBI group. The subgroup of patients with systemic injuries involving the spine, lung, viscera, pelvis, or extremities showed an even higher mortality rate of 25%. Associated systemic injuries can also affect the average total cost of care over the first year after injury. These costs increase (in 1998 dollars) from $59,000 in isolated severe TBI to $90,000 when additional systemic injuries are present. The patient's long-term level of recovery may be affected by the presence of associated injuries.

A longer duration of coma has been reported in TBI patients with multiple injuries along with greater problems with long-term psychosocial functioning, memory, attention, and learning. Masson and co-workers (1996) looked at a group of 149 patients 5 years after a mild-to-moderate TBI and found that the majority of disabilities reported were related to their systemic injuries. Similar findings have been reported in the pediatric population. A study of 95 pediatric patients found that those with TBI plus multiple trauma had a 2.5 times greater frequency of poor outcome, even though the severity of head injury was greater in the patients with isolated TBI.

Postinjury Factors

Emergency Department and Intensive Care Unit Management

A delay in care or transportation to a facility that is not prepared to manage a trauma patient can have a negative long-term effect. The primary injury after TBI is the biomechanical damage that occurs directly to the CNS. As emphasized above, trauma-related secondary insults of hypotension, hypoxia, hypovolemia, and elevated ICP can result in the secondary injuries of ischemia and diffuse cerebral edema. The focus of early TBI management should include minimizing any secondary insults. Wald and co-workers (1993) grouped patients by the presence or absence of secondary brain injury and found no significant differences in the mortality rates between a rural setting and an urban community with access to trauma centers. In a comparative analysis of TBI survival in New Delhi, India, and Charlottesville, VA, it was found that early management might affect outcome. The availability of better critical care improved the mortality rate of the Virginia patients who localized to painful stimuli (GCS motor score = 5). The combination of prehospital variables with clinical and radiographic findings has shown predictive power on mortality and outcome (Fearnside et al. 1993). Systemic complications after injury can also influence TBI recovery; postinjury pulmonary, cardiovascular, hematologic, or infectious problems are associated with poor outcomes. Increased efforts by emergency department and ICU staff to prevent secondary insults and systemic complications may result in improved survival with less disability.

There is an emphasis in the neurosciences on developing multidisciplinary approaches to patient care. The TBI population is a patient group that may benefit from this treatment approach. Trauma teams, neurosurgeons, and emergency department staff work closely together to coordinate the initial care. After the acute stabilization, the treatment team expands to include orthopedic surgery, neurology, rehabilitation services (including the physiatrist, physical and occupational therapists, and speech-language pathologist), respiratory therapy, nursing, nutrition, and social services. The use of a formalized team approach of aggressive early intervention has recently been compared with a traditional, nonformalized program. Patients in the formalized program had a significant decrease in both coma duration and length of stay in the inpatient rehabilitation setting. Improvements were also seen in discharge impairment scores and motor, sensory, and cognitive function. This resulted in 94% of the formalized program patients being discharged to their home compared with only 57% of patients in the nonformalized program. Specialized "acute TBI units" may actually provide an optimal treatment setting with cost-effective medical care, resulting in improved outcomes.

Hemodynamic Factors

Increased mortality and morbidity have been associated with early postinjury episodes of systolic blood pressure less than 90 mm Hg or respiratory compromise (apnea, cyanosis, or PO_2 <60 mm Hg). One or both of these parameters have been reported at some time after injury and through resuscitation in 57% of comatose TBI patients (Chesnut et al. 1993b). Another study found that only 23% of the patients with a history of hypotension or hypoxia had a good recovery compared with 56% of the patients who had neither factor. In addition, the presence of either factor doubled the mortality rate (Wald et al. 1993).

Many researchers have confirmed that hypotension has a negative impact on TBI survival and recovery (Chesnut et al. 1993b; Fearnside et al. 1993; Pigula et al. 1993; Winchell et al. 1996). Mortality rates are doubled (55% versus 27%) in patients that are hypotensive on admission, and they have shown a significant increase in morbidity compared with normotensive patients. Transient episodes of hypotension may commonly occur in the ICU after TBI. The total number of these episodes has been associated with increased mortality and a decrease in the number of patients discharged home, with the most detrimental effects occurring in patients having an initial GCS of 8 (Winchell et al. 1996). The Traumatic Coma Data Bank review found that 32% of 493 patients developed late hypotension, and 24% had hypotensive episodes only in the ICU. This group showed a very poor outcome: 66% were in a vegetative state or dead compared with only 17% of the group without late hypotension who fell into these categories (Chesnut et al. 1993a). Hypotension that occurs intraoperatively during the first 72 hours after injury has been associated with a higher mortality rate compared with normotensive TBI patients (82% versus 25%). In the pediatric TBI population, the development of hypotension resulted in a fourfold increase in mortality (Pigula et al. 1993). The use of small-volume hypertonic saline solutions for blood pressure resuscitation provides a therapeutic effect that may help to improve outcome from severe TBI (Vassar et al. 1993; Wade et al. 1997).

The detrimental effects of hypoxemia after TBI are recognized in animal models of injury and in humans. Information on the balance between cerebral oxygen delivery and consumption may be obtained by monitoring jugular venous oxyhemoglobin saturation ($SjvO_2$) (Robertson et al. 1995). Desaturation ($SjvO_2$ <50%) has been reported to occur at least once in 39% of TBI patients, and it was related to both intracranial hypertension and systemic causes (Robertson et al. 1995). Episodes of desaturation have been correlated with poor outcomes, which supports the thought that reductions in oxygen delivery contribute to secondary neurological injury (Robertson et al. 1995). Other tools for detecting early ischemic secondary injury include brain tissue partial pressure of O_2 (ti-PO_2) and cerebral arteriovenous oxygen difference ($AVDO_2$). Falls of ti-PO_2 below 10 mm Hg for more than 15 minutes is consistent with ischemia and has been associated with unfavorable outcomes (Kiening et al. 1997). Late cerebral infarction and poor outcome can also be predicted by the failure of $AVDO_2$ to fall in response to treatment interventions (LeRoux et al. 1997). A constant, noninvasive means of monitoring cerebral oxygenation may be provided by NIRS, but the validity of this tool has not been proved. A multimodality recording system has allowed the comparison of NIRS with other monitoring parameters. NIRS was found to correlate with 97% of the cerebral hemodynamic changes; this was compared to only a 53% correlation provided by $SjvO_2$ measures. At this time, NIRS should not be used in isolation, but it can supply information regarding clinical trends (Kirkpatrick et al. 1995). Hyperbaric oxygen therapy has been used in efforts to improve oxygenation after TBI. A benefit in mortality was seen, with only 17% of the treatment group dying compared with 32% of the control group. This benefit did not carry through to long-term results because there was no increase in the number of survivors with favorable outcomes.

Cerebral vasculature and CBF are altered after TBI, and this can lead to changes in cerebral oxygen metabolism ($CMRO_2$). Not maintaining adequate CBF increases the risk of secondary ischemia. Cerebral ischemia (CBF <18 ml/100 g/min) occurs in up to 30% of TBI patients in the first hours after injury (Bouma and Muizelaar 1995). Hypovolemic shock associated with TBI has a mortality rate of 62%, and there is a direct relationship between mortality and the volume of blood required for resuscitation in the first 24 hours (Siegel 1995). In severe TBI, there may be an association between low CBF and 3-month mortality; patients with CBF values of 29 ml/100 g per minute had a mortality rate of 32% versus 20% for CBF values of 62 ml/100 g per minute. In addition, an increased need for inpatient rehabilitation has been shown when hypovolemic shock occurs after TBI. The relationship between blood flow changes and outcome after TBI has been assessed with xenon-133–CBF studies. CBF is lowest on the day of injury; flow increases over the next 1–5 days. Favorable outcome at 6 months after injury has been reported in 58.8% of the patients who consistently maintained a CBF of 33 ml/100 g per minute, but favorable recovery occurred in no patients whose rate fell below that level.

This suggests that a phasic elevation in CBF after TBI is necessary for functional recovery (Kelly D et al. 1997). The combination of increased CBF with an elevated ICP may indicate the loss of cerebral autoregulation, whereas increased CBF with a normal ICP suggests an appropriate relationship between metabolism and CBF, thus improving the chance for a favorable outcome (Kelly D et al. 1997; Kelly D et al. 1996). Although the early changes in postinjury CBF are uncertain in the pediatric patient, the contribution of hypovolemia and CBF to mortality and morbidity has been established in this population.

$CMRO_2$ is a stronger predictor of outcome than CBF. A significant association was seen between low $CMRO_2$ values and death or persistent vegetative state at 6 months after injury. In most children, cerebral metabolism is initially normal. At 1–3 days after injury, however, a fall in both $CMRO_2$ and $AVDO_2$ can be observed. The likelihood of an unfavorable GOS outcome was greater in children who had a lower mean $CMRO_2$ over the first 24 hours (Sharples et al. 1995). Diaspirin cross-linked hemoglobin (DCLHb) has been used in efforts to increase MAP and improve CBF. In animals, this agent also raises the CPP and results in lower fluid loads for MAP maintenance. The effects on long-term outcome have not been assessed, but DCLHb may prove to be beneficial in the early treatment of hypovolemia and CBF (Chappell et al. 1996). The physiological effects of alterations in CBF after TBI remain unclear because one study suggests a better outcome when isolated focal hyperemia is seen near intraparenchymal or extracerebral lesions. This information is confounded by the possibility that these patients may have initially sustained a less severe injury. The variations in CBF and $CMRO_2$ after a brain injury may actually represent a continuum of hemodynamic responses to injury; mild changes could be part of the normal recovery process, but extreme fluctuations may result in secondary insults to the brain that further injury and worsen outcome.

Intracranial Pressure

The normal ICP is between 0 and 10 mm Hg, and most centers involved in TBI management define an elevated ICP as any value greater than 20 mm Hg. Sustained episodes of an ICP of 25 mm Hg have been associated with increased mortality and poor outcome by many researchers (Fearnside et al. 1993; Gopinath et al. 1993; Resnick et al. 1997). Although ICP elevations can have a negative influence, a prognosis should not be made on this information alone. Favorable GOS outcomes have been reported in 38% of severe TBI patients with prolonged (>96-hour) ICP elevations. This percentage increased to 60% in younger patients and rose even further when the GCS was 5 or more (Resnick et al. 1997).

A measure that may be more important than absolute ICP is CPP. A low CPP can lead to cerebral ischemia and contribute to further neurological injury. One of the most important strategies in providing adequate cerebral oxy-

Table 56B.10:   Computed tomography findings and clinical effects

Author, year	Patient population	Computed tomography findings	Effects
Narayan et al. 1981	Adults	High-density mass lesion	Unfavorable outcome by GOS
Marshall et al. 1983	Adults	Midline shift, subdural hematoma	Clinical deterioration, mortality
Toutant et al. 1984	Adults	Compressed cisterns	Increased mortality, severe disability
Eisenberg et al. 1990	Adults	Midline shift, mass lesion, compressed cisterns, SAH	Increased mortality, elevated intracranial pressure
Marshall et al. 1991	Adults	Midline shift, mass lesion, brainstem lesion	Increased mortality
Fearnside et al. 1993	Adults	Midline shift, cerebral edema, IVH, compressed cisterns	Increased mortality
		Intracerebral contusion, SAH, hematoma	Unfavorable outcome by GOS
Aldrich et al. 1992b	Adults, penetrating injury	Midline shift, compressed cistern, SAH, IVH, hyperdense lesion	Unfavorable outcome by GOS
Aldrich et al. 1992a	<16 years	Diffuse swelling	Increased mortality

IVH = intraventricular hemorrhage; GOS = Glasgow Outcome Scale; SAH = subarachnoid hemorrhage.
Source: R Narayan, R Greenberg, J Miller, et al. Improved confidence of outcome prediction in severe head injury. A comparative analysis of the clinical examination, multimodality evoked potentials, CT scanning and intracranial pressure. J Neurosurg 1981;54:751–762; LF Marshall, DP Becker, SA Bowers, et al. The National Traumatic Coma Data Bank. J Neurosurg 1983;59:276–284; S Toutant, M Klauber, L Marshall, et al. Absent or compressed basal cisterns on first CT scan: ominous predictors of outcome in severe head injury. J Neurosurg 1984;61:691–694; LF Marshall, T Gautille, MR Klauber, et al. The outcome of severe closed head injury. J Neurosurg 1991;71(Suppl.):S28–S36; M Fearnside, R Cook, P McDougall, et al. The Westmead Head Injury Project outcome in severe head injury. A comparative analysis of pre-hospital, clinical and CT variables. Br J Neurosurg 1993;7:267–279; E Aldrich, E Eisenberg, C Saydjari, et al. Diffuse brain swelling in severely head-injured children. A report from the NIH Traumatic Coma Data Bank. J Neurosurg 1992a;76:450–454; EF Aldrich, HM Eisenberg, C Saydjari, et al. Predictors of mortality in severely head-injured patients with civilian gunshot wounds: a report from the NIH Traumatic Coma Data Bank. Surg Neurol 1992b;38:418–423.

genation is maintaining the CPP above 50 mm Hg. Rosner et al. (1995) reported on the benefits of keeping the CPP at a minimum of 70 mm Hg. Patients treated to maintain this CPP level had a 29% mortality rate. Favorable GOS outcomes ranged from 35% in patients with an initial GCS of 3 up to 75% for patients with a GCS of 7. Volume expansion, ventriculostomy drainage, vasopressors, and mannitol were used to maintain the CPP. Another study has shown the adverse effect of a CPP below 60 mm Hg (Gopinath et al. 1993). However, one study showed that, although maintaining a higher CPP resulted in a 20% reduction in the frequency of jugular oxygen desaturation, there was also a substantial increase in the frequency of acute respiratory distress syndrome, which canceled out any positive effect on outcome.

Morphological Variables

CT and MRI can provide information on injury morphology and severity. Researchers have identified specific findings on imaging studies that correlate with outcome (Table 56B.10). Abnormalities that are predictive of mortality and disability include midline shift, compression or obliteration of the mesencephalic cisterns, subarachnoid blood, intraventricular hemorrhage, large-volume mass lesions, and diffuse edema or bilateral swelling. The use of CT findings combined with prehospital and clinical variables can predict mortality with 84.4% accuracy; the same information can differentiate good from poor outcome with an accuracy

of 72.5% (Fearnside et al. 1993). The appearance of the basal cisterns on the initial CT can provide significant prognostic information. The mortality rate has been reported at 77% if the perimesencephalic cisterns are obliterated, 39% if they are compressed, and 22% if they are normal. In addition, patients with a GCS of 6–8 and obliterated cisterns had a much higher risk of unfavorable outcome than did those with normal cisterns. Diffuse hemispheric edema on CT has been associated with early hypoxia and hypotension. In children age 16 or younger, diffuse edema carries a high mortality rate (53%) compared with a rate of 16% in children without this finding. CT imaging can also be beneficial in the chronic stage after TBI. Enlargement of the width of the third ventricle suggests diencephalic atrophy and has been correlated with persistent cognitive deficits, behavioral problems, and vocational outcome (Reider-Groswasser et al. 1993). Widening of the septum-caudate distance indicates loss of the deep gray nuclei and catastrophic injury; it has been correlated with the overall prognosis for recovery from a vegetative state after severe TBI (Reider-Groswasser et al. 1997).

MRI provides greater imaging detail and may reveal lesions not seen on CT. One study found that MRI detected a greater number of lesions than did CT studies in 85% of patients with mild or moderate TBI. Decreases in brain volume and expansion of CSF spaces, as measured by MRI volumetric studies, have been correlated with poor neuropsychological outcome. This suggests that MRI volumetrics may be a useful tool in efforts to predict long-term cognitive outcome. SPECT and PET can provide information on the functional state and metabolic activity of brain tissue. These tools are beginning to have a role in the evaluation of TBI patients. SPECT shows promise in the assessment of mild-to-moderate TBI. Alterations identified on SPECT images in this population have correlated well with injury severity, and a negative early study is thought to predict a good outcome. SPECT may become a useful tool in attempts to objectify sequela in patients with persistent postconcussion complaints. PET can show focal abnormalities of uptake in regions beyond those identified by MRI and CT, which may allow for diagnostic localization of both structural and functional lesions. Dynamic and functional neuroimaging may have a future role in TBI management by providing information about cerebral function.

Duration of Coma or Post-Traumatic Amnesia

After a severe brain injury, patients can have a variable amount of time in an unresponsive and confusional state. The importance of this period has been recognized since 1932, when Ritchie Russell proposed that the sum of the comatose and confusional periods was the most useful predictor of outcome. The duration of coma provides useful information on injury severity, and in 1928, Symonds described the significant prognostic implications of this measure. When DAI is the primary injury, there is almost a linear relationship between the duration of coma and recovery time. The length of coma also has been correlated with the presence of residual impairments. One study found that none of the patients who remained comatose for more than 2 weeks had a good outcome. It was suggested that increasing periods of coma might have a proportional relationship to functional outcome. Another study suggests that the GOS is a direct reflection of whatever process determines the length of coma. Cognitive function after TBI (including memory, attention, and learning skills) has been associated with coma duration. The length of coma also relates to the ability to return to work or school (Ruff et al. 1993). In addition, the recovery of motor function after TBI has been correlated with the duration of coma. The adequate assessment and documentation of coma length should be emphasized in TBI management to provide assistance with long-term decision making and prognostic efforts.

The recovery of consciousness can proceed along a different timeline for each patient. During this process, the TBI patient demonstrates a period of PTA, or the period from injury until the patient shows continuous memory for ongoing events. PTA has been identified as the best yardstick by which to measure the severity of a head injury. The presence of PTA is often assessed prospectively by using the Galveston Orientation and Amnesia Scale, with a score of 75 marking the end of PTA. It can also be estimated retrospectively with good validity. Many researchers have reported on the powerful prognostic value of PTA duration as a measure of injury severity (Katz and Alexander 1994,

Zafonte et al. 1997b). Patients with prolonged PTA have shown more extensive tissue damage on MRI, with lesions present in both central structures and hemispheric areas. PTA has a strong predictive relationship to GOS in patients with DAI, with a direct correlation between longer duration of PTA and worse outcomes. No patients having PTA longer than 12 weeks had a good recovery, whereas 80% of patients with PTA that lasted less than 2 weeks had a good recovery (Katz and Alexander 1994). Another study found that the duration of PTA was predictive of acute rehabilitation function independence measure scores, as well as both admission and discharge disability rating scale results (Zafonte et al. 1997b). Monitoring of PTA can provide a global measurement of brain damage and is a key element in prognostic efforts after TBI.

Neurophysiological Variables

Evoked potentials can be used in the assessment of the TBI patient to evaluate the responsiveness of the CNS to external stimuli. They also provide information that can assist in outcome predictions. However, they require some expertise and are not widely used for outcome prediction. Evoked potentials that have been assessed after TBI include the somatosensory (SSEP), visual (VEP), auditory (BAEP), and P300 responses. One study found that the combined multimodality evoked potentials were the single best prognostic indicator compared with the clinical examination, CT, and ICP. Combining the multimodality evoked potentials with the clinical examination provided the greatest predictive accuracy. Many researchers have found a high predictive accuracy for poor prognosis when there is bilateral loss of the SSEP due to diffuse injury. The reliability of SSEP data increases with serial recordings. During hourly ICU monitoring, one study found that deterioration in the SSEPs often occurred before elevations of ICP, and the final summed SSEP correlated with the GOS (Konasiewicz et al. 1994). VEPs are easy to perform and interpret, but they do not have the predictive accuracy of SSEPs. Prolongation of the VEP has shown a linear relationship with changes in ICP and thus may have some relationship to outcome (Kane et al. 1996). Although generally less reliable than SSEP findings, BAEPs may be a useful monitoring tool in the acute phase after injury because these responses are the least likely to be affected by barbiturates. A potential problem in their clinical effectiveness is that they rely on an intact peripheral auditory system. Serial BAEPs can potentially give an early warning of uncal herniation because changes in the responses have been seen before pupillary changes. Often, early after injury, the TBI patient cannot undergo direct cognitive testing; at that time, these modalities can help to provide information on cognitive function. In this setting, evoked responses are best used in a serial fashion to monitor for change and assist in rehabilitation planning. In the chronic phase, the SSEP and BAEP can continue to provide predictive information, but SSEPs maintain a higher predictive value for functional recovery (Goldberg and Karazim 1998). Long-latency somatosensory and cortical auditory evoked potentials may give better prognostic information in the chronic phase after TBI. The combination of testing all three sensory modalities has demonstrated a high correlation with the patient's clinical condition in the rehabilitation setting and outcome at 1 year after injury.

An evoked potential paradigm has been used to assess cognition and neuropsychological activity. Long-latency event-related potentials are obtained in response to the infrequent presentation of a novel, brief stimulus within a background of brief, frequently repeating stimuli. The modality for the stimuli may be the same (i.e., two auditory tones) or different (i.e., visual and auditory). The long-latency event-related potential is a positive deflection that occurs approximately 300 ms (P300) after presentation of the novel stimuli, and it can be seen passively or with the patient actively counting the stimuli. This testing technique provides a means for cognitive assessment in unresponsive patients; it is thought to reflect the cortical processing of information and can be used as a measure of cognitive recovery. A prolonged latency of this response has been shown with both PTA and severe TBI (Rappaport and Clifford 1994). It has shown a very significant correlation with 3-month outcome (Kane et al. 1996), and absence of this response suggests that a patient will not regain consciousness (Rappaport and Clifford 1994).

A conventional electroencephalogram (EEG) has limited value in predicting acute events or outcome from TBI. In the early postinjury phase, there are a few EEG findings that can provide some clinical information. The presence of normal sleep spindles 48 hours or more after injury has been associated with a favorable outcome. In addition, death has been associated with the presence of an isoelectric study or repeated isoelectric intervals, nonreactive alpha, or a theta pattern of EEG activity. Late in the clinical course, a low-voltage, nonreactive EEG suggests a poor outcome. The combination of EEG reactivity with SSEP data can predict a good or bad outcome with 98% accuracy (Gutling et al. 1995). A variation of the conventional EEG called compressed spectral array has shown good prognostic accuracy for brain injury. The combination of compressed spectral array EEG with GCS at the time of the EEG has reportedly been able to discriminate between death and good outcome at 1 year with 95.8% accuracy. In general, these neurophysiological studies are most useful for predicting survival in the acute unresponsive period after severe TBI.

CONCLUSION

TBI remains a major public health problem. Since the 1970s, significant improvements have been made in the emergency care of the trauma patient. Along with better critical care, this appears to have resulted in a substantial decline in the mortality and morbidity associated with this condition. Although much has been learned about the pathophysiology of TBI, to date no single effective agent has been found for the treatment of the injured brain. Several approaches are being explored and will no doubt ultimately prove helpful. Nevertheless, meticulous attention to detail in maintaining normal homeostasis in the injured patient remains the cornerstone of management. Some key principles of in-hospital care include early and liberal use of CT scanning; prompt evacuation of intracranial mass lesions; aggressive correction of hypotension and hypoxia; avoiding hyperglycemia, hyponatremia and hyperthermia; maintaining cerebral perfusion by continuous monitoring of ICP and blood pressure; and the use of all available measures to keep ICP under control.

REFERENCES

Asikainen I, Kaste M, Sarna S. Patients with traumatic brain injury referred to a rehabilitation and re-employment programme: social and professional outcome for 508 Finnish patients 5 or more years after injury. Brain Inj 1996;10:883–899.

Bouma G, Muizelaar J. Cerebral blood flow in severe clinical head injury. New Horiz 1995;3:384–394.

Bullock R, Chesnut R, Clifton G, et al. Guidelines for the management of severe head injury. J Neurotrauma 1996;13:639–734.

Chappell J, McBride W, Shackford S. Diaspirin cross-linked hemoglobin resuscitation improves cerebral perfusion after head injury and shock. J Trauma 1996;41:781–788.

Chesnut RM, Marshall LF, Klauber MR, et al. The role of secondary brain injury in determining outcome from severe head injury. J Trauma 1993a;34:216–222.

Chesnut RM, Marshall LF, Piek J, et al. Early and late systemic hypotension as a frequent and fundamental source of cerebral ischemia following severe brain injury in the Traumatic Coma Data Bank. Acta Neurochir Suppl (Wien) 1993b;59: 121–125.

Cifu D, Kreutzer J, Marwitz J, et al. Functional outcomes of older adults with traumatic brain injury: a prospective, multicenter analysis. Arch Phys Med Rehabil 1996;77:883–888.

Clifton GL, Allen S, Barrodale P, et al. A phase II study of moderate hypothermia in severe brain injury. J Neurotrauma 1993; 10:263–271.

Corrigan JD. Substance abuse as a mediating factor in outcome from traumatic brain injury. Arch Phys Med Rehabil 1995; 76:302–309.

Fearnside M, Cook R, McDougall P, et al. The Westmead Head Injury Project outcome in severe head injury. A comparative analysis of pre-hospital, clinical and CT variables. Br J Neurosurg 1993;7:267–279.

Goldberg G, Karazim E. Application of evoked potentials to the prediction of discharge status in minimally responsive patients: a pilot study. J Head Trauma Rehabil 1998;13:51–68.

Goldstein F, Levin H, Presley R, et al. Neurobehavioral consequences of closed head injury in older adults. J Neurol Neurosurg Psychiatry 1994;57:961–966.

Gopinath S, Contant C, Robertson C, et al. Critical thresholds for physiological parameters in patients with severe head injury. Congress of Neurological Surgeons Annual Meeting. Vancouver, British Columbia, 1993.

Greene K, Jacobowitz R, Marciano F, et al. Impact of traumatic subarachnoid hemorrhage on outcome in non-penetrating head injury. Part II: Relationship to clinical course and outcome variables during acute hospitalization. J Trauma 1997; 42:964–971.

Gutling E, Gonser A, Imhof H, et al. EEG reactivity in the prognosis of severe head injury. Neurology 1995;45:915–918.

Heinzelmann M, Platz A, Imhof H. Outcome after acute extradural haematoma, influence of additional injuries and neurological complications in the ICU. Injury 1996;27:345–349.

Hsiang J, Yeung T, Yu A, et al. High risk mild head injury. J Neurosurg 1997;87:234–238.

Jennett B. Epidemiology of head injury. J Neurol Neurosurg Psychiatry 1996;60:362–369.

Jordan B, Relkin N, Ravdin L, et al. Apolipoprotein E episolon4 associated with chronic traumatic brain injury in boxing. JAMA 1997;278:136–140.

Kane N, Curry S, Rowlands C, et al. Event-related potentials-neurophysiological tools for predicting emergence and early outcome from traumatic coma. Intensive Care Med 1996;22: 39–46.

Katz D, Alexander M. Traumatic brain injury: predicting course of recovery and outcome for patients admitted to rehabilitation. Arch Neurol 1994;51:661–670.

Kelly D, Kordestani R, Martin N, et al. Hyperemia following traumatic brain injury: relationship to intracranial hypertension and outcome. J Neurosurg 1996;85:762–771.

Kelly D, Martin N, Kordestani R, et al. Cerebral blood flow as a predictor of outcome following traumatic brain injury. J Neurosurg 1997;86:633–641.

Kelly M, Johnson C, Knoller N, et al. Substance abuse, traumatic brain injury and neuropsychological outcome. Brain Inj 1997;11:391–402.

Kiening K, Hartl R, Unterberg A, et al. Brain tissue pO_2 monitoring in comatose patients: implications for therapy. Neurol Res 1997;19:233–240.

Kilaru S, Garb J, Emhoff T, et al. Long term functional status and mortality of elderly patients with severe closed head injury. J Trauma 1996;41:957–963.

Kirkpatrick P, Smielewski P, Czoynka M, et al. Near-infrared spectroscopy use in patients with head injury. J Neurosurg 1995;83:963–970.

Konasiewicz S, Moulton R, Shedden P. Somatosensory evoked potentials and intracranial pressure in severe head injury. Can J Neurol Sci 1994;21:219–226.

Kraus JF, McArthur DL, Silverman TA, Jayaraman M. Epidemiology of Brain Injury. In RK Narayan, JE Wilberger, JT Povlishock (eds), Neurotrauma. New York: McGraw-Hill, 1996.

LeRoux P, Newell D, Lam A, et al. Cerebral arteriovenous oxygen difference: a predictor of cerebral infarction and outcome in patients with severe head injury. J Neurosurg 1997;87:1–8.

Levin H. Outcome from Mild Head Injury. In RK Narayan, JE Wilberger, JT Povlishock (eds), Neurotrauma. New York: McGraw-Hill, 1996.

Levy M, Masri L, Levy K, et al. Penetrating craniocerebral injury resultant from gunshot wounds: gang-related injury in children and adolescents. Neurosurgery 1993;33:1018–1024.

Lu W, Rhoney D, Boling WB, et al. A review of stress ulcer prophylaxis in the neurosurgical intensive care unit. Neurosurgery 1997;41:416–426.

Marion DW, Penrod LE, Kelsey SF, et al. Treatment of traumatic brain injury with moderate hypothermia. N Engl J Med 1997;336:540–546.

Masson F, Maurette P, Salmi L, et al. Prevalence of impairments 5 years after a head injury, and their relationship with disabilities and outcome. Brain Inj 1996;10:487–497.

Meagher RJ, Narayan RK. The triage and acute management of severe head injury. Clin Neurosurg 1999;46:in press.

Narayan RK, Wilberger JE, Povlishock JT (eds). Neurotrauma. New York: McGraw-Hill, 1996.

Pigula FA, Wald SL, Shackford SR, et al. The effect of hypotension and hypoxia on children with severe head injuries. J Pediatr Surg 1993;28:310–314.

Quigley MR, Vidovich D, Cantella D. Defining the limits of survivorship after very severe head injury. J Trauma 1997;42:7–10.

Rappaport M, Clifford J. Comparison of passive P300 brain evoked potentials in normal and severely traumatically brain injured patients. J Head Trauma Rehabil 1994;9:94–104.

Reider-Groswasser I, Cohen M, Costeff H, et al. Late CT findings in brain trauma: relationship to cognitive and behavioral sequelae and to vocational outcome. AJR Am J Roentgenol 1993; 160:147–152.

Reider-Groswasser I, Costeff H, Sazbon L, et al. CT findings in persistent vegetative state following blunt traumatic brain injury. Brain Inj 1997;11:865–870.

Resnick D, Marion D, Carlier P. Outcome analysis of patients with severe head injuries and prolonged intracranial hypertension. J Trauma 1997;42:1108–1111.

Robertson CS, Gopinath SP, Goodman JC, et al. $SjvO_2$ monitoring in head-injured patients. J Neurotrauma 1995;12:891–896.

Roof R, Duvdevani R, Heyburn J, et al. Progesterone rapidly decreases brain edema: treatment delayed up to 24 hours is still effective. Exp Neurol 1996;138:246–251.

Rosner MJ, Rosner SD, Johnson AH. Cerebral perfusion pressure: management protocol and clinical results. J Neurosurg 1995; 83:949–962.

Sharples P, Stuart A, Matthews D, et al. Cerebral blood flow and metabolism in children with severe head injury. Part I: relation to age, Glasgow Coma Score, outcome, intracranial pressure, and time after injury. J Neurol Neurosurg Psychiatry 1995;58: 145–152.

Siegel JH. The effect of associated injuries, blood loss, and oxygen debt on death and disability in blunt traumatic brain injury: the need for early physiologic predictors of severity. J Neurotrauma 1995;12:579–590.

Sosin DM, Sniezek JE, Waxweiler RJ. Trends in death associated with traumatic brain injury, 1979 through 1992. Success and failure. JAMA 1995;273:1778–1780.

Vassar M, Fischer R, O'Brien P, et al. A multicenter trial for resuscitation of injured patients with 7.5% sodium chloride. The effect of added dextran 70. The Multicenter Group for the Study of Hypertonic Saline in Trauma Patients. Arch Surg 1993;128:1003–1011.

Wade C, Grady J, Kramer G, et al. Individual patient cohort analysis of the efficacy of hypertonic saline/dextran in patients with traumatic brain injury and hypotension. J Trauma 1997;42: S61–S65.

Wald S, Shackford S, Fenwick J. The effect of secondary insults on mortality and long-term disability after severe head injury in a rural region without a trauma system. J Trauma 1993;34: 377–381.

Winchell R, Simons R, Hoyt D. Transient systolic hypotension. A serious problem in the management of head injury. Arch Surg 1996;131:533–539.

Zafonte RD, Mann NR, Mills SR, et al. Posttraumatic amnesia: its relation to functional outcome. Arch Phys Med Rehabil 1997b;78:1103–1106.

Chapter 56
Trauma of the Nervous System

C. SPINAL CORD TRAUMA
Charles H. Tator and Ghassan S. Skaf

Recognition of spinal cord injury (SCI) can be difficult in the acute phase, especially in the context of multiple traumas or multiple metastatic disease. Patients with congenital anomalies and spinal arthropathies, including cervical spondylosis, ankylosing spondylitis, and spinal stenosis, are predisposed to develop SCI. Effective management of the acute SCI patient depends on an appreciation of how the injury occurred, knowledge of the epidemiology of SCI, and accurate clinical examination and classification of the neurological injury. Also important are detailed radiological assessment of the injuries to the vertebral column, spinal cord, and nerve roots, and an understanding of the principles of medical and surgical treatment. Based on accurate clinical and radiological assessments, a rational treatment plan can be made and a reasonable prediction of prognosis offered.

The most useful classification for clinical purposes is based on assessment of the neurological deficit based on the clinical examination rather than on other criteria, such as the pathological, electrophysiological, or imaging features. The neurological assessment and classification must be robust and reliable so that serial observations by the same or different observers will provide reliable sequential comparisons. Reliability is essential for the management of individual patients, for longitudinal studies at one institution, and for comparison with other institutions in research projects. The American Spinal Injury Association (ASIA) and the International Medical Society of Paraplegia (IMSOP) published the International Standards for Neurological and Functional Classification of Spinal Cord Injury in 1992.

This classification is now the international standard and should be used by all physicians and surgeons managing patients with acute SCI, just as the Glasgow Coma Scale is used to assess head injuries.

High-resolution imaging of patients with spinal injuries is fundamental to the detection, classification, and management of these injuries and is also essential for the determination of spinal stability. Accurate imaging is an important step in preventing further neurological compromise, which can result from spinal instability. Noninvasive imaging techniques have undergone a remarkable evolution since the 1970s with the introduction of multiplanar computerized reconstruction techniques, such as computed tomography (CT) and magnetic resonance imaging (MRI). These noninvasive techniques allow rapid diagnosis and provide the patient with the best chance for recovery by facilitating early management based on precise imaging information about the spinal column and neurological injuries.

Advances in the understanding of the pathophysiological processes underlying acute SCI have led to significant improvements in clinical management. The treatment of acute SCI has three primary goals: maximized neurological recovery, spinal stabilization, and early mobilization and rehabilitation. Achieving these goals requires a logical management scheme that begins in the prehospital phase and includes careful extrication, stabilization, immobilization, and transportation of victims to the hospital and continues through the in-hospital imaging studies, acute management, and surgical treatment. This chapter focuses on clinical

Table 56C.1:   Age and gender of patients with spinal cord injury

Age (yrs)	Percentage of patients
Birth–10	10
11–20	20
21–30	25
31–40	15
41–50	10
51–60	10
Over 60	10
Total	100
Gender	
Male	80–85
Female	15–20

Source: Reprinted with permission from CH Tator, EG Duncan, VE Edmonds, et al. Changes in epidemiology of acute spinal cord injury from 1947 to 1981. Surg Neurol 1993;40:207–215.

manifestations and radiographic findings and provides a comprehensive overall management approach to the acute care of SCI.

EPIDEMIOLOGY AND CAUSES OF SPINAL CORD INJURY

Acute SCI is relatively uncommon, affecting about 1 in 40 patients who present to a major trauma center. Significant head injuries are five to 10 times more common than SCIs, but a considerable number of patients have both. About 5–10% of head-injured patients have an associated spinal injury, and about 25% of SCI patients have an associated head injury. Estimates of the annual incidence of SCI in developed countries vary from 11.5 to 53.4 per million people. There are about 10,000 new acute SCI cases per year in the United States. Spinal injuries without neurological deficit are much more common than those with neurological deficits.

Males compose 80–85% of patients with SCI. Although SCI occurs at all ages, patients younger than age 30 compose the majority of victims (Table 56C.1). In 1975, the case fatality rate was almost 50%, with 80% of the fatalities occurring at the scene of the accident or by the time of arrival at the hospital. For those who survive to reach the hospital, reported mortality rates range from 4.4% to 16.7%. SCI patients experience multiple ongoing neurological and medical problems that may require prolonged hospitalization or several stays in acute treatment units and rehabilitation centers (Tator et al. 1993a). Often associated with these physical injuries is significant damage to the social and psychological well-being of patients and their families. The financial burden of SCI to the patient, the health care system, and society is great (Tator et al. 1993a). Added to the expenses for acute and long-term management are indirect costs from lost income and lost productivity. In 1990, the cost to the United States of caring for all SCI patients was estimated to be $4 billion.

Approximately 55% of injuries to the spinal cord occur in the cervical spine region, with approximately 15% of injuries in each of the other three regions: thoracic, lumbar, and sacral. The areas most liable to spinal trauma are those with the greatest mobility: the cervical spine (C5-C7) and the thoracolumbar spine (T10-L2).

There are considerable differences among countries, and even among regions within one country (e.g., urban and rural), with respect to the causes of SCI. In addition, the causes and effects of SCI differ among various age groups; for example, younger victims have a greater preponderance of injuries due to high-velocity, high-impact forces due to high-risk activities, such as traffic accidents, motor sports, and diving. Younger victims are subject to physiological factors that affect the spine, such as undeveloped paraspinal musculature and more elastic ligaments. Older victims tend to have more rigid spines and additional pathological features, such as osteoporosis or pre-existing cervical or lumbar spondylosis.

In developed countries, traffic accidents are the most common causes of SCI, accounting for about 50% of all SCIs. Alcohol is a contributing factor in approximately 25% of all cases of SCI. Other drugs are a factor in a much smaller number of patients (Tator et al. 1993b). Sports and recreational causes of injury have increased in many developed countries, and in some countries they have replaced work-related injuries as the second most frequent cause of SCI. The sports and recreational activities that are responsible for this increase combine risk-taking and very high physical forces on the vertebral column, such as rock climbing, parachuting, surfing, and diving. In some locations, sports and recreational causes account for up to 25% of SCI. Diving results in about 1,000 SCIs per year in the United States, with 95% of these resulting in quadriplegia. Conversely, work accidents in some countries have diminished as safer practices have been promulgated and targeted prevention programs instituted, especially in the mining, logging, and construction industries. Falls (especially at home) are the third most common cause of SCIs. Indeed, in individuals older than 65 and in many less-developed countries, falls may even exceed traffic accidents as a cause of SCI. Violence (including homicide, suicide, and war) as a cause of SCI has shown a substantial increase in the past 10 years, especially in some developed countries. Indeed, in some locations, violence has become the most common cause of SCI (Sutherland 1993).

SEVERITY OF NEUROLOGICAL INJURY: AMERICAN SPINAL INJURY ASSOCIATION/INTERNATIONAL MEDICAL SOCIETY OF PARAPLEGIA IMPAIRMENT SCALE

The ASIA/IMSOP scale contains five grades of impairment (Table 56C.2). *Completeness* in grade A is defined as absence of sensory and motor function in the lowest sacral segment. Grade B describes a patient who has only sensory preservation below the level of injury. The scale defines the function in grades C and D on the basis of the Medical

Table 56C.2: American Spinal Injury Association/International Medical Society of Paraplegia Impairment Scale*

Grade A—complete	No motor or sensory function is preserved in the sacral segments S4 and S5.
Grade B—incomplete	Sensory but not motor function is preserved below the neurological level and extends through the sacral segments S4 and S5.
Grade C—incomplete	Motor function is preserved below the neurological level, and the majority of key muscles below the neurological level have a muscle grade <3.
Grade D—incomplete	Motor function is preserved below the neurological level, and the majority of key muscles below the neurological level have a muscle grade ≥3.
Grade E—normal	Motor and sensory functions are normal.

*Classification of spinal cord injury is based on the International Standards for Neurological and Functional Classification of Spinal Cord Injury by the American Spinal Injury Association and the International Medical Society of Paraplegia.

Research Council muscle grading system. Grade E denotes a patient with normal motor and sensory spinal cord function.

Effect of Associated Spinal Pathological States

The most common pre-existing abnormality of the spinal column that predisposes to SCI is cervical spondylosis. In some series, this condition is present in about 10% of patients with SCI (Tator et al. 1993b). Less common pathological entities include congenital anomalies, such as congenital fusion (Klippel-Feil syndrome); metastatic spinal disease with pathological fractures; and spinal arthropathies, such as ankylosing spondylitis or rheumatoid arthritis. When trauma is superimposed on a pre-existing condition, such as an acute flexion injury in a patient with a congenital os odontoideum or with Down syndrome contributing to atlantoaxial dislocation, much less force than normal is required to produce SCI.

Effect of Multiple Trauma

Isolated SCI is present in only about 20% of SCI patients. About 20% of patients with SCI have other major injuries, such as cerebral contusion or flail chest, which reduce neurological recovery and increase mortality. The reduced neurological recovery in multiple trauma may be related to systemic hypoxia or hypotension, which are frequent in patients with multiple trauma. In addition, the SCIs in multiple-trauma patients tend to be more severe than in those with isolated SCI.

The management of patients with SCI in the presence of multiple trauma is a great challenge because of the many difficulties and potential pitfalls. For example, intubation to maintain adequate airway may be extremely hazardous in

Table 56C.3: Etiology, vertebral level, severity of neurological injury, and type of bony injury in adult spinal cord injury

	Percentage of injuries
Cause of injury	
Traffic accidents (motor vehicle, bicycle, pedestrian)	40–50
Work	10–25
Sports and recreation	10–25
Falls (home, elsewhere)	20
Violence	10–25
Level of injury	
Cervical (C1 to C7-T1)	55
Thoracic (T1-T11)	15
Thoracolumbar (T11-T12 to L1-L2)	15
Lumbosacral (L2-S5)	15
Severity of neurological injury (ASIA/IMSOP scale)	
Complete	
Grade A	45
Incomplete	
Grade B	15
Grade C	10
Grade D	30
Type of bony injury	
Minor fracture (including compression)	10
Fracture dislocation	40
Dislocation only	5
Burst fracture	30
SCIWORA	5
SCIWORET(including osteoarthritis and cervical spondylosis)	10

ASIA/IMSOP = American Spinal Injury Association/International Medical Society of Paraplegia; SCIWORA = spinal cord injury without radiological abnormality; SCIWORET = spinal cord injury without radiological evidence of trauma.
Source: Reprinted with permission from CH Tator, EG Duncan, VE Edmonds, et al. Changes in epidemiology of acute spinal cord injury from 1947 to 1981. Surg Neurol 1993;40:207–215.

the presence of a cervical SCI. Hypoxia due to diaphragmatic or intercostal muscle paralysis is common in patients with cervical SCI. Abdominal distention, ileus, vomiting, and aspiration may add to the hypoxia. Hypotension is often present in SCI with multiple trauma due to a combination of spinal neurogenic shock with systemic shock. Patients with SCI, especially those with cervical injuries, lose sympathetic activity (Kiss and Tator 1993), and unopposed vagotonia may cause cardiac arrhythmia or even reflex cardiac arrest. Intra-abdominal hemorrhage or visceral rupture in patients with SCI may be overlooked because lost spinal cord transmission prevents the development of the typical symptoms and physical findings associated with those conditions.

Effect of Level and Type of Vertebral Column Injury

Table 56C.3 shows the types and levels of vertebral column injuries encountered in patients with SCI. In thoracic injuries there is a higher frequency of complete neurological injury than in cervical or thoracolumbar cord injuries. In the senior author's analysis of 358 patients with SCI, the 71 thoracic injuries showed a significantly higher frequency of complete injuries (77.5% complete) than did the 202 cases of cervical injuries (60.4% complete) or the 85 cases of thoracolumbar cord injuries from T11-T12 to L1-L2 (64.7% complete) (Tator 1993b). In complete injuries, neurological recovery was greatest in patients with cervical injuries, second in those with thoracic injuries, and lowest in those with thoracolumbar injuries. In all three regions, the ability of patients with incomplete injuries to recover was related to the severity of the initial neurological deficit: The greater the deficit at admission, the less the neurological recovery.

Anterior dislocations and fracture dislocations are more likely to cause complete cord injuries than are compression fractures or burst fractures. Improved imaging by CT and MRI has reduced markedly the relative frequency of patients previously described as having SCI without radiological abnormality (SCIWORA) and has increased the recognition of burst fractures and intracanalicular bone and disc material compressing the spinal cord. There is still a significant number of patients, especially children, with true SCIWORA. Improved imaging, particularly high-resolution bone window CT, also has improved the ability to diagnose the offending associated lesion in patients with acute SCI without radiological evidence of trauma (SCIWORET) (Tator 1996a). The majority of these patients have cervical spondylosis, and the remainder have congenital anomalies.

CLINICAL MANIFESTATIONS OF ACUTE SPINAL CORD INJURY

Level of Spinal Cord Injury

In the past, clinicians used many different ways of defining the level of an SCI. The ASIA/IMSOP classification provides precise definitions for the neurological level, sensory level, skeletal level, and zone of partial preservation (Figure 56C.1). The neurological level is the most caudal segment of the spinal cord having normal sensory and motor function on both sides of the body. Because normal segments may differ on the two sides and in terms of motor and sensory function, up to four different segments may be identified in determining the neurological level (i.e., right sensory, left sensory, right motor, and left motor). The terms *sensory level* and *motor level* are defined as the most caudal segment of the cord having normal sensory or motor function on both sides of the body. These levels are determined by neurological examination of a key sensory point in each of the 28 right and 28 left dermatomes and a key muscle in each of the 10 right and 10 left myotomes. The *zone of partial preservation* is defined as encompassing the dermatomes and myotomes caudal to the neurological level that remain partially innervated in complete injuries. The *skeletal level* of an injury is defined as the level of greatest

vertebral damage on radiological examination. The skeletal and neurological levels may be similar or may differ by one or more segments.

Complete versus Incomplete Injury

The ASIA/IMSOP grading scale (see Table 56C.2) is very precise, especially with respect to the important distinction between *complete* and *incomplete*. For this designation, it is absolutely essential for the clinician to test touch and pinprick sensation in the lowest sacral dermatomes, perianally at the mucocutaneous junction, and deep anal sensation. Also, voluntary motor contraction of the external anal sphincter must be tested by digital examination. The distinction between complete and incomplete is crucial for planning treatment and predicting outcome.

Until about 1970, approximately two-thirds of patients with acute SCI had clinically complete injuries on admission to tertiary care facilities. Since then, there has been a reversal, so that in the 1990s, approximately two-thirds of patients arriving have incomplete injuries. The reasons for this significant epidemiological change are likely related to earlier referral and time of arrival; better prehospital first-aid care, including better management of systemic and neurogenic shock; less mishandling by untrained people; and increased use of seat belts.

For cervical, thoracic, and thoracolumbar cord injuries, the prognosis for neurological recovery is vastly better in incomplete than in complete injuries. Nevertheless, reports of large series of acute SCI patients have almost always included a small percentage of initially complete cases with significant recovery of distal cord function: Approximately 1–2% of patients with complete injuries become ambulatory. Nihilists might argue that complete injuries that recover always represent difficulties encountered in performing the initial neurological assessment due to inebriation, sedative or other drug effects, spinal shock, lack of cooperation, or a concomitant head injury. We believe that approximately 1–2% of patients with complete cord injuries recover some distal cord function, even in the absence of all the factors just noted that interfere with precise, early classification, and that early appropriate treatment can increase the number. Some physiologically intact fibers can be detected in the subacute or chronic stage by electrical stimulation in SCI patients who were initially thought to have complete lesions (the so-called dis-complete syndrome), which supports our theory. Pathological studies of the cord in the majority of complete cases show some preserved neural tissue at the injury site (Bunge et al. 1993).

Spinal Shock

Spinal shock occurs in major SCI and can be a source of considerable confusion. It must be distinguished from sys-

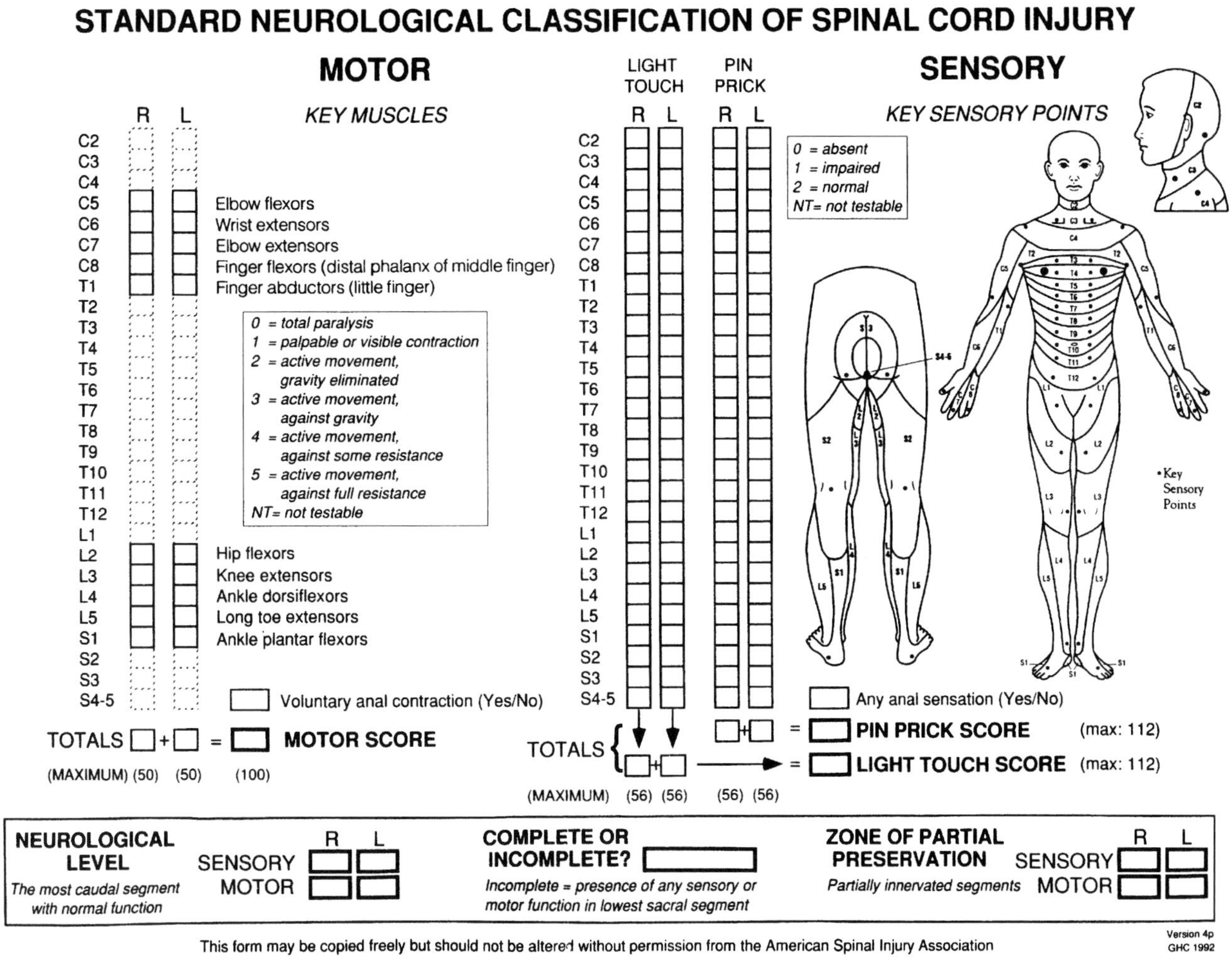

STANDARD NEUROLOGICAL CLASSIFICATION OF SPINAL CORD INJURY

MOTOR

KEY MUSCLES

R L

C2
C3
C4
C5 Elbow flexors
C6 Wrist extensors
C7 Elbow extensors
C8 Finger flexors (distal phalanx of middle finger)
T1 Finger abductors (little finger)
T2
T3
T4
T5
T6
T7
T8
T9
T10
T11
T12

0 = total paralysis
1 = palpable or visible contraction
2 = active movement, gravity eliminated
3 = active movement, against gravity
4 = active movement, against some resistance
5 = active movement, against full resistance
NT= not testable

L1
L2 Hip flexors
L3 Knee extensors
L4 Ankle dorsiflexors
L5 Long toe extensors
S1 Ankle plantar flexors
S2
S3
S4-5

☐ Voluntary anal contraction (Yes/No)

TOTALS ☐ + ☐ = ☐ **MOTOR SCORE**

(MAXIMUM) (50) (50) (100)

LIGHT TOUCH PIN PRICK

R L R L

C2
C3
C4
C5
C6
C7
C8
T1
T2
T3
T4
T5
T6
T7
T8
T9
T10
T11
T12
L1
L2
L3
L4
L5
S1
S2
S3
S4-5

Any anal sensation (Yes/No)

TOTALS { ☐+☐ = ☐ **PIN PRICK SCORE** (max: 112)
        { ☐+☐ → = ☐ **LIGHT TOUCH SCORE** (max: 112)

(MAXIMUM) (56) (56) (56) (56)

SENSORY

KEY SENSORY POINTS

0 = absent
1 = impaired
2 = normal
NT= not testable

• Key Sensory Points

NEUROLOGICAL LEVEL		**COMPLETE OR INCOMPLETE?**	**ZONE OF PARTIAL PRESERVATION**	
The most caudal segment with normal function	SENSORY R ☐ L ☐ MOTOR R ☐ L ☐	Incomplete = presence of any sensory or motor function in lowest sacral segment	Partially innervated segments	SENSORY R ☐ L ☐ MOTOR R ☐ L ☐

This form may be copied freely but should not be altered without permission from the American Spinal Injury Association

Version 4p
GHC 1992

FIGURE 56C.1 Neurological classification of spinal cord injury by the American Spinal Injury Association/International Medical Society of Paraplegia. This diagram contains the principal information about motor, sensory, and sphincter function necessary for accurate classification and scoring of acute spinal cord injuries. The 10 key muscles to be tested for the motor examination are shown on the left, along with the Medical Research Council grading system. The 28 dermatomes to be tested on each side for the sensory examination are shown on the right. The system for recording the neurological level, the completeness of the injury, and the zone of partial preservation (in complete injuries) is shown at the bottom.

temic shock, which can also occur in spinal cord–injured patients (e.g., in a thoracic cord injury with a concomitant aortic injury). Spinal shock involves the loss of somatic motor, sensory, and sympathetic autonomic function due to SCI (Kiss and Tator 1993). The more severe and the higher the level of SCI, the greater the severity and duration of spinal shock. Thus, spinal shock is most severe in complete upper cervical cord injuries, less severe in incomplete thoracic injuries, and minimal in all lumbar cord injuries. The somatic motor component of spinal shock consists of paralysis, flaccidity, and areflexia with respect to deep tendon reflexes and cutaneous reflexes. The sensory component of spinal shock is anesthesia to all modalities; the autonomic component is systemic hypotension, skin hyperemia and warmth, and bradycardia due to loss of sympathetic function with persisting parasympathetic function (unopposed vagotonia). The exact mechanism of spinal shock is unknown but may be related to temporary electrolyte or neurotransmitter effects on impulse conduction. The major difficulty in clinical examination occurs in the first few hours and days after SCI, when there is an admixture of the physiological, temporary effects of spinal shock and the pathological, more permanent effects of the SCI. Another problem is the variable duration of spinal shock. It is recommended that clinicians use the following guidelines: The somatic motor and sensory components of spinal shock last only an hour or less and thus have ended by the time most patients are examined in the first hospital reached. (In most countries, a hospital is now within 1–4 hours of injury.) In contrast, the reflex and autonomic components of spinal shock may last days to months, depending on the level and severity of SCI. In practical terms, this means that motor and sensory deficits detected 1 hour or longer after SCI are due to physical cord injury rather than to spinal shock. Fol-

Table 56C.4:   Acute spinal cord injury syndromes in trauma patients

Complete spinal cord injury: ASIA/IMSOP grade A
Unilevel—no zone of partial preservation
Multiple level—with zone of partial preservation
Incomplete spinal cord injury—ASIA/IMSOP grades B, C, and D
Cervicomedullary syndrome
Central cord syndrome
Anterior cord syndrome
Posterior cord syndrome
Brown-Séquard's syndrome
Conus medullaris syndrome
Complete cauda equina injury: ASIA/IMSOP grade A
Incomplete cauda equina injury: ASIA/IMSOP grades B, C, and D

ASIA/IMSOP = American Spinal Injury Association/International Medical Society of Paraplegia.
Source: Reprinted with permission from CH Tator, EG Duncan, VE Edmonds, et al. Changes in epidemiology of acute spinal cord injury from 1947 to 1981. Surg Neurol 1993;40:207–215.

lowing these guidelines will help eliminate the possible error of missing a serious SCI that occurs because the observed deficits were presumed to be due to spinal shock.

Incomplete Acute Spinal Cord Injury Syndromes

Table 56C.4 shows the large variety of incomplete acute neurological syndromes occurring in SCI. In general, these syndromes are named according to the presumed location of the injury in the transverse plane of the spinal cord (Tator 1994). It is very helpful to categorize the patients with incomplete injury according to the location of the cord injury for two reasons. First, recognition of the type of incomplete syndrome gives some information about the mechanism of injury, which provides useful information for selection of treatment. Second, the various categories of incomplete injury have different prognoses for recovery.

Cervicomedullary Syndrome
(Upper Cervical Cord to Medulla)

A high proportion of injuries to the upper cervical cord also includes damage to the medulla. These injuries may extend down to C4 or even lower in the cord and up to the pons, either due to direct injury or vascular injury to the vertebral arteries. *Cervicomedullary syndrome* is a useful term to describe these syndromes, which involve the upper cervical cord and brainstem, although several other terms have been used, including *bulbar-cervical dissociation pattern*. The essential features of these syndromes in their severe forms include respiratory arrest, hypotension, tetraplegia, and anesthesia from C1 to C4 with sensory loss over the face conforming to the onionskin or Dejerine pattern of perioral sparing. The higher the lesion, the more severe the manifestations, such as those present in patients with atlanto-occipital dislocation. The mechanisms of cord injury include traction injury from severe dislocation, anteroposterior compression from burst fracture, ruptured disc, or odontoid displacement.

Accurate physical examination and knowledge of the neuroanatomy of this region aid in our understanding of the clinical manifestations of this syndrome. The highest fibers to cross the midline from the descending trigeminal nucleus and tract are those carrying perioral sensation. Fibers carrying sensation from the ear cross at the most caudal region of the descending trigeminal nucleus. This results in the onionskin or Dejerine pattern of sensory impairment on the face due to medullary and high cervical lesions. A high central medullary lesion can produce loss of pinprick sensation in the perioral region. A lesion in the lower medulla and upper cervical cord produces a more peripheral facial distribution of sensory loss involving the forehead, ear, and chin, with perioral sparing.

Cervicomedullary injuries may mimic the central cord syndrome because of the presence of greater arm than leg weakness. Classically, this feature has been attributed to the anatomical arrangement of the decussating fibers in the pyramidal tract at the cervicomedullary junction, accounting for the syndrome of cruciate paralysis of Bell. It is postulated that the pyramidal decussation in the ventrolateral aspect of the cervicomedullary junction is anatomically susceptible to compression by the odontoid process and the anterior rim of the foramen magnum. Therefore, it is thought that the motor fibers to the upper extremities decussate rostral and ventral to those of the lower extremities and then assume a medial position in the lateral corticospinal tract between the medulla and C1 (Figure 56C.2). Conversely, the lower-extremity fibers that lie lateral to the arm fibers in the medulla continue caudally in this position to decussate between C1 and C2. By the time these fiber pathways reach the C2 level, they have crossed completely, to assume a lateral position in the lateral corticospinal tract (Figure 56C.3; see also Figure 56C.2). Thus, an injury at the medulla-C1 junction would damage the fibers from the upper limb that are crossing at this level and spare the uncrossed lower limb fibers of the corticospinal tract, to produce selective bilateral arm paralysis. There is considerable controversy about this anatomical explanation for the syndrome of cruciate paralysis because several authors have found no evidence for the presumed different sites of decussation of the arm and leg fibers in the corticospinal tract. Evidence suggests that the arm and leg fibers intermingle in the pyramidal decussation (Levi et al. 1996). In monkeys, there is anatomical evidence for alternative explanations, such as the finding that arm fibers only are present in the uncrossed ventral corticospinal tract, which suggests that injury confined to this tract might account for the arms being preferentially affected.

Acute Central Cord Syndrome

Schneider described the acute central cervical SCI syndrome, which is characterized by a disproportionately greater loss of

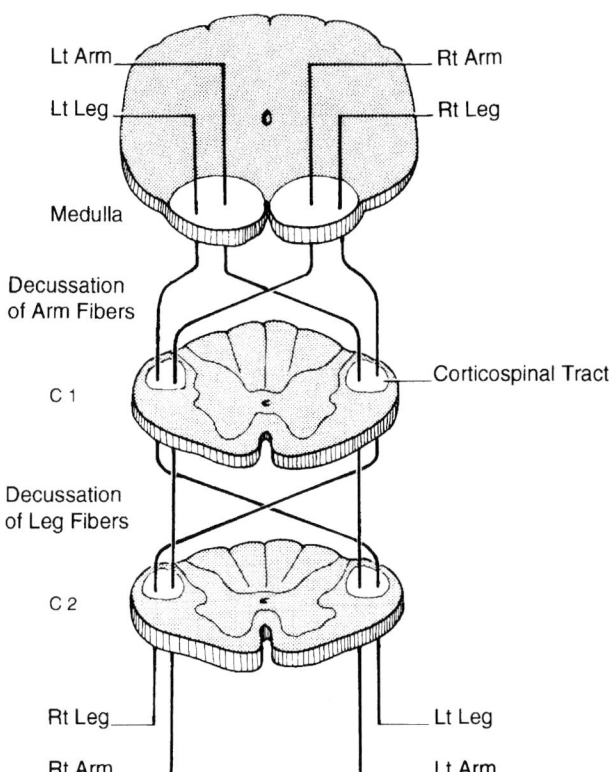

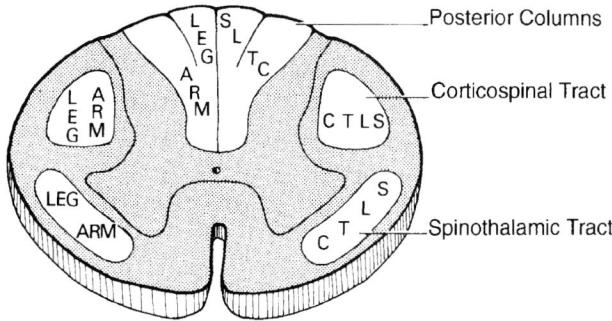

FIGURE 56C.3 Topographic distribution in the posterior columns, corticospinal, and spinothalamic tracts. The locations of the axons subserving arm and leg function are shown in the three tracts. Similarly, the locations of the axons subserving sacral (S), lumbar (L), thoracic (T), and cervical (C) function in the three tracts are indicated. (Reprinted with permission from CH Tator. Classification of Spinal Cord Injury Based on Neurological Presentation. In RJ Narayan, JE Wilberger Jr, JT Povlishock [eds], Neurotrauma. New York: McGraw-Hill, 1994;1059–1073.)

FIGURE 56C.2 The crossing of the axons in the corticospinal tracts. The upper, middle, and lower cross sections show the medulla, the spinal cord at C1, and the spinal cord at C2, respectively. The axons subserving arm function cross the midline between the medulla and C1, whereas those subserving leg function cross between Cl and C2. As noted in the text, recent evidence does not support the lamination concept in the corticospinal tract. (Reprinted with permission from CH Tator. Classification of Spinal Cord Injury Based on Neurological Presentation. In RJ Narayan, JE Wilberger Jr, JT Povlishock [eds], Neurotrauma. New York: McGraw-Hill, 1994;1059–1073.)

motor power in the upper extremities than in the lower extremities, with varying degrees of sensory loss. Many cases recovered spontaneously without surgical treatment, even though he hypothesized that acute compression was often an etiological factor. For example, he theorized that this syndrome in many older people who also had cervical spondylosis was due to central hematomyelia and surrounding "edematomyelia" due to anterior-posterior compression of the cord during hyperextension injury. In the hyperextension injury, the cord was compressed between bony bars or spurs anteriorly and enfolded ligamentum flavum posteriorly, a mechanism suggested by Taylor (Figure 56C.4). Table 56C.5 compares the central cord syndrome with the syndrome of cruciate paralysis. Clinically, it may be very difficult to make this distinction. Fortunately, the combination of plain films, CT, and MRI can usually localize the lesion accurately to either the mid- to lower cervical spine in the central cord syndrome or to the cervicomedullary junction in the syndrome of cruciate paralysis.

To explain why the arms are affected more than the legs in the central cord syndrome, Schneider cited the presumed lamination of the corticospinal tract with the leg fibers lateral and the arm fibers medial in the cord (see Figure 56C.3). This concept of the lamination of the corticospinal fibers, as originally postulated by Foerster in 1936, was challenged by Nathan and Smith in 1956. Nathan and Smith found that the motor fibers subserving upper and lower limb movements were intermingled in the corticospinal tract, similar to what has been found in the pyramidal decussation. The central necrotic areas in pathological specimens appeared to involve principally the presumed location of the medial arm fibers of the corticospinal tracts bilaterally, with relative sparing of the lateral leg fibers. In 1958, Schneider and colleagues attributed the upper limb predilection to the involvement of the anterior horn cells in the necrotic center of the cord and postulated a vascular etiology in cases of central cord syndrome without cervical spondylosis or other bony compression. Schneider implicated a number of possible ischemic mechanisms to account for central infarction, including watershed infarcts between zones of medullary artery perfusion, vertebral artery interruption or stretching, anterior spinal artery spasm or occlusion at the site of maximal hyperextension, and venous infarction. Any of these mechanisms might underlie the central infarction of the medially located upper limb fibers of the corticospinal tract, which are supplied by the anterior sulcal arterial branches of the anterior spinal artery. Conversely, the laterally located leg fibers of the corticospinal tract might survive these ischemic mechanisms of injury because they are supplied by the arteriae coronae or the pial mesh, which derives its feeders from branches of both the anterior and posterior spinal arteries. Schneider and colleagues also implicated selective damage to the microcircu-

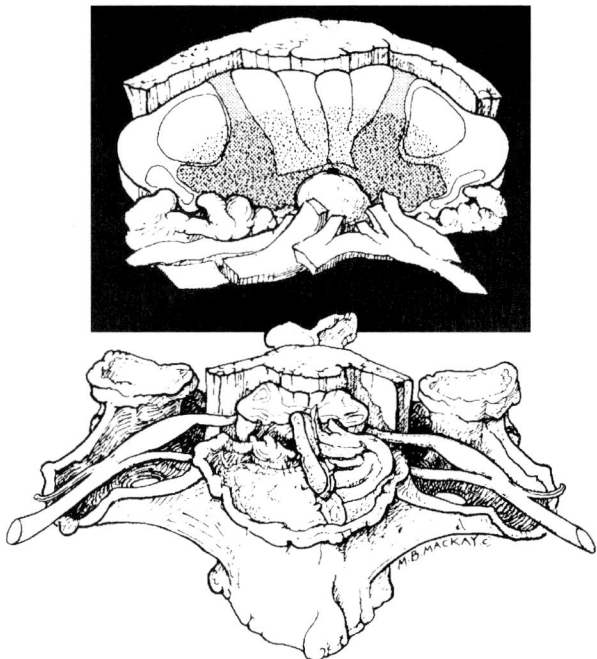

FIGURE 56C.4 Central cord syndrome. The drawing depicts a case of cervical spondylosis with osteoarthritis of the cervical spine, including anterior and posterior osteophytes and hypertrophy of the ligamentum flavum. Superimposed is an acute hyperextension injury that has caused rupture of the intervertebral disc and infolding of the ligamentum flavum. The spinal cord is compressed anteriorly and posteriorly. The central portion of the cord (*rough stippling*) sustained the greatest damage. The damaged area includes the medial segments of the corticospinal tracts presumed to subserve arm function. (Reprinted with permission from CH Tator. Classification of Spinal Cord Injury Based on Neurological Presentation. In RJ Narayan, JE Wilberger Jr, JT Povlishock [eds], Neurotrauma. New York: McGraw-Hill, 1994;1059–1073.)

lation in the center of the cord, with anterior horn cell ischemia as a mechanism for producing the central cord syndrome. They thought that "the higher perfusion demands of the gray matter" might account for "the selective vulnerability of the central gray matter to ischemia."

In 1992, Quencer and coworkers analyzed the correlations between the clinical, MRI, and pathological findings in 11 patients with central cord syndrome. Most of these were elderly patients with cervical spondylosis or stenosis, although some of the younger patients had disc herniations or subluxation. All 11 patients underwent MRI, at 18 hours to 2 days after SCI in seven patients and at 3–10 days after injury in the remaining four patients. Autopsy studies of the central cord syndrome were available in three patients, two of whom had had MRI. Surprisingly, these studies did not find any evidence of blood in the cord, either on T1- or T2-weighted images or in the pathological specimens. All patients showed hyperintense signals within the cord on gradient-echo MRI, which the investigators interpreted as edema. The histological specimens did not show central necrosis but, rather, that the "central gray matter was intact." The histological changes were primarily edema and separation of the axon myelin units in the earlier intervals after SCI, followed at the later stages by demyelination and myelin breakdown of mainly large axons, especially in the corticospinal tracts but also affecting other areas of the white matter. These investigators concluded that the central cord syndrome is primarily due to "direct mechanical compression of the cord, maximal along its posterolateral aspect," which causes damage to the white matter consisting of edema, myelin breakdown, and axonal disintegration, especially in the corticospinal tracts but also elsewhere in the white matter. Furthermore, the damage to the corticospinal tracts was diffuse and not concentrated centrally in the presumed location of the arm fibers, as postulated by Foerster. There-

Table 56C.5: Comparison of central cord syndrome with cruciate paralysis with arms weaker by site, manifestations, and prognosis

	Central cord syndrome	*Cruciate paralysis*
Site of lesions	Mid- to lower cervical cord Anterior horn cells Lateral corticospinal tract (medial part)	Lower medulla and upper cervical cord, anterior aspect Corticospinal decussation caudal to the pyramids
Clinical manifestations	Arms weaker than legs; flaccid arms acutely; legs normal or variably weak; lower motor neuron deficits in upper limbs persists	Arms weaker than legs; flaccid arms acutely; legs normal or variably weak; upper motor neuron deficits develop in upper limbs ± Trigeminal sensory deficit (onionskin, spinal tract of cranial nerve V) ± Cranial nerve dysfunction (IX, X, or XI)
Prognosis for neurological recovery	Variable	Usually good

Source: Reprinted with permission from CH Tator, EG Duncan, VE Edmonds, et al. Changes in epidemiology of acute spinal cord injury from 1947 to 1981. Surg Neurol 1993;40:207–215.

fore, Quencer and colleagues favored the conclusion of Nathan and Smith that the arm and leg fibers intermingle in the corticospinal tract.

Although it is true that many patients with central cord syndrome do make a substantial recovery without surgery, many nevertheless retain significant deficits, especially with severe impairment of the hands, due to a combination of weakness and severe proprioceptive loss. When persisting compression, instability, or neurological deterioration are factors, patients with central cord syndrome should be considered surgical candidates, similar to other patients with other incomplete syndromes. With persisting compression, it is preferable to decompress the lesion early, but even late decompression has been helpful in this syndrome. The overall prognosis for patients with central cord syndrome is relatively good. In patients with cord contusion without hematomyelia, approximately 50% of patients recover enough lower extremity strength and sensation to walk independently, although typically with significant spasticity. Recovery of upper extremity function is usually not as good, and fine motor control is usually poor. Bowel and bladder control often recovers.

Anterior Cord Syndrome

Anterior cord syndrome was originally described in the setting of acute cervical trauma by Schneider, who presented two cases of "immediate complete paralysis with hyperesthesia at the level of the lesion and an associated sparing of touch and some vibration sense." These two patients had ruptured discs and bone fragments in the canal, and both made a substantial recovery after operative removal of the intracanalicular space-occupying lesions (Figure 56C.5). This syndrome has the poorest prognosis of the incomplete injuries. Only 10–20% of patients recover functional motor control, although sensation may partially return enough to prevent injuries such as burns or decubitus ulcers. In Schneider's view, it was "a syndrome for which early operative intervention is indicated."

Posterior Cord Syndrome

This is an extremely rare type of incomplete SCI syndrome, and indeed many, including the authors, have doubted its existence. Supposedly, it occurs after major destruction of the posterior aspect of the cord, leaving some residual functioning spinal cord tissue anteriorly (Figure 56C.6). Thus, clinically, the patient retains spinothalamic function but loses movement and proprioception due to damage to the posterior half of the cord, including the corticospinal tracts and posterior columns.

Brown-Séquard's Syndrome

Brown-Séquard's syndrome is caused by a lesion of the lateral half of the spinal cord (Figure 56C.7) and is characterized by

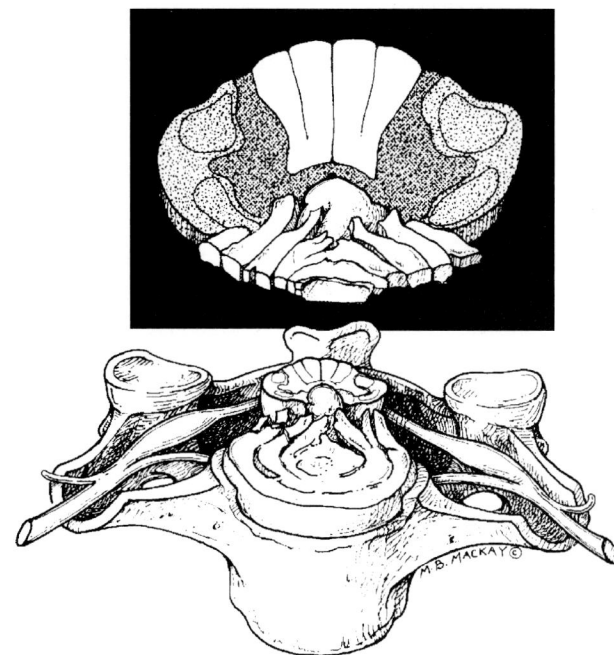

FIGURE 56C.5   Anterior cord syndrome. A large disc herniation is shown compressing the anterior aspect of the cord and resulting in damage (*rough stippling*) to the anterior and lateral white matter tracts and to the gray matter. The posterior columns remain intact. (Reprinted with permission from CH Tator. Classification of Spinal Cord Injury Based on Neurological Presentation. In RJ Narayan, JE Wilberger Jr, JT Povlishock [eds], Neurotrauma. New York: McGraw-Hill, 1994;1059–1073.)

ipsilateral motor and proprioceptive loss and contralateral pain and temperature loss. The syndrome can be associated with a variety of mechanisms of injury, including hyperextension, flexion, locked facets, compression fractures, and a herniated disc. Brown-Séquard's syndrome may be present from the start in some cases, but in others it may become apparent within days after injury as a gradual evolution from a bilateral incomplete injury. Hybrid combinations of Brown-Séquard's and other incomplete syndromes are frequent. Brown-Séquard's syndrome occurs most often after cervical injuries, less frequently in the thoracic cord and conus medullaris. In milder cases, there may be no sphincter deficit. This syndrome has the best prognosis of any incomplete SCI. Approximately 90% of patients regain the ability to walk independently as well as anal and urinary sphincter control.

Conus Medullaris Syndrome

In most patients, almost all the lumbar cord segments are opposite the T12 vertebral body and almost all the sacral cord segments are opposite the L1 vertebral body, with the cord ending opposite the L1-L2 disc space (Figure 56C.8). Because injuries at T11-T12 and T12-L1 are relatively common due

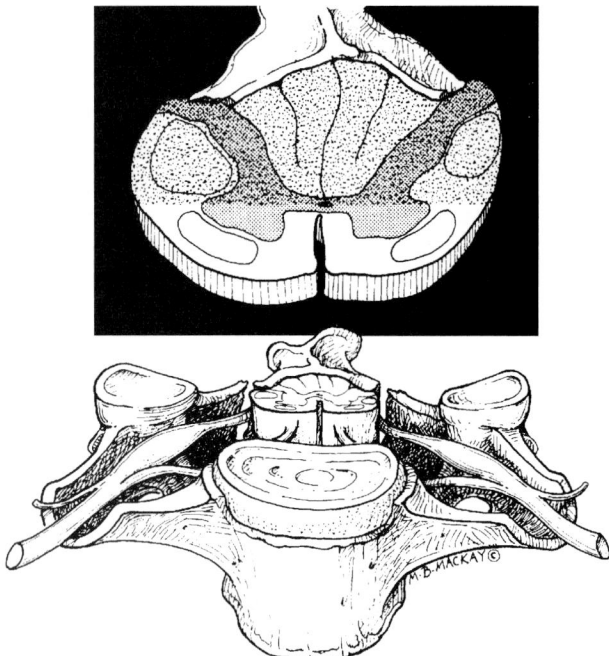

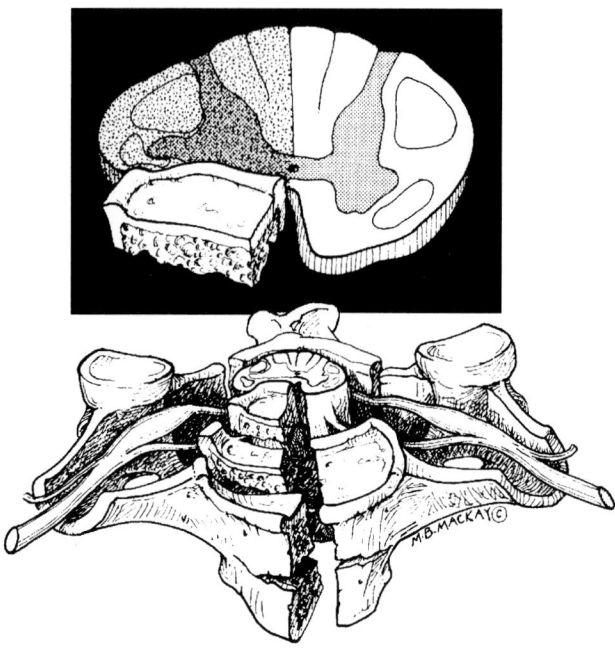

FIGURE 56C.6   Posterior cord syndrome. A laminar fracture is depicted with anterior displacement of the fractured bone and compression of the posterior aspect of the spinal cord. The damaged area of the cord (*rough stippling*) includes the posterior columns and the posterior half of the lateral columns along with the corticospinal tracts. (Reprinted with permission from CH Tator. Classification of Spinal Cord Injury Based on Neurological Presentation. In RJ Narayan, JE Wilberger Jr, JT Povlishock [eds], Neurotrauma. New York: McGraw-Hill, 1994;1059–1073.)

FIGURE 56C.7   Brown-Séquard's syndrome. A burst fracture is depicted with posterior displacement of bone fragments and disc, resulting in unilateral compression and damage (*rough stippling*) to one-half of the spinal cord. (Reprinted with permission from CH Tator. Classification of Spinal Cord Injury Based on Neurological Presentation. In RJ Narayan, JE Wilberger Jr, JT Povlishock [eds], Neurotrauma. New York: McGraw-Hill, 1994;1059–1073.)

to the mobility of these segments compared with the relatively immobile thoracic segments above, injuries to the conus medullaris are frequent. Indeed, in the senior author's experience, these conus medullaris injuries composed approximately 24% of SCI. These injuries usually produce a combination of lower motor neuron deficits with initial flaccid paralysis of the legs and anal sphincter, followed in the chronic phase by a combination of some degree of muscle atrophy and spasticity or reflex hyperactivity with possibly an extensor plantar response. The sensory picture may be variable; in some cases, the only evidence of incompleteness is retention of some perianal sensation, which is an example of sacral sparing. In the more severe conus lesions, the bowel and bladder deficits may be profound, with the ultimate development of a low-pressure, high-capacity neurogenic bladder.

Cauda Equina Injuries

With the cord terminating normally opposite the L1-L2 disc space (see Figure 56C.8), injuries at this level or below involve the roots of the cauda equina, although injuries one or two levels above also involve the origins of some of the

roots comprising the cauda equina. Clinically, these injuries may be complete, in which case they would be grade A on the ASIA/IMSOP scale. Incomplete injuries have varying severity, ranging from grades B to D. As with cord injuries, the motor fibers tend to be more susceptible to trauma, so that incomplete cases always have sensory preservation with or without some motor preservation. Cases with motor preservation only are extremely rare. The degree of bowel and bladder deficit parallels that of SCI. Cauda equina injuries may have a much better prognosis for neurological recovery than SCI does because the lower motor neuron has greater inherent resilience to trauma, with fewer secondary injury mechanisms and greater regenerative capacity than the upper motor neuron and its tracts.

One of the most interesting and dangerous cauda equina syndromes is associated with acute central disc herniation at L4-L5 or L5-S1, causing major damage to the sacral roots lying centrally within the dural sac (Figure 56C.9). There may be partial or complete sparing of the lumbar roots and often the S1 roots as well. Thus, these patients may have total preservation of strength in the legs but have complete bowel and bladder paralysis and perianal anesthesia. This syndrome constitutes a surgical emergency because recovery

FIGURE 56C.8 Conus medullaris syndrome. A burst fracture of T12 is depicted with posterior dislocation of bone fragments from the vertebral body into the spinal canal, resulting in compression of the conus medullaris. Almost all the lumbar cord segments are opposite the T12 vertebral body, so that a severe compression injury at this level could affect all the lumbar and sacral segments of the cord. (Reprinted with permission from CH Tator. Classification of Spinal Cord Injury Based on Neurological Presentation. In RJ Narayan, JE Wilberger Jr, JT Povlishock [eds], Neurotrauma. New York: McGraw-Hill, 1994;1059–1073.)

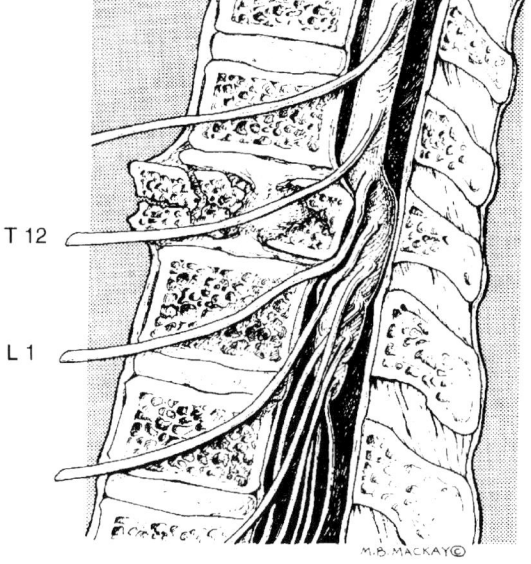
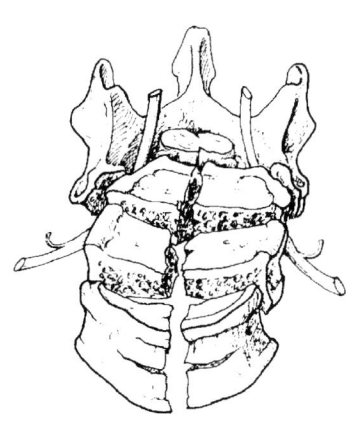

FIGURE 56C.9 Cauda equina syndrome. The drawing shows an acute central disc herniation of L4-L5 with major compression of the central aspect of the cauda equina. The medially placed sacral roots from S2 downward sustain the maximal compression, whereas the more laterally located L5 and S1 roots are completely or partially spared. (Reprinted with permission from CH Tator. Classification of Spinal Cord Injury Based on Neurological Presentation. In RJ Narayan, JE Wilberger Jr, JT Povlishock [eds], Neurotrauma. New York: McGraw-Hill, 1994;1059–1073.)

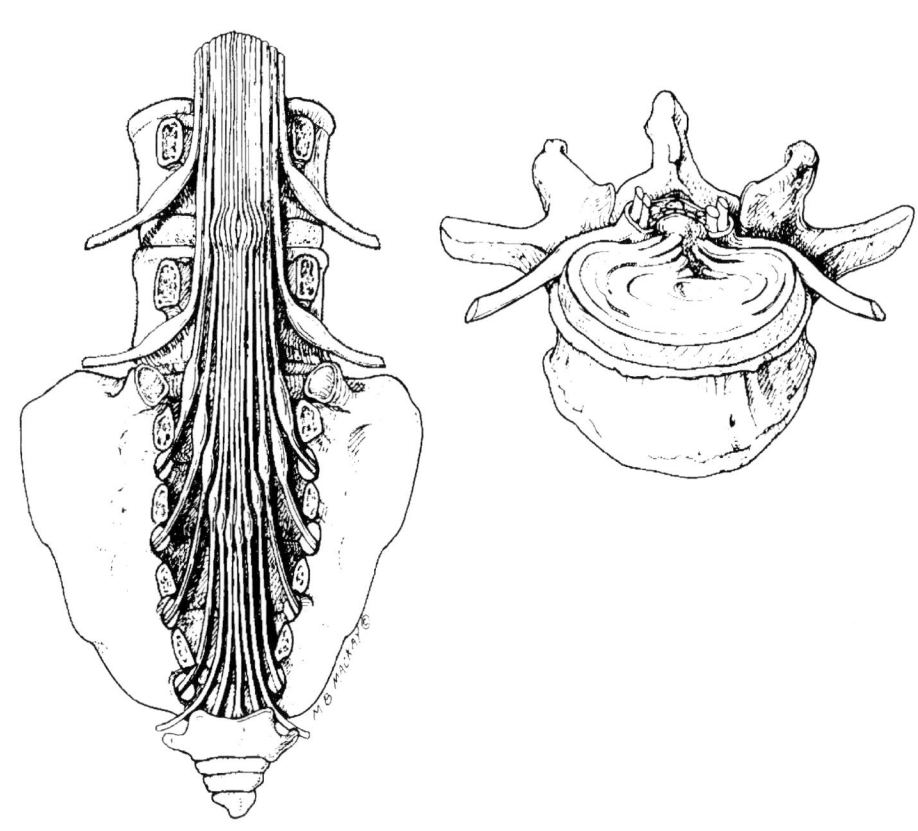

of function is more likely with early decompression. However, the sacral roots are very delicate and sometimes never recover, even if decompressed expeditiously.

Reversible or Transient Syndromes

A number of complete or incomplete SCI syndromes (Table 56C.6) are reversible or transient, one of the most interesting of which is the "burning hands" syndrome, which frequently occurs in athletes. The syndrome is characterized by transient paresthesias and dysesthesias in the upper limbs, especially the hands. It may exist with or without long tract signs, which, if present, are usually evanescent. There may be pathological changes in the posterior horns, and intramedullary lesions and spinal abnormalities, such as ligamentous instability, disc disease, and spinal stenosis, may be demonstrable by MRI. Hyperextension may be the most

Table 56C.6: Reversible transient syndromes of traumatic spinal cord injury

Burning hands syndrome
Contusio cervicalis
Cord concussion
Hysteria

Source: Reprinted with permission from CH Tator. Spinal Cord Syndromes with Physiologic and Anatomic Correlations. In AH Menezes, VKH Sonntag (eds), Principles of Spinal Surgery. New York: McGraw-Hill, 1996;769–799.

Table 56C.7: Acute traumatic spinal cord injury syndromes without radiological abnormality (SCIWORA) or evidence of trauma (SCIWORET)

SCIWORA—in children (less commonly in adults)
SCIWORET—in adults (less commonly in children)

Occurs in:	Cervical spondylosis
	Spinal stenosis
	Ankylosing spondylitis
	Other arthropathies
	Disc herniation
	Nucleus pulposus embolism

Source: Reprinted with permission from CH Tator. Spinal Cord Syndromes with Physiologic and Anatomic Correlations. In AH Menezes, VKH Sonntag (eds), Principles of Spinal Surgery. New York: McGraw-Hill, 1996;769–799.

frequent mechanism of injury. These transient syndromes in athletes are usually bilateral, which distinguishes them from the other syndrome of "stingers" or "burners" in athletes due to unilateral nerve root or brachial plexus lesions (especially traction injury), most of which are also transient.

Spinal cord concussion is a transient loss of motor or sensory function of the spinal cord that usually recovers within minutes but always within hours. In almost all instances, the initial clinical examiner learns that the symptoms are rapidly diminishing and finds a normal neurological examination. The exact pathophysiology of spinal cord concussion is unknown but most likely represents a biochemical lesion, such as leakage of potassium from the intracellular to the extracellular space, either due to direct mechanical injury or secondary to a vascular mechanism.

Acute Spinal Cord Injury Syndrome without Radiological Evidence of Trauma

In the pediatric population, the syndrome of SCIWORA is more common than in adults and represents a significant percentage of pediatric SCI. Children with SCIWORA tend to be less severely injured than those with definite evidence of bony injury, but complete SCIs have been described. By definition, the negative radiological examination includes only plain films and tomography, either conventional or CT. If a negative MRI were also included in the syndrome, the number of cases would diminish dramatically because of MRI's extreme sensitivity in detecting mild cord or spinal column injuries, which are usually not detected by plain films or CT. Children are more susceptible to these injuries than are adults, presumably because of the laxity of their spinal ligaments and the weakness of their paraspinal muscles. True SCIWORA can also occur in adults (Table 56C.7), but it is much less common than the syndrome of SCIWORET. Patients with SCIWORET have abnormal radiological examinations, but the radiographs show no evidence of trauma. Before the use of CT in spinal trauma, the incidence of SCIWORET in adults with SCI was approximately 14%. The addition of CT has reduced the incidence of SCIWORET to about 5%. It is likely that very few SCIs will remain undetected by MRI because of the high sensitivity of

MRI for detecting mild SCI and spinal column lesions not involving bone, such as ligamentous injuries and hematomas. Cervical spondylosis is the most common associated condition in adults with SCIWORET, but other arthropathies may on rare occasion be associated with SCI and not show radiological evidence of trauma. An example is a minor, radiologically undetectable fracture in a patient with ankylosing spondylitis who develops an epidural hematoma. Acute traumatic disc herniations often are not detected by older-generation CT scanners but can be easily diagnosed by MRI. Some patients with spinal stenosis, especially in the cervical region, may develop major SCI without traumatic changes on plain films or CT. Patients with nucleus pulposus embolism may have profound spinal cord deficits without any radiological evidence of trauma, even when trauma was an antecedent factor. MRI in these cases usually shows evidence of spinal cord infarction.

Post-Traumatic Acute Spinal Cord Injury without Direct Trauma to the Spine

Post-traumatic acute SCI without direct trauma to the spine is a relatively rare syndrome. It differs from SCIWORET and SCIWORA in that these patients sustain a lesion of the spinal cord that manifests as an acute spinal cord syndrome and is associated with trauma, but the trauma is not to the spine (Table 56C.8). The syndrome can occur in both children and adults. In 1974, Keith and co-workers described several cases in children with major abdominal, thoracic, or limb trauma and concluded that many of them had sustained an aortic injury that caused occlusion of intercostal or lumbar arteries, with subsequent occlusion of medullary arteries and spinal cord infarction. Rarely, penetrating injuries, such as gunshot wounds, can interrupt major arterial feeders to the cord without direct trauma to the spine. Severe hypotension and systemic shock in trauma patients can also result in spinal cord ischemia and infarction, even without causing concomitant cerebral ischemia.

Table 56C.8: Trauma patients with an acute spinal cord syndrome but without direct trauma to the spine

With hypotension and systemic shock
With vascular injury to feeding artery, aorta, or vertebral artery
Anterior spinal artery syndrome

Source: Reprinted with permission from CH Tator. Spinal Cord Syndromes with Physiologic and Anatomic Correlations. In AH Menezes, VKH Sonntag (eds), Principles of Spinal Surgery. New York: McGraw-Hill, 1996;769–799.

Table 56C.9: Chronic post-traumatic spinal cord syndromes

Post-traumatic syringomyelia
Post-traumatic microcystic myelomalacia ("marshy cord syndrome")
Arachnoiditis
Deafferentation pain syndromes (neurogenic, myelogenic, and cephalogenic)
"Dis-complete" syndrome

Source: Reprinted with permission from CH Tator. Spinal Cord Syndromes with Physiologic and Anatomic Correlations. In AH Menezes, VKH Sonntag (eds), Principles of Spinal Surgery. New York: McGraw-Hill, 1996;769–799.

Penetrating Injuries to the Spine

The pathology of gunshot wounds from World War I was first described by Holmes in 1915. Missile and bone fragments may come to rest in the epidural space, subdural space, or spinal cord or among roots of the cauda equina. Fragments of clothing, skin, or other debris may be carried into the spinal canal. Furthermore, missile fragments may remain mobile within the spinal canal, and migration of bullets has been reported. Epidural or subdural hematomas rarely occur, but intramedullary hemorrhage is frequent, particularly in the gray matter. Post-traumatic progressive cystic myelopathy (progressive syringomyelia or myelomalacia) may cause late deterioration of neurological function. Brachial and lumbosacral plexus injuries are frequently associated with penetrating SCIs. Fistula formation may occur between the spine and the bowel, bladder, or pleural cavity, and arteriovenous fistulas may also occur. In the majority of cases, stab wounds result in incomplete injuries. The configuration of the spine tends to force the blade to one side of the spinal canal, resulting in Brown-Séquard's syndrome. Epidural hematomas, infections, cerebrospinal fluid leakage, and delayed neurological deficits have been reported more frequently after spinal stab wounds.

The management of patients with penetrating injuries follows the same principles applied to all SCI victims (see Management of Acute Spinal Cord Injury, later in this chapter). It is our practice to start patients with penetrating injuries on broad-spectrum antibiotics in the emergency room and continue the treatment for 10–14 days after injury. Corticosteroids are used only if the penetrating injury is not associated with major visceral injury, such as penetration of the intestine, because of significantly increased risk of infection.

Chronic Post-Traumatic Spinal Cord Syndromes

Several important clinical syndromes develop in the subacute and chronic stages after acute SCI (Table 56C.9). Cystic degeneration at the epicenter of the cord injury, mainly in the central region of the cord but also spreading rostral and caudal, is a frequent sequela of hemorrhagic necrosis and ischemia of the cord in the acute stage. The greater the acute injury, the greater the tendency to subsequent cyst formation at the injury site and beyond. The exact pathophysiology of progressive post-traumatic syringomyelia is unknown, but cord disruption and arachnoiditis are common antecedents. This clinical syndrome occurs in about 3% of cord injuries and begins months to years later, usually with the onset of causalgia-type differentiation pain. Subsequently, there is further loss of sensory or motor function, or both. The motor deficits usually comprise a lower motor neuron type at the level of the injury or above, an upper motor neuron type below the level of the injury (if the injury was incomplete), and further loss of bowel or bladder function. The sensory loss tends to be of the spinothalamic type because the cyst formation usually begins centrally, which damages the crossing sensory afferents in the anterior white commissure on their way to the spinothalamic tract.

The syndrome of post-traumatic microcystic myelomalacia is similar to post-traumatic syringomyelia in that it can cause late deterioration of spinal cord function months to years after SCI due to a progressive lesion in the cord. The new clinical deficits can be identical to post-traumatic syringomyelia. Based on radiology, MRI, and surgical data (because there is no comprehensive pathological study of this condition), the cord shows *microcystic degeneration*, a term that the authors prefer to "marshy cord syndrome." Arachnoiditis is a constant accompaniment and may play a causative role.

Arachnoiditis occurs after SCIs of all types and severity. Even minor injuries may result in florid arachnoiditis, whereas some major disruptive injuries may cause little. The propensity to spread from the site of injury also varies widely, from cases in which it is confined to the epicenter of the lesion to those in which there is extensive involvement in the rostrocaudal direction. Connective tissue bridging from the dura to the arachnoid and from the arachnoid into the injured cord itself tends to be greater in cases with pial disruption or dural laceration (Tator 1996b). Otherwise, the etiology of this rare, late post-traumatic syndrome is unknown. Post-traumatic arachnoiditis can cause progres-

Table 56C.10:   Findings in hypovolemic shock versus neurogenic shock

	Hemorrhagic shock	*Neurogenic shock*
Pulse	Tachycardia	Bradycardia
Skin	Cool, clammy	Warm, dry
Mental status	Altered	Normal
Urine output	Low	Normal

sive neurological deterioration, either slowly or stepwise. The latter course suggests a vascular component due to fibrotic strangulation of subarachnoid arteries and veins supplying or draining the spinal cord.

Various pain syndromes can be present immediately after SCI, but the majority of them ultimately abate. Approximately 25% of patients with SCI continue to have significant pain syndromes, the most important of which are the neuropathic pain states of the deafferentation type. These are classified as neurogenic, myelogenic, or cephalogenic, depending on whether the abnormal painful impulses are generated from the damaged nerve roots, spinal cord, or brain (Tator 1996c).

Dimitrijevic has defined a clinical syndrome in which clinically complete cases have some evidence of impulse conduction across the lesion site, as shown by evoked potential testing or some other neurophysiological means. The relevance of this "dis-complete" syndrome to clinical management or prognosis is uncertain.

MANAGEMENT OF ACUTE SPINAL CORD INJURY

In recent years, the management of acute SCI has evolved due to advances in understanding of the pathophysiological processes in acute SCI. A logical management scheme that begins at the scene of the accident in the prehospital phase and continues through neurological assessment, radiographic diagnosis, acute management, and surgical treatment is essential to maximize neurological recovery and achieve spinal stabilization.

All victims of significant trauma, especially those who have had loss of consciousness, should be treated as having an SCI until proved otherwise. The same goes for all victims of minor trauma with complaints referable to the spine (e.g., neck or back pain or spinal tenderness) or to the spinal cord (e.g., numbness or tingling, weakness, or paralysis in an extremity) as well as victims with abdominal breathing (paradoxical respiration) or priapism. Management should proceed in association with routine treatment of other injuries.

Management in the Field

As a basic tenet of trauma management, airway establishment or protection takes precedence. If there is no sign of respiratory distress, the airway can be protected with a nasal or oral airway and supplemental oxygen provided. If the patient is unconscious, the respiratory effort is poor, or the upper airway is obstructed, intubation is usually necessary. Traditionally, nasal intubation was advised, but there is some controversy over the preferred route of intubation (oral or nasal). Most recent studies (e.g., Wright and colleagues in 1992) have indicated that the method of intubation should depend on the skill and expertise of the individuals involved rather than the concerns of inducing or worsening neurological injury. Efforts should be directed at keeping the neck in as neutral a position as possible during the establishment of an airway.

If possible, intravenous access should be established and vigorous circulatory support provided to avoid hypotension, which may be caused by SCI itself and may further injure the spinal cord due to decreased oxygen or blood supply. It is vitally important at this stage to attempt to differentiate hypovolemic from neurogenic shock (Table 56C.10), especially in the patient with multiple injuries. The heart rate may provide a clue as to the etiology of the hypotension. Hypovolemic shock is typically accompanied by tachycardia, whereas the sympathetic denervation of neurogenic shock due to SCI is often accompanied by bradycardia due to relative vagal overactivity (unopposed vagotonia). In neurogenic shock, vasopressors are indicated when fluid replacement is ineffective in restoring blood pressure. Fluids should be given as necessary to replace losses, but overhydration should be avoided, especially in associated head injury. The application of medical antishock trousers may increase peripheral resistance in the lower extremities and ameliorate the hypotension of neurogenic shock.

Once the patient has been resuscitated and is physiologically stable, consideration must be given to extraction from the vehicle and transportation. During this process, adequate immobilization must be maintained at all times by using logrolling techniques or by the application of scoop stretchers or spine boards (short spine boards are easier to apply inside the confining spaces of vehicles). A hard cervical collar should also be applied while the patient is still inside the vehicle. On extrication, efforts should be exerted to maintain neutral alignment of the head, thorax, and pelvis. Once outside the vehicle, the patient can be positioned on a long spine board and firmly secured before any further movement or transport is attempted. Further stabilization of the head by using sandbags or generous taping is necessary to supplement the cervical collar. In unintubated patients, continued attention must be focused on the airway during transport. Vomiting and subsequent aspiration is not an infrequent occurrence in this setting. Thus, strong consideration should be given to placement of a nasogastric tube. If this is not feasible, the patient should be transported with the head of the backboard in a slight Trendelenburg's position.

Before transportation, an attempt should be made to establish the extent and level of any motor or sensory loss to identify the deficits and document any delayed deterioration. If possible, the patient should be asked about symptoms of pain, numbness, or weakness. The initial evaluation of motor function should ascertain whether the patient is able to move the upper and lower limbs voluntarily. The initial sensory examination should attempt to establish whether there is a relative loss of appreciation of painful sensation below a certain level and, if time permits, to perform a careful testing of the sacral sensory areas.

Management in the Hospital

Because of the significant frequency of associated injuries, the emergency room evaluation and treatment of the patient with an SCI requires a multidisciplinary team. A focused history should be obtained from witnesses at the scene or from ambulance personnel to help establish the nature of the activity that caused the injury and the mechanism of injury (e.g., hyperflexion, extension, axial loading). It is important to determine whether there was loss of consciousness, weakness, numbness, or tingling in any extremity at any time after the injury.

The injured patient should be maintained on the backboard to facilitate transfer to radiology or CT table, but once studies are completed, the backboard should be removed by logrolling the patient. Early removal of the board reduces the risk of decubitus ulcers in injured patients. SCI patients who lie on a hard surface for longer than 2 hours without being logrolled may develop a pressure sore that can last a lifetime.

While logrolling the injured patient in the emergency room evaluation, it is very important to palpate the spine for tenderness or "step-off." However, the number of times a patient with SCI is moved for such an evaluation should be minimized. Local tenderness, if present, suggests underlying bony, muscular, or ligamentous injury. A focal hematoma suggests a direct blow to the spine and may be associated with posterior element fractures. Widening of the spaces between two spinous processes (or a "gap") suggests a significant ligamentous injury to the spine secondary to extreme flexion and may be associated with compression fracture, subluxation, or dislocation.

Neurological Assessment

In contrast to the brief prehospital spinal and neurological evaluation, the initial examination in the emergency room should be as thorough and complete as the associated injuries allow and should follow the ASIA system (see Figure 56C.1). The neurological examination should be directed to determining whether the SCI is complete or incomplete and at what spinal cord level the injury has occurred.

Ten muscle groups are examined for strength. These are graded on the standard 6-point scale:

0 = Total paralysis

1 = Palpable or visible muscle contraction
2 = Active muscle movement, full range of motion of the involved joint with gravity eliminated
3 = Active muscle movement, full range of motion of the involved joint against gravity
4 = Active muscle movement, full range of motion of the involved joint against moderate resistance
5 = Normal active muscle movement, full range of motion of the involved joint against full resistance

The sensory examination involves thorough testing of perception of pinprick and light touch modalities in all 28 dermatomes from C2 to S5. The responses are reported as normal, impaired, or absent. Sacral sensation is best assessed at the anal mucocutaneous junction, and the external anal sphincter should be evaluated based on the presence or absence of voluntary contraction around the examiner's finger (see Complete versus Incomplete Injury, earlier in this chapter). It is not unusual to find preserved sacral function in an otherwise apparently complete injury.

A number of factors may make the neurological examination incomplete and unreliable: associated head injury or altered level of consciousness from drugs, alcohol or hypotension, spinal shock, and the presence of peripheral nerve or brachial plexus injury.

Evaluation of the level of the lesion requires familiarity with the relationship between the bony spinal canal and the spinal cord and nerves. Due to the disproportionately greater growth of the spinal column than the spinal cord during development, to determine which segment of the cord underlies a given vertebra, one should add 2 to the number of the vertebrae from C2 to T1. In general, the lumbar cord segments L1 through L5 are opposite the T12 vertebral body, and the S1 through S5 segments are opposite the L1 vertebral body. In the adult, the conus medullaris lies at about L1 vertebral body. Cervical nerves 1–7 exit above the pedicles of their like-numbered vertebrae, the C8 nerve root exits above the first thoracic pedicle, and the remainder of the nerve roots caudal to C8 exit below the pedicles of their like-numbered vertebrae.

Radiographic Evaluation

Once an appropriate baseline neurological status has been established, radiographs should be obtained. Techniques include plain radiographs, dynamic flexion-extension films, conventional tomography, CT, myelography with and without CT, and MRI. MRI provides the best assessment for cord injuries and in most centers is performed after plain films.

Plain Radiographs. Despite the availability of newer imaging techniques, plain-film radiographs remain indispensable in the initial assessment of acute SCI. *The Advanced Trauma Life Support Instructor Manual* of the American College of Surgeons recommends a lateral cervical spine radiograph on *every* patient with multiple trauma as part of the initial assessment (Figure 56C.10A). Its value lies in providing a

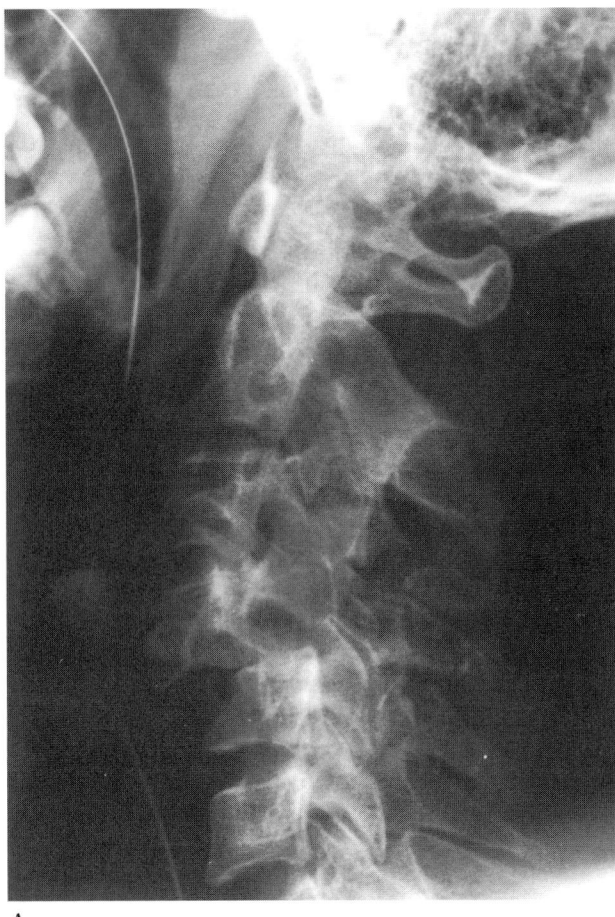

A

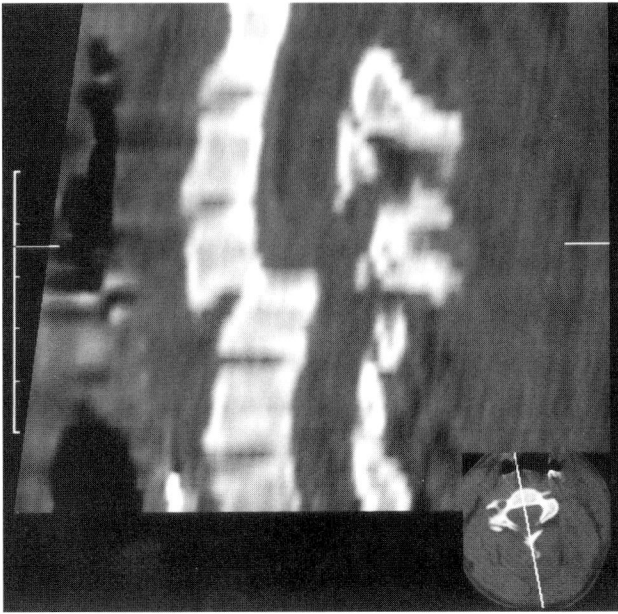

B

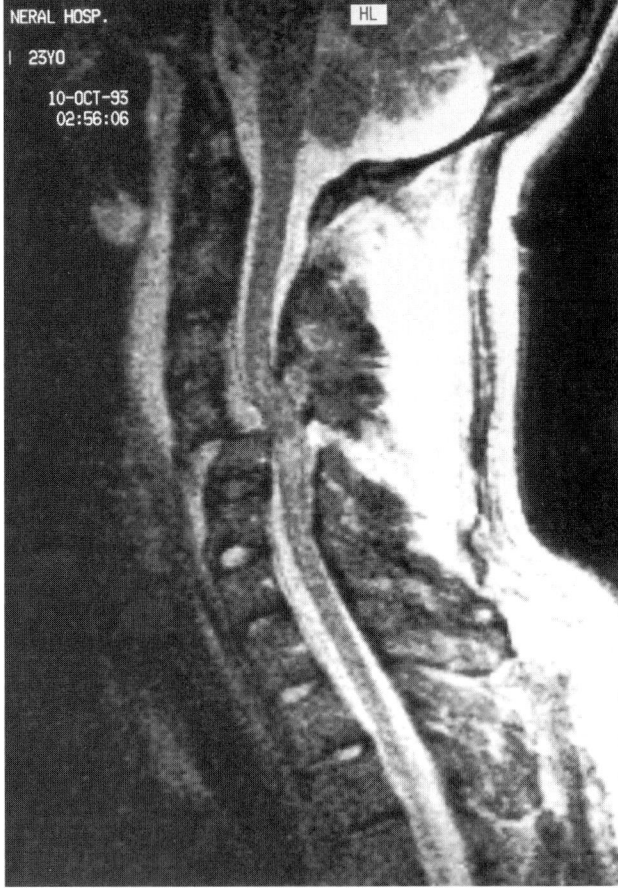

C

FIGURE 56C.10 (A) Lateral radiograph of the cervical spine, shows significant malalignment (anterolisthesis) of C4 vertebral body on C5 and bilateral facet dislocation. (B) Reformatted mid-sagittal computed tomographic image demonstrates the severity of the fracture dislocation and identifies the presence of fractures of the posterior elements. (C) Sagittal long recovery time–long echo delay time (T2-weighted) spin-echo magnetic resonance image shows increased signal (brightness) within the cervical spinal cord at the level of the fracture dislocation. There is effacement of the cerebrospinal fluid space both anterior and posterior to the cord and increased signal involving the interspinous ligaments, indicating posterior ligamentous disruption.

rapid evaluation of the contour and alignment of the vertebral bodies. Adjunctive findings, such as loss of vertebral body height, widening or fracture of the posterior elements, or soft tissue swelling, may be important in documenting the presence or absence of injury. The lateral film can be obtained during the initial assessment because it requires no patient movement. Once the patient is stabilized, several additional views are necessary to complete the evaluation of the cervical spine. The anteroposterior view provides additional information on spinous process alignment and the posterior elements, whereas oblique views allow for evaluation of the pedicles, laminae, neural foramina, and facet alignment. The open-mouth odontoid view is most useful in evaluating odontoid fractures and C1 injuries.

Indications for thoracolumbar films include spinal pain or tenderness, any neurological symptoms or positive neurological findings, presence of head injury or any alteration of consciousness, a specific injury mechanism (i.e., ejection or fall), and any evidence of multiple injury. Samuels and Kerstein (1993) found a 2% frequency of thoracolumbar injury in a consecutive series of 756 such patients. They concluded that routine thoracolumbar films are not indicated unless there is a positive clinical examination or a significant mechanism of injury. However, because the frequency of noncontiguous simultaneous spinal fractures may approach 15%, it is essential to survey the entire spine if one area of injury is initially identified.

Dynamic Radiographs.   Ligamentous damage after spinal injury can occur in the absence of bony injury, thus giving rise to "normal" initial radiographs. However, the presence of ligamentous damage may become manifest on dynamic flexion-extension views. The upper limits of physiological motion between vertebral bodies in the horizontal plane is 3.5 mm. Caution must be exercised in interpreting flexion-extension films after acute trauma because significant muscle spasm may be present and may compensate for incompetent ligaments. In acute situations, the dynamic views are indicated only when the plain films are negative and there are no neurological complaints.

Conventional Tomography.   With the advent of CT, conventional tomography has become less available in many radiology departments and is no longer used in the acute evaluation of spinal injury. However, it remains an excellent modality to assess bony alignment and spatial relationship of bone fragments. It is superior to CT in detecting horizontally oriented fractures, such as odontoid fractures, even with computer reformations. Its disadvantages include the need to move the patient into the decubitus position, which requires close supervision, and the higher overall radiation dose.

Computed Tomography.   CT has greatly improved the diagnosis and management of patients presenting with spinal trauma. It is the optimum method for viewing the bony central spinal canal and any impingement by osseous fragments, particularly at the thoracolumbar junction. Plain radiographs often underestimate encroachment on the canal in this area.

The CT examination should be tailored by the use of preliminary plain radiographs and clinical symptomatology. It is the best imaging modality for visualizing vertically oriented fractures. Sagittal or coronal computer reformations (Figure 56C.11B; see also Figure 56C.10B) and three-dimensional surface renderings allow assessment of gross bony displacement but produce poor resolution. Woodring

and Lee (1993) concluded that most of the abnormalities not detected on plain films occurred at the C1 and C7 levels. The following reasons prompted CT evaluation in patients who were initially thought to have normal plain spine films: less than optimal demonstration of the lower cervical spine (48%), less than optimal demonstration of the upper cervical spine (25%), unexplained neurological complaints or findings (10%), and prevertebral soft tissue swelling (18%) (Woodring and Lee 1993).

CT is limited in its ability to evaluate the thecal sac and intraspinal soft tissues. Its ability to assess acute disc rupture is also imperfect. Except in relation to spinal canal compromise, subluxation is not well demonstrated on CT. If CT slices are too far apart, abnormalities may be missed (this is particularly important in evaluating the facets). In spite of these drawbacks, CT is an important tool to better define the bony anatomy after known or suspected spinal injury. It is our practice to obtain a routine CT scan of the head and additional thin cuts through the craniocervical junction, down to C2-C3 disc space level, on all head-injured patients with decreased level of consciousness.

Myelography.   Myelography provides relatively nonspecific information on the patency of the subarachnoid space (i.e., the presence of a subtotal or complete block). When supplemented with CT scanning, it represents an excellent method to delineate the spinal cord and nerve roots and their relationship to surrounding structures. This technique is still useful for detecting dural lacerations with extravasation of cerebrospinal fluid and nerve root avulsion. In many institutions, MRI has supplanted myelography with CT for diagnosing SCI.

Magnetic Resonance Imaging.   MRI has substantially improved the ability to assess SCI because it is the only imaging modality capable of directly imaging the spinal cord parenchyma noninvasively. MRI has indeed replaced myelography for the assessment of most acute SCIs because it produces higher-quality images in a shorter period. MRI provides information on ligamentous injury and spinal canal compromise due to bone fragments, traumatic disc herniations, and epidural hematoma. It is also possible to visualize cord transection, hematomyelia, contusion, ischemia, and edema. MRI is useful in assessing the transverse dental ligament, the anterior and posterior longitudinal ligaments, and the interspinous ligaments. Some authors even feel that MRI may be as sensitive as CT in imaging traumatic bony abnormalities (Duh et al. 1993).

MRI-compatible traction devices, ventilators, and monitoring equipment are all available. In our opinion, MRI should be made available for emergent evaluation of SCI patients and should be performed after immobilization in a collar, halo, or tongs. Extra caution is advised in evaluating patients with penetrating spinal injuries because many bullet fragments possess ferromagnetic properties that cause extreme artifact on images or may torque (move) during the procedure. It is our practice to perform myelography

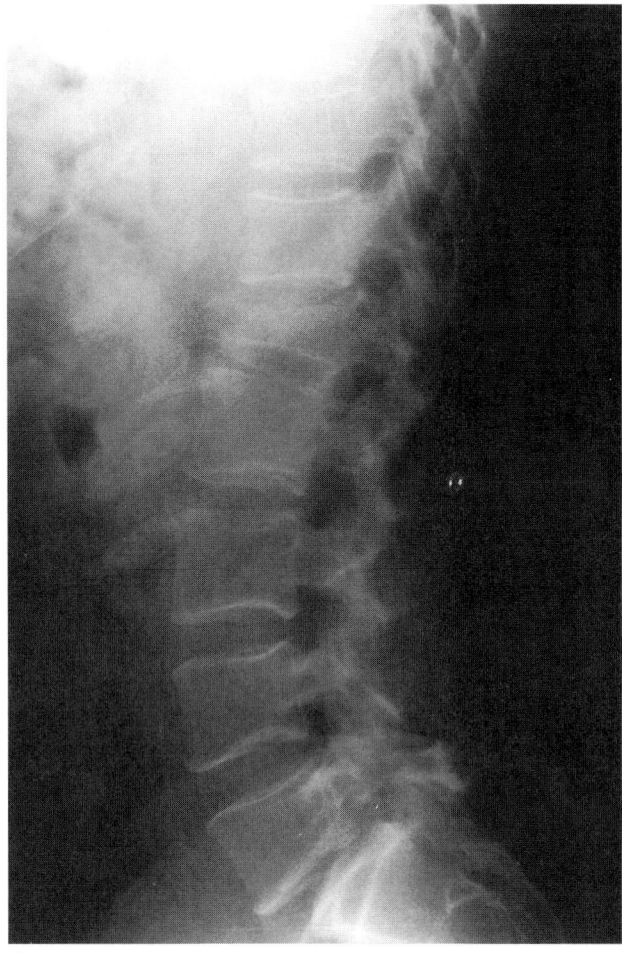

A

FIGURE 56C.11   (A) Lateral radiograph of the thoracolumbar spine shows a burst fracture of L1 vertebral body. There is a significant loss of height of L1 vertebral body due to disruption of the superior endplate. A mild retrolisthesis into the spinal canal is also seen. (B) Reformatted midsagittal computed tomographic images show a burst fracture of L1 with a retropulsed fragment that causes severe compromise of the spinal canal. (C) Midsagittal T2-weighted spin-echo magnetic resonance images show severe distal conus and proximal cauda equina compression due to the retropulsed bone fragment. A ventral subdural hematoma within the thecal sac at this level and extending inferiorly is also seen.

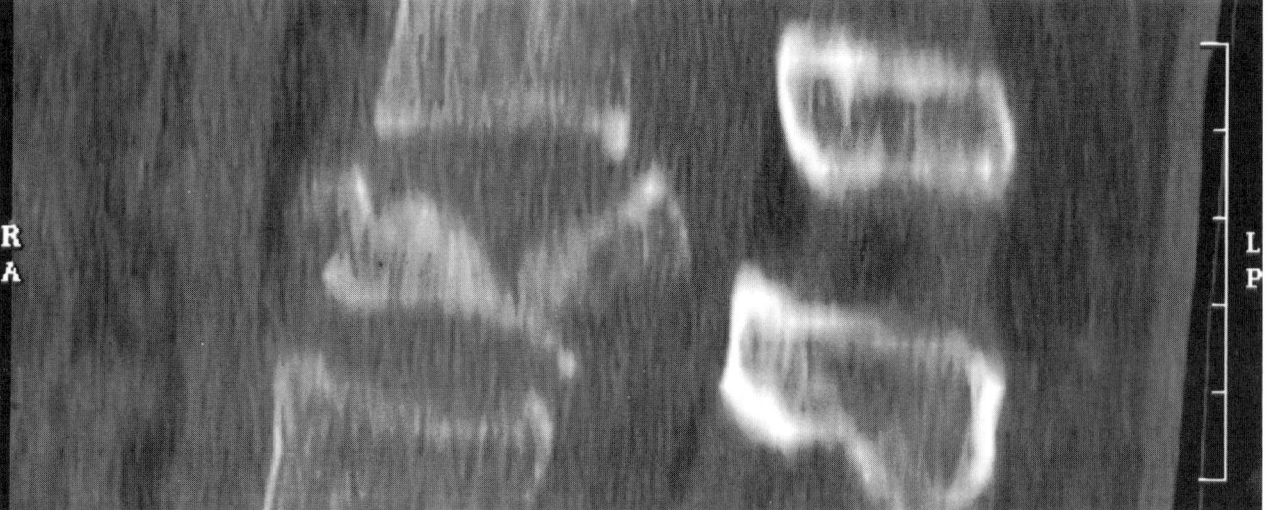

B

followed by CT images if retained metal fragments produce MRI artifact that interferes with adequate imaging.

MRI is most commonly performed in the sagittal and axial planes using spin-echo sequences with 3- to 4-mm slice thickness. Sagittal images give excellent visualization of spondylolisthesis and any cord compression. Axial images aid in lateralizing abnormalities and determining canal cross section. Coronal images are occasionally obtained in patients with scoliotic curves. The short recovery time (TR)–short echo delay time (TE) (T1-weighted) sequence generally gives the best anatomical detail, showing spinal cord caliber and cord compression. The long TR–long TE

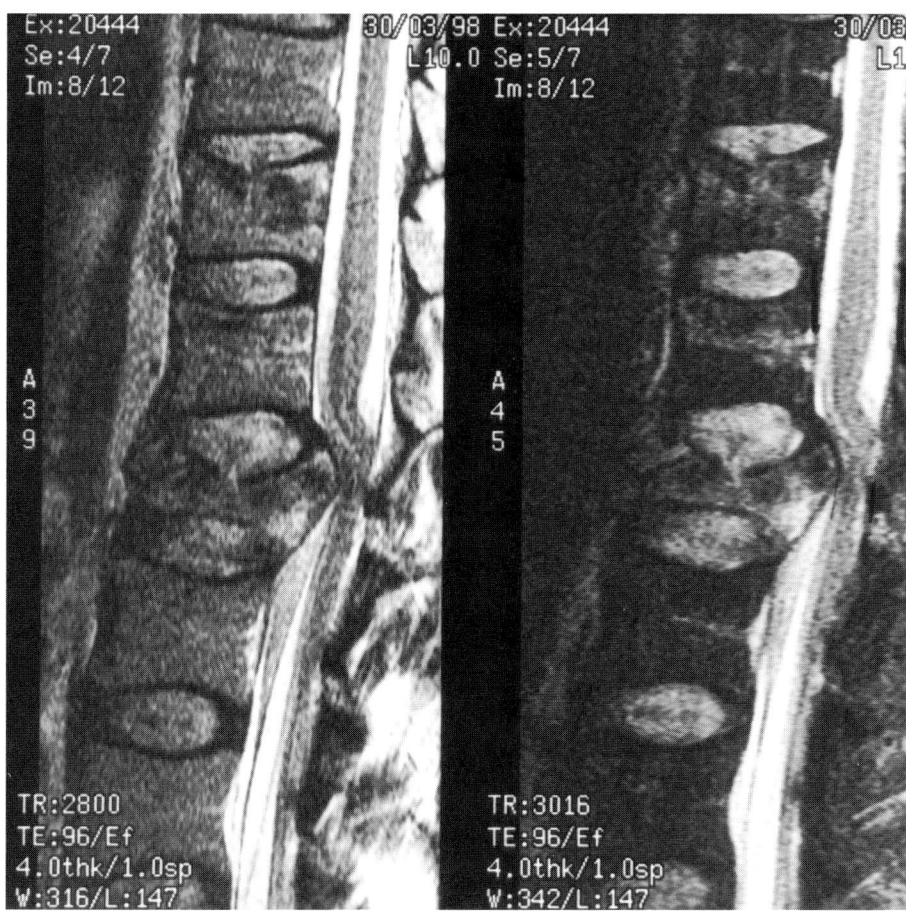

C

(T2-weighted) and long TR–short TE (proton density weighted) series are best at showing subtle changes in soft tissue contrast within cord parenchyma (Figure 56C.12).

Cord edema in acute injuries is seen as an area of increased signal (brightness) on the T2-weighted sequence and may spread along several segments, making it an excellent indicator of the extent of injury but less reliable for determining the exact level of injury.

Cord hemorrhage may vary in appearance, depending on the dominant state of the hemoglobin metabolites in the clot. The T2-weighted sequence is best at detecting clot. A hyperacute clot imaged within minutes or a few hours of injury may appear bright because of oxyhemoglobin. After several days, the clot may acquire brightness on both the T1- and T2-weighted series due to accumulation of methemoglobin. Most commonly, the clot appears as a focus of decreased signal (darkness), representing deoxyhemoglobin formation, during the first few days after injury. In 1992, Flanders and co-workers found that a hematoma tends to be more focal and correlates better with the site of trauma and instability. The pattern of cord edema and hemorrhage, as demonstrated by Schaefer and co-workers and Silberstein and co-workers in 1992 on T2-weighted MRI, correlates with the degree of initial neurological deficit and with the ultimate neurological outcome.

Epidural hematoma may have a variable appearance on T2-weighted MRI (high, low, or mixed signal) depending on the age of the clot and its dominant biochemical composition (oxy-, deoxy-, or methemoglobin) and can extend over several segments of the spinal canal.

MRI has shown that traumatic disc herniation is a surprisingly common occurrence in conjunction with spinal fracture or ligamentous injury. According to Flanders et al., it can accompany up to 54% of traumatic SCIs, and its demonstration is important for determining the necessity for surgical decompression and the type of surgical approach chosen to achieve adequate decompression and stabilization. Signs of disc injury on MRI include the following:

1. Widened disc space
2. Relative hyperintensity of one disc on T2-weighted sequence
3. Outer annular fiber or longitudinal ligament discontinuity
4. Posterior protrusion of disc material into the epidural space
5. Posterior deviation of the posterior longitudinal ligament (see Figures 56C.10C, 56C.11C, and 56C.12)

The sensitivity and the role of MRI in defining isolated bony injuries remain debatable. Many clinicians maintain

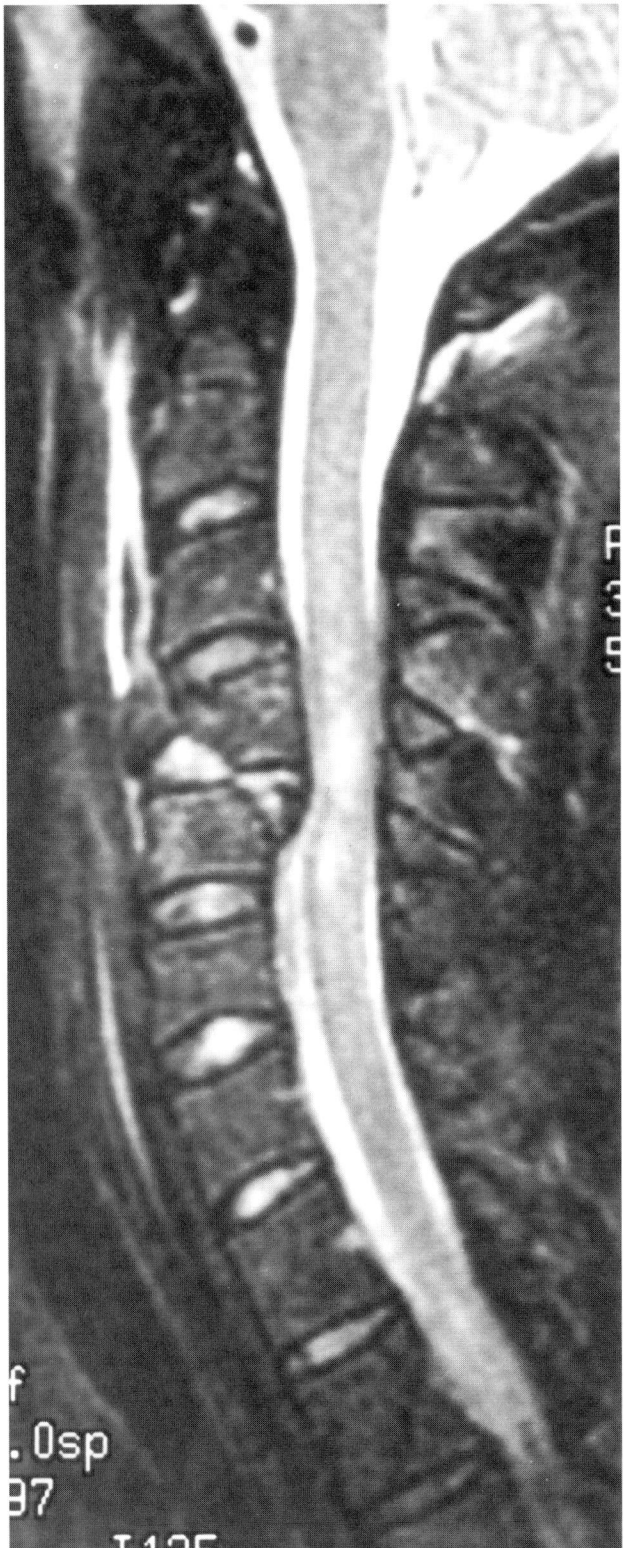

FIGURE 56C.12 Sagittal long recovery time–long echo delay time (T2-weighted) magnetic resonance image of the cervical spine shows C4 vertebral burst fracture with anterior displacement of C5 vertebral body on C4 and avulsion fracture of the superior-posterior aspect of C5, adding to the spinal canal compromise. Increased signal within the spinal cord and in the posterior ligaments is also demonstrated.

that CT scanning is a more sensitive technique, particularly to identify fractures of the posterior elements or other abnormalities of the vertebral column, such as ossification of the posterior longitudinal ligament. However, MRI is extremely sensitive to the pathological marrow changes (edema and hemorrhage) that occur in association with bony fractures. MRI is also the current modality of choice in the diagnosis and follow-up of long term complications of SCI, such as syringomyelia, myelomalacia, and cord atrophy.

Medical Treatment

The best current acute medical and pharmacological therapy of SCI is based on the potentially reversible pathophysiological changes (e.g., ischemia, hypoxia, and lipid peroxidation) that occur after SCI. In patients with severe multiple trauma who require extensive or prolonged resuscitation or rapid transport to the operating room to treat associated life-threatening injuries, it may not be possible to obtain all the necessary radiographs. In such situations, efforts should be exerted to maintain strict immobilization of the neck and back until the patient is stable enough to undergo further imaging. It is essential to ensure hemodynamic stability before proceeding with further imaging or surgical treatment of the spinal injury. The description and treatment of delayed complications of SCI, such as deep venous thrombosis, are beyond the scope of this chapter.

Systemic Assessment and Care.   To assess the patient appropriately, all clothing should be cut away or otherwise removed, and vital signs monitored (respiratory rate, blood pressure, heart rate, and body temperature). Blood samples should be obtained for routine hematological and biochemical investigations, for typing and cross-match, and for arterial blood gas analysis.

The first concern during these initial stages of care is the maintenance of adequate ventilation and oxygenation. The frequency and severity of respiratory deficiency are related to the level and severity of SCI, with the more severe instances occurring in complete cervical SCI, especially above C5. Hypoxia in the injured regions of the cord worsens the damaging pathophysiological cascade, leading to secondary injury. Artificial ventilation is started if PO_2 is less than 70 mm Hg, PCO_2 exceeds 45 mm Hg, respiratory rate exceeds 30 breaths per minute, or vital capacity is less than 500 cc. Aspiration of vomitus, abnormal breathing patterns, or increased work of breathing due to the level of SCI may be relative indications for artificial ventilation. Pneumothorax, hemothorax, or (less frequently) hemopneumothorax are common injuries (occurring in approximately 15%) and may require chest tube insertion (Ryan et al. 1993). Pulmonary contusion is present in about 1% of SCI and is detectable with arterial blood gas measurement and chest radiograph.

The blood pressure should be vigorously supported, with normotension as the goal to ensure adequate spinal cord blood flow in the first hours after injury. Fluid resuscitation is thus a keystone in the initial therapy and should consist of an appropriate combination of crystalloid and colloid solutions, depending on the presence of any associated injuries. Extreme care is needed to prevent overhydration that may lead to pulmonary edema and may increase the intracranial pressure in patients with concomitant head injury. Insertion of a central line to monitor the central venous pressure or, better, a pulmonary artery catheter to maintain a pulmonary capillary wedge pressure of 18 mm Hg can help prevent overhydration. If, despite adequate fluid replacement, the blood pressure cannot be normalized or elevated slightly, assuming that there are no systemic contraindications, vasopressors (e.g., dopamine) should be considered. Intravenous atropine may be needed in SCI with severe bradycardia.

Hypothermia is another problem in SCI patients due to the loss of sympathetic control, which causes vasodilatation below the level of injury and may produce poikilotherm. Therefore, patients with SCI depend on the environmental temperature for control of their body temperature (Gutierrez et al. 1993).

Acute gastric dilatation and paralytic ileus frequently occur in direct response to spinal cord trauma. The ileus resolves usually within the first 3 or 4 days but may last somewhat longer in cervical injuries. Furthermore, the loss of large volumes of fluid and electrolytes into the gastrointestinal tract may accentuate hypovolemia, induce electrolyte disturbances, and push the abdominal wall outward and the diaphragm upward, making breathing extremely difficult. It may also induce vomiting with a high risk of aspiration, especially in cervical SCI patients who have lost their protective reflexes. Thus, most patients with SCI need early insertion of a nasogastric tube and avoidance of oral intake until the ileus and the acute gastric dilatation resolve. Hydration is maintained with intravenous fluids, but if the period of ileus continues beyond a few days, total parenteral nutrition should be instituted.

In the acute period, an indwelling 16–18-Fr Foley catheter is used to monitor urinary output and to prevent detrusor overdistention after SCI. The initial aim is to have a functioning bladder that stores well and empties easily with a minimum of urinary tract infections and no urinary incontinence or autonomic dysreflexia. Baseline blood urea, creatinine, and urine culture should be obtained. The evaluation of pre-existing problems, such as incontinence, prostate enlargement, or renal pathology, is important for decisions about long-term management. Any associated trauma to the urinary tract should be properly investigated and treated. In most cases, intermittent catheterization can be commenced within a few days of injury; it produces less infection and trauma to the urinary tract than does continuation of an indwelling catheter.

Pharmacotherapy. Optimal acute management of SCI includes pharmacological intervention with methylprednisolone (MPS), as established by the National Acute Spinal Cord Injury Study II (NASCIS II) in 1990 and further

defined by NASCIS III in 1997 (Bracken et al. 1997). The first study compared placebo versus MPS (30-mg/kg bolus and then 5.4 mg/kg/hour for 23 hours) versus naloxone (5.4-mg/kg bolus and then 4.0 mg/kg/hour for 23 hours). It was a randomized, prospective, double-blinded, multicenter study. The randomization, which was performed within 12 hours of injury, separated patients into two groups, according to their entry time of less than or more than 8 hours from injury. Neurological examinations were obtained on admission and then at 6 weeks, 6 months, and 12 months after injury. Their conclusion was that patients treated with MPS within 8 hours of injury had significantly increased recovery of neurological function. Patients treated after 8 hours in both the MPS and naloxone groups recovered less motor function than did those in the placebo group. The medical complications were the same for all three groups. The NASCIS III study compared the efficacy of MPS administered for 24 hours with MPS administered for 48 hours or tirilazad mesylate administered for 48 hours in patients with acute SCI. The conclusion was that patients who receive MPS within 3 hours of injury should be maintained on the treatment regimen for 24 hours, but when MPS is initiated 3–8 hours after injury, patients should be maintained on corticosteroid therapy for 48 hours. In a small number of patients, GM_1 ganglioside was effective for improving neurological outcome. A trial in a much larger number of patients is ongoing.

Immobilization and Traction. Once the radiographic diagnosis of the bony injury has been established, consideration must be given to acute spinal stabilization and, if appropriate, spinal realignment. Gardner-Wells tongs and the halo ring are the two most commonly used devices. The majority of these devices are compatible with CT and MRI, but contraindications to their use include comminuted skull fractures, extensive scalp lacerations, and the anticipated need for emergency craniotomy. Penetration of the skull by tongs has been reported, with associated serious infectious complications. Realignment of the spine can be accomplished in some patients by the application of traction. If the spine is already aligned, the amount of traction needed to maintain stabilization is no more than 5–10 lb. In the cases of severe ligamentous injury with distraction already present, the application of traction is contraindicated. As a general rule, no more than 5 lb per level of injury should be applied in the first few hours (i.e., a C5-C6 dislocation would require 30 lb of traction), although the maximum weight allowed and the allowable speed of escalation of weight application are highly controversial. Depending on the nature of the bony injury, slight flexion or extension of the neck may aid in achieving realignment. Some advocate the use of muscle relaxants, analgesics, sedatives, or general anesthesia. In 1992, Hadley and coworkers found in a nonrandomized series that the most important factor in neurological recovery was the time from injury to the decompression and alignment of the spinal canal. The few cases in which there was significant neurological improvement were all realigned

Table 56C.11:   Indications for emergency decompression or débridement

---

Incomplete lesions with extrinsic compression in patients who, after maximal possible reduction of subluxation, show:
  Progression of neurological signs
  Bone fragments or soft tissue elements (disc, hematoma) in the spinal canal on computed tomography, magnetic resonance imaging, or myelogram
  Necessity for decompression of a vital cervical root
  Compound fracture or penetrating trauma of the spine (rarely for decompression)
  Acute anterior spinal cord syndrome
  Unreducible fracture dislocations from locked facets causing spinal cord compression

---

Table 56C.12:   Contraindications to emergent operation (but may later require surgery)

Complete spinal cord injury more than 24 hrs after the injury
Medically unstable patient
Central cord syndrome without cord compression

---

within 8 hours of injury. Once realignment has been achieved, the patient may be maintained in traction until definitive management of the spinal injury is undertaken or fitted in a halo vest to allow early immobilization and lessen the risk of neurological deterioration. However, neurological deterioration during the application of traction or after halo vest placement is always possible. In that case, the authors recommend discontinuing traction and obtaining urgent radiological studies (CT, myelogram, or MRI) to evaluate the presence of spinal cord compression. The NASCIS II study documented a 5% frequency of neurological deterioration after hospitalization in the 487 patients studied. Thus, even though the frequency of neurological deterioration is not high during traction and immobilization, continued vigilance must be maintained.

Surgical Treatment

The traditional neurosurgical approach to acute SCI has been to stabilize the patient medically for a period that may last weeks before considering surgical intervention. This approach is based on the need to reduce both neurological and systemic complications from early surgery. A 1992 study of 1,019 thoracolumbar fractures by the Scoliosis Research Society reported a 3% overall complication rate in patients treated nonsurgically compared with a 25% rate in operated patients. However, most complications in the surgical group were related to wound, instrumentation, and graft problems, with only a 0.6% rate of neurological deterioration attributed directly to surgical intervention. Early surgical intervention on the cervical spine should be performed only under one circumstance: to avoid further deterioration in neurological function. The severity of the pathological changes and the degree of recovery are directly related to the duration of acute compression, as demonstrated by experimental studies in which longer compression times produced less clinical recovery (Carlson et al. 1997; Delamarter et al. 1995). In contrast, the clinical evidence of the relationship between duration of compression and recovery of spinal cord function is not well established

and depends largely on anecdotal accounts of improved recovery after rapid decompression by traction or surgery. There is a need for well-designed experimental and clinical studies of the timing and neurological results of surgical decompression of acute SCI. Furthermore, there has been controversy about whether surgery, especially early surgery, increases the rate of complications in patients with SCI. In one study from our center in 1987, the only difference in morbidity between the surgical and nonsurgical cases was a slight increase in the frequency of deep venous thrombosis in the operated group. In another study, those operated on in the first 24 hours had a lower rate of complications than those operated on at later times. In the randomized trial of the timing of surgery by Vaccaro et al. (1997), there was no significant difference in the length of acute postoperative intensive care stay or length of inpatient rehabilitation between the early and late surgery groups. Thus, with respect to complications, there is no compelling evidence that early surgery enhances the rate of complications.

We advocate early surgical intervention within the limits of patient stability. The indications for surgical intervention are (1) the promotion of neurological recovery and (2) the restoration of spinal stability. Spinal stability can be accomplished with external orthoses, such as the halo, or by internal fixation techniques. The issue of promotion of neurological recovery and the benefits and timing of surgery are highly controversial. The single widely accepted indication for immediate surgical intervention is documented neurological deterioration in association with ongoing spinal cord compression from disc or bone fragments, hematoma, or unreduced subluxation. Early aggressive surgical intervention has been advocated for incomplete lesions (excluding the central cord syndrome) for the reasons outlined in Table 56C.11. In general, emergency decompressive surgery is contraindicated in *complete* lesions after 24 hours from the injury, in central cord syndrome without cord compression, and in medically unstable patients (Table 56C.12). A few authorities argue that early aggressive surgical intervention is warranted, even in the face of an initially complete SCI. They believe that persistent compression may exacerbate the secondary injury cascade after SCI that has been shown to occur experimentally.

Nevertheless, even in the presence of an initially incomplete SCI, there is no clear, compelling evidence of neurological benefits from surgical intervention. In the only prospective, randomized, controlled trial of the timing of surgical decompression, early decompression (<72 hours after injury) did not produce significantly improved neurological recovery compared with late decompression (5 days or longer after injury) (Vaccaro et al. 1997). All other studies were retrospective and were not randomized. Randomized prospective studies are required to assess the value of early decompression, and until such studies are done, early surgical treatment of SCI will remain controversial.

Neurological Rehabilitation

The long-term management of SCI, especially in which the deficit remains severe or complete, is complex and specialized. A great deal of expertise is now available for the rehabilitation of such patients, who should be treated in a specialized SCI rehabilitation unit (see Chapter 54).

REFERENCES

Bracken MB, Shepard MJ, Holford TR, et al. Administration of methylprednisolone for 24 or 48 hours or tirilazad mesylate for 48 hours in the treatment of acute spinal cord injury. Results of the third national acute spinal cord injury randomized controlled trial. JAMA 1997;277:1597–1604.

Bunge RP, Puckett WR, Becerra JL, et al. Observations on the pathology of human spinal cord injury: a review and classification of 22 new cases with details from a case of chronic cord compression with extensive focal demyelination. Adv Neurol 1993;59:79–89.

Carlson GD, Warden KE, Barbeau JM, et al. Viscoelastic relaxation and regional blood flow response to spinal cord compression and decompression. Spine 1997;22:1285–1291.

Delamarter RB, Sherman J, Carr JB. Pathophysiology of spinal cord injury: recovery after immediate and delayed decompression. J Bone Joint Surg Am 1995;77(A):1042–1049.

Duh MS, Bracken MD, Shepard MJ, Wilberger JE. Surgical treatment of spinal cord injury—the National Acute Spinal Cord Injury Study II experience [abstract]. American Association of Neurological Surgeons Annual Meeting, Boston, April 1993.

Gutierrez PA, Young RR, Vulpe M. Spinal cord injury—an overview. Urol Clin North Am 1993;20:373–382.

Kiss ZHT, Tator CH. Neurogenic Shock. In ER Geller (ed), Shock and Resuscitation. New York: McGraw-Hill, 1993;421–440.

Levi ADO, Tator CH, Bunge RP. Clinical syndromes associated with disproportionate weakness of the upper versus the lower extremities after cervical spinal cord injury. Neurosurgery 1996;38:179–185.

Ryan M, Klein S, Bongard F. Missed injuries associated with spinal cord trauma. Am Surg 1993;59:371–374.

Samuels LE, Kerstein MD. Routine radiologic evaluation of the thoracolumbar spine in blunt trauma patients: a reappraisal. J Trauma 1993;34:85–89.

Sutherland MW. The prevention of violent spinal cord injuries. Spinal Cord Inj Nurs 1993;10:91–95.

Tator CH. Classification of Spinal Cord Injury Based on Neurological Presentation. In RJ Narayan, JE Wilberger Jr, JT Povlishock (eds), Neurotrauma. New York: McGraw-Hill, 1994; 1059–1073.

Tator CH. Pain following Spinal Cord Injury. In RH Wilkins, SS Rengachary (eds), Neurosurgery (2nd ed). New York: McGraw-Hill, 1996c;3975–3977.

Tator CH. Pathophysiology and Pathology of Spinal Cord Injury. In RH Wilkins, SS Rengachary (eds), Neurosurgery (2nd ed). New York: McGraw-Hill, 1996b;2847–2859.

Tator CH. Spinal Cord Syndromes with Physiologic and Anatomic Correlations. In AH Menezes, VKH Sonntag (eds), Principles of Spinal Surgery. New York: McGraw-Hill, 1996a; 769–799.

Tator CH, Duncan EG, Edmonds VE, et al. Changes in epidemiology of acute spinal cord injury from 1947 to 1981. Surg Neurol 1993b;40:207–215.

Tator CH, Duncan EG, Edmonds VE, et al. Complications and costs of management of acute spinal cord injury. Paraplegia 1993a;31:700–714.

Vaccaro AR, Daugherty RJ, Sheehan T, et al. Neurologic outcome of early versus late surgery for cervical spinal cord injury. Spine 1997;22:2609–2613.

Woodring JH, Lee C. Limitations of cervical radiography in the evaluation of acute cervical trauma. J Trauma 1993;34:32–39.

Chapter 56
Trauma of the Nervous System

D. PERIPHERAL NERVE TRAUMA
Robert L. Tiel and David G. Kline

The human peripheral nerve has significant regenerative potential. Injured axons have immense ability to regrow, and they do so over great distances. By comparison, the response of the connective tissue of nerve to serious injury is often poorly structured and may prevent effective and thus functional axonal growth. Nonetheless, advances over the last century have permitted useful repair of some nerve injuries. The use of antibiotics has greatly reduced the specters of infection and inflammation that were so devastating in previous generations. More recently, improved surgical optics and illumination have made the internal structure of the nerve accessible to direct surgery. Development of intraoperative neurophysiological methods to assess the presence or absence of useful regeneration has also improved the results of repair. It is hoped that further advances in neurophysiology, coupled with progress in cellular, genetic, and molecular neurobiology, will continue until the potential of human nerve regeneration can be directed, controlled, and maximized. Unfortunately for those obliged to treat in the present, optimal benefits remain in the future. We must content ourselves with a clear understanding of current principles and apply them as appropriately as possible to the problems of nerve injury and repair.

ANATOMY

Understanding nerve injury and repair is predicated on a clear and concise comprehension of the macro- and microscopic anatomy of the nerve. The peripheral nerve is in continuity with the central nervous system (CNS), and no discontinuity is observed as the nerve changes from the CNS to the peripheral nervous system (Figure 56D.1). The outer layer of the CNS is the dura mater, which joins with the outer layer of connective tissue of the peripheral nervous system to become the epineurium. The epineurium forms an external sheath for the nerve, which gives it a cordlike appearance and consistency. This sheath is then set in loose areolar connective tissue and fat, allowing easy separation of nerve from adjacent tissue while reducing local traction on nervous tissue. In healthy nerve, the tissue attaching nerve to surrounding structures is fine and transparent and is termed by some the *mesoneurium*.

At the lateral aspects of the spinal theca, around the exiting rootlets, the subarachnoid space is obliterated, the outer layer of the nerve root sheath is reflected, and the inner layer becomes continuous with the perineurium of nerve. This layer provides a lamellated sheath of cells interspersed with fine collagen fibers arranged in oblique, circular, and longitudinal directions. The perineurium encloses the basic subunit of nerve fibers within a nerve, the fasciculus. The perineurium also provides most of the elasticity and tensile strength to the peripheral nerve. It also constitutes, together with the endoneural capillaries, the blood-nerve barrier and maintains intrafascicular pressure.

Within the fasciculus, each nerve fiber is supported by a framework of collagen fibrils known as the *endoneurium*. This connective tissue structure begins at the junction of rootlets with the spinal cord. The endoneurium provides additional tensile strength to the nerve but also maintains an endoneural space that opens on the subarachnoid space proximally and the interstitial space of the end organ dis-

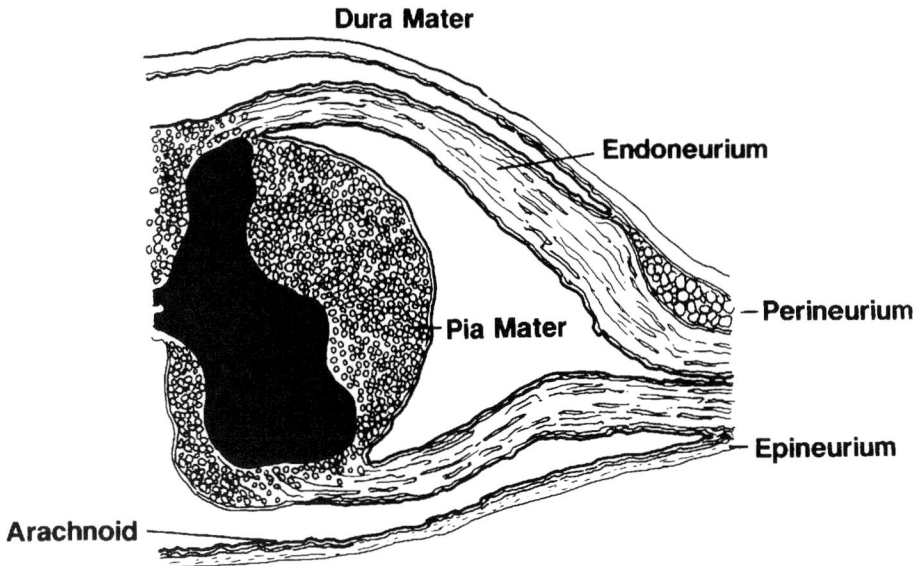

FIGURE 56D.1 The transition of connective tissue coverings of the central nervous system to layers of the peripheral nervous system. (Adapted from FR Haller, FN Low. The fine structure of the peripheral nerve root sheath in the subarachnoid space in the rat and other laboratory animals. Am J Anat 1974;131:1–20.)

tally. Each myelinated fiber is surrounded by a Schwann cell sheath or neurilemma. In myelinated fibers a Schwann cell ensheathes only one axon. In unmyelinated fibers, one Schwann (or Remak) cell encloses multiple nerves.

A transverse section of a nerve suggests a static separation of the aforementioned components. When viewed longitudinally, however, no fasciculus runs an independent, unaltered course. The process of fascicular redistribution, dispersal, and intermingling continues along the length of a nerve. There are repeated changes in size, number, and arrangement of the fasciculi so that within a few centimeters fascicular patterns are recognizably different. Fasciculi tend to take a more longitudinal or layered course in the distal extremity. The number of fasciculi varies depending on nerve and level studied and may range from 1 to 100.

The vascular supply of nerves demonstrates the following underlying properties:

1. It is predominately a longitudinal system with feeding branches joining spinal nerves proximally and branches of the nerve distally.
2. It has variability of nutrient arteries.
3. It possesses a large number of anastomotic connections and collaterals from epineurial, mesoneural, and endoneural networks.

The nutrient artery usually comes from a major artery, runs parallel with the nerve, and projects into a number of branches that interconnect; arterioles penetrate the perineurial covering and form an anastomosing capillary network within the endoneurium. Through this plexiform arrangement, the redundancy of the vascular supply is ensured over long distances. The veins in the epineurium arise from the intraneural capillary beds and, after short courses, connect with the draining veins of neighboring structures. The endothelium of the intrafascicular capillaries and the basal membrane that surrounds them form the

blood-nerve barrier in conjunction with the perineurium and maintains the homeostasis of the endoneural space.

NERVE INJURY

Seddon Classification

Significant trauma to nerve originates when force applied to a nerve is sufficient to cause a persistent loss of function. The clinical features of nerve injury vary with the geometry, nature, and duration of the deforming force. Seddon recognized three basic ways in which a nerve can respond to trauma.

Neurapraxia is the result of a mild degree of compression or stretch, which produces a block in conduction (probably metabolic) rather than axonal loss. It affects large fibers in preference to small fibers. Recovery occurs over a period of hours to days. Dysfunction of peroneal or ulnar nerve due to a blow or pressure and radial nerve ("Saturday night") palsy due to compression are common clinical examples. Complete recovery is the rule.

Axonotmesis occurs when the axon has lost continuity while its endoneural nerve sheath remains intact. Distal wallerian degeneration ensues, and retrograde degeneration of the first few internodes occurs proximal to the divided nerve fiber. Because of the intact nerve sheath, regeneration occurs with the axon regrowing down its proper course. Fidelity of reconnection is excellent, and a good functional recovery can be expected. Therapeutic crush of the phrenic or obturator nerve is an iatrogenic example of this type of injury, although these procedures are rarely performed anymore. Most, but not all, serious radial palsies associated with humeral fracture are due to axonotmesis.

Neurotmesis is caused by greater degrees of injury. There are endoneural, perineurial, and frequently epineurial disruptions as well as axonal damage, and useful regrowth is unusual. Some neurotmetic injuries result in transection, but most leave the nerve in continuity with severe intraneural damage. In either case, surgical repair is required for recovery in this category of injury.

Sunderland Classification

Many nerve injuries leave the nerve in gross continuity with varying degrees of intraneural damage. The Sunderland grading method is oriented toward the lesion in continuity and is anatomically based on the structure of the nerve, with progressive grades reflecting more severe damage.

Grade 1 is a metabolic dysfunction of the myelin sheath, axon, or both. This manifests itself electrophysiologically as a conduction block and corresponds to a neurapraxic injury.

Grade 2 is the loss of axon continuity with preservation of all layers of the connective tissue framework; the endoneural, perineurial, and epineurial layers all remain intact. In the Seddon system, this is an axonotmetic injury.

Grade 3 is loss of axon continuity with the additional loss of endoneural integrity. In this setting, internal endoneural scarring can prevent reinnervation, and disruption of the endoneural sheath may cause a "mismatch" as regenerating axons stray from their proper endoneural sheaths. Using the Seddon system, in our interpretation, the Sunderland grade 3 corresponds to a combined axonotmetic and neurotmetic injury.

Sunderland grade 4 injury is loss of perineural integrity and thus disruption of the fascicle. This is associated with more intraneural scarring and consequently less effective nerve regeneration. As in grade 3 injuries, the connective tissue disruption allows mismatch to occur with a type of regeneration that falls short of producing functional recovery. In the Seddon system, this corresponds to a neurotmetic injury in continuity.

Grade 5 is loss of epineural, perineural, and endoneural continuity and thus transection of the nerve. This is by definition a neurotmetic injury.

The Sunderland classification can be correlated with the Seddon system (Figure 56D.2). There are conceptual advantages to each.

MANAGEMENT OF PERIPHERAL NERVE INJURIES

The proper management of traumatic peripheral nerve injuries is based on both localization and gradation of nerve injury (Kline and Hudson 1995). Localization depends on inspection of the injured site, neurological examination, and deductive reasoning. At the time of injury, examination often is impaired by pain, edema, and associated injuries. These factors must be handled appropriately; analgesics should be given as necessary, and patience must be practiced in the examination of traumatized patients. An electromyogram (EMG) is no substitute for thoughtful clinical exami-

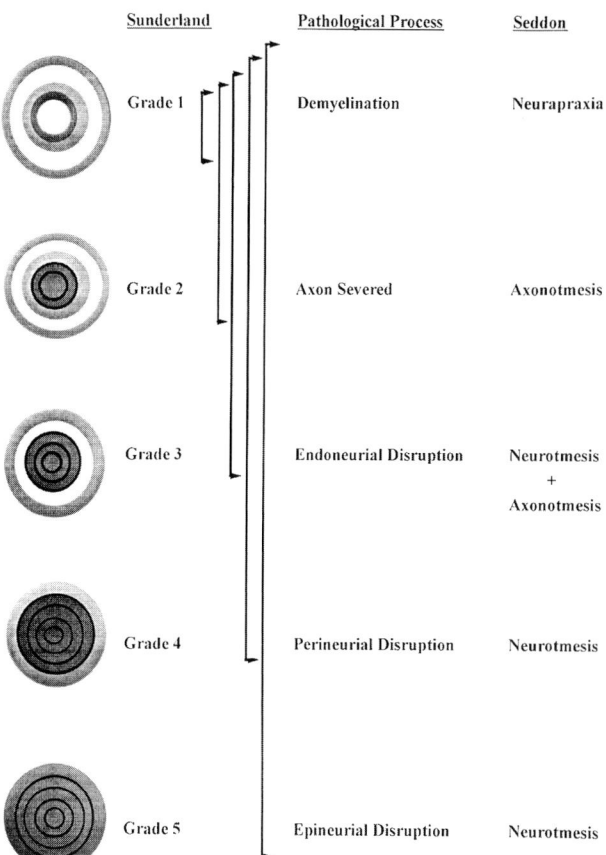

FIGURE 56D.2 A comparison of the Seddon and Sunderland classification systems.

nation. Gradation of injury is more difficult. Loss of function is no guide; all grades of injury by definition impair function. Grading systems are based on the pathology of the damage, which is usually not available in a definitive fashion without surgical exploration of the nerve. Nonetheless, an understanding of the mechanisms of injury and the temporal course of nerve recovery provide guidance in this regard.

Mechanisms of Nerve Injury

Most serious nerve injuries are a result of four basic mechanisms of trauma: laceration, compression, stretch, or high-velocity-missile injury.

Laceration

Laceration to nerve occurs in the setting of knife wounds but also may be seen with injuries caused by shattered glass and by more blunt mechanisms, such as chain saws, propeller blades, automobile metal, and animal bites. Even though 15–20% of "transection" injuries leave the nerve in continuity and some of these may recover without surgery, most lesions due to these mechanisms are neurotmetic, or

Sunderland grade 4 or 5, and consequently require surgical intervention. There is always the possibility of partial laceration. Surgical repair is the mainstay of treatment and should be done acutely for sharp transection, if logistically feasible. Delay in repair of sharp lesions can result in nerve retraction, requiring secondary grafting, which may result in reduced functional recovery. Conversely, blunt transections are best repaired 2–3 weeks after injury. At this point, internal demarcation between healthy and damaged tissues is obvious to inspection of proximal and distal stumps.

Compression

Compressive neural injuries usually result from the patient being immobilized for a prolonged period. In patients previously well, this immobility is usually due to coma from alcohol intoxication, drug abuse, or general anesthesia. The type of injury is usually neurapraxic, axonotmetic, or both, but on occasion endoneural damage does occur. The recovery time is the major indicator of the degree of injury; because spontaneous recovery is the rule, these injuries do not usually require surgical intervention. Large motor and position sense fibers are the most susceptible to compression. They are the first to fail and the last to recover and in mild injuries may be the only fibers to have function disrupted. As with most nerve injuries, a spectrum of damage can be seen, and there are cases in which effective regeneration without surgical repair is impossible.

Stretch

Stretch is the most common mechanism of serious injury to peripheral nerves. Stretch involving a limb and nerve decreases the cross-sectional area of nerve and increases intraneural pressure. As stretch approaches the elastic limit of 20%, nerve function also starts to fail. Nerve injury proceeds, starting at a Sunderland grade 1 level, and progresses grade by grade until the 30% limit is achieved. At this juncture, the perineurium and then the epineurium give way, and the nerve ruptures. As a consequence, all grades of injury may occur with this mechanism of injury. The 20% elastic limit is an average; significant damage may occur with as little as a 6% stretch. In mixed motor and sensory nerves, stretching may affect all function, or sensation alone, but seldom results in motor disability without sensory impairment. Given the lengths over which stretching forces may take place, the damage tends to spread over a section or length of nerve rather than occurring at a precise point. As discussed later, this makes successful surgical repair difficult and significantly prolongs the time course of recovery.

Stretch-Avulsion

Because the perineurium provides significant strength to peripheral nerve, the absence of this layer at the nerve rootlet level contributes significantly to the propensity for nerve

root avulsion to occur at this location. Clinically, this may be suspected by an associated Brown-Séquard spinal cord injury, Horner's syndrome, phrenic palsy, severe paraspinal denervation, or other indications of very proximal nerve root injury. Myelography with the demonstration of torn dural sheaths and extradural pooling of contrast (Figure 56D.3) serves to indicate the proximal location of trauma but cannot establish with certainty either the presence or the extent of avulsion. Sensory nerve conduction studies show preservation of sensory nerve action potentials (SNAPs) because the lesion is proximal to the dorsal root ganglion. Combined with the clinical picture of complete motor and sensory loss, the presence of SNAPs can substantiate the diagnosis of preganglionic injury. Such testing works better for lower-plexus than higher-plexus spinal nerves. Where there is pre- and postganglionic injury, SNAPs are absent, just as with postganglionic lesions alone.

High-Velocity Missile Injury

High-velocity missiles generate shock-wave pressures on impact, high-pressure regions in front of and lateral to the projectile, and pressure associated with the formation of a temporary explosive cavity in the track of the missile. Consequently, structures adjacent to and distant from the missile path may be abruptly stretched and deformed. Nerves directly in the path may be severed or torn. As a consequence of these stretching and disruptive mechanisms, all grades of injury may occur with missile injuries. In addition, there may be severe injury to associated vessels, bone, and muscles. Often, surgery is required for vascular repair, and then damaged or severed nerves are identified. Severed ends should be tagged and sutured to the operative bed to avoid retraction. Formal repair should be delayed for several weeks because this is a blunt injury to nerves. Where nerve continuity is more likely, as with most missile wounds, the injury is followed for several months by clinical examination and EMG. Then, if spontaneous recovery is not evident by either clinical or EMG examination, exploration and intraoperative recording is necessary to grade the injury and to determine proper management.

Time Course of Spontaneous Nerve Recovery

The time course of recovery after nerve injury reflects many stages. The first stage is the period of proximal stump degeneration with retrograde demyelination of the first few internodes. The next stages are axonal sprouting and then axonal regeneration. Next, the injury must be bridged, neurotization of the distal stump achieved, and finally axonal connection to the end organ accomplished. This process must be repetitive enough to create a neural pool large enough to elicit muscle activity and may take years to complete if the lesion is proximal. The recovery time depends not only on level of injury in relation to muscles to be

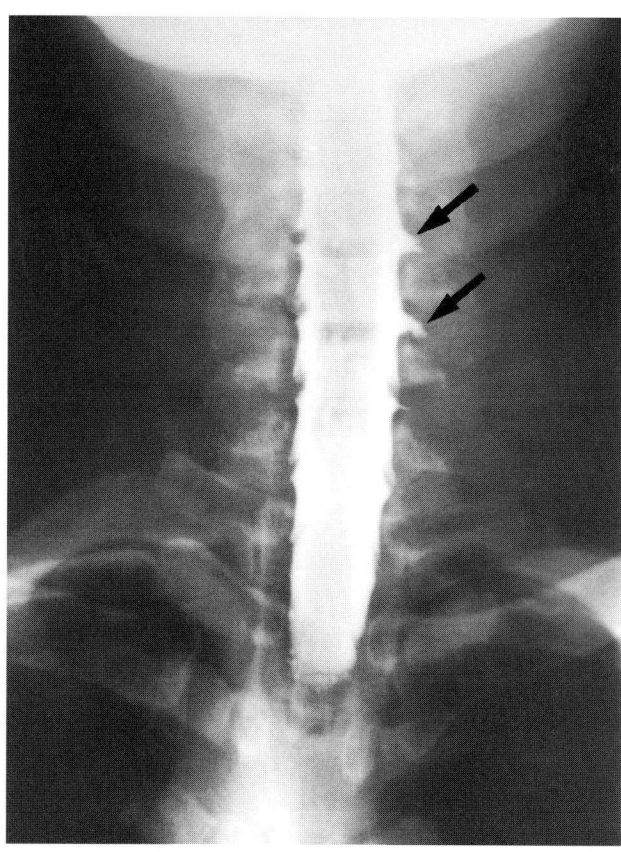

FIGURE 56D.3 The torn dural sheath allows the creation of a pseudomeningocele (*arrows*), seen here (**A**) by myelography and (**B**) by computed tomography. (Reprinted with permission from DG Kline, AR Hudson. Nerve Injuries. Philadelphia: Saunders, 1995.)

A

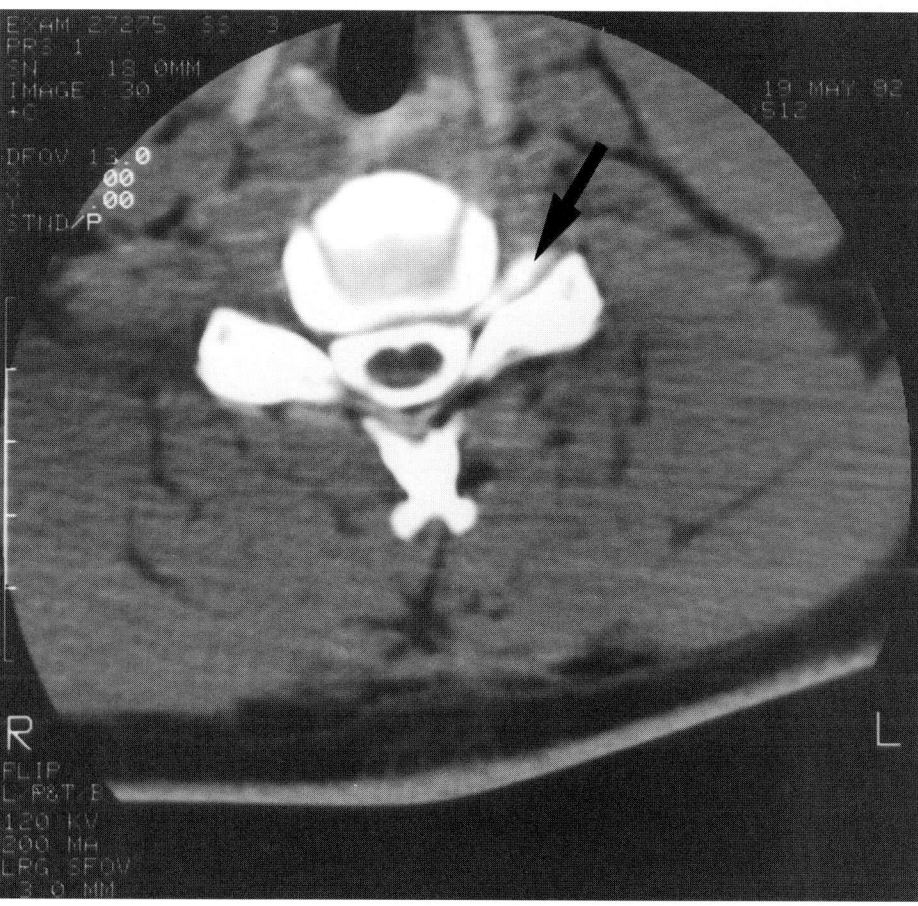

B

innervated but also on the specific nerve or plexal element involved. Consequently, we cannot afford to wait for a spontaneous recovery in many serious injuries because if recovery fails, it will be too late to undertake a repair. Often, the geometry of nerve injury is such that the most proximal muscle is 6–8 in. below the level of nerve injury. Waiting the requisite period to judge clinical recovery biases against the better clinical results achievable when the injured nerve is explored earlier.

When an axon is discontinuous, the time necessary to overcome retrograde degeneration, sprouting, and spanning of the injury site increases the time necessary for recovery. This may be 2 weeks with axonotmetic injuries and may extend to 4 weeks with sutured neurotmetic injuries. There is a similar expenditure of time once axons reach their end organ until enough maturation occurs to provide function. In general, the regenerative rate for axons is faster in the proximal than in the distal limb. A useful clinical approximation for recovery of motor function is an overall growth rate of 1 in. per month. Exceptions are lengthy stretch injuries and lesions that have undergone operative repair, particularly those using grafts and two suture lines. In those instances, growth rates for axons are much slower.

The time course of nerve recovery ultimately indicates the degree of injury. A severe neurapraxic injury may require several weeks to recover; rarely, this process takes as long as 6 weeks. No clinical recovery 8 weeks after nerve injury usually indicates a higher grade of injury. The clinical determination of recovery focuses on the most proximal muscles served by the injured nerve.

Temporal Limits of Regeneration

The functional potential of nerve recovery decreases with the passage of time. Although there is variation in the intrinsic recoverability of nerves and the percentage of strength necessary for useful function in associated muscles, most muscles are subject to a 24- to 36-month limit of denervation, after which little useful motor recovery is expected from reconnection. The exceptions to the rule regarding motor recovery are large muscles, such as biceps, triceps, gastrocnemius-soleus, and quadriceps. Surprisingly, the facial muscles, despite being smaller and carrying out a finely coordinated function, sometimes show a potential for recovery even years after losing neural input. When sensory function is considered, the period of effective repair may be increased by several years.

Management of Delayed or Failed Recovery

A challenge to management occurs with complete loss of function, without suspicion of transection, which does not show recovery by 8 weeks. Some of these injuries recover spontaneously in weeks to months with function superior to that achieved by resection and grafting; others recover with less function than is achieved by suturing; some segments do not recover spontaneously and should be resected and repaired. Proper clinical management depends on methods that allow timely determination of the degree of injury.

For lesions in which proximal muscles are within 3 in. of the injury site, observation alone may be adequate to determine useful clinical response. Unfortunately, many serious lesions affect nerve levels for which the closest distal innervated muscle is 6–18 in. away. Awaiting clinical evidence of recovery in such cases can be disastrous because if recovery does not occur, it would be too late for the repair to be effective. In any case, care must be exercised in the clinical examination to avoid the pitfalls of anomalous innervation and "trick" movements. If successive branches of a nerve show reinnervation, the decision against operative intervention is straightforward. Similarly, if no functional recovery is observed or potential inputs are far downstream, or both, operative assessment is warranted. Peripheral electrophysiological studies provide additional methods of assessment.

Nerve stimulation can be achieved either by surface electrodes or needle electrodes. The demonstration of contraction in the distribution of the injured nerve indicates adequate regeneration and eliminates the need for surgical investigation. Negative surface electrode examinations should be followed by needle electrode examination. Similarly, during operative exposure the involved nerve may be stimulated directly and the limb observed for muscular contractions distal to the level of injury. Care must be taken to avoid false interpretation. Obviously, contraction of muscles proximal to the injury site or contractions in the distribution of adjacent nerves do not provide evidence of recovery of the injured nerve.

EMG, if performed in a serial and thorough manner, is a useful tool in the management of peripheral nerve injuries. Early in the course of injury, the EMG may demonstrate retained motor units and thus assist in the determination of partial injury. Because the changes of denervation take several weeks, the full pattern of denervation after serious injury may not be evident. Loss of insertional activity; onset of spontaneous activity at rest, including fibrillations and positive sharp waves; and loss or distortion of the muscle action potential define the denervation pattern. With the passage of time, EMGs reveal the presence of reinnervation manifested by restoration of some insertional activity, decreased numbers of fibrillations, and sometimes the addition of nascent potentials. Unfortunately, the EMG cannot predict the overall quality of reinnervation. When EMG does demonstrate reinnervation, an additional short period of observation is indicated; during this period, if some spontaneous muscle contraction does not occur, surgery becomes necessary.

Operative Examination and Electroneurography

If recovery is not evident within the first 2 months of focal injury or during the first 3–4 months after a stretch injury,

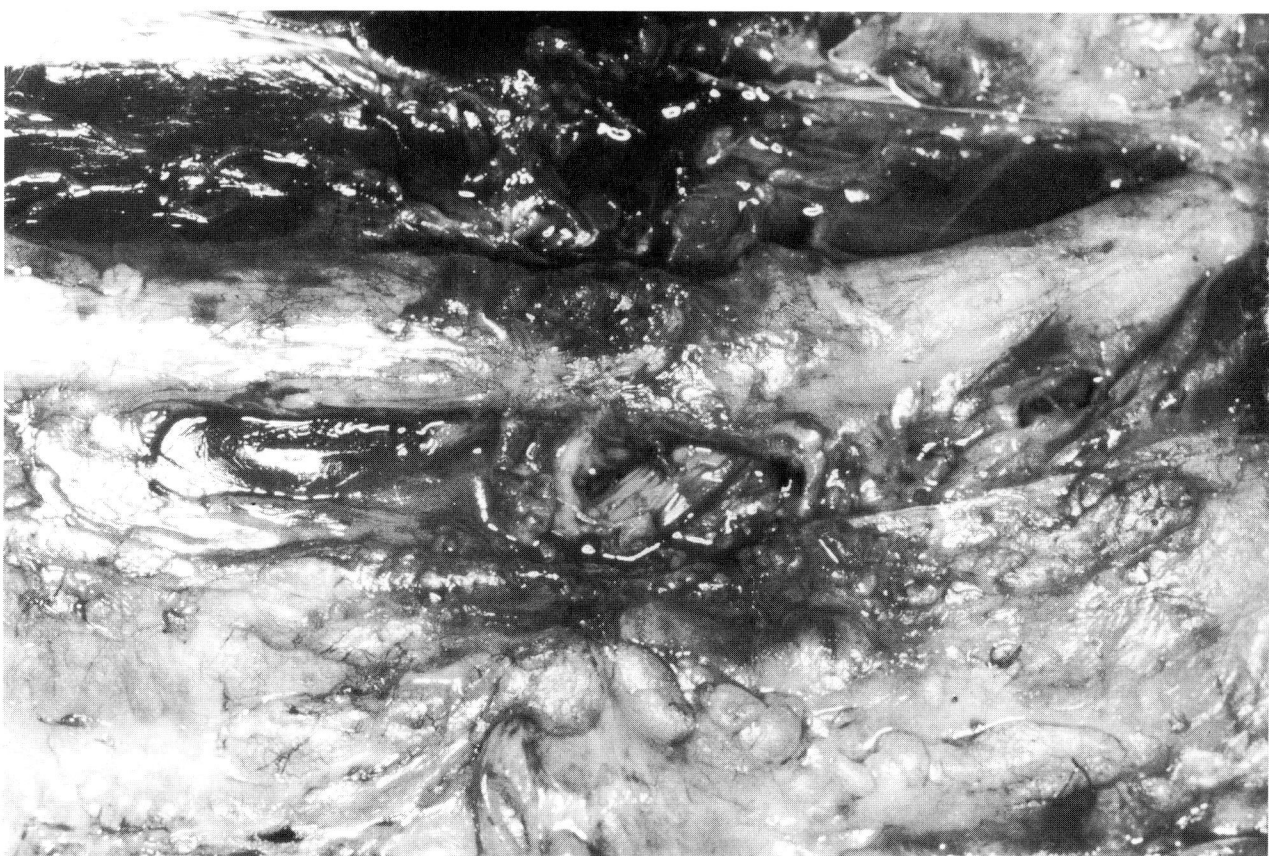

FIGURE 56D.4   Neuroma in continuity of the median nerve in the forearm after a gunshot injury.

direct operative examination of the nerve injury site is warranted. The diagnostic portion of the operation starts with an external neurolysis, whereby the segment of nerve is freed from surrounding tissue. This segment is viewed, palpated, and assessed electrophysiologically, across as well as distal to the level of injury. With this information, nerve injury grading can be completed. Once grading is achieved, surgical repair, if indicated, can be undertaken; otherwise, the incision is closed and the operation terminated.

Nerve rupture or transection is the most obvious condition that may be discovered. After dissection of the scarred bed, both damaged nerve ends are identified and freed. Occasionally, the ends have retracted a significant distance from the original site of rupture or transection. As a result of retraction and neuromas involving the ruptured nerve stumps, end-to-end repair is impossible without undue tension on the suture line. Grafts are required for repair when simple end-to-end or epineurial repair is impossible.

Often during exploration, the epineurium is intact, but a distinctly abnormal and usually firm section of nerve is identified. This represents a neuroma in continuity (Figure 56D.4). Visual and tactile inspection has proved unreliable in determining regenerative potential. The essential question is whether there has been significant growth of functional axons through the site of injury and distal to

the damaged segment. The presence of distal contraction on direct stimulation above the injury resolves the question immediately. In many instances, no contraction is evident and then NAP recording (electroneurography) is required to evaluate the regenerative potential of the damaged nerve.

Electroneurography is the direct recording of NAPs from a nerve (Figure 56D.5). It is the method used to demonstrate the regeneration of axons across a damaged segment before reinnervation of the target muscle can occur (Kline and Happel 1993). This ability to determine return of function across a damaged segment is especially important in instances in which clinical recovery may not be evident for 6–18 months and in which temporal limitations of reinnervation may significantly affect outcome. The recording of an adequate NAP beyond the injured segment reflects the presence of 3,000–4,000 regenerated moderate- to large-diameter nerve fibers at the recording site, thereby indicating a good potential for recovery and eliminating the need for operative repair (Figure 56D.6).

In the case of root avulsion, the diagnosis is usually suspected preoperatively. The presence of a high-amplitude, fast-conducting NAP in a nerve with total loss of function indicates preganglionic injury with sensory fiber sparing. Such a response should not be confused with a NAP of

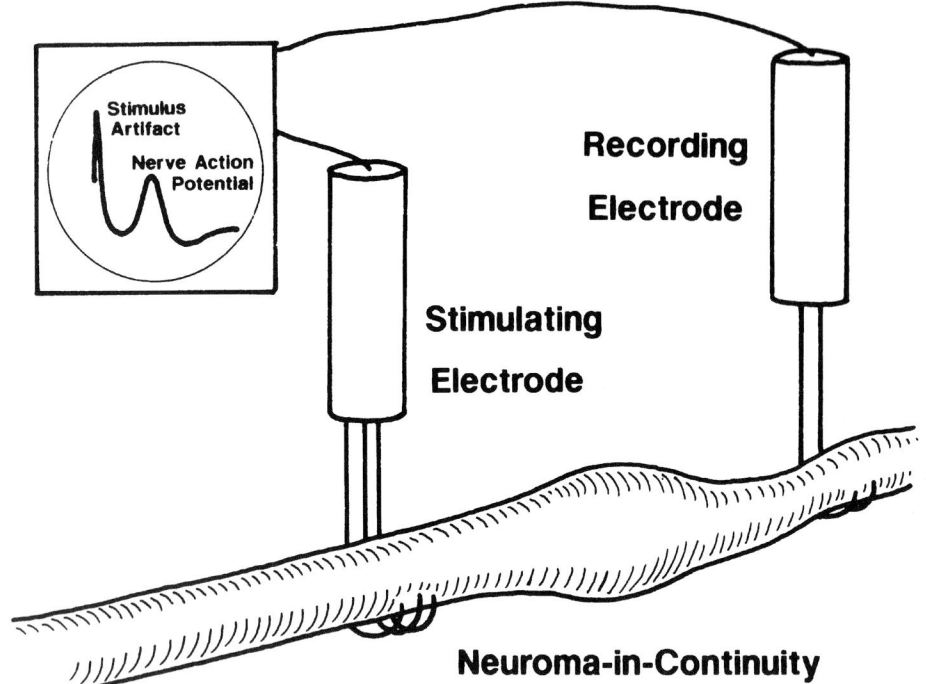

Neuroma-in-Continuity

FIGURE 56D.5   The intraoperative recording of a nerve action potential requires mobilization of the nerve (neurolysis), proximal stimulation, and distal recording.

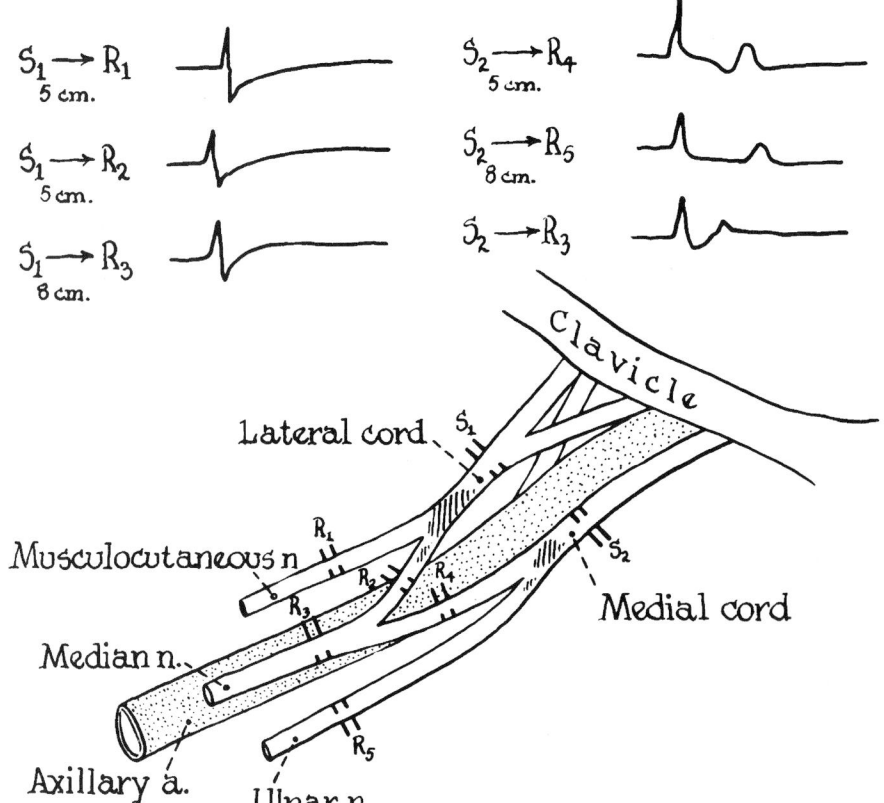

FIGURE 56D.6   Diagram shows location of nerve action potentials (NAPs) in a brachial plexus exploration for a gunshot injury. The absence of NAPs from S1 to R1, R2, and R3 indicates a complete lateral cord injury, and resection and grafting are indicated. The presence of NAPs from S2 to R3, R4, and R5 indicates a functioning medial cord, which should be considered for split repair or simply neurolysed. (a = artery; n = nerve.) (Reprinted with permission from DG Kline. Evaluation of the Neuroma in Continuity. In G Omer, M Spinner (eds), Management of Peripheral Nerve Problems. Philadelphia: Saunders, 1980.)

FIGURE 56D.7 Epineurial repair showing suture of the epineurium after fascicular alignment.

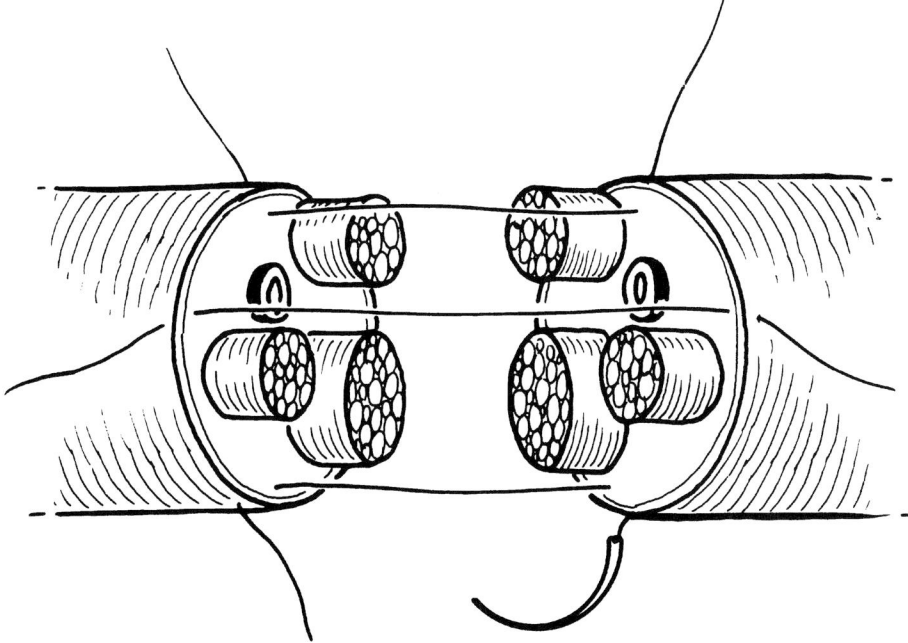

smaller amplitude and slower conduction velocity that is characteristic of relatively recent regeneration.

REPAIR OF NERVE INJURIES

Once the decision for resection and suturing has been made, the surgeon has a variety of options in the management of nerve repair. The goal of nerve repair is to achieve the proper reapproximation of nerve ends so as to ensure maximum fidelity of nerve regeneration.

Epineurial Repair

In the case of simple laceration, the nerve ends are inspected and the contused margins are cut back sharply with a razor or scalpel until a normal fascicular pattern is identified. Opposing ends are aligned carefully to ensure proper realignment of fascicles (Figure 56D.7). The course of the epineurial blood vessels provides additional information for orientation. The process is greatly facilitated by magnification, either by loupes or the operating microscope. The epineurium of opposing stumps is then sutured together. Suture material must be strong and inert. In general, a 6-0 monofilament nylon or proline suture is adequate.

Sutureless anastomotic techniques have been investigated for more than 50 years; these include various wrapping techniques, plasma clot, fibrin glue, and, more recently, carbon dioxide laser–assisted anastomosis. In our opinion, there is no method or material superior to a fine, relatively inert suture.

Care must be taken to ensure that tension on the suture line is minimized. Because the cut ends of nerve retract, there is always tension on an end-to-end nerve repair. Tension can be minimized by additional mobilization of the nerve intraoperatively, judicious positioning of the limb at surgery, and postoperative use of a sling or splint. If these measures fail, nerve grafting should be considered. The use of "stay" sutures should be avoided. The repaired nerve should be returned to a soft bed of viable tissue as free of scar tissue as possible. There is no current role for the wrapping of suture lines with "protective material."

Fascicular Repair

Because fascicular matching is one of the goals of nerve repair, end-to-end fascicular repair has attracted much attention. This is based on theoretical merit and the availability of magnification, which, along with use of stimulation in an awake patient, allows identification of fascicles. Fascicular repair requires dissection of the distal and proximal stumps, identification and correlation of individual fascicles, and then their suturing (Figure 56D.8). A 9-0 or 10-0 monofilament nylon suture is used. This technique requires an internal dissection of the cut ends and an internal placement of suture material, resulting in a lengthier neuroma and more intraneural scar tissue. In sharp lacerations, fascicular realignment can usually be achieved by epineurial repair (see Epineurial Repair, earlier in this chapter). In cases in which there has been significant stump trimming, the fascicular pattern can change dramatically even within short distances. Suturing of fascicles in these cases cannot ensure an accurate match, and results are less successful than epineurial repair. Complete fascicular repair should be used only for ulnar and median injuries at the wrist level.

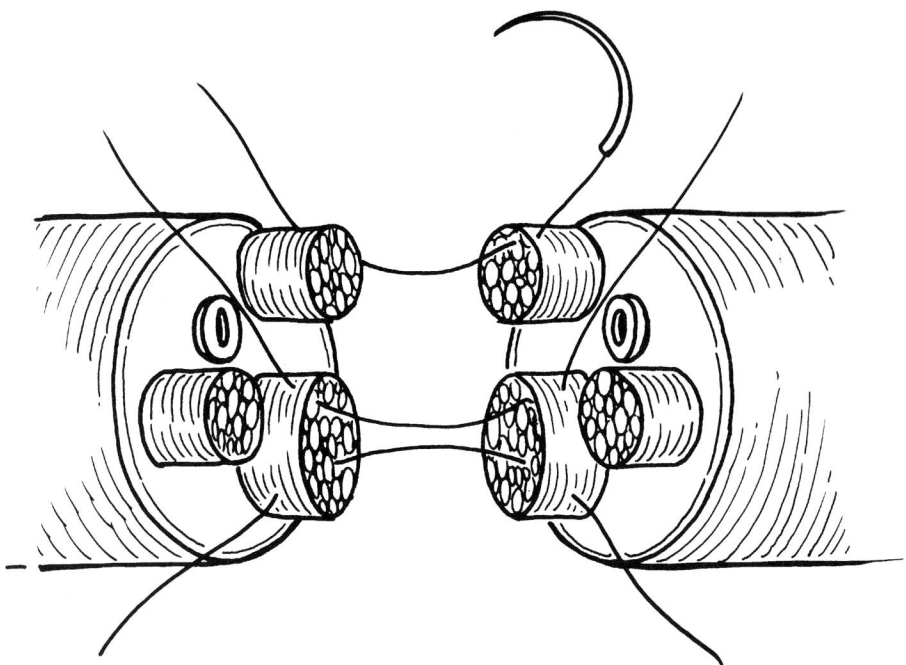

FIGURE 56D.8 Fascicular repair showing suture of the perineurium after fascicular alignment.

Nerve Grafts and Grouped Interfascicular Repair

Nerve grafts should be considered when the length of the damaged segment or the anatomy of the branching pattern prevents end-to-end approximation and suture. The method of grouped interfascicular repair consists of the isolation of fascicles or groups of fascicles over a distance of 1–2 cm on each stump. Multiple cables are then created after harvest of the sural, antebrachial cutaneous, superficial radial, or other appropriate nerve. In most instances, the use of autogenous grafts suffices. There are extreme cases in which the supply of autogenous grafts is exhausted or unavailable. In these instances, the use of allografts, as demonstrated by MacKinnon and Hudson in 1992, may prove useful. The necessity of temporary immunosuppression, however, limits the widespread adoption of this method.

Sections of the donor nerve are trimmed and then sutured to the grouped fascicles at each end of the gap (Figures 56D.9 and 56D.10). Growth through grafts takes much longer than through end-to-end repair. The regenerating nerve fibers must cross two fascicular interfaces and, consequently, the chance that axons may reach extrafascicular sites is increased. Nonetheless, the results with well-done graft repairs are surprisingly good. The length of the graft will affect the clinical outcome. Grafts with lengths up to 20 cm have been successfully used. The quality of the operative bed and the thickness of the donor nerve will also affect the outcome. Grafts are revascularized at the ends first, then from the outside in. A healthy soft tissue bed surrounding the graft will facilitate revascularization and decrease the development of central necrosis. Donor grafts of high caliber are more likely to undergo central necrosis than grafts of low caliber.

The use of grafts represents an advancement in operative repair but is not a replacement for end-to-end or epineurial repair. Consequently, the method should be reserved for situations in which repair cannot be accomplished by end-to-end reapproximation and suturing that is often the case with serious nerve injuries in which nerve grafting is frequently used.

Split Repair

Despite the presence of a NAP across a lesion-in-continuity, a portion of the nerve may look better than the rest. In this case, the nerve should be internally dissected and the more normal section split from the more scarred section. However, splitting apart of injured plexus elements or of injured tibial from peroneal divisions in sciatic injuries is always indicated. Partial injuries may require split repair of fascicles. This is often required with larger brachial plexus elements and is routine with the sciatic nerve at the buttock level, where it is split into its tibial and peroneal divisions. These split sections are then tested for NAPs. Nonconductive segments or fascicles are then resected and repaired, usually by grafts. This is termed a *split repair*; functional outcome with such a repair is usually better than with either end-to-end or graft repair of the whole nerve.

Neurotization

Neurotization is the process of using alternative neural outputs to substitute for irrevocably lost neural tissue. The sit-

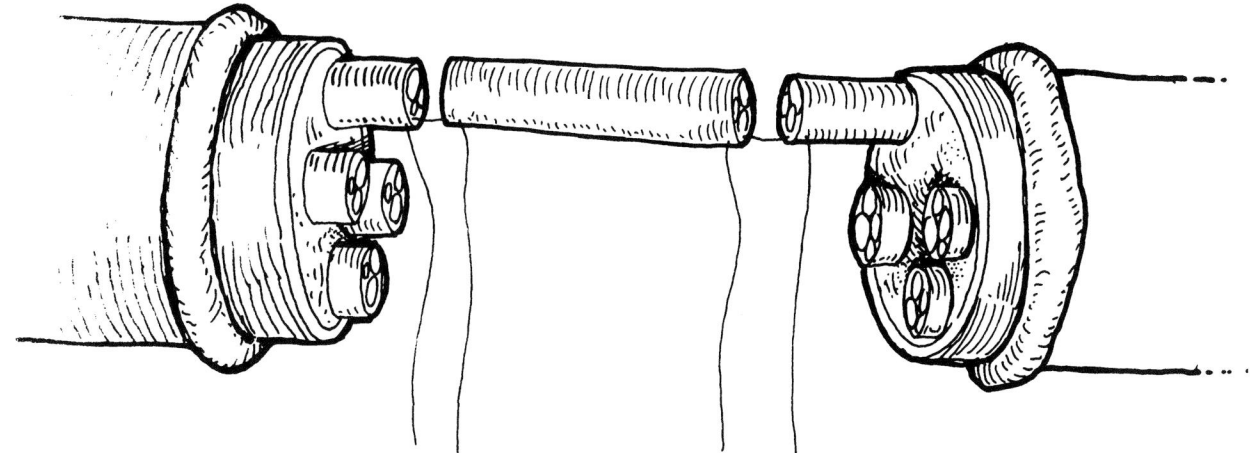

FIGURE 56D.9   Diagram of grouped fascicular repair shows interposed graft.

FIGURE 56D.10   Operative photograph of a grouped fascicular repair using multiple grafts. (Reprinted with permission from DG Kline, AR Hudson. Nerve Injuries. Philadelphia: Saunders, 1995.)

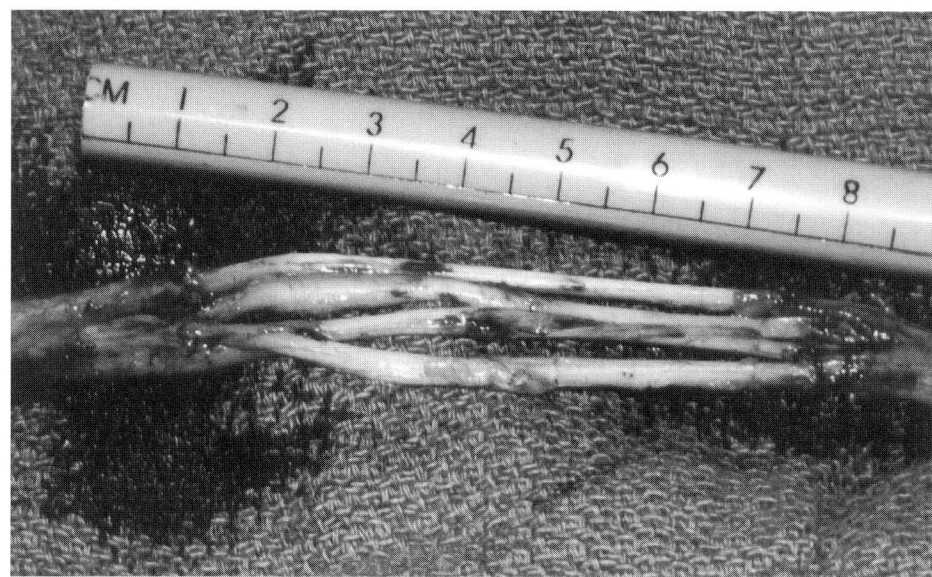

uation presents itself most commonly in the case of nerve root avulsions or complete damage to the spinal nerves in their proximal parts. Various procedures have been described in which the cervical plexus, the contralateral C7 spinal nerve, spinal accessory nerve, phrenic nerve, pectoral nerves, or intercostal nerves have been used as proximal outflow donors. These nerves are directly connected to distal nerves, such as the musculocutaneous. Sural interposition grafts may be required, depending on the distances involved and the donor nerves. In some series, the results have been encouraging. Success in achieving flexion at the elbow joint against gravity using neurotized elements has been reported in 25–50% of patients. When lower elements are spared, as in an upper trunk avulsion, the substitution of the medial pectoral nerve for the musculocutaneous has also proved very useful. We are currently coupling this neu-

rotization with that of the distal spinal accessory nerve into the suprascapular nerve to allow some degree of arm abduction as well as elbow flexion.

Recently, the central motor reorganization that allows the neurotization to be functionally useful has been demonstrated. In patients in whom the intercostal nerves were used to innervate the biceps brachii, Mano et al. (1995) used motor evoked potentials to demonstrate a migration of the motor stimulation area of the intercostals controlling biceps function to a more lateral area of the cortex. This finding gives insight into a latent central plasticity that may allow useful neurotization to occur without the need for excessive rehabilitation. The process of neurotization is still undergoing modification. It should not be considered to lie within the province of the occasional operator, and it should be limited to centers experienced in these techniques.

Nerve Root Reimplantation

At present, the clinical potential for reimplantation of avulsed ventral roots remains essentially unproved. There is experimental evidence of re-established continuity between motoneurons and reimplanted ventral roots in cats (Hoffmann et al. 1993). In humans, ventral roots have been reimplanted and reinnervation in distal muscles demonstrated (Carlsteadt 1995), but unambiguous demonstration that the reimplanted roots were responsible for the reinnervation was in our view unproved. Consequently, it still remains to be seen whether the quantity and quality of this type of reconnection is enough for the restitution of function in humans with root avulsions.

REHABILITATION

Pre- and postoperatively, there is a great need for maintenance of range of motion in the involved extremity. The treatment for a frozen joint is far more painful than its prevention. The physician must be sure that the patient understands and accepts both the importance and the responsibility for range-of-motion exercises three to four times per day. The physical therapist can assist in the education of the patient, monitor progress, and encourage compliance but cannot substitute for poor patient-doctor communication, poor motivation, or poor compliance. A one-time visit to the physical therapist serves little purpose.

With the recovery of early function, both physical therapy and occupational therapy become very important to help the patient maximize functional return. In some cases, splints, braces, and other assistive devices are also important, especially while awaiting neural recovery.

MANAGEMENT OF FAILED REGENERATION

The goal of nerve repair is the return of function via the restitution of continuity between neurons and their end organs. Unfortunately, there are instances when recovery is not possible or is unsuccessful. For example, there are some instances of referral past the 2- to 3-year time limit of effective reinnervation. In these instances, appropriate tendon transfers and joint stabilization procedures should not be overlooked. In general, secondary reconstructive procedures are performed in a distal-proximal direction. This is especially true in the upper extremity because effectiveness of the hand is a major criterion for usefulness. If appropriate tendon transfers cannot be of help, more proximal reconstruction may not be indicated. Most wrist and hand surgery is made more difficult by proximal shoulder arthrodesis or elbow flexion contractures. Prosthetic devices may be considered, but their long-term use has been disappointing. Finally, amputation may have to be considered in the case of a flail extremity without hope for meaningful recovery, even though many patients elect to retain their paralyzed limb. The patient must understand that removal of the paralyzed limb usually does not alleviate any associated pain.

CONCLUSION

The management of nerve injury requires an understanding of anatomy, an appreciation of neurophysiology, and intimate knowledge of nerve regeneration. There are rewards to both patient and physician if these educational goals are met. For the patient, there can be recovery of motor function, return of sensation, and reduction of pain. For the clinician who has patience born of experience, the management of nerve injury offers a diagnostic challenge and, on many occasions, therapeutic satisfaction.

REFERENCES

Carlsteadt T, Grane P, Halin RG, Noren G. Return of function after spinal cord implantation of avulsed spinal roots. Lancet 1995;346:1323–1325.

Hoffmann CF, Thomeer RT, Marani E. Reimplantation of ventral rootlets into the cervical spinal cord after their avulsion: an anterior surgical approach. Clin Neurol Neurosurg 1993;95 (Suppl.):S112–S118.

Kline D, Happel L. A quarter century of experience with intraoperative nerve active potential recording. Can J Neurol Sci 1993;20:3–10.

Kline DG, Hudson AR. Nerve Injuries. Philadelphia: Saunders, 1995.

Mano Y, Nakamuro T, Tamura R, et al. Central motor reorganization after anastomosis of the musculocutaneous and intercostal nerves following cervical root avulsion. Ann Neurol 1995;38:15–20.

Chapter 57
Vascular Diseases of the Nervous System

A. ISCHEMIC CEREBROVASCULAR DISEASE
José Biller and Betsy B. Love

EPIDEMIOLOGY AND RISK FACTORS

Every year, at least 500,000 Americans experience a new or recurrent stroke. Despite gradual declines in overall stroke death rates in many industrialized countries, stroke remains the third leading cause of death, with 150,000 fatalities annually in the United States. Stroke is also the leading cause of disability in adults. Of the 350,000 survivors each year, approximately 31% require assistance with activities of daily living, 20% require assistance with ambulation, and 16% require institutional care. The human and financial costs of stroke are immense, and its estimated annual economic impact on our society, both directly in health care and indirectly in lost income, is approximately $40.9 billion.

Steep decreases in stroke incidence and mortality have occurred in industrialized nations in recent years. The reduction in U.S. stroke mortality has been attributed to a declining stroke incidence, with suggestive evidence favoring a trend in declining stroke severity. Despite these trends in developed countries, stroke mortality and incidence are still high in many other countries. Socioeconomic factors, dietary and lifestyle behaviors, different patterns of risk factors, and environmental conditions may explain the different incidences of stroke observed in different parts of the world.

A number of factors that may be classified as modifiable and unmodifiable increase the risk of ischemic stroke (Table 57A.1). Risk factors for stroke include older age, male gender, African-American ethnicity, low socioeconomic status, family history, arterial hypertension, diabetes mellitus, dyslipidemia, heart disease, cigarette smoking, excessive alcohol intake, and body mass index. Clinicians cannot assume that these risk factors express themselves exclusively by accelerating atherosclerosis. There are also considerable data implicating hemostatic and microcirculatory disorders in stroke as well as circadian and environmental factors.

The incidence of stroke increases dramatically with advancing age, and increasing age is the most powerful risk factor for stroke. Men develop ischemic strokes at higher rates than women up to the age of 75 years. The rate of cerebral infarction is higher in blacks than in whites; this could be partially explained by the higher prevalence of diabetes and arterial hypertension experienced by blacks. The stroke incidence and case fatality rates are also markedly different among the major ethnic groups in Auckland, New Zealand. Maori and Pacific Islands people have a higher mortality within 28 days of stroke when compared with Europeans, especially men (Bonita et al. 1997).

Heredity seems to play a minor role in the pathogenesis of cerebral infarction. However, an increased risk is seen with a family history of stroke among first-degree relatives, a maternal history of death from stroke, and a paternal or maternal history of stroke. A positive parental history of stroke is also an independent predictor of stroke risk. There

Table 57A.1: Risk factors for ischemic stroke

Nonmodifiable	Modifiable
Age	Arterial hypertension
Race/ethnicity	Transient ischemic attacks
Gender	Prior stroke
Family history	Asymptomatic carotid bruit/stenosis
Genetics	Cardiac disease
	Aortic arch atheromatosis
	Diabetes mellitus
	Dyslipidemia
	Cigarette smoking
	Alcohol consumption
	Increased fibrinogen
	Elevated homocyst(e)ine
	Low serum folate
	Elevated anticardiolipin antibodies
	Oral contraceptives
	Obesity

are also a number of genetic causes of stroke. Some inherited diseases, such as the hereditary dyslipoproteinemias, predispose to accelerated atherosclerosis. A number of inherited diseases are associated with nonatherosclerotic vasculopathies, including Ehlers-Danlos (especially type IV) syndrome, Marfan's syndrome, Rendu-Osler-Weber disease, and Sturge-Weber syndrome. Familial atrial myxomas, hereditary cardiomyopathies, and hereditary cardiac conduction disorders are examples of inherited cardiac disorders that predispose to stroke. Deficiencies of protein C and S or antithrombin III are examples of inherited hematological abnormalities that can cause stroke. Finally, rare inherited metabolic disorders that can cause stroke include MELAS (*m*itochondrial *e*ncephalopathy, *l*actic *a*cidosis, and *s*trokelike episodes), Fabry's disease, and homocystinuria. Controversial evidence shows that the presence of the apolipoprotein ε2 allele in elderly individuals and deletion of the gene for the angiotensin-converting enzyme may increase the risk of stroke (Slooter et al. 1997).

At least 25% of the adult population has arterial hypertension, defined as systolic blood pressure greater than 140 mm Hg, or diastolic blood pressure greater than 90 mm Hg. Arterial hypertension predisposes to ischemic stroke by aggravating atherosclerosis and accelerating heart disease, increasing the relative risk of stroke three- to fourfold. It is also the most important modifiable risk factor for stroke. Blood pressure treatment resulting in a reduction in systolic blood pressure of 10–12 mm Hg and 5–6 mm Hg diastolic, is associated with a 38% reduction in stroke incidence (MacMahon et al. 1996). Treatment of isolated systolic hypertension in the elderly is also effective in reducing stroke risk. The Systolic Hypertension in the Elderly Program showed a 36% reduction in nonfatal plus fatal stroke over 5 years in the age 60 and older group, with isolated systolic hypertension treated with active medication. Treating systolic hypertension also slows the progression of carotid artery stenosis.

Diabetes mellitus increases the risk of ischemic cerebrovascular disease two- to fourfold compared with the risk in nondiabetics. In addition, diabetes mellitus increases morbidity and mortality after stroke. Macrovascular disease is the leading cause of death among patients with diabetes mellitus. The mechanisms of stroke secondary to diabetes may be caused by cerebrovascular atherosclerosis, cardiac embolism, or rheological abnormalities. The excess stroke risk is independent of age or blood pressure status. Diabetes associated with arterial hypertension or hyperlipidemia adds significantly to stroke risk. Diabetic persons with retinopathy and autonomic neuropathy appear to be a group at particularly high risk for ischemic stroke. High insulin levels increase the risk for atherosclerosis and may represent a pathogenetic factor in cerebral small vessel disease. However, presently no evidence exists that tighter diabetic control or normal HbA1c levels over time decrease the risk of stroke or stroke recurrence.

High total cholesterol and high low-density lipoprotein concentration are correlated with atherosclerosis. Although overwhelming evidence relates low levels of high-density lipoprotein cholesterol with coronary heart disease, the association with cerebrovascular disease is less clear. Some studies have shown a positive relationship between serum cholesterol levels and death resulting from nonhemorrhagic stroke. The relationship has not been consistent, however, possibly because different risks are associated with different lipoprotein subtypes. People with high serum lipoprotein (a) levels appear to have a higher risk of ischemic stroke. Lipid-lowering agents may slow progression of atherosclerotic plaque growth and may possibly cause a regression in plaque formation.

An estimated 1–2 million Americans have chronic nonvalvular arterial fibrillation (NVAF), a condition that is associated with an overall risk of stroke of approximately fivefold and a mortality of approximately twice that of age- and sex-matched individuals without atrial fibrillation. The prevalence of atrial fibrillation increases with advancing age. Approximately 70% of individuals with atrial fibrillation are between 65 and 85 years of age. NVAF is associated with a substantial risk of stroke. Recent congestive heart failure, arterial hypertension, and prior thromboembolism increase the risk of embolism in patients with NVAF. The use of oral anticoagulation therapy decreases the relative risk of stroke in patients with NVAF by approximately two-thirds. Left atrial enlargement increases the risk of stroke in men. Likewise, left ventricular hypertrophy by electrocardiography (ECG) in men with pre-existing ischemic heart disease is a major risk for stroke.

Cigarette smoking is an independent risk factor for ischemic stroke in men and women of all ages, and a leading risk factor of carotid atherosclerosis in men. The risk of stroke in smokers is two to three times greater than in nonsmokers. The mechanisms of enhanced atherogenesis promoted by cigarette smoking are incompletely understood. More than 5 years may be required before a reduction in stroke risk is observed after cessation of smoking. Switching to pipe or cigar smoking is of no benefit. There is a J-shaped association between alcohol consumption and ischemic stroke; light to moderate use (up to two drinks a day) evenly distributed throughout the week offers a reduced risk, whereas heavy drinking is associated with an increased risk of total stroke. Moderate alcohol intake may elevate high-density lipoprotein concentration.

Obesity, particularly abdominal or truncal, is an important risk factor for cardiovascular disease in men and women of all ages. There is some evidence that physical activity can reduce the risk of stroke. Habitual snoring increases the risk of stroke and adversely affects outcome of patients admitted to the hospital with stroke.

Atherosclerotic lesions of the carotid bifurcation are a common cause of stroke. Persons with an asymptomatic carotid bruit have an estimated annual risk of stroke of 1.5% at 1 year and 7.5% at 5 years. Asymptomatic carotid artery stenosis less than 75% carries a stroke risk of 1.3% annually; with stenosis greater than 75%, the combined transient ischemic attack (TIA) and stroke rate is 10.5% per year, with most events occurring ipsilateral to the stenosed carotid artery. Plaque composition may be an important factor in the pathophysiology of carotid artery disease. Plaque structure rather than degree of carotid artery stenosis may be a critical factor in determining stroke risk. Ultrasonographic carotid artery plaque morphology may identify a subgroup of patients at high risk of stroke. Ulcerated, echolucent, and heterogeneous plaques with a soft core represent unstable plaques at high risk for arterioarterial embolism.

Patients who suffer TIAs are at greater risk than normal controls for stroke or death from vascular causes. The risk of stroke is approximately three times higher. Approximately 10–15% of those experiencing a stroke have TIAs before their stroke. Patients with hemispheric TIAs are at greater risk of ipsilateral stroke than patients with retinal TIAs. Patients with a first stroke are at greater risk of recurrent stroke, especially but not exclusively, early after the first stroke. Those who suffer a recurrent stroke have a higher mortality than patients with first stroke. If the recurrence is contralateral to the first stroke, prognosis for functional recovery is poor. The risk of stroke recurrence is increased also by the presence of underlying dementia.

The aorta is the most frequent site of atherosclerosis. Protruding aortic arch atheromas are associated with otherwise unexplained TIAs or strokes. Aortic arch atheromatosis detected by transesophageal echocardiography is an independent risk factor for cerebral ischemia; the association is particularly strong with mobile and thick atherosclerotic plaques measuring greater than or equal to 4 mm in thickness (The French Study of Aortic Plaques in Stroke Group 1996).

Hemostatic factors may be important in assessing the risk of cerebrovascular disease. Elevated hematocrit, hemoglobin concentration, and increased blood viscosity may be indicators of risk for ischemic stroke. Elevation of plasma fibrinogen is an independent risk factor for the development of cerebral infarction. An elevated plasma fibrinogen level may reflect progression of atherogenesis. Compared with white Americans, black Americans have higher mean levels of fibrinogen, factor VIII, von Willebrand's factor, and antithrombin III, and lower mean levels of protein C. Fibrinogen levels are closely correlated with other stroke risk factors such as cigarette smoking, arterial hypertension, diabetes, obesity, hematocrit levels, and spontaneous echocardiographic contrast. Antiphospholipid antibodies are a marker for an increased risk of thrombosis, including TIAs and stroke, particularly in those younger than 50 years of age. Whether elevated anticardiolipin antibodies contribute causally to the risk of stroke or are merely a marker of increased risk because of an association with other precursors of stroke remains unknown. Elevated levels of plasma homocyst(e)ine have been associated with an increased risk of stroke and thrombotic events in case-controlled studies, but further corroboration is needed from prospective studies. Conversely, serum folate concentrations less than or equal to 9.2 nmol/liter have been associated with elevated plasma levels of homocyst(e)ine, and a decreased folate concentration alone may be a risk factor for ischemic stroke, particularly among blacks (Giles et al. 1995).

Stroke is uncommon among women of childbearing age. The relative risk of stroke is increased among users of high-dose estrogen oral contraceptives, particularly with coexistent arterial hypertension, cigarette smoking, and increasing age. New agents containing lower doses of estrogen and progestogen have reduced the frequency of oral contraceptive–related cerebral infarction. Conversely, postmenopausal hormone replacement with estrogens reduces the risk and mortality of stroke. The risk of thrombosis associated with pregnancy is high in the postpartum period. The risk of cerebral infarction is increased in the 6 weeks after delivery but not during pregnancy. The factor V Leiden mutation is associated with deep venous thrombosis in otherwise healthy individuals with additional prothrombotic risk factors. An overall association of the factor V Leiden mutation and arterial thrombosis has not been found. Elevated von Willebrand's factor is a risk factor for myocardial infarction and ischemic stroke.

A diurnal and seasonal variation of ischemic events occurs. Circadian changes in physical activity, catecholamine levels, blood pressure, blood viscosity, platelet aggregability, blood coagulability, and fibrinolytic activity may explain the circadian variations in onset of myocardial and cerebral infarction. Although an early morning peak occurs for all subtypes of stroke, most clinical trials on the use of platelet antiaggregants or other antithrombotic agents do not take these circadian variations into account. Rhythmometric analyses support the notion that stroke is a chronorisk disease, in which cold temperatures also represent a risk factor. A history of recent infection, particularly of bacterial origin and within 1 week of the event, is also a risk factor for ischemic stroke in patients of all ages.

PATHOPHYSIOLOGY OF CEREBRAL ISCHEMIA

The cerebral arteries are either conducting or penetrating. Except for the lack of an external elastica lamina in the intracranial arteries, the morphological organization of the cerebral vessels is similar to those in other vascular beds. The arterial wall consists of three layers: the outer layer, or adventitia; the middle layer, or media; and the inner layer, or intima. The intima is a smooth monolayer of endothelial cells providing a nonthrombotic surface for blood flow. One of the major functions of the endothelium is active inhibition of coagulation and thrombosis.

The brain microcirculation comprises the smallest components of the vascular system, including arterioles, capillaries, and venules. The arterioles are composed primarily of smooth muscle and are the major sites of resistance to blood flow in the arterial tree. The capillary wall consists of a thin monolayer of endothelial cells. Nutrients and metabolites diffuse across the capillary bed. The venules are composed of a fragile muscle wall and function as collecting tubules. The cerebral microcirculation distributes blood to its target organ by regulating blood flow and distributing oxygen and glucose to the brain while removing by-products of metabolism.

A cascade of complex biochemical events occurs seconds to minutes after cerebral ischemia. Cerebral ischemia is caused by reduced blood supply to the microcirculation. Ischemia causes impairment of brain energy metabolism, loss of aerobic glycolysis, intracellular accumulation of sodium and calcium ions, release of excitotoxic neurotransmitters, elevation of lactate levels with local acidosis, free radical production, cell swelling, overactivation of lipases and proteases, and cell death. Many neurons undergo apoptosis after focal brain ischemia (Choi 1996). Ischemic brain injury is exacerbated by leukocyte infiltration and development of brain edema. Exciting new treatments for stroke target these biochemical changes.

Complete interruption of cerebral blood flow causes suppression of the electrical activity within 12–15 seconds, inhibition of synaptic excitability of cortical neurons after 2–4 minutes, and inhibition of electrical excitability after 4–6 minutes. Normal cerebral blood flow at rest in the normal adult brain is approximately 50–55 ml/100 g per minute, and the cerebral metabolic rate of oxygen is 165 mmol/100 g per minute. There are certain ischemic flow thresholds in experimental focal brain ischemia. When blood flow decreases to 18 ml/100 g per minute, the brain reaches a threshold for electrical failure. Although these cells are not functioning normally, they do have the potential for recovery. The second level, known as the *threshold of membrane failure*, occurs when blood flow decreases to 8 ml/100 g per minute. Cell death can result. These thresholds mark the upper and lower blood flow limits of the ischemic penumbra. The ischemic penumbra or area of misery perfusion is the condition of the ischemic brain between these two flow thresholds in which there are some neurons that are functionally silent but structurally intact and potentially salvageable.

PATHOLOGY OF ISCHEMIC STROKE

The pathological characteristics of ischemic stroke are dependent on the mechanism of stroke, the size of the obstructed artery, and the availability of collateral blood flow. There may be advanced changes of atherosclerosis visible within arteries. The surface of the brain in the area of infarction appears pale. With ischemia caused by hypotension or hemodynamic changes, the arterial border zones may be involved. A wedge-shaped area of infarction in the center of an arterial territory may result if there is occlusion of a main artery in the presence of collateral blood flow. In the absence of collateral blood flow, the entire territory supplied by an artery may be infarcted. With occlusion of a major artery, such as the internal carotid artery, there may be a multilobar infarction with surrounding edema. There may be evidence of flattening of the gyri and obliteration of the sulci caused by cerebral edema. A lacunar infarction in subcortical regions of the brainstem may be barely visible, with a size of 1.5 cm or less. Emboli to the brain tend to lodge at the junction between the cerebral cortex and the white matter. Early reperfusion of the infarct when the clot lyses may occur, leading to hemorrhagic transformation.

The microscopic changes after cerebral infarction are well documented. The observed changes depend on the age of the infarction. The changes do not occur immediately and may be delayed up to 6 hours after the infarction. There is neuronal swelling initially, which is followed by shrinkage, hyperchromasia, and pyknosis. Chromatolysis appears and the nuclei become eccentric. Swelling and fragmentation of the astrocytes and endothelial swelling occur. Neutrophils infiltrate as early as 4 hours after the ischemia and become abundant by 36 hours. Within 48 hours, the microglia proliferate and ingest the products of myelin breakdown and form macrophages. There is neovascularity with proliferation of capillaries and increased prominence of the existing capillaries. The elements in the area of necrosis are gradually reabsorbed and a cavity, consisting of glial and fibrovascular elements, forms. In a large infarction, there are three distinct zones: an inner area of coagulative necrosis; a central zone of vacuolated neuropil, leukocytic infiltrates, swollen axons, and thickened capillaries; and an outer marginal zone of hyperplastic astrocytes and variable changes in nuclear staining.

CLINICAL SYNDROMES OF CEREBRAL ISCHEMIA

A number of syndromes result from ischemia involving the central nervous system (Brazis et al. 1996).

Transient Ischemic Attacks

Approximately 80% of ischemic strokes occur in the carotid or anterior circulation, and 20% occur in the vertebrobasilar or posterior circulation. A TIA is a prognostic indicator of stroke, with one-third of untreated TIA patients having a stroke within 5 years. The interval from the last TIA is an important predictor of stroke risk; of all patients who subsequently experience stroke, 21% do so within 1 month and 51% do so within 1 year of the last TIA. Cardiac events are the principal cause of death in patients who have had a TIA. The 5–6% annual mortality after TIAs is mainly caused by myocardial infarction, similar to the 4% annual cardiac mortality in patients with stable angina pectoris.

A TIA is a temporary, focal, and "nonmarching" neurological deficit of sudden onset; related to ischemia of the brain, retina, or cochlea; and lasting less than 24 hours. Yet, most TIAs last only 5–20 minutes. Episodes that last longer than 1 hour are usually caused by small infarctions. The onset of symptoms is sudden, reaching maximum intensity almost immediately. To qualify as a TIA, the episode should be followed by complete recovery. TIAs involving the anterior or carotid circulation should be distinguished from those involving the posterior or vertebrobasilar circulation. Headache is a frequent symptom in patients with TIAs. The following symptoms are considered typical of TIAs in the carotid circulation: ipsilateral amaurosis fugax, contralateral sensory or motor dysfunction limited to one side of the body, aphasia, contralateral homonymous hemianopia, or any combination thereof. The following symptoms represent typical TIAs in the vertebrobasilar system: bilateral or shifting motor or sensory dysfunction, complete or partial loss of vision in both homonymous fields, or any combination of these symptoms. Perioral numbness also occurs. Isolated diplopia, vertigo, dysarthria, and dysphagia should not be considered TIAs, unless they occur in combination with one another, or with any of the other symptoms just listed (Table 57A.2).

Occlusive disease in the subclavian arteries or the innominate artery can give rise to extracranial steal syndromes. The most defined syndrome is the subclavian steal syndrome. In this syndrome, reversal of flow in the vertebral artery is caused by a high-grade subclavian artery stenosis or occlusion proximal to the vertebral artery and symptoms of brainstem ischemia. Ischemic symptoms may be precipitated by actively exercising the arm. The left side is involved most frequently. With innominate occlusion, the origin of the right carotid is also subject to the consequences of reduced pressure. The presence of a subclavian steal syndrome can be suspected in the presence of a reduced or delayed radial pulse and diminished blood pressure in the affected arm relative to the contralateral arm. A subclavian steal may be symptomatic or asymptomatic. Many patients have angiographic evidence of reversed vertebral blood flow without ischemic symptoms. Transcranial Doppler sonography may detect transient retrograde basilar blood flow. Retrograde vertebral artery flow is a benign entity. Brainstem infarction is an uncommon complication of the subclavian steal syndrome.

Transient global amnesia (TGA) is characterized by a reversible antegrade and retrograde memory loss, except for

Table 57A.2: Recognition of carotid and vertebrobasilar transient ischemic attacks

Symptoms suggestive of carotid transient ischemic attacks
    Transient ipsilateral monocular blindness (amaurosis fugax)
    Contralateral body weakness or clumsiness
    Contralateral body sensory loss or paresthesias
    Aphasia with dominant hemisphere involvement
    Various degrees of contralateral homonymous visual field defects
    Dysarthria (not in isolation)
Symptoms suggestive of vertebrobasilar transient ischemic attacks
    Usually bilateral weakness or clumsiness, but may be unilateral or shifting
    Bilateral, shifting or crossed (ipsilateral face and contralateral body) sensory loss or paresthesias
    Bilateral or contralateral homonymous visual field defects or binocular vision loss
    Two or more of the following symptoms: vertigo, diplopia, dysphagia, dysarthria, and ataxia
Symptoms not acceptable as evidence of transient ischemic attack
    Syncope, dizziness, confusion, urinary or fecal incontinence, and generalized weakness
    Isolated occurrence of vertigo, diplopia, dysphagia, ataxia, tinnitus, amnesia, drop attacks, or dysarthria

a total amnesia of events that occur during the attacks, and inability to learn newly acquired information. During the attacks, patients remain alert without motor or sensory impairments and often ask the same questions repeatedly. Patients are able to retain personal identity and carry on complex activities. TGA most commonly affects patients in their 50s and older. Men are affected more commonly than women. The attacks begin abruptly and without warning. A typical attack lasts several hours (mean, 3–6 hours) but seldom longer than 12 hours. Onset of TGA may follow physical exertion, sudden exposure to cold or heat, or sexual intercourse. Although a large number of conditions have been associated with transient episodes of amnesia, in most instances TGA is primary or of unknown cause. TGA has been documented in association with intracranial tumors, overdose of diazepam, cardiac arrhythmias secondary to digitalis intoxication, and as a complication of cerebral and coronary angiography. Many reports have suggested a vascular etiology for this heterogeneous syndrome. Bilateral hippocampal and parahippocampal complex ischemia, possibly of migrainous origin, in the distribution of the posterior cerebral arteries is a potential mechanism. Acute confusional migraine in children and TGA have a number of similar features. Others have suggested an epileptic etiology for a minority of patients. Transient amnesias have been divided into pure TGA, probable epileptic amnesia, and probable transient ischemic amnesia. In contrast to patients with TIAs, the prognosis of persons with pure TGA is benign, with no apparent increased risk for vascular end points. Recurrences are uncommon. Extensive evaluations are not required. Treatment with platelet antiaggregants is not indicated in most patients unless there is a suspicion for transient ischemic amnesia. The use of prophylactic calcium-channel blockers may be justified in patients with a potential migrainous etiology.

Drop attacks are characterized by the sudden loss of muscle tone and strength. The attacks cause the patients to unexpectedly fall to the ground. Consciousness is preserved. Most attacks occur while standing or walking and often follow head or neck motion. Drop attacks have been considered a symptom of vertebrobasilar ischemia, but many of these patients have other coexistent disorders that could otherwise explain their symptoms. In rare instances, drop attacks may indeed be caused by ischemia of the corticospinal tract or reticular formation. However, isolated drop attacks are seldom a manifestation of vertebrobasilar occlusive disease. In most instances these attacks are secondary to akinetic seizures, high cervical spine or foramen magnum lesions, postural hypotension, Tumarkin's otolithic crises (in Ménière's disease), or near syncope.

TIAs may result from an atherothromboembolism that originates from ulcerated extracranial arteries, emboli of cardiac origin, occlusion of small penetrating arteries that arise from the large surface arteries of the circle of Willis, altered local blood flow caused by severe arterial stenosis, nonatherosclerotic vasculopathies, or hypercoagulable states. Preceding TIAs occur in large numbers of patients with brain infarction. In published series of cases of stroke, TIAs occurred before 25–50% of atherothrombotic infarcts, in 11–30% of cardioembolic infarcts, and in 11–14% of lacunar infarcts. Lacunar TIAs in general share the same pathogenetic mechanisms of lacunar infarcts and are associated with a substantially better prognosis than are nonlacunar TIAs.

Crescendo episodes of cerebral ischemia that increase in frequency, severity, or duration may be most threatening. A small subset of crescendo TIAs is the capsular warning syndrome, characterized by restricted episodes of capsular ischemia, causing contralateral symptoms involving face, arm, and leg. When capsular infarction develops, it is usually a lacunar-type stroke and involves a single penetrating vessel. Occasionally, striatocapsular or anterior-choroidal artery territory infarction occurs. Typically, these patients are refractory to conventional forms of therapy (Donnan et al. 1993).

Rational treatment of patients with TIAs depends on a careful history and detailed physical examination. The neurovascular examination may disclose a well-localized bruit in the mid- or upper cervical area. Bruits arise when normal laminar blood flow is disturbed. However, the presence of a cervical bruit does not necessarily indicate underlying carotid atherosclerosis. Correlation with angiography or ultrasound studies show only 60% agreement with cervical auscultation in predicting the presence of arterial stenosis. Radiated cardiac murmurs, hyperdynamic states, nonatherosclerotic carotid arterial lesions, and venous hums can produce cervical murmurs. The absence of a bruit has little diagnostic value. The bruit may disappear when the stenosis is advanced. Conversely, a cervical bruit may be heard contralateral to an internal carotid artery occlusion.

Different types of microemboli (e.g., cholesterol crystals, platelet fibrin, calcium, and so forth) can be seen in the retinal arterioles during or between attacks of transient monocular visual loss. Engorgement of conjunctival and episcleral vessels, corneal edema and rubeosis iridis, and anterior chamber cells flare are indicative of an underlying ischemic oculopathy. Asymmetrical hypertensive retinal changes noted on funduscopy are suggestive of a high-grade carotid artery stenosis or occlusion on the side of the less severely involved retina. Venous stasis retinopathy may occur with high-grade carotid stenosis or occlusion and is characterized by diminished or absent venous pulsations, dilatated and tortuous retinal veins, peripheral microaneurysms, and blossom-shaped hemorrhages in the midperipheral retina. Corneal arcus senilis may be less obvious or absent on the side of low perfusion.

Many conditions can resemble a TIA. Space-occupying lesions; subdural, intracerebral, or subarachnoid hemorrhage; seizures; hypoglycemia; migraine; syncope; and labyrinthine disorders are among the diverse conditions in the differential diagnosis when TIA is considered. Symptoms of a transient neurological dysfunction that resolve indistinctly should lead the physician to question the diagnosis of TIA. Similarly, a migration or march of symptoms from one part of the body to another is rare during a TIA and more indicative of a focal seizure or migraine. Fortification phenomena or scintillating bright visual symptoms are suggestive of migraine. In rare instances, involuntary limb shaking movements can occur, but, in general, involuntary movements reflect convulsive activity rather than a TIA.

Carotid Artery System Syndromes

Amaurosis fugax may be described as a sudden onset of a fog, haze, scum, curtain, shade, blur, cloud, or mist. A curtain or shade pattern with the loss of vision moving superiorly to inferiorly is described only in 15–20% of patients. Less commonly, a concentric vision loss presumed to be caused by marginal perfusion can diminish blood flow to the retina. The vision loss is sudden, often brief, and painless. The length of vision loss is usually 1–5 minutes and rarely lasts more than 30 minutes. After an episode of amaurosis fugax, the vision is usually fully restored, although some patients may have permanent vision loss caused by a retinal infarction (see Chapters 14 and 15).

The sole feature that distinguishes the middle cerebral artery (MCA) syndrome from the carotid artery syndrome is amaurosis fugax. An MCA infarction is one of the most common manifestations of cerebrovascular disease. The clinical picture with an MCA infarction is varied and depends on whether the site of the occlusion is in the stem, superior division, inferior division, or lenticulostriate branches, and whether there is good collateral blood flow.

When the stem of the MCA is occluded, there is usually a large infarction with contralateral hemiplegia, conjugate eye deviation toward the side of the infarct, hemianesthesia, and homonymous hemianopia. Associated global aphasia occurs if the dominant hemisphere is involved and hemineglect with nondominant hemispheric lesions. The difference between an upper division MCA infarction and an MCA stem lesion is that the hemiparesis usually affects the face and arm more than the leg with upper division infarction. A Broca-type aphasia is more common in upper division infarcts because of the preferential involvement of the anterior branches of the upper division in occlusions. With lower division MCA syndromes, a Wernicke-type aphasia is seen with dominant hemisphere infarction and behavioral disturbances are seen with nondominant infarction. A homonymous hemianopia may be present. A lenticulostriate branch occlusion may cause a lacunar infarction with involvement of the internal capsule producing a syndrome of pure motor hemiparesis. These syndromes are variable and are dependent on the presence of collaterals of whether brain edema is present.

Alexia with agraphia may occur with left angular gyrus involvement. Gerstmann's syndrome, which consists of finger agnosia, acalculia, right-left disorientation, and agraphia may be seen with dominant hemisphere parietal lesions. The aphasias with dominant hemispheric infarctions may be of the Broca, Wernicke, conduction, or global type, depending on the site and extent of involvement. Anosognosia, the denial of hemiparesis, most commonly is associated with right hemispheric strokes. Nondominant infarction may cause hemi-inattention, tactile extinction, visual extinction, anosognosia, anosodiaphoria, apraxia, impaired prosody, and rarely acute confusion and agitated delirium. A contralateral homonymous hemianopia or contralateral inferior quadrantanopia can occur with infarctions in either hemisphere.

Anterior cerebral artery (ACA) territory infarctions are uncommon (Figure 57A.1). They occur in patients with vasospasm after subarachnoid hemorrhage caused by ACA or anterior communicating artery aneurysm. Excluding these causes, the percentage of acute cerebral infarcts that are in the ACA territory is less than 3%. The characteristics of ACA infarction vary according to the site of involvement and the extent of collateral blood flow. Contralateral weakness involving primarily the lower extremity, and to a lesser extent, the arm, is characteristic of infarction in the territory of the hemispheric branches of the ACA. Other characteristics include abulia, akinetic mutism (with bilateral mesiofrontal damage), impaired memory or emotional disturbances, transcortical motor aphasia (with dominant hemisphere lesions), deviation of the head and eyes toward the lesion, paratonia (gegenhalten), discriminative and proprioceptive sensory loss (primarily in the lower extremity), and sphincter incontinence. An anterior disconnection syndrome with left arm apraxia caused by involvement of the anterior corpus callosum can be seen. Pericallosal branch

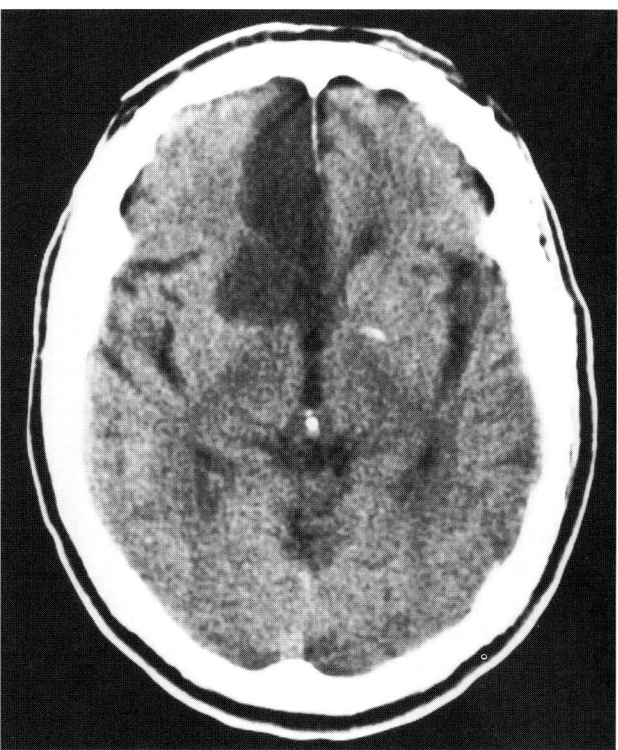

FIGURE 57A.1 Nonenhanced axial computed tomographic scan of a 63-year-old man with left-sided weakness and abulia demonstrates a right anterior cerebral artery (ACA) territory infarction. More superior images showed the entire ACA distribution was infarcted.

involvement can cause apraxia, agraphia, and tactile anomia of the left hand. Infarction of the basal branches of the ACA can cause memory disorders, anxiety, and agitation. Infarction in the territory of the medial lenticulostriate artery (artery of Heubner) causes more pronounced weakness of the face and arm without sensory loss caused by this artery's supply of portions of the anterior limb of the internal capsule.

The anterior choroidal artery syndrome is often characterized by hemiparesis caused by involvement of the posterior limb of the internal capsule, hemisensory loss caused by involvement of the posterolateral nucleus of the thalamus or thalamocortical fibers, and hemianopia secondary to involvement of the lateral geniculate body or the geniculo-localcarine tract. The visual field defect with anterior choroidal artery syndrome infarcts is characterized by a homonymous defect in the superior and inferior visual fields that spares the horizontal meridian. In a small number of patients left spatial hemineglect with right hemispheric infarctions and a mild language disorder with left hemispheric infarctions may occur. With bilateral infarctions in the anterior choroidal artery syndrome territory, there can be pseudobulbar mutism, and a variety of other features including facial diplegia, hemisensory loss, lethargy, neglect, and affect changes.

Lacunar Syndromes

Ischemic strokes resulting from small vessel or penetrating artery disease (lacunes) have unique clinical, radiological, and pathological features. Lacunar infarcts are small ischemic infarctions in the deep regions of the brain or brainstem that range in diameter from 0.5 to 15.0 mm. These infarctions result from occlusion of the penetrating arteries, chiefly the anterior choroidal, middle cerebral, posterior cerebral, and basilar arteries. Lacunes may be single or multiple, symptomatic or asymptomatic. At least 20 lacunar syndromes have been described. The five best recognized syndromes are (1) pure motor hemiparesis, (2) pure sensory stroke, (3) sensory motor stroke, (4) homolateral ataxia and crural paresis (ataxic hemiparesis), and (5) dysarthria–clumsy hand syndrome. Multiple lacunes may be associated with acquired cognitive decline. Headaches are uncommon in patients with lacunar infarcts.

Pure motor hemiparesis is often caused by an internal capsule, basis pontis, or corona radiata lacune and is characterized by a contralateral hemiparesis or hemiplegia involving the face, arm, and to a lesser extent, the leg, accompanied by mild dysarthria, particularly at onset of stroke. There should be no aphasia, apraxia, or agnosia, and there are no sensory, visual, or other higher cortical disturbances. Pure sensory stroke is often caused by a lacuna involving the ventroposterolateral nucleus of the thalamus. It is characterized by paresthesias, numbness, and a unilateral hemisensory deficit involving the face, arm, trunk, and leg. Sensory motor stroke is often caused by a lacuna involving the internal capsule and thalamus or posterior limb of the internal capsule; large striatocapsular infarcts also can cause a similar syndrome. It is characterized by a contralateral unilateral motor deficit with a superimposed hemisensory deficit. Homolateral ataxia and crural paresis is often caused by a lacuna either in the contralateral posterior limb of the internal capsule or the contralateral basis pontis. It is characterized by weakness, predominantly in the lower extremity, and ipsilateral incoordination of the arm and leg. Dysarthria–clumsy hand syndrome is often caused by a lacuna involving the deep areas of the basis pontis and is characterized by supranuclear facial weakness, dysarthria, dysphagia, loss of fine motor control of the hand, and Babinski's sign.

Vertebrobasilar System Syndromes

The areas of the cerebellum supplied by the posterior inferior cerebellar artery (PICA) are variable. There are several different patterns of PICA territory cerebellar infarctions. If the medial branch territory is affected, involving the vermis and vestibulocerebellum, the clinical findings include prominent vertigo, ataxia, and nystagmus. If the lateral cerebellar hemisphere is involved, patients can have vertigo, gait ataxia, limb dysmetria and ataxia, nausea, vomiting, conjugate or dysconjugate gaze palsies, miosis, and dysarthria. If the infarction is large, altered consciousness or confusion may occur. Hydrocephalus or herniation may develop. There is also a syndrome of combined dorsolateral medullary and cerebellar infarction that may be caused by a vertebral artery occlusion or a medial PICA occlusion. Although a PICA occlusion can be the cause of Wallenberg's (lateral medullary) syndrome, this syndrome is more often caused by an intracranial vertebral artery occlusion.

The anterior inferior cerebellar artery syndrome causes a ventral cerebellar infarction. The signs and symptoms include vertigo, nausea, vomiting, and nystagmus caused by involvement of the vestibular nuclei. There may be ipsilateral facial hypalgesia and thermoanesthesia and corneal hypesthesia because of involvement of the trigeminal spinal nucleus and tract. Ipsilateral deafness and facial paralysis occurs because of involvement of the lateral pontomedullary tegmentum. An ipsilateral Horner's syndrome is present because of compromise of the descending oculosympathetic fibers. Contralateral trunk and extremity hypalgesia occurs and thermoanesthesia caused by involvement of the lateral spinothalamic tract. Finally, ipsilateral ataxia and asynergia is caused by involvement of the cerebellar peduncle and cerebellum.

Infarction in the territory of the superior cerebellar artery produces a dorsal cerebellar syndrome (Figure 57A.2). Vertigo may be present, although it is less common with superior cerebellar artery infarcts than with the other cerebellar syndromes. Nystagmus is caused by involvement of the medial longitudinal fasciculus and the cerebellar pathways. An ipsilateral Horner's syndrome is caused by involvement of the descending sympathetic tract. Ipsilateral ataxia and asynergia and gait ataxia are caused by involvement of the superior cerebellar peduncle, brachium pontis, superior cerebellar hemisphere, and dentate nucleus. There is an intention tremor caused by involvement of the dentate nucleus and superior cerebellar peduncle. Choreiform dyskinesias may be present ipsilaterally. Contralaterally, there is hearing loss caused by lateral lemniscus disruption and trunk and extremity hypalgesia and thermoanesthesia caused by spinothalamic tract involvement.

Weber's syndrome is caused by infarction in the distribution of the penetrating branches of the posterior cerebral artery (PCA) affecting the cerebral peduncle, especially medially, with damage to the fascicle of cranial nerve III and the pyramidal fibers. The resultant clinical findings are contralateral hemiplegia of the face, arm, and leg caused by corticospinal and corticobulbar tract involvement and ipsilateral oculomotor paresis, including a dilated pupil. A slight variation of this syndrome is the midbrain syndrome of Foville in which the supranuclear fibers for horizontal gaze are interrupted in the medial peduncle, causing a conjugate gaze palsy to the opposite side. Benedikt's syndrome is caused by a lesion affecting the mesencephalic tegmentum in its ventral portion, with involvement of the red nucleus, brachium conjunctivum, and fascicle of cranial nerve III. This syndrome is caused by infarction in the dis-

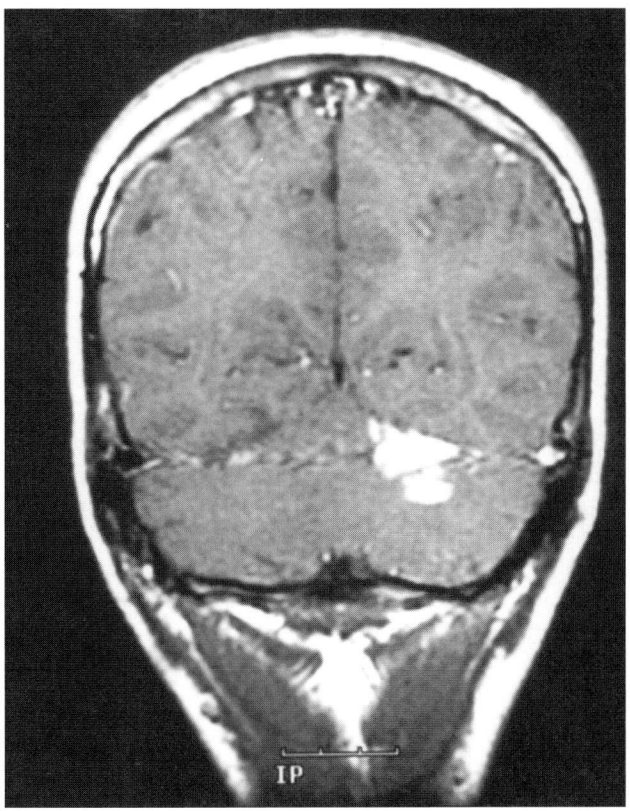

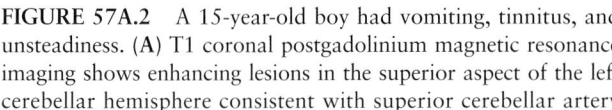

A

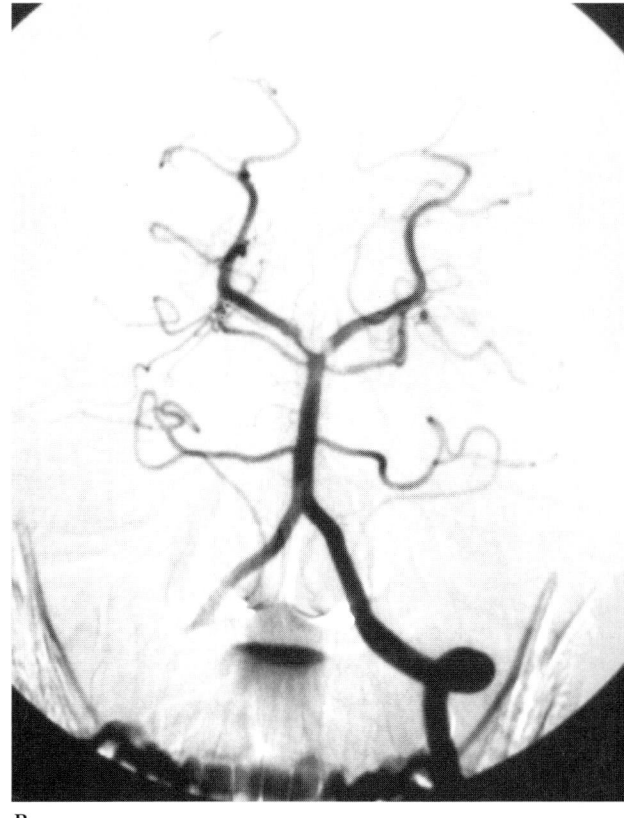

B

FIGURE 57A.2 A 15-year-old boy had vomiting, tinnitus, and unsteadiness. (A) T1 coronal postgadolinium magnetic resonance imaging shows enhancing lesions in the superior aspect of the left cerebellar hemisphere consistent with superior cerebellar artery infarct. (B) Anteroposterior view left vertebral artery injection shows a filling defect of the basilar apex also involving the proximal left superior cerebellar artery consistent with thromboembolus.

tribution of the penetrating branches of the PCA to the midbrain. The clinical manifestations are ipsilateral oculomotor paresis, usually with pupillary dilation and contralateral involuntary movements, including intention tremor, hemiathetosis, or hemichorea. Claude's syndrome is caused by lesions that are more dorsally placed in the midbrain tegmentum than with Benedikt's syndrome. There is injury to the dorsal red nucleus, which results in more prominent cerebellar signs without the involuntary movements. Oculomotor paresis occurs (see Table 74.1 for variations of these syndromes). Nothnagel's syndrome is characterized by an ipsilateral oculomotor palsy with contralateral cerebellar ataxia. Infarctions in the distribution of the penetrating branches of the PCA to the midbrain is the cause of this syndrome. Parinaud's syndrome can result from infarctions in the midbrain territory of the PCA penetrating branches. This syndrome is characterized by supranuclear paralysis of eye elevation, defective convergence, convergence-retraction nystagmus, light-near dissociation, lid retraction, and skew deviation (see Chapter 23).

Top of the basilar syndrome (see Chapter 23) is caused by infarction of the midbrain, thalamus, and portions of the temporal and occipital lobes. It is caused by occlusive vascular disease, often embolic in nature, of the rostral basilar artery. The following signs may occur:

- Behavioral abnormalities include somnolence, peduncular hallucinosis, memory disturbances, or agitated delirium.
- Ocular findings include unilateral or bilateral paralysis of upward or downward gaze; impaired convergence; pseudoabducens palsy; convergence-retraction nystagmus; abnormalities of abduction; Collier's sign, which consists of elevation and retraction of the upper eyelids; skew deviation; and oscillatory eye movements. Visual defects that may be present include hemianopia, cortical blindness, and Balint's syndrome.
- Pupillary abnormalities that may be seen include either small and reactive pupils, large or midposition and fixed pupils, and occasionally corectopia.
- Motor and sensory deficits may occur.

Although there are many named pontine syndromes, the most beneficial categorization is based on neuroanatomical divisions. Locked-in syndrome is the result of bilateral ventral pontine lesions that produce quadriplegia, aphonia, and impairment of the horizontal eye movements in some

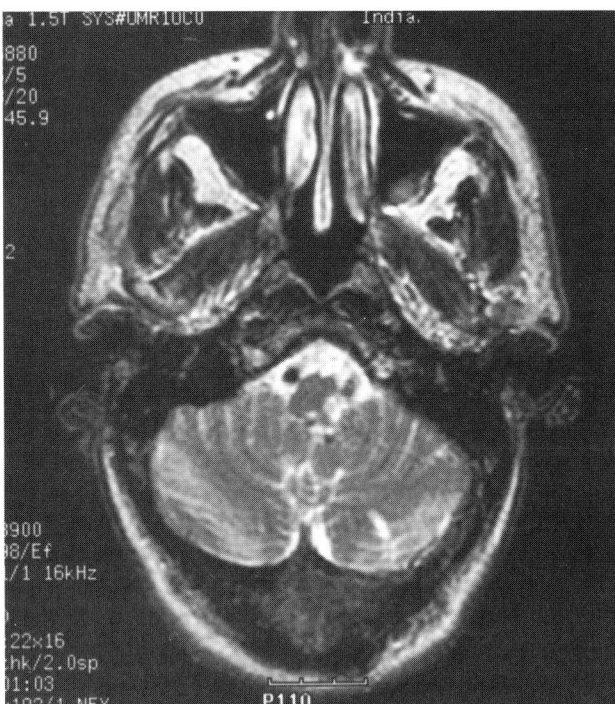

FIGURE 57A.3 A 74-year-old man had sudden onset of vertigo, vomiting, and gait unsteadiness. T2-weighted axial magnetic resonance imaging of the brain demonstrates an infarct in the posterolateral side of the medulla and a small cerebellar infarct in the distribution of the left posterior inferior cerebellar artery. There is poor flow void seen in the left vertebral artery.

patients. Wakefulness is maintained because of sparing of the reticular formation. The patient can move his or her eyes vertically and can blink because the supranuclear ocular motor pathways lie more dorsally. In some patients, there is a herald hemiparesis that makes the lesion appear to be cortical in nature. However, within a few hours, there is progression to bilateral hemiplegia and cranial nerve findings associated with the locked-in syndrome. Pure motor hemiparesis and ataxic-hemiparesis caused by pontine lesions are discussed with the lacunar syndromes.

Occlusion of the anterior inferior cerebellar artery can lead to the lateral inferior pontine syndrome. Findings with this syndrome include ipsilateral facial paralysis, impaired facial sensation, paralysis of conjugate gaze to the side of the lesion, deafness, tinnitus, and ataxia. Contralateral to the lesion, there is hemibody impairment to pain and temperature, which in some instances includes the face. There may be horizontal and vertical nystagmus and oscillopsia. The medial inferior pontine syndrome is caused by occlusion of a paramedian branch of the basilar artery. With this syndrome, there is ipsilateral paralysis of conjugate gaze to the side of the lesion, abducens palsy, nystagmus, and ataxia. Contralateral to the lesion, there is hemibody impairment of tactile and proprioceptive sensation and paralysis of the face, arm, and leg. An occlusion of the anterior inferior cerebellar artery may lead to the total unilateral inferior pontine

syndrome, a combination of the symptoms and signs seen with the lateral and medial pontine syndromes.

The lateral pontomedullary syndrome can occur with occlusion of the vertebral artery. The manifestations are a combination of the medial and lateral inferior pontine syndromes. Occlusion of the paramedian branch of the mid-basilar artery can lead to ipsilateral impaired sensory and motor function of the trigeminal nerve with limb ataxia, characteristics of the lateral midpontine syndrome. Ischemia of the medial midpontine region is caused by occlusion of the paramedian branch of the midbasilar artery and can lead to ipsilateral limb ataxia. Contralateral to the lesion, eye deviation and paralysis of the face, arm, and leg occur. Although there are predominant motor symptoms, variable impaired touch and proprioception may occur. The lateral superior pontine syndrome may occur with occlusion of the superior cerebellar artery and produces a characteristic syndrome of ipsilateral Horner's syndrome, horizontal nystagmus, paresis of conjugate gaze, occasional deafness, and severe ataxia of the limbs and gait. Contralateral to the lesion, there is hemibody impairment to pain and temperature, skew deviation, and impaired tactile, vibratory, and proprioceptive sensation in the leg greater than in the arm.

The lateral medullary syndrome (Wallenberg's syndrome) is most often caused by occlusion of the intracranial segment of the vertebral artery (Figure 57A.3). Less commonly, it is caused by occlusion of PICA. This syndrome produces an ipsilateral Horner's syndrome; loss of pain and temperature sensation in the face; weakness of the palate, pharynx, and vocal cords; and cerebellar ataxia. Contralateral to the lesion, there is hemibody loss of pain and temperature sensation. The medial medullary syndrome is less common and may be caused by occlusion of the vertebral artery, a branch of the vertebral artery, or the lower basilar artery. The findings with this syndrome include an ipsilateral lower motor neuron paralysis of the tongue and contralateral paralysis of the arm and leg. In addition, there is contralateral hemibody loss of tactile, vibratory, and position sense. Occlusion of the vertebral artery can lead to a total unilateral medullary syndrome, a combination of medial and lateral medullary syndromes.

The manifestations with PCA territory infarctions are variable, depending on the site of the occlusion and the availability of collateral blood flow. Occlusion of the precommunal P1 segment causes midbrain, thalamic, and hemispheric infarction. Occlusion of the PCA in the proximal ambient segment before branching in the thalamogeniculate pedicle causes lateral thalamic and hemispheral symptoms. Occlusions also may affect a single PCA branch, primarily the calcarine artery, or cause a large hemispheric infarction of the PCA territory. Unilateral infarctions in the distribution of the hemispheral branches of the PCA may produce a contralateral homonymous hemianopia caused by infarction of the striate cortex, the optic radiations, or the lateral geniculate body. There is partial or complete macular sparing if the infarction does not reach the occipital pole. The visual field defect may be limited to a quadrantanopia. A superior quadrantanopia is caused by infarction of the striate cortex inferior to the calcarine fissure or the inferior optic radiations in the temporo-occipital lobes. An inferior quadrantanopia is the result of an infarction of the striate cortex superior to the calcarine fissure or the superior optic radiations in the parieto-occipital lobes.

More complex visual changes may occur, including formed or unformed visual hallucinations, visual and color agnosias, or prosopagnosia. Finally, some alteration of sensation with PCA hemispheral infarctions occurs, including paresthesias or altered position, pain, and temperature sensations. Infarction in the distribution of the callosal branches of the PCA involving the left occipital region and the splenium of the corpus callosum produces alexia without agraphia (Figure 57A.4). In this syndrome, patients can write, speak, and spell normally, but are unable to read words and sentences. The ability to name letters and numbers may be intact, but there can be inability to name colors, objects, and photographs. Right hemispheric PCA territory infarctions may cause contralateral visual field neglect. Amnesia may be present with PCA infarctions that involve the left medial temporal lobe or when there are bilateral mesiotemporal infarctions. In addition, an agitated delirium may occur with unilateral or bilateral penetrating mesiotemporal infarctions. Large infarctions of the left posterior temporal artery territory may produce an anomic or transcortical sensory aphasia.

Infarctions in the distribution of the penetrating branches of the PCA to the thalamus can cause aphasia if the left pulvinar is involved, akinetic mutism, global amnesia, and the Dejerine-Roussy syndrome. In the latter syndrome, the patient has contralateral sensory loss to all modalities, severe dysesthesias on the involved side (thalamic pain), vasomotor disturbances, transient contralateral hemiparesis, and choreoathetoid or ballistic movements. A number of syndromes that can result from infarctions in the distribution of the penetrating branches of the PCA to the midbrain were previously discussed with the midbrain syndromes.

Bilateral infarctions in the distribution of the hemispheric branches of the PCAs may cause bilateral homonymous hemianopias. Bilateral occipital or occipitoparietal infarctions can cause cortical blindness, often with denial or unawareness of blindness (Anton's syndrome). Another syndrome, Balint's syndrome, seen with bilateral occipital or parieto-occipital infarctions, consists of optic ataxia, psychic paralysis of fixation with inability to look to the peripheral field and disturbance of visual attention, and simultanagnosia.

Syndromes of Thalamic Infarction

The main thalamic blood supply comes from the posterior communicating arteries and the perimesencephalic segment of the PCA. Thalamic infarctions typically involve one of four major vascular regions: posterolateral, anterior, para-

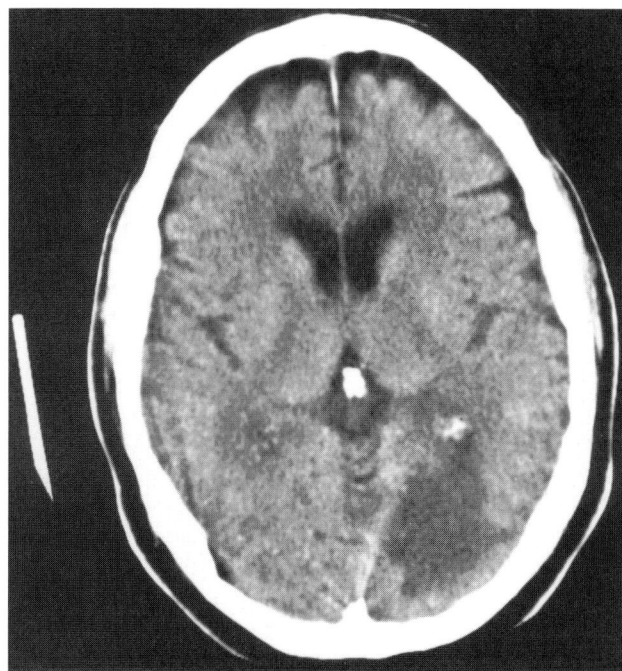

FIGURE 57A.4 A 77-year-old man had alexia without agraphia, right homonymous hemianopia, and antegrade amnesia. Nonenhanced axial cranial computed tomography demonstrates an area of decreased parenchymal attenuation in the left occipitoparietal region.

median, and dorsal. Posterolateral thalamic infarctions result from occlusion of the thalamogeniculate branches arising from the P2 segment of the PCA. Three common clinical syndromes may occur: pure sensory stroke, sensorimotor stroke, and the thalamic syndrome of Dejerine-Roussy. Anterior thalamic infarction results from occlusion of the polar or tuberothalamic artery. The main clinical manifestations consist of neuropsychological disturbances, emotional-facial paresis, occasional hemiparesis, and visual field deficits. Left-sided infarcts are associated with dysphasia, whereas neglect is seen primarily in patients with right-sided lesions. Paramedian thalamic infarctions result from occlusion of the paramedian or thalamic and subthalamic arteries. The main clinical manifestations include the classic triad of decreased level of consciousness, memory loss, and vertical gaze abnormalities. Dorsal thalamic infarctions result from occlusion of the posterior choroidal arteries. These infarctions are characterized by the presence of homonymous quadrantanopia or horizontal sectoranopias. Involvement of the pulvinar may account for thalamic aphasia.

Watershed Ischemic Syndromes

During or after cardiac surgery or after an episode of severe arterial hypotension, prolonged hypoxemia, or bilateral severe carotid artery disease, ischemia may occur in the watershed areas between the major circulations. Watershed

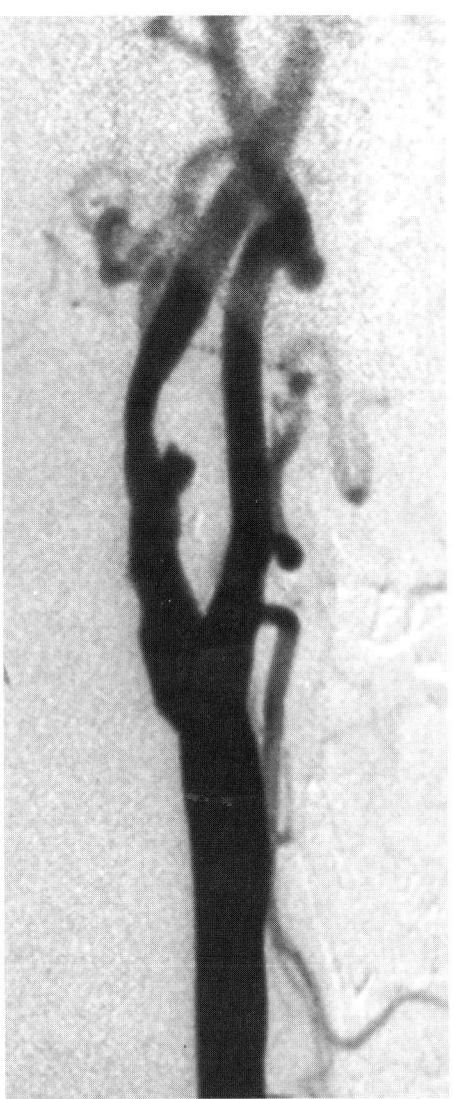

FIGURE 57A.5   Right common carotid angiogram shows 17% right internal carotid artery stenosis (North American Symptomatic Carotid Endarectomy Trial criteria) just superior to a large carotid ulceration. (Courtesy of Vincent Mathews, MD.)

infarctions also may be unilateral when there is some degree of hemodynamic failure in patients with underlying severe arterial stenosis or occlusion. Watershed infarcts also may be caused by microembolism or hyperviscosity states.

Ischemia in the border zone or junctional territory of the ACA, MCA, and PCA may result in bilateral parieto-occipital infarcts. There can be a variety of visual manifestations, including bilateral lower altitudinal field defects, optic ataxia, cortical blindness, and difficulty in judging size, distance, and movement. Ischemia between the territories of the ACA and MCA bilaterally may result in bibrachial cortical sensorimotor impairment (man-in-a-barrel), and impaired saccadic eye movements caused by compromise of the frontal eye fields. Ischemia on the border zone regions between the MCA and PCA may cause bilateral parietotemporal infarctions. Initially there is cortical blind-ness that may improve, but defects such as dyslexia, dyscalculia, dysgraphia, and memory defects for verbal and nonverbal material may persist.

DIAGNOSIS AND TREATMENT OF THREATENED ISCHEMIC STROKE

An ischemic stroke develops when there is interrupted cerebral blood flow to an area of the brain. Ischemic strokes account for approximately 80–85% of all strokes. Ischemic strokes may result from (1) large artery atherosclerotic disease resulting in stenosis or occlusion, (2) small vessel or penetrating artery disease (lacunes), (3) cardioembolism, (4) nonatherosclerotic vasculopathies, (5) hypercoagulable disorders, and (6) infarcts of undetermined causes. However, a rigid classification of ischemic stroke subtypes is difficult to establish because of the frequent occurrence of mixed syndromes.

Large Artery Atherothrombotic Infarctions

Large artery atherothrombotic infarctions almost always occur in patients who already have significant risk factors for cerebrovascular atherosclerosis (see Table 57A.1). Atherothrombosis is multifactorial, comorbidities frequently overlap, and risk factors are often additive. For example, arterial hypertension is often associated with hyperlipidemia, hyperglycemia, elevated fibrinogen levels, excessive weight, and left ventricular hypertrophy on ECG. A resting ankle-brachial index less than 0.90 is indicative of generalized atherosclerosis (Zheng et al. 1997). Persons with a stroke are at high risk for development of other vascular complications. After a stroke, there is a 25% chance of a fatal thrombotic event in 3 years. Many of these deaths are caused by myocardial infarction. The mechanisms of large artery atherothrombotic infarction often reflect plaque complication; ulceration with artery-to-artery embolization (Figure 57A.5), or thrombosis in the setting of pre-existing arterial stenosis. Artery-to-artery embolism is a common mechanism of cerebral ischemia. Embolism from ulcerated carotid artery atherosclerotic plaques is a common cause of cerebral infarction. In situ thrombosis occurs in the proximal carotid, distal vertebral artery, and lower or middle basilar artery (Figures 57A.6A and B). Atherosclerotic involvement of the intracranial portion of the vertebrobasilar system frequently occurs in tandem and is the common pathological mechanism associated with the syndrome of vertebrobasilar territory infarction; this may arise in association with hypercoagulable states. Hemodynamic alterations also may trigger these events. Whether the pathogenesis of stroke caused by intracranial arterial stenosis is different from that caused by extracranial arterial disease is unsettled.

In patients with risk factors for atherosclerosis, the cholesterol-rich minimally raised fatty streak may progress

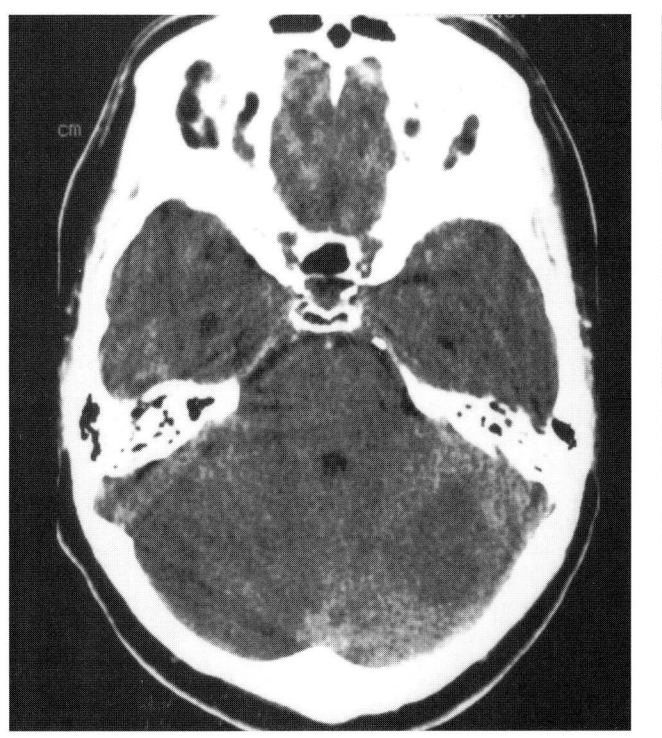
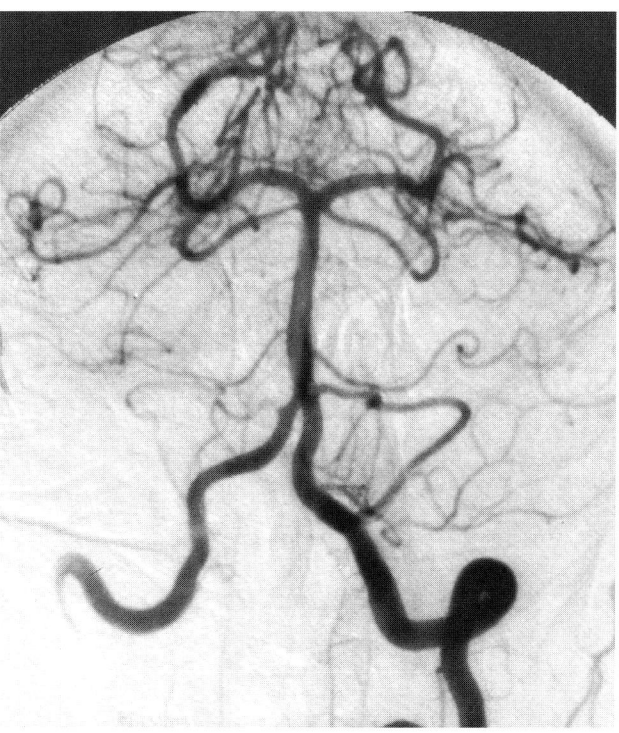

A   B

FIGURE 57A.6   (A) Nonenhanced axial computed tomographic scan shows bilateral cerebellar and pontine infarcts. (B) Anteroposterior view of vertebrobasilar angiogram shows a large filling defect on the basilar artery, consistent with partial thrombosis. (Courtesy of Vincent Mathews, MD.)

to a fibrous plaque that can evolve into a complicated plaque with intraplaque hemorrhage, extensive necrosis, calcification, and subsequent thrombosis (Figure 57A.7). The infiltration of the fibrous cap by foam cells may contribute to the rupture of the atherosclerotic carotid artery plaque. Atherosclerosis is often segmental and asymmetric, and earlier lesions tend to occur in areas of low shear stress, such as the outer aspect of the carotid artery bulb. Atherosclerosis primarily affects the larger extracranial and intracranial vessels, particularly the carotid siphon, MCA stem, origin of the vertebral arteries (V_1), intracranial segment of the vertebral arteries (V_4), and basilar artery. The distribution of cerebral atherosclerosis is different in certain ethnic groups. Stenosis of major intracranial arteries is more prevalent among blacks and Asians than in whites.

Small Vessel or Penetrating Artery Disease

Lacuna usually occur in patients with long-standing arterial hypertension, current cigarette smoking, and diabetes mellitus. The most frequent sites of involvement are the putamen, basis pontis, thalamus, posterior limb of the internal capsule, and caudate nucleus. Multiple lacuna are associated strongly with arterial hypertension and diabetes mellitus. Diastolic rather than systolic blood pressure seems to be a major determinant of multiple lacuna. Available evidence suggests that

structural changes of the cerebral vasculature caused by arterial hypertension are characterized by fibrinoid angiopathy, lipohyalinosis, and microaneurysm formation. Accelerated hypertensive arteriolar damage of the small penetrating arteries is operative in a large number of patients with lacunar infarction. Microatheroma of the ostium of a penetrating artery, embolism, or changes in hemorrheology are pathophysiologically operative in the remainder of cases. However, the mere association of a lacunar syndrome in a patient with arterial hypertension and diabetes is not sufficient for a diagnosis of a lacunar infarct, and other causes of ischemic stroke must be excluded. Large striatocapsular infarctions should be distinguished from lacunar infarcts, because they frequently have potential cardioembolic sources or coexistent severe carotid artery stenosis and often present with signs and symptoms of cortical dysfunction (Nicolai et al. 1996). Control of hypertension, prevention of microangiopathy, a better understanding of the ideal hemodynamic profile, and judicious use of platelet antiaggregants are essential in the management of patients with lacunar infarcts.

Cardiogenic Embolism

Cerebrovascular events are a serious complication of a diverse group of cardiac disorders. Cardioembolic strokes are associated with substantial morbidity and mortality.

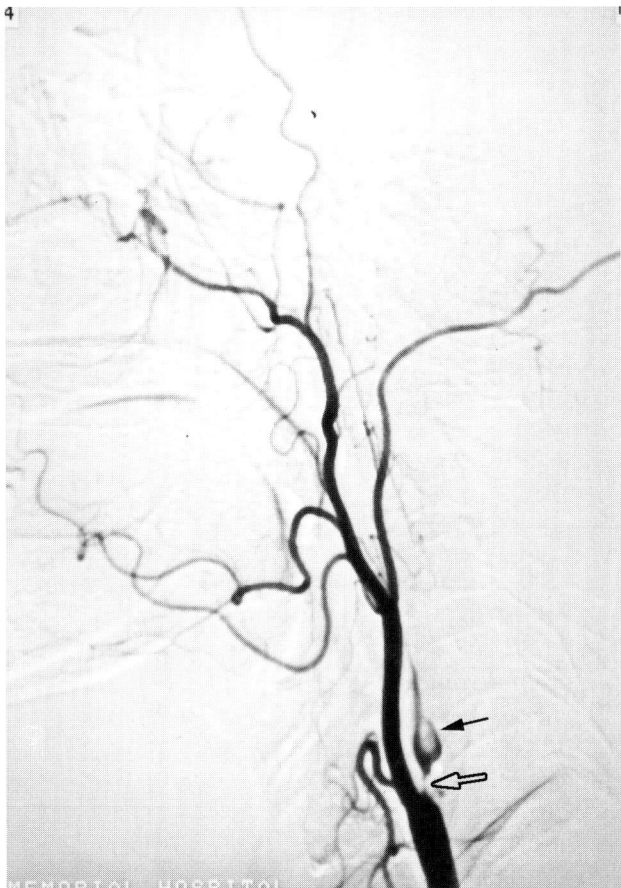

FIGURE 57A.7   Left carotid angiogram (lateral view) shows severe stenosis (*open arrow*) of origin of the left internal carotid artery with an intraluminal thrombus (*arrow*). The artery was occluded in other images. (Courtesy of Vincent Mathews, MD.)

Table 57A.3:   Sources of cardioembolism

Acute myocardial infarction
Left ventricular aneurysm
Dilatated cardiomyopathy
Cardiac arrhythmias
   Atrial fibrillation
   Sick sinus syndrome
Valvular heart disease
   Rheumatic mitral valve disease
   Calcific aortic stenosis
   Mitral annulus calcification
   Mitral valve prolapse
   Infective endocarditis
   Nonbacterial thrombotic endocarditis
   Prosthetic heart valves
   Filamentous strands of the mitral valve
   Giant Lambl's excrescences
   Aneurysms of the sinus of Valsalva
Intracardiac tumors (atrial myxoma, rhabdomyoma, papillary
   fibroelastoma)
Intracardiac defects with paradoxical embolism
   Patent foramen ovale
   Atrial septal aneurysm
   Atrial septal defect
Cyanotic congenital heart disease
Fontan procedure
Mitochondrial encephalomyopathies (mitochondrial encephalop-
   athy, lactic acidosis, and strokelike episodes; myoclonic
   epilepsy and ragged-red fibers; Kearns-Sayre)
Coronary artery bypass grafting
VVI pacing
Heart transplantation
Artificial hearts
Cardioversion for atrial fibrillation
Balloon angioplasty
Ventricular support devices
Extracorporeal membrane oxygenator

Embolism of cardiac origin accounts for approximately 15–20% of all ischemic strokes. The most common substrate for cerebral embolism in older individuals is NVAF accounting for two-thirds of emboli of cardiac origin. Other cardiac conditions with high embolic potential include acute myocardial infarction, infective endocarditis, mitral stenosis, and mechanical prosthetic heart valves. Congenital heart disease is probably the most common cardiac disorder causing ischemic stroke in children. Emboli from cardiac sources may be silent or cause severe neurological deficit or death. Although most types of heart disease may produce cerebral embolism, certain cardiac disorders are more likely to be associated with emboli (Table 57A.3). Cardioembolic cerebral infarcts are often large, multiple, bilateral, and wedge shaped. Sudden, unheralded, focal neurological deficits worse at onset are often presenting manifestations. Any vascular territory may be affected. Ischemic strokes with a potential cardiac source are more often associated with Wernicke's aphasia, hemianopia without hemiparesis or hemisensory disturbances, and ideomotor apraxia. Other features suggestive of a potential cardiac source of embolism included posterior division of the MCA, ACA, or cerebellar compromise; involvement of multiple vascular territories; or a hemorrhagic component of the infarction. Reliable clinical determination of a cardioembolic source of stroke may be hampered by a variety of problems. Identification of a potential embolic cardiac source is not by itself sufficient to diagnose a brain infarct as cardioembolic because (1) many cardiac problems may coexist with cerebrovascular atherosclerosis, (2) cardiac arrhythmias may occur after arrhythmogenic lesions such as parietoinsular and brainstem infarcts, (3) computed tomographic (CT) scan differentiation between cardioembolic and atherosclerotic causes of cerebral infarction is not always reliable, and (4) cardiac changes detected by echocardiography are prevalent in control populations.

An embolic stroke occurs in approximately 1% of hospitalized patients with acute myocardial infarction. Left ventricular thrombi are commonly associated with recent anterior wall transmural myocardial infarction. Echocardiographical studies have demonstrated that approximately one-third to one-half of acute anterior myocardial infarctions, but less than 4% of acute inferior myocardial infarctions, develop left ventricular thrombi. Almost all episodes of embolism occur within 3 months following acute myocardial infarction, with 85% of emboli developing in the first 4 weeks. A decreased ejection fraction is an independent predictor of an increased risk of stroke following myocardial infarction (Loh et al. 1997). Patients with acute myocardial infarction who receive thrombolytic therapy have a small risk of stroke. A direct comparison of tissue plasminogen activator and streptokinase shows an excess of strokes with tissue plasminogen activator. Myocardial infarction is rare in young adults. Although the prevalence of left ventricular thrombi in individuals with left ventricular aneurysms is high, the frequency of systemic embolism is low. Dilatated or congestive cardiomyopathy may result from arterial hypertension or a variety of inflammatory, infectious, immune, metabolic, toxic, and neuromuscular disorders. The global impairment of the ventricular performance predisposes to stasis and thrombus formation. Patients commonly have signs of impaired left ventricular systolic function, and less than one-half have diastolic heart failure. Occasionally, patients have atrial fibrillation. A systemic embolism may be the presenting manifestation. Embolism occurs in approximately 18% of patients with dilated cardiomyopathy not receiving anticoagulants. Patients with idiopathic hypertrophic subaortic stenosis may present with stroke. Thromboembolism is uncommon in patients with congestive heart failure. Mitochondrial disorders are seldom associated with dilated cardiomyopathies. Cerebral infarction is a complication of mitochondrial encephalomyopathies (MELAS; myoclonic epilepsy and ragged-red fibers; Kearns-Sayre syndrome). Stroke in Kearns-Sayre syndrome is likely secondary to embolism. Apical aneurysms complicate Chagas' cardiomyopathy.

Most cases of mitral stenosis are caused by rheumatic heart disease. Systemic emboli occur in 9–14% of patients with mitral stenosis, with 60–75% having cardioembolic cerebral ischemia. Systemic embolism may be the first symptom of mitral stenosis, particularly if it is associated with atrial fibrillation. Aortic valve calcification with or without stenosis is not a risk factor for stroke (Boon et al. 1996). Cerebral embolism is a rare occurrence in patients with bicuspid aortic valves. Individuals with mitral annular calcification have twice the risk of stroke. Mitral valve prolapse affects 3–4% of adults, and when uncomplicated, does not seem to have an increased risk of stroke. Neurological ischemic events appear to occur more commonly among men older than 50 years with auscultatory findings of a systolic murmur and thick mitral valve leaflets on echocardiography. Thromboembolic phenomena complicating infective endocarditis may be systemic (left-sided endocarditis) or pulmonary (right-sided endocarditis). Vegetations are detected by transthoracic echocardiography in 54–87% of patients with infective endocarditis and are associated with an increased risk of embolism (Eishi et al. 1995). Systemic emboli may occur in nearly one-half of patients with nonbacterial thrombotic endocarditis, a condition characterized by the presence of multiple, small, ster-

ile thrombotic vegetations most frequently involving the mitral and aortic valves. The risk of thromboembolism is higher with mechanical prosthetic heart valves than with biological prosthetic heart valves. Thromboemboli are more common with prosthetic heart valves in the mitral position than with prosthetic heart valves in the aortic position. The rate of systemic embolism in patients with mechanical heart valves receiving anticoagulant therapy is 4% per year in the mitral position, and 2% per year in the aortic position. Filamentous strands attached to the mitral valve appear to represent a risk for cerebral embolism, particularly in young patients, but the risk of recurrent cerebral ischemia is incompletely understood. The association of giant Lambl's excrescences or aneurysms of the sinus of Valsalva and cerebral embolism is low.

Patients with NVAF, the leading source of cardioembolic infarctions in older adults, have a fivefold increase in stroke incidence, with a cumulative risk of 35% over a lifetime. Patients with rheumatic atrial fibrillation have a sevenfold increase in stroke incidence. However, individuals younger than 65 years with lone atrial fibrillation have a low embolic potential. Stroke patients with atrial fibrillation are also at high risk of death during the acute phase of stroke and during the subsequent year after stroke. A dramatic increase in the rate of atrial fibrillation occurs with age, from 0.2 cases per 1,000 patients aged 30–39 years to 39 cases per 1,000 patients aged 80–89 years. The proportion of strokes caused by atrial fibrillation also steadily increases, from 6.7% of all strokes in patients aged 50–59 to 36.2% in those aged 80–89.

Cerebral and systemic embolism may occur also in the setting of the sick sinus syndrome. Patients at greatest risk for embolization have bradytachyarrhythmias; left atrial spontaneous contrast and decreased atrial ejection force increase stroke risk (Mattioli et al. 1997). Patients with sick sinus syndrome may experience cerebral ischemia or systemic embolism, even after pacemaker insertion. VVI pacing is associated with a higher risk of embolic complications than atrial or dual-chamber pacing.

Atrial myxomas are rare cardiac tumors complicated by postural syncope and systemic and embolic manifestations. Embolic complications are a presenting symptom in one-third of patients with atrial myxoma. Recurrent emboli before surgery are common. Peripheral and multiple cerebral arterial aneurysms also have been diagnosed years following the initial embolic manifestations from atrial myxoma. Treatment of atrial myxomas consists of prompt surgical resection of the cardiac mass. Cardiac rhabdomyomas are associated closely with tuberous sclerosis; systemic embolism is unusual. Mitral valve papillary fibroelastoma, an uncommon valvular tumor, is complicated rarely by stroke.

A paradoxical embolism caused by a right-to-left shunt through a patent foramen ovale (PFO) or atrial septal aneurysm (ASA) can be responsible for stroke and other ischemic cerebral events. A PFO is present in 35% of subjects between the ages of 1 and 29 years, in 25% of people between ages 30 and 79, and in 20% between ages 80 and 99 years. A PFO provides opportunity for right-to-left shunting during transient increases in the right atrial pressure. PFO is more common in patients with stroke than in matched controls. Patients with no identifiable cause for ischemic stroke and PFO usually have a larger PFO with more extensive right-to-left shunting than patients with stroke of determined etiology. Platelet antiaggregants, oral anticoagulants, transcatheter closure of the PFO, or surgical closure of the PFO have been recommended. ASA also might be a source of cerebral emboli. The coexistence of PFO and ASA increases the risk of embolic stroke. PFO and ASA have been associated also with mitral valve prolapse. Strokes are often severe but recurrences are uncommon. Pulmonary arteriovenous malformations occur in 15–20% of patients with Rendu-Osler-Weber syndrome and can be the source of paradoxical embolism causing cerebral ischemia.

Spontaneous echocardiographic contrast is associated with elevated fibrinogen levels and plasma viscosity and is a potential risk factor for cardioembolic stroke. Spontaneous echocardiographical contrast is highly associated with previous stroke or peripheral embolism in patients with atrial fibrillation or mitral stenosis and increased left atrial size. The risk of cerebrovascular events is increased in adults with cyanotic congenital heart disease in the presence of arterial hypertension, atrial fibrillation, history of phlebotomy, and particularly with microcytosis (Perloff et al. 1993).

The preponderance of posterior circulation ischemia following cardiac catheterization is unexplained. Stroke occurs after coronary artery bypass grafting with a frequency ranging between 1% and 5% (Figure 57A.8). The etiology of postoperative stroke is multifactorial; hypoperfusion, ventricular thrombus, and emboli are probable etiologies, although embolic causes are the most likely mechanisms. Clamp manipulation during coronary artery bypass surgery also may favor the release of aortic atheromatous debris. Carotid artery occlusion, but not carotid artery stenosis, increases the risk for stroke following coronary artery bypass grafting (Mickleborough et al. 1996). Thromboembolic phenomena can complicate cardiac surgery using cardiopulmonary bypass with deep hypothermia and cardiac arrest. Stroke is a potential complication of cardioversion for atrial fibrillation. Strokes may follow heart transplantation, the use of ventricular support systems and artificial hearts, and the use of the extracorporeal membrane oxygenator. Stroke following inadvertently placed left-sided heart pacemaker leads is an unusual complication.

Nonatherosclerotic Vasculopathies

Although the majority of arterial disorders leading to stroke is caused by atherosclerosis, several nonatherosclerotic vasculopathies can be responsible for a minority of ischemic strokes. These vasculopathies include cervicocephalic arte-

rial dissections, traumatic cerebrovascular disease, radiation vasculopathy, moyamoya, fibromuscular dysplasia (FMD), and cerebral vasculitis (Tables 57A.4 and 57A.5). Together, these uncommon conditions represent 5% of all ischemic strokes. They are relatively more common in children and young adults.

Cervicocephalic arterial dissections are one of the most frequent nonatherosclerotic vasculopathies causing ischemic stroke in young adults. A dissection is produced by subintimal penetration of blood in a cervicocephalic vessel with subsequent longitudinal extension of the intraluminal hematoma between its layers. Most dissections involve the extracranial segment of the internal carotid artery. Intracranial carotid and vertebrobasilar dissections are less common. The recurrence rate of cervicocephalic arterial dissections is approximately 1% per year. The risk of recurrent dissections is increased in younger patients and in patients with family history of arterial dissections.

Cervicocephalic arterial dissections have been reported after blunt or penetrating trauma and also are associated with FMD, Marfan's syndrome, Ehlers-Danlos syndrome type IV, pseudoxanthoma elasticum, coarctation of the aorta, Menkes' disease, α_1-antitrypsin deficiency, cystic medial degeneration, elevated arterial elastase content (Thal et al. 1997), lentiginosis, atherosclerosis, extreme vessel tortuosity, moyamoya, pharyngeal infections, sympathomimetic drug abuse, and luetic arteritis. Not infrequently, cervicocephalic arterial dissections occur spontaneously.

Dissection of the cervicocephalic vessels may cause transient retinal, hemispheric, or posterior fossa ischemia, Horner's syndrome, hemicranial pain, cranial nerve palsies, cerebral infarction, or subarachnoid hemorrhage. Ischemic symptoms result from arterial occlusion or secondary embolization. Dissections should be considered in the differential diagnosis of stroke in any young adult, particularly when traditional risk factors are absent.

Diagnosis is based on arteriographical findings although high-resolution magnetic resonance imaging (MRI) and magnetic resonance angiography (MRA) and extracranial and transcranial ultrasound are rapidly replacing contrast angiography for the diagnosis of cervicocephalic arterial dissections, particularly in cases of carotid artery involvement. Arteriographical features include the presence of a pearl and string sign; double-lumen sign; short, smooth, tapered stenosis; vessel occlusion; or pseudoaneurysm formation. MRI demonstrates the intramural hematoma and the false lumen of the dissected artery (Figure 57A.9). Ultrasound studies can be helpful in monitoring their course.

Therapeutic interventions have included immediate anticoagulation with heparin followed by a 3- to 6-month course of warfarin; platelet antiaggregants; or surgical correction for selected individuals with pseudoaneurysms or those who fail to respond to medical therapy. Although anticoagulants are often empirically recommended, their value in patients with extracranial cervicocephalic arterial

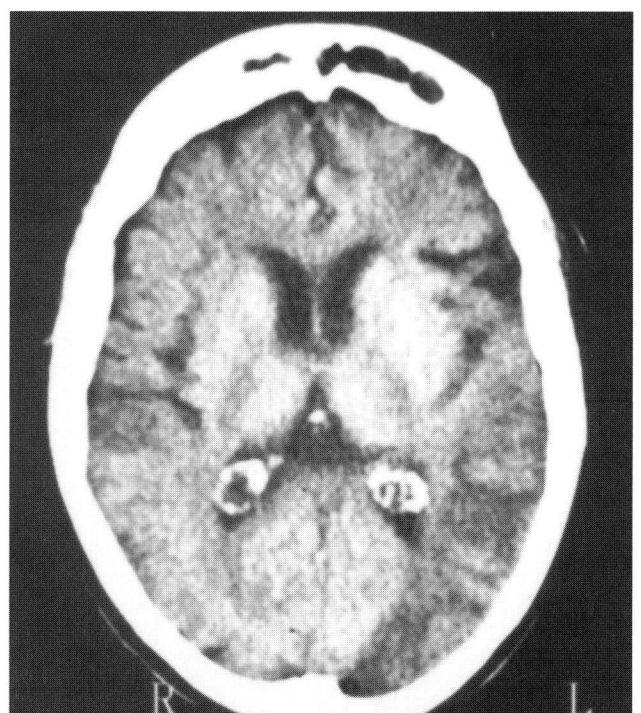
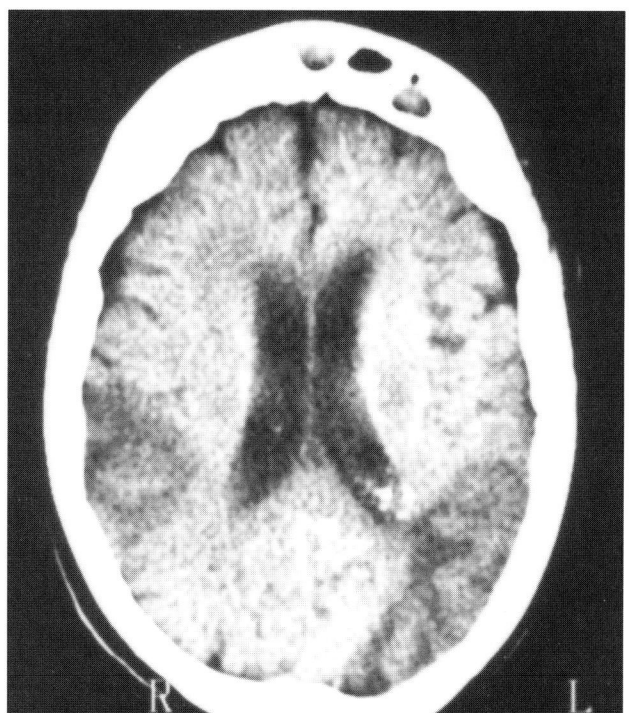
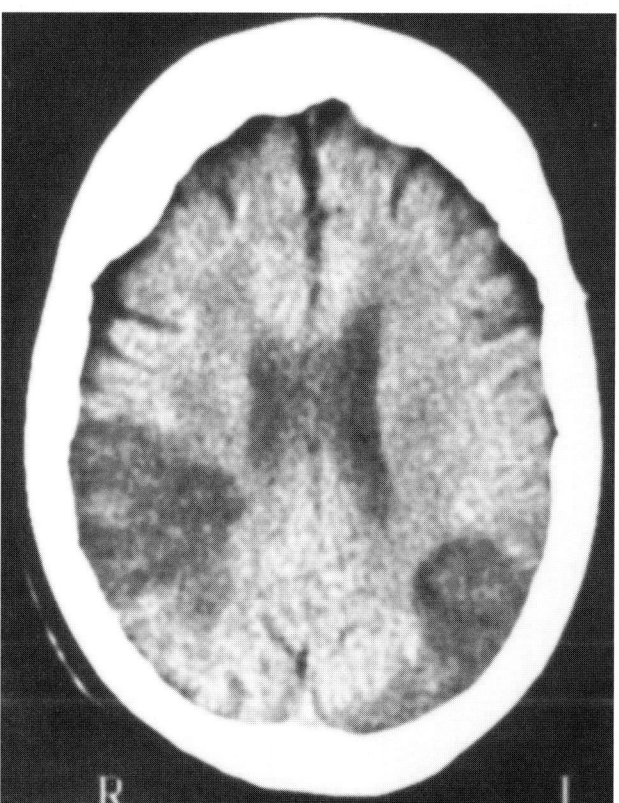

FIGURE 57A.8 An 80-year-old woman remained unresponsive with left-sided hemiplegia and right-sided hemiparesis after coronary artery bypass grafting and aortic valve replacement. Nonenhanced axial computed tomography demonstrates large left temporo-parieto-occipital and right frontoparietal infarctions.

Table 57A.4:   Selected nonatherosclerotic vasculopathies

Cervicocephalic arterial dissections
Traumatic cerebrovascular disease
Radiation-induced vasculopathy
Moyamoya disease
Fibromuscular dysplasia
Vasculitis
Migrainous infarction

Table 57A.5:   Classification of cerebral vasculitides

Infectious vasculitis
    Bacterial, fungal, parasitic
    Spirochetal (syphilis, Lyme disease)
    Viral, rickettsial, mycobacterial
    Cysticercosis, free-living amebae
Necrotizing vasculitides
    Classic polyarteritis nodosa
    Wegener's granulomatosis
    Allergic angiitis and granulomatosis (Churg-Strauss)
    Necrotizing systemic vasculitis-overlap syndrome
    Lymphomatoid granulomatosis
Vasculitis associated with collagen vascular disease
    Systemic lupus erythematosus
    Rheumatoid arthritis
    Scleroderma
    Sjögren's syndrome
Vasculitis associated with other systemic diseases
    Behçet's disease
    Ulcerative colitis
    Sarcoidosis
    Relapsing polychondritis
    Köhlmeier-Degos disease
Giant cell arteritides
    Takayasu's arteritis
    Temporal (cranial) arteritis
Hypersensitivity vasculitides
    Henoch-Schönlein purpura
    Drug-induced vasculitides
    Chemical vasculitides
    Essential mixed cryoglobulinemia
Miscellaneous
    Vasculitis associated with neoplasia
    Vasculitis associated with radiation
    Cogan's syndrome
    Dermatomyositis polymyositis
    X-linked lymphoproliferative syndrome
    Thromboangiitis obliterans
    Kawasaki's syndrome
Primary central nervous system vasculitis

Source: Reprinted with permission from J Biller, LH Sparks. Diagnosis and Management of Cerebral Vasculitis. In HP Adams Jr (ed), Handbook of Cerebrovascular Diseases. New York: Marcel Dekker, 1993;549–567.

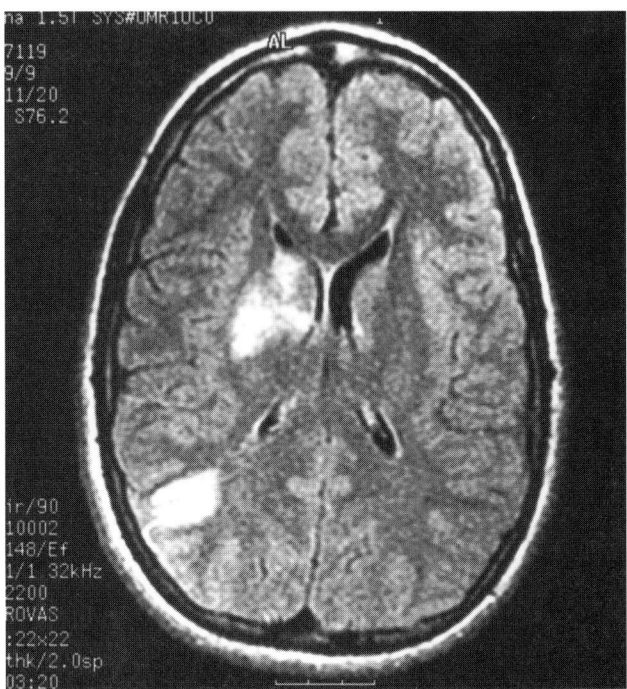

A

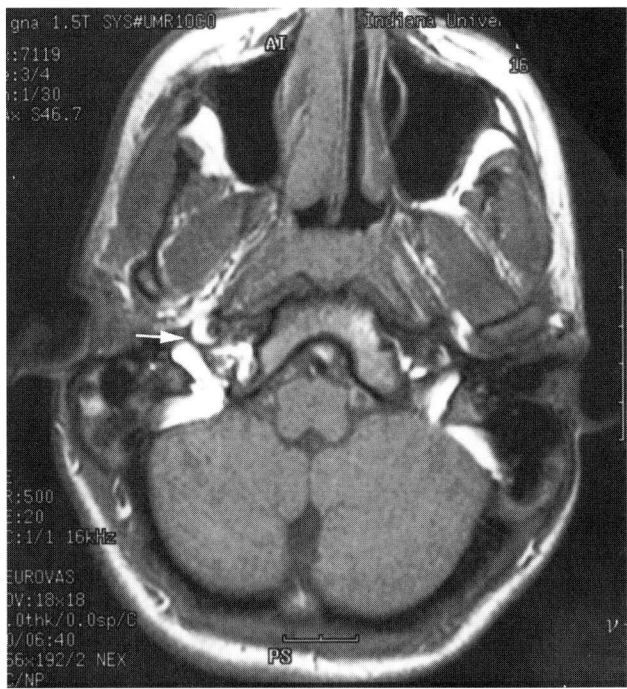

B

FIGURE 57A.9   A 16-year-old boy collapsed to the ground after experiencing right eye pain and left-sided weakness. (**A**) Axial T2-weighted magnetic resonance imaging of the brain shows ischemic areas in the right basal ganglia and right posterior parietal region, (**B**) associated with a crescent sign (*arrow*) of high signal consistent with intraluminal blood products on the right internal carotid artery suggestive of a dissection.

dissections has not been firmly established. Anticoagulation should be withheld in patients with intracranial dissections because of the risk of subarachnoid hemorrhage.

Trauma is a leading cause of mortality in the United States. Blunt or penetrating traumatic cerebrovascular disease may result in cervicocephalic arterial dissection, arterial thrombosis, arterial rupture, pseudoaneurysm formation, or development of an arteriovenous fistula. Internal carotid artery thrombosis also may follow maxillary and mandibular angle fractures. Carotid artery trauma may cause hematoma formation of the lateral neck, retinal or hemispheric ischemia, and a Horner's syndrome. Neurological deficits may be mild or devastating. Comatose patients with carotid arterial injuries with a Glasgow Coma Scale score less than 8 do poorly regardless of management (see Chapter 5, Table 5.4). Missing the diagnosis may lead to devastating results. A thorough evaluation of the airway, oropharynx, and esophagus is needed. Arteriography is indicated in most instances and surgical repair may be needed.

Injury to the endothelial cells by high-intensity radiation may cause accelerated atherosclerotic changes, particularly in the presence of hyperlipidemia. These changes may occur months to years after completion of radiation therapy. Radiation vasculopathy correlates with radiation dose and age at time of radiation therapy. Lesions develop in locations that are unusual for atherosclerosis and may involve the extracranial or intracranial vessels. Patients who receive therapeutic radiation therapy for lymphoma, Hodgkin's disease, or thyroid carcinoma are at risk for involvement of the extracranial circulation. Follow-up ultrasound carotid and MRI studies are recommended in these patients. Radiation therapy also may cause an occlusive vasculopathy of small and large intracranial arteries following irradiation of craniopharyngiomas, germinomas, pituitary tumors, or other intracranial neoplasms. Intracranial arterial stenosis also may follow stereotactic radiosurgery.

Moyamoya is a chronic progressive noninflammatory occlusive intracranial vasculopathy of unknown pathogenesis. There is fibrocellular intimal thickening and smooth muscle cell proliferation and increased elastin accumulation in cultured smooth muscle cells derived from patients with moyamoya (Yamamoto et al. 1997). Cases have been associated with neonatal anoxia, trauma, basilar meningitis, tuberculous meningitis, leptospirosis, cranial radiation therapy, neurofibromatosis, tuberous sclerosis, brain tumors, FMD, polyarteritis nodosa, Marfan's syndrome, pseudoxanthoma elasticum, hypomelanosis of Ito, Williams syndrome, cerebral dissecting and saccular aneurysms, sickle cell anemia, β-thalassemia, Fanconi's anemia, factor XII deficiency, type I glycogenosis, reduced form of nicotinamide-adenine dinucleotide phosphate-coenzyme Q reductase deficiency, renal artery stenosis, Down syndrome, Graves' disease, and coarctation of the aorta.

Moyamoya may cause TIAs, including hemodynamic paraparetic TIAs secondary to watershed paracentral lobule ischemia, headaches, seizures, movement disorders, mental

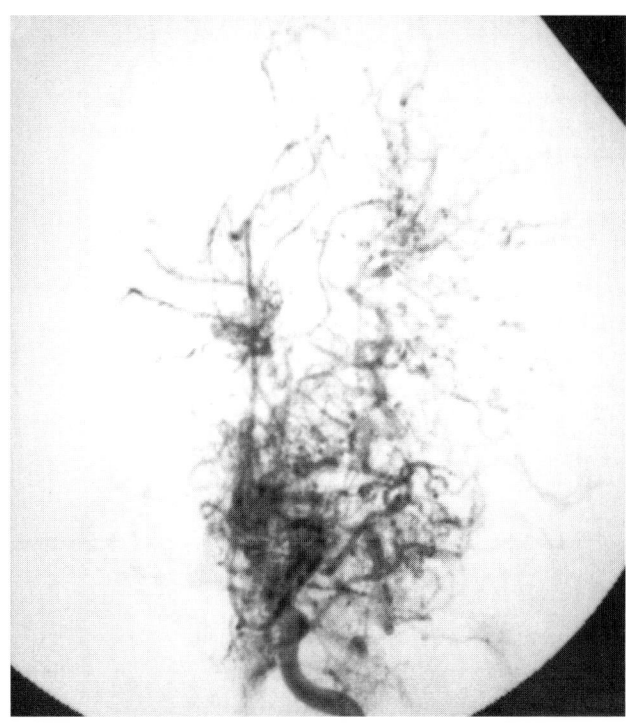

FIGURE 57A.10 Left carotid angiogram (anteroposterior view) shows occlusion of the supraclinoid internal carotid artery and innumerable moyamoya vessels. (Courtesy of Vincent Mathews, MD.)

deterioration, cerebral infarction, or intracranial hemorrhage. It most frequently affects children, adolescents, and young adults. Diagnosis is based on a distinct arteriographical appearance (Figure 57A.10). Moyamoya is characterized by progressive, bilateral stenosis of the distal internal carotid arteries extending to the proximal ACA and MCA, often with involvement of the circle of Willis and development of an extensive collateral network at the base of the brain like a cloud or puff of smoke (moyamoya). Intracranial aneurysms, particularly located in the posterior circulation, may be present.

The optimal treatment of moyamoya has not been determined. Platelet antiaggregants, calcium-channel blockers, and corticosteroids have been used with variable results. Anticoagulants are not useful. Good results have been reported with superficial temporal artery to MCA anastomosis and other revascularization procedures.

FMD is a segmental, nonatheromatous dysplastic, noninflammatory angiopathy affecting predominantly young and middle-aged women. Cervicocephalic FMD affects less than 1% of the population, occurs more often in whites than in blacks, and predominantly involves the cervical carotid arteries at the C1 to C2 level. FMD of the intracranial arteries is rare and mainly limited to the intrapetrosal internal carotid artery or carotid artery siphon. The etiology of FMD is unknown. Immunological and estrogenic effects on the arterial wall may be etiological mechanisms. Four distinct histological types are recognized: intimal fibroplasia, medial hyperplasia, medial fibroplasia, and perimedial dysplasia. Medial fibroplasia is the most frequent form of FMD, followed by perimedial dysplasia, and intimal fibroplasia. The majority of cases of FMD involves the renal arteries, followed by the carotid and iliac arteries. Some cases are familial. Most often, patients with cervicocephalic FMD are asymptomatic or present with headaches, neck pain, carotidynia, tinnitus, vertigo, asymptomatic carotid bruits, transient retinal or cerebral ischemia, cerebral infarction, or subarachnoid hemorrhage. Cervicocephalic FMD may be associated with arterial dissection. Hypertensive patients may have concomitant renal FMD. Cerebral ischemia is usually related to the underlying arterial stenosis or arterial thromboembolism.

The diagnosis of cervicocephalic FMD is made on the basis of cerebral angiography. Cervicocephalic FMD occurs most often in the extracranial carotid artery and is bilateral in approximately two-thirds of cases. The lesions of medial fibroplasia account for the characteristic "string of beads" angiographical appearance seen in approximately 90% of cases.

The optimal treatment of symptomatic cervicocephalic FMD has not been determined. In view of the benign natural history of this condition, platelet antiaggregants are recommended. Surgical intervention with angioplasty or interposition grafting is seldom warranted.

Inflammatory vasculitides can involve any size of vessel, including the precapillary arterioles and postcapillary venules. Many infectious and multisystem noninfectious inflammatory diseases cause cerebral vasculitis (see Table 57A.5). Cerebral vasculitis is a consideration in young patients with ischemic or hemorrhagic stroke; patients with recurrent stroke; patients with stroke associated with encephalopathic features; and patients with stroke accompanied by fever, multifocal neurological events, mononeuritis multiplex, palpable purpura, or abnormal urinary sediment. Other manifestations of cerebral vasculitis include headaches, seizures, and cognitive deterioration. Laboratory studies typically show anemia of chronic disease, leukocytosis, and an elevated erythrocyte sedimentation rate. The diagnosis of vasculitis usually requires confirmation by arteriography or biopsy. Overall, these disorders have a poor prognosis. Corticosteroids and alkylating agents have improved the survival rate.

Intracranial vasculitis and stroke can result from meningovascular syphilis; prodromal manifestations are common before stroke. The MCA territory is most commonly affected. Spinal cord infarction may result from meningomyelitis. Other neurological manifestations in patients with secondary syphilis include headaches, meningismus, mental status changes, and cranial nerve abnormalities. The cerebrospinal fluid (CSF) may show a modest lymphocytic pleocytosis, elevated protein content, and a positive VDRL test result. Concurrent human immunodeficiency virus (HIV) infection can lead to rapid progression of early syphilis to neurosyphilis. Luetic aneurysms of the ascending aorta can extend to involve the origin of the great vessels and can lead to stroke. Treatment schedules for syphilis are listed in standard textbooks; patients with concurrent HIV infection and meningovascular syphilis may require prolonged antibiotic treatment. Worldwide, an estimated 1 billion people are infected with *Mycobacterium tuberculosis*. Strokes can result from tuberculous endarteritis. The exudative basilar inflammation entraps the cranial nerves at the base of the brain, most frequently the third, fourth, and sixth cranial nerves. The basilar arteriolitis most commonly involves penetrating branches of the ACA, MCA, and PCA (medial and lateral lenticulostriate, anterior choroidal, thalamoperforators, and thalamogeniculate arteries). There is usually a modest lymphocytic and mononuclear pleocytosis. The CSF protein is usually elevated, and the glucose level is depressed. In the early stages, a predominantly neutrophilic response may be noted. Smears of CSF demonstrate *M. tuberculosis* in 10–20% of cases. Repeated CSF examinations increase the yield considerably.

Fungal arteritis may result in aneurysms, pseudoaneurysms, thrombus formation, and cerebral infarction. Complications of acute purulent meningitis include intracranial arteritis and thrombophlebitis of the major sinuses and cortical veins. Intracranial arterial stenoses have been associated with a complicated clinical course. Varicella zoster may cause a virus-induced necrotizing arteritis similar to granulomatous angiitis. Cerebral infarction is a complication of the acquired immunodeficiency syndrome and may result from vasculitis, meningovascular syphilis, infective endocarditis, aneurysmal dilation of major cerebral arteries, nonbacterial thrombotic endocarditis, anticardiolipin antibodies, or other hypercoagulable states. Large artery cerebrovascular occlusions have been found in association with meningoencephalitis caused by free living amebae. Other infectious agents known to produce cerebral infarcts include *Mycoplasma pneumoniae*, coxsackie 9 virus, California encephalitis virus, mumps paramyxovirus, hepatitis C virus, *Borrelia burgdorferi*, *Rickettsia typhi* group, cat-scratch disease, *Trichinella* infection, and the larval stage (cysticercus) of *Taenia solium*. Unilateral or bilateral carotid artery occlusion can complicate necrotizing fasciitis of the parapharyngeal space.

Ischemic stroke is a complication of illicit drug use and over-the-counter sympathomimetic drugs. The substances implicated most commonly are the amphetamines, cocaine (free-base or "crack"), phenylpropanolamine, pentazocine (Talwin) in combination with pyribenzamine (T's and blues), phencyclidine, heroin, anabolic steroids, and glue sniffing. Ischemic or hemorrhagic strokes may follow within hours of cocaine use, whether the drug is smoked, snorted, or injected (Figure 57A.11) (see Chapter 57G).

Ischemic stroke is also a complication of a variety of multisystem vasculitides. Stroke in patients with systemic lupus erythematosus may be attributable to cardiogenic embolism (nonbacterial verrucous or Libman-Sacks endocarditis, which occurs in the ventricular surface of the mitral valve), antiphospholipid antibodies, underlying vasculopathy, or less often to an immune-mediated vasculitis (Figure 57A.12) (see Chapter 55A).

Behçet's syndrome may involve vessels of any size. Venous thrombosis is more frequent than occlusive arterial compromise. Affected patients are mainly of Mediterranean or East Asian origin and may have a history of iritis, uveitis, and oral, genital, and mucocutaneous ulcerations. Cerebrovascular complications include strokes, carotid aneurysm formation, and cerebral venous thrombosis. Cogan's syndrome is a rare condition characterized by nonsyphilitic interstitial keratitis, vestibular dysfunction, and deafness. Complications include aortic insufficiency and mesenteric ischemia. The angiitic form of sarcoidosis primarily affects the eyes, meninges, and cerebral arteries and veins. Köhlmeier-Degos or malignant atrophic papulosis is a multisystem occlusive vasculopathy characterized by cutaneous, gastrointestinal, and neurological manifestations; it may be complicated by ischemic or hemorrhagic strokes. Cerebral vasculitis may also complicate the course of children with acute poststreptococcal glomerulonephritis. The multisystem vasculitides are described in more detail in Chapter 55A.

Takayasu's arteritis is a chronic inflammatory arteriopathy of the aorta and its major branches. The cause is unknown, but an immune mechanism is suspected. The disease is suspected in young women of Asian, Mexican, or Native American ancestry. The disease develops insidiously causing stenosis, occlusion, aneurysmal dilatation, or coarctation of the involved vessels. The disease has two phases. In the acute or prepulseless phase, nonspecific systemic manifestations are present. Patients have skin rashes, fever,

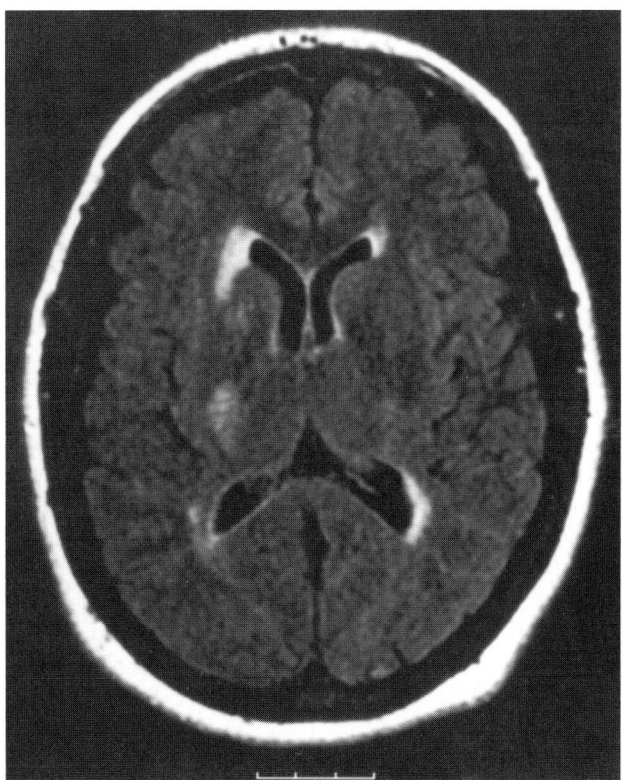

FIGURE 57A.11   A 41-year-old woman with a history of cocaine abuse had acute onset of left-sided hemiplegia, left hemibody sensory deficit, and a left homonymous visual field deficit. Axial fluid-attenuated inversion recovery images of the brain demonstrates an area of infarction in the posterior limb of the right internal capsule in the distribution of the anterior choroidal artery territory. There is associated periventricular ischemia.

FIGURE 57A.12   Lateral carotid angiogram demonstrates irregular beading appearance (arrowheads) of large and medium branches of the anterior, middle, and posterior cerebral arteries in a patient with systemic lupus erythematosus. (Courtesy of Vincent Mathews, MD.)

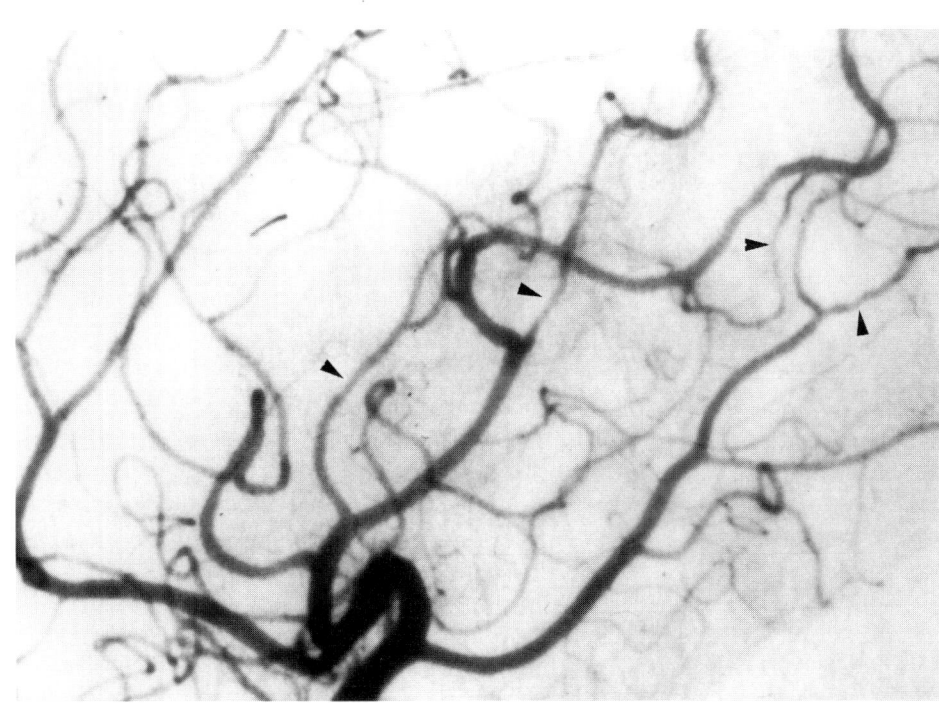

myalgias, arthritis, pleuritis, and elevated erythrocyte sedimentation rate. Months or years later, the second or occlusive phase develops and is characterized by multiple arterial occlusions. Patients may have cervical bruits, absent carotid or radial pulses, asymmetric blood pressure recordings, and arterial hypertension. Neurological symptoms result from central nervous system or retinal ischemia associated with stenosis or occlusion of the aortic arch and arch vessels, or arterial hypertension caused by aortic coarctation or renal artery stenosis. The diagnosis can be confirmed by MRA, but the most accurate assessment still requires aortography.

Cranial (giant cell or temporal) arteritis is a polysymptomatic systemic large vessel arteritis with a predilection to involve carotid artery branches (see Chapter 73). Thromboangiitis obliterans, also known as *Buerger's disease*, is a rare, segmental inflammatory, obliterative angiopathy of unknown cause. The condition involves small and medium arteries and veins. It is suspected in young men who smoke and have a history of superficial migratory thrombophlebitis presenting with distal limb ischemia accompanied by digital gangrene. The disorder is characterized by remissions and exacerbations. Cerebral involvement is uncommon. Strokes can result from isolated angiitis of the central nervous system. Symptoms of large-vessel involvement include stroke-like presentations. Small-vessel involvement may be manifested as a mass lesion or multifocal encephalopathy. The erythrocyte sedimentation rate is usually normal or minimally elevated (see Chapter 57G).

Epidemiological studies suggest a nonrandom association of both headache and migraine with stroke, particularly among young women. This rare association was limited to women younger than age 35 in a large Italian case-controlled study (Carolei et al. 1996). The possible association between migraine headache and stroke was also evaluated by the Physician's Health Study; physicians reporting migraine had increased risks of subsequent total stroke and ischemic stroke compared with those not reporting migraines (Buring et al. 1995).

The International Headache Society classification and diagnostic criteria for headache disorders, cranial neuralgias, and facial pain requires that one or more migrainous aura symptoms must be present and not fully reversed within 7 days from onset, associated with neuroimaging confirmation of ischemic infarction to establish a diagnosis of migrainous infarction (see Chapter 73). This definition implies that a firm diagnosis of migraine with aura has been made in the past. Also, the clinical manifestations judged to be the result of a migrainous infarction must be those typical of previous attacks for that individual, and finally, other causes of infarction, including those related to migraine therapy, need to be excluded by appropriate investigations.

Headache accompanies a number of embolic or thrombotic causes of stroke, including cervicocephalic arterial dissections. Migraines also can be a prominent symptom in the antiphospholipid antibody syndrome. Symptomatic migraine attacks are more frequent than migraine-induced ischemic insults. The presence of headache with a stroke is therefore not sufficient to make the diagnosis of migraine as the cause of the patient's symptoms. Furthermore, patchy subcortical abnormalities on MRI in patients with migraine with aura should be interpreted with caution. In other words, migrainous infarction remains a diagnosis of exclusion.

The pathogenesis of migrainous infarction is controversial. Cerebral infarcts complicating migraine are mostly cortical and involve the distribution of the PCA. The usual scenario of migrainous infarction is one of recurrent episodes of gradual buildup of unilateral throbbing headaches, associated with stereotyped visual phenomena occurring in both visual fields simultaneously, in one of which the vision loss becomes permanent. Migrainous infarctions have been subdivided as definite when all the International Headache Society criteria are fulfilled, and possible when some, but not all criteria, are fulfilled. Patients with migrainous infarction are at increased risk for recurrent stroke.

Cerebral autosomal dominant arteriopathy with subcortical infarcts and leukoencephalopathy (CADASIL) is a familial nonarteriosclerotic, nonamyloid arteriopathy characterized by recurrent subcortical ischemic strokes starting in midadulthood, leading to pseudobulbar palsy, subcortical dementia, and early MRI abnormalities. The disease has been mapped to chromosome 19q12. A subtype of migraine, known as familial hemiplegic migraine, characterized by transient weakness or frank paralysis during the aura, has also been mapped close to the CADASIL locus (Hutchinson et al. 1995). The newer acronym, cerebral autosomal dominant arteriopathy with subcortical infarcts, leukoencephalopathy, and migraine (CADASILM), refers to a subvariety of CADASIL characterized by the high frequency of migraine (Verin et al. 1995).

Inherited and Miscellaneous Disorders

Homocystinuria, an inborn error of amino acid metabolism, is an unusual cause of stroke (Table 57A.6). Three specific enzyme deficiencies responsible for homocystinuria have been identified: cystathionine β-synthetase, homocysteine methyltransferase, and methylene tetrahydrofolate reductase. The accumulation of homocyst(e)ine in the blood leads to endothelial injury and premature atherosclerosis. Patients with homocystinuria may display a marfanoid habitus, malar flush, livedo reticularis, ectopia lentis, myopia, glaucoma, optic atrophy, psychiatric abnormalities, mental retardation, spasticity, seizures, osteoporosis, and a propensity for intracranial arterial or venous thrombosis. Death may result from pulmonary embolism, myocardial infarction, or stroke. Raised levels of plasma homocyst(e)ine may be an independent risk factor for cerebrovascular disease, coronary, and peripheral arterial occlusive disease. Elevated levels of homocyst(e)ine can be effectively reduced with the administration of folate, occasionally requiring the addition of pyridoxine (vitamin B_6), vitamin B_{12}, choline, or betaine.

Fabry's disease is an X-linked disorder of glycosphingolipid metabolism characterized by deficient lysosomal α-galactosidase activity. As a result, deposits of ceramide trihexosidase accumulate in endothelial and smooth muscle cells. Patients have a painful peripheral neuropathy, renal disease, hypertension, cardiomegaly, autonomic dysfunction, and corneal opacifications. Characteristic dark-red or blue lesions, that do not blanch on pressure, called *angiokeratoma corporis diffusum*, are found between the umbilicus and knees. Stroke and myocardial infarction are common. Female carriers may have mild disease or are asymptomatic.

Marfan's syndrome is an autosomal dominant inherited connective tissue disease associated with qualitative and quantitative defects of fibrillin. Histopathological studies of aortic segments show cystic medial necrosis. This disorder is characterized by a variety of skeletal, ocular, and cardiovascular findings. Patients with Marfan's syndrome may display arachnodactyly, extreme limb length, joint laxity, pectus excavatum or carinatum, subluxation of the lens, and aortic valvular insufficiency. Marfan's syndrome is associated with a high incidence of dilatation of the aortic root. Other cardiovascular abnormalities include coarctation of the aorta, mitral valve prolapse, and mitral annulus calcification with regurgitation. Progressive dilatation of the aortic root may lead to dissection of the ascending aorta, resulting in ischemia to the brain, spinal cord, or peripheral nerves. Saccular intracranial aneurysms or dissection of the carotid artery can occur. Annual echocardiographic studies are recommended. Patients should avoid contact sports.

Patients with Ehlers-Danlos syndrome, a fairly common heritable connective tissue disorder, display hyperextensibility of the skin, hypermobile joints, and vascular fragility leading to a bleeding diathesis. Arterial complications have been reported in association with Ehlers-Danlos syndrome types I, III, and IV, especially type IV. Complications include dissections, arteriovenous fistulae, and aneurysms. Other cardiovascular abnormalities in patients with type IV Ehlers-Danlos syndrome include ventricular and atrial septal defects, aortic insufficiency, bicuspid aortic valve, mitral valve prolapse, and papillary muscle dysfunction. Arteriography carries special risks and should be avoided if possible.

Patients with pseudoxanthoma elasticum, an inherited group of disorders of elastic tissue, often display loose skin and small, raised, orange-yellowish papules resembling "plucked chicken skin" in intertriginous areas. Patients with pseudoxanthoma elasticum have a higher risk of coronary artery disease and myocardial infarction. These patients may also have arterial hypertension, angioid streaks of the retina, retinal hemorrhages, arterial occlusive disease, and arterial dissections. Women with pseudoxanthoma elasticum should avoid estrogens.

Sneddon's syndrome consists of widespread livedo reticularis and ischemic cerebrovascular manifestations. A number of reports have documented a hereditary transmission and a

Table 57A.6:   Inherited and miscellaneous disorders causing cerebral infarction

Homocystinuria
Fabry's disease
Marfan's syndrome
Ehlers-Danlos syndrome
Pseudoxanthoma elasticum
Sneddon's syndrome
Rendu-Osler-Weber syndrome
Neoplastic angioendotheliomatosis
Susac's syndrome
Eales disease
Reversible cerebral segmental vasoconstriction
Hypereosinophilic syndrome
Cerebral amyloid angiopathy
Coils and kinks
Arterial dolichoectasia
Complications of coarctation of the aorta
Air, fat, amniotic fluid, bone marrow, and foreign particle embolism

link between Sneddon's syndrome and antiphospholipid antibodies. However, the etiopathogenesis remains unknown, although an immune mechanism is suspected. Endothelial cells could be the primary target tissue. Antiendothelial cell antibodies may be present (Frances et al. 1995).

Hereditary hemorrhagic telangiectasia (Rendu-Osler-Weber) is a familial disorder transmitted as an autosomal dominant trait. Ischemic stroke as a presenting manifestation of Rendu-Osler-Weber has been reported infrequently. Paradoxical venous emboli passing through a pulmonary arteriovenous malformation can be the source of cerebral ischemia. Other potential causes leading to cerebral ischemia include air embolism and hyperviscosity secondary to polycythemia.

Neoplastic angioendotheliomatosis, also called *intravascular malignant lymphomatosis or angiotropic lymphoma*, is a rare disease characterized by multiple, small and large vessel occlusion by neoplastic cell of lymphoid origin without an obvious primary tumor. Simultaneous involvement of blood vessels throughout the body and compromise of different cerebral arterial territories is common with this disorder. Patients may present with recurrent multifocal cerebral infarctions, dementia, or myelopathy. Diagnosis requires skin, liver, renal, meningeal, or brain biopsy. Combination chemotherapy has been recommended.

Microangiopathy of brain, retina, and inner ear (Susac's syndrome) is a rare microcirculatory syndrome that affects mainly adult women (Petty et al. 1998). The syndrome is unrelated to arterial hypertension or diabetes and is characterized by arteriolar branch occlusions of the brain, retina, and inner ear, with resultant encephalopathy, vision loss, vestibular dysfunction, and asymmetrical sensorineural hearing loss. Brain biopsy may show multifocal brain microinfarcts in both gray and white matter. The etiology is unknown but has been attributed to a disturbance of coagulation, microembolism, or both. Treatment with corticosteroids, cyclophosphamide, or anticoagulant therapy is empiric, but branch retinal artery occlusions and central nervous system infarctions recur despite the treatment. Hyperbaric oxygen treatment may be an option for refractory visual symptoms.

Eales disease, commonly reported in India and the Middle East, is a rare, noninflammatory occlusive disease of the retinal vasculature characterized by repeated retinal and vitreous hemorrhages. The disorder affects mainly young men. Brain infarctions are rare.

Idiopathic reversible cerebral segmental vasoconstriction is an unusual clinical angiographical syndrome characterized by recurrent headaches, and transient motor and sensory findings associated with reversible arterial narrowing and dilatation involving predominantly the arteries round the circle of Willis. The etiology is unknown.

The hypereosinophilic syndrome is a rare disorder caused by bone marrow overproduction of eosinophils that lodge in endothelial cells in the microcirculation primarily of heart, brain, kidney, lungs, gastrointestinal tract, and skin. Neurological complications include emboli from involved endocardium and heart valves, and neurological manifestations may result also from a hypercoagulable state with cerebral thromboses, and microcirculatory inflammation and occlusion by eosinophils. Cerebral infarction is a rare complication.

Cerebral amyloid angiopathy occurs both sporadically or in rare instances as a hereditary disorder. Cerebral amyloid angiopathy is characterized by the localized deposition of amyloid in the media and adventitia of small arteries and arterioles of the cerebral cortex and meninges in the elderly. Cerebral amyloid angiopathy is more commonly associated with lobar hemorrhage than with ischemic stroke, but has been associated with an increased frequency of cerebral infarction in patients with Alzheimer's disease (Olichney et al. 1995). Biopsy of the involved cortex and leptomeninges is the only definitive way to diagnose cerebral amyloid angiopathy.

Redundant length of the cervical carotid artery causes coils and kinks and other forms of tortuosity. Occasionally associated with FMD, kinks and coils of the carotid artery are an infrequent cause of cerebral ischemia. Arterial kinking seldom affects the vertebrobasilar circulation. Cerebral ischemia associated with kinking is attributable to a combination of flow reduction caused by obstruction, neck rotation, and distal embolization. Dolichoectasia is an unusual vascular disease that causes enlargement and elongation of arteries, particularly the basilar artery. This arteriopathy causes false aneurysm that leads to stroke, brainstem compression, and cranial nerve palsies. The mechanisms of stroke are penetrating artery occlusion, basilar artery thrombosis, or embolism from the dolichoectatic artery.

Ischemic stroke and intracranial hemorrhage, the latter caused by arterial hypertension or ruptured intracranial aneurysm, are important complications of coarctation of the aorta. Neurological complications can result also from aortic rupture, infective aortitis or endarteritis, associated aortic bicuspid valve, and dissection of the aorta proximal to the coarctation.

Atheromatous emboli (cholesterol emboli syndrome) may follow manipulation of an atherosclerotic aorta during catheterization or surgery. Clinical presentation may include TIAs, stroke, retinal embolism pancreatitis, renal failure, and livedo reticularis. Purple toes may occur also as a result of small cholesterol emboli lodging in the digital arteries. Pedal pulses are normal. Patients also have a low-grade fever, eosinophilia, anemia, elevated erythrocyte sedimentation rate, and elevated serum amylase. Anticoagulation may exacerbate further embolization, and its use should be discouraged.

Accidental introduction of air into the systemic circulation can be a cause of cerebral or retinal ischemia. Air embolism is a dreaded complication of surgical procedures, including intracranial operations in the sitting position; open heart surgery; surgery of the lungs, pleura, sinuses, neck and axilla; hemodialysis; thoracocentesis; arteriography; central venous catheters; and scuba diving. Symptoms include seizures and multifocal neurological findings such as cerebral edema, confusion, memory loss, and coma. CT scan may be useful in visualizing the gaseous bubbles. Treatment includes prompt resuscitative measures, placement of the patient in the left lateral position, inotropic agents, anticonvulsants, antiedema agents, and hyperbaric oxygen. Caisson disease can occur in persons who are scuba diving. Neurological features are caused by multiple small nitrogen emboli leading to ischemia of the brain and spinal cord; signs of spinal cord dysfunction are prominent. Hyperbaric oxygen therapy is the usual treatment.

Fat embolism to the brain complicates long bone fractures, sickle cell disease, cardiopulmonary bypass, soft tissue injuries, and blood transfusions. This syndrome occurs suddenly within hours to 3 or 4 days after injury and is characterized by dyspnea, fever, tachycardia, tachypnea, cyanosis, cutaneous petechiae, and coagulopathy. Neurological manifestations are confusion, disorientation, delirium, hemiparesis, aphasia, and coma. Petechial hemorrhages may be apparent on funduscopy, conjunctivae, base of the neck, and axillary region. Vigorous respiratory supportive therapy is essential.

Amniotic fluid embolism is a rare catastrophic obstetrical complication caused by the entry of amniotic fluid into the maternal bloodstream during parturition. Vigorous supportive therapy with intravenous fluids and blood replacement to treat shock, correction of respiratory distress syndrome, disseminated intravascular coagulation, and underlying fibrinolytic state are essential. Among other causes of emboli are large intracranial saccular aneurysms or extracranial false aneurysms of the internal carotid artery. Tumor emboli to the brain have been reported with osteosarcoma, atrial myxoma, and with carcinoma of the lung, breast, pharynx, or esophagus. Talc, cornstarch, and other foreign particles injected as adulterants in illicit drugs can embolize to the brain or retina. Paradoxical embolism during bone marrow infusion is an infrequent complication.

Hypercoagulable Disorders

Alterations in hemostasis are associated with an increased risk of cerebrovascular events, particularly those of an ischemic nature and may account for a considerable number of cryptogenic strokes (Table 57A.7). These disorders account for 1% of all strokes and for 2–7% of ischemic strokes in young patients (Kitchens 1994).

Primary Hypercoagulable States

Inherited disorders predisposing to thrombosis especially affect the venous circulation. These disorders include antithrombin III (AT-III) deficiency, protein C and protein S deficiencies, activated protein C (APC) resistance, abnormalities of fibrinogen (dysfibrinogenemia), and abnormalities of plasminogen or tissue plasminogen activator. Inherited thrombophilia should be suspected in patients with recurrent episodes of deep venous thrombosis, recurrent pulmonary emboli, family history of thrombotic events, unusual sites of venous (mesenteric, portal, or cerebral) or arterial thromboses, or in patients with thrombotic events occurring during childhood, adolescence, or early adulthood. Approximately one-half of all thrombotic episodes occur spontaneously, although these patients are at greatest risk when exposed to additional risk factors such as pregnancy, surgery, trauma, or oral contraceptive therapy.

AT-III deficiency is inherited in an autosomal dominant fashion, thus affecting both sexes. There are three categories of inherited AT-III deficiency: classic or type I characterized by decreased immunological and biological activity of AT-III; type II or AT-III deficiency characterized by low biological activity of AT-III but essentially normal immunological activity; and type III characterized by normal AT-III activity in the absence of heparin, but reduced in heparin-dependent assays. Acquired AT-III deficiency may follow acute thrombosis and disseminated intravascular coagulation. It has been associated also with nephrotic syndrome, liver cirrhosis, eclampsia, various malignancies, the use of estrogens or oral contraceptives, L-asparaginase, tamoxifen, and heparin therapy. A normal level of AT-III activity obtained at the time of an acute thrombotic event is sufficient to exclude a primary deficiency. However, a low level of AT-III activity must be confirmed by repeat testing, after resolution of the thrombotic episode and discontinuation of anticoagulant therapy. Confirmation of a low plasma level of AT-III activity on repeat testing is compatible with a primary deficiency and is an indication to investigate other family members. Thrombotic episodes associated with AT-III deficiency are treated acutely with heparin with or without adjunctive AT-III concentrate. Prophylactic therapy in patients with recurrent thrombosis

Table 57A.7: Hypercoagulable states

Primary hypercoagulable states
Antithrombin III deficiency
Protein C deficiency
Protein S deficiency
Activated protein C resistance with or without factor V Leiden mutation
Afibrinogenemia
Hypofibrinogenemia
Dysfibrinogenemia
Hypoplasminogenemia
Abnormal plasminogen
Plasminogen activators deficiency
Lupus anticoagulant and anticardiolipin antibodies
Secondary hypercoagulable states
Malignancy
Pregnancy/puerperium
Oral contraceptives
Ovarian hyperstimulation syndrome
Other hormonal treatments
Nephrotic syndrome
Polycythemia vera
Essential thrombocythemia
Paroxysmal nocturnal hemoglobinuria
Diabetes mellitus
Heparin-induced thrombocytopenia
Homocystinuria
Sickle cell disease
Thrombotic thrombocytopenic purpura
Chemotherapeutic agents

consists of long-term warfarin administration, keeping the therapeutic international normalized ratio (INR) range between 2.0 and 3.0.

Protein C deficiency is inherited in an autosomal dominant fashion. Homozygous protein C deficiency presents in infancy as purpura fulminans neonatalis. Heterozygotes are predisposed to recurrent thrombosis. Thrombotic manifestations are predominantly venous. Acquired protein C deficiency has been associated with the administration of L-asparaginase, warfarin therapy, liver disease, disseminated intravascular coagulation, postoperative state, bone marrow transplantation, and the adult respiratory distress syndrome. Testing for immunological and functional assays of protein C should be performed after oral anticoagulation has been discontinued for at least a week. Heparin does not modify the levels of protein C. Warfarin-induced skin necrosis is a serious potential complication of protein C–deficient patients at the initiation of warfarin therapy; this syndrome often occurs in association with large loading doses of warfarin. The acute management of thrombosis associated with protein C deficiency consists of prompt administration of heparin followed by incremental doses of warfarin, starting with low doses until adequate anticoagulation is achieved. Long-term management requires the administration of warfarin.

Protein S deficiency also has an autosomal dominant mode of inheritance. Protein S exists in plasma in two forms;

approximately 40% of the total protein S is functionally active or free, and the remaining is complexed to a binding protein. Homozygous protein S deficiency presents with venous thromboembolic disease. Heterozygotes are prone to recurrent thrombosis including cerebral venous thrombosis. Acquired protein S deficiency occurs during pregnancy, in association with acute thromboembolic episodes, disseminated intravascular coagulation, nephrotic syndrome, systemic lupus erythematosus, and with the administration of oral contraceptives, oral anticoagulants, and L-asparaginase. Testing for immunological assays of total and free protein S, and functional assay of protein S, should be confirmed after resolution of the thrombotic episode and discontinuation of oral anticoagulants. Heparin therapy is effective in the management of acute thrombotic events associated with protein S deficiency, whereas warfarin is advocated for patients with recurrent thromboembolism.

Resistance to APC is one of the most common identifiable risk factors for venous thromboembolic disease, including cerebral venous thrombosis. The relation of APC resistance to arterial disease is not well established. APC resistance has been identified as five to 10 times more common than deficiencies of AT-III, protein C, or protein S. APC resistance also has an autosomal dominant mode of inheritance. APC resistance is associated in most patients with a single point mutation in the factor V gene (factor V Leiden), which involves the replacement of arginine 506 with glutamine 506 (Arg 506 Gln). Testing for resistance to APC must be done after discontinuation of anticoagulants. There are conflicting results about factor V Leiden gene mutation and the risk for acute cerebral arterial thromboses.

Abnormalities of fibrinogen account for approximately 1% of all inherited thrombotic disorders. Fibrinogen cross-links platelets during thrombosis and is an important component of atherosclerotic plaques. High concentrations of fibrinogen increase the risk for stroke and myocardial infarction. Afibrinogenemia is probably transmitted as an autosomal recessive trait; complications include umbilical cord bleeding, gastrointestinal hemorrhage, and intracranial hemorrhage. Hypofibrinogenemia represents the heterozygous form of afibrinogenemia; bleeding is rare. Dysfibrinogenemia reflects a qualitative disorder in the fibrinogen molecule and may be associated with hemorrhagic or thrombotic episodes. Hereditary dysfibrinogenemia is inherited in an autosomal dominant fashion. Decreased concentrations of fibrinogen are associated with disseminated intravascular coagulation, liver failure, snake bite, treatment with L-asparaginase, ancrod, fibrinolytic drugs, and valproate. Treatment consists of infusions of cryoprecipitate.

Decreased levels of plasminogen (hypoplasminogenemia), qualitative abnormalities in the plasminogen molecule (dysplasminogenemias), and defective release of plasminogen activators occur in families with recurrent thrombotic events. Cerebral venous thrombosis occurs with disorders of plasminogen. Prophylactic therapy in patients with recurrent thrombosis consists of lifelong anticoagulation.

Lupus anticoagulants and anticardiolipin antibodies are known collectively as *antiphospholipid antibodies* and have a pathogenetic role in arterial and venous thrombosis. However, whether these antibodies are a primary cause of these vascular events or a consequence of a previous clinical event remains controversial. Antiphospholipid antibodies are present in patients with systemic lupus erythematosus and related autoimmune disorders, Sneddon's syndrome, acute and chronic infections (including HIV), neoplasias, inflammatory bowel disease, administration of certain drugs, early onset severe preeclampsia, liver transplantation, and also in individuals without demonstrable underlying disorders. A distinct group of patients have a *primary* antiphospholipid antibody syndrome; its association with ischemic cerebrovascular disease is rare.

Antiphospholipid antibodies are associated with recurrent fetal loss, a prolongation of the activated partial thromboplastin time (aPTT) that does not correct on 1 to 1 mixing with normal plasma, thrombocytopenia, a false-positive VDRL test result, and livedo reticularis. They may also be associated with cerebral and ocular ischemia, cerebral venous thrombosis, migraine, vascular dementia, chorea, transverse myelopathy, myocardial infarction, peripheral arterial thromboembolism, venous thrombosis, pulmonary embolism, and Degos' disease. Multiple cerebral infarctions are common in patients with antiphospholipid antibodies; a subset of patients may present with vascular dementia (Figure 57A.13). Still another group may have an acute or progressive thrombotic ischemic encephalopathy. Pathological studies of cerebral arteries involved in association with antiphospholipid antibodies demonstrate the presence of a chronic thrombotic microangiopathy, but no evidence of vasculitis. Patients with antiphospholipid antibodies have an increased frequency of mitral and aortic vegetations. There are findings resembling verrucous endocarditis (Libman-Sacks). Left ventricular thrombus formation is a rare occurrence. Treatment for arterial thrombosis associated with antiphospholipid antibodies is not well established. One case-controlled study found that high-intensity warfarin (INR >3.0), with or without aspirin, was more effective in preventing thrombotic recurrences than low-intensity warfarin, with or without aspirin, or aspirin alone (Khamashta et al. 1995). Pregnant patients are often treated with prednisone and low-dose aspirin.

Secondary Hypercoagulable States

Strokes may complicate the clinical course of malignancies. In rare instances, stroke may be the initial manifestation of cancer. Cerebral infarction mostly complicates lymphomas, carcinomas, and solid tumors. Cerebral hemorrhages are more common with leukemia. Hypercoagulability is not an uncommon finding in patients with malignancy, especially with mucin-producing carcinomas of the pancreas, gastrointestinal tract, and lung; myeloproliferative disorders; acute promyelocytic leukemia; and brain tumors. Mucinous

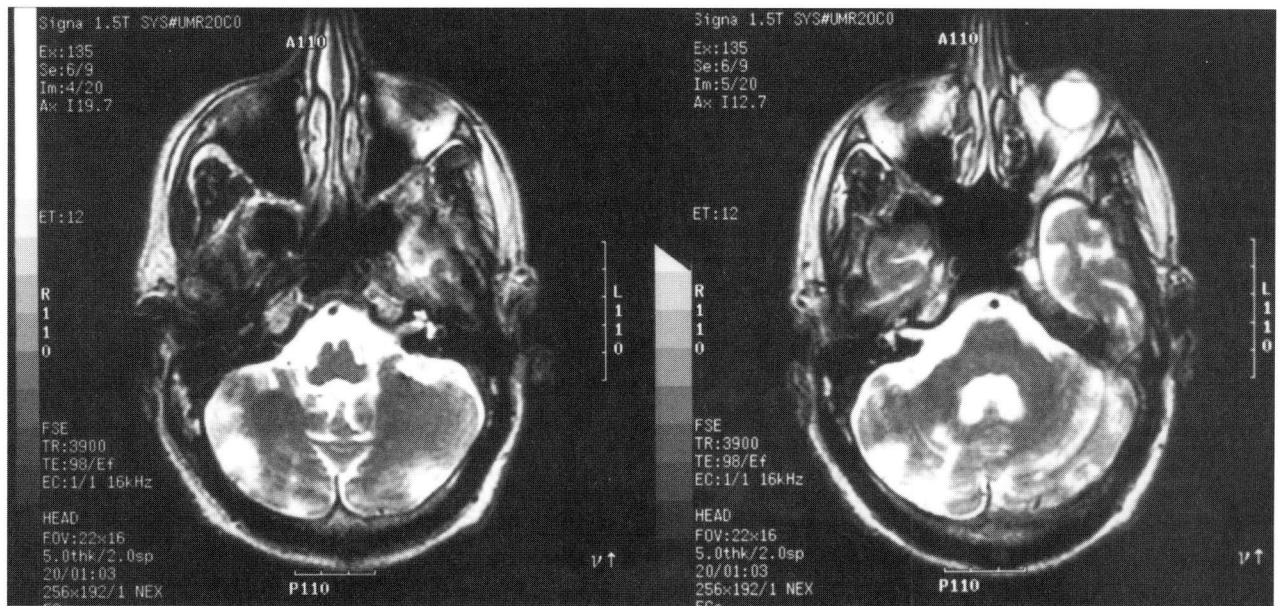

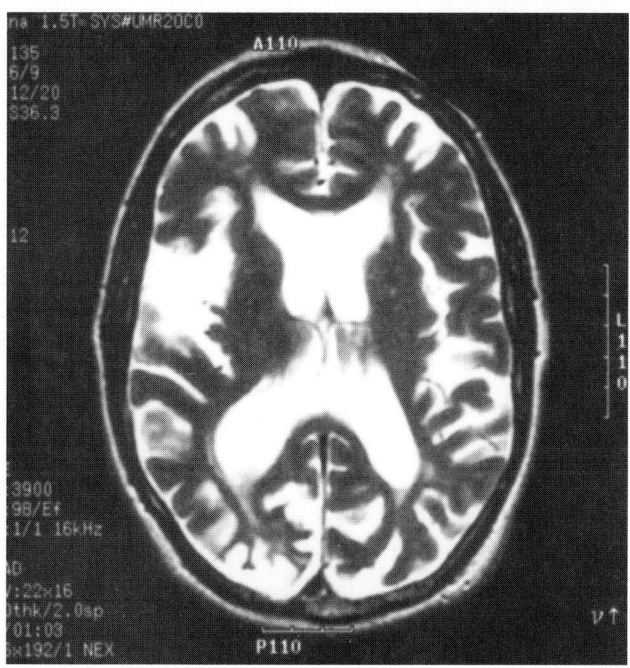

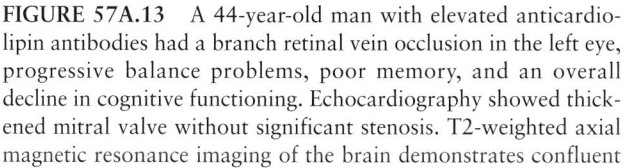

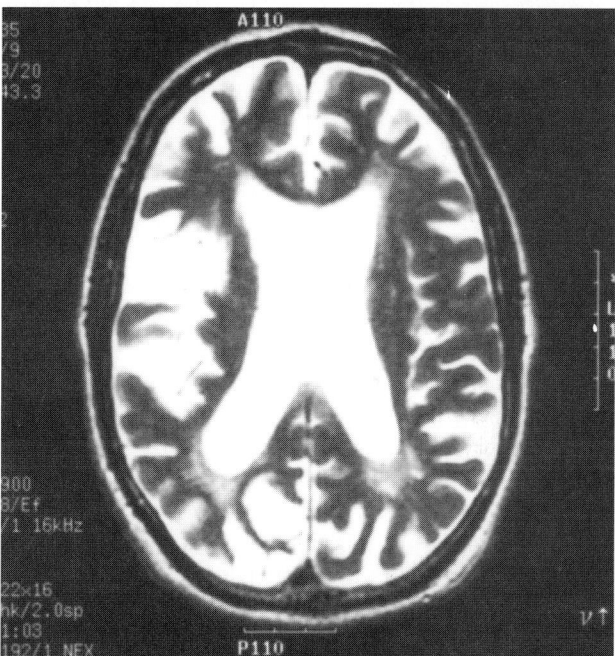

FIGURE 57A.13   A 44-year-old man with elevated anticardiolipin antibodies had a branch retinal vein occlusion in the left eye, progressive balance problems, poor memory, and an overall decline in cognitive functioning. Echocardiography showed thickened mitral valve without significant stenosis. T2-weighted axial magnetic resonance imaging of the brain demonstrates confluent hyperintensities in the periventricular region and basal ganglia consistent with ischemia. There are also bilateral hyperintensities in the cerebellum consistent with infarcts. Cortical ischemic changes are also present bilaterally in the occipital lobes and in the right frontal lobe.

adenocarcinomas of the gastrointestinal tract, lung, and ovary may produce infarcts from widespread cerebral arterial occlusions by mucin. The etiology of the hypercoagulable state is often multifactorial. The pathophysiology is believed to be a state of low-grade disseminated intravascular coagulation and secondary fibrinolysis, but with the balance shifted toward clotting. Atherosclerosis is still the leading cause of infarction in patients with malignancy. Cerebral infarction in patients with malignancy also may be caused by tumor emboli, bone marrow embolization, emboli originating from mural thrombi, or emboli arising from marantic vegetations associated with nonbacterial thrombotic endocarditis. Many patients with nonbacterial thrombotic endocarditis have associated disseminated

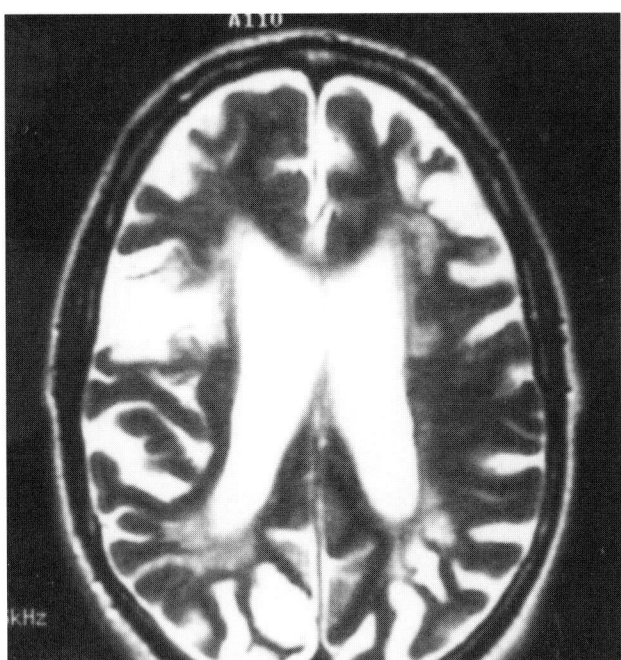

FIGURE 57A.13   *(continued)*

intravascular coagulation, which may cause capillary occlusion of multiple organs, especially the lungs, kidneys, gastrointestinal tract, heart, and brain. Neurological manifestations produce a diffuse encephalopathy secondary to disseminated microinfarcts. Other patients with malignancy and cerebral infarction may have cerebral venous occlusive disease caused by thrombi, tumor invasion, or stroke associated with chemotherapy. In addition, cancer-enhanced atherothrombosis, neoplastic angioendotheliomatosis, arterial compression by tumor, occlusive vascular disease secondary to irradiation, intercurrent angiitis, and arterial rupture also may be responsible for cerebral infarction in some patients. Treatment consists of management of the underlying malignancy. Anticoagulants and platelet antiaggregants are used with variable success.

The postpartum period is a hypercoagulable state. Characteristically, arterial causes of stroke are more common during pregnancy, whereas venous causes of stroke are more common during the puerperium (see Chapter 85).

Oral contraceptives cause alterations of the vessel wall with intimal hyperplasia. They also increase blood viscosity. These are decreased levels of protein S, antithrombin III activity, and plasminogen activator content in women taking oral contraceptives. There also may be an increase in the levels of fibrinogen, factors VII and X. Oral contraceptive therapy may enhance arterial hypertension. Women taking oral contraceptives have an estimated ninefold increased risk of thrombotic stroke. This risk is increased by prolonged use, high dosage of the estrogen component, cigarette smoking, concomitant diabetes, arterial hypertension, hyperlipidemia, and age older than 35 years. Current users of oral contraceptives are at increased risk of stroke.

One study showed that oral contraceptives containing 30–40 µg of estrogen are associated with a one-third reduced risk compared with preparations containing 50 µg. The occurrence of intracranial venous thrombosis as a complication of oral contraceptives is well recognized. A patient on oral contraceptives occasionally presents with stroke caused by paradoxical embolism associated with deep venous thrombosis. Oral contraceptives also increase the risk of subarachnoid hemorrhage.

Oral contraceptives probably should be avoided in women with arterial hypertension. They should also be avoided in the first 2 weeks after delivery. Women older than 35 years of age who smoke cigarettes probably should be advised to choose a different contraceptive method. As part of primary stroke prevention efforts, women who smoke should not use oral contraceptives. The ovarian hyperstimulation syndrome occurs in women after induction of ovulation with clomiphene, human menopausal gonadotropin, human follicle-stimulating hormone extracted from human pituitary, and human chorionic gonadotropin. Evidence of body fluid shifts and hypercoagulability exist with this syndrome, reflected in thromboembolic events. Stroke is a rare but serious consequence of severe ovarian hyperstimulation syndrome.

Thromboembolic events are a feared complication of hormone treatment in transsexuals. Cerebral infarction has occurred as a side effect of exogenous estrogen in a male-to-female transsexual. Likewise, TIAs and cerebral infarction may follow the administration of anabolic steroids for the treatment of hypogonadism and hypoplastic anemias. Cerebral ischemia has occurred also following the use of human recombinant erythropoietin in the treatment of anemia of patients on hemodialysis.

The nephrotic syndrome may be accompanied by venous and arterial thromboses, including cerebral arterial and venous occlusive disease. Ischemic stroke can be the presenting manifestation. The mechanism by which nephrotic syndrome causes hypercoagulability is multifactorial and includes elevated levels of fibrinogen, raised levels of factors V, VII, VIII, and X, thrombocytosis, enhanced platelet aggregation, and reduced levels of AT-III and protein S. The exact role of hyperlipidemia, corticosteroids, and diuretic use is uncertain. Nephrotic syndrome should be considered as a contributing mechanism in any patient with ischemic stroke and pre-existing renal disease. A urinalysis is the initial clue to the diagnosis. The presence of severe proteinuria and a low serum albumin should prompt consideration of a hypercoagulable state. Treatment of thromboembolism associated with nephrotic syndrome consists of anticoagulants until remission of the renal condition.

Polycythemia vera and primary or essential thrombocythemia are typically disorders of middle-aged or elderly patients. Polycythemia vera is characterized by increased red blood cell mass and normal arterial oxygen saturation. Patients have ruddy cyanosis, painful pruritus, hypertension, splenomegaly, elevated hemoglobin, high hematocrit value, thrombocytosis, leukocytosis, and elevated serum B_{12} levels. Typically, the bone marrow is hypercellular. Secondary polycythemia may occur in association with cerebral hemangioblastoma, hepatoma, hypernephroma, uterine fibroids, benign renal cysts, carbon monoxide exposure, and administration of androgens. Cerebral blood flow is reduced and cerebral hemorrhage, and arterial or venous thrombosis, can complicate the condition. The majority of the intracranial events are thrombotic in origin, the larger cerebral arteries being the most frequently involved. The risk of stroke parallels the hemoglobin level: The higher the hemoglobin and hematocrit values, the greater the risk of stroke. Headaches, dizziness, vertigo, tinnitus, visual disturbances, carotid and vertebrobasilar TIAs, chorea, and fluctuating cognitive impairment are well-recognized features of patients with polycythemia vera. Spinal cord infarction is a rare complication. Cautious lowering of the hematocrit is a reasonable therapeutic approach. Because of the potential risk of hemorrhagic intracranial complications, aspirin therapy should be used cautiously.

Cerebral thrombotic and hemorrhagic complications are not uncommon in primary or essential thrombocythemia. Patients may have splenomegaly, mucocutaneous hemorrhagic diathesis, persistently elevated platelet count, usually in excess of 1 million per μL, giant platelets, and a bone marrow megakaryocyte hyperplasia. Neurological complications are common. Headaches, dizziness, amaurosis fugax, and TIAs of the brain are relatively frequent. Cerebral arterial thrombosis caused by platelet-fibrin thrombi is a rare but serious complication of essential thrombocythemia. Papilledema secondary to cerebral venous thrombosis may be a complication in patients whose platelet levels have not been controlled. Cerebral infarctions also have been reported in patients with secondary thrombocythemia caused by iron deficiency anemia. Iron deficiency anemia with or without thrombocytosis also has been implicated as a cause of intraluminal thrombus of the carotid artery, intracranial venous thrombosis, and intracranial hemorrhage (Hartfield et al. 1997). Thrombocytosis is common after splenectomy, but does not seem to carry an increased thromboembolic risk. However, reactive thrombocytosis following cardiopulmonary bypass surgery may be involved in the etiology of stroke in the late recovery period after surgery. The role of rebound thrombocytosis in ischemic stroke among heavy alcohol drinkers is uncertain. Treatment of primary thrombocythemia includes hydroxyurea, plateletpheresis, recombinant interferon-α, and aspirin. Vigorous correction of the anemia is indicated for those patients with thrombocytosis associated with iron deficiency anemia.

Paroxysmal nocturnal hemoglobinuria is an acquired clonal stem cell disorder characterized by severe hemolytic anemia and hemosiderinuria. A feared complication is cerebral venous thrombosis. Thrombosis of major cerebral veins or dural sinuses and portal vein thrombosis are the most frequent causes of death. Acute thrombotic episodes involving the cerebral veins may be treated with thrombolytic agents, unless contraindicated, or anticoagulant therapy. High-dose cyclophosphamide and granulocyte-colony stimulating factor are being studied for the treatment of paroxysmal nocturnal hemoglobinuria.

Diabetes is a well-established risk factor for ischemic stroke. Diabetes associated with arterial hypertension or hyperlipidemia adds significantly to stroke risk. There are a variety of platelet, rheological, coagulation, and fibrinolytic abnormalities that may play a role in the pathogenesis of stroke in diabetic patients. Numerous hemorrheological disturbances appear to affect the development of diabetic microvascular disease and may contribute to cerebrovascular ischemic events. Hemorrheological alterations producing increased blood viscosity may include increased fibrinogen values, increased hematocrit, elevated factors V and VII, increased platelet aggregation, increased platelet adhesion, increased release of β-thromboglobulin, decreased red blood cell deformability, and decreased fibrinolytic activity.

Heparin-induced thrombocytopenia can cause high morbidity and mortality from thrombotic complications. Heparin therapy may induce two types of thrombocytopenia. The most frequently observed is type I heparin-induced thrombocytopenia, which is a mild and benign condition with platelet counts around 100,000 per μl. This thrombocytopenia tends to occur early and resolve spontaneously. Complications are rare. Type II heparin-induced thrombocytopenia is a major, albeit infrequent, adverse side effect of heparin therapy, more common with the use of bovine heparin. An immune-mediated disorder characterized by increased levels of platelet-associated IgG and IgM, it increases the risk for venous and arterial thrombotic complications involving the brain, heart, and limbs. Fatalities are high, and hemorrhagic complications are rare. Prevention is paramount, requiring an optimal reduction of the time of exposure to heparin to less than 5 days when possible, and daily platelet counts during heparin administration. Treatment requires immediate discontinuation of heparin. If anticoagulant therapy is still needed, the use of low-molecular-weight heparinoids, ancrod, dextran, recombinant hirudin, prostacyclin analogues, or warfarin should be considered.

Elevated plasma homocyst(e)ine levels are an independent risk factor for atherosclerotic disease. Diagnosis of hyperhomocyst(e)inemia may be made by demonstrating elevated basal plasma levels of homocyst(e)ine or raised levels after methionine loading. Homocystinuria is covered earlier in this chapter under Inherited and Miscellaneous Disorders).

Cerebrovascular disease is a major cause of morbidity and mortality in sickle cell disease. Strokes in sickle cell anemia (HbSS) patients manifest as ischemic strokes in children and as intracerebral and subarachnoid hemorrhage in adults. The most common presentations of stroke in patients with sickle cell disease are hemiparesis, seizures, language or visual impairments, and coma. Cognitive impairment may result from silent infarcts. Coma is more suggestive of intracranial hemorrhage rather than cerebral infarction. Patients at greatest risk of stroke are those with (HbSS) severe anemia, higher reticulocyte white blood cell counts, and lower hemoglobin F levels. Sickle cell disease leads to a hyperviscous condition within the microvasculature. At low oxygen tensions, erythrocytes containing hemoglobin S assume a sicklelike appearance. Sludging in small vessels occurs, resulting in microinfarctions in the affected organs. Although there is pathological evidence that microvascular occlusion and sludging caused by sickling does occur in the brain, the clinical and neurodiagnostic findings are consistent with a large vessel arterial occlusive (intimal hyperplasia with superimposed thrombosis) disease affecting the major intracranial arteries, frequently involving the arterial border zones between major cerebral arteries and adjacent deep white matter. Infarcts are more common in the anterior–MCA boundary zone. Sickle cell disease commonly causes a moyamoyalike angiographical pattern. Sickle cell disease may be accompanied by thrombotic cerebral infarction, cerebral venous occlusive disease, or subarachnoid, intracerebral, or intraventricular hemorrhage. Delayed intracranial hemorrhage may follow cerebral infarction and has been described as a complication of bone marrow transplantation. Spinal cord infarction is extremely rare. Neurological symptoms may be triggered by hypoxia, sepsis, dehydration, or acidosis.

The evaluation of the stroke patient with sickle cell anemia must be carefully individualized. Blood cell count, peripheral blood smear, hemoglobin electrophoresis, and sickling test are essential. MRI, MRA, and transcranial Doppler studies are valuable investigations in sickle cell patients; transcranial Doppler is useful in detecting the intracranial vasculopathy and may make it possible to detect patients at highest risk for cerebral infarction and to initiate treatment prior to stroke. Cerebral angiography can be done safely with the use of low-osmolar contrast media after partial exchange transfusion is performed to avoid complications associated with contrast material. Maintenance of hemoglobin S at a level less than 30% appears to be effective in reducing the rate of recurrent cerebral infarction (Pagelow et al. 1995). Meticulous hydration, adequate oxygenation, and analgesia are necessary.

Thrombotic thrombocytopenic purpura is a life-threatening, generalized microcirculatory condition of undetermined etiology, characterized by fever, thrombocytopenic purpura, microangiopathic hemolytic anemia, renal dysfunction, and fluctuating neurological signs. Thrombotic thrombocytopenic purpura is exceedingly rare, with a reported incidence of 1 person in 1 million annually. Most cases are idiopathic, but thrombotic thrombocytopenic purpura also may be caused by drug exposure or it may be associated with pregnancy and the postpartum state, connective tissue disorders, infective endocarditis, or neoplasms. The pathological response is caused by widespread segmental hyaline microthrombi in the microvasculature. Neurological symptomatology is protean and fleeting.

Patients frequently have headaches, visual disturbances, cranial nerve palsies, delirium, seizures, aphasia, paresis, and coma. Treatment is with infusions of fresh frozen plasma, plasmapheresis, corticosteroids, and platelet antiaggregants singly or in combination have been used also. If plasma exchange fails, splenectomy combined with corticosteroids and intravenous vincristine may be used.

Infarcts of Undetermined Cause

Despite an extensive workup, in up to 40% of persons with ischemic stroke an etiology cannot be determined. This percentage is possibly higher in patients younger than 45 years of age. Some of these ischemic strokes may result from asymptomatic episodes of paroxysmal atrial fibrillation; electrophysiological testing may be useful under those circumstances. The role of thrombophilia is also often underrecognized and warrants more detailed investigation in selected patients. The risk of recurrence of stroke of undetermined etiology appears to be slightly less than that of ischemic strokes of other types.

ESSENTIAL INVESTIGATIONS FOR PATIENTS WITH THREATENED STROKES

A basic workup, to be done in all patients with TIAs or evolving ischemic stroke, includes full blood cell count with differential and platelet count, erythrocyte sedimentation rate, prothrombin time (PT), PPT, plasma glucose level, blood urea nitrogen, serum creatinine, lipid analysis, luetic serology, urinalysis, chest roentgenography, and ECG. Nonenhanced cranial CT is also being done in all patients because it may detect hemorrhagic or mass lesions that can present as a TIA or evolving stroke (Biller 1994). Approximately 10–40% of patients with TIAs have evidence of cerebral infarction on CT. Attention to early CT signs of ischemic stroke in the MCA territory such as loss of gray–white matter differentiation, sulcal effacement, effacement of the Sylvian fissure, and obscuration of the lentiform nucleus is critical. The horizontal part of the MCA is occasionally hyperdense in the noncontrast CT (dense MCA sign) before the infarction becomes visible (Figures 57A.14A and B). This finding is indicative of a thrombotic or embolic occlusion of the MCA. The dense MCA sign often predicts a large cortical infarct, but is not always a poor prognostic indicator. MRI and intracranial and extracranial MRA improve the localization of acute stroke and provide powerful noninvasive means to evaluate the pathological changes that occur following acute ischemic stroke (Figures 57A.15 and 57A.16). MRI is superior to CT in cerebral ischemia. The sensitivity of MRI in differentiating infarction or other lesions from normal tissue depends primarily on changes in tissue T1 and T2 relaxation times, which are related to tissue water content. The

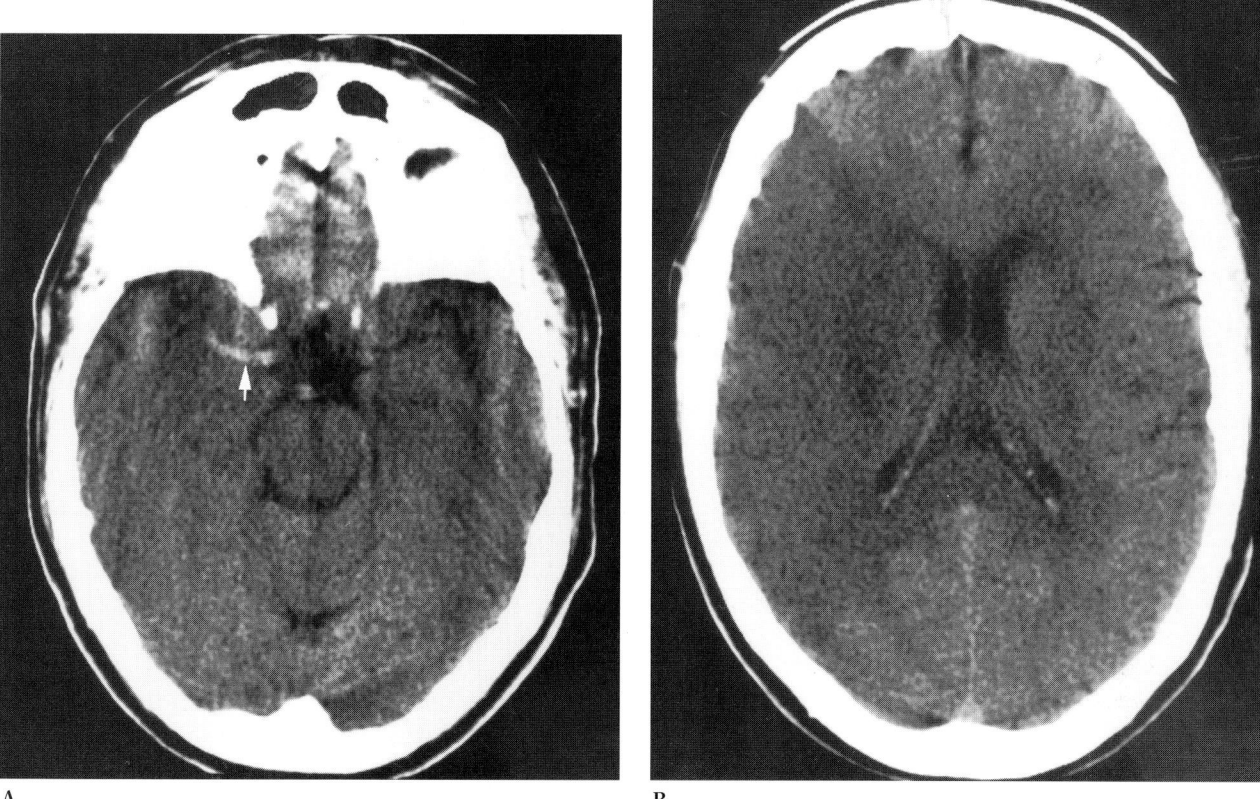

A   B

FIGURE 57A.14   Nonenhanced axial computed tomographic scans show (**A**) a dense right middle cerebral artery (MCA) sign (*arrow*) on the M1 segment and (**B**) a complete right MCA territory infarction. (Courtesy of Vincent Mathews, MD.)

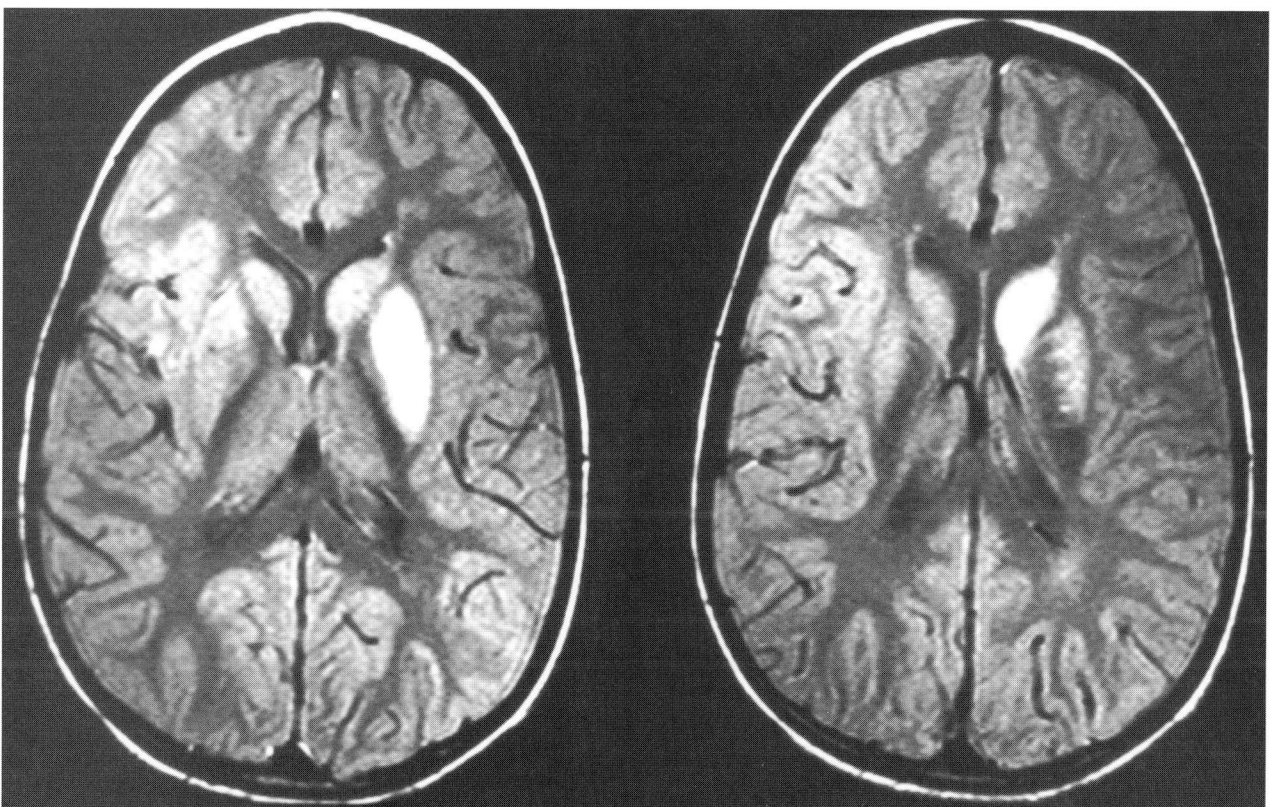

FIGURE 57A.15   Axial proton density magnetic resonance imaging demonstrates areas of increased signal intensity involving the head of the left caudate nucleus and the left lenticular nucleus consistent with infarction. The internal portion of the globus pallidus is spared.

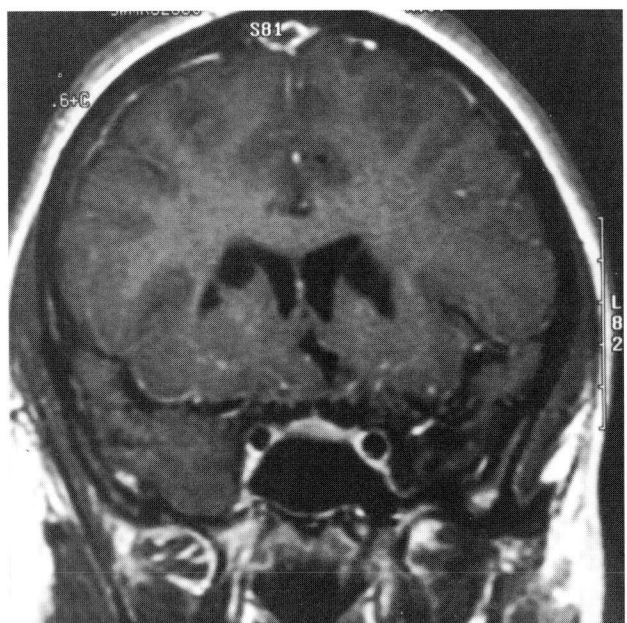

FIGURE 57A.16 Coronal T1-weighted magnetic resonance imaging with contrast of a 14-year-old boy demonstrates bilateral recurrent artery of Heubner territory infarcts with involvement of the head of the caudate nucleus and anterior limb of the internal capsule. (Courtesy of Vincent Mathews, MD.)

usefulness of diffusion-weighted MRI and perfusion imaging in differentiating ischemia from infarction in the early phase of stroke is under active investigation.

The emphasis in screening is on noninvasive testing, including Doppler imaging, B-mode scanning, duplex scanning, and transcranial Doppler imaging (see Chapter 38D). In studies of duplex Doppler ultrasonography, sensitivity for detection of greater than 50% diameter stenosis ranged from 87–96% and specificity ranged from 81–96%. Clinicians, however, need to be aware of the practical limitations of the ultrasound techniques. Severe stenosis or occlusion of an artery cannot be determined confidently by sonography. These methods also may fail to detect an intraluminal thrombus or a small atherosclerotic plaque, and some lesions are anatomically beyond the reach of the scanner. Transcranial Doppler sonography assists in the evaluation of blood flow velocities and patency of the main intracranial arteries and in the identification of high-intensity transient microembolic signals.

Cardiac investigations to determine whether emboli have a cardiac source are advised in selected circumstances. Noninvasive cardiac imaging has expanded the ability to diagnose and assess a variety of cardiac conditions, many of which have been implicated as potential causes of TIA and evolving stroke. These imaging techniques differ widely in the information they provide about the morphology, function, and metabolic status of the heart. Most institutions currently use serial two-dimensional echocardiography to detect left ventricular thrombus. The morphology of the thrombus predicts its embolic potential; left ventricular thrombi that have a protruding and mobile appearance on echocardiography are most likely to embolize. The sensitivity of two-dimensional echocardiography in detecting left ventricular thrombi varies from 77% to 92%; specificity varies from 84% to 94%, and predictive accuracy is 79%.

Patients with atrial fibrillation are likely to develop atrial thrombi caused by stasis of blood in the left atrium or left atrial appendage. Atrial thrombi are not always well visualized with routine studies. The left atrium, and in particular, the left atrial appendage, is often difficult to visualize with M-mode echocardiography. Left atrial thrombi can be detected successfully with two-dimensional echocardiography, but sensitivity and specificity of this technique are difficult to ascertain. Transesophageal echocardiography is used in selected individuals, particularly when the transthoracic images are technically inadequate for the evaluation of mitral and aortic prosthetic valves or vegetations; whenever there is a need for better visualization of the left atrial appendage or interatrial septum; or when a right-to-left shunt, left atrial spontaneous contrast, or aortic atherosclerosis is suspected. Continuous (Holter) ECG monitoring is seldom indicated, except when the history suggests paroxysmal disturbances of cardiac rhythm.

Most patients with TIAs or evolving stroke have cerebrovascular atherosclerosis. The gold standard for establishing the extent of vascular disease remains conventional angiography or intra-arterial digital subtraction angiography. Either method can accurately determine the size and location of atherosclerotic lesions and aid in reliably assessing the vasculature, detecting tandem arterial lesions and the collateral circulation.

Angiography is not without complications, and its use is being challenged by the increasingly improving quality of MRA. Although the risks associated with cerebral angiography have been gradually decreasing, the risk of any complication is approximately 1–5%, of which one-half are minor groin hematomas. The risk of permanent neurological disability is approximately 0.2%, and the risk of death has been estimated to be 0.05%.

Cerebral angiography is indicated in the following circumstances:

- The diagnosis remains uncertain. When a patient's workup fails to confirm the diagnosis, angiography is recommended to differentiate between atherosclerotic cerebrovascular occlusive disease and nonatherosclerotic vasculopathies, such as FMD, cervicocephalic arterial dissections, vasculitis, as well as intracranial aneurysms or vascular malformations (Figure 57A.17).
- Surgical treatment is planned. A full display of the extracranial and intracranial vasculature is important once potential surgical candidates are identified.

- Distinctions affecting treatment are unclear; for example, angiography can assist in cases in which differentiation between carotid and vertebrobasilar TIA or evolving stroke is unclear on clinical grounds only.
- Patients have very early evolving stroke symptoms or frequent TIAs.

PREVENTING STROKE RECURRENCE: MEDICAL THERAPY

At present, general measures, including control of associated risk factors such as hypertension, hyperlipidemia, cigarette smoking, and the use of antithrombotic agents (platelet antiaggregants and anticoagulants), remain the mainstays of medical therapy for stroke prevention. A large proportion of strokes should be preventable by controlling blood pressure, treating atrial fibrillation, and stopping cigarette smoking.

Platelet Antiaggregants

Evidence from several clinical studies favors the use of platelet antiaggregants as the first line of therapy in patients at high risk for stroke. These agents are indicated for secondary prevention of stroke. There is no evidence to support the use of aspirin in primary prevention of stroke among low-risk, middle-aged people. Although aspirin offered a long-term protective effect among 372 asymptomatic patients with carotid bruits and greater than 50% carotid stenosis on duplex ultrasonography, many physicians continue its use in patients with carotid bruits or asymptomatic carotid stenosis under the assumption that it may be effective. Data regarding intraplaque hemorrhage caused by platelet antiaggregants are conflicting.

Aspirin is the standard medical therapy for prevention of stroke and recurrent stroke. Aspirin, started within 48 hours of an acute ischemic stroke, is also safe and effective (International Stroke Trial Collaborative Group 1997; CAST 1997). The mechanism of action of aspirin is the irreversible inhibition of platelet function by inactivation of cyclo-oxygenase. Meta-analyses have shown that aspirin reduces the combined risk of stroke, myocardial infarction, and vascular death by approximately 25%. The optimal dose of aspirin remains a source of controversy among neurologists. The range of acceptable management includes daily doses of 30–1,300 mg of aspirin. The main side effect is gastric discomfort. Gastrointestinal hemorrhage occurs in 1–5% of cases. Enteric-coated preparations are generally the best tolerated.

Ticlopidine reduces the relative risk of death or nonfatal stroke by 12% in comparison with aspirin. Ticlopidine acts primarily by irreversibly inhibiting the adenosine diphosphate pathways of the platelet membrane. Ticlopidine also

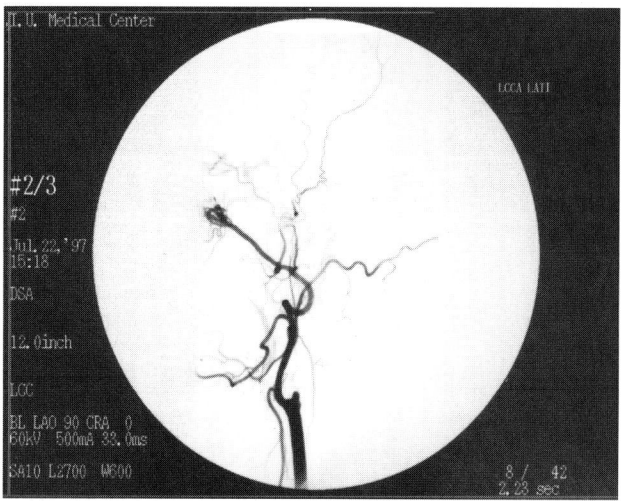

FIGURE 57A.17 A 43-year-old woman with a history of hypertension, hypercholesterolemia, and tobacco use had right-sided hemiparesis. Cerebral angiogram demonstrates an occlusion of the left internal carotid artery just past the bifurcation. There is partial reconstitution via ethmoid collaterals.

reduces plasma fibrinogen levels and increases erythrocyte deformability. The recommended dosage of ticlopidine is 250 mg twice a day. Ticlopidine has more side effects than aspirin, including diarrhea, nausea, dyspepsia, and rash. These side effects tend to occur during the first few months of therapy. The dosage can be temporarily reduced to lessen the side effects for a few weeks, then brought back to 250 mg twice a day administered with food. A more worrisome adverse reaction is reversible neutropenia, which occurs in 2.4% of cases and is severe in 0.85%. This reaction can be encountered during the first 3 months of treatment, and for this reason a complete blood cell count must be obtained every 2 weeks during this period. The drug must be discontinued if the neutrophil count falls below 1,200 per μL. Rarely, thrombocytopenia and thrombotic thrombocytopenic purpura may occur.

The Clopidogrel versus Aspirin in Patients at Risk of Ischemic Events (CAPRIE) study assessed the relative efficacy of clopidogrel (75 mg daily) and aspirin (325 mg daily) in reducing the incidence of ischemic stroke, recent myocardial infarction, or symptomatic atherosclerotic peripheral arterial disease. The results of this study showed that clopidogrel was more effective (8.7% relative risk reduction) than aspirin in reducing the combined risk of ischemic stroke, myocardial infarction, or vascular death in patients with atherosclerotic disease. Clopidogrel is a platelet adenosine diphosphate receptor antagonist. Overall, the tolerability of clopidogrel was excellent, with no increased incidence of neutropenia, and a lower incidence of gastrointestinal hemorrhage and peptic, gastric, or duodenal ulcers when compared with aspirin. The rate of diarrhea, rash, and pruritus was higher than with aspirin (CAPRIE Steering Committee 1996).

Whether dipyridamole in combination with aspirin achieves any additional benefit over aspirin alone in patients with threatened stroke is still a matter of controversy. The European Stroke Prevention Study 2 (ESPS-2) randomized patients with prior stroke or TIA to treatment with aspirin alone (25 mg twice a day), modified-release dipyridamole alone (200 mg twice a day), the two agents in combination, or placebo. The ESPS-2 investigators concluded that both low-dose aspirin and high-dose dipyridamole in a modified-release form alone were superior to placebo, and that the combination was significantly superior to each drug alone. Dipyridamole is a phosphodiesterase inhibitor that increases the levels of the cyclic adenosine monophosphate. The ESPS-2 investigators reported an additive effect of dipyridamole when prescribed with aspirin. The main side effects of dipyridamole are gastrointestinal distress, headaches, and vasodilation. The use of low-dose aspirin did not reduce the risk of bleeding (Diener et al. 1996).

There is no persuasive evidence from current or past trials that patients benefit from the use of sulfinpyrazone or suloctidil. Drugs that block the glycoprotein IIb/IIIa receptor are currently under investigation.

Oral Anticoagulants

Oral anticoagulation with warfarin is indicated for primary and secondary prevention of stroke in patients with NVAF. Six randomized studies evaluated the primary and secondary prevention of stroke in patients with NVAF. Three of these studies also evaluated aspirin at a daily dose of 75, 300, and 325 mg. These six studies demonstrated that the relative risk of stroke is reduced by 68% with the use of warfarin (Koefoed et al. 1997). Advancing age increases the risk of major hemorrhage in patients given warfarin for stroke prevention; patients older than 75 years are at greater risk of hemorrhagic complications. The relative risk reduction with aspirin therapy was 21% (18–44%) (The Atrial Fibrillation Investigators 1997). Therefore, NVAF patients at high risk of stroke should be treated with dose-adjusted warfarin (INR 2.0–3.0); INR values less than 2.0 and greater than 4.0 should be avoided. Patients younger than 65 years without other risk factors can be given aspirin 325 mg per day. Low-intensity, fixed-dose warfarin plus aspirin is inadequate for stroke prevention in high-risk patients with NVAF. Anticoagulation is also recommended for patients with atrial fibrillation and hyperthyroidism. Patients who cannot tolerate pharmacological cardioversion may benefit from electrophysiological or surgical procedures. Anticoagulant therapy has a protective effect against stroke following acute myocardial infarction. To prevent arterial embolism, immediate anticoagulation with heparin is initiated followed by oral anticoagulation for 3 months following an anterior wall myocardial infarction, or a myocardial infarction with apical wall motion abnormalities or left ventricular thrombus. Patients with mechanical prosthetic heart valves should receive long-term oral anticoagulants to prolong the INR to 2.5–3.5. Patients undergoing cardioversion for atrial fibrillation should receive anticoagulation for 3 weeks before and 4 weeks after cardioversion. Use of long-term anticoagulation in patients with left ventricular aneurysms and mural thrombi is not indicated because of the low risk of embolization. Uncertainty persists about the use of warfarin in the management of patients with symptomatic stenosis of a major intracranial artery.

TREATMENT OF ACUTE ISCHEMIC STROKE

Modern therapy for acute ischemic stroke is currently being approached in four different ways. First, and most important, are general measures aimed at prevention and treatment of complications. Second are those reperfusion strategies directed at arterial recanalization. Third are cytoprotective strategies aimed at cellular and metabolic targets. The fourth approach aims at the inhibition of the inflammatory processes associated with cerebral ischemia. Eventually, combined therapy will be used for acute ischemic stroke treatment: evaluated low-molecular-weight heparins and heparinoids and unfractionated subcutaneous heparin for the treatment of acute ischemic stroke.

Results are available from one completed randomized double-blind controlled trial of nadroparin-calcium (Fraxiparin), a low-molecular-weight heparin. In this trial, 312 patients were randomized within 48 hours of stroke to receive nadroparin-calcium 4,100 antifactor Xa IU subcutaneously either once or twice daily, or placebo. Treatment was continued for 10 days. After 10 days, all patients received aspirin, 100 mg per day. There was no difference between the groups at 3 months. However, after 6 months, there was a significant dose-dependent reduction in the rate of poor outcome among the three study groups in favor of patients treated with nadroparin-calcium twice daily compared with those who received treatment once daily or placebo (Kay et al. 1995).

The International Stroke Trial studied approximately 20,000 patients who were randomized within 48 hours of ischemic stroke onset to receive fixed dose 10,000 or 25,000 units of heparin subcutaneously daily (compared with no heparin). Treatment was continued for 14 days or until hospital discharge if shorter. There was no significant difference in the rate of death or recurrent ischemic or hemorrhagic stroke at 2 weeks (11.7% with heparin and 12.0% without heparin). Patients receiving heparin had significantly fewer recurrent ischemic stroke at 2 weeks, but this was negated by a similar increase in hemorrhagic strokes (International Stroke Trial Collaborative Group 1997). This trial used subcutaneous rather than intravenous heparin.

Definite data regarding the safety and efficacy of intravenous heparin for acute ischemic stroke or cardioembolic stroke are lacking, but intravenous heparin is given to some patients with nonseptic cardioembolic stroke to prevent recurrence. In a small trial, performed by the Cerebral Embolism Study Group, 45 patients with acute cardioembolic stroke who presented within 48 hours of symptom onset were randomized to receive either early or delayed treatment. The early treatment group received an intravenous heparin bolus of 5,000–10,000 units followed by a maintenance infusion for at least 96 hours before the patient was switched to warfarin. Patients in the control group received no heparin and were given platelet antiaggregants or warfarin 10 days poststroke. None of the 24 patients who received heparin experienced stroke recurrence or hemorrhage within the 96-hour treatment period. Of the 21 patients who received delayed anticoagulation, two experienced early recurrent embolic cerebral infarcts, one had a deep venous thrombosis, two had hemorrhagic transformations, and three died. The study suggested that heparin might be helpful, but it was terminated prematurely. The use or not of intravenous heparin remains the physician's preference. Heparin should not be used if a patient has a septic embolus or if the CT shows a hemorrhagic or large infarction. When intravenous heparin is given, many physicians do not use an intravenous bolus and aim for a target aPTT of 55–75 seconds, or 1.5–2.0 times control.

Intravenous unfractionated heparin appears to be ineffective in patients with acute partial stable stroke. A large randomized study evaluated unfractionated heparin in 225 patients with noncardioembolic stroke. Patients who had progressing deficit in the first hour of observation were excluded from the study because of the prevailing belief, at that time, that stroke in evolution should be anticoagulated. There was no significant difference in stroke progression or death at 7 days.

Although convincing statistical proof is still lacking, anecdotal evidence supports early initiation of intravenous unfractionated heparin to prevent stroke recurrence in several uncommon situations. These indications include cerebral infarction in the setting of inherited or acquired hypercoagulable states, intraluminal arterial thrombus, extracranial cervicocephalic arterial dissections, and aseptic cerebral venous sinus thrombosis.

Aggregate data from randomized and nonrandomized studies on the use of anticoagulants in stroke in evolution suggest that intravenous heparin reduces the rate of progression of cerebral infarction. However, some studies have not demonstrated a beneficial effect of intravenous heparin in these patients. Despite such controversy, many physicians continue to use intravenous heparin in selected patients with stroke in evolution caused by large vessel atherothrombosis. However, no cause-and-effect relationship between heparin administration and clinical improvement can be established.

Thrombolytic Therapy

If patients meet appropriate criteria, thrombolytic therapy may be administered. Thrombolytic therapy is able to recanalize acute intracranial occlusions. A strong correlation has been shown between recanalization and neurological improvement in acute cerebral ischemia. The National Institute of Neurological Disorders and Stroke rt-PA [recombinant tissue plasminogen activator] Stroke Study Group showed that treatment with intravenous tissue plasminogen activator within 3 hours of onset of ischemic stroke improved clinical outcome (minimal or no disability on the clinical assessment scales) at 3 months (The National Institute of Neurological Disorders and Stroke rt-PA Stroke Study Group 1995). Treatment did not lessen death rates or account for an excess mortality. The frequency of symptomatic intracerebral hemorrhage was 10 times greater in patients given tissue plasminogen activator (6.4% in the treatment group compared with 0.6% in the placebo group). Most hemorrhages occurred within 36 hours of treatment. Intravenous tissue plasminogen activator should be administered only by physicians with experience in the diagnosis and management of stroke and with familiarity with the potential hemorrhagic complications associated with thrombolytic therapy.

In the National Institute of Neurological Disorders and Stroke rt-PA trial, exclusion criteria for administration of tissue plasminogen activator were rapidly improving or isolated mild neurological deficits, seizure at onset of stroke, prior intracranial hemorrhage, blood glucose level less than 50 mg/dl or greater than 400 mg/dl, gastrointestinal or genitourinary bleeding within the 3 weeks before stroke, recent myocardial infarction, current use of oral anticoagulants (PT >15 seconds or INR >1.7), a prolonged aPTT or previous use of heparin in the previous 48 hours, platelet count less than 100,000 per µL, another stroke or serious head injury in the previous 3 months, major surgery within the previous 14 days, or pretreatment systolic blood pressure greater than 185 mm Hg or diastolic blood pressure greater than 110 mm Hg.

In spite of a consistently lower frequency of intracerebral hemorrhage with the use of streptokinase (SK) rather than tissue plasminogen activator, in patients with acute myocardial infarction, current data do not support the use of intravenous streptokinase, 1.5 million units, in acute ischemic stroke. The potential therapeutic benefit of intra-arterial thrombolysis and of the combination of thrombolytic neuroprotectant agents is being studied. Whether the combined use of intravenous and intra-arterial rt-PA in acute ischemic stroke is safe or effective has yet to be determined.

Defibrinogenating Agents

Ancrod, an enzyme extracted from the venom of the Malayan pit viper, lowers fibrinogen and blood viscosity, inhibits erythrocyte aggregation, indirectly stimulates thrombolysis, and possibly causes local vasodilatation. It also has a weak anticoagulant effect at high dosages. Its potential as a treatment for ischemic stroke is being evaluated.

Inhibitors of Neutrophil Adhesion and Migration

Inflammation may be an important phenomenon during cerebral ischemia, and attention is given to the cytokines as possible targets for specific therapeutic intervention. The cytokines are hormonelike proteins or glycoproteins that are produced by a variety of cells. The major classes of cytokines are the interferons, interleukins, tumor necrosis factors, and colony-stimulating factors. Based on the encouraging information of many preclinical results, a multicenter study investigating the clinical therapeutic potential of anti-intercellular adhesion molecule–1 antibodies (enlimomab) as therapy for acute ischemic stroke (<6 hours) has been completed. The study was a double-blinded, randomized, placebo-controlled, parallel group trial. Study results were negative. Mortality at 90 days was 16% in the placebo group (308 patients) compared with 22% in the enlimomab-treated group (317 patients). Among survivors, functional outcome (measured with modified Rankin Scale and Barthel Index) was also better among the placebo-treated patients. The sudden decrease in blood flow after ischemia provokes a cascade of events eventually leading to cell death (see section on Pathophysiology of Cerebral Ischemia, earlier in this chapter). Several cytoprotective agents, in vitro and in animal studies, interfere at one step or another with this cascade, thus potentially protecting the cells from ischemia.

Selective cerebroselective calcium-channel blockers such as nimodipine have been tested in acute stroke. The benefits of nimodipine administration for patients with acute ischemic stroke remain unproved. Endogenous excitatory amino acid neurotransmitters play a major role in the pathogenesis of cerebral ischemia. In animals, excitatory amino acid antagonists have been shown to reduce the size of an infarct. From preliminary studies, some of these compounds appear to be safe in humans, but their efficacy has not been demonstrated. Several clinical trials of excitatory amino acid antagonists are under way. Optimal protective regimens may require blockading of both N-methyl-D-aspartate (NMDA) and non-NMDA receptors. Despite widespread interest in neuroprotective drug therapy and positive results in experimental animals, no neuroprotective agent has been approved, as yet, by the U.S. Food and Drug Administration for acute ischemic stroke. Free radicals produced during ischemia can degrade polyunsaturated lipids, which are building blocks of cellular membranes by lipid peroxidation. Tirilazad, a 21-aminosteroid compound, decreases damage secondary to global ischemia in animals. Clinical trial results in humans with stroke, however, were negative.

Citicoline, an intermediary in the biosynthesis of phosphatidylcholine, improved functional outcome when started within 24 hours of stroke onset (Clark et al. 1997). The benefits and safety of lubeluzole therapy, a neuroprotective agent studied in patients within 6 hours of stroke onset, include greater functional recovery among survivors, but no significant changes in mortality, which was the primary efficacy end point. Other agents, such as neurotrophins, calpain inhibitors, glycine site antagonists, naftidrofuryl, aptiganel hydrochloride, and fosphenytoin, are under investigation. Treatments with gangliosides, dextrorphan, selfotel (CGS-19755), barbiturates, prostacyclin, pentoxifylline, opiate antagonists, aminophylline, β-adrenergic receptor blockers, vasopressor therapy, glycerol, and isovolemic, hypovolemic, and hypervolemic hemodilution have been ineffective.

Surgical Therapy

Symptomatic Carotid Artery Stenosis

Stroke is often caused by atherosclerotic lesions of the carotid artery bifurcation; approximately 15% of ischemic strokes are caused by extracranial internal carotid artery stenosis. Echolucent and ulcerated carotid artery plaques may be associated with an increased risk of stroke. Carotid endarterectomy (CEA), by removing the atherosclerotic plaque, restores cerebral blood flow and reduces the risk of cerebral ischemia. Results from three major prospective contemporary studies provide compelling evidence of the benefit of CEA performed by experienced surgeons in improving the chance of stroke-free survival in high-risk symptomatic patients. Timely surgical intervention in selected patients with hemispheric TIAs, amaurosis fugax, or completed nondisabling carotid territory strokes within the previous 6 months associated with 70–99% diameter-reducing carotid stenosis can reduce the risk of recurrent cerebral ischemia or death. Other factors that increase the risk of ipsilateral stroke are hemispheric (rather than retinal) site of ischemia, ulcerative nature of the stenosis, presence of contralateral carotid artery occlusion, and vascular risk factors. Benefits of CEA are similar for men and women. Advanced age by itself should not be considered a contraindication for properly selected patients with symptomatic high-grade carotid artery stenosis.

The North American Symptomatic Carotid Endarterectomy Trial (NASCET) confirmed the effectiveness of CEA for preventing stroke in 659 symptomatic patients with TIAs or minor strokes with high-grade (70–99%) diameter-reducing carotid artery stenosis. A uniform and strict technique measured carotid artery stenosis from an arteriogram. For different end points, absolute risk reductions in favor of surgery were 17.0% for ipsilateral stroke; 15.0% for all strokes; 16.5% for the combined outcomes of all strokes and death; 10.6% for major ipsilateral stroke; 9.4% for all major strokes; and 10.1% for major stroke and death. CEA was also beneficial and not more dangerous in symptomatic patients with atheromatous carotid artery pseudo-occlusion (carotid string sign). Longer term outcome was also better for surgically treated patients despite an occluded contralateral carotid artery. Morbidity and mortality of early CEA was similar to that of delayed surgery. The European Carotid Surgery Trial (ECST) also indicated the benefit from CEA compared with medical therapy in patients with mild carotid territory ischemic events associated with a diameter-reducing proximal internal carotid stenosis between 70% and 99%. The cumulative risk of any ipsilateral stroke at 3 years was 10.3% for the surgical group and 16.8% for the medical group. The ECST trial used different criteria than NASCET for measurement of carotid artery stenosis on angiography. These methodological differences were more important with mild carotid artery stenosis. The Veterans Administration Trial of Carotid Endarterectomy in Symptomatic Carotid Stenosis was terminated early because of the positive results of NASCET and ECST. The Veterans Administration study also showed that CEA improved outcome in selected symptomatic patients with high-grade extracranial carotid artery stenosis. Among symptomatic patients with less than 30% stenosis, results from the ECST trial favor the use of medical therapy with platelet antiaggregants. The utility of CEA for symptomatic patients with 30–69% carotid artery stenosis has not yet been determined. Results were analyzed separately for those patients with 30–49% and those with 50–69% stenosis. Analysis from 1,599 patients suggests that CEA is not indicated in most of these patients (European Carotid Surgery Trialists' Collaborative Group 1996). Recent results from NASCET-2 (30–69% stenosis) showed a relative modest benefit in favor of surgery among patients with 50–69% stenosis (Barnett HJM, personal communication, 1998).

The benefit of CEA is highly dependent on surgical risk. Mortality and morbidity caused by CEA are significantly lower for asymptomatic patients. The acceptable level of surgical risk varies with the indication for carotid artery surgery. Acceptable guidelines are 3% risk for asymptomatic patients, 5% for patients with TIAs, 7% for patients with stroke, and 10% for patients with recurrent stenosis.

Whether selected patients should undergo CEA on the basis of duplex scanning alone (without cerebral angiography), or duplex scanning complemented by MRA remains controversial. Carotid artery angioplasty and stenting may offer an alternative treatment to CEA, but there are concerns regarding the risk and clinical consequences of distal embolization. Carotid artery angioplasty and stenting is an experimental intervention being developed and tested in a few centers for its potential effectiveness. Randomized trials are needed before these techniques can be recommended.

Asymptomatic Carotid Artery Stenosis

Asymptomatic carotid artery atherosclerosis is prevalent in the general population, especially in the elderly. Compared with symptomatic stenosis, asymptomatic carotid artery stenosis is associated with a relatively low risk of ipsilateral cerebral infarction. Data from four randomized clinical trials concerning the efficacy of CEA in patients with asymptomatic carotid artery stenosis are now available. Results of the first three trials were negative. The Carotid Artery Surgery Asymptomatic Narrowing Operations Versus Aspirin trial enrolled asymptomatic patients with 50–90% carotid artery stenosis. Patients with greater than 90% carotid artery stenosis were excluded on the basis of presumed surgical benefit. Overall, the trial showed no difference between the medically and surgically treated groups. The Veterans Affairs Asymptomatic Carotid Endarterectomy Trial evaluated 444 asymptomatic patients with angiographically proven carotid stenosis of 50–99%. The study showed a relative risk reduction in the incidence of ipsilateral neurological events in favor of surgery when both TIA and stroke were included as composite end points. However, when ipsilateral stroke was considered alone, only a nonsignificant trend favoring surgery was noted. For the combined outcome of stroke and death, no significant differences were found between the two treatment arms (Hobson et al. 1993). The fourth randomized clinical trial, the Asymptomatic Carotid Atherosclerosis Study (ACAS), found that CEA combined with aspirin and risk-factor reduction is superior to aspirin and risk-factor reduction alone in preventing ipsilateral stroke in patients younger than 80 years who had three 60% asymptomatic carotid artery stenoses. The ACAS angiographical methods were similar to NASCET. The aggregate morbidity and mortality of the ACAS participating surgeons was extremely low. Based on a 5-year projection, ACAS showed that CEA reduced the absolute risk of stroke by 5.9% (which corresponds to an absolute risk reduction of only 1% per year), and the relative risk of stroke and death by 53%. The surgical benefit incorporated a perioperative stroke and death rate of 2.3% including a permanent arteriographical complication rate of 1.2%.

In spite of these results, controversy surrounds the selection of asymptomatic patients for CEA. Based on the low risk of stroke for all deciles until 80–89% carotid artery stenosis demonstrated by the European Carotid Artery Surgery Trialists (The European Carotid Surgery Trialists' Collaborative Group 1995), some experts recommend surgery only when the degree of stenosis is greater than 80%, provided that the operation is performed by an experienced surgeon with a complication rate (combined arteriographical and surgical) of 3% or less. The value of impaired cerebral vasomotor reactivity using intravenous administration of acetazolamide as a predictor of stroke risk in patients with asymptomatic carotid artery stenosis is controversial. The necessity for widespread screening of patients with asymptomatic carotid artery stenosis is not supported by available data. Although concomitant CEA and coronary artery bypass grafting can be achieved with acceptably low operative risk, the best management for symptomatic carotid stenosis patients with coexisting severe carotid and coronary artery disease is still unknown. The risk seems to be low for asymptomatic carotid stenosis patients, and the available data do not justify preoperative prophylactic CEA.

GENERAL MANAGEMENT OF ACUTE ISCHEMIC STROKE

Rapid diagnosis of stroke and initiation of treatment are important to maximize recovery, prevent recurrence of stroke, and prevent complications. Patients with an acute stroke should be admitted to the hospital for emergency evaluation and treatment, preferably in a stroke unit or intensive care unit where close medical and nursing observation is available. Treatment of unselected acute stroke patients in specialized stroke units correlated with a lower mortality, reduced length of hospital stay, reduced frequency of discharge to a nursing home, and potentially reduced cost. Development of a stroke team is advantageous to expedite emergency care. Emergency care involves attention to the protection of the airway to avoid obstruction, hypoventilation, and aspiration pneumonia. Pulse oximetry or arterial blood gases may be indicated. Supplemental oxygen and ventilatory assistance should be added if needed. Mild hypothermia protects the brain from ischemic injury; mild hyperthermia worsens ischemic outcome. Prevention of pulmonary complications is necessary in the bedridden patient or in the patient with impaired oropharyngeal function. The mortality from pneumonia is as high as 15–25%. Aspiration was documented by videofluoroscopical modified barium swallow examination in more than one-third of patients with brainstem strokes, in one-fourth with bilateral hemispheric, and in one-tenth of patients with unilateral hemispheric strokes. It is important to place a temporary enteral feeding tube if there is evidence of oropharyngeal dysfunction to minimize the risk of aspiration. Patients with oropharyngeal dysfunction, even if it appears to be mild, should receive nothing by mouth until evaluation by an experienced speech pathologist and until appropriate swallowing studies are completed. Good pulmonary toilet is needed, including chest pulmonary toilet, frequent turning, and volumetrics.

The next step is assessment of the circulation. This involves evaluation of cardiac function and blood pressure. Because of the high frequency of cardiac dysfunction associated with stroke, cardiac monitoring is recommended for the first 24–48 hours after stroke. An immediate ECG should be obtained. Concomitant cerebral and myocardial ischemia can occur in approximately 3% of cases. Ischemic stroke can be complicated by a variety of cardiac arrhythmias. If ischemic ECG changes occur, serial creatine kinase and lactate dehydrogenase isoenzymes are indicated. In patients with stroke, the blood pressure should be monitored frequently or even continuously for the first 48–72 hours. It is not unusual for the blood pressure to be transiently elevated after a stroke. One study showed that pharmacological elevation of systolic blood pressure to a mean of 156 mm Hg appeared to be safe and may improve neurological symptoms in some patients with thrombotic stroke (Rordorf et al. 1997). Within a few days, the blood pressure may return to prestroke levels. Whether transient elevations should be treated is controversial. It is important not to overtreat the blood pressure and cause hypotension. The most important objective is to maintain adequate cerebral blood flow in the presence of impaired autoregulation. If urgent lowering of the blood pressure is indicated, intravenous labetalol can be given (e.g., 10 mg over 1–2 minutes, repeated or doubled every 10–20 minutes until the desired response has been achieved or a maximum dosage of 300 mg has been administered). Contraindications to the use of labetalol include congestive heart failure, asthma, or second- or third-degree heart block.

Immediately after the patient's arrival in the emergency room, blood should be sent for appropriate studies including a complete blood cell count, prothrombin time (INR), aPTT, and a general chemistry screen. A focused neurological examination should be performed to assess neurological stability and to determine the extent of infarction. General signs that point toward a large infarction are forced eye deviation, hemiplegia, and altered consciousness. A National Institutes of Health stroke scale value of greater than 15 is another general indicator of a large infarction. Once stability of the airway, breathing, and circulation is determined and a focused neurological examination is performed to assess neurological stability, the patient should be sent immediately for an emergent cranial CT scan without contrast.

Attention should be directed not only to the treatment of the stroke, but also to the prevention of complications. A variety of neurological and medical complications can arise after a stroke. During the first week after an acute cerebral infarction, the most common cause of deterioration is development of brain edema. Brain edema begins to develop within the first several hours after an ischemic event. The edema reaches its peak after stroke. Ischemic edema is initially cytotoxic and later vasogenic. Cytotoxic edema involves predominantly the gray matter, whereas vasogenic edema involves predominantly the white matter. Those at the greatest risk for development of edema are younger patients and those with large infarctions, often caused by large artery occlusions. There is no specific pharmacological agent that has been proven effective against ischemic cerebral edema. Traditional treatment of increased intracranial pressure associated with acute ischemic stroke is shown in Table 57A.8. For cerebellar strokes with edema and herniation, posterior fossa decompression or ventriculostomy may be life saving.

In the second through the fourth weeks, pneumonia is the most common cause of non-neurological death. Many cases of pneumonia are caused by aspiration of toxic fluids, inert substances, or bacterial pathogens. Basal ganglia infarcts might predispose patients to pneumonia because of frequent aspiration during sleep. Other potential complications include seizures, cardiac arrhythmias, myocardial infarction, deep venous thrombosis, electrolyte disturbances, decubitus ulcers, and urosepsis. Cardiac dysfunction can manifest as ECG changes, arrhythmias, or myocardial ischemia.

Frequent neurological checks are vital to the early recognition of neurological changes associated with herniation, recurrent or progressive stroke, or complications such as seizures. Seizures occur in a small percentage (<5%) of patients after an ischemic stroke. Anticonvulsant medications may be initiated if a seizure occurs.

Lower extremity deep venous thrombosis in the hemiparetic limb is common if prophylaxis is not initiated. If there are no contraindications, low-dose subcutaneous heparin is used at a dosage of 5,000 units twice a day. If heparin is contraindicated, intermittent pneumatic compression of the lower extremities is recommended.

The patient's nutritional status and fluid requirements should be assessed. Patients with a large ischemic stroke may need a fluid restriction of two-thirds maintenance during the first few days. Swallowing function should be assessed before intake of fluid or food is initiated. Patients who have significant oropharyngeal dysfunction require parenteral or tube feeding.

Although urinary incontinence is not uncommon in the acute phase of stroke, indwelling catheters should be placed only if absolutely necessary and should be removed at the earliest possible time to avoid urosepsis. The chronic use of an indwelling catheter should be limited to patients with incontinence or urinary retention that is refractory to other treatments. In the presence of an indwelling catheter, treatment of asymptomatic bacteriuria is usually not indicated. However, for significant clinical infections with pyuria and fever, treatment is recommended.

Approximately 15% of patients develop pressure sores after a stroke. Steps to avoid this complication include frequent inspection of the skin, skin cleansing, frequent turning, use of special mattresses and protective dressings, maintaining adequate nutritional status, and trying to improve the patient's mobility early on.

One of the most common causes of injury to the patient with a stroke is falling. Assessments of the risk for falling should be made at regular intervals during the acute hospitalization and also during the chronic rehabilitation phase. Reduction of postprandial systolic blood pressure has been associated with a higher incidence of falls and syncope. Measures should be instituted to minimize the risk of falls. Shoulder subluxation can occur in hemiplegic patients. Chronic sequelae can be minimized if therapy is initiated before severe restriction of movement develops.

Rehabilitation after stroke begins as soon as the diagnosis of stroke is established and as soon as any life-threatening neurological or medical complications have been stabilized (see Chapter 54). Patients are screened to evaluate whether they are candidates for rehabilitation. The criteria used to make this decision, including the stroke survivor's clinical and neurological status and social and environmental factors are complex (Post-Stroke Rehabilitation Guideline Panel 1995). The available evidence on the effectiveness of rehabilitation suggests that rehabilitation is beneficial to some patients, but the supe-

Table 57A.8: Medical management guidelines for elevated intracranial pressure in patients with acute ischemic stroke

Correction of factors exacerbating increased intracranial pressure
Hypercarbia
Hypoxia
Hyperthermia
Acidosis
Hypotension
Hypovolemia
Positional
Avoid head and neck positions compressing jugular veins
Avoid flat supine position; elevate head of the bed 15–30 degrees
Medical therapy
Endotracheal intubation and mechanical ventilation, if Glasgow Coma Scale <8
Hyperventilate to a P_{CO_2} of 30 mm Hg (if herniating); gradual withdrawal
Mannitol (20% solution), 1 g/kg over 30 mins (bolus); followed by 0.25–0.50 g/kg over 30–60 mins every 4–6 hrs, depending on clinical status, serum osmolality, volume status, and intracranial pressure measurements (gradual withdrawal)
Fluid restriction
Maintenance of euvolemia with isotonic solutions. Use normal saline. Avoidance of glucose-containing solutions. Replacement of urinary losses with normal saline in patients receiving mannitol.

riority of one type or the characteristics of patients most likely to benefit are not clear.

Depressive symptoms are common after stroke, occurring in over 25% of patients. Stroke patients should be questioned and screened for depression. Depression is more common following left hemispheric infarcts, especially in the frontal lobe, possibly caused by disruption of catecholamine pathways. Treatment with antidepressants is often successful in ameliorating symptoms.

CEREBRAL VENOUS THROMBOSIS

Intracranial sinovenous occlusive disease is an infrequent condition with a variety of causes. The increasing recognition of this condition is probably because of an enhanced clinical awareness and the use of MRI. Intracranial venous thrombosis can be aseptic or septic. Septic intracranial venous thrombosis, relatively infrequent in modern times, most often involves the cavernous sinus. Cavernous sinus thrombosis is typically a complication of a facial or orbital infection and often presents with proptosis, chemosis, and painful ophthalmoplegia. Septic lateral sinus thrombosis is an infrequent complication of otitis media or mastoiditis and often presents with headaches, fever, otalgia, vertigo, papilledema, and abducens nerve palsy (Figure 57A.18).

Aseptic intracranial venous thrombosis is divided into dural venous sinus thrombosis, deep venous thrombosis, and superficial or cortical vein thrombosis. The superior sagittal

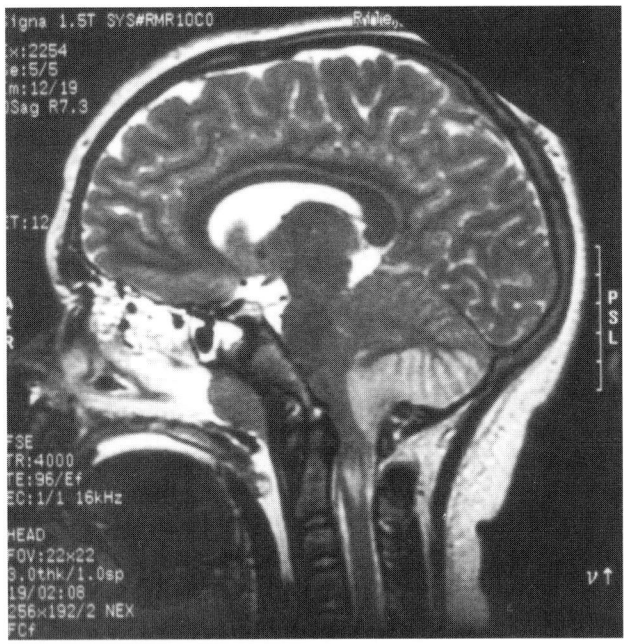

A

FIGURE 57A.18 A 10-year-old girl with otomastoiditis was evaluated because of unresponsiveness. Magnetic resonance imaging shows areas of increased signal in the right cerebellum greater than the left cerebellum, consistent with infarctions. The cerebellar tonsils are herniated. (A) Associated edema occurs in the superior cervical cord and inferior medulla. Phase contrast magnetic resonance angiographical images demonstrate lack of flow in the straight sinus and the right transverse sinus. Only a small amount of signal in the region of the right sigmoid and internal jugular vein is seen. (B) Some arterial flow is represented in the examination.

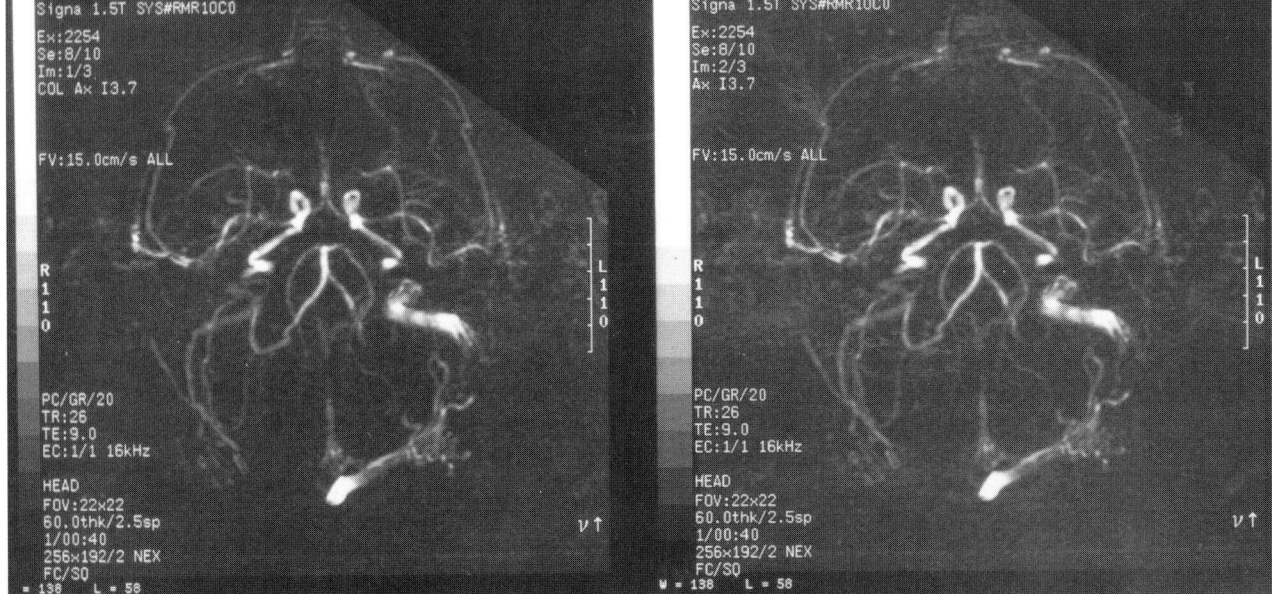

B

sinus is most frequently involved (Figure 57A.19). Etiologies are protean and the onset often insidious. The most common etiologies are listed in Table 57A.9. However, in approximately 20% of cases, no cause is found (Bousser et al. 1997).

Intracranial venous thrombosis may occur at any time from infancy to old age, but most reported modern cases have been in adult women in association with the puerperium. Onset of symptoms may be acute, subacute, or chronic. Cerebral venous infarction is the most serious consequence of cerebral venous thrombosis. Intracranial venous thrombosis should be considered a potential cause for pseudotumor cerebri or unexplained hemorrhagic infarctions. Venous infarctions are often multifocal and bilateral,

affecting both the gray matter and the subcortical white matter. Evidence of cerebral edema is unusual. Cerebral venous thrombosis may present without focal signs. Chief complaints are headaches, vomiting, transient visual obscurations, focal or generalized seizures, lethargy, or coma. Papilledema is common. There may be alternating focal deficits, hemiparesis or paraparesis, or other focal neurological deficits according to the location of the venous structure involved. Salient radiological features are the presence of low-density areas of infarction, hemorrhages, and small ventricles. There may be visualization of thrombus within the sinus on postcontrast images (empty-delta sign) or direct visualization of the clot (cord sign). The availabil-

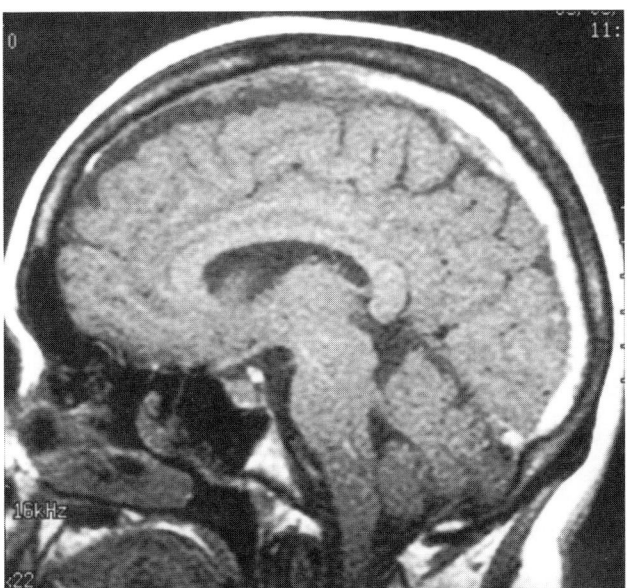

FIGURE 57A.19   Unenhanced sagittal T1-weighted magnetic resonance imaging shows an area of increased signal and enlargement of the superior sagittal sinus throughout most of its course consistent with superior sagittal sinus thrombosis. It also involves the region of the torcula.

ity of MR venography makes it possible to diagnose early and atypical cases. MR venography is a reliable diagnostic tool and has replaced angiography for the diagnosis of cerebral venous thrombosis, patients with intracranial venous occlusive disease should be screened for thrombophilia.

Accepted therapeutic measures include reduction of increased intracranial pressure. Prophylactic anticonvulsants, and antibiotics in cases involving a septic etiology. Several investigators have reservations about using anticoagulants in the treatment of intracranial venous thrombosis, because of concerns of hemorrhagic complications. Other investigators recommend anticoagulants for the treatment of intracranial venous thrombosis, ostensibly to prevent the extension of thrombus, to allow the development of collateral circulation, and to prevent pulmonary embolism.

REFERENCES

The Atrial Fibrillation Investigators. The efficacy of aspirin in patients with atrial fibrillation. Analysis of pooled data from 3 randomized trials. Arch Intern Med 1997;157:1237–1240.

Biller J. Essential investigations for patients with transient ischemic attacks and evolving stroke. J Stroke Cerebrovasc Dis 1994;4:S11–S13.

Biller J, Sparks LH. Diagnosis and Management of Cerebral Vasculitis. In HP Adams Jr (ed), Handbook of Cerebrovascular Diseases. New York: Marcel Dekker, 1993;549–567.

Bonita R, Broad JB, Beaglehole R. Ethnic differences in stroke incidence and case fatality in Auckland, New Zealand. Stroke 1997;28:758–761.

Boon A, Lodder J, Cheriex E, Kessels F. Risk of stroke in a cohort of 815 patients with calcification of the aortic valve with or without stenosis. Stroke 1996;27:847–851.

Bousser MG, Ross Russsell R. Cerebral Venous Thrombosis. In Major Problems in Neurology (Vol. 33). Philadelphia: Saunders 1997.

Brazis PW, Masdeu JC, Biller J. Localization in Clinical Neurology. Vascular Syndromes of the Cerebrum (3rd ed). Boston: Little, Brown, 1996;535–564.

Buring JE, Hebert P, Romero J, et al. Migraine and subsequent risk of stroke in the Physician's Health Study. Arch Neurol 1995;52:129–134.

CAPRIE Steering Committee. A randomised, blinded, trial of clopidogrel versus aspirin in patients at risk of ischaemic events (CAPRIE). Lancet 1996;348:1329–1339.

Carolei A, Marini C, De Matteis G. History of migraine and risk of cerebral ischemia in young adults. The Italian National

Table 57A.9:   Etiologies of intracranial sinovenous occlusive disease

Facial/orbital/paranasal sinuses/middle ear infections
Pregnancy and puerperium
Carcinoma
Dehydration
Marasmus
L-Asparaginase therapy
Androgen therapy
Cisplatin and etoposide therapy
ε-Aminocaproic acid therapy
Intravenous catheters, cardiac pacemakers
Polyarteritis nodosa
Systemic lupus erythematosus
Wegener's granulomatosis
Behçet's disease
Degos' disease (malignant atrophic papulosis)
Inflammatory bowel disease
Sarcoidosis
Osteoporosis
Congestive heart failure
Nephrotic syndrome
Budd-Chiari syndrome
Chronic lung disease
Trichinosis
Diabetes mellitus
Cerebral arterial occlusions
Homocystinuria
Head injury
Paroxysmal nocturnal hemoglobinuria
Sickle cell disease and trait
Polycythemia vera
Essential thrombocythemia
Iron deficiency anemia
Hypoplasminogenemia
Afibrinogenemia
Cryofibrinogenemia
Antiphospholipid antibody syndrome
Disseminated intravascular coagulation
Antithrombin III deficiency
Protein S deficiency
Protein C deficiency
Combined deficiencies (protein C, protein S, and antithrombin III)
Activated protein C resistance
Factor V Leiden mutation
Heparin-induced thrombocytopenia
Arteriovenous malformations
Sturge-Weber syndrome
Idiopathic

Research Council Study Group on Stroke in the Young. Lancet 1996;347:1053–1506.

CAST. Randomised placebo-controlled trial of early aspirin use in 20,000 patients with acute ischaemic stroke. CAST (Chinese Acute Stroke Trial). Lancet 1997;349:1641–1649.

Choi DW. Ischemia-induced neuronal apoptosis. Curr Opin Neurobiol 1996;6:667–672.

Clark WM, Warach SJ, Pettigrew LC, et al. A randomized dose-response trial of citicoline in acute ischemic stroke patients. Citicoline Stroke Study Group. Neurology 1997;49:671–678.

Diener HC, Cunha L, Forbes C, et al. The European Stroke Prevention Study II. Dipyridamole and acetylsalicylic acid in the secondary prevention of stroke. J Neurol Sci 1996;143:1–13.

Donnan GA, O'Malley HM, Qaung L, et al. The capsular warning syndrome: pathogenesis and clinical features. Neurology 1993;43:957–962.

Eishi K, Kawazoe K, Kuriyama Y, et al. Surgical management of infective endocarditis associated with cerebral complications. Multi-center retrospective study in Japan. J Thor Cardiovasc Surg 1995;110:1745–1755.

European Carotid Surgery Trialists' Collaborative Group. Risk of stroke in the distribution of an asymptomatic carotid artery. Lancet 1995;345:209–212.

European Carotid Surgery Trialists' Collaborative Group. Endarterectomy for moderate symptomatic carotid stenosis: interim results from the MRC European Carotid Surgery Trial. Lancet 1996;347:1591–1593.

Frances C, Le Tonqueze M, Salohzin KV, et al. Prevalence of anti-endothelial cell antibodies in patients with Sneddon's syndrome. J Am Acad Dermatol 1995;33:64–68.

The French Study of Aortic Plaques in Stroke Group. Atherosclerotic disease of the aortic arch as a risk factor for recurrent ischemic stroke. N Engl J Med 1996;334:1216–1221.

Giles WH, Kittner SJ, Anda RF, et al. Serum folate and risk for ischemic stroke. First National Health and Nutrition Examination Survey epidemiologic follow-up study. Stroke 1995;26:1166–1170.

Hartfield DS, Lowry NJ, Keene DL, Yager JY. Iron deficiency anemia: a cause of stroke in infants and children. Pediatr Neurol 1997;16:50–53.

Hobson RW II, Weiss DG, Fields WS, et al. Efficacy of endarterectomy for asymptomatic carotid stenosis. N Engl J Med 1993;328:276–279.

Hutchinson M, O'Riordan J, Javed M, et al. Familial hemiplegic migraine and autosomal dominant arteriopathy with leukoencephalopathy (CADASIL). Ann Neurol 1995;38:817–824.

The International Stroke Trial Collaborative Group. The International Stroke Trial (IST): a randomised trial of aspirin, subcutaneous heparin, both, or neither among 19435 patients with acute ischaemic stroke. Lancet 1997;349:1569–1581.

Kay R, Wong KS, Yu YL, et al. Low-molecular-weight heparin for the treatment of acute ischemic stroke. N Engl J Med 1995;33:1588–1593.

Khamashta MA, Cuadrado MJ, Mujic F, et al. The management of thrombosis in the antiphospholipid antibody syndrome. N Engl J Med 1995;332:993–997.

Kitchens GS. Thrombophilia and Thrombosis in Unusual Sites. In RW Colman, J Hirsh, VJ Marder, et al. (eds), Hemostasis and Thrombosis: Basic Principles and Clinical Practice (3rd ed). Philadelphia: Lippincott–Raven, 1994;1255–1273.

Koefoed BG, Gullov AL, Petersen P. Prevention of thromboembolic events in atrial fibrillation. Thromb Haemostasis 1997;78:377–381.

Loh E, Sutton MS, Wun CC, et al. Ventricular dysfunction and the risk of stroke after myocardial infarction. N Engl J Med 1997;336:251–257.

MacMahon S, Rodges A. Primary and secondary prevention of stroke. Clin Exp Hyperten 1996;18:537–546.

Mattioli AV, Castellani ET, Fusco A, et al. Stroke in paced patients with sick sinus syndrome: relevance of atrial mechanical function, pacing mode and clinical characteristics. Cardiology 1997;88:264–270.

Mickleborough LL, Walker PM, Takagi Y, et al. Risk factors for stroke in patients undergoing coronary artery bypass grafting. J Thorac Cardiovasc Surg 1996;112:1250–1258.

Moore TB, Chow VJ, Ferry D, Feig SA. Intracardiac right-to-left shunting and the risk of stroke during bone marrow infusion. Bone Marrow Transplant 1997;19:855–856.

The National Institute of Neurological Disorders and Stroke rt-PA Stroke Study Group. Tissue plasminogen activator for acute ischemic stroke. N Engl J Med 1995;333:1581–1587.

Nicolai A, Lazzarino LG, Biasutti E. Large striatocapsular infarcts: clinical features and risk factors. J Neurol 1996;243:44–50.

Olichney JM, Hansen LA, Hofstetter CR, et al. Cerebral infarction in Alzheimer's disease is associated with severe amyloid angiopathy and hypertension. Arch Neurol 1995;52:702–708.

Pagelow CH, Adams RJ, McKie V, et al. Risk of recurrent stroke in patients with sickle cell disease treated with erythrocyte transfusions. Pediatrics 1995;126:896–899.

Perloff JK, Marelli AJ, Miner PD. Risk of stroke in adults with cyanotic congenital heart disease. Circulation 1993;87:1954–1959.

Petty GW, Engel AG, Younge BR, et al. Retinocochleocerebral vasculopathy. Medicine 1998;77:12–40.

Post-Stroke Rehabilitation Guideline Panel: Post-Stroke Rehabilitation. Clinical Practice Guideline. No. 16. U.S. Department of Health and Human Services, Rockville, MD, AHCPR Pub. No. 95-0662, May 1995.

Rordorf G, Cramer SC, Efird JT, et al. Pharmacological elevation of blood pressure in acute stroke. Clinical effects and safety. Stroke 1997;28:2133–2138.

Slooter AJ, Tang MX, van Duijn CM, et al. Apolipoprotein E epsilon 4 and the risk of dementia with stroke. A population-based investigation. JAMA 1997;277:818–821.

Teehan EP, Padberg FT Jr, Thompson PN, et al. Carotid arterial trauma: assessment with the Glasgow Coma Scale (GCS) as a guide to surgical management. Cardiovasc Surg 1997;5:196–200.

Thal DR, Schober R, Sclote W. Carotid artery dissection in a young adult: cystic medial necrosis associated with an increased elastase content. Clin Neuropathol 1997;16:180–184.

Verin M, Rolland Y, Landgraf F, et al. New phenotype of cerebral autosomal dominant arteriopathy mapped to chromosome 19: migraine as the prominent clinical feature. J Neurol Neurosurg Psychiatry 1995;59:579–585.

WHO Collaborative Study of Cardiovascular Disease and Steroid Hormone Contraception. Ischaemic stroke and combined oral contraceptives: results of an international, multicentre, case-control study. Lancet 1996;348:498–505.

Yamamoto M, Aoyagi M, Tijima S, et al. Increase in elastin gene expression and protein synthesis in arterial smooth muscle cell derived from patients with moyamoya disease. Stroke 1997;28:1733–1738.

Zheng ZJ, Sharrett AR, Chambless LE, et al. Association of ankle-brachial index with clinical coronary heart disease, stroke and preclinical carotid and popliteal atherosclerosis: The Atherosclerosis Risk in Communities (ARIC) Study. Atherosclerosis 1997;131:115–125.

Chapter 57
Vascular Diseases of the Nervous System

B. INTRACEREBRAL HEMORRHAGE
Carlos S. Kase

Intracerebral hemorrhage (ICH) accounts for approximately 10% of strokes. Its clinical importance derives from its frequency and high mortality. Although the latter is strongly dependent on hematoma size and, to a lesser extent, location, the overall mortality for this stroke subtype varies between 25% and 60%. There has been a general decline since the 1980s in the incidence of stroke, including ICH, as a result of improved detection and treatment of hypertension. However, ICH continues to be a major public health problem, especially in populations at high risk, such as young and middle-aged African-Americans and Hispanics (Bruno et al. 1996), in whom this stroke subtype occurs significantly more frequently than in whites. Furthermore, the management of ICH is controversial, as the value of surgical or nonsurgical treatment of the various types of ICH has not been defined by properly designed prospective clinical trials.

MECHANISMS OF INTRACEREBRAL HEMORRHAGE

Hypertension

The main cause of ICH is hypertension. The primary role of hypertension is supported by a high frequency (72–81%) of history of hypertension, significantly higher admission blood pressure measurements as compared with patients with other stroke subtypes, and a high frequency of left ventricular hypertrophy.

Broderick et al. (1993), studying 188 patients with primary ICH (i.e., with exclusion of patients with hemorrhage associated with ruptured arteriovenous malformations [AVMs], tumor, anticoagulant and thrombolytic therapy, and cocaine ingestion), determined the cause to be hypertension in 72%. Further support for the importance of hypertension in the pathogenesis of ICH is the steady increase in ICH incidence with advancing age, which is associated also with an increase in the prevalence of hypertension.

The actual vascular lesion produced by chronic hypertension that leads to arterial rupture and ICH is probably lipohyalinosis of small intraparenchymal arteries (Caplan 1994a). The role of microaneurysms of Charcot and Bouchard is uncertain, although their anatomical location at sites preferentially affected by ICH supports their etiological importance.

The nonhypertensive causes of ICH are listed in Table 57B.1.

Vascular Malformations

Because a detailed discussion of intracranial aneurysms and AVMs (see Chapter 57C) is provided elsewhere, we limit the analysis here to the role of small vascular malformations in the pathogenesis of ICH. These lesions are often documented

Table 57B.1:   Nonhypertensive causes of intracerebral hemorrhage

---

Vascular malformations (saccular or mycotic aneurysms, arteriovenous malformations, cavernous angiomas)
Intracranial tumors
Bleeding disorders, anticoagulant and fibrinolytic treatment
Cerebral amyloid angiopathy
Granulomatous angiitis of the central nervous system and other vasculitides, such as polyarteritis nodosa
Sympathomimetic agents
Hemorrhagic infarction
Trauma

---

by either magnetic resonance imaging (MRI), after pathological examination of specimens obtained at the time of surgical drainage of ICHs, or at autopsy. However, cerebral angiography also plays an important role in the diagnosis of these lesions. In a group of 38 young ICH patients (mean age, 46 years) subjected to angiography, Halpin et al. (1994) documented AVMs in 23 patients and aneurysms in nine (a total of 32 of 38, or 84%). The ICH in these 38 patients had computed tomographic (CT) characteristics suggestive of an underlying structural lesion (associated subarachnoid or intraventricular bleeding, calcification, prominent vascular structures, atypical ICH location). However, in 42 patients lacking these CT features, angiography still documented vascular abnormalities in 10 (AVMs in eight, aneurysm in two).

ICHs caused by small AVMs or cavernous angiomas are frequently located in the subcortical white matter of the cerebral hemispheres. Less commonly, basal ganglionic and pontine ICHs occur as a result of ruptured small vascular malformations. The clinical presentation of the ICH in this setting has few distinctive characteristics. The hematoma is generally smaller and symptoms develop more slowly compared with hypertensive ICH. The presence of associated subarachnoid hemorrhage on CT scan suggests an aneurysm or AVM as the cause in a case of lobar ICH. In addition, those ICHs associated with small vascular malformations tend to occur in generally younger patients, when compared with those with hypertensive ICH (Kase 1994a), and have a female preponderance.

Cavernous angiomas are being increasingly recognized as a cause of ICH in the subcortical portions of the cerebral hemispheres and in the pons, as a result of the high diagnostic yield of MRI. This technique demonstrates a characteristic pattern on T2-weighted images, with a central nidus of irregular bright signal intensity mixed with mottled hypointensity, surrounded by a peripheral hypointense ring corresponding to hemosiderin deposits (Figure 57B.1), reflecting previous episodes of bleeding. These lesions are predominantly supratentorial, favoring the temporal, frontal, and parietal lobes, whereas the less frequent infratentorial locations favor the pons. They are generally single lesions, but multiplicity is not uncommon, especially in patients with familial cavernous angiomas. The latter is common among individuals

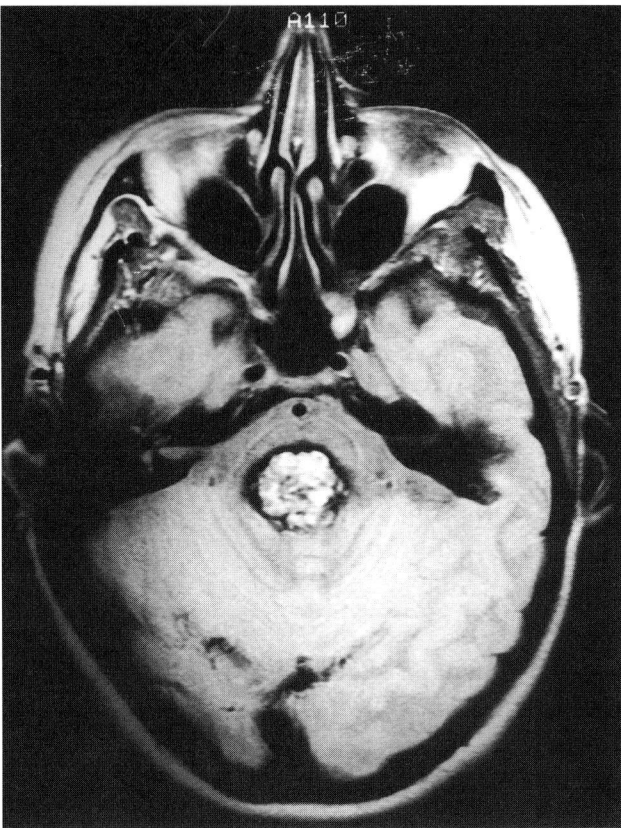

FIGURE 57B.1   Magnetic resonance imaging (proton density) of large cavernous angioma of the midpons in axial view, showing mixed signal central nidus with peripheral hemosiderin ring.

of Mexican-American descent, in whom cavernous angiomas are inherited in an autosomal dominant pattern, linked to a mutation in chromosome 7q (Gil-Nagel et al. 1996). Their clinical presentation is with either seizures (27–70%), ICH (10–30%), or progressive neurological deficits (35%). Seizures are the most common presenting feature of supratentorial cavernous angiomas; ICH occurs in both the supratentorial and infratentorial varieties; and progressive neurological deficits are a more common presentation of posterior fossa (especially pontine) malformations. A progressive course, caused by recurrent small hemorrhages within and around the malformation, can evolve over protracted periods, at times suggesting a diagnosis of multiple sclerosis or a slowly growing brainstem glioma.

A clinical profile thus can be suggested for cases of ICH caused by small vascular malformations. These occur in generally young, predominantly female patients, who present with a progressive syndrome of lobar ICH, in which CT scan can document a superficial lobar hematoma with adjacent local subarachnoid hemorrhage or MRI demonstrates the characteristic features of a small AVM or cavernous angioma. Lack of documentation of the vascular malformation on angiography is not uncommon, and definite diagnosis requires either MRI or the histological examination of a sample of the hematoma and its wall.

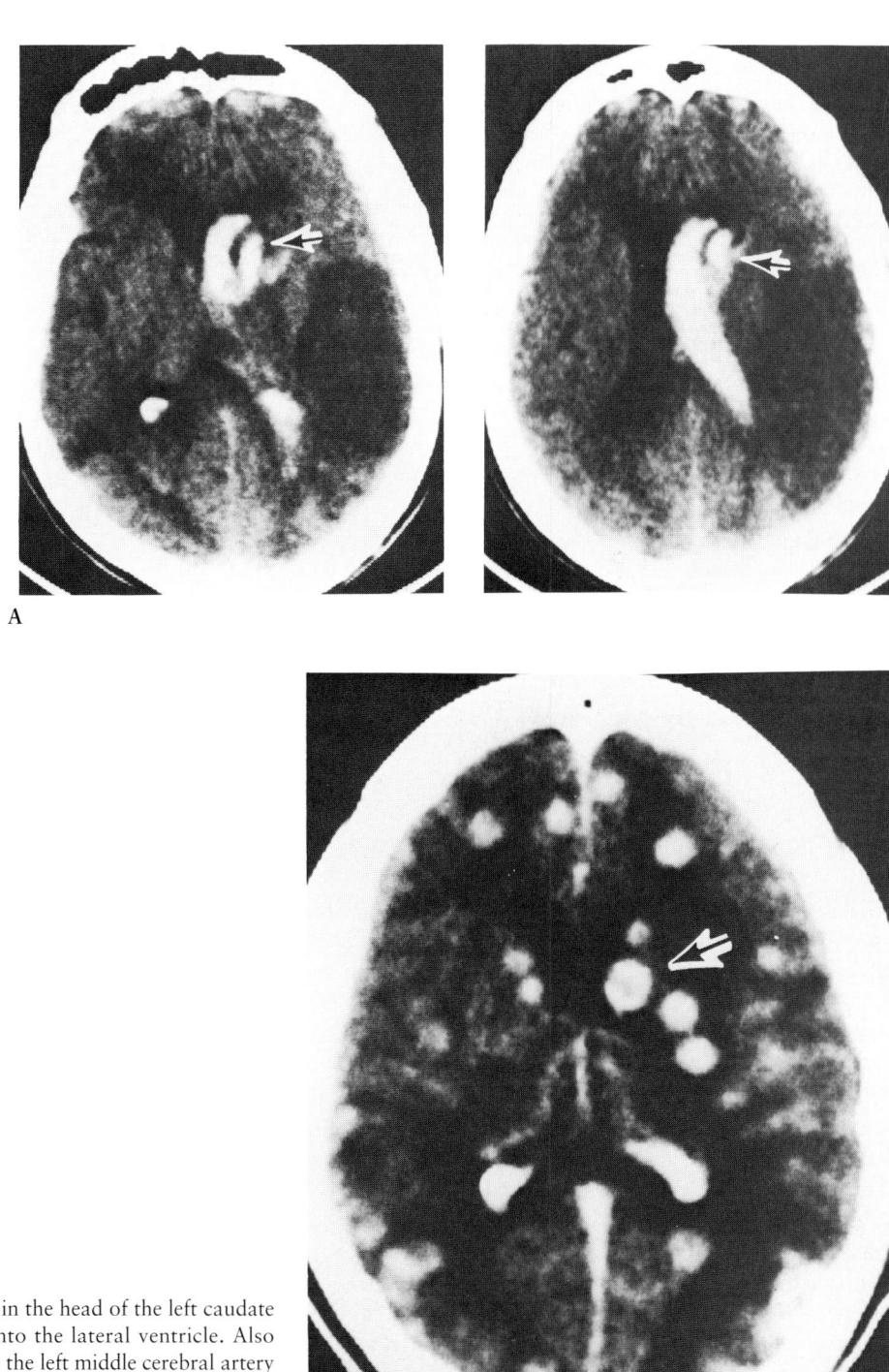

FIGURE 57B.2   **(A)** Hemorrhage in the head of the left caudate nucleus (*arrow*), with extension into the lateral ventricle. Also shown is an unrelated old infarct in the left middle cerebral artery distribution. Noncontrast computed tomographic (CT) scan. **(B)** Postcontrast infusion CT scan of the same case, showing multiple enhancing metastases from bronchogenic carcinoma. The lesion shown in the area of the head of the caudate nucleus (*arrow*) was related to the hemorrhage shown in **(A)**.

Intracranial Tumors

Bleeding into an underlying brain tumor is relatively rare in series of patients presenting with ICH, accounting for less than 10% of the cases. The tumor types most likely to lead to this complication are glioblastoma multiforme or metastases from melanoma, bronchogenic carcinoma, choriocarcinoma, or renal cell carcinoma (Figure 57B.2). The ICHs produced in this setting may have clinical and imaging characteristics that should raise the suspicion of an underlying brain tumor, including (1) the presence of papilledema on presentation; (2) the location of ICH in sites that are rarely affected in hypertensive ICH, such as the corpus callosum, which in turn is commonly involved in malignant gliomas; (3) the presence of ICH in multiple sites simultaneously; (4) a CT scan characterized by a ring of high-density hemorrhage surrounding a low-density center in a noncontrast study; (5) a disproportionate amount of surrounding edema and mass effect associated with the acute hematoma; (6) enhancing nodules adjacent to the hemorrhage on contrast CT scan; and (7) an MRI pattern of heterogeneous signal changes within a mass lesion, surrounded by a hemosiderin hypointense ring and bright signal edema at the periphery on T2-weighted sequences. In these circumstances, a search for a primary or metastatic brain tumor should follow, including evaluation for systemic malignancy and, if there is none, cerebral angiography, and eventually craniotomy for biopsy of the hematoma cavity. The confirmation of the diagnosis of ICH secondary to malignant brain tumor carries a dismal prognosis, with a short-term mortality in the 90% range.

Bleeding Disorders, Anticoagulants, and Fibrinolytic Treatment

Bleeding disorders caused by abnormalities of coagulation are rare causes of ICH. Hemophilia caused by factor VIII deficiency leads to ICH in approximately 2.5–6.0% of patients, one-half with ICH and one-half with subdural hematomas. The majority of these hemorrhages occur in young patients, generally under age 18, and their mortality is high, on the order of 10% for subdural hematomas and 65% for ICH. Immune-mediated thrombocytopenia, especially idiopathic thrombocytopenic purpura, is associated with life-threatening ICH in approximately 1% of patients. Bleeding can occur when the platelet count drops below 10,000/µl, and the hemorrhages may occur anywhere in the brain. Acute leukemia, especially the acute lymphocytic variety, is a common cause of ICH, which favors the lobar white matter of the cerebral hemispheres. The occurrence of ICH frequently coincides with systemic bleeding, mostly mucocutaneous and gastrointestinal. These bleeding complications of acute lymphocytic leukemia are often accompanied by both thrombocytopenia (platelet counts of 50,000/µl or less) and rapidly increasing numbers of abnormal circulating leukocytes of 300,000/µl, or more (blastic crisis). Acute promyelocytic leukemia, a variant of acute myelogenous leukemia, has a particular propensity to produce ICH as a result of disseminated intravascular coagulation, caused by the release of a procoagulant factor from the promyelocyte granules.

Treatment with oral anticoagulants increases the risk of ICH by eightfold to 11-fold, in comparison with nonanticoagulated individuals with otherwise similar risk factors for ICH. Anticoagulant-related cases account for 9–11% of ICHs. Potential risk factors for intracranial bleeding in anticoagulated patients include advanced age, hypertension, preceding cerebral infarction, head trauma, and excessive prolongation of the prothrombin time. The latter factor plays a major role in the pathogenesis of ICH in patients receiving oral anticoagulants. In the secondary stroke prevention trial SPIRIT (The Stroke Prevention in Reversible Ischemia Trial Study Group, 1997), 651 patients assigned to warfarin were maintained at an international normalized ratio of 3.0–4.5, resulting in 24 instances of ICH (14 fatal), in comparison with three ICHs (one fatal) in the group of 665 patients treated daily with 30 mg of aspirin. These data further support the recommendation that oral anticoagulation in patients with cerebrovascular disease should aim at an international normalized ratio of 2–3 to reduce the frequency of this complication.

These hemorrhages have certain distinctive clinical characteristics. They tend to present with a slowly progressive course, at times over periods as long as 48–72 hours, in contrast with the usually more rapidly evolving presentation of hypertensive ICH. Because of this longer course, hematomas in anticoagulated patients tend to reach volumes that are, on average, larger than those of hypertensive ICH, in turn resulting in the higher mortality of approximately 65%. Signs of systemic bleeding rarely accompany ICH. Anticoagulant-related ICH may represent bleeding from vessels different from those involved in ICH of hypertensive origin (Hart et al. 1995).

In addition to the anticoagulants, other substances with the potential for altering clot formation mechanisms are occasionally associated with ICH. These include drugs with fibrinolytic properties such as streptokinase and tissue-type plasminogen activator (t-PA). The use of these substances for coronary thrombolysis in the early phases of myocardial infarction has been associated with a small but nonetheless consistent risk of ICH. In the case of t-PA, this complication seems to be partially dose related. A 1.5% rate of ICH followed the use of a total t-PA dose of 150 mg, whereas the rate fell to 0.5–0.6% with the currently recommended dose of 100 mg. There is evidence to suggest that this complication of thrombolytic therapy may be favored by pre-existent vasculopathies with bleeding potential, such as cerebral amyloid angiopathy (CAA) (Sloan et al. 1995). The role of other factors, such as the simultaneous use of heparin anticoagulation and aspirin to prevent coronary reocclusion, is uncertain.

The ICHs that follow treatment with t-PA in acute myocardial infarction generally start early after onset of thrombolytic treatment, approximately 40% of them occurring during the drug infusion. The site of bleeding is most commonly the subcortical (lobar) white matter of the cerebral hemispheres, where sometimes multiple hematomas occur and are occasionally associated with a subdural hematoma (Figure 57B.3). The prognosis of this complication is dismal, with a mortality of 44.0–87.5% in different series.

Recombinant t-PA for the treatment of acute ischemic stroke has a rate of ICH (6.4%), which is 10 times higher than in untreated patients. The high frequency of ICH par-

FIGURE 57B.3 Sites of intracranial hemorrhage in nine patients treated with tissue-type plasminogen activator for acute myocardial infarction. (**A**) Left temporal lobar hematoma (left panel) and chronic and acute subdural hematoma (*arrow*; right panel). (**B**) Right parasagittal frontoparietal lobar hemorrhage. (**C**) Bilateral multiple occipital lobar hematomas. (**D**) Left frontal and occipital hematomas (*arrows*). (**E**) Right cerebral hemorrhage (*arrows*; right panel), with extension to the vermis and fourth ventricle (left panel). (**F**) Left posterior temporal lobar hemorrhage. (**G**) Left frontoparietal lobar hemorrhage with ventricular extension. (**H**) Small right posterior parietal parasagittal hematoma. (**I**) Left temporoparietal lobar hemorrhage. (Reprinted from CS Kase, MS Pessin, JA Zivin, et al. Intracranial hemorrhage after coronary thrombolysis with tissue plasminogen activator. Am J Med 1992;92:384–390. With permission from Excerpta Medica, Inc.)

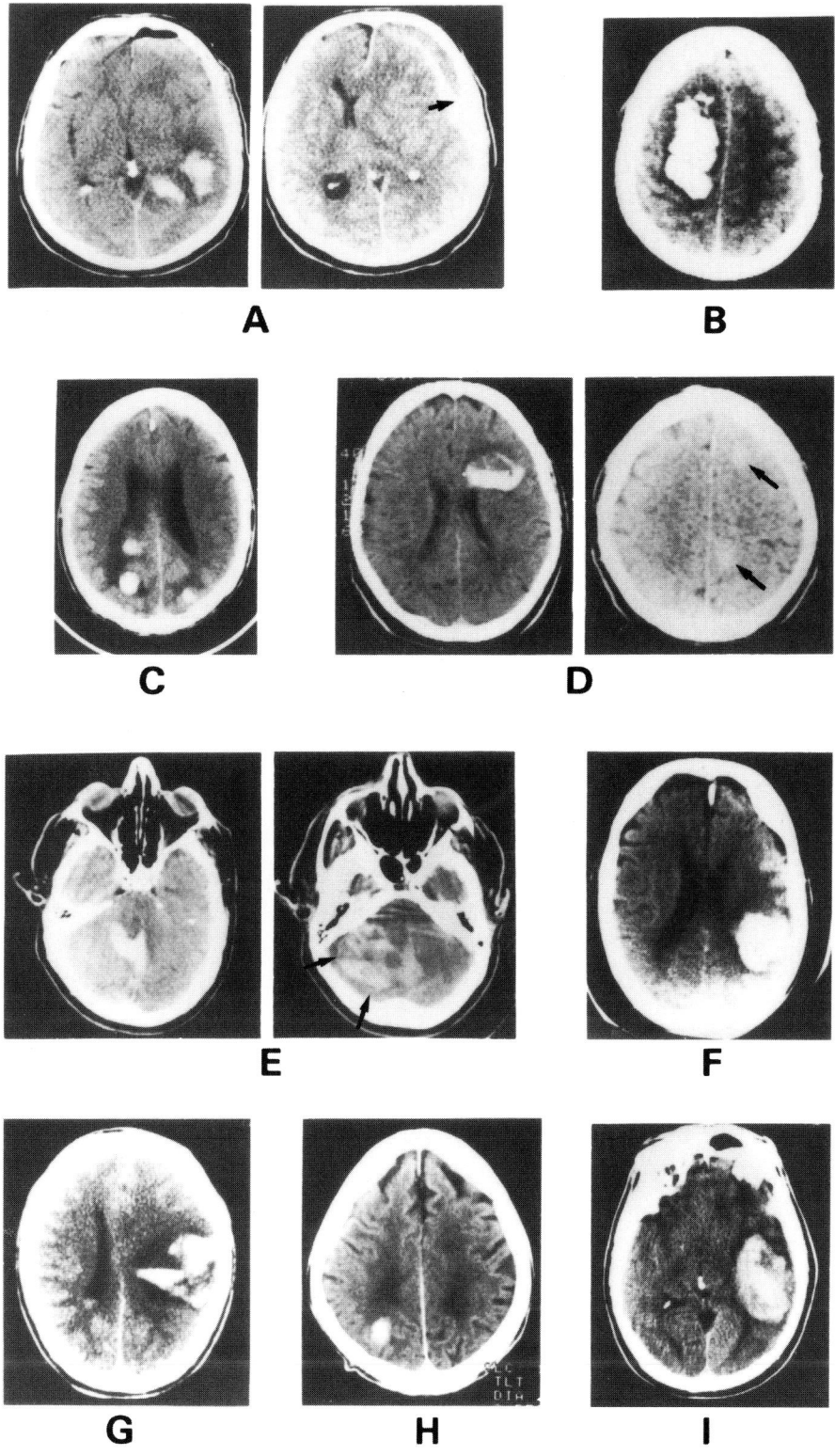

tially limits the usefulness of this therapy, and exclusion of patients at high risk of this complication should improve its risk-to-benefit ratio. Risk factors for ICH in this setting include a severe neurological deficit at presentation, and documentation of hypodensity or mass effect on CT before treatment (The NINDS t-PA Stroke Study Group 1997).

Cerebral Amyloid Angiopathy

CAA is characterized by selective deposition of amyloid in cerebral vessels, primarily small and medium-sized arteries of the cortex and leptomeninges. Because the frequency of CAA increases steadily with age, reaching 60% in unselected autopsies of individuals older than 90 years, it characteristically causes ICH in the elderly but is rarely documented before the age of 55 years. In addition, the superficial location in the cortex and leptomeninges of the affected vessels is responsible for a predominantly lobar location of the ICHs and a high frequency of local subarachnoid hemorrhage. The widespread character of the angiopathy is responsible for the observation of both recurrent and multiple simultaneous, predominantly lobar hemorrhages in elderly nonhypertensive patients. An additional characteristic of CAA is its association with histopathological features of Alzheimer's disease, with clinical and progressive dementia in 10–30% of patients with CAA, and demonstration of neuritic plaques in approximately 50% of the cases. CAA may present with features other than ICH, such as episodes of transient focal neurological deficit clinically suggestive of either transient ischemic attacks or focal seizures. These often occur days, weeks, or months before the episode of major lobar ICH and may correspond to small foci of hemorrhage that may be documented at multiple cortical sites by gradient-echo MRI sequences.

The histological lesion in CAA is deposition of Congo red–positive, birefringent amyloid material in the media and adventitia of cortical and leptomeningeal arteries (Figure 57B.4). The actual mechanism of rupture of an affected artery may be either a weakening of the wall or the formation of microaneurysms at sites of amyloid deposition, particularly when hypertensive fibrinoid necrosis develops in the same location. Other conditions may combine with CAA to produce rupture of affected vessels, including head trauma, neurosurgical procedures, concomitant granulomatous angiitis of the central nervous system (CNS), and use of fibrinolytic agents in the treatment of acute myocardial infarction.

Granulomatous Angiitis of the Central Nervous System and Other Vasculitides

Granulomatous angiitis of the CNS, also referred to as *isolated angiitis of the CNS*, is characterized by mononuclear inflammation with giant cell formation in the media and adventitia of small and medium-sized intracranial arteries and veins (see Chapter 57G). An associated element of intimal hyperplasia leads frequently to cerebral infarcts and occasionally ICH.

Among the vasculitides, the other variety that is known to present with ICH is polyarteritis nodosa. As opposed to granulomatous angiitis of the CNS, this form of necrotizing vasculitis depicts prominent signs of systemic involvement, including fever, malaise, weight loss, anemia, elevated sedimentation rate, and renal impairment with hypertension (see Chapter 55A).

Sympathomimetic Agents

Amphetamines cause ICH after intravenous, oral, or intranasal use (see Chapter 64). The hemorrhages have occurred within minutes to a few hours after drug use, and the majority have been located in the subcortical white matter of the cerebral hemispheres. In approximately one-half of the reported cases, transient hypertension has been documented, as well as multifocal areas of spasm and dilatation (beading) of intracranial arteries on angiography. Although the latter is frequently referred to as a *vasculitis* or *arteritis*, histological proof is lacking, and this angiographic picture probably represents multifocal spasm secondary to the drug. This view is supported by finding the same angiographical abnormalities following use of other sympathomimetic agents, including ephedrine, pseudoephedrine, and phenylpropanolamine. Phenylpropanolamine is found in approximately 70 over-the-counter decongestants and appetite suppressants and has been associated with ICH in more than 20 reported cases. These have occurred in young patients (median age in the early 30s), predominantly women, usually without a history of hypertension but with acute hypertension on admission in one-third of patients. Most hemorrhages have occurred within minutes to a few hours from the first-time ingestion of the drug, usually in recommended doses. Beading of intracranial arteries is frequent on angiography. These ICHs related to phenylpropanolamine may result from a direct vascular effect of the drug with production of multifocal segmental spasm or, less commonly, a true vasculitis combined with transient hypertension in individuals particularly susceptible to the drug's sympathomimetic effect.

Cocaine (see Chapter 64) has become the most common sympathomimetic agent associated with ICH (Nolte et al. 1996). Both ICH and subarachnoid hemorrhage can occur within short periods (generally minutes) from use of both the alkaloidal (free-base) form of cocaine and its precipitate form known as *crack*. The ICHs favor the subcortical white matter, but occasionally occur in the deep portions of the hemispheres (Figure 57B.5). There may be multiple simultaneous ICHs, both deep and superficial, the mechanism of which remains unknown. In some instances, the origin of the ICH can be traced to a coexistent AVM or aneurysm, whereas the remainder are probably associated with either cocaine-induced vasoconstriction followed by reperfusion, heavy alcohol intake, or rarely, a drug-induced cerebral vasculitis.

Hemorrhagic Infarction

Hemorrhagic infarction is pathologically and pathogenically different from ICH in that it results from arterial or venous occlusion, rather than from the vascular rupture that causes ICH. As a result, its pathological aspect is one of multifocal petechial hemorrhagic staining of an area of the brain primarily affected by ischemic necrosis (i.e., infarction). Hemorrhagic infarction characteristically occurs in the setting of cerebral embolism or, less frequently, cerebral infarction secondary to venous occlusion (e.g., superior sagittal sinus thrombosis); in both, the bleeding reflects

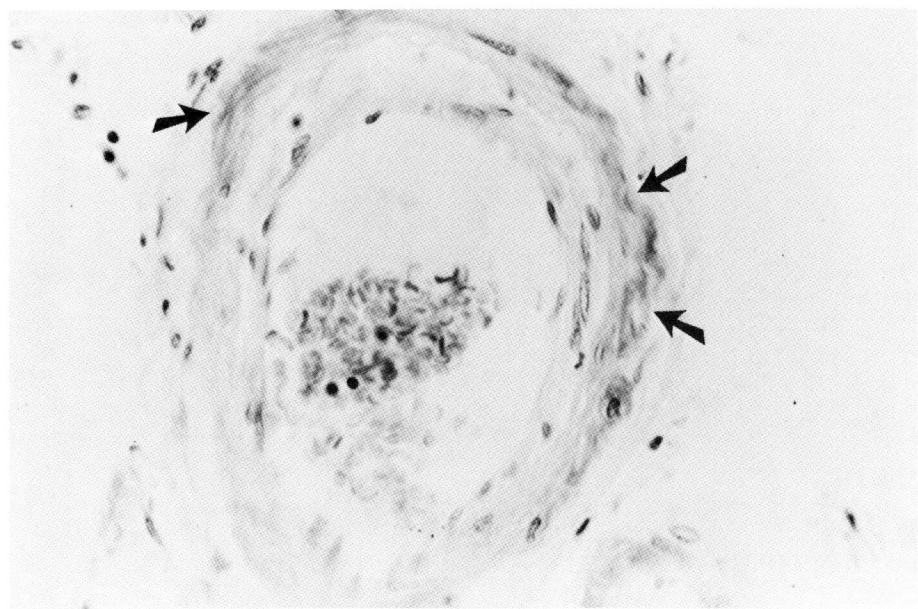

A

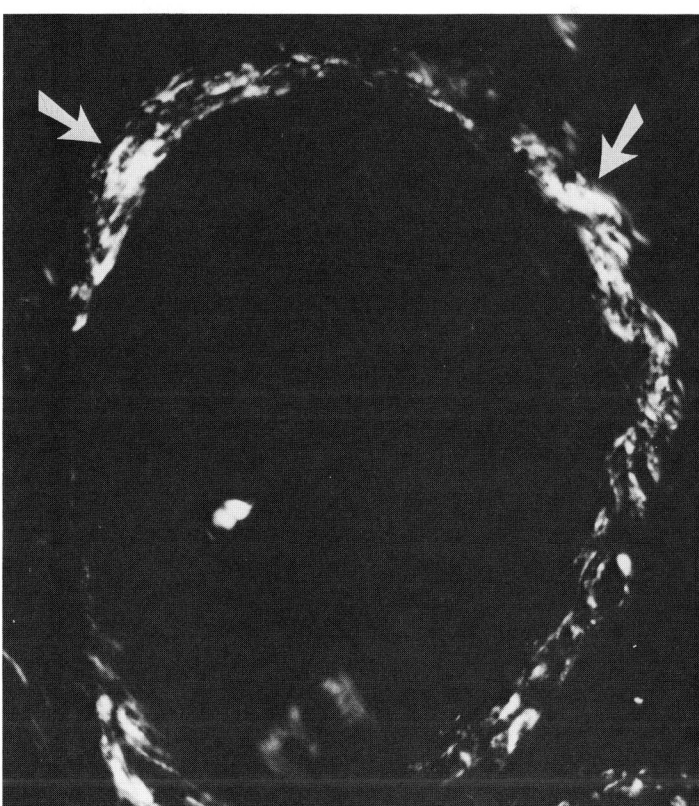

B

FIGURE 57B.4   (A) Medium-sized leptomeningeal artery with amyloid infiltration (*arrows*); Congo red staining. (B) Positive birefringence (*arrows*) under polarized light, characteristic of amyloid deposition; Congo red staining.

the mechanism of the infarct and is not the result of therapeutic measures such as anticoagulant drugs.

Clinical differences between hemorrhagic infarction and ICH usually permit their clear distinction (Table 57B.2), but severe and confluent foci of hemorrhagic infarction may be difficult to distinguish from foci of primary ICH.

Trauma

ICH caused by cerebral contusion characteristically occurs in the surface of the brain, because its mechanism is one of direct brain trauma against its bony covering at the time of an acceleration-deceleration head injury (see Chapter 56A).

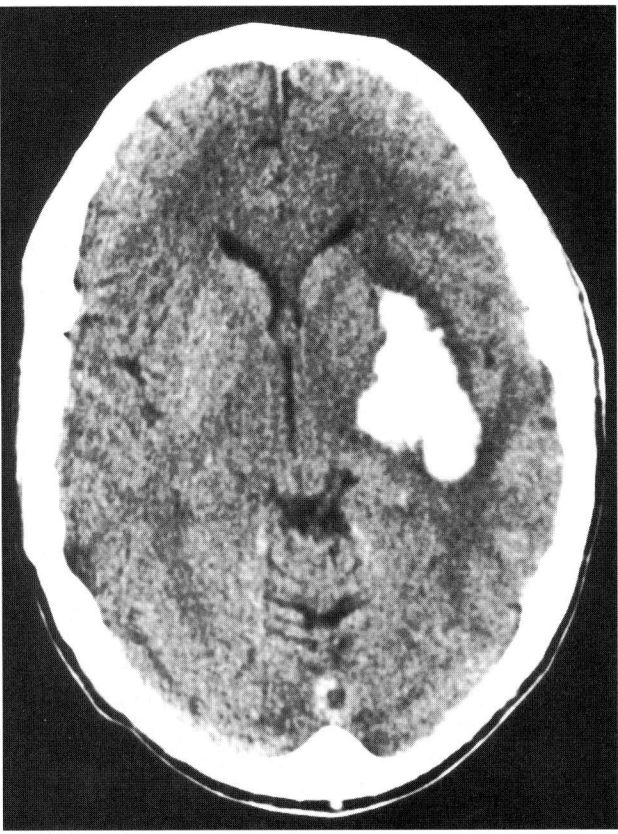

FIGURE 57B.5 Left putaminal hemorrhage after use of crack cocaine. (Courtesy of Susan S. Pansing, MD, Boston VA Medical Center, Boston, MA.)

This explains the sites of predilection for traumatic brain hemorrhages in the basal frontal, anterior temporal, and occipital areas, resulting from the coup and contrecoup mechanisms. Thus, traumatic brain hemorrhages are frequently multiple.

CLINICAL FEATURES OF INTRACEREBRAL HEMORRHAGE

The clinical presentation of ICH has two main elements: symptoms that reflect the effects of intracranial hypertension, and those that are specific for the location of the hematoma. The general clinical manifestations of ICH related to increased intracranial pressure (ICP) (headache, vomiting, and depressed level of consciousness) are variable in their frequency at onset of ICH. The correlation of these symptoms, especially abnormal level of consciousness, with hematoma size applies to all anatomical varieties of ICH, which, in turn, relates directly to mortality.

A characteristic of ICH at presentation is the frequent progression of the focal neurological deficits over periods of hours. This early course reflects the progressive enlargement of the hematoma (Figure 57B.6), which at times amounts to volume increments of over 300%, as measured by serial CT scans (Brott et al. 1997). Seizures at the time of presentation of ICH are rare, except for lobar ICH, which occur in as many as 28% of patients. The subcortical hemorrhage probably creates an area of partially isolated cortex, which reacts with sustained paroxysmal activity.

Table 57B.2: Differences between intracerebral hemorrhage and hemorrhagic infarction

	Intracerebral hemorrhage	*Hemorrhagic infarction (embolic)*
Clinical		
Onset	Sudden followed by progression	Maximal from onset
Raised intracranial pressure	Prominent	Absent
Embolic source	No	Yes
Computed tomographic scan		
High attenuation	Dense, homogeneous	Spotted, mottled
Mass effect	Prominent	Absent or mild
Location	Subcortical, deep (gray nuclei)	Cortex more than subcortical white matter
Distribution	Beyond arterial territories	Along branch distribution
Late enhancement	Ring-type	Gyral-type
Ventricular blood	Yes	No
Magnetic resonance imaging*		
Hypointense blood (T2)	Homogeneous	Patchy, mottled
Hyperintense edema (T2)	Thin peripheral halo	Extensive, in vascular territory
Angiogram/magnetic resonance angiography	Mass effect (avascular)	Branch occlusion

*Magnetic resonance imaging depicts the same features as computed tomographic (CT) scanning in regard to mass effect, location, distribution, late enhancement, and ventricular blood. This table lists only the features that magnetic resonance imaging adds to those of CT.
Source: Reprinted with permission from CS Kase, JP Mohr, LR Caplan. Intracerebral Hemorrhage. In HJM Barnett, JP Mohr, BM Stein, et al. (eds), Stroke: Pathophysiology, Diagnosis, and Management. Philadelphia: Saunders, 1998;649–700.

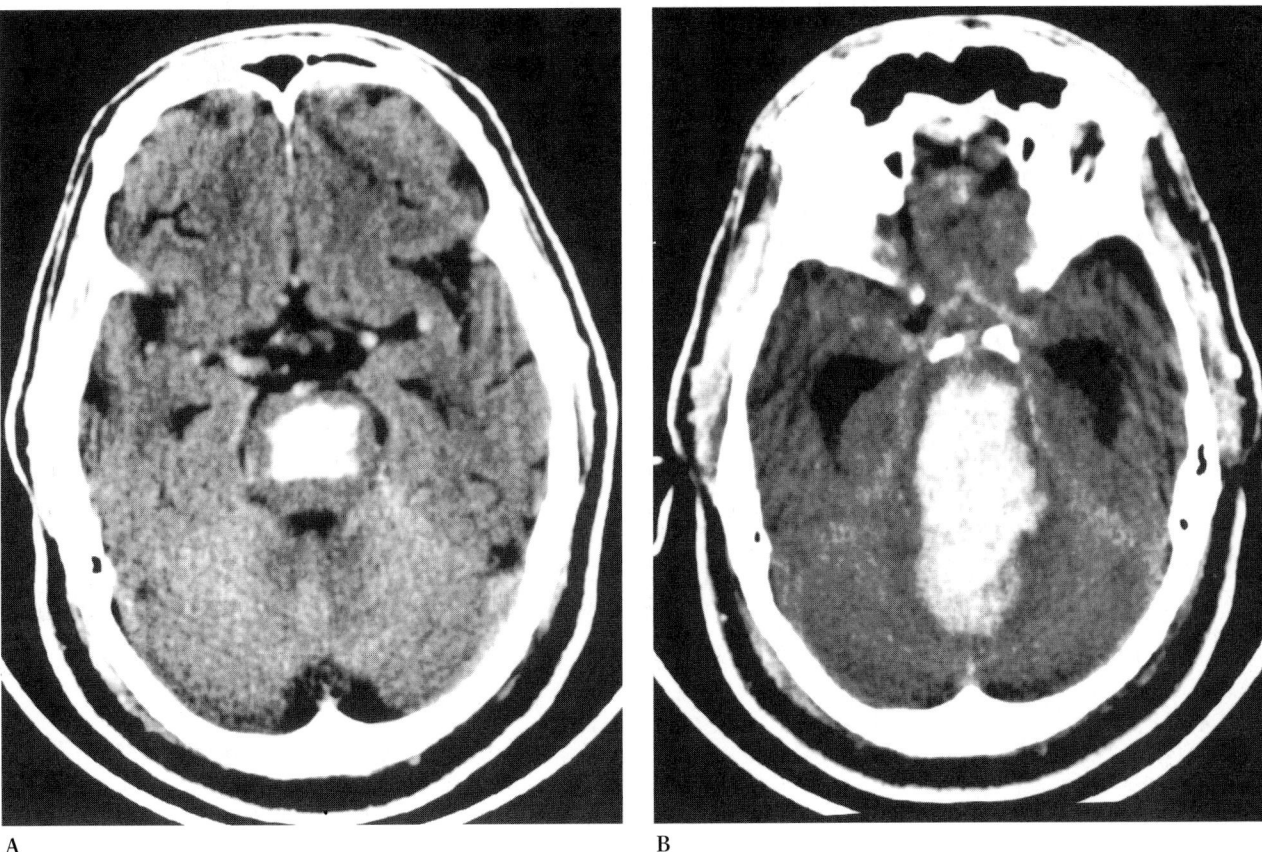

A   B

FIGURE 57B.6   (A) Basal-tegmental pontine hemorrhage at the time of admission. (B) Massive enlargement of hemorrhage with extension into the fourth ventricle and hydrocephalus of temporal horns, 6 hours later.

Table 57B.3:   Temporal changes in magnetic resonance imaging features of intracerebral hemorrhage

Stage of intracerebral hemorrhage	Type of hemoglobin	Magnetic resonance imaging signal intensity	
		T1-weighted	T2-weighted
First hours	Oxyhemoglobin	Same or ↓	↑
Hours to days	Deoxyhemoglobin	Same or ↓	↓↓
First days	Methemoglobin, intracellular	↑	↓
Several days to months	Methemoglobin, extracellular	↑↑	↑↑
Several days to indefinitely	Ferritin/hemosiderin	Same or ↓	↓↓

Same = equal signal with surrounding brain; ↓ = hypointense to brain; ↑ = hyperintense to brain; ↓↓ = marked hypointensity; ↑↑ = marked hyperintensity.

The CT scan is sensitive to the high-density fresh blood in the brain parenchyma, along with associated features of local mass effect and ventricular extension. MRI adds further precision, especially in determining the time elapsed between onset and time of MRI examination. The type of signal intensity change depicted by T1- and T2-weighted MRI sequences can be correlated with the hyperacute, acute, subacute, and chronic stages of evolution of an intracerebral hematoma (Table 57B.3).

The physical examination findings that relate to the different anatomical locations of ICH are summarized in Table 57B.4.

Putaminal Hemorrhage

The most common variety of ICH, putaminal hemorrhage, represents approximately 35% of the cases (Kase et al. 1998) (Figure 57B.7). A wide spectrum of clinical severity relates to hematoma size, from minimally symptomatic cases presenting with pure motor hemiparesis, slight hemiparesis, and dysarthria, to the extreme of coma with decerebrate rigidity in instances of massive hematomas with rupture into the ventricles. Modern CT scan series of putaminal hemorrhage document a mortality of 37%, in

Table 57B.4: Clinical features of anatomical forms of intracerebral hemorrhage

Type of intracerebral hemorrhage	Hemiplegia	Hemisensory syndrome	Aphasia	Homonymous visual field defects	Gaze palsy Horizontal	Vertical	Brainstem signs
Putaminal	Generally dense	Frequent	Global > motor > conduction	In larger hematomas	Contralateral	No	No (only present with herniation)
Caudate	Absent or mild, transient	Absent	No	No	Generally absent	No	No
Thalamic	Generally dense	Frequent, prominent	Occasional, thalamic variety	In larger hematomas	Contralateral, occasionally ipsilateral	Yes, upward	Skew deviation, Horner's syndrome, Parinaud's syndrome
Lobar	Prominent in fronto-parietal location	Prominent in fronto-parietal location	In dominant temporo-parietal location	In occipital hematomas	Contralateral in frontal hematomas	No	No (only present with herniation)
Cerebellar	Absent	Absent	No	No	Ipsilateral	No	Ipsilateral fifth through seventh nerve palsy, Horner's syndrome
Pontine	Variable, usually bilateral	Variable, usually bilateral	No	No	Bilateral	No	Pinpoint reactive pupils, ocular "bobbing," decerebrate rigidity, respiratory rhythm abnormalities
Mesencephalic	Variable, usually present	Rare	No	No	No	Occasional, upward	Unilateral or bilateral third nerve palsy
Medullary	Generally absent	Occasional	No	No	No	No	Nystagmus, ataxia, hiccups, facial hypesthesia, dysarthria, dysphagia, twelfth nerve palsy, Horner's syndrome
Intraventricular	Generally absent	Rare	No	No	Occasional	Occasional	Rare (decerebrate rigidity)

contrast to 65–75% from pre-CT data. This difference reflects the description of the full spectrum of hematoma size in recent reports, including smaller hematomas with benign outcomes, which were misdiagnosed as infarcts in the pre-CT scan era.

Ventricular extension carries an invariably poor prognosis in putaminal hemorrhage. This feature, however, probably reflects the larger size of hematomas that track from the laterally placed putamen to the medially placed ventricular system, rather than the presence of intraventricular blood *per se*. This view is supported by the generally good prognosis in cases of caudate nucleus hemorrhage that are almost invariably associated with ventricular extension, as their paraven-

tricular location allows early entrance of blood into the ventricular space, even when the hematoma is small.

Caudate Hemorrhage

Caudate hemorrhage is a rare variety of ICH that accounts for only approximately 5% of the cases (Kase et al. 1998) (Figure 57B.8). It results from rupture of penetrating arteries from the anterior and middle cerebral arteries, and its most common cause is hypertension. Presentation is similar to that of subarachnoid hemorrhage in that the clinical picture is dominated by signs of intracranial hypertension and meningeal irritation, with focal neurological deficits (hemiparesis, horizontal gaze palsy, Horner's syndrome) being minimal and transient or altogether absent. The main differential diagnosis of caudate ICH is ruptured anterior communicating artery aneurysm with bleeding through the septum pellucidum into the ventricular system. In this instance, CT scan shows blood in the interhemispheric fissure and in the lowermost frontal cuts, as opposed to the higher location of the unilateral clot in the head of one caudate nucleus in primary caudate ICH. Ventricular extension of the hemorrhage is a regular feature in caudate ICH, and hydrocephalus is usually present. Nevertheless, the outcome is generally good. The majority of patients recover without neurological sequelae, because this type of ICH causes minimal parenchymal destruction, as compared with other forms of supratentorial ICH.

Thalamic Hemorrhage

Thalamic hemorrhage represents 10–15% of the cases of ICH (Kase et al. 1998) (Figure 57B.9). Its onset tends to be more abrupt than that of putaminal hemorrhage, and slow progression of deficits is less common. These features may reflect early communication of the medially located hematoma with the third ventricle. The prognosis in thalamic hemorrhage relates to hematoma size. There is a lack of correlation between survival and ventricular extension of the hemorrhage, again documenting that hematoma size, not ventricular extension *per se*, is the most crucial factor related to the vital prognosis in ICH. Another reliable sign of poor prognosis in thalamic ICH is the presence of hydrocephalus, a complication that occasionally occurs abruptly, as a result of aqueductal obstruction by an intraventricular clot.

Lobar Hemorrhage

Lobar hemorrhage is second to putaminal hemorrhage in frequency, accounting for approximately 25% of the cases (Kase et al. 1998) (Figure 57B.10). Nonhypertensive mechanisms, including AVMs, sympathomimetic agents (in

FIGURE 57B.7 Right putaminal hemorrhage.

young patients), and CAA (in elderly patients) are frequent causes. The peripheral (subcortical) location of these hematomas explains the lower frequency of coma at onset, as compared with the deep ganglionic forms of supratentorial ICH. The clinical features reflect location: hemiparesis of upper limb predominance in frontal hematomas, sensorimotor deficit and hemianopia in parietal hemorrhages, fluent aphasia with relatively preserved repetition in dominant temporal hematomas, and homonymous hemianopia in occipital lobe hemorrhages. The mortality rate in lobar ICH is lower than in hematomas in other locations, and the long-term functional outcome may be better also.

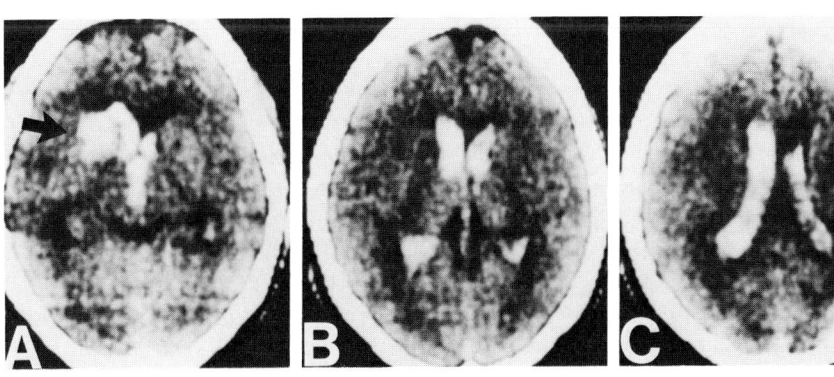

FIGURE 57B.8 Left caudate hemorrhage (*arrow*) (**A**), with extension into the lateral and third ventricles (**A–C**).

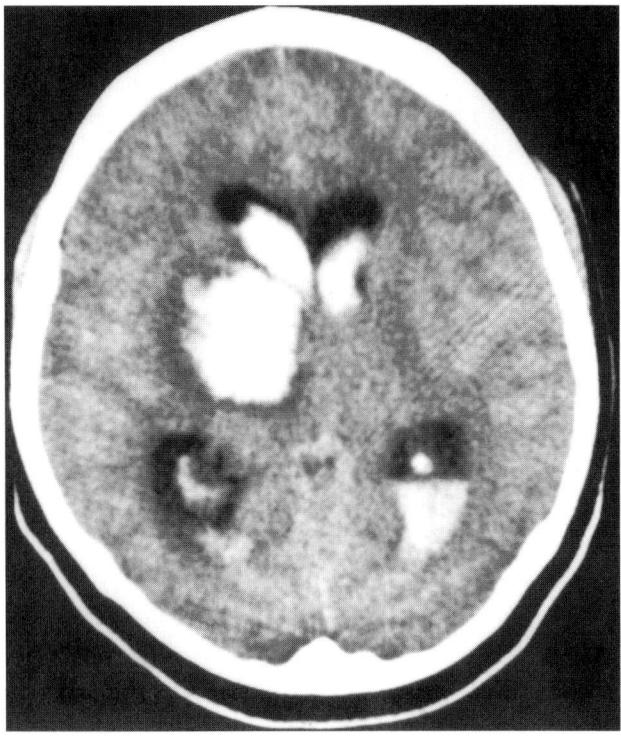

FIGURE 57B.9   Right thalamic hemorrhage with ventricular extension.

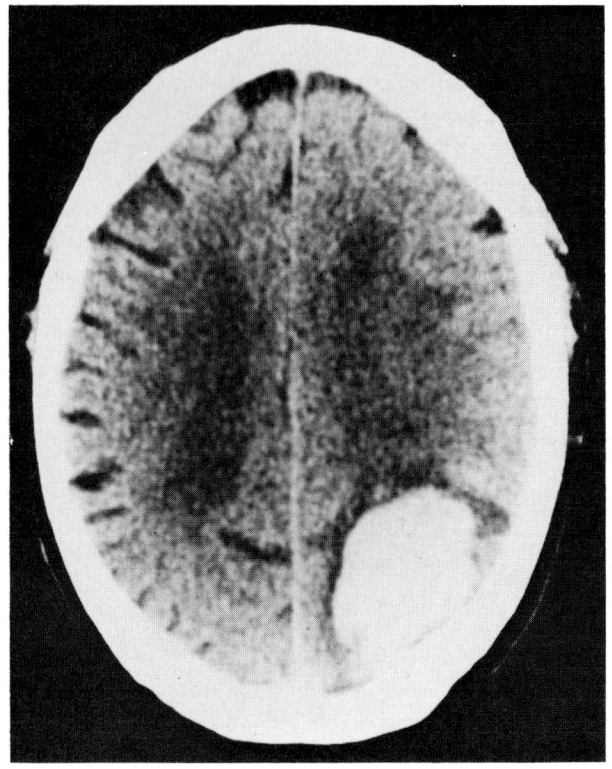

FIGURE 57B.10   Right parieto-occipital lobar hemorrhage.

Cerebellar Hemorrhage

Cerebellar hemorrhage represents approximately 5–10% of the cases (Kase et al. 1998) (Figure 57B.11). Its clinical presentation is characteristic, with abrupt onset of vertigo, headache, vomiting, and inability to stand and walk, with absence of hemiparesis or hemiplegia. The physical findings that allow its clinical diagnosis are the triad of ipsilateral appendicular ataxia, horizontal gaze palsy, and peripheral facial palsy (Kase 1994b).

The clinical course in cerebellar hemorrhage can be difficult to predict at onset. There is a notorious tendency for abrupt deterioration to coma and death, after a period of clinical stability under hospital observation. This unpredictable course has stimulated a search for early clinical or CT signs that may separate patients with benign outcome from those who deteriorate clinically with onset of brainstem compression and high mortality.

Pontine Hemorrhage

Pontine hemorrhage represents approximately 5% of the cases (Kase et al. 1998) (Figure 57B.12). The massive, bilateral basal-tegmental variety produces the classic picture of coma, quadriplegia, decerebrate posturing, horizontal ophthalmoplegia, ocular bobbing, pinpoint reactive pupils (for which a magnifying glass may be required to allow detec-

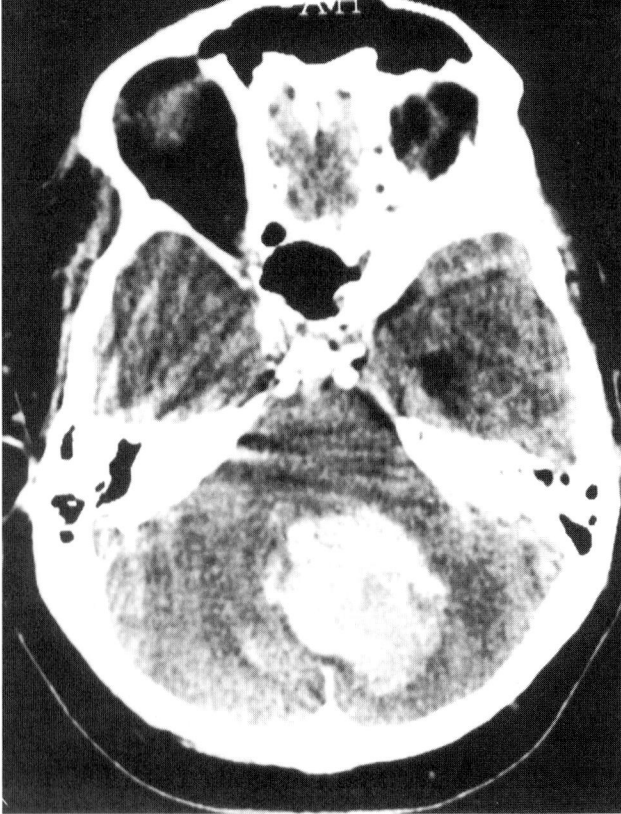

FIGURE 57B.11   Large midline and left-sided hemispheric cerebellar hemorrhage.

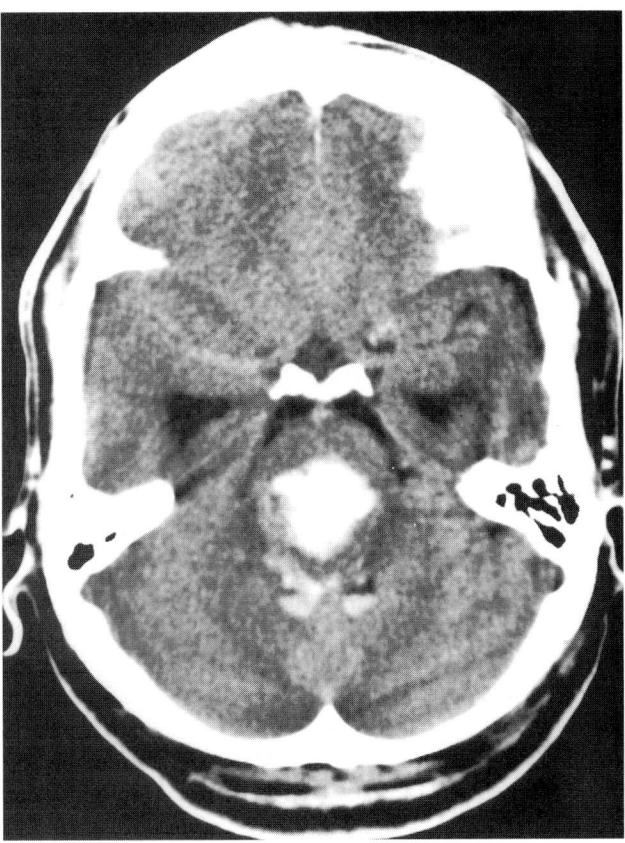

FIGURE 57B.12   Large tegmento-basal pontine hemorrhage with hydrocephalus of temporal horns.

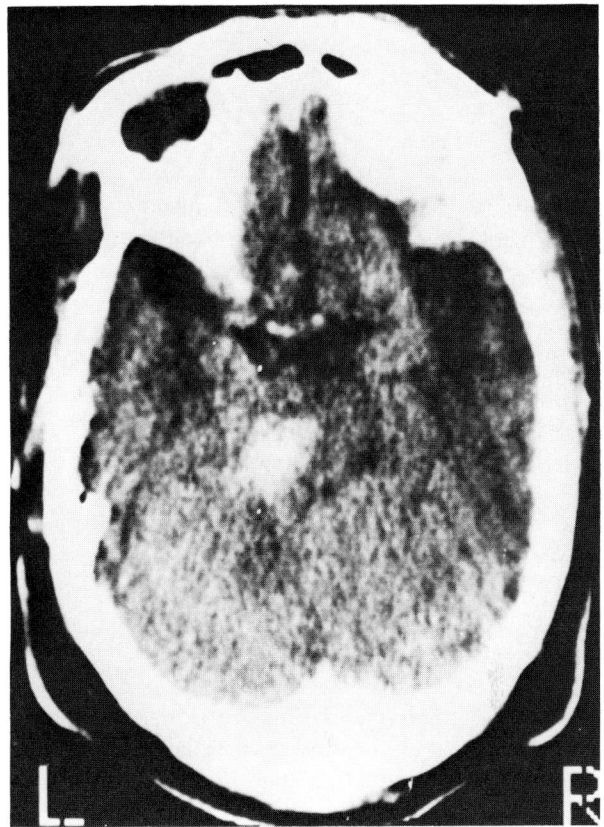

FIGURE 57B.13   Left tegmental pontine hemorrhage.

tion of the light reflex), abnormalities of respiratory rhythm, and preterminal hyperthermia. Since the introduction of CT and MRI scanning, less severe forms of pontine hemorrhage are recognized that are compatible with survival. These hemorrhages are frequently located in the tegmentum, lateral to the midline (Figure 57B.13), and thus produce syndromes of predominantly unilateral pontine cranial nerve involvement ("one-and-a-half" syndrome, internuclear ophthalmoplegia, fifth and seventh nerve palsies), with variable degrees of long-tract interruption. These hematomas probably result from rupture of distal tegmental branches of a long circumferential artery originating from the basilar trunk.

Mesencephalic Hemorrhage

Mesencephalic hemorrhage is exceptionally rare (Kase et al. 1998). The etiological mechanism is hypertension or ruptured AVM in one-half of the reported cases, the others being of undetermined cause. Occasional unilateral hematomas (Figure 57B.14) can present with ipsilateral third nerve palsy and cerebellar ataxia, with contralateral hemiparesis. Bilateral cases frequently have prominent tectal-tegmental signs, with bilateral ptosis, paralysis of upward gaze, and small pupils with light-near dissociation

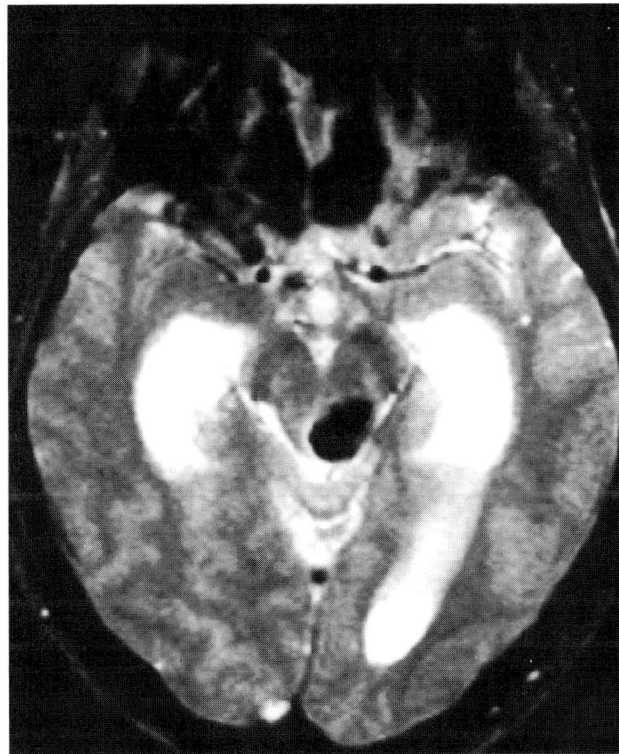

FIGURE 57B.14   Gradient-echo (T2) magnetic resonance imaging scan of left tegmental midbrain hemorrhage.

(see Chapter 23). Most patients survive without surgical treatment, but with persistent sequelae.

Medullary Hemorrhage

Examples of pure primary ICH involving the medulla alone are rare, with most reported cases representing medullary extension of caudal pontine hematomas. The clinical presentation of primary medullary hemorrhage reflects the location of the lesion on one-half of the medulla, generally extending beyond the dorsolateral region, both medially (resulting in ipsilateral hypoglossal nerve palsy) and ventrally (resulting in contralateral hemiparesis) (Barinagarrementeria and Cantu 1994). These two features distinguish most examples of medullary hemorrhage from the classical presentations of Wallenberg's lateral medullary syndrome, caused by infarction rather than hemorrhage (see Chapter 23).

Intraventricular Hemorrhage

Extension of hemorrhage into the ventricular system is a common feature of caudate and thalamic hemorrhages and of large putaminal and lobar hemorrhages. As a primary form, not associated with a component of intraparenchymal bleeding, intraventricular hemorrhage is rare, accounting for only approximately 3% of ICHs (Caplan 1994b). The site of origin of the hemorrhage is thought to be the vasculature of the subependymal region, but rarely the source can be identified in the choroid plexus.

The causes of intraventricular hemorrhage are similar to those of ICH elsewhere, including hypertension, aneurysm, AVM, coagulation disorders, cerebral tumors, cocaine use, and rare vasculopathies, such as moyamoya disease. Those from aneurysm rupture are generally caused by an anterior communicating artery aneurysm that ruptures in an upward direction, bleeding directly into one of the lateral ventricles; in these instances, basal frontal subarachnoid hemorrhage and interhemispheric hemorrhage accompany the intraventricular hemorrhage and should always raise the diagnostic suspicion of a ruptured aneurysm. AVMs that cause purely intraventricular hemorrhage are generally small and located in the medial aspect of the basal ganglia or thalamus. Rarely, an intraventricular AVM or cavernous angioma may cause a primary intraventricular hemorrhage.

The clinical presentation of intraventricular hemorrhage is of acute onset of headache, nausea, vomiting, and decreased level of consciousness, with focal neurological deficits either minimal or altogether absent. This presentation is identical to that of subarachnoid hemorrhage from ruptured aneurysm or AVM. If focal deficits such as hemiparesis or ocular motor disturbances are prominent, the picture is not strictly that of a pure intraventricular hemorrhage, but rather one of primary ICH with ventricular extension.

Intraventricular hemorrhage can be diagnosed reliably with CT and MRI, the latter being more sensitive for the detection of a small component of subependymal, intraparenchymal hemorrhage. Also, MRI can suggest a diagnosis of aneurysm, AVM, or cavernous angioma as the mechanism of the hemorrhage. Even after extensive testing, many intraventricular hemorrhages remain of unknown mechanism.

The prognosis of intraventricular hemorrhage is strongly dependent on the severity of the initial presentation and its mechanism. Patients who are comatose as a result of the initial hemorrhage generally succumb, especially if they have early signs of brainstem involvement (ophthalmoparesis, loss of pupillary reflexes, decerebrate rigidity). Those who remain alert or obtunded, without signs of parenchymal involvement, tend to recover without neurological sequelae, although memory disturbances may be a relatively frequent residual deficit (Caplan 1994b). Patients with the idiopathic form of intraventricular hemorrhage have the best prognosis.

TREATMENT OF INTRACEREBRAL HEMORRHAGE

Issues related to treatment of ICH have been dominated by two main considerations: (1) the type and intensity of medical interventions required to improve the functional and vital prognosis, and (2) the choice between medical and surgical therapy. To a great extent, these two important aspects of treatment remain unclarified, largely as the result of a remarkable paucity of prospective clinical trials. These two issues are discussed separately.

General Management of Intracerebral Hemorrhage

Because ICH is associated frequently with increased ICP, most of the therapies used in this setting are directed at lowering ICP or preventing its increase. Among the many medications and procedures available, a small group has come into customary use in most institutions, despite their value not being proven in properly controlled studies.

Initial Evaluation

On arrival in the emergency department, patients with ICH need to be immediately evaluated for stabilization of vital signs and airway protection. If the patient has a depressed level of consciousness, with a Glasgow Coma Scale score of 8 or less, endotracheal intubation should follow (see Chapter 5, Table 5.4). This is best performed by using short-acting agents such as thiopental (1–5 mg/kg) or lidocaine (1 mg/kg) to block the increases in ICP that result from tracheal stimulation.

Laboratory test data on presentation with ICH should include coagulation studies, especially in instances of hemorrhage in patients receiving anticoagulants or previously treated with thrombolytic agents. Coagulation abnormalities in patients receiving anticoagulants should be treated emergently, because if anticoagulation is not reversed it can lead to progressive enlargement of the hematoma. Patients with ICH in the setting of heparin anticoagulation should be treated with protamine sulfate, 1 mg per 100 units of heparin estimated in plasma (Olson 1993), whereas those on warfarin should receive 5–25 mg of parenteral vitamin K_1 and, most important, fresh frozen plasma (10–20 ml/kg) or prothrombin complex concentrate. Instances of ICH after thrombolytic therapy are best treated with 4–6 units of cryoprecipitate, or fresh frozen plasma, as well as 1 units of single donor platelets. The use of the antifibrinolytic agent aminocaproic acid is controversial because of its increasing the risk of deep vein thrombosis and pulmonary embolism.

Following emergent evaluation of the vital signs and laboratory studies, clinical examination and CT are needed to establish the topography and size of the ICH, which in turn determine the plan for further management. These decisions generally are made in conjunction with a neurosurgical consultant.

General Measures for Prevention of Further Elevation of Intracranial Pressure

General measures include control of hypertension and treatment of seizures. The former can be necessary because persistent hypertension, by causing increased cerebral perfusion pressure, may produce an increase in cerebral edema around the ICH, with further elevation of ICP. However, this potential benefit of antihypertensive therapy must be balanced against the possible harmful effects of drug-induced hypotension with resulting cerebral ischemia and further neurological deterioration. This difficult clinical problem is compounded by the lack of knowledge concerning optimal balance between adequate cerebral perfusion and control of ICP. Pharmacological correction of severe hypertension is mandatory in the acute phases of ICH, with the aim being maintenance of normal cerebral perfusion pressure levels, on the order of 50–70 mm Hg (Ropper 1993), and a mean arterial pressure below 130 mm Hg (Diringer 1993). The antihypertensive agent of choice in this setting is the intravenous beta- and alpha-blocking agent labetalol, often used in combination with loop diuretics. Although theoretically contraindicated because of their cerebral vasodilator properties, nitroprusside and hydralazine are the most appropriate choices when labetalol fails to control the blood pressure. These agents, in particular nitroprusside, have the advantage of being very effective and easy to titrate, and the feared side effect of increased ICP caused by cerebral vasodilation is rarely, if ever, of clinical consequence.

Seizures, a feature of the lobar rather than deep ganglionic varieties, typically occur at ICH onset. In patients who did not have early seizures, there is a negligible risk of late epilepsy. Thus, the routine prophylactic use of anticonvulsants in patients with ICH is not justified. Early tonic-clonic convulsions need immediate control because they can contribute to increased ICP. The major anticonvulsants are of comparable value in this situation.

Specific Treatment of Increased Intracranial Pressure

The mainstays of treatment of intracranial hypertension have been hyperventilation, diuretic therapy, and corticosteroids. Hyperventilation is most effective in rapidly lowering intracranial hypertension, usually within minutes of achieving levels of hypocapnia in the range of 25–30 mm Hg. Intravenous mannitol (0.25–1.00 g/kg), a rapid and reliable way of lowering ICP, is frequently used along with hyperventilation in situations of neurological deterioration with impending herniation. The value of corticosteroids has not been proved, although dexamethasone is used frequently with the hope of decreasing intracranial hypertension by reducing cerebral edema.

Intensive monitoring of ICP with aggressive medical treatment of intracranial hypertension appears to improve the outcome of comatose patients with ICH. In addition, failure to control raised ICP with these measures can be used as an objective indicator that surgical evacuation of the hematoma is required, because persistently elevated ICP under these circumstances results invariably in progression to coma and death.

Choice between Medical and Surgical Therapy in Intracerebral Hemorrhage

A direct surgical approach is considered frequently in patients with superficial (lobar) hematomas of the cerebral hemispheres or with cerebellar hemorrhage, whereas patients with deep hemorrhages (caudate, thalamic, pontine, mesencephalic, and medullary in location) are rarely, if ever, surgical candidates. Putaminal hemorrhage occupies an intermediate position and is most controversial. Few scientific data are available to assist the clinician in this therapeutic choice.

Four randomized clinical trials compared surgical with nonsurgical treatment of ICH, and the results were generally inconclusive, mostly because of methodological issues (Kase and Crowell 1994). A well-designed, prospective, multicenter clinical trial is required to answer this important clinical question, and at the same time evaluate conventional craniotomy against other newer surgical approaches.

A promising technique for surgical treatment of intracerebral hematomas involves the stereotactic drainage of the hemorrhage with the aid of local instillation of a fibrinolytic agent (urokinase). The introduction of the draining

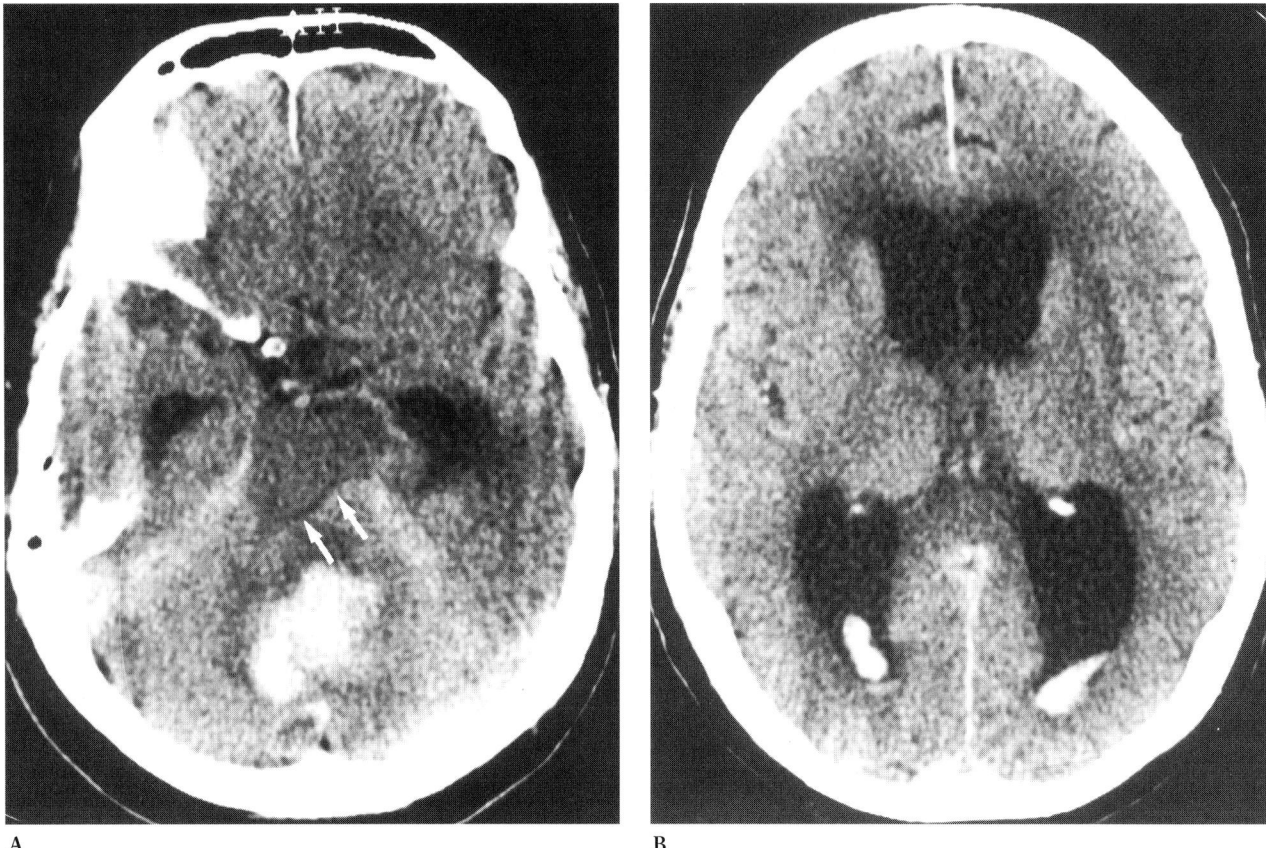

A   **B**

FIGURE 57B.15   Midline cerebellar hemorrhage with brainstem distortion, obliteration of quadrigeminal cistern (*arrows*) (**A**), and supratentorial hydrocephalus (**B**).

cannula is done under local anesthesia and CT guidance, and the procedure allows repeated drainage of liquefied portions of the hematoma following local urokinase infusion. This can achieve the removal of as much as 80% of the hematoma, without the need for craniotomy. This technique may have a role in the surgical management of deep-seated thalamic or putaminal hematomas, as well as in patients considered to be too high-risk for hematoma drainage through a craniotomy under general anesthesia.

Because of the lack of prospective data on randomized trials of therapy in ICH, most patients are currently treated nonsurgically, with the exception of those with putaminal and lobar hemorrhage with progressive deterioration in the level of consciousness, and most instances of cerebellar hemorrhage. Patients with putaminal and lobar ICH who undergo a steady decline in level of consciousness, with onset of coma, have a mortality of 100% with medical therapy. On the basis of this consideration, occasional patients with putaminal ICH are treated surgically, with a slight improvement in survival rates, but without any demonstrated improvement in functional outcome. This raises a difficult ethical dilemma of improved survival with poor quality of life in patients with massive basal ganglionic ICHs, in whom severe hemiplegia, hemisensory loss, and aphasia or hemi-inattention syndromes are the expected permanent sequelae. A somewhat less pes-

simistic picture exists in the case of lobar ICH with progressing mass effect. The surgically more accessible superficial hematomas suggest the potential for less devastating neurological sequelae, thus justifying surgery in selected cases. The most likely candidates for surgery are patients with lobar hemorrhages of intermediate size (hematoma volumes between 20 and 40 ml), who have a decline in level of consciousness or marked mass effect by CT scan.

The other group for whom surgery is frequently considered includes patients with cerebellar hemorrhage. Although a benign outcome without surgical evacuation is well documented in small cerebellar hemorrhages, the potential for sudden deterioration to coma and death, not infrequently after a clinically stable course under hospital observation, is well recognized. CT criteria for early selection of candidates for surgical therapy are large hematomas (diameter of 3 cm or more), presence of hydrocephalus, and obliteration of the quadrigeminal cistern (Figure 57B.15). In addition to these CT features, early signs of pontine tegmental compression and development of obtundation and extensor plantar responses constitute indications for emergency surgical therapy, because the outcome is otherwise uniformly fatal.

In addition to direct evacuation of a hematoma, there is the option of ventricular drainage for the relief of hydrocephalus and increased ICP in cases of cerebellar, thalamic, and caudate ICH. In cerebellar hemorrhage, massive hydrocephalus can be a major cause of clinical deterioration, and ventricular drainage may provide dramatic improvement. Because ventricular drainage does not diminish compression of the brainstem, however, and because of the potential for upward transtentorial cerebellar herniation following decompression of the supratentorial ventricular system, this approach can be only rarely the sole form of surgical treatment. It may, however, be used immediately before occipital craniectomy for wide decompression of the posterior fossa and hematoma drainage. Patients with thalamic hemorrhage occasionally show a prompt reversal of ocular motor signs, coma, or both, after ventricular drainage.

The value of these methods of management of ICH needs assessment by a prospective, multicenter, randomized trial of surgical versus nonsurgical treatment of ICH.

REFERENCES

Barinagarrementeria F, Cantu C. Primary medullary hemorrhage: report of four cases and review of the literature. Stroke 1994;25:1684–1687.

Broderick J, Brott T, Tomsick T, et al. Lobar hemorrhage in the elderly: the undiminishing importance of hypertension. Stroke 1993;24:49–51.

Brott T, Broderick J, Kothari R, et al. Early hemorrhage growth in patients with intracerebral hemorrhage. Stroke 1997;28:1–5.

Bruno A, Carter S, Qualls C, et al. Incidence of spontaneous intracerebral hemorrhage among Hispanics and non-Hispanic whites in New Mexico. Neurology 1996;47:405–408.

Caplan LR. Hypertensive Intracerebral Hemorrhage. In CS Kase, LR Caplan (eds), Intracerebral Hemorrhage. Stoneham, MA: Butterworth–Heinemann, 1994a;99–116.

Caplan LR. Primary Intraventricular Hemorrhage. In CS Kase, LR Caplan (eds), Intracerebral Hemorrhage. Stoneham, MA: Butterworth–Heinemann, 1994b;383–401.

Diringer MN. Intracerebral hemorrhage: pathophysiology and management. Crit Care Med 1993;21:1591–1603.

Gil-Nagel A, Dubovsky J, Wilcox KJ, et al. Familial cerebral cavernous angioma: a gene localized to a 15-cM interval on chromosome 7q. Ann Neurol 1996;39:807–810.

Halpin SFS, Britton JA, Byrne JV, et al. Prospective evaluation of cerebral angiography and computed tomography in cerebral haematoma. J Neurol Neurosurg Psychiatry 1994;57: 1180–1186.

Hart RG, Boop BS, Anderson DC. Oral anticoagulants and intracranial hemorrhage: facts and hypotheses. Stroke 1995;26:1471–1477.

Kase CS. Aneurysms and Vascular Malformations. In CS Kase, LR Caplan (eds), Intracerebral Hemorrhage. Stoneham MA: Butterworth–Heinemann, 1994a;153–178.

Kase CS. Cerebellar Hemorrhage. In CS Kase, LR Caplan (eds), Intracerebral Hemorrhage. Stoneham, MA: Butterworth–Heinemann, 1994b;425–443.

Kase CS, Crowell RM. Prognosis and Treatment of Patients with Intracerebral Hemorrhage. In CS Kase, LR Caplan (eds), Intracerebral Hemorrhage. Stoneham, MA: Butterworth–Heinemann, 1994;467–489.

Kase CS, Mohr JP, Caplan LR. Intracerebral Hemorrhage. In HJM Barnett, JP Mohr, BM Stein, et al. (eds), Stroke: Pathophysiology, Diagnosis and Management (3rd ed). Philadelphia: Saunders, 1998;649–700.

Kazui S, Minematsu K, Yamamoto H, et al. Predisposing factors to enlargement of spontaneous intracerebral hematoma. Stroke 1997;28:2370–2375.

Nolte KB, Brass LM, Fletterick CF. Intracranial hemorrhage associated with cocaine abuse: a prospective autopsy study. Neurology 1996;46:1291–1296.

Olson JD. Mechanisms of hemostasis: effect on intracerebral hemorrhage. Stroke 1993;24(Suppl. I):109–114.

Ropper AH. Treatment of Intracranial Hypertension. In AH Ropper (ed), Neurological and Neurosurgical Intensive Care (3rd ed). New York: Raven, 1993;29–52.

Sloan MA, Price TR, Petito CK, et al. Clinical features and pathogenesis of intracerebral hemorrhage after rt-PA and heparin therapy for myocardial infarction: the Thrombolysis in Myocardial Infarction (TIMI) II Pilot and Randomized Clinical Trial combined experience. Neurology 1995;45:649–658.

The NINDS t-PA Stroke Study Group. Intracerebral hemorrhage after intravenous t-PA therapy for ischemic stroke. Stroke 1997;28:2109–2118.

The Stroke Prevention in Reversible Ischemia Trial (SPIRIT) study group. A randomized trial of anticoagulants versus aspirin after cerebral ischemia of presumed arterial origin. Ann Neurol 1997;42:857–865.

Wijdicks EFM, Jack CR. Intracerebral hemorrhage after fibrinolytic therapy for acute myocardial infarction. Stroke 1993; 24:554–557.

Chapter 57
Vascular Diseases of the Nervous System

C. INTRACRANIAL ANEURYSMS AND SUBARACHNOID HEMORRHAGE
Warren R. Selman, Robert W. Tarr, and Robert A. Ratcheson

The importance of proper management of patients with intracranial aneurysms cannot be overestimated. The spectrum of neurological disorders produced by aneurysms ranges from the asymptomatic unruptured aneurysm to the ruptured aneurysm that produces debilitating stroke and death. The most devastating consequences of intracranial aneurysms are from the complications of subarachnoid hemorrhage (SAH). This chapter emphasizes strategies to prevent or ameliorate these complications.

CLINICAL SIGNS

Although intracranial aneurysms are the most common cause of SAH, not all aneurysms rupture. With the increased use of noninvasive imaging capable of visualizing the intracranial vasculature, many aneurysms are discovered incidentally. With better understanding of the natural history of aneurysms and improvement in surgical and anesthetic management, the attitude regarding proper management of these incidental aneurysms has evolved toward a greater inclination to obliterate the aneurysm electively.

The classic signs of a major aneurysmal rupture include a sudden explosive headache, loss of consciousness, photophobia, meningismus, nausea, and vomiting. Because the prognosis is better if treatment occurs before these signs develop, it is important that the signs and symptoms associated with aneurysmal expansion or a minor hemorrhage

become equally well known. Warning signs are frequently present hours, days, weeks, or longer before catastrophic hemorrhage. Sentinel headaches occur in approximately one-half of patients before rupture, and many others have nausea, neck ache, lethargy, or photophobia. These symptoms are presumably caused by a noncatastrophic leak of the aneurysm and may be confirmed by demonstrating red blood cells or xanthochromia in the cerebrospinal fluid.

Localized headache may accompany expansion of an aneurysm before rupture. Hemorrhage into the wall of an aneurysm can produce thunderclap headache associated with aneurysmal enlargement in the absence of red blood cells in the cerebrospinal fluid (Ostergaard 1993). Thus, the absence of blood in the cerebrospinal fluid in a patient with a characteristic history may not be enough to exclude the possibility of a symptomatic aneurysm. Such patients should undergo, at least, noninvasive imaging of the cerebral vessels with magnetic resonance angiography (MRA) or spiral computed tomographic (CT) angiography, and if these studies are inadequate or if questions remain, then formal cerebral angiography.

Aneurysms may give evidence of growth before rupture. Premonitory signs, which may be attributable to aneurysmal enlargement, include visual field deficits, extraocular movement abnormalities, orbital or facial pain, or localized head pain (Weir 1994). The difficulty of diagnosing an aneurysm before a major hemorrhage occurs can be appreciated by considering the common occurrence of the alternative diag-

Table 57C.1: Hunt and Hess and World Federation of Neurological Surgeons Scales

Hunt and Hess Scale
    Grade 0: Asymptomatic
    Grade I: Slight headache, no neurological deficit
    Grade II: Severe headache but no neurological deficit other
      than perhaps a cranial nerve palsy
    Grade III: Drowsiness and mild deficit
    Grade IV: Stupor, moderate to severe hemiparesis, and
      possible early rigidity and vegetative disturbances
    Grade V: Deep coma, decerebrate rigidity, and moribund
      appearance
World Federation of Neurological Surgeons Scale
    Grade I: GCS 15; motor deficit absent
    Grade II: GCS 13 or 14; motor deficit absent
    Grade III: GCS 13 or 14; motor deficit present
    Grade IV: GCS 7–12; motor deficit absent or present
    Grade V: GCS 3–6; motor deficit absent or present

GCS = Glasgow Coma Scale.

noses, including migraine headache, meningitis, tension headache, sinusitis, and influenza. The high morbidity and mortality associated with SAH mandate a high degree of suspicion to allow appropriate treatment of patients whose symptoms indicate they may harbor intracranial aneurysms.

PHYSICAL FINDINGS

The physical findings in patients with unruptured aneurysms may be determined in part by the size and location of the aneurysm, although few aneurysms can be diagnosed with confidence on the basis of clinical presentation alone. Thus, aneurysms arising from the anterior communicating artery can produce visual field defects, endocrine dysfunction, or localized frontal headache. Aneurysms of the internal carotid artery can produce oculomotor paresis, visual field deficits, impaired visual acuity, endocrine dysfunction, and localized facial pain. Aneurysms arising from the internal carotid artery in the cavernous sinus, unless they rupture to produce a carotid cavernous fistula, can be responsible for the cavernous sinus syndrome. Intracavernous aneurysms greater than 1 cm in diameter account for 15% of all symptomatic unruptured aneurysms. Those of the middle cerebral artery can produce dysphasia, focal arm weakness, or paresthesias. Basilar bifurcation aneurysms can be associated with oculomotor paresis, although the clinical features of posterior circulation aneurysms seldom permit diagnosis before they rupture.

Of primary importance is altered oculomotor nerve function. This nerve is affected most commonly by an internal carotid artery aneurysm arising at or near the origin of the posterior communicating artery. Much less frequently, an aneurysm of the posterior circulation may affect this nerve. Because the pupilloconstrictor fibers and levator palpebrae fibers lie superficially, a third nerve palsy secondary to an aneurysm usually is associated with a dilated pupil and pto-

sis, whereas an ischemic lesion of the nerve, such as in patients with diabetes, usually spares the pupil. However, this point is not clinically reliable, and in most cases angiography should be performed.

The physical findings in patients with ruptured aneurysms depend in part on the amount and location of the hemorrhage. Aneurysmal rupture can result in hemorrhage into the subarachnoid space alone or in combination with subdural hematoma, intracerebral hematoma, or intraventricular hemorrhage. Thus, the immediate physical findings can vary from slight meningismus and headache to profound neurological deficits with coma or death.

Disturbances of higher functions, which may vary from lethargy to coma, occur commonly with SAH. Memory disturbances usually do not occur early but may be seen in later stages. Dysphasia is seen rarely in uncomplicated SAH, and its presence suggests an intracerebral hematoma. Dementia and emotional lability are well known, especially with bilateral frontal lobe damage from rupture of an anterior communicating artery aneurysm.

Cranial nerve dysfunction can occur secondary to (1) direct compression by the aneurysm, (2) direct pressure by extravasated blood, or (3) raised intracranial pressure. The optic nerve and its connections are frequently affected by SAH. In a patient with a sudden headache, the finding of subhyaloid hemorrhages is pathognomonic of SAH. These lesions are dark red globular hemorrhages at the posterior pole of the eye, thought to be caused by rapid venous engorgement. They may have a horizontal fluid level in the erect patient. Intraocular hemorrhages occur in approximately 20% of patients with SAH. The optic tract is compromised frequently by internal carotid or large middle cerebral artery aneurysms. Anterior communicating artery aneurysms can affect the optic chiasm, whereas internal carotid aneurysms usually affect the optic nerve.

Disturbances of motor function can be associated with a major SAH. Paralysis can occur as a result of extension of the hemorrhage into the parenchyma, or as a result of extra-axial pressure from a hematoma.

Because treatment and prognosis depend to a great extent on the clinical status of the patient, a grading system based on the neurological presentation of the patient is used routinely. Such systems have been proposed by several authors. The two systems that are in most common use are the Hunt and Hess classification and the World Federation of Neurological Surgeons proposed universal grading scale (Table 57C.1), which is based in part on the Glasgow Coma Scale (see Chapter 5, Table 5.4).

LABORATORY STUDIES

The laboratory evaluation of patients suspected of having a ruptured or unruptured intracranial aneurysm uses a combination of CT scan, magnetic resonance imaging (MRI), lumbar puncture, and angiography.

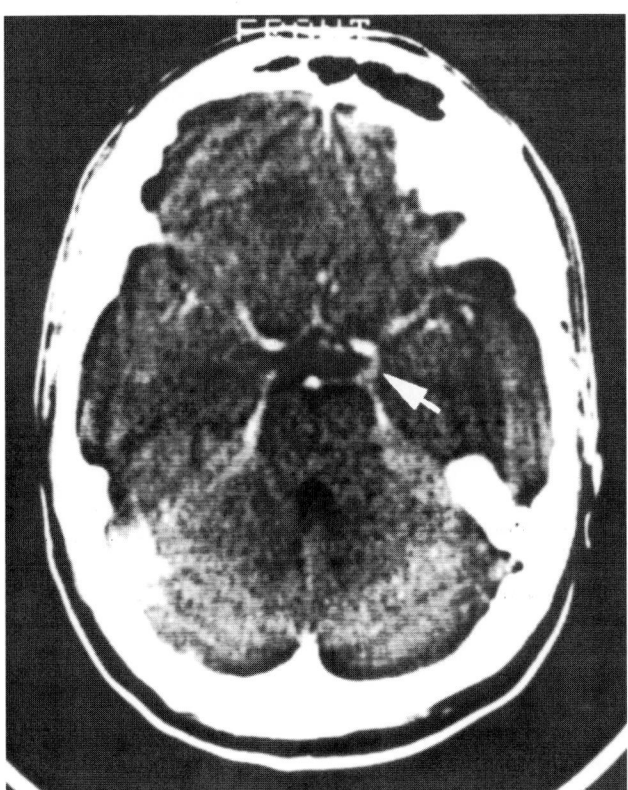

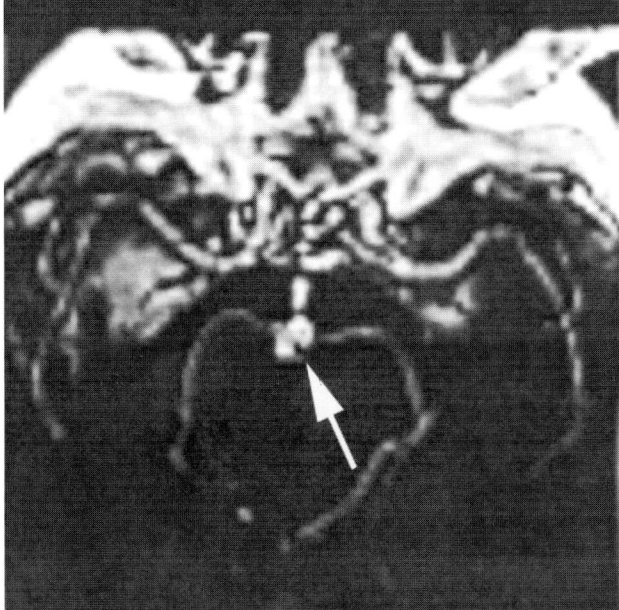

FIGURE 57C.2   Computed tomographic angiogram demonstrating the anatomical relation of the basilar tip aneurysm (*arrow*) to adjacent vascular and skull base structures.

FIGURE 57C.1   Postcontrast computed tomographic scan demonstrating a left posterior communicating artery aneurysm (*arrow*).

The CT scan may, on occasion, demonstrate an intracranial aneurysm. Most frequently, these are large or giant aneurysms with peripheral calcification on an unenhanced scan and central dense enhancement on contrasted studies (Figure 57C.1). Such aneurysms may be quite large and mimic intracranial neoplasms. Smaller aneurysms also have been detected with high-resolution CT.

CT angiography with three-dimensional reconstruction can be a useful aid to understanding the morphology of the aneurysm and its relationship to adjacent normal vessels (Figure 57C.2). Because CT angiography uses intravascular contrast it is not hampered to the extent that MRA is by flow-related artifacts. CT angiography has another advantage over MRA in that it is able to detect calcium within the wall of the aneurysm. Such a finding may have an effect on the therapy.

MRI also can detect intracranial aneurysms (Figure 57C.3). The recent development of different pulse sequences has made MRA possible. MRA has the ability to visualize aneurysms as small as 4 mm, and unlike CT angiography, does not require administration of contrast material. Both of these studies are considered noninvasive and are not associated with the risks of invasive conventional cerebral angiography. With improved resolution, these studies may become a practical screening test for unruptured intracranial aneurysms.

The CT scan is indispensable for delineating the amount and location of blood in the subarachnoid space (Figure 57C.4). The sooner the CT scan is performed in relation to the suspected hemorrhage, the greater the likelihood of visualizing blood. In the setting of a suspected acute SAH, CT, not MRI, remains the procedure of choice because MRI is less effective in detecting blood early after the rupture of an aneurysm. The location of the blood can indicate the site of aneurysmal rupture. Blood in the basal cisterns is seen with ruptured aneurysms in any location, but is most common with those of the internal carotid and basilar artery. Blood in the sylvian fissure is most common in middle cerebral artery aneurysms. Intraventricular blood is associated with anterior communicating and basilar artery aneurysms. Intracerebral hemorrhages of the frontal lobe can be seen with anterior communicating artery aneurysms, and those of the temporal lobe with middle cerebral artery aneurysms.

SAH is not always detected by CT scan. The amount of extravasated blood and the time interval between the SAH and the scan affect the percentage of negative study results. Modern-generation CT scanners can detect the presence of acute SAH in 90–95% of patients who undergo a scan within 24 hours after the hemorrhage. The sensitivity decreases to 80% at 72 hours. A negative CT scan result in a patient with the appropriate history of SAH should be followed by a lumbar puncture. If the CT scan demonstrates a characteristic SAH, there is little to be gained by performing a lumbar puncture.

If either the CT scan or the lumbar puncture is positive for SAH, an angiogram should be obtained. Angiography

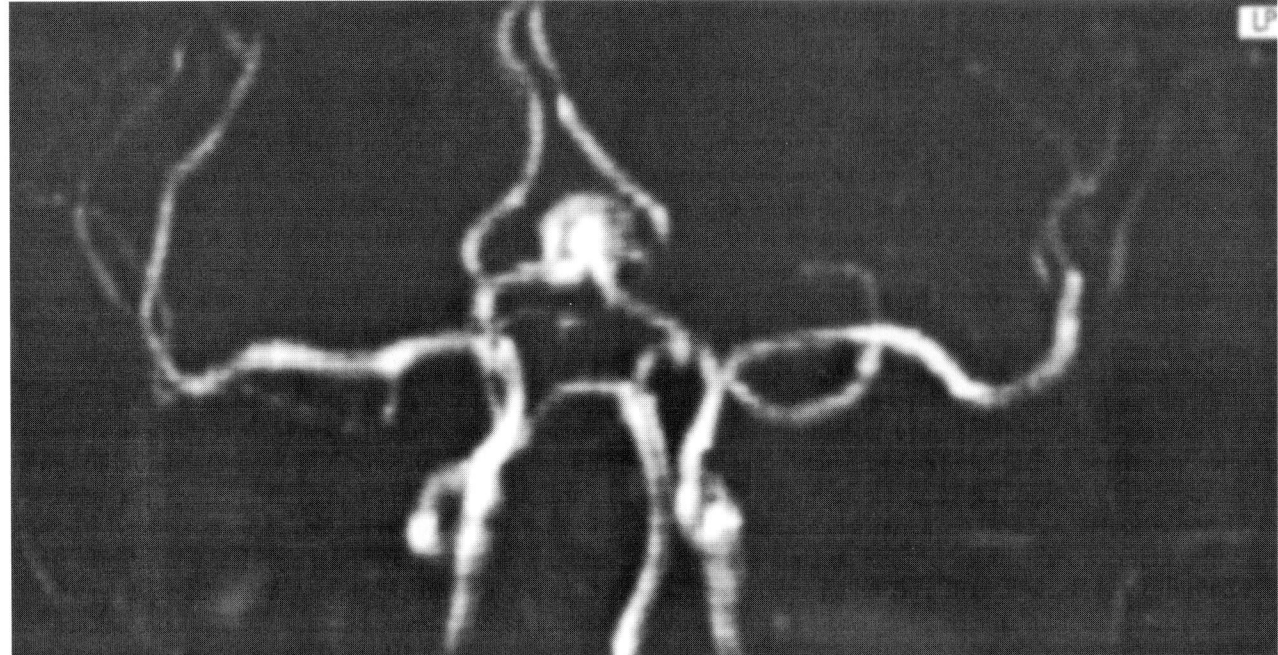

A

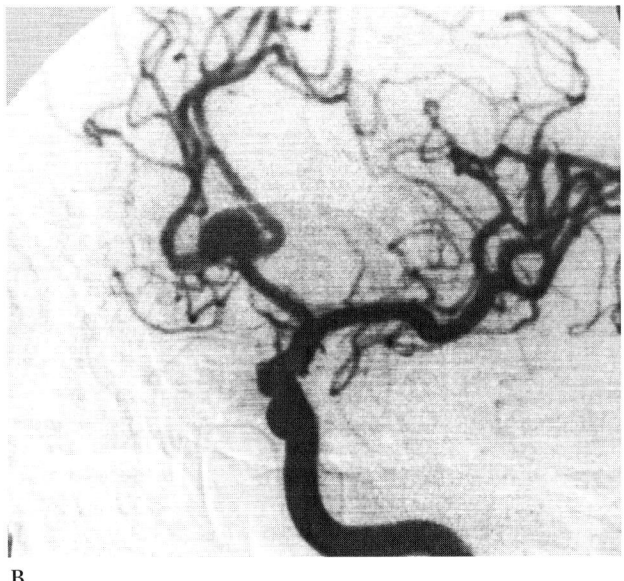

B

FIGURE 57C.3 (A) Three-dimensional time-of-flight magnetic resonance angiogram reveals an aneurysm of the anterior communicating artery. (B) Left internal carotid artery angiogram, which confirmed the anterior communicating artery aneurysm demonstrated on the magnetic resonance angiogram.

should be performed as soon as reasonably possible so that appropriate therapeutic measures can be undertaken. Four-vessel angiography should be carried out because multiple aneurysms occur in approximately 20% of patients. The goals of angiography are to identify the cause of the hemorrhage and, if an aneurysm is present, to delineate its neck and the relationship to surrounding vessels. Several views may be required to fulfill these goals. The aneurysm is named according to its vessel of origin. Approximately 80–85% of aneurysms arise from arteries located in the anterior circulation, the majority of which occur on the posterior communicating artery, the

anterior communicating artery, or the trifurcation of the middle cerebral artery. Between 15% and 20% of aneurysms arise from the posterior circulation, the majority of which occur at the bifurcation of the basilar artery or at the origin of the posterior inferior cerebellar artery on the vertebral artery.

ANEURYSM PATHOGENESIS AND ETIOLOGY

Several classifications of aneurysms have been proposed. That suggested by Weir is summarized in Table 57C.2. This

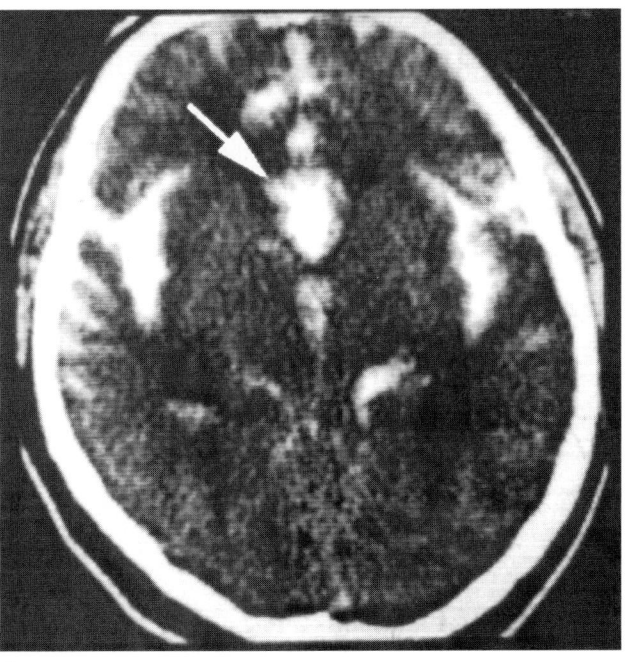

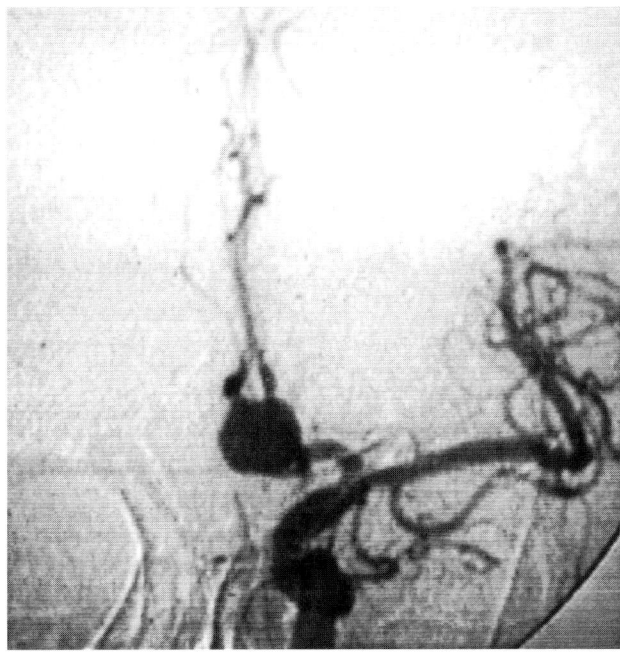

A   B

FIGURE 57C.4 (A) Uncontrasted computed tomography shows diffuse subarachnoid hemorrhage. Note blood in the septum pellucidum indicative of an anterior communicating artery aneurysm. (B) Left internal carotid artery angiogram confirmed the location of the anterior communicating artery aneurysm.

morphological classification is helpful in defining the different natural history of these lesions. Intracranial aneurysms are classified on the basis of their morphology as either saccular, fusiform, or dissecting. Further classification on the basis of presumed cause is also possible.

Saccular Aneurysms

Saccular or berry aneurysms are the most common form of aneurysms and are most often responsible for aneurysmal subarachnoid hemorrhage. Saccular aneurysms may arise from defects in the muscular layer of cerebral arteries that occur at vessel bifurcations and from degenerative changes that damage the internal elastic membrane, resulting in weakness of the vessel wall. They usually occur on the first- or second-order arterial branches of the vessel emanating from the circle of Willis. Evidence suggests that both genetic and environmental factors contribute to the development of saccular aneurysms. The evidence that genetic factors are important comes from the documented association of intracranial aneurysms with heritable connective tissue disorders such as autosomal dominant polycystic kidney disease, Ehlers-Danlos syndrome type IV, neurofibromatosis type I, and Marfan's syndrome. The familial occurrence of intracranial aneurysms also points to a role for genetic factors. In those patients who have a first-degree relative with an aneurysmal SAH, the risk of a ruptured aneurysm is four times higher than the risk in the general population. A role

for acquired factors in the pathogenesis of saccular aneurysm is suggested by the mean age of 50 for patients with aneurysmal SAH, and the increase in the incidence of hemorrhage that occurs with age. Cigarette smoking has been identified consistently as a risk factor in all population studies, and a role for systemic hypertension, although not as strong as that of cigarette smoking, in the etiology of aneurysm formation appears likely.

Saccular aneurysms also may result from infection, trauma, or neoplasm. Mycotic aneurysms result from infected emboli that lodge in the arterial intima or the vasa vasorum and account for approximately 5% of all intracranial aneurysms. They are seen most frequently in patients with subacute bacterial endocarditis, congenital heart disease, or a history of intravenous drug use. Such aneurysms usually occur on more distal branches of the cerebral vasculature. Proper management includes appropriate intravenous antibiotic therapy, with surgery in selected cases. Fungal aneurysms, which are much rarer than bacterial, usually are associated with arteritis and thrombosis and have been uniformly fatal.

Traumatic aneurysms are rare but can be associated with either blunt or penetrating head injury. Such aneurysms occur at sites other than bifurcations. Because angiograms are not routinely performed following head trauma, these lesions may not be detected, but they should be considered in patients who suffer delayed deterioration. Early operative repair has been suggested because of the high mortality associated with these lesions.

Table 57C.2:   Surgical classification of intracranial arterial aneurysms

Morphology
  Saccular
  Fusiform
  Dissecting
Size
  <3 mm
  3–6 mm
  7–10 mm
  11–25 mm
  >25 mm (giant)
Location
  Anterior circulation arteries
    Internal carotid
      Carotid canal
      Intracavernous
      Paraclinoid (ophthalmic)
      Posterior communicating region
      Anterior choroidal region
      Carotid bifurcation
    Anterior cerebral
      A1 (main branch)
      Anterior communicating region
      A2 (distal): callosomarginal region or distal
        pericallosal
    Middle cerebral
      M1 (main branch): lenticulostriate or temporal branch
        regions
      Bifurcation
      Peripheral
  Posterior circulation arteries
    Vertebral
      Main trunk
      Posterior inferior cerebellar artery region
    Basilar
      Bifurcation
      Superior cerebellar artery region
      Anterior inferior cerebellar artery region
      Basilar trunk
      Vertebrobasilar junction region
    Posterior cerebral
      P1 (first branches of basilar—distal to apex)
      P2 (distal posterior cerebral)

Source: Reprinted with permission from B Weir. Intracranial Aneurysms and Subarachnoid Hemorrhage: An Overview. In RH Wilkins, SS Rengachary (eds), Neurosurgery. New York: McGraw-Hill, 1985;1309.

Neoplastic embolization, in rare cases, may produce an aneurysm in patients with choriocarcinoma, atrial myxoma, and undifferentiated carcinoma. In forming an aneurysm, the tumor embolus may remain viable, penetrate the endothelium, grow subintimally, and eventually destroy the arterial wall.

Fusiform Aneurysms

Fusiform or dolichoectatic aneurysms are classified separately from saccular aneurysms, although in some patients these types may overlap. The basilar artery is most commonly affected, although these aneurysms also can be seen in the anterior circulation. Only rarely are these lesions associated with SAH. Their presentation is characterized by cranial nerve or brainstem dysfunction secondary to direct compression or by embolization from intraluminal thrombus.

Dissecting Aneurysms

Dissecting aneurysms result from cystic medial necrosis or a traumatic tear in the endothelium and subadjacent layers of the artery, with blood coursing through a false lumen while the true lumen is collapsed on itself. The false lumen may connect with the true lumen distally or may burst through the remaining external arterial wall. Such aneurysms can occur in any portion of the extracranial or intracranial arterial circulation. Trauma is a common cause in the neck and anterior circulation, but is a rare cause in the posterior circulation. Connective tissue diseases such as Marfan's syndrome and other disorders such as fibromuscular dysplasia predispose to arterial dissections. The treatment of these lesions has not been standardized; parent artery occlusion with or without bypass grafting using conventional microsurgical or neuroendovascular techniques may be necessary.

EPIDEMIOLOGY

The incidence and prevalence of intracranial aneurysms and aneurysmal SAH should be considered separately. Intracranial aneurysms are found on postmortem examination in between 1% and 6% of adults in large autopsy series (Schievink 1997). The prevalence of intracranial aneurysm seen during angiography for patients not suspected of harboring an aneurysm is between 0.5% and 1.0%. The overall incidence of SAH from aneurysms is approximately seven per 100,000 people per year (Menghini et al. 1998). Nearly one-half of these individuals die from their SAH.

Various reviews have noted a slight female predominance in series of SAH from aneurysms, with a mean age of hemorrhage of approximately 50 years. Ruptured aneurysms rarely occur in children, and there is a steady increase in the incidence of rupture from 0.3 per 10,000 persons per year between 25 and 34 years of age to 3.7 per 10,000 persons per year for patients 65 years of age or older.

A special category of patients have been defined as those who have a family history of aneurysms and SAH. Familial occurrence of intracranial aneurysms is defined by the presence of aneurysms in two or more first- to third-degree relatives without any known hereditary disease. It is not known whether the pathogenesis of familial intracranial aneurysms differs from that of the general population (Ronkainen et al. 1998). In a community-based study from

Rochester, MN, it was determined that the relative risk of SAH among first-degree relatives of patients with the familial form of SAH was four times higher than the general population. Other studies have shown that in patients with familial intracranial aneurysms, there is a lower mean age at the time of rupture compared with SAH in the general population (Ronkainen et al. 1998). Screening studies, with either MRA, CT angiography, or conventional angiography, for the presence of aneurysms in this group of patients appears warranted.

COURSE OF ANEURYSMAL SUBARACHNOID HEMORRHAGE

The International Cooperative Study on the Timing of Aneurysm Surgery used the Glasgow Outcome Scale to report on outcomes at 6 months following SAH for 3,521 patients and noted the following: 57.6% had good recovery; 9.1% were moderately disabled; 5.5% were severely disabled; 1.8% had vegetative survival; and 26.0% died. Approximately 12% of patients die before reaching a hospital, and approximately 40% of patients who are hospitalized die within 30 days (Olafsson et al. 1997). The total mortality rate in the first year is 63%, and within the first 5 years is 72%. The authors noted little change in the initial mortality and morbidity of patients suffering a SAH over the past several decades and concluded that only the detection and treatment of intracranial aneurysms prior to rupture has any influence on the frequency of sudden death from SAH. The subject of detection and treatment of unruptured aneurysms is discussed in the following section of this chapter.

The outlook for long-term survival is not good. In a study of late morbidity and mortality in patients treated nonoperatively following SAH from a single aneurysm, the main cause of death in patients surviving 6 months was recurrent hemorrhage. Rebleeding occurred at a rate of 3.5% per year during the first decade, and the mortality associated with late rebleeding was 67%.

Functional outcome also must be considered when assessing patient management. Subtle cognitive dysfunction and psychosocial impairment can prevent the return to premorbid lifestyle in up to 20% of survivors. Neuropsychological deficits in fact are common among survivors after SAH. Neuropsychological testing performed 6 months after SAH and craniotomy produced abnormal results in 13 of 15 patients, including 10 patients who had a "good recovery" (Beristain et al. 1996). A prospective study of 89 patients who were alert enough to undergo neuropsychological testing during their initial hospitalization for SAH found cognitive deficits in 76% of patients. Long-term quality of life may be diminished in many SAH survivors in that 41% have memory problems, 35% experience fatigue, 48% undergo personality changes, and 26% complain of insomnia (Ogden et al. 1997). The combination of these changes appears to adversely affect the ability of patients who suffer a SAH to return to work because approximately one-half of SAH survivors do not return to previous full-time employment.

TREATMENT AND PROGNOSIS

Surgery is the cornerstone of therapy. In few other situations in medicine is it as clear that surgery plays such a definitive role. The risk reduction for subsequent SAH afforded by surgery has been well documented in population-based studies (Olafsson et al. 1997). Every effort should be made to direct appropriately selected patients toward surgery as soon as possible. In general, patients in good condition are best managed by *early operative intervention to secure the aneurysm.* The neurosurgeon is able to consider such early intervention because of advances in both microsurgical and neuroendovascular techniques. The benefits of early treatment include prevention of rebleeding, improved prevention and management of delayed ischemic deficits from vasospasm, and a shorter hospital course with potentially fewer complications.

The frequency of major complications as following SAH is as follows: ischemic deficits, 27%; hydrocephalus, 12%; brain swelling, 12%; recurrent hemorrhage, 11%; intracranial hematoma, 8%; pneumonia, 8%; seizures, 5%; gastrointestinal hemorrhage, 4%; syndrome of inappropriate antidiuretic hormone secretion, 4%; and pulmonary edema, 1%. As detailed in the following section, the initial management of patients suffering SAH must proceed rapidly and comprehensively to prevent or lessen the chance of demise because of any of these conditions, but especially the two that produce the greatest morbidity and mortality, rebleeding and delayed ischemic deficits.

Aneurysm rupture can be responsible for a multitude of events that can have severe consequences with respect to systemic and neurological function. Many systems besides the central nervous system (including the cardiovascular system, respiratory system, and endocrine system) can be affected by aneurysm rupture. Both immediate and delayed effects must be anticipated and treated. The initial management of SAH has been detailed (Ratcheson and Wirth 1994). The importance of appropriate intensive care management of patients suffering a hemorrhage has been highlighted by confirmation that secondary insults are associated with a negative effect on clinical outcome (Enblad and Persson 1997).

Although aneurysm rupture almost universally results in SAH, the location of the hemorrhage is not confined to the subarachnoid space. The location of the hemorrhage can affect outcome, and patients with massive intraventricular hemorrhage or intracerebral hematomas tend to die earlier than those with blood in other locations. The consequences of bleeding into the brain parenchyma or ventricles include an elevation of intracranial pressure caused by mass effect and acute hydrocephalus. Either of these conditions may require immediate treatment separately or in combination with definitive aneurysm treatment.

Central Nervous System Complications

Hydrocephalus caused by SAH can be classified as either immediate or delayed. Pertuiset and colleagues in 1972 examined 91 cases of ruptured supratentorial aneurysms. Forty-three percent were associated with ventricular enlargement. Acute dilatation occurs in 20% of patients; it is caused by increased ventricular outflow resistance, appears within 3 days of the SAH, and requires immediate treatment. Delayed ventricular dilatation usually occurs after the tenth day and is seen in 23% of patients. Subsequent studies have shown that the development of acute hydrocephalus appears to be related to the degree of intraventricular blood, whereas the development of delayed hydrocephalus can be correlated with the amount of SAH. Deterioration from hydrocephalus was observed in 22% of 660 patients followed during the first 28 days after admission in a study by Vermeij and colleagues (1994). The sum score of cisternal blood on the initial CT, the presence of ventricular blood, and long-term treatment with antifibrinolytic agents were significantly related to the development of hydrocephalus.

Three percent to 5% of patients with SAH have seizures during their hospitalization. The use of anticonvulsants in the acute stage is considered standard therapy for the prevention of seizures, although there is no documentation that prophylactic anticonvulsant therapy during the acute phase after SAH has any influence on the development of chronic seizures. Epilepsy develops in approximately 15% of patients who suffer a SAH, and it develops within the first 18 months in over 90% of these patients. The greatest risk factors for the development of late epilepsy are poor neurological grade on admission, rupture of a middle cerebral artery aneurysm, cerebral infarction secondary to vasospasm, and shunt-dependent hydrocephalus.

Systemic Complications

Neurogenic pulmonary edema, considered to be a mixed pressure and permeability edema characterized by the rapid onset of respiratory failure with a protein concentration greater than 4.5 g/dl in the edema fluid, may develop in patients who suffer a SAH. Most patients with neurogenic pulmonary edema from SAH are comatose. Although it was initially believed that a massive sympathetic discharge produced generalized vasoconstriction, more recent studies suggest that a direct neurogenic effect on the lungs results in pulmonary capillary endothelial damage. Treatment of this condition includes monitoring, and if possible, reduction of intracranial pressure, mechanical ventilation with positive end-expiratory pressure, and monitoring the cardiovascular status with a Swan-Ganz catheter to attain the lowest pulmonary wedge pressure that maintains an effective cardiac output (Mayer et al. 1994).

Alterations of the electrocardiogram are the most frequent cardiac abnormality in patients with SAH. The most common changes include prolongation of the QT interval, ST-segment elevation or depression, and increased amplitude or deep inversion of the T waves (neurogenic T waves). These abnormalities are believed to result from disturbances of ventricular repolarization caused by a derangement of autonomic control of the heart. These changes are considered to represent epiphenomena that reflect intracranial abnormalities without contributing directly to morbidity or mortality, though at death subendocardial hemorrhages are common.

Hyponatremia usually is associated with the syndrome of inappropriate antidiuretic hormone secretion, but in some patients with SAH, a true natruresis or cerebral salt-wasting syndrome may occur. Assessment of the intravascular volume status, body weight, and blood volume can differentiate these disorders and allow proper treatment. Patients with a true natruresis have evidence of postural hypotension and tachycardia, decreased blood and intravascular volume, elevated hematocrit, and decreased body weight. Sodium and volume replacement are needed for proper treatment. The syndrome of inappropriate antidiuretic hormone secretion (SIADH), on the other hand, is associated with a normal cardiovascular status, a normal or low hematocrit, and normal or increased body weight. The hyponatremia seen in this condition is dilutional or false, as opposed to the true hyponatremia seen with cerebral salt wasting. Symptoms of SIADH depend on both the level of hyponatremia and the rate at which it develops. Although the best therapy is fluid restriction, this is often balanced by the need to maintain a high intravascular volume to prevent the development of delayed ischemic deficits secondary to vasospasm. In either case, it must be remembered that rapid correction is rarely needed, and no more than one-half the sodium deficit should be replaced over the first 24 hours.

Prevention of Repeat Hemorrhage and Delayed Ischemic Deficits

Rebleeding

Historically, the most feared complication for survivors of the initial hemorrhage had been recurrent bleeding, which occurred in approximately 20% of patients and was usually fatal. In recent years, a tendency toward early operation has substantially reduced the risk of rebleeding (Figure 57C.5). Although it appeared that this reduced rate of rebleeding did not result in a decline in overall mortality or an increase in favorable outcome, it must be remembered that this appearance would be based on patients who were treated in the 1970s and 1980s. More recent experience in most major centers with early operative intervention and improved perioperative care would substantiate a much better outcome in patients who undergo early operation.

The improved outcome may be caused not only by a decrease in the devastating consequences of rehemorrhage,

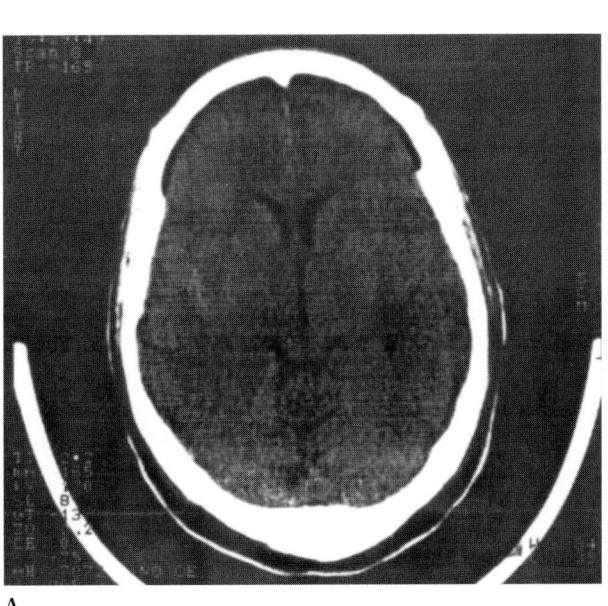
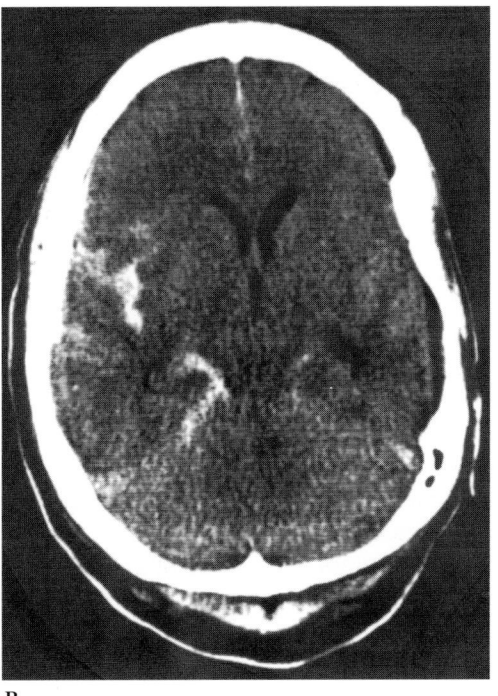

A   B

FIGURE 57C.5   (**A**) Uncontrasted computed tomography shows a subarachnoid hemorrhage in the right sylvian fissure. (**B**) The patient suffered a deterioration in neurological status, and a repeat uncontrasted computed tomographic scan performed 2 hours later shows increased blood indicative of aneurysmal rebleeding.

but also by the ability to provide more effective treatment of vasospasm after the aneurysm has been obliterated. Some studies suggest that cerebral vasospasm and ischemia, the leading causes of death and disability among survivors of an initial aneurysm rupture, negate the benefits of reduced rebleeding following early operation. New treatment options for the prevention and treatment of vasospasm following SAH were not considered in such conclusions. According to the International Cooperative Study on the Timing of Aneurysm Surgery, 13.5% of all patients who experience aneurysmal SAH suffer delayed cerebral ischemia resulting in permanent disability or death. Of the 1,494 patients in that study who died or became disabled, delayed ischemia caused by cerebral vasospasm accounted for 32% of the total; in comparison, the direct effect of aneurysmal rupture resulted in 25% and rebleeding in 17.6% of such outcomes. Nonetheless, it must be remembered that rehemorrhage can be an immediate, devastating, and irreversible event. The consequences of vasospasm evolve more slowly and are now more predictable, preventable, and treatable.

Initial attempts to improve management mortality (i.e., death while awaiting surgery) used medical measures to decrease the incidence of rehemorrhage while waiting for definitive surgery to secure the aneurysm. The control or prevention of systemic hypertension is vital. Mild blood pressure reduction to keep the systolic pressure below 160 mm Hg, or a 10% reduction from known prehemorrhagic values, can usually be tolerated with safety. These mea-

sures alone, however, are not adequate for the prevention of rebleeding.

Pharmacological means to prevent rebleeding have been used, although their role is becoming less important as early operative intervention is more widely practiced. ε-Aminocaproic acid is an antifibrinolytic drug that competitively inhibits the activator that converts plasminogen to plasmin. Inhibition of the breakdown of the blood clot around and within the ruptured aneurysm wall should lessen the chance of rehemorrhage. Antifibrinolytic agents can reduce the rebleeding rate by 25–50% during the second week following the initial hemorrhage, but are associated with various complications, the most serious being related to the development of delayed thrombotic events. There is no change in the overall mortality from SAH when antifibrinolytic agents are used in anticipation of delayed surgery because the decrease in mortality from rebleeding is offset by an increased mortality from ischemic complications. The use of short-term (<24–48 hours) antifibrinolytic therapy may prevent rebleeding before "early" (within 48 hours) surgery without provoking increased ischemic complications, but this treatment regimen remains to be fully evaluated.

As the pathophysiological alterations following aneurysmal SAH have become more clearly defined (Bederson 1997), the role of early surgery for the management of SAH is becoming clearly established. The majority of patients should be considered for this form of management because, in combination with aggressive prevention and management of vasospasm, improved overall management morbidity can be expected. A prospective study from three centers that attempts early surgery demonstrated that rebleeding is still a significant problem, because only approximately one-half of the patients were operated on within 72 hours, and 35% of the patients with a poor outcome had had rebleeding (Roos et al. 1997). Surgical obliteration is the treatment of choice for most intracranial aneurysms. Early surgery to secure an aneurysm can decrease the complications associated with prolonged bed rest, avoid the need for antifibrinolytic therapy and its attendant complications, and permit more aggressive treatment of ischemic complications with blood volume and blood pressure manipulation. To decrease overall mortality, the elimination of rebleeding in the preoperative period by early surgery would be beneficial. Advances in surgical techniques and perioperative management have made early operation safer, so that the incidence of ischemic complications is not increased by surgery performed on the day of aneurysmal rupture or within the next 2 days. There is ample evidence that surgery can be performed safely in the time immediately following aneurysmal rupture. The results of a multicenter prospective study on the influence of timing of surgery on outcome showed a definite reduction in rehemorrhage with early surgery (early surgery group, 6%; late surgery group, 13%).

Early surgery may not be appropriate for every patient with an aneurysmal SAH, but every attempt should be made to secure the aneurysm as soon as possible to prevent rebleeding. Although the pendulum has swung toward early surgery for ruptured intracranial aneurysms, patient selection with respect to grade and timing of intervention is still a matter to be decided by the individual surgeon. Some consider operation only for patients with good grade aneurysms, whereas others believe the high management mortality associated with patients with grades IV and V aneurysms, especially younger patients, can be lowered only by early surgical intervention and aggressive postoperative management. There is clear support for the expeditious conduct of surgery on ruptured aneurysms. The data also confirm previous observations that timing of surgery alone is not the sole determinant of outcome.

Delayed Cerebral Ischemia

As indicated earlier, a major cause of morbidity and mortality after SAH is delayed ischemic deterioration. Approximately 5 days after SAH, any or all of the major branches of the circle of Willis that are exposed to blood may develop vasospasm, which may last for 1–2 weeks or longer.

SAH can alter the mechanisms that control cerebral blood flow and metabolism (Bederson 1997). Chemical control of blood flow by carbon dioxide is altered in patients with SAH. Autoregulation is commonly lost after SAH. Because the degree of impairment of autoregulation may be different in different regions of the brain, a reduction in cerebral perfusion pressure may cause extreme ischemia in some areas but not in others. These changes in the intrinsic control of cerebral blood flow are particularly deleterious because several factors may operate to reduce cerebral blood flow after SAH, including decreased cerebral perfusion pressure from the raised intracranial pressure as a result of acute hydrocephalus or clot formation.

Blood in the subarachnoid space triggers a pathological process that results in spasm of the vessels of the major branches of the circle of Willis. This vasospasm can dramatically decrease the caliber of the cerebral vessels and result in a decreased cerebral blood flow. Because flow in a vessel is inversely proportional to the fourth power of the radius, small changes in vessel caliber can have profound effects. If regional flow decreases below the critical thresholds for membrane integrity, ischemic edema formation and infarction can occur. Focal regions of edema can further impair local blood flow despite an overall normal intracranial pressure.

The precise cause of vasospasm is not well defined, but the presence of blood in the subarachnoid space is the event that triggers the pathological response. Correlation of pathological specimens from patients with angiographical narrowing has demonstrated changes in vessel morphology, including subintimal cellular proliferation. Specimens obtained the second week after SAH demonstrate thickening of the arterial wall with medial necrosis. However, angiographical narrowing is reversible and, on the basis of experimental studies, is more likely to be caused by prolonged but reversible smooth muscle contraction.

The term *vasospasm* is often used interchangeably to refer to the clinical condition of delayed ischemic deterioration and to the vascular narrowing seen on angiography. This terminology is unfortunate, in that angiographic findings do not invariably correlate with the clinical picture. Whether such discrepancies are caused by different thresholds of ischemic tolerance or to other factors is not clear. This lack of strict correlation should not detract from an appreciation of the importance of delayed ischemic deterioration as a cause of serious morbidity and mortality, for its prevention and treatment are clearly a matter of life or death.

Ischemic complications have been reported to occur in 24–32% of patients after SAH. The amount of blood in the subarachnoid space is an important prognostic factor, and thus the CT scan has become an important means of predicting the occurrence of vasospasm. A study of 47 patients with aneurysmal SAH who had CT evaluation within 4 days of the initial bleed found that the amount of blood present on the CT scan correlated well with the location and severity of vasospasm. Of the 18 patients with no blood in the subarachnoid space, only one developed spasm. In the presence of subarachnoid blood clots larger than 5 by 3 mm or layers of blood greater than 1 mm thick in the fissures and basal cisterns, severe spasm occurred in 23 of 24 patients.

Numerous protocols have been proposed as a treatment for vasospasm. One of the most successful was intravascular volume expansion. Fluid administration with or without induced hypertension is fundamental to the management of SAH in combating the effects of cerebral arterial spasm. Hemodynamic monitoring for the prevention and reversal of neurological deficits following SAH is important. Unoperated neurologically normal patients should have the pulmonary wedge pressures kept to 10–12 mm Hg and the cardiac index and blood pressure at normal levels. For the unoperated patient with stable or evolving neurological deficits, the pulmonary wedge pressure is increased until the deficit is reversed or the cardiac index decreases. Although initially it was suggested that systemic blood pressure be augmented for the therapy of vasospasm, neurological deficits in some patients can be reversed with pulmonary wedge pressure manipulations alone without inducing hypertension.

Medical therapy for the prevention and treatment of vasospasm is now standard in the management of patients with SAH and includes a regimen of volume expansion, additional augmentation of cardiac index with dobutamine, and induced systemic hypertension (Ratcheson and Wirth 1994). The current management of cerebral vasospasm is based on the optimization of volume status and cardiac output (Findlay 1997).

Vasospasm appears to be related to an inhibition of reuptake of calcium, which leads to continued vascular smooth muscle contraction. A cooperative clinical trial of nimodipine, a relatively selective cerebral vasculature calcium channel blocker, in the treatment of patients at risk for cerebral arterial spasm included 116 patients who were neurologically intact at the time of entry. Spasm with neurological deficits was seen in 16 of 60 placebo-treated patients and in 13 of 56 nimodipine-treated patients. Severe deficits, however, such as death, coma, or major loss of motor function, occurred in eight placebo-treated patients but in only one treated patient. The efficacy of nimodipine for the prevention of delayed ischemia has been confirmed through a subsequent meta-analysis of published reports (Barker and Ogilvy 1996), although despite a decrease in severe neurological deficits, there is no reduction in the degree of angiographical vasospasm. It is not clear whether this implies action on smaller vessels than those visualized angiographically or other direct anti-ischemic effects of this agent. Later studies with intravenously administered calcium-channel–blocking agents have reported a reduction of the incidence of delayed ischemic deterioration, with a permanent deficit rate of less than 5%.

Despite improvements in hemodynamic augmentation and medical treatment, the development of vasospasm is still a harbinger of potential deterioration from ischemic deficits. New methods of predicting and detecting vasospasm permit the use of more aggressive treatment modalities such as endovascular balloon dilatation of spastic arteries. Transcranial Doppler studies permit bedside evaluation of blood flow velocity (which increases with a reduction in vessel diameter) in the intracranial portion of the internal carotid artery and proximal branches of the circle of Willis. With this early detection of velocity changes, it is possible to select patients who should be considered for treatment prior to the development of fixed neurological deficits.

Endovascular treatment, such as angioplasty with a silicone balloon to treat vasospasm, has become an indispensable treatment modality in the comprehensive management of patients suffering a SAH and can provide dramatic improvement in the function of patients who would otherwise suffer from ischemic neurological deterioration (Eskridge et al. 1998) (Figure 57C.6).

SPECIAL TREATMENT CONSIDERATIONS

Unruptured Aneurysms

Because of the poor overall outcome of patients with intracranial aneurysms after SAH and the low morbidity and mortality associated with operation for unruptured aneurysms, a strong case can be made for surgical treatment of asymptomatic aneurysms. Some authors, however, emphasize the relatively benign prognosis, especially for aneurysms less than 10 mm (The International Study of Unruptured Intracranial Aneurysms Investigators 1998). Olafsson and colleagues (1997) reported that the occurrence rate of an initial hemorrhage in patients with aneurysms larger than 1 cm in diameter was 1.5% per year, of whom one-half experienced their bleeding episode within the first few months after identification of the aneurysm. However, the large number of ruptured aneurysms that are smaller than 1 cm argues strongly against accepting a benign prognosis for lesions below this size (Caplan 1998). The only method of lowering the initial mortality from SAH is to detect and treat unruptured aneurysms (Schievink et al. 1995).

The decision to operate or not depends on several factors and is complicated because the rupture of an incidental aneurysm is a long-term risk spread out over many years, whereas the risk of surgery is immediate. Some have used the process of decision analysis in an attempt to optimize the management of incidental aneurysms. Factors to be considered are the size of the aneurysm, the morbidity and mortality after SAH, the surgical morbidity and mortality, the life expectancy of the patient, and the attitude of the patient toward short-term and long-term risk. With a surgical mortality of 2% and morbidity of 6%, a life expectancy of 12 years appears to be the break-even value. Decision analysis highlights areas of relative ignorance. The management of patients with incidental aneurysms would be improved by more accurate knowledge of the natural history of specific aneurysms with respect not only to size, but to configuration and location, and comparison with institutional and surgeon-specific results.

The natural history of unruptured aneurysms was examined in 142 patients by Juvela and colleagues (1993). They noted an average annual rupture rate of 1.4%, with a

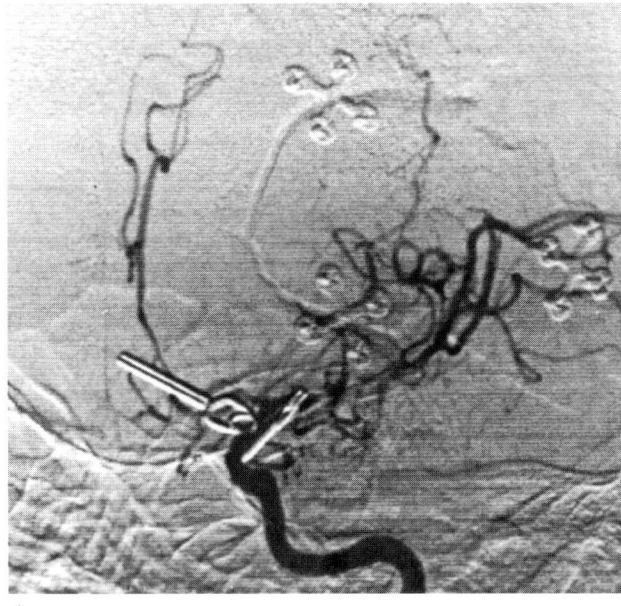 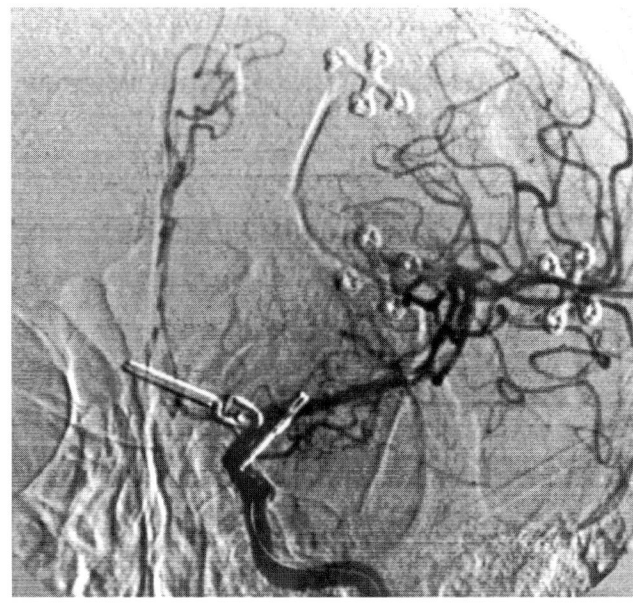

A   B

FIGURE 57C.6   (**A**) Left internal carotid artery angiogram demonstrates severe left middle cerebral artery vasospasm. (**B**) Left internal carotid artery angiogram following angioplasty shows increased diameter of the left middle cerebral artery.

cumulative rate of bleeding of 10% at 10 years, 26% at 20 years, and 32% at 30 years after the diagnosis. Because 67% of the 27 aneurysms that later ruptured were 6 mm or less in diameter, the size of the aneurysm could not be used as a predictor for the risk of rupture. These investigators could find no critical diameter above which the risk of rupture increases, but did note a linear association between the risk of rupture and aneurysm size. In patients with multiple aneurysms, the risk of rupture was inversely associated with age. The authors concluded that an unruptured aneurysm should be operated on, irrespective of its size, if it is technically possible and if the patient's age and concurrent diseases do not preclude surgical intervention.

A meta-analysis of 28 surgical series containing 733 patients undergoing elective surgery for asymptomatic, unruptured intracranial aneurysms found a morbidity of 4.1% (95% confidence interval 2.8, 5.8%), and a mortality of 1.0% (95% confidence interval 0.4, 2.0%) (King et al. 1994). Elective aneurysm surgery has been demonstrated to be cost-effective provided that the surgical morbidity and mortality remain at low levels, that patient life expectancy is at least 13 years, and that the patient's quality of life is decreased by the knowledge of the aneurysm (King et al. 1995). In view of the devastating consequences of aneurysmal rupture, there must be strong contraindications not to consider the surgical treatment of incidentally discovered aneurysms.

Neuroendovascular Techniques in the Treatment of Cerebral Aneurysms

Although the role of endovascular techniques in the management of vasospasm has become well established, the use

of these techniques in the treatment of aneurysms themselves continues to be defined (Viñuela et al. 1997). There are currently two major categories of endovascular treatment of intracranial aneurysms: occlusion of parent artery and aneurysm, and direct embolization or coil induction of thrombosis of the aneurysms with parent artery preservation. Aneurysms that are fusiform or giant and those without a well-defined neck may require parent artery occlusion. The morbidity of this procedure has been reported to be 15%, with 3% permanent complications. Direct balloon occlusion of aneurysms in which occlusion could not be obtained by craniotomy has been reported to provide obliteration in 75%, with a mortality of 18% and stroke in 11%. A major difficulty with direct balloon occlusion is that the wall of the aneurysm may be exposed to an increase in pressure while adapting to the shape of the balloon, and in the preceding report, 10 of the 15 deaths were due to aneurysmal rupture.

Newer techniques have evolved in the direct endovascular embolization of intracranial aneurysms, including the use of detachable coils and electrothrombosis for obliteration of the aneurysm sac (Viñuela et al. 1997) (Figures 57C.7 and 57C.8). The results of aneurysm occlusion using this method suggest that it is most effective in treating aneurysms smaller than 25 mm in diameter, and with neck width smaller than 4 mm in diameter. In a series of 403 patients with acute SAH treated at eight centers in the United States, complete aneurysm obliteration was achieved in 70.8% of aneurysms with a small neck and 35.0% of large aneurysms, and there was an 8.9% immediate procedural morbidity (Viñuela et al. 1997). Neuroendovascular therapy appears to have an expanding role in the management of poor-grade patients, as well as in patients harboring aneurysms that have been

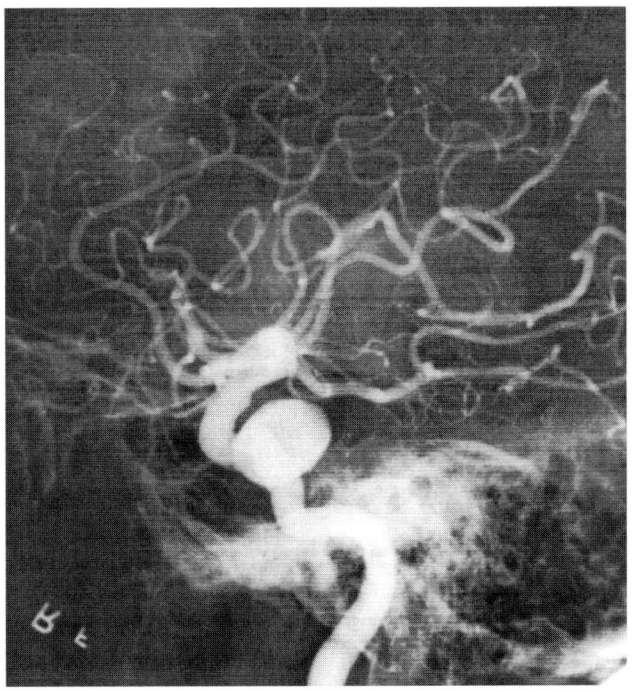 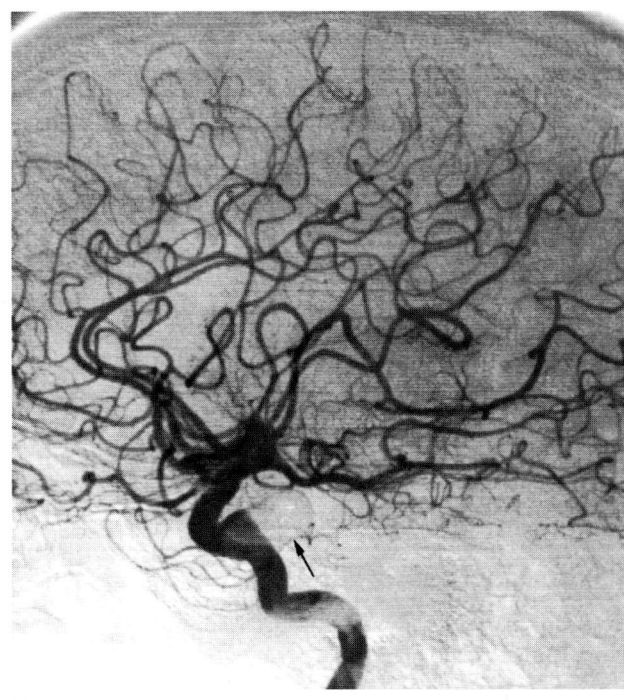

A   B

FIGURE 57C.7 (A) Lateral right internal carotid angiogram reveals a large cavernous carotid artery aneurysm. (B) Lateral right internal carotid artery angiogram following balloon embolization (*arrow*) shows almost complete obliteration of the aneurysm.

determined to be difficult to treat by microsurgical techniques. The role of these techniques in the management of the majority of intracranial aneurysms can only be determined after more experience is gained and long-term follow-up is available for comparison with the published reports with microsurgical neurosurgical techniques.

Subarachnoid Hemorrhage in Pregnancy

Special consideration needs to be given to the management of SAH during pregnancy (see Chapter 85). The frequency of discovery of cerebral aneurysms is increased during pregnancy. SAH is the third most common nonobstetrical cause of maternal death. SAH accounts for approximately one-half of all intracranial bleeding in pregnancy and if untreated carries a grave prognosis. The incidence of aneurysmal bleeding parallels the elevation in cardiac output and blood volume, increasing throughout gestation, and extending into the early postpartum period. The risk of recurrent hemorrhage is between 35% and 75%, with a mortality of 50–75%. In patients suffering a SAH, neurosurgical considerations generally take precedence over obstetrical considerations, but the management of patients with incidentally discovered aneurysms is not well defined and treatment should be individualized. The time of aneurysm rupture in normal pregnancies is as follows: 8% ruptured in the first 3 months, 22% in the next 3 months, 59% between the seventh and tenth month, 3% during labor, and 8% in the puerperium. Ruptured aneurysms

should probably be clipped as soon as possible, regardless of the state of the pregnancy. If the patient is near term, an expeditious cesarean section may prevent the burden of labor being added to the difficult course following aneurysm rupture and repair.

Subarachnoid Hemorrhage of Unknown Etiology

A normal angiogram can be seen in patients with SAH, because occasionally localized hemorrhage with intense spasm or thrombosis can prevent filling of an intracranial aneurysm. Because of the drastic consequences of missing a ruptured aneurysm, repeat angiography 7–10 days later is recommended. Repeat angiography has been shown to reveal an aneurysm in 19% of patients in whom the initial angiogram failed to demonstrate an aneurysm (Kaim 1996). Despite a thorough and complete angiographical evaluation, diagnostic studies fail to reveal an etiology for the SAH in a substantial number of patients (see Perimesencephalic Hemorrhage, later in this chapter). Although trauma is the most common cause for SAH, the difference in distribution of blood and the antecedent history rarely make the distinction from aneurysmal SAH difficult. Other causes for nonaneurysmal subarachnoid hemorrhage include angiographically occult vascular malformations, hemorrhagic infarctions, and hypertensive hemorrhages. SAH of unknown cause is not associated with the high morbidity and mortality of aneurysmal SAH, and the risk of fatal rebleeding is well under 1% per year.

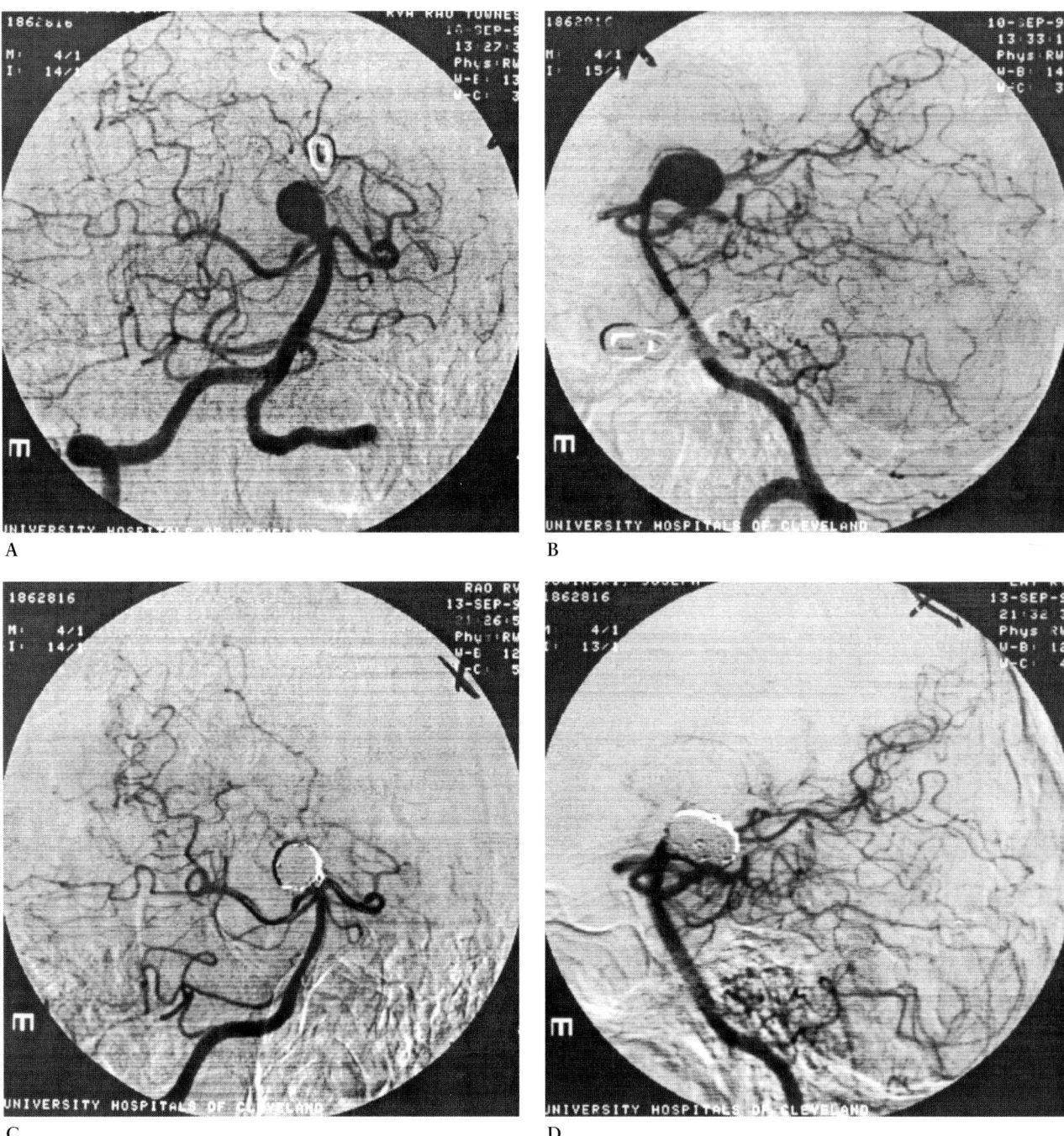

FIGURE 57C.8   (A) Right anterior oblique and (B) lateral left vertebral artery angiogram demonstrating a large basilar tip aneurysm. (C) Right anterior oblique and (D) lateral following treatment with Guglielmi detachable coils show obliteration of the aneurysm.

Perimesencephalic Hemorrhage

A distinct pattern of SAH that can occur without a detectable aneurysm is perimesencephalic hemorrhage. This entity may be caused by rupture of a capillary telangiectasia of the pons (Wijdicks and Schievink 1997). Although knowledge of this condition can provide an explanation for a negative angiogram result in the presence of definitive SAH, it should not be used as an reason to omit angiography because localized perimesencephalic hemorrhage can be seen with aneurysmal rupture. Patients with this pattern of hemorrhage and a normal angiogram result should be considered to have a distinct subset of SAH and generally do not suffer from repeat hemorrhage. These patients have a relatively benign clinical course, although symptomatic vasospasm may occur.

REFERENCES

Barker FG II, Ogilvy CS. Efficacy of prophylactic nimodipine for delayed ischemic deficit after subarachnoid hemorrhage: a meta-analysis. J Neurosurg 1996;84:405–409.

Bederson J. Pathophysiology of Subarachnoid Hemorrhage. Park Ridge, IL: American Association of Neurological Surgeons, 1997.

Beristain X, Gaviria M, Dujovny M, et al. Evaluation of outcome after intracranial aneurysm surgery: the neuropsychiatric approach. Surg Neurol 1996;45:422–429.

Caplan LR. Should intracranial aneurysms be treated before they rupture? N Engl J Med 1998;339:774–775.

Enblad R, Persson L. Impact on clinical outcome of secondary brain insults during the neurointensive care of patients with subarachnoid haemorrhage: a pilot study. J Neurol Neurosurg Psychiatry 1997;62:512–516.

Eskridge JM, McAuliffe W, Song JK, et al. Balloon angioplasty for the treatment of vasospasm: results of the first 50 cases. Neurosurgery 1998;42:510–517.

Findlay JM. Current management of cerebral vasospasm. Contemp Neurosurg 1997;19:1–6.

The International Study of Unruptured Intracranial Aneurysms Investigators. Unruptured intracranial aneurysms—risk of rupture and risks of surgical intervention. N Engl J Med 1998;339:1725–1733.

Juvela S, Porras M, Heiskanen O. Natural history of unruptured intracranial aneurysms: a long-term follow-up study. J Neurosurg 1993;79:174–182.

Kaim A. Value of repeat angiography in cases of unexplained subarachnoid hemorrhage (SAH). Acta Neurol Scand 1996;93:366–373.

King JT Jr, Berlin JA, Flamm ES. Morbidity and mortality from elective surgery for asymptomatic, unruptured, intracranial aneurysms: a meta-analysis. J Neurosurg 1994;81:21–26.

King JT Jr, Glick HA, Mason TJ, et al. Elective surgery for asymptomatic, unruptured, intracranial aneurysms: a cost-effective analysis. J Neurosurg 1995;83:403–412.

Mayer SA, Fink ME, Hommas S, et al. Cardiac injury associated with neurogenic pulmonary edema following subarachnoid hemorrhage. Neurology 1994;44:815–820.

Menghini VV, Brown RD Jr, Sicks JD, et al. Incidence and prevalence of intracranial aneurysms and hemorrhage in Olmsted County, Minnesota, 1965 to 1995. Neurology 1998;51:405–411.

Ogden JA, Utley T, Mee EW. Neurological and psychosocial outcome 4 to 7 years after subarachnoid hemorrhage. Neurosurgery 1997;41:25–34.

Olafsson E, Hauser A, Gudmundsson G. A population-based study of prognosis of ruptured cerebral aneurysm: mortality and recurrence of subarachnoid hemorrhage. Neurology 1997;48:1191–1195.

Ostergaard JR. Unruptured Vascular Malformation and Subarachnoid Hemorrhage. In J Olesen, P Tfelt-Hansen, KMA Welch (eds), The Headaches. New York: Raven, 1993;647–652.

Ratcheson RA, Wirth P (eds). Ruptured Cerebral Aneurysms: Perioperative Management. Baltimore: Williams & Wilkins, 1994.

Ronkainen A, Vanninen R, Hernesniemi J. Familial aneurysms. Headache Q 1998;9:34–38.

Roos YB, Beenen LF, Groen RJ, et al. Timing of surgery in patients with aneurysmal subarachnoid haemorrhage: rebleeding is still the major cause of poor outcome in neurosurgical units that aim at early surgery. J Neurol Neurosurg Psychiatry 1997;63:490–493.

Schievink WI. Intracranial aneurysms. N Engl J Med 1997;336:28–40.

Schievink WI, Wijdicks EFM, Parisi JE, et al. Sudden death from aneurysmal subarachnoid hemorrhage. Neurology 1995;45:871–874.

Vermeij FH, Hasan D, Vermeulen M, et al. Predictive factors for deterioration from hydrocephalus after subarachnoid hemorrhage. Neurology 1994;44:1851–1855.

Viñuela F, Duckwiler G, Mawad M. Guglielmi detachable coil embolization of acute intracranial aneurysm: perioperative anatomical and clinical outcome in 403 patients. J Neurosurg 1997;86:475–482.

Weir B. Headaches from aneurysms. Cephalalgia 1994;14:79–87.

Wijdicks EFM, Schievink WI. Perimesencephalic nonaneurysmal subarachnoid hemorrhage: first hint of a cause? Neurology 1997;49:634–636.

Chapter 57
Vascular Diseases of the Nervous System

D. ARTERIOVENOUS MALFORMATIONS
Warren R. Selman, Robert W. Tarr, and Robert A. Ratcheson

Arteriovenous malformations (AVMs) are developmental abnormalities of blood vessels in which one or more primitive direct communications between otherwise normal arterial and venous channels are preserved. The most devastating consequences of these lesions occur as a result of intracranial hemorrhage. These lesions may be found also in patients with seizures or may be discovered fortuitously during evaluation for an unrelated disorder. The proper management of AVMs is complex and requires an understanding of their natural history and their effect on cerebral circulation and metabolism. Microsurgical resection, neuroendovascular embolization, and stereotactic radiosurgery may be used alone or in combination to eliminate the risk of subsequent hemorrhage.

PATHOLOGY

Vascular malformations may be divided into four major types: (1) venous malformations, (2) cavernous malformations, (3) telangiectases, and (4) AVMs.

Venous angiomas, which are the most common type of vascular malformation, are composed entirely of venous structures and are almost always clinically silent. The presence of a large dilated enhancing vein extending to the cortical or ependymal surface with a radial configuration of smaller veins as seen on a contrast-enhanced computed tomography (CT) or magnetic resonance imaging (MRI) is diagnostic (Figure 57D.1). Angiography is rarely needed to confirm the diagnosis.

Cavernous malformations are low-flow vascular anomalies consisting of sinusoidal vascular channels lined by a single layer of endothelium. The walls of the dilated vessels are thin and contain no smooth muscle or elastic tissue. Marked hyalinization of the vascular channels is common. There is no intervening brain parenchyma within the collagenous stroma separating the individual vascular channels. Of all the vascular anomalies, cavernous malformations are most likely to occur with other lesions. The most common association is that of a cavernous malformation and a venous angioma. As noted later, the cavernous malformation is responsible for the clinical presentation in these mixed lesions.

Capillary angiomas or telangiectases are small solitary groups of abnormally dilated capillaries. They rarely give rise to spontaneous hemorrhage and usually are detected only in postmortem examinations. There is one case report that suggests that capillary telangiectasia may be associated with the syndrome of perimesencephalic hemorrhage (see Chapter 57C), but this finding needs to be confirmed in a larger series (Wijdicks and Schievink 1997).

True AVMs generally are believed to be congenital lesions that arise from aberrant connections within the primitive arterial and venous plexus overlying the developing cortical mantle. This area of altered vasculature becomes incorporated into the brain parenchyma. The AVM itself is composed of abnormal arteries and veins. Larger vessels resemble veins in that they contain a small amount of muscularis and lack elastica. The amount of gliotic tissue that intervenes between the abnormal vessels varies greatly between specimens. Most AVMs show evidence of microscopic hemorrhage in this tissue regardless of whether the patient has experienced a symptomatic hemorrhage. There is no normal capillary bed in the nidus of an AVM.

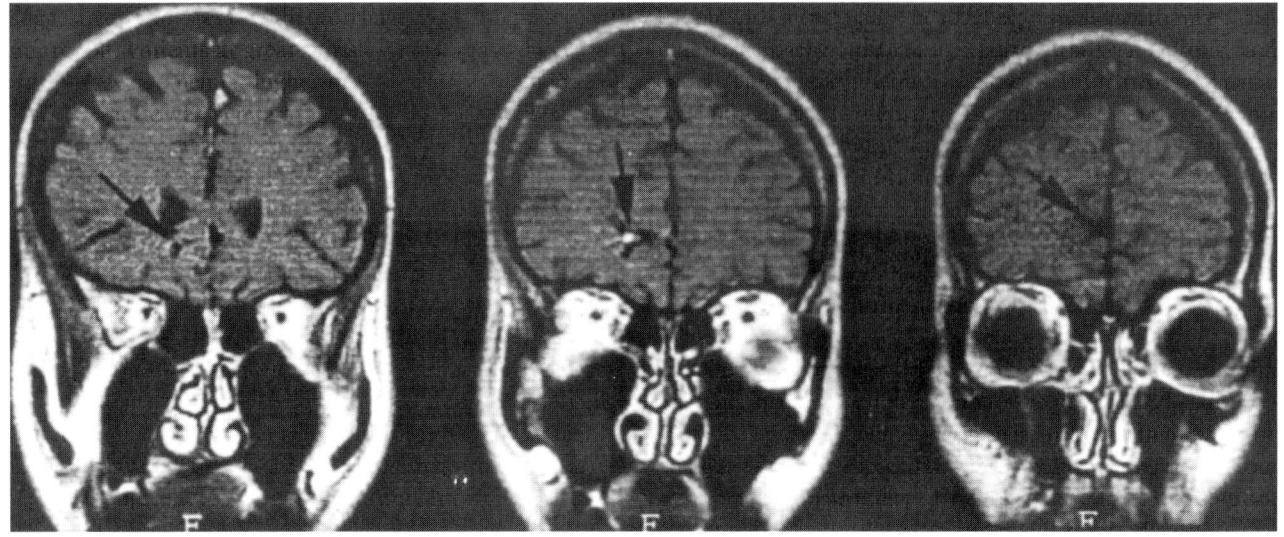

A

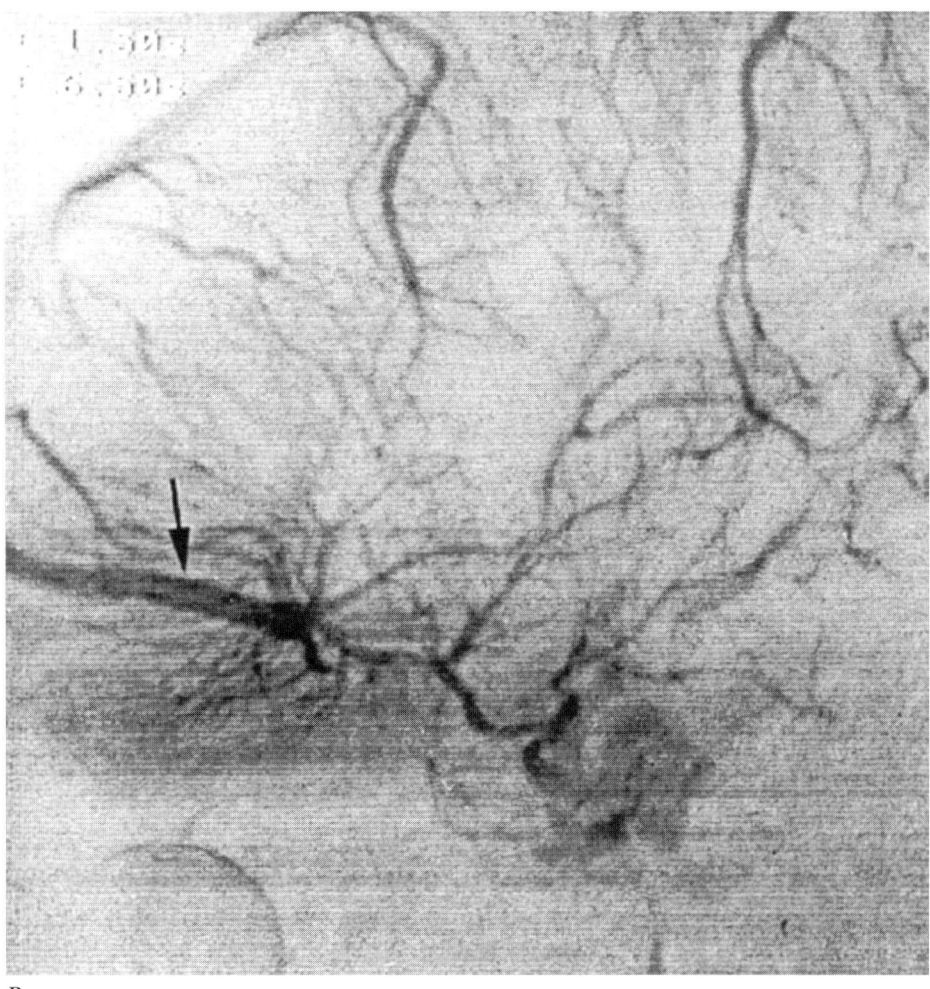

B

FIGURE 57D.1 (A) Coronal T1-weighted magnetic resonance images demonstrate the venous tributaries and large draining vein characteristic of a venous angioma (*arrows*). (B) Lateral venous phase from a right internal carotid artery angiogram confirms the right frontal venous angioma (*arrow*) draining toward the anterior portion of the superior sagittal sinus.

FIGURE 57D.2 Sagittal T1-weighted magnetic resonance image demonstrates a cavernous angioma involving the dorsal midbrain (*arrow*). Note the characteristic surrounding areas of high signal intensity caused by walled-off microhemorrhages.

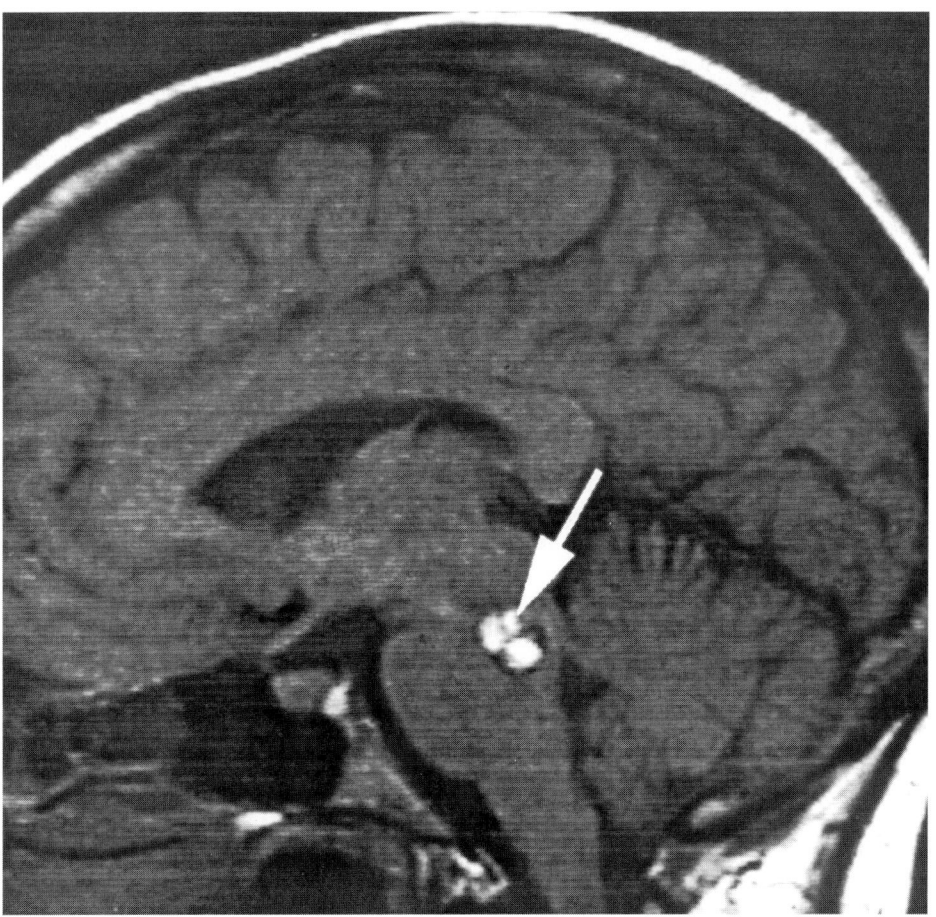

EPIDEMIOLOGY AND CLINICAL SIGNS

Cavernous Malformations

The prevalence of cavernous malformations depends on the nature of the study. In major autopsy series, the prevalence is 0.02–0.53%. Studies based on MRI have reported a higher prevalence of 0.4–0.9% (Maraire and Awad 1997). Familial forms of cavernous malformations, characterized by multiple lesions, appear to be transmitted in an autosomal dominant fashion (Notelet et al. 1997). Cavernous malformations occur in all age groups, but the majority of patients present in the second to fourth decade of life. Most cavernous malformations are solitary lesions, but multiple lesions occur in approximately one-third of sporadic cases, and in over two-thirds of familial cases.

Cavernous malformations are dynamic lesions, and intralesional hemorrhage, thrombosis, organization, calcification, cyst formation, and involution of the caverns all contribute to the changes in these lesions. Cavernous malformations, unlike venous angiomas, have no distinctive CT scan appearance, but do have a characteristic MRI signature (Figure 57D.2). It is the MRI pattern of a central core of increased intensity surrounded by a rim of decreased intensity on T2-weighted sequences, or multiloculated rounded areas of increased signal on T1-weighted sequences, that allows radiographic identification of these lesions. Although the MRI picture is characteristic, the differential diagnosis should include cryptic or partially thrombosed arteriovenous malformations, primary hemorrhagic or metastatic tumors, infectious and granulomatous diseases, and inflammatory lesions (Perl and Ross 1993).

Cavernous malformations are rarely visualized on angiography because of the small size of the afferent vessels, the presence of thrombosis, and the relatively low flow in these lesions. *Cryptic malformation* is a term used to describe a small malformation that is undetectable by angiography but is demonstrated by pathological examination to be responsible for intracranial hemorrhage. Cavernous malformations account for 25–50% of occult lesions. The remainder are considered to be angiographically occult AVMs. Because the natural history of the two lesions is different, in the presence of a new hemorrhage, follow-up angiography after the resolution of any mass effect may be needed to exclude the presence of a small AVM.

Solitary and multiple lesions may be clinically silent. The most common clinical manifestations of cavernous malformations are seizures, hemorrhage, and progressive neurological deficit (Aiba et al. 1995). Cavernous malformations have almost twice the frequency of seizures as AVMs and have been reported in between 38% and 100% in clinical series. Those lesions with calcification, evidence of chronic intralesional hemorrhage with thrombus organization, and thick pseudocapsules are more likely to present with seizures than gross hemorrhage. Women are more likely to present with gross hemorrhage and neurological deficits, whereas men are more likely to present with seizures. Clinically significant hemorrhage has been reported in between 8% and 37% of lesions in large clinical series (Maraire and Awad 1997). The annualized risk of hemorrhage has been estimated to be between 0.1% and 2.7% per lesion per year. In contrast to primary hemorrhage occurring from an AVM, the clinically significant bleeding noted with cavernous malformations is rarely life threatening, and the initial bleed is self-limited and patients usually have a good or fair outcome. There is, nonetheless, an increased risk of recurrent hemorrhage after an initial bleeding episode, which has been estimated to be between 20% and 85%. The signs and symptoms of the hemorrhage depend on the location of the lesion. Brainstem hemorrhages have a high rate of recurrent symptomatic hemorrhage, noted in up to 69%, and a significant morbidity (Fritschi et al. 1994).

Arteriovenous Malformations

The incidence of AVMs varies depending on the source material examined, but has been estimated to be between one-seventh and one-tenth that of intracranial aneurysms, or 1.4 per 10,000 individuals per year. True AVMs rarely produce clinical symptoms before the first decade and commonly present in the second and third decades of life. They occur with equal frequency in men and women.

Patients with AVMs may seek medical attention for one or a combination of the following problems: (1) intracranial hemorrhage, (2) seizures, (3) focal neurological deficits, (4) impairment of higher cortical function, (5) headache, and (6) bruit. With greater use of noninvasive imaging techniques, it has become apparent that many such lesions may remain asymptomatic and are discovered only incidentally.

Headaches, usually of migrainous type, may occur in 5–35% of patients with AVMs. They characteristically begin during the second decade of life; they may be generalized, unilateral, focal, continuous, or intermittent; and they are not specific for the presence or location of an AVM. In the absence of hemorrhage or hydrocephalus, the relation of the headache to the AVM is not always apparent (Lance 1993).

AVMs typically produce an intracerebral hemorrhage, but intraventricular, or subarachnoid hemorrhage also may be present. In contrast to aneurysms, which produce predominantly subarachnoid hemorrhage, AVMs tend to produce localized intracerebral hemorrhage. The resulting neurological deficit depends on the location and size of the hemorrhage. There is no characteristic clinical picture that is specific for AVM hemorrhage. In most cases there is nothing remarkable about the history other than the sudden onset of severe headache, which is characteristic of any intracerebral hemorrhage.

Seizures may occur in patients at any age. Seizures have been reported as a presenting feature in 28–67% of patients with AVMs. More than 50% of patients found to have an AVM are likely to have had at least one seizure by the age of 30. A seizure is more common as an initial symptom between the ages of 11 and 20 years and hemorrhage between the ages of 21 and 30 years. It has been suggested that patients with large AVMs are twice as likely to have seizures in contrast to hemorrhage as their presenting symptom, with the converse relation holding for smaller lesions.

In addition to headaches, seizures, and hemorrhage, less frequent clinical manifestations of AVMs include focal neurological deficits caused by ischemia (steal phenomenon), cardiomegaly, and high-output congestive failure caused by the high-volume shunt, obstructive hydrocephalus, communicating hydrocephalus, and cranial nerve compression. The occurrence of these problems is in part related to the patient's age. Cardiomegaly and cardiac failure are usually manifested only during infancy and early childhood in a patient with a vein of Galen aneurysm, which is something of a misnomer because the underlying lesion is an AVM. Similarly, obstructive hydrocephalus is usually a disease of childhood secondary to aqueductal compression from an enlarged vein of Galen aneurysm or AVM, but communicating hydrocephalus may occur at any age from an intraventricular hemorrhage.

PHYSICAL FINDINGS

The physical examination should be tailored to the age of presentation. In infancy, evidence of a hyperdynamic cardiovascular state should be sought. It is necessary to measure head circumference and check for funduscopical evidence of papilledema. At any age, auscultation of the head may reveal a bruit, which may often be of some help in localization. Finally, the presence and character of a neurological deficit can localize the site of hemorrhage.

PHYSIOLOGY AND METABOLISM

In 1928, Cushing and Dandy both described alterations of normal blood flow patterns in the brain surrounding AVMs. These authors reasoned, on the basis of finding red blood (arterialization) in the venous channels, that the brain was not using the flow for metabolic purposes. The paucity of filling of surrounding cortex in the presence of an AVM as noted on angiography was described as cerebral steal.

Blood flow to and from AVMs is conducted through normally located channels. Because there is not a separate AVM circulation, the relationship between cortical nutrient branches and the arteries diverting blood into an AVM is important. A simplified model to describe the relationship of pressure in nutrient branches of a feeding vessel to AVM flow is depicted in Figure 57D.3. A decrease in pressure along a feeding artery is directly proportional to the time-average velocity of flow and the length of the artery. Thus, the higher the flow to the AVM, the less the pressure in the nutrient arteries. Increased venous pressure associated with an AVM also leads to a further decrease in nutrient flow.

Although many high-flow AVMs demonstrate angiographical cerebral steal, not all produce ischemic symptoms. This is explained in part by the autoregulatory response of the normal cerebral vasculature to a decrease in local perfusion pressure. In addition, neurons maintain normal electrophysiological function until flow is reduced from normal levels of 50 ml/100 g per minute to less than 20 ml/100 g per minute. Nonetheless, chronic hypoperfusion in the nutrient vessels surrounding an AVM may result in maximal dilation such that autoregulation is lost in this area. Such changes make the territory involved susceptible to alterations in systemic pressure and could result in cerebral ischemia.

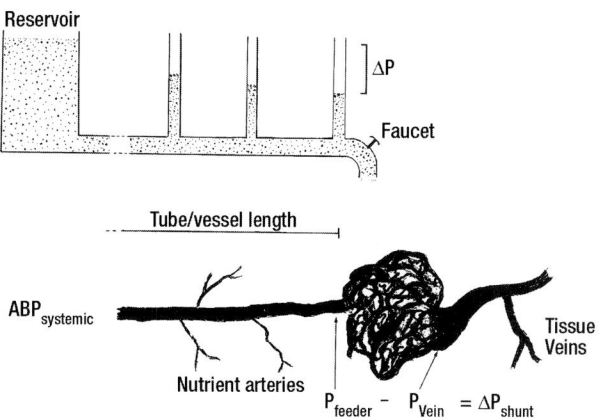

FIGURE 57D.3   Relationship of pressure (P) in the nutrient branches (those supplying surrounding normal cortex) to the flow in the feeding vessel supplying an arteriovenous malformation. (ABP= arterial blood pressure.) (Adapted from Nornes H, Grip A. Hemodynamic aspects of cerebral arteriovenous malformation. J Neurosurg 1980;53:456.)

LABORATORY STUDIES

The identification of patients suspected of having an AVM has been made easier by the development of modern noninvasive diagnostic imaging techniques. CT, MRI, and MR angiography (see Chapter 38B) are useful in determining the presence of vascular malformations. If an AVM is found, conventional angiography (see Chapter 38C) is essential in determining the optimal treatment. An AVM may receive arterial input from any of the major cerebral arteries. If the AVM is located solely within the territory of a single cerebral artery, then the blood supply to the malformation may come solely from that artery. In larger AVMs, or those bordering more than one territory, the arterial supply is usually from more than one arterial distribution. Thus, complete four-vessel angiography is needed to define these lesions. The venous drainage may be through the superficial or deep venous system, or directly into a major sinus, or some combination of these patterns.

The CT scan is often the first study that suggests the presence of a vascular malformation in a patient with headaches, seizures, or a neurological deficit. Information can be gained from both noncontrast and contrast-enhanced scans. The noncontrast scan can establish the presence and location of hemorrhage. A lobar hemorrhage should increase the suspicion of a vascular malformation as the underlying cause. Other diagnostic considerations include hypertensive hemorrhage, aneurysmal rupture, and hemorrhage into a tumor. Enhancement occurs because of collection of the contrast material in the intravascular compartment as well as in surrounding areas with altered blood-brain barrier permeability. The presence of a serpentine enhancement pattern is highly characteristic. High-resolution (2.0-mm slice thickness) dynamic CT imaging after contrast administration allows accurate measurement of the size of the AVM nidus (Figure 57D.4).

Standard sequences such as T1- and T2-weighted MRIs provide precise information on the size and location of an AVM (Figure 57D.5). The relation of feeding arteries and draining veins can be appreciated using MR angiography. Three-dimensional time-of-flight techniques are especially helpful for visualizing arterial flow, and two-dimensional time-of-flight is best for showing the slower flow in the venous drainage (Figure 57D.6).

Functional imaging (see Chapter 38E) is helpful in determining the effects of the AVM on the blood flow and regulatory capacity of the surrounding brain. Stable xenon CT scanning has been used to delineate the response to acetazolamide. The presence of a steal phenomenon may indicate a loss of autoregulation in the brain surrounding the AVM (Figure 57D.7). The relation of the AVM to vital cortical areas can be appreciated by the use of functional MRI (Figures 57D.8 and 57D.9). These newer imaging modalities provide information that influences therapeutic planning.

COURSE AND PROGNOSIS

Intracranial hemorrhage is the most significant clinical manifestation of an AVM. All studies have demonstrated a relatively constant and high risk of hemorrhage associated with AVMs. It is important to stress that the cumulative rate of hemorrhage is the same regardless of the presentation. Even an unruptured AVM carries a 4% yearly risk of hemorrhage. The mortality from the first hemorrhage varies between 6% and 14%. Once an AVM has bled, the likelihood of recurrent hemorrhage is approximately 6% for the first year and 4% for the subsequent years. Any estimate of the risk of hemorrhage for an individual patient must take into account specific considerations that may not be entirely reflected in

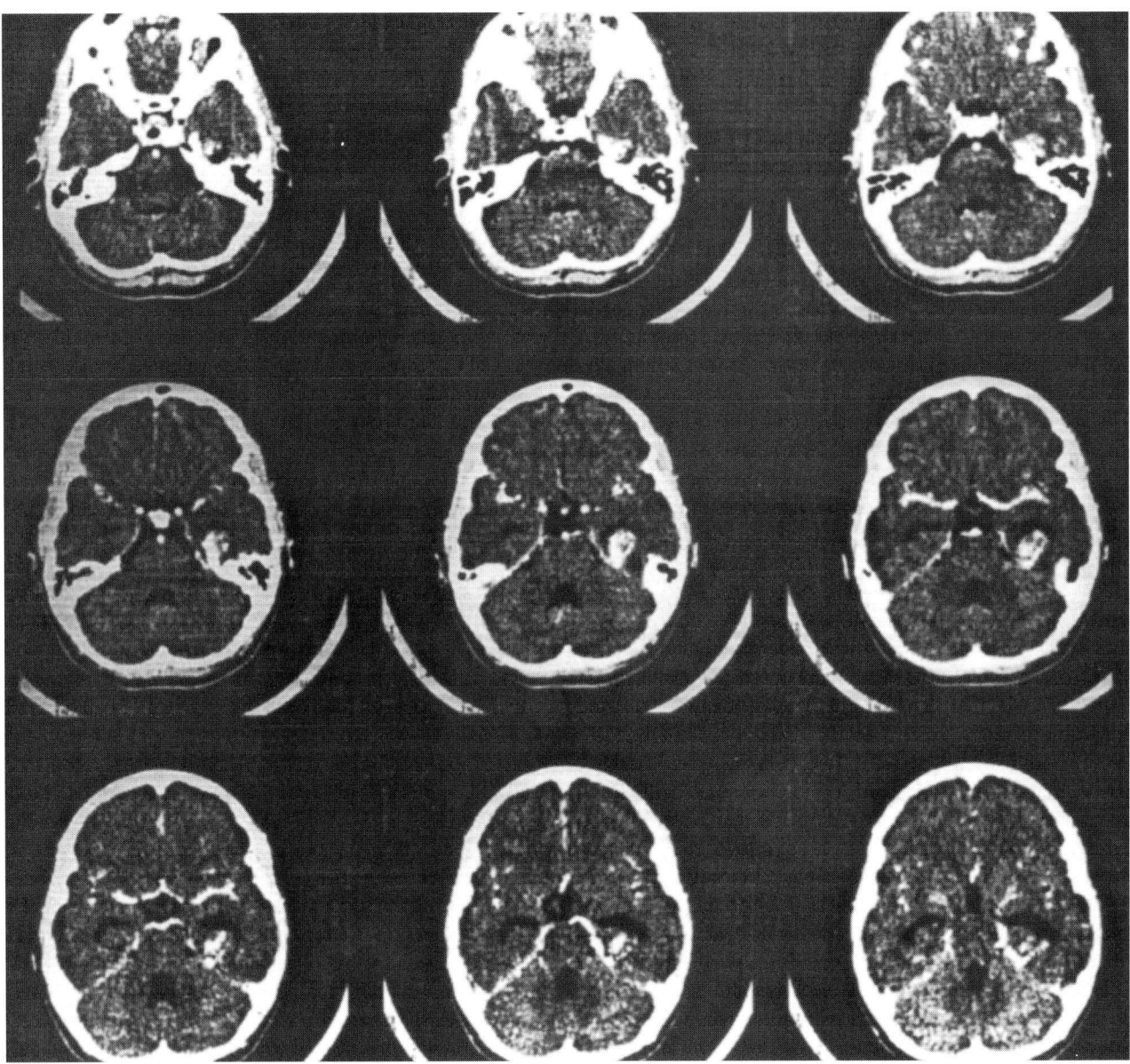

FIGURE 57D.4   Dynamic contrast enhanced computed tomography (2-mm slice thickness) delineates the nidus of a left posterior temporal lobe arteriovenous malformation.

cumulative data. For example, untreated AVMs in the posterior fossa appear to have a particularly poor prognosis. Children are at relatively greater long-term risk for rehemorrhage in that the period of increased risk of hemorrhage is entirely before them. Patients with smaller AVMs, because of differences in the flow patterns and pressure within the nidus, may be more likely to hemorrhage than large AVMs. Systemic hypertension increases the risk of AVM hemorrhage. It is also apparent that AVMs that have aneurysms on intranidal vessels and those that have areas of venous outflow restriction are more prone to hemorrhage (Figure 57D.10).

The overall course of patients harboring an AVM is not benign. In addition to the effects of a major hemorrhage,

neuronal damage from repeated minor hemorrhages or ischemia of adjacent brain from cerebral steal can result in progressive neurological deterioration. The yearly mortality reported by Ondra and coworkers in their large, 1990 series with long-term follow-up was 1–2%; the rate of mortality plus morbidity was 5%; the rate of morbidity alone was 3.5%. Other series have reported a mortality of approximately 0.9% per year. It has been suggested that these rates are not constant in that symptoms appear more commonly during the third and fourth decades of life. Thus, the mortality and morbidity for individuals younger than 20 years and older than 40 may be lower than in the intervening age group.

FIGURE 57D.5 Coronal T1-weighted magnetic resonance image demonstrates a left frontal arteriovenous malformation nidus that extends to the ventricular surface.

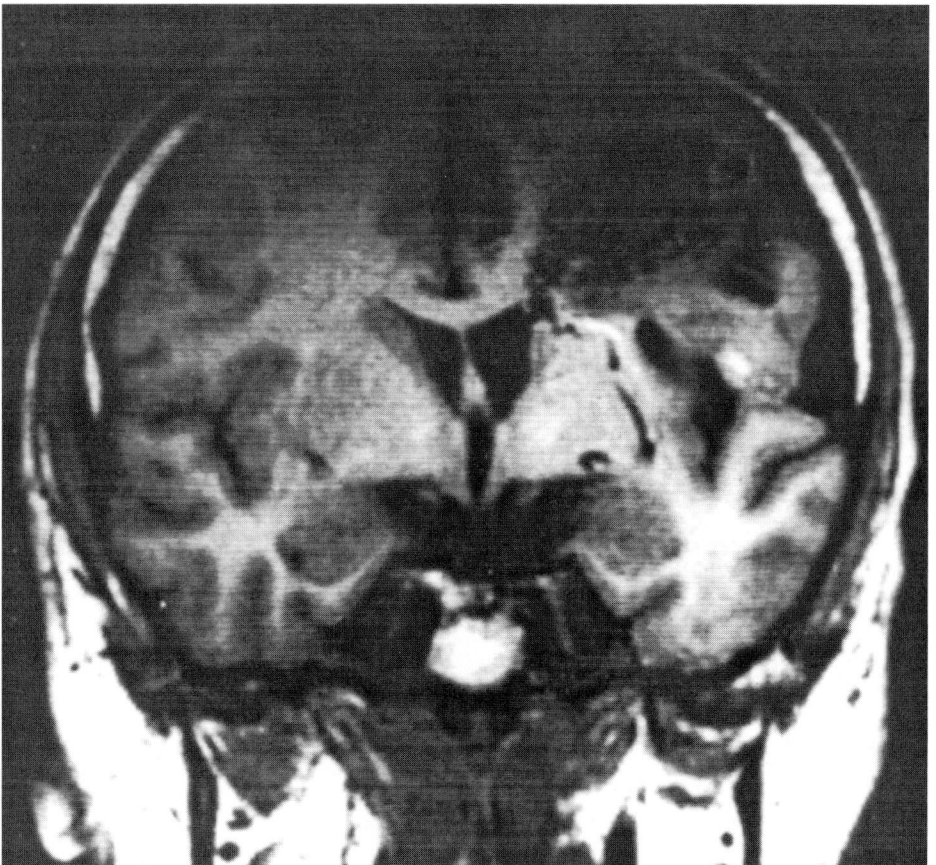

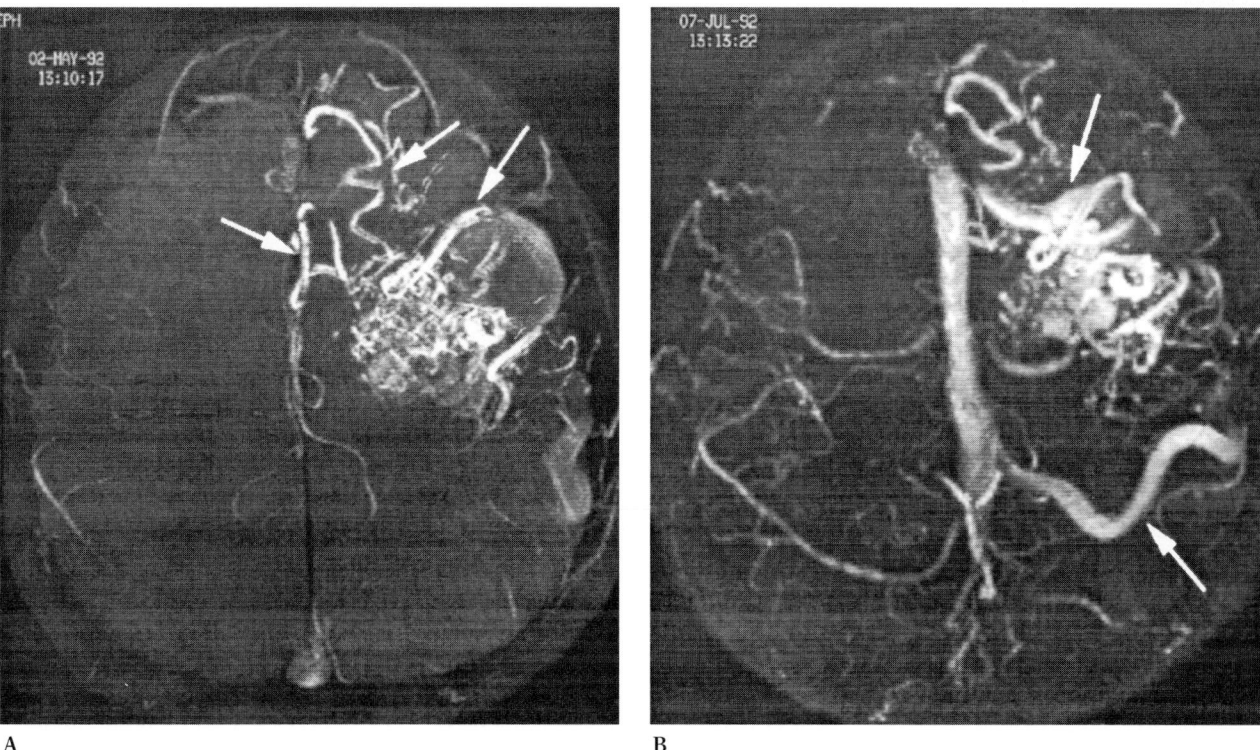

A

B

FIGURE 57D.6 **(A)** Three-dimensional time-of-flight magnetic resonance angiography demonstrates arterial pedicles (*arrows*) as well as a venous varix. The entire venous drainage pattern cannot be defined on this study. **(B)** Two-dimensional time-of-flight magnetic resonance angiography of the same patient details the venous drainage of the arteriovenous malformation into the superior sagittal sinus (*arrows*).

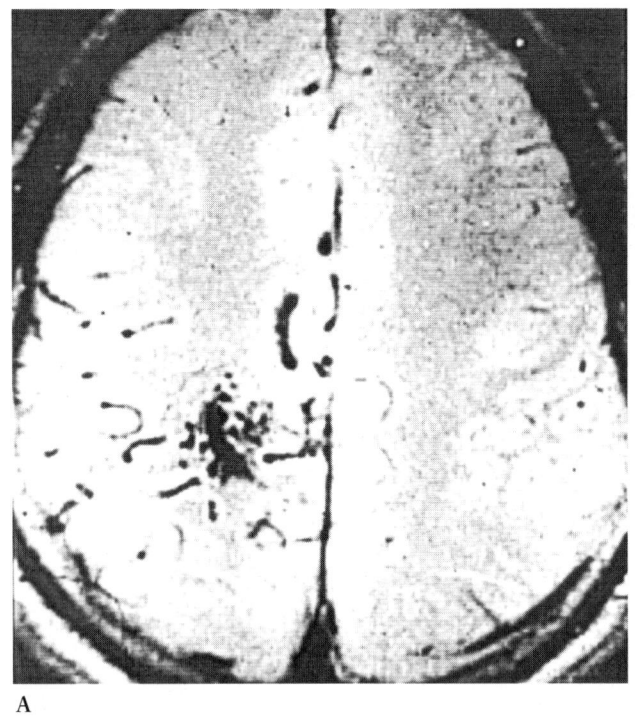

A

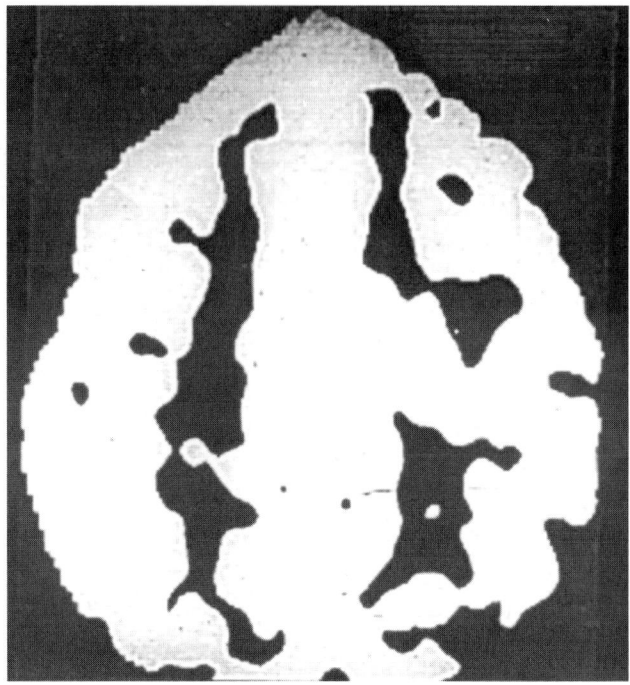

B

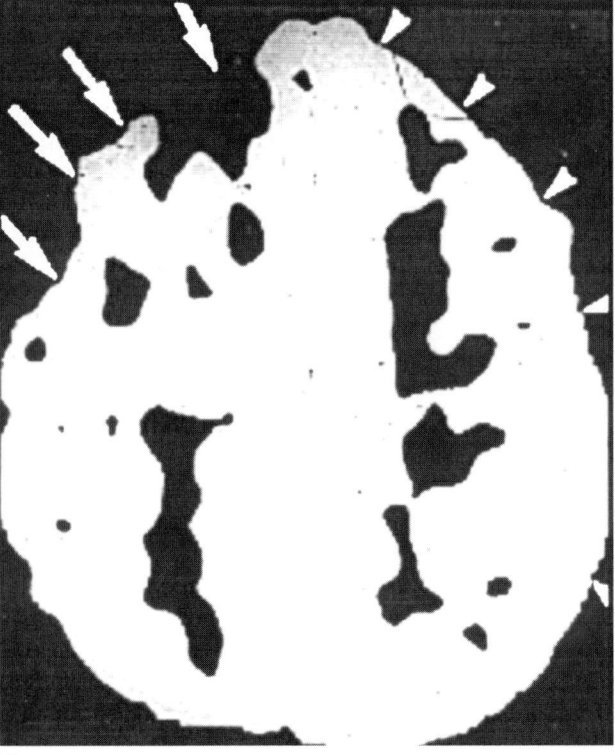

C

FIGURE 57D.7   (**A**) Axial proton density–weighted magnetic resonance image shows a right parietal lobe arteriovenous malformation. Xenon computed tomographic scan cerebral blood flow analysis (**B**) before and (**C**) after the administration of acetazolamide (Diamox) demonstrates normal augmentation of blood flow with acetazolamide in the left hemisphere (*arrowheads*), but a diminution of flow or vascular steal phenomenon (*arrows*) in the right frontal lobe.

TREATMENT

Cavernous Malformations

The therapeutic options for cavernous malformations include medical management of seizures, surgical excision for control of seizures, or prevention of hemorrhage or recurrent bleeding. The use of stereotactic radiosurgical therapy is being investigated, but at this point the standard doses used for true AVMs are associated with a poor clinical response and a high complication rate. With lower doses, there are fewer complications reported, but the end points

FIGURE 57D.8 Functional magnetic resonance imaging with arm motor activation outlines the motor cortex.

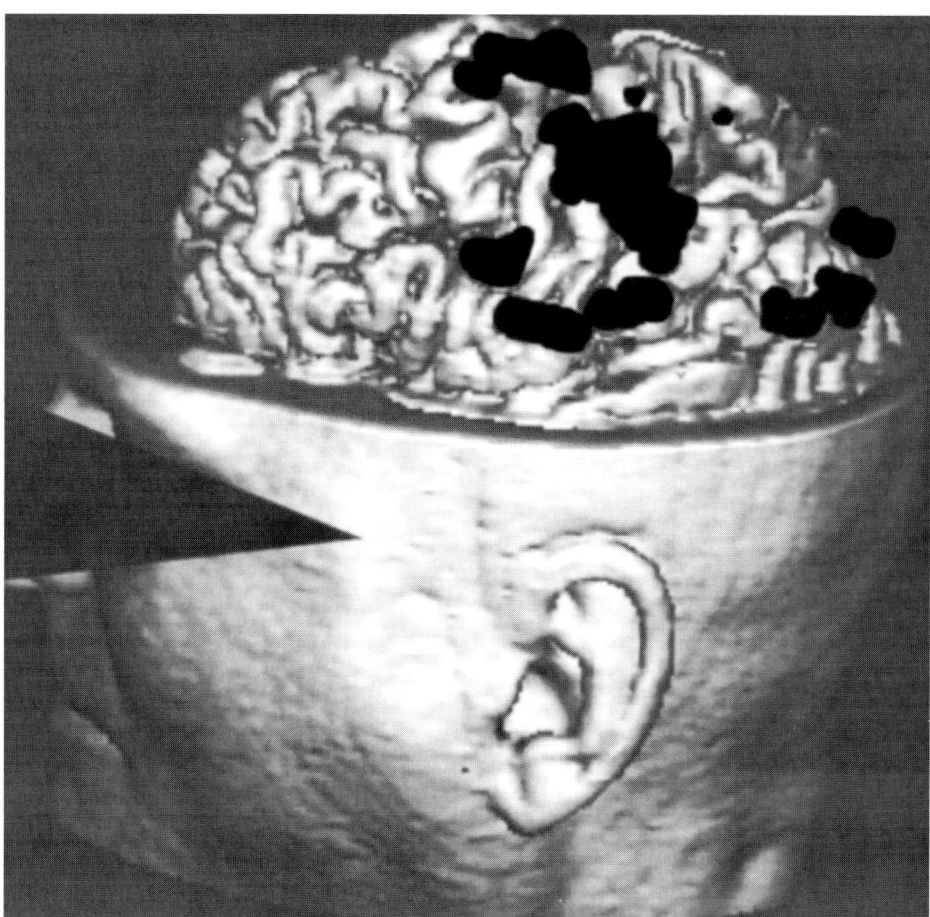

for therapeutic success are harder to define than with the criteria of angiographical obliteration used for true AVMs.

With respect to seizures, surgical therapy is used only if medical management is unsuccessful. Because of the risk of hemorrhage, however, consideration for resection should be given to any lesion that is surgically accessible. In patients presenting with a hemorrhage, in light of the high risk of recurrent hemorrhage, surgical resection should be considered for any accessible lesion in the supratentorial region, and for any brainstem lesion that has a presentation on the pial surface (Maraire and Awad 1997).

Arteriovenous Malformations

In light of a better understanding of the natural history of AVMs, and with refinements in therapeutic options, consideration of treatment should be given to most patients who harbor an AVM. With respect to which mode of therapy is optimal, microsurgery, radiosurgery, and endovascular surgery are all comparable and complementary.

Although the main indication for treatment is prevention of neurological morbidity caused by hemorrhage, a reduction in the occurrence of seizures with successful AVM extirpation has been demonstrated (Hwa-Shain et al. 1993). As noted in the previous section, however, the major morbidity and mortality from an AVM result from hemorrhage, and surgical excision is the most direct and immediate method of eliminating the risk of subsequent hemorrhage.

To facilitate surgical decision making, grading systems for predicting the operative risks in patients with different AVMs have been proposed. The factors to be considered in determining the difficulty of removing an AVM include the size of the lesion, number of feeding arteries, amount of flow through the lesion, degree of steal from the surrounding brain, location of the lesion, functional importance of the surrounding brain, and path of the venous drainage. Some of these variables are interrelated; for ease of grading, the proposed systems focus on size, pattern of venous drainage, and the function of the surrounding brain. Both retrospective and prospective experience with these systems has demonstrated a correlation between the grade of the AVM and the surgical risk.

The decision to pursue treatment must be made in light of a comparison between the natural history of AVMs and the risks of therapy for each individual. The wide variations both in the natural history discussed in the previous section and in treatment outcomes make this a controversial deci-

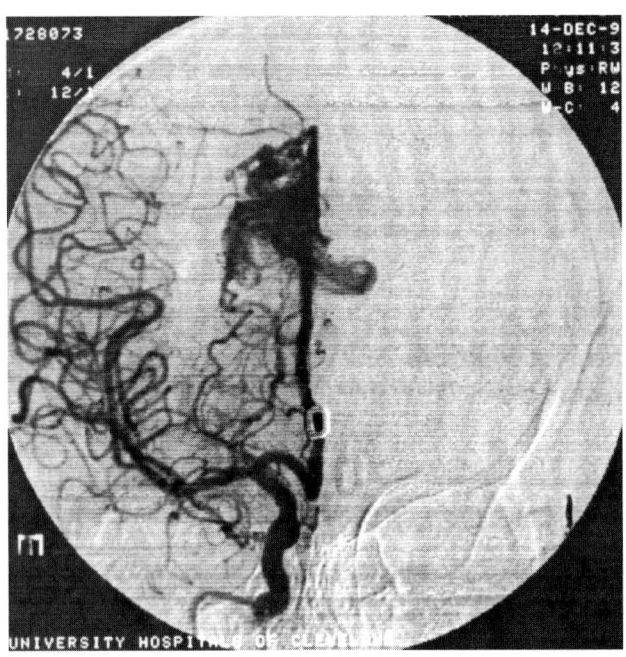
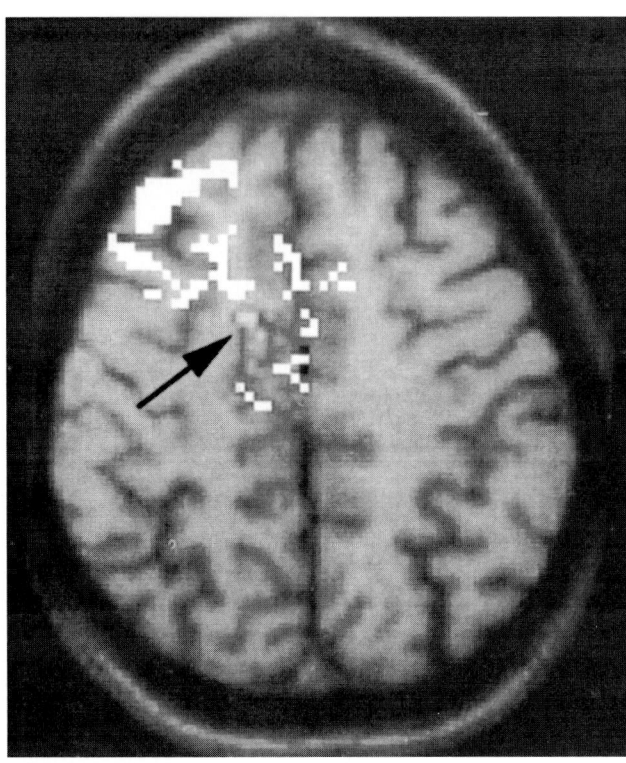

A   B

FIGURE 57D.9   (A) Right internal carotid artery angiogram shows a right frontal arteriovenous malformation. (B) Functional magnetic resonance imaging with left leg activation. Note the proximity of the arteriovenous malformation nidus (*arrow*) to the left leg motor cortex.

sion. If a hemorrhage has occurred from a small, accessible AVM located in a noncritical area of the brain, therapeutic intervention is clearly warranted. A large lesion, with a complex blood supply, located in a critical area, and that has never bled, generates considerably more controversy with regard to its best management.

Decision analysis has been used to determine the role of microsurgical excision in the management of patients with AVMs. The hazards of an uncritical use of decision analysis are evident when applied to AVM treatment. Decision-analysis techniques suggest that unless surgical mortality is on the order of 1% and surgical morbidity no more than 7%, nonoperative therapy is the preferred method of management. For these calculations, a 20-year follow-up was used, and the bleeding rate was assumed to be 1% per year. There are several problems with this application of decision analysis to AVM management. First, the probability of bleeding is a critical issue. With longer periods of follow-up, it has become apparent that the rate of rebleeding is higher than previously believed. Thus, a 1% rate of bleeding severely underestimates the 4% per year rate of hemorrhage now known to occur in patients who present with or without hemorrhage. Second, an observation period of 20 years may be too short for general application. As stated previously, most AVMs are detected in the second, third, and fourth decades of life. Longer periods of observation,

compatible with a normal life expectancy in the nonoperated group, would necessarily increase the overall probability of hemorrhage. Furthermore, the likelihood of hemorrhage appears to be increased during these early decades, whereas patients in this age group, in general, would be considered low-risk surgical candidates. Individual factors that may influence the incidence of hemorrhage and microsurgical outcome are not always considered in treatment algorithms. For example, small lesions are more likely to bleed, and these lesions also are associated with a lower surgical morbidity and mortality. Finally, surgical series of between 70 and 100 patients each have reported immediate favorable outcomes compatible with decision analyses favoring operative intervention, with mortalities of approximately 1% and morbidity of less than 12%. Thus, although decision-analysis schemes may help to provide a framework for considering the optimal management of AVMs, care must be taken to include all the variables that can influence the decision for each individual.

The role of surgery in the management of AVMs is expanding. Sisti and colleagues (1993) reviewed their experience with 67 AVMs less than 3 cm in diameter and reported angiographical obliteration in 94%, with a surgical morbidity of 1.5% and no operative mortality. Forty-five percent of these lesions were in regions that in some reports would be considered surgically inaccessible, such as the thalamus,

FIGURE 57D.10 Left vertebral artery angiogram shows several intranidal aneurysm (*arrows*) associated with this arteriovenous malformation nidus.

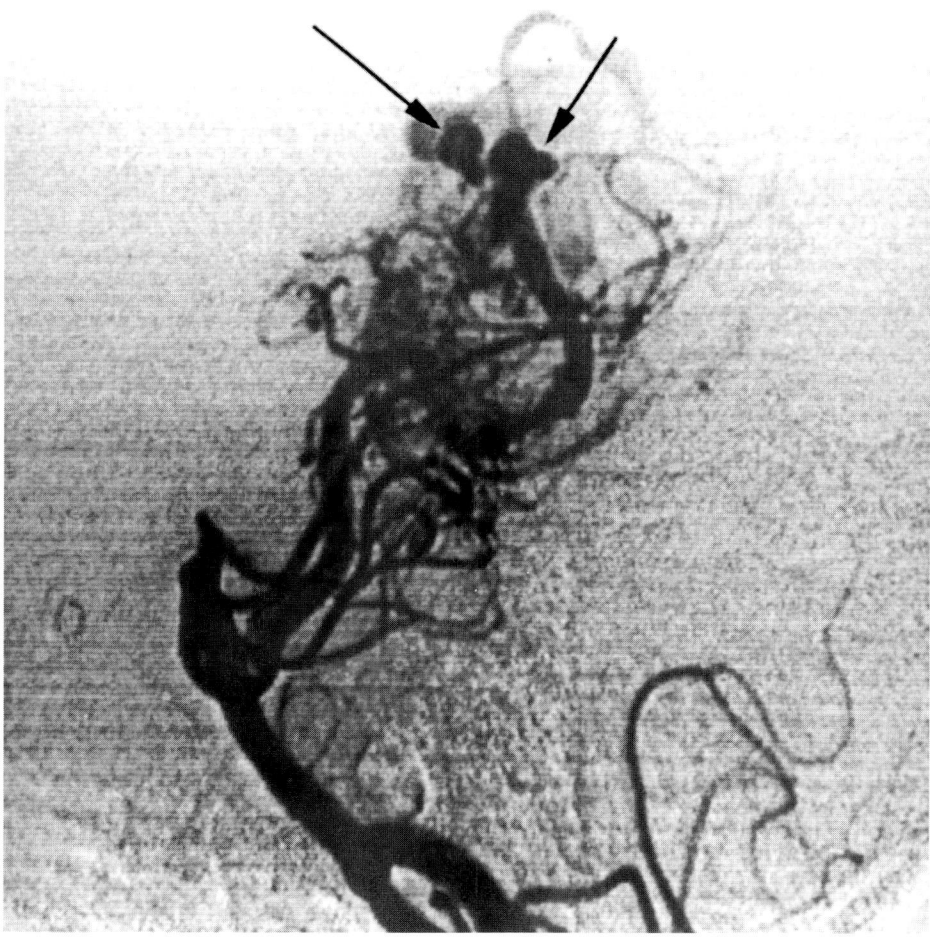

brainstem, medial hemisphere, and paraventricular regions. The immediate protection against hemorrhage provided by microsurgical removal and the avoidance of any risk of development of delayed radiation-related brain injury are distinct advantages over stereotactic radiosurgery. The results of this series emphasize that small size and location should not dictate which form of treatment is offered to a patient.

Special consideration must be given to the management of AVMs in pregnant women (see Chapter 85). Intracranial hemorrhage in pregnancy is caused as often by AVMs as by aneurysms. Although increased blood volume and venous pressure may be important in the pathogenesis of AVM hemorrhage, the time of hemorrhage does not always occur with the peak in cardiovascular changes of pregnancy. Labor and delivery is a high-risk period for AVM-associated hemorrhage, when 11% of these incidents occur. The decision about the diagnostic workup, time of surgery, and preoperative management should be based on neurosurgical rather than obstetrical criteria. If a hemorrhage has occurred during pregnancy, the risk of repeat hemorrhage is higher than in the nonpregnant patient. Because of this high rate of rebleed, some authors have suggested that surgical excision of AVMs that have ruptured should be undertaken as soon as the patient is stable. The stage of the pregnancy must be

considered also; for those near term, an elective cesarean section at 38 weeks' gestation may carry the smallest combined risk to mother and child.

Large lesions previously classified as unresectable also may be managed surgically by using a regimen of preoperative embolization and staged resection. Preoperative embolization can cause thrombosis of much of the vascular nidus and decrease the number of feeding arteries. The role of endovascular techniques in the management of AVMs is continuing to expand with the development of improved catheters and embolization material. In particular, the preoperative use of both diagnostic and therapeutic endovascular techniques has allowed safer and more effective use of microsurgery and radiosurgery for the treatment of complex AVMs (Dion and Mathis 1994).

Radiosurgery has become a major form of therapy for AVMs. The role of stereotactic radiation in the treatment of AVMs is both expanding and being better defined (Figure 57D.11). The results of the previous series demonstrate that stereotactic radiation is most effective in the obliteration of small AVMs. Because of the delayed reaction of the vessels, the patient remains at risk for bleeding until complete thrombosis is attained. The patient also should be advised of the possibilities of incomplete AVM

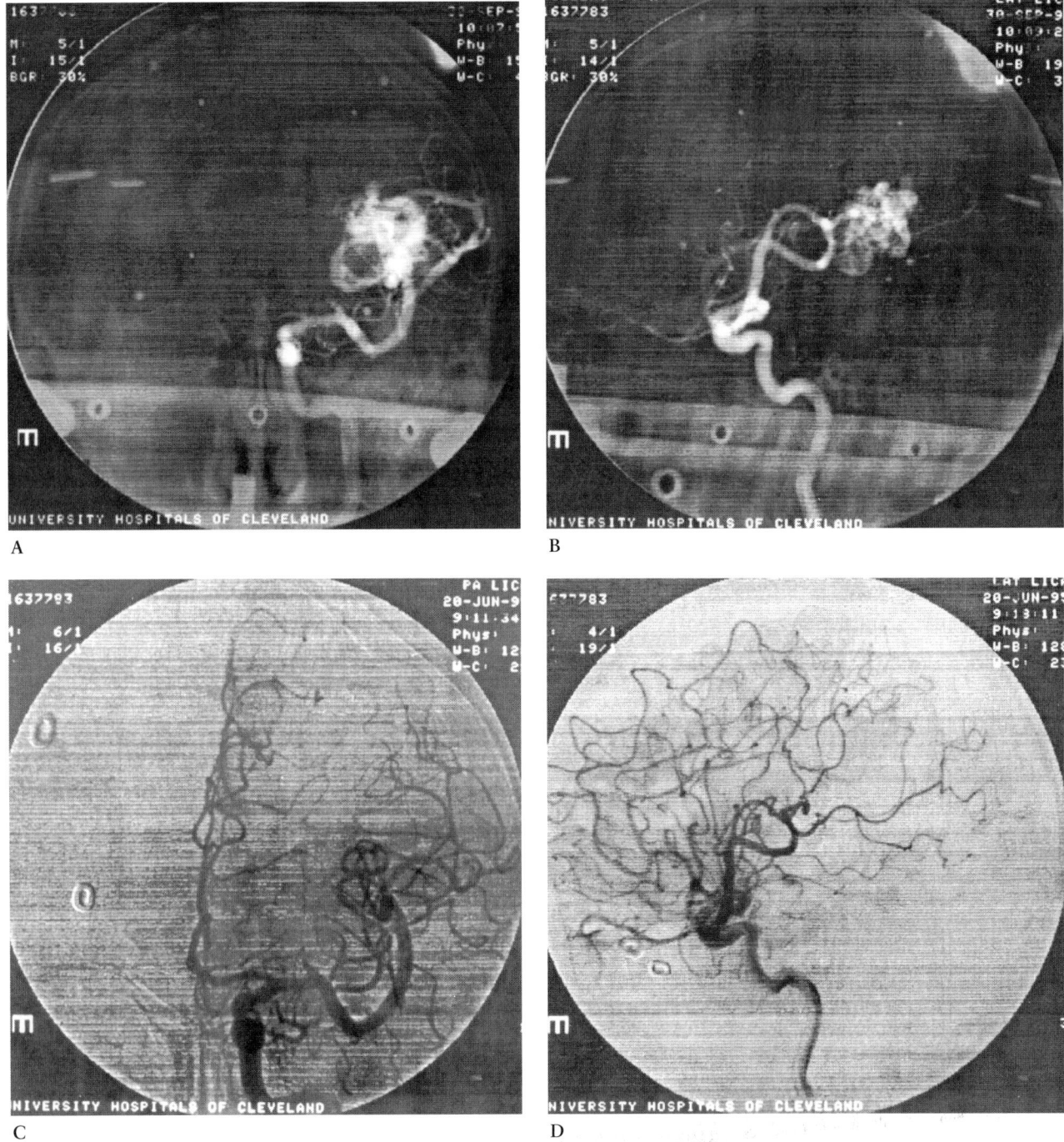

FIGURE 57D.11   (A) Posteroanterior and (B) lateral stereotactic left internal carotid artery angiogram demonstrates a left temporal arteriovenous malformation supplied by the left middle cerebral artery. Two-year follow-up (C) posteroanterior and (D) lateral left internal carotid artery angiogram after radiosurgery show obliteration of the arteriovenous malformation.

obliteration and the risk of delayed development of radiation-induced brain injury. Even in the most favorable circumstances with a lesion less than 3 cm in diameter, the percent of lesions completely obliterated after 3 years is approximately 85%. An analysis of microsurgical and radiosurgical treatments concluded that microsurgical treatment of AVMs of grades I through III was associated with significantly fewer postoperative hemorrhages, fewer

post-treatment neurological deficits, and fewer deaths. A life-table analysis confirmed the statistically significant difference in hemorrhage-free survival time between the microsurgical and stereotactic radiosurgical treatment groups (Pikus et al. 1998).

The risks and benefits of the therapeutic options for patients with AVMs can be appreciated by direct comparison (Table 57D.1).

Table 57D.1: Comparison of treatment modalities

Treatment modality	Advantages	Disadvantages
Microsurgical excision	Immediate elimination of risk of hemorrhage	Risk of immediate new neurological deficit
Endovascular embolization	Immediate reduction in size of AVM; immediate closure of intranidal aneurysms; no general anesthesia; short hospitalization	Rarely achieves total and permanent obliteration of AVM; risk of immediate new neurological deficit from hemorrhage or ischemia
Stereotactic radiosurgery	Noninvasive treatment; short hospitalization	Latency of 1–3 yrs with risk of hemorrhage until complete obliteration of AVM; risk of delayed neurological deficit from radiation damage

AVM = arteriovenous malformation.
Source: Adapted from GK Steinberg, MP Marks. Intracranial Arteriovenous Malformation: Therapeutic Options. In HH Batjer, LR Caplan, L Friberg. (eds), Cerebrovascular Disease. Philadelphia: Lippincott–Raven, 1997;727–742.

The importance of a comprehensive team approach, which includes specialists in microvascular neurosurgery, endovascular neuroradiology, and stereotactic radiation, cannot be overemphasized to ensure that patients receive appropriate therapy. Large lesions previously classified as unresectable may be safely managed with a combination of endovascular techniques, followed by surgical excision, and small lesions can be immediately and effectively eliminated with microsurgery.

REFERENCES

Aiba T, Tanaka R, Koike T, et al. Natural history of intracranial cavernous malformations. J Neurosurg 1995;83:56–59.

Dion JE, Mathis JM. Cranial arteriovenous malformations: the role of embolization and stereotactic surgery. Neurosurg Clin North Am 1994;5:459–474.

Fritschi JA, Reulen HJ, Spetzler RF, et al. Cavernous malformations of the brain stem. A review of 139 cases (review). Acta Neurochir 1994;130:35–46.

Hwa-Shain Y, Tew JM Jr, Gartner M. Seizure control after surgery on cerebral arteriovenous malformations. J Neurosurg 1993;78: 12–18.

Lance JW. Mechanism and Management of Headache (5th ed). London: Butterworth–Heinemann, 1993;217–219.

Maraire JN, Awad IA. Cavernous Malformations: Natural History and Indications for Treatment. In HH Batjer, et al. (eds), Cerebrovascular Disease. Philadelphia: Lippincott–Raven, 1997; 669–677.

Notelet L, Chapon F, Khoury S, et al. Familial cavernous malformations in a large French kindred: mapping of the gene to the CCMI locus on chromosome 7q. J Neurol Neurosurg Psychiatry 1997;63:40–45.

Perl J, Ross J. Diagnostic Imaging of Cavernous Malformations. In I Awad, D Barrow (eds), Cavernous Malformations. Park Ridge, IL: American Association of Neurological Surgeons, 1993;7–48.

Pikus HJ, Beach ML, Harbaugh RE. Microsurgical treatment of arteriovenous malformations: analysis and comparison with stereotactic radiosurgery. J Neurosurg 1998;88:641–646.

Sisti MB, Kader A, Stein BM. Microsurgery for 67 intracranial arteriovenous malformations less than 3 cm in diameter. J Neurosurg 1993;79:653–660.

Steinberg GK, Marks MP. Intracranial Arteriovenous Malformation: Therapeutic Options. In HH Batjer, LR Caplan, L Friberg (eds), Cerebrovascular Disease. Philadelphia: Lippincott–Raven, 1997; 727–742.

Wijdicks EFM, Schievink WI. Perimesencephalic subarachnoid hemorrhage: first hint of a cause? Neurology 1997;49: 634–636.

Zabramski JM, Wascher TM, Spetzler RF, et al. The natural history of familial cavernous malformations: results of an ongoing study. J Neurosurg 1994;80:422–432.

Chapter 57
Vascular Diseases of the Nervous System

E.   STROKE IN CHILDHOOD
Richard S. K. Young

Sigmund Freud provided one of the earliest descriptions of stroke in childhood in 1887. It was the natural history of acute hemiplegia of childhood in which a previously healthy child became acutely ill with hemiparesis, convulsions, and fever. Sequelae included impaired intelligence, intractable seizures, and growth failure of the affected limbs.

The annual incidence of cerebral infarction in children after the newborn period is 1.2 per 100,000 and the combined incidence of nontraumatic intracerebral and subarachnoid hemorrhage is 1.5 per 100,000 (Broderick et al. 1993). The incidence is slightly higher in black than in white children. Approximately 66% of strokes in children are associated with a known risk factor (Kerr et al. 1993).

Stroke in childhood has both differences from and similarities to stroke in adults. Stroke in children differs primarily because of the predominance of congenital and genetic causes. There are also notable differences with regard to incidence, etiology, clinical presentation, and course. As is true in adults, disorders of the heart and great vessels are responsible for many strokes in children. Atherosclerosis may be associated with nonhemorrhagic stroke in as many as one-fourth of affected children.

CLINICAL SYMPTOMS AND SIGNS

The presentation of stroke in children differs from that in adults in the following ways: (1) seizures at onset are more frequent in children whether the stroke is hemorrhagic or ischemic infarction; and (2) stroke in the dominant hemisphere produces loss of expressive language, usually presenting as mutism in younger children; fluent aphasia is uncommon in childhood stroke.

Acute hemiplegia of childhood usually occurs before age 2 years. The cause is presumed to be vascular occlusion. Seizures are the initial symptom in 80% of cases. The seizures may be multiple or single, focal or generalized. Fever and alteration of consciousness are common at the onset. Residual hemiparesis, epilepsy, mental impairment, and hyperactive behavior are common sequelae. Prognosis is least favorable when there are multiple seizures at the onset of illness.

PATHOGENESIS AND ETIOLOGY

The common causes of childhood stroke are summarized in Table 57E.1 and are discussed here. Occlusive vascular disease is only slightly more common (55%) than intracranial hemorrhage (45%). Cyanotic congenital heart disease is the most frequent cause of ischemic strokes, accounting for 26%. Other common causes of stroke are sickle cell disease, intracranial infection, vascular malformations, and occlusive vascular disease. Inborn errors of metabolism are a rare cause of stroke that are a consideration in children but not adults. Acquired immunodeficiency disease is becoming an increasingly important cause of stroke in children.

Trauma to the neck may predispose to arterial dissection. Cerebellar infarction may occur also as a result of trauma. Subluxation between the first and second cervical vertebrae caused by abnormal neck movements may result in arterial injury.

DIFFERENTIAL DIAGNOSIS

The differential diagnosis of hemiplegia caused by stroke includes three major entities: transient postictal hemiparesis

Table 57E.1: Major causes of stroke in children

Cardiac
    Cyanotic congenital disease
    Catheterization
    Intraoperative or postoperative
    Bacterial endocarditis
    Atrial myxoma
    Rhabdomyoma
    Mitral valve prolapse
Hematological
    Sickle cell disease
    Leukemia
    Disseminated intravascular coagulation
    Thrombocytopenia
    Polycythemia
    Hemophilia
Infection
    Meningitis—bacterial, tuberculous, fungal
    Parameningeal
    Viral
Trauma
    Arterial occlusion
    Intracerebral hematoma
    Shaken baby syndrome
Vascular
    Major vessel occlusion with telangiectasia (moyamoya)
    Major vessel occlusion without telangiectasia
    Fibromuscular dysplasia
    Collagen vascular disease
    Migraine
Metabolic
    Homocystinuria
    Diabetes
    Mitochondrial encephalomyopathy
Toxic
    Phencyclidine
    Methamphetamine
    Phenylpropanolamine
    Cocaine
Hemorrhagic
    Arteriovenous malformation
    Aneurysm

(Todd's paralysis), hemiplegic migraine, and the syndrome of alternating hemiplegia. Transient postictal hemiparesis usually lasts less than 24 hours. Electroencephalography may disclose epileptiform activity in postictal hemiparesis and slow-wave activity in cases of stroke. In contrast to stroke, imaging studies in postictal hemiparesis do not show edema, mass effect, or infarction.

Patients with complicated migraine often develop symptoms and signs referable to a vascular territory. These include hemiplegia, hemidysesthesia, hemianopia, and aphasia. Complicated migraine differs from stroke in several respects. First, hemiplegic migraine is preceded by severe headache. Second, the neurological deficits are tran-

sient, generally lasting more than 60 minutes but less than a week. Third, neuroimaging studies are normal. In unusual circumstances, complicated migraine may be associated with cerebral infarction, but the prognosis for complete or near-complete recovery is good.

Alternating hemiplegia is an unusual syndrome of young children (onset <18 months) characterized by frequent episodes of hemiplegia involving both sides of the body, progressive developmental delay, and ocular motor and autonomic disturbances (Bourgeois et al. 1993). Although the children frequently have seizure disorders, the attacks of hemiplegia are not associated with epileptogenic discharges. Cerebral blood flow studies with single-photon emission computed tomography have not documented cerebral ischemia. Similarly, the normal lactate and pyruvate levels in children with alternating hemiplegia differentiate the disorder from the syndrome of MELAS (*m*itochondrial *e*ncephalopathy, *l*actic *a*cidosis, and *s*trokelike episodes).

EVALUATION OF THE CHILD WITH STROKE

Cranial magnetic resonance imaging is the cornerstone of evaluation of stroke in children. Standard laboratory tests to rule out infection and hematological or collagen vascular disease should be obtained in all children with stroke (Table 57E.2). More sophisticated laboratory and imaging studies may be indicated depending on the results of the magnetic resonance imaging.

Magnetic resonance angiography can often replace conventional arteriography and digital subtraction angiography. ^{99m}Tc-HMPAO single-photon emission computed tomography is a sensitive, complementary diagnostic measure in the early detection and localization of regional cerebral blood flow alterations in childhood stroke.

CAUSES OF STROKE IN CHILDHOOD

Cardiac Disorders

The frequency of stroke in children with cyanotic congenital heart disease, especially tetralogy of Fallot or transposition of the great vessels, is 1.6–3.8%. Children with these types of cyanotic heart disease are most likely to develop cerebrovascular complications before 2 years of age. The mechanism of stroke is often thrombosis as a result of polycythemia and reduced cerebral blood flow during periods of diminished cardiac output.

Cardiogenic emboli should be presumed when there is evidence of multiple infarctions (Figures 57E.1 and 57E.2). Cardiac emboli may be infectious or noninfectious. Septic emboli from bacterial endocarditis cause focal neurological deficits because of infarction or rupture of mycotic aneurysms.

Noninfectious cardiogenic emboli may break off from apical clots in poorly contractile ventricles. Marantic endo-

Table 57E.2:   Evaluation of stroke in children

Standard evaluation
  Imaging studies
    Magnetic resonance imaging
    Chest roentgenography
    Carotid ultrasound
    Cardiac ultrasound
  Hematological studies
    Complete blood cell count and platelet count
    Electrolytes, blood urea nitrogen, and creatinine
    Glucose
    Total bilirubin, serum glutamic oxaloacetic transaminase,
      lactic dehydrogenase, serum glutamic pyruvate transami-
      nase, CK
    Total protein
    Uric acid
    Calcium, phosphate
    Cholesterol, triglycerides
    Prothrombin test, partial thromboplastin time
    Erythrocyte sedimentation rate and serum viscosity
    Hemoglobin electrophoresis (if indicated)
    Blood cultures
  Other
    Electrocardiography and Holter monitoring
    Urinalysis
Optional (pending initial assessment)
  Imaging studies
    ^{99m}Tc single-photon emission computed tomography
    Digital subtraction angiography
    Angiography
  Hematological studies
    CK isoenzymes
    Fibrinogen
    VDRL
    Platelet function test
    Magnesium
    Thyroid function tests
  Other
    Exercise tolerance test
    Electroencephalography
    Lumbar puncture
  Collagen vascular screen
    Protein C and protein S
    Antithrombin III
    Rheumatoid factor
    Antinuclear antibody
    Lupus anticoagulant
    Serum protein electrophoresis
    C3, C4, CH50

CK = creatine kinase.

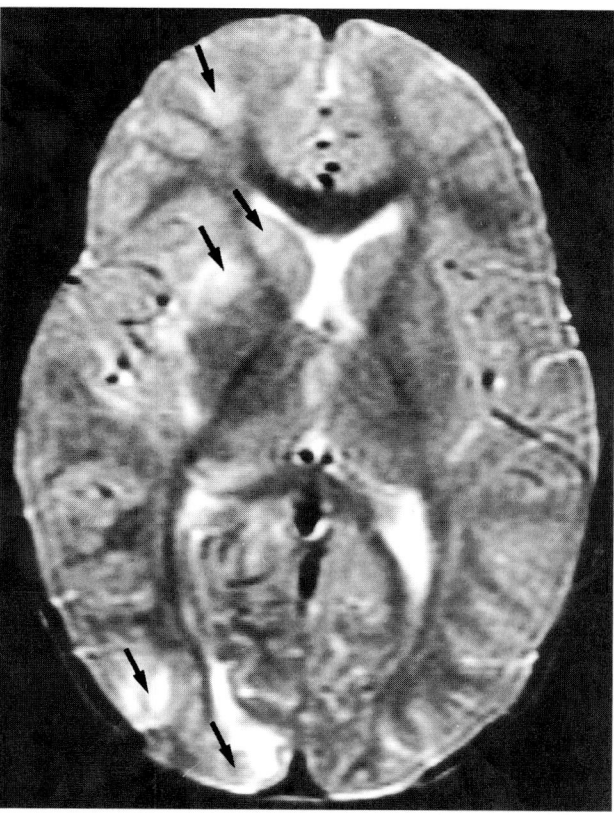

FIGURE 57E.1   Multiple cerebral emboli. T2-weighted magnetic resonance image of this 2-year-old child with presumed embolic disease shows multiple areas of infarction in the frontal, parietal, and occipital regions as well as in the basal ganglia (*arrows*).

in 5% of patients undergoing valve replacement who are not anticoagulated. The use of anticoagulants reduces the frequency of embolization by one-half. The frequency of stroke during cardiac catheterization correlates with the efficacy of heparinization during the procedure. Rhabdomyoma of the heart associated with tuberous sclerosis is a rare cause of cerebral emboli (see Chapter 69).

Arterial hypertension may play an important role in the pathogenesis of stroke in black patients. The increased prevalence of hypertension, hypertensive intracerebral hemorrhage, and lacunar infarction among young black patients with stroke suggests accelerated hypertensive arteriolar damage.

Hematological Disorders

Stroke is a frequent complication of hematological disorders, especially sickle cell disease, leukemia, thrombocytopenia, and hemophilia. The occlusions associated with sickle cell disease can occur in small vessels or large arteries, including the carotid. Carotid occlusions provoke the development of collateral vessels of the moyamoya telangiectatic type (see discussion of moyamoya disease in Occlusive Vascular Disease, later in this chapter).

carditis (Figure 57E.3) occurs most commonly with coagulopathies or malignancies. Other types of noninfective emboli are fat emboli from long bone fractures. Paradoxical cerebral emboli cross from the right side of the heart to the left through a patent foramen ovale or atrial septal defect.

Embolic stroke is a complication of cardiac surgery in the intraoperative and immediate postoperative periods. The usual sources of emboli are thrombi on damaged or prosthetic heart valves. Thromboembolic complications occur

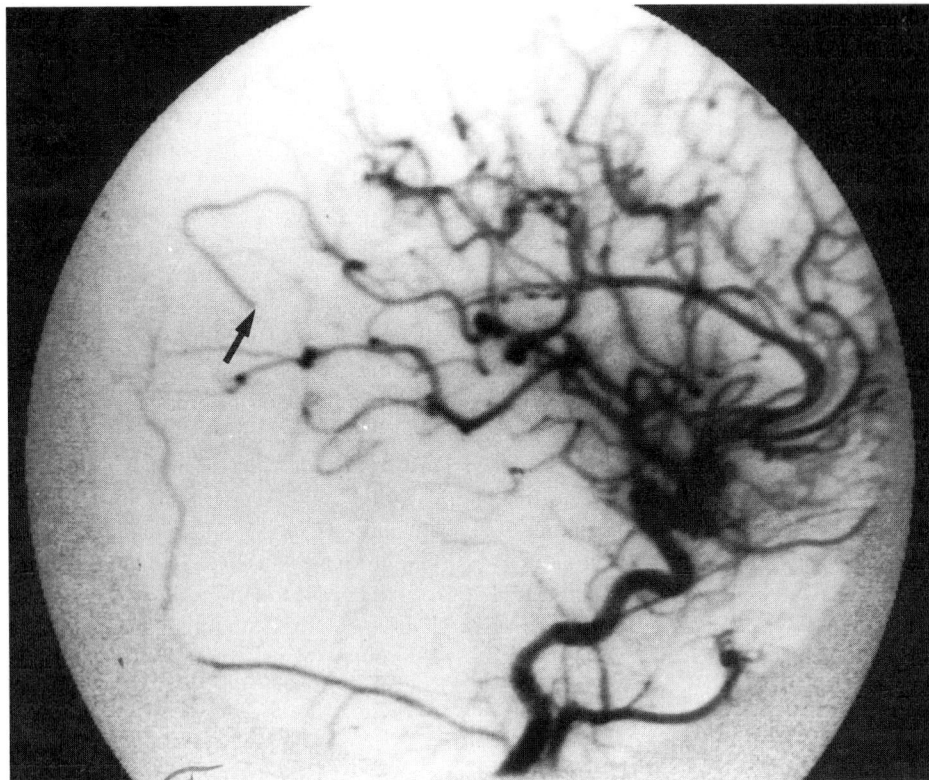

FIGURE 57E.2 Multiple cerebral emboli. The angiogram discloses abrupt cessation of the posterior parietal branch of the middle cerebral artery (*arrow*).

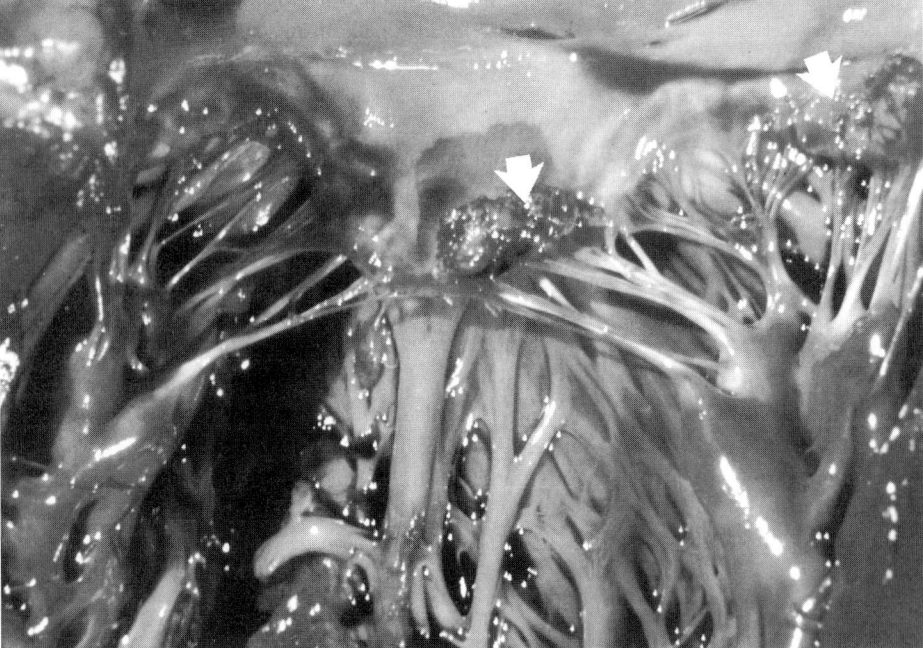

FIGURE 57E.3 Marantic endocarditis. Cardiac vegetations (*arrows*) in this teenager with leukemia are noninfective.

Factors responsible for stroke in homozygotes for sickle cell disease include diffuse sickling with vascular occlusion, perfusion failure, intra-arterial embolization, and intimal hyperplasia and thrombosis with partial recanalization. The abnormal erythrocytes clog large and small vessels, decreasing total, hemispheric, or regional blood flow. Cere-

bral infarction usually occurs in the region of arterial border zones.

Stroke occurs in as many as 17% of persons with sickle cell disease. The mean age of stroke is 7.7 years and the risk of recurrence is 67%. Asymptomatic cerebral infarction may occur in another 25% of affected children. Intracere-

FIGURE 57E.4 Factor IX deficiency. Both lobar and petechial hemorrhages are present in this child with factor IX deficiency.

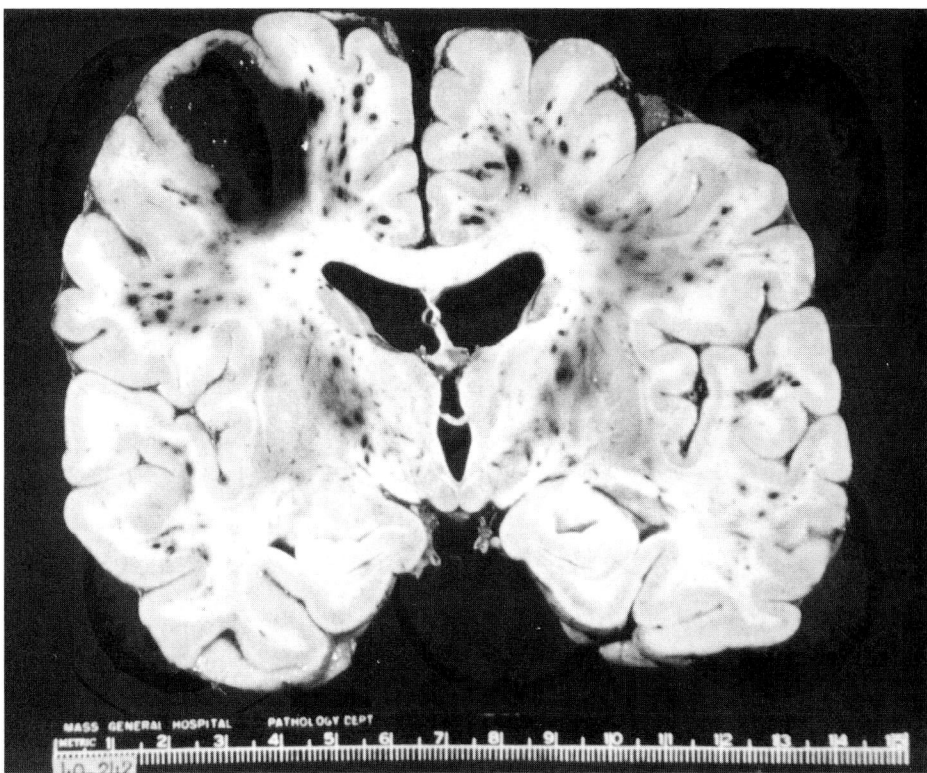

bral hemorrhage, when it occurs, is caused usually by a ruptured aneurysm. Elevated homocysteine levels may be a risk factor for the development of stroke in patients with sickle cell disease (Houston et al. 1997). Periodic prophylactic hypertransfusion of red blood cells (hypertransfusion therapy) has decreased stroke recurrence by increasing cerebral blood flow. Even hypertransfusion therapy does not change the angiographic picture of an existing vascular occlusion, and strokes often recur within months of terminating hypertransfusion therapy. Transcranial ultrasonography identifies those children with sickle cell disease who are at highest risk for cerebral infarction.

Coagulation factor deficiencies, such as hemophilia or thrombocytopenia, predispose children to intracranial hemorrhage after minor trauma (Figure 57E.4). Disorders of coagulation inhibition (antithrombin III and protein C or protein S deficiency) or fibrinolysis, whether genetic or acquired, cause thrombotic occlusions.

Cancer and Its Treatment

Children with leukemia and other forms of cancer have a 14% risk for stroke, usually within the first year after diagnosis. Vascular thrombosis occurs with leukocytosis over 100,000 white blood cells per liter, neoplastic infiltration of vessels, central nervous system infection, and secondary to chemotherapeutic drugs (e.g., L-asparaginase, cytosine arabinoside). Secondary thrombocytopenia causes intra-

parenchymal hemorrhage, and radiation therapy produces a progressive vasculopathy that results in large vessel occlusion.

Disseminated intravascular coagulation is a complication of the acute leukemias, especially acute promyelocytic leukemia. Disseminated intravascular coagulation may be associated with focal neurological features or generalized encephalopathy.

Venous sinus occlusion occurs most commonly in the torcula in association with metastatic neuroblastoma, in which case radiation therapy may be beneficial. Other vascular complications include emboli from cardiac or pulmonary tumors, marantic endocarditis, and drug-induced cardiomyopathy.

Infectious Disease

Cerebrovascular disease occurs in up to 25% of children with human immunodeficiency virus infection and is equally divided between hemorrhagic and nonhemorrhagic infarcts. In the former, the pathological findings are hemorrhage caused by thrombocytopenia, arteriopathy, and aneurysms. Dystrophic calcification of blood vessels is identified in 80% of patients on postmortem examination.

Carotid arteritis can occur in children with chronic tonsillitis and cervical adenitis, and retropharyngeal abscess. Unilateral and bilateral occlusions of the cervical portion of the internal carotid arteries may develop.

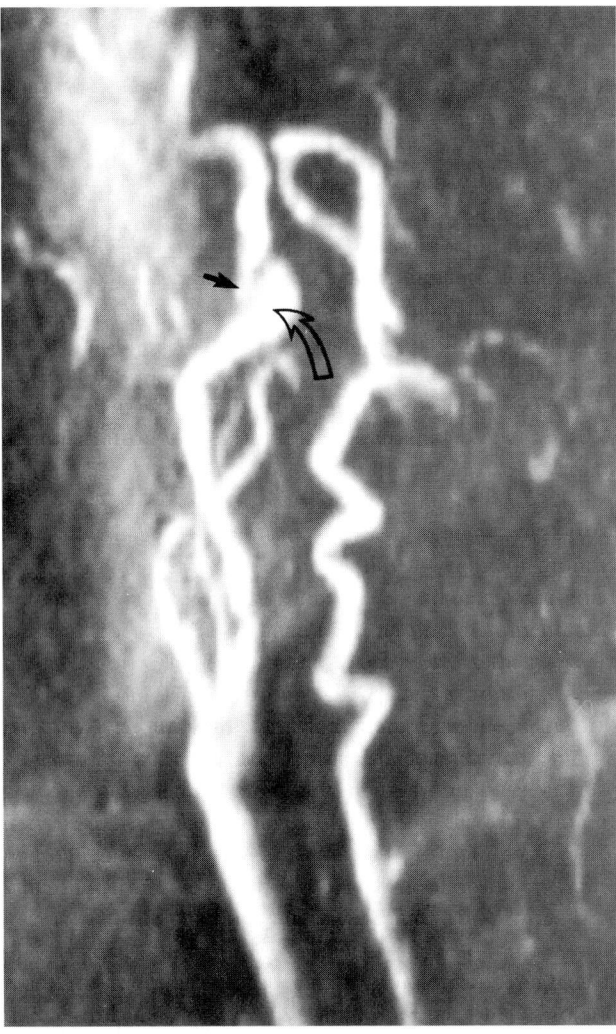

FIGURE 57E.5 Carotid artery trauma. Narrowing of the proximal internal carotid artery (*arrow*) is seen. A false aneurysm is present (*curved arrow*).

Occlusive Vascular Disease

Occlusion of major vessels occurs not only in association with adjacent infection but also from trauma to the neck and fibrous dysplasia of bone. The usual sites of occlusion are the carotid or the vertebral arteries (Figures 57E.5 and 57E.6). Children may experience carotid thrombosis and dissection from apparently trivial injuries sustained in grabbing and shaking the neck or during exercise and sports. The carotid artery may be injured in the tonsillar fossa when a child falls with either a sharp or blunt object (e.g., pencil, lollipop) in the mouth. Vertebral artery thrombosis or dissection may follow minor neck trauma, especially rapid neck rotation. The site of occlusion is usually at the C1 to C2 level.

No cause can be determined in approximately 20% of children with acute hemiplegia secondary to cerebral infarction. Vascular occlusive disease may occur with and without secondary telangiectasia. The syndrome with telangiectasia is called *moyamoya disease* and is characterized by obstruction or narrowing of the supraclinoid internal carotid artery or the proximal portion of the anterior or middle cerebral artery. A prominent unilateral or bilateral telangiectatic network of collaterals forms, especially in the vessels to the basal ganglia. The initial symptoms vary from recurrent headache to abrupt hemiparesis. Recovery follows, but before it is complete, new episodes of focal neurological dysfunction occur either ipsilaterally or contralaterally.

Vascular occlusion without telangiectasia may be associated with inflammatory arteritis, stenosis of the internal carotid artery, distal branch occlusion over the convexity, and very small artery disease. Fibromuscular dysplasia is an idiopathic segmental nonatheromatous disorder of the internal carotid artery that occurs in children and adults. The cervical portion of the artery is most often affected. Transient ischemic attacks and stroke are the only neurological features, whereas hypertension results from renal artery involvement. Arteriography reveals an irregular contour of the internal carotid artery in the neck, resembling a string of pearls (Figure 57E.7).

Several metabolic disorders cause stroke in children (see Chapter 68). Homocystinuria causes vascular thrombosis by a combination of intimal thickening, intimal fibrosis, and increased platelet adhesiveness. Fabry's disease, an X-linked disorder of α-galactosidase, causes occlusion of large and small vessels by the accumulation of glycosphingolipids in endothelial cells, hypertensive hemorrhage, and cerebral aneurysms. Dyslipoproteinemias, such as high-density lipoprotein deficiency and triglyceride disorders, lead to thrombotic strokes and transient ischemic attacks in children. Cerebral infarction occurs in conjunction with diabetic ketoacidosis or hypoglycemic episodes. Mitochondrial disorders such as MELAS (Figure 57E.8) and Leigh disease are associated with acute hemiplegia and other focal dysfunction. The mechanism is probably impaired oxidative metabolism of the brain and cerebral vessels.

Systemic lupus erythematosus and polyarteritis nodosa are causes of vascular occlusions. The lupus anticoagulant, a circulating antiphospholipid antibody, is associated with thromboembolism in as many as 50% of patients who are anticoagulant positive.

Substance abuse leads to an increased frequency of stroke. Amphetamine, phenylpropanolamine, cocaine, and phencyclidine acutely increase blood pressure and cause intracranial hemorrhage. Cocaine and amphetamine are potent vasoconstrictors that cause infarction by vasculitis and vasospasm. Stroke occurs mainly in young adults and may follow any route of administration but takes place more often when "crack" cocaine is smoked. The interval from administration to stroke is unknown in most cases, but may be minutes to hours. Infarction may be caused by vasospasm or vasculitis. Cerebral infarction is a possible consequence of in utero exposure to cocaine.

Venous occlusion of cerebral veins or major intracranial sinuses is caused by hemoconcentration from dehydration and

FIGURE 57E.6 Carotid artery trauma. Following carotid artery trauma, the magnetic resonance image demonstrates carotid dissection with a stenotic true lumen (*arrow*) and a clot in the false lumen (*curved arrow*).

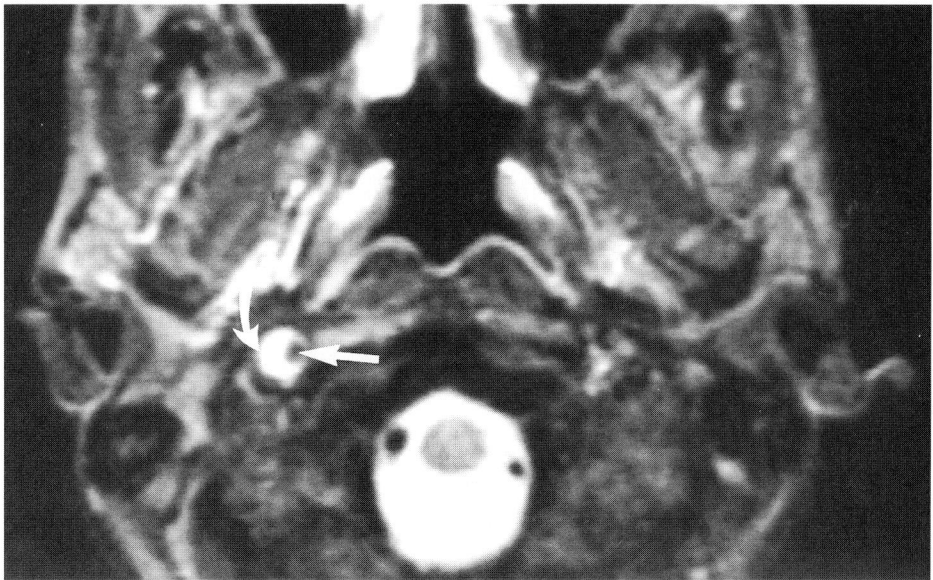

FIGURE 57E.7 Fibromuscular dysplasia. No flow occurs in the middle cerebral artery. A string of pearls can be seen consistent with fibromuscular dysplasia (*arrow*).

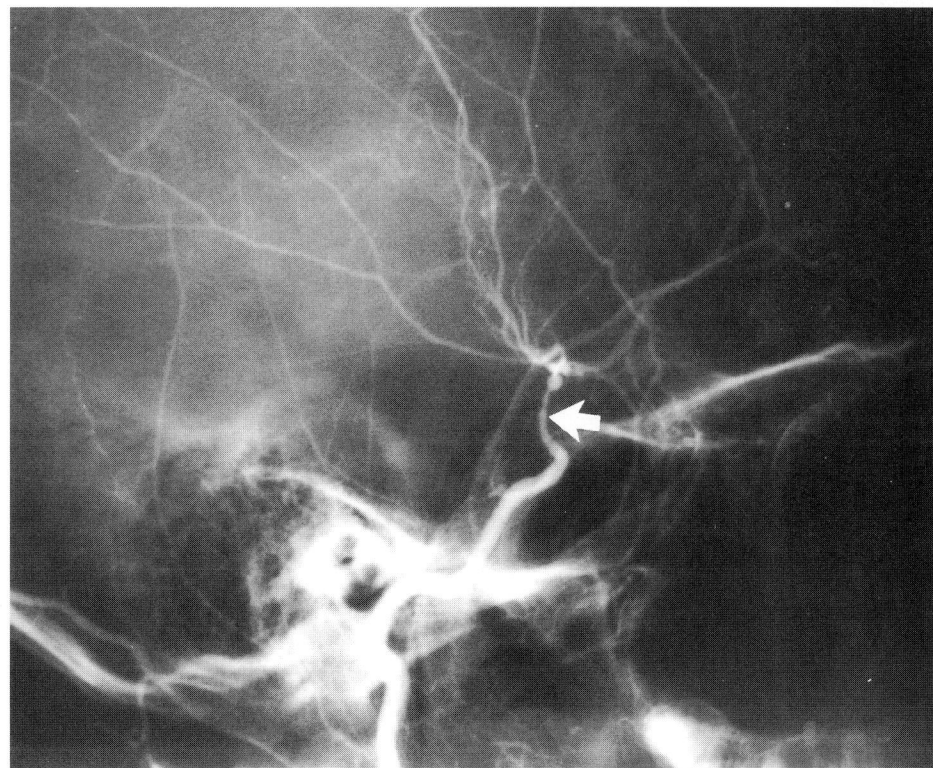

polycythemia with cyanotic heart disease. Intracranial infection, especially acute bacterial meningitis, but also tuberculous meningitis, fungal meningitis, and viral infections, may cause arteritis or thrombophlebitis. Thrombophlebitis also occurs secondary to parameningeal infections including sinusitis, mastoiditis, or subdural empyema, and systemic infections. The initial features are usually focal seizures, focal headache, and focal neurological signs.

Hemorrhage

Arteriovenous malformations (AVMs) are the third most common cause of intracranial hemorrhage in children after cranial trauma and coagulopathies. Small AVMs may present as a focal seizure, whereas very large AVMs often are associated with an intracranial bruit, seizures, and focal neurological signs. Intense headache caused by subarach-

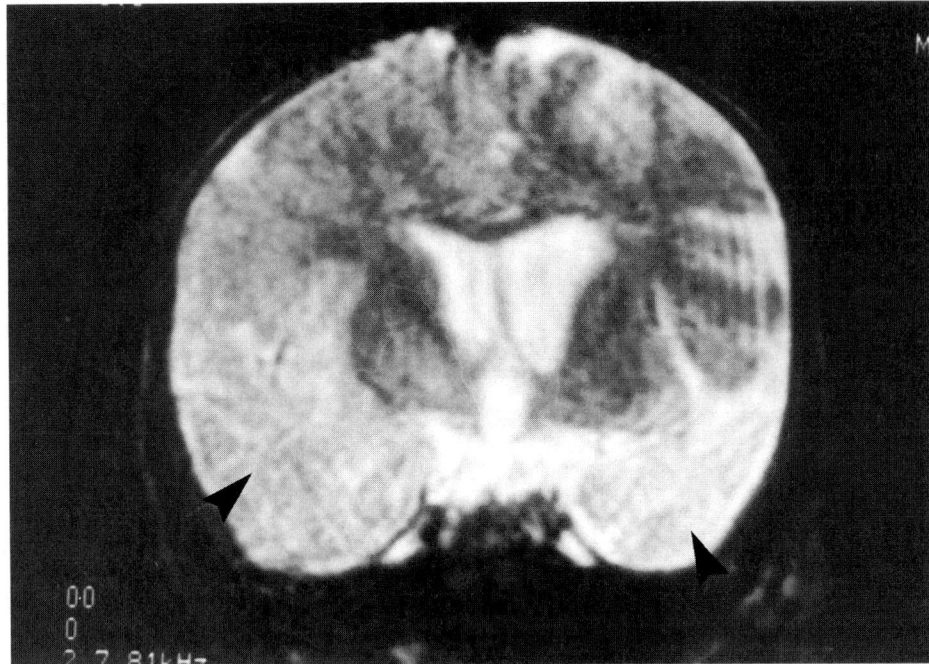

FIGURE 57E.8 MELAS (*m*itochondrial *e*ncephalopathy, *l*actic *a*cidosis, and *s*troke). Magnetic resonance imaging discloses multiple areas of cerebral infarction (*arrows*) and ventricular dilatation.

noid hemorrhage may be present with either small or large AVMs. The mortality may be as high as 20%. Thrombosis of the AVM may cause focal infarction.

Saccular aneurysms are rarely symptomatic in childhood and are considerably less frequent than AVMs. Congenital aneurysms are associated sometimes with coarctation of the aorta and polycystic kidneys. Aneurysms in children are more often of the giant type, rather than the smaller saccular variety in adults. Large or giant aneurysms, when present, are usually in the middle cerebral artery and posterior circulations.

Massive extracerebral hemorrhage, either subdural or subarachnoid, may occur in the shaken baby syndrome. Sudden acceleration or deceleration of the infant's head may rupture bridging veins, leading to extracerebral collections of blood. Classic physical findings in the shaken baby syndrome include retinal hemorrhages and pressure marks on the infant's shoulders.

Intracerebral hemorrhage is a serious complication of leukemia, idiopathic thrombocytopenia, or hemophilia. In some instances, the trauma may be trivial. In idiopathic thrombocytopenia, the platelet count is usually below 20,000 per μl at the time of hemorrhage.

STROKE IN THE NEWBORN

Stroke in the newborn is usually caused by intrauterine or perinatal vascular occlusion (see Chapter 84). Porencephalic cysts may be a consequence of stroke in utero (Figure 57E.9). Infarction caused by hypoxic-ischemic encephalopathy is usually bilateral, resulting in quadriparesis, whereas single-vessel occlusion causes hemiplegia (see Figure 57E.9). Maternal use of cocaine during the prepartum period may lead to vasoconstriction and cerebral infarction.

Cerebral infarction from arterial occlusion occurs more often in full-term newborns than in premature newborns (Figure 57E.10). Three patterns of infarction occur: (1) Arterial border zone infarction is usually associated with resuscitation and probably results from hypotension; (2) multiarterial infarction is less often associated with perinatal distress and may be caused by congenital heart disease, disseminated intravascular coagulation, and polycythemia; and (3) single-artery infarction can be caused by injury to the cervical portion of the carotid artery during a difficult delivery because of either misapplication of obstetrical forceps or hyperextension and rotation of the neck with stretching of the artery over the lateral portion of the upper cervical vertebrae. Because birth-related trauma is currently infrequent, the cause of most single-artery infarctions may be more likely to be related to cardiogenic emboli.

COURSE AND PROGNOSIS

Mortality after stroke in children ranges from 20–30%, depending on the location and the underlying cause. Hemorrhagic stroke has a higher mortality than ischemic stroke. There is increased risk of immediate death if hemorrhagic infarction is accompanied by coma (Keidan et al. 1994). Residual neurological dysfunction is present in more than 50% of survivors and is more common after ischemic stroke. The prognosis is poor for infants whose initial features are seizures and hemiplegia. Most continue to have

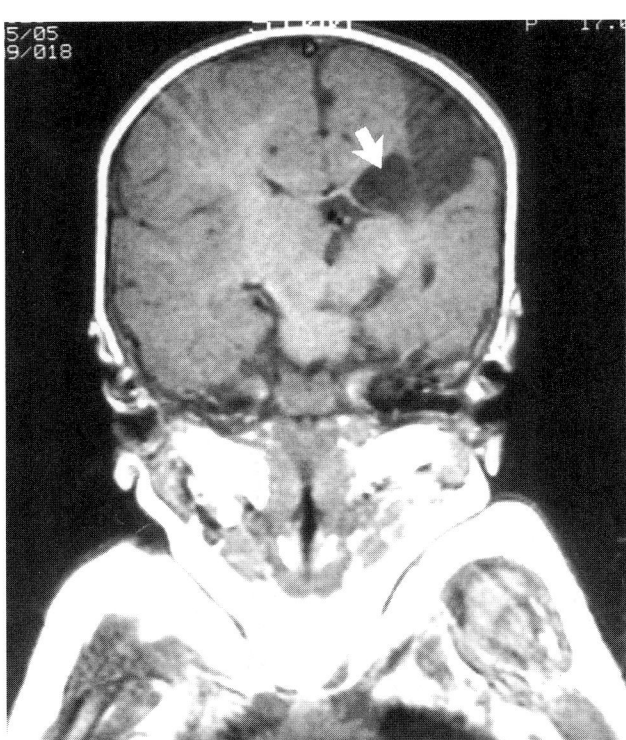

FIGURE 57E.9 Porencephaly. A coronal magnetic resonance image demonstrates an area of infarction in the territory supplied by the middle cerebral artery. There is dilatation of the lateral ventricle (*arrow*).

seizures, motor dysfunction, or cognitive impairment. In contrast, the risk of later epilepsy in children who do not have seizures at onset is only 20%. When seizures develop, it is usually within 1 year of the stroke.

Most children with residual hemiparesis walk. The onset of hemiplegia during the first year is usually not associated with permanent facial weakness. Persistent mirror movements and atrophy of the involved limbs are seen after strokes in young children. Chorea, dystonia, and other movement disorders also occur. The outcome of vertebrobasilar stroke is variable; prognostic factors include patency of one vertebral artery and an adequate collateral blood flow.

The plasticity of the immature nervous system has its greatest effect on the development of higher cognitive functions. Recovery of language is the rule in children with unilateral stroke younger than age 8 years, although some abnormalities persist when the left hemisphere is affected. The overall intelligence quotient (IQ) of children with proven unilateral strokes is measurably reduced. Children with left hemisphere lesions acquired after the first year have lower verbal than performance IQs, whereas children with right hemisphere lesions have lower performance IQs. Attention problems, changes in dichotic listening performance, and academic difficulties in organizational skills (right-sided lesions) and in reading and writing (left-sided lesions) also occur.

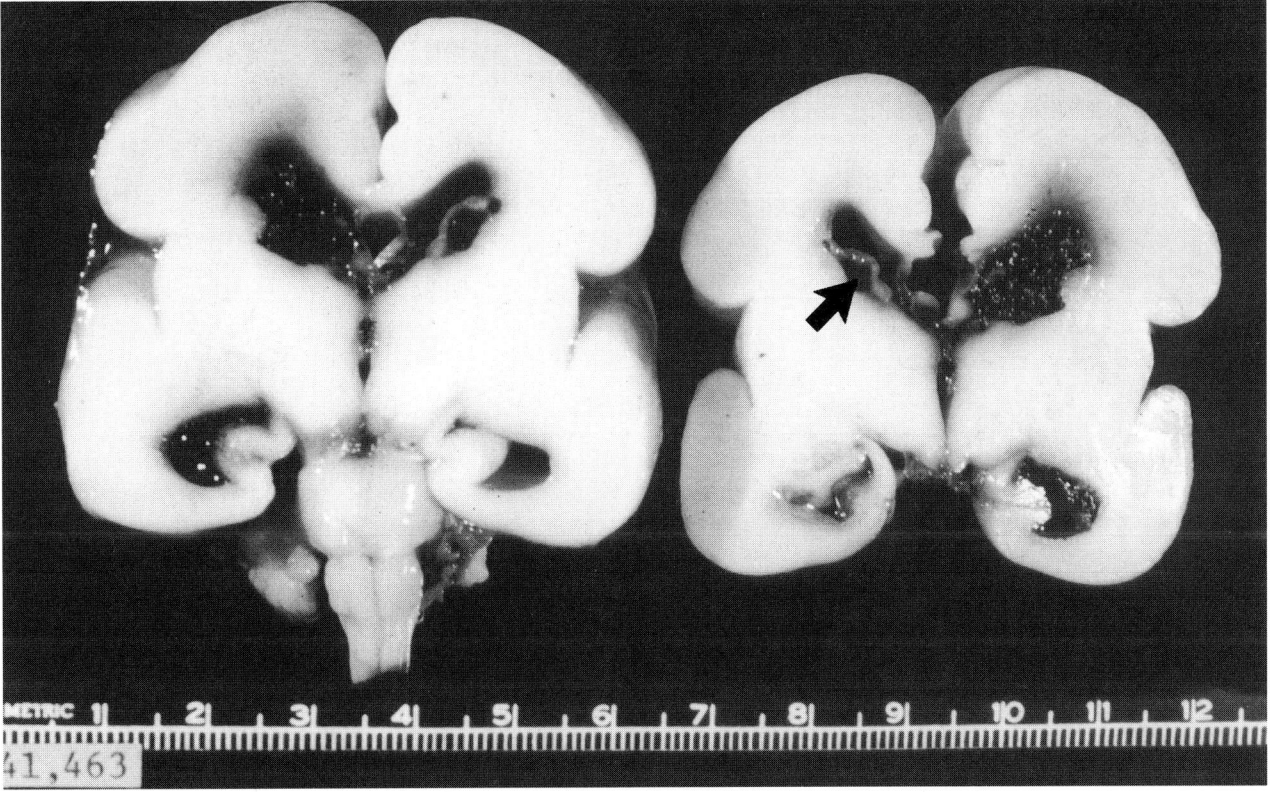

FIGURE 57E.10 Intraventricular hemorrhage in the neonate. Subependymal hemorrhage (grade 1) exists in the left germinal plate (*arrow*). A more extensive hemorrhage (grade 2) has ruptured into the ventricle on the right.

TREATMENT OF STROKE IN CHILDHOOD

Treatment of childhood stroke depends on the underlying cause. Many of the management strategies are the same as for adults (see other sections in Chapter 57).

Because of the low incidence, there have been few randomized, prospective studies of the pharmacological treatment of stroke in childhood. Oral anticoagulation may play a role in preventing cardiogenic embolization. One caveat in chronically anticoagulating toddlers is the danger of cerebral hemorrhage caused by frequent falls. In these circumstances, treatment with platelet antagonists may be the most judicious course.

Aneurysms are treated primarily surgically. Small AVMs over the cortex of the brain may be surgically removable if they are in a silent area of brain. Larger AVMs may respond to proton-beam radiation or embolization.

REFERENCES

Bourgeois M, Aicardi J, Goutieres F. Alternating hemiplegia of childhood. J Pediatr 1993;122:673–679.

Broderick J, Talbot T, Prenger E, et al. Stroke in children within a major metropolitan area: the surprising importance of intracerebral hemorrhage. J Child Neurol 1993;8:250–255.

Houston PE, Rana S, Sekhsaria S, et al. Homocysteine in sickle cell disease: relationship to stroke. Am J Med 1997;103: 192–196.

Keidan I, Shahar E, Barzilay Z, et al. Predictors of outcome of stroke in infants and children based on clinical data and radiologic correlates. Acta Pediatr 1994;83:762–765.

Kerr LM, Anderson DM, Thompson JA, et al. Ischemic stroke in the young: evaluation and comparison of patients six months to thirty-nine years. J Child Neurol 1993;8:266–270.

Rivkin MJ, Volpe JJ. Strokes in children. Pediatr Rev 1996;17: 265–278.

Chapter 57
Vascular Diseases of the Nervous System

F. SPINAL CORD VASCULAR DISEASE
David S. Geldmacher

The spinal cord is subject to many of the same vascular diseases that involve the brain, but its anatomy and embryology render it susceptible to some syndromes that do not have intracranial counterparts.

VASCULAR ANATOMY OF THE SPINAL CORD

The embryonic arterial supply to the spinal cord derives from radicular arteries that enter at each spinal level and divide to follow the dorsal and ventral roots. The ventral radicular branches join along the midline to form the anterior spinal artery. Irregular anastomoses among the dorsal roots, as they enter the cord on each side, form paired posterior spinal arteries. The anterior and posterior spinal arteries constitute longitudinal arterial plexuses. Circumflex vessels (arteria vasocorona) connect the anterior and posterior arterial systems around the lateral margins of the cord (Figure 57F.1).

During development, a few predominant radicular arteries provide most of the flow to the spinal cord through the anterior spinal artery. Five to eight large anterior radicular arteries and a similar number of posterior radicular arteries exist in adults. The largest and most frequently identified of the anterior vessels is the arteria radicularis magna or great artery of Adamkiewicz, which courses along one of the lower thoracic or upper lumbar anterior roots to join the anterior spinal artery. It provides a major portion of the blood flow to the lower thoracic cord and the lumbar enlargement. The sacral cord, conus medullaris, and cauda equina are supplied by small lower segmental arteries. The cervical and upper thoracic spinal cord is richly vascularized by a plexus arising from branches of the ascending cervical and vertebral arteries.

In contrast to the lumbar and cervical regions, the blood supply to the midthoracic cord is relatively tenuous, often consisting of only one significant radicular vessel. At thoracic levels, the anastomotic network is less intricate, and the anterior spinal artery may become discontinuous. The midthoracic region of the spinal cord is considered traditionally to be the most vulnerable to compromise from hypoperfusion or occlusion of a single artery, but more recent evidence suggests that the lower thoracic cord is at greatest risk (Cheshire et al. 1996) (Figure 57F.2).

The main blood supply to spinal gray matter, as well as to anterior and lateral funiculi, is derived from anterior sulcal arteries. These arise from the anterior spinal artery in the midline and course into the ventral median fissure. Each anterior sulcal artery distributes blood to only the left or right half of the spinal cord. The greatest distance between sulcal arteries is in the thoracic segments; the vascularity is proportional to the numbers of neurons located throughout the cord at that level. The dorsal columns and extreme dorsal horns (approximately one-third of the cord cross section) are supplied by penetrating branches from the posterior spinal arteries. The superficial white matter also receives blood flow via the circumflex anastomotic vessels.

The venous system of the spinal cord parallels the arterial supply. A group of radial veins flows outward to the surface of the cord, ending in a coronal plexus, and deep parenchymal veins empty into central sulcal veins in the median fissure. Unlike the arteries, however, each parenchymal vein drains both the right and left sides of the cord. There are few venous anastomoses within the substance of the cord, but sulcal veins often have intersegmental anastomoses. The anterior median spinal vein, which lies external to its corresponding artery, is filled from the sulcal veins. As with the other spinal veins, the

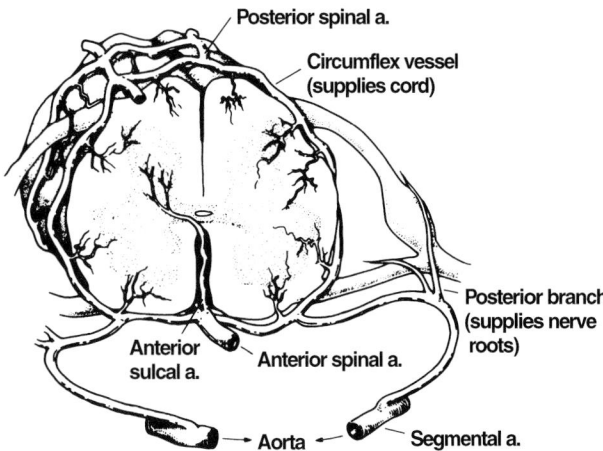

FIGURE 57F.1   Arterial supply to the spinal cord and nerve roots at the level of a radicular artery (a). (Adapted from RA Henson, M Parsons. Ischaemic lesions of the spinal cord: an illustrated review. QJM 1967;36:205–222.)

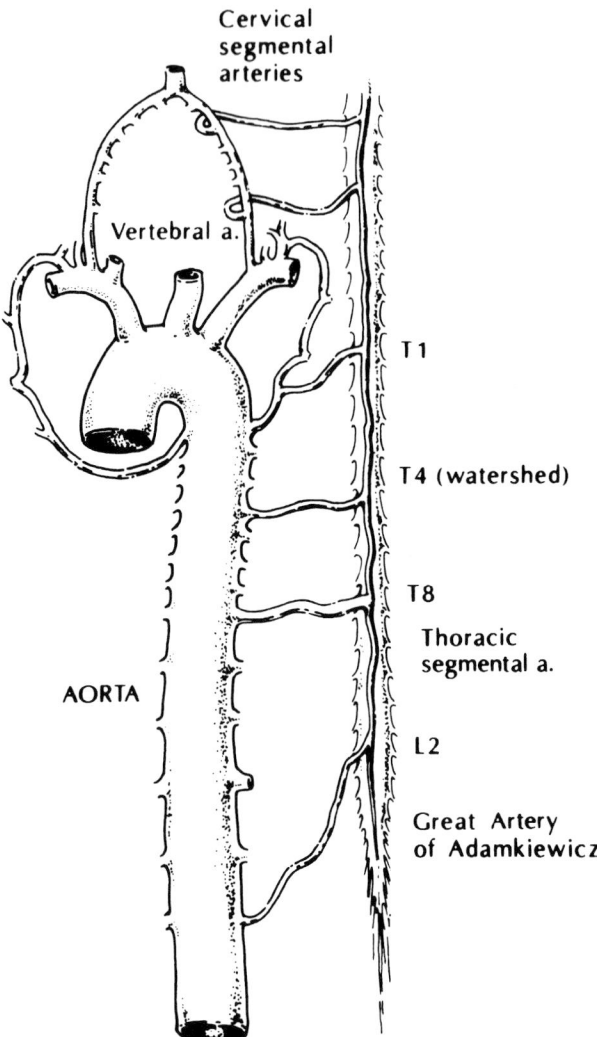

FIGURE 57F.2   Relationship of typical anterior radicular arteries and spinal cord segments. The midthoracic cord is the region most at risk for ischemia during hypoperfusion.

median spinal vein is more irregular than the corresponding artery and may be doubled. Extramedullary venous channels are also prominent along the dorsal cord, but do not consistently form vessels directly corresponding to the posterior spinal arteries. Eight to 12 major anterior radicular veins arise from the anterior median spinal vein. They are joined by anterolateral anastomoses from the coronal venous plexus at the nerve roots before passing through the dura. There is typically a large vein that drains the levels of the lumbar enlargement (vena radicularis magna). Posterior radicular veins are present throughout, but are particularly prominent in the cervical region. Venous blood from the entire cord runs into the epidural and paravertebral venous plexuses, forming a large valveless system from sacrum to occiput (Batson's plexus). The absence of valves to resist retrograde flow in this continuous venous network may be a factor in the pathogenesis of some spinal cord vascular disease.

SPINAL CORD ISCHEMIA

Animal studies of aortic compression resulting in paralysis were reported as early as 1667, and, clinically, paraparesis resulting from aortic obstruction was recognized in the mid-1800s. By the early twentieth century, cardiac embolism, atheromatous disease, and decompression sickness were described as causes of spinal cord ischemia. Although it is less common than cerebral vascular disease, the true prevalence of spinal cord infarction is not known. It probably represents less than 1% of all acute strokes.

Clinical Presentation and Course

Weakness, numbness, pain, and urinary complaints are common presenting symptoms of spinal cord ischemia. The weakness may progress gradually over hours or be maximal at onset. Because of the vulnerability of the thoracic cord to flow-related ischemia, paraparesis is more frequent than quadriparesis. Numbness, accompanied by paresthesias, often parallels the weakness and occasionally precedes it. Back pain in a radicular distribution is common. Visceral referred pain can mistakenly suggest an intra-abdominal process. Urinary dysfunction is typical, usually in the form of retention, but bladder and bowel incontinence may develop after the initial spinal shock resolves.

Examination of the patient initially reveals flaccid paresis with diminished superficial (abdominal, cremasteric) and tendon reflexes below the level of ischemia. Spasticity and hyperreflexia, accompanied by extensor plantar responses, usually evolve with ischemia above the lumbar segments. A posterior spinal artery syndrome only occurs rarely and is notable for preservation of strength and reflexes (Mascalchi et al. 1998).

Sensory loss is nearly universal in spinal cord ischemia. The location of a lesion may be predicted by the cutaneous distribution of sensory loss and the modalities involved. Occlusion of the anterior spinal artery impairs pain and temperature perception below the lesion, whereas in a posterior spinal syndrome there is derangement of touch, vibration, and proprioceptive senses below the lesion. A smaller lesion, such as that from the occlusion of a central sulcal artery, can present with a partial Brown-Séquard's syndrome or a suspended dissociated sensory loss (loss of pain and temperature sensation over the segment affected by the lesion, with preserved sensation above and below the lesion).

The course of spinal ischemic syndromes is variable. Transient ischemic attacks of the cord may occur, with weakness and numbness lasting 15 minutes. A slowly progressive myelopathy attributed to chronic constriction of radicular vessels in the neck has been suggested, but not established. Infarction of the spinal cord typically becomes evident as paresis within minutes of the initial symptoms or precipitating event. Intervals of many hours from the onset of pain, however, are recognized. Pain is often persistent and is a major contributor to long-term disability in spinal cord vascular syndromes (Pelser and van Gijn 1993). Return of function depends on the degree of parenchymal damage; there may be complete recovery. The duration of dysfunction is useful in determining prognosis. Unless significant motor recovery occurs in the first 24 hours, the likelihood of major improvement is low. The clinical presentation of spinal cord syndromes is presented in more detail in Chapter 28.

Investigations

Magnetic resonance imaging (MRI) is the imaging procedure of choice for diagnosing spinal cord ischemia, but the results can be normal even in the presence of significant symptoms. The pattern of signal changes, and their time course, are very similar to those for cerebral infarction (Mascalchi et al. 1998; Rovira et al. 1998). Other laboratory and radiographic studies are not diagnostic in noncompressive spinal cord ischemia. Although an ischemic spinal cord may occasionally appear swollen, myelography is usually normal. In many cases, the cerebrospinal fluid (CSF) protein is elevated, but CSF pleocytosis is rare.

Causes of Spinal Cord Ischemia

The causes are summarized in Table 57F.1. Regional hemodynamic compromise from mechanical disruption of the aorta is the most common cause of spinal cord infarction, accounting for nearly 40% of one series of 44 patients (Cheshire et al. 1996). Complications of aortic aneurysm repair represent the largest proportion of those cases. Clamping of the aorta above the renal arteries for more than

Table 57F.1: Causes of spinal cord ischemic syndromes

Regional hemodynamic compromise
Systemic hypotension
Occlusive vascular disease
Embolism
Vasculitis
Arterial dissection
Thrombosis
Venous occlusion

20–30 minutes or operative ligation of lower thoracic intercostal vessels places the cord at risk for ischemia and infarction. Either procedure can abolish effective flow via the artery of Adamkiewicz. Similarly, aneurysmal aortic dissection causes spinal ischemia by diversion of blood flow around the ostia of intercostal and segmental arteries. In this condition, there is infarction of gray matter with preservation of superficial white matter. The longitudinal anastomotic network is apparently able to maintain sufficient blood supply to perfuse the perimeter of the cord, but not its central zones. Vertebral artery dissection may also lead to posterior cervical cord infarction (Bergqvist et al. 1997). Nonpenetrating aortic trauma may cause torsional occlusion of vessels supplying the cord, with resultant ischemia.

Systemic hypotension produces cord ischemia, but because encephalopathy is common after resuscitation, isolated spinal cord syndromes are infrequent. Low thoracic levels are especially susceptible to hypoperfusion. If there is prolonged hypoxemia, however, the pathological lesions are distributed diffusely throughout the spinal gray matter. Localized thoracic cord ischemia may result from disordered autoregulation following percutaneous radiofrequency spinal rhizotomy.

Atherosclerotic plaques in the aorta may overlie the origin of branches to the spinal cord and diminish their blood flow or be a source of embolism. Transesophageal echocardiography may identify such plaques in the descending aorta. The spinal cord vessels are of a size that is generally not subject to occlusive atheromatous disease, but they are prone to luminal narrowing from arteriosclerotic hyalinization. Either of these conditions may result in intermittent claudication of the spinal cord manifested by activity-induced, transient symptoms of myelopathy. As with cerebral vascular disease, these transient ischemic attacks may precede spinal cord infarction. Intermittent spinal claudication may respond positively to aortobifemoral bypass.

Radiotherapy may produce myelopathy in part from occlusive changes in parenchymal spinal cord arterioles. The degree of myelopathy depends on the total radiation dose, dose per fraction, and the length of the irradiated segment of the cord.

Embolism causes both acute and stepwise spinal cord dysfunction. Fibrocartilaginous emboli from intervertebral disks are the cause of an ischemic syndrome unique to the spinal cord. The anterior portion of the cervical cord is the site of multiple arterial and venous microemboli from a ruptured intervertebral disk in up to 70% of such cases. Women are affected twice as often as men. Fragments of disk material are traumatically forced into bone marrow sinusoids by local fracture and increased tissue pressure may introduce the emboli into the spinal vertebral plexus and arterial channels. Approximately one-half of these events are purely arterial. The other one-half have mixed arterial and venous involvement (Toro et al. 1994).

Emboli arising from the mitral valve in rheumatic heart disease and from acute bacterial endocarditis may cause acute paraplegia. Similarly, thromboembolism from an atrial myxoma may cause multiple spinal cord infarcts. Myelopathy associated with decompression sickness (see Chapter 64) results from circulating nitrogen bubbles that block small spinal arteries. Spinal cord ischemia also may complicate therapeutic renal or bronchial artery embolizations.

Vasculitic and thrombotic causes of spinal cord ischemia are well known. Before the antibiotic era, meningovascular syphilis was a common cause of anterior spinal artery ischemic syndromes and spinal meningitis continues to be occasionally associated with paraplegia of vascular origin. Systemic inflammatory conditions such as Crohn's disease, polyarteritis nodosa, and giant cell arteritis may also lead to myelopathy. Sickle cell disease, intrathecal chemical irritants, angiographic contrast material, the postpartum state, and intravascular neoplastic invasion all predispose to thrombosis and spinal cord infarction.

Venous infarction without hemorrhage is clinically indistinguishable from the arterial ischemic syndromes. There may be an associated systemic thrombophlebitis, which propagates into the spinal canal via the venous plexus. A subacute necrotizing myelitis (Foix-Alajouanine syndrome), causing stepwise spinal cord dysfunction, may occur with extensive spinal cord thrombophlebitis and no systemic foci of venous inflammation, or in association with chronic obstructive pulmonary disease, or a neoplasm (usually of the lung). This condition may also be the result of spinal cord vascular malformations and dural venous fistulae. Polycythemia rubra vera may be associated with noninflammatory spinal venous thrombosis that results in cord ischemia.

Treatment

The general medical management of spinal cord ischemia is the same as for cerebral vascular disease, including maintenance of adequate blood pressure, early bed rest, and reversal of proximate causes such as hypovolemia or arrhythmias. The role of acute anticoagulation with heparin has not been studied, nor has thrombolytic therapy. Such interventions will continue to be difficult to study because of the low incidence of spinal cord infarction and the variability of its natural course. Supportive care is directed toward minimizing the complications of autonomic dysfunction and immobility. Physical and occupational therapy are useful in promot-

ing functional recovery. Overall mortality is approximately 20%, and more than minimal improvement can be expected in only 35–40% of spinal infarction (Cheshire et al. 1996). Nonetheless, with appropriate rehabilitation, most patients are able to return to home and live without professional assistance (Pelser and van Gijn 1993).

SPINAL VASCULAR MALFORMATIONS

Spinal angiomas are tortuous, dilated arteries and veins without an intervening capillary network; they may involve the spinal cord, leptomeninges, or both. Nomenclature is based on the relative contribution of each vessel type. If veins predominate, the lesion is called a *venous angioma*; if arteries are more prominent, the lesion is called an *arteriovenous malformation*.

Distribution and Prevalence

Patients with spinal angiomas are often included as a subgroup of patients with manifestations of spinal tumors. The reported frequency of spinal angiomas in patients with spinal tumors ranges from 3–11%. The frequency may be higher, because an unknown number never become symptomatic and are never diagnosed. Spinal angiomas usually occur in men, with reported sex ratios of up to 9 to 1. The diagnosis is made most frequently between ages 30 and 70, but symptoms can develop during childhood. Lower thoracic and lumbar angiomas, situated posteriorly or posterolaterally, are the most common, but cervical lesions tend to produce symptoms and are diagnosed earlier.

Clinical Presentation and Course

Spinal angiomas are frequently misdiagnosed. The onset of manifestations can be acute or insidious and the course may include remissions and relapses. The most common complaints at onset are pain, weakness, and sensory symptoms. The predilection of spinal angiomas for the lower thoracic and lumbar regions results in complaints referable to those levels. Later, the initial signs and symptoms persist and are joined by bowel and bladder complaints. The onset of symptoms is frequently associated with trauma, exercise, pregnancy, or menstruation. Misdiagnosis, especially as demyelinating disease, was common before MRI of the spine. Nonetheless, the interval between symptom onset and accurate diagnosis may be years. Severe locomotor disability develops in approximately 20% by 6 months after onset of symptoms and in 50% by 3 years. Once leg weakness or gait difficulties start, they tend to progress rapidly.

The signs and symptoms of spinal vascular malformations are attributable to mass effect and ischemia. Although it is unusual for an unruptured spinal angioma to cause sufficient mass effect to cause spinal cord dysfunction, epidural, subdural, and intramedullary hemorrhage can occur and produce spinal cord compression. Dural arteriovenous malformations may present also as a slowly progressive myelopathy, which may be related to a vascular steal phenomenon.

Pain may be local, radicular, diffuse, or any combination of these. There may be upper motor neuron weakness, lower motor neuron weakness, or both. A spinal bruit is a highly specific, though uncommon, finding that is diagnostic of a spinal angioma. Angiomas may coexist in the skin or paraspinal muscles. In cutaneomeningospinal angiomatosis (Cobb's syndrome), dural angioma may coexist with a cutaneous angioma in the corresponding dermatome. Foix-Alajouanine syndrome (see Causes of Spinal Cord Ischemia, earlier in this chapter) also may be caused by thrombosis of a vascular malformation. Spinal hemorrhage usually has an abrupt onset and may be associated with the typical symptoms of spinal subarachnoid hemorrhage (SAH), including headache, meningeal infection, and cord and nerve root damage.

Vascular malformations may cause increased local venous pressure, decreased perfusion pressure, decreased tissue perfusion, and finally tissue ischemia. This explains the coexistence of deficits in more than a single arterial territory and the symptomatic improvement that results from ligation of feeding vessels. The sometimes confusing and widely varied presentation of spinal vascular malformations results in a large differential diagnosis, which includes neoplasms, herniated discs, multiple sclerosis, intracranial SAH, subacute combined degeneration, meningovascular syphilis, and transverse myelitis (see Chapter 28).

Investigations

MRI is the highly sensitive and specific diagnostic procedure of choice in the initial evaluation of spinal angiomas. In addition to identifying the angioma, MRI can discriminate extramedullary from intramedullary lesions, document thrombosis of the malformation following ligation or embolization of the feeding vessels, and show areas of decreased signal intensity extending beyond the limits of the angioma, presumably from edema.

Even in the absence of SAH, the CSF may be abnormal, with mild pleocytosis and elevated protein. Plain radiography is rarely helpful. The classic appearance on myelography is of serpentine filling defects representing the dilated mass of blood vessels within the spinal canal. Partial or complete block to the flow of contrast or enlargement of the cord may occur. Most lesions are dorsal in the spinal canal and are best visualized when myelography is obtained in the supine position. However, ventral lesions may not be seen unless the patient is placed in the prone position.

The definitive radiological procedure is selective spinal angiography using digital subtraction techniques. Most institutions perform this procedure while the patient is intubated and under general anesthesia. Selective spinal angiography is tedious and requires that each segmental artery in the region being examined be injected. A positive study result provides useful information about the malformation, including its location, size, configuration, and blood flow. MR angiography is increasingly replacing invasive catheter angiography.

Treatment

The treatment of spinal angiomas is by surgical resection or angiographically directed embolization into the malformation. Once lodged within the angioma, these iatrogenic emboli promote thrombosis and decrease blood flow. A sequential approach of embolization, followed by definitive surgical therapy, is common.

SPINAL HEMORRHAGE

Subarachnoid, intramedullary, subdural, and epidural hemorrhage may affect the spinal cord and its meninges. The onset is usually sudden and painful and most commonly is related to trauma or vascular malformations.

Subarachnoid Hemorrhage

Spinal SAH accounts for less than 1% of all SAHs. The most common cause is a spinal angioma, but these account for only approximately 10% of the total. Other associated conditions include coarctation of the aorta, rupture of a spinal artery, mycotic and other aneurysms of the spinal artery, polyarteritis nodosa, spinal tumors, lumbar puncture, blood dyscrasias, and therapeutic thrombolytics and anticoagulants.

Clinical presentation of spinal SAH is characterized by the sudden onset of severe back pain, which is often localized near the level of the hemorrhage. Within minutes, the pain becomes diffuse and signs of meningeal irritation become prominent. Multiple radiculopathies and myelopathy may be present. Headache, cranial neuropathies, and a decreased level of consciousness are associated with diffusion of blood above the foramen magnum. The CSF is grossly bloody, intracranial pressure is frequently elevated, and papilledema may be present.

Correct diagnosis requires a strong clinical suspicion. The evaluation of spinal SAH frequently follows negative radiological studies of the intracranial structures. History may reveal the initial severe back pain or prior anticoagulant use. Physical examination may reveal a spinal bruit, cutaneous angioma, sensory level, the stigmata of collagen vascular disease, or evidence suggesting septicemia. Radiological studies are discussed under spinal vascular malformations. Treatment is directed toward the underlying cause.

Hematomyelia

Intramedullary spinal hemorrhage most often results from trauma. Hematomyelia may follow direct trauma to the spinal column or hyperextension injuries of the cervical spine. Spontaneous hematomyelia is caused usually by bleeding of a spinal vascular malformation, hemorrhage into a spinal tumor or syrinx, a bleeding diathesis, anticoagulant drugs, or venous infarction. The hemorrhage tends to disrupt spinal gray matter rather than white matter. There are no recognized intraspinal counterparts to intracerebral hypertensive hemorrhage and amyloid angiopathy. Hematomyelia most commonly presents as spinal shock associated with the sudden onset of severe back pain, which is often radicular. Spasticity develops below the level of the lesion and fasciculations, atrophy, and areflexia may occur in the myotomes corresponding to the lesion.

MRI is the best imaging modality to detect intramedullary hemorrhage. Lumbar puncture may be consistent with SAH. The initial treatment is supportive. Laminectomy and drainage of the hematoma, followed by resection of the tumor or vascular malformation, can be performed if neurological deficits are incomplete or progressive.

Spinal Epidural and Subdural Hemorrhage

Spinal epidural hemorrhage (SEH) occurs more frequently than spinal subdural hemorrhage (SSH). SEH is more commonly observed in men and has a bimodal distribution, with peaks during childhood and the fifth and sixth decades of life. Cervical lesions are more common in childhood, whereas thoracic and lumbar lesions predominate in adults. Hemorrhages can be spontaneous but often occur following trivial exertion or minor trauma. SEH is a complication of both lumbar puncture and epidural anesthesia and is more likely in anticoagulated patients. Other causes include blood dyscrasia, thrombocytopenia, neoplasms, and vascular malformations.

SSH is most common in women. It may occur at any age but tends to predominate in the sixth decade. Most occur in the thoracic and lumbar regions. Hemorrhagic diatheses, including treatment with anticoagulants, blood dyscrasias, and thrombocytopenia, are the precipitating factors most commonly associated with SSH. Other factors include trauma, lumbar puncture, vascular malformation, and spinal surgery.

The clinical presentations of SEH and SSH are indistinguishable. The initial symptom is severe back pain at the level of the bleed. Myelopathy or cauda equina syndrome with motor and sensory findings corresponding to the level of the lesion develops over hours to days. The diagnosis should be suspected in patients with disorders of coagulation who have undergone recent lumbar puncture and develop back pain or signs of spinal cord or root dysfunction. Patients with a rapidly decreasing platelet count or less than 20,000 platelets/μl are at particular risk of developing SEH or SSH with a spinal tap and should receive a platelet transfusion prior to lumbar puncture. Clotting studies and a platelet count are important in the initial evaluation. In SEH and SSH, the CSF may be normal, xanthochromic, or contain increased protein.

MRI, the imaging modality of choice, delineates the hematoma and its location referable to the dura. In addition, gadolinium-enhanced MRI and MR angiography may show an underlying vascular malformation. In patients unable to tolerate MRI or where it is unavailable in the acute phase of the illness, myelography with CT scanning provides an alternative. Myelography reveals a filling defect or complete blockage to the flow of contrast material at the level of the lesion. The myelographical appearances of SEH and SSH may be indistinguishable.

Treatment is directed toward the underlying defect. Laminectomy with evacuation of the clot should be performed as soon as possible. The prognosis for recovery is better when surgery is performed early and the preoperative deficits are not severe.

REFERENCES

Bergqvist CA, Goldberg HI, Thorarensen O, Bird SJ. Posterior cervical spinal cord infarction following vertebral artery dissection. Neurology 1997;48:1112–1115.

Cheshire WP, Santos CC, Massey EW, Howard JF Jr. Spinal cord infarction: etiology and outcome. Neurology 1996;47:321–330.

Mascalchi M, Cosottini M, Ferrito G, et al. Posterior spinal artery infarct. Am J Neuroradiol 1998;19:361–363.

Pelser A, van Gijn J. Spinal infarction: a follow-up study. Stroke 1993;24:896–898.

Rovira A, Pedraza S, Comabella M, et al. Magnetic resonance imaging of acute infarction of the anterior spinal cord. J Neurol Neurosurg Psychiatry 1998;64:279–281.

Toro G, Roman GC, Navarro-Roman L, et al. Natural history of spinal cord infarction caused by nucleus pulposus embolism. Spine 1994;19:360–366.

Chapter 57
Vascular Diseases of the Nervous System

G. CENTRAL NERVOUS SYSTEM VASCULITIS
James W. Schmidley

Isolated vasculitis of the central nervous system (CNS) is rare, but not so rare that one or two cases are not encountered each year in large medical centers. The diagnosis of this disorder puts the neurologist on the horns of a dilemma. There are no characteristic clinical features; the results of routine laboratory investigations, both medical and neurological, are either normal or nonspecific. The single test, short of a biopsy, that is sometimes helpful in establishing the diagnosis is catheter angiography. This invasive test has the drawbacks of low sensitivity and specificity: The result may be negative in pathologically documented cases of CNS vasculitis. The consequence of missing the diagnosis is the death of the patient; the consequence of delay in diagnosis is likely to be severe disability. The only therapies that appear to be effective are also highly toxic, and one should feel uneasy administering them without solid evidence supporting vasculitis.

TYPES OF CENTRAL NERVOUS SYSTEM VASCULITIS

When vasculitis is clinically and pathologically restricted to the CNS, it is referred to as a *primary* or *isolated* CNS vasculitis. Early, classic descriptions of this disorder included the term *granulomatous*, but this histological feature, although frequent, is not required for diagnosis. This section covers isolated CNS vasculitis and the CNS vasculitides associated with cutaneous herpes zoster infections, drug abuse, lymphomas, and amyloid angiopathy.

The CNS also may be involved by widespread systemic vasculitis, usually polyarteritis nodosa or Wegener's granulomatosis. These disorders, which are discussed in Chapter 55A, rarely present with isolated CNS manifestations.

ISOLATED CENTRAL NERVOUS SYSTEM VASCULITIS

The mode of onset is acute or subacute. Although the classic picture is one of progressive, cumulative, and multifocal neurological dysfunction, there are abundant exceptions, including patients whose presentation suggests cerebral tumor, chronic meningitis, demyelinating disease, acute encephalitis, myelopathy, simple dementia, and degenerative disorders. When isolated CNS angiitis presents as a stroke, it is usually because of intracerebral hemorrhage, which occurs in approximately 15% of patients at some time in the illness. The disease rarely causes cerebral infarcts or transient ischemic attacks in the absence of clinical or laboratory evidence of a widespread CNS inflammatory disorder, such as a cerebrospinal fluid (CSF) pleocytosis.

Nonfocal symptoms such as headache and confusion are the most common presentation. Aside from confusion, the most common sign at presentation is hemiparesis. Ataxia of limbs or gait, focal cortical dysfunction including aphasia, and seizures are also frequent. Virtually every neurological sign or symptom has been reported at least once (Calabrese et al. 1997). Nonspecific visual complaints occur in approximately 15% of patients, but disorders of specific oculomotor nerves, optic nerve, or visual fields are much less common. Systemic symptoms are generally absent. Fully developed cases almost invariably show signs and symptoms of progressive, widespread neurological dysfunction; however, occasional patients present with a multiple sclerosis–like course of early relapses and remissions, or clinical manifestations largely restricted to one part of the nervous system, such as the spinal cord or cerebellum.

Pathology of Isolated Central Nervous System Vasculitis

The vascular inflammation is usually of a chronic granulomatous nature, with monocytes and histiocytes, lymphocytes, and plasma cells infiltrating the walls of small (200 μm) arteries and veins, particularly in the leptomeninges. Larger vessels may be involved but never to an extent exceeding that of smaller ones. Although present in most autopsy cases, giant cells are not required to make a diagnosis. There is no predilection for bifurcations, as in polyarteritis nodosa, although fibrinoid necrosis can occur; eosinophils are not present in large numbers. Small, clinically silent foci of vasculitis are occasionally present in one or more viscera but, by definition, produce neither laboratory or symptomatic evidence of organ dysfunction.

Etiology and pathogenesis are unknown. Many vasculitis syndromes are a result of deposition of immune complexes, but there is little support for this mechanism in isolated CNS vasculitis. The infiltrating cells have been CD4+ T lymphocytes in the few cases in which leukocyte typing has been done. There is no convincing evidence of infection with *Mycoplasma*, or any other microorganism, in human CNS vasculitis, although *Mycoplasma* does cause CNS vasculitis in animals.

Laboratory Findings in Isolated Central Nervous System Vasculitis

General medical laboratory investigations are usually unremarkable. Some patients have an elevated sedimentation rate, but usually not to the degree seen in temporal arteritis. The laboratory is of use only in eliminating systemic vasculitis, neoplasm, infection, or other alternate diagnoses. Electroencephalography and computed tomographic scan are not specific, although they are usually abnormal; there is less experience with magnetic resonance imaging (MRI), but it is unlikely to be any more specific. Although some literature has stressed the contrary, the CSF has been abnormal (in some way) in almost all autopsy-documented cases. Unfortunately, the abnormalities are totally nonspecific, namely a mild lymphocytic pleocytosis and a mild to moderate elevation in protein. Oligoclonal bands and elevated IgG index are occasionally encountered, as are low glucose values and leukocyte counts of several hundred per μl. The major value of CSF examination in investigating suspected CNS vasculitis is to rule out infections, including syphilis, or neoplastic infiltration of the meninges.

Although some publications emphasize the value of angiography in making the diagnosis, (1) cerebral angiography has been entirely normal in many pathologically documented cases, and (2) the arteriographic changes of vasculitis, when seen, are not specific (Alhalabi and Moore 1994). Given its lower spatial resolution, MR angiography is unlikely to be useful.

The typical changes of vasculitis in cerebral angiography are widespread segmental changes in the contour and caliber of vessels. Small aneurysms, usually on vessels much smaller than those bearing congenital saccular aneurysms, are occasionally present, but cannot be distinguished from aneurysms complicating atrial myxoma or infective endocarditis. Occlusion of large cerebral vessels is rare.

It is my opinion that many published cases of angiographically diagnosed CNS vasculitis, including the so-called isolated, benign variant, represent misinterpretation or overinterpretation of nonspecific angiographic changes, unconfirmed by a tissue diagnosis. Until the pathological processes underlying these cases are established, the use of more circumspect terms such as *reversible cerebral vasoconstriction* or *cerebral angiopathy* is appropriate.

Approach to Diagnosis

All patients in whom CNS vasculitis is suspected should be evaluated thoroughly to exclude a systemic vasculitis. A careful history and physical examination, with attention to the skin, eyes, testicles, paranasal sinuses, and lungs, are likely to be more revealing than a "shotgun" laboratory approach. The CSF should be examined in all cases to exclude infectious and neoplastic meningitis. An MRI scan should be performed to exclude other diagnoses such as multiple cerebral metastases, multicentric primary CNS tumors, hydrocephalus, or demyelinating diseases. Other conditions mimicking CNS vasculitis may include atrial myxoma, cholesterol embolization to the CNS, infectious endocarditis, Sneddon's syndrome, the antiphospholipid-antibody syndrome, encephalitis, neoplastic angioendotheliosis, malignant hypertension, and eclampsia.

Patients whose neurological illness is compatible with isolated CNS vasculitis, but which resists diagnosis by physical examination, routine laboratory testing, imaging, and CSF analysis, should be studied with catheter angiography. Although nonspecific and present in only a minority of proven cases, the classic angiographic picture can be supportive of a diagnosis of CNS vasculitis provided that the many other conditions capable of producing an identical appearance have been excluded. In my opinion, if therapy with cyclophosphamide or another potent immunosuppressive agent is contemplated, then the diagnosis must be confirmed by biopsy. If possible, the biopsy should be directed to lesions visible on MRI, and the specimen should include leptomeninges. If no lesion is available for biopsy, then the nondominant frontal or temporal pole should be sampled, again taking care to ensure that leptomeninges are included.

Therapy

High-dose prednisone plus cyclophosphamide is currently the treatment of choice (Calabrese et al. 1997). Some patients recover or stabilize on corticosteroid therapy alone, but more progress while only on corticosteroid therapy. The results of therapy are difficult to interpret because of the rarity of the disorder, so that even tertiary centers do not accumulate large numbers of patients; the difficulty of unequivocally establishing the diagnosis, other than by biopsy; and the inclusion of patients with the so-called benign form of CNS vasculitis, and of patients with diagnoses based only on angiography. Intravenous immunoglobulin has been administered with success a few times, but in poorly documented cases.

CENTRAL NERVOUS SYSTEM VASCULITIS ASSOCIATED WITH SYSTEMIC DISORDERS

Cutaneous Herpes Zoster Infection

CNS vasculitis associated with herpes zoster usually presents as a severe hemispheric stroke, in the weeks or months following an ipsilateral ophthalmic division infection in an elderly patient (Amlie-Lefond et al. 1995). Angiography shows ipsilateral segmental stenoses of proximal middle and anterior cerebral arteries. Evidence of varicella zoster virus is found in the same segments of these vessels, although histologically, necrosis has been more prominent than inflammation. Presumably, the virus reaches the affected arterial segments via intracranial projections of the ophthalmic division of the trigeminal nerve. The effectiveness of acyclovir and corticosteroids for this syndrome is unknown, but their use seems reasonable. A second type of cerebral vasculitis associated with herpes zoster is less common and less well understood. It is a diffuse, small-vessel vasculitis, in the absence of parenchymal infection, which can follow noncephalic, as well as ophthalmic, eruptions of zoster.

Intravenous Drug Abuse

The usual scenario in CNS vasculitis associated with intravenous drug abuse is subarachnoid or intracerebral hemorrhage following the use of intravenous, or even oral, methamphetamine or another sympathomimetic, including "look-alike" diet pills. It is uncertain whether the "vasculitis" reported in the angiograms of these patients is a true inflammatory process or a vasculopathy induced by an unusual reaction to the drug, hypertension, or other factors. When the case reports are examined critically, it becomes obvious that (1) in only one has vasculitis been pathologically documented; (2) the "vasculitis" has sometimes occurred after first use of the drug, an event unlikely to be immunologically mediated; and (3) the course is usually monophasic rather than progressive and multifocal, as one would expect in a true vasculitis. Because drug abusers (to say nothing of dealers) are famously unreliable, it is sometimes difficult to be certain what illicit drugs actually were used and in what doses, and it is virtually impossible to trace inert substances used as fillers, which nonetheless might be responsible for the clinical events in some cases.

Experimental animals given sympathomimetic drugs chronically do not, in most models, develop a CNS vasculitis. Many case reports claim cure using corticosteroids, but I remain unconvinced that this represents anything other than the natural history of the syndrome. Before entertaining this diagnosis in intravenous drug users, it is also important to exclude the other, definitely treatable causes of stroke in this population, subacute and acute bacterial endocarditis being the most important. Additional causes of cerebral embolization in drug abusers include talc and air emboli, the latter caused by inadvertent injection of air into the internal or common carotid artery while attempting to puncture the internal jugular vein in the neck. Intravenous drug abusers are at risk for hepatitis-associated polyarteritis nodosa, which can involve either the peripheral or the CNS. A rather nonspecific cerebral vasculitis may occur in cocaine users, although vasculitis is not present in the brains of most patients with cocaine-associated strokes (Aggarwal et al. 1996).

Lymphoma

Rare patients with systemic lymphoma, nearly always Hodgkin's disease, also have an isolated CNS vasculitis, in the absence of parenchymal or meningeal involvement by lymphoma (Yuen and Johnson 1996). This association, not noted for other malignant neoplasms, naturally leads to speculation that the Hodgkin's disease somehow triggers or provokes the vasculitis. In some patients, the CNS vasculitis has developed concurrent with, or following, disseminated herpes zoster infection, further confounding the picture. In the nonzoster cases, the CNS disorder improves with remission of the Hodgkin's disease brought about by chemotherapy or radiotherapy.

Amyloid

Cerebrovascular amyloid seems on rare occasions to coexist with a CNS vasculitis (Fountain and Eberhard 1996). In most instances, the vascular amyloid is the same type that accumulates in senile plaques as well as vessels in Alzheimer's disease. The relationship, if any, between these two, usually distinct, processes is not clear. Amyloid deposited in any location frequently evokes a limited degree of giant cell macrophage response and may elicit a sparse lymphocytic infiltrate as well. Therefore, the vasculitis may just represent an excessive degree of inflammatory response to the vascular amyloid. The vasculitis also could cause amyloid deposition. Cytokines such as interleukin-1 increase production of amyloid precursor protein by endothelium, at least in vitro. If cytokines or other by-products of inflammation cause amyloid deposition in vessel walls, it is curious that they seem to do so only in the vasculature of the CNS. When they occur independently, both amyloid and vasculitis preferentially affect cortical and leptomeningeal vessels; the fact that the two are found together in approximately the same distribution makes it difficult to draw conclusions as to which is cause and which is effect. In some cases, amyloid deposits are found in the walls of noninflamed vessels, suggesting they cannot be the result of the inflammation. However, even these cases have not been studied in serial histological sections.

Most patients have presented with a progressive clinical picture consistent with vasculitis, including abnormal spinal fluid. Although cerebrovascular amyloid angiopathy without vasculitis almost always presents with intraparenchymal hemorrhage (see Chapter 57B), this is true in only approximately 30% of patients with amyloid-associated CNS vasculitis. In the absence of a better understanding of this disorder, treatment should be the same as for isolated CNS vasculitis.

REFERENCES

Aggarwal SK, Williams V, Levine SR, et al. Cocaine-associated intracranial hemorrhage: absence of vasculitis in 14 cases. Neurology 1996;46:1741–1743.

Alhalabi M, Moore PM. Serial angiography in isolated angiitis of the CNS. Neurology 1994;44:1221–1226.

Amlie-Lefond C, Kleinschmidt-DeMasters BK, Mahalingham R, et al. The vasculopathy of varicella-zoster virus encephalitis. Ann Neurol 1995;37:784–790.

Calabrese LH, Duna GF, Lie JT. Vasculitis in the central nervous system. Arthritis Rheumatism 1997;40:1189–1201.

Fountain NB, Eberhard DA. Primary angiitis of the central nervous system associated with cerebral amyloid angiopathy. Neurology 1996;46:190–197.

Yuen RW, Johnson PC. Primary angiitis of the nervous system associated with Hodgkin's disease. Arch Pathol Lab Med 1996;120:573–576.

Chapter 58
Primary and Secondary Tumors of the Central Nervous System

Section Editor:
Michael E. Cohen

This chapter presents an overview of current state-of-the-art treatment of adults and children with central nervous system (CNS) neoplasms. Individual chapters focus on pathology, rationale of radiation and chemotherapy, molecular biology, clinical presentation, management, and clinical consequences.

Metastases by far account for most of the tumors identified in the CNS. Eighteen percent to 25% of all patients with cancer who undergo postmortem examinations are found to have metastasis to the CNS. Metastasis is much less common in children than in adults. Although tumors of the CNS represent the second most common neoplasm in children, their incidence is only 3.2–4.4 per 100,000. Whereas there are approximately 17,000–18,000 newly diagnosed cases of primary CNS tumors in adults each year in the United States, there are fewer than 3,000 newly diagnosed primary benign and malignant tumors in children (Surawicz et al. 1999).

Despite remarkable progress in recent decades in understanding the disease and the biology of tumors, there has been little progress in the fight against CNS cancers. However, advances in molecular biology and immune modulation, use of monoclonal antibodies, recognition of abnormal karyotypes, and knowledge of oncogenes and their products all raise the expectation that biological approaches in the future will herald a new and more definitive approach to therapy.

Treatment of CNS neoplasia remains operative intervention followed by radiation and adjuvant chemotherapy. Although these approaches are the same regardless of where cancer occurs in the body, the CNS does present unique problems. Because neoplasia occurs in a fixed space, a tumor is apt to be more symptomatic when it is considerably smaller than a tumor presenting elsewhere in the body. Furthermore, as a result of the diversity and compactness of neural structures, small, strategically placed lesions are likely to cause significant functional disabilities. This results in significant disability earlier in the course of the disease than that from a tumor elsewhere in the body. The direct effects of the tumor on elegant neural structures are problematic, and the mass associated with tumor and the consequent edema also give rise to problems of increased intracranial pressure. The neurologist therefore must be prepared to handle the complications of herniation and structural compromise.

Compounding the anatomical and mechanical problems of the nervous system are concerns that surgery, radiation, or chemotherapy can damage normal tissue. All of these approaches have a narrow risk-to-benefit ratio. Debulking surgery by definition requires removal of as much tumor as possible. Even in skilled hands, aggressive surgery may result in the sacrifice of normal tissue. Adjuvant treatment, such as radiation, although it preferentially destroys rapidly dividing cells, does not separate normal from abnormal tissue. Even with the most aggressive tumors, the mitotic index and turnover rate of abnormal tissue does not significantly differ from that of some elements of normal CNS tissue. As a result, the amount of radiation necessary to destroy malignant cells is invariably associated with the potential to injure normal tissue.

There are similar problems with chemotherapy. In addition, the blood-brain barrier acts to limit the entry of drugs given systemically and so limits the effectiveness of many chemotherapeutic agents.

The brain-adjacent tumor is the non-necrotic leading edge of a tumor that grows in fingerlike projections into normal tissue. Because this region generally has an intact blood-brain barrier, chemotherapy has limited ability to reach the periphery of a tumor. Similarly, drugs given intrathecally are effective only for tumors located near the ependymal lining of the ventricle or along the meningeal surfaces. Drugs given via the cerebrospinal fluid do not penetrate into more deeply situated sites. Selective arterial infusion of drugs that have a high first-pass extraction ratio eliminates systemic side effects while providing a method of presenting large amounts of drug directly to the tumor. Although theoretically attractive, arterial infusion, in addition to presenting more chemotherapy to the tumor bed, increases the tendency to destroy normal tissue.

Perhaps the single most important advance in the armamentarium of the neuro-oncologist has been diagnostic rather than therapeutic. No longer does the discovery of a tumor represent a diagnostic tour de force. Once the suspicion of a cranial neoplasm is raised, magnetic resonance imaging (MRI) or computed tomography (CT) readily confirms the diagnosis. This technology is accurate in more than 90% of cases. In fact, MRI is rapidly replacing CT as the neuroimaging technique of choice. Increasingly, MR angiography is being used as a noninvasive means of identifying the vascularity and blood supply of neoplasms.

The inability to define the margins of a tumor because of edema and the insinuation of abnormal tissue into normal tissue has limited the ability to definitively predict the response to treatment. MR spectroscopy, positron emission tomography, functional MRI, blood-flow techniques, and three-dimensional imaging, although they hold promise for determining size, volume, and normal metabolism, still do not define with precision the margins of a tumor. Unfortunately, imaging techniques have far outstripped the ability to react in a positive therapeutic way to the information obtained. Early diagnosis may lead to more aggressive treatment, but whether this produces better results is still conjectural.

Only in a few cases has early diagnosis proved to alter long-term prognosis. In adults, this has been the case with an isolated metastatic lesion, meningiomas, and extra-axial tumors that produce symptoms by compression rather than destruction. For the more malignant tumor, such as glioma, early identification has not proved as beneficial. The situation with childhood tumors is better. There is evidence to suggest that changes in treatment since Cushing's time have markedly improved the survival of children with medulloblastomas. In select cases in which tumors have been stratified according to age, location, and extent of CNS seeding, 5-year survival rates of children with medulloblastomas approach 50–70%. Germinomas are also highly chemosensitive and radiosensitive tumors. Prolonged progression-free survival rates in children with low-grade tumors in the absence of cure have increased. Whether this improvement relates to a different biology of tumors in children and adults or to improved treatment remains conjectural.

Despite these successes, the effect of treatment of most CNS neoplasms continues to be limited. Unfortunately, an increasing price is paid for aggressive approaches to treatment. As the last chapter in this section suggests, dementia, endocrinopathies, leukoencephalopathies, vasculopathies, and secondary oncogenesis have been unwanted complications of both radiation and chemotherapy. In patients in whom mean survival time is measured in months, the decision to commit to aggressive and sometimes painful therapy increasingly remains a question of quality of life and is the province of the patient as well as the treating physician.

These caveats notwithstanding, much is being done for the patient with CNS tumor. The future, as suggested by the section on molecular biology, and its application to the treatment of human neoplasia suggest that definitive and sustained cures may be close at hand.

REFERENCE

Surawicz TS, McCarthy BJ, Kupelian V, et al. Descriptive epidemiology of primary and CNS tumors: results from the Central Brain Tumor Registry of the United States, 1990–1994. J Neuro-Oncol 1999;1:14–25.

Chapter 58
Primary and Secondary Tumors of the Central Nervous System

A. PATHOLOGY OF NERVOUS SYSTEM TUMORS
Reid R. Heffner, Jr.

CLASSIFICATION OF TUMORS

The first comprehensive classification of nervous system tumors, formulated by Percival Bailey and Harvey Cushing in 1926, was founded on the science of embryology. Each tumor type was portrayed as having an embryological cell of origin. In 1949, Kernohan contributed a tumor-grading system for the purpose of assessing prognosis. Russell and Rubinstein, in a long-running effort, modified Bailey and Cushing's original system to make it more current and scientific. Their system is still preferred by many American and British neuropathologists. The World Health Organization (WHO) classification, completed in 1979 and revised in 1993 (Kleihues et al. 1993), is an attempt to consolidate and reconcile several different classifications. Although it is not universally adopted, the WHO classification is used widely by neuropathologists (Table 58A.1).

TECHNIQUES

Frozen Sections and Touch Imprints

Frozen sections performed during surgery are more difficult to interpret than fixed tissue but are useful to ensure that a representative sample was obtained for permanent sections. Another advantage is the opportunity to prepare touch imprints from fresh tissue (Sidawy and Jannotta 1997). Touch imprints resemble ordinary cytological specimens, but more tumor cells are usually seen because the neoplas-

Table 58A.1: Histological classification of tumors of the central nervous system

Tumors of neuroepithelial origin
  Astrocytic tumors
    Diffuse astrocytoma
    Astrocytoma
    Anaplastic astrocytoma
    Glioblastoma multiforme
      Gliosarcoma
    Circumscribed astrocytoma
      Juvenile pilocytic astrocytoma
      Pleomorphic xanthoastrocytoma
      Subependymal giant cell astrocytoma
  Oligodendroglial tumors
    Oligodendroglioma
    Anaplastic oligodendroglioma
  Ependymal tumors
    Ependymoma
    Myxopapillary ependymoma
    Anaplastic ependymoma
    Subependymoma
  Mixed gliomas
    Oligoastrocytoma
    Astroependymoma
  Choroid plexus tumors
    Choroid plexus papilloma
    Choroid plexus carcinoma
  Neuronal tumors
    Ganglioglioma
    Gangliocytoma
    Dysembryoplastic neuroepithelial tumor
    Central neurocytoma
    Paraganglioma
  Primitive neuroectodermal (embryonal) tumors
    Medulloepithelioma
    Medulloblastoma
    Pineoblastoma
    Neuroblastoma
    Ependymoblastoma
Meningeal tumors
  Meningioma
  Papillary meningioma
  Anaplastic meningioma
Nerve sheath tumors
  Schwannoma (neurilemoma)
  Neurofibroma
  Neurofibrosarcoma
Tumors of blood vessel origin
  Hemangioblastoma
  Hemangiopericytoma
Germ cell tumors
  Germinoma
  Embryonal carcinoma
  Choriocarcinoma
  Teratoma
Malignant lymphomas
  Hodgkin's disease
  Non-Hodgkin's lymphoma
Malformative tumors
  Rathke's cleft cyst
  Craniopharyngioma
  Epidermoid cyst
  Dermoid cyst
  Neuroepithelial (colloid) cyst
  Enterogenous cyst
  Lipoma
Local extension from regional tumors
  Glomus jugulare tumor
  Chordoma
  Chondroma
  Chondrosarcoma
  Osteoma
  Rhabdomyosarcoma
  Fibrous histiocytoma
Metastatic tumors
  Carcinoma
  Sarcoma
  Lymphoma
  Leukemia

Source: Modified with permission from P Kleihues, PC Burger, BW Scheithauer. The new WHO classification of brain tumors. Brain Pathol 1993;3:255–268.

tic tissue makes direct contact with the glass and cellular detail may be improved.

Electron Microscopy

The use of electron microscopy in the diagnosis of tumors is labor intensive, time consuming, and expensive; interpretation is delayed by 1–2 weeks. Nevertheless, it is valuable in the diagnosis of certain tumors. Electron microscopy is used to gain insight into cell specialization by visualizing the components of the cell cytoplasm (neurofilaments, neurosecretory granules, and other organelles) that reflect cell type. Further information can be derived by inspection of the basement membranes, desmosomes, and microvilli of the cell membrane.

Immunocytochemistry

Monoclonal antibody technology has expanded the role of immunohistochemistry. A relatively specific antibody to a cellular constituent is produced and then labeled with a marker that can be identified microscopically. The limiting step is the production of high-quality antibodies that are specific for a target cell antigen.

Most diagnostic pathologists use the immunoperoxidase staining technique with horseradish peroxidase. Staining is permanent and stable, and the reaction is visible by conventional light microscopy. Several antibodies applied to the study of central nervous system (CNS) tumors are intended to detect cellular antigens in normal and tumor cells. Tumors cannot be distinguished by the detection of tumor-specific antigens that are not present in normal cells (Table 58A.2).

Table 58A.2:   Immunohistochemistry of common central nervous system neoplasms*

	GFAP	Vimentin	S-100 protein	Neurofilaments/ synaptophysin	Cytokeratin/ EMA
Astrocytoma	+++	+	+	−	−
Oligodendroglioma	+/−	+/−	+	−	−
Ependymoma	+	+/−	+	−	+
Ganglioglioma	+	+	+	+++	−
PNET	+	+/−	+	+	−
Meningioma	−	++	−	−	+
Schwannoma	−	++	+++	−	−
Metastatic carcinoma	−	+/−	+/−	−	+++

+ = weakly positive; ++ = moderately positive; +++ = strongly positive; − = negative staining; EMA = epithelial membrane antigen; GFAP = glial fibrillary acidic protein; PNET = primitive neuroectodermal tumor.
*The reactions listed represent typical staining characteristics of each tumor type. Staining reactions may vary among tumors of the same type and, in the diagnosis of an individual tumor, a profile of histochemical stains generally is obtained.

Glial Cell Markers

Testing for glial fibrillary acidic protein (GFAP) is the best-known immunohistochemical method for identifying glial cells, particularly astrocytes. GFAP derives from glial intermediate filaments, measuring 10–12 nm in diameter, that are antigenically different from cytokeratins found in epithelial cells and neurofilaments. Well-differentiated astrocytomas stain intensely; ependymomas and anaplastic astrocytomas stain less intensely because fewer filaments are present.

Neuronal Markers

Neurofilaments are heteropolymers composed of three subunits, with molecular weights of 68, 150, and 200 kD, that are unique to neurons. Each triplet protein is immunochemically distinct and is the product of a different gene. Normal neurons and neuronal tumors (gangliogliomas and differentiating medulloblastomas) stain for neurofilaments. Another neuronal cell marker is synaptophysin, a 38-kD glycosylated polypeptide, which is a component of presynaptic vesicle membranes. Thought to be an oligomeric protein that avidly binds calcium within the neurotransmitter vesicles, synaptophysin is important in the calcium ion–dependent release of neurotransmitter molecules. It is a reliable marker of neuroectodermal differentiation and is found in all neuroectodermal tumors, including neuroendocrine tumors, such as carcinoids and paragangliomas.

Epithelial Cell Markers

Cytokeratins are a class of intermediate filaments with molecular weights of 40–67 kD, primarily located in epithelial cells. Antibodies against cytokeratin are most commonly used in the diagnosis of carcinomas but can also be used to identify craniopharyngiomas and meningiomas. Epithelial membrane antigen (EMA) is a nonfibrous glycoprotein constituent of most normal and neoplastic epithelial cells. In the CNS, EMA is a known marker of metastatic carcinoma and chordomas. Many meningiomas also stain for EMA, but glial neoplasms do not.

S-100 Protein

S-100 protein is a soluble protein, composed of three antigenically distinct portions, that has a molecular weight of 21 kD. It is common to neuroectodermal cells, including melanocytes and glia. The S-100 protein has questionable value as a diagnostic marker in CNS tumors, but it does distinguish nerve sheath tumors from tumors of mesenchymal origin, such as fibrosarcoma.

Methods of Assessing Cell Proliferation

A crude estimate of cellular proliferation can be made from the mitotic index (i.e., the number of mitoses/1,000 tumor cell nuclei). Routine histological sections should not be used to derive the mitotic index because mitoses are difficult to distinguish from pyknotic nuclei, and the cells undergoing mitosis represent only a small fraction of cycling cells.

Genes situated on the short arms of the five acrocentric chromosomes (chromosomes 13, 14, 15, 21, and 22) are regulators in the transcription of ribosomal RNA. This group of genes and their associated proteins, such as RNA polymerase I and nucleolin, comprise the nucleolar organizer regions (AgNOR). After silver colloid impregnation, which is specific for sulfhydryl-rich proteins, AgNOR can be recognized in the interphase nuclei of tumor cells from formalin-fixed, paraffin-embedded tissue. The correlation between the number of AgNOR in the nuclei and the proliferative activity of the tumor is relatively good in several tumor types. This technique is useful to assess cell proliferation in astrocytomas and medulloblastomas.

Flow cytometry (FCM) is a method by which cells suspended in fluid move in single file past sensors that record selected physical or chemical characteristics. Tumor assessment by FCM uses mainly fresh or frozen tissues and body fluids, but newer modifications allow the use of fixed or paraffin-embedded specimens.

FCM is used to evaluate tumor DNA ploidy, including diploid, triploid, tetraploid, and polymorphic patterns. The clinical value of FCM studies is greatest when they complement the histological diagnosis, but they may be a predictive indicator when histological diagnosis fails. The FCM of most benign tumors shows a diploid histogram with a low percentage of S-phase cells. Cells from aggressive malignant tumors are often aneuploid, with an increased or decreased amount of DNA. Aneuploid tumors display additional G_0 and G_1 peaks, which correspond to tumor cells having a DNA content that is different from the diploid standard. The proliferation index, or number of S-phase cells, in such tumors tends to be higher than that of diploid cells.

Meningiomas, nerve sheath tumors, and low-grade astrocytomas have a lower proliferation index than do glioblastomas. However, FCM data for aneuploid astrocytomas and medulloblastomas is paradoxical and correlates with a longer mean patient survival than diploid tumors. Patients with hypertriploid astrocytomas survive longer than those with other DNA histographic types do (Salmon and Kiss 1993). Not only are 90% of metastatic tumors aneuploid, but also more than 30% of meningiomas and schwannomas are aneuploid. Therefore, determining ploidy in tumors of meningeal and nerve sheath origin has little value in assessing prognosis.

Proliferation Antigens

Most proliferation antigens are nuclear constituents that manifest during one or more proliferative phases in the cell cycle, allowing the recognition of cycling cells. Their value in the management and prognosis of brain tumors is beginning to gain recognition. The detection of proliferation antigens permits an estimation of the growth fraction in both normal and neoplastic cells. They do not provide information on the duration of the cell cycle from which the doubling time of cell proliferation can be calculated. Most proliferation antigens are unstable and are denatured by formalin. The murine monoclonal antibody Ki-67 binds to a human nuclear protein in the growth fraction (G_1, S, G_2, and M phases of the cell cycle), with maximum expression in the M phase but not in the G_0 phase. MiB-1, a variant of Ki-67 that recognizes Ki-67 epitopes in paraffin sections, is being used in place of Ki-67. In most tumors, including brain tumors, Ki-67 or MiB-1 expression increases with malignancy. This is important therapeutically because proliferating cells are most affected by irradiation and chemotherapy. Of all brain tumors, glioblastomas exhibit the greatest growth fraction (15–20%). The growth fraction of meningiomas, ependymomas, oligodendrogliomas, and schwannomas is less than 2%.

Proliferating cell nuclear antigen, a 261–amino acid auxiliary protein of DNA polymerase delta, a nuclear enzyme involved in DNA repair, may also have diagnostic value. First discovered in patients with systemic lupus erythematosus, this antigen is demonstrated in S-phase cells and the growth fraction of the cell cycle. The Ki-S1 antigen (molecular weight of 160 kD) increases from the G_1 to the M phase and may offer certain advantages over some other proliferation antigens (Kreipe et al. 1993).

MOLECULAR PATHOLOGY

Small amounts of tumor-specific proteins cannot be detected by immunohistochemistry, but molecular probes can detect the increased messenger RNA (mRNA) that encodes the gene product. Anaplastic tumors, in particular, may transcribe excessive levels of mRNA without further translation into protein products. Diagnostic elevations of prolactin mRNA are present in prolactinomas, and the same techniques should be useful in primary CNS tumors. Other gene products, such as proliferation antigens, growth factors, and their receptors, are identifiable by molecular probes.

Molecular probes are well suited to the study of chromosomes and genes, structures that are central to the development of neoplasia. Many tumors are associated with cytogenetic abnormalities, such as chromosomal translocations and deletions. The most familiar example is deletions in chromosome 22 in many meningiomas. However, abnormalities at the submicroscopic or molecular levels, such as gene rearrangements and single gene defects that may affect oncogenes and tumor suppressor genes, cannot be detected by karyotyping.

Gene rearrangements have been extensively studied in lymphomas. Because cancer is considered a clonal process in which all cells comprising a given tumor arise from a single cell, the gene rearrangement in a lymphoma should be identical in every tumor cell, thus serving to establish the lesion as a monoclonal proliferation. Gene rearrangement studies have also been essential in detecting residual tumor during clinical relapse or remission and in comparing the clonality of the original neoplastic cells and a recurrence. Gene rearrangements have not been adequately studied in tumors of the nervous system.

Neurofibromatosis type 1 (NF-1) is associated with loss of the *NF-1* gene, a tumor-suppressor gene that maps to chromosome 17q11.2. Another suppressor gene, *p53* on chromosome 17p, also has considerable potential for pathological diagnosis; it is composed of 11 exons encoding a 53-kD nuclear phosphoprotein that regulates normal cell growth. The wild-type *p53* gene is a tumor suppressor that can reverse the phenotype of transformed cells. Mutations of the *p53* gene occurring in "hot spots" in exons 5–8 are found in many human tumors. The most frequent abnormalities are mis-sense mutations.

The half-life of wild-type *p53* gene product is 20–30 minutes; normal cells have only trace amounts, which cannot be detected by immunohistochemistry. Mutant *p53* proteins have a longer half-life and accumulate sufficiently in the cell nucleus to be detected in several types of brain tumors by immunohistochemistry. In astrocytomas and glioblastomas, a significant proportion of tumors show mutations of the *p53* gene (Louis et al. 1993). Screening for *p53* mutations is now being systematically applied to other CNS tumors in an effort to better determine prognosis.

Pathology of the Future

Laboratory techniques applied to the diagnosis of CNS neoplasia are becoming increasingly sophisticated, providing greater accuracy but at greater cost. Assessing the proliferative capacity of tumors will improve when more informative proliferation antigens are discovered. Better understanding of growth factors and their receptors may provide additional insight into tumor proliferation and spread, so that the aggressiveness of a tumor subtype can be predicted. Also, apoptosis as it relates to prognosis appears to have some practical applications. The apoptotic index tends to be higher in malignant tumors.

Future advances in automated FCM may include determinations of cellular DNA to assess ploidy and chromosome evaluation using slit-scanning measurements. Further adaptation of FCM to paraffin-embedded tissue is allowing retrospective studies of archival material. Monoclonal antibodies may be used not only as in vitro markers in tissue specimens but also as in vivo agents, by radioactively labeling antibodies. This would permit novel pathological studies of tumor tissue after it is surgically removed.

Because cytogenetic analysis shows both numerical and structural abnormalities in chromosomes of brain tumor cells, karyotyping is being revived as a technique for the study of astrocytomas and other CNS neoplasms. In areas where conventional karyotyping is not routinely done, other techniques, such as interphase cytogenetics, can provide karyotype-related information (Perry et al. 1997), such as the presence of monosomy and trisomy.

Gene structure and the localization of genes in chromosomes by means of molecular probes have important implications for the diagnosis of CNS tumors. Using the newer technique of comparative genomic hybridization, for example, DNA technology can be applied to tissue specimens of CNS tumors to examine tumor-specific changes, including deletions and gene amplification. Another promising approach involves telomere loss and telomerase activity that reflects malignancy in brain tumors (Nakatani et al. 1997). The opportunities offered by molecular biology parallel the growth of information on the functional properties of nucleic acids in brain tumors.

Principles of Interpretation

Many neuropathological terms are borrowed from the discipline of general pathology. The lexicon that follows includes the terms most frequently used in clinical practice.

Anaplasia

Anaplasia or backward growth suggests that tumor cells have gone from a more differentiated to a less differentiated state. Dedifferentiation probably does not occur; rather, the cells of an anaplastic tumor are primitive compared to normal cells. Anaplasia is recognized by a histological appearance characterized by lack of cytoplasmic differentiation. Anaplastic astrocytes cannot make normal quantities of intermediate filaments. Techniques that show cytoplasmic contents, such as electron microscopy and immunocytochemistry, are coming to be of less importance than nuclear aberrations in the evaluation of anaplastic tumors. A high nucleus-to-cytoplasm ratio, reflecting increased nuclear size, and pleomorphism are common characteristics of anaplasia.

Tumor Grading

The fundamental concept of tumor grading is that histological differentiation predicts biological behavior. Most systems assign a numerical value to each grade; grade 1 is most benign and grade 4 most malignant. Astrocytomas have been graded this way for decades, and a similar system has been developed for other gliomas and nonglial tumors.

Grading, which depends on histological differentiation, should not be confused with tumor staging, which depends on gross characteristics and extent of tumor spread. Staging of CNS tumors has been defined and systematized for use in clinical trials. Computed tomography (CT) and magnetic resonance imaging have increased the accuracy of tumor staging.

Palisading and Pseudopalisading

Palisading is diagnostic of schwannomas. The term describes a collection of fusiform neoplastic Schwann cells arranged in parallel arrays or palisades, like a palisade fence constructed of parallel stakes. Necrosis never occurs in true palisading, but pseudopalisades consist of zones of serpiginous necrosis surrounded by linear stacks of neoplastic cells. Pseudopalisading is the *sine qua non* of glioblastoma multiforme and may rarely be seen in other malignant gliomas.

Rosettes

The term *rosette* is confusing because it has been applied to several histological formations. The two major kinds of rosettes are Homer Wright rosettes and perivascular rosettes. A Homer Wright rosette is a ring of cells around a central point toward which the delicate fibrillary processes converge. Some fibrillary processes are argyrophilic, which favors the notion that Homer Wright rosettes are evidence of neuroblastic differentiation. They are associated with primitive neuroectodermal tumors (PNETs), such as medulloblastoma, neuroblastoma, and pineoblastoma, but are frequently few and difficult to locate in the pathological specimen.

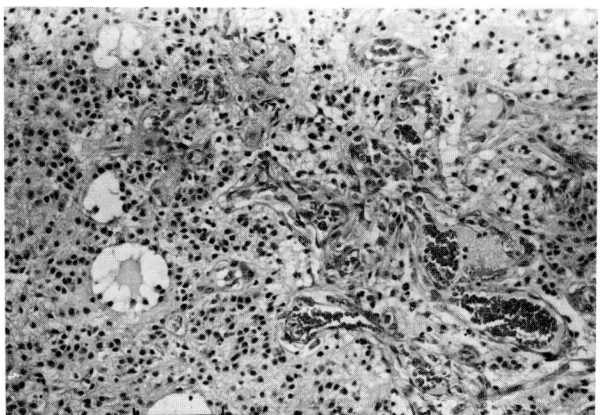

FIGURE 58A.1   Glioblastoma multiforme. Small vessels with endothelial proliferation partially occlude several vascular lumina (hematoxylin-eosin stain; calibration bar = 125 μm).

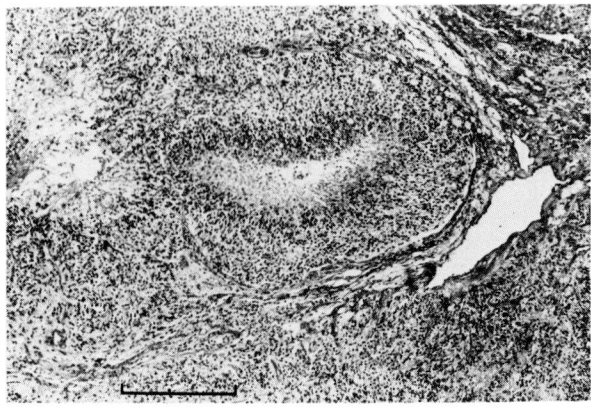

FIGURE 58A.2   Glioblastoma multiforme. Pseudopalisading with central necrosis (hematoxylin-eosin stain; calibration bar = 400 μm).

Perivascular rosettes surround a thin-walled vascular channel from which groups of cells radiate in a roselike configuration. The cells are elongated, with their nuclei oriented away from the central vessel. The blood vessel is immediately surrounded by a nucleus-free zone containing tapering cellular processes attached to the vessel. Most ependymomas contain perivascular rosettes.

Desmoplasia

Desmoplasia is the induction of mesenchymal tissue by tumors in the CNS parenchyma or the induced proliferation of normal mesenchymal tissue in regions such as the meninges. Desmoplasia is a reactive rather than a neoplastic change but does not necessarily signify a better prognosis. Gangliogliomas and medulloblastomas typically stimulate a desmoplastic response.

Endothelial Proliferation

Endothelial and smooth muscle cell proliferation most often occurs in capillaries that tend to become partially occluded and therefore resemble renal glomeruli. Endothelial proliferation and neovascularity are stimulated by soluble tumor angiogenesis factors produced by several different tumors.

NEUROEPITHELIAL TUMORS

Tumors of the astrocytic series are the largest and most heterogeneous group of neuroepithelial tumors from both a clinical and a pathological standpoint. Historically, the term *astrocytoma* has been applied broadly, but only four types have clinical importance: diffuse astrocytoma, juvenile pilocytic astrocytoma, pleomorphic xanthoastrocytoma (PXA),

and subependymal giant cell astrocytoma. Each has a distinctive topography, histology, and natural history.

Diffuse Astrocytomas

Astrocytoma, anaplastic astrocytoma, and glioblastoma multiforme form a continuum of the same process. Well-differentiated astrocytomas regularly undergo malignant change to anaplastic astrocytoma and glioblastoma multiforme. The grading system now in general use is three-tiered: Astrocytoma is a low-grade, well-differentiated tumor; glioblastoma multiforme has striking anaplasia, endothelial proliferation (Figure 58A.1), and pseudopalisading (Figure 58A.2); and anaplastic astrocytoma is intermediate between astrocytoma and glioblastoma multiforme. The absence of necrosis is the principal criterion separating anaplastic astrocytoma from glioblastoma. Chromosome 17p losses and mutations of *p53* are early events, followed by 9p deletions. Loss of chromosome 10 and amplification of epidermal growth factor receptor gene are late developments.

Diffuse astrocytomas are most common in the cerebral hemispheres, usually deep. A smaller proportion of diffuse astrocytomas occur in the spinal cord and brainstem. Despite its size, the cerebellum is a relatively uncommon location for diffuse astrocytomas. Brainstem gliomas warrant special attention because they occur predominantly in children and typically involve the pons. Exophytic and calcified lesions suggest a better prognosis.

Astrocytomas are solitary, poorly circumscribed tumors in which the tissue is homogeneous and solid. Cystic degeneration may occur (Figure 58A.3) but less often than in juvenile pilocytic astrocytomas of the cerebellum. Widespread infiltration (called *gliomatosis cerebri*) is rare. Both hemispheres are involved and may be replaced by tumor. The histological appearance of gliomatosis shows cells that

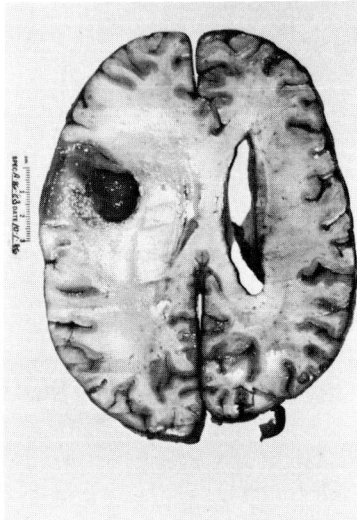

FIGURE 58A.3 Cystic astrocytoma located in left cerebral hemisphere. Tumor is poorly demarcated and has gelatinous appearance.

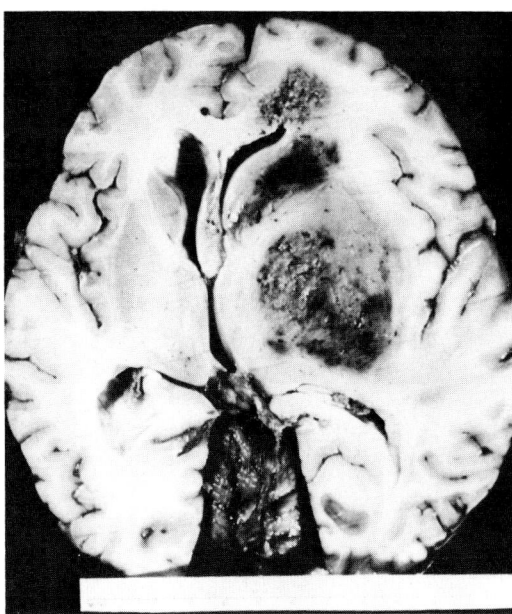

FIGURE 58A.4 Glioblastoma multiforme. Large, necrotic, and hemorrhagic tumor replaces many of the deep structures in the right cerebrum. The affected hemisphere is swollen, with a shift in midline structures to the left.

are gemistocytic, protoplasmic, or most often fibrillary. The cell type and architectural pattern have less impact on the prognosis than does the degree of anaplasia.

Astrocytic derivation is easily established in routine microscopic sections and confirmed by immunohistochemical studies. Astrocytoma cells contain numerous cytoplasmic filaments of the intermediate type that stain intensely for GFAP.

Anaplastic Astrocytoma

Anaplastic astrocytomas are as common as low-grade astrocytomas. The mean age at onset is about 10 years younger than for glioblastoma multiforme. They are usually located in the cerebral hemispheres. The average survival time from diagnosis is about two to three times longer than for glioblastoma multiforme. Features that help to distinguish astrocytomas from anaplastic astrocytomas are greater numbers of Ki-67 or MiB-1 reactive nuclei in immunostains (Kirkegaard et al. 1998), loss of the *CDKN2* gene locus, and reduced levels of Rb protein in tumor cells.

Glioblastoma Multiforme

Glioblastoma multiforme is the most common primary brain tumor in adults, comprising about 50% of all gliomas. It is the most aggressive, malignant, and lethal primary tumor of the CNS parenchyma. The peak age at onset is 40–60 years.

Glioblastoma multiforme most commonly occurs in the deep white matter, basal ganglia, or thalamus and is rarely found in the cerebellum or spinal cord. As the name implies, the gross and microscopic appearance is heterogeneous. The affected portion of brain is usually replaced by a

single, well-circumscribed lesion that infiltrates the cerebral cortex and spreads to the opposite hemisphere via the corpus callosum. Multiple tumors also occur. In advanced stages, the tumor may extend into the meninges or the ventricle. Seeding of the neuraxis as multiple implants on the brain or ventricular surfaces is an atypical growth pattern. Non-CNS metastases are extremely rare.

The cut surface has a variegated appearance (Figure 58A.4) characterized by yellow or white zones of necrosis and hemorrhage in varying stages of decomposition, which range in color from red to green. In areas where the tumor is less distorted, it has a gray, gelatinous appearance and may show cystic change. Adjuncts to diagnosis include amplification of epidermal growth factor receptor and *CDK4* genes.

Circumscribed Astrocytomas

Pilocytic astrocytoma, PXA, and subependymal giant cell astrocytoma are circumscribed astrocytomas. These tumors are more common in children than in adults and generally have a better prognosis than diffuse, poorly demarcated tumors (Burger et al. 1997).

Juvenile Pilocytic Astrocytomas

Juvenile pilocytic astrocytomas are usually well circumscribed and slow growing. They are most commonly found in the cerebellum, hypothalamus, and optic nerve

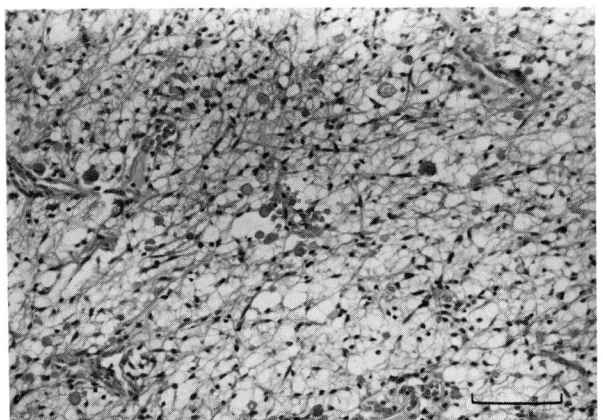

FIGURE 58A.5   Juvenile pilocytic astrocytoma. The tumor is composed of fusiform cells and microcytic areas. Rosenthal fibers appear as large, round, somewhat granular structures (hematoxylin-eosin stain; calibration bar = 125 μm).

but may involve the cerebrum, where they represent a diagnostic problem in some cases. Outcome depends on the surgical accessibility of tumor location. The gross appearance varies somewhat with anatomical location. A cerebellar tumor, which is more often hemispheric than vermal, is typically a large single cyst containing clear xanthochromic fluid. Solid tumor may surround the cyst or form a mural nodule in the cyst cavity. Hypothalamic and optic nerve tumors are usually solid. Optic nerve gliomas appear as a focal, segmental nerve swelling. Both unilateral and bilateral optic nerve gliomas are associated with NF-1.

The distinctive histological feature of juvenile pilocytic astrocytoma is a biphasic pattern with compact pilocytic areas interspersed among microcytic, spongy areas. Dense portions contain piloid (hairlike) or bipolar astrocytes with elongated, spindle-shaped nuclei. Rosenthal fibers are common. These are masses of intracellular astrocytic filaments that are round to fusiform in shape, with a hyaline or granular appearance (Figure 58A.5).

Pleomorphic Xanthoastrocytomas

PXA is a variant of astrocytoma. The average age at diagnosis is 10 years. A history of seizures often precedes diagnosis. PXA usually involves the cerebral cortex and overlying meninges, and the preferred site is the temporal lobe. The histological features are hypercellularity with many atypical and pleomorphic tumor astrocytes. Bizarre giant cells are present, but mitoses are unusual. Neoplastic astrocytes are strongly immunoreactive for GFAP. Also present are large numbers of xanthomatous cells (lipidized astrocytes) with foamy, lipid-filled cytoplasm. Despite a histological appearance and FCM data (Rostomily et al. 1997) that suggest malignant behavior, PXA has a relatively favorable prognosis. Postoperative survival times range from 2

to 17 years (Kepes 1993). Malignant transformation to glioblastoma multiforme is unusual.

Subependymal Giant Cell Astrocytomas

Most subependymal giant cell astrocytomas are associated with tuberous sclerosis (see Chapter 69). They resemble tallow gutterings (the drippings of tallow from a burning candle) on the wall of the lateral ventricle when the brain is imaged in coronal section. An elongated, sausagelike, or lobulated gross appearance is typical. The lateral ventricles are enlarged when the tumors block the foramen of Monro.

The rich vascularity of the tumor gives the cut surfaces a red and beefy appearance. Calcification is almost invariable and is at times so extensive that the mass becomes stone hard. The tumors are very cellular, consisting of closely packed giant astrocytes with abundant cytoplasm that are often arranged around a blood vessel. Giant astrocytes may have a gemistocytic or fusiform morphology. Despite the large size, the cell nuclei are uniform and not anaplastic.

Some giant cells are clearly of astrocytic origin; the cytoplasm is filled with intermediate filaments of the astrocytic type. Other tumor cells resemble neurons having prominent nucleoli and Nissl substance (rough endoplasmic reticulum). Neuronal differentiation is suggested by positive immunohistochemical staining for 68-kD neurofilament protein. Because tuberous sclerosis is characterized by hamartomas of many organs, giant cell astrocytomas may also be hamartomas rather than neoplasms. This is consistent with the benign behavior of these tumors.

Oligodendroglial Tumors

Oligodendroglial tumors comprise only 1% of brain tumors in children and less than 5% of brain tumors in all ages. Most are located in the cerebrum, especially in the frontal lobe. They are often well demarcated. Almost 25% of tumors are hemorrhagic and sometimes bleed sufficiently to have a strokelike presentation.

The histological features are a lobular architecture, in which clusters of relatively uniform neoplastic cells are separated by vascular septa. Spontaneous hemorrhage may arise from this network of delicate capillaries. Calcification is the rule, probably secondary to changes in tissue pH from hemorrhage. The most distinctive histological feature is the "fried-egg" appearance of the tumor cell nucleus and cytoplasm caused by fixation (Figure 58A.6).

Tissue prepared for electron microscopy lacks the artificial cytoplasmic clearing seen in paraffin-embedded tissue and contains a paucity of organelles. The cytoplasm tends to be free of filaments, although occasional microtubules may be encountered. Intercellular junctions are typically absent.

Necrosis and mitotic activity are the most reliable measures of poor prognosis. Of possible prognostic value are reports of chromosomal abnormalities involving 1p and 19q.

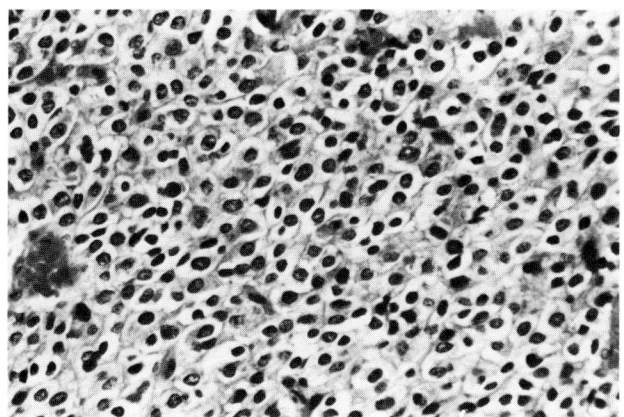

FIGURE 58A.6 Oligodendroglioma. Cells have uniform nuclei surrounded by clear cytoplasm, producing a fried-egg appearance.

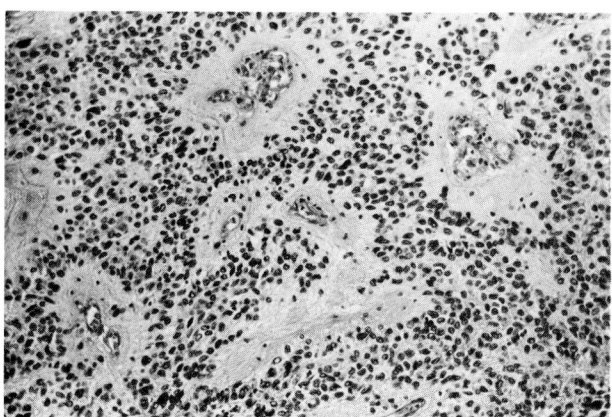

FIGURE 58A.7 Ependymoma. Perivascular rosettes with nucleus-free zones around blood vessels.

Ependymal Tumors

Ependymomas comprise 4% of all brain tumors and are the third most common CNS tumors in children. They may occur at any age, but in children they are most frequent in the first decade. Ninety percent of tumors are in the brain, with an infratentorial site twice as common as a supratentorial site, and 10% are in the spinal cord. The typical ependymoma projects from an ependymal surface to occupy the ventricle. Obstructive hydrocephalus develops when tumors are large enough to obstruct the flow of cerebrospinal fluid (CSF). A small number of ependymomas are unrelated to the ventricular system but arise within the deep cerebral white matter, presumably from ependymal cell rests.

Ependymomas are well-circumscribed masses that tend to compress rather than infiltrate the adjacent parenchyma. Cystic tumors are more likely to be found in the cerebrum. Ependymomas in contact with CSF pathways may seed ventricular surfaces and subarachnoid spaces; seeding is associated with a poor prognosis. The histological appearance is characterized by sheets of cells interrupted by two distinctive structures that are randomly dispersed within the neoplastic tissue: perivascular rosettes (Figure 58A.7) and canals (i.e., glandlike structures lined by cells resembling those that line the ventricles). Perivascular rosettes are very common, but canals, which are virtually pathognomonic, occur in fewer than 10% of cases. Electron microscopy shows an epithelial appearance with numerous microvilli and prominent zonulae adherentes. Cilia and their basal attachments, known as basal bodies or blepharoplasts, are easily identified. Sheaves of 10- to 12-nm intermediate filaments are detectable in the cytoplasm. They appear to be immunologically identical to astrocytic filaments and react positively for GFAP using immunocytochemical methods. Unlike astrocytomas, few tumor cells react intensely to GFAP because most cells have very few filaments.

Myxopapillary Ependymoma

Myxopapillary ependymoma is a subtype of ependymoma that is almost exclusively restricted in location to the cauda equina and conus medullaris. These tumors also occur in the presacral region and the subcutaneous tissue of the back. They are more common in adults than in children, tend to be red because of their lush vascularity, and are sometimes frankly hemorrhagic and gelatinous in their gross appearance. They have a papillary histological architecture. Mucoid material can be identified within tumor cells and in the supporting stroma.

Anaplastic Ependymoma

The concept of anaplastic ependymoma is poorly defined because biological behavior is equally dependent on tumor location and histological evidence of anaplasia. Three criteria are most important in determining prognosis: hypercellularity leading to overlapping of nuclei, nuclear hyperchromasia and pleomorphism, and the presence of more than five mitoses per high-power field. All three criteria must be met to justify the diagnosis of anaplastic ependymoma. FCM DNA analysis may be an additional way to determine anaplasia (Kotylo et al. 1997).

Subependymoma

Subependymomas are being detected with increasing frequency by CT and magnetic resonance imaging in the absence of clinical manifestations. Ninety percent of subependymomas occur in adults. These are small and not aggressive. In children, subependymomas are more likely to be large, symptomatic, and biologically aggressive. Subependymomas appear as a glistening, pearly white, intraventricular protuberance, most often in the fourth ventricle. Large tumors may obstruct the fourth

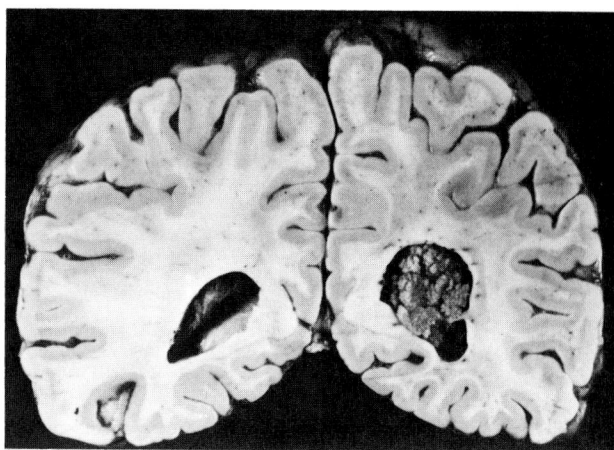

FIGURE 58A.8 Choroid plexus papilloma. Polypoid lesion with a nodular surface is located in the right lateral ventricle.

ventricle and cause hydrocephalus. Between cell clusters are bands of fibrils, numerous microcysts, and foci of calcification. This appearance suggests that the tumor is actually an astrocytoma derived from subependymal astrocytes.

CHOROID PLEXUS TUMORS

Choroid Plexus Papilloma

Choroid plexus papillomas comprise only 0.5% of intracranial tumors. As a rule, they are confined to the portion of the ventricular system that contains a choroid plexus. Approximately half are in the fourth ventricle. Tumors in the lateral ventricle are more common in children than in adults and may cause hydrocephalus by excessive CSF production. Males are more often affected than females. The onset of symptoms is usually in the first decade and may occur at birth.

Choroid plexus papillomas have a pink or red, highly vascular polypoid appearance with a granular surface (Figure 58A.8). Large tumors in the third or fourth ventricles may occlude or even distend the ventricle, causing hydrocephalus.

Histologically, choroid plexus papillomas resemble normal choroid plexus; they have a distinctly papillary structure, with the surface of each papilla covered by a layer of cuboidal or columnar epithelium that lacks cilia. Unlike the normal choroid plexus, the epithelium of papillomas tends to pile up into multiple layers, nuclear pleomorphism is greater, and the nucleus to cytoplasm ratio is higher. The epithelial cells are supported by a fibrovascular stroma, which sometimes contain focal calcification or psammoma bodies.

Electron microscopic examination of the neoplastic epithelial cells shows that they possess prominent surface microvilli and variable numbers of cilia. Within the cyto-

plasm are abundant glycogen granules and small numbers of intermediate filaments. The cells rest on a basement membrane with the basal surfaces juxtaposed to capillaries lined by fenestrated endothelium. Immunocytochemical reactions show that some tumors contain cells that stain positively for low-molecular-weight cytokeratin and for GFAP.

Choroid Plexus Carcinoma

The diagnosis of choroid plexus carcinoma in adults should be made only after metastatic adenocarcinoma, most often from the lung, is excluded. Carcinoma of the choroid plexus tends to arise in the lateral ventricle and then invade the adjacent brain parenchyma and seed throughout the subarachnoid spaces. Systemic metastases occur occasionally. Histologically, choroid plexus carcinoma is a papillary adenocarcinoma that does not secrete mucin, an important distinction from the majority of metastatic adenocarcinomas.

NEURONAL TUMORS

Neuronal tumors, in contrast to PNETs, are well differentiated and have a relatively favorable prognosis. The most common neuronal tumors are ganglioglioma, dysembryoplastic neuroepithelial tumor (DNT), and neurocytoma.

Ganglioglioma

Most gangliogliomas occur before age 21 and comprise 4–8% of pediatric brain tumors. They grow slowly and tend to show benign biological behavior. The most common site is the temporal lobe. Other lobes of the cerebral hemispheres, cerebellum, and spinal cord are less often affected. The tumors are cystic and well circumscribed, extending to the surface of the brain, expanding and flattening its contours. The solid portions are firm, gray, and gritty due to calcific deposits that are evident on CT scanning.

The histological appearance of large portions of the tumor resembles low-grade astrocytoma; sheets or bundles of spindle cells are seen. A small number of neurons in the tumor have a dysplastic appearance because they lack polarity and congregate in clusters. This is unlike the normal-appearing neurons that may be trapped in an infiltrating astrocytoma. Some neurons are binucleated or multinucleated, whereas others have very large and eccentric nuclei. The cytoplasmic borders are typically irregular and vacuolated. Within the cytoplasm, there are prominent Nissl bodies and neurofilaments, which are best demonstrated by immunohistochemical reactions for neurofilament protein. The astrocytic component is mainly composed of piloid astrocytes, often associated with Rosenthal fibers. GFAP activity is abundant.

Dysembryoplastic Neuroepithelial Tumors

DNTs are benign and may be hamartomas rather than neoplasms. They occur throughout childhood, with a mean age of onset of 9 years. DNTs are usually supratentorial and intracortical in location and are often associated with a long history of intractable seizures (Daumas-Duport 1993). The temporal lobe is the most common location for DNTs. They are multinodular and associated with cortical dysplasia. Cellular heterogeneity is characteristic; DNTs contain astrocytes as well as oligodendroglial cells and neuronal elements, which are frequently surrounded by clear halos or vacuoles and may lie in pools of mucinlike material.

Central Neurocytomas

Central neurocytomas are slow-growing tumors that are usually located in the lateral or third ventricle near the foramen of Monro, frequently within the septum pellucidum (Hassoun et al. 1993). Age at onset is usually in the second or third decade. They are usually sharply demarcated, sometimes lobulated masses that fill the ventricular space without infiltration of the surrounding brain, which makes them amenable to surgical resection.

The main histological feature is a monotonous appearance of uniform tumor cells that mimic oligodendroglioma. Their cytoplasm contains microtubules, synapses, and neurosecretory granules. Further, central neurocytomas are immunoreactive for synaptophysin.

Primitive Neuroectodermal Tumors

PNETs of the CNS are medulloblastoma, neuroblastoma, and pineoblastoma (Schild et al. 1993). Non-CNS PNETs are adrenal neuroblastoma, retinoblastoma, and perhaps Ewing's sarcoma. The common attributes of PNETs are occurrence predominantly in children and young adults and high rate of malignancy.

Histologically, all PNETs appear to be alike, mainly composed of primitive, undifferentiated dark cells devoid of any distinctive architecture. Their nuclei are hyperchromatic, vary from round to fusiform, and are surrounded by little discernible cytoplasm. Mitoses are generally more abundant than in other types of CNS tumors. PNETs that originate in the CNS often show extensive leptomeningeal spread. Despite the histological similarities of PNETs, a unifying concept remains controversial because proof of a common histogenesis is lacking. This does not invalidate the phenotypic similarities of PNET cells based on mor-

phological, cytogenetic, immunohistochemical, and biochemical parameters.

The causes and pathogenesis of PNET probably are multifactorial. Tumors resembling PNET can be induced in animals exposed to avian sarcoma virus. In humans, the importance of genetic factors is exemplified by retinoblastoma, in which there is a variable deletion in chromosome 13. Until more is known about the biology of PNET, it is convenient to consider it a neoplasm of undifferentiated, multipotential stem cells with the ability for differentiation into more mature elements. In the CNS, this process may take the path of neuronal or glial maturation. The glial line may be represented by cells with astrocytic (spongioblastoma), oligodendroglial, or ependymal (ependymoblastoma) features.

Medulloblastoma

The name *medulloblastoma* is misleading because it is doubtful that any cell identifiable as a medulloblast exists during histogenesis. In theory, the medulloblast represents an interim phase of cellular differentiation, when primitive elements of the embryonic mantle layer are still capable of maturation along glial and neuronal lines.

Medulloblastoma is the most common PNET of the CNS and serves as the prototype for the group. More than 50% of medulloblastomas occur in children younger than 10 years of age. A second, smaller frequency peak occurs between the ages of 18 and 25. Medulloblastoma, by definition, originates in the cerebellum, usually the midline. It is generally well defined, soft, friable, and focally necrotic. Medulloblastomas have a proclivity to invade the ventricle and disseminate along CSF pathways. The aggressiveness of medulloblastomas is affirmed by reports of metastases to bone, lymph nodes, and other extracranial sites.

Medulloblastomas resemble other PNETs histologically. Sheets of small, poorly differentiated cells are punctuated by occasional Homer Wright rosettes (Figure 58A.9). True neuronal differentiation is rare, but when it occurs, the tumor cells contain neurotubules and dense-core vesicles. Glial differentiation is more common but is difficult to see in routine paraffin sections. The best way to show astrocytic maturation is by the immunoperoxidase methods for GFAP. Amplification of c-myc oncogene distinguishes medulloblastoma from other PNETs.

Cerebral Primitive Neuroectodermal Tumors

Cerebral PNETs occur in children and young adults and have an aggressive course and recurrence rate. Death occurs within 8–24 months of diagnosis. These tumors disseminate throughout the CSF pathways and metastasize to lungs and other systemic organs. A variant of this tumor, cerebral neuroblastoma, undergoes neuroblastic differentiation; astrocytic differentiation is inconspicuous or absent.

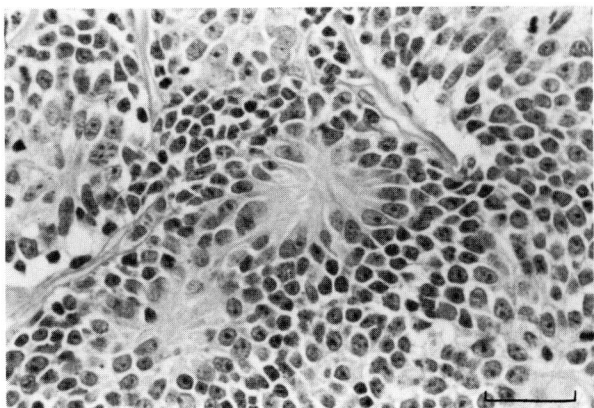

FIGURE 58A.9   Medulloblastoma. Cellular tumor composed of small, poorly differentiated cells with Homer Wright rosette formation (hematoxylin-eosin stain; calibration bar = 125 μm).

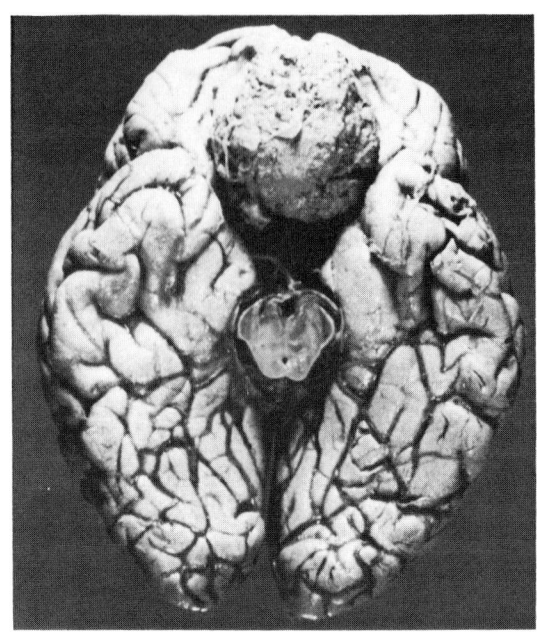

FIGURE 58A.10   Meningioma. Large, discrete, extra-axial tumor located in the inferior frontal region.

MENINGEAL TUMORS

Meningiomas comprise 10–15% of all intracranial tumors. They are most prevalent after age 50 and constitute less than 2% of CNS tumors in children. The female to male ratio is 3 to 2 in adults and 1 to 1 in children. More than 90% of meningiomas are associated with abnormalities of chromosome 22. The abnormality is reminiscent of the Philadelphia chromosome described in chronic myelocytic leukemia. A gene on chromosome 22 may be responsible for the development of meningioma. Progesterone receptors are present in up to 50% of cases, and estrogen receptors are present in approximately 20% of tumors. Their significance is unclear, other than that meningiomas sometimes enlarge dramatically with pregnancy and regress after delivery.

The locations of meningiomas, in descending order of frequency, are the cerebral convexity, parasagittal region, sphenoid wing, parasellar region, and spinal canal. Posterior fossa and lateral ventricle locations are more common in children. Multiple meningiomas suggest neurofibromatosis type 2 (NF-2).

Meningiomas tend to be well demarcated from the adjacent brain or spinal cord, which they compress rather than invade (Figure 58A.10). Cerebral edema is common and frequently extensive. The pattern of tumor spread includes growth along the brain or dural surface (referred to as *meningioma-en-plaque*), infiltration of the dura, and extension into the bone, which may stimulate hyperostosis. Meningiomas are generally firm in consistency and often gritty because of the presence of psammoma bodies. Macrocystic lesions are more likely to occur in children.

Most meningiomas develop in the meninges, but all tumors arising in the meninges are not meningiomas. Arachnoidal elements, specifically the cap cells derived from the neural crest and from various mesenchymal components, such as fibroblasts, are thought to be the cells of origin. Meningiomas are mixed tumors, and their diverse histology has led to descriptions of at least 20 histological variants. The WHO has proposed nine morphological types, but from a practical standpoint, most meningiomas do not exist in pure form, and each tumor is a composite of several types. Except for the papillary meningioma, the correlation between histological type and prognosis is poor. Therefore, we view meningiomas as having two basic histological patterns: meningothelial or fibroblastic. Meningothelial or syncytial tumors are composed of arachnoidal cap cells and have an epithelial appearance. The cells are arranged in sheets or lobules, often with prominent whorls and psammoma bodies. Fibroblastic meningiomas are distinguished by the spindle appearance of cells that produce abundant collagen and reticulin fibers. Both patterns frequently coexist in the same tumor. Ultrastructural examination shows that some cells are epithelial, possessing basement membranes and joined by desmosomes. One of the most remarkable features is the complex interdigitations of cell processes extending from neighboring cells. Collections of filaments measuring 10 nm in diameter are conspicuous within the cytoplasm of many cells. Cytokeratin and EMA, markers for epithelial cells, are shown in 38% and 100%, respectively, of meningiomas.

Anaplastic Meningiomas

The concept of anaplastic meningioma is controversial; even histologically benign meningiomas recur in 15–20% of cases. Recurrence is abetted by incomplete surgical excision and invasion of the dura or bone. Histologically, anaplastic meningiomas are characterized by hypercellularity, a high nucleus-to-cytoplasm ratio, numerous mitoses, and necrosis. The mitotic rate is the single most important indicator of aggressive behavior and is associated with rapid recurrence and metastases. A high proliferative index based on immunostaining for Ki-67 or MiB-1 is emerging as important in determining outcome (Prayson 1996). Increased anaplasia is likely in recurrent tumors. Deletions in chromosome 14 are reported to correlate with poor prognosis.

Nerve Sheath Tumors

Schwannomas and neurofibromas derive from nerve sheaths. Both are composed of Schwann cells and endoneural fibroblasts. Despite an intracranial or intravertebral location, they are extra-axial tumors of the peripheral nervous system. Multiple nerve sheath tumors should suggest NF-1. Most are slow growing and benign. Neurofibrosarcoma may develop de novo or in a pre-existing benign tumor, much less frequently in schwannoma than in neurofibroma.

Schwannomas (Neurilemomas)

The frequency of schwannomas peaks in the fourth and fifth decades. Most are located on the vestibular portion of the eighth cranial nerve. Other cranial nerves, particularly the trigeminal, are much less frequent sites. Vestibular schwannomas (acoustic neuroma) are more common in women, which may relate to the female predominance of estrogen binding in these tumors. Bilateral lesions are diagnostic of NF-2.

Vestibular schwannomas erode the internal auditory meatus and occupy the cerebellopontine angle; with increasing size, they compress and deform the pons. Spinal schwannomas comprise about 30% of intraspinal tumors. Most arise from the dorsal roots, preferring sensory nerves, like their cranial counterparts. Spinal schwannomas may extend through the dura or, in some cases, through the intervertebral foramen as a dumbbell-shaped mass that is partly within and partly outside the spinal canal.

Schwannomas are composed of two distinct types of tissue. Cellular, dense zones, known as Antoni A areas, contain spindle-shaped cells arranged in palisades. Antoni B areas are myxoid and microcytic in appearance. Hemorrhage often occurs in highly vascular regions. Electron microscopy reveals basement membranes adjoining tumor cells, which substantiate their Schwann cell lineage.

Neurofibromas

Neurofibromas are less common than schwannomas on spinal nerve roots. They usually originate from nerve terminals in the dermis and from large nerve trunks, such as the brachial plexus. Neurofibromas on spinal roots and other peripheral nerves look different from schwannomas. The involved nerve is focally swollen, but the entire nerve segment is infiltrated, rendering surgical excision difficult. A plexiform pattern of spread is pathognomonic of NF-1. On gross inspection, neurofibromas are gray and gelatinous. Histologically, bundles of uniform, fusiform cells are suspended haphazardly in a myxoid background.

TUMORS OF BLOOD VESSEL ORIGIN

Hemangioblastomas

Hemangioblastomas are benign, vasoformative tumors. About 10% of patients with hemangioblastoma have von Hippel–Lindau disease. The age at diagnosis ranges from adolescence to the sixth decade, with the peak frequency at 40 years. Hemangioblastomas are more common in males. The tumor usually arises in the cerebellum, vermis more often than hemisphere, and is the most common primary cerebellar neoplasm in adults. Hemangioblastomas are sometimes located in the cerebrum or spinal cord, where they occur in association with syringomyelia.

Hemangioblastomas are cystic, sharply demarcated, and noninfiltrative, often allowing total surgical resection. The cyst contents are usually clear and yellow; a rusty color indicates previous bleeding. Solid portions of the tumor are dark red because of an elaborate vascular supply, which predisposes to spontaneous hemorrhage. Histological examination shows abundant capillaries coursing throughout the tumor mass. Hemangioblastomas and so-called supratentorial angioblastic meningiomas are histologically similar and may be variants of the same tumor.

An erythropoietinlike substance is identified in the cyst fluid of 20% of tumors. It may be associated with pure red cell hyperplasia.

Hemangiopericytomas

Hemangiopericytoma, once considered a variant of meningioma, is now generally accepted to be a vasogenic tumor that occurs anywhere in the body, most often in soft tissues. Most CNS hemangiopericytomas occur in the meninges, where they account for about 5% of meningeal tumors. They occur at all ages, peaking in the fourth to sixth decades. Hemangiopericytoma is an aggressive tumor; the recurrence rate after surgery is 80%, and the likelihood of systemic metastases is 20%. At surgery, hemangiopericytoma is often misdiagnosed as meningioma because of its location and its tendency to compress the CNS parenchyma. Histologically, the tumor is extremely cellular and vascular. Mitoses are abundant, reflecting the tumor's malignant nature. Its pericytic derivation is confirmed by electron microscopic examination, in which smooth muscle–like cells containing intermediate filaments are evident.

GERM CELL TUMORS

Germ cell tumors are most common in school-aged children. CNS germ cell tumors are similar to those arising from the gonads. Like their counterparts in the retroperitoneum and mediastinum, CNS germ cell tumors have a midline location. The pineal region is the most common site, followed by the base of the brain in the vicinity of the pituitary gland, where they are sometimes referred to as *ectopic pinealomas*. Germ cell tumors as a group grow rapidly, with a propensity to seed the subarachnoid space. Cytological examination of the CNS may be diagnostic.

Most authorities believe that germ cell tumors arise from totipotential germ cells that are capable of producing several different cell subtypes. Tumors are often composed of more than one tumor type, and the prognosis is determined by the most malignant component in the tumor. Histologically, most CNS germ cell tumors are identical to testicular seminoma, which is composed of two distinct cell populations. The larger germ cells have abundant cytoplasmic glycogen and alkaline phosphatase activity, and the stroma contains lymphocytes that are both T cells and B cells.

Embryonal carcinoma is the most primitive, undifferentiated germ cell tumor. α-Fetoprotein is present in the tumor cells and in the CSF. Endodermal sinus tumors form structures resembling the yolk sac. Choriocarcinoma, characterized by differentiation into trophoblastic tissue, is highly vascular, prone to massive hemorrhage, and contains chorionic gonadotropin.

Teratomas have the ability to differentiate into elements from all three germ layers. They may contain mature components, such as teeth, hair, muscle, cartilage, and bronchial wall. These are arranged in a haphazard, nonfunctional manner but are benign. Immature anaplastic elements may be found alongside the benign elements or may comprise the entire tumor. Teratomas often contain other tumor types, particularly embryonal carcinoma.

MALIGNANT LYMPHOMAS

Lymphomas arise in lymph nodes and other somatic organs and spread to the CNS. CNS involvement occurs in 25–30% of systemic non-Hodgkin's lymphomas but is exceptional in Hodgkin's disease. Systemic lymphomas tend to infiltrate the leptomeninges and spare the parenchyma. The spine is a favored site, and spinal compression is a common complication.

Primary CNS lymphomas, which account for less than 1% of CNS tumors, differ from systemic lymphoma in three ways. In lymphoma, (1) the tumor originates in the parenchyma and spares the meninges, which explains why the CSF cytologic examinations contain tumor cells in only 25% of patients; (2) the spinal cord is the least common site of involvement; and (3) tumor rarely spreads from the brain to other organs.

The incidence of lymphoma is increased in immunodeficient patients, such as patients with acquired immunodeficiency syndrome and organ transplant recipients. Primary lymphoma is mainly a disease of the middle-aged and elderly. Survival without treatment is only 2–5 months. Tumor locations, in descending order of frequency, are the cerebrum, cerebellum, and brainstem. Tumors tend to be multiple, well demarcated, and centrally necrotic.

Most CNS lymphomas are B-cell tumors, usually large cell or immunoblastic sarcoma. Regardless of cell type, lymphomas typically show a perivascular pattern in which malignant cells surround blood vessels in concentric layers. This arrangement resembles the inflammatory responses of encephalitis, for which it may be mistaken.

MALFORMATIVE TUMORS

Craniopharyngiomas

Craniopharyngiomas comprise 2–5% of CNS tumors. Most become symptomatic in the first two decades but can occur at any age. Craniopharyngiomas are thought to arise from cell rests of Rathke's pouch, an evagination of the primitive stomatodeum. Remnants of Rathke's pouch may be identified as nests of squamous epithelium on the anterior surface of the infundibulum and the pars tuberalis in infants and adults. Craniopharyngiomas may be intrasellar or more frequently suprasellar in location, involving the hypothalamus and the optic nerve. The expanding mass causes hydrocephalus by encroaching on the third ventricle.

The advancing margins of the craniopharyngioma are relatively sharp, but a distinct surgical tissue plane may not be present. Both solid and cystic areas are intermingled. The cysts can become large and are typically filled with a dark, viscous fluid. Irregularly shaped calcific deposits, varying in size from grains of sand to fine gravel, are found in approximately 75% of cases. The microscopic appearance has been compared to that of adamantinoma, a tumor of the jaw derived from ameloblastic epithelium.

Epidermoid and Dermoid Cysts

Epidermoid and dermoid cysts are implantation or sequestration cysts derived from misplaced ectoderm. They may be congenital or acquired. The congenital type is caused by inclusion of ectodermal tissue during embryonic closure of the neural groove (see Chapter 66) or during coalescence of epithelial fusion lines in the cranium. Sequestration cysts accompany dysraphism, such as spina bifida, and may communicate with the skin surface through a sinus tract.

Acquired cysts may be caused by performing a lumbar puncture with a needle that has no trocar, which causes fragments of epidermis to be transplanted into the spinal canal.

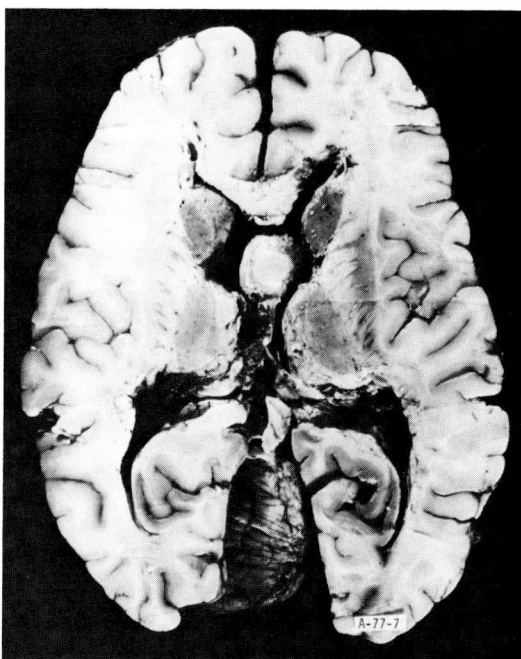

FIGURE 58A.11   Colloid cyst. Spherical tumor occupies the third ventricle, causing hydrocephalus.

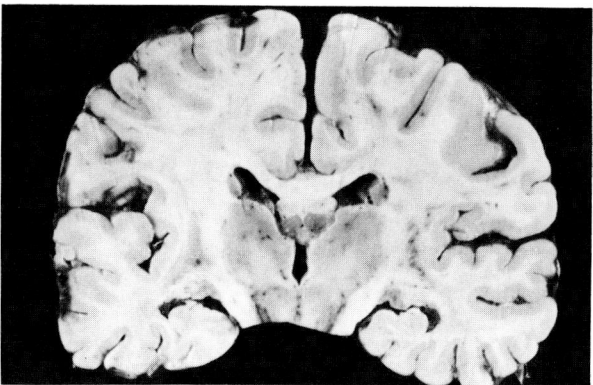

FIGURE 58A.12   Lipoma. Lesion resembling normal adipose tissue beneath corpus callosum and fornices.

Epidermoid cysts occur in young adults and are usually found in the cerebellopontine angle and skull. Dermoids are more common in children and tend to occur near the midline in the cerebellar vermis, parasellar or parapontine region, and spinal canal, especially in the lumbosacral region. Intact tumors are enveloped by a fibrous capsule that has a glistening white surface, like mother-of-pearl, and are called *pearly tumors*. The lining and contents of the epidermoid are composed of keratin-producing squamous epithelium that may be attenuated or focally stratified. The adjacent collagenous wall is often partially calcified, producing a linear or speckled pattern in CT images. The inner layer of a dermoid is also composed of squamous epithelium, but the presence of hair follicles and skin appendages distinguishes dermoid cysts from epidermoid cysts. The cyst contents, once introduced into the meninges by spontaneous rupture or during surgery, can incite severe chemical meningitis that is typically granulomatous.

Neuroepithelial (Colloid) Cysts

Cysts lined by epithelial cells usually occur in the third ventricle and may arise in the choroid plexus, in the periventricular brain parenchyma, and rarely in the meninges. Colloid cysts are thought to be developmental rather than neoplastic, but their precise origin has not been established. The ependyma, choroid plexus, and embryonic glandular paraphysis are all possible progenitors of later cyst formation.

Colloid cysts are larger than neuroepithelial cysts in other locations and become symptomatic by causing obstructive hydrocephalus. Onset of symptoms usually occurs in childhood. Cysts vary in size from tiny tumors found only incidentally at postmortem examination to structures up to 4 cm in diameter that totally fill or distend the third ventricle. They project from the choroid plexus in the roof of the third ventricle as a spherical mass with a smooth exterior surface (Figure 58A.11). The cut surface shows a fibrous outer capsule enclosing an amorphous mucoid material. Regardless of location, neuroepithelial cysts are lined by uniform epithelial cells, which usually form a single layer but may be stratified. The cells are cuboid or columnar and often vacuolated. The vacuoles contain a mucinlike substance that is secreted into the cyst, causing progressive enlargement.

Lipomas

Most lipomas are located in the midline and are sometimes associated with other developmental abnormalities, such as agenesis of the corpus callosum. Typical locations include the dorsal aspect of the midbrain, cerebellar vermis, and spinal cord. The most common location is the surface of the corpus callosum. Lipomas of the spinal cord often become symptomatic by causing cord compression, but lipomas of the brain are usually asymptomatic and are incidental findings during neuroimaging studies and on postmortem examination.

Lipomas are yellow and resemble normal fat. Histologically, they are vascular or exhibit smooth muscle elements, or both, giving rise to the terms angiolipoma and angiomyolipoma. Tumors of the brain, particularly those adjacent to the corpus callosum, may seem to infiltrate the parenchyma (Figure 58A.12) but are benign in histological appearance and biological behavior. Lipomas of the spinal canal are almost invariably in an epidural or subdural position and are well demarcated from the adjacent spinal cord. Some lipomas contain peripheral calcifications, cartilaginous regions, or osseous foci with evidence of extramedullary hematopoiesis.

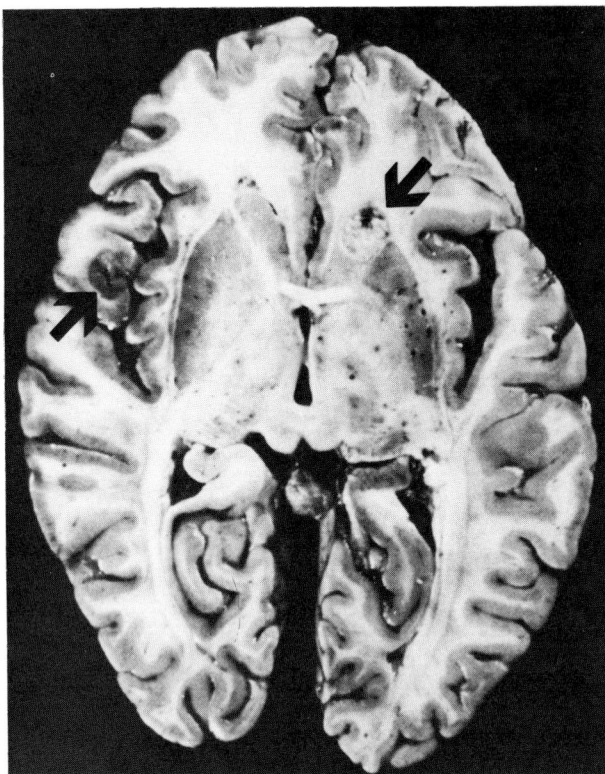

FIGURE 58A.13 Metastatic carcinoma. Note the arrow that points to well-demarcated tumor, with focal eccentric necrotic area, located in the right caudate nucleus. A second darker, infiltrative lesion in the left temporal cortex is more difficult to discern (*arrow* on left).

METASTATIC TUMORS

The frequency of metastatic tumors to the CNS is difficult to determine. Approximately one-fourth of CNS tumors found on postmortem examination are metastatic. Most occur in middle-aged and older adults. Multiple CNS metastases are detected in at least 75% of cases. The location of parenchymal metastases is directly related to tissue volume. Cerebral metastases are eight times as common as cerebellar metastases, and brainstem and spinal cord metastases are relatively uncommon. Metastases seek out the corticomedullary junction, perhaps because of a reduction or alteration in blood flow at the interface between gray and white matter.

The typical metastasis is round and well demarcated, with central necrosis or hemorrhage (Figure 58A.13). Spontaneous bleeding indicates choriocarcinoma, melanoma, or kidney carcinoma. A zone of edema customarily surrounds even small metastatic lesions. The histological appearance is variable and recapitulates the morphology of the primary tumor. Most metastatic lesions are carcinomas rather than sarcomas or lymphomas.

REFERENCES

Burger PC, Scheithauer BW, Lee RR, et al. An interdisciplinary approach to avoid the overtreatment of patients with central nervous system lesions. Cancer 1997;80:2040–2046.

Daumas-Duport C. Dysembryoplastic neuroepithelial tumors. Brain Pathol 1993;3:283–295.

Hassoun J, Soylemezoglu F, Gambarelli D, et al. Central neurocytoma: a synopsis of clinical and histological features. Brain Pathol 1993;3:297–306.

Kepes JJ. Pleomorphic xanthoastrocytoma: the birth of a diagnosis and a concept. Brain Pathol 1993;3:269–274.

Kirkegaard LJ, DeRose PB, Yao B, et al. Image cytometric measurement of nuclear proliferation markers (MIB-1, PCNA) in astrocytomas. Am J Clin Pathol 1998;109:69–74.

Kleihues P, Burger PC, Scheithauer BW. The new WHO classification of brain tumors. Brain Pathol 1993;3:255–268.

Kotylo PK, Robertson PB, Fineberg NS, et al. Flow cytometric DNA analysis of pediatric intracranial ependymomas. Arch Pathol Lab Med 1997;121:1255–1258.

Kreipe H, Heidebrecht HJ, Hansen S, et al. A new proliferation-associated nuclear antigen detectable in paraffin-embedded tissues by the monoclonal antibody Ki-S1. Am J Pathol 1993;142:3–10.

Louis DN, von Deimling A, Chung RY, et al. Comparative study of p53 gene and protein alterations in human astrocytic tumors. J Neuropathol Exp Neurol 1993;52:31–38.

Nakatani K, Yoshimi N, Mori H, et al. The significant role of telomerase activity in human brain tumors. Cancer 1997;80:471–476.

Perry A, Tonk V, McIntire DD, et al. Interphase cytogenetic (in situ hybridization) analysis of astrocytomas using archival, formalin-fixed, paraffin-embedded tissue and nonfluorescent light microscopy. Am J Clin Pathol 1997;108:166–174.

Prayson RA. Malignant meningioma. Am J Clin Pathol 1996; 105:719–726.

Rostomily RC, Hoyt JW, Berger MS, et al. Pleomorphic xanthoastrocytoma. DNA flow cytometry and outcome analysis of 12 patients. Cancer 1997;80:2141–2150.

Salmon I, Kiss R. Relationship between proliferative activity and ploidy level in a series of 530 human brain tumors including astrocytomas, meningiomas, schwannomas, and metastases. Hum Pathol 1993;24:329–335.

Schild SE, Scheithauer BW, Schomberg PJ, et al. Pineal parenchymal tumors. Cancer 1993;72:870–880.

Sidawy MK, Jannotta FS. Intraoperative cytologic diagnosis of lesions of the central nervous system. Am J Clin Pathol 1997; 108(Suppl. 1):556–566.

Chapter 58
Primary and Secondary Tumors of the Nervous System

B. MOLECULAR BIOLOGY OF NERVOUS SYSTEM TUMORS
Steven J. Greenberg and Michael E. Cohen

Neoplasia represents the emergence of a relatively autonomous form of cell replication, independent of the external host environment, largely as a result of somatic mutations in the genomic DNA. The molecular mechanisms of checks and balances that regulate and limit normal cellular proliferation form the basis of our current understating of cancer development. These mechanisms involve the activation of dominant oncogenes and the inactivation of tumor-suppressor genes. With the expanding field of molecular genetics of cancer, new paradigms have been developed to characterize individual central nervous system tumors and to define their origins on the basis of a sequence of genetic mutations. This section reviews the essential concepts of cell growth and death, introduces oncogenes and tumor-suppressor genes, and covers recent advances in our understanding of the molecular biology of nervous system tumors.

CELL GROWTH AND CELL DEATH

Normal homeostasis is maintained by a balance between cell birth and cell death. Tumor growth can be thought of as an imbalance in which cell birth exceeds cell death. This can result from an increased rate in proliferation, a decreased death rate, or both.

Growth arrest may be reversible or irreversible. Normally, the majority of stem cells or basal cells are growth arrested in a reversible state. Arrest is maintained by soluble growth-inhibitory cytokines (i.e., transforming growth factors [TGFs], interferons, interleukins [ILs], tumor necrosis factors [TNFs], and antiangiogenesis factors) or by intrinsic signals that block signal transduction and thus cell cycle progression. Growth-arresting signals, or negative signals, can be suppressed, as when required for regeneration after tissue injury. Irreversible growth arrest takes one of four forms: terminal differentiation, necrosis, apoptosis, and senescence. Conversely, cells that resist the constraints imposed by the various mechanisms of growth arrest may become "immortal." Immortalization removes the normal constraints on tumor cell growth and allows for malignant progression.

Terminal Differentiation

Terminal differentiation is associated with the expression of a very specialized function or product of a tissue (e.g., neuronal development). Rejuvenation is severely restricted, and progression to terminal differentiation usually precludes the ability to undergo subsequent mitoses. This may partially explain why neuronal tumors are uncommon.

Apoptosis is programmed cell death. It is a normal process during fetal development, in the newborn, and continuously throughout life. In contrast to necrosis, apoptosis may be selective for single cells and reflect a natural order. The cell shrinks and fragments, but the lysosomes and cell membranes remain intact. The chromatin condenses, and DNA fragments produce a characteristic 180– to 200–base pair ladder on agarose gel electrophoresis. Apoptotic cells are removed by phagocytosis with little, if any, evidence of inflammation. Cell death by apoptosis or necrosis occurs in many tumors. Apoptosis can be initiated by effects mediated extracellularly (paracrine) or by functions internal to the cell (autocrine). Lymphotoxins and TNFs are powerful paracrine agents. Upsetting the balance between oncogenes and tumor-suppressor genes is an autocrine process that influences cell survival and death.

Necrosis describes a pathological form of cell death resulting from ischemic, metabolic, or toxic injury or trauma. Necrosis involves groups of cells and is often accompanied by inflammation. Cellular necrosis is characterized by dilatation of the endoplasmic reticulum, swelling of mitochondria, and breakdown of the plasma membrane with consequent loss of ion transport. The nuclear chromatin becomes flocculent, and release of lysosomal enzymes causes nonspecific degradation of DNA. The cell swells and dies. Release of cellular contents into the extracellular milieu may incite an inflammatory response.

Senescence is nonrandom cellular death caused by the inherent constraints of aging. Normal human cells undergo a fixed number of cell divisions in vitro and then stop proliferating. Embryonic human fibroblasts undergo 50–60 population doublings and cannot exceed this limit. The number of doublings, not the length of time in culture, determines the life span. Normal cells transplanted serially also undergo a limited number of cell divisions, so that senescence is not an in vitro artifact. Further, the doubling potential of cells in culture is inversely proportional to the age of the donor. Donors with premature aging, such as those with progeria or Down syndrome, senesce prematurely. Finally, interspecies variations in doubling reflect the maximum life spans of the different species: Fibroblasts of rodents, humans, and tortoises have maximum doublings of 40, 60, and 125, respectively. Collectively, these observations suggest that senescence is an intrinsic property of individual cells. Escape from senescence, or "immortality," is a necessary but insufficient alteration that predisposes a cell to neoplastic transformation.

Aging is a well-orchestrated program of genetic events rather than the random accumulation of mutations in DNA and RNA or damage to proteins. This claim is supported by the observation that the hybrid products between fusion of cells with finite life spans and immortalized cells are senescent. Also, hybridizations formed between two different immortalized cell lines can produce senescence. These results suggest that growth arrest by senescence is a dominant process encoded by multiple genetic loci that function in a complementary fashion. Several putative senescence genes have been mapped to different chromosomes by intraspecies and interspecies hybridization experiments, and by microscopic cell-injected chromosomal transfer techniques.

CELL CYCLE

The multistep path leading to oncogenesis involves the disruption of regulatory events that act either to promote growth (positive signals) or to induce growth arrest (negative signals). These signals are orchestrated by proteins that are the products of oncogenes. The proteins promote growth- or tumor-suppressor genes that act to inhibit unbridled growth. For each cancer, a different constellation of oncogenes and tumor-suppressor genes is involved. The final common pathway by which the resultant malignant genotype deregulates growth is a subversion of normally occurring processes that characterize the cell cycle.

The successful transfer of genetic information from parental cells to progeny requires that DNA be duplicated and that the genetic information, along with other cell products, be efficiently packaged and partitioned. To accomplish cell division, a cell in the resting state, G_0, progresses through G_1, S, G_2, and M phases of a proliferative cycle (Figure 58B.1). The synthetic phase (S) denotes the complete duplication of nuclear DNA. The mitotic phase (M) encompasses the condensation of chromosomes, attachment to the spindles, and segregation of chromosomes into two equal compartments. These events are separated by two transitional gaps, G_1 (between M and S) and G_2 (between S and M). A number of essential biochemical processes (obligatory molecular pathways) occur during the gap transitions. For example, the transcription and translation of enzymes required to synthesize deoxyribonucleotide triphosphate precursors for DNA synthesis in S phase occurs in late G_1. Perhaps even more important are the critical checkpoints concentrated within G_1 and G_2 that serve to monitor the competency of cell cycle progression.

Obligatory molecular pathways define essential functions that are necessary for cell cycle progression. Therefore, mutations in genes that regulate essential functions are usually lethal. Transition checkpoints, Gap-1 and Gap-2 (G_1 and G_2), negatively regulate the cell cycle, are nonlethal, and result in defective cell cycle progression if mutated or deleted. Checkpoints are shown in Figure 58B.1 in captioned areas. Checkpoints have tumor-suppressor gene activity. Activities in the signal transduction pathways drive the cell cycle and are proto-oncogenes. Oncogenesis results from a series of events characterized by the loss of tumor-suppressor genes and the mutation and deregulated expression of proto-oncogenes that result in oncogene expression.

Obligatory Molecular Pathways

Anything but precise execution of the steps of cell division may result in cell death, the development of cancer, or the production of sterile offspring. It is useful to think of the cell cycle as inter-related mechanisms composed of obligatory positive regulatory pathways and negative surveillance pathways.

The first level of the cell cycle consists of all biosynthetic reactions for the elaboration of structural molecules and enzymatic proteins necessary to accomplish cell division. These are needed for the cell to reach appropriate size and mass and to accumulate sufficient high-energy substrates and structural components needed for DNA duplication

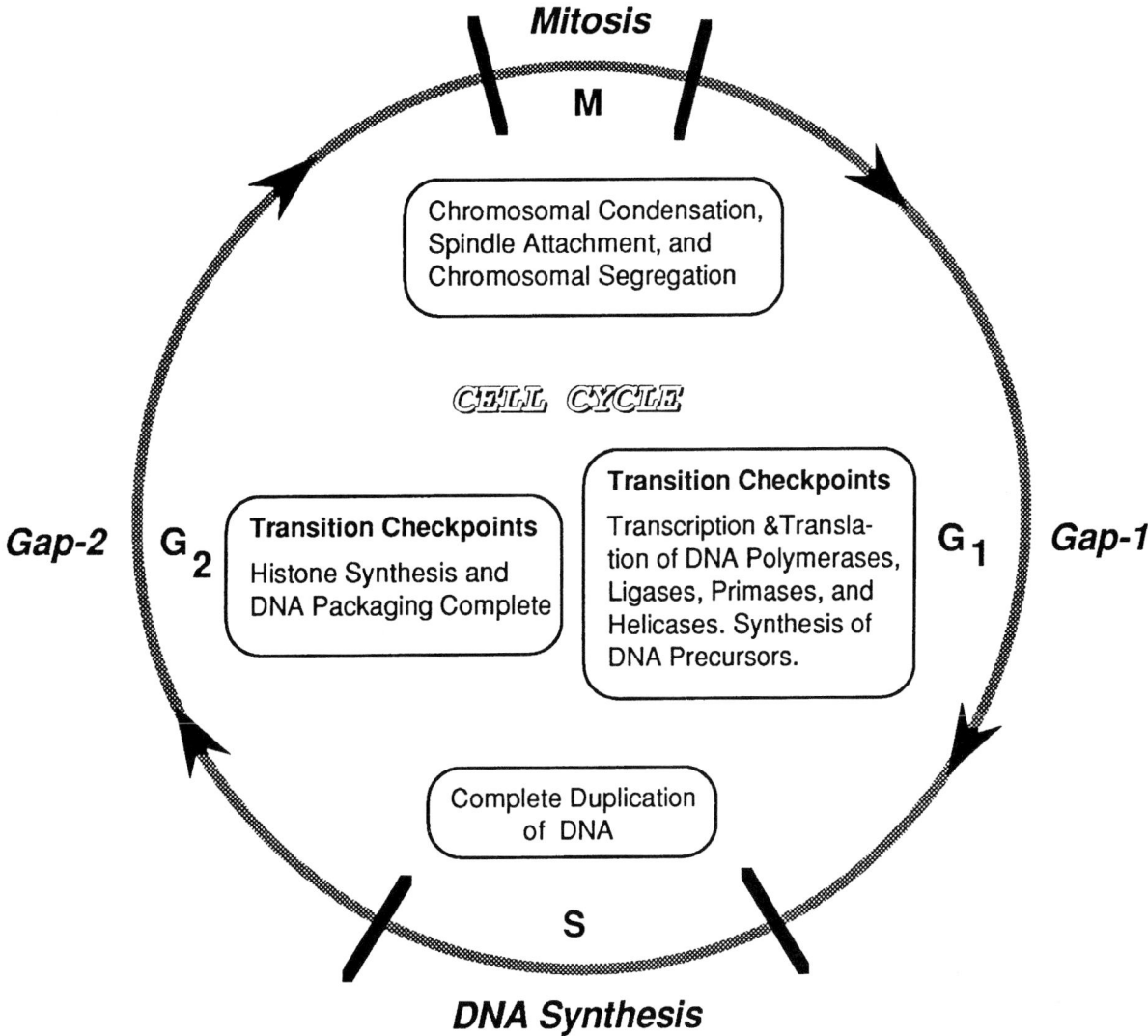

FIGURE 58B.1   Schematic representation of the cell cycle divided into the four phases: G_1, S, G_2, and M.

and packaging. These biosynthetic reactions are obligatory; deletion of any one pathway usually results in termination of the cell cycle and programmed cell death by apoptosis.

Regulatory Pathways

At a second pathway, a complex network of biochemical signals promotes specific transitions in the cell cycle. The chief mediators of cell-cycle regulation are proteins called *cyclins* and their associated enzymes, cyclin-dependent kinases. Passage through gap transitions depends on the activity of certain cyclin–protein kinase complexes. Twelve families of human protein kinases have been described. Multicellular eukaryotes also express multiple cyclins. Each cyclin-kinase complex is regulated by phosphorylation or dephosphorylation of specific amino acid residues on the kinase. Thus, the possibilities produced by different cyclin-

kinase associations as well as post-translational modifications of kinase and cyclin molecules create a spectrum of enzyme activities that can provide for regulation of many targets in a tissue-specific fashion.

Activation of cyclin-kinase complexes is regulated by proteins that function to link the external cellular environment with the cell cycle via signal transduction pathways. These positive regulators include growth hormones and their receptors, G proteins, protein kinases, and transcription factors. Altered genes that produce the dysregulated expression of analogous positive effectors of cell growth are termed oncogenes (see Oncogenes, later in this chapter).

Surveillance Pathway

A biological quality-assurance system monitors the cell cycle as it progresses from G_1 to S to G_2 to M. At various checkpoints, cell sufficiency is assessed for cell size and mass, adequacy of environmental nutrients, and competence of structural subcomponents. The DNA template is examined to determine whether there has been damage or modification. If surveillance detects a problem, the cell cycle is halted, and repair is attempted. The surveillance pathways are not obligatory, and deletion of any single checkpoint function is usually not directly lethal but may permit abnormal progression of the cell cycle. Potential consequences include the development and propagation of chromosomal abnormalities and genetic mutation (translocations, amplifications, point mutations, or aneuploidy) that support the emergence of rare cancerous cell clones.

A properly functioning surveillance system has tumor-suppressor effects. Tumor-suppressor genes function by inducing protein products that arrest the cell cycle (see Tumor-Suppressor Genes, later in this chapter). The molecular basis of cancer is explained by the sequential loss of tumor-suppressor gene function and the accumulation of genetic abnormalities, resulting in oncogene expression.

ONCOGENES

The transfer and processing of external stimuli via cytoplasmic messengers that influence nuclear events are fundamental to normal cell growth and proliferation. Proto-oncogenes are normal cellular genes that encode certain proteins. These proteins promote the cascade of events that induce orderly cell division by activation of cyclin-kinase complexes. Proto-oncogene expression, when subverted by gene mutation, amplification, or chromosomal translocation, becomes oncogenic and contributes to the induction or progression of cancer by participating in dysregulated cell growth. Thus, oncogenes are dominant, mutated proto-oncogenes that participate in the transformation of cells to a malignant state. Oncogenes encode proteins with diverse functions, including growth factors, growth factor receptors, transducers of growth factor responses, and nuclear transcription factors.

The transfer and processing of external growth stimuli via cytoplasmic messengers (i.e., proto-oncogenes) to influence nuclear events are fundamental to the physiological response of proliferation. Growth signals are transduced to cells by growth factors that bind specific receptors. Growth factor receptors convey signals to the cytoplasm via intrinsic tyrosine kinase moieties or related enzymatic constructs or by association with a membrane transducer, such as the nonreceptor protein tyrosine, serine, or threonine kinases; or guanosine triphosphatase (GTPase)-activating proteins (GAP). Ultimately, activation of second messengers and the release of nuclear transcription factors cause induction and expression of cellular genes that result in progression of the cell cycle and proliferation. The uncoupling of proto-oncogenes from normal physiological regulation may result in unrestrained growth stimulation (oncogene expression) and thereby potentiate the development of cancer.

The mutations with the greatest oncogenic potential are those that increase expression of a normal growth-related factor, deregulate production of an altered growth-related factor, or elaborate a dominant negative translational product. Dominant negative mutations inactivate the function of the wild-type proteins produced by tumor-suppressor genes, which function normally to control cell growth by competing for essential interacting molecules. Dominant negative mutations may therefore function as tumor-suppressor gene antagonists.

Growth Factors

Physiological environmental growth signals are transduced to cells by growth factors that bind specific receptors. Hormones, ILs, and colony-stimulating factors diffuse to the cell, whereas other factors are associated with the cell surface. Genetic incorporation into a viral genome that infects the human genome is another mechanism that provides for the deregulated expression of a growth factor in the infected host.

Genetic amplification occurs frequently in gliomas and is another mechanism that accounts for overexpression of growth factors. Levels of expression of TGF-α and -β, acidic and basic fibroblast growth factors (FGFs), and platelet-derived growth factor (PDGF) A and B chains are increased in all grades of gliomas compared to normal brain tissue. Growth factor–related oncogene activity represents a regulatory defect that permits the sustained or constitutive expression of its gene product, in contrast to an inducible gene that is activated in response to a physiological growth stimulus.

A deregulated cell may respond intrinsically to a growth factor oncogene product (autocrine process), or the growth factor may stimulate a near-neighbor cell population to proliferate (paracrine process). For example, vigorous angiogenesis is needed to support tumor growth larger than 1–2 mm in diameter in gliomas. FGFs and TGFs are potent paracrine stimulators of neoplasm-associated angiogenesis. Although unrestrained proliferation from growth factor expression may promote and support neoplasia, this is probably not responsible for actual cancer transformation.

Receptors

Growth factor receptors link the external environment with the cell interior. Receptors span the plasma membrane and are transduced by ligand binding. Growth factor–related receptors, as well as receptor oncogenes, convey signals to the cytoplasm via an intrinsic tyrosine kinase activity, but others operate without a tyrosine kinase moiety.

Upregulation of wild-type cell surface receptors does not induce the same proliferative response as increased expression of growth factor unless the receptor binds with its appropriate factor. However, the mutational alterations contained within oncogenic receptors tend to uncouple the tyrosine kinase activity from the binding of external ligand, causing the receptor to function independently from the influence of its growth factor. Both epidermal growth factor receptor (EGF-R) and PDGF-R are activated and overexpressed in gliomas. Gene amplifications with mutated EGF-R are present in approximately 50% of glioblastoma multiforme. PDGF-R is also amplified and overexpressed in gliomas and may represent a more aggressive tumor phenotype.

Signal Transducers

A growing body of evidence suggests that tyrosine kinases, serine or threonine kinases, or a separate family of proteins (GAP) that activates *ras p21* GTPase, are involved in signal transduction mediated by cytokine receptors that lack intracytoplasmic tails.

Tyrosine phosphorylation of cellular substrates is believed to play a crucial role in the intracellular transduction pathways that regulate cellular activation and differentiation. Many of the nonreceptor protein tyrosine kinases (PTKs) are intimately associated with growth receptors that lack this enzymatic activity and are localized on the inner surface of the plasma membrane. In this way, engagement of growth receptors by growth-factor ligands results in the increased tyrosine phosphorylation of cellular substrates, including, in many instances, the receptors themselves.

The catalytic activities of the PTKs are normally under strict regulation, being subject to self-phosphorylation on tyrosine and serine or threonine residues. In contrast, oncogenic tyrosine kinases uncouple protein phosphorylation from the hierarchy of cellular restraints governing these events.

Transcription Factors

Transcription and replication regulate all aspects of cellular activity and are the final targets of the cascade of events leading from growth factor–receptor interaction to intracytoplasmic signal transduction. Transcription factors are proteins that recognize certain motifs in promoter regions that bind to the DNA, thereby promoting transcription by stimulating RNA polymerase activity. Similar motifs in promoters of different genes permit the coordinate induction of multiple genes by a single transcription factor. Further complicating this process may be various combinations of motifs in a single promoter, each motif interacting with different transcription factors, the product of which may exert negative or positive control over gene expression. A number of oncogenes represent mutated transcription factor proto-oncogenes (*fos, jun, myc*) that control the transcription of growth factor–related genes. Alternatively, normal transcription factor–promoter interaction can be neutralized by recombination of promoter with mutant proteins. If the wild-type (normal) transcription factor activates a tumor-

suppressor gene function, thus inhibiting growth, complex formation between a promoter and a mutated transcription factor (a dominant-negative mutation) can abolish normal growth regulation and lead to malignant transformation. Dominant-negative mutations of transcription factors that act this way (*erb* A, *rel*, and *p53*), for all intents and purposes, are nuclear oncogenes.

TUMOR-SUPPRESSOR GENES

Tumor-suppressor genes impart negative signaling that suppresses cell division. The characterized tumor-suppressor genes are the retinoblastoma (*RB*), Wilms' tumor (*WT-1*), neurofibroma (*NF-1*), adenomatous polyposis coli (*APC*), and *p53* genes.

The *p53* tumor-suppressor gene is the most frequently affected in human cancers. The *p53* gene product resembles a transcriptional activator factor, is susceptible to phosphorylation, and functions in a cell cycle–dependent manner. The *p53* gene promotes the expression of a protein that binds to cyclin-dependent kinases and inhibits their action. In this manner, *p53* expression halts the cell cycle, preventing G_1-to-S progression and allowing time for DNA repair before dividing, thereby preventing replication of damaged DNA. In addition, wild-type *p53* induces apoptosis triggered by extensive DNA damage, whereas mutant *p53* mitigates programmed cell death. Loss of tumor-suppressive function may occur by gene deletions and by products of dominant negative mutations that antagonize wild-type *p53* activity (Table 58B.1).

GENETIC BASIS OF CANCERS OF THE NERVOUS SYSTEM

Gliomas

The development of human gliomas is a complex, multistep process in which clonal genetic aberrations subvert normal growth regulatory mechanisms. There is no known premalignant condition associated with the development of human gliomas, but an increasing number of genetic alterations correlate with increasing histopathological malignancy. Progression from low-grade to higher-grade gliomas is associated with consistent mutations, deletions, and amplifications that represent either inactivation of tumor-suppressor function or activation of gene products that promote growth (oncogenic).

By comparing glial tumor DNA with a patient's non-neural DNA, such as that from peripheral leukocytes, loss of tumor-associated genetic material in one or both alleles from multiple chromosomal loci can be detected. Genetic analysis of glial tumors suggests several interesting associations between detectable genetic alterations and progression from astrocytoma to anaplastic astrocytoma to glioblastoma.

Table 58B.1:   Human tumor-suppressor genes

Gene	Chromosomal location	Tumor type
Adenomatous polyposis coli (*APC*)	5q21	Familial polyposis, colorectal carcinoma
Neurofibroma type 1 (*NF-1*)	117q11.2	von Recklinghausen's neurofibromatosis, neurofibromas, Lisch nodules, optic glioma, plexiform neurofibroma, neurofibrosarcoma
p53	17p13	A vast array of human tumors, including colorectal, small cell lung, and breast carcinomas, gliomas, Hodgkin's and non-Hodgkin's lymphomas, and others
Retinoblastoma (*RB*)	13q14.1	Retinoblastoma, osteosarcoma, and small cell lung, ductal breast, stomach, bladder, and colon carcinomas
Wilms' tumor (*WT-1*)	11p13	Wilms' tumor, rhabdomyosarcoma, breast carcinoma, hepatoblastoma, transitional cell bladder carcinoma, and lung carcinoma
Probable tumor-suppressor genes		
Neuroblastoma	1p36.1	Neuroblastoma, melanoma, multiple endocrine neoplasia type 2, medullary thyroid carcinoma, pheochromocytoma, ductal cell carcinoma
Deleted in colorectal carcinoma (*DCC*)	18q21	Colon carcinoma
Mutated in colorectal cancer (*MCC*)	5q	Colon carcinoma
Neurofibroma type 2 (*NF-2*)	22q12.2	Meningioma, acoustic neuroma, pheochromocytoma

Deletions from chromosomes 13, 17, and 22 occur with similar frequency in all glial tumors and probably reflect early events in glioma pathogenesis. Deletions at region 17p are seen in approximately 35% of all gliomas. The suggested candidate genes lost in gliomas (*p53* on 17p, *NF-2* on 22q, and *RB* on 13q) are established or putative tumor-suppressor genes. Point mutations also may occur. Mutations in *p53* occur in approximately 31% of anaplastic gliomas and glioblastoma tumors and in 12% of low-grade astrocytomas. In these cases, mutant *p53* probably behaves like a dominant negative mutation.

Additional genetic loss occurs at region 9p near the interferon-α and -β loci in grade III and IV gliomas; more extensive biallelic loss occurs only in glioblastomas. The hemizygous or homozygous loss of the interferon alleles may facilitate progression to a more malignant state by loss of putative anticancer-promoting cytokines, or deletion of these genes may confer a growth advantage. Another candidate tumor-suppressor gene on 9p, known as *p16* or *cdkn2*, encodes a 16-kD protein initially isolated as an inhibitor of *CDK4*, a cyclin-dependent kinase whose normal action is to promote cell division (Serrano et al. 1993). Deletion of *cdkn2* occurs with high frequency in human glial cell lines and in glial tumors.

Loss of alleles at loci on chromosome 19q also occurs in anaplastic gliomas and glioblastomas. Glioblastoma multiforme alone is associated with additional genetic deletion from chromosome 10, probably causing loss of an additional tumor-suppressor gene locus.

Additive genetic rearrangements are also associated with a progressively malignant glial phenotype (Collins 1993). Amplification of the *EGF-R* gene is a frequent event found almost exclusively in grade III or IV gliomas, and overex-pression of *EGF-R* occurs with a frequency of 40–50% in glioblastomas. Mutations in the amplified *EGF-R* genes are common, but it is not known if these genetic alterations serve to uncouple receptor-signal transduction from normal growth-regulatory controls. Multiple double-minute chromosomes are observed cytogenically in approximately 50% of glioblastomas and indicate gene amplifications. Other genes that are amplified in glioblastomas include *PDGF-Ra* and, to a lesser degree, *myc*, *myb*, and K-*ras*.

Retinoblastoma

Retinoblastoma may be hereditary (40%) or sporadic. The hereditary form occurs in young infants, with multiple bilateral tumors. The nonhereditary form occurs in older children and is always a single unilateral tumor. This hereditary pattern led to the prediction of a retinoblastoma susceptibility gene inherited as a mutant allele. Subsequent mutation in the remaining wild-type gene disables both alleles and results in cancer. In the nonhereditary form, two independent, spontaneous mutations, one in each RB locus in the same retinoblast, are required. This would be expected to occur infrequently, and, indeed, is found in 1 per 30,000 people. The *RB* gene on chromosome 13q14.1 was the first tumor-suppressor gene cloned. Loss of *RB* gene function has since been reported in other human cancers and may contribute to the initiation or progression of osteosarcoma, soft tissue sarcoma, prostate cancer, breast carcinomas, small cell lung carcinoma, and bladder carcinoma.

The retinoblastoma gene encodes a 105-kD nuclear phosphoprotein (pRB). In G_1, pRB shifts from a hypophosphorylated form to a progressively hyperphosphorylated state just before G_1-S transition; it remains phosphorylated in S, G_2, and most of M, and it reverts to a nonphosphorylated protein just before G_1. Nonphosphorylated pRB is believed to inhibit growth and to act as a checkpoint control at the G_1-S transition of the cell cycle (Wiman 1993). This periodicity is reminiscent of the cell cycle dependence of cyclin synthesis, and the candidate upstream modifier of pRB phosphorylation is a G_1-specific cyclin :p34cdc2 kinase complex. The target of nonphosphorylated pRB appears to be the downregulation of certain growth-related transcription factors, particularly EGF, *myc*, and *fos*. Therefore, the loss of pRB function may uncouple proto-oncogene transcription factor expression from negative upstream regulators, thereby mimicking the constitutive expression of transcription factor oncogenes.

Direct evidence that *RB* mutations and deletions lead to cancer comes from gene transfer experiments (see Gene Transfer Therapy, later in this chapter). In these experiments, the wild-type *RB* complementary DNA is inserted into a retroviral expression vector and introduced for expression in cells via retroviral infection or plasmid transfection. Such introduction of the normal *RB* gene, in cancer cells lacking RB function, causes potent growth suppression.

Neuroblastoma

Neuroblastoma is the most common solid tumor found in children in the United States. N-*myc* amplification and overexpression are frequently associated with advanced stages of disease and indicate a poorer prognosis. Deletion of the short arm of chromosome 1 is a consistent cytogenic alteration, and introduction of functional chromosome 1p fragments into overexpressing N-*myc* neuroblastoma cells induces some degree of differentiation. Transfer of chromosome 17 into neuroblastoma in vitro also suppresses the tumorigenic phenotype without affecting growth of cultured neuroblastoma cells. The oncogene *p53*, located on chromosome 17, is not thought to be the candidate tumor-suppressor function conveyed in these experiments. These experiments suggest that when deleted or mutated, tumor-suppressor genes on chromosome 1p or 17, other than *p53*, contribute to the development of neuroblastoma.

Neurofibromatosis Types 1 and 2

Neurofibromatosis type 1 is an autosomal dominant disorder that affects 1 per 3,500 individuals of all ethnic groups (see Chapter 69). The *NF-1* gene is located on 17q11.2. As with retinoblastoma, tumors arise after a germline mutation is accompanied by a new allelic mutation, which supports the notion that the *NF-1* gene is also a tumor-suppressor gene.

NF-1 is massive, spanning 300 kD and comprising 50 exons. The protein product of *NF-1*, neurofibromin, is found in all tissues, but its greatest expression is in brain and spinal cord. Two isoforms exist, of which one is felt to play a role in differentiation. Neurofibromin is a member of the GAP family and interacts with a *ras p21* to convert the active *p21:GTP* complex to the inactive *p21:GDP* form. Neurofibromin functions as a tumor suppressor by blocking *ras*-mediated mitogenic signaling, thereby promoting terminal differentiation.

Neurofibromatosis type 2 is an autosomal dominant disorder whose frequency is 1 per 50,000. Familial linkage analysis suggests that the gene causing neurofibromatosis type 2, *NF-2*, is localized to chromosome 22q12.2. Analyses of meningiomas and acoustic neuromas have shown a propensity for the hemizygous state. One-half of all cases represent acquired new mutations. The *NF-2* gene encodes for the protein merlin, which contains a 587–amino acid cytoskeletal protein. The mechanism by which this protein functions is not understood, although a tumor-suppressor role is postulated.

GENE THERAPY

Antisense Technology

Selective inhibition of transcription has become feasible by the use of antisense technology. An antisense nucleic acid sequence is one that interacts with a complementary nucleic acid sequence to block the biological effect mediated by the targeted sequence (Tari and Lopez-Berestein 1993). The application of antisense technology as a modulator of gene expression has evolved in two ways.

The transcript-targeted approach arrests translation using an antisense oligomer with nucleotide sequences complementary to the protein coding or sense sequence. Methodology designed to inhibit messenger copy should be more efficient than technology designed to inhibit its protein product because a single messenger RNA molecule makes multiple peptide copies. Natural, phosphodiester-linked antisense oligoribo- and oligodeoxy-ribonucleotides effectively inhibit gene expression but have short half-lives and penetrate poorly into cells. These disadvantages have been circumvented by the synthesis of several classes of phosphate-modified oligonucleotides that are nuclease resistant and have greater cell permeability than oligodeoxynucleotides.

The second approach in antisense technology has been to target sequence-specific sites in double-stranded genomic DNA by triple-helix formation. Triple-helix formation may effectively suppress DNA replication, inhibit transcription, or, by occupying a binding site, prevent recognition of a nuclear transcription factor.

Transfection of rat C6 glioma with an episome-based vector encoding antisense insulinlike growth factor–1 complementary DNA prevented the formation of subcutaneous C6 tumors (Trojan et al. 1993). Pathologically, implanted lesions contained few tumor cells and large mononuclear infiltrates.

Another cancer-related gene target involves the phenomenon of multiple drug resistance. Most neoplasms respond initially to chemotherapeutic agents, but resistance invariably develops. Many chemotherapeutic agents that derive from naturally occurring substances, such as fungi, bacteria, or plants, upregulate the multiple drug–resistant (MDR) gene. This gene codes for a 170-kD protein, which functions to actively transport chemotherapeutic agents out of the cell, thereby conferring resistance on this class of drugs. Just as it is possible now to confer methotrexate resistance to stem cells by genetic transfer of the dihydrofolate reductase gene, it may be feasible to circumvent unwanted multiple drug resistance in cancer cells by antisense down-modulation of the MDR gene.

Gene Transfer Therapy

Gene transfer technology is an efficient and promising method of transferring genetic information into nucleated mammalian cells. The proper expression of a gene transferred into a cell is regulated by multiple, spatially related genetic sequences found upstream and downstream from the gene of interest. These genetic sequences are called cis-acting DNA elements. Every gene is accompanied by promoter and enhancer sequences, splice signals, polyadenylation signals, and elements that determine messenger RNA half-life. These elements may be manipulated experimentally to cause the induction and expression of a particular gene inserted in a given recombinant construct. Such systems of recombinant elements are called expression vectors. The most widely used vectors for the purpose of gene transfer include the retrovirus-, herpes-, and adenovirus-mediated expression vectors and recombinant viruses. Efficient gene transfer therapy is accomplished by gene incorporation into a molecularly engineered expression vector that preferentially results in expression of the inserted gene. Subsequently, the gene-vector construct is assembled into a vehicle, usually a highly infectious viral particle, which transports the genetic information into the cell.

The first human therapy experiments were designed to reconstitute the function of the immune system by administering autologous lymphocytes transduced with a normal human adenosine deaminase (ADA) gene. This provided the enzymatic activity lacking in patients with ADA-deficient severe combined immunodeficiency. Human cancer gene therapy was inaugurated in 1991 as an extension of the gene marker experiments with tumor-infiltrating lymphocytes (TIL). However, the goal in these experiments was to enhance the killing capabilities of TIL against cancer (in this case, malignant melanoma) by adding the human gene for TNF to the retroviral expression vector. TNF possesses potent anticancer effects, but toxic levels are reached at 8 mg/kg of body weight. Using gene transfer, reconstituted TILs migrate to the cancer and secrete into the microenvironment constitutively expressed TNF. Delivered in this manner, effective high doses of TNF could be provided at specific tumor sites without causing systemic side effects. It is not established that TIL is a useful TNF delivery system for the central nervous system.

Another cancer gene transfer strategy targets cancer cells as recipients of molecularly engineered cytokine genes. This approach is based on the premise that the elaboration of certain cytokines boosts the host's T-lymphocyte antitumor immune-mediated response. The TNF gene has been inserted into tumor cells that were first surgically extracted and cultured in vitro. The transduced, TNF-secreting tumor cells were used as a cell vaccine and transferred back into the patient. The injection sites and draining lymph nodes were surgically excised and the putative tumor-reactive T cells expanded in vitro and ultimately reinfused into the patient. TIL immunotherapy also has been accomplished by inserting the IL-2 gene into tumor cells, at which point the cells are grown in culture and then transplanted back to the patient. Secretion of IL-2 is intended to augment the antitumor, cell-mediated response.

Defective suppressor genes can be replaced by gene transfer therapy. Replacement of lost pRB or p53 tumor-suppressor gene function into several tumors causes reversal of the neoplastic nature of the cells both in vitro and in vivo.

Certain herpes simplex viral mutants are able to replicate in dividing cells only, but they retain herpes-induced cytopathic effects. This bias in viral replication can be used to selectively kill human gliomas inoculated into nude mice. Thymidine kinase-deficient herpes simplex viral mutants injected directly into gliomas significantly reduces tumor growth and prolongs survival in mice who harbor systemic and intracerebral tumors.

Alternatively, the herpes simplex thymidine kinase gene can be inserted into a retroviral expression vector and the kinase gene subsequently transduced into murine fibroblasts. In 1992, Culver and coworkers inoculated mice with a mixture of fibrosarcoma cells and cells transduced with murine fibroblasts expressing herpes simplex thymidine kinase and were then treated with the antiherpes drug ganciclovir. Cells modified to contain the herpes simplex thymidine kinase gene become sensitive to treatment with the antiviral agent ganciclovir. Tumors produced from a mixture of tumor cells and herpes simplex thymidine kinase retroviral vector–producing fibroblasts regressed rapidly and completely with ganciclovir treatment. Rats carrying intracerebral gliomas, subsequently injected intratumorally with the thymidine kinase retroviral vector–producing murine fibroblasts, and thereafter treated with ganciclovir, responded with macroscopic and microscopic tumor regression.

The use of genetically modified viruses and retrovirus-mediated viral gene transfer in these studies is striking for the relative effectiveness of the therapies and the lack of overt undesirable effects in cancers with an otherwise universally fatal outcome. These approaches form the framework of recently initiated molecular genetic therapeutic protocols for the treatment of brain tumors in humans by recombinant viral gene therapy.

Immunotherapy

Unconjugated monoclonal antibodies (MAbs) produce anti-tumor effects by complement activation, antibody-dependent cell-mediated cytotoxicity, opsonization, or phagocytosis. MAbs directed against the growth factor receptors EGF-R, bombesin, and IL-2R have been employed in several cancer therapy protocols with variable results. Antibodies generated to a tumor marker are themselves antigenic. Antibodies that recognize the hypervariable combining site of the antitumor antibody are termed *anti-idiotype* antibodies. The original tumor epitope and the recognition site of the anti-idiotype antibody may share peptide configurations. Anti-idiotype antibodies that mimic tumor-associated antigens have been used as anticancer vaccines.

Strategies using conjugated antibodies deliver a tissue-specific, high-dose antitumor effect. Cancer chemotherapeutic agents, including doxorubicin, idarubicin, bleomycin, methotrexate, cytosine arabinoside, chlorambucil, cisplatin, vinca alkaloids, and mitomycin C, have been conjugated to tumor-directed MAbs to deliver a selective dose of drug. Recombinant toxins are hybrid cytotoxic proteins made by recombinant DNA technology. Antibody-toxin fusion products are used to selectively kill cancer cells and are derived from the bacterial and plant toxins of *Pseudomonas*, diph-theria, and ricin. Growth factor–toxin fusion products can target cancers that overexpress growth factor receptors. In 1992, Fitzgerald and coworkers showed that a chimeric toxin consisting of recombinant TGF-α and modified *Pseudomonas* exotoxin selectively binds to and kills cells with EGF-R expression, rendering this an attractive agent for treatment of high-grade gliomas. Radio-immunoconjugates deliver high-energy radionuclides to specific cell targets to induce cancer killing; and iodine-125–labeled anti–EGF-R MAb has been used to treat glial tumors.

REFERENCES

Collins VP. Amplified genes in human gliomas. Semin Cancer Biol 1993;4:27–32.

Serrano M, Hannon GJ, Beach D. A new regulatory motif in cell-cycle control causing specific inhibition of cyclin D/CDK4. Nature 1993;366:704–706.

Tari AM, Lopez-Berestein G. Antisense oligonucleotides and carriers for gene therapy. Cancer Bull 1993;25:164–170.

Trojan J, Johnson TR, Rudlin SD, et al. Treatment and prevention of rat glioblastoma by immunogenetic C6 cells expressing antisense insulin-like growth factor-1 RNA. Science 1993;259:94–97.

Wiman KG. The retinoblastoma gene: role in cell cycle control and cell differentiation. FASEB J 1993;7:841–845.

Chapter 58
Primary and Secondary Tumors of the Central Nervous System

C. CLINICAL PRESENTATION AND THERAPY OF NERVOUS SYSTEM TUMORS

Kurt A. Jaeckle, Michael E. Cohen, and Patricia K. Duffner

Each year in the United States, approximately 17,000 patients are newly diagnosed with primary central nervous system (CNS) tumors and another 150,000 patients develop metastatic CNS malignancies. Over the last decade, these numbers have steadily increased. Despite considerable progress in the understanding of brain tumor biology and improved diagnostic neuroimaging, surgical techniques, and radiotherapeutics, management of most malignant CNS tumors remains largely supportive. CNS neoplasms typically cause a progressive evolution of neurological dysfunction. The patient may disregard initial transitory symptoms, but persistent symptoms usually prompt medical consultation, at which point the clinician must recognize that the situation requires further attention. This chapter provides an approach to the clinical diagnosis and management of primary and metastatic nervous system tumors.

The clinical features of intracranial nervous system tumors can be broadly categorized into three groups: (1) generalized, (2) localizing, and (3) false localizing.

GENERALIZED CLINICAL FEATURES

Generalized symptoms and signs are usually caused by increased intracranial pressure, diffuse infiltration of tumor, edema, or hydrocephalus. The more common generalized clinical features are headache, altered mental status, seizures, lightheadedness, papilledema, and nausea and vomiting.

In general, malignant tumors have a briefer duration of clinical symptoms than do benign tumors. In patients with frontal lobe glioblastomas, the average duration of symptoms before histological diagnosis is only 5 months, and an apoplectic onset, usually due to intratumoral hemorrhage, occurs in approximately 4%. In contrast, occasional patients with well-differentiated astrocytomas may have a seizure history spanning decades. The location of the tumor can also influence the duration of symptoms. Tumors in the anterior temporal or frontal lobes can grow silently to considerable size and cause generalized symptoms as an initial feature, whereas tumors in the posterior fossa or the posterior frontal, parietal, and occipital lobes often cause focal symptoms before generalized dysfunction develops.

Headache

Headache is an initial feature in 20% of patients with brain tumors but develops during the course in 60%. The pain is typically dull, localized, and intermittent, and it often varies in severity. A discriminating feature, present in only 15% of adults, is nocturnal or early morning occurrence. Headaches may be precipitated by changing position, coughing, Valsalva's maneuver, and exertion. Nausea or vomiting accompanies the headache at some point in 50% of patients.

The headache is ipsilateral to the tumor in approximately 80% of patients. Because supratentorial pain-sensitive structures are primarily supplied by trigeminal nerve afferents, the headache is often referred to frontal retro-orbital or anterior temporal locations. Posterior fossa tumors irritate pain-sensitive structures innervated by sensory branches of cranial nerves IX and X and the upper cervical nerves, resulting in referred pain to the occiput and neck. Pain is the result of traction on the large cerebral arteries, circle of Willis, major venous sinuses, or proximate portions of the cortical venous tributaries. It may also result from distention of extracranial vessels, third ventricle dilatation, inflammation of pain-sensitive intra- or extracranial structures, or direct pressure on one of the pain-sensitive cervical or cranial nerves.

Severe headache may be caused by a sudden increase in intracranial pressure (pressure or plateau waves). Sudden pressure changes are usually prompted by changes of position, such as standing or initiating ambulation after prolonged sitting or recumbency. The headache is abrupt in onset, reaches peak intensity quickly, and may be relieved by modification of position. It may be associated with blurring of vision, instability or collapse of gait, impaired consciousness, vomiting, or incontinence. Pressure-wave headache usually suggests a significant mass effect, raised intracranial pressure, or obstruction of cerebrospinal fluid (CSF) flow. However, elevation of CSF pressure alone does not account for all brain tumor headaches. Infusions of saline that elevate CSF pressure above 500 mm H_2O in normal volunteers do not cause headache, and the frequency of headache is similar in patients with and without raised intracranial pressure.

Altered Mental Status

Disturbed concentration, forgetfulness, personality changes, mood swings, and decreased initiative are especially common in patients with frontal or temporal lobe tumors. Problems with abstract reasoning, logical judgment, and stream of thought become noticeable to family and friends. Initially, these symptoms may be attributed to other factors, but symptoms become worse with time and include a shortened attention span, distractibility, blunted affect, disinhibition, apathy, memory disturbances, irritability, and disturbed sleep patterns. If left untreated, confused or disoriented states progress to prolonged somnolence and coma.

Seizures

Seizures occur in approximately one-third of patients and are more common with slow-growing tumors, such as astrocytomas, oligodendrogliomas, and meningiomas. Seizures are most common with (in order of frequency) frontal, parietal, and temporal lobe tumors and are slightly less common in children, possibly because of a higher frequency of posterior fossa tumors.

Papilledema

Papilledema, once a feature in 60–70% of patients with primary brain tumor, is now seen in only 10–20%. The decrease may result from neuroimaging techniques that permit earlier tumor detection, wide use of corticosteroids to reduce intracranial pressure, and generally more aggressive treatment. Posterior fossa tumors cause papilledema by obstructing ventricular outflow, but supratentorial tumors may cause papilledema without pathological evidence of ventricular obstruction.

Early papilledema does not cause symptomatic loss of visual acuity, but advanced papilledema enlarges the blind spot, restricts peripheral vision, is associated with dyschromatopsia, and ultimately may cause optic atrophy. Retinal hemorrhages, when present, cause scotomas and decreased acuity, particularly when the hemorrhage is located near the macula. Ipsilateral optic atrophy with contralateral papilledema (Foster Kennedy syndrome) suggests a large olfactory groove tumor, typically a meningioma.

Nausea and Vomiting

Nausea is a common complaint. Vomiting usually suggests a large tumor producing mass effect and cerebral displacement. The recurrent nature of the vomiting should distinguish increased intracranial pressure from benign causes. Recurrent early morning or nocturnal vomiting and projectile (forceful) vomiting not preceded by nausea increases the suspicion of an intracranial mass. As with migraine, vomiting may occur during a severe headache. Sudden vomiting, lasting hours and then remitting, may indicate intratumoral hemorrhage, transient CSF pathway obstruction, or a temporary elevation of intracranial pressure. Vomiting is especially common with posterior fossa tumors, presumably because of compression of brainstem emetic centers (e.g., area postrema) or hydrocephalus with raised intracranial pressure.

LOCALIZING CLINICAL FEATURES

Focal symptoms may result from tumor-induced parenchymal destruction, infarction, or edema. The distinction is clinically relevant because symptoms due to edema are potentially reversible with corticosteroid treatment. Factors released into the local tumor environment (e.g., peroxidases, H^+ ions, proteolytic enzymes, and cytokines) may also produce potentially reversible focal dysfunction.

Cortical Tumors

Frontal lobe tumors produce focal symptoms when the tumor infiltrates or causes edema in the adjacent brain. Simple motor or generalized seizures followed by postictal paralysis are often clues to a frontal location. Parasagittal or convexity meningiomas and frontal gliomas are especially associated with seizures. Localizing signs of frontal tumors include cortical dysarthria, contralateral weakness, apraxia, and aphasia. Unilateral frontal lobe release reflexes, such as contralateral palmomental and grasp reflexes, may be present. Unilateral anosmia suggests an infiltrative olfactory groove tumor, usually a subfrontal meningioma.

The features of temporal lobe tumors are contralateral corticospinal tract dysfunction, homonymous (particularly superior quadrantanopic) visual field deficits, aphasia, and partial complex seizures. Seizures occur in one-third of patients. Conductive and anomic aphasias are particularly common with posterosuperior dominant temporal lobe tumors. Cognitive and personality changes and memory dysfunction are frequently identified. Occasionally, paranoia, disinhibition, depression, and psychopathic behavior occur.

Sensory disturbances and attention deficit are the most prominent features of parietal lobe tumors. Two-thirds of patients have signs of contralateral corticospinal tract dysfunction. Involvement of the parietal optic radiations causes contralateral homonymous inferior quadrantanopia or hemianopia. Contralateral visual extinction of simultaneous stimulation within a quadrant or hemifield may be an early feature. Almost one-half of patients with parietal tumors develop seizures during the course of illness, which are usually simple motor or sensory in type. Other possible features, depending on the hemisphere affected, are contralateral motor or sensory neglect, constructional and dressing apraxia, finger agnosia, right-left confusion, and acalculia.

Visual symptoms suggest an occipital lobe tumor. The most common visual field defect is a congruous homonymous hemianopia that spares the macula. Focal occipital seizures are usually characterized by episodic contralateral flashing lights, colors, or formed geometric patterns. Color anomia, visual agnosias, and optic alloesthesia (displacement of images from one visual field to another) may also be present, as may metamorphopsia (distortion of the shape of visual images).

Third Ventricle and Pineal Region Tumors

Tumors in or near the third ventricle often obstruct the ventricles or aqueduct and cause hydrocephalus. Positional changes may abruptly increase ventricular pressure and produce severe frontal or vertex headache, vomiting, and occasionally syncope. Third ventricular region tumors also cause memory disturbances, diabetes insipidus, amenorrhea, galactorrhea, and disturbances of satiation or thermoregulation.

Tumors in the pineal region cause hydrocephalus by obstructing the posterior third ventricle. Parinaud's syndrome (pupillary light-near dissociation, disturbances in upward gaze, and convergence-retraction nystagmus) is caused by pressure on the tectum of the midbrain and the posterior commissure. Precocious puberty may occur in boys with pineal region tumors.

Brainstem Tumors

Focal neurological dysfunction is a prominent feature of midbrain tumors. Intra-axial signs develop before the general features of increased intracranial pressure from aqueductal obstruction. Tumors involving the quadrigeminal plate cause disorders of vertical gaze, Parinaud's syndrome, and hearing difficulties. Tumors in the tegmentum may cause weakness, by placing pressure on the corticospinal pathways, and internuclear ophthalmoplegia. Ataxia indicates involvement of the dentatorubrothalamic projections.

The initial features of pontine and medullary tumors are usually those of intra-axial dysfunction. Early extra-axial signs, such as cranial neuropathies, followed by brainstem dysfunction, are characteristic of tumors of the cerebellopontine angle, cranial nerves, cerebellum, meninges, and base of skull. Pontine or medullary gliomas are more common in children. Presentation consists of varying combinations of cranial neuropathies, long tract signs, and ataxia. Compression of the fourth ventricle causes obstructive hydrocephalus and generalized symptoms. Preterminal features of brainstem tumors are disturbances of respiratory patterns and blood pressure homeostasis.

Cerebellar Tumors

Cyclical vomiting and occipital headache are common among patients with cerebellar tumors. The headache is usually bilateral and may radiate into the retro-orbital or temporal regions and neck and shoulders. Stiffness and limitation of neck motion and a head tilt may be associated and may suggest incipient tonsillar herniation. Dizziness or vertigo and horizontal and rotatory nystagmus may also be prominent. Appendicular or truncal ataxia is characteristic. Tendon reflexes and tone are diminished ipsilateral to the lesion. Cranial nerve palsies and corticospinal tract findings occur late in the course and indicate secondary invasion or compression of the brain-

Table 58C.1:   Primary intracranial neoplasms

Tumor	Frequency (%)
Glioblastoma	25.1
Astrocytoma	11.9
Other gliomas	4.2
Ependymoma	3.2
Oligodendroglioma	2.7
Mixed gliomas	1.7
Meningiomas	24.0
Pituitary adenomas	6.8
Sarcomas	6.2
Hemangiomas	6.5
Hemangioblastomas	3.0
Craniopharyngiomas	2.5
Neurinomas	2.4

Source: Modified with permission from HM Zimmerman, MG Netsky, LM Davidoff. Atlas of Tumors of the Nervous System. Philadelphia: Lea & Febiger, 1956.

stem. Ventricular outflow obstruction causes hydrocephalus and generalized features of increased intracranial pressure.

FALSE LOCALIZING FEATURES

False localizing features are those that suggest involvement of the neuraxis remote from the actual tumor location. They are usually caused by raised intracranial pressure, shifts of intracranial structures, or vascular events. Abducens nerve palsy is the best-recognized false localizing sign. It develops when increased intracranial pressure causes compression of the nerve against the petrous ligament or bony floor of the base of the skull.

Diffuse tumor invasion of the frontal lobe or corpus callosum causes ataxia of gait (frontal ataxia) that may be indistinguishable from cerebellar ataxia. Dysmetria from corticospinal limb weakness and cortical dysarthria can also be mistaken for evidence of cerebellar disease, and retropulsion may be present.

Compression of the cerebral peduncle by the free edge of the tentorium cerebelli contralateral to the herniating cerebral hemisphere (Kernohan's notch syndrome) may cause a falsely localizing hemiparesis ipsilateral to the lesion. Compression or invasion of vessels by tumor and hypercoagulable states associated with the malignancy or its treatment may cause infarction or hemorrhage distant from the tumor site. A typical example is infarction of the occipital cortex after compression of the posterior cerebral artery during transtentorial herniation.

PRIMARY BRAIN TUMORS

Table 58C.1 lists primary intracranial neoplasms and their incidence.

Astrocytoma: Low Grade and Well Differentiated

Astrocytomas constitute 25% of all intracranial gliomas and 10% of all CNS tumors. Median age of onset is in the third to fourth decade. Low-grade astrocytomas may occur in all parts of the CNS, but the most common sites are the frontal and temporal lobes. They infiltrate along white matter paths and extend considerable distances from their original focus. The typical durations of symptoms before diagnosis of grades 1 and 2 astrocytomas are 21 and 11 months, respectively. Seizures occur in 30% of cases.

Diagnosis is made by computed tomography (CT) or magnetic resonance imaging (MRI). Low-grade gliomas often do not enhance and are best detected with T2-weighted MRI sequences. Their presence is also suggested by calcification or, in cerebellar astrocytoma, by a characteristic cyst with an enhancing mural nodule. Pilocytic astrocytomas and pleomorphic xanthoastrocytomas usually enhance and look malignant but often have a prolonged clinical course.

The usual therapy for astrocytoma is maximal surgical resection. Surgery alone is rarely curative because of the diffusely infiltrative nature of hemispheric tumors, but it has the additional benefit of establishing a definitive diagnosis on which rational treatment can be planned. Five-year survival rates are better in patients who receive radical subtotal resection. A 90–95% cure rate can be achieved by resection of cerebellar astrocytomas. Surgery alone is also beneficial in many cases of subependymal giant cell astrocytomas and well-differentiated gangliogliomas in tuberous sclerosis. In children, the prognosis depends in part on tumor type and location (Table 58C.2).

The 5-year survival rate of children with low-grade supratentorial astrocytomas approaches 70%. Concern about the long-term effects of radiation in children less than 3 years old has led to the recommendation to reoperate and use local radiation when the tumor increases in size (Cohen and Duffner 1994). In adults with low-grade supratentorial astrocytomas, 5-year survival rates are 21–55%, and 10-year rates are 10–43%. Although generally considered benign, biopsy and autopsy studies have shown that approximately 50% of astrocytomas transform into more anaplastic tumors eventually, and only 16% of patients with supratentorial low-grade glioma are alive at 15 years.

Adjuvant radiotherapy may be beneficial in the management of incompletely resected tumors. On average, the 5- and 10-year survival rates for irradiated patients are 48% and 26%, respectively, compared with 26% and 12% for patients who did not receive radiation (Berger et al. 1996).

There is evidence that higher doses (>50 Gy) produce significantly longer survival than lower doses, and older patients appear to benefit most from postoperative radiation. Generally, limited-field radiotherapy is used. There is controversy over the optimal timing of postsurgical radiotherapy, particularly when there has been complete radiographic resection of low-grade supratentorial astrocytoma. Some feel that

Table 58C.2: Prognosis of well-differentiated astrocytomas in children according to location

Tumor	Location	Survival	Treatment
Low-grade astrocytoma	Hemisphere	<40–50% 5 yrs	No consensus
Brainstem glioma	Brainstem	<20–30% 5 yrs	Radiation + surgery
Juvenile astrocytoma	Midline	5–20 yrs	Radiation + surgery
Optic pathway glioma	Optic pathway	Variable	No consensus
Cerebellar astrocytoma	Cerebellum	Curable	Surgery

immediate radiotherapy delays progression and increases survival; others feel that treatment should be delayed until recurrence because the benefit of early radiation may result in long-term toxicity, such as dementia, brain necrosis, secondary malignancies, and tumor dedifferentiation.

Chemotherapy has no established benefit in the treatment of low-grade astrocytomas. The use of nitrosourea (BCNU or CCNU) adds no additional benefit to radiation alone in the management of grade 1 and 2 astrocytomas. However, certain subsets, such as progressive pilocytic astrocytomas, may be sensitive to chemotherapy. Because of concerns of toxicity due to radiation in young children with recurrent low-grade astrocytoma, the role of chemotherapy with some agents, such as cyclophosphamide, etoposide, carboplatin, and vincristine, is being explored.

Malignant Astrocytoma: Anaplastic Astrocytoma and Glioblastoma Multiforme

Clinical Course and Prognosis

Most primary brain tumors are malignant (see Table 58C.1). The age at onset is usually 40–60 years, with a male-to-female ratio of 2 to 1. Malignant astrocytomas can occur anywhere in the neuraxis and affect both hemispheres with equal frequency. The average duration from symptom onset to diagnosis is approximately 3–5 months. Occasional patients have a long history of seizures, which suggests that the tumor dedifferentiated from a lower-grade astrocytoma.

Several prognostic variables have been identified. Glioblastomas (exhibiting histological evidence of tumor necrosis) have a worse prognosis than anaplastic astrocytomas. Age correlates inversely with survival; the death rate for patients younger than age 48 is one-third that of patients older than 65. In children, survival is poorest under 3 years of age. Duration of symptoms longer than 6 months, the presence of seizures, and a high postoperative performance status correlate with a better prognosis. Debulking surgery is generally believed to promote a more favorable prognosis than biopsy, but patient benefit may have been preselected for good outcome by operative candidacy and favorable tumor location (e.g., lobar versus deep). The amount of postoperative residual tumor on CT or MRI correlates inversely with prognosis.

Survival of children with anaplastic astrocytomas and glioblastoma multiforme is consistently better than for adults. One-year survival for all ages ranges from 60% to 73% for malignant astrocytomas and from 36% to 44% for glioblastoma. The presence of necrosis, regardless of grade, is always a poor prognostic sign in malignant gliomas (Figure 58C.1).

Young age and good functional performance status, as defined by Karnofsky's performance scale, suggest a better prognosis. The median survival time of patients with a Karnofsky's performance scale score of 70–100 is 12 weeks, and 34% survive 18 months. The median survival time with a Karnofsky's rating of 40–60 is only 6 weeks, and 13% survive 18 months.

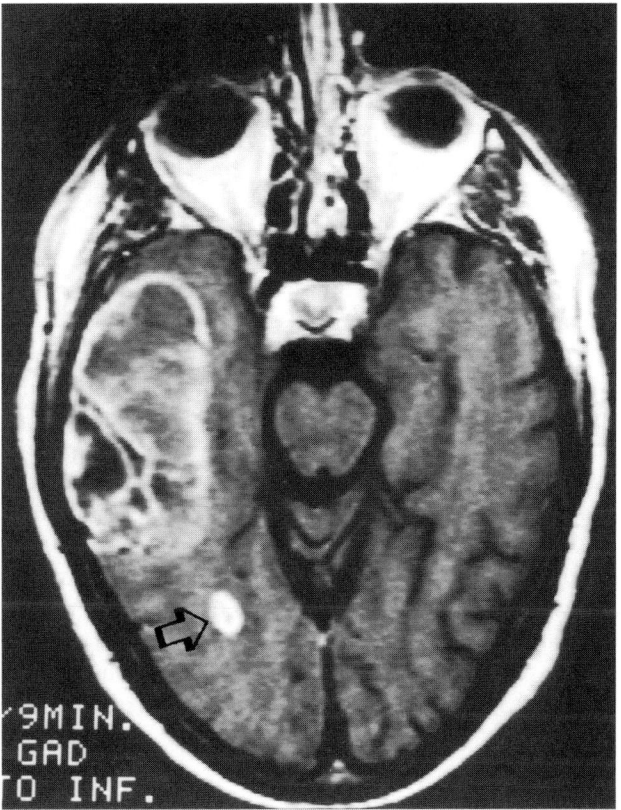

FIGURE 58C.1 Glioblastoma. Gadolinium-enhanced T1-weighted axial magnetic resonance image of a 73-year-old man shows the characteristic heterogeneous densities within the temporal lobe tumor and a satellite lesion (*arrow*).

Radiotherapy

A benefit of radiotherapy for malignant astrocytoma was shown in prospective randomized trials conducted by the Brain Tumor Study Group (BTSG) and Scandinavian Glioblastoma Study Group. The mean survival rate for patients who receive only supportive care after surgery is 17 weeks; the mean survival for those also receiving 6,000 cGy to the whole brain is 42 weeks. No difference in survival is seen with 6,000-cGy whole-brain irradiation versus 6,000-cGy whole-brain plus a focal 1,000-cGy boost to the tumor. Equal success is achieved when limited-field radiotherapy to the enhancing tumor with a 2.5- to 3.0-cm margin is compared to whole-brain treatment and the risk of late injury to normal tissue is avoided. The risks of cognitive decline associated with whole-brain radiotherapy exceed that of local field therapy. Most standard approaches now use limited-field treatment, with approximately 40–50 Gy to the enhancing lesion with large margins, followed by a coned-down boost to the tumor bed to a total dose of approximately 60 Gy, administered in 180- to 200-cGy fractions, 5 days per week.

Hyperfractionation or accelerated fractionation schemes, in which radiation treatments are divided into several fractions per day, or with larger doses per fraction, may produce similar survival rates to standard radiation schedules with acceptable toxicity. Hyperfractionation provides no additional benefit in the treatment of malignant astrocytomas, and accelerated treatment with twice-a-day fractionation at 160 cGy per fraction to a total dose of 54.4 Gy produces survival rates equivalent to that of standard treatment (Curran et al. 1993).

New radiotherapy techniques used in clinical trials include radioactive implants, stereotactic radiosurgery (linear accelerator or gamma knife), charged and heavy particles, radiation with radiosensitizers, hyperthermia, and boron neutron capture therapy. None have proved superior to standard radiotherapy. The BTSG showed a marginal benefit of iodine-125 interstitial brachytherapy in treatment of malignant gliomas. Stereotactic radiosurgery is a method for administering focal irradiation by using a stereotactic coordinate device in conjunction with the radiation source. This type of treatment has been designated stereotactic radiosurgery, if modified linear accelerators or charged particle beams are used, and gamma knife, if multiple cobalt beams are used. The procedure can allow administration of high doses of focal radiotherapy and minimization of radiation to adjacent normal tissues in a single session (radiosurgery) or multiple sessions (fractionated stereotactic radiation). Evaluation of radiosurgery compared to conventional treatment, or as a boost to conventional radiotherapy, is an area of active research and offers considerable promise. However, as with brachytherapy, acute and long-term complications related to edema or necrosis of tissue are significant, and the actuarial risk of a need for reoperation for removal of necrotic elements is approximately 48%

at 24 months (Alexander and Loeffler 1998). The potential for acute toxicity increases with lesions larger than 3 cm in diameter. Three-dimensional conformal photon radiation therapy is another method designed to enhance the confirmation of radiation dose to a target volume, with 30% or greater reduction in volume of normal brain irradiated. The benefit of this approach over conventional radiotherapy has yet to be proved.

Chemotherapy

Chemotherapy has some benefit in the treatment of young patients of good performance status with anaplastic gliomas. Nitrosoureas are the standard treatment to which new agents are compared. They have the theoretical advantages of high lipid solubility, limited ionization at physiological pH, and low plasma protein affinity. Several nitrosoureas (BCNU, CCNU, methyl-CCNU, ACNU, and PCNU) have a modest effect in patients with malignant gliomas. In the first BTSG trial, patients with malignant astrocytomas were randomized postoperatively to (1) supportive care, (2) radiotherapy alone, (3) BCNU alone, or (4) BCNU plus radiotherapy. The median survival was 17 weeks for the supportive care group, 25 weeks for BCNU, 37.5 weeks for radiotherapy, and 40.5 weeks for BCNU plus radiotherapy. In addition, survival at 18 months was increased for the group treated with BCNU plus radiotherapy. Most other chemotherapeutic regimens or corticosteroids alone have not proved superior to BCNU in prospective randomized clinical trials. In anaplastic astrocytoma, the combination of procarbazine, CCNU, and vincristine increases time to progression and survival compared with BCNU. A meta-analysis compared the benefits of prospective treatment with radiotherapy to radiation and chemotherapy in patients with malignant astrocytomas and found a significant benefit of adjuvant chemotherapy. However, most of the benefit occurred in the group of younger patients with anaplastic astrocytoma (Fine et al. 1993).

The limited effectiveness of systemic chemotherapy has prompted the testing of alternative delivery techniques, such as systemic administration with blood-brain barrier modification, intra-arterial infusion, and intratumoral administration in biodegradable polymers. These approaches are not yet superior to standard therapy.

Immunotherapy

Patients with malignant gliomas have known impairments in the following immunological functions: antibody-mediated cytotoxicity, delayed hypersensitivity reactions, cell-mediated cytotoxicity, and lymphocyte blastogenesis to mitogens (Jaeckle 1994). Attempts to boost immunity with nonspecific stimulants, such as bacillus Calmette-Guérin and levamisole, have shown no benefit. Immunization of patients with tumor tissues, cell lines, or tumor antigens has also been without clear value. Passive administration of interleukins and interferons has been attempted; interferon-β appears to have the most promising activity. Transfer of sensitized lymphocytes or interleukin-2–activated killer cells to the resected tumor bed has been largely unsuccessful. Antiglioma monoclonal antibodies have been conjugated to radioactive isotopes, chemotherapy, and plant or bacterial toxins, but the delivery of these relatively large molecules and their fragments through the blood-brain barrier has limited their effectiveness. Although immunotherapy may have a theoretical role in the maintenance of remission, it has yet to be useful in the treatment of glial neoplasms.

Genetic Modification

Genetic modification is the most promising future approach to the treatment of gliomas. An understanding of the derangements in molecular events governing cell growth, differentiation, signaling, transcription, and translation in malignant gliomas will probably lead to rational approaches to therapy. Genetic abnormalities are common in malignant gliomas; amplification of the epidermal growth factor receptor gene occurs in 30–40%, and deletion of the long arm of chromosome 10 occurs in a significant number of glioblastomas. Deletion of an important tumor suppression gene (*MMAC/PTEN*) on chromosome 10 occurs in the majority of glioblastomas.

Cotransplantation of tumor transfected with vectors encoding antisense oligonucleotides that act at the level of DNA or messenger RNA may inhibit specific production of important growth factors, receptors, kinases, or signaling elements. Antisense oligonucleotides to glioma transforming growth factor–β2 decrease tumor growth and augment local immune response in animals with implanted gliomas. Gene therapy studies have been initiated with intratumoral transfer of murine cells producing herpes simplex thymidine kinase vector, after which systemic ganciclovir is administered to effectuate tumor cytotoxicity. Ongoing studies are evaluating the potential advantages of adenovirus vectors and other gene therapy strategies.

Promising work is in progress with agents that block cell growth factor receptor (e.g., epidemal growth factor receptor, platelet-derived growth factor receptor) function; agents that inhibit or disrupt tumor angiogenesis, metalloproteinase-induced cell invasion, extracellular matrix function, or intracellular kinase-related signal transduction; and agents that potentiate cellular differentiation.

Cerebellar Astrocytomas

Cerebellar astrocytomas and brainstem gliomas have very different prognoses, despite their pathological similarities. Cerebellar astrocytomas have the best prognosis of all brain tumors. They represent 12% of brain tumors in children, and although the peak frequency is at 5–9 years of age, they also occur in adolescents and adults. The tumors usually

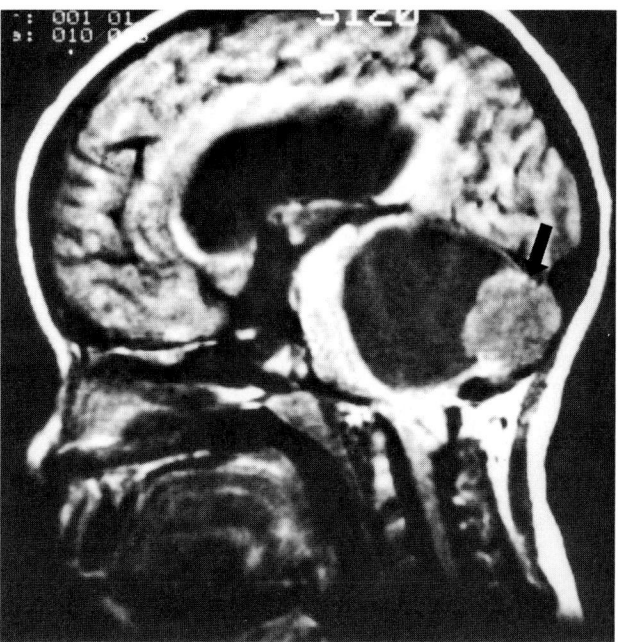

FIGURE 58C.2 Large cystic pilocytic astrocytoma with mural nodule (*arrow*). Gadolinium-enhanced T1-weighted sagittal magnetic resonance image in a 10-year-old girl with ataxia and vomiting.

grow slowly in the cerebellar hemisphere and consist of a large cyst with a mural nodule. Solid or diffuse cerebellar astrocytomas occur in 30% of cases and are usually located in the midline (Figure 58C.2).

The 5-year survival after surgical removal approaches 95%. The mural nodule must be located and removed at surgery, or the tumor may recur. The need for adjuvant radiotherapy has not been established. Diffuse astrocytomas of the cerebellum have a worse prognosis: The 25-year cumulative survival is only 38%, compared with 94% for juvenile cystic cerebellar astrocytoma. Glioblastoma multiforme may occur in the cerebellum and has the same poor prognosis as when located elsewhere. Radiation therapy is recommended for cerebellar glioblastoma, as for cerebral glioblastoma (approximately 60 Gy). The role of chemotherapy is not established.

Brainstem Tumor

Brainstem gliomas account for 10–20% of tumors seen in the pediatric age group (Figure 58C.3). Peak frequency is between 5 and 10 years of age. They are rare before 2 years of age, but a significant number may occur in adults. Genders are affected equally. The anatomical localization of these tumors is defined as the region of the brain traversed by the fourth ventricle and aqueduct of Sylvius. Neoplasms found rostral to the mesencephalon and caudal to the medulla are not considered brainstem tumors.

Stereotactic biopsy is used to prevent damage to vital brainstem structures and the possibility of brainstem

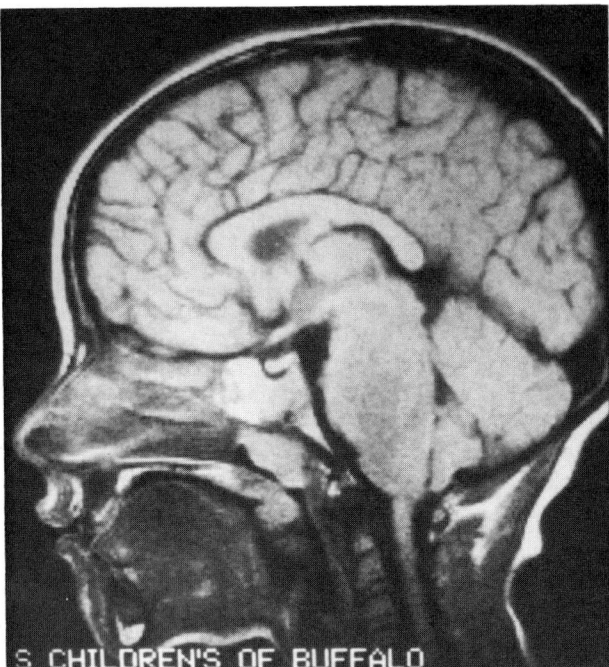

FIGURE 58C.3   Brainstem astrocytoma. Magnetic resonance scan, unenhanced T1-weighted sagittal image. The tumor produces elliptical expansion of the pons and medulla.

swelling. Unfortunately, these small biopsies cannot be used as definitive confirmation because of sampling errors and potential for malignant dedifferentiation. Thus, many authors now reject the need for confirmation by pathology and approach treatment based solely on imaging criteria.

A small group of tumors that may be surgically accessible and may have a relatively benign course include masses that present in an exophytic location (i.e., the floor of the fourth ventricle, lateral recesses, cerebellar pontine angle, or cervical medullary junction). Unlike intrinsic parenchymatous masses, fungating portions of the tumor are surgically accessible and are associated with long-term survival. Evacuation of tumor cysts may also enhance survival and relieve symptoms.

In most series, 5-year survivals range from 5% to 30%. Examination of actuarial survival curves suggests two different populations. The first group represents the majority of brainstem tumors and has a short period from symptoms to diagnosis. The flat portion of the survival curve represents a small group of long-term survivors who have a relatively benign course and, for the most part, represent those with exophytic lesions. Patients with neurofibromatosis (NF) may have a better prognosis. There are reports of long progression-free survivals regardless of location or imaging findings.

The best treatment for brainstem tumors is radiotherapy. Despite many trials using hyperfractionation or radiation with chemotherapy as a radiosensitizer, survival rates continue to be no more than 20–30%. Currently, standard dictum dictates radiation in doses of 5,500 cGy over 5–6 weeks. Poor outcomes have influenced the decision to treat children with brainstem tumors aggressively and to consider treatment on experimental protocols.

Optic Nerve and Chiasmatic Gliomas

Optic pathway tumors represent 3–5% of all childhood tumors. Chiasmatic lesions are more frequent in adolescents than in children. The association of optic pathway tumors with NF is well recognized. The frequency of gliomas in children 2–9 years of age with NF may be as high as 10%. Conversely, approximately 50% of children with optic gliomas have NF type 1. Virtually all children with bilateral orbital tumors have NF type 1. Most of these tumors are pilocytic astrocytomas. Anaplastic astrocytomas and glioblastomas in this area are less common. Although tumors of the optic pathway are found in adults, visual pathway tumors are found primarily in childhood. Optic pathway gliomas may be limited to the optic nerve, extend posteriorly to involve the optic chiasm or tracts, or invade the anterior hypothalamus, causing obstructive hydrocephalus. Occasionally, a visual pathway tumor may outline the entire anterior extent of the visual pathway from the orbit to the lateral geniculate body.

Diminished visual acuity is a common initial feature but may not be noted until late in the course because children are usually not aware of gradual vision loss. Proptosis suggests intraorbital involvement, whereas nystagmus should suggest chiasmatic involvement with disturbed visual fixation. Optic pathway tumors should be considered in any infant with a diagnosis of congenital nystagmus or spasmus nutans. Visual field defects may be quite variable, depending on location of the tumor. Field defects may be monocular, bilateral, central, or centrocecal. Papillitis and central vision loss suggest an orbital lesion. Papilledema should suggest involvement of the hypothalamus and secondary obstruction of the foramen of Monro with subsequent hydrocephalus.

Optic pathway tumors are readily identified by MRI or CT (Figure 58C.4). Coronal, sagittal, and axial studies outline the entire course of the visual pathway and permit complete anatomical visualization. Although visual evoked potentials may help to establish the functional integrity of a visual pathway, they are not useful as a prognostic tool. Repeat MRI and visual acuity with field measurement should allow early identification of progression.

Treatment of optic nerve gliomas remains controversial. Histologically, they are invariably pilocytic astrocytomas. Because the natural history of this tumor is indolent, the current wisdom is to commit to treatment only on evidence of progression. The decision to perform a biopsy on or remove a tumor from a sighted eye is recommended only in situations in which malignant behavior is likely to lead to vision loss or death.

Adjuvant therapy is recommended when visual deterioration occurs or neuroimaging indicates posterior extension of an intraorbital mass into the optic canal or chiasm. Under 5 years of age, patients are treated with chemotherapy, usually a platinum-based regimen, either carboplatin alone or carboplatin and vincristine. Radiotherapy is considered when total resection is not possible. Unfortunately, radiation has been associated with vasculitis, endocrinopathies, and intellectual deterioration. The recurrence rate of optic gliomas after complete intraorbital excision is 5%. Radiation is reserved for patients over 5 years of age in whom the tumor is intracranial rather than intraorbital. Listernick et al. (1997) outlined the current approach to children with optic pathway tumors.

Oligodendroglioma

Oligodendrogliomas account for less than 5% of primary brain tumors. The median age of onset is approximately 40 years. These tumors are slow growing, and often symptoms date back months to years. Seizures are a common initial feature and may predate the diagnosis by years. Oligodendrogliomas are typically frontal lobe in location but may occur in the posterior fossa or spinal cord. Approximately 6% are histologically malignant (anaplastic oligodendroglioma). The prognosis of mixed tumors containing oligodendroglioma and astrocytoma is primarily determined by the astrocytic component.

Oligodendrogliomas are best treated with maximal surgical resection. Postoperative radiation is controversial, particularly in completely resected low-grade oligodendroglioma. Variable benefit of postoperative radiotherapy has been reported, but most data suggest a beneficial effect of radiotherapy for incompletely resected tumors. A 5-year survival rate of 27% has been reported with surgery and 36% with surgery and radiation. The value of chemotherapy, particularly procarbazine-vincristine-lomustine, for the anaplastic tumor is being explored, with preliminary data suggesting high response rates but unclear evidence for survival benefit to date (Cairncross et al. 1994).

Ependymoma

Ependymomas account for 8% of all childhood brain tumors. Most are in the posterior fossa, but a substantial number, especially in children, are supratentorial. Their peak frequency is from birth to 4 years of age, but adults are also affected. Myxopapillary ependymomas are usually located in the filum terminale (Figure 58C.5). Tumors occurring in this location have a favorable prognosis. Two-thirds are infratentorial, and one-third are supratentorial. Infratentorial tumors are found in the roof, floor, or lateral recesses of the fourth ventricle. Tumor may occlude the fourth ventricle or aqueduct. Tumor may extend from the

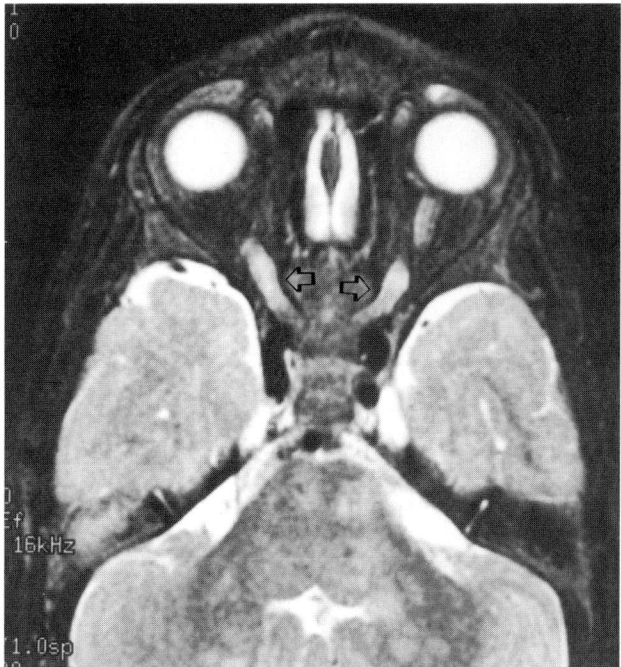

FIGURE 58C.4 Bilateral optic nerve gliomas. T2-weighted axial magnetic resonance image of a 21-year-old man with neurofibromatosis. Nodular enlargement of both optic nerves is shown (*arrows*).

fourth ventricle and encase the brainstem within the tumor mass. Supratentorial ependymomas may be entirely within lateral third ventricles or may be partially intraventricular or extraventricular. Tumors are not exclusively limited to the ventricular surface and may be found anywhere in the cerebral hemispheres (Cohen and Duffner 1994).

The treatment of ependymomas is debulking surgery followed by radiation. Survival directly relates to effectiveness of surgical removal followed by either radiation or chemotherapy (Pollack et al. 1995). Postoperative radiation is considered standard therapy for older children with ependymomas. The Pediatric Oncology Group has demonstrated that treatment failure is related to the primary location of the tumor rather than spread throughout the neuraxis. As such, neuraxis radiation is not recommended unless leptomeningeal disease is recognized at diagnosis (Kovalic et al. 1993). In a series that excluded postoperative deaths, the 5-year survival rate after radiation was 43–53%. Poor prognostic features include age less than 2–5 years at diagnosis, brainstem invasion, and radiation dose less than 4,500 cGy. Degree of malignancy has not been established as a significant risk factor.

Although radiation continues be the best treatment, there is some suggestion that this tumor may be, in part, chemosensitive. Duffner et al. (1993) showed that postoperative chemotherapy consisting of cyclophosphamide and vincristine for children less than 3 years of age was associated with a 48% response rate. Needle et al. (1997) reported a 5-year, progression-free survival of 74% using a

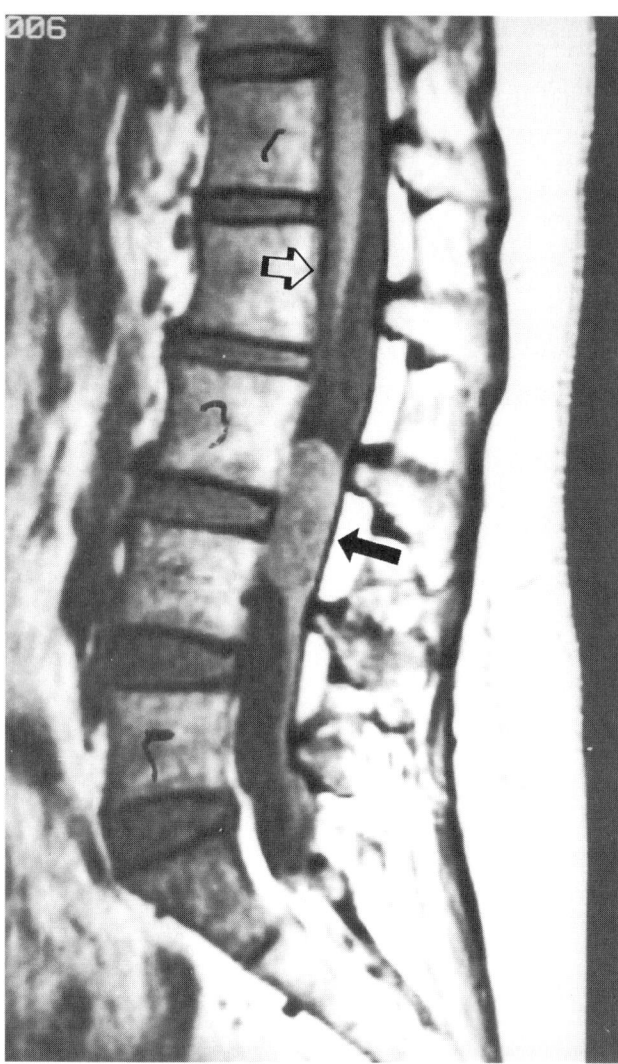

FIGURE 58C.5 Myxopapillary ependymoma. Unenhanced sagittal T1-weighted magnetic resonance scan. The capsule-shaped lesion of the filum terminale (*black arrow*) clearly originates below the caudal aspect of the spinal cord (*open arrow*).

chemotherapy regimen of carboplatin and vincristine and then ifosfamide and etoposide after surgery and radiation.

Complete resection alone is usually curative for myxopapillary tumors of the cauda equina unless residual postoperative tumor persists, thus requiring radiotherapy. The role of chemotherapy in this tumor group has not been established.

Ganglioglioma

Gangliogliomas account for 0.6% of intracranial tumors and are usually located in the temporal lobe. Onset is usually in children and young adults. The initial features are psychomotor seizures and focal neurological signs. Calcification is common. Histologically, both gliomatous and neuronal elements are present. Surgery remains the primary mode of therapy. Radiotherapy is often recommended for persistent or recurrent tumor, but the actual benefit has not been determined.

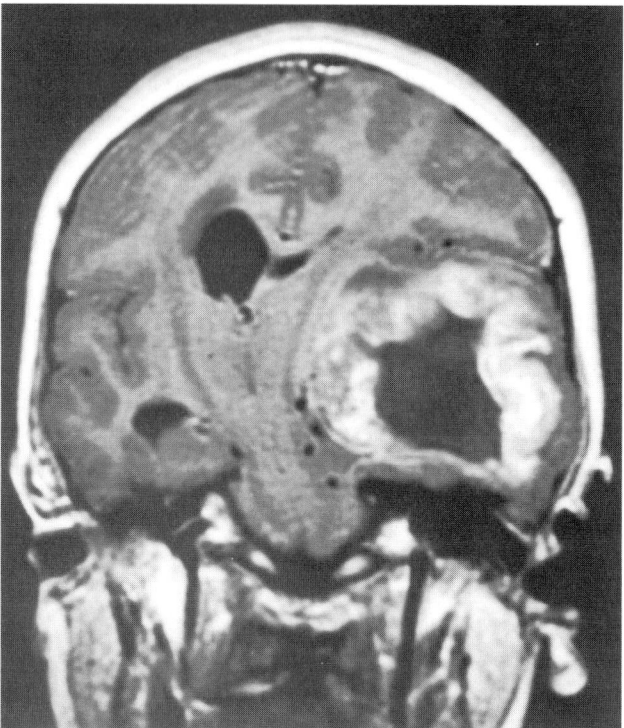

FIGURE 58C.6 Primitive neuroectodermal tumor in an 11-year-old girl. Enhanced coronal magnetic resonance scan. Large cystic mass produces midline shift and compression of the mesencephalon.

Primitive Neuroectodermal Tumors

Cerebral primitive neuroectodermal tumors (PNETs) are a group of tumors with common pathological and clinical features found in the cerebrum of children and young adults. Most occur during infancy. PNETs metastasize through the CSF, and extracranial metastases occur. Focal neurological features can be mild despite massive tumor bulk. Seizures, headaches, nausea, and vomiting are common initial symptoms. The duration of symptoms before diagnosis is often less than 6 months. Increased intracranial pressure and long tract signs are often present. CT and MRI often show calcification and cyst formation in the tumor (Figure 58C.6).

PNETs are radiosensitive and may respond transiently to chemotherapy. Their propensity to metastasize requires radiation of the entire craniospinal axis. Unlike children with medulloblastoma, in whom 5-year survival may be as high as 70%, children with PNETs usually survive less than 1 year.

Medulloblastoma

Medulloblastomas account for 23% of brain tumors in children. Although they are pathologically indistinguishable from PNETs, medulloblastomas differ from PNETs in clinical presentation, location, and predilection for children rather than infants. However, they occur in all age groups. Medulloblastomas tend to arise in the vermis, filling and infiltrating the floor of the fourth ventricle. CSF dissemination is unusual at onset of symptoms in older children but is common before 2 years of age. Systemic metastases to bone marrow, bone, lymph nodes, and other organs may occur. Patients with ventriculoperitoneal shunts may develop peritoneal metastases.

Baseline staging evaluations include enhanced craniospinal MRI, CSF cytology, bone marrow aspiration, and a bone scan. Polyamines may be elevated in the CSF and can be useful in diagnosis and monitoring of response. Infrequently, ventriculoperitoneal shunting may be warranted to control symptoms of increased intracranial pressure before decompressive surgery. The overall 5-year survival rate is better than 50%, which compares well with the 3-year survival rate of 1.6% reported by Cushing in 1930. Survival is most favorable in those who undergo gross total tumor resection followed by radiation rather than partial resection. After surgery, the recommended dose of radiation is 50–60 Gy to the posterior fossa and 36 Gy to the neuraxis. This level of radiation is recommended, despite the strong possibility of adverse side effects, because the recurrence rate is 80%. The two pediatric cancer consortiums in the United States are currently evaluating the benefits of reduced radiation coupled with chemotherapy in good-risk patients (i.e., those who have had total tumor resection, are older than 3 years at the time of diagnosis, and have no evidence of extraneural metastases or subarachnoid seeding). These trials are predicated on the premise that the adverse affects of radiation can be eliminated while favorable survival rates are maintained.

Several chemotherapy trials have demonstrated a significant advantage to chemotherapy in children who are younger than 2 years of age, who have brainstem involvement, and who have had partial resection or biopsy. A study that randomized children with medulloblastoma to receive radiotherapy with or without chemotherapy (CCNU, vincristine, and prednisone) found that survival significantly improved in those receiving adjuvant chemotherapy. The nitrosoureas methotrexate, vincristine, and procarbazine have had a beneficial effect in uncontrolled trials of patients with tumor recurrence.

Meningioma

Meningiomas account for 10–15% of all brain tumors. Intracranial meningiomas are twice as common in women as in men. Their frequency may be increased after ionizing radiation and in NF type 2 (NF-2). A substantial number of meningiomas show a deletion on chromosome 22.

Meningiomas occur most frequently in the parasagittal regions, followed by the lateral convexity and the sphenoid ridge. Other common sites include the olfactory groove, tuberculum sella area, cerebellopontine angle, petrous ridge, foramen magnum, lateral ventricle, and optic nerve sheath. Multiple meningiomas may be present (Figure 58C.7), particularly in NF-2 (see Chapter 69). Parasagittal and convexity lesions can reach massive size before causing clinical symptoms, but optic nerve sheath or chiasm tumors impair vision early and ultimately cause blindness.

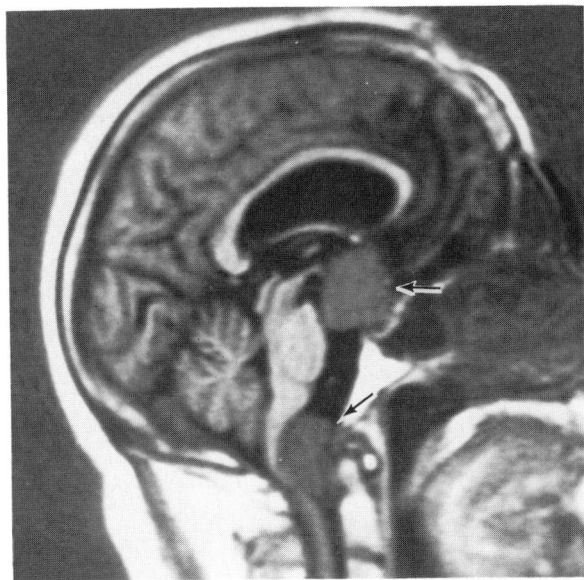

FIGURE 58C.7   Multiple meningiomas. Unenhanced sagittal T1-weighted magnetic resonance image. A 56-year-old woman with suprasellar and foramen magnum tumors (*arrows*).

The diagnosis of meningioma is established by CT or MRI, which shows a densely enhancing mass connected to the dura (see Figure 58C.7). Meningiomas cause varying degrees of edema. Angiography is useful before surgery to define the vascular supply, which often derives from the external carotid circulation.

Surgical resection is the primary treatment mode and provides a median 5-year survival rate of 55%. Sex, age, and tumor site do not correlate with survival. Patients who have had a gross total resection and dural attachments live the longest.

The efficacy of adjunctive radiotherapy after surgery is not established. In 1974, the recurrence rate after surgery but without radiotherapy was 74%, as compared with 29% after treatment with 50–55 Gy alone. In 1992, Miralbell and colleagues reported survival at 8 years of 88% for patients irradiated after subtotal resection, compared with 48% in historical controls not receiving irradiation; this difference did not reach significance. Radiotherapy is often used in unresectable malignant meningioma, invasive angioblastic meningioma, and recurrent meningioma when further surgery is not feasible. Newer techniques being investigated are proton irradiation and stereotactic radiosurgery. Chemotherapy is not recommended in the treatment of meningioma.

Approximately 76% of meningiomas have progesterone receptors, 19% have estrogen receptors, 96% have somatostatin receptors, and 89% have epidermal growth factor receptors. The finding of membrane receptors on meningiomas has led to therapeutic studies of progesterone and estrogen receptor (mifepristone and tamoxifen) inhibitors and growth factors (trapidil).

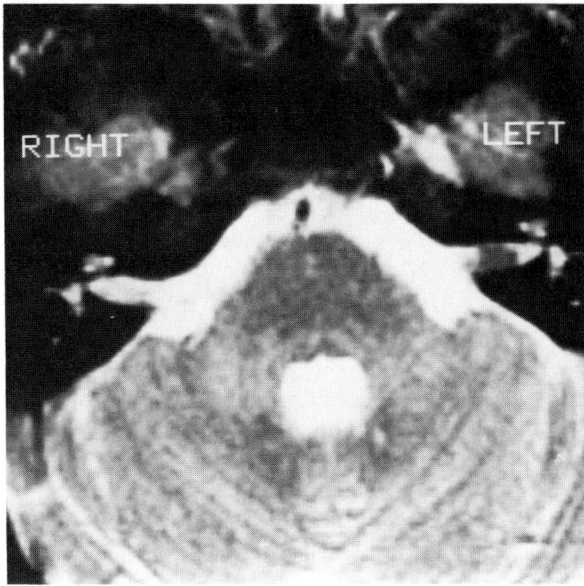

FIGURE 58C.8 Intracanalicular acoustic neuroma. T2-weighted axial magnetic resonance image showing small, dark lesion in the left internal auditory canal.

Vestibular Schwannoma (Acoustic Neurinoma)

Acoustic schwannomas usually originate from the vestibular portion of cranial nerve VIII. They are frequently bilateral in NF-2, in which an abnormality of chromosome 22 is linked to the disease. The initial features are tinnitus, hearing impairment, and compression of brainstem structures and cranial nerves VII and V. Vertigo is a late feature. Pain mimicking trigeminal neuralgia may occur. The diagnosis is suggested by sensorineural hearing loss and abnormal auditory evoked responses. MRI is the diagnostic procedure of choice and allows the identification of even small intracanalicular acoustic neuromas (Figure 58C.8).

A consensus statement by the National Institutes of Health concluded that (1) the term *vestibular schwannoma* was preferred, (2) treatment must be individualized and requires a multidisciplinary approach, (3) surgery is the procedure of choice, (4) facial nerve intraoperative monitoring should be performed, and (5) NF-2 should be considered in all such patients.

The use of the operating microscope, intraoperative facial and cochlear nerve monitoring, and laser and ultrasonic instruments has reduced postoperative morbidity in patients with vestibular schwannomas. Preservation of facial nerve function was previously possible in only one-third of patients, and nearly all developed postoperative hearing loss. Postoperative preservation of facial nerve function is now possible in 86% of patients, with some preservation of cochlear nerve function in 26% and retention of normal hearing in 8% (Cerullo et al. 1993).

Pineal Region Tumors

Pineal region tumors are divided into those derived from pineal parenchymal cells (pineocytomas and pineoblastoma) and germ cell tumors (germinomas and teratomas). They account for less than 1% of all intracranial tumors. Germinomas are more common in Asians than in whites. Other tumors that occur in this region are astrocytomas, ependymomas, glioblastomas, meningiomas, gangliogliomas, and cystic structures, including dermoid, epidermoid, and simple pineal cysts. Ectopic pineal tumors may present as suprasellar masses.

More than 50% of pineal region tumors are germinomas. Less common tumors of germ cell origin are embryonal carcinoma, endodermal sinus tumor, choriocarcinoma, and teratoma. Embryonal cell carcinoma and endodermal sinus tumors may be associated with elevated CSF concentrations of serum α-fetoprotein. Choriocarcinoma, malignant teratoma, and embryonal cell carcinoma are associated with increased CSF concentrations of β-human chorionic gonadotropin. These nongerminomas, particularly those producing high β–human chorionic gonadotropin or α-fetoprotein concentrations, have a worse prognosis than germinomas.

Germinomas are very radiosensitive and are associated with significant operative morbidity. Radiotherapy without pathological confirmation was advocated. Further, presurgical radiation therapy may prevent leptomeningeal spread. However, improvements in stereotactic biopsy technique have decreased morbidity and support the practice of establishing a definitive histological diagnosis before therapy.

Spinal neuraxis radiotherapy is suggested for poor-risk patients who have CSF, MRI, or myelographic evidence of spinal metastases. Germ cell tumors are highly chemosensitive, particularly to cisplatin-containing regimens.

Primary Central Nervous System Lymphoma

The incidence of primary CNS lymphomas (PCNSLs) is increasing independent of the expected increase associated with organ transplant and human immunodeficiency virus infection. Most PCNSLs show monotypic surface immunoglobulin and are positive for the CD20 B-cell marker. Tumors associated with HIV are usually small, multiple, and predominantly located in the temporal lobes and basal ganglia. Tumors not associated with HIV are larger (>2 cm) and are usually located in the parietal lobe (Figure 58C.9).

The initial features are headache, vomiting, mental status changes, focal signs, and occasionally papilledema. Orbital involvement is associated in 10–20%, and leptomeningeal meningeal dissemination is associated in 10–60%.

The prognosis is poor. Median survival without treatment is approximately 2 months but is extended to 25 months by radiotherapy. The 5-year survival rate for patients receiving more than 50 Gy is 42%, as opposed to 13% when less than 50 Gy is used. An additional dose of 40 Gy to the spinal neuraxis is recommended when there is evidence of CSF spread. Relapse usually occurs within 2 years. The median time to progression has been extended to 41 months by the combination of chemotherapy with systemic and intrathecal methotrexate, followed by cranial irradiation (40 Gy to whole brain and a 14.4-Gy local field boost), followed by high-dose cytarabine. Survival is 10 months in patients receiving radiation alone.

Craniopharyngioma

Craniopharyngiomas are more common in children than in adults and often reach substantial size before detection. They may extend into the hypothalamus, third ventricular region, optic chiasm, and frontal lobes. Craniopharyngiomas are typically calcified and cystic. These features permit preliminary radiographic diagnosis by MRI or CT. The usual initial features are headache, visual disturbances, visual field deficits, endocrinopathies, diabetes insipidus, and somnolence. Surgical resection is the treatment of choice, but the recurrence rate is 50%, and radiotherapy is then indicated. The 5- and 10-year survival rates after postoperative radiotherapy are 84% and 72% for children and 54% and 51% for adults (Regine et al. 1993). Radiation provides better than 30% improvement in visual field defects and visual acuity without causing optic atrophy. Despite the excellent survival rates, treatment causes significant endocrine disturbance (diabetes insipidus, panhypopituitarism, and obesity), radionecrosis, and intellectual impairment.

Glomus Jugulare Tumors

Most glomus jugulare tumors originate in the middle ear and consist of cells in the adventitia of the jugular bulb near the exit of the glossopharyngeal nerve. The initial features may be deafness, otalgia, otorrhea, and pulsatile tinnitus. The squamous portion of the temporal bone is often destroyed, with subsequent referral of neurological symptoms to the posterior cranial fossa. Histologically, the tumor mimics a capillary hemangioblastoma or angioblastic meningioma.

Surgical excision is curative, with bleeding as a major feature, because the tumor is extremely vascular. Recurrences follow incomplete removal. Radiation, either alone or combined with surgery, may be equally satisfactory. Metastases are rare.

Chordomas

Chordomas are slow-growing neoplasms of notochordal origin. Small remnants of notochordal tissue are sometimes identified as a normal variant embedded in the dorsum sel-

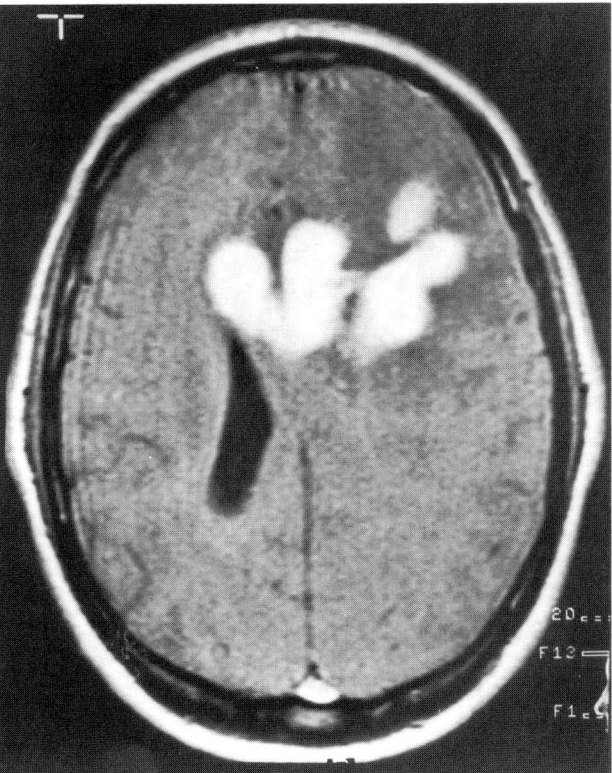

FIGURE 58C.9 Primary central nervous system lymphoma. T1-weighted enhanced axial magnetic resonance image of a 16-year-old woman. There is coalescence of multiple homogeneously enhancing nodules in the frontal periventricular region with surrounding edema.

lae, clivus, or roof of the nasopharynx. The mean age of onset of intracranial chordoma is 45 years, and men are slightly more commonly affected than are women (Watkins et al. 1993). Intracranial chordomas are commonly found at the spheno-occipital synchondrosis and may grow into the sella turcica, optic chiasm, and parasellar structures, compressing the pons or cranial nerves. The initial features are headache and palsies of cranial nerves VI, IX, or X. Brainstem dysfunction develops later. Sacral chordomas cause localized lumbosacral pain and radiculopathies.

Metastases, although uncommon, can spread to meninges, lymph nodes, liver, and lungs. MRI shows low T1 and high T2 signal and heterogeneous gadolinium pentetic acid enhancement. Surgical resection (and re-resection at recurrence) is the only beneficial treatment. Metastases are resistant to radiotherapy and chemotherapy. The 5- and 10-year survival rates are 58% and 35%, respectively.

TUMORS IN CHILDREN YOUNGER THAN 2 YEARS

Thirteen percent of childhood brain tumors occur before age 2 years. This group is considered separately from older children and adults because treatment is generally less effective, survivals are shorter, and infants are at increased risk for radiation-induced neurotoxicity. One cause for poor survival is the higher incidence of malignant tumors. Cerebellar astrocytoma, which has the best prognosis among childhood CNS tumors, is unusual before age 2, whereas PNETs, which have the worst prognosis, are frequent (Duffner et al. 1993).

Clinical Features

Before age 6 months, supratentorial tumors are common; afterward, a gradual transition in location occurs, so that by the second year, most tumors are in the posterior fossa. Because cranial sutures are not fused in infants, skull expansion and molding occurs in response to increased intracranial pressure. Sutural diastasis can delay diagnosis because the features of increased intracranial pressure are lacking. Rapid head growth during infancy may be the first suggestion of increased pressure. The usual initial features of congenital brain tumors are congenital hypotonia and macrocephaly. Leptomeningeal dissemination of tumor is likely to occur early in the course.

Vomiting and failure to thrive are early features of brain tumors in infants. A gastrointestinal evaluation may precede consideration of CNS tumor. However, vomiting rarely occurs without other signs of increased intracranial pressure. Developmental delay is sometimes the reason for medical consultation; a history of deterioration in function is much more common. The diencephalic syndrome is an unusual but characteristic syndrome in infants with tumors in and around the hypothalamus. The infants have severe emaciation despite a voracious appetite, and they have a bright, alert appearance.

Infantile hemiplegia is usually caused by malformations or perinatal stroke (see Chapters 66 and 84) but may also be caused by tumor. In general, children with hemiparetic cerebral palsy lateralize handedness during the first year and have never used the affected hand normally. A history of normal use of both hands followed by strong hand dominance before 18 months should suggest a progressive CNS disorder.

Seizures are a common symptom of supratentorial tumors in infants. The seizures are usually partial, with and without secondary generalization. Electroencephalograms may show focal slowing. Infantile spasms are sometimes caused by brain tumors, most frequently in association with tuberous sclerosis (see Chapter 69).

Treatment

Successful treatment of infants with brain tumors requires an experienced pediatric neurosurgeon and anesthesiologist and a properly equipped pediatric intensive care unit. Surgical mortality approaches 10%. Young children are more prone to hypothermia and excessive blood loss than are older children. Preoperative ventricular shunting may be necessary to relieve pressure and stabilize the child's condition but carries the risk of peritoneal dissemination of tumor. Radiation has severe long-term sequelae, including intellectual deterioration, growth failure, hypothyroidism, leukoencephalopathy, vasculopathy, spinal deformities, and oncogenesis. As a result, the tendency is to monitor children until definite symptomatic progression occurs.

Debulking surgery followed by longitudinal evaluation with serial CT or MRI is recommended in young children with low-grade supratentorial astrocytomas. Reoperation is considered for tumor recurrence. Chemotherapy is often recommended in children less than 5 years old who have inoperable tumors to delay the administration of radiotherapy. This approach is often well tolerated, and overall survival rates are often comparable to or better than those treated with radiation alone. Children who develop progressive disease on chemotherapy can be salvaged with radiation, even when radiation has been postponed for more than 12 months after initial diagnosis.

Neurofibromatosis

Infants with NF-2 (see Chapter 69) are at particular risk for brain tumors. The diagnosis is often difficult without a family history because the cutaneous manifestations are mild. Optic nerve glioma is the most common brain tumor in children with NF who are less than 10 years of age. Routine CT screening is often required for diagnosis. The diagnosis is sometimes suggested by exophthalmos. Assessment of visual acuity may be difficult in young children because of poor cooperation, and in such cases, visual evoked potentials may be substituted. MRI can be confusing in children with NF. More than one-half of children have increased T2 signals of unclear significance in the basal ganglia, optic pathways, brainstem, and cerebellum.

SECONDARY NEOPLASMS OF THE CENTRAL NERVOUS SYSTEM

Approximately 20% of cancer patients have neurological dysfunction at some point in their course (Table 58C.3). These patients are some of the most challenging in the field of neurology. Advanced cancer may cause neurological dysfunction by multilevel metastases; metabolic effects of systemic organ system dysfunction; infection; vascular diseases, including thrombosis, embolism, and hemorrhage; and nonmetastatic (remote, paraneoplastic) disorders. The toxic effects of anticancer drugs can also cause neurological dysfunction. The role of the clinician is to identify the cause, remedy situations that threaten vital function, outline a plan for the evaluation and management of reversible conditions, and provide palliation and psychological support when cure is not possible.

Table 58C.3: Classification of nervous system metastases

Skull
  Calvarium
  Skull base
Intracranial
  Dura
  Intraparenchymal central nervous system
Leptomeningeal
Spinal
  Epidural
  Intramedullary
  Vertebra and sacrum
Plexus
  Brachial
  Lumbosacral

Table 58C.4: Central nervous system metastases: most common location in order of frequency*

Cerebrum
Cerebellum
Brainstem
Leptomeninges
Base of brain
Spinal cord

*47% are single; 53% are multiple.

Skull Metastases

Breast and prostate carcinomas are the most common source of skull metastases, followed by lung carcinoma, neuroblastoma, lymphoma, and myeloma. Such metastases are often asymptomatic and do not require treatment unless intracranial structures are invaded. Radiotherapy may be necessary if the metastases are associated with severe headache, tumor invasion and thrombosis of the sagittal sinus, or evidence of cerebral extension.

Base-of-skull metastases usually spread from the breast, lung, and prostate. Clinical syndromes correlate with the location of the metastasis. The orbital syndrome is dull supraorbital pain accompanied by blurred vision and diplopia. External ophthalmoplegia and proptosis may be present. The parasellar syndrome of unilateral frontal headache and extraocular palsies is caused by infiltration of the cavernous sinus and cranial nerves. In both syndromes, tumor is proximate to the optic nerve sheath, and corticosteroids are warranted before radiotherapy to avoid acute vision loss from radiation-induced edema. The gasserian ganglion syndrome is pain and sensory disturbances referable to the second and third divisions of the trigeminal nerve. Most patients complain of numbness of the face and a dull ache in the jaw. Pterygoid or masseter weakness and other cranial nerve palsies (especially abducens) are late complications. The jugular foramen syndrome is hoarseness and dysphagia from involvement of the glossopharyngeal and vagus nerves. Pain may be present in the submandibular area or behind the ear. Unilateral vocal cord paralysis is seen on laryngoscopy. The occipital condyle syndrome is ipsilateral neck and posterior head pain that can be reproduced by extending and tilting the head to the involved side or by applying pressure over the occipital area. Dysarthria and dysphagia from hypoglossal palsy occur in one-half of cases.

The diagnosis of base-of-skull lesions is made clinically and confirmed by thin-slice (2- to 3-mm) CT with bone windows. MRI may show the tumor mass more clearly but does not show bony erosion as well as CT does. Isotope bone scan may show uptake in the appropriate area. Most patients obtain symptomatic relief after base-of-skull irradiation.

Dural Metastases

Dural metastases are most common with breast and prostate carcinoma and lymphoma. A subdural effusion containing tumor cells may be associated. These tumors may cause headache or venous sinus thrombosis or may secondarily invade the subdural space and underlying brain.

Intraparenchymal Central Nervous System Metastases

More common sources of intraparenchymal metastases are lung carcinoma (27%), melanoma (22%), and breast carcinoma (15%). Less common sources (<10%) are tumors of the ovary, gastrointestinal tract, pancreas, and cervix, as well as Hodgkin's disease and sarcomas. Approximately 80% of CNS metastases are in the cerebrum, 16% in the cerebellum, and 3% in the brainstem. Approximately one-half are single and one-half multiple (Table 58C.4). Approximately 12–25% of cancer patients have CNS metastases at postmortem examination, and most are symptomatic some time during the course of illness. Metastases usually reach the brain through the blood and have a predilection for the gray matter–white matter interface.

The initial feature in many patients is a focal neurological abnormality referable to the tumor location (or locations) or seizures. Headache is the most common symptom of CNS metastases, and mental status changes are second. About 5–10% of patients experience an apoplectic event or a transitory neurological disturbance similar to a stroke or focal seizure. Multiple tumors may cause an agitated delirium.

The diagnosis is readily established by enhanced CT or MRI in a patient with known cancer. Biopsy is needed for diagnosis only when the primary is unknown (approximately 10%). The standard treatment for brain metastases is reduction of edema with corticosteroids, along with radiotherapy. The administration of 40 Gy in 4 weeks to whole brain and 20 Gy in 1 week to whole brain was evaluated in two sequential studies. Median survivals were 15 and 18 weeks, respectively. Forty-nine percent died of progressive brain metastases; the rest died of systemic disease. Eighty percent of the survival

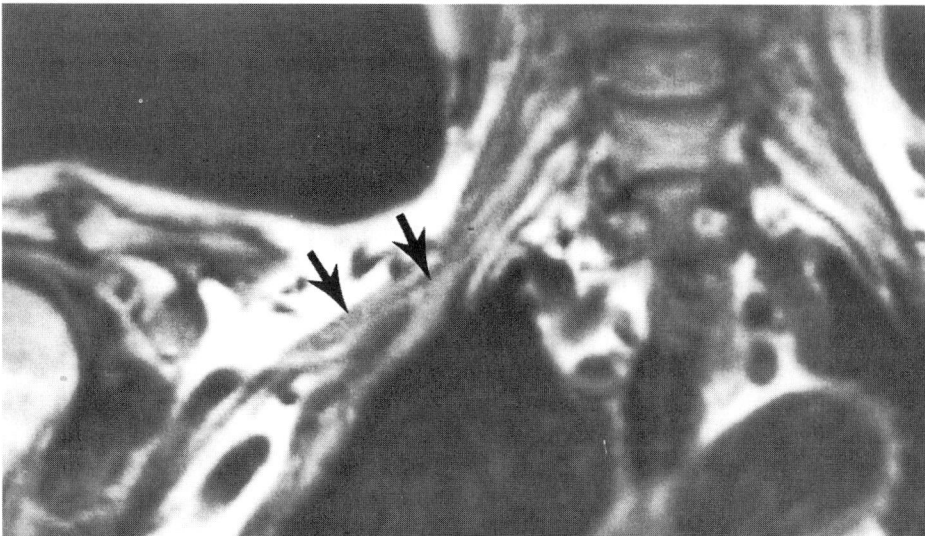

FIGURE 58C.10   Metastatic brachial plexopathy. Sagittal magnetic resonance image of the brachial plexus in a 78-year-old woman with breast carcinoma, shoulder pain, and arm weakness. Metastatic tumor invasion has produced diffuse thickening of the cords (*arrows*) of the brachial plexus, in the absence of a well-defined tumor mass.

time was spent in a stable or improved neurological state. Surgery alone was associated with a median survival of approximately 6 months. Important features associated with better prognosis include controlled systemic cancer, solitary metastases, and lack of significant neurological deficit. In 1992, Patchell and coworkers found that resection of single brain metastasis followed by radiotherapy significantly prolongs survival over radiation alone in patients with controlled systemic disease and good performance status. Promising radiotherapeutic techniques under study include accelerated or hyperfractionated radiotherapy and stereotaxic radiosurgery. In patients with multiple metastases, poor performance status, and overwhelming systemic cancer, palliative treatment with short courses of radiation, such as 20 Gy in 1 week or 30 Gy in 2 weeks, may be a reasonable compromise.

Increased survival in patients treated with chemotherapy for small cell lung carcinoma (SCLC) has created interest in the use of prophylactic cranial radiation to prevent the development of late-stage cerebral metastases. The frequency of brain metastases in SCLC is approximately 5% with prophylactic cranial irradiation and 23% without it. However, nonirradiated patients who develop late-stage brain metastases respond equally well to radiation therapy, and a difference in overall survival has not been established. The potential late-stage toxic effects of prophylactic irradiation are a concern, as is the unnecessary treatment of some patients who might never develop brain metastases.

Chemotherapy with cisplatin, doxorubicin (Adriamycin), bleomycin, methotrexate, nitrosoureas, and other drugs has produced brief responses without increase in survival, regardless of the mode of delivery. Certain chemosensitive metastatic tumors, such as SCLC, appear to be highly responsive in nonirradiated patients. Overall, chemotherapy is palliative, and should be guided by tumor sensitivity, consideration of blood-brain barrier penetrability, and clinical condition of the patient.

PLEXUS METASTASES

Brachial Plexopathy

Systemic tumors may invade the brachial plexus by direct extension from lung, breast, or axillary lymph nodes, and less commonly by lymphatic or hematogenous spread. Pain is the initial feature in 80% of patients. The pain is typically severe and located primarily in the shoulder, with radiation down the ulnar aspect of the arm, forearm, and hand. Weakness, atrophy, sensory loss, dysesthesias, and hyporeflexia in the C8 to T1 distribution may be associated. The diagnosis can be established by CT or MRI of the plexus region (Figure 58C.10). It is useful to include the upper thoracic and cervical spine in the scan because concomitant epidural extension of tumor is present in more than one-third of patients. The finding of a Horner's syndrome, or weakness with atrophy of the rhomboids or serratus anterior, suggests that tumor invasion is close to the spine. Radiotherapy usually relieves the pain. Surgical neurolysis is beneficial in selected cases.

Radiation-induced plexopathy must be considered in previously treated patients. This complication occurs 3 years or more after treatment in approximately 5% of breast cancer patients treated with more than 50 Gy to the region. Paresthesias, hypesthesia, weakness, hyporeflexia, arm edema, and causalgic pain are present. Weakness involves the upper or whole plexus in contrast to the more common lower plexopathy involvement with tumor plexopathy.

Lumbosacral Plexopathy

Tumors often involve the lumbosacral plexus by direct extension from contiguous pelvic structures or by metastasis to regional lymph nodes or bone with secondary inva-

FIGURE 58C.11 Metastatic lumbosacral plexopathy. Axial computed tomographic scan of the pelvis in a 68-year-old woman with metastatic breast carcinoma. The tumor has produced diffuse invasion of the lumbosacral plexus, iliac wing, and gluteal and paraspinal musculature.

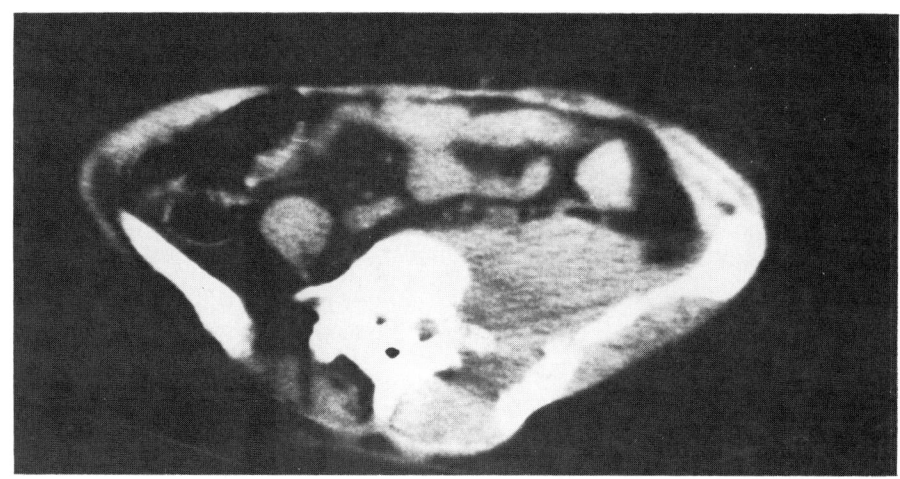

sion. The tumors most commonly associated are colorectal tumors, lymphomas, and retroperitoneal sarcomas. Pain is the initial feature and is followed 2–4 weeks later by numbness, weakness, and paresthesias in the leg, and occasionally incontinence or impotence. Common clinical signs are leg weakness, sensory loss, reflex asymmetry, focal back or sciatic notch tenderness, positive straight-leg–raising tests, and leg edema. On occasion, a rectal mass may be palpated. The tumor typically involves the lower plexus (L5-S1). A quintet of leg pain, weakness, leg edema, a rectal mass, and hydronephrosis suggests plexopathy due to cancer.

CT or MRI establishes the diagnosis (Figure 58C.11). Nearly one-half of patients develop epidural extension, usually at sacral or lower lumbar levels, often below the conus medullaris. Lumbosacral plexopathy is treated with radiotherapy to the area of visualized tumor, taking into account the expected area of involvement based on the neurological examination. The syndrome may be difficult to distinguish clinically from leptomeningeal metastases in the absence of a well-defined pelvic mass.

Radiation injury to the lumbosacral plexus also occurs but is less frequent than its brachial plexus counterpart, occurring in approximately 0.1% of patients with carcinoma of the cervix or endometrium treated to the pelvis (Georgiou et al. 1993). Leg weakness, edema, and paresthesias are commonly observed. Electromyography evidence of myokymia, which is uncommon in tumor plexopathy, helps to confirm this diagnosis. The clinical course is usually one of slow progression, but significant benefit can be obtained from rigorous rehabilitative therapy and proper use of orthotics.

REFERENCES

Alexander E, Loeffler GS. Radiosurgery for primary malignant tumors. Semin Surg Oncol 1998;14:43–52.

Berger MS, Leibel SA, Bruner JM, et al. Primary Central Nervous System Tumors of the Supratentorial Compartment. In VA Levin (ed), Cancer in the Nervous System. New York: Churchill Livingstone, 1996;86–87.

Cairncross JG, Macdonald D, Ludwin S, et al. Chemotherapy for anaplastic oligodendroglioma. National Cancer Institute of Canada Clinical Trials Group. J Clin Oncol 1994;12:2013–2021.

Cerullo LJ, Grutsch JF, Heiferman K, et al. The preservation of hearing and facial nerve function in a consecutive series of unilateral vestibular nerve schwannoma surgical patients (acoustic neuroma). Surg Neurol 1993;39:485–493.

Cohen ME, Duffner PK. Brain Tumors in Children: Principles of Diagnosis and Treatment (2nd ed). New York: Raven, 1994.

Curran WJ, Scott CB, Weinstein AS, et al. Survival comparison of radiosurgery eligible and ineligible malignant glioma patients treated with hyperfractionated radiotherapy and carmustine: a report of the Radiation Therapy Oncology Group 8302. J Clin Oncol 1993;11:857–862.

Duffner PK, Horowitz ME, Krischer JP, et al. Postoperative chemotherapy and delayed radiation in children less than three years of age with malignant brain tumors. N Engl J Med 1993;328:1725–1731.

Fine HA, Dear KB, Loeffler JS, et al. Metaanalysis of radiation therapy with and without adjuvant chemotherapy for malignant gliomas in adults. Cancer 1993;71:2585–2597.

Georgiou A, Grigsby PW, Perez CA. Radiation-induced lumbosacral plexopathy in gynecologic tumors: clinical findings and dosimetric analysis. Int J Radiat Oncol Biol Phys 1993;26:479–482.

Jaeckle KA. Immunotherapy of malignant gliomas. Semin Oncol 1994;21:249–259.

Kovalic JJ, Flaris N, Grigsby PW, et al. Intracranial ependymoma: long-term outcome, patterns of failure. J Neurooncol 1993;15:125–131.

Listernick R, Louis DN, Packer RJ, et al. Optic pathway gliomas in children with neurofibromatosis 1: consensus statement from the NF1 Optic Pathway Glioma Task Force. Ann Neurol 1997;41:143–149.

Needle MN, Goldwein SW, Grass J, et al. Adjuvant chemotherapy for the treatment of intracranial ependymoma of childhood. Cancer 1997;80:341–347.

Pollack LF, Gerszten PC, Martinez AJ, et al. Intracranial ependymomas of childhood: long-term outcome and prognostic factors. Neurosurgery 1995;37:655–667.

Regine WF, Mohiuddin M, Kramer S. Long-term results of pediatric and adult craniopharyngiomas treated with combined surgery and radiation. Radiother Oncol 1993;27:13–21.

Watkins L, Khudados ES, Kaleoglu M, et al. Skull base chordomas: a review of 38 patients, 1955–88. Br J Neurosurg 1993;7:241–248.

Chapter 58
Primary and Secondary Tumors of the Central Nervous System

D. CLINICAL PRESENTATION AND THERAPY FOR SPINAL TUMORS
Laszlo L. Mechtler and Michael E. Cohen

EXTRADURAL TUMORS

Epidural Metastasis

Epidemiology

Epidural spinal cord compression (ESCC) by metastases is more common than compression by primary spinal tumors. It occurs in 5% of patients who die of cancer, which represents more than 25,000 cases annually of spinal cord compression in the United States. Moreover, prolonged survival time from improved cancer treatment is expected to increase the incidence of ESCC. Approximately one-half of ESCCs in adults are metastases from breast, lung, or prostate cancer; the primary tumor is not identified in 10% of cases (Table 58D.1).

Distribution

The overall frequency of metastases to any portion of the spine is a function of length: 70% involve the thoracic spine, 20% the lumbosacral spine, and 10% the cervical spine. Lung and breast carcinomas tend to metastasize to the thoracic spine and colon or pelvic tumors to the lumbosacral spine. Approximately 10–38% of epidural metastases involve multiple noncontiguous levels—an important consideration in evaluation and treatment.

The anatomical site of metastasis is an important factor in patient management. Bony lesions occur in more than 90% of patients with spinal metastasis, of which 71% are osteolytic, 8% are osteoblastic, and 21% are mixed. Eighty-five percent of metastases arise in the vertebral body

and invade the epidural space anteriorly. Laminectomy can be effective in decompressing the spinal cord but fails to remove the tumor, which arises from the anterior body of the vertebrae. Metastatic lesions never involve the intravertebral disc or transgress the dura.

Pathogenesis

Metastases cause ESCC by three mechanisms. The first and most common is hematogenous spread to the vertebra, which contains highly vascularized hematopoietic bone marrow and rich growth factors. Second is spread of tumor cells to the vertebral column through the vertebral venous (Batson's) plexus. Batson's veins are valveless and have low intraluminal pressure that allows retrograde tumor seeding when intrathoracic or intra-abdominal pressure increases (i.e., through coughing, sneezing, or Valsalva's maneuver). The third mechanism of direct invasion of tumor through the intravertebral foramina is responsible for approximately 15% of ESCCs. Lymphoma accounts for about 75% of these cases, in which radioisotope studies and radiographs are typically normal.

Clinical Features

Pain, the most common initial feature, occurs in 95% of adults and 80% of children. Pain is usually localized to the site of metastasis and is caused by stretching the pain-sensitive bony periosteum. Radicular pain is less frequent but is also localizing. It is often bilateral in thoracic ESCC and unilateral in cervical and lumbosacral ESCC. Segmental or funicular pain, indicating intrinsic spinal cord damage, is

Table 58D1:   Types of primary tumors causing metastatic epidural spinal cord compression in men and women

	Men (%)	Women (%)
Lung	53	12
Breast	0	59
Prostate	8	—
Kidney	3	3
Melanoma	0	1
Gastrointestinal	5	3
Female reproductive	—	6
Miscellaneous	31	16

Source: Modified with permission from RJ Stark, RA Henson, SJW Evans. Spinal metastases—a retrospective survey from a general hospital. Brain 1982;105:189–213.

uncommon and is continuous, burning, dull, and diffuse. As in degenerative disc disease, Valsalva's maneuver, straight-leg raising, and neck flexion aggravate back pain. Unlike a herniated disc, ESCC pain is characteristically aggravated by recumbency (which is worse at night). Epidural metastasis is the initial manifestation of malignancy in about 10% of patients. The primary is usually lung cancer, myeloma, lymphoma, or renal cell cancer (Figure 58D.1).

Common clinical features at the time of diagnosis are bilateral weakness (76%), autonomic dysfunction (57%), and sensory complaints (51%). Weakness (caused by anterior compression of the spinal cord) precedes the sensory symptoms. At the time of diagnosis, 50% of patients are ambulatory, 35% are paraparetic, and 15% are paraplegic. As many as one-half of those who are paraplegic at diagnosis had deteriorated abruptly or within the previous 24- to 48-hour period. Rapid progression is mostly seen in patients with lung cancer, lymphoma, or renal tumors. Autonomic dysfunction is never the presenting symptom. Sensory complaints are almost always painful. Lhermitte's sign, herpes zoster, gait ataxia, and Brown-Séquard's syndrome are unusual in ESCC.

Neuroimaging

On plain radiographs of the spine, metastases cause changes in the pedicles, which are compact bone, before the vertebral

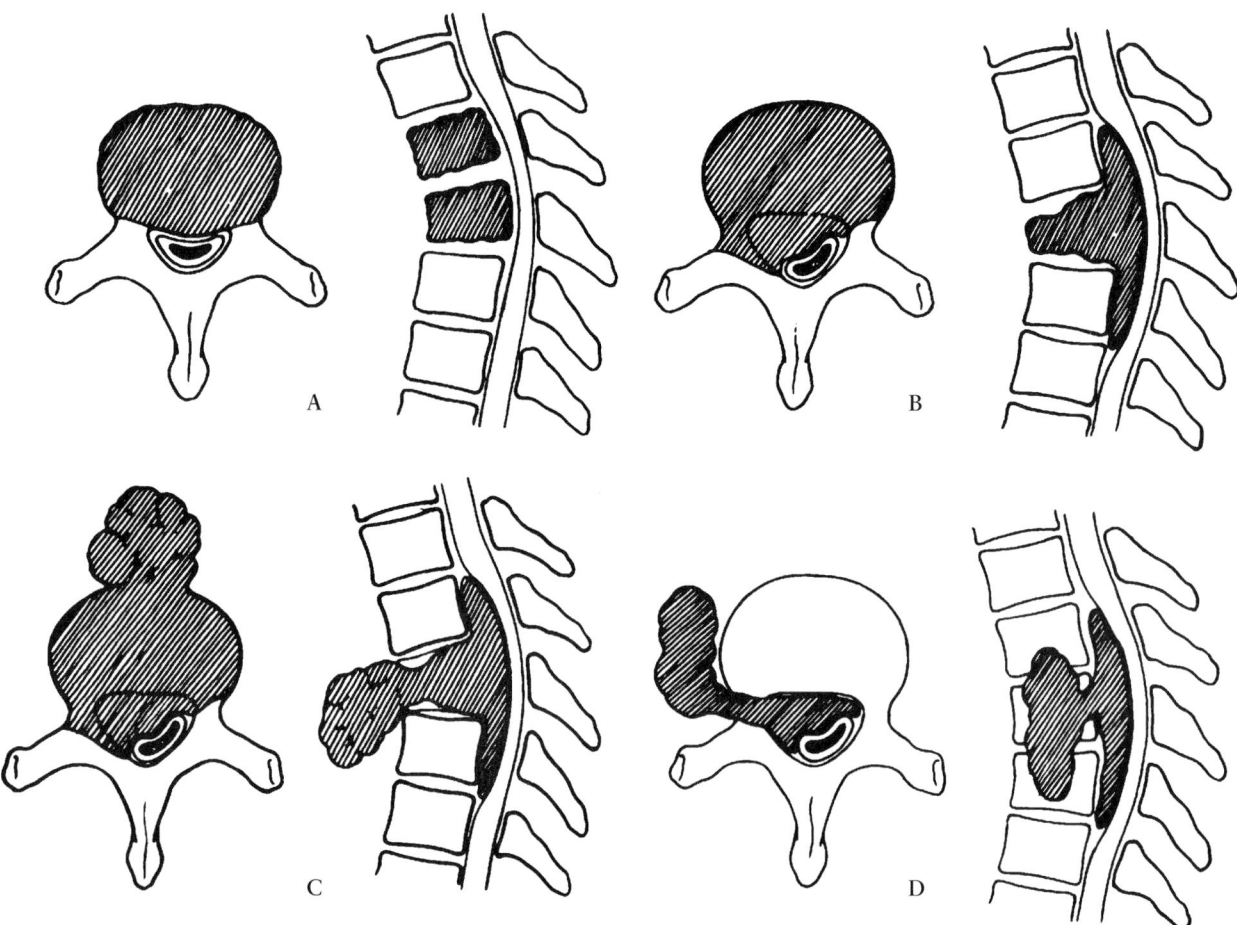

FIGURE 58D.1   Epidural spinal cord compression. Tumor spread into the epidural space expands the vertebral body (**A**), or a sleeve-like extension compromises the spinal cord (**B**). Direct extension from a prevertebral focus (**C**) through the vertebral body occurs with lung cancers. Radiographs may be normal when tumors extend through the neural foramina (**D**). (Reprinted with permission from JP Constans. Spinal metastases with neurological manifestations: review of 600 cases. J Neurosurg 1983;59:111.)

FIGURE 58D.2 Metastatic breast cancer to the lumbar spine on a T1-weighted sagittal magnetic resonance image demonstrating multiple well-circumscribed areas of decreased signal intensities (*open arrows*) within the vertebral body (**A**). Several of these lesions become isointense or hyperintense when enhanced (*arrows*), making detection more difficult (**B**).

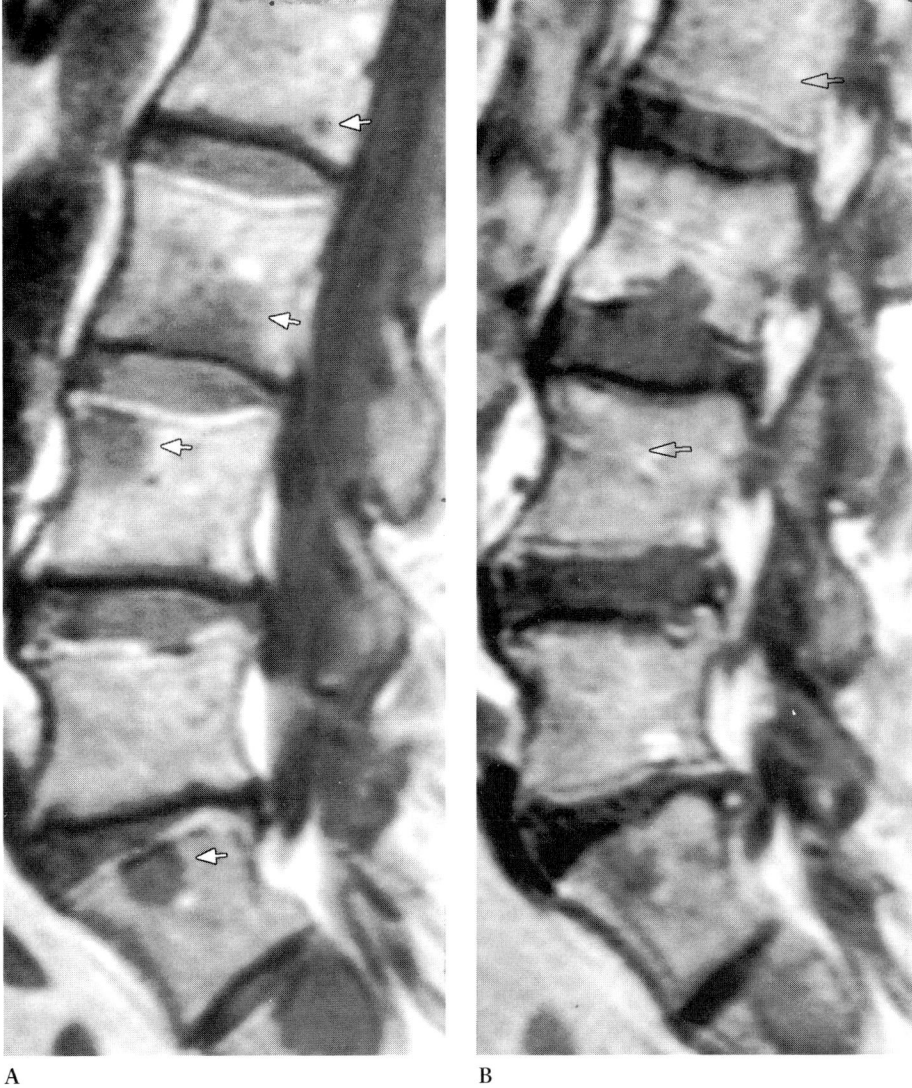

A   B

bodies, which must be 50% destroyed before changes can be identified. Abnormal radiographs at the time of presentation are seen in 85% of patients with ESCCs from epithelial tumors but in only 33% of patients with lymphoma. The most common findings are pedicle erosion ("winking owl" sign), paravertebral soft tissue shadow, vertebral collapse, and pathological fracture dislocation. The likelihood of epidural tumor is 87% when vertebral compression is greater than 50%. ESCC is present in only 7% of patients with radiological evidence of vertebral metastases without collapse.

The sensitivity of bone scanning approaches 91%, but its specificity is limited, with a high false-positive rate. Computed tomography (CT) of the spine is more sensitive and specific than plain radiographs or radionuclide scanning for ESCC. The combination of myelography followed by CT was the study of choice but is being replaced by magnetic resonance imaging (MRI). MRI is as sensitive as bone scans for detecting vertebral metastasis and is more specific.

MRI provides detailed anatomical resolution of the vertebrae and surrounding structures and permits direct visualization in multiplanar sections along the entire length of the spinal column. Unenhanced T1-weighted sagittal images are obtained first because contrast enhancement might obscure subtle vertebral metastases (Figure 58D.2). This is followed by a T2-weighted or enhanced T1-weighted scan. The characteristic findings on MRI are multiple foci of low signal intensity on T1-weighted images. Collapse and destruction of the vertebral body sparing the adjacent disc spaces are common. Short T1 inversion recovery, which is a fat-suppression technique, increases the sensitivity of MRI. Although gadolinium enhancement may mask vertebral lesions, it is helpful in the detection and characterization of epidural, intradural, and intramedullary processes. Conventional myelography is preferred to MRI in patients who cannot lie still because of claustrophobia or severe pain and in patients with severe scoliosis, ferromagnetic implants, aneurysm clips, or a cardiac pacemaker. In cases in which MRI does not yield the diagnosis, myelography should be performed.

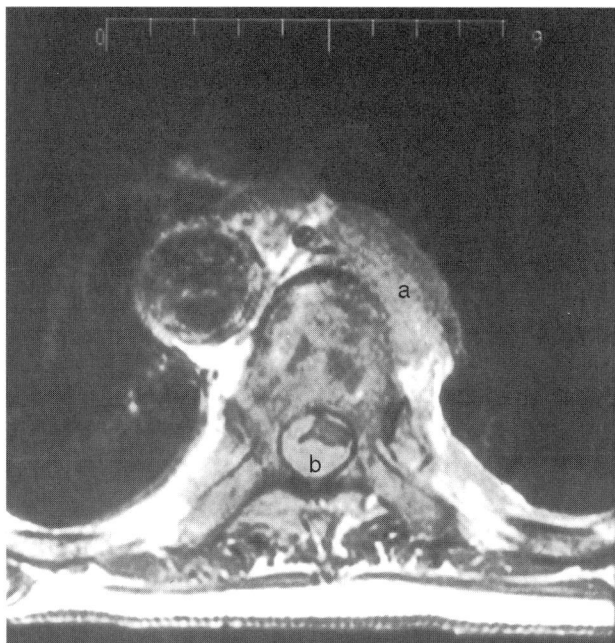

FIGURE 58D.3   A T1-weighted axial post–gadolinium-pentetic acid contrast magnetic resonance image at the level of the midthoracic spine demonstrates a contrast-enhanced paravertebral mass (a) consistent with non–small cell lung cancer. Spinal cord compression is secondary to epidural extension of this paravertebral mass (b).

Prognostic Variables

Severity of weakness at time of diagnosis is the most significant prognostic variable for recovery of neurological function. Ninety percent of patients who are ambulatory at diagnosis remain ambulatory after treatment. After radiation, 75% of paraparetic patients with radiosensitive tumors remain ambulatory, whereas only 34% with radioresistant tumors remain ambulatory. In contrast, only 13% of paraplegic patients with radiosensitive tumors and none with radioresistant tumors become ambulatory. Rate of onset and progression of symptoms correlate better with outcome than does duration. Outcome also depends on the radiosensitivity of the primary tumor. Myeloma, lymphoma, neuroblastoma, and to a lesser degree, breast and prostate cancer, have a more favorable prognosis; non–small cell lung cancer, renal cancer, and melanoma have a poor prognosis. The extent and location of epidural disease also influence the response to treatment. Vertebral collapse and anterior location of the metastasis is less favorable because surgical access is limited, and a partial myelographic block has a more favorable prognosis for neurological recovery than a complete block.

Treatment

ESCC is usually associated with inadequate control of the primary tumor, and survival time is short. Treatment of ESCC is palliative and directed at maintaining ambula-

tion, decreasing tumor bulk, and relieving pain. Patients with advanced cancer and poor performance status are treated conservatively. In those without advanced disease, expeditious diagnosis and treatment should improve or at least maintain neurological function. High-dose corticosteroids are started immediately, followed by radiotherapy and sometimes chemotherapy. Corticosteroids rapidly decrease spinal cord vasogenic edema and promote clinical improvement in relation to dose administered. Dexamethasone, 100 mg intravenously followed by 24 mg every 6 hours, is recommended. The usual maintenance dose is 4 mg every 6 hours. An intravenous bolus of high-dose dexamethasone may cause severe but transitory (5-minute) dysesthesias of the genitalia. Other side effects include hiccoughs, psychosis, hallucinations, hyperglycemia, gastrointestinal bleeding, and drug interaction (phenytoin and warfarin).

Recommendations conflict for the treatment of ESCC. Historically, decompressive laminectomy had been the most common treatment for ESCC. Improved outcomes have also been obtained with the combination of laminectomy and radiotherapy. Other studies showed no difference between radiotherapy and laminectomy plus radiotherapy. Radiotherapy alone is now the treatment of choice. Patients with radiosensitive tumors (e.g., lymphoma, seminoma, myeloma, Ewing's sarcoma, and neuroblastoma) respond, but patients with radioresistant tumors (e.g., lung, colon, renal, and melanoma) also respond as well to radiotherapy alone as to combined surgery and radiation. The recommended radiation fields are two normal vertebral bodies above and below the margins of epidural tumor. Because epidural metastasis may occur at multiple levels, the entire spinal cord must be visualized by MRI or myelography (Figure 58D.3). The frequency of local recurrence after initial response, independent of histology, is approximately 10%. Most radiation oncologists recommend 3,000 cGy over 10 fractions. If the irradiated volume is large or if the tumor is highly radiosensitive, a smaller daily dose is usually used.

Decompressive laminectomy is indicated in patients with a posteriorly situated epidural metastasis in the absence of vertebral disease. ESCC in children is often from tumors (e.g., neuroblastoma) that invade the spinal canal through the neural foramen. In this situation, decompressive laminectomy may be effective. Because metastatic tumor is anterior to the cord in 85% of cases, vertebral body resection followed by stabilization offers the best results. The reported surgical morbidity is 9%, but the ambulation rate increased from 28% to 80% postoperatively, and median survival is 16 months. Postoperation radiation therapy is required (Table 58D.2).

With few exceptions, ESCCs do not respond to chemotherapy rapidly enough to prevent neurological deterioration. Systemic chemotherapy can be used to treat chemosensitive tumors with stable or slowly progressive neurological deficits because such epidural tumors are not protected by the blood-brain barrier. The best results have occurred with small cell tumors, such as lymphoma, germ cell tumors, neuroblastoma, or Ewing's sarcoma. Chemotherapy or hormonal therapy also may be effective in breast and prostate cancer. Some promising results have been achieved with systemic chemotherapy in children with chemosensitive tumors, but further studies are needed.

Overall, tumor type is a more important determinant of the functional outcome than type of treatment. The life expectancy of patients with bronchogenic carcinoma is 87 days; for breast cancer, it is 7 months; and for hematological malignancies, it is 12 months.

Extradural Primary Spinal Neoplasms

Tumors of the vertebral column, unlike tumors of all other bones, are more often malignant than benign. Myeloma is the only common primary tumor of the spine in adults. Neuroblastoma and Ewing's sarcoma are the main malignant spinal tumors of childhood, and despite substantial morbidity with early treatment, the outcome is often favorable because these tumors are relatively sensitive to radiation and chemotherapy.

Multiple myeloma is a plasma cell neoplasm that accounts for up to 33% of bone tumors. The peak incidence is in the sixth through eighth decades. It is twice as common in African-Americans as in Americans of European ancestry. Polyneuropathy is sometimes associated and confuses the diagnosis of spinal cord compression. ESCC occurs in 10–15% of people with multiple myeloma. The median age of onset of plasmacytomas is 50 years, and the male-to-female ratio is 3 to 1. Most plasmacytomas evolve into multiple myeloma after 10 years. Radiation and chemotherapy remain the treatments of choice.

Ewing's sarcoma accounts for nearly 20% of spinal cord compression in children. Osteosarcoma and neuroblastoma are next in frequency. Neuroblastoma is the most common cause of spinal cord compression in children less than 5 years of age. Intensive chemotherapy and radiotherapy are beneficial in the treatment of Ewing's sarcoma, neuroblastoma, and osteosarcoma. Chordomas arise from notochordal remnants. Their location is the sacrococcygeal area in 50% of cases and the skull base in 35%. Chordomas are the second most common tumors of the spine. Peak incidence is the fifth through seventh decades (the same as that for metastatic cancer). Hematogenous dissemination occurs in 33% of cases. Surgery, the primary therapy, is followed by radiation when resection is incomplete.

INTRADURAL TUMORS

Leptomeningeal Metastasis

Leptomeningeal metastasis (LM) occurs when tumor cells infiltrate the arachnoid and the pia mater (leptomeninges),

Table 58D.2: Indications for surgical intervention in epidural spinal cord compression

Need for tissue diagnosis
Spinal instability
Progressive deterioration during chemotherapy or radiotherapy
Recurrent disease in previously irradiated site
Rapidly progressive cord compression by a known radio-
    resistant tumor

Source: Modified with permission from N Sundaresan, HH Schmidek, AL Schiller, et al. Tumors of the Spine: Diagnosis and Clinical Management. Philadelphia: Saunders, 1990.

causing focal or multifocal infiltration. LM develops in approximately 5–8% of patients with non-Hodgkin's lymphoma and up to 70% of patients with leukemia. Adenocarcinomas are the most common solid tumors causing LM. Breast cancer is first, followed by lung, melanoma, and gastrointestinal cancers. The prevalence of LM is increased in long-term survivors of melanoma and small cell lung cancer.

Untreated primary central nervous system (CNS) tumors, such as medulloblastoma, ependymoma, and glioma, also have a high frequency of LM. CNS prophylaxis has markedly decreased the risk of LM in leukemia. The risk factors for leptomeningeal lymphomatosis in non-Hodgkin's lymphoma are bone marrow and testicular involvement, extranodal disease, epidural invasion, diffuse histology, Burkitt's syndrome, and lymphoblastic histology. Most primary CNS lymphomas are parenchymal, often leading to leptomeningeal spread, whereas systemic lymphomas are primarily meningeal with secondary parenchymal invasion.

Pathology

The characteristic pathologic features of LM are thin, sheetlike layers of tumor cells, multifocal nodules, infiltration of cranial or spinal nerve roots (or both), and superficial invasion of the brain and spinal cord through the Virchow-Robin spaces. Tumor infiltration is more prominent along the ventral surface of the brain and the dorsal surface of the spinal cord. LM is associated with a high frequency of brain metastasis (42%) and dural metastasis (16–37%). ESCC is seen in 1–5% of patients with LM. Most breast or lung cancers that cause LM have spread directly from vertebral or paravertebral metastasis, whereas gastrointestinal cancer invades through the perineural spaces. Deep CNS parenchymal metastasis occurs through hematogenous spread.

Clinical Features

The clinical features of LM are referable to the cerebrum, cranial nerves, or spinal nerve roots, individually and in combination. The features of cranial nerve involvement, in order of decreasing frequency, are ocular motor palsies,

Table 58D.3: Leptomeningeal metastases from solid tumors in 90 patients: cerebrospinal fluid (CSF) findings

	Initial (%)	Subsequent (%)
Pressure >160 mm CSF	50	71
Cells >5/µl	57	70
Protein >50 mg/dl	81	89
Glucose <40 mg/dl	31	41
Positive cytology	54	91
Normal	3	1

Source: Reprinted with permission from WR Wasserstrom, JP Glass, JB Posner. Diagnosis and treatment of leptomeningeal metastases from solid tumors: experience with 90 patients. Cancer 1982;49:549–772.

facial weakness, hearing loss, vision loss, facial numbness, and tongue deviation. Headache and encephalopathy are common. Seizures occur in 6% of patients. In the spine, the lumbosacral roots are most commonly involved. This results in a cauda equina syndrome of asymmetrical weakness, dermatomal sensory loss, and paresthesias. Pain is an initial symptom in 25% of patients.

The pathophysiology of clinical symptoms and signs of LM may be due to hydrocephalus, parenchymal invasion, ischemia, metabolic competition, immune responses, and disruption of the blood-brain barrier.

Examination of the cerebrospinal fluid (CSF) is the most important test for LM. Only 3% of initial lumbar punctures yield normal CSF. The abnormalities, in order of decreasing frequency, are increased protein concentration, lymphocytic pleocytosis, increased CSF pressure, and positive cytology. The glucose concentration is decreased in 31% of patients. Cytological examination is the most specific test. Positive cytology is seen on initial CSF examination in 54% of cases, and the yield increases to above 90% when three separate spinal taps are performed (Table 58D.3). The best yield is obtained when CSF is taken from the symptomatic area. False-negative CSF cytology results are common, but they can be minimized by good technique. This involves withdrawing at least 10.5 ml of CSF for cytological analysis, processing the CSF specimen immediately, obtaining CSF from the site of known leptomeningeal disease, and repeating the procedure at least once after initial cytology is negative (Glantz et al. 1998). CSF markers, such as carcinoembryonic antigen, β-glucuronidase, β₂-microglobulin, and lactate dehydrogenase are more useful for following the response to treatment than for initial diagnosis.

Newer techniques for diagnosing LM include flow cytometry and monoclonal antibodies. Polymerase chain reaction techniques have increased the sensitivity in diagnosis of lymphomatous meningitis. This technique is based on detection of clonal rearrangements of the immunoglobulin or T-cell receptor genes (Rhodes et al. 1996).

Neuroimaging

Gadolinium-enhanced MRI is the modality of choice and has almost twice the sensitivity of CT myelography. MRI

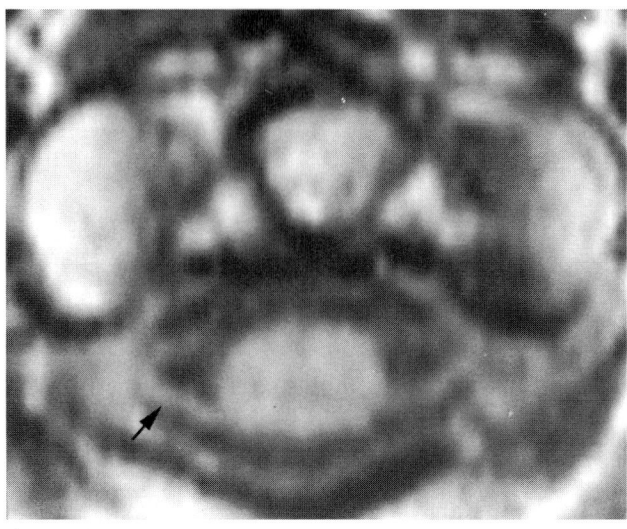

A

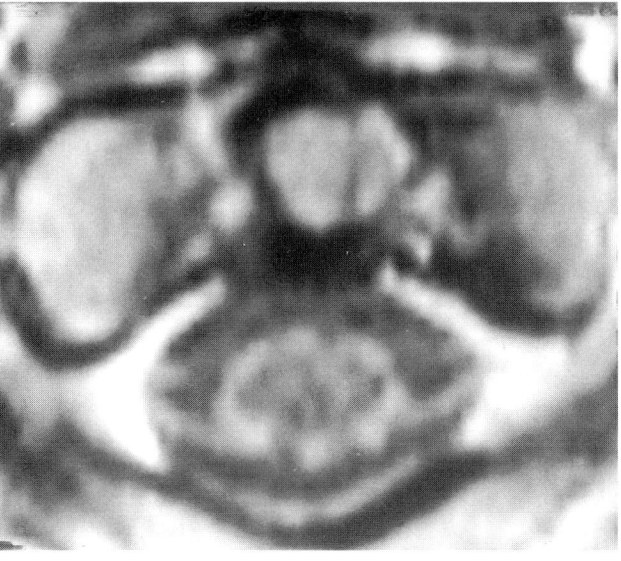

B

FIGURE 58D.4 Leptomeningeal metastasis. T1-weighted axial magnetic resonance images at C1 show thickened nerve roots (*arrow*) (**A**). Leptomeningeal enhancement with gadolinium shows "sugar coating" of the spinal cord and nerve roots (**B**).

shows thin, linear enhancement on the surface of nerve roots and the spinal cord (Figure 58D.4). Sensitivity may be increased with high-dose contrast studies. Enhanced spinal MRI may detect LM in about one-half of patients who are at high risk of CSF seeding with a negative initial CSF cytology or no spinal symptoms. Treatment should be initiated on the basis of MRI even when CSF cytology is normal, if the clinical setting is supportive of LM (Gomori et al. 1998).

Treatment

The median survival of untreated patients with LM is 4–6 weeks. Most patients die from progressive neurological dysfunction. Radiotherapy is combined with intrathecal and systemic chemotherapy. Radiation therapy is delivered to the symptomatic site at a dose of 2,000–3,000 cGy in 10–15 fractions. Total cranial-spinal axis radiotherapy is used only for meningeal leukemia because of myelosuppression. Intrathecal therapy is favored because systemic chemotherapy is probably not as effective in treating LM from solid tumors. An intraventricular reservoir is the recommended method to deliver intrathecal chemotherapy because it provides a more uniform distribution of drug in the CSF. It also allows frequent repetitions of low dosages of chemotherapeutic agents by means of a "concentration × time" regimen, which theoretically improves effectiveness without increasing toxicity. This is especially important when using methotrexate and cytosine arabinoside because they are cell cycle–specific agents and need fairly constant CSF levels to be effective. Methotrexate, 12–20 mg reconstituted in preservative-free sterile normal saline, is the mainstay of intrathecal chemotherapy for solid tumors. Cytosine arabinoside (ara-C), 30–100 mg, is substituted or added to methotrexate in LM from lymphoma or leukemia. Among patients with leukemia and lymphoma, 75–80% show a CSF response or clinical response to intrathecal chemotherapy, but patients with solid tumors, such as breast cancer, have a 40–80% response rate and a median survival of 6–7 months. The overall response rate for non–small cell lung cancer and melanoma is less than 20%.

With radioisotope ventriculography, more than 60% of patients show ventricular outlet, spinal, or convexity blocks due to leptomeningeal seeding. CSF flow blocks, when untreated, increase morbidity by increasing neurotoxicity (high-concentration effect), increase CSF tumor progression (protective site effect), and increase systemic toxicity (reservoir effect). These flow abnormalities may be corrected with appropriately directed radiotherapy. Intrathecal chemotherapy should be preceded by a radionuclide flow study and should be delayed if abnormal flow is documented until appropriate radiotherapy re-establishes normal flow (Chamberlain and Kormanik 1996).

Intradural Extramedullary Primary Neoplasms

Most primary intradural extramedullary neoplasms are histologically benign tumors, such as meningiomas (25%), nerve sheath tumors (29%), and developmental tumors (epidermoids, dermoids, lipomas, and teratomas) (Table 58D.4).

Meningiomas

Most meningiomas arise from arachnoid cells. More than 90% are intradural, 6% are both intradural and extradural, and 7% are only extradural. Multiple meningiomas are rare except in patients with neurofibromatosis type 2. The peak incidence of meningiomas is between ages 40 and 70 years; 85% are in women, and 80% are located in the thoracic spine. Meningiomas in men are commonly located in the cervical spine, tend to grow rapidly, and have an intradural and extradural component.

Table 58D.4: Mayo Clinic classification of 1,322 primary tumors of the spinal canal

Type	Frequency (%)
Neurilemomas (schwannomas)	29.0
Meningioma	25.5
Glioma (astrocytoma, ependymoma)	22.0
"Sarcoma" (lipoma, fibrosarcoma, chondromas, lymphomas)	11.9
Vascular tumors	6.2
Chordoma	4.0
Epidermoid, dermoid, teratoma	1.4

Source: Modified with permission from JL Sloof, JW Kernohan, CS MacCarty. Primary Intramedullary Tumors of the Spinal Cord and Filum Terminale. Philadelphia: Saunders, 1964.

The initial symptom of spinal meningiomas, like other spinal tumors, is usually pain followed by paraparesis and sensory disturbances. The average duration of symptoms from onset to diagnosis is 23 months. Bone is not often affected, and only 10% have radiographic abnormalities. Myelography shows a characteristic displacement of the spinal cord away from the mass and enlargement of the subarachnoid space above and below the tumor. Meningiomas have a homogeneous appearance on MRI and are usually isointense to spinal cord on T1-weighted and T2-weighted sequences. Surgery is the treatment of choice. The recurrence rate is 13% after 10 years (see Table 58D.4 for frequency of spinal cord tumors of all types).

Nerve Sheath Tumors

Nerve sheath tumors are schwannomas and neurofibromas. Schwannomas (neurilemomas) are composed of Schwann cells and produce an eccentric enlargement of the involved nerve root. Neurofibromas are a mixture of Schwann cells and fibroblasts with abundant collagen fibers and cause diffuse enlargement of the nerve root. Nerve sheath tumors comprise 29% of primary spinal cord tumors (Figure 58D.5).

Nerve sheath tumors are evenly distributed along the spinal axis. Men and women are equally affected. Age at onset is usually between 31 and 60 years; average age is 43.5 years for nerve sheath tumors and 53 years for spinal meningiomas. Two-thirds of tumors are intradural, and of the remainder, one-half are dumbbell-shaped (intra-extradural) and one-half are extradural.

Pain is the initial feature in 75% of patients. It may be axial, radicular, or referred (distant nondermatomal pain). Pain is exacerbated by Valsalva's maneuver, coughing, sneezing, and recumbency. Mean duration of symptoms before diagnosis averages 1–4 years. Weakness and sensory symptoms predominate at the time of diagnosis; sphincter dysfunction is uncommon. Malignant deterioration of a neurofibroma (neurofibrosarcoma) occurs in 3–13% of all cases; one-half of those are people with neurofibromatosis.

Radiographs of the spine are abnormal in 50% of cases. The usual finding is widening of the intervertebral foramen, erosion of the pedicle or vertebral body, and widening of

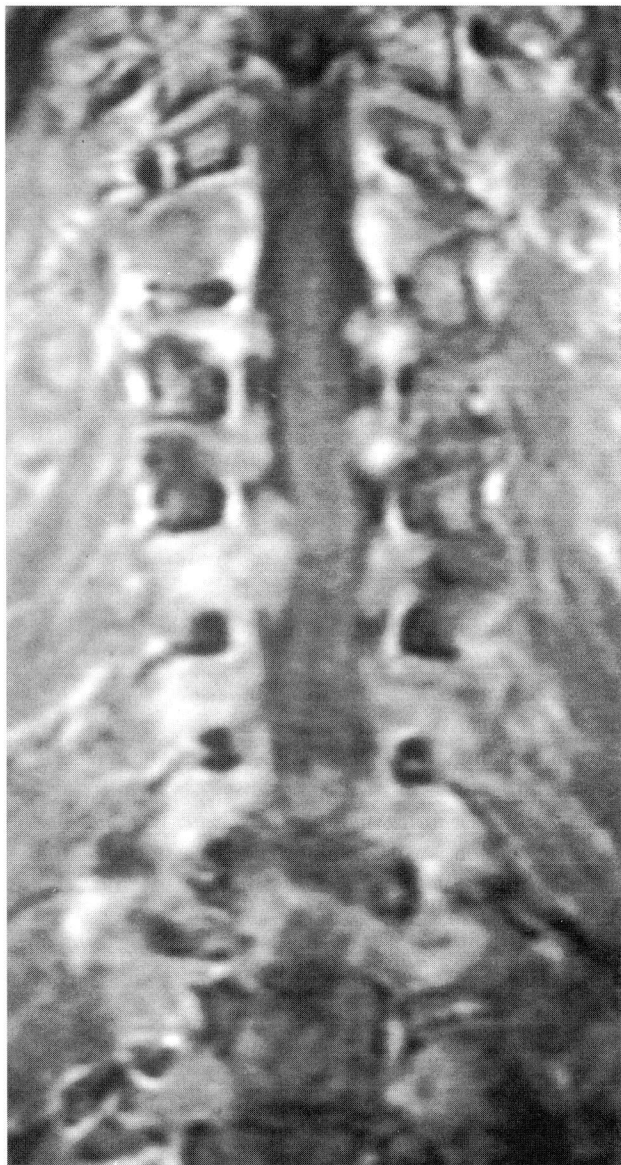

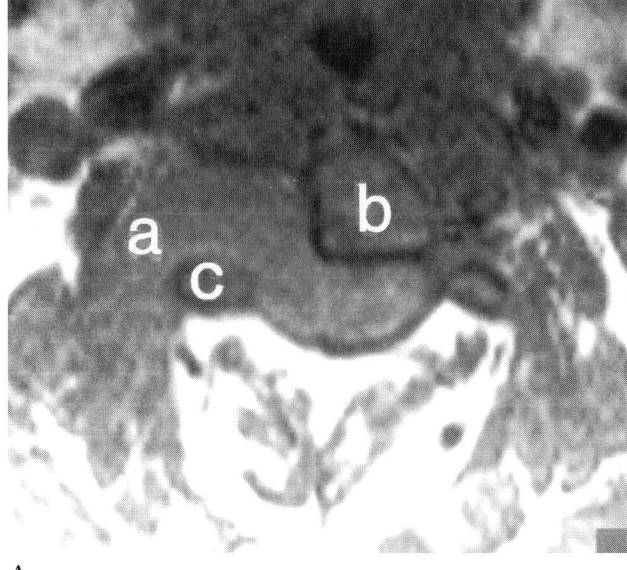

A

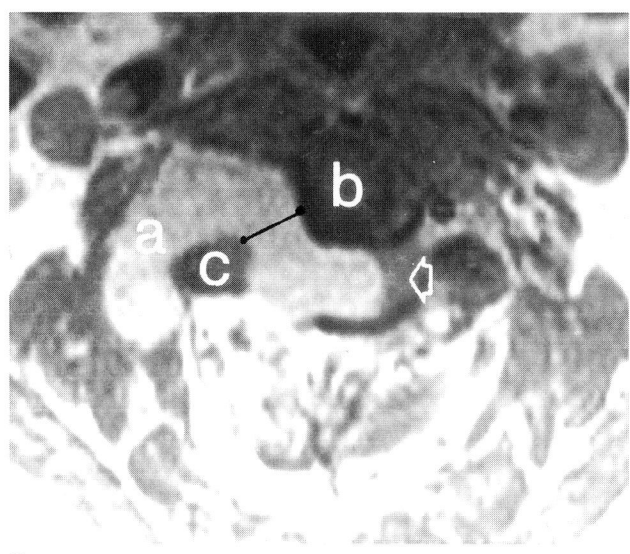

B

FIGURE 58D.5 Contrast T1-weighted coronal magnetic resonance image of the cervical spine shows multiple bilateral enhancing neurofibromas with distortion of the spinal cord in a patient with neurofibromatosis.

FIGURE 58D.6 Axial T1-weighted magnetic resonance images with and without gadolinium. (A) Unenhanced study shows an isointense dumbbell-shaped schwannoma that extends through the intervertebral foramina of C2-C3. (B) Contrast enhancement shows a hyperintense mass (a) compressing the spinal cord and enlarging the foramen between the vertebral body (b) and the pedicle (c). The arrow points to the compressed spinal cord.

the interpedicular distance (Figure 58D.6). CT, myelography, or MRI provides a definitive image. Intradural schwannomas are usually hypointense on T1-weighted images and hyperintense on T2-weighted images. Ringlike enhancement is considered a sign of cystic degeneration and is more consistent with schwannoma than meningioma.

Embryonal Tumors

Embryonal tumors (epidermoid, dermoid cysts, teratomas, and lipomas) comprise 1–2% of primary spinal tumors. They are usually found in the lumbar region and associated with spina bifida occulta, posterior dermal sinuses, syringomyelia, or diastematomyelia. Associated cutaneous abnormalities may

be found, including hypertrichosis, pigmented skin, sacral dimple, and cutaneous angiomas. Most lipomas are in the cervicothoracic region and are intramedullary as well as intradural-extramedullary. MRI shows high signal intensity on T1-weighted and low signal–intensity T2-weighted images.

Intramedullary Spinal Cord Tumors

Intramedullary spinal cord tumors, both primary and metastatic, account for 2–4% of adult and 10% of pedi-

Table 58D.5: McCormick clinical/functional classification scheme

Grade	Definition
I	Neurologically normal; mild focal deficit not significantly affecting function of involved limb; mild spasticity or reflex abnormality; normal gait.
II	Presence of sensorimotor deficit affecting function of involved limb; mild to moderate gait difficulty; severe pain or dysesthetic syndrome impairing patient's quality of life; still functions and ambulates independently.
III	More severe neurological deficit requires cane or brace for ambulation or significant bilateral upper extremity impairment; may or may not function independently.
IV	Severe deficit; requires wheelchair or cane or brace with bilateral upper extremity impairment; usually not independent.

atric CNS tumors. Glial tumors account for 22% of primary intraspinal tumors, the third most common after schwannomas and meningiomas. Astrocytomas and ependymomas account for 80–90% of all intramedullary tumors at all ages; in adults, ependymomas are more common than astrocytomas, whereas in children, ependymomas are more common than astrocytomas. Pediatric intramedullary astrocytic tumors are usually in the cervical cord, but some tumors extend the entire length of the cord (holocord astrocytomas). The McCormick Clinical and Functional Classification Scheme is used to prognosticate and quantify the results of treatment (Table 58D.5).

Ependymoma

One-half of all ependymomas are located below the foramen magnum and involve either the spinal cord (55%) or the cauda region (45%), which includes the conus medullaris, filum terminale, and cauda equina. Myxopapillary ependymomas are characteristically seen in the region of the filum terminale and originate from islands of ependymal cells within this fibrous band. The male-to-female ratio of spinal ependymomas is 2 to 1, and the median age of onset is 36 years. MRI has reduced the duration from symptom onset to diagnosis from 24–36 months to 14 months, and as a consequence, the frequency of weakness and sphincter involvement has decreased. The main complaint (95%) at the time of diagnosis is back pain. Most patients have dysesthesias without sensory loss. This is attributed to the location of spinal ependymomas around the central canal: The symmetrical expansion of the central canal causes an interruption of the crossing spinothalamic tracts (central cord syndrome). When pain and numbness occur in a radicular pattern involving the legs, the underlying tumor is usually a myxopapillary ependymoma involving either the filum or the conus.

MRI, with and without contrast, is the imaging modality of choice for detecting intramedullary tumors. Ependymomas have a homogeneous enhancement pattern with

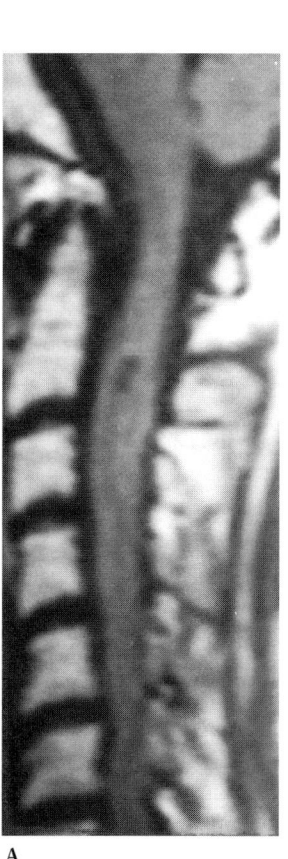
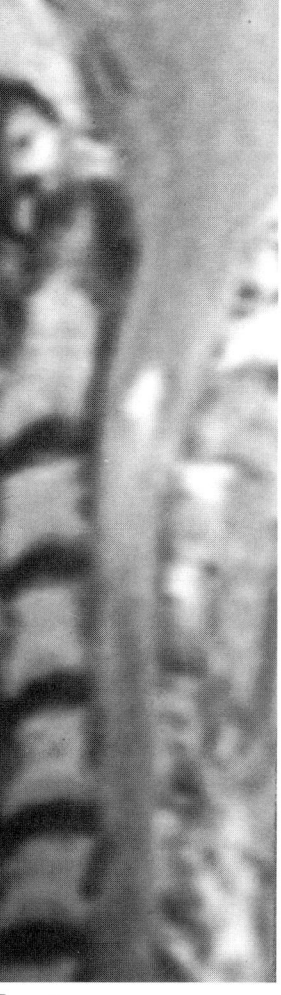

A   B

FIGURE 58D.7 Sagittal T1-weighted magnetic resonance images with and without gadolinium of the cervical spine. (**A**) Nonenhanced study shows an enlarged cervical spinal cord opposite C2-C3 with rostral cyst. (**B**) Contrast enhancement is seen within the intramedullary mass. Pathology confirmed the diagnosis of ependymoma.

sharply defined rostral and caudal poles; 30% have rostral-caudal cysts (Figure 58D.7). Hypointensity at the tumor margins on both T1- and T2-weighted images indicates a relatively firm pseudocapsule, which should suggest ependymomas. Transverse T1-weighted gadolinium-enhanced MRI shows symmetric cord enlargement and intense, homogeneous enhancement.

Ependymomas, unlike astrocytomas, have a cleavage plane and tend not to invade normal tissue. Most ependymomas can be debulked with minimal morbidity. Patients with leg weakness usually show significant spinal cord thinning at surgery, which makes further excision hazardous. The common postoperative complications are a temporary increase in dysesthesias and a loss of proprioception. Postoperative radiotherapy is not indicated after total resection but should be done when MRI shows residual tumor or the histology indicates an anaplastic ependymoma. The 10-year survival rate is greater than 90%, with especially good results in patients with myxopapillary tumors.

Astrocytoma

Excluding cauda equina tumors, astrocytoma is the most common intramedullary spinal tumor in all ages; in children, astrocytoma is twice as common as ependymoma. The peak incidence is in the third to fifth decade of life. The average age at onset is 40 years for low-grade astrocytoma and 31 years for malignant astrocytoma. Overall, more than 75% are low-grade gliomas. Malignancy is more common in adults than in children. The distribution of astrocytomas is consistent with the length of cord segments; most are in the thoracic region. Up to 40% of astrocytomas have an associated intratumoral cyst or syringomyelia.

The clinical features of spinal cord astrocytoma are localized back pain initially, followed by progressive weakness. Unlike ependymomas, paresthesias are more common than dysesthesias. The duration of symptoms before diagnosis is 41 months for low-grade astrocytomas and 4–7 months for malignant astrocytomas. Unlike most intracranial low-grade astrocytomas, spinal astrocytomas enhance with gadolinium. MRI shows a patchy, heterogeneous pattern of enhancement consistent with a diffusely infiltrating tumor. Axial MRIs usually show asymmetric expansion of the cord. Astrocytomas are solitary, except in patients with NF-2. Malignant astrocytomas spread through the subarachnoid pathways and seed the leptomeninges. The complete spine and brain must be fully imaged to establish a treatment plan.

Therapy for intramedullary astrocytomas is controversial. Innovations in neurosurgery, such as bipolar coagulating forceps, operating microscopes, intraoperative ultrasonography, and the Cavitron ultrasonic surgical aspirator, have greatly increased the resectability of astrocytomas. However, the small number of cases and the indolent natural history of the tumor make evaluation of treatment efficacy difficult. Postoperative adjuvant therapy is not needed when gross total resection is achieved, but postoperative radiation is recommended after subtotal resection. Tumor recurs in children receiving 4,500 cGy of radiation, which suggests that this dose is not curative. The 5-year survival rate with low-grade astrocytoma is greater than 90%. The mean survival time for anaplastic astrocytoma and glioblastoma multiforme is less than 1 year, despite surgery, radiotherapy, and chemotherapy. Radical surgery is not indicated.

Intramedullary Metastasis

Intramedullary spinal cord metastasis accounts for 6% of myelopathies in cancer patients (Schiff and O'Neill 1996). The primary cancers responsible for intramedullary metastasis are lung (49%), breast (15%), lymphoma (9%), colorectal (7%), head and neck (6%), and renal (6%) (Figure 58D.8). There is a relative tendency for small cell lung carcinoma to metastasize to the spinal cord.

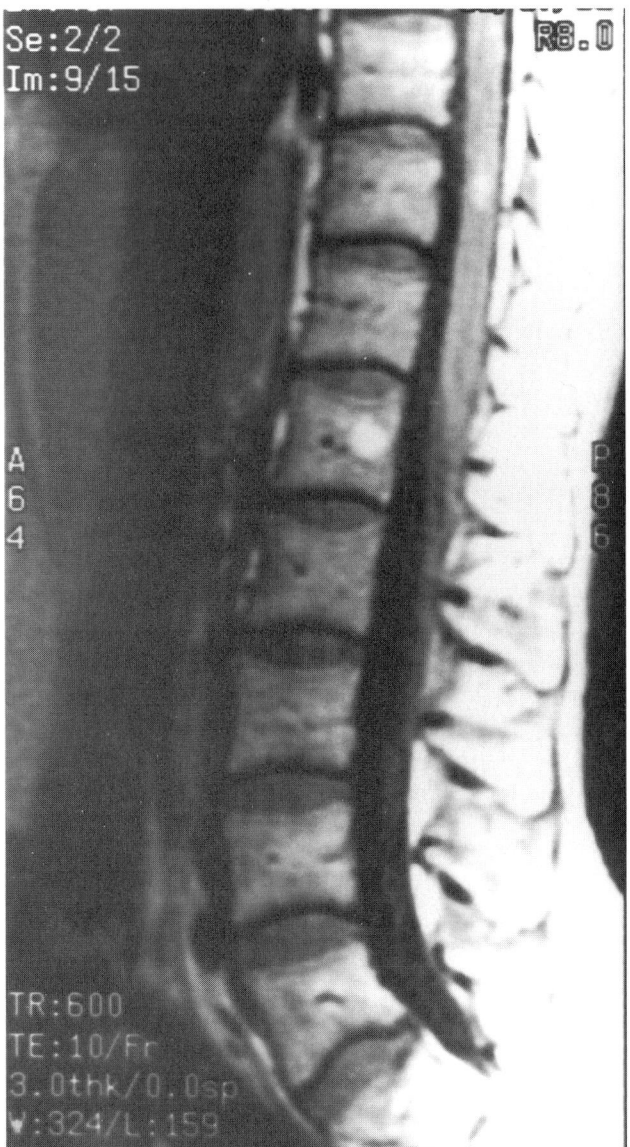

A

FIGURE 58D.8   Breast metastases to the lower thoracic spinal cord. (A) Sagittal T1-weighted noncontrast image shows an intramedullary hyperintensity, representing either hemorrhagic or mucinous metastases. (B) Sagittal T1-weighted image after gadolinium-pentetic acid administration shows an enhancing intramedullary lesion opposite the T11 vertebral body. (C) Sagittal T2-weighted image shows the metastasis as an area of relative hypointensity. In addition, there is evidence of cord edema rostral or caudal to the metastasis.

Intramedullary spinal metastases are thought to be arterially disseminated, a notion that is supported by the fact that one-half of patients have brain metastases. The conus medullaris is the most commonly affected segment, with 12.5% of patients having multilevel disease.

Three-fourths of patients develop significant neurological deficits within 1 month. The most common initial features are weakness, sensory deficits, urinary incontinence, and

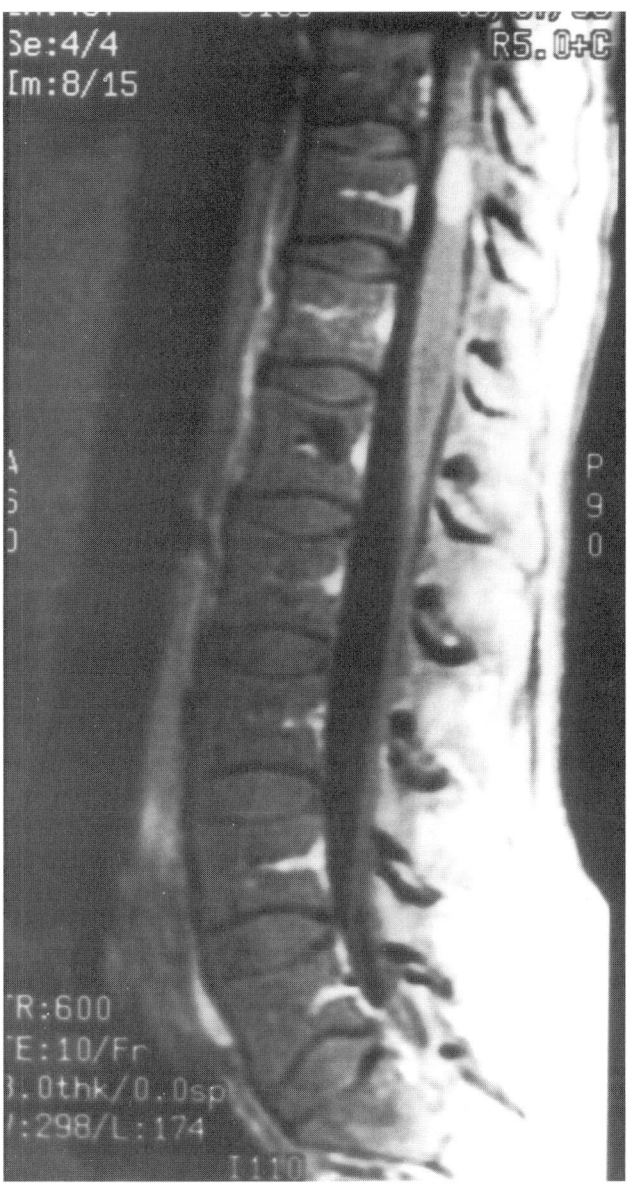

B

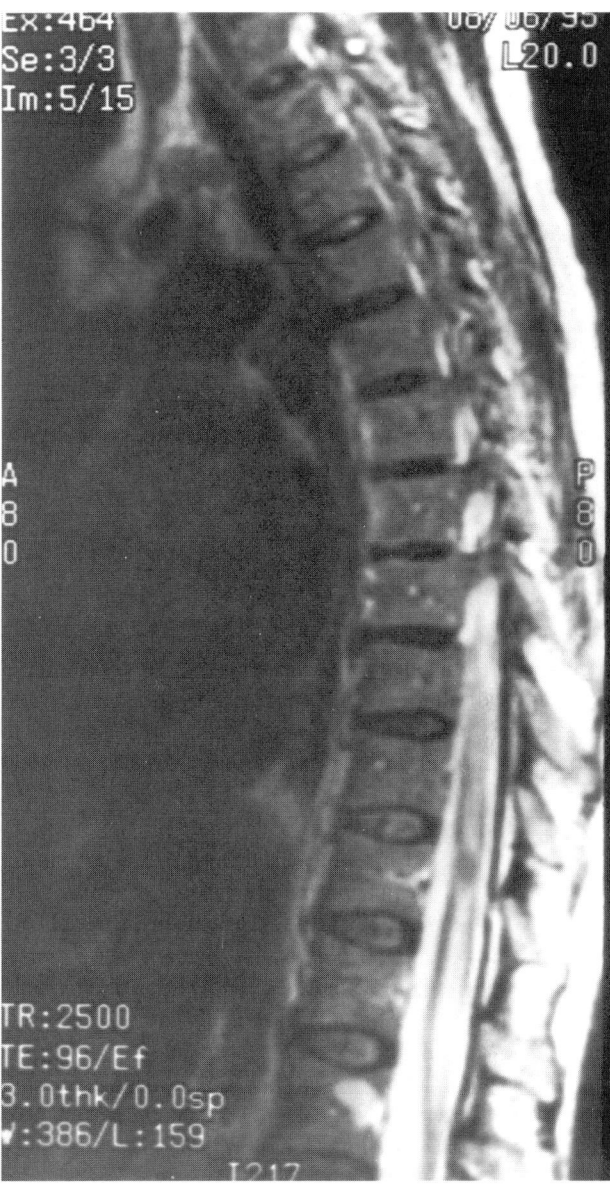

C

pain. Weakness from intramedullary metastasis is usually asymmetrical, whereas weakness from ESCC is relatively symmetrical. MRI is the investigation of choice. Focal beam radiation is recommended. The prognosis is poor, with 80% expected to die within 3 months (Schiff and O'Neill 1996).

REFERENCES

Chamberlain MC, Kormanik PA. Prognostic significance of III-indium-DTPA CSF flow studies in leptomeningeal metastases. Neurology 1996;46:1674–1677.

Glantz MJ, Cole BF, Glantz LK, et al. Cerebrospinal fluid cytology in patients with cancer: minimizing false negative results. Cancer 1998;82:733–739.

Gomori JM, Heching N, Siegal T. Leptomeningeal metastases: evaluation by gadolinium-enhanced spinal magnetic resonance enhanced imaging. J Neurooncol 1998;36:55–60.

Rhodes CH, Glantz MJ, Glantz LK, et al. A comparison of polymerase chain reaction examination of cerebrospinal fluid and conventional cytology in the diagnosis of lymphomatous meningitis. Cancer 1996;77:543–548.

Schiff D, O'Neill BP. Intramedullary spinal cord metastasis: clinical features and treatment outcome. Neurology 1996;47:906–912.

Chapter 58
Primary and Secondary Tumors
of the Central Nervous System

E. CLINICAL PRESENTATION AND THERAPY
OF PERIPHERAL NERVE TUMORS

Laszlo L. Mechtler and Michael E. Cohen

Peripheral nerve tumors are located on cranial nerves, spinal nerve roots, peripheral nerves, and the sympathetic chain. The cells of origin are neurons or nerve sheath cells. Tumors of neuronal origin, whether central or peripheral, are rare. Tumors of nerve sheath origin are composed of Schwann cells, perineural cells, or fibroblasts. The Schwann cell, like oligodendroglia in the central nervous system, forms myelin sheaths. It originates from the neural crest, as do sensory and autonomic neurons, meningocytes, melanocytes, chromaffin cells, and perineural cells. The endoneurium is the content of the nerve fascicles, comprising the connective tissue of the nerve fascicle, the individual nerve fibers with their Schwann cell sheaths, and the endoneurial capillaries. The smallest connective tissue unit of the nerve is the endoneurium, which encircles individual nerve fibers. The Schwann cell is the innermost component of the endoneurium; other components are capillaries, collagen fibers, and fibroblasts. The endoneurium is surrounded by the perineurium, which is composed of flattened specialized cells, each with a basal lamina. This perineurial layer is in direct continuity with the pia-arachnoid. The epineurium is the outermost sheath of the nerve, and it encompasses several nerve fascicles. The gross anatomical structure is recognized as the nerve, including blood vessels and connective tissue that are mesodermal in origin (Figure 58E.1).

Electron microscopy and immunohistochemistry are necessary for accurate diagnosis of peripheral nerve tumors. S-100 protein, Leu-7, myelin basic protein, and glial fibrillary acidic protein are immunohistochemical markers of Schwann cells. Perineural cells stain with antibodies that react to the epithelial membrane antigen but not to the S-100 protein, and they function as a diffusion barrier. Schwann cells and perineural cells have basal laminae that are absent in fibroblasts. Schwann cells probably synthesize their basal laminae. Immunohistochemical staining and ultrastructural findings are most helpful in differentiating malignant peripheral nerve sheath tumors (MPNSTs) from other soft tissue sarcomas, such as fibrosarcomas, synovial sarcomas, and leiomyosarcomas.

The World Health Organization classifies anaplastic peripheral nerve tumors as MPNSTs instead of individually referring to neurogenic sarcomas, anaplastic neurofibromas, or malignant schwannomas (Wanebo et al. 1993). Schwannomas and neurofibromas are the most common benign peripheral nerve tumors. The Schwann cell is thought to be the cell of origin in both. Other benign peripheral nerve growths are hamartomas, cysts, and neuromas (Table 58E.1).

SCHWANNOMAS

Schwannomas account for 8% of all intracranial primary tumors in adults. Eighty percent to 90% of those occur in the cerebellopontine angle. They are also the most common spinal nerve tumor. Previously, schwannomas were described as either neurilemomas or neurinomas, although *schwannoma* is now the preferred terminology. The salient

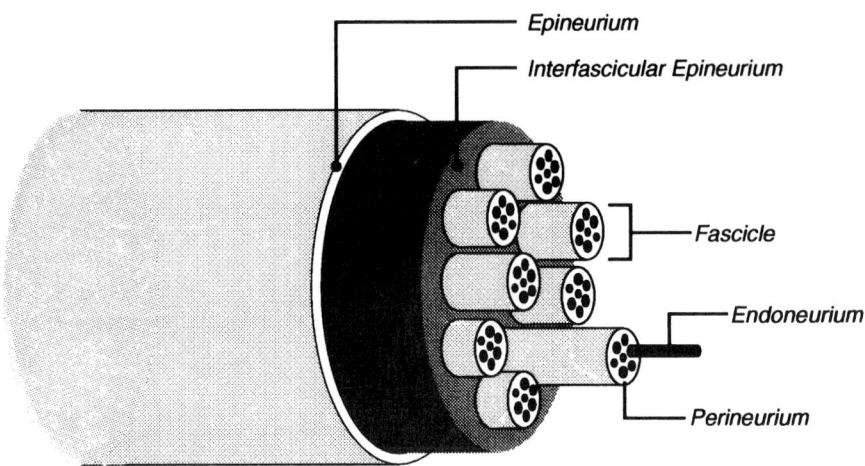

FIGURE 58E.1   A cross-sectional diagram of a peripheral nerve demonstrating the endoneurium, which contains the neural elements. Bundles of nerve fibers are bound by the perineurium to form fascicles. The epineurium surrounds and lies between the fascicles and forms a barrier, creating an endoneurial microenvironment.

feature of neurofibromatosis type 2 (NF-2) is the vestibular schwannoma that occurs bilaterally in more than 95% of patients. Two-thirds of patients with NF-2 develop spinal or subcutaneous schwannomas, which may precede the development of vestibular schwannomas. *Schwannomatosis* is the term used to describe multiple schwannomas without evidence of NF-1 or NF-2 (MacCollin et al. 1996).

Histology

Schwannomas are benign encapsulated tumors with two characteristic components: a highly cellular type (Antoni type A) and a loose myxoid type (Antoni type B). Degenerative changes are prominent in large tumors and in deep locations, such as the retroperitoneum. These changes include cyst formation, calcification, hemorrhage, and hyalinization. Schwannomas are immunoreactive for S-100 protein and to a lesser degree for Leu-7 (Figure 58E.2).

Clinical Features

Schwannomas have a predilection for flexor surfaces of the limbs and main nerve trunks. The age at presentation is 20–50 years. They are almost always solitary and arise eccentrically from within the nerve; therefore, nerve bundles are stretched over the surface of the tumor. Weakness and sensory symptoms are unusual unless the tumor is in a confined space, such as the carpal tunnel. The initial symptom is usually a painful swelling, although deep-seated tumors, especially those in the mediastinum, may grow very large before detection.

The most characteristic diagnostic feature is shooting pain and paresthesias induced by palpation of the nerve. Spontaneous pain is unusual. About 10% of schwannomas are predominantly Antoni type A and are designated *cellular schwannomas*. These are misinterpreted as malignant because of hypercellularity, hyperchromasia, and abundant mitoses in 30% of cases. Despite these features, the tumor is benign and forms a painless mass, usually in the paravertebral region of the retroperitoneum, pelvis, and mediastinum.

Plexiform or multinodular schwannomas comprise 5% of the total and occur predominantly in the subcutaneous tissue of young adults. These are also benign. Melanotic schwannomas are the rarest form of schwannoma. They originate from Schwann cells that are capable of melanogenesis and involve the nerve roots. Melanotic schwannomas are also benign but are associated with cardiac myxomas, which are the main cause of morbidity.

Diagnosis

Magnetic resonance imaging is the most specific study for evaluating peripheral nerve sheath tumors. Schwannomas

Table 58E.1:   Tumorlike conditions of the peripheral nerves

Lesion type	Signs and symptoms
Morton's neuroma (plantar neuroma)	Fibrosing process of plantar digital nerve with pain between the third and fourth metatarsals
Amputation neuroma	Disorganized proliferation of a proximal nerve after transection; tender to pressure
Nerve sheath ganglion (nerve cyst)	Mucin-filled cyst in perineurium; most commonly seen affecting the peroneal nerve
Neuromuscular hamartoma (benign triton tumor)	Mosaic tumor with mature striated muscle intermingled within nerve bundles; rare
Mucosal neuroma	Nodular thickening of lips, tongue, and eyelids of patients associated with type 2b multiple endocrine neoplasia

Source: Modified from JM Woodruff. The pathology and treatment of peripheral nerve tumors and tumor-like conditions. CA Cancer J Clin 1993;43:290–308.

FIGURE 58E.2 Classic schwannoma, composed of compact interwoven bundles of bipolar spindle cells. Note palisading. (Courtesy of RR Heffner, State University of New York, Albany.)

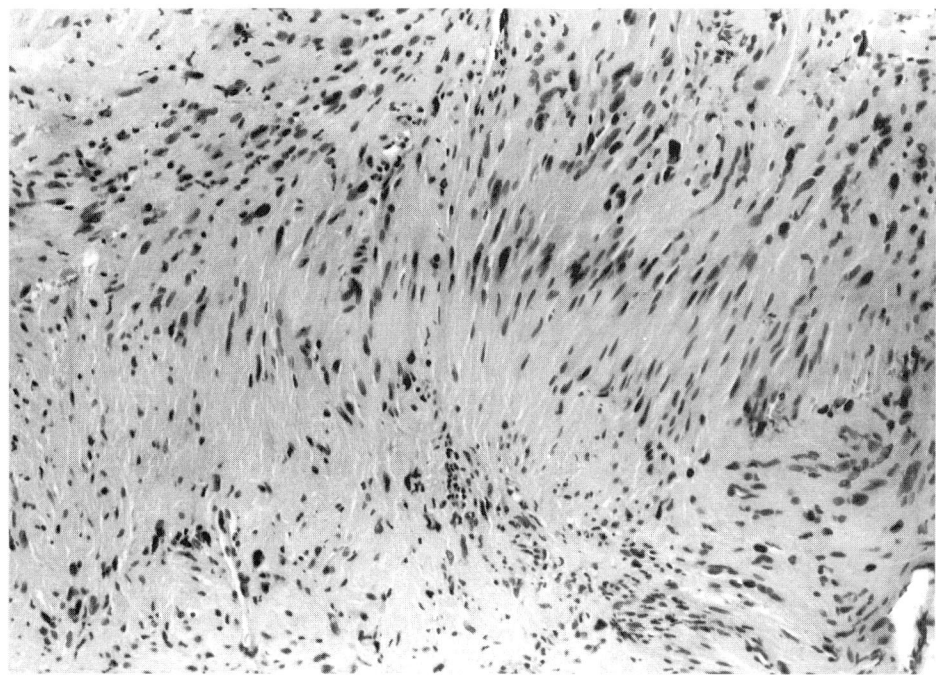

FIGURE 58E.3 Neurofibroma consisting of a mixture of proliferated Schwann cells and fibroblasts between dispersed nerve fibers. (Courtesy of RR Heffner, State University of New York, Albany.)

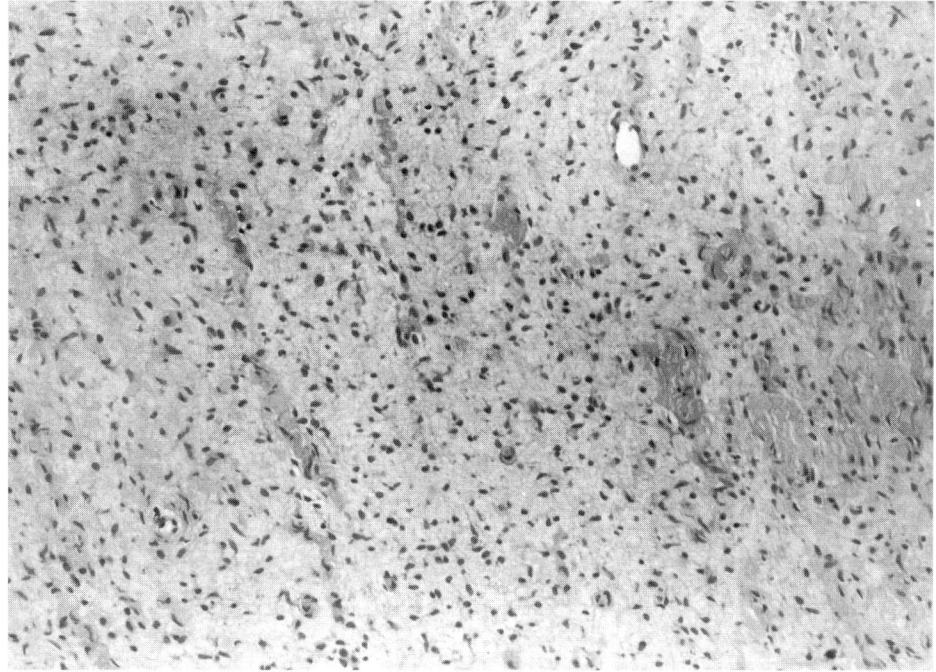

are hyperintense on T2-weighted images and isointense with muscle on T1-weighted images. Schwannomas tend to be situated at the periphery of the nerve. The development of magnetic resonance neurography has enhanced both the resolution and conspicuousness of the peripheral nerve and surrounding structures. In NF-1, two-thirds of patients can undergo complete excision of a neurofibroma, with a small percentage requiring graft repair at nerves (Donner et al. 1994). Magnetic resonance neurography is useful in assess-

ing the resectability of neurofibromas preoperatively (Kuntz et al. 1996) (Figure 58E.3).

Treatment

The goals of treatment are tumor resection with preservation of nerve function. Malignant transformation does not occur, and even after partial resection, most patients do not

Table 58E.2:   Comparison of schwannomas and neurofibromas

	Schwannoma	*Neurofibroma*
Peak age	20–50 yrs	20–30 yrs, younger in NF
Gross appearance	Encapsulated, rarely plexiform	Nonencapsulated, more often plexiform
Cut surface	Tan-brown; may be cystic hemorrhagic	Homogeneous gray and gelatinous
S-100 immunostaining	Staining relatively uniform and intense	Staining variable
Relation to NF-1	Uncommon	Predominant type
Malignant transformation	Almost never	Rare in solitary form; 4% in NF-1
Clinical symptoms	Palpation produces pain and paresthesias; motor/sensory deficits uncommon	Palpation does not commonly produce pain or paresthesias; motor/sensory deficits prominent

NF = neurofibromatosis.

experience symptomatic regrowth. Nerve function may be monitored intraoperatively by intermittently measuring nerve action potentials. Large, histologically benign schwannomas (classic, cellular, plexiform, and melanotic) should not be totally excised if removal would cause neurological deficits.

NEUROFIBROMAS

In 90% of cases, neurofibromas are solitary tumors. The age of onset is 20–30 years. Multiple tumors are seen in people with NF.

Histology

Neurofibromas have fewer Schwann cells and more collagen and reticulin fibers than schwannomas do (see Figure 58E.3). Myelinated and unmyelinated axons are characteristically included in the substance of the tumor. Tumor cells are immunoreactive for S-100 protein but not for epithelial membrane antigen.

Clinical Features

Solitary neurofibromas are located predominantly on cutaneous nerves. Patients may complain of painful swelling, but palpation of a mass does not reproduce the shooting pain and paresthesias characteristic of schwannomas. Neurofibromas more often cause weakness and sensory symptoms when noncutaneous sites are involved. Malignant transformation of solitary neurofibromas is rare.

NF is a complex disorder that affects both the neuroectoderm and mesoderm (see Chapter 69). NF-1 is subclassified into three groups: (1) multiple neurofibromas, which are usually large and involve deep and major nerves; (2) plexiform neurofibromas, which form solitary, tortuous, fusiform enlargements of nerves; and (3) diffuse neurofibromas, seen in children and young adults, forming a subcutaneous or cutaneous plaquelike elevation of the skin. NF-2 is characterized by bilateral acoustic schwannomas, peripheral neurofibromas, meningiomas, and gliomas.

Diagnosis

Magnetic resonance imaging distinguishes neurofibromas from schwannomas (Table 58E.2). Although both tumors are hyperintense on T2-weighted images and isointense with muscle on T1-weighted images, two-thirds of neurofibromas showed a target pattern of increased peripheral signal intensity and decreased central signal intensity on T2-weighted studies. Unlike schwannomas, neurofibromas are in a central position and may not be distinguishable from the nerve.

MALIGNANT PERIPHERAL NERVE SHEATH TUMORS

Most neuropathologists believe that MPNSTs arise from the Schwann cell (malignant schwannoma) but prefer the term *MPNST* because it is noncommittal in defining the cell of origin. The prevalence of MPNSTs is 0.001% in the general population and 4% in patients with NF. NF accounts for approximately 50% of MPNSTs (Wanebo et al. 1993). These usually arise from transformed solitary neurofibromas or plexiform neurofibromas. Irradiation of neurofibromas has also been implicated in malignant transformation.

Histology

MPNSTs arise as large fusiform or eccentric masses, which suggests that tumor spreads both proximally and distally along the nerve sheath. The average size at diagnosis is 5 cm. Unlike benign nerve sheath tumors, 50% of MPNSTs show large areas of necrosis. The characteristic histology is hypermitotic, densely packed, polychromatic, interlacing spindle cells with slender or curved nuclei and indistinct cytoplasm. One-half of the cells express S-100 protein (Figure 58E.5). Schwann cells, because of their origin in the neural crest,

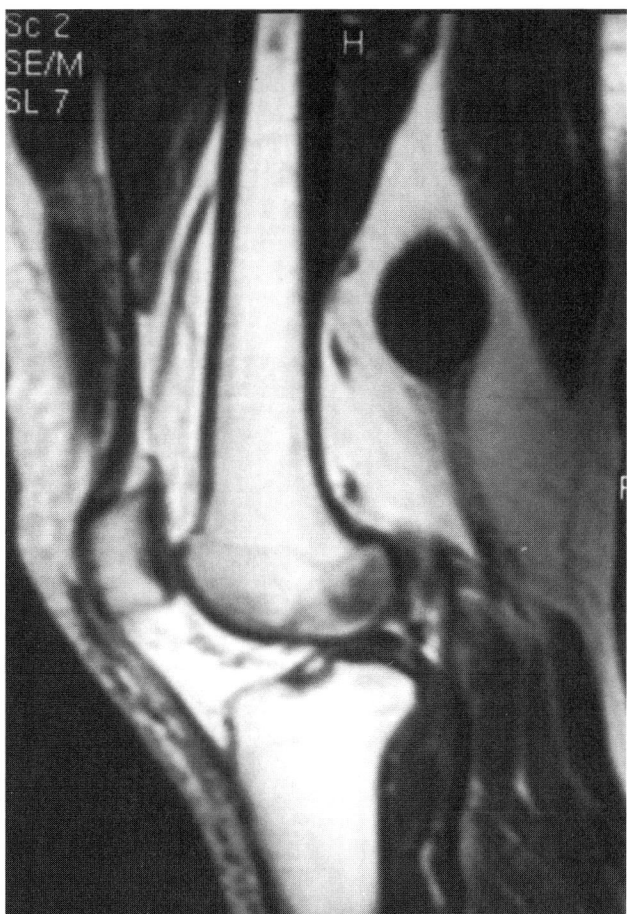

FIGURE 58E.4 A noncontrast T1-weighted sagittal image shows an eccentric, ball-like enlargement of the sciatic nerve displacing the nerve trunk posteriorly.

retain the capacity to differentiate into other cell types. This divergent differentiation occurs in 15–28% of MPNSTs.

Peripheral nerve sheath tumors with foci of rhabdomyosarcoma are called *malignant triton tumors*. Mature islands of cartilage and bone are common elements, but mucin-secreting glands are rare in these tumors.

Clinical Features

MPNSTs cause spontaneous pain, swelling, and marked motor and sensory disturbances. The swelling is firm and immovable. MPNSTs should be suspected in patients with NF-1 who experience rapid increases in size of neurofibromas, especially when associated with pain and new neurological disturbances. The sciatic nerve is the one most often involved, followed by tumors of the brachial plexus and sacral plexus (Figure 58E.4).

Treatment

MPNSTs are highly malignant tumors with a propensity for recurrence (at a rate of 45%) and metastasis, usually to the lung, liver, or bone. Median survival time from diagnosis is about 3 years. The 5-year survival rate is 34–39%. Surgical resection is the most effective treatment, usually requiring amputation of the limb or wide en bloc excision followed by adjuvant radiation therapy. Chemotherapy is ineffective. Prognosis is adversely affected by a large tumor (>5 cm), presence of NF-1, and a centrally located tumor (Hajdu 1993) (Table 58E.3).

FIGURE 58E.5 Malignant peripheral nerve sheath tumors showing pleomorphic, densely packed cells, generally configured in parallel bundles. (Courtesy of RR Heffner, State University of New York, Albany.)

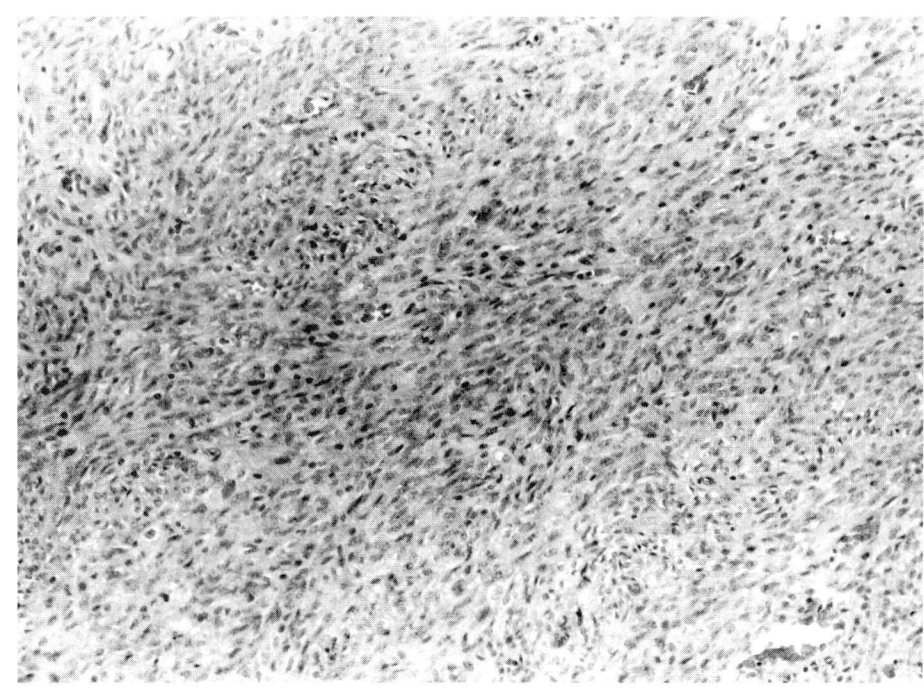

Table 58E.3:   Primary peripheral nerve sheath tumors

Schwannoma (neurilemoma)
    Classic
    Cellular
    Plexiform
    Melanotic
Neurofibroma
    Solitary
    Multiple
    Plexiform
    Diffuse
Malignant peripheral nerve sheath tumor
    Malignant triton tumors
    Glandular malignant schwannoma
    Malignant epithelioid schwannoma

REFERENCES

Donner TR, Voorhies RM, Kline DG. Neural sheath tumors of major nerves. J Neurosurgery 1994;81:362–373.

Hajdu SI. Peripheral nerve sheath tumors. Histogenesis classification and prognosis. Cancer 1993;72:3549–3552.

Kuntz C, Blake L, Britz G, et al. Magnetic resonance neurography of peripheral nerve lesions in the lower extremity. Neurosurgery 1996;39:750–756.

MacCollin M, Wardfin W, Dronn D, Short MP. Schwannomatosis: a clinical and pathologic study. Neurology 1996;46:1072–1079.

Wanebo JE, Malik JM, VandenBerg SR, et al. Malignant peripheral nerve sheath tumors: a clinicopathologic study of 28 cases. Cancer 1993;71:1247–1253.

Chapter 58
Primary and Secondary Tumors of the Central Nervous System

F.   PARANEOPLASTIC SYNDROMES
Jerome B. Posner

Paraneoplastic syndromes are disorders associated with cancer but are not a direct effect of the tumor mass or its metastases (Posner 1995). Although all nonmetastatic complications of cancer are, strictly speaking, paraneoplastic, most neurologists restrict the term *paraneoplastic syndromes* to disorders listed as remote effects of cancer (Table 58F.1).

GENERAL CONSIDERATIONS

Frequency

The frequency of paraneoplastic syndromes depends on how they are defined. Mild nervous system dysfunction, either clinical or electrophysiological, is common in patients with cancer. Proximal muscle weakness or a mild peripheral neuropathy (PN) occurs in at least 6% of patients with cancer. The frequency is higher when quantitative sensory examinations, electrophysiological assessments, or muscle biopsy are added to clinical examination. Many of these mild or subclinical abnormalities are caused by metabolic or nutritional disturbances associated with advanced cancer.

Disabling paraneoplastic disorders are uncommon in patients with cancer. In one series of more than 1,400 cancer patients, only three had cerebellar degeneration, three had myelopathy, and none had significant sensory neuronopathy. Among 3,843 patients with lung cancer, only 14 developed paraneoplastic encephalomyelitis syndrome, and the frequency of cerebellar degeneration was even lower.

Clinically significant paraneoplastic syndromes probably affect fewer than 3% of patients with small cell lung and ovarian cancers, which are the tumors with the highest frequency of paraneoplastic syndromes.

Pathogenesis

An autoimmune-mediated mechanism accounts for most, if not all, paraneoplastic syndromes. Lambert-Eaton myasthenic syndrome (LEMS) (see Chapter 82) is the only paraneoplastic disorder that is unequivocally established as immune–mediated. However, the presence of serum autoantibodies in many patients with paraneoplastic syndromes involving the central nervous system (CNS) suggests that immune mechanisms also participate in these disorders (Table 58F.2). For example, in paraneoplastic cerebellar degeneration (PCD), antibodies that react selectively with Purkinje's cells, the pathological target of the syndrome, and with the cells of the causal cancer are found in the serum and cerebrospinal fluid (CSF). Antibody titers are higher in CSF than in serum, which suggests CNS synthesis. Inflammatory infiltrates found in the CNS also suggest immune-mediated mechanisms. Similar infiltrates in the tumors of patients with paraneoplastic syndromes suggest that the immune response is directed against the tumor as well. This may explain why patients with paraneoplastic syndromes usually have small and indolent cancers. For example, high titers of anti-Hu antibody are found in patients with small

Table 58F.1:   Nonmetastatic (paraneoplastic) effects of cancer on the nervous system

Disorder	Mechanisms	Examples
Metabolic, nutritional, and hormonal	Organ failure	Hepatic encephalopathy
	Tumor makes hormones	Cushing's syndrome
	Substrate competition	Hypercalcemia, hypoglycemia
Vascular	Hyper- or hypocoagulability	Cerebral emboli (nonbacterial thrombotic endocarditis)
Infections	Immune suppression	Progressive multifocal leukoencephalopathy
Side effects of therapy	Several	Radiation myelopathy
		Cis-platinum neuropathy
Remote effects	Autoimmune	Lambert-Eaton myasthenic syndrome

Source: Modified with permission from JB Posner, HM Furneaux. Paraneoplastic Syndromes. In BH Waksman (ed), Immunologic Mechanisms in Neurologic and Psychiatric Disease. New York: Raven, 1990;187–219.

Table 58F.2:   Paraneoplastic antibodies, their associated cancer(s), and neurological findings

Antibody	Associated cancer	Syndrome	Antigen	Onconeuronal antigen
Anti-Hu	SCLC Neuroblastoma	Encephalomyelitis, sensory neuropathy	All neuronal nuclei 35–40 kD	HuD, HuC, Hel-N1, HuR
Anti-Yo	Gynecological, breast	Cerebellar degeneration	Purkinje's cytoplasm 34, 62 kD	CDR 34 CDR 62-1, 62-2
Anti-Ri	Breast, gynecological, SCLC	Cerebellar ataxia, opsoclonus	Neuronal nuclei CNS, 55, 80 kD	NOVA1, NOVA2
Anti-amphiphysin	Breast	Stiff-man syndrome	Synaptic vesicles 128 kD	Amphiphysin
Anti-VGCC	SCLC	LEMS	Presynaptic VGCC	α_1 subunit
Anti-MysB	SCLC	LEMS	Presynaptic VGCC	β subunit VGCC
Anti-Ma	Multiple	Cerebellar, brainstem dysfunction	Neuronal nuclei and cytoplasm, 37, 40 kD	Ma1
Anti-Ta	Testicular	Limbic encephalitis	Cytoplasm neurons 40, 50 kD	Ta (Ma2)
Anti-Tr	Hodgkin's lymphoma	Cerebellar degeneration	Cytoplasm neurons and Purkinje's spiny dendrites	—
Anti-CAR	SCLC, others	Photoreceptor degeneration	Retinal photoreceptor 23 kD	Recoverin
Anti-VGKC	Thymoma and others	Neuromyotonia (Isaac's syndrome)	Several VGKC (peripheral nerves, central neurons, glia, dorsal root ganglia)	α subunit of several VGKC
Anti-CV2	SCLC, others	Encephalomyelitis Cerebellar degeneration	Glia (subset) 66 kD	POP66

CNS = central nervous system; Lambert-Eaton myasthenic syndrome; SCLC = small cell lung cancer; VGCC = voltage-gated calcium channel; VGKC = voltage-gated potassium channel.

cell lung cancer and paraneoplastic encephalomyelitis or sensory neuronopathy. Low-titer anti-Hu antibodies are found in approximately 20% of patients with small cell lung cancer without neurologic dysfunction. The presence of low-titer antibodies predicts a more indolent course for the cancer than does their absence (Graus et al. 1997a).

The antibodies found in paraneoplastic syndromes are different from each other but have some common characteristics. Most are polyclonal immunoglobulin G (IgG) that fix complement. They react predominantly or exclusively with both target neurological tissue (e.g., neuromuscular junction in LEMS or Purkinje's cells in PCD) and underlying tumor. Antibodies often identify a subset of patients with a specific clinical syndrome and a specific tumor. For example, the anti-Yo antibody is found in patients with

PCD and gynecological tumors; the anti-Tr antibody is found in patients with PCD due to Hodgkin's disease. The detection of any of several paraneoplastic antibodies suggests, first, that the neurological disorder is a paraneoplastic syndrome and, second, that the patient has a specific underlying cancer that may be occult and potentially curable (see Table 58F.2).

Diagnosis

Neurological disorders associated with cancer often become symptomatic before the underlying cancer is discovered. Several clues help a neurologist decide if a neurological syndrome is paraneoplastic:

1. Most paraneoplastic syndromes evolve subacutely, often over days or weeks, and stabilize by the time the patient seeks neurological consultation.
2. Paraneoplastic syndromes usually cause substantial disability by the time of the first neurological consultation; mild or waxing and waning symptoms are unlikely to be paraneoplastic.
3. Paraneoplastic syndromes are often stereotypical, making other causes unlikely. However, none of the paraneoplastic syndromes, even the most characteristic, is invariably associated with cancer. Only two-thirds of patients with LEMS have cancer (almost always a small cell lung cancer), one-half of patients with PCD have cancer, and only 10% of patients with dermatomyositis have cancer, although the proportion is much higher in elderly patients.
4. Paraneoplastic syndromes are often associated with CSF pleocytosis and elevated concentrations of protein and IgG.
5. Paraneoplastic syndromes predominantly affect one part of the nervous system, with only subtle or minor findings in other parts. For example, PCD mainly causes severe ataxia, dysarthria, and nystagmus, but some patients exhibit mild dementia and extensor plantar responses. The term *encephalomyelitis* is often used when the CNS is widely involved. The term *neuromyopathy* is applied when peripheral nerves and muscle are involved.
6. Elevated concentrations of antibodies specific to the neurological disorder and the cancer are sometimes found in serum and CSF.

Treatment

Most paraneoplastic syndromes are untreatable, and their course depends on the course of the tumor. Successful treatment of the underlying cancer rarely leads to resolution of neurological symptoms. Treatment of the paraneoplastic syndrome with vitamins, plasmapheresis, Ig, immunoadsorbative columns, and immunosuppression using corticosteroids or other drugs does not help most patients.

SPECIFIC NEOPLASTIC SYNDROMES

Table 58F.3 lists the paraneoplastic syndromes affecting the nervous system. The most characteristic syndromes are described in the next section.

Paraneoplastic Cerebellar Degeneration

PCD may complicate any malignant tumor but is most common with small cell lung cancer, gynecological cancers, and Hodgkin's disease (Graus et al. 1997b). Males and females are equally affected, and the age incidence reflects

Table 58F.3: Paraneoplastic syndromes affecting the nervous system

I. Brain and cranial nerves
   A. Subacute cerebellar degeneration
   B. Opsoclonus-myoclonus
   C. Limbic encephalitis and other dementias
   D. Brainstem encephalitis
   E. Optic neuritis
   F. Photoreceptor degeneration
II. Spinal cord and dorsal root ganglia
   A. Necrotizing myelopathy
   B. Subacute motor neuronopathy
   C. Motor neuron disease
   D. Myelitis
   E. Sensory neuronopathy
III. Subacute peripheral nerve
   A. Subacute or chronic sensorimotor peripheral neuropathy
   B. Acute polyradiculoneuropathy (Guillain-Barré syndrome)
   C. Mononeuritis multiplex and microvasculitis of peripheral nerve
   D. Brachial neuritis
   E. Autonomic neuropathy
   F. Peripheral neuropathy with islet cell tumors
   G. Peripheral neuropathy associated with paraproteinemia
IV. Neuromuscular junction and muscle
   A. Lambert-Eaton myasthenic syndrome
   B. Myasthenia gravis
   C. Dermatomyositis, polymyositis
   D. Acute necrotizing myopathy
   E. Carcinoid myopathies
   F. Myotonia
   G. Cachectic myopathy
   H. Stiff man syndrome
V. Multiple levels of central and peripheral nervous system or unknown site
   A. Encephalomyelitis
   B. Neuromyopathy

the age distribution of the cancer. Neurological manifestations precede cancer symptoms in more than one-half of these patients. The interval between neurological and cancer symptoms may be as much as 4 years, and in some cases the tumor is not found until autopsy.

The initial sign of cerebellar dysfunction is usually gait ataxia. The ataxia becomes progressively severe over weeks or months. The result is disabling symmetrical truncal and appendicular ataxia and dysarthria. Nystagmus, frequently downbeating, is associated. Vertigo is a common symptom, and many patients complain of diplopia. Alternate presenting features are a sudden onset, suggesting a stroke, or a slow progression, suggesting cerebellar degenerative disease. The cerebellar deficit usually stabilizes at a time when the patient is severely incapacitated. Spontaneous improvement is rare.

Some patients with PCD are mildly demented, but the dementia does not correlate with pathological changes in the cerebral cortex. Less common associated features are dysphagia, extensor plantar responses, and sensory abnormalities. PCD and LEMS are sometimes concurrent conditions in patients with small cell lung cancer (Mason et al.

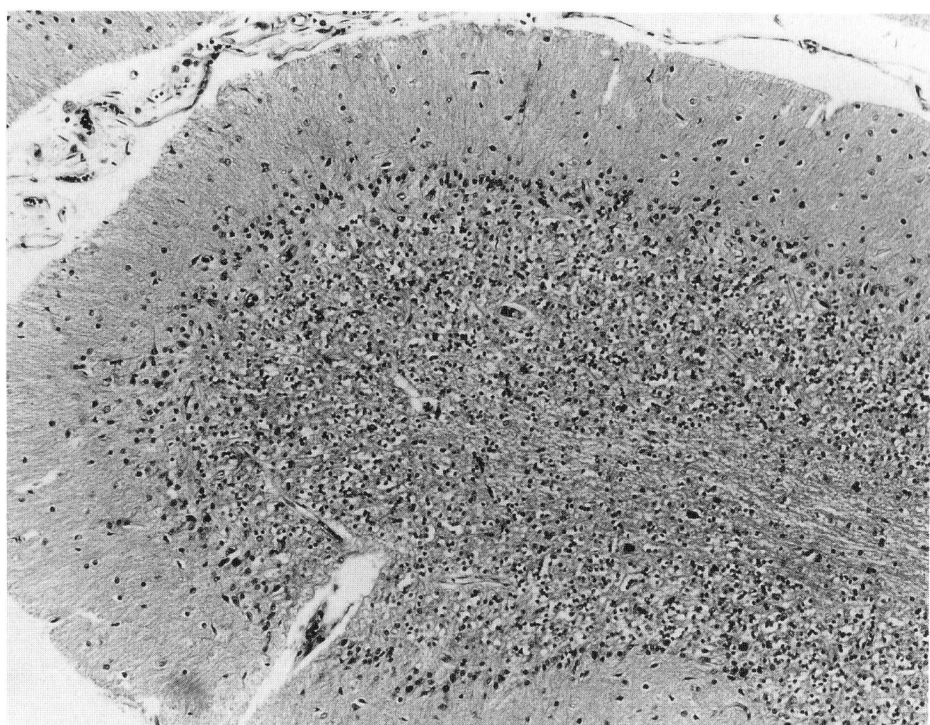

FIGURE 58F.1   A section of cerebellum from a patient with paraneoplastic cerebellar degeneration associated with ovarian cancer. The molecular layer appears normal, the granule cell layer is slightly thinned, Purkinje's cells are completely absent, and there is mild gliosis of the Purkinje's cell layer (hematoxylin-eosin stain).

1997). The CSF examination may be normal or may show a few white blood cells, a mildly increased protein concentration, an increased IgG concentration, and oligoclonal bands. Careful cytological examination of the CSF is required to rule out leptomeningeal metastases. Computed tomography and magnetic resonance imaging (MRI) are usually normal early in the course of the disease but show cerebellar atrophy with prominent cerebellar folia and a dilatated fourth ventricle later on.

Many patients have autoantibodies against Purkinje's cells in the serum and CSF. The most characteristic antibody is anti-Yo, which reacts with the patient's Purkinje's cells and cancer (usually ovarian). Genes coding for the Purkinje's cell antigen recognized by the serum have been cloned.

The characteristic pathology of PCD is severe loss of Purkinje's cells in all parts of the cerebellum (Verschuuren et al. 1996) (Figure 58F.1). Other, less constant abnormalities are thinning of the molecular layer of the cerebellar cortex with variable microglial proliferation and astrocytic gliosis, proliferation of Bergmann astrocytes, and decreased numbers of granule cells. Basket cells and tangential fibers are usually normal (Figure 58F.2). The cerebellar white matter reflects the loss of Purkinje's axons; myelinated fibers are decreased, and reactive gliosis is seen in the cerebellar folia and in the white matter surrounding the dentate nucleus. The deep nuclei of the cerebellum and the brainstem nuclei with cerebellar connections are usually preserved.

The clinical features of PCD are usually so characteristic as to be diagnostic. When not characteristic, PCD must be distinguished from a primary or metastatic cerebellar tumor and from leptomeningeal metastases. This is accomplished by cranial imaging studies and CSF examination, respectively. Other diagnostic considerations include nonparaneoplastic cerebellar degenerative disorders, cerebellar hemorrhage and infarction, abscess, viral infections, drug-induced cerebellar ataxia, and alcoholic cerebellar degeneration. In alcoholic cerebellar degeneration, ataxia involves gait predominantly, and dysarthria and nystagmus are unusual.

Partial or near-complete remission of PCD may occur after treatment of the primary tumor. The presence of ocular flutter or opsoclonus as part of the paraneoplastic syndrome increases the likelihood of improvement after removal of the primary cancer, but these symptoms may indicate a specific paraneoplastic syndrome. Corticosteroids do not affect the course of illness, and plasmapheresis or intravenous immunoglobulin is rarely beneficial. Theoretically, immunosuppressive therapy could be beneficial before Purkinje's cells are irreversibly damaged.

Opsoclonus-Myoclonus Syndrome

Opsoclonus is an eye movement disorder characterized by almost continuous arrhythmic, multidirectional, involuntary, high-amplitude conjugate saccades that may be associated with synchronous blinking of the lids (see Chapter 16). It is a feature of neuroblastoma in children and some tumors in adults. The movements persist when the eyes are closed and during sleep. Opsoclonus increases with attempts at visual pursuit or voluntary refixation. It may be an isolated finding, but it is often accompanied by myoclonus of the trunk, limbs, head, diaphragm, larynx, pharynx, and palate. The result of trunk and limb myoclonus is ataxia. Opsoclonus in adults is often part of PCD.

The differential diagnosis of opsoclonus-myoclonus is discussed in Chapter 16.

A neuroblastoma can be identified in more than one-half of children with opsoclonus-myoclonus, but among all children with neuroblastoma, only 2% develop opsoclonus-myoclonus. The neurological syndrome precedes tumor identification in at least one-half of patients. Tumor location is equally likely in the chest or the abdomen, and evaluation should include careful palpation of the abdomen, MRI of chest and abdomen, and measurement of the urinary excretion of homovanillic acid and vanillylmandelic acid.

In most children, the course is prolonged, with waxing and waning of neurological dysfunction. Either adrenocorticotropic hormone or oral corticosteroids provide partial or complete relief of symptoms in 80% of patients with neuroblastoma after 1–4 weeks of therapy. Relapses occur when therapy is discontinued but may also occur while treatment is in progress.

Opsoclonus-myoclonus also occurs in adults. Approximately 20% have an underlying cancer, usually of the lung. Neurological symptoms often precede tumor diagnosis and usually progress for several weeks. The opsoclonus is associated with truncal ataxia, dysarthria, myoclonus, vertigo, and encephalopathy. The CSF may show a mild pleocytosis and elevation of protein concentration.

Antibodies against CNS tissue have been reported in children with opsoclonus-myoclonus (Connolly et al. 1997). An antibody that is designated *anti-Ri* has been found in the serum and, at relatively higher concentrations, in the CSF of adults. Anti-Ri reacts with the nuclei of neurons throughout the nervous system and with either the nuclei or cytoplasm of cancers from patients with opsoclonus-myoclonus. The anti-Ri antigens have relative molecular weights of 55 and 80 kD, and one responsible gene has been cloned. Only a small number of patients with anti-Ri syndrome have been identified, and the usefulness of anti-Ri as a marker of disease is not established. The neuropathological findings in adult opsoclonus-myoclonus are variable. Some have no specific abnormalities; others resemble those of PCD. Those with findings resembling PCD may have PCD as well as opsoclonus. One anti-Ri patient had inflammatory infiltrates throughout the brain that were most severe in the brainstem. The absence of neuropathological changes in some patients with opsoclonus-myoclonus indicates that the site of the pathology is not yet identified.

The prognosis for neurological recovery or partial remission is better for opsoclonus-myoclonus than for PCD. Improvement may occur after treatment of the underlying tumor and may occur spontaneously. Clonazepam sometimes provides symptomatic relief. Symptoms of opsoclonus-myoclonus were relieved in one adult with an anaplastic lung tumor after administration of thiamine, which suggests

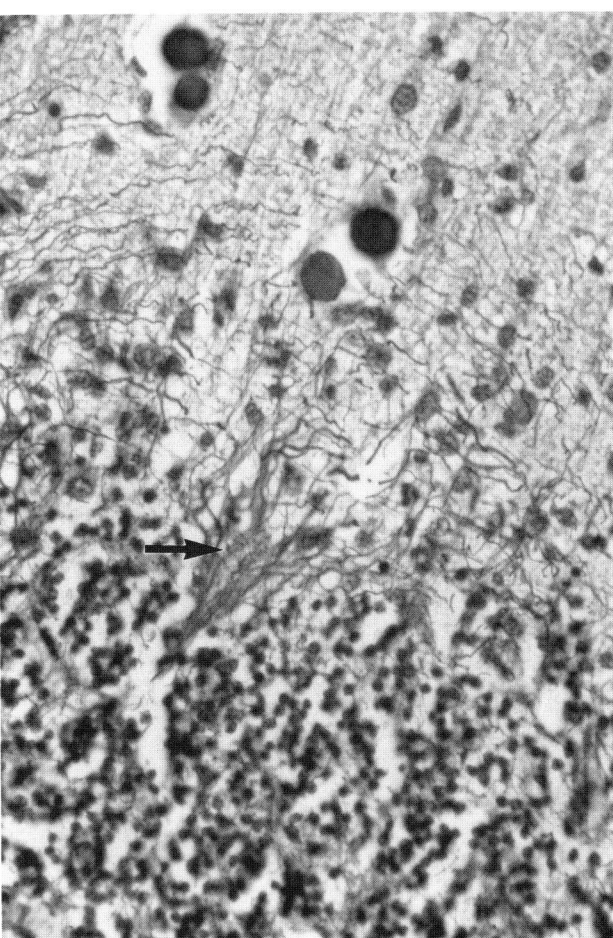

FIGURE 58F.2 Cerebellar cortex of a patient with paraneoplastic cerebellar degeneration showing the endings of a basket cell. The basket cell should enclose a Purkinje's cell, but the Purkinje's cell has disappeared (*arrow*) (Bodian stain).

a nutritional deficiency. Other patients have failed to respond to thiamine. Protein A immunoadsorptive column has also been effective (Cher et al. 1995).

Encephalomyelitis–Sensory Neuronopathy

The clinical features of encephalomyelitis–sensory neuronopathy syndrome are sensory neuropathy or encephalomyelitis, or both (Table 58F.4). When encephalomyelitis-sensory neuronopathy is associated with small cell lung cancer, an autoantibody called anti-Hu is detected in the blood, and the syndrome is called *anti-Hu syndrome*.

Paraneoplastic Sensory Neuronopathy

Probably fewer than 20% of patients with subacute sensory neuronopathy have an underlying cancer. The condition is

Table 58F.4: Encephalomyelitis–sensory neuronopathy syndrome

Syndrome	Symptoms
Limbic encephalopathy	Amnestic dementia
Brainstem encephalitis	Dysphagia, respiratory difficulties
Cerebellar encephalitis	Ataxia
Myelitis	Motor weakness
Autonomic neuropathy	Postural hypotension, obstipation
Sensory neuropathy	Loss of all sensory modalities and reflexes

rare: Not a single case was found in two large series of more than 2,000 cancer patients. A similar sensory neuronopathy occurs in patients with Sjögren's syndrome and in those with no definable cause.

Two-thirds of patients with paraneoplastic sensory neuronopathy (PSN) have lung cancer, particularly small cell cancer. The neuronopathy precedes the diagnosis of cancer in approximately two-thirds of patients, and at times the neoplasm is not diagnosed until autopsy. In at least one instance, a lung tumor identified by biopsy disappeared spontaneously as the sensory neuropathy developed.

The initial features are symmetrical pain, paresthesias, dysesthesias, and numbness in the distal limbs. The sensory loss occasionally begins asymmetrically in arms, legs, or face. Wherever it starts, it usually progresses to loss of all sensation in the arms and legs over several weeks, and then spreads proximally to involve the trunk and sometimes the face. Rapid symptom evolution over hours or days may occur. Loss of joint position sensation results in a severe sensory ataxia and pseudoathetosis of the hands. Tendon reflexes are depressed or absent. Motor power is normal or only mildly impaired. Muscle wasting and weakness, if prominent, is caused by anterior horn cell involvement from an accompanying myelitis.

Electrodiagnostic studies show that sensory nerve action potentials are either absent or have an abnormally low amplitude; motor conduction velocities are normal or only minimally reduced; and needle electromyography does not indicate denervation. Examination of the CSF shows elevated protein concentration, mild pleocytosis, and oligoclonal bands.

Pathological changes are mainly confined to the dorsal root ganglia; most are affected, but in some patients the involvement is patchy. The first changes in the dorsal root ganglia are neuronal degeneration and infiltration by lymphocytes and macrophages (Figure 58F.3). The inflammatory changes are confined to the ganglia, with little or no extension into the nerve roots. As the disease progresses, inflammatory cells disappear, neurons are lost, and capsule cells proliferate, forming residual nodules of Nageotte. The loss of neurons in the dorsal root ganglia causes secondary degeneration of the posterior nerve roots, peripheral sensory nerves, and posterior columns of the spinal cord. Minor loss of neurons in the posterior horns of the spinal cord occurs in long-standing cases. The lateral and anterior columns and anterior horns of the spinal cord and the anterior nerve roots are usually well preserved. Skeletal muscle may show changes consistent with minimal neurogenic

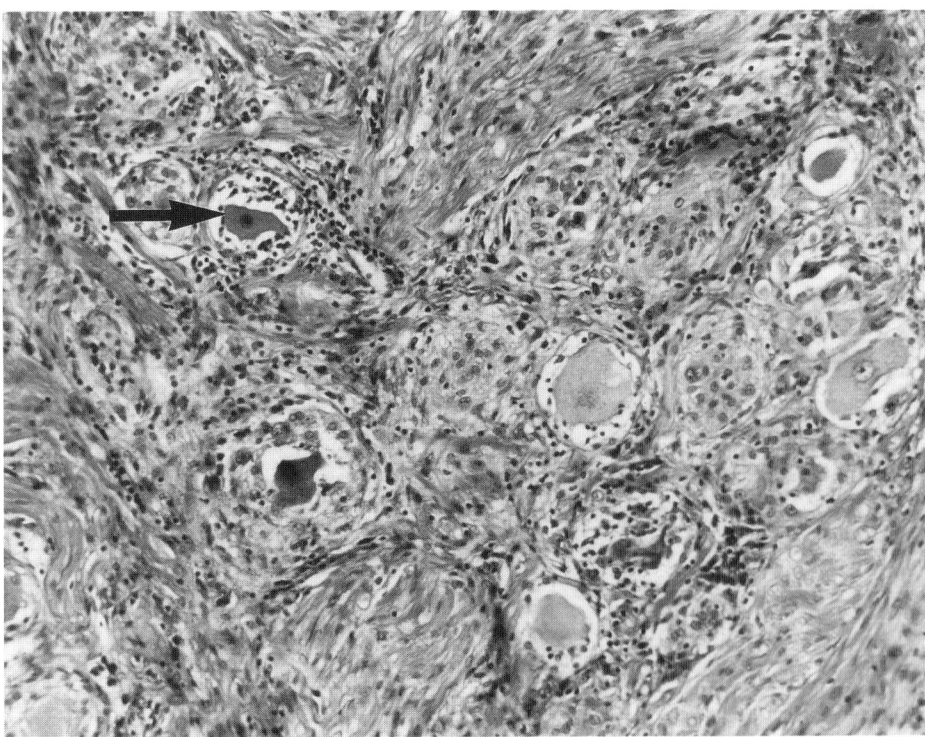

FIGURE 58F.3 The dorsal root ganglion from a patient with paraneoplastic sensory neuronopathy–encephalomyelitis. Most of the dorsal root ganglion cells have disappeared, and the obviously damaged cell in this section is surrounded by lymphocytes (*arrow*) (hematoxylin-eosin stain).

atrophy. These changes are not prominent and resemble disuse atrophy. Approximately one-half of patients with PSN also have inflammatory lesions elsewhere in the spinal cord and brain.

The course of the neurological disorder is independent of the course of the associated neoplasm. The course is occasionally indolent (Graus et al. 1994). Treatment of the primary tumor, corticosteroids, immunosuppressive drugs, and plasmapheresis are not beneficial in treating PSN.

Limbic Encephalitis

Limbic encephalitis is a rare complication of cancer (Alamowitch et al. 1997). Middle-aged men and women are equally affected. Limbic encephalitis is associated with lung tumors, especially small cell cancer, in at least 70% of cases. Other carcinomas and Hodgkin's disease are occasionally associated, but the clinical and pathological features of limbic encephalitis are rare in the absence of an underlying cancer.

The neurological symptoms may precede diagnosis of the tumor by up to 2 years; sometimes the cancer is not detected until autopsy. Symptoms usually progress over several weeks, but the course may be more insidious. Anxiety and depression are common early symptoms, but severe impairment of recent memory is the most striking feature. Other manifestations include agitation, confusion, hallucinations, partial or generalized seizures, and hypersomnia. Progressive dementia is the rule, but spontaneous remissions may occur. Examination of the CSF shows pleocytosis and elevated protein concentration. The electroencephalogram may be normal, show generalized slow-wave abnormalities, or show unilateral or bilateral temporal slow-wave or spike foci. Cranial computed tomography and MRI are usually normal, but medial temporal abnormalities are sometimes reported.

Pathological changes are seen in the gray matter of the hippocampus, cingulate gyrus, pyriform cortex, orbital surfaces of the frontal lobes, insula, and amygdaloid nuclei. The caudate nucleus, putamen, globus pallidum, thalamus, hypothalamus, and subthalamic nucleus are sometimes affected. The pathological changes consist of (1) extensive loss of neurons, (2) reactive gliosis and microglial proliferation, and (3) perivascular lymphocytic cuffing, which is less prominent late in the course of illness. Some patients with clinical features of limbic encephalitis have no pathological changes in the brain.

No treatment is uniformly beneficial. Occasional patients have spontaneous remissions, and others improve after treatment of the underlying tumor.

Brainstem Encephalitis

Paraneoplastic brainstem, or bulbar, encephalitis is usually associated with clinical and pathological evidence of encephalomyelitis elsewhere in the central and peripheral nervous systems. It is often associated with small cell lung cancer, but an identical syndrome may occur without malignancy.

Neurological symptoms may precede or follow discovery of the malignancy and may develop when the tumor is in remission. The clinical features vary according to the brainstem structures involved. The more common features are vertigo, ataxia, nystagmus, vomiting, bulbar palsy, ocular motor disorders, and corticospinal tract dysfunction. Less common are deafness, myoclonus of the branchial musculature, hypoventilation, and movement disorders, including parkinsonism.

The pathological changes are similar to those observed in other forms of paraneoplastic encephalomyelitis: lymphocytic perivascular cuffing, gliosis, microglial proliferation, and loss of neurons. No treatment is beneficial, including treatment of the underlying tumor.

Myelitis

Myelitis is usually a part of the encephalomyelitis syndrome. Inflammation is also present in the brain and dorsal root ganglia. The major clinical feature is patchy wasting and weakness of muscles, sometimes combined with fasciculations. The arms are more severely affected than the legs because the predominant involvement is in the cervical spinal cord. Severe weakness of neck and intercostal muscles may cause respiratory failure. Sensory symptoms are usually a manifestation of an associated sensory neuronopathy, but the clinical picture in patients with severe posterior horn involvement resembles syringomyelia. Corticospinal tract signs may be caused by lesions in the spinal cord or brainstem, and autonomic dysfunction may result from involvement of autonomic neurons.

Retinal Degeneration

Paraneoplastic retinal degeneration is usually associated with small cell lung cancer. Visual symptoms often precede detection of the underlying tumor. Symptoms may begin in one eye. Episodic visual obscurations and night blindness are followed by rapidly progressive, painless loss of visual acuity. Early in the course, examination shows ringlike scotomata, retinal arteriolar narrowing, and relative preservation of visual acuity, but later, large central scotomata and loss of visual acuity become evident. The CSF is normal. The electroretinogram is abnormal, but the latencies of visual evoked potentials are normal. One patient's visual symptoms improved after treatment with corticosteroids, but others have not benefited from corticosteroids or from treatment of the underlying tumor.

Pathological features of paraneoplastic retinal degeneration are (1) widespread degeneration and loss of photoreceptor cells, (2) loss of nuclei from the outer nuclear layer, and (3) macrophages containing melanin granules in the outer retinal layers and the retinal pigment epithelium. The other layers of the retina, the microvasculature, and the optic nerves are preserved. In one patient, who survived for more than a year after the onset of symptoms, the outer retinal layers were replaced completely by glial tissue containing pigment-filled cells.

Antibodies have been detected in the sera of several patients with paraneoplastic retinal degeneration. The underlying tumor is usually small cell lung cancer, but other tumors also provoke similar antibodies. Immunoglobulin deposits have been detected in the retina of patients with antibody-positive retinal degeneration.

Subacute Motor Neuronopathy

Subacute motor neuronopathy is usually associated with Hodgkin's disease or other malignant lymphomas. Neurological symptoms begin any time during the course of the malignancy but usually after diagnosis of the tumor, at a time when the tumor is in remission, and often after mantle or para-aortic radiation therapy. Patients develop subacute, progressive, painless, and often patchy lower motor neuron weakness, which usually affects the legs more than the arms. Involvement is limited to the spinal lower motor neurons and spares the bulbar musculature. Sensory loss, if present, is mild, despite profound weakness. Motor and sensory nerve conduction velocities are normal or only mildly decreased, but needle electromyography shows denervation. The CSF is usually acellular with a mildly elevated protein concentration. MRI of the spinal cord is normal. The course of the neuropathy is independent of the activity of the underlying neoplasm. The weakness is generally not totally incapacitating and stabilizes or improves spontaneously after months or years. No treatment is effective.

The main pathological characteristics of subacute motor neuronopathy are (1) degeneration of anterior horn cells; (2) demyelination and probably axonal loss in anterior nerve roots, associated with large hyperchromatic Schwann cells; and (3) neurogenic atrophy of muscle. Patchy, mild demyelination of the spinal cord white matter may occur, particularly in the dorsal columns. Other features are a minor loss of neurons from Clarke's columns, the intermediolateral cell column, and commissural nuclei. Significant inflammation is unusual, but neuronophagia with proliferation of microglia, astrocytes, and lymphocytes in the anterior horns of the spinal cord was reported in two patients. Changes in lateral columns typical of motor neuron disease are not seen.

Subacute motor neuronopathy may be caused by an opportunistic viral infection of anterior horn neurons. The strong association between subacute motor neuronopathy and lymphomas, tumors associated with immunosuppression, supports the opportunistic viral infection hypothesis. The pathological abnormalities seen in subacute motor neu-

ronopathy resemble those of burnt-out poliomyelitis. Virus-like particles were identified in the spinal anterior horns of one patient, but a virus was not isolated. A similar anterior horn cell disorder in mice is caused by a murine leukemic virus. The virus causes a subacute, progressive paralysis associated with anterior horn cell degeneration without significant inflammation and lymphoma.

Gordon and co-workers (1997) question whether a specific lower motor neuron syndrome is associated with lymphoma. They found that many patients had either definite or suggestive upper motor neuron signs, either clinically or at autopsy (see next section).

Motor Neuron Disease (Amyotrophic Lateral Sclerosis)

The evidence supporting a paraneoplastic form of amyotrophic lateral sclerosis is inconclusive, but in an occasional patient the association seems more than coincidental (Forsyth et al. 1997). Patients are described with slowly progressive motor neuron disease with tumors in different sites. The neurological illness develops before the cancer is identified in almost half of the patients. It has been suggested that primary lateral sclerosis may sometimes be a paraneoplastic syndrome, and that anti-Hu encephalomyelitis may begin with clinical findings that mimic motor neuron disease. However, most patients with motor neuron disease and cancer have the two coincidentally, although an association may exist between amyotrophic lateral sclerosis and lymphoma (Gordon et al. 1997).

Peripheral Neuropathy

Nondisabling mild distal sensorimotor PN is common in patients with cancer. Many cancer patients have metabolic and nutritional disturbances that cause neuropathy, and the existence of a true paraneoplastic PN is disputed. Among patients with small cell lung cancer, the frequency of PN is not increased during the early stages of illness, but it is present in all patients by the time they have lost 15% or more of their body weight. Poor nutrition probably causes or aggravates PN in most patients with cancer; a true paraneoplastic PN also occurs but is less common.

Approximately 5–10% of patients who present to a neurologist for PN, and who are not known to have cancer or other systemic illness, eventually prove to have cancer if the initial evaluation does not reveal another cause (e.g., vitamin deficiency or diabetes).

Lambert-Eaton Myasthenic Syndrome

LEMS is characterized by proximal muscle weakness, particularly in the pelvic girdle. This disorder is described in detail in Chapter 82.

Dermatomyositis or Polymyositis

Dermatomyositis or polymyositis may be associated with cancer at all ages, but the frequency of malignancy is more striking in patients older than 40. These disorders are described in detail in Chapter 83.

REFERENCES

Alamowitch S, Graus F, Uchuya M, et al. Limbic encephalitis and small cell lung cancer—clinical and immunological features. Brain 1997;120:923–928.

Cher LM, Hochberg FH, Teruya J, et al. Therapy for paraneoplastic neurologic syndromes in six patients with protein A column immunoadsorption. Cancer 1995;75:1678–1683.

Connolly AM, Pestronk A, Mehta S, et al. Serum autoantibodies in childhood opsoclonus-myoclonus syndrome: an analysis of antigenic targets in neural tissues. J Pediatr 1997;130:878–884.

Forsyth PA, Dalmau J, Graus F, et al. Motor neuron syndromes in cancer patients. Ann Neurol 1997;41:722–730.

Gordon PH, Rowland LP, Younger DS, et al. Lymphoproliferative disorders and motor neuron disease: an update. Neurology 1997;48:1671–1678.

Graus F, Bonaventura I, Uchuya M, et al. Indolent anti-Hu-associated paraneoplastic sensory neuropathy. Neurology 1994;44:2258–2261.

Graus F, Dalmau J, René R, et al. Anti-Hu antibodies in patients with small-cell lung cancer: association with complete response to therapy and improved survival. J Clin Oncol 1997a;15:2866–2872.

Graus F, Dalmau J, Valldeoriola F, et al. Immunological characterization of a neuronal antibody (anti-Tr) associated with paraneoplastic cerebellar degeneration and Hodgkin's disease. J Neuroimmunol 1997b;74:55–61.

Mason WP, Graus F, Lang B, et al. Small-cell lung cancer, paraneoplastic cerebellar degeneration and the Lambert-Eaton myasthenic syndrome. Brain 1997;120:1279–1300.

Posner JB. Neurologic Complications of Cancer. Philadelphia: Davis, 1995.

Verschuuren J, Chuang L, Rosenblum MK, et al. Inflammatory infiltrates and complete absence of Purkinje cells in anti-Yo associated paraneoplastic cerebellar degeneration. Acta Neuropathol 1996;91:519–525.

Chapter 58
Primary and Secondary Tumors of the Central Nervous System

G. QUALITY OF LIFE AND LATE EFFECTS OF TREATMENT
Patricia K. Duffner and Michael E. Cohen

As the survival rate of patients with brain tumors improves, the long-term effects of central nervous system (CNS) treatment are of increasing importance. Quality-of-life issues have been raised in regard to such treatment across all age groups, but the greatest concern is for children, particularly those who are very young at the time of treatment with radiation to the neuraxis.

INTELLECTUAL FUNCTION

The long-term effects of cranial irradiation on intellectual function have been studied most thoroughly in children treated for acute lymphoblastic leukemia. The largest retrospective study included 104 children who had received three forms of CNS prophylaxis. One group had been treated with intrathecal methotrexate alone, the second received intrathecal methotrexate plus cranial irradiation (2,400 cGy), and the third received intrathecal methotrexate and intermediate-dose intravenous methotrexate. Radiated children had significantly lower full-scale IQs than the other two groups of patients. Furthermore, radiated children did worse on wide-range achievement tests and other tests of neuropsychological function. Although these differences were statistically significant, IQ scores of the radiated children were generally within normal ranges.

Several retrospective studies have been used to evaluate the neuropsychological function of children who were radiated for brain tumors. Most of these studies showed that 30–50% of these patients had IQs less than 80, and only 10–20% had IQs exceeding 90.

Prospective evaluations have also been performed. Significant intellectual decline occurred over time, but unlike the retrospective analyses, IQ scores at the end of 2 years were still greater than 90. Children in both the retrospective and prospective studies had a high frequency of learning disabilities and attention-deficit disorder. The differences in intellectual function reported in prospective and retrospective studies were likely due to the disproportionate effect of risk factors on small populations of patients. Risk factors for intellectual decline include age at radiation, volume and dose of radiation, location of tumor, and chemotherapy, particularly with methotrexate.

Hydrocephalus, which was initially suggested as a cause for the intellectual limitations in children with brain tumors, is not a significant risk factor. One of the most important risk factors for intellectual problems is age at time of radiation. Several studies have documented that the children most severely affected by radiation are those who are less than 5 years old. Recent studies have suggested that the baseline intelligence of infants with brain tumors is often abnormal. Although children older than 8–10 years may have relative intellectual preservation, it is not clear when it is safe to irradiate a young child.

Large-volume radiation is another significant risk factor for intellectual dysfunction. Significant decline in intellectual function occurs in children who receive whole-brain radiation but not in those who receive local radiation.

The location of tumor is a risk factor independent of treatment. Thus, the child who has a supratentorial tumor is more likely to have a lower baseline IQ than is the child whose tumor is located in the posterior fossa. After treatment, IQs decline in both groups. Because the child with the supratentorial tumor is already functioning at a lower level, further decline may place the child in the frankly retarded range. There is debate about whether children with midline tumors are also at increased risk for intellectual deterioration.

Another risk factor is the concomitant use of intrathecal methotrexate and cranial irradiation for brain tumors. Complications associated with intrathecal methotrexate and cranial irradiation were first identified in a leukemic population. Patients with acute lymphoblastic leukemia who were treated with intrathecal methotrexate and cranial radiotherapy for CNS prophylaxis had a greater than 50% frequency of basal ganglia calcifications, hypodense areas, and widened sulci on computed tomography (CT) scan. Other studies suggested that it was not methotrexate alone but rather the combination of methotrexate and radiation that caused the high proportion of children with leukoencephalopathy. The group at highest risk for developing leukoencephalopathy was children who had a history of CNS leukemia and who had been treated with intrathecal or intraventricular methotrexate in addition to radiation.

During the 1970s, some children with brain tumors were treated with intraventricular methotrexate. Because of abnormal cerebrospinal fluid (CSF) dynamics, severe necrotizing leukoencephalopathy was reported in one child, who became vegetative. Because many patients with brain tumors have altered CSF dynamics secondary to either communicating or obstructive hydrocephalus, the clearance of methotrexate may be abnormally slowed. The toxicity of methotrexate relates not only to peak levels but also to duration of exposure. Because of its complications, intrathecal methotrexate has not been used in the United States for children with brain tumors for several years. Intrathecal methotrexate, however, is still given to children with medulloblastoma in Europe, and concerns about the effects of this treatment continue.

The intellectual deterioration associated with radiation is progressive. In a series of 120 children with medulloblastomas operated on between 1967 and 1987, studied 5 years after treatment, 58% had IQs above 80; but at 10 years after treatment, only 15% had IQs above 80. Also, 5 years after treatment, 40% of the children were at a normal level in school, whereas after 10 years only 11% of the children were at grade level.

Thus, cranial irradiation clearly is associated with a significant and progressive decline in intellectual function. Risk factors, including young age at time of treatment, large volume and dose of radiation, and concomitant use of methotrexate, all exacerbate the process. The majority of irradiated children develop learning disabilities, including attention-deficit disorder, perceptual problems, and fine-motor coordination difficulties, which necessitate placement in special classes or extra help and resource rooms.

ENDOCRINE FUNCTION

Growth

The most common endocrine complication of CNS irradiation is growth failure. The causes of short stature in radiated children include growth hormone deficiency (GHD), decreased vertebral body height, precocious puberty, and hypothyroidism. GHD is a direct result of cranial irradiation, which has an immediate suppressive effect on the hypothalamic-pituitary axis. Moreover, radiation-induced GHD is not a transient phenomenon. Patients tested as late as 8–10 years after radiation treatment have been found to have GHD. Although the exact dose of radiation required to produce GHD is not known, a minimum of 2,500–2,900 cGy is probably necessary. An inverse relationship between dose and peak growth hormone response has been recognized. GHD relates not only to the total dose but also to the size and number of fractions.

The speed of onset of GHD may relate to the age at which a child receives radiation. In one study, a child less than 3 years of age had the least initial disturbance of growth hormone secretion after irradiation and the mildest alteration in growth patterns. Both the dose and the time elapsed since radiation also significantly influence peak growth hormone response. Although the speed of onset is increased in the group receiving higher radiation doses, ultimately all children have approximately the same frequency of GHD, about 85%.

The putative site of radiation-induced GHD is believed to be the ventromedian nucleus of the hypothalamus. Damage to this site occurs even with posterior fossa radiation alone because the anterior limit of the radiation port to the posterior fossa is the posterior clinoid. Although the port excludes the pituitary, the ventromedian nucleus is within the radiated region. It appears that GHD in irradiated children is primarily due to failure of synthesis or delivery of growth hormone–releasing factor to the pituitary.

The clinical implications of radiation-induced GHD have been studied in children with leukemia and in those with brain tumors. Originally, the literature suggested that radiated children with leukemia had generally normal growth patterns. This was based in part on one very large study. Re-evaluation of this same group of children in 1992, after most had undergone pubertal growth spurts, brought into question the earlier results. Brecher and colleagues found that the mean height for irradiated males was 166.7 cm compared with 179.1 cm in nonirradiated males. Similar results were found in females (154.0 cm vs. 162.2 cm). Thus, the earlier report suggesting normal growth patterns may have been overly optimistic.

The likelihood of GHD in irradiated children is so high that some authors have suggested that when growth deviation greater than 1 standard deviation is identified, growth hormone treatment can be given without first performing formal tests of growth hormone production and secretion.

Although patients with GHD are being treated increasingly with exogenous growth hormone, growth rates during treatment are inferior to those achieved in nonirradiated children with idiopathic GHD. Although growth during the first year of therapy is generally good, a normal growth rate is not maintained over a 3-year period. In one study, a comparison was made among three groups: short children, children with idiopathic GHD, and children who had received cranial irradiation for brain tumors. The irradiated children grew well during the first year but less well than the idiopathic GHD children. These authors found that children could attain catch-up growth with both a higher dose and increased frequency of growth hormone administration.

Hypothyroidism is another factor that contributes to poor growth and a suboptimal response to growth hormone treatment. Appropriate treatment with thyroxine in hypothyroid children with GHD is necessary for maximum efficacy of the growth hormone treatment trial. Another reason for less than optimal response is the tendency for irradiated children to develop precocious puberty.

Abnormal spinal growth after neuraxis radiation is one of the major contributors to short stature among irradiated children. The effects of irradiation on the vertebral bodies relate to both dose and age at irradiation. The younger the children are at time of irradiation, the greater the loss in growth potential. Children irradiated at 1 year of age have a potential 9-cm loss of adult height compared to children irradiated at 10 years, in whom a 5.5-cm loss has been reported. Unfortunately, on current growth hormone dosage schedules, growth hormone replacement therapy improves only leg growth. The final result is a child with short stature and marked skeletal disproportion.

Thyroid Function

Hypothyroidism is another common complication of the treatment of brain tumors that occurs in approximately 30% of children who receive radiation to the neuraxis. Primary hypothyroidism occurs because the thyroid gland lies within the radiation port to the cervical spine. Secondary hypothyroidism is much less common, with a 3% frequency in one study, compared with 28% for primary hypothyroidism. Although the time of onset is not yet defined, most patients develop hypothyroidism within 4–8 years of radiation treatment. The combination of chemotherapy and craniospinal radiation increases the likelihood of hypothyroidism to 68% in one study.

Recognition and treatment of hypothyroidism is important because the condition adversely affects growth, learning abilities, and general health. Moreover, treatment of euthyroid children with compensated hypothyroidism is necessary because there is an increased risk of thyroid carcinoma in patients with chronic elevations of thyroid-stimulating hormone. Thyroid function should be assessed serially because some of these children may not require lifelong therapy.

Gonadal Function

Gonadal dysfunction has been reported in children treated for brain tumors. At one time, gonadal dysfunction was considered an extremely unusual complication of CNS therapy. Subsequent studies have shown that these optimistic views are not supported when patients are monitored for a long time. Abnormal gonadotrophin levels may develop during the peripubertal years. Gonadal dysfunction is due to radiation as well as chemotherapy. Radiation to the spinal axis may be associated with scatter to the gonads. Although radiation scatter to the testes is small, doses of radiation to the ovaries may be significantly higher and, as such, contribute to ovarian dysfunction. In one study, 35% of girls treated with spinal radiation had primary ovarian dysfunction, as determined by elevated gonadotrophin levels. Of interest, the addition of chemotherapy did not significantly increase the frequency of these abnormalities. However, agents such as cyclophosphamide may damage the testicular germinal epithelium. Even when pubertal development is normal, patients have a high frequency of dose-related oligo- or azoospermia. Recovery may occur many years later. Because Leydig cell function is less affected, patients undergo normal puberty and have normal androgen production. The ovaries are less sensitive than are the testes to chemotherapeutic agents. Although girls are less susceptible to cyclophosphamide damage, they may undergo premature menopause.

ONCOGENESIS

The oncogenic potential of chemotherapy and radiation therapy is well known. As more patients survive brain tumors, the potential for the development of a treatment-induced second primary cancer becomes of increasing concern. The likelihood that a survivor of childhood cancer will develop a second malignancy is 10 times higher than that of age-matched controls. Genetic predisposition, susceptibility of the host, and previous CNS therapy all may play a role in the development of second malignancies. Most children develop malignancies in tissues previously exposed to radiation.

The dose of radiation required to induce second malignancies is unknown. Radiation in low, moderate, and high doses have all been associated with the development of second tumors. Perhaps the best-known example is the experience with children who received low-dose radiation for "status thymicolymphaticus," which was common in the United States in the 1950s. Tumors of the head and neck have been identified in children who received therapeutic radiation for tinea capitis. In a follow-up study, a 30-year relative risk assigned among these patients for the development of tumors of the head and neck was 8.4. There was a direct relationship between dose and risk. The most common brain tumor identified was meningioma.

As with low-dose radiation, moderate-dose radiation has also been associated with oncogenesis. The bulk of reported cases occurred in children with leukemia and lymphoma who received cranial radiation as part of CNS prophylaxis. Whereas most patients developed meningiomas after low-dose radiation, those treated with moderate-dose radiation have also developed astrocytic tumors.

As might be expected, high-dose radiation for CNS neoplasia has also been associated with second malignancies. In reference to this cohort of patients, the definition of a second primary tumor is a tumor that occurs in a previous radiation port, develops after a sufficient latent period, is of a different histology from the primary tumor, and is not found in patients with a neurocutaneous syndrome, such as neurofibromatosis or tuberous sclerosis. The duration from irradiation to diagnosis of the second tumor has ranged from 2 to 47 years, with a mean of 20 years. In patients who have developed meningiomas and astrocytomas, the tumors are apt to behave in a highly malignant fashion. More benign second tumors have tended to occur later than more aggressive tumors (i.e., 20 years versus 6 years after radiation).

PATHOLOGICAL CONSEQUENCES OF TREATMENT

The pathological consequences of treatment are not uniformly accepted. The most widely recognized pathological effects of radiation and chemotherapy treatment have been leukoencephalopathy and vasculopathy. Unfortunately, these bear little direct relationship to the previously described clinical effects. Whereas dementia is a common late effect of radiation, gray matter pathology has infrequently been reported. Leukoencephalopathy, on the other hand, is widely reported and has been attributed to radiation, methotrexate, and other chemotherapeutic agents. Total dose of radiation greater than 5,000 cGy, in fractions exceeding 200 cGy per dose, or radiation in combination with chemotherapeutic agents have been responsible for most reported cases of leukoencephalopathy. Radiation necrosis is similar to leukoencephalopathy but of a more intense nature. The areas of white matter most frequently involved have been the centrum semiovale, periventricular regions, and basal ganglia. Involvement is usually multifocal and asymmetrical, consisting of loss of oligodendroglia, myelin, axonal swelling, fragmentation, coagulative necrosis, and mineralizing angiopathy. Although pathological findings tend to be dose related, changes have been found after moderate-dose radiation in patients with CNS leukemia who received as little as 1,800 cGy radiation to the craniospinal axis. Demyelination has been reported in patients given methotrexate by intraventricular, intrathecal, or—when given in extremely high doses—intravenous routes. In addition to methotrexate, cytosine arabinoside and BCNU have also been identified with leukoencephalopathy.

Disruption of the blood-brain barrier and the CSF barrier is thought to be instrumental in causing leukoencephalopathy. Radiation and drugs can alter the tight junctions of the barriers. This allows egress of intrathecally or intraventricularly administered drugs to pass from the ventricular spinal fluid into brain parenchyma, with resulting high concentrations of drugs in deep white matter. Additionally, altered CSF clearance, secondary to a communicating or obstructive hydrocephalus, results in retention of toxic drug levels in the spinal fluid. This potentially provides more time for toxic agents to diffuse back from the ventricles into deep cerebral white matter.

Neuroimaging has helped to define the emergence of in vivo manifestations of leukoencephalopathy. CT features of leukoencephalopathy are hypodense areas in the white matter, cerebral atrophy, increased sulci with enlargement of ventricles, and calcification. These features have been related to total dose of radiation and dose per fraction. However, there are no precise quantitative correlations.

Changes of leukoencephalopathy seen with magnetic resonance imaging are characteristic and differ somewhat from those seen with CT. Findings consist of diffuse white matter abnormalities manifested by increased T2-weighted signals extending from the ventricles to the cortical medullary junction. The changes in the white matter consist of scalloped lateral margins extending from the ventricle with sparing of the arcuate fibers and overlying cortex. As with CT, these changes have been correlated with dose, patient age, and volume of radiation. Because of the sensitivity but limited specificity of magnetic resonance imaging, the changes of leukoencephalopathy can also be seen in asymptomatic individuals, particularly in elderly subjects.

Positron emission tomography (PET) scanning provides another dimension for evaluating adverse effects of therapy. PET scanning identifies altered metabolism and provides the potential for identifying areas of cerebral diaschisis. Diaschisis is defined as abnormalities of function remote from the diseased site, presumably secondary to metabolic and anatomical changes at the site of treatment. Thus, findings in local metabolism on PET as well as metabolic changes distant from the lesion are beginning to permit correlations between structure and function. PET scanning is also used to distinguish radiation necrosis from tumors. In patients with evidence of an edematous mass lesion months to years after radiation, hypometabolism on PET may suggest radiation necrosis rather than recurrent tumor. Glucose metabolism in low-grade astrocytomas may also be hypometabolic and stands in marked contrast to the hypermetabolism seen in glioblastomas. This may lead to confusion in differentiating a low-grade tumor from radiation necrosis.

Occlusive arterial disease has been identified in patients who have received injections of L-asparaginase as well as radiation. Large-vessel disease is readily identified by angiography. Small blood vessels may also develop angiopathic features and luminal occlusion. Histopathologically, there is deposition of calcium, mucopolysaccharides, and necrotic material in and around small vessels. These features are most commonly seen in the basal ganglia, and they accompany leukoencephalopathy. Cerebral and cerebellar vessels are less frequently involved.

In sum, all anatomical levels of the nervous system can be adversely affected by treatment. Demyelination is the most consistently observed neuropathological sequela, followed by mineralizing angiopathy with occlusion of small vessels. Dystrophic calcification, when identified, is usually seen in deep gray matter nuclei. Most of these changes are associated with radiation rather than chemotherapy and are dose related. Isolated reports have suggested that the changes of leukoencephalopathy may be reversible, but for the moment, the knowledge of delayed CNS effects of treatment should temper enthusiasm for radical and aggressive treatments.

CHANGES IN TREATMENT

In recent years, interest in the long-term effects of CNS therapies has led to increased understanding of the toxicities of the regimens employed. Whereas in the 1970s and early 1980s it was sufficient to document these abnormalities, it now behooves us to recognize these risk factors and alter treatment accordingly. As such, various alterations in treatment have been proposed. Large-volume neuraxis irradiation, for example, increases the risks of intellectual deterioration, endocrinopathies, spinal shortening, and second malignancies. As such, the neuro-oncology community has tried to develop treatment regimens that reduce the volume of irradiation. This is reflected in the change in approach to children with ependymomas. Previously, most radiation therapists treated children with ependymomas with craniospinal radiation. Currently, children whose ependymomas have not metastasized by the time of diagnosis are treated with local radiation alone. This approach was an outgrowth of studies demonstrating that failure in most cases occurred in the primary site and that isolated neuraxis dissemination was quite rare. Another attempt to reduce volume of irradiation has been made for children with germinomas. Although these are exquisitely radiosensitive tumors, they are also sensitive to certain chemotherapeutic agents, particularly cisplatin and its analogues. In current trials, patients diagnosed as having germinomas are treated with several courses of chemotherapy before irradiation in an attempt to eliminate tumor bulk. If there is no evidence of residual disease after chemotherapy, both volume and dose of radiation are reduced.

Another important risk factor is high-dose radiation. An attempt to reduce the dose to the neuraxis is being explored in a study of children with standard- or good-risk medulloblastoma. It is anticipated that reducing the dose of radiation to the neuraxis will cause less adverse effect on intelligence, vertebral body growth, and endocrine function (including hypothyroidism) and possibly a lower frequency of gonadal dysfunction. Whether the lower dose will also reduce the risk of the development of thyroid cancer is conjectural.

Another important risk factor is young age at the time of irradiation. In an attempt to address these concerns, young children are treated with regimens of prolonged postoperative chemotherapy in an attempt to delay or eliminate radiation therapy (Duffner et al. 1993). Whether the prolonged chemotherapy will also cause serious long-term damage is not yet known.

Finally, the role of chemotherapy as a risk factor has only recently been assessed. As a result of the recognition of methotrexate leukoencephalopathy, the use of this agent has been markedly reduced in the United States. A variety of other chemotherapeutic agents are under trial. The cooperative groups must closely assess the long-term toxicity of adjuvant chemotherapy to better determine the most appropriate use for these agents.

In the first century BC, Publius Syrus said, "There are some remedies worse than the disease." Because children with brain tumors are now surviving into adulthood, it is important to recognize the toxicities of treatment regimens and to alter therapy, where necessary, to improve the quality of life of long-term survivors.

ETHICAL CONSIDERATIONS

Despite much progress in the diagnosis and treatment of cancer of the nervous system, cures for most tumors that invade the CNS, whether primary or secondary, remain out of reach. Current treatments pose some risk, and in up to 50% of patients, there is a significant impact on quality of life. These concerns and the fact that health care has moved from 5% of the gross national product 40 years ago to close to 15% have put risk-to-benefit and cost-to-benefit issues on the national agenda.

Despite the pragmatism dictated by economic considerations, there is optimism based on advances in applied molecular biology that the enigma of cancer can be recognized and cured. The current understanding of the biology of cancer suggests that clonal selection is a process by which cancer evolves. Tumor-suppressor genes are inactivated, and oncogenes are activated, in a cascade of events that favor cell division. This process confers a survival advantage on clones of cells that favor growth, invasion, metastasis, and adverse immune modulation in defense of normal host mechanisms. Ultimately, these cells destroy the host. This approach is the cellular extension of Darwinian evolution by natural selection and suggests that cancer is fundamentally a biological problem. Only recently have cancer biologists begun to understand how this process takes place. The hope is that in the coming decades this knowledge will translate into improvement in the diagnosis, treatment, and subsequently, cure of cancer.

The identification of cancer-suppressor genes, such as the retinoblastoma gene, neurofibromatosis gene, and *p53* gene, raises the possibility that patients at high risk may be identified long before the inevitable path of oncogenesis begins. This increases the potential for detection and even prevention. Unfortunately, in the short run, identification without the ability to prevent or treat may lead to undue anxiety, loss of insurance, disruption of family units, loss of income, and, in less stable patients, a potential increase in suicides. Confronted with long-term therapy and an uncertain future, it is understandable that patients may react with disbelief, anger, hostility, or depression. Many patients may feel despair that their lives are out of control. Young people, because of interruption in careers and family responsibilities, may develop severe psychological problems. The middle-aged may regard cancer as disruptive, and the elderly may become withdrawn or hostile.

The diagnosis of cancer should not necessarily be identified with loss of hope. There are approximately 3 million cancer patients cured of their diagnosis living today in the United States and another 3 million living active lives whose cancer is under control. The 5-year survival rates for cancer of all types have dramatically increased in recent decades. Sixty percent of all children with cancer of the nervous system will survive to adulthood, and 30% of adults will survive for more than 5 years. Today, more than any other time in the past, there is a favorable climate for outcome after diagnosis of cancer. These facts should form the basis of a philosophical approach to all patients who are initially diagnosed with cancer of the nervous system. Patients who believe that their cancer is treatable, if not curable, are most likely to comply with therapeutic treatments and recommendations.

All patients, regardless of age, have a right to receive complete information about their diagnoses, treatment options, and probable outcomes. Part of the art of medicine is the insight to know how much the patient should learn about the diagnosis. In our opinion, all patients initially should be given hope for improvement, if not complete cure. For all malignancies, regardless of how dismal the prognosis, there is a statistical possibility for cure. Initial treatment should begin with this philosophy in mind. Access should be readily available to information networks that provide patients with the most recent information about their diagnoses.

Because most chemotherapy and radiotherapy regimens affect normal as well as abnormal tissue, the potential for adverse consequences, independent of the potential for cure, exists for all treatment protocols. Thus, the risk-to-benefit ratio must be spelled out in a forthright and factual manner. For children, cognitive abnormalities and effects on growth should be clearly discussed with responsible parents and, where appropriate, with patients. For adults, the impact of treatment on neurological function must be clearly elucidated, along with subsequent loss of earning potential and impact on family dynamics.

Recommendations for entry into randomized clinical trials should be undertaken with the knowledge that there is no known therapy superior to the one that is being offered. One must question whether clinical trials benefit patients. In the absence of known treatment, a well-designed clinical trial offers access to the best standard therapy or known treatments that may be equivalent or superior to standard treatment. As suggested by Levine (1993), physicians should recommend the therapy they believe is best for the patient. Patients should be assured that if they are enrolled in a randomized clinical trial they are receiving one of the best-known therapies for their condition. This is an underlying principle of the World Health Organization's declaration at Helsinki: "Concern for the interest of the subject must always prevail over the interest of science and society." Justification for participation in a clinical trial may simply be limited to the knowledge that patients are likely to get the best-known treatment at participating institutions and that the staff at these institutions is the most qualified. This observation, independent of the expectation of cure, argues for treatment at comprehensive cancer centers (Levine 1993).

In recommending participation in a clinical trial, a balance must be struck between the perception that all trials are benign and beneficial and the knowledge that research is dangerous. Although absence of therapy, in all probability, is associated with continued growth of tumor, the treatment itself may be associated with untoward side effects that have significant impact on the quality of life experienced by those with limited time remaining. When patients have a disease associated with a limited life span, they should be given the choice of pursuing a cure or remission, maximizing comfort, or maintaining current function. The decision to pursue a course of treatment need not necessarily be associated with cure but with other options, such as maintenance of quality of life or biological function. Clinical trials must be designed that offer the patient better therapy or therapy similar to that used in current medical practice. The patient's interests must always be foremost in the design of any treatment protocol.

Perhaps the skill and judgment of a physician is most tested when a patient enters a terminal phase. Home care and hospital-based programs have increasingly become part of patient care plans. Terminal care is often protracted, complex, and expensive. Decisions on when to withhold treatment of the disease or to recommend do-not-resuscitate orders should be the patient's, working in concert with a sympathetic, well-informed physician and appropriate family members and advisors. If the patient is judged psychologically able to deal with the information, the patient and the family have the right to know about the nature and duration of the patient's remaining life.

REFERENCES

Duffner PK, Horowitz ME, Krischer JP, et al. Postoperative chemotherapy and delayed radiation in children less than three years of age with malignant brain tumors. N Engl J Med 1993;328:1725–1731.
Levine RJ. Ethics of clinical trials. Cancer 1993;72:2805–2810.

Chapter 59
Infections of the Nervous System

Section Editor:
Marylou V. Solbrig

Infectious diseases will always be a part of human existence. Historically, transmissible diseases acquired names that described the affliction (yellow fever, scarlet fever) or place of origin (Lassa fever, Ebola hemorrhagic fever, Japanese encephalitis, Four Corners virus). Over time, some names were changed or dropped in deference to regional sensibilities or political correctness; yet none of the responsible agents, excepting the smallpox virus, has gone away. New microbes are still being discovered and, sooner or later, many infect the nervous system.

The new pathogens are challenges, and so are the old ones. As a group, infections of the nervous system occur often and figure in the differential diagnosis of many neurological syndromes. All require urgent care, especially the bacterial meningitides, cerebral malaria, subdural empyemas, or epidural abscesses; some are true medical or medical and surgical emergencies.

There was a time when neurology and plagues were rarely considered together. Now, however, old pathogens such as pneumococcus, tuberculosis, and malaria have returned with multidrug-resistant genotypes. A pandemic strain of group A *Neisseria meningitidis* swept Asia in the 1980s, traveled with pilgrims on the hajj in Saudi Arabia in 1987, then moved on to Africa, where it is still in circulation. Iatrogenic or virus-induced immunosuppression has rendered rare infections of the central nervous system common, and the acquired immunodeficiency syndrome epidemic will be remembered as one of the great tragedies of the twentieth century.

Things can get better. There is today better understanding of infectious diseases. The presence and expression of human disease is a consequence of the agent's biology, genotypic variation, host factors, ecology, and human behavior, in combination. As a result, there is better tracking of diseases, the ability to target preventive services to vulnerable populations, and the translation of biomedical advances into new diagnostic, therapeutic, and vaccine developments. The wider availability of computed tomography scanning and nuclear magnetic resonance imaging has improved diagnosis and treatment of all neurological infectious diseases, focal and parasitic diseases in particular. Improved antiretroviral treatments have extended the lives of many.

However, things can also get worse. The newest drugs, vaccines, and diagnostic tests remain beyond the reach of large portions of the world's population. Optimism based on biomedical progress is being offset by growing fears that emerging infections (infections new to humanity) or re-emergent infections (for which existing antimicrobials are obsolete) may pose some of the greatest dangers facing our world in the future. Xenotransplantation, or cross-species organ transplantation, now in its planning and pilot stages, is almost certain to be a method of cross-species transfer of viruses. The ever-increasing mobility of the human population means that any transmissible disease spread by person-to-person contact can be disseminated globally. Acquired immunodeficiency syndrome knows no national boundaries. Tuberculosis consistently ranks as a leading cause of death by a single pathogen in the world, and epidemics of meningococcal meningitis menace sub-Saharan Africa every 8–14 years.

Not only rapid travel, but population growth, habitat destruction, global warming, even changes in the food chain, have consequences in the clinic and in the demographics of infectious diseases.

The subject of infectious diseases of the nervous system is a large one, spanning several medical and scientific disciplines. The body of information necessary to support treatment decisions, which includes (1) a history of travel or immigration, (2) the geography of endemic, epidemic, and resistant strains, (3) the context of the systemic disease, and (4) a knowledge of the diagnostic, therapeutic, containment, and preventive measures, is also large.

As in previous editions of *Neurology in Clinical Practice*, bacterial diseases appear together in one section of this chapter (A). Diseases caused by conventional DNA and RNA viruses appear together in the viral section (B). Fungal and parasitic diseases are now separated (C and D), a consequence of the expanded clinical experience and documentation of the care and treatment of these diseases. Human immunodeficiency virus–related disease has its own section (E), and, in keeping with the Nobel Selection Committee's decision in 1997, the spongiform encephalopathies ("protein only" diseases, or disorders of protein conformation), have their own section (F).

Chapter 59
Infections of the Nervous System

A. BACTERIAL INFECTIONS
Marylou V. Solbrig, John F. Healy, and Cheryl A. Jay

As a group, bacterial infections of the nervous system figure in the differential diagnosis of many neurological syndromes. Under circumstances ideal for a given micro-organism, nearly any human bacterial pathogen can cause meningitis. Some, such as *Borrelia* and Ehrlichiae, have crossed species barriers from other mammals to cause serious meningeal or encephalitic disease, whereas others, such as the mycobacteria and pneumococci, have begun to outdistance standard antibiotics. The potency of clostridial neurotoxins are well known to intensive care unit (ICU) personnel and military researchers. Moreover, because of their potential as biological weapons, even the most exotic of bacterial infections, such as anthrax, plague, and tularemia, are widely recognized. Antibiotics granted modern medicine treatment capabilities of unprecedented scope and success, but such therapies can no longer be taken for granted. Although spe-cific antibiotic or antitoxin treatments have been identified for most of the infections reviewed here, significant morbidity and mortality from bacterial infections of the nervous system remain.

PYOGENIC BACTERIA

Bacterial Meningitis

Bacterial meningitis is an inflammatory response to infection of the leptomeningeal cells and subarachnoid space, producing a clinical syndrome of fever, headache, meningismus, and cerebrospinal fluid (CSF) pleocytosis. Bacterial meningitis was a fatal disease from its recognition in 1805 by Gaspard Vieusseux as "epidemic cerebrospinal fever" to the early 1900s. In 1932, the antimicrobial effects of the sulfonamides were appreciated, and in 1941, penicillin was isolated. With modern antibiotics, bacterial meningitis is a more treatable disease. Still, in the United States, bacterial meningitis causes at least 2,000 deaths annually and mortality is estimated at 10–30%.

Epidemiology and Recent Trends

Acute bacterial meningitis occurs throughout the world. Three main pathogens, *Haemophilus influenzae*, *Streptococcus pneumoniae*, and *Neisseria meningitidis*, account for 75–80% of cases after the neonatal period. The relative contribution of each organism to the epidemiology of bacterial meningitis varies with the age of the patient and geography.

Before the introduction of the conjugate vaccines, *H. influenzae* type b was the most common cause of bacterial meningitis in the United States, causing 45% of cases. *S. pneumoniae* accounted for 18% of cases, and *N. meningitidis* for 14%. Widespread vaccination against *H. influenzae* type b since 1987 has markedly reduced the frequency of *H. influenzae* meningitis in children. With the resulting 82% reduction in *H. influenzae* meningitis between 1985 and 1991 among children under age 5 in the United States, *S. pneumoniae* and *N. meningitidis* have become the principal causes of meningitis in children older than 1 month (Quagliarello and Scheld 1997). However, *H. influenzae* bacteremia and meningitis are increasing in frequency among adults who test positive for human immunodeficiency virus (HIV) (Munoz et al. 1997).

In Africa, the meningococcal A + C polysaccharide vaccine has modified the cyclic pattern of epidemic meningococcal meningitis. The sub-Saharan (Sahel) regions of Africa between 5 and 15 degrees north latitude, with annual rainfall of 30–110 cm, constitute the African meningitis belt. Regional prevalence of meningococcal meningitis in epidemic years is 400–1,000 cases per 100,000 population. Used for prophylaxis and outbreak control, the vaccine has broken the 8- to 14-year patterns of recurrence of meningococcal meningitis. Smaller epidemics, with shortened interepidemic intervals in some countries, have resulted, in addition to outbreaks of meningitis in countries outside the belt (Varaine et al. 1997).

Simultaneously, there has been a worldwide increase in infection with strains of *S. pneumoniae* resistant to penicillin and other β-lactam antibiotics (second- and third-generation cephalosporins). Altered penicillin-binding proteins, and not β-lactamase production, mediate resistance. Early reports from Spain, Hungary, and South Africa were followed by similar reports from Japan and multiple centers in the United States. In 1994, isolates from 25% of patients with invasive pneumococcal infection in Atlanta, GA, hospitals were resistant to penicillin. Moreover, 9% of pneumococci from this study group also were resistant to cefotaxime, another antibiotic commonly used to treat meningitis, highlighting the growing problem of antibiotic resistance (Quagliarello and Scheld 1997).

Pathogenesis

S. pneumoniae, *N. meningitidis*, and *H. influenzae* are spread by droplets or exchange of saliva. Bacterial meningitis develops most commonly when pathogens colonizing the nasopharynx cause bacteremia and breech the blood-brain barrier. However, meningitis also arises as a consequence of parameningeal infection (ear, sinus, dental, or paraspinal sites), after traumatic or surgical disruption of the blood-brain barrier, or when a cerebral abscess ruptures into the ventricular or subarachnoid spaces.

Clinical Features

Bacterial meningitis presents as an acute febrile illness with prominent headache, neck stiffness, photophobia, and altered mental status. Infants, the elderly, and immunocompromised patients may show only mild behavioral changes with low-grade fever and little clinical evidence of meningeal inflammation. Approximately 15% of all patients, and 40% of older patients, demonstrate focal cerebral findings, and 20–50% of patients develop seizures at some time during the course. The likelihood of infection with a specific pathogen relates, in large part, to age (Table 59A.1). Group B streptococci, *Listeria*, and gram-negative bacilli cause meningitis and invasive disease at the extremes of life, in neonates and the elderly. In the United States, *N. meningitidis* is now the predominant pathogen among children aged 2–18 years and *S. pneumoniae* among adults (Schuchat et al. 1997).

Diagnosis

The patient with suspected bacterial meningitis requires blood cultures and urgent lumbar puncture (LP). Cranial computed tomography (CT) before LP is indicated when focal findings or clinical evidence of raised intracranial pressure (ICP) are present. When the need for CT scanning significantly delays LP, blood cultures should be obtained and empiric antibiotic therapy administered appropriate to the clinical setting. LP is then performed as soon as possible following CT.

CSF examination reveals elevated pressure (200–500 mm H_2O) and protein (100–500 mg/dl, normal 15–45 mg/dl), decreased glucose (<40% serum glucose), and marked pleocytosis (100–10,000 white blood cells [WBC]/μl, normal <5) with 60% or greater polymorphonuclear leukocytes. The CSF Gram's stain result is positive in at least 60% of cases, and CSF culture results are positive in approximately 75%. The likelihood of finding Gram's stain or culture-positive CSF may decrease 5–40% if antibiotics were administered before the LP. However, antibiotics given 1–2 hours before the spinal tap do not decrease diagnostic sensitivity of CSF culture done in conjunction with blood cultures and latex particle agglutination and counterimmunoelectrophoresis testing of CSF for

Table 59A.1: Antibiotics recommended for empiric therapy of suspected bacterial meningitis when the Gram's stain is nondiagnostic and when an organism is identified by cerebrospinal fluid culture

Clinical setting	Likely organism	Empiric treatment	Identified organism	Type-specific treatment
Immunocompetent <3 mos	Group B streptococcus	Ampicillin + broad-spectrum cephalosporin	Group B streptococcus	Ampicillin + gentamicin (neonates)
	Escherichia coli		Enterobacteriaceae	Broad-spectrum cephalosporin + aminoglycoside
	Listeria monocytogenes		L. monocytogenes	Ampicillin + gentamicin
3 mos to 18 yrs	Neisseria meningitidis	Broad-spectrum cephalosporin*	N. meningitidis	Penicillin G
	Streptococcus pneumoniae		S. pneumoniae	Vancomycin + broad-spectrum cephalosporin*
	Haemophilus influenzae		H. influenzae	Ceftriaxone
18–50 yrs	S. pneumoniae	Broad-spectrum cephalosporin*		
	N. meningitidis			
>50 yrs	S. pneumoniae	Ampicillin + broad-spectrum cephalosporin*		
	L. monocytogenes			
	Gram-negative bacilli		Pseudomonas aeruginosa	Ceftazidime + aminoglycoside
			Group B streptococcus	Penicillin G (adult)
Head trauma, cerebrospinal fluid shunt, neurosurgery	Staphylococci Gram-negative bacilli S. pneumoniae	Vancomycin + ceftazidime	Methicillin-resistant S. aureus or S. epidermidis	Vancomycin ± gentamicin ± rifampin
Immunocompromised	L. monocytogenes Gram-negative bacilli, also S. pneumoniae and H. influenzae	Ampicillin + ceftazidime		
			Nocardia asteroides	Trimethoprim-sulfamethoxazole
Epidemics	N. meningitidis		N. meningitidis	Penicillin G or centriaxone (IM tifomycine under some circumstances [see text])
			Yersinia pestis	Chloramphenicol
Others			Mycobacterium tuberculosis	Isoniazid, rifampin, pyrazinamide, ethambutol
			Brucella spp.	Doxycycline + aminoglycoside + rifampin

*Add vancomycin or rifampin if significant local prevalence of resistant pneumococcus exists.
Source: Adapted from NE Bharucha, EP Bharucha, SK Bhabha. Bacterial Infections. In WG Bradley, RB Daroff, GM Fenichel, CD Marsden (eds), Neurology in Clinical Practice. Boston: Butterworth–Heinemann, 1996;1181–1243; and VJ Quagliarello, WM Scheld. Treatment of bacterial meningitis. N Engl J Med 1997;336:708–716.

bacterial antigens. Latex agglutination detects the antigens of *H. influenzae* type b, *S. pneumoniae*, *N. meningitidis*, *Escherichia coli* K1, and group B streptococci. Some test kits may not include tests for group B meningococci because its coat polysaccharide is weakly antigenic. Because antibiotic therapy takes longer than 12 hours to sterilize CSF, culture results are often positive for the first several hours after antibiotics. Early in disease, 10–20% of patients have CSF cell counts less than 1,000 cells/μl. Otherwise, cell counts below 1,000 cells/μl in a patient with a compatible clinical syndrome indicate partially treated meningitis, concurrent immunosuppression, or a nonbacterial cause. Rarely, cell counts of less than 100 cells/μl are seen in the apurulent bacterial meningitis syndrome of pneumococcal meningitis, with overwhelming bacterial meningeal infection and absent CSF neutrophil response. Blood cultures reveal the causative organism in 50% of bacterial meningitis cases, consistent with the importance of bacteremia in pathogenesis. Petechial or purpuric rash suggests *N. meningitidis*, or, less often, *Staphylococcus aureus*, pneumococcus, or the rickettsiae. Neuroimaging studies may be normal or reveal complications of bacterial meningitis, such as cerebral edema, communicating or obstructive hydrocephalus, infarction, or venous sinus thrombosis.

The differential diagnosis includes viral, rickettsial, tubercular, fungal or parasitic meningitis, subarachnoid hemorrhage, and neuroleptic malignant syndrome. When meningeal signs are less prominent, cerebral or epidural abscess, subdural empyema, and viral encephalitis are additional diagnostic considerations.

Treatment

Antibiotic selection depends on clinical setting in conjunction with allergies, local resistance patterns, and CSF results. When LP is delayed or the Gram's stain result is nondiagnostic, empiric therapy is initiated. Ampicillin or penicillin G and a third-generation cephalosporin are typical first-line agents. Until recently, empiric coverage included ampicillin to cover most pneumococcus, meningococcus, and *Listeria* and a third-generation cephalosporin, such as cefotaxime, ceftriaxone, or ceftazidime, to cover gram-negative organisms and ampicillin-resistant *H. influenzae*. However, with the emergence of resistant pneumococcus, these recommendations are changing, and local resistance patterns influence empiric antibiotic coverage in adults with community-acquired meningitis. In patients with recent head trauma or neurosurgery, vancomycin should be added to a broad-spectrum cephalosporin to cover *S. aureus*. Ceftazidime, unlike other third-generation cephalosporins, covers *Pseudomonas* and is reserved for situations in which meningitis with this organism is suspected or proven. Current recommendations for empiric therapy, based on patient's age and immune status, are summarized in Table 59A.2.

When CSF Gram's stain result or culture reveals a particular bacterial pathogen, treatment is directed toward the specific pathogen. In meningitis caused by *S. pneumoniae* of unknown antibiotic sensitivity, vancomycin or rifampin (RIF), combined with a broad-spectrum cephalosporin that achieves adequate CSF levels should be given, because of the emergence of penicillin-resistant pneumococcus. Therefore, bacterial meningitis with gram-positive cocci is treated with vancomycin plus a broad-spectrum cephalosporin. Gram-negative cocci are treated with penicillin G. Gram-positive bacilli are treated with ampicillin (or penicillin G) plus an aminoglycoside. Gram-negative bacilli are treated with a broad-spectrum cephalosporin and an aminoglycoside. Current antibiotic recommendations, when culture results reveal a specific pathogen, are listed in columns four and five of Table 59A.2.

Because bacterial meningitis develops at an immunologically privileged site lacking a lymphatic system, bactericidal, rather than bacteriostatic, antibiotics that rapidly achieve adequate CSF levels should be selected. Therefore,

antibiotic selection and reevaluation are made in the context of several general pharmacological observations and principles. Meningeal inflammation increases permeability of the blood-brain barrier to β-lactam antibiotics from 0.5–2.0% to 5–10% of serum concentration. For more lipid-soluble antibiotics, such as chloramphenicol, RIF, and trimethoprim (TMP), CSF levels reach 30–40% of serum concentrations even without meningeal inflammation. The low pH of infected CSF impairs aminoglycoside activity, and increased CSF protein reduces the concentrations of active free drug for the β-lactams, which are highly protein-bound. Antibiotics used in meningitis, their relevant properties, and specific indications appear in summary form in Table 59A.2.

Optimal duration of therapy is not known for bacterial meningitis. Parenteral antibiotics are administered for 7–10 days for meningococcal and *H. influenzae* meningitis, 10–14 days for pneumococcus, and longer courses of 14–21 days for *Listeria* monocytogenes, Group B streptococci, and 21 days for gram-negative bacilli other than *H. influenzae* (Quagliarello and Scheld 1997). Treatment of bacterial meningitis sometimes extends to include family, medical personnel, and other contacts who may require chemoprophylaxis. In many instances, proven or suspected bacterial meningitis requires notification of public health authorities, to ensure accurate surveillance.

Adjunctive Therapy

Accumulating experimental evidence from animal models supports a role for inflammatory cytokines in the pathophysiology of bacterial meningitis. The proinflammatory cytokines, interleukin 1 and 6, and tumor necrosis factor-α, produced by CSF leukocytes in response to a bacterial stimulus, whether whole organism, component, or toxin, mediate central nervous system (CNS) inflammation, cerebral edema, and cerebrovascular dysregulation in these models. Because corticosteroids may interrupt the inflammatory cascade, their use in bacterial meningitis has been proposed. The available evidence on adjunctive dexamethasone therapy confirms benefit for *H. influenzae* type b meningitis in reducing audiological sequelae and suggests benefit in reducing audiological and neurological sequelae in pneumococcal meningitis in children. Adjunctive dexamethasone therapy, recommended in children over 2 months of age with bacterial meningitis, should be started intravenously at the same time as, or shortly before, the first dose of antibiotic as 15 mg/kg body weight and administered every 6 hours for 2 days (McIntyre et al. 1997).

Indications for corticosteroid therapy for meningitis in adults are less clear. In a single 1989 study, dexamethasone, 12 mg intravenously every 12 hours for 3 days, was beneficial in patients with pneumococcal meningitis. However, with increasing pneumococcal resistance to antibiotics, the effect of corticosteroids on CSF antibiotic penetration influences evolving recommendations for management of pneumococ-

Table 59A.2: Antibiotic treatment for bacterial meningitis[a]

Antibiotic	Bactericidal/ bacteristatic	Therapeutic to toxic ratio	Cerebrospinal fluid penetration	Organism	Intravenous dose (adult)	Remarks
Penicillins						
Penicillin G	Cell wall damaged; bactericidal	Wide, except in renal failure and the elderly	3+	Neisseria meningitis, some Streptococcus pneumoniae, group B Streptococcus	24 million U/day (q4h)	Some S. pneumoniae and N. meningitidis may be resistant
Ampicillin	Bactericidal	Wide	3+	As for penicillin G + some Haemophilus influenzae, Listeria monocytogenes, 60–70% Escherichia coli	12 g/day (q4h)	Inactivated by β-lactamase[b]
Extended-spectrum penicillins	Bactericidal	Wide	3+	As for ampicillin + Pseudomonas aeruginosa, Klebsiella pneumoniae, indolepositive Proteus, Serratia	Carbenicillin, 18–30 g/day (q4h) Ticarcillin, 12–20 g/day (q4h) Azlocillin, piperacillin, and mezlocillin, 10–15 g/day (q4h)	Used in combination with an aminoglycoside; β-lactamase sensitive[b]
Antistaphylococcal penicillins	Bactericidal	Wide	2+	Staphylococcus aureus, Staphylococcus epidermidis	Methicillin, nafcillin, and oxacillin, 8–12 g/day (q4h)	Except methicillin-resistant strains
Vancomycin	Bactericidal	Narrow	3+	S. aureus including methicillin-resistant strains, S. epidermidis, penicillin-resistant pneumococci, enterococci, diphtheroids, and Flavobacterium meningosepticum	3 g/day (q6h)	Ototoxic, nephrotoxic effects additive with aminoglycoside; can be used in penicillin allergy
Third-generation cephalosporins	Bactericidal	Wide	3+	Broad-spectrum; some gram-positive and especially gram-negative E. coli, Klebsiella, Proteus, Serratia, N. meningitidis, H. influenzae (including β-lactamase-secreting strains)	Cefotaxime, 8–12 g/day (q4h) Ceftriaxone, 4 g/day (q12h) Ceftazidime, 8 g/day (q6h)	Inactive against enterococci, many penicillin-resistant pneumococci, L. monocytogenes, Clostridium difficile[c] Ceftazidime, not cefotaxime/ceftriaxone, active against Pseudomonas
Chloramphenicol	Bacteristatic; bactericidal in therapeutic concentrations against Haemophilus, S. pneumoniae, and meningococcus	Narrow; peak serum levels should be maintained between 15 and 25 mg/liter	4+	H. influenzae, S. pneumoniae, N. meningitidis	4 g/day (q6h) PO administration > IV provided no vomiting	H. influenzae resistance occurs; drug superseded by third-generation cephalosporins in developed countries[d]
Aminoglycosides	Bactericidal but not uniformly so because of acidic pH and low CSF levels	Narrow	1+; consider intrathecal or intraventricular administration	Gram-negative enteric organisms, P. aeruginosa	Netilmicin, tobramycin, and gentamicin, 200 mg/day (q8h) Kanamycin, amikacin, 1 g/day (q8h)	Dose-related vestibular, hearing and renal toxicity[e]

Table 59A.2: *(continued)*

Antibiotic	Bactericidal/ bacteriostatic	Therapeutic to toxic ratio	Cerebrospinal fluid penetration	Organism	Intravenous dose (adult)	Remarks
Trimethoprim-sulfamethoxazole	Bacteristatic or bactericidal	Narrow	4+	Broad-spectrum *S. pneumoniae*, *H. influenzae*, meningococcus, gram-negatives, *Staphylococcus*, *L. monocytogenes*, *Nocardia*	Trimethoprim, 1.2 g/day sulfamethoxazole, 6 g/day (q12h) (trimethoprim 15 mg/kg/day PO q12h)	Not widely used (cause of kernicterus in newborns)
Metronidazole	Bactericidal	Narrow	4+	Anaerobes	1.5 g/day (q8h)	With large doses, prolonged therapy causes seizures, peripheral neuropathy
Rifampin	Bactericidal	Narrow	4+	Prophylaxis for meningococcus and *H. influenzae*; given with vancomycin for resistant *Staphylococcus* and *Flavobacterium meningosepticum*	600 mg/day PO	Avoid widespread use in areas where tuberculosis is endemic, as it produces resistant strains
Fluoroquinolones	Bactericidal	Narrow	Ciprofloxacin 1+ Ofloxacin 2+ Pefloxacin 3+	Gram-negative including *P. aeruginosa* and *Staphylococcus*; use selectively for multidrug-resistant gram-negative bacteria and *Mycobacterium tuberculosis*; prophylaxis for meningococcus	Ciprofloxacin, 1.5 g/day (q12h) Pefloxacin and ofloxacin, 800 mg/day (q12h)	Not in prepubertal children or pregnant women; neuropsychiatric side effects; lowers seizure threshold; raises theophylline level
Unique β-lactams	Bactericidal	Narrow	2+ 3+	Broad-spectrum most gram-positive and gram-negative nosocomial *Fonterobacter* and *Acinetobacter*, polymicrobial bacteremia	Imipenem, 2 g/day (6qh)	Except methicillin-resistant *S. aureus*, enterococcus; not often used in meningitis[f] if alternative exists

4+ = excellent; 3+ = very good; 2+ = good; 1+ = poor; CSF = cerebrospinal fluid.

[a]Readers should check the product information sheet included in the package of each drug and follow those instructions.

[b]β-lactamase inhibitors (e.g., clavulanate or sulbactam) may be used with ampicillin, amoxicillin, or ticarcillin to inhibit β-lactamases. They are not always effective.

[c]Ceftriaxone can be administered once a day if necessary. It is eliminated by kidneys and liver, and impaired function of either organ does not lead to excess drug accumulation. Ceftazidime is especially effective against *Pseudomonas* species. As single agents, ceftriaxone and cefotaxime are the most frequently used in childhood meningitis. Avoid ceftriaxone in babies younger than 3 months because it displaces bilirubin.

[d]Avoid in newborns (gray baby syndrome). Serum levels should be monitored in infants and toddlers. Levels greater than 40 mg/liter are toxic. Levels greater than 25 mg/liter can cause dose-related reversible marrow suppression. Idiosyncratic irreversible marrow aplasia (1 in 20,000 patients) is the most feared complication. Shock and liver dysfunction interfere with excretion. Phenytoin, phenobarbital, and rifampin interact. Serum level monitoring is essential.

[e]Also weak neuromuscular blockers; caution in myasthenia gravis, lung disease, respiratory failure, and postoperatively when curare has been used. It should be avoided in renal failure. If used, modify dosage interval according to creatinine level, and monitor blood levels. Controlled studies in newborns showed that intrathecal administration did not improve outcome and intraventricular administration was detrimental. Drug given intrathecally may not reach ventricles, and direct intraventricular administration is traumatic and toxic. Similar controlled studies in adults have not been done, and the intrathecal route or intraventricular administration via percutaneous reservoir may be necessary with resistant strains. Third-generation cephalosporins and antipseudomonal penicillins have made these routes less necessary.

[f]May be epileptogenic.

Source: Adapted from NE Bharucha, EP Bharucha, SK Bhabha. Bacterial Infections. In WG Bradley, RB Daroff, GM Fenichel, CD Marsden (eds), Neurology in Clinical Practice (2nd ed). Boston: Butterworth-Heinemann, 1996;1181–1243.

cal meningitis. For example, experimental evidence in animal models of meningitis shows that concurrent corticosteroid administration reduces vancomycin penetration into CSF. As a result, currently recommended treatment of pneumococcal meningitis in adults receiving adjuvant dexamethasone, pending antibiotic sensitivities, consists of ceftriaxone plus RIF. In treating penicillin-resistant pneumococcal meningitis, a second LP in 24–48 hours is recommended to document bacteriological improvement, because adjuvant dexamethasone may mask clinical signs of poor antibiotic response (Quagliarello and Scheld 1997).

Complications

Focal cerebral signs such as hemiparesis usually imply arteritis, septic venous thrombophlebitis, or cerebritis. Meningeal inflammatory processes, including bacterial meningitis, also can cause cranial neuropathies. A cranial nerve VI palsy and deteriorating level of consciousness within the first 48 hours usually indicates an increase in ICP. ICP monitoring may be necessary in patients with depressed consciousness to guide treatment of intracranial hypertension. Subdural effusions may develop in children, particularly with *H. influenzae* or other gram-negative meningitis. Indications for tapping and culturing a subdural effusion include persistent fever, rapidly enlarging head circumference in the absence of hydrocephalus, or focal neurological signs related to the effusion. Subdural effusions are aspirated under CT guidance. Sterile effusions often resolve spontaneously; subdural empyemas require more aggressive neurosurgical management. Depending on clinical circumstances, hydrocephalus may require intervention with serial LPs (if communicating) and external ventricular drainage. Obstructive hydrocephalus may be monitored expectantly with serial CTs.

Some Specific Pathogens and Public Health Issues

Pneumococcus.   Meningitis occurs in approximately 4% of patients with invasive *S. pneumoniae*. Associated conditions include otitis media, skull fractures, alcoholism, and sickle cell disease. Pneumovax, the pneumococcal vaccine composed of polysaccharides of 23 pneumococcal types, is recommended for patients with surgical or functional asplenia (such as sickle cell disease) and chronic illnesses. Of all blood culture isolates of pneumococci in the United States, 88% are contained in the 23-valent vaccine.

Rare pneumococcal meningitis cases have been classified as apurulent by the absence of CSF pleocytosis. Turbid CSF, masses of pneumococci, elevated protein, fewer than 100 cells/μl, and low CSF glucose are characteristic. Twenty-four hours after initiating antibiotic treatment, CSF cell counts can increase to more than 2,000 cells/μl and pneumococci disappear from the CSF.

Penicillin G and ampicillin are equally effective in treating meningitis caused by penicillin-sensitive strains of *S. pneumoniae*. For patients with *S. pneumoniae* resistant to

both penicillin and ceftriaxone, treatment is by ceftriaxone combined with either vancomycin or RIF.

Meningococcus.   *N. meningitidis* infection may manifest as fever and bacteremia without sepsis, meningococcemia without meningitis, or meningitis with or without meningococcemia. Meningitis occurs in an estimated 48% of cases of invasive disease. Rare isolates produce β-lactamase or have altered penicillin-binding proteins. In the event of poor initial response to penicillin or ampicillin, isolates should be tested for sensitivities and therapy changed to ceftriaxone or cefotaxime. Treatment of systemic infection may not eliminate nasopharyngeal carriage. During widespread outbreaks or epidemics, when up to 1% of the population may be affected, a single injection of long-acting oily preparation of chloramphenicol (Tifomycine) at a dose of 3 g intramuscularly has been used successfully.

Current commercial vaccines include the quadrivalent vaccine with activity against serogroups A, C, Y, and W135. Protective antibodies persist for up to 5 years in adults, but only 1–2 years in children younger than 4. Vaccination is recommended for patients with complement deficiency or asplenia, as well as military recruits and travelers to hyperendemic or epidemic areas such as Nigeria, Niger, and Cameroon. Most vaccinations are given during outbreaks. Vaccine against serogroup B has been developed in Cuba and used in some areas of South America.

Prophylaxis for meningococcal meningitis is recommended for all household members who may have had saliva-exchange contact and for medical personnel with mouth-to-mouth contact. A 2-day course of oral RIF is given in doses of 600 mg every 12 hours for adults, 10 mg/kg every 12 hours for children 1 month to 12 years old, and 5 mg/kg every 12 hours for infants younger than 1 month of age. Alternatives include ceftriaxone intramuscularly (250 mg for adults, 125 mg for children), recommended for pregnant and lactating women or children younger than 2 years, or minocycline or ciprofloxacin.

Haemophilus influenzae.   Meningitis complicates approximately 10% of *H. influenzae* infections, often in the setting of a parameningeal ear or nose infection or basal skull fracture. The *H. influenzae* type b conjugate vaccine series is administered at 2, 4, and 12–18 months. Chemoprophylaxis with oral RIF is recommended for all household members in which there are susceptible children under 4 years of age. The doses are the same as for meningococcal prophylaxis, but treatment is given for 4 days.

Listeria monocytogenes.   *Listeria*, a common meningeal pathogen in immunosuppressed hosts and neonates, also causes meningitis in the normal host. Meningitis develops in 36% of cases of invasive listeriosis. Ampicillin plus gentamicin is recommended for patients of all ages with *Listeria* meningitis, because neither ampicillin nor penicillin is bactericidal for *Listeria* in vitro and third-generation cephalosporins are inactive against *Listeria*. TMP in combination with sulfamethoxazole (SMX) may be used in penicillin-allergic patients.

Listeria cerebritis or rhombencephalitis is a distinct nonmeningitic syndrome, which presents as headache, fever, nausea, and vomiting, followed by cranial nerve palsies, decreased consciousness, seizures, and focal deficits. The CSF may contain few or no WBCs. CSF Gram's stain and culture results are negative, but blood culture results are positive. *Listeria* cerebritis requires 6 weeks of treatment.

Nosocomial Agents

Increasing numbers of nosocomially acquired infections, including meningitis, are disturbing facts of hospital life. Gram-negative bacteria of the Enterobacteriaceae family (*E. coli, Klebsiella pneumoniae*), *Pseudomonas* species, and gram-positive cocci (staphylococci, pneumococcus) frequently cause hospital-acquired meningitis. Members of the genus *Acinetobacter*, especially multiresistant strains of *Acinetobacter baumannii*, increasingly cause nosocomial pneumonia, bacteremia, and meningitis in the ICU. Associated systemic features include petechial rash in 30% of patients and Waterhouse-Friderichsen syndrome. *Acinetobacter* and meningococcus thus share clinical, as well as microbiological, features, leading to diagnostic confusion. *Acinetobacter* are rod-shaped gram-negative organisms during rapid growth and coccoid in the stationary stage. Most *A. baumannii* are now resistant to ampicillin, carbenicillin, cefotaxime, chloramphenicol, gentamicin, and other aminoglycosides. Imipenem, carbenicillin plus an aminoglycoside, or amoxicillin-clavulanic acid are treatment alternatives.

Brain Abscess

Brain abscess is a focal suppurative process of brain parenchyma, accounting for an estimated 1 in 10,000 general hospital admissions. Brain abscesses develop most frequently by spread from a contiguous infected cranial site, such as ear, sinus, or teeth. Other predisposing causes include open head trauma, previous neurosurgery, and craniofacial osteomyelitis. Hematogenous spread from a remote source also can cause brain abscesses, particularly in the setting of congenital heart disease with right-to-left shunt or pulmonary disorders such as lung abscess, bronchiectasis, or arteriovenous fistula. Metastatic, or blood-borne abscesses, usually are found at gray and white matter junctions, in the distribution of the middle cerebral artery, and are often multiple. However, 20% of abscesses are occult, with no source of infection ever found (Anderson 1993). Classifying brain abscesses by likely entry point of infection allows physicians to predict likely pathogens and choose appropriate empiric therapy. Frontal abscesses arise most often from paranasal sinus infection, temporal or cerebellar abscesses from an otogenic source, and multi-

ple abscesses from a remote source. Experimental evidence suggests that bacteria require damaged brain, such as the microscopic or macroscopic area of necrosis resulting from septic thrombophlebitis, emboli, or hypoxemia, to establish infection. The predilection of metastatic abscesses for gray and white matter junctions, for example, may be a consequence of the fluctuations in blood supply to those areas. Once infection is established, the abscess passes through the stages of cerebritis, central necrosis, capsular development, and maturity over a period of approximately 14 days.

Clinical Features

Patients with brain abscess present with signs and symptoms of an expanding mass lesion, with progressive headache, altered mentation, or focal deficit. Approximately one-half of patients develop nausea and vomiting. Approximately the same proportion have fever, and hence the diagnosis should not be excluded based on normal temperature alone. Acute worsening of headache and nuchal pain, together with an increase in temperature, can signify rupture of the abscess into the subarachnoid space, a serious event.

Diagnosis

Neuroimaging studies reveal one or more ring-enhancing masses with slight surrounding edema. The ring of enhancement may be thicker near the cortex and thinner near the ventricle (Figure 59A.1); large abscesses tend to have thin, enhancing rings of relatively uniform thickness. Associated sinus or ear infection also may be identified by cranial imaging, though dedicated sinus or temporal bone CT may be necessary as well, in order to better visualize the primary site of infection. An early lesion in the cerebritis stage appears an a nonenhancing focal low-density area on CT scan or hypointensity on magnetic resonance imaging (MRI). Air within a brain mass, in the absence of recent neurosurgery, suggests an abscess. An indium-labeled leukocyte scintillation scan demonstrating an active inflammatory focus may complement CT or MRI studies.

Peripheral leukocytosis may be mild or absent and should not be relied on for considering the diagnosis. Because of the risk of herniation or precipitating rupture, LP is contraindicated in suspected or proven brain abscesses. CSF reveals only nonspecific findings of elevated protein and lymphocytic pleocytosis with normal glucose and rarely yields positive culture results unless the abscess has ruptured into the subarachnoid space.

Pathogens

Occurring as mixed infections 30–60% of the time, brain abscess pathogens vary with the clinical setting. In immunocompetent patients the most commonly encountered aerobic organisms are the alpha-hemolytic and nonhemolytic streptococci (such as *Streptococcus milleri*), *S. aureus*, and

Enterobacteriaceae. Other important pathogens include anaerobes such as *Bacteroides*, *Fusobacterium*, *Peptostreptococcus*, and *Propionibacterium*; and gram-negative bacteria such as *Eikenella*, *Actinobacillus*, *Cardiobacterium*, and *Haemophilus*; and enteric gram-negative bacteria such as *E. coli*, *Klebsiella*, and *Pseudomonas*. Several important associations include *S. milleri* or pneumococcus with a sinus source; *Bacteroides*, *Enterobacter*, *Proteus*, streptococci, or *Pseudomonas* with an ear source; anaerobic streptococci with pulmonary infections; *Actinomyces* with dental procedures; and *S. aureus* in the patient with head trauma, recent neurosurgery, or cranial osteomyelitis. Various other bacteria may occasionally be found in brain abscesses, including *Clostridium* spp. after trauma and wound contamination by soil, *Citrobacter diversus* in neonates, *Salmonella* spp., *Streptobacillus moniliformis* (the agent of rat-bite fever), and *Brucella* spp. Except for pneumococcus and *H. influenzae*, typical bacterial meningitis pathogens infrequently cause brain abscess (Case Records 1993).

Geography and immune status are other important determinants of brain abscess microbiology. Tuberculomas frequently cause space-occupying lesions in countries with high tuberculosis (TB) prevalence. *Amebae* spp., toxoplasmosis, cysticercosis, or other helminths, including schistosomal species, *Paragonimus* spp., trichinosis, sparganosis, and echinococcosis cause parasitic cerebral abscesses. *Pseudallescheria boydii* fungal abscess may follow a near-drowning episode by 2–4 weeks.

In immunocompromised patients with T-cell or mononuclear phagocyte defects, causes of brain abscesses include *Listeria monocytogenes*, *Nocardia asteroides*, *Gordona terrae* (an environmental actinomycete), *Mycobacterium* spp., and parasites such as *Toxoplasma*, *Acanthamoeba*, *Cryptococcus*, and *Trypanosoma cruzi*. In HIV-infected patients, polymicrobial pyogenic abscesses with *S. bovis*, *Fusobacterium*, *Peptostreptococcus*, and group G streptococcus have been reported, along with abscesses with unusual combinations of organisms, such as *Candida* and staphylococci (Maniglia et al. 1997). Neutrophil abnormalities lead to an increased incidence of Enterobacteriaceae and *Pseudomonas* abscesses; fungal abscesses caused by *Aspergillus*, *Mucor*, or *Candida*; and *Strongyloides*.

Differential Diagnosis

In the febrile patient with headache, altered mentation, and lateralizing findings, the differential diagnosis includes other infectious etiologies, such as subdural empyema, epidural abscess, viral encephalitis, bacterial or acute aseptic meningitis, and endocarditis with septic embolism or mycotic aneurysm rupture. When fever is low grade or absent, primary or metastatic brain tumor is a consideration. Occasionally, demyelinating lesions present as focal deficits or seizures and appear as ring-enhancing masses on neuroimaging studies. Resolving cerebral hemorrhages also appear as ring-enhancing lesions on neuroimaging studies, particularly

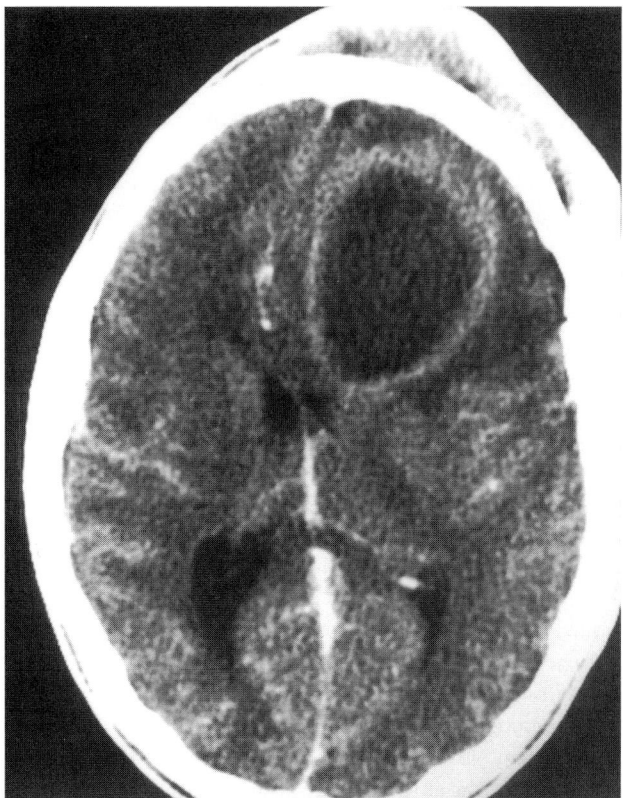

FIGURE 59A.1 Brain abscess. Contrast-enhanced computed tomographic scan showing a ring-enhancing lesion with surrounding edema in the left frontal lobe. The appearance is typical for an abscess, with the ring of enhancement thicker adjacent to the well-vascularized gray matter and thinner along its border with the white matter near the ventricle. Forehead edema is consistent with the primary infection in the frontal sinus.

CT. Brainstem infection with *L. monocytogenes* or *Propionibacterium acnes* may produce a brainstem encephalitis (rhombencephalitis) that clinically mimics brainstem abscess.

Treatment

Successful treatment of brain abscess requires antibiotics in all patients and surgery in many. Antibiotics must not only penetrate brain tissue, but also reach the abscess cavity and retain activity at its characteristically low pH. For years, standard brain abscess therapy combined high-dose penicillin (24 million U/day intravenously) with chloramphenicol (1 g every 6 hours). Because metronidazole (1 g loading dose, followed by 500 mg every 6 hours) provides excellent anaerobic coverage and penetrates well into brain abscesses, it has replaced chloramphenicol, which carries the additional risk of aplastic anemia. Hence, empiric antibiotic therapy for brain abscess usually includes metronidazole and either penicillin or a third-generation cephalosporin (cefotaxime, ceftriaxone, or ceftazidime), which covers the streptococci and aerotolerant anaerobes resistant to metronidazole. Following head trauma or neurosurgical procedures, when *S. aureus* is a concern, an anti-staphylococcal penicillin (nafcillin, methicillin) or vancomycin is added.

Current recommendations for empiric therapy, based on location of abscess and inferred source of infection, are metronidazole with either penicillin or a third-generation cephalosporin for frontal abscesses; penicillin, metronidazole, and ceftazidime for temporal or cerebellar abscesses; nafcillin, metronidazole, and cefotaxime for multiple (metastatic) abscesses; nafcillin and cefotaxime for penetrating wounds; and vancomycin and ceftazidime for postoperative abscesses (Mathisen and Johnson 1997). Intravenous treatment continues for 6–8 weeks and may be followed by oral therapy for 2–3 months. Surgical excision may shorten the time course of intravenous therapy by 1 or 2 weeks.

Optimal therapy usually requires neurosurgical intervention. Although controversy continues as to whether aspiration under stereotactic CT guidance or total excision yields better results, excision is recommended for gas-containing, multiloculated, or fungal abscesses. Patients for whom medical management alone may be the better choice include patients with multiple, deep, or dominant hemisphere abscesses; simultaneous meningitis or ependymitis; abscesses measuring less than 3 cm; or abscesses that shrink after antimicrobial therapy. Surgery is not performed in the cerebritis stage until a capsule forms. Ear, nose, sinus, and dental infections should be evaluated by the appropriate surgical specialists.

Adjunctive medical therapy for medical or surgical cases includes corticosteroids for mass effect, hyperosmolar agents for worsening cerebral edema and ICP, and prophylactic or symptomatic anticonvulsants. Decreased mortality from brain abscesses over the last two decades, from more than 50% to less than 10%, reflects improvements in neuroimaging and neurosurgical techniques. One-half of survivors are neurologically normal. Rapid disease progression before hospitalization and poor level of consciousness at the time of admission portend poor outcome. Intraventricular rupture of a brain abscess is associated with mortality exceeding 80%.

After treatment, patients are followed with neuroimaging studies at monthly intervals for approximately 6 months or until contrast enhancement disappears. Persistent contrast enhancement predicts recurrence in up to 20% of patients. Seizures occur in 25–50% of patients during their early period of hospitalization, and anticonvulsants initiated during hospitalization are continued for 6–12 months. When administered prophylactically, anticonvulsants are continued for a minimum of 3 months after surgery.

Subdural Empyema

Subdural empyema is a collection of pus between the dura and arachnoid. It develops most commonly as a consequence of ear or sinus infection. Other causes include cranial osteomyelitis, penetrating head trauma or neurosurgery, infection of subdural effusions in childhood meningitis, and hematogenous spread from a remote source. Purulent material tracks over the brain surface over the hemispheres (Figure 59A.2), along the falx or adjacent to the primary focus. Posterior fossa involvement is unusual; spinal subdural empyemas are rare and always metastatic.

Clinical Features

Patients typically present acutely with prominent headache, fever, stiff neck, seizures, focal neurological symptoms and signs, and rapid deterioration. The diagnosis should be considered in patients with meningeal signs and deficits indicating extensive, unilateral hemispheric dysfunction or in patients with sinusitis who develop meningeal signs. A parafalcine collection would be indicated by leg weakness, paraparesis, or sphincter disturbance. Children younger than 5 years may develop subdural empyemas after *H. influenzae* or gram-negative bacterial meningitis and present with irritability, poor feeding, and increasing head circumference. Radicular pain and signs of cord compression in the absence of vertebral tenderness suggest spinal subdural empyema.

Diagnosis

Because there are similarities between subdural empyema and bacterial brain abscess with regard to pathogenesis and clinical presentation, the disorders share many aspects of diagnosis and management. Bacterial pathogens for both disorders are similar, although subdural empyemas are less often mixed. Neuroimaging studies help establish the diagnosis, but may underestimate the size of the empyema. In infants, the diagnosis may be made by subdural taps. The empyema fluid is usually too turbid to transilluminate. Spinal cases are examined by MRI or myelography.

Treatment

Because subdural empyema progresses rapidly, combined medical and surgical management should proceed emergently. Untreated, subdural empyemas are uniformly fatal. Whether craniotomy or burr hole aspiration is the better surgical treatment remains controversial. Burr holes work well for early cases, but pus may reaccumulate. Craniotomy is recommended in posterior fossa cases or if cranial osteomyelitis coexists. Otitis or sinusitis may require simultaneous surgical therapy. Empyema fluid should be cultured, and antibiotic treatment is continued for at least 3 weeks. In as many as one-fourth of cases, no organism can be cultured from pus (Anderson 1993).

Overall mortality is 14–18%. Poor prognosis is associated with rapid disease progression before hospitalization and depressed level of consciousness at admission. Mortality is 75% in comatose patients. An estimated 42% of survivors develop seizures within 16 months.

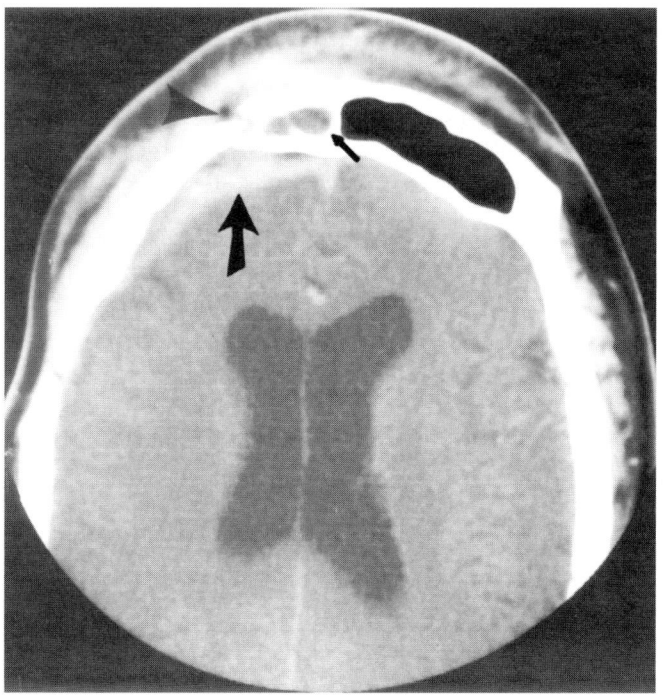

A

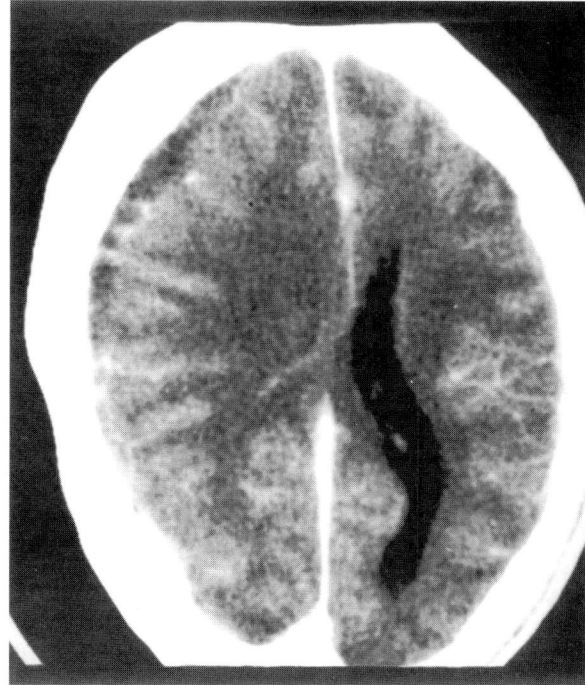

B

FIGURE 59A.2   Subdural empyema. **(A)** Contrast-enhanced computed tomographic scan showing right frontal sinus infection (*short arrow*) that has spread to the right subdural space (*long arrow*) and forehead (*arrowhead*). **(B)** In a second patient, the contrast-enhanced computed tomographic scan shows an extra-axial fluid collection and midline shift disproportionately greater than the size of the subdural collection in a second patient.

Cranial Epidural Abscess

Cranial epidural abscess, an infection in the space between dura and skull, begins as cranial osteomyelitis complicating ear, sinus (Figure 59A.3), or orbital infection, and nasopharyngeal malignancy. Diagnosis, urgent management, and prognosis are similar to subdural empyema. Because *S. aureus* is a frequent isolate, particularly after trauma or surgery, antibiotics should cover staphylococcus, as well as the aerobes, anaerobes, and gram-negative organisms encountered in brain abscesses and subdural empyemas. Brain abscess, subdural empyema, and epidural abscess may occur simultaneously in the same patient.

Septic Venous Sinus Thrombosis

Septic thrombosis of cerebral veins or venous sinuses may complicate meningitis or epidural or subdural abscesses or develop during the intracranial spread of infection from extracerebral veins. Once established, infection and clot spread through the venous system, aided by the absence of valves in intracranial veins. Fortunately, antibiotics have rendered this grim complication of facial, sinus, ear, dental infection, or bacterial meningitis itself less common.

Clinical Features

Thrombosis may develop in the cavernous, superior sagittal, or lateral sinuses, depending on the site of primary infection. Specific presenting features vary with the site involved, and include headache, altered mentation, cranial neuropathies, seizures, fluctuating focal deficits, nonarterial distribution strokes, and increased ICP. Cavernous sinus thrombosis is indicated by ipsilateral proptosis and facial edema, retinal vein engorgement, retinal hemorrhages or papilledema, and clinical involvement of the third, fourth, sixth, and ophthalmic division of the fifth cranial nerves. Lateral (transverse) sinus thrombosis is accompanied by papilledema, extension to the jugular bulb by involvement of cranial nerves IX, X, and XI, and extension to petrosal sinuses by involvement of cranial nerves V and VI. Sagittal sinus thrombosis is associated with papilledema, focal or generalized seizures, leg weakness, aphasia, or cortical sensory deficits.

Diagnosis

CT scan or MRI may demonstrate the primary infection or clot within the sinus. Clot within the sinus may appear as hyperdensity in the sinus on noncontrast CT, but may be

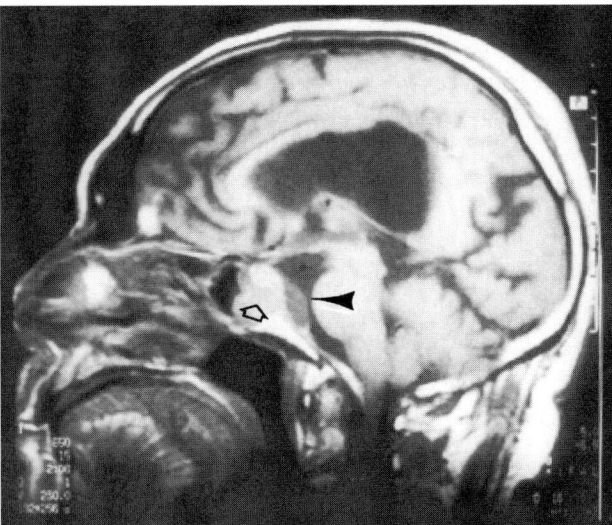

FIGURE 59A.3   Epidural abscess. T1 magnetic resonance image showing sphenoid sinus disease (*open arrow*) that has eroded into the epidural space along the posterior border of the clivus. The abscess is seen as an area of low signal with convex border (*closed arrow*).

missed by MRI, because acute thrombus may appear hypointense on T2-weighted images. MR venography or cerebral angiography with venous phase studies may be necessary to confirm the diagnosis.

Treatment

Treatment is directed toward the primary infection. Anticoagulants are considered by some as being contraindicated because venous infarcts are often hemorrhagic. However, they may help prevent clot propagation, particularly in early cases. Polycythemia, if present, is treated with volume expansion.

Spinal Epidural Abscess

Spinal epidural abscess follows infection elsewhere in the body in most cases. Infection develops in the epidural space by direct extension of vertebral osteomyelitis or soft tissue infections (retroperitoneal, mediastinal, perinephric, psoas, or paraspinal abscess), following penetrating trauma or decubitus ulcers or by hematogenous spread from skin or parenteral drug use. Rarely, back or abdominal surgery, LP, or epidural anesthesia have been contributory.

Clinical Features

Localized back pain and radicular pain are common early symptoms, frequently overshadowed by rapid evolution of paraparesis or quadriparesis. The thoracic spine is involved in 50–80% of cases, lumbar in 17–38%, and cervical in 10–25%.

Diagnosis

The combination of fever, back pain with local spine tenderness, and radiculopathy or myelopathy mandates emergent evaluation. Peripheral WBC count and erythrocyte sedimentation rate are usually elevated. Plain film findings, apparent in approximately one-half of cases, include intervertebral disc space narrowing or lytic changes. The diagnosis depends on MRI or myelography if MRI is not available. MRI is the test of choice because it is noninvasive and provides images of the cord and epidural space in sagittal and transverse planes, as well as direct visualization of inflammatory tissue (Figure 59A.4). LP risks spinal herniation or spreading infection to the subarachnoid space should the needle pass through the abscess. Even so, because outcome depends so heavily on early diagnosis, myelography should be performed in suspected cases when MRI cannot be obtained emergently. Blood culture results are often positive and correlate well with abscess pathogens. Differential diagnosis includes transverse myelitis, spinal osteomyelitis, or, less commonly, spinal subdural empyema, epidural hematoma or metastases, primary spinal tumors, spinal artery syndromes, and discitis. More chronic cases may resemble the hypertrophic spinal pachymeningitis (progressive dural fibrosis with motor root compression) associated with TB or syphilis.

Treatment

Once MRI or myelography has established the diagnosis, urgent surgical decompression and antibiotic therapy are needed. Antibiotics to cover *S. aureus* and gram-negative bacilli are administered, pending definitive identification by cultures of blood or intraoperative specimens. *S. aureus* is the most common pathogen, detected in 50–90% of cases, followed by streptococci and gram-negative enteric bacilli in 10–20% of cases. Other pathogens include *Mycobacterium tuberculosis, Salmonella, Listeria, Brucella, Actinomyces* spp., *Nocardia*, fungi (cryptococcosis, aspergillosis, mucormycosis, coccidiomycosis, blastomycosis), and parasites (cysticercosis, *echinococcosis* schistosomiasis). Corticosteroids are frequently administered preoperatively and postoperatively, during the first week of treatment. Antibiotic treatment continues 3–4 weeks in uncomplicated spinal epidural abscess, and for 6–8 weeks if osteomyelitis is apparent. Prognosis for recovery is good if surgery is performed in the early stages. Neurological recovery is unlikely if surgery is performed more than 24 hours after the onset of paralysis. Medical management alone is considered in patients with complete paralysis of greater than 3 days' duration or extensive multisegmental disease.

Shunt Infections

Staphylococcus epidermidis, followed by *S. aureus*, causes most infections of external ventricular catheters, ICP mon-

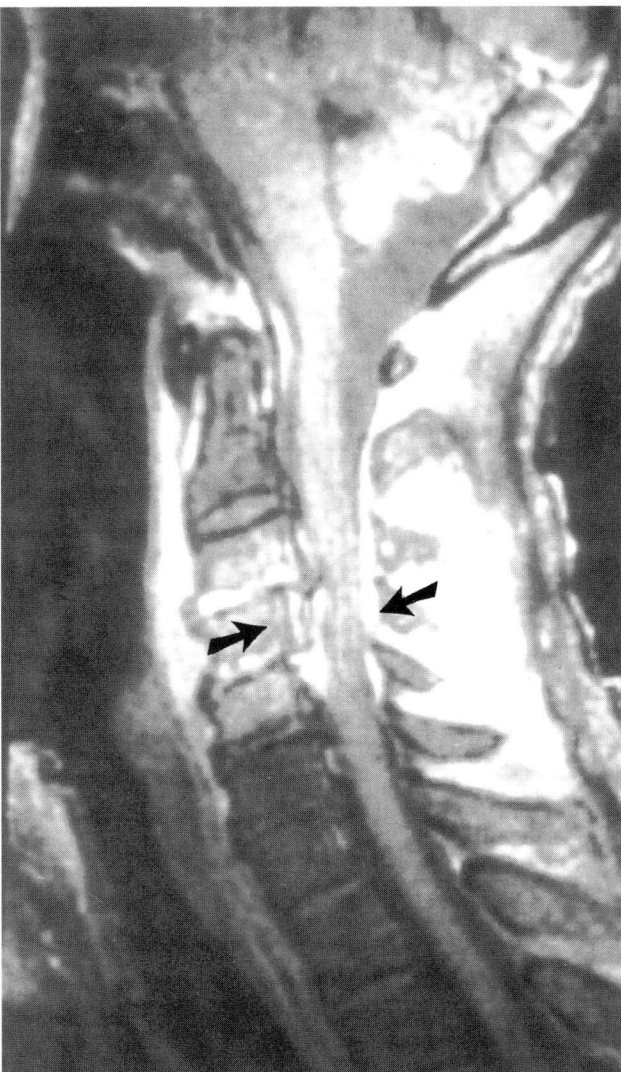

FIGURE 59A.4 Spinal epidural abscess. T1 gadolinium-enhanced sagittal magnetic resonance image of the spine showing enhancing inflammatory tissue compressing the spinal cord at C2 and C3. Enhancement of prevertebral soft tissues and C2, C3, and C4 vertebral bodies is also seen (*arrows*).

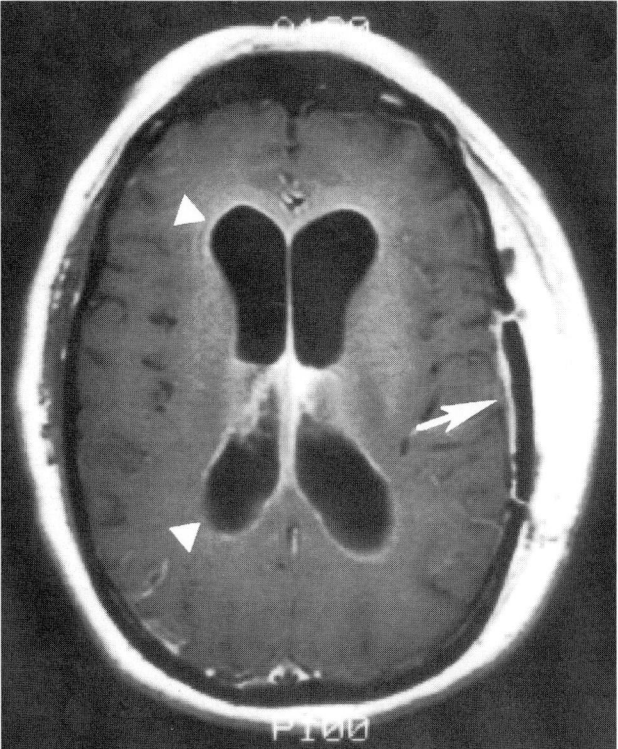

FIGURE 59A.5 Ependymitis secondary to shunt infection. Gadolinium-enhanced T1 magnetic resonance image showing abnormal contrast enhancement of ependymal lining of dilatated lateral ventricles (*arrowheads*); swollen, infected contrast-enhancing craniotomy site; and dural enhancement (*long arrow*) after removal of shunt.

itors, shunt devices, and Ommaya reservoirs. Infection, often within 2 weeks of installation, is signaled by fever, shunt malfunction, and wound infection (Figure 59A.5). Meningeal signs may be absent, but CSF pleocytosis is present. Although greater CSF cell counts may be anticipated in ventricular compared with lumbar CSF, both should be examined and cultured. Because most infections are hospital-acquired, the organism is assumed to be methicillin resistant, and initial treatment is with vancomycin, combined with a third-generation cephalosporin, and sometimes an aminoglycoside, to cover gram-negative bacilli. Intrathecal vancomycin and aminoglycoside are often also necessary, along with removal of the shunt (Kim and Pons 1994).

MYCOBACTERIAL DISEASES

Tuberculosis

Although TB most commonly involves the lungs, it can produce disease in nearly every organ system. Approximately 1% of cases are complicated by neurological disease such as meningitis, tuberculoma, or tuberculous involvement of the spine with myelopathy (Pott's disease). The TB complex consists of obligate aerobic organisms infecting humans and other animals. Two main species are recognized, *Mycobacterium tuberculosis* and *Mycobacterium bovis*. Other less common species include *Mycobacterium africanum* in West and Central Africa and *Mycobacterium ulcerans*. The atypical or nontuberculous mycobacteria, *Mycobacterium avium-intracellulare*, are widely distributed saprophytes and cause multisystem infections, including meningitis, in immunocompromised patients.

Current Trends

TB is the most important infectious disease in the world, with an estimated one-third of the population infected. No single factor accounts for the large numbers of new or complicated cases encountered each year. As is the case for other infections introduced to new, susceptible populations, TB occurs in epidemic waves. Unfortunately, this wave is taking 300 years to pass and has not yet crested in many countries of Asia and Africa. HIV infection has been associated with large numbers of new cases and with a high risk of extrapulmonary TB. Currently, extrapulmonary disease is responsible for approximately 20% of reported cases of TB in the United States. In numerically decreasing order, pleural and lymphatic disease is followed by bone and joint disease, genitourinary disease, miliary disease, meningitis, and peritonitis. As a consequence of worldwide neglect of TB as a public health problem, large numbers of patients now harbor resistant or multiresistant tubercle bacilli.

Pathogenesis

Neurological TB may develop during primary infection or reactivate as a consequence of immunosuppression. TB meningitis develops most commonly after a two-stage process. Tubercle bacilli spread hematogenously from the lung or other organs, form tubercles in the brain parenchyma, and, at a later stage, rupture into the subarachnoid or ventricular space. In other instances, meningitis may arise in the course of miliary TB or from parameningeal infection. In contrast to bacterial meningitis, the meninges are the primary site of infection. Inflammatory exudate spreads along the subarachnoid space and pial vessels to the brain. Pott's disease, or spinal TB, develops when hematogenous spread of tubercle bacilli to the spine causes vertebral osteomyelitis, adjacent joint space infection, and subsequent paravertebral abscess.

Tuberculosis Meningitis

Clinical Features.   TB meningitis typically follows a subacute course with low-grade fever, headache, and intermittent nausea and vomiting, followed by more severe headache and fever, neck stiffness, drowsiness, and cranial (usually oculomotor, but also II, VII, and VIII) nerve palsies. Progressive disease is associated with more pronounced meningeal signs, seizures, and focal neurological deficits, including hemiparesis and involuntary movements, increasing lethargy, and signs of increased ICP. Other presentations of tuberculous meningitis include acute meningitis, behavioral or intellectual disturbances without meningeal signs, encephalopathy, seizures, isolated cranial neuropathies, stroke, increased ICP, and recurrent serous or aseptic meningitis. Meningeal signs are present in approximately 70% of cases, cranial nerve palsy in 25%, and focal neurological findings in 16–18%. Purified protein derivative testing is positive in 50% of affected patients.

Diagnosis.   Identifying tubercle bacilli on CSF acid-fast bacilli (AFB) smear or culture establishes the diagnosis. Ser-

ial LPs and centrifugation of specimens increases the yield of the AFB smear, a test that is diagnostic in only 10–30% of cases. CSF culture results are positive for *M. tuberculosis* in 45–70% of patients but may take 6–8 weeks to become positive. Because a negative CSF AFB smear result does not rule out TB meningitis and culture may not yield organisms for weeks, a presumptive diagnosis is often made based on other clinical criteria so that empiric anti-TB therapy can be started as early as possible.

CSF examination demonstrates normal or elevated opening pressure, elevated protein (80–400 mg/dl), low glucose (<40 mg/dl), and pleocytosis (averaging 200–400 WBC/μl with lymphocytic predominance. However, patients with miliary TB or CNS tuberculomas may have a normal CSF result initially. CSF WBC counts of less than 5/μl have been reported in up to 11% of HIV-seropositive patients and 5% of HIV-seronegative patients. In other instances, an early polymorphonuclear or eosinophilic CSF cellular response may be seen. The lack of sensitivity and specificity of standard CSF analysis and AFB smears has prompted the search for additional diagnostic tests. As a result, polymerase chain reaction (PCR) techniques have been applied to the diagnosis of TB meningitis, with reported sensitivities of 70–75%. Enzyme-linked immunosorbent assay (ELISA) and radioimmunoassay tests for antimycobacterial antigens in the CSF have also been developed (LoBue and Catanzaro 1997).

Additional investigations should include chest radiography, tuberculin test, brain neuroimaging study, retinal examination for choroidal tubercles, and general examination for lymphadenopathy and hepatosplenomegaly. Cranial CT or MRI showing basal meningeal and sylvian enhancement with hydrocephalus suggests the diagnosis.

Differential diagnosis includes untreated or partially treated bacterial meningitis, other causes of granulomatous meningitis (spirochetes, *Brucella*, most fungi, and parasites such as *Amebae*, *Toxoplasma*, and trypanosomes), other conditions that elicit a subacute or chronic granulomatous response (CNS sarcoid, lupus, Behçet's, Vogt-Koyanagi-Harada disease, granulomatous angiitis), and lymphomatous or carcinomatous meningitis. TB should be considered also when suspected bacterial meningitis fails to resolve with antibacterial therapy.

Tuberculomas

Tuberculomas, the parenchymal form of CNS TB, occur as single or multiple brain or spinal cord lesions and present with signs and symptoms of space-occupying lesions. On CT or MRI scan, the lesions may be of low or high intensity, with ring enhancement. Miliary disease is characterized by multiple small (1–2 mm) lesions. Open or stereotactic biopsy may be necessary if definitive diagnosis of TB cannot be made at an extraneural site. Single lesions are removed commonly and anti-TB drugs administered. In regions where TB is prevalent, the decision to initiate anti-TB therapy may be made without histological confirmation.

Spinal Tuberculosis

The most common site of involvement by TB of the spine is T10. Back pain is the chief complaint and paraspinal muscle spasms or angling of the spine caused by collapse of a vertebra (a gibbus) may be found on examination. Plain films show decreased radiodensity of bone and joint space destruction in long-standing disease, but may be normal in early disease. Radionuclide bone scanning improves detection of spinal TB, but the best modality is MRI, which simultaneously visualizes the spinal cord. Progressive paraparesis requires urgent surgical intervention. Surgery also may be indicated for biopsy if the diagnosis is in doubt or to obtain cultures for sensitivities. The differential diagnosis of vertebral bacterial diseases includes infections with staphylococci, streptococci, and typhoid and other gram-negative bacilli; paratyphoid disease; and brucellosis. Compared with other bony infections, there is less sclerosis in tuberculous spondylitis. Skeletal TB appears to be rare in HIV-infected patients.

Treatment. Chemotherapy for TB requires several bactericidal drugs to sterilize lesions and avoid inducing resistance. Optimal drug combinations vary with region, clinical setting, and local resistance patterns (Dutt and Stead 1997). One recommended regimen for initial treatment of CNS TB is with isoniazid (INH, single oral dose 10 mg/kg/day), RIF (single oral dose 10 mg/kg/day), pyrazinamide (single oral dose 35 mg/kg/day), and ethambutol (single oral dose 25 mg/kg/day) or streptomycin (SM, single intramuscular dose 10 mg/kg/day). RIF, SM, and INH (when there is meningeal inflammation) penetrate to the CSF well. If there is satisfactory clinical improvement after 2 months, three- or four-drug regimens can be consolidated to two agents, usually INH and RIF, for an additional 10 months. In areas with high prevalence of drug-resistant disease and HIV infection, treatment begins with five to seven drugs until drug-susceptibility results are known. Additional agents include ethionamide, which penetrates CSF well, cycloserine, para-aminosalicylic acid, thiacetazone, clofazimine, ofloxacin, and rifabutin, which is active against *M. avium* infections and penetrates CSF well. Oral pyridoxine (25–50 mg/day) is given concurrently with INH to prevent neuropathy. Monthly vision and color identification studies are recommended for patients taking ethambutol, to monitor for toxic optic neuropathy. Monthly hearing evaluations are necessary when SM is used, and the drug should be stopped at signs of vestibular toxicity. Liver enzyme levels are monitored also, because INH, RIF, and pyrazinamide are hepatotoxic. Treatment can be continued with elevated liver enzyme levels if the patient remains anicteric or without other signs of liver toxicity. RIF induces cytochrome P450, and thus can alter levels of concurrently administered phenytoin. RIF also accelerates methadone metabolism and may precipitate withdrawal symptoms in patients receiving maintenance therapy.

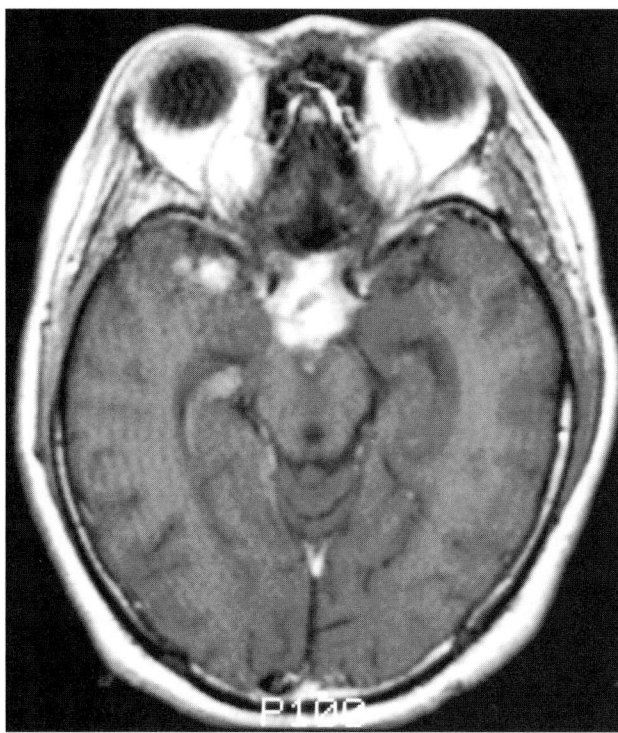

FIGURE 59A.6 Tubercular meningitis. T1 gadolinium-enhanced axial magnetic resonance image showing marked enhancement of the suprasellar cistern and right sylvian fissure, consistent with granulomatous infection.

During treatment CSF is re-examined to monitor treatment efficacy of drug level. Neuroimaging studies are performed 2–3 months after the start of treatment, and again at 3- to 6-month intervals to verify improvement in lesions. Two years of treatment may be necessary for tuberculomas. Chemotherapy alone is effective treatment for most spinal TB without cord involvement.

Complications. TB meningitis, particularly when advanced, can be an acute, life-threatening illness. Untreated it is nearly always fatal, usually within 3–6 weeks of presentation. Even with treatment, a 21% mortality for immunocompetent patients and 33% for HIV-infected patients has been reported. Complications of untreated, late, or incompletely treated CNS TB include progressive hydrocephalus, which may require shunting; blindness caused by damage to the optic nerves and chiasm in the suprasellar cistern (Figure 59A.6); the syndrome of inappropriate secretion of antidiuretic hormone, treated with fluid restriction; tuberculoma-associated edema; vasculitis; arachnoiditis; spinal cord atrophy; and syringomyelia. Arachnoid adhesions may lead to abnormal CSF circulation or ventricular trapping (Figure 59A.7); CSF flow studies before shunt placement may be beneficial.

Although definitive clinical trial data are lacking, corticosteroid therapy has been generally accepted for spe-

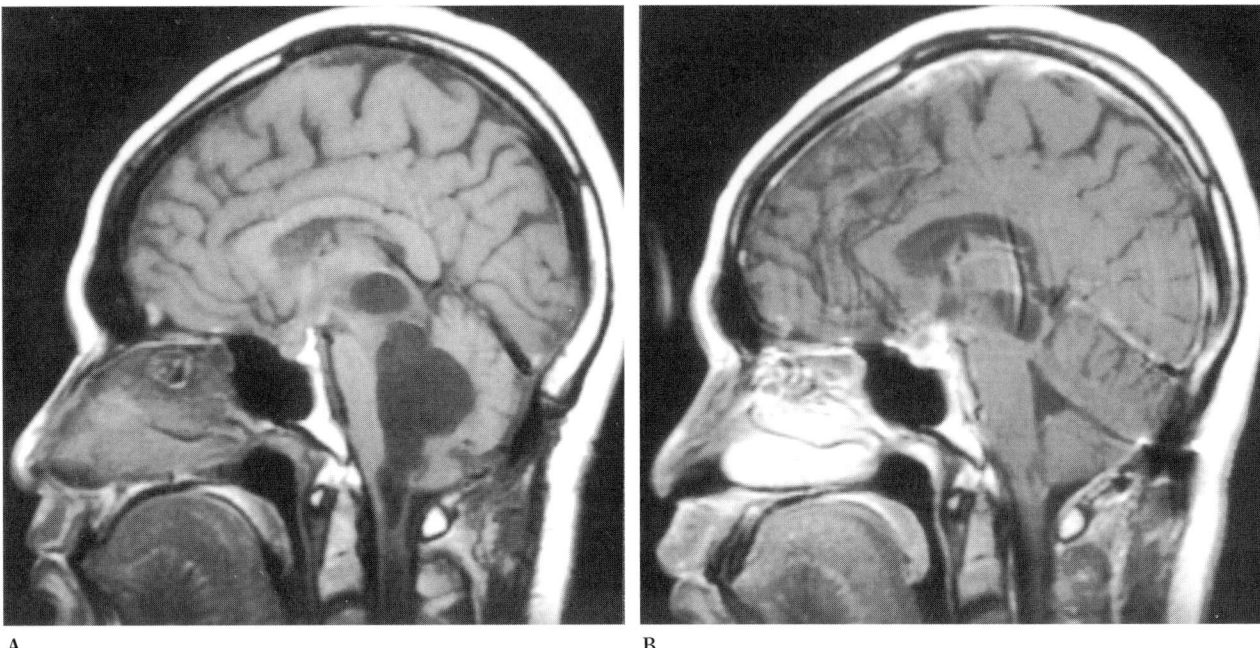

A   B

FIGURE 59A.7   Tuberculosis meningitis with arachnoid adhesions and trapped fourth ventricle. Preoperative (**A**) and postoperative (**B**) T1-weighted sagittal magnetic resonance images showing dilatation of the fourth ventricle, posterior third ventricle, and a syrinx, resolving (**B**) after placement of right lateral and fourth ventricular shunts.

cific indications: (1) increased ICP; (2) complicated meningitis with hydrocephalus, vasculitis, or arachnoiditis; (3) very high CSF protein with impending spinal block; (4) tuberculoma with surrounding edema; (5) destructive ocular lesions; (6) replacement therapy for adrenal insufficiency; and (7) severely debilitated patients with drug-sensitive strains. Dooley et al. (1997) analyzed data from seven studies conducted from 1955–1991 and concluded that adjuvant corticosteroids improve neurological outcome in patients with tuberculous meningitis of moderate severity (drowsiness, cranial nerve palsies, or hemiparesis, but not coma). Specifically, a regimen of dexamethasone at 8–12 mg per day (or prednisone equivalent) tapered over 6–8 weeks, hastened resolution of CSF abnormalities, reduced the appearance of new neurological complications, and improved long-term neurological and general function of patients with intermediate meningeal disease. Less benign treatment modalities include intrathecal streptomycin for meningitis and intrathecal hyaluronidase for spinal arachnoiditis.

Prevention.   Vaccination is by intracutaneous injection of bacille Calmette-Guérin (BCG) vaccine. Enormous variation in protection, from 6–77%, has been reported, but BCG is thought to help in preventing meningitis in children in developed countries. As a live vaccine derived from *M. bovis*, BCG is contraindicated in immunocompromised patients and should not be administered with other live vaccines.

Leprosy (Hansen's Disease)

Current Status

Leprosy, caused by the acid-fast bacterium *Mycobacterium leprae*, is an infection of superficial tissues, primarily peripheral nerves and skin. Leprosy has been the most common cause of crippling hand disease in the world and a frequent cause of blindness. There were an estimated 10–12 million cases worldwide in the early 1980s. By 1994, following the widespread use of multidrug therapy, numbers were reduced to 2.4 million.

Leprosy cases are distributed nonhomogeneously across South and Southeast Asia, Africa, Central and South America, with India, Indonesia, Myanmar, Nigeria, and Brazil collectively contributing nearly all registered cases. BCG vaccination, background prevalence of *M. tuberculosis*, and the atypical environmental mycobacteria influence leprosy epidemiology. In East Africa, for example, a reciprocal relationship between numbers of cases of TB and leprosy exists. Insufficient data exist to support the comorbidity of HIV and leprosy, but lepromatous leprosy patients may have falsely positive HIV ELISA and Western blot test results.

Leprosy is spread by the respiratory route or skin-to-skin contact, although transmission by insects has not been completely excluded. Most exposed individuals are naturally immune. Susceptible individuals develop one of three forms: lepromatous, borderline, or tuberculoid. All patients with leprosy manifest some degree of nerve involvement that varies with the immune response to the infection. Lepromatous leprosy is more common in Africa and Mexico, and tuberculoid leprosy is more frequent in India.

Clinical Features

The unique clinical features of leprosy result from the peripheral nerve tropism of *M. leprae* and its preference for temperatures 7–10°C lower than core body temperature. The long incubation period varies from 6 months to 40 years and is a consequence of its very slow growth, doubling only once every 11–13 days. Early signs include a hypopigmented anesthetic patch, areas of cutaneous sensory loss without skin patches, and multifocal or diffuse skin infiltration. Sensory impairment proceeds in a predictable sequence, with loss of temperature sensation first, followed by pain, and then touch, with sparing of proprioception and vibration. Sweating is diminished also.

Patients with impaired cell-mediated immunity develop lepromatous leprosy. Bacilli distribute widely through skin and nerves, producing a symmetrical dermal and neural syndrome. Multiple small macules, infiltrations, papules, and nodules appear, affecting cooler areas of the body first. Peripheral nerves thicken in the superficial, and thus cooler, portions of their course, but the strict correlation between skin lesions and anesthetic areas, characteristic of early and tuberculoid forms, does not apply in lepromatous cases. As disease progresses, sensory disturbances worsen, with sparing of sensation in the palms and soles and midchest and midback until late in the course, and motor involvement begins. Visual impairment and blindness may result from exposure keratitis caused by lagophthalmos or corneal anesthesia, iritis, or cataracts, caused by intraocular bacteria or use of corticosteroids. Destructive lesions of the respiratory tract above the larynx, testes, and structures of hands and feet develop, and diffuse systemic disease may cause lymphedema, hepatosplenomegaly, nephritis, and renal amyloidosis. Lucio reactions, sloughing ulcerations on the lower extremities or throughout the body, a consequence of arteriolar vasculitis and infarction, has been described in untreated Central or South American lepromatous patients.

Patients with good resistance develop tuberculoid leprosy, with multifocal, often asymmetrical, lesions of nerve and sometimes skin. Compared with lepromatous leprosy, infection is less disseminated, and anesthesia is confined to a few well-defined widely scattered hypopigmented or erythematous areas with palpable outer edges, hair loss, and anhidrosis. Thickening of the nerve supplying sensation to the affected area may be found nearby. Nerve damage results from bacterial multiplication within Schwann cells or granulomatous damage to the perineurium. When more proximal nerve trunks are involved, a clinical syndrome resembling mononeuritis multiplex results. In tuberculoid leprosy, the ulnar nerve is involved most frequently, and more vulnerable than usual to trauma and pressure palsies. Radial motor involvement occurs late, owing to its deep course in the arm and forearm, whereas its distal superficial sensory portion may become thickened and palpable earlier. Painful granulomas or abscesses in the course of affected nerves may occur and require urgent medical and surgical attention. Loss of protective sensation in the hands and feet leads to traumatic, nonhealing injuries of the fingers and toes. Sympathetic nerve injury also contributes to trophic and osteoporotic changes in the small bones of the hands and feet.

Borderline (dimorphous) leprosy, an intermediate form with features of both tuberculoid (localized) and lepromatous (widespread) disease, includes the polyneuritic form of leprosy.

Diagnosis

The diagnosis of leprosy should be considered in patients with transient, recurrent, or persistent numbness or paresthesias or when a chronic, asymptomatic, atypical skin rash does not respond to standard treatments. Palpable nerves commonly identified include greater auricular nerve in the neck, ulnar at the elbow, median at the wrist, terminal branch of the radial near the wrist, peroneal at the head of the fibula or in front of the ankle, posterior tibial below the inner malleolus, and sural on the lateral foot. Electromyography and nerve conduction studies demonstrate focal or multifocal neuropathy in tuberculoid cases or a more diffuse sensory neuropathy in lepromatous cases. Radial nerve sensory conduction study is one of the more sensitive indicators of disease. Absence of response to sweat tests or to intradermal pilocarpine or histamine confirms dermal sympathetic nerve involvement.

Demonstrating *M. leprae* in skin, nasal mucous membrane, or biopsy establishes the diagnosis. In the slit-scrape method, smears of scrapings from skin lesions are stained for AFB. Skin biopsy facilitates correct classification and may be repeated to assess treatment response. Nerve biopsy is performed in purely neural cases or when a skin biopsy has not been diagnostic. The lepromin test can be used to classify the type of leprosy and to assess resistance to disease. Lepromin reagent, a suspension of killed *M. leprae* and cellular material from host tissue, is injected intradermally in a dose of 0.1 ml. The early Fernandez reaction, read at 48 hours, is an allergic reaction similar to the tuberculin reaction. The degree of erythema and induration are assessed. The Fernandez reaction is positive in all forms of leprosy. The Mitsuda reaction, read at 4–5 weeks, is an indicator of resistance. It is positive in tuberculoid patients, weakly positive or negative in borderline patients, and negative in lepromatous patients. Because healthy individuals with no exposure to leprosy may have positive Mitsuda reactions, the test is not used for diagnosis.

The differential diagnosis includes other causes of hypertrophic neuropathy (Refsum's disease, Dejerine-Sottas disease, primary amyloidosis, sarcoidosis, neurofibromatosis, chronic inflammatory demyelinating polyneuropathy), conditions causing distal anesthesia with ulcers and loss of digits (syringomyelia, tabes, diabetic pseudotabes, yaws, congenital insensitivity to pain), and other causes of peripheral and multifocal neuropathies.

Treatment

Therapy should consist of two or more drugs and begins as soon as the diagnosis is made and classification as multibacillary or paucibacillary is determined. Multibacillary leprosy is treated with RIF, 600 mg once a month; dapsone (a folate antagonist), 100 mg daily; and clofazimine, 50 mg daily plus 300 mg once a month for a minimum of 2 years, or until skin-smear results are negative, which typically takes approximately 5 years. Dapsone neuropathy, a symmetrical distal sensory neuropathy, may arise during long-term treatment, and clofazimine has been associated with retinopathy. Paucibacillary leprosy is treated with RIF, 600 mg once a month, and dapsone, 100 mg daily for 6 months. Additional drugs include the thioamides, fluoroquinolones, minocycline, and clarithromycin. Hemolytic reaction to dapsone is a concern in patients with glucose-6-phosphate dehydrogenase deficiency.

Reactions and Complications

Reversal (type 1) reactions develop after the initial therapy for borderline leprosy releases *M. leprae* antigen. Augmented cell-mediated immunity upgrades the disease toward the tuberculoid end of the clinical spectrum, and patients develop fever, inflammation within existing skin lesions, and neuritis. Urgent therapy prevents permanent nerve damage and consists of prednisone, 40–60 mg daily, tapered over 2–3 months. Antileprosy treatment is continued. Declining cell-mediated immunity in a patient with borderline leprosy leads to lepromatous disease, known as the *downgrading response.*

Erythema nodosum leprosum, or type 2 reaction, may be precipitated by treatment of lepromatous disease, intercurrent infection, or stress. Ninety percent of lepromatous leprosy patients experience erythema nodosum leprosum reactions after starting therapy. Antigen release from dying mycobacteria in the face of high circulating antibodies to *M. leprae* antigens provokes an Arthus-type reaction. Clinical manifestations include painful papules, neuritis, fever, uveitis, and lymphadenitis. Mild reactions may be treated with chloroquine or salicylates, and more severe reactions with a short course of corticosteroids. Recurrent erythema nodosum leprosum reactions are treated with thalidomide, which inhibits tumor necrosis factor-α secretion, starting with 200–400 mg as a single oral bedtime dose, and followed by 50–100 mg daily after 1–2 weeks. Thalidomide is not used in women of childbearing age, because of the risk of producing phocomelia in the fetus. Eye reactions,

such as acute iridocyclitis, should be treated with topical atropine and corticosteroids.

Hands and feet require careful, regular monitoring for swelling, ulceration, and functional or sensory loss during treatment. Protective footwear and wound care are provided as needed. Nerve abscesses may occur in tuberculoid or neural leprosy patients and require surgical decompression and drainage. Because relapses have been reported more than 8 years after triple-drug therapy, patients require long-term follow-up.

Prevention

Chemoprophylaxis of household contacts is not routine, although exceptions have been made for children in contact with a lepromatous patient, who then receive monthly RIF for 6 months. BCG or vaccines derived from killed or chemically modified *M. leprae* and research strains have been used. BCG's protective effect varied from 80% in Uganda to 20–30% in Myanmar and India.

SPIROCHETES

Spirochetes belonging to the genera *Treponema*, *Borrelia*, and *Leptospira* are important human pathogens. Except for the endemic treponemal diseases (yaws, pinta, bejel), all produce multiphasic or relapsing diseases with multifocal neurological involvement. Diagnosis and management of these infections, which are increasing in frequency throughout the world, are hampered by suboptimal diagnostic methods, incomplete treatment, and potential relapses despite therapy.

Syphilis

Syphilis, a chronic multisystem disease caused by the spirochete *T. pallidum*, is spread venereally or vertically (i.e., mother to child). Venereally acquired disease is characterized by episodes of active disease separated by periods of latency, with neurological disease in secondary and later stages. An estimated 4–9% of patients with untreated syphilis develop symptomatic neurosyphilis, with meningovascular syphilis in 2–3%, general paresis in 2–5%, and tabes dorsalis in 1–5%.

Clinical Features

Primary syphilis is characterized by one or more primary skin lesions, called *chancres*, which develop at the site of inoculation from 3–90 days (average, 20) after exposure. Spirochetes can be demonstrated in the lesions by darkfield microscopy. Neurological disease is not a feature of primary syphilis, although asymptomatic spread to the CNS has been documented in 30% of cases of early syphilis.

Secondary syphilis occurs 2–12 weeks after contact. Disseminated infection manifests clinically by constitutional symptoms such as fever, malaise, generalized lymphadenopathy, rash, and neurologically as syphilitic meningitis or cranial neuropathies, including hearing loss, and ocular changes. Approximately 30% of secondary syphilis patients develop CSF profiles indicating meningeal infection, but only 1–2% of patients are symptomatic. CSF shows lymphocytic pleocytosis, elevated protein, and low-to-normal glucose. Spirochetes can be detected by dark-field microscopic examination of secondary skin lesions, and occasionally, in CSF and the anterior chamber of the eye. After the second stage resolves, the patient enters a latent, asymptomatic period, with disease apparent only by serology. CSF at this stage is usually normal; abnormalities indicate asymptomatic neurosyphilis.

Up to one-third of untreated patients develop late syphilis (tertiary syphilis), a slowly progressive inflammatory disease that includes gummatous (granulomatous), cardiovascular, and neurological forms. Early manifestations of tertiary neurosyphilis include pure meningeal or meningovascular disease, with a 5- to 10-year latency from primary infection, and parenchymal forms, which occur 10–30 years after initial infection. *General paresis* refers to parenchymal cerebral involvement, and *tabes dorsalis* to syphilitic myeloneuropathy. Syphilitic gummas, granulomas that present as space-occupying lesions in brain or cord, may occur at any stage of disseminated disease.

Actually, neurosyphilis spans all stages of disseminated disease. Meningeal, meningovascular, and parenchymal syndromes are perhaps best viewed as a continuum of disease, rather than as discrete disorders. Syphilitic meningitis, meningovascular syphilis, general paresis, and tabes are different clinical expressions of the same fundamental pathological events, specifically meningeal invasion, obliterative endarteritis, and parenchymal invasion. Especially in the antibiotic era, symptomatic neurosyphilis may present, not as one classic syndrome, but as mixed, subtle, or incomplete disease (Cintron and Pachner 1994). All of the neurological complications of syphilis have been reported in HIV disease, which may accelerate the onset and progression of neurosyphilis.

Syphilitic meningitis typically occurs earlier than other forms of neurosyphilis and is often asymptomatic. Rare complications of acute syphilitic meningitis include hydrocephalus, myelitis, or lumbosacral radiculitis. Meningovascular syphilis usually occurs 4–7 years after primary infection (range, 6 months to 12 years). In addition to stroke, involvement of large and small cerebral vessels also causes headache, vertigo, insomnia, and psychiatric or personality disorders.

General paresis, the encephalitic form of neurosyphilis, typically presents as progressive dementia beginning 15–20 years after original infection (range, 3–30 years). The clinical picture also may include delusional or apathetic states, dysarthria, myoclonus, intention tremor, seizures, hyperreflexia, and Argyll Robertson pupils (small, irregular pupils that constrict with accommodation but not light). Disease manifestations correspond to the mnemonic *paresis*: personality, affect, reflexes, eye, sensorium, intellect, and speech.

Tabes dorsalis, the spinal form of syphilis, also develops approximately 15–20 years after the original infection (range, 5–50 years). Tabes is characterized by lightning pains, autonomic dysfunction (urinary incontinence), and sensory ataxia. Affected patients have normal strength and lack reflexes in the legs; a positive Romberg's sign accompanies impaired proprioception. Pupils are abnormal in more than 90% of cases, with Argyll Robertson pupils observed in approximately one-half. Other associated features include optic atrophy, ophthalmoplegia, ptosis, gastric or other visceral crises (pharyngeal, laryngeal, genitourinary, intestinal, rectal), impotence, fecal incontinence, and pain and temperature loss leading to trophic changes such as Charcot's (neuropathic) joints and perforating foot ulcers.

Syphilitic inflammatory diseases of the eye include uveitis, chorioretinitis, and vasculitis. Each may accompany acute syphilitic meningitis or present as an isolated complication of secondary syphilis. Optic atrophy evolves over months to years and may coexist with other forms of neurosyphilis, particularly tabes. Optic nerve degeneration usually begins peripherally and extends to the center of the nerve, producing progressive constriction of the visual fields with preserved acuity. Syphilitic otitis, an unusual manifestation, presents as unexplained hearing loss or vestibular abnormalities, with positive treponemal serology.

At birth, congenitally infected infants may show signs of serous nasal discharge (snuffles), rash, condylomas, hepatosplenomegaly, or osteochondritis. Left untreated, the classic stigmata of Hutchinson's teeth, saddle nose, interstitial keratitis, saber shins, mental retardation, hearing loss, and hydrocephalus develops.

Diagnosis

Syphilis can be diagnosed by demonstration of spirochetes in lesions of primary, secondary, or early congenital syphilis. More commonly, however, treponemal and nontreponemal serologic tests are used to make the diagnosis. Treponemal tests include fluorescent treponemal antibody absorption, microhemagglutination assay, fluorescent treponemal antibody-absorption double staining, hemagglutination treponemal test for syphilis, and *T. pallidum* immobilization. Treponemal test results become positive 3–4 weeks after inoculation and usually remain positive for life. Nontreponemal or reagin tests detect antibodies to membrane lipids of *T. pallidum*, using antigens such as cardiolipin, lecithin, or cholesterol, and include the VDRL test and rapid plasma reagin test. More sensitive but less specific than treponemal serologies, nontreponemal test results become positive 5–6 weeks after exposure and usually become negative in the year following adequate treatment.

Clearly, patients with classic neurosyphilis syndromes require serum serologies and CSF examination. Because syphilitic eye disease often is associated with neurosyphilis, patients with syphilis and ocular manifestations should also undergo LP. The Centers for Disease Control and Prevention recommend CSF examination for all patients with syphilis who have neurological or ophthalmic symptoms and signs or active tertiary disease (aortitis, gumma, iritis) or have failed therapy. In addition, the Centers for Disease Control and Prevention advise that HIV-infected patients with late latent syphilis or latent syphilis of unknown duration undergo LP prior to treatment (Centers for Disease Control 1998).

The diagnosis of neurosyphilis depends on clinical evidence, CSF findings, and serology. CSF mononuclear pleocytosis (>5 cells per μl) and elevated protein support the diagnosis of neurosyphilis. CSF-VDRL is very specific; it is more sensitive in meningovascular syphilis and general paresis than in asymptomatic neurosyphilis and tabes. False-positive CSF-VDRL may occur if blood contaminates CSF, as occurs with traumatic LP, and was reported in a single case of carcinomatous meningitis. Intrathecal *Treponema pallidum* antibody production, oligoclonal antibodies, IgM antibodies, or PCR-amplified products may increase sensitivity of CSF examination (Cinque et al. 1997). Serum VDRL may be negative in up to 25% of patients with late neurosyphilis, but specific treponemal tests remain reactive. The CSF of patients with tabes may show less pronounced inflammatory changes than other forms of neurosyphilis.

False-positive serum treponemal tests in serum occur in Lyme borreliosis, nonvenereal treponematoses, genital herpes simplex, pregnancy, lupus, alcoholic cirrhosis, scleroderma, and mixed connective tissue disease. Transient false-positive reactions to nontreponemal tests can result from mycoplasma or enterovirus infection, mononucleosis, pregnancy, parenteral drug use, advanced TB, scarlet fever, subacute bacterial endocarditis, viral pneumonia, brucellosis, rat-bite fever, relapsing fever, leptospirosis, measles, mumps, lymphogranuloma venereum, malaria, trypanosomiasis, and varicella. Chronic false-positive reactions may be caused by malaria, leprosy, lupus, other connective tissue disorders, parenteral drug use, Hashimoto's thyroiditis, rheumatoid arthritis, reticuloendothelial malignancy, and advanced age.

The differential diagnosis of neurosyphilis includes other inflammatory meningovascular or CNS granulomatous diseases, such as TB or cryptococcal meningitis, brucellosis, Lyme disease, CNS sarcoid, and cerebral vasculitides.

Treatment

Optimal treatment of neurosyphilis is aqueous penicillin G at doses of 18–24 million units per day intravenously (3–4 million units every 4 hours) for 10–14 days. The alternative, procaine benzyl penicillin, 2.4 million units intramuscularly daily, with probenecid, 500 mg orally four times daily, both for 10–14 days, has been associated with treatment failures. In penicillin-allergic patients, alternatives include oral doxycycline, 200 mg twice daily for 4 weeks, or skin testing to confirm allergy and consideration of desensitization. A patient with a positive serum treponemal antibody test result and neurological disease compatible with neurosyphilis should be treated with penicillin in doses adequate for neurosyphilis, even in the absence of CSF confirmation. Because of sequestration of spirochetes in the inner ear and poor antibiotic penetration to that area, syphilitic otitis may require a longer duration of therapy, from 6 weeks to 3 months.

Patients with documented neurosyphilis should be followed after therapy. Clinical symptoms or signs of syphilis should prompt consideration of re-treatment, as should fourfold increase of serum titers or failure of titers greater than 1 to 32 to decrease at least fourfold by 12–24 months. If pleocytosis was present, LP should be performed every 6 months until cell count normalizes. Patients in whom CSF cell count does not decrease after 6 months, or in whom CSF does not return to normal after 2 years, may require retreatment.

Complications of Treatment

Jarisch-Herxheimer reactions occur most frequently in patients with early syphilis. Clinical features of this systemic response to release of heat-stable pyrogens from spirochetes include rigors, fever, hypotension, and leukopenia. In meningovascular syphilis, signs that remain after 6 months usually persist indefinitely. Treatment of general paresis may improve the cognitive or psychiatric disease in relatively early cases or arrest disease progression in approximately one-half of advanced cases. Residual symptoms of tabes continue after the CSF has normalized and require symptomatic treatment of joint deformities with orthotics, visceral crises with atropine, and pain with anticonvulsants or amitriptyline. Pre-existing optic atrophy and extensive perioptic meningeal infiltrate may presage progressive vision loss during treatment. Adequate treatment of the mother before the sixteenth week of gestation prevents congenital syphilis.

Lyme Disease (Borreliosis)

Lyme disease, a systemic disease with dermatological, rheumatological, neurological, and cardiac manifestations, is caused by *Borrelia burgdorferi* and transmitted by the hard-shelled deer ticks: *Ixodes dammini* in the eastern United States, *Ixodes pacificus* in the western United States, and *Ixodes ricinus* in Europe.

Clinical Features

The existence of both early and late neurological manifestations, diagnostic uncertainty, and potential for relapse despite therapy fuel continuing debate over the spectrum of Lyme-related neurological disease. Best agreement exists for the early neurological syndromes, which include lymphocytic meningitis, cranial neuropathy (commonly unilateral or bilateral Bell's palsy), and painful radiculoneuritis, which can occur alone or in combination. Optic neuritis, mononeuritis multiplex, and Guillain-Barré syndrome are other, less frequent manifestations of early neurological involvement. Neurological complications of more advanced Lyme disease include encephalomyelitis, with predominant white matter involvement, and peripheral neuropathy. Lymphocytic meningitis is usually acute, but may cause a chronic or relapsing meningitis and communicating hydrocephalus. Radiculoneuritis, beginning as a painful limb disorder, may continue with exacerbations and remissions for up to 6 months. Encephalopathy with memory or cognitive abnormalities, confusional states, accelerated dementia, and normal CSF study results may occur. Other psychiatric or fatigue syndromes appear less likely to be causally related (Halperin et al. 1996).

Several systemic disorders support the diagnosis of Lyme borreliosis. Dermatological manifestations include erythema chronicum migrans, a painless expanding macular lesion present shortly after initial infection in approximately two-thirds of patients, and acrodermatitis chronicum atrophicans, a bluish red discoloration of the legs that occurs after the first year of infection. Other extraneural features include *Borrelia* lymphocytoma, occurring 6–12 months after infection, recurrent monoarthritis or polyarthritis, and second- or third-degree cardiac conduction block.

Diagnosis

The best clinical marker for the disease is the erythema chronicum migrans rash that occurs in 60–80% of patients. The diagnosis of active neuroborreliosis is made by the presence of consistent history, signs and symptoms, together with CSF pleocytosis, serum anti–*B. burgdorferi* antibodies, and evidence of intrathecal antibody production. Serologic testing by ELISA is performed as an initial screen, followed by Western blot confirmation. Culture of organisms and PCR testing of CSF are also available.

The most common form of neuroborreliosis in Europe, radiculoneuritis (lymphocytic meningoradiculitis, Bannwarth's syndrome), is rare in the United States. The meningitic forms of borreliosis may resemble CNS lymphoma, because the CSF may contain atypical lymphocytes. The differential diagnosis of *Borrelia* encephalomyelitis includes a first episode of multiple sclerosis. Bites from uninfected ticks may produce similar neuropathies (Garcia-Monco and Benach 1995).

Treatment

Borrelia is treated with parenteral antibiotics if there is evidence that infection has crossed the blood-brain barrier. Ceftriaxone (2 g once daily intravenously) or penicillin (3–4 million units intravenously every 3–4 hours) for 2–4 weeks are first-line drugs. Tetracycline or chloramphenicol are alternatives in penicillin- or cephalosporin-allergic patients. Jarisch-Herxheimer reactions may occur within 2 hours of initiating therapy. Meptazinol, a drug with mixed opiate agonist and antagonist properties, may mitigate the attack. Routine use of corticosteroids is not indicated. Recommendations for the use of corticosteroids in neuroborreliosis generally have been limited to patients treated aggressively with intravenous antibiotics with evidence of severe inflammation that fails to improve with time.

CSF examination should be performed toward the end of the 2- to 4-week treatment course to assess the need for continuing treatment, and again 6 months after the conclusion of therapy. Intrathecal antibody production may persist for years following successful treatment and in isolation does not indicate active disease. Patients in whom CSF pleocytosis fails to resolve within 6 months, however, should be retreated.

Peripheral or cranial nerve involvement without CSF abnormalities may be treated with oral agents, either doxycycline, 100 mg twice daily for 14–21 days, or amoxicillin, 500 mg every 8 hours for 10–21 days.

Relapsing Fever

The term *relapsing fever* applies to two distinct borrelial diseases, louse-borne relapsing fever and tick-borne relapsing fever. Both are characterized by episodic fever and spirochetemia, systemic symptoms, and variable presence of neurological complications. The human body louse transmits *Borrelia recurrentis* and soft ticks of the genus *Ornithodoros* transmit other *Borrelia* spp., including *Borrelia duttoni*.

Clinical Features

Overcrowding and poor hygiene predispose to louse-borne relapsing fever. Clinical features may be mild, but severe febrile illness with mortality reaching 40% in epidemic situations also is seen. Hepatosplenomegaly, jaundice, respiratory symptoms (cough and dyspnea), and myocarditis are more common than in the tick-borne syndrome, and neurological manifestations, including meningitis, meningoencephalitis, cerebral hemorrhage, or neuropathy, develop in approximately 30% of patients.

Neurological syndromes associated with tick-borne relapsing fever appear at the end of the first bout of fever or with relapses. Cranial neuritis is the most common neurological manifestation of tick-borne disease, with facial weakness affecting up to 22% of patients. Lymphocytic meningitis, subarachnoid hemorrhage, encephalitis, transient or permanent focal deficits, iritis, iridocyclitis, optic atrophy, and sciatic neuralgias also have been described.

Diagnosis

Demonstrating borreliae in the peripheral blood of febrile patients using dark-field microscopy, Wright's or Giemsa's stained blood smears establishes the diagnosis. *Proteus* OX-K agglutinin titers are elevated in relapsing fever. Nervous system disease is accompanied by CSF lymphocytic pleocytosis and elevated protein. Spirochetes may be detected in CSF by smear or animal inoculation in approximately 12% of patients with CNS signs. In the western United States, the differential diagnosis of tick-borne relapsing fever includes Colorado tick fever and Rocky Mountain spotted fever.

Treatment

Louse-borne relapsing fever is treated with a single oral dose (500 mg) of tetracycline; erythromycin in the same dose is also effective. Tick-borne relapsing fever is treated with either oral tetracycline or erythromycin, 500 mg every 6 hours for 5–10 days.

Leptospirosis

Many wild and domestic animals carry *Leptospira interrogans*. Leptospirosis is a worldwide zoonotic infection transmitted directly to humans by contact with urine of infected rodents or domestic animals, or indirectly via water or soil contaminated by infected urine. The severity of disease varies widely; jaundice, hemorrhage, and renal failure develop in severe cases. Approximately 15% of patients develop signs and symptoms of meningitis, and many more have lymphocytic CSF.

Clinical Features

The illness often follows a biphasic course. The first bacteremic phase is characterized by fever, headache, myalgias, nausea, vomiting, and abdominal pain. Dissemination of the organism in the acute phase leads to meningeal invasion, during which leptospirae may be cultured from blood and CSF but not urine. A second immune phase develops in the second week, once the patient has mounted an antibody response to the organism. This stage is characterized by more severe systemic illness, with meningitis, uveitis, rash, and in severe cases, hepatorenal and hemorrhagic syndromes. Eighty percent to 90% of patients have CSF abnormalities consistent with aseptic meningitis. CSF examination reveals lymphocytic pleocytosis, elevated protein, and normal glucose levels, but the leptospirae have been cleared from the CSF by this stage. CSF pressure is usually normal, yet LP may improve the headache. More severe forms of illness are accompanied by conjunctival suffusion, myositis with rhabdomyolysis, meningoencephalitis, or myelitis. In Weil's disease, the most severe form, hepatorenal dysfunction and myocarditis accompany depressed consciousness and, occasionally, intracerebral hemorrhage. Cerebral arteritis is an unusual late complication, and a form of moyamoya disease has been thought to occur as a result of obstruction

of the internal carotid arteries near the circle of Willis. Mononeuritis multiplex and Guillain-Barré syndrome have been reported. Invasion of the eyes by leptospirae during the acute phase may produce uveitis weeks or months after recovery.

Diagnosis

Jaundice, renal failure, and elevated serum creatine kinase (CK) following a febrile illness suggest the diagnosis. Organisms can be isolated from blood or CSF during the first 10 days of illness and from urine during the first month of illness. Serological test results, based on macroscopic or microscopic agglutination procedures, are positive after the first week.

Treatment

Severe leptospirosis is treated with penicillin G, 1.5 million units intravenously every 6 hours for at least 7 days. Less severe cases are treated with doxycycline, 100 mg twice daily for 5–7 days.

TOXIN-PRODUCING BACTERIA

Neurotoxigenic *Clostridia:* Botulism and Tetanus

Clostridia, strictly anaerobic gram-positive bacilli, form highly resilient spores that are ubiquitous in the environment. Unlike pathogens that cause neurological disease by forming mass lesions or inducing inflammation and subsequent cellular injury, several clostridial species elaborate exotoxins that gain access to the nervous system by avid and specific binding to motor nerve terminals. The resulting clinical syndromes are motor disorders that often are accompanied by autonomic dysfunction. Botulism and tetanus require notification of public health authorities, both to obtain therapeutic antisera and to initiate appropriate epidemiological investigation. Knowledge of their characteristic clinical features facilitates early diagnosis of these rare, but treatable, disorders.

Botulism

An unusual cause of acute generalized weakness, botulism develops when the extremely potent neurotoxin secreted by *Clostridium botulinum* blocks peripheral cholinergic transmission. *C. botulinum* spores are widespread in soil and aquatic sediment. Eight botulinum toxin serotypes define the various *C. botulinum* strains (Case Records 1997). Types A, B, E, and, rarely, F cause human disease. Types C and D cause botulism in animals, and type G does not appear to cause human or veterinary illness. Food-borne botulism, described in 1895 by van Ermengen, develops when preformed toxin is ingested from contaminated food. Wound botulism, first recognized in 1942, occurs when *C. botulinum* in an infected wound secretes botulinum toxin directly into the bloodstream. Toxin production by *C. botulinum* colonizing the gut causes infantile botulism. Less commonly, gut colonization causes botulism in adults with pre-existing gastrointestinal disorders, such as intestinal surgery or inflammatory bowel disease (Midura 1996).

Pathogenesis and Pathophysiology. Botulinum toxin blocks acetylcholine release at peripheral synapses, leading to the paralytic and autonomic clinical manifestations of botulism (Montecucco and Schiavo 1994). With a median lethal dose as low as 1 ng/kg in mice, it is the most potent toxin known. Unlike *C. botulinum* spores, the toxin is heat-labile. Botulinum toxin is initially synthesized as a single 150-kD protein chain and contains a single disulfide bond. Proteolysis forms heavy (100 kD) and light (50 kD) chains. The C-terminal region of the heavy chain binds tightly and specifically to presynaptic membranes, whereas the N-terminal domain governs internalization of the toxin into the motor neuron. Once internalized, botulinum toxin cannot be neutralized by therapeutically administered antibodies. After translocation across vesicular membranes into the cytosol, cleavage of the disulfide bond liberates the light chain, which contains the catalytic activity of botulinum toxin. The light chain is a zinc endopeptidase that targets various proteins mediating exocytosis. Hence, botulinum toxin causes irreversible blockade at peripheral cholinergic synapses. Recovery requires sprouting of new nerve terminals, accounting for the protracted clinical course of botulism.

Current Status. First reported in 1976, infant botulism is now the most common form in the United States. Among adults, food-borne botulism is much more common than wound botulism. Since the late 1980s, injection drug use, specifically "skin popping" heroin, has been linked to wound botulism. *Skin popping* refers to subcutaneous injection, typically by chronic addicts whose poor venous access precludes intravenous administration. Since 1990, a sharp increase in wound botulism in California has been associated with skin popping "black tar" heroin (Centers for Disease Control 1995). Whether the outbreak will spread to other western states in which black tar heroin is distributed also remains to be seen.

Clinical Features. Whether toxin is ingested or elaborated in situ from gut colonization or an infected wound, common early symptoms of botulism include diplopia, ptosis, dysarthria, and dysphagia. Extraocular and bulbar muscle weakness progresses rapidly to the limbs, typically symmetrically, and also to respiratory muscles. Alertness and cognition are normal, unless hypoxemia or hypercarbia supervene because of respiratory failure. Reflexes are depressed or absent, and sensation is normal. These symptoms and signs all indicate neuromuscular blockade. In botulism, impaired cholinergic transmission also involves autonomic synapses, as indicated by large, poorly reactive pupils, dry mouth, paralytic ileus, and occasionally bradycardia.

In food-borne botulism, nausea, vomiting, and diarrhea often accompany early neurological symptoms, typically 12–36 hours after toxin ingestion. Gastrointestinal symptoms may be less prominent in early wound botulism. Clinical features of infantile botulism vary widely (Midura 1996). Constipation, poor suck, weak cry, and listlessness are common, and the baby often appears floppy. The incubation period may be as brief as a few days or as long as a month. A small percentage of cases of sudden infant death syndrome result from infant botulism. Honey has been implicated as the source of *C. botulinum* spores in infantile botulism. Dust is another important environmental source of spores; however, in most cases of infantile botulism, a source cannot be identified.

Diagnosis. The differential diagnosis includes other causes of acute generalized weakness. Preserved alertness and lack of sensory or upper motor neuron signs help exclude acute brainstem disorders such as stroke, demyelinating syndromes, and encephalitis. The descending paralysis of botulism closely resembles the Miller-Fisher variant of Guillain-Barré syndrome and overlaps with the clinical features of diphtheritic polyneuropathy. However, in botulism, sensation is normal, as is CSF. Electromyography and nerve conduction study results reveal changes indicating presynaptic neuromuscular blockade, in contrast to the often elevated CSF protein and electrophysiological features that suggest the demyelinating neuropathies of Guillain-Barré syndrome or diphtheria. Pupillary involvement and ileus help distinguish botulism from myasthenia gravis presenting in crisis. In addition, peripheral electrophysiological studies, particularly repetitive nerve stimulation, in myasthenia reveal a postsynaptic defect in neuromuscular transmission (decrement on repetitive stimulation; see Chapter 37B), rather than the presynaptic electrophysiological abnormalities that characterize botulism (increment on slow repetitive stimulation). False-positive edrophonium test results have been noted in botulism. Normal CSF and prominent ocular signs differentiate botulism from poliomyelitis, in which pleocytosis is the rule and extraocular weakness and ptosis are rare. Tick paralysis also causes acute generalized weakness caused by impaired presynaptic neuromuscular transmission, but weakness typically ascends and spares extraocular muscles. Paralytic shellfish toxicity and organophosphate poisoning are other considerations; the latter causes a syndrome in which cholinergic, rather than anticholinergic, features predominate. The differential diagnosis of infantile botulism includes sepsis, pneumonia, failure to thrive, myasthenia, polio, Guillain-Barré syndrome, brainstem encephalitis, meningitis, hypothyroidism, and metabolic disorders.

Electromyography and nerve conduction studies with repetitive stimulation and CSF examination help narrow the differential diagnosis of acute generalized weakness. An important, and sometimes overlooked, study is measurement of bedside pulmonary function tests, particularly vital capacity and negative inspiratory pressure, in order to assess the need for mechanical ventilation. Symptoms and signs suggesting cholinergic blockade at both autonomic and neuromuscular synapses suggest the diagnosis of botulism. History of similar symptoms in family or acquaintances or of eating home-canned foods should be specifically sought, as should evidence of recent trauma or chronic infection. Although many patients with wound botulism have a clinically obvious site of infection, it should be emphasized that the extremely high potency of botulinum toxin means that small, seemingly trivial abscesses can cause botulism.

In a patient with a compatible clinical syndrome, the diagnosis of botulism is confirmed by toxin assay or by culturing *C. botulinum*. Toxin detection requires mouse bioassay, which can be arranged through state health departments or the Centers for Disease Control and Prevention. Appropriate samples for toxin assay include suspected food sources, blood and stool in most instances, as well as gastric contents, and enema fluid in infant botulism. Rapid determination of the source of toxin helps identify individuals at risk in food-borne cases. Because *C. botulinum* is a strict anaerobe, culture specimens require special collection, transport, and culture procedures. Appropriate culture materials include suspected contaminated foods, wound specimens, and stool.

Treatment. Once taken up by neurons, botulinum toxin is invulnerable to antibody inactivation and irreversibly blocks exocytosis. Hence efforts to neutralize circulating antitoxin and eradicate its source often begin before toxin or culture results, which take days, are known (Burningham et al. 1994). In adults, trivalent (types A, B, E) equine antitoxin is given if initial testing reveals no hypersensitivity reaction. Nasogastric suctioning and enemas may help remove toxin in food-borne cases. In wound botulism, infected wounds, even if minor, should be débrided. Because the procedure could liberate more toxin, it may be prudent to débride wounds after antitoxin administration. Whether antibiotics active against *C. botulinum* should be given is controversial, because of the concern that bacterial lysis could release more toxin. If other intercurrent infections require antibiotic therapy, aminoglycosides are probably best avoided whenever possible, because they also impair presynaptic neuromuscular transmission.

Meticulous supportive care plays a critical role. Close monitoring in an ICU is important, even in patients who do not require intubation at presentation, because respiratory decompensation can develop precipitously. Serial bedside pulmonary function tests are more sensitive than blood gas parameters in determining the need for mechanical ventilation, because vital capacity decreases before hypoxemia and hypercarbia develop. Complications of prolonged immobility, such as stress ulcer, malnutrition, pneumonia, urosepsis, deep venous thromboembolism, and depression should be anticipated and managed appropriately. In infants, supportive care, including mechanical ventilation in many patients, is the mainstay of therapy. Treatment of infant botulism usually does not include antitoxin administration or antibiotics (Midura 1996).

Botulism is a notifiable condition. Public health authorities provide assistance and advice in obtaining appropriate diagnostic studies and antitoxin, when appropriate. Epidemiological investigation in food-borne cases helps determine and eradicate the source and identify other individuals who may be at risk.

Modern critical care has decreased mortality from 60% to 20% (Case Records 1997). Because botulinum toxin irreversibly destroys the cellular apparatus responsible for acetylcholine release at neuromuscular junctions, motor recovery depends on motor axon sprouting, which takes weeks to months. Long-term ventilatory support and tracheostomy may be necessary. Full recovery can take years.

Tetanus

Clostridium tetani secretes tetanospasmin, also known as tetanus toxin, and tetanolysin. The function of tetanolysin remains uncertain; tetanospasmin blocks release of inhibitory neurotransmitters by spinal interneurons, causing the dramatic muscle contractions that characterize tetanus. *C. tetani* spores can survive for years in soil and house dust. When introduced into the anaerobic environment of a suitable wound, conversion to the toxin-producing vegetative form may cause tetanus. Neonatal tetanus complicates umbilical sepsis, which is usually related to improper umbilical stump care. Septic procedures during pregnancy or abortion can cause maternal tetanus. Other circumstances favoring the growth of *C. tetani* include deep puncture wounds, chronic skin or dental infections, decubitus ulcers, and other contaminated, necrotic wounds. Although trauma precedes most cases, a responsible wound is not identified in 20% of patients. Tetanus, a preventable disease, is an important international public health problem, particularly in the developing world.

Pathogenesis and Pathophysiology. Tetanospasmin inhibits release of γ-aminobutyric acid and glycine, which are inhibitory neurotransmitters in the brainstem and spinal cord (Ernst et al. 1997). A single type of tetanus neurotoxin exists, in contrast to the multiple serotypes of botulinum toxin. Interestingly, though botulinum and tetanus toxins cause dramatically different clinical syndromes, they share many biochemical features (Montecucco and Schiavo 1994). Both are 150-kD zinc endopeptidases consisting of light and heavy chains connected by a disulfide bond. Specificity and translocation reside in the heavy chain, in the C- and N-termini, respectively. The light chain is the zinc endopeptidase, which blocks exocytosis. Unlike botulinum toxin, which remains in the motor axon terminal, tetanus toxin travels to the anterior horn cell by retrograde axonal transport, moves into the intersynaptic space, and enters inhibitory neurons. Impaired exocytosis in these spinal inhibitory neurons causes uncontrolled muscle contraction, a prominent clinical feature of tetanus. Similar disinhibition in the intermediolateral column of the spinal cord is thought to produce autonomic dysfunction.

Current Status. Underreporting is the rule for all forms of tetanus in both industrial and developing countries (Galazka and Gasse 1995). Neonatal tetanus remains a significant public health problem in the developing world. In industrialized nations, tetanus is rare, owing to toxoid immunization programs, which usually target children. As a result, tetanus has become particularly rare in children and young adults and is primarily a disease of the elderly in industrialized countries. Interestingly, immunization efforts also decrease mortality from neonatal tetanus. Since the 1980s, tetanus outbreaks have developed among heroin addicts in Hong Kong, reminiscent of similar outbreaks in New York City during the 1960s (Sun et al. 1994).

Clinical Features. The typical incubation period is 2 weeks but can range from hours to a month or more. Cardinal features include muscle rigidity and spasms, which may be accompanied by sympathetic hyperactivity. Local tetanus, in which symptoms remain limited to a limb, is a rare form. Far more common is generalized tetanus, also called *lockjaw*, as trismus heralds the disorder in over 75% of cases. Tetanus resulting from infected head and neck wounds may present with facial or ocular muscle spasms, so-called cephalic tetanus. Sustained contraction of facial muscles causes a sneering grimace known as *risus sardonicus*. Other early symptoms include dysphagia and axial muscle involvement, such as neck stiffness, abdominal rigidity, and back pain. Early involvement of face, neck, and trunk muscles has been ascribed to the shorter axons of motor neurons supplying cranial and axial muscles, as compared with the limbs. Laryngospasm compromises ventilation and makes intubation extremely difficult. Sustained contraction of back muscles causes opisthotonos, an arching posture of the back.

As tetanus progresses, reflex muscle spasms develop, triggered by sensory stimuli, movement, or emotion. Tetanospasms cause pain, further threaten respiration, and can be severe enough to cause fractures. Manifestations of autonomic dysfunction include fever, profuse diaphoresis, hypertension, marked tachycardia, and other manifestations of sympathetic hyperactivity. Examination can be difficult, as it may prompt spasms. Major neuro-

logical signs include rigidity, spasms, and hyperreflexia. General physical examination helps localize the source of infection.

Diagnosis. Differential diagnosis includes hypocalcemia, strychnine poisoning, dystonic reactions to neuroleptics or antiemetics, meningitis, encephalitis (including rabies), status epilepticus, and the acute abdomen. Oral infection or mandibular fracture or dislocation may cause isolated trismus, without the generalized features of tetanus. Immunization status should be established, if possible, and a history of chronic infection should be sought. The characteristic muscle contractions elevate serum CK, but there are no pathognomonic laboratory abnormalities in tetanus. CSF is normal. Wound cultures must be interpreted cautiously. Positive culture results may indicate wound colonization, rather than true infection with subsequent toxin production. Moreover, in most established cases, wound cultures do not yield *C. tetani*.

Treatment. Therapeutic goals include protecting the airway, neutralizing circulating tetanospasmin and preventing its further production, managing spasms and dysautonomia, and general supportive care (Ernst et al. 1997). The risk for precipitous respiratory decompensation, even in mild cases, warrants ICU management for all patients with tetanus.

Initial management of most patients with generalized tetanus includes endotracheal intubation, because laryngospasm may appear abruptly even in mild cases. Human tetanus immune globulin, given as a single dose of at least 500 IU intramuscularly, neutralizes circulating toxin. Infected wounds should be débrided after human tetanus immune globulin administration, because the procedure may release further toxin. Metronidazole or penicillin should be given to eradicate *C. tetani*. Because minute amounts of tetanospasmin can produce clinical disease, affected patients frequently do not mount a protective immune response. Hence tetanus toxoid should be administered, either primary immunization series or booster injection as appropriate, to all patients with tetanus.

A quiet, dark environment minimizes sensory stimulation that may precipitate spasms or hypertensive crises. Benzodiazepines, such as parenteral diazepam, lorazepam, or midazolam, reduce rigidity and spasms. Such agents also provide effective sedation, an important consideration because severe tetanus typically requires weeks or months of ICU care. Most patients also require treatment with neuromuscular blockers, such as pancuronium or vecuronium, to control spasms. Intravenous dantrolene and intrathecal baclofen also have been used successfully to manage muscle rigidity and spasms in tetanus.

A paucity of randomized clinical trial data means that treatment recommendations for tetanus depend heavily on clinical experience. This is particularly true for managing sympathetic hyperactivity. Hypertension and tachycardia often respond to beta blockers such as propranolol or labetalol, although treatment may be complicated by cardiac arrest or hypotension. Other agents used to manage autonomic dysfunction include clonidine, morphine, constant infusions of magnesium sulfate or atropine, or intrathecal bupivacaine. As with all critically ill patients, optimal supportive care includes attention to nutritional status and measures to prevent stress ulcers, deep venous thrombosis, and decubitus ulcers.

Even in situations in which ICU care and mechanical ventilation are not available, early tracheotomy is still performed for generalized tetanus for airway protection during laryngeal spasms and removal of upper airway secretions. Chlorpromazine and other phenothiazines are used in conjunction with diazepam in severe cases for muscle spasm control.

Tetanus is a reportable illness whose complex management poses considerable challenges for neurointensivists. It is worth noting that tetanus could be largely prevented with simple modifications in peripartum and neonatal care and more widespread use of tetanus toxoid, which is both inexpensive and safe. In the United States, primary immunization consists of four doses, separated by intervals of 4–8 weeks between for the first three doses, with the fourth dose given 6–12 months later.

Complications. Without treatment, generalized tetanus is uniformly fatal. The overall case-fatality rate in the United States from 1991 through 1994 was 25%, with substantially higher rates among older patients (Izurieta et al. 1997). Complications include acute respiratory failure from laryngospasm, long bone fractures from severe tetanospasm, and cardiac arrest from dysautonomia. Patients with protracted courses may require tracheostomy or develop seizures or other evidence of withdrawal related to long-term use of benzodiazepines. Most survivors recover fully. Because disease is caused by the binding of tetanus toxin to receptors, immunodeficiency neither lengthens nor shortens the pure tetanus-related disease.

Diphtheria

Diphtheria is an acute infectious disease of the tonsils, pharynx, larynx, nose, other mucous membranes, or skin, caused by *Corynebacterium diphtheriae*. The potentially fatal effects of diphtheria depend on the production of an exotoxin, by a lysogenic tox⁺ phage. Although toxic to all tissues, the exotoxin's most dramatic activity is against heart and peripheral nerves. Approximately 20% of patients develop myocarditis and neuritis.

Clinical Features

Faucial diphtheria is the most common form, presenting with fever, sore throat, membranous pharyngitis, cervical lymphadenopathy, and edema. In North America and Europe, skin infections with *C. diphtheriae* are now more common than nasopharyngeal disease. Cutaneous diphtheria appears as a pustule or nonhealing ulcer with a gray, dirty membrane. Toxic complications of cutaneous infections are rare, with neuritis more likely than myocarditis.

The toxin inhibits protein synthesis, causing segmental demyelination of motor and sensory fibers producing a toxic cranial and peripheral polyneuritis. Early signs and symptoms, within 2 weeks of the appearance of faucial disease, suggest vagal dysfunction with paralysis of the soft palate, nasal speech, and nasal regurgitation of fluids. Blurred vision, caused by ciliary paralysis of accommodation, or diplopia, caused by oculomotor nerve paralysis, appear in the third or fourth week of the disease. Peripheral polyneuritis, more likely in severe cases, typically begins between the sixth and seventh week of illness, when the patient may appear otherwise stable. The neuropathy varies widely in severity. Phrenic and further vagal nerve involvement may produce a rapidly descending paralysis of pharynx, larynx, and diaphragm. A subacute motor neuropathy, involving proximal groups first, sometimes evolves slowly, halting after 1–2 weeks, or rapidly generalizes to quadriplegia and respiratory paralysis. Vibratory, proprioceptive, and other cutaneous sensory loss may be limited to the hands and feet or extend over much of the body. Sphincter dysfunction sometimes develops; cardiac vagal denervation can result in arrhythmias or baroreceptor abnormalities. Conduction abnormalities may follow the onset of neurological symptoms by several weeks and peak after clinical recovery has begun. CSF may be normal or reveal elevated protein, which is not a poor prognostic sign, when there is radicular involvement. CNS manifestations such as encephalopathy or chorea have been reported. Primary cutaneous diphtheria is characterized by early localized anesthesia surrounding the skin ulcer, followed by weakness of surrounding muscles, before progression to generalized disease.

Diagnosis

Diagnosis of early diphtheria should be considered in patients with tonsillitis or pharyngitis with pseudomembrane, hoarseness, stridor, palatal paralysis, cervical adenopathy, or swelling. Definitive diagnosis requires isolation and identification of the organism from infected sites, but treatment with diphtheria antitoxin (equine hyperimmune serum) should be started as soon as a presumptive diagnosis is made. Anesthetic skin next to a chronic ulcer suggests cutaneous diphtheria.

Treatment

Diphtheria antitoxin can only neutralize circulating toxin before it enters cells. Antitoxin dose depends on the site of primary infection: 20,000–40,000 units for faucial diphtheria of less than 48 hours, 40,000–80,000 units for faucial diphtheria of longer than 48 hours, and 80,000–100,000 units for extensive disease or neck swelling. Patients with sensitivity to horse serum receive a 1 to 10 dilution test dose first and can be desensitized with increasing doses of antiserum, with epinephrine readily available. Bulbar, ciliary weakness and delayed sensorimotor neuropathy are characteristic of diphtheria. Neuropathy after antitoxin administration may indicate a serum sickness reaction.

Antibiotics terminate toxin production and prevent further proliferation of the organism. Either parenteral or oral penicillin G, 100,000 U/kg twice daily, or erythromycin, 5 mg/kg four times daily for 14 days, are recommended. Additional treatment is largely supportive, with respiratory and cardiac monitoring. Neurological recovery is the rule, although arrhythmias or heart failure may be fatal.

Diphtheria is included in the triple vaccine DPT (diphtheria, pertussis, and tetanus), which is administered as three primary doses at 2-month intervals beginning at 6–8 weeks of age. A fourth dose is given 6–12 months after the third, and DT is given at school entry.

RICKETTSIAE AND RELATED ORGANISMS

Typhus and spotted fevers are caused by members of the Rickettsiaceae family, obligate intracellular bacteria transmitted to humans by insects. All share the clinical triad of high fever, skin rash, and headache, with meningoencephalitis developing during the second week of illness in a proportion of cases. *Rickettsia* infect small blood vessels throughout the body causing endothelial infection, endothelial wall proliferation, thrombosis, and perivascular inflammation. The vasculitis is most prominent in skin, heart, skeletal muscle, kidney, and CNS.

Epidemic (Louse-Borne) Typhus

Rickettsia prowazekii is transmitted by the human body louse from person to person, causing epidemic louse-borne typhus. A nonhuman reservoir, the southern flying squirrel in the eastern and south-central United States, has been recognized as an alternative source of infection, but the vector insect is not known.

Clinical Features

Illness begins within 12 days of a louse bite with abrupt fever, headache, limb pain, nausea, vomiting, facial swelling, and rash. The rash appears first in the axillae and upper trunk, spreading to become confluent and hemorrhagic, but sparing the face, palms, and soles. Vacant, placid expressions or agitation are described during the

high, unremitting fever, whereas meningitis or meningoencephalitis with focal neurological deficits, delirium, or coma accompany severe disease and complicate up to 50% of cases. Tinnitus, hyperacusis, deafness, dysphagia, and midbrain stroke syndromes are recognized consequences of brainstem microinfarction. Transverse myelitis, hemiparesis, painful peripheral neuropathy, akinetic mutism, and psychiatric disturbances have been reported in survivors. Systemic complications include vascular occlusions and gangrene, myocarditis, shock, and secondary infections.

Diagnosis

The combination of a cold weather environment, crowded conditions, and infrequent bathing and changing of clothes provides an ideal setting for louse-borne typhus. Clinical suspicion and serological demonstration of heterophile antibodies to *Proteus* mirabilis OX-19 and OX-2 strains, the Weil-Felix reaction, assist in diagnosis. CSF may show modest elevations in protein and lymphocyte count, with normal glucose. Specialized laboratories can make a diagnosis by organism isolation, agglutination or ELISA serologic tests, or PCR amplification.

Treatment

Early and specific treatment is indicated to avoid a potentially fatal outcome. Effective therapies include oral or intravenous chloramphenicol, 500 mg every 6 hours intravenously for 7 days; oral or intravenous tetracycline, 500 mg every 6 hours intravenously for 7 days; or doxycycline in a single oral dose of 200 mg for adults. Relapses are retreated with the same regimen. Formaldehyde-inactivated *R. prowazekii* vaccine is recommended for persons with occupational exposure.

Murine Typhus

Rickettsia typhi, harbored by rats worldwide and transmitted to humans by flea bites, causes murine typhus. Early disease is characterized by fever, headache, myalgia, nausea, plus truncal rash in 18% of patients. Neurological symptoms, including confusion, drowsiness, seizures, ataxia, and focal deficits affect 1–45% of patients. Diagnosis is based on clinical suspicion, and the Weil-Felix reaction is the same as for louse-borne typhus. Serologic tests diagnose the disease retrospectively. Treatment is with chloramphenicol, tetracycline, or doxycycline.

Scrub Typhus

Scrub typhus is a febrile disease in East and Southeast Asia with headache, painful adenopathy, eschars, trunk, and thigh rash. *Rickettsia tsutsugamushi*, the causative agent, is transmitted by the bite of larval-stage trombiculid mites (chiggers). Meningoencephalitis or myocarditis accompany severe cases. Neurological manifestations include tremors, nervousness, dysarthria, deafness, delirium, apathy, and meningitis. Specific serological or PCR tests are used for diagnosis when available. Treatment is with a single oral dose of doxycycline, 200 mg for adults and 100 mg for children. Other forms of tick typhus, some in geographically overlapping areas, include *Rickettsia japonica* in Japan, *Rickettsia australis* in Australia, Mediterranean spotted fever (*Rickettsia conorii*) in Asia, Africa, and the Mediterranean, and Siberian tick typhus (*R. siberica*).

Rocky Mountain Spotted Fever

Rocky Mountain spotted fever, a tick-borne infection caused by *Rickettsia rickettsii*, is the most virulent of the spotted fevers, with fatality of 20% when treatment is delayed. Rocky Mountain spotted fever is present in the northwestern and eastern United States, Canada, Mexico, Columbia, and Brazil. Seasonality is predicted by activity of local ixodid tick species, including *Dermacentor andersoni* (wood tick) and *Dermacentor variabilis* in the western United States, *Amblyomma americanum* (lone-star tick) in the southern United States, *Rhipicephalus sanguineus* in Mexico, and *Amblyomma cajennense* in Brazil and Columbia, predicts seasonality. In the United States, there are approximately 700 cases per year.

Clinical Features

Illness begins with fever, headache, myalgia, and gastrointestinal symptoms 2–14 days after the tick bite. Rash appears first around the wrist and ankles from days 3–5 of the illness and spreads to the soles of the feet and forearms. Petechial and ecchymotic rashes, indicating microcirculatory injury, may foreshadow gangrene of the digits or rhabdomyolysis. Other complications include renal failure and pulmonary edema. CNS manifestations accompany severe cases. Meningitis or meningoencephalitis with microinfarcts causes focal neurological deficits, transient deafness, depressed consciousness, or coma. CSF examination reveals elevated protein and lymphocytic or polymorphonuclear pleocytosis in approximately 30% of patients, with low glucose in fewer than 10%. Electroencephalography shows diffuse abnormalities, which may persist into convalescence. Flame hemorrhages, venous engorgement, or arterial occlusion on ophthalmoscopic examination indicate retinal vasculitis.

Diagnosis

R. rickettsii can be demonstrated by direct immunofluorescence or immunoperoxidase staining of skin biopsy in patients with rash, but acute diagnosis may be difficult.

Other laboratory tests may indicate anemia, thrombocytopenia, coagulopathy, hyponatremia, and muscle tissue breakdown. Serology retrospectively confirms the diagnosis.

Rocky Mountain spotted fever and the other rickettsial diseases should be distinguished from other causes of meningoencephalitis with rash, insect exposure, or recurrent fever by tests specific for the alternative diagnoses: from meningococcemia by blood and CSF culture, viral hemorrhagic fevers or hemorrhagic measles by serology, relapsing fever and tularemia by blood culture, typhoid fever by blood or bone marrow culture, leptospirosis by clinical or laboratory evidence of myositis and hepatitis, Lyme disease by serology, malaria by blood films, secondary syphilis by serology, toxic shock syndrome by blood wound or vaginal culture, and thrombocytopenic purpuras and immune-mediated vasculitis by serological markers of collagen-vascular disease.

Treatment

Treatment is with oral or intravenous tetracycline (25–50 mg/kg/day) or chloramphenicol (50–75 mg/kg/day) in four divided doses or oral doxycycline, 100 mg twice a day for 7 days and continued for 2 days once the patient has become afebrile.

Q fever

Q fever, an acute or chronic febrile illness that occurs worldwide, is caused by *Coxiella burnetii* acquired by aerosol spread from cattle, sheep, and goats or through unpasteurized milk. *C. burnetii* is in the rickettsial family, but differs from the other rickettsial infections by the aerosol route of transmission, absence of rash, and lack of cross-reacting antibodies to *Proteus* OX species. Characteristic clinical syndromes include atypical pneumonias or hepatitis. Also seen are endocarditis, vertebral osteomyelitis, and neurological syndromes, including aseptic meningitis, encephalitis, delirium, dementia, extrapyramidal syndrome, and manic psychosis. Diagnosis depends on ELISA or indirect fluorescent antibody serologic tests. Rarely, *C. burnetii* has been isolated from the CSF. Early, uncomplicated Q fever is treated with chloramphenicol, tetracycline, or doxycycline. Endocarditis requires therapy with RIF and cotrimoxazole or tetracycline and cotrimoxazole for several months. A formalinized vaccine is available for individuals with occupational exposure.

Ehrlichiosis

Ehrlichioses are tick-borne zoonotic infections caused by an intraleukocytic bacterium closely related to Rickettsiae. First recognized as a canine pathogen, two species of *Ehrlichia* have been associated with human disease, including a summertime meningitis, in the United States, and a third species with a mononucleosislike illness in Japan.

Clinical Features

In the United States, incidence peaks from spring through autumn. Patients present with fever, headache, myalgia, rash, and history of tick bite. Occasionally, patients present with meningitis only. Renal failure, disseminated intravascular coagulation, cardiomegaly, opportunistic infection, seizures, encephalopathy, or coma are among the serious complications that develop in a portion of cases (Fishbein et al. 1994).

Diagnosis

Most patients have varying degrees of leukopenia, thrombocytopenia or anemia, and mild to moderate hepatic enzyme abnormalities. Diagnosis depends on epidemiological and clinical features, plus a high index of suspicion. Acute and convalescent sera confirm the diagnosis. PCR-based tests are available for early confirmation of acute infection.

Treatment

Treatment is with oral or intravenous doxycycline, 100 mg twice daily for 7 days.

Bartonella

Oroyo fever and verruga peruana are two forms of the same disease, bartonellosis, caused by *Bartonella bacilliformis*. Oroyo fever is associated with encephalitis and cerebral venous thromboses and verruga peruana with intracranial nodules. These diseases occur in river valleys along the western slopes of the Andes in Peru, Ecuador, and Columbia at altitudes of 2,000–8,000 feet. Sandfly bite transmits the disorder. Oroyo fever is a syndrome of fever, rapid anemia, joint and long bone pain, headache, and delirium. *Bartonella* may invade the brain or spinal cord in red cells with parasites, producing meningoencephalitis, venous thrombosis, or myelitis. CSF shows elevated protein, pleocytosis, and intracellular organisms. Verruga peruana, usually a sequel to Oroyo fever, is a rheumatic syndrome with cutaneous miliary or nodular eruptions over exposed parts of the body, and occasionally over mucous membranes and internal organs, including the brain.

B. bacilliformis can be seen in red blood cells in the acute febrile stage and in smears from verruga. The two clinical forms of bartonellosis were linked by the fatal self-inoculation experiment of the Peruvian medical student, Daniel Carrion, who, with the help of a colleague, injected himself with material from verruga peruana cutaneous lesions and gave himself Oroyo fever. Bartonellosis also is referred to as *Carrion's disease*, in his honor.

The differential diagnosis for Oroyo fever includes malaria, typhus, and typhoid. The verruga stage resembles yaws or secondary syphilis. Chloramphenicol (4 g daily in divided doses) for at least 7 days is the drug of first choice. Penicillin, tetracycline, streptomycin, and cotrimoxazole are alternatives.

ZOONOSIS PATHOGENS AND RELATED ORGANISMS

Brucellosis

Brucellosis, a zoonosis caused by several *Brucella* species (*B. melitensis*, *B. abortus*, and *B. suis*), is a multisystem illness characterized by fever, frequent bone and joint disease (arthritis, sacroiliitis, spondylitis, osteomyelitis), and respiratory, gastrointestinal, or cardiac disease. Infrequent but important manifestations of disease include an extremely wide range of neurological conditions, affecting approximately 5% of patients. Normally a disease of domestic and wild animals, *Brucella* is transmitted to humans by ingestion of infected unpasteurized milk, aerosol spread, or by contact with infected animals or animal products. The disease exists worldwide, but is especially prevalent in Mediterranean regions, the Middle East, the Indian subcontinent, and Latin America.

Early complaints may include fatigue, sensations of malodorous sweat or abnormal taste, and symptoms of depression. Untreated, an undulant fever pattern emerges in 2- to 4-week cycles. Meningitis can be the presenting manifestation, or it may occur late in disease. Acute or chronic meningitis, encephalitis, meningovascular disease, multifocal white matter disease, intracerebral or epidural abscess, subdural empyema, intracranial hypertension, ruptured mycotic aneurysms, hydrocephalus, papilledema, cranial neuropathies, psychosis, parkinsonism, radiculopathies (usually lumbosacral) or myelopathy associated with spondylitis, peripheral neuropathies, and myositis have been reported. Vertebral, paravertebral, or psoas abscesses may complicate sacroiliitis or vertebral osteomyelitis. Endocarditis occurs in approximately 2% of cases.

Brucellosis figures in the differential diagnosis of nearly any neurological disease in endemic areas. Definitive diagnosis depends on isolation of brucellae from blood, bone marrow, or other tissues. Because the organism is difficult to culture, diagnosis usually depends on (1) positive *Brucella* agglutination or ELISA test results with high titers of antibody in blood and CSF; (2) abnormal CSF with a lymphocytic pleocytosis, elevated protein, and low to normal glucose; and (3) response to therapy. CSF may be turbid, hemorrhagic, or clear and may also be positive by Coombs' test and contain oligoclonal bands. Rare findings include acellular CSF or positive *Brucella* culture during meningitis.

Uncomplicated brucellosis is treated with oral doxycycline, 200 mg daily, with streptomycin, 1 g intramuscularly daily for 12 weeks, or another aminoglycoside for the first 4 weeks, then followed by RIF (10–15 mg/kg/day) for an additional 4–8 weeks. Neurobrucellosis, endocarditis, skeletal, and other severe organ involvement are treated with three-drug therapy with doxycycline, an aminoglycoside, and RIF for at least 12 weeks. Children under 8 years of age are treated with TMP-SMX in combination with an aminoglycoside and RIF. The end point of treatment is normalization of CSF cell counts. Adjunctive corticosteroid therapy has been used for concurrent vasculitic or demyelinating disease.

Anthrax

Anthrax, caused by the gram-positive sporulating bacillus *Bacillus anthracis*, is usually a disease of herbivores, acquired from contact with soil containing spores. Less commonly, anthrax causes hemorrhagic meningitis in humans, after exposure to infected animals or their products. The three main forms of disease are cutaneous, respiratory, and gastrointestinal. Meningitis is seen in less than 5% of cases. For a diagnosis of anthrax meningitis, there should be a primary site of infection, such as a malignant pustule or pulmonary syndrome, plus CSF and blood containing *B. anthracis*. Treatment is with penicillin G, 4 million units every 4–6 hours for 7–10 days. Intubation may be necessary, because of facial, oropharyngeal, and neck edema.

Plague

Plague, caused by *Yersinia pestis*, is a zoonotic infection of wild rodents, transmitted by the bites of infected fleas to humans, an accidental host. Meningitis is an unusual manifestation of plague, usually complicating bubonic plague, particularly if buboes are located in the axilla. Human infection takes the clinical forms of febrile lymphadenitis (bubonic plague), septicemic, pneumonic, or meningeal plague. Most meningitis cases follow inadequately treated bubonic plague by 9–15 days, but primary plague meningitis also occurs. *Y. pestis* can be found on CSF Gram's stain and culture. Treatment of the primary infection is with streptomycin, 30 mg/kg per day intramuscularly in two divided doses for 10 days. Meningitis is treated with intravenous chloramphenicol, 25 mg/kg initially, followed by 60 mg/kg per day in four divided doses for 10 days, either alone or in combination with streptomycin. Because of its excellent penetration, chloramphenicol is recommended also for endophthalmitis and myocarditis.

Tularemia

Tularemia (rabbit fever, deer fly fever, Ohara's disease, yatobyo) is an infectious disease of rodents caused by *Francisella tularensis*. Virulent in susceptible species, including the accidental human host, tularemia may cause meningitis or encephalitis as complications of disseminated infection. Tularemia is transmitted to humans by insect bite, handling infected animals, ingesting infected meat or water, or inhaling contaminated aerosols or dust. *F. tularensis* causes an acute febrile illness; classic forms include ulceroglandular, oculoglandular, pneumonic, pharyngeal, abdominal, or typhoidal (septicemic) disease. Dissemination may lead to meningitis with mononuclear pleocytosis, elevated protein, and low glucose. Encephalitis and Guillain-Barré syndrome accompanying the pneumonic and pleuritic form have been reported also. Clinical suspicion and serological studies aid in the diagnosis, although antibodies detected by agglutination tests cross-react with *Brucella* spp., *Yersinia* spp., and the *Proteus* OX-19 strain that identifies typhus. A microagglutination test with greater sensitivity is now available. Culture and isolation of *F. tularensis* are difficult. Streptomycin, 1 g intramuscularly daily for 10–14 days, treats the infection. Gentamicin is an alternative. Resolution of symptoms and convalescence are slow. Debilitating fatigue continues for months after acute illness in up to one-third of cases.

Pasteurellosis

Pasteurellae, primarily animal pathogens carried in the nasopharynx or gastrointestinal tract of many domestic and wild mammals and birds worldwide, are rare causes of meningitis or brain abscess in humans during disseminated infections. Human *Pasteurella* infections, usually *P. multocida*, are either focal soft tissue infection after an animal bite, respiratory infection, or bacteremia. Diagnosis is by demonstration or culture of the organism from wound, sputum, or CSF, and treatment is with penicillin.

Glanders

Glanders, primarily an equine infection by *Pseudomonas mallei*, occasionally produces human disease consisting of suppurative infections, lymphadenopathy, and pulmonary disease. Meningitis or brain abscesses occur in up to one-fourth of patients. A history of contact with horses, mules, or donkeys is typical, and transmission occurs through contamination of broken skin or mucosal surfaces by draining ulcers of an infected animal. Diagnosis is by microscopic examination of exudates. A 3-week course of sulfadiazine, 100 mg/kg daily in divided doses, is recommended.

Melioidosis

Melioidosis, caused by the ubiquitous soil saprophyte *Pseudomonas pseudomallei*, is a glanderslike infectious disease of animals and humans, with meningitis or brain abscess complicating disseminated forms. Melioidosis is endemic in Southeast Asia and northern Australia, with most cases occurring during the annual rainy season. Clinical forms include pneumonitis, hemorrhagic pneumonitis, and respiratory failure, septicemia, pustular or necrotic skin lesions, focal adenitis, and chronic suppurative visceral abscesses. Parotid abscesses may cause local injury, by rupture into the auditory canal or facial nerve compression. A role for a neurological toxin in the development of aseptic meningitis or brainstem encephalitis, bulbar and respiratory weakness, and peripheral motor neuropathy of Guillain-Barré type, in the absence of direct CNS infection, has been suggested but not proven.

The diagnosis should be considered in patients with a radiological pattern of TB from which AFB-staining bacteria cannot be found. Melioidosis is diagnosed by identifying organisms with bacteriological staining and culture techniques. Patients are seropositive by indirect fluorescent antibody or ELISA tests. Septicemic forms are treated with TMP, 8 mg/kg, and SMX, 40 mg/kg per day, plus ceftazidime, 120 mg/kg per day, with intravenous therapy for 2 weeks, and oral treatment for 6 months.

Cat-Scratch Disease

Cat-scratch disease, a slowly progressive regional adenitis caused by *Bartonella* (formerly *Rochalimaea*) *henselae* or less often, *Afipia felis*, is associated with aseptic meningitis in immunocompetent individuals and encephalitis, myelitis, or radiculoneuritis in HIV-infected patients. Several clinical patterns have been recognized. Immunocompetent individuals may have one or several bacteremic episodes with fever, arthralgias, headache, and aseptic meningitis, but the illness is self-limited in the majority of cases. HIV-infected patients with disseminated *B. henselae* infection may have bacillary angiomatosis (neovascular proliferative skin lesions), which resemble the cutaneous stigmata of verruga peruana or Kaposi's sarcoma, oculoglandular syndrome with preauricular adenitis, palpebral or conjunctival granulomas, anemia, hepatosplenomegaly, or encephalomyelitis. Direct plating of homogenized tissue of accessible lesions has yielded bacteria, but cultivation of *Bartonella* spp. is technically difficult and slow. ELISA tests and PCR amplification from infected tissues are available. Intravenous gentamicin is recommended for encephalitis and oral doxycycline, erythromycin, or ciprofloxacin for bacillary angiomatosis, but controlled treatment trials have not been completed.

Rat-Bite Fever

Rat-bite fever is a systemic febrile illness caused by *S. moniliformis*, which is transmitted by the bite of a rat or other small rodents. Patients develop rash or even purpuric skin lesions, asymmetrical polyarthralgias, or septic arthritis, with the additional complications of meningitis, brain abscesses, endocarditis, or myocarditis. Diagnosis is by visualization or culture of organisms from blood, joint fluid, or purulent

material. Treatment is with penicillin, streptomycin, or a cephalosporin in penicillin-allergic patients.

ENTERIC BACTERIA

Salmonellosis

A common cause of neonatal meningitis, *Salmonella* species are associated also with brain abscess, subdural empyema, and recurrent bacteremia in HIV-infected patients. *S. typhi* and *S. paratyphi* are recognized agents of enteric fever, vascular (endothelial) infection leading to aortoduodenal fistulas, and chronic carrier states. Disseminated intravascular coagulation complicates severe infections. Atypical manifestations include pneumonitis, pericarditis, sacroiliitis, arthritis, and osteomyelitis, the last being particularly common in patients with sickle cell hemoglobinopathies.

Until fairly recently, chloramphenicol was used to treat typhoid fever. However, because of outbreaks associated with resistant strains in Latin America, the Middle East, South and Southeast Asia, ciprofloxacin for adults (500 mg orally twice a day for 10–14 days) or ceftriaxone for children (100 mg/kg/day intravenously or intramuscularly for 10–14 days) or adults (1–2 g daily) are considered better choices for patients in these areas. One study found that chloramphenicol therapy, combined with corticosteroids for the first 48 hours of illness, improved outcome in critically ill patients with delirium, stupor, coma, or shock.

Shigellosis

Shigella species, members of the Enterobacteriaceae family and agents of bacillary dysentery, are postulated to cause a fatal, toxic encephalopathy in children by elaboration of Shiga toxin according to Goren and colleagues in 1992. The encephalopathy is a syndrome of sudden headache, cerebral edema, and rapid neurological decompensation, beginning several hours to 6 days after onset of diarrheal illness. Shigellosis is diagnosed by stool culture. Enteric and systemic disease is treated with ciprofloxacin (500 mg orally twice daily for adults for 1–5 days) or TMP-SMX (160 mg of TMP and 800 mg of SMX orally twice daily in adults) and rehydration, but antibiotics may not influence the neurological disease.

Campylobacteriosis

Campylobacter, among the most frequent bacterial infections of humans worldwide, causes both acute enteric and systemic illnesses. Sources of infection include raw milk, water, and poultry. *Campylobacter jejuni* has been identified as the most common antecedent pathogen for the Guillain-Barré syndrome, accounting for an estimated 20–40% of all cases. The onset of Guillain-Barré syndrome is usually 2–3 weeks after the diarrheal illness and follows an estimated 1 per 1,000–2,000 *Campylobacter* infections. The presence of anti-GM$_1$ antibodies in Guillain-Barré patients infected with *C. jejuni* Penner serogroup 19, and anti-GQ1b ganglioside antibodies in Miller-Fisher variant patients infected with *C. jejuni* Lior serogroup 7, has led to the hypothesis that lipopolysaccharides of these *Campylobacter* isolates induce neuropathic disease by molecular mimicry (Yuki 1997; Yuki et al. 1997). *Campylobacter* infection is diagnosed by isolation and identification of the organism from stool or blood. Most strains are treated adequately with erythromycin, 250 mg orally four times daily for 5–7 days.

Whipple's Disease

Whipple's disease, caused by *Tropheryma whippleii*, is a multisystem disorder characterized by gastrointestinal disease (abdominal pain, diarrhea, weight loss), arthritis, lymphadenopathy, addisonian symptoms (hypotension, asthenia, cutaneous hyperpigmentation), and protean neurological manifestations including dementia, oculofaciomasticatory myorhythmia (slow, repetitive, synchronous, rhythmic contractions of ocular, facial, masticatory, or limb muscles), supranuclear ophthalmoplegia, meningitis, neuropathy, and myopathy. Classically, the disease occurs as coexisting neurological and gastrointestinal disease, and the diagnosis is made by identifying periodic acid–Schiff-positive macrophages and bacilli on duodenal or jejunal biopsy. Brain biopsy, demonstrating periodic acid–Schiff-positive material, has been used to establish the diagnosis in the absence of intestinal disease. For its numerous other presentations, sarcoidosis, collagen vascular disease, malabsorption syndromes, Addison's disease, frontotemporal dementia, Creutzfeldt-Jakob disease, progressive supranuclear palsy, or Wernicke's encephalopathy are differential diagnostic considerations. Treatment is with oral double-strength TMP-SMX twice daily for 1 year. Severely ill patients are treated with thrice daily TMP-SMX for the first 2 weeks, together with folinic acid. CNS relapse, occurring in 35% of patients several years after treatment, is retreated with oral TMP-SMX. Oral chloramphenicol, parenteral ceftriaxone, or penicillin are other treatment options for those who respond poorly.

RESPIRATORY PATHOGENS

Chlamydial Diseases

Each of the three chlamydial species, *C. psittaci*, *C. trachomatis*, and *C. pneumoniae* are human pathogens, with *C. psittaci* most consistently associated with neurological complications.

Psittacosis (or ornithosis), caused by *C. psittaci*, is transmitted from bird to humans by the aerosol route. Fever, cough, myalgia, headache, and hepatomegaly are presenting clinical features, occasionally accompanied by cranial nerve palsy, myelitis, meningoencephalitis, seizures, or cerebellar ataxia. CSF contains few or no lymphocytes, and normal protein, although elevated protein has been reported with myelitis. Psittacosis is diagnosed by serology and treated with oral tetracycline or erythromycin, 500 mg four times per day for 10–14 days. In the absence of a firm diagnosis, erythromycin may be preferable, because it also covers other *Legionella* and *Mycoplasma*, which also cause atypical pneumonias with neurological symptoms.

C. trachomatis causes ocular and venereal disease. Trachoma presents as follicular conjunctivitis with inflammatory infiltrates. The conjunctivae scar as the disease progresses, and eventually the eyelashes turn inward and abrade the cornea. Treatment is with erythromycin or tetracycline.

C. pneumoniae (TWAR agent) is associated with pneumonia, bronchitis, and sinusitis and may predispose to early arteriosclerotic disease.

Mycoplasma Syndromes

The human mycoplasmas are *M. pneumoniae*, *M. hominis*, *Ureaplasma urealyticum*, and *M. genitalium*. *M. pneumoniae*, responsible for most clinical disease, causes respiratory infections. Systemic illness with cough is the most consistent clinical presentation. Extrapulmonary involvement includes rash, cardiac abnormalities, arthralgias, vascular diseases (Raynaud's phenomenon, internal carotid artery occlusion, stroke), and neurological syndromes (aseptic meningitis, meningoencephalitis, leukoencephalitis, transverse myelitis, brainstem syndromes, Guillain-Barré, and peripheral neuropathy). Neurological manifestations are more frequent in hospitalized patients. Diagnosis depends on recognizing the clinical syndrome and may be confirmed by demonstration of cold agglutinins or complement-fixing antibodies. Erythromycin, 500 mg every 6 hours in adults, 1 g per day in older children, and 30–50 mg/kg per day in young children for 21 days is the recommended treatment. Tetracycline is an alternative in adults and children older than 8 years. *U. urealyticum* and *M. hominis*, present in the genital tract, cause neonatal meningitis.

Legionellosis

Legionella pneumophila causes Legionnaires' disease, which is associated with myositis and with cerebral manifestations ranging from headache to coma. *L. pneumophila* is transmitted to humans from its natural aquatic habitat by aerosol or airborne droplets, particularly where humidifiers or air conditioners are used. Legionnaires' disease is characterized by mild to severe pulmonary disease, gastrointestinal disease, hyponatremia, myalgias or myositis, and neurological symptoms. Encephalopathy, manifesting as altered mental status, is the most common neurological abnormality; ataxia, cranial nerve palsy, motor neuropathy, mild inflammatory CSF changes, and electroencephalographical abnormalities have been reported. The diagnosis is suspected in patients with pneumonia and purulent sputum with few or no organisms seen on Gram's stain or in patients who fail to respond to β-lactam or aminoglycoside antibiotics. Diagnosis is made by culture, serology, or DNA probe. Treatment is with erythromycin, 1 g intravenously every 6 hours until clinical improvement, followed by 2 g orally in divided doses for 3 weeks. Reversible ototoxicity may occur with total daily doses of 4 g. Alternative agents include clarithromycin, doxycycline, ciprofloxacin, and RIF. The disease is not contagious from person to person.

Pertussis

Bordetella pertussis causes pertussis (whooping cough), an upper respiratory catarrhal infection followed by paroxysmal coughing in a series of short expiratory bursts and an inspiratory gasp. Pertussis is a severe disease in children younger than 1 year, associated with seizures and encephalopathy. Subconjunctival, scleral, or CNS hemorrhages can follow the increased intrathoracic and intraabdominal pressures during violent coughing at any age. Definitive diagnosis is by isolation of *B. pertussis*, but because the organism is difficult to culture, a clinical case definition (cough of 2 weeks' duration in the setting of a community outbreak) is used. A vaccine composed of one or more components of the organism combined with diphtheria and tetanus toxoids (DPT) is used for immunization. Three primary doses are administered at 2-month intervals beginning at 6–8 weeks of age. Treatment is with erythromycin at doses of 40–50 mg/kg per day for 14 days, and erythromycin for prophylaxis of household contacts may be necessary. Infants should be cared for in an ICU.

CARDIAC INFECTIONS

Endocarditis

When cerebral emboli from all sources are counted, approximately 3% result from infective endocarditis. Common pathogens include enterococci, *Streptococcus viridans*, *S. aureus*, *S. epidermidis*, or *Pseudomonas aeruginosa*. Cerebral embolization occurs in at least one-third of all infective endocarditis cases, commonly in middle cerebral artery territory. Bland or hemorrhagic cerebral infarcts, arteritis, single or multiple abscesses, mycotic aneurysms (often at bifurcation points of distal branches of the middle cerebral artery), intraparenchymal or subarachnoid hemorrhage, cerebritis, meningitis, and asymptomatic CSF pleocytosis can develop during active endocarditis.

Blood culture, a critical diagnostic test for endocarditis, may give negative results in 2.5–31.0% of cases. Reasons for culture-negative endocarditis include (1) fungal endocarditis; (2) slow growth of fastidious organisms such as *Haemophilus*, variant streptococci, *Brucella*; (3) failure to culture intracellular pathogens such as chlamydiae or rickettsiae; (4) right-sided endocarditis; and (5) recent antibiotic use. CSF examination, if clinically indicated, most consistently shows increased numbers of polymorphonuclear leukocytes, red cells, elevated protein, and normal glucose levels. Treatment is with parenteral antibiotics for at least 4 weeks. Indications for valve replacement include more than one significant embolic episode or failure of antibiotic therapy; mycotic aneurysms may require neurosurgical intervention. Mycotic aneurysms may follow treatment by months or years.

Rheumatic Fever

Rheumatic fever, a sequelae of group A streptococcal infection, is diagnosed by one or more clinical criteria (carditis, migratory polyarthritis, subcutaneous nodules, erythema marginatum, chorea), plus culture evidence of recent group A streptococcal infections or elevated antistreptolysin O titers. The childhood chorea, Sydenham's chorea, occurs in less than 10% of patients. Onset may be immediate or several months after the index infection. Even patients with chorea only are treated, according to the American Heart Association guidelines, which advise prophylactic monthly intramuscular injections of 1.2 million units of benzathine penicillin G or daily oral penicillin V to prevent recurrent attacks.

STAPHYLOCOCCAL SYNDROMES

Toxic Shock Syndrome

Toxic shock syndrome (TSS), epidemiologically linked to several toxigenic *S. aureus* strains, is a multisystem disorder characterized by desquamating skin rash, especially on the palms and soles, high fever, hypovolemic shock, vomiting or diarrhea, renal failure, hyperemic mucosal surfaces, thrombocytopenia, liver enzyme abnormalities, myalgias, and encephalopathy. Several related toxic exoproteins, most often TSS toxin 1 (TSST-1), produced by isolates of *S. aureus* from patients, cause the disease. TSS has been reported in children, in menstruating women using hyperabsorbent tampons, and following gynecological and other surgical procedures. CNS complications may be more frequent in nonmenstrual TSS.

Confusion, disorientation, agitation, or somnolence independent of anoxic or metabolic changes are described. Other features include headache, generalized electroencephalographic abnormalities, persistent amnestic syndrome, poor concentration, and difficulty with calculations. CSF is usually normal. Serum CK levels, elevated in over one-half of patients, reflect the severity of myositis and convalescent-stage weakness. Although blood, vaginal fluid, or wounds may be cultured for *S. aureus* and isolates tested for production of TSST-1, TSS remains a clinically defined syndrome. Other febrile exanthems with hypotension, such as Rocky Mountain spotted fever, leptospirosis, meningococcemia, gram-negative sepsis, viral exanthems, and drug reaction, should be excluded. Management requires aggressive fluid replacement and treatment with a β-lactamase–resistant antistaphylococcal antibiotic or clindamycin, 900 mg intravenously every 8 hours for 10–14 days.

Pyomyositis

Tropical pyomyositis is a subacute syndrome caused by staphylococcal infection, characterized by the spontaneous appearance of bacterial abscesses within the fascial boundaries of skeletal muscles, usually muscles of large bulk. Tropical pyomyositis accounts for 3–4% of surgical admissions to hospitals in sub-Saharan Africa. Although early staphylococcal pyomyositis may respond to an antistaphylococcal penicillin or vancomycin alone, drainage of abscess cavities is usually necessary. In temperate regions, a different, hyperacute pyomyositis, caused by group A betahemolytic streptococcal infection, is recognized. When it occurs, it is usually the earliest sign of critical, potentially fatal, disseminated infection, designated *streptococcal TSS*. Therapy includes penicillin or ampicillin, a third-generation cephalosporin, surgical drainage, and blood pressure support with volume expansion. For both syndromes, ultrasound, CT, or MRI of the affected area often demonstrates the infection.

ACTINOMYCETES (FILAMENTOUS BACTERIA)

Nocardiosis

Nocardiosis is a locally invasive or disseminated infection caused by the aerobic actinomycetes *Nocardia asteroides*, *N. otitidiscaviarum*, and *N. brasiliensis*. Disseminated disease commonly involves the CNS. The organisms are soil saprophytes, spread to humans by inhalation, through broken skin, from the gut, or after dental procedures. Primary infection typically manifests as pneumonia with cavitary pulmonary lesions, but sinusitis, keratitis, cutaneous abscesses and fistulas, septic arthritis, or vertebral osteoarthritis are seen also. Disseminated disease occurs in immunosuppressed patients. CNS syndromes, including cerebral abscesses, meningitis, and, rarely, hemorrhagic meningitis develop in approximately one-third of all pulmonary cases, and primary CNS infection in another 5–7%. Cerebral abscesses often appear as complex multiloculated structures with satellite extensions on neuroimaging studies. Brain

abscesses tend to burrow into a ventricle or out to the subarachnoid space, so meningitis is often associated with abscesses.

Nocardia spp. appear as weakly gram-positive, branching filaments in sputum, drainage from fistulas, or histological specimens. Dense bacterial concentrations resemble Chinese calligraphy. *Nocardia*, when stained with modified acid-fast procedures, are partially acid fast. Because nocardiosis is an infection with a variable, often chronic, course, treatment with sulfonamides (TMP-SMX) may extend for months to years. The recommended intravenous dose is TMP (15 mg/kg/day) and SMX (75 mg/kg/day), the equivalent of two double-strength tablets every 8 hours. Second-line drugs include minocycline, imipenem, or an aminoglycoside in combination with a third-generation cephalosporin. Small cerebral abscesses may resolve with medical management alone.

Actinomycosis

Actinomycosis, characterized by abscesses that cross fascial planes to form sinuses, is a rare cause of brain abscesses. Actinomycosis is caused by a variety of gram-positive anaerobic or microaerophilic rods of the genera *Actinomyces* (most commonly *A. israelii*) and *Arachnia*, normal mouth and female genital tract flora. Most infections are either cervicofacial, thoracic, abdominal, or pelvic. Cervicofacial actinomycosis or "lumpy jaw" is the most common form and may develop following dental procedures or oral mucosa trauma, as a complication of dental caries or periodontal disease, or without antecedent trauma or predisposing infection. Abscesses and draining sinuses form and exudates contain *sulfur granules*, so named because they are yellow. Actinomyces reach the brain by direct extension of oral-cervicofacial disease or hematogenous spread. Brain abscess is the most common CNS presentation. Abscesses may be single or multiple and may appear multiloculated with ring enhancement (Figure 59A.8) or more homogeneous enhancement on neuroimaging studies. Abscess rupture into the subarachnoid space produces acute meningitis. Chronic meningitis may develop as a consequence of spread from a parameningeal site, such as the middle ear or sinus or paraventricular or parameningeal parenchymal abscess. Spinal epidural abscess may follow vertebral osteomyelitis. Cavernous sinus thrombosis and spinal cord subdural empyema also have been reported.

Macroscopic and microscopic examination of pus and granules, followed by culture, establishes the diagnosis. Bacteriological identification from sulfur granules or a sterile site confirms the diagnosis. Actinomycosis resembles nocardiosis, but the latter does not form granules in visceral organs. Actinomycosis occurs in immunocompetent patients, whereas nocardiosis is a disease of immunosuppressed patients. Treatment is with penicillin, initially 18–24 million units in divided doses intravenously per day

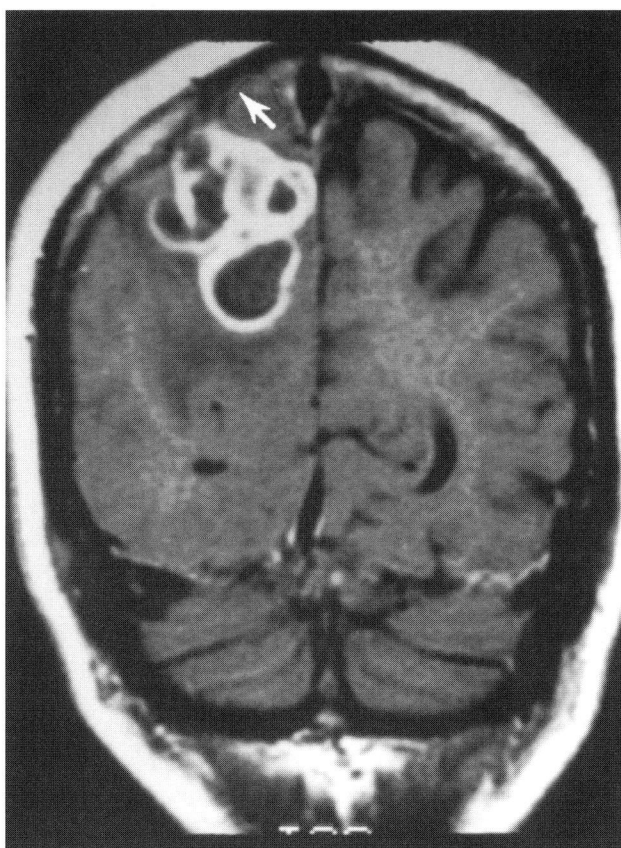

FIGURE 59A.8 Actinomycosis. Coronal T1 gadolinium-enhanced magnetic resonance image showing multiloculated, ring-enhancing lesion in a patient with intracerebral spread of actinomycosis abscesses from a skull infection. Skull involvement is indicated by resorption of normal fatty marrow signal (*arrow*).

for 2–6 weeks, followed by oral penicillin or amoxicillin for 6–12 months. Surgical drainage and excision may be indicated. Clindamycin penetrates bone well and may be the drug of choice if there is bony involvement.

REFERENCES

Anderson M. Management of cerebral infection. J Neurol Neurosurg Psychiatry 1993;56:1243–1258.

Bharucha NE, Bharucha EP, Bhabha SK. Bacterial Infections. In WG Bradley, RB Daroff, GM Fenichel, CD Marsden (eds), Neurology in Clinical Practice (2nd ed). Boston: Butterworth–Heinemann, 1996;1181–1243.

Burningham MD, Walter FJ, Mechem C, et al. Wound botulism. Ann Emerg Med 1994;24:1184–1187.

Case Records of the Massachusetts General Hospital. A 71-year-old woman with confusion, hemianopia, and an occipital mass. N Engl J Med 1993;329:1335–1341.

Case Records of the Massachusetts General Hospital. A 58-year-old woman with multiple cranial neuropathies. N Engl J Med 1997;335:184–190.

Centers for Disease Control. 1998 guidelines for treatment of sex-ually transmitted diseases. MMWR Morb Moral Wkly Rep 1998;47(No. RR-1):28–49.

Centers for Disease Control. Wound botulism—California, 1995. MMWR Morb Moral Wkly Rep 1995;44:889–892.

Cinque P, Scarpellini P, Vago L, et al. Diagnosis of central nervous system complications of HIV-infected patients: cerebrospinal fluid analysis by the polymerase chain reaction. AIDS 1997;11: 1–17.

Cintron R, Pachner AR. Spirochetal diseases of the nervous system. Curr Opin Neurol 1994;7:217–222.

Dooley DP, Carpenter JL, Rademacher S. Adjunctive corticosteroid therapy for tuberculosis: a critical reappraisal of the literature. Clin Infect Dis 1997;25:872–887.

Dutt AK, Stead W. Tuberculosis. Part II. The treatment of tuberculosis. Dis Mon 1997;43:247–276.

Ernst MD, Klepser ME, Fouts M, Marangos MN. Tetanus: pathophysiology and management. Ann Pharmacother 1997;31: 1507–1513.

Fishbein DB, Dawson JE, Robinson LE. Human ehrlichiosis in the United States, 1985–1990. Ann Intern Med 1994;120:736–743.

Galazka A, Gasse F. The present status of tetanus and tetanus vaccination. Curr Topics Micro Immunol 1995;195:31–53.

Garcia-Monco JC, Benach JL. Lyme Neuroborreliosis. Ann Neurol 1995;37:691–702.

Halperin JJ, Logigian EL, Finkel MF, Pearl RA. Practice parameters for the diagnosis of patients with nervous system Lyme borreliosis (Lyme disease). Neurology 1996;46:619–627.

Izurieta HS, Sutter RW, Strebel PM, et al. Tetanus surveillance—United States, 1991–1994. In CDC Surveillance Summaries (February). MMWR CDC Surveill Summ 1997;46(SS-2):15–25.

Kim YS, Pons VG. Infections in the neurosurgical intensive care unit. Neurosurg Clin North Am 1994;5:741–754.

LoBue PA, Catanzaro A. Tuberculosis. Part II. The diagnosis of tuberculosis. Dis Mon 1997;43:185–246.

Maniglia RJ, Roth T, Blumberg EA. Polymicrobial brain abscess in a patient infected with human immunodeficiency virus. Clin Infect Dis 1997;24:449–451.

Mathisen GE, Johnson JP. Brain abscess. Clin Infect Dis 1997;25: 763–781.

McIntyre PB, Berkey CS, King SM, et al. Dexamethasone as adjunctive therapy in bacterial meningitis: a meta-analysis of randomized clinical trials since 1988. JAMA 1997;278:925–931.

Midura TF. Update: infant botulism. Clin Micro Rev 1996;9: 119–125.

Montecucco C, Schiavo G. Microreview: mechanism of action of tetanus and botulinum neurotoxins. Mol Microbiol 1994;13:1–8.

Munoz P, Miranda ME, Llancaqueo A, et al. Haemophilus species bacteremia in adults. The importance of the human immunodeficiency virus epidemic. Arch Intern Med 1997;157:1869–1873.

Quagliarello VJ, Scheld WM. Treatment of bacterial meningitis. N Engl J Med 1997;336:708–716.

Schuchat A, Robinson K, Wenger JD, et al. Bacterial meningitis in the United States in 1995. N Engl J Med 1997;337:970–976.

Sun KO, Chan YW, Cheung RTF, et al. Management of tetanus: a review of 18 cases. J R Soc Med 1994;87:135–137.

Varaine F, Caugant DA, Riou JY, et al. Meningitis outbreaks and vaccination strategy. Trans R Soc Trop Med Hygiene 1997;91:3–7.

Yuki N. Molecular mimicry between gangliosides and lipopolysaccharides of Campylobacter jejuni isolated from patients with Guillain-Barré syndrome and Miller Fisher syndrome. J Infect Dis 1997;176(Suppl. 2):S150–153.

Yuki N, Takahashi M, Tagawa Y, et al. Association of Campylobacter jejuni serotype with antiganglioside antibody in Guillain-Barré syndrome and Fisher's syndrome. Ann Neurol 1997;42:28–33.

Chapter 59
Infections of the Nervous System

B. VIRAL INFECTIONS
Marylou V. Solbrig

The clinical spectrum of viral diseases is very wide. Signs of primary infection range from subclinical infection, detected only by the presence of antibodies, to systemic febrile illness with nervous system symptoms (headache, lethargy, photophobia), or unequivocal meningeal or parenchymal central nervous system (CNS) disease. Acute CNS viral syndromes are mostly meningitis or encephalitis. Yet viruses also establish latent or persistent infections and, therefore, are associated with recrudescent infections such as herpes zoster or chronic progressive nervous system syndromes, such as subacute sclerosing panencephalitis (SSPE).

By virtue of their existence as antigen, parasite, or genetic element, viruses also influence or exacerbate CNS inflammatory, autoimmune, malignant, metabolic, or deficiency diseases. For example, human herpesvirus 6 (HHV-6) is now linked to multiple sclerosis (Sola et al. 1993; Wilborn et al. 1994) and Epstein-Barr virus (EBV) is associated with CNS B-cell lymphomas. Any virus worsens lactic acidemic metabolic or mitochondrial disorders, and an enterovirus cofactor has been implicated in a nutritional neuropathy in Cuba (Mas et al. 1997).

A growing understanding of the relation between infection, systemic virulence, and neurovirulence translates into more antiviral therapies in the future. As more specific drugs become available, the ability to distinguish among viral CNS infections will have greater therapeutic implications. However, at present, viruses, small pieces of DNA or RNA wrapped in a protein, when spread to humans, provide many sobering examples of the extreme vulnerability of the CNS to infection.

VIRAL SYNDROMES

Meningitis (Aseptic Meningitis)

Viral meningitis, an inflammatory response to viral infection of leptomeningeal cells and the subarachnoid space, is one form of aseptic meningitis. *Aseptic meningitis*, defined in the 1920s, applies to the patient who acutely develops signs, symptoms, and a cerebrospinal fluid (CSF) profile suggesting meningeal inflammation, but evidence of typical bacterial, parasitic, fungal pathogens, or parameningeal infection cannot be found. A brief clinical illness with no evidence of CNS parenchymal dysfunction and good prognosis is implied.

Viruses account for the majority, at least 70%, of cases of aseptic meningitis. Although most patients with viral meningitis present with fever, malaise, headache, nausea, vomiting, nuchal rigidity, and photophobia, age, immune status, and viral etiology may influence the clinical features. Children under 2 years of age show fever, irritability, or seizures secondary to fever or the infection itself, but may never develop signs of meningeal irritation. In Europe and the United States, nonpolio enteroviruses (coxsackie and enteric cytopathogenic human orphan virus [echovirus]), are the most common causal agents, either as sporadic cases or in summertime outbreaks, followed by mumps, arboviruses, herpesviruses, lymphocytic choriomeningitis virus (LCMV), and human immunodeficiency virus (HIV) at the time of seroconversion.

Diagnosis is based on CSF samples, patient history, epidemiological trends, and supportive laboratory tests. Lumbar CSF shows a mild to moderate pleocytosis with 10–500 white blood cells (WBC)/μl, predominantly lymphocytes, mildly elevated protein (<100 mg/dl), glucose usually greater than 40% of a simultaneous serum sample, and slightly elevated opening pressure. Polymorphonuclear pleocytosis may be seen in up to 40% of patients with viral meningitis initially, changing to a lymphocytic CSF profile within approximately 12 hours. Polymorphonuclear cells may persist in meningitis due to eastern equine encephalitis virus (EEEV), La Crosse virus, enterovirus, or rarely, with adult human cytomegalovirus (CMV) when there is concurrent HIV infection. CSF cell counts in excess of 500 WBC/μl may be seen with mumps, LCMV, herpes simplex virus (HSV), Japanese encephalitis, EEEV, and California serogroup of viruses. CSF glucose may be depressed in patients with mumps, HSV-2, varicella zoster virus (VZV), and LCMV; but CSF glucose levels below 25 mg/dl should prompt a search for bacteria, fungi, sarcoid, or carcinomatous meningitis. Gram's stain and bacterial and fungal antigen test results are negative; computed tomography or magnetic resonance imaging (MRI) scans are normal.

Viral meningitis should be distinguished from aseptic meningitis caused by spirochetes, *Chlamydia*, *Rickettsia*, mycoplasma, *Brucella*, *Ehrlichiae*, partially treated bacterial meningitis, parameningeal infection, tuberculosis, fungal meningitis, endocarditis, postviral or vaccination meningeal reaction, drugs, leaking epidermoid cyst, collagen vascular diseases including Kawasaki's syndrome, and subarachnoid hemorrhage, based on CSF, serum, and neuroimaging studies. For most patients, sending CSF for routine studies, bacterial culture, and Gram's stain; VDRL; cryptococcal antigen; acid-fast bacilli; fungal and viral cultures; plus drawing and freezing acute phase serum for comparison with convalescent sera is reasonable. Polymerase chain reaction (PCR)-based tests for amplifying and detecting viral nucleic acid in CSF are available for HSV, VZV, human CMV, EBV, HIV, some enteroviruses, and measles (Tyler 1994). Definitive diagnosis of other agents depends on CSF viral culture, elevated serum or CSF virus-specific IgM antibodies, or an increase (usually a fourfold increase) in virus-specific IgG antibodies in paired serum samples obtained early in illness and approximately 10–14 days later. In certain cases with initial polymorphonuclear pleocytosis, the physician may elect empiric antibiotic coverage, pending culture results. It has not been established whether antiviral treatment alters the course of mild meningitis caused by HSV-2 in the normal host, but primary genital herpes is treated with acyclovir. Persistence of headache, meningeal signs, and CSF lymphocytic pleocytosis beyond 2–4 weeks, or recurrence of meningitis, prompts evaluation for other infectious, neoplastic, or vasculitic etiologies. Examples of viral meningitides that become chronic are the herpesviruses, LCMV, and enteroviruses in hypoglobuline-

mic patients. Persistent headache also may point to ventriculitis or ependymitis with secondary hydrocephalus.

Encephalitis

Viral encephalitis, the manifestation of brain parenchymal viral infection, is caused by approximately 100 DNA and RNA viruses. The worldwide burden of encephalitic disease is not precisely known. There are over 50,000 deaths from rabies each year worldwide, and at least 35,000 cases and 10,000 deaths from Japanese encephalitis (JE) each year in Asia. Passive reporting retrieves less than 2,000 of the estimated 20,000 cases of encephalitis in the United States each year.

Neurotropic viruses reach the CNS by hematogenous or by neuronal spread in the case of herpes, rabies, and occasionally, polio virus. Viral encephalitis is characterized by acute fever, headache, altered mentation, and evidence of parenchymal brain involvement: seizures, focal cerebral symptoms or signs, stupor or coma, and signs of increased intracranial pressure. A prodromal phase of systemic symptoms may or may not precede the onset of neurological signs. The prodrome may include parotitis (mumps), rash (measles, rubella, parvovirus), or myalgias (arboviruses); no prodrome is seen with HSV encephalitis. Neurological signs reflect CNS cellular dysfunction following direct viral invasion and associated inflammatory changes. Encephalitis, accompanied by signs of meningeal or spinal cord infection, is designated meningoencephalitis or encephalomyelitis, respectively.

In the United States, the most common pathogens are HSV-1, arboviruses, enteroviruses, measles, and mumps. Diagnosis requires a detailed history with attention to recent travel, insect or animal bites, immunization, or exposures. Arbovirus infections occur more frequently in the summer in the northern hemisphere, mumps in winter, and HSV encephalitis occurs year-round. HSV-1 is the most common etiological agent of focal viral encephalitis in the United States and JE virus the most common cause in Asia. Other viruses causing focal encephalitis are VZV, HHV-6, the enteroviruses, Powassan's virus, La Crosse virus, the equine encephalitis viruses, and measles.

Neuroimaging studies, particularly MRI, may show temporal or orbitofrontal cortex enhancement or edema in HSV encephalitis. In most other acute viral encephalitides, neuroimaging findings are nonspecific. Brain MRI or computed tomographic scans serve to exclude brain abscess, subdural empyema, cranial extradural abscess, or septic venous thrombosis and establish the safety of proceeding with the lumbar puncture.

The CSF is under normal or elevated pressure, with elevated protein (usually <200 mg/dl), normal glucose, and up to several hundred white cells, usually lymphocytic or mononuclear. Xanthochromia and red cells may occur in HSV encephalitis. Meningeal inflammation increases the passage of serum proteins and immunoglobulins into the subarachnoid space, increasing antibody concentration above the usual CSF to serum IgG ratio of 1 to 200 in the absence of infection. Oligoclonal bands, evidence of intrathecal IgG antibody synthesis, can be found during acute viral encephalitides caused by mumps or occasionally HSV and VZV. More often, oligoclonal bands develop in response to protracted CNS antigenic stimulation and indicate chronic infections. Oligoclonal bands reactive with specific viral antigens are detected in the CSF of patients with SSPE, progressive rubella panencephalitis, or human T-cell leukemia virus (HTLV-I)-associated tropical spastic paraparesis.

Electroencephalography (EEG) in acute viral encephalitis is usually abnormal with diffuse slowing, but may show patterns suggesting specific diagnoses. Repetitive sharp wave complexes over the temporal lobes or periodic lateralized epileptiform discharges are recorded with HSV-1 encephalitis and in rare cases of infectious mononucleosis encephalitis. Periodic slow-wave complexes occur in SSPE, and triphasic waves at higher periodic frequency in Creutzfeldt-Jakob disease. The EEG of acute measles encephalitis may be abnormal while the patient is cognitively fine, in contrast to mumps encephalitis, in which patients with profoundly depressed consciousness may have relatively normal EEGs.

The differential diagnosis of the acutely ill, febrile patient with signs of parenchymal brain involvement includes brain abscess; subdural empyema; cranial epidural abscess; atypical bacterial, fungal, and parasitic infections; parainfectious or postinfectious encephalomyelitis; Reye's syndrome; other toxic metabolic encephalopathies; endocarditis; septicemia; and collagen vascular disorders. Parainfectious or postinfectious encephalomyelitis appears as multifocal white matter lesions with increased signal intensity on T2-weighted images on MRI scans and usually follows the acute viral illness by 1–3 weeks. The clinical signs and symptoms of postviral encephalomyelitis—sudden fever, seizures, loss of consciousness, or focal deficits—can be identical to acute viral encephalitis, but onset of the postinfectious disease is often more abrupt.

Cultures and serology are important diagnostic tools for identifying specific viral agents and excluding other nonviral pathogens. Diagnosis may be confirmed by virus isolation from CSF or brain in HSV-1; from brain or oropharynx in rabies; from stool in polio or other enteroviruses; from vesicles in VZV; from blood early in arboviral infections; from blood in arenavirus infections (LCMV and Lassa) and mumps; from sputum or oropharynx in the viral exanthems, influenza, adenovirus, Venezuelan equine encephalitis, and some enterovirus infections; and from urine in human CMV and mumps. Specimens for virus isolation should be kept chilled or frozen. Herpes viral (human CMV, HSV, VZV, EBV), HIV, enteroviral, JC virus, and measles viral nucleic acid can be detected by PCR from CSF specimens (Tyler 1994; Cinque et al. 1997).

Because intravenous acyclovir is well tolerated and improves outcome in HSV encephalitis, initiation of treatment of all patients with sporadic, primary viral encephalitis with intravenous acyclovir, pending diagnosis or exclusion of HSV by PCR, culture, or serology, has become the standard of care in many areas. Presently, HSV accounts for approximately 10% of viral encephalitis cases in the United States.

Prognosis is improved by early treatment and expectant care. Raised intracranial pressure should be considered in patients with deepening coma, whereas seizures may be anticipated and treated if they develop. Hyponatremia secondary to inappropriate antidiuretic hormone secretion is managed with water restriction. Hyperthermia associated with rabies or the arboviruses tropic for central deep gray structures (JE, EEEV, the California serogroup, or Rocio) is treated with external cooling techniques, and not aspirin (because of the risk of Reye's syndrome). Little evidence supports using corticosteroids as adjunctive treatment in acute encephalitis. Corticosteroids do not improve outcome and may prolong the presence of the virus in the CNS. Agent-specific treatments and prophylaxis are summarized in Tables 59B.1 and 59B.2 and discussed in later sections.

Myelitis

Myelitis, caused by viral infection of the spinal cord, presents as monoplegia, paraplegia, or quadriplegia; sensory loss; or sphincter paralysis. Viral myelitis follows poliovirus or other enterovirus infection of anterior horn cells; VZV infection of dorsal root ganglia and adjacent cord; or cord parenchymal infection by rabies, HSV, or CMV in patients with acquired immunodeficiency syndrome (AIDS), HTLV-I and -II, EBV, simian B virus, JE, or the tick-borne encephalitis (TBE) virus subtypes. MRI may reveal cord swelling and intramedullary enhancement. The diagnosis of direct viral myelitis is based on (1) exclusion of compressive lesions by a spine neuroimaging study, (2) exclusion of treponemal, tubercular, schistosomal, and other infectious, parainfectious, demyelinating, or vasculitic syndromes by CSF, serological, and autoimmune studies, and MRI scanning, and (3) confirmation of viral etiology by virus isolation, serology, or detection of PCR-amplified viral nucleic acid in the CSF. A history of preceding illness, particularly influenza or measles, or recent vaccination, suggest a paraviral or postviral etiology.

Radiculoneuritis

Radiculitis or neuritis, root or nerve inflammation, are rare complications of systemic infection by many common viruses or follow direct viral invasion by specific agents. Acute radiculitis is the typical presentation of VZV infection, myeloradiculitis follows the initial febrile phase of the central European subtype of TBE, and lumbosacral radiculitis is seen with human CMV infection in patients with

Table 59B.1: Treatment and prophylaxis of viral infections

Antivirals	Dose	Indications	Toxicity or cautions
Nucleoside analogues			
Acyclovir	10 mg/kg (IV) q8h × 10–14 days	HSV-1, HSV-2, or primary immunocompromised VZV	Renal impairment
	15 mg/kg (IV) q8h × 10–14 days	B virus	
Acyclovir	800 mg (PO) 5× daily × 7 days	Dermatomal zoster or primary immunocompromised VZV	Low solubility
Famciclovir	500 mg (PO) 3× daily × 7 days	Dermatomal zoster or primary immunocompromised VZV	Headache, nausea
Valacyclovir	2 g (PO) 4× daily × 7 days	Dermatomal zoster or primary immunocompromised VZV	Thrombotic thrombocytic purpura/hemolytic uremic syndrome in human immunodeficiency virus patients
Ganciclovir	5 mg/kg (IV) q12h × 14 days (initially)	HCMV, B virus	Bone marrow suppression
Ribavirin	2 g (IV) ×1, then 1 g (IV) q6h × 4 days, then 0.5 g (IV) q8h × 6 days	Lassa fever	Anemia
Cytarabine	2 mg/kg (IV) × 5 days q4wk	PML	Bone marrow suppression
Trifluridine	1% ophthalmic solution	Herpetic keratoconjunctivitis	
Pyrophosphate analogue			
Foscarnet	60 mg/kg (IV) q8h × 14 days	Acyclovir-resistant VZV or HSV HCMV	Hypocalcemia, renal impairment
Other			
Amantadine	100 mg (PO) twice daily × 2–4 wks	Influenza A	CNS + anticholinergiclike side effects
Cytokines			
Interferon-α	3 million U/day (SC)	PML, acyclovir-resistant VZV, or hepatitis C	Flulike side effects
	10^5–10^6 U/m^2 body surface (IT)	SSPE	
Supplements			
Vitamin A	400,000 IU (IM)	Acute measles in vitamin A deficiency	

CNS = central nervous system; HCMV = human cytomegalovirus; HSV = herpes simplex virus; PML = progressive multifocal leukoencephalopathy; SSPE = subacute sclerosing panencephalitis; VZV = varicella zoster virus.

AIDS or HSV-2. Lower motor neuropathies accompany polio, other enteroviral infections, and HTLV-I and -II infections. Mixed sensorimotor neuropathies are reported with HTLV-I, human CMV, and HIV-1; sensory, motor, and autonomic neuropathies are reported with EBV.

The sequelae of two historic hemorrhagic fever outbreaks also included neuropathic syndromes. Marburg fever caused lower extremity pain and paresthesias in recovered patients, and dengue fever caused epidemic mononeuritis multiplex during World War II in the Pacific Theater. Today, mixed cryoglobulinemia neuropathies or mononeuritis multiplex are associated with hepatitis C infection.

Nerve conduction velocity and electromyographic testing, followed by CSF examination and viral culture, PCR-based tests, or serology may be indicated to establish a diagnosis and exclude other infectious causes (diphtheria, leprosy, syphilis, *Borrelia*, leishmaniasis), and the Guillain-Barré syndrome. Nerve biopsy can demonstrate direct infection of nerve by EBV or human CMV, as well as other infectious agents: *Mycobacterium leprae*, African or American trypanosomes, and filarial worms (*Dracunculus medinensis*).

Myositis

Myalgia is a prominent prodrome or early symptom in many acute viral diseases. Serum creatine kinase elevations have been recorded during influenza A2 epidemics, but bear no close relation to the degree of myalgia. Chest pain, trunk and abdominal muscle pain, and intercostal muscle swelling are characteristic of pleurodynia (known also as *epidemic myalgia*, *Bornholm's disease*, and *devil's grip*), caused by coxsackie A and B and viruses and echovirus. Rhabdomyolysis and myoglobinuria can accompany influenza A and B, coxsackie, echovirus, HSV, EBV, parainfluenza, and adenovirus infections. Inflammatory myopathies are seen in HIV and HTLV-I. Culture, biopsy, or serological evaluation may be indicated to exclude the treatable bacterial and parasitic infections of muscle: leptospirosis; trichinosis; toxoplasmosis; cysticercosis; sar-

Table 59B.2:   Immunotherapy of viral infections*

Immunotherapy	Dose or route	Indications
Immunoglobulins (IG)		
VZIG (varicella zoster)	One vial (125 U) per 10 kg of body weight (IM)	For hypoglobulinemic patients after exposure
RIG (rabies)	Human RIG, 20 IU/kg, or equine RIG, 40 IU/kg (divided between wound and IM injection)	After exposure
Central European encephalitis hyperimmunoglobulin	IM	Following multiple tick bites in endemic area
Human cytomegalovirus hyperimmunoglobulin	IV	Prophylaxis after bone marrow transplantation
Polyvalent IG or hyperimmunoglobulin	IV	Treatment of chronic enterovirus meningo-encephalitis in hypoglobulinemic patients
Polyvalent IG		Treatment of human T-cell leukemia virus I myelopathy
Measles hyperimmunoglobulin	IV	Treatment of measles inclusion body encephalitis in immunocompromised patients
Cytotoxic T cells		
Epstein-Barr virus (EBV)-specific cytotoxic T lymphocytes		Prophylaxis of EBV lymphoproliferative disease in bone marrow transplant recipients

*Live vaccines include yellow fever, measles, mumps, rubella, smallpox, polio, and varicella zoster virus. Killed vaccines include polio, rabies, influenza, arboviruses (Japanese encephalitis, tick-borne encephalitis, Kyasanur Forest, Rift Valley, eastern equine encephalitis, western equine encephalitis, and Venezuelan equine encephalitis). Soluble protein includes hepatitis B.

cocystosis; trypanosomiasis; filariasis; and staphylococcal, streptococcal, or gram-negative bacterial pyomyositis.

Congenital Infections

Several viral, bacterial, and protozoan pathogens, linked conceptually by the TORCH acronym (*Toxoplasma gondii*, other micro-organisms, rubella, CMV, HSV), cross the placenta and injure the developing fetus. Of the viral pathogens, members of the herpesvirus family (HSV, human CMV, VZV) are responsible for the largest number of congenital infections. Other agents include rubella, HIV, nonpolio enteroviruses, LCMV, western equine and Venezuelan equine encephalitis virus, mumps, human parvovirus B19, Lassa, and Ebola viruses (Wright et al. 1997).

The developing nervous system, retina, cochlea, and reticuloendothelial system are the particular targets of intrauterine infection. Signs of meningoencephalitis, such as lethargy or irritability, poor feeding, seizures, opisthotonic posturing, hypotonia, or bulging fontanelle, may be seen in isolation, or as one element of a multifocal, disseminated infection that may include microcephaly, chorioretinitis, hearing loss, hepatosplenomegaly, jaundice, thrombocytopenia, and rash. Bacterial meningitis and neonatal sepsis should be excluded by CSF examination and serum and CSF cultures.

A CSF lymphocytic pleocytosis and elevated protein is consistent with congenital CNS viral infection. Neuroimaging studies may reveal ventriculitis, hydrocephalus, intracranial calcifications, delayed myelination, multicystic encephalomalacia, or lissencephaly. Prenatal fetal ultrasound can detect intracra-

nial calcifications or hydrocephalus. Microbiological evaluation includes viral cultures, serological studies for suspect viruses, and studies for *Treponema pallidum* and *Toxoplasma gondii*. Diagnosis can be confirmed by virus isolation from urine or saliva in human CMV; from oropharynx, CSF, conjunctiva, or skin lesions in HSV; from urine, CSF, nasopharynx, or blood in rubella; or by PCR evaluation of CSF samples. Detection of virus-specific IgM antibodies in neonatal serum, CSF, or both, or, in some cases, maternal serum, supports a specific diagnosis. In cases in which isolated progressive ventriculomegaly is recognized in utero, early delivery as soon as fetal lung maturity allows might achieve a better long-term neurological prognosis (Kirkinen et al. 1996). Periodic sight, hearing, and developmental evaluations are recommended because of high rates of neurodevelopmental, visual, and auditory sequelae. Progressive hearing loss is a particular feature of congenital human CMV and rubella infections.

VIRUSES

Herpesviruses

Herpesviruses are highly disseminated in nature among most mammalian, bird, reptile, and amphibian species. These viruses cause acute infections, but also share the biological capacity of latency, the ability to remain quiescent for periods of time in the host and to be reactivated at or near the site of original infection. Neurological diseases in humans are caused by the HHV HSV type 1 and type 2, VZV, CMV, EBV, and HHV-6; and the simian herpes ("monkey") B-virus.

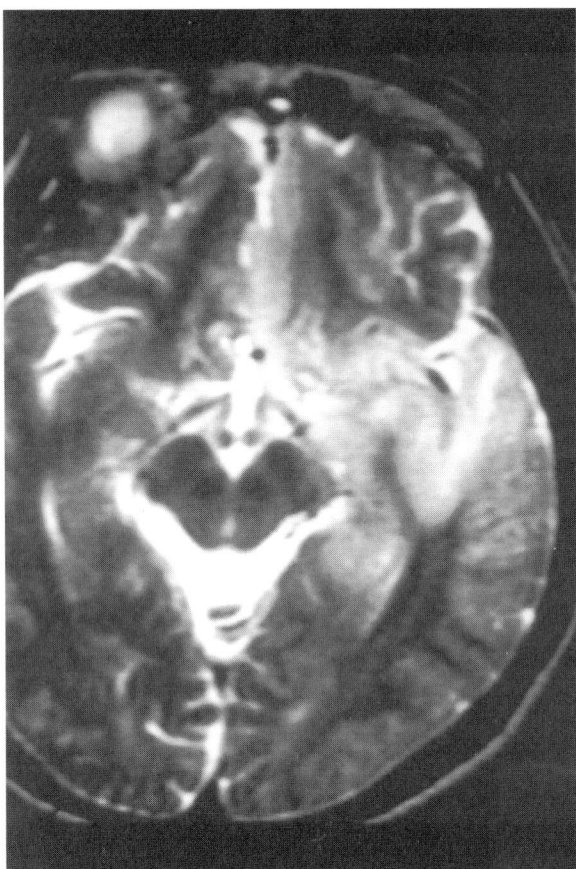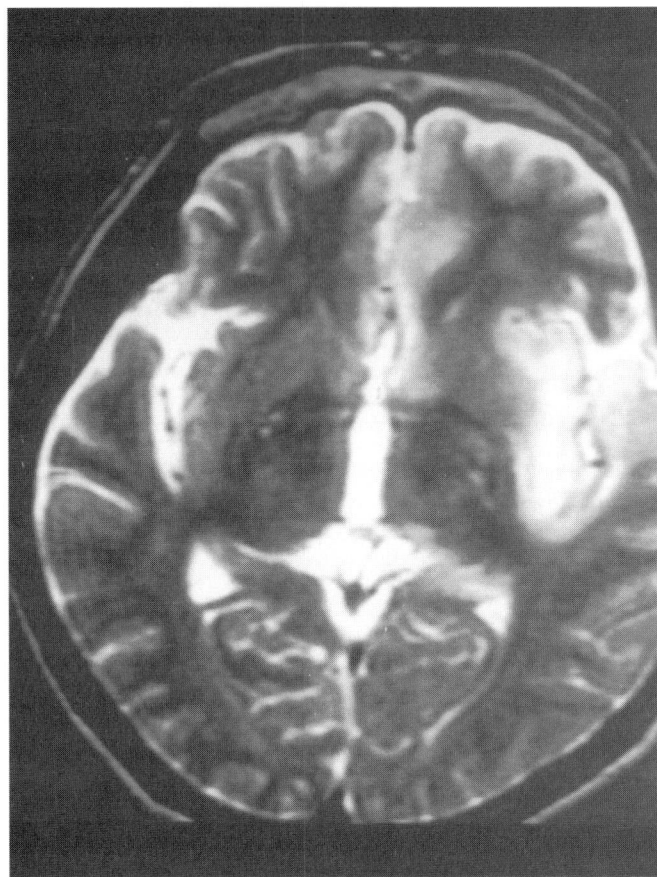

FIGURE 59B.1   Herpes simplex encephalitis. Axial T2-weighted magnetic resonance image showing increased signal in left medial temporal lobe, inferior frontal lobe, and insula cortex. (Courtesy of J. Healy.)

Herpes Simplex Encephalitis Virus Type 1

HSV-1 encephalitis is the most common cause of sporadic, fatal encephalitis in the United States, accounting for approximately 10% of encephalitis cases. Early recognition is important because of the efficacy of the antiviral drug acyclovir in reducing morbidity and mortality. Mortality in untreated cases is 70%. HSV-1 strains cause nearly all cases of herpes simplex encephalitis in adults and cause oral herpes. Type 2 strains cause genital disease, aseptic meningitis, and congenitally acquired encephalitis in the neonate. Both types 1 and 2 have been associated with myelitis. HSV-1 and -2 related diseases in immunosuppressed hosts are discussed in Chapter 59E.

HSV-1 is acquired by respiratory or salivary contact. Up to 33% of HSV-1 encephalitis cases may occur as part of the primary infection, with spread of virus across the primary olfactory areas to orbitofrontal cortex and temporal lobes. In the majority of cases, however, encephalitis is probably a consequence of reactivation and centripetal spread of virus latent in the trigeminal ganglia since infection earlier in life. It is estimated that 50% of the population has antibodies to HSV-1 by age 15, and 90% by adulthood.

Fever and headache are consistent features. The onset may be abrupt, with focal or generalized seizures, or more protracted, with behavioral changes, an amnestic syndrome, aphasia, or other focal signs. There is no pathognomonic set of clinical findings for HSV encephalitis. Focal signs, hemiparesis, hemisensory loss, ataxia, or focal seizures are seen in approximately one-half of patients when first examined.

The diagnosis is suspected in febrile patients with a deteriorating level of consciousness. The CSF may be under increased pressure, with lymphocytic pleocytosis, and cell counts of 10–1,000 WBC/μl. Red blood cells also may be present. CSF protein is elevated, and glucose is normal or low. Virus is rarely recovered from the CSF but HSV DNA can be detected in the CSF by PCR techniques. CSF PCR testing has an estimated sensitivity of greater than 95% and a specificity of nearly 100% (Whitley and Lakeman 1995). EEG and MRI studies may both be abnormal early in the disease. The EEG shows diffuse slowing, focal temporal region changes, or periodic lateralized epileptiform discharge. MRI scans show focal abnormalities as areas of high signal intensity on T2-weighted images in frontotemporal regions (Figure 59B.1).

Conditions that mimic the clinical presentation of HSV encephalitis include other viral and postviral encephalitides; other CNS infections with acute presentations and focal features, such as cryptococcal abscesses, adult toxoplasmosis, bacterial endocarditis, and *Naegleria*; sagittal sinus or other cerebral vein thromboses; and mitochondrial encephalopathy, lactic acidosis, and strokelike episodes (MELAS).

Because of its safety and favorable effect on outcome in HSV encephalitis, empiric therapy with acyclovir is used without brain biopsy in most cases. Treatment is with intravenous acyclovir (10 mg/kg every 8 hours) for 10–14 days. Renal insufficiency is the major serious, although infrequent and reversible, side effect. Brain biopsy is reserved for atypical cases or those who respond poorly to treatment. Accumulations of viral particles forming acidophilic intranuclear inclusion bodies in neurons (Cowdry type A inclusions) are seen on biopsy (Plate 59B.I). Vidarabine, as a slow intravenous infusion of 15 mg/kg per day for 14 days, is an alternative for patients with allergies to acyclovir or acyclovir-resistant strains. Vidarabine's low solubility requires high fluid volumes for administration and may cause difficulties in patients with cerebral edema. PCR evaluations of CSF may be used to follow therapeutic response.

Treatment with acyclovir reduces mortality from 70% to 20%. Over one-third of patients recover with mild or no neurological impairment. Relapses following treatment with acyclovir are reported, and choreoathetosis may be the first sign of relapse in children. Biopsy is necessary to document continued infection, thus distinguishing relapse caused by active viral replication from immune-mediated disease. Relapse caused by direct viral effect is treated with an increased dose of acyclovir, 15 mg/kg every 8 hours for 21 days, and intravenous vidarabine.

Neonatal Herpes Simplex Virus Type 2

Of all infants with neonatal HSV-2 infections, approximately 50% have CNS disease, which presents as either disseminated disease with signs of brain involvement at age 1 week or as encephalitis at 2 weeks of age. The diagnosis is suspected when skin vesicles are present. CSF PCR diagnostic tests, which use primer sequences common to both HSV-1 and -2, can specify the diagnosis in the absence of a rash. Treatment is with intravenous acyclovir, 10 mg/kg every 8 hours for 10–14 days. Vidarabine is considered equally effective (Whitley and Lakeman 1995).

Varicella Zoster Virus

Chickenpox is caused by primary infection with VZV. A self-limited cerebellar ataxia is often seen in otherwise healthy children. Primary VZV may produce encephalitis in immunocompromised patients and, rarely, a progressive, fatal encephalitis in healthy children. Postinfectious encephalomyelitis follows an estimated 1 in 2,500 cases.

Reye's syndrome (2.5 per 10,000 cases) and congenital varicella are other known complications.

Treatment of immunocompromised children with intravenous acyclovir (500 mg/m² per dose every 8 hours for 7 days) should begin within the first 24–72 hours after onset of the rash. Oral acyclovir treats varicella in healthy children and adults. VZV immunoglobulin is used for prophylaxis of immunocompromised patients and pregnant women. VZV immunoglobulin, one vial (125 units) per 10 kg of body weight intramuscularly, should be given within 96 hours, and preferably, within 48 hours of exposure (Arvin 1996).

Following primary infection, the virus becomes latent in cells of the dorsal root ganglia. Reactivation of endogenous latent virus produces herpes zoster, or shingles. The virus can reactivate after injury or trauma to the spine or roots or in response to waning cell-mediated immunity to VZV, caused by age or immunosuppression related to HIV infection, cancer, cytotoxic drugs, or systemic illness.

Herpes zoster typically begins with pain and paresthesias in one or two adjacent spinal or cranial dermatomes. Pain is followed in 3–4 days by a pruritic vesicular eruption in the area supplied by the affected root. The eruption can last 10 days to 2 weeks. Occasionally, a few lesions outside the primary dermatome appear in healthy hosts. Herpes zoster most often involves the thoracic dermatomes, usually T5-T12. Fourteen percent to 20% of patients have disease in the distribution of a cranial nerve, and 16% in lumbosacral dermatomes, usually L1 or L2. Involvement of the first division of the trigeminal ganglion produces ophthalmic zoster and may be associated with conjunctivitis, keratitis, anterior uveitis, or iridocyclitis. Vision loss following herpes zoster ophthalmicus is rare, however, and more commonly caused by retrobulbar neuritis. Involvement of the geniculate ganglion produces otic zoster, or the Ramsay Hunt syndrome: facial paresis plus tympanic membrane and external auditory canal rash. Older age and cranial nerve involvement are risk factors for zoster encephalitis, so all cases of ophthalmic zoster should be treated with antivirals. Herpes zoster involving lumbosacral ganglia may be accompanied by bladder dysfunction or ileus. The clinical variant, zoster *sine herpete*, applies to syndromes of prolonged radicular pain without zoster rash but with detectable VZV DNA in the CSF.

Herpes zoster is frequently the first clinical presentation of underlying HIV infection; it may be protracted and multidermal. In Africa, herpes zoster has a positive predictive value for HIV infection of 95%.

Herpes zoster is considered in the differential diagnosis of patients with acute radicular pain. A lymphocytic pleocytosis, with cell counts to several hundred per microliter, may antedate the rash. Approximately 40% of healthy individuals with herpes zoster have elevated CSF cell and protein counts, and VZV can be isolated from the CSF of these patients. VZV DNA can be detected in the CSF by PCR techniques, and VZV may be cultured from vesicles or detected by microscopic examination of vesicular scrapings.

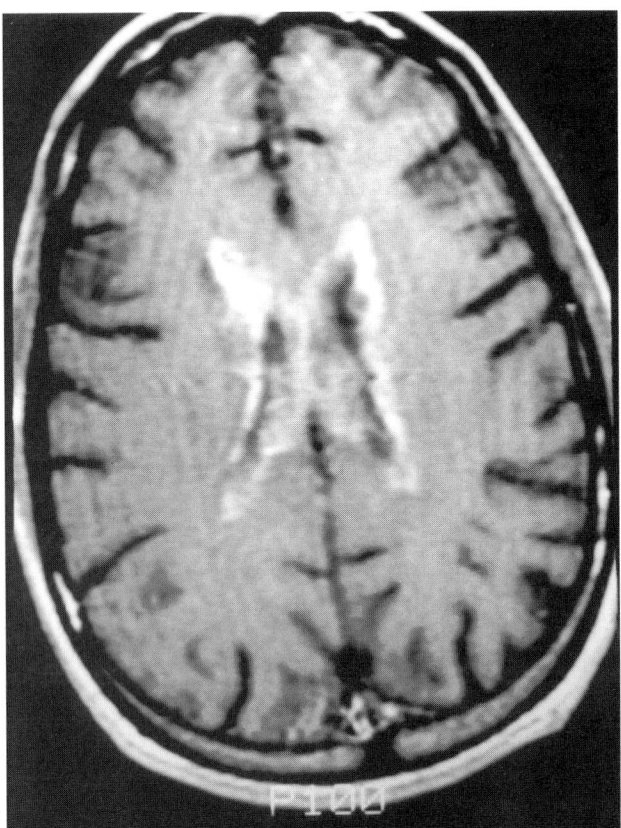

FIGURE 59B.2   Human cytomegalovirus ventriculitis. Axial gadolinium-enhanced T1 magnetic resonance image showing contrast enhancement of ependyma of lateral ventricles. (Courtesy of J. Healy.)

Complications include postherpetic neuralgia, segmental motor atrophy in the affected dermatome, meningitis, myelitis, large vessel vasculitis (usually involving the carotid or its branches on the side of zoster ophthalmicus), and multifocal leukoencephalitis or encephalitis with generalized cerebral vasculopathy. VZV encephalitis with vasculopathy has been reported in AIDS and cancer patients and individuals treated with cyclophosphamide or corticosteroids. The syndrome may occur without any signs of cutaneous infection or may progress after cutaneous lesions have healed. Mixed ischemic and hemorrhagic infarcts in subcortical gray and white matter, plus ischemic, demyelinative, or both kinds of lesions in deep white matter are noted radiologically and pathologically (Amlie-Lefond et al. 1995).

Risk factors for postherpetic neuralgia are age over 50 years and prodromal sensory symptoms. Treatments are directed toward lessening pain, reducing virus shedding, and shortening healing time. Acyclovir (800 mg orally five times daily for 7 days), famciclovir (500 mg orally three times daily for 7 days), or valacyclovir, a pro-acyclovir with improved oral absorption (2 g orally four times daily for 7 days) accelerate cutaneous healing and decrease acute zoster pain if begun within 72 hours of onset of rash. Famciclovir may

prove to be the best drug because of its great bioavailability after oral doses and convenient administration schedule (Stein 1997). Whether these agents significantly decrease the incidence, duration, or severity of postherpetic neuralgia is less certain. In patients without contraindications, a short course of corticosteroids, such as 40 mg prednisolone per day, tapered over 3 weeks, also may be prescribed. Compared with acyclovir therapy alone, combined therapy has been shown to improve comfort levels (pain reduction during the acute phase) following herpes zoster, but not prevent the development of postherpetic neuralgia (Wood et al. 1994). Antiviral treatment of zoster myelitis and encephalitis is as described for herpes simplex encephalitis. Foscarnet and interferon-α, drugs unrelated to the nucleoside analogues, are used for acyclovir-resistant zoster infections (Arvin 1996).

Corticosteroids are often used for sight-threatening complications (optic neuritis, orbital apex syndrome) and postviral cerebral (large vessel) vasculitic complications. Corticosteroids may be used for exaggerated inflammatory response to simultaneous acute VZV, such as an aggressive myelitis. Postviral inflammatory conditions are discussed in other chapters. Brief corticosteroid use, to treat the small and large vessel vasculopathy that accompanies persistent VZV encephalitis in immunocompromised patients, is controversial but has a few advocates. A live attenuated varicella vaccine boosts VZV immune responses in adults, raising hope that, in the future, it may be possible to prevent dermatomal zoster.

Human Cytomegalovirus

Human CMV infection is one of the more common congenital viral infections, with an incidence of up to 2% per live birth in the United States. Persistent, high levels of viral replication in the eye and brain of the maturing fetus produce retinitis, encephalitis, and ependymitis, a pattern similar to that seen with human CMV infection of patients with AIDS (Figure 59B.2). Mild or subclinical congenital infections are recognized later in childhood because of deafness or developmental delay. Congenital human CMV infection is the most common, nonheritable cause of hearing loss in the United States. Infection by passage through the birth canal or following breast-feeding accounts for additional infantile cases. Sexual transmission accounts for virus spread in the adult population. In immunocompetent adults, CMV may cause inapparent infection, a mononucleosis syndrome, aseptic meningitis, encephalitis, or the Guillain-Barré syndrome.

Diagnosis of congenital CMV infection depends on the detection of virus by culture or by PCR of viral nucleic acid in urine, saliva, or CSF during the first 2 weeks of life. CMV inclusion-bearing cells are found in affected organs (Plate 59B.II) and in stained preparations of urinary sediment and saliva. Acute CMV infection in immunocompetent adults usually relies on serology, because patients may excrete virus in urine for variable periods. Serological and

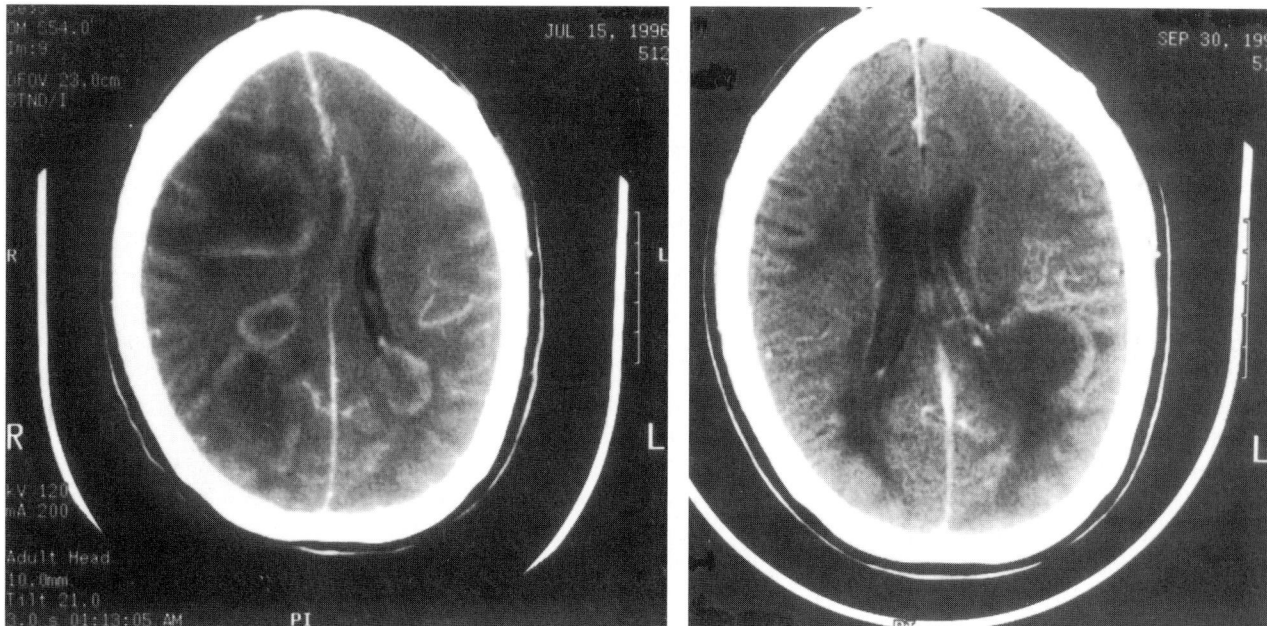

FIGURE 59B.3 Concurrent human herpesvirus 6 and human immunodeficiency virus disease. Contrast computed tomographic scans showing multiple, ring-enhancing frontal, parietal, and occipital lesions. The second image shows parietal recurrence 3 months later. Pathology demonstrated perivascular lymphocytic infiltrates, demyelination, and axonal sparing. (Courtesy of S. Busono.)

virus detection methods are currently being extended to focus on quantitation of viral burden for patients with persistent infections. PCR evaluations of CSF offer a means of evaluating therapeutic response.

Hearing can improve in patients with symptomatic congenital infections treated with intravenous ganciclovir, 4–6 mg/kg every 12 hours for 6 weeks. Treatment of CMV retinitis, encephalitis, or lumbosacral radiculitis in immunocompromised patients begins with intravenous ganciclovir, 5 mg/kg every 12 hours for 2 weeks for induction, followed by 5 mg/kg per day, 5 days per week for maintenance. An extended discussion of CMV treatment in HIV-infected patients is presented in Chapter 59E. Because of the frequency of subclinical infection in the adult population, bone marrow transplant recipients should receive human CMV hyperimmune globulin as prophylaxis.

Epstein-Barr Virus

Primary infection occurs as infectious mononucleosis. Nervous system disease occurs in less than 1% of EBV infectious mononucleosis cases as aseptic meningitis, encephalitis, cerebellitis, transverse myelitis, optic neuritis, cranial neuropathies, the Guillain-Barré syndrome, small fiber sensory, or autonomic neuropathy syndromes. A diagnosis is made by serum heterophile antibodies, serum and CSF EBV-specific antibodies, or EBV DNA in CSF. Immunomodulation with intravenous immunoglobulin may improve small fiber sensory or autonomic neuropathies if treatment begins during acute disease (Bennett et al. 1996). One case of EBV

meningoencephalitis following bone marrow transplantation has been treated successfully with ganciclovir.

As a B-cell transforming virus, EBV is associated also with CNS lymphomas. Nucleic acid footprints of latent EBV infection are found in the jaw, orbit, and CNS malignancies of endemic Burkitt's lymphoma and the CNS lymphomas of AIDS and Burkitt's lymphoma cases. EBV DNA may be demonstrated in the CSF by PCR techniques before CNS lymphoma is clinically apparent. Vaccine and immune therapies in development for these conditions include the use of virus-specific cytotoxic T lymphocytes as prophylaxis for EBV lymphoproliferative disease in bone marrow transplant patients (Heslop and Rooney 1997).

Human Herpesvirus Type 6

HHV-6 is a prevalent, T-lymphotropic virus, causing a spectrum of diseases ranging from inapparent to disseminated, fatal infection. Exanthem subitum (or sixth disease) of infants or lymphadenopathy syndromes are the most common associated illnesses, but early life infection also can cause meningoencephalitis. HHV-6 is increasingly recognized as an opportunistic infection in immunocompromised patients (Figure 59B.3) or perhaps as the causative agent of T-cell immunodeficiency, as HHV-6 can replicate in various cells of the immune system: lymphocytes, macrophages, and natural killer cells. A possible role for HHV-6 in multiple sclerosis has been suggested by the presence of higher antibody levels in patients with multiple sclerosis, the presence of HHV-6 DNA in patient CSF, and the differential distribution of HHV-6 in brains of patients with multiple sclerosis compared with disease-free adult brains. The B variant of HHV-6, the variant most commonly isolated from immunocompromised patients, has a susceptibility to ganciclovir that is similar to the susceptibility of CMV in vitro.

Cercopithecine Herpes Virus 1 (B Virus)

B virus of Old World monkeys is known and respected by all veterinarians and primate handlers because it is highly pathogenic for humans and fatal in 70% of cases. Disease is transmitted by direct contact with the virus, usually by animal bite, or by virus-containing fomites. Fever, myalgia, herpetiform rash, meningismus, and early stage nystagmus or diplopia are followed by an ascending encephalomyelitis causing flaccid paralysis, urinary retention, and signs of CNS involvement, including seizures, progressive lethargy, and coma. Diagnosis is by wound or contact site culture and demonstration of increasing antibodies in paired acute and convalescent sera. Median nerve somatosensory evoked potential may identify early brainstem and cervical cord involvement and aid in differentiating B virus from HSV encephalitis.

Immediate wound care, by soaking or scrubbing the contact area with soap or detergent for 15 minutes, or rinsing of eyes or mucous membranes, is recommended for all exposures. Symptomatic patients are treated with intravenous acyclovir, 15 mg/kg every 8 hours for 10–14 days. The regimen may then be changed to oral acyclovir, 800 mg five times per day. Treatment often continues for months or years, with regular cultures of the conjunctiva, oropharynx, and genital area. Intravenous ganciclovir at doses of 5 mg/kg every 12 hours is an alternative for initial treatment (Holmes et al. 1995).

Rabies

Rabies, a significant global human encephalitic disease with nearly 100% mortality, is enzootic in all continents except Australia and Antarctica, and absent from certain island states or nations: Great Britain, Ireland, Iceland, Japan, New Zealand, Hawaii, the Bahamas, and Bermuda. Reservoirs of infection are nonimmunized dogs, wild carnivores (skunks, foxes, raccoons, wolves, jackals, wild dogs, merkats, the mongoose), and bats.

Human rabies cases are almost always attributable to a bite, but rare nonbite (aerosol) exposures have been documented. Head and face bites carry the highest risk of fatal disease. The incubation period is usually from 1–2 months, but may vary from 1 week to several years. A prodrome of headache, fever, paresthesias, and pain at the inoculation site is followed by an acute neurological phase, then coma. Cases in which hyperactivity dominates have been called *furious* rabies. Characteristic neuropathological intraneuronal inclusions (Negri's bodies) (Plate 59B.III) and inflammatory changes are maximal in the brainstem and limbic system. Up to 80% of patients exhibit hydrophobia or aerophobia: spasms of pharyngeal and nuchal muscles lasting from 1–5 minutes, triggered by swallow attempts or tactile, auditory, visual, and olfactory stimuli. The spasms are thought to be an exaggerated respiratory tract protective reflex. As the disease progresses, attacks increase in frequency and are accompanied by agitation, hallucinations, autonomic hyperactivity, and seizures. Body temperature may reach 105° to 107°F.

Paralytic, myelitic, or "dumb" rabies, accounting for 20% of patients, is characterized by paresthesias, weakness, and flaccid paralysis in the bitten extremity progressing to quadriplegia. Paralytic rabies is most often associated with bat rabies virus strains.

The diagnosis of rabies is suspected in any patient with a history of exposure and clinical picture of agitated or paralytic encephalitic illness. When no history can be obtained, rabies is included in the differential diagnosis of any encephalitis progressing rapidly to coma, particularly if the patient has been to an endemic area. Other differential diagnostic considerations include intoxications, postvaccination encephalitis, tetanus, which has a shorter (<2 week) incubation period and normal spinal fluid, or rabies phobia (a hysterical response to an animal bite).

Intracerebral inoculation of mice with patient saliva or examination of skin from the face or neck within the hairline for the presence of rabies antigen, are the most rapid methods of antemortem diagnosis. Neuralizing antibodies in serum and CSF are present in the nonimmunized patient. Active disease produces high titers (>1 to 5,000), which is helpful for diagnosing acute rabies in previously immunized individuals. High titers also distinguish acute rabies from postvaccination encephalomyelitis associated with vaccines derived from animal neural tissue. PCR protocols for detection of viral sequences in brain specimens have been established (Kamolvarin et al. 1993).

Transdermal bites or scratches and mucous membrane contact with saliva constitute exposure. In rabies, CSF and other body fluids are highly infectious, and appropriate precautions should be taken. Postexposure treatment and prophylaxis of rabies includes wound care and the immediate administration of multiple doses of rabies vaccine and of antirabies immunoglobulin to individuals who were never immunized. Wounds are washed with soap and water, followed by benzalkonium chloride and ethanol or iodine. Then, tissue-culture or purified duck-embryo vaccines, at least 2.5 IU per dose, are administered intramuscularly on days 0, 3, 7, 14, and 28 into the deltoid or anterolateral thigh muscles. Previously immunized individuals are given vaccine on days 0 and 3. Human diploid cell vaccines, in use in many areas of the world, are improvements over the biological products derived from animal (usually sheep) neural tissue, which caused the Guillain-Barré syndrome or acute disseminated encephalomyelitis approximately once per 2,000 vaccinations, and other less severe neurological complications as often as once in 120 vaccinations (Johnson 1997).

Human rabies immunoglobulin, 20 IU/kg, or equine rabies immunoglobulin, 40 IU/kg, is administered once at the beginning of prophylaxis to patients never previously vaccinated. At least one-half the dose is administered in the area of the wound, and the rest given intramuscularly in the gluteal region. A skin test must be performed before the use of the equine rabies immunoglobulin. Because human rabies immunoglobulin may partially suppress active production of antibody, no more than the recommended dose should be given.

A dog or cat immunized within the previous 3 years is considered an unlikely source of infection, but should be confined and observed for 10 days. If ill, the animal is killed, and the brain is examined at a regional health laboratory by immunohistochemistry for rabies virus antigen. Wild animals belonging to known infected species, based on area health department data, should be considered as rabid until laboratory test results are negative. Treatment can be stopped if the animal remains healthy for the 10-day observation period or if the killed animal is confirmed antigen-negative.

Pre-exposure prophylaxis is available to veterinarians, animal handlers, laboratory workers, or travelers to endemic areas. One-milliliter injections of human diploid cell rabies vaccine administered intramuscularly or 0.1 ml intradermally is given on days 0, 7, and 21 or 28 (Johnson 1997).

Poliovirus and Other Nonpolio Enteroviruses

The most common forms of infection by any of the enteroviruses are subclinical or mild febrile illness. Collectively, the enteroviruses are the leading causes of aseptic meningitis for which a pathogen can be identified. Severe clinical syndromes are associated with some of these agents.

Poliovirus

Poliovirus, one of the most virulent members of the enterovirus group, is the agent of acute anterior poliomyelitis (infantile paralysis). The virus is worldwide in distribution, more prevalent in temperate regions, and most common in late summer and early fall. Polio is transmitted by fecal-oral contact, and during epidemics, also by pharyngeal spread. Three antigenically distinct types of poliovirus have been defined. All can cause paralytic disease through destruction of motor neurons in the spinal cord and brainstem.

Clinically apparent infection with poliovirus results in aseptic meningitis (8% of cases) or paralytic illness (1% of all cases). A 7- to 14-day incubation period is followed by headache, signs of meningeal irritation, drowsiness, and seizures in infants. Asymmetric flaccid weakness of limbs, diaphragm, or cranial nerve–innervated muscles develops within days and progresses, on average, for 3–5 days. Cerebellitis, transverse myelitis, and facial paresis also have been reported.

Diagnosis is based on CSF pleocytosis and the clinical picture. Polymorphonuclear cells are predominant early, with a shift to lymphocytes after several days. CSF protein is slightly elevated; levels of 100–300 mg/dl may accompany cases of severe paralysis. Confirmation is by isolation of virus from CSF, stool, or throat washings, along with a fourfold increase in antibody titer. The differential diagnosis of nonparalytic polio is aseptic meningitis caused by other pathogens. The differential diagnosis of an acute, pure motor neuronopathy with cellular spinal fluid includes CMV and carcinomatous meningitis. Bulbospinal disease with inflammatory spinal fluid is seen in the Russian spring and summer encephalitis variant of TBE and rabies. The Guillain-Barré syndrome is distinguished by antecedent rather than concurrent febrile illness, CSF albuminocytological dissociation, absent reflexes, more common facial nerve involvement, and nerve conduction patterns and late responses consistent with proximal demyelination.

Treatment is supportive, with particular attention to ventilatory assistance. Mortality from paralytic poliomyelitis is less than 10%, but bulbar forms have poorer prognoses, in which mortality may approach 50%.

Primary immunization is with three doses of trivalent oral (live attenuated/Sabin) vaccine within the first year of life and a fourth dose before school entry. The advantages of oral polio vaccine are ease of administration and induction of intestinal immunity. The disadvantage is the risk of reversion to neurovirulence and production of paralytic disease in vaccinees and contacts. Vaccine-related cases of paralytic polio have included infants receiving their first oral polio vaccine dose, nonimmune adults in contact with recipients of oral polio vaccine, and immunocompromised individuals. Inactivated polio vaccine should be administered to persons with immunodeficiency diseases.

The Advisory Committee on Immunization Practices has recommended that inactivated polio vaccine may be substituted for live attenuated vaccine for the entire series or that a sequential series be used in which the first two immunizations are with inactivated vaccine and the second two with live attenuated vaccine.

The postpolio syndrome describes the approximately one-quarter of polio patients who develop progressive lower motor neuron weakness 30–40 years after acute polio. Atrophy, fasciculations, and electromyographic evidence of active denervation are found in previously involved motor groups.

Nonpolio Enteroviruses

Outbreaks of polio in communities who refuse vaccination for religious reasons are known. Where high herd immunity to poliovirus exists, other enteroviruses account for most cases of viral-induced paralytic disease. Coxsackie A and B viruses cause aseptic meningitis and, rarely, encephalitis, paralytic disease, or acute cerebellar ataxia. Coxsackie A9 was isolated from patients' CSF in the 1991–1993 Cuban epidemic of peripheral and optic neuropathy, in which it may have precipitated a nutritional neuropathy. Group B coxsackieviruses cause myocarditis, epidemic myalgia, newborn encephalitis from in utero–acquired infection, and congenital CNS defects. Echoviruses cause syndromes of aseptic meningitis, acute cerebellar ataxia, cranial polyneuritis, and chronic (persistent) meningoencephalitis plus dermatomyositis in children with agammaglobulinemia. The encephalitic syndrome is treated with immune globulin. Echovirus 9 may cause a petechial rash resembling meningococcemia. Meningitis caused by coxsackievirus produces CSF cell counts typically up to 250 WBC/μl with 10–50% polymorphonuclear cells. Echovirus infections are associated with CSF pleocytosis from several hundred to greater than 1,000 WBC/μl, 90% of which may be polymorphonucleocytes early in infection.

Enterovirus type 70 is the etiological agent of a syndrome of conjunctivitis and motor neuron disease. Epidemic acute hemorrhagic conjunctivitis first appeared in Ghana, West Africa, in 1969, and spread across Africa, Asia, and Europe in 1970 and 1971 to involve tens of millions of people. The eye disease was characterized by severe eye pain, photophobia, blurred vision, and varying degrees of subconjunctival hemorrhage. In a minority of patients, usually young men, a neurological (poliolike) phase developed 2 weeks after the conjunctivitis as acute asymmetric hypotonic or flaccid weakness of the lower extremities. Isolated facial nerve palsy, upper limb weakness, radicular, myelopathic, dysautonomic syndromes or multiple cranial neuropathies were reported also.

Acute hemorrhagic conjunctivitis surfaced again in 1981 in many of the same countries, in French Polynesia and other Pacific Islands, was imported to the United States, and spread among household contacts. A similar disease caused by enterovirus type 71 has occurred in Bulgaria and moved around the world. The other agent of epidemic hemorrhagic conjunctivitis, coxsackie A24, has not been associated with motor neuron disease. Each of these are highly contagious viruses for which there is no specific antiviral treatment, underscoring the importance of surveillance, public health measures, and sanitation in limiting disease.

Arboviruses

Arboviruses, a group of over 500 arthropod-borne RNA viruses, belong to several different taxonomic families. More than 100 are known to infect humans, causing limited febrile illness, encephalitis, or hemorrhagic fever. Considered together, arboviruses represent the leading cause of encephalitis worldwide.

St. Louis Encephalitis Virus (Flavivirus)

St. Louis encephalitis (SLE) virus is a cause of late summer encephalitis outbreaks in North America. In epidemic years,

SLE accounts for the largest number of viral encephalitis cases reported in the United States. Because SLE virus cycles between *Culex* mosquitoes and birds each summer, all components of the SLE virus cycle and hence, an epidemic, are contained in the backyards and birdbaths of many North American homes. In the United States, there are an average of 135 cases per year, but SLE also occurs in the Caribbean and Central and South America.

The illness is characterized by febrile headache only, aseptic meningitis, or encephalitis. Signs and symptoms of CNS infection progress over several days to a week. The incidence of encephalitis is higher in the elderly; in this population, case-fatality rates reach 30%. Season, place of residence, exposure, and presence of similar cases in the community are important considerations in the diagnosis. CSF cell counts are generally less than 200 WBC/μl, with lymphocytic predominance. Protein in the CSF is mildly elevated. Although virus may be isolated from serum or CSF, specific diagnosis usually relies on serological testing. IgM antibodies may be present in the CSF as early as day 3 of illness. The slower evolution of neurological symptoms, the presence of generalized weakness and tremor, and the absence of focal findings and seizures favor a diagnosis of SLE over HSV encephalitis.

No specific antiviral treatment exists. Treatment, as for all the arboviral encephalitides, is supportive, with control of cerebral edema, hyperthermia, and seizures.

Japanese Encephalitis Virus (Flavivirus)

Widely distributed in Asia, through Japan, China, Taiwan, Korea, the Far Eastern former Soviet Union, Southeast Asia, and India, JE virus accounts for the greatest number of arboviral encephalitis cases and deaths each year. Virus cycles between *Culex*, *Aedes*, or *Anopheles* species of mosquitoes, pigs, and birds.

An incubation period of 6–16 days is followed by a febrile headache syndrome, aseptic meningitis, or encephalitis. The encephalitic form is characterized by a 2- to 4-day viremic prodrome of headache, fever, nausea, vomiting, dizziness, drowsiness, and abdominal symptoms in children, progressing to meningoencephalitis with signs of cortical, subcortical, extrapyramidal, bulbar, cerebellar, and spinal cord involvement. Excitability or delirium, seizures, hyperthermia, expressionless facies, axial rigidity, limb tremors and other involuntary movements, erratic eye movements, cranial nerve palsies, ataxia, limb paresis, including lower motor neuron type weakness in the arms, and segmental sensory disturbance are reported.

The CSF may be subject to elevated pressure, with 10–500 (rarely up to 1,000) WBC/μl, with an early polymorphonuclear pleocytosis later replaced by lymphocytes. CSF protein is elevated (50–100 mg/dl). Specific diagnosis is made by demonstrating a fourfold increase in IgG antibodies between acute and convalescent sera, or IgM antibodies in serum and

CSF. Virus isolation from the blood is infrequent, but may be isolated from the CSF in one-third of patients. MRI studies may show areas of abnormal signal in thalamus and basal ganglia. The differential diagnosis includes HSV encephalitis and the bulbar paretic form of polio.

Poor prognosis is associated with prolonged fever, seizures, coma, or respiratory complications, and high CNS virus load. The case-fatality rate is 30–40%. Sequelae include parkinsonism, seizure disorders, paresis, mental retardation, and psychiatric disorders.

Formalin-inactivated vaccine is recommended for resident populations and travelers. The risk of disease among travelers has been estimated to be between 1 in 5,000 and 1 in 20,000 per week of travel. Primary immunization is with two doses, separated by 7–14 days, and a single booster dose at 1 year. Revaccination is recommended at 3-year intervals.

Murray Valley Encephalitis Virus (Australian X Disease; Flavivirus)

Murray Valley encephalitis virus has caused epidemics in Australia, primarily the Murray Valley region of New South Wales and Victoria, and sporadic cases in New Guinea. Outbreaks occur in summer months, after years of heavy rainfall. The virus cycles between *Culex* and *Aedes* mosquito species and large water birds.

A 2- to 5-day viral prodrome is followed by rapid progression to an encephalitic illness. Most patients are in a coma when first examined. Treatment is supportive. Neurological sequelae are seen in 40% of milder cases and all patients who recover from coma. These include cognitive impairment, paraplegia, or ataxic gait. No vaccine is available. Surveillance of virus activity in mosquitoes and birds and targeted insect control efforts are practiced in areas of recurrent epidemics.

Tick-Borne Encephalitis Virus (Flavivirus)

TBE occurs over a wide area of Europe and the former Soviet Union, corresponding to the distribution of ixodid tick vectors. Central European encephalitis virus and Russian spring-summer encephalitis virus, subtypes of the same virus, cycle between ticks and several wild rodent species and domestic livestock. Transmission also occurs by consumption of unpasteurized goat's milk.

The Central European form is a biphasic illness with systemic febrile illness followed by second-stage aseptic meningitis, encephalitis, myelitis, or radiculitis and a case-fatality rate of 1–2%. Russian spring-summer encephalitis is an indolent or more protracted febrile illness progressing to a meningoencephalitis, with a case-fatality rate of 20%. Bulbospinal form may dominate. Neurological sequelae occur in 30–60% of survivors of Russian spring-summer encephalitis, particularly a bibrachial paresis. Serum antibodies can be detected

by the time neurological disease is apparent. Vaccines and TBE-immunoglobulin for pre-exposure or postexposure prophylaxis are available. Immunoglobulin should be given within 4 days of the tick bite. The TBE vaccine is also protective against Omsk hemorrhagic fever, a tick-borne hemorrhagic illness with geographical overlap to Russian spring-summer encephalitis.

Louping Ill Virus (Flavivirus)

Louping ill was first recognized as a neurological disease in sheep in Scotland in the late 1800s. The virus is distributed among several domestic livestock species in the United Kingdom and spreads to humans by tick bites or to abattoir workers or veterinarians by direct exposure to sick sheep. The human illness is biphasic, with an initial influenzalike illness followed by remission, and then a meningoencephalitis. Diagnosis is by CSF virus isolation or high antibody titers in the CSF. The western subtype TBE vaccine may confer cross-protection.

Negishi virus (flavivirus), antigenically related to louping ill, is a recognized cause of encephalitis in Japan and China.

Kyasanur Forest Disease Virus (Flavivirus)

Kyasanur Forest disease is a tick-borne biphasic illness in which an initial hemorrhagic fever is followed by remission and then meningoencephalitis. A formalin-inactivated vaccine is in use in the Mysore state of India, its endemic area.

Powassan's Virus (Flavivirus)

Powassan's encephalitis has been reported in Russia, Canada, and the United States. The virus cycles between ticks and small mammals. Powassan's virus has been called the most herpeslike of the arboviruses because of some cases with temporal lobe involvement. Neurological sequelae affect an estimated 35% of patients.

West Nile Virus (Flavivirus)

West Nile virus is distributed throughout Africa, the Middle East, parts of Europe, the former Soviet Union, India, and Indonesia, where it is transmitted to humans by mosquitoes or ticks. Rash, lymphadenopathy and pharyngitis may be followed by aseptic meningitis, encephalitis, myelitis, radiculitis, or papillitis. Treatment is supportive.

Rocio Virus (Flavivirus)

Rocio virus caused an encephalitis epidemic in the Sao Paolo state of Brazil in 1975–1976. The case-fatality rate was 4%. Sequelae, including cerebellar, motor, and neuropsychiatric signs, were reported in 20% of survivors. The virus is presumed to cycle between *Aedes* species and wild birds.

Modoc Virus (Flavivirus)

Modoc virus has caused aseptic meningitis in an individual exposed to deer mice in Modoc County, CA. Virus has been isolated from the same rodent species in Oregon, Montana, and Alberta, Canada.

California Serogroup of Viruses (Family Bunyaviridae)

The California serogroup contains several viruses with mosquito vectors, small mammal or deer hosts, and limited geographical range. Among this group, La Crosse virus is an endemic cause of summer encephalitis in the midwestern United States. Most cases are in children, who have seizures and polymorphonuclear or mononuclear pleocytosis on CSF examination. Children who recover may have epileptic (10%), cognitive (2%), or paretic (<2%) sequelae. Jamestown Canyon virus (Michigan, New York) and Snowshoe hare virus (Alaska, Canada, and the northern United States) are other causes of aseptic meningitis.

Rift Valley Fever Virus (Bunyavirus)

Rift Valley fever is usually an influenzalike illness, but hemorrhage, hepatitis, meningoencephalitis, and retinitis are reported. Common complaints are of fever, headache, retroorbital pain, and loss of vision. Macular and perimacular retinitis, with retinal hemorrhage and edema are seen. The virus cycles between a wide variety of mosquito species and large domestic animals. The disease is found in Egypt, Sudan, East Africa, southern Africa, and Mauritania, West Africa, at times of high mosquito density related to wet seasons or new dam constructions. Formalin-inactivated vaccines have been developed to protect laboratory and veterinary personnel working in disease areas.

Equine Encephalitis Viruses (Family Alphaviridae)

EEEV is the most severe of the arboviral encephalitides, with encephalitis mortality of 50–70%. Younger children are more susceptible to EEEV as judged by higher case-infection ratios and more severe sequelae. EEEV is a summertime epizootic encephalitis in the eastern United States. A prodrome of fever, headache, nausea, and vomiting progresses rapidly to delirium and coma. Meningeal signs and excessive salivation are common. Children show opisthotonus, generalized rigidity, or focal findings. The CSF may be subject to elevated pressure, with 500–3,000 WBC/µl, with polymorphonuclear leukocyte predominance and elevated protein. The virus cycles in *Culex* mosquitoes and birds in the eastern United States. Horse or pheasant deaths in the area suggest virus circulation in that region. The diagnosis is made by virus isolation from sera or the presence of antibodies. There are approximately five cases per year in the United States.

Western equine encephalitis (WEE) is seen in mid-June through late September in the western United States. WEE is less virulent, with 5–10% mortality. Seizures, altered sensorium, rigidity, tremor, and other involuntary movements are noted during disease. CSF contains few to 500 WBC/µl, with monocytes being the predominant cell type. Motor or intellectual sequelae are common in infants. There are an average of five cases per year in the United States.

Highlands J virus, a WEE complex virus, cycles between birds and mosquitoes in freshwater swamp habitats of the Atlantic coast and is a rare cause of encephalitis in the eastern United States.

Venezuelan equine encephalitis is a febrile illness with myalgias progressing to encephalitis and coma in a small proportion of cases. Epilepsy, paralysis, tremor, hallucinations, and emotional lability may persist as permanent sequelae in children, and occasional cases of residual epilepsy or tremor have been reported in adults. Outbreaks have accompanied equine epidemics in Venezuela and other northern latitude areas of South America. Other favored ecological zones are tropical or subtropical forest of both Americas. Because the clinical presentation of Venezuelan equine encephalitis infection is rarely overtly encephalitic, the diagnosis may be missed unless recent travel in an area of disease activity in tropical America is taken into account. Both saliva and blood are infectious early in the disease.

The equine vaccine combining EEEV, WEE, or Venezuelan equine encephalitis antigens are used to protect laboratory workers or others in high-risk occupations.

Other alphaviruses, Semliki Forest virus (Uganda, Central Africa) and a close antigenic relative, Me Tri virus (Vietnam) (Ha et al. 1995) cause febrile headaches and infrequent encephalitis.

Colorado Tick Fever Virus (Orbivirus)

Colorado tick fever virus causes an aseptic meningitis in persons exposed to wood ticks in the Rocky Mountains in spring and summer. Diagnosis is by virus isolation from blood or by serology.

Measles

Despite the availability of an effective vaccine, measles, a highly contagious respiratory-borne disease, is still an important cause of childhood mortality in developing countries, childhood blindness, and sporadic outbreaks in industrialized nations. Measles causes four major CNS syndromes: acute encephalitis, postviral encephalomyelitis, measles inclusion body encephalitis, and SSPE.

Fever, maculopapular rash, cough, coryza, and Koplik's spots are characteristic of acute measles. CSF pleocytosis and EEG slowing may be documented in otherwise uncomplicated cases, but true encephalitis is infrequent. Keratitis and corneal ulceration accompany measles in children with preexisting malnutrition, particularly vitamin A deficiency. High-dose vitamin A supplementation, a single intramus-

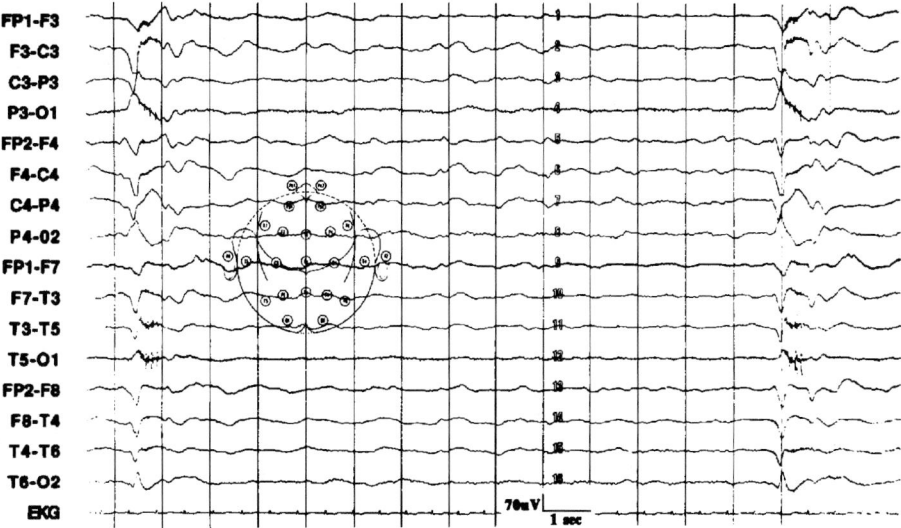

FIGURE 59B.4 Electroencephalogram of a 23-year-old man with subacute sclerosing panencephalitis showing generalized slow-wave complexes occurring approximately every 12 seconds. (Courtesy of K. Nudleman.)

cular dose of 400,000 IU for all ages, is recommended in regions with vitamin A deficiency or measles fatality rates greater than 1%.

Postinfectious encephalomyelitis follows an estimated 1 in 1,000 cases, usually within 2 weeks of the rash.

Measles inclusion body encephalitis is a rapidly progressive dementing illness, with behavior changes, myoclonus, refractory focal or generalized seizures, delirium, or coma developing 1–6 months after measles exposure, in individuals with deficiencies in cell-mediated immunity. Patients are afebrile and CSF analysis is normal. Treatment consists of supportive care, the withholding of immunosuppressive therapy if possible, and passive immunoglobulin therapy.

SSPE is a rare late complication of measles, caused by persistent, nonproductive measles virus infection of neurons and glia. The pathogenesis of SSPE is related to defective measles virus maturation in neural cells. Aberrant M (matrix) protein as well as other envelope proteins interfere with assembly and budding of infectious virus. The virus remains in intracellular form and spreads by cell-to-cell contact.

SSPE has an annual incidence from under 0.1 cases to 5 or 6 cases per million in nonimmunized populations. In areas of high early-life attack rates, SSPE accounts for a proportion of childhood neurodegenerative conditions. Children infected in the first 2 years of life are at greater risk, and case-series consistently show SSPE to be more frequent in boys. The median interval between acute measles infection and SSPE is 8 years, with a range from 2–12 years. The early stage is marked by behavioral or personality changes and declining school performance. Myoclonus, seizures, spasticity, choreoathetoid or ballistic movements, ataxia, and chorioretinitis follow in the second stage. Optic atrophy, quadriparesis, autonomic instability, akinetic mutism, and coma are seen in the final stage. The majority of cases follow a progressive downhill course to death

within a few years, some temporarily plateau or improve, and possibly 5% remit spontaneously.

At the time neurological symptoms occur, neurons and glia contain nuclear and cytoplasmic viral inclusion bodies (Plate 59B.IV), and antibodies to virus are high in both serum and CSF. The diagnosis can be established by high measles-specific IgG antibody in CSF or serum to CSF ratios consistent with intrathecal measles antibody synthesis. CSF pleocytosis is absent, glucose is normal, and total protein is normal or elevated. Acute symptoms together with increased intracranial pressure are poor prognostic signs. The earliest MRI findings are high signal intensity on T2-weighted images of gray and subcortical white matter in posterior portions of the hemispheres. During the second stage of disease, the EEG shows a pattern of generalized slow-wave complexes with a regular periodicity (Figure 59B.4). The complexes may last up to 3 seconds and occur at regular intervals, between 4 and 14 seconds, against a background of depressed activity.

Some patients have improved or stabilized after one or several 6-week treatments of intraventricular interferon-α through an Ommaya reservoir, starting at 105 U/m^2 body surface area per day, with daily increments, up to 106 U/m^2 per day on the fifth day, 5 days per week, combined with oral isoprinosine (asinosiplex), 100 mg/kg per day. CSF measles antibody and renal and hepatic function are followed during treatment. Courses may be repeated up to six times, at 2- to 6-month intervals (Anlar et al. 1997). The laboratory enpoint of treatment is the eradication of detectable measles antibody from the CSF. Systemic (subcutaneous) interferon-α, in daily doses of up to 5 million units, has been used with intrathecal interferon-α, to simultaneously treat peripheral reservoirs of measles virus, lymphoid and glandular tissue. Prolonged or repeated treatments carry the risks of meningitis, interferon-α–induced encephalopathy, and interferon-α upper and lower motor neuron toxicity.

Immunization with attenuated live measles vaccine is recommended for infants between 6 and 15 months of age. In areas where measles circulates widely, immunization is performed early, at 6 or 9 months. Fatal infection has followed measles vaccine in severely immunocompromised children, but there is no epidemiological evidence that vaccination causes SSPE.

Rubella

Rubella virus infection in childhood or adult life is usually a mild illness. Maculopapular rash, fever, and lymphadenopathy characterize clinically apparent infection. Postinfectious encephalomyelitis is estimated to complicate 1 of 6,000 cases, with onset 1–6 days after the appearance of the rash.

Gestational rubella, especially infection acquired during the first trimester, has serious consequences for the fetus. Eighty percent of children with a congenital rubella syndrome have some form of nervous system involvement. Signs in infancy include bulging fontanelle, lethargy, irritability, and tone abnormalities. CSF protein is elevated, and virus may be isolated from the CSF. Sequelae in survivors include mental retardation, sensorineural hearing loss, motor and posture abnormalities, cataracts, pigmentary retinopathy, and congenital heart disease.

An uncommon, late-onset rubella encephalitis, progressive rubella panencephalitis, may follow congenital rubella or natural childhood rubella. There is a prolonged asymptomatic period, followed by the onset of neurological deterioration during the second decade of life. Symptoms include behavioral changes, intellectual decline, ataxia, spasticity, and seizures. Although progressive rubella panencephalitis may exhibit some of the clinical features of SSPE, patients with progressive rubella panencephalitis tend to be older, have more protracted clinical courses, and be without generalized myoclonus or periodic burst-suppression EEG patterns. Although a few spontaneous remissions have been reported, the typical course is one of progressive neurological decline, leading to death within 8 years. Sera and CSF from affected children contain antirubella IgG antibodies. Diffuse brain atrophy may be found on MRI.

Where live attenuated virus vaccines have been administered to preschool children, rubella-associated acute disseminated encephalomyelitis has vanished. However, the rubella virus vaccine is not free of problems because of secondary arthritis in adult vaccine recipients. Postexposure vaccination is not recommended.

Mumps

Mumps virus causes a mild childhood illness with parotitis but has the capacity for widespread invasion of visceral organs, the vestibular labyrinths, and the CNS. In unimmunized populations, mumps is a common cause of aseptic meningitis and encephalitis. In the United States in the 1960s, mumps was a leading cause of viral encephalitis.

The incidence of mumps meningitis and encephalitis varies with different epidemics from less than 1% to 70%. Mumps meningitis may precede parotitis and can occur without salivary gland enlargement in 40–50% of patients. In the rest, mumps meningitis or encephalitis develops approximately 5 days after the onset of parotitis. Seizures occur in 20–30% of patients with CNS symptoms, but follow-up EEGs are usually normal. Even obtunded patients may have relatively mild EEG changes and recover with few sequelae. Complications include deafness from labyrinth membrane and sensory transducer damage, myelitis, or hydrocephalus following viral replication in choroidal and ependymal cells.

In mumps meningoencephalitis, the CSF pressure is slightly increased; cell counts, usually 25–500 WBC/μl with lymphocytic predominance, may reach 3,000 WBC/μl; protein is normal or moderately elevated and may include mumps-specific oligoclonal IgG; glucose is depressed in 29% of cases. Mumps virus can be cultured from the CSF.

Postinfectious encephalomyelitis follows an estimated 1 in 6,000 cases and develops 7–15 days after parotitis.

Mumps prevention is by vaccination with live attenuated virus at 15 months of age; mumps vaccine is one component of the trivalent measles-mumps-rubella vaccine. Infrequent reports of mumps meningitis had been reported from some strains of mumps vaccine that are no longer in use.

Arenaviruses

Arenaviruses are rodent-borne viruses and textbook examples of zoonoses, infections originating from animal sources that have escaped from their historic cycles in nature and emerged as human infections. Transmission is by contact with rodent excreta or saliva. The arenaviruses of neurological consequence are LCMV, Lassa fever, and Argentine hemorrhagic fever viruses.

The CNS disease usually seen with LCMV is aseptic meningitis, but encephalitis has been diagnosed in 5–34% of serologically confirmed LCMV cases. CSF cell counts in excess of the 10–500 WBC/μl range usually accepted for viral meningitis may be present with LCMV. Ascending or transverse myelitis, bulbar syndromes, parkinsonism, and sensorineural hearing loss also have been reported. Hydrocephalus may arise as a sequelae of ependymitis or ventriculitis. LCMV infection of the fetus has produced hydrocephalus, diffuse parenchymal disease, mental retardation, and chorioretinitis.

Lassa fever, the West African viral hemorrhagic fever with high mortality, produces a multisystem disease with fever, pharyngitis, hemorrhage, hepatic involvement, shock, plus neurological syndromes in 40% of hospitalized patients. Imported cases have occurred in Europe, Israel,

Canada, the United States, Japan, and Australia. Encephalitis with seizures, depressed consciousness, amnestic syndromes, dystonia or tremor, convalescent ataxic syndromes, and neuropsychiatric sequelae have been described. One-third of all patients with Lassa fever develop hearing impairments, two-thirds of whom are left with significant sensorineural hearing loss.

Acute ataxia may accompany Argentine hemorrhagic fever and abnormal brainstem evoked potential waveforms have been reported in patients treated with immune plasma.

Arenaviral diagnosis is by viral culture and serology. IgM antibody to LCMV is present in serum, CSF, or both during acute meningitic disease. Ribavirin, a guanosine analogue, has proven efficacy in arenaviral hemorrhagic fever animal models. For the treatment of Lassa fever in humans, intravenous ribavirin is administered as a 2-g loading dose, followed by 1 g every 6 hours for 4 days, then 0.5 g thrice daily for six additional days. Anemia is the major side effect. Oral ribavirin is available through the Centers for Disease Control and Prevention (Atlanta, GA) for the prophylaxis of contacts (Solbrig 1997).

Other Hemorrhagic Fever Viruses

Arboviral Agents of Hemorrhagic Fevers

Just as the arboviral encephalitides already found in the United States are each spreading as a result of vector proliferation and susceptible population exposure, so are the arboviral hemorrhagic fevers.

Dengue (Flavivirus).
In terms of size of epidemics and severity of disease, dengue fever and dengue hemorrhagic fever are the most important arthropod-borne viral diseases of humans. Up to 100 million cases of dengue fever and 250,000 cases of dengue hemorrhagic fever occur each year in tropical Asia, Africa, Australia, and the Americas. Dengue virus cycles between humans and mosquitoes. *Aedes aegypti*, the most important vector, is a mosquito that has evolved to live in proximity to humans and breed well in manufactured throwaway containers holding stagnant water. The expansion of *Aedes aegypti* throughout the Americas and the inadvertent import of another competent vector, *Aedes alboticus*, to the United States and Brazil from Asia, has established dengue on all continents with tropical and subtropical areas.

Dengue fever begins, after a 2- to 7-day incubation period, as a sudden febrile illness with headache, myalgias, arthralgia, prostration, abdominal discomfort, and rash. Over the next 2–3 days the rash clears while the patient defervesces. A second, maculopapular rash appears, first on the trunk, and bleeding may follow. Dengue hemorrhagic fever is the severe form of disease, occurring in persons, usually children, previously sensitized by infection with a heterologous dengue serotype.

Neurological complications including encephalopathy, encephalitis, mononeuritis multiplex involving cranial and peripheral nerves, and Guillain-Barré and Reye's syndromes have been associated with both self-limited (classic) dengue fever and dengue hemorrhagic fever. Diagnosis depends on virus isolation from blood in the early stages, or serological tests. The CSF may contain few (<30) or no WBC. The differential diagnosis of fever with rash, petechiae, or purpura includes malaria, typhoid fever, the viral exanthems (measles, rubella, enteroviruses), viral hemorrhagic fevers, syphilis, scarlet fever, meningococcemia, rickettsial diseases, gram-negative sepsis, drug reactions, and noninfectious causes of disseminated intravascular coagulation. Specific antiviral treatment has not been evaluated for dengue and care is supportive. Salicylates are contraindicated because of the risk of hemorrhagic exacerbation and Reye's syndrome.

Yellow Fever (Flavivirus).
Yellow fever occurs in tropical South America and sub-Saharan Africa. The return of yellow fever to the Americas in large urban epidemics is predicted because of the large numbers of susceptible people and successful expansion of *Aedes aegypti*. Asians have been spared yellow fever, perhaps because of cross-protection by dengue immunity. Vaccination with yellow fever 17D, a live viral vaccine developed by the World Health Organization, has been associated with rare encephalitis cases in infants. Because of the risk of encephalitis, the vaccine is contraindicated for infants under 6 months of age. A French vaccine, produced from infected mouse brains was associated with a 1% incidence of post-vaccine encephalitis and is no longer manufactured.

Filoviruses

Ebola and Marburg viruses are the two known members of the Filoviridae. Both viruses cause fulminating hemorrhagic fever with severe shock and high mortality. Early headache and additional signs of a meningeal or encephalitic process are rapidly eclipsed by complications of hemorrhage, hypotension, hepatic failure, and disseminated intravascular coagulopathy. Muscle necrosis caused by disseminated intravascular coagulopathy and intramuscular hemorrhage follows early myositis or muscle pain. A low-grade (<25 WBC) CSF pleocytosis has been reported in patients with Marburg virus early in their illnesses. Treatment is supportive. No therapeutic role for convalescent sera or interferon has been established by controlled clinical trial. Blood and all body fluids are highly infectious.

Papovavirus and Progressive Multifocal Leukoencephalopathy

Progressive multifocal leukoencephalopathy (PML), a subacute, demyelinating disease of the CNS, is presently the only human central demyelinating disease of proven viral etiology.

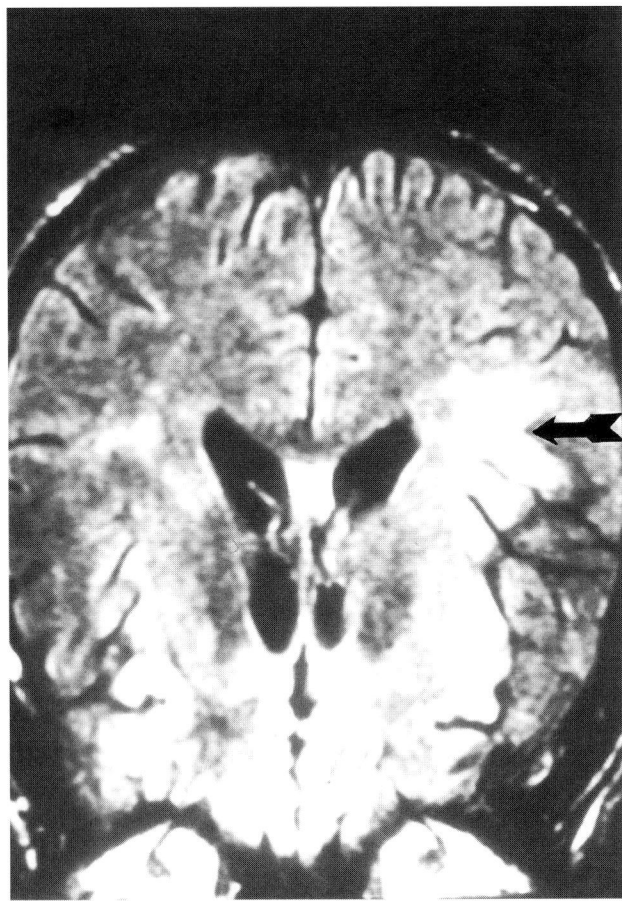

FIGURE 59B.5 Progressive multifocal leukoencephalopathy. Coronal magnetic resonance imaging fluid attenuation inversion recovery sequence, with arrow showing hyperintense temporal white matter. (Courtesy of J. Healy.)

PML is a result of infection of oligodendrocytes by an opportunistic papovavirus (Plate 59B.V). Most cases have been caused by the JC strain and a few by the SV-40 strain. JC virus, when contracted in early childhood, is not associated with illness. JC virus persists in the host and is reactivated in cases of diseases or medical treatments known to impair cell-mediated immunity: lymphoproliferative disorders, tuberculosis, sarcoidosis, prolonged immunosuppression, and inherited and acquired immunodeficiency diseases. Rare until the 1980s, PML is now encountered more frequently because of its association with AIDS. In a small number of cases, no underlying disease can be identified.

Onset is subacute, with signs and symptoms of multifocal, asymmetric white matter involvement. In non–AIDS-associated PML, early lesions tend to be in subcortical white matter of the occipital lobes, causing visual field deficits or cortical blindness. Motor weakness, behavior changes, cognitive impairment, cerebellar ataxia, dysarthria, and sensory abnormalities also are seen, whereas headache, seizures, and extrapyramidal syndromes are rarer. The disease progresses to dementia as the number of lesions increases.

CSF cell counts and protein levels are usually normal. Neuroimaging can establish the diagnosis in a noninvasive fashion. MRI studies show focal or multifocal lesions of subcortical white matter, sometimes the cerebellum, brainstem, and spinal cord, without mass effect or contrast enhancement. Fluid attenuation inversion recovery sequences, which null CSF signals, are particularly good for demonstrating paraventricular disease (Figure 59B.5). White matter lesions are larger and more confluent than those of multifocal leukoencephalitis of VZV. Bland spinal fluid and an indolent course distinguish PML from paraviral and postviral encephalomyelitis. If necessary, brain biopsy reveals PML's unique histopathology: oligonucleocytes with enlarged nuclei that contain inclusion bodies, as well as viral particles, antigen or viral DNA. JC virus has never been cultured from CSF, but JC virus DNA may be detected in CSF using PCR amplification (Cinque et al. 1997). Intrathecal antibodies can be detected in non-AIDS patients. One treatment protocol uses repeated courses of intravenous cytarabine (2 mg/kg/day) for 5 days every 4 weeks (Moreno et al. 1996); intrathecal cytarabine and interferon-α may be used in conjunction. A further discussion of PML and its treatment appears in Chapter 59E. Patients most likely to benefit from therapy are those with relatively intact immune systems in whom it may be possible to reduce or eliminate iatrogenic immunosuppression.

Non–Human Immunodeficiency Virus Retroviruses: Human T-Cell Leukemic Viruses

The Retroviridae is a large family of viruses, grouped initially by pathogenic features, but later revised on the basis of nucleotide sequence and genome structure. HTLV types I and II belong to the HTLV-bovine leukemia group; HIV belongs to the lentivirus group.

HTLV, the etiological agent of adult T-cell leukemia, was serologically linked to a progressive spastic paraparesis, known as *tropical spastic paraparesis*, in West Indies patients in 1985. Later, in Japan, a similar syndrome with elevated HTLV-I antibodies was named *HTLV-I associated myelopathy* (HAM).

HTLV-I is endemic in southern Japan, Taiwan, Okinawa, the Caribbean basin (including northeast South America), central and West Africa, southern India, and the Seychelles. In the United States and Western Europe, the incidence of HTLV infection is higher among intravenous drug users and homosexuals. Ten to 20 million people around the world are estimated to be infected with HTLV-I. Most seropositive individuals are asymptomatic; fewer than 1% of infected patients develop spastic paraparesis. Spread of HTLV-I, as other retroviruses, is by sexual, parenteral, or vertical transmission. In the United States, all blood supplies have been screened for HTLV-I since 1988.

With an incubation period of approximately 20 years, HAM is usually recognized in the fifth decade of life as a progressive spastic paraparesis or myeloneuropathy. Occasionally, acute cases, resembling transverse myelitis, also occur. Neurological findings include lower extremity weakness and spasticity that is usually symmetric, impotence, urinary and fecal incontinence, and generalized hyperreflexia except in cases of concomitant sensory neuropathy. Inflammatory myositis, cerebellar ataxia, nystagmus, vertigo, deafness, optic neuritis, adult T-cell leukemia, uveitis (as vitreous opacities, iritis, retinal vasculitis), sicca syndrome, inflammatory arthropathy, and lymphocytic alveolitis may be present. HTLV-II is associated with atypical hairy cell leukemias, mycosis fungoides, other lymphocytic or leukemoid malignancies, and a similar myelopathy.

Serological testing using an enzyme-linked immunosorbent assay, followed by Western blot confirmation, is used for diagnosis. False-positive serologic test results for syphilis and Lyme disease and antiphospholipid antibodies have been reported with HAM. The CSF contains mild elevations in lymphocytes and protein; elevated gamma-globulin fraction, oligoclonal bands, and CSF antibody levels, reflecting intrathecal synthesis. HTLV-I is usually not found in cells of the CSF, but has been detected in small populations of lymphocytes in the CSF by PCR. Spine MRI studies may show normal cord, hyperintense signal abnormalities on T2-weighted images, or atrophy in late disease. The patterns of signal enhancement tend to be diffuse in HAM, in contrast to discreet or multifocal abnormalities seen in MS. Periventricular gray or white matter lesions may be seen also.

Conditions clinically similar to the subacute spastic paraparesis of HTLV-I include HIV-associated vacuolar myelopathy, idiopathic inflammatory conditions, hereditary spastic paraplegia, and toxic-metabolic disorders such as vitamin B_{12} deficiency, lathyrism (India), cycad poisoning (Pacific Islands), or konzo (Central Africa).

Because the progression of disease is most rapid during the first year, early treatment during this time has the best chance of improving outcome. Treatments have been directed against the inflammatory components of disease. Primary therapy has been with initial intravenous injections of 1 g of methylprednisolone per day, followed by oral prednisone, 80 mg on alternate days for 2 months, then tapering by 10 mg each month for the next 6 months. Patients who fail prednisone therapy may receive intravenous immunoglobulin at 400 mg/kg for 5 days; repeated monthly for three or more cycles, intramuscular interferon-α, or plasmapheresis. The anabolic corticosteroid danazol, 400 mg thrice daily, has been reported to slow or reverse bladder symptoms.

Influenza

Influenza has been associated with myositis, Reye's syndrome, and with two other CNS syndromes: influenza encephalopathy and postinfluenza encephalitis 2–3 weeks after recovery from influenza A. The encephalitic syndrome, accompanied by an inflammatory spinal fluid, is transient, with full recovery in most cases. Oral amantadine at doses of 100 mg twice daily is approved for use in treatment and prophylaxis of influenza A.

Thought to be a late sequelae of the 1917–1918 influenza, encephalitis lethargica and postencephalitic parkinsonism have been historically linked to the influenza pandemic of those years. The parkinsonian syndrome was distinguished from idiopathic Parkinson's disease by younger age of onset, hyperkinetic movements, oculogyric crises, respiratory tics, and behavior disorders. However, a complete appreciation of the relation between the diseases is hindered by the absence of serological specimens from the time and the inability to apply contemporary microbiology techniques to the postmortem specimens.

Adenovirus

Adenoviruses cause acute respiratory disease in children and military recruits, conjunctivitis, hemorrhagic cystitis, and gastroenteritis. Meningoencephalitis or unilateral deafness coincident with nasopharyngeal infection are rare complications in normal hosts; fatal meningoencephalitis was reported in a bone marrow transplant patient. Diagnosis is by isolation of virus from extraneural sites or by serology.

Parvovirus

Acute infection with B19 parvovirus causes the fifth exanthem of childhood, erythema infectiosum (fifth disease), transient aplastic crises, or arthritis in adults. Chronic parvovirus infection has been found in patients with necrotizing vasculitis resembling polyarteritis or Wegener's granulomatosis. Neurological manifestations have included encephalitis with fifth disease, brachial plexitis, abnormal pupillary reflexes, and recurrent paresthesias.

Hepatitis Viruses

The viral causes of hepatitis are hepatitis A, B, C, D (delta), and E viruses. Hepatitis C and occasionally hepatitis B have been associated with a systemic vasculitic disease and mixed cryoglobulinemia, and hepatitis B has been associated with polyarteritis nodosa. Extrahepatic manifestations of hepatitis C viral infection include cranial and peripheral neuropathies, mononeuritis multiplex, polymyositis, and anterior spinal artery stroke. A brain autopsy specimen of a patient with progressive encephalomyelitis with rigidity yielded hepatitis C viral DNA by reverse transcription PCR. Interferon-α treats the liver and renal involvement and may either help or exacerbate the peripheral neuropathy. Plasma exchange is an alternative for patients whose neuropathy is worsened by interferon-α.

Other Syndromes

Recurrent Meningitis

Recurrent meningitis, or discreet episodes of meningitis, has been linked to viruses, other infectious agents, and idiopathic inflammatory conditions. Viral causes of recurrent aseptic meningitis include HIV, HSV-1 and -2, and EBV. HSV-1 and EBV have been isolated from CSF in cases of Mollaret's meningitis, a febrile, meningitic syndrome with Mollaret's cells, pathologically distinct large cells of monocyte-macrophage lineage resembling endothelial cells, in the CSF. Recurrences of Mollaret's meningitis have been reported at intervals of several weeks to several months, and episodes may recur for decades. Recurrent bacterial meningitis suggests CSF leak, dermal sinus, parameningeal infection, or impaired B-cell immunity. Other causes of recurrent aseptic meningitis include partially treated or atypical bacterial or fungal pathogens, particularly *Borrelia*, rupture of dermoid cysts into CSF spaces, nonsteroidal anti-inflammatory or sulfa drugs, intravenous immunoglobulin and monoclonal antibodies, sarcoidosis, and the other uveomeningitic syndromes. Behçet's disease is suggested by the combination of mucosal ulcerations, orchitis, and meningitis and Vogt-Koyanagi-Harada syndrome by deafness, vitiligo, and alopecia.

Viliuisk Encephalomyelitis

Viliuisk encephalomyelitis is a biphasic illness of the Iakut people of Siberia, in whom an acute meningoencephalitis is followed weeks or months later by a progressive dementia with pyramidal, extrapyramidal, or amyotrophic lateral sclerosis–like features. The acute febrile onset, CSF pleocytosis, epidemiology, geographical clusters, and inflammatory neuropathology have suggested an infectious etiology, but no agent has been identified.

Rasmussen's Encephalitis

Rasmussen's encephalitis is a subacute focal encephalitis with epilepsy of children and young adults. Human CMV has been detected by PCR in brain biopsy specimens in some cases, and clinical improvement after ganciclovir has been reported (McLachlan et al. 1996). HSV-1 has been implicated in additional cases, based on PCR and in situ hybridization studies (Jay et al. 1995). Nonviral treatments have been directed toward the immunological aspects of the disease, such as the presence of glutamate receptor antibodies in some patients. Epilepsy surgeries, including hemispherectomy or subpial intracortical transection if hemiplegia has not developed (Dulac 1996), are undertaken in patients with poor response to medical treatments.

Progressive Encephalomyelitis with Rigidity

Progressive encephalomyelitis with rigidity is a syndrome of limb and trunk rigidity and stimulus-sensitive muscle spasms, cellular spinal fluid, and inflammatory pathology in cervical cord and brainstem. Early descriptions of progressive encephalomyelitis with rigidity noted clinical and pathological similarities between this syndrome and spinal forms of encephalitis lethargica described by von Economo. The pathology is consistent with either previous viral infection or an immunopathology. Some cases are paraneoplastic or manifest antineuronal autoantibodies and have been treated with plasmapheresis and prednisone. The differential diagnosis of progressive encephalomyelitis with rigidity includes other syndromes with involuntary motor symptoms: tetanus, stiff man syndrome, cramps, tetani, and hemifacial spasm. The electromyographic silent period is usually absent in patients with tetanus, but normal in the stiff man syndromes.

Epidemic Neuromyasthenia (Benign Myalgic Encephalomyelitis)

Descriptions of epidemic neuromyasthenia (benign myalgic encephalomyelitis) were of a syndrome of protracted fatigue, following an initial "viral" syndrome that may include respiratory or gastrointestinal complaints, headache, muscle pain, and lethargy. Using today's terminology, such patients would be considered to have chronic fatigue syndrome, the contemporary syndrome of disabling fatigue, constitutional symptoms, and neuropsychiatric complaints, often depression. One or several viruses have been etiological candidates, based on the findings of elevated antibodies to the herpesviruses, coxsackie B, measles, and rubella viruses, but a completely satisfying hypothesis of pathogenesis and recommendations for treatment has not been developed.

REFERENCES

Amlie-Lefond C, Kleinschmidt-DeMasters BK, Mahalingam R, et al. The vasculopathy of varicella-zoster virus encephalitis. Ann Neurol 1995;37:784–790.

Anlar B, Yalaz K, Oktem F, Kose G. Long-term follow-up of patients with subacute sclerosing panencephalitis treated with intraventricular alpha-interferon. Neurology 1997;48:526–528.

Arvin AM. Varicella-zoster virus. Clin Microbiol Rev 1996;9:361–381.

Bennett JL, Mahalingam R, Wellish MC, Gilden DH. Epstein-Barr virus-associated acute autonomic neuropathy. Ann Neurol 1996;40:453–455.

Berger JR. HTLV-1 associated myelopathy. In RT Johnson, JW Griffin (eds), Current Therapy in Neurologic Disease (5th ed). St. Louis: Mosby–Year Book, 1997.

Cinque P, Scarpellini P, Vago L, et al. Diagnosis of central nervous system complications in HIV-infected patients: cerebrospinal fluid analysis by the polymerase chain reaction. AIDS 1997;11:1–17.

Dellemijn PL, Brandenburg A, Niesters HG, et al. Successful treatment with ganciclovir of presumed Epstein-Barr meningoencephalitis following bone marrow transplant. Bone Marrow Transplant 1995;16:311–312.

Dulac O. Rasmussen's syndrome. Current Opin Neurol 1996;9:75–77.

Fogan L. Progressive encephalomyelitis with rigidity responsive to plasmapheresis and immunosuppression. Ann Neurol 1996;40:451–453.

Ha DQ, Claisher CH, Tien PH, et al. Isolation of a newly recognized alphavirus from mosquitoes in Vietnam and evidence for human infection and disease. Am J Trop Med Hyg 1995;53:100–104.

Heslop HE, Rooney CM. Adoptive cellular immunotherapy for EBV lymphoproliferative disease. Immunol Rev 1997;157:217–222.

Holmes GP, Chapman LE, Stewart JA, et al. Guidelines for the prevention and treatment of B-virus infections in exposed persons. Clin Infect Dis 1995;20:421–439.

Jay V, Becker LE, Otsubo H, et al. Chronic encephalitis and epilepsy (Rasmussen's encephalitis): detection of cytomegalovirus and herpes simplex virus 1 by the polymerase chain reaction and in situ hybridization. Neurology 1995;45:108–117.

Johnson RT. Rabies. In RT Johnson, JW Griffin (eds), Current Therapy in Neurologic Disease (5th ed). St. Louis: Mosby–Year Book, 1997.

Kamolvarin N, Tirawatnpong T, Rattanasiwamoke R, et al. Diagnosis of rabies by polymerase chain reaction with nested primers. J Infect Dis 1993;167:207–210.

Kirkinen P, Serlo W, Jouppila P, et al. Long-term outcome of fetal hydrocephaly. J Child Neurol 1996;11:189–192.

Knox KK, Pietryga D, Harrington DJ, et al. Progressive immunodeficiency and fatal pneumonitis associated with human herpesvirus 6 infection in an infant. Clin Infect Dis 1995;20:406–413.

Mas P, Pelegrino JL, Guzman MG, et al. Viral isolation from cases of epidemic neuropathy in Cuba. Arch Pathol Lab Med 1997;121:825–833.

McLachlan RS, Levine S, Blume WT. Treatment of Rasmussen's syndrome with ganciclovir. Neurology 1996;47:925–928.

Moreno S, Miralles P, Diaz MD, et al. Cytarabine therapy for progressive multifocal leukoencephalopathy in patients with AIDS. Clin Infect Dis 1996;23:1066–1068.

Mustafa MM, Weitman SD, Winick NJ, et al. Subacute measles encephalitis in the young immunocompromised host: report of two cases diagnosed by polymerase chain reaction and treated with ribavirin and review of the literature. Clin Infect Dis 1993;16:661–666.

Sola P, Merelli E, Marasca R, et al. Human herpesvirus 6 and multiple sclerosis: survey of anti-HHV-6 antibodies by immunofluorescence analysis and of viral sequences by polymerase chain reaction. J Neurol Neurosurg Psychiatry 1993;56:917–919.

Solbrig MV. Lassa fever and central nervous system diseases: a review. Neurol Infect Epidemiol 1997;2:13–18.

Stein GE. Pharmacology of new antiherpes agents: famciclovir and valacyclovir. J Am Pharmacol Assoc 1997;NS37:157–163.

Stott GA. Famciclovir: a new systemic antiviral agent for herpesvirus infections. Am Fam Physician 1997;55:2501–2504.

Tyler KL. Polymerase chain reaction and the diagnosis of viral central nervous system diseases. Ann Neurol 1994;36:809–811.

Whitley RJ, Lakeman F. Herpes simplex virus infections of the central nervous system: therapeutic and diagnostic considerations. Clin Infect Dis 1995;20:414–420.

Wilborn F, Schmidt CA, Brinkman V, et al. A potential role for human herpesvirus type 6 in nervous system disease. J Neuroimmunol 1994;49:213–214.

Wood MJ, Johnson RW, McKendrick RW, et al. A randomized trial of acyclovir for 7 days with and without prednisolone for treatment of acute herpes zoster. N Engl J Med 1994;330:896–900.

Wright R, Johnson D, Neumann M, et al. Congenital lymphocytic choriomeningitis virus syndrome: a disease that mimics congenital toxoplasmosis or cytomegalovirus infection. Pediatrics 1997;100:E9.

Chapter 59
Infections of the Nervous System

C. FUNGAL INFECTIONS
Jody Corey-Bloom and Marylou V. Solbrig

Fungi, causes of superficial, subcutaneous, or systemic (deep tissue) disease, are found throughout the world, with distributions influenced by climate, geography, host exposure, and immunity. Fungal infections of the central nervous system (CNS), previously accounting for relatively few instances of disease worldwide, are now encountered with increasing frequency, because of the expanded use of immunosuppressive medical treatments, broad-spectrum antibiotics, CNS invasive procedures, and the acquired immunodeficiency syndrome (AIDS) epidemic.

Fungi, eukaryotic organisms with polysaccharide-based cell walls, are categorized as yeasts or molds on the basis of their reproductive habits. Yeasts are single round cells that bud, giving rise to daughter cells. The mold (or mycelia) fungi form hyphae, extensions of chains of cells. Most of the major respiratory pathogens are dimorphic, existing as yeasts or molds at different stages of their life cycle. Fungi cause disease in humans either by direct tissue invasion or by noninvasive means, such as allergic mechanisms or toxin production. Well-known mycotoxins include ergotamine, a product of the rye ergot (a fungus of cereal plants), and the trichothecene mycotoxins, allegedly used in aerosol form in biological warfare as yellow rain to produce a systemic illness characterized by weakness, ataxia, hypothermia, and shock.

Cryptococcus neoformans, Coccidioides immitis, Paracoccidioides brasiliensis, Histoplasma capsulatum, and *Blastomyces dermatitidis* are known as pathogenic, or endemic, fungi for their ability to cause invasive disease in normal hosts. In patients with simultaneous immunosuppression, the likelihood of CNS complications of disseminated disease by these agents may increase. *Candida albicans,*

Aspergillus fumigatus, and *Zygomycetes rhizopus (Mucor)* are considered opportunistic fungi and are almost exclusively pathogens of immunocompromised patients.

Fungal infections of the CNS in AIDS are considered elsewhere in this chapter (Chapter 59E).

FUNGAL SYNDROMES

Subacute or Chronic Meningitis

The clinical syndrome of chronic fungal meningitis is a 4-week or longer course of headache, fever, neck stiffness, nausea, vomiting, or weight loss, with a cerebrospinal fluid (CSF) profile demonstrating elevated protein, low or normal glucose, and lymphocytic pleocytosis. Patients may come to medical attention earlier than 4 weeks. They may have been given a presumptive diagnosis of tuberculous meningitis and receive empiric therapy for tuberculosis (TB), particularly if cognitive or behavioral changes, cranial neuropathies, or other neurological symptoms develop. Chronic meningitis is one presentation of CNS fungal infection, but it may be caused by a large number of infectious and noninfectious diseases.

The discovery of hydrocephalus in association with cranial neuropathies suggests an infectious process with basilar meningitis; however, the stereotyped clinical presentation of chronic meningitis usually provides few clues as to precise etiology. Cognitive changes, apraxia, gait difficulties, or other signs of communicating hydrocephalus may occur without clinical symptoms of antecedent meningitis.

CSF examination reveals a mild or moderate mixed cell pleocytosis, elevated protein, and low to normal glucose. The

CSF white blood count (WBC) is usually 500/μl or less, except in blastomycosis, in which it may be greater than 1,000 cells/μl. Predominant early polymorphonuclear pleocytosis suggests infection with *Coccidioides* or *Aspergillus*. CSF eosinophilia and even oligoclonal banding are more likely with coccidioidomycosis. In general, fewer cells are seen in immunocompromised patients, although opportunistic meningeal infection by *Candida* produces CSF cell counts that average 600 WBC/μl. Low CSF glucose is also a frequent concomitant of *Candida* infection.

Identification of specific fungi relies on direct smears, culture, or serologic testing. Cryptococcal polysaccharide antigen can be detected by latex agglutination in over 90% of patients with cryptococcal meningitis, whereas India ink smear of CSF sediment is positive in approximately 50% of patients. False-positive results occur if yeasts are confused with artifact or lymphocytes. CSF antigen detection for *Candida* and CSF antibody detection by complement fixation for *Histoplasma* and *Coccidioides* are also available. Most cases of cryptococcal meningitis have positive CSF culture results; approximately one-third of coccidioidal meningitis and one-half of candidal meningitis cases have positive CSF culture results. The diagnostic yield by culture, staining, and cytology is increased with high volume and repeated CSF studies, but *Histoplasma*, *Blastomyces*, and *Sporothrix* CSF culture results may remain negative.

Magnetic resonance imaging studies may demonstrate parameningeal sites of infection, concurrent parenchymal disease, or hydrocephalus. Extraneural evidence of fungal infection should be sought in the general physical and ophthalmological examinations and on chest roentgenography. Mycosis should be considered in any patient with a respiratory infection living in an endemic area, or if the patient is immunosuppressed, long after residence there. Residual pulmonary nodules, coin lesions, or calcifications on chest roentgenography suggest histoplasmosis, coccidioidomycosis, or TB. Signs of associated systemic disease such as skin lesions, subcutaneous nodules, abscesses, or draining sinuses should be cultured, biopsied, or stained with India ink. Skin tests for TB and serological testing for human immunodeficiency virus, histoplasmosis, and coccidioidomycosis may be undertaken in select patients.

The differential diagnosis of chronic meningitis includes TB, neurosyphilis, brucellosis, actinomycetes infections, protozoal infections, meningeal carcinomatosis or lymphoma, benign lymphocytic meningitis, parameningeal bacterial infection, the uveomeningitic syndromes (sarcoid, Behçet's disease, Vogt-Koyanagi-Harada syndrome), granulomatous angiitis, collagen vascular disorders, hemosiderosis, resolving subarachnoid hemorrhage, subdural hematoma, and drug reactions.

Because tuberculous meningitis is the most common cause of chronic meningitis, an empiric trial of anti-TB drugs is appropriate in cases of undiagnosed chronic meningitis. As experience with oral antifungal agents increases, empiric use of one of the oral agents, such as fluconazole, may be recommended in the future. Empiric therapy with amphotericin B should be restricted to cases of chronic meningitis undiagnosed despite meningeal tissue biopsy. Neurosurgical intervention is indicated for ventricular shunting, exploration of a mass or focal lesion, and for brain or meningeal biopsies in undiagnosed patients with clinical deterioration.

Parenchymal Syndromes

All the major fungi can produce either meningitis or focal CNS lesions. Fungal CNS infections may present as subacute syndromes with headache and localizing signs, seizures, decrements in mentation or consciousness, and evidence of increased intracranial pressure, with or without fever. Fungal CNS infections cause diffuse granulomatous infiltrates, solitary abscess, multiple microabscesses or macroabscesses, or vasculitis disease, spanning several neuropathological categories of meningeal and parenchymal brain or spinal cord disease. There is often overlap between meningeal, vasculitic, and parenchymal disease (Figure 59C.1).

Large space-occupying abscesses or granulomas are associated with *Cryptococcus*, *Aspergillus*, *Mucor*, *Candida*, *Blastomyces*, *Pseudallescheria*, and the dematiaceous fungi. Biopsy is indicated for solitary or accessible brain lesions when a diagnosis cannot be made by less invasive means. A polysaccharide capsule around the cell wall is characteristic of only one pathogen for humans, *Cryptococcus neoformans*, but occasionally *Sporothrix schenkii* in the brain or eye may be encapsulated when examined in neuropathology specimens. Resection is required for dematiaceous fungi cases.

Acute syndromes, such as the rhinocerebral syndrome, stroke, or epidural cord compression, also are associated with fungal infections. The rhinocerebral syndrome is a progressive fungal infection affecting the sinuses, orbit, and brain (DeShazo et al. 1997). An acute, invasive fungal sinusitis, beginning with nasal stuffiness and discharge, is followed by the development of a painless, necrotic black palatal or nasal septal ulcer or eschar, and rapid spread of infection to contiguous soft tissue, orbit, skull, and intracranial sites. Spread of infection is signaled by face pain and headache, fever, orbital cellulitis, proptosis, eye movement abnormalities, orbital apex syndrome, or cavernous sinus or internal carotid artery thromboses.

The rhinocerebral syndrome is caused by saprophytic fungi of the order Mucorales; also by *Aspergillus*, *Fusarium*, *Pseudallescheria*, and the dark-walled dematiaceous fungi. The syndrome is seen in diabetics, particularly with ketoacidosis, leukemic patients who have been neutropenic for long periods of time and receive broad-spectrum antibiotics, organ transplant recipients, patients receiving deferoxamine chelation therapy for hemochromatosis, individuals with protein-calorie malnutrition or lactic acidosis, and, rarely, in previously healthy people. The diagnosis is suspected in diabetic patients in whom depressed consciousness fails to improve after metabolic abnormalities have been corrected, or in diabetic patients with very high CSF glucose concentrations reflecting uncontrolled diabetes.

Neuroimaging studies are indicated to visualize sinus, soft tissue, or orbit infection and to guide to areas of potential surgical exploration. Mucosal thickening or air–fluid levels on sinus roentgenography, or erosion of bone in the walls of the sinus or orbit on computed tomographic scan suggest the diagnosis. Magnetic resonance imaging can show soft tissue, sinus, orbit, or contiguous cerebral infection or infarction (see Figure 59C.2). Diagnosis is made by demonstration of the organism in the biopsied tissue specimen. The differential diagnosis includes aggressive orbital tumors and bacterial sinus or periorbital infection with septic venous thrombosis. Treatment includes surgical débridement, correction of underlying medical conditions, and amphotericin B. Untreated, the fungus may disseminate rapidly by vascular routes, causing death within days.

Cerebrovascular complications of systemic fungal infection arise in several settings. *Aspergillus* and members of the order Mucorales are infarctive as a consequence of hyphal invasion and subsequent occlusion or thrombosis of large cerebral blood vessels. Small vessel thromboses formed by pseudohyphae or hyphae, or microinfarcts surrounding areas of vasculitis, account for smaller infarcts in association with *Candida* or *Cryptococcus*, for example. Meningeal and subarachnoid inflammatory reactions may contribute to vasculitic occlusion of passing vessels. Fungal endocarditis, most commonly caused by *Candida*, may produce emboli; vessel wall erosion and, less commonly, subarachnoid hemorrhage caused by a ruptured mycotic aneurysm, may occur. Spinal syndromes may result from direct extension of vertebral infection caused by *Blastomyces*, *Coccidioides*, *Cryptococcus*, or *Aspergillus*, and less often, emboli.

PATHOGENS

Cryptococcus neoformans

Cryptococcus is the most common cause of clinically recognized fungal meningitis and meningocerebral syndromes. Cryptococcosis is a systemic infection caused by the encapsulated yeast fungus, *Cryptococcus neoformans*, which is present in soil and pigeon excreta worldwide. Infection occurs by inhalation. Although mild pulmonary symptoms may be the first sign of cryptococcal infection, the most common presentation in the normal (immunocompetent) host is meningitis. Others may present with cerebral abscesses or an isolated granulomatous lesion, a cryptococcoma. Rarely, chronic cases of cryptococcal meningitis may masquerade as a progressive dementia. Whether a patient's course is indolent or rapid may correlate with the degree of simultaneous immunosuppression. In cases of longer survival, cystic lesions, hydrocephalus, and hyponatremia may

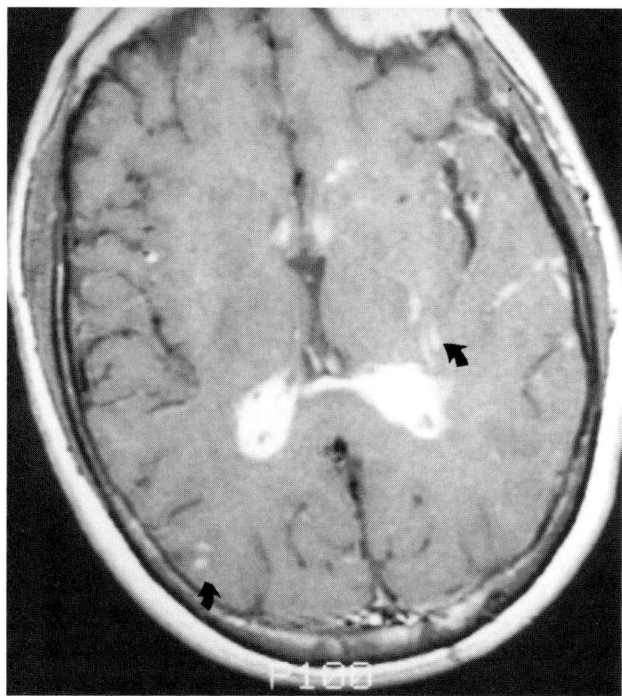

FIGURE 59C.1 Cryptococcal meningitis. Axial T1 gadolinium magnetic resonance image showing abnormal enhancement of subarachnoid space, perivascular spaces (*arrows*), and ventricles. (Courtesy of J. Healy.)

develop. Signs of disseminated disease include papular or ulcerative skin changes, lytic bone lesions, or prostatitis.

Diagnosis of CNS cryptococcal infection relies on detection of cryptococcal polysaccharide antigen by latex agglutination, demonstration of the organism in India ink preparations of CSF (Figure 59C.3), or CSF culture. Approximately 50% of CSF India ink preparations and 75% of CSF culture results are positive in cases of cryptococcal meningitis. The latex agglutination test for cryptococcal polysaccharide antigen is sensitive and specific for cryptococcal infection; initial CSF cryptococcal antigen titers of less than 1 to 256 often predict a better therapeutic response. In some cases, elevated CSF pressure is associated with vision loss and may be a poor prognostic sign.

Standard therapy for cryptococcal CNS infection in immunocompetent patients is intravenous amphotericin B (0.3–0.5 mg/kg/day) with oral flucytosine (150 mg/kg/day in four daily divided doses). The response in most patients is good, with success rates of 75–85%, but therapy is required for 4–6 weeks or longer (Sanchez and Noskin 1996). In the immunosuppressed host without AIDS, amphotericin B dosing is often increased to 0.7 mg/kg per day (Sarosi and Davies 1994). If used as monotherapy, treatment with amphotericin B is extended to 10 weeks or until blood and CSF culture results are negative for a minimum of 4 weeks. Before treatment is stopped, it should be demonstrated that the CSF glucose is normal and that

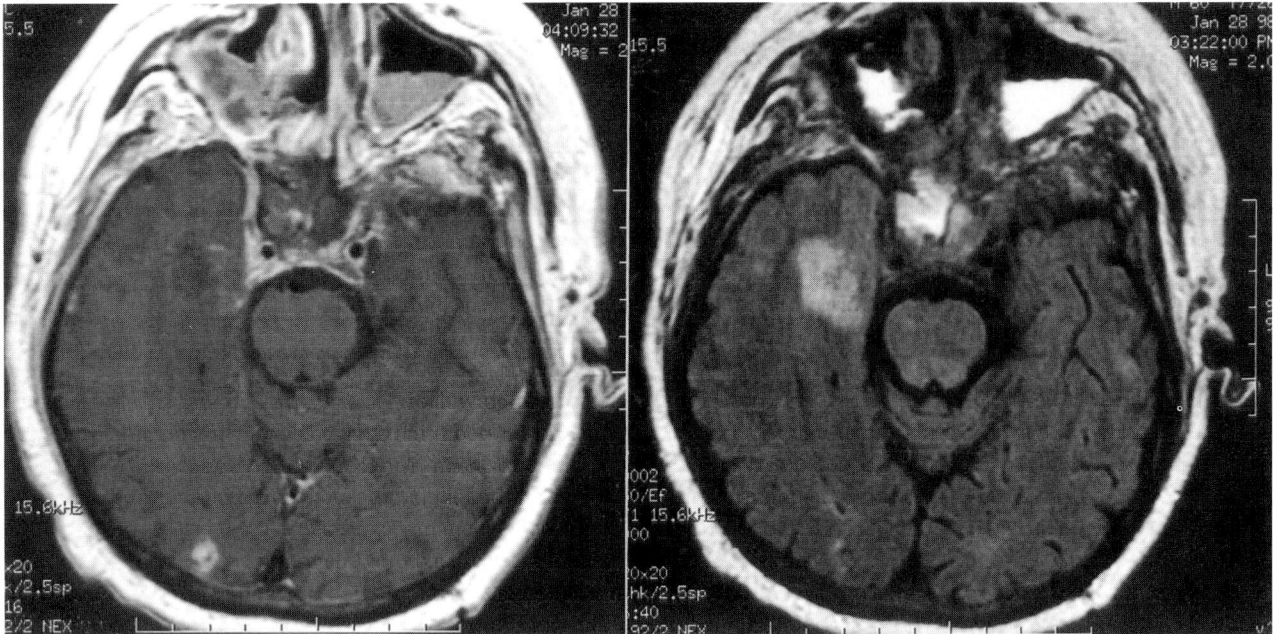

FIGURE 59C.2 *Mucor* sinusitis/mucormycosis. Gadolinium-enhanced T1 axial image showing perineural invasion of right cavernous sinus, breakdown of the blood-brain barrier in the right temporal lobe and right occipital lobe, and subtle pial enhancement around the pons. Axial magnetic resonance fluid attenuation inversion recovery image, on right, shows air–fluid levels in both maxillary sinuses as well as opacification of the sphenoid sinuses. Edema is seen in the medial temporal lobe. (Courtesy of T. Shimamoto.)

CSF protein should be declining (but need not be normal). India ink smear results may remain positive after culture results become negative, so positive smear results do not necessarily indicate active disease. Oral fluconazole, at doses of 400–800 mg per day, has been suggested as an alternative treatment for cryptococcal meningitis, but its efficacy in non-AIDS patients has not been well established. Because relapse rates of 20–25% have been described in the first year after therapy, patients should be followed with urine, sputum, and CSF cultures for at least 1 year after treatment.

Coccidioides immitis

Coccidioidomycosis, an infrequent cause of meningeal or vertebral infection, is a disease that follows inhalation of airborne spores of *Coccidioides immitis*, a highly infectious fungus that exists in soils in the arid zones of the western and southwestern United States (the San Joaquin Valley or Lower Sonoran Deserts), and similar geological areas of Central and South America. Although the majority of cases are self-limited, chronic pulmonary disease, skin disease, or disseminated disease occur in approximately 1% of patients. Male subjects, the very old and very young, noncaucasian races, pregnant women, and immunosuppressed individuals appear to be at a higher risk for dissemination. Osteoarticular disease including lytic skull and vertebral lesions is seen in approximately one-third of patients with disseminated disease. Portions of the vertebral arch are involved initially, which is distinct from TB, in which the vertebral body and disc space are first infected.

Meningitis usually occurs within 6 months of symptomatic or asymptomatic primary infection and may be the initial manifestation of disease. Signs and symptoms of CNS involvement are often subtle or nonspecific. Headache is common, but frank meningeal signs are usually absent. Fever, weakness, behavior changes, mental slowness, ataxia, vomiting, seizures, cranial nerve palsies, or focal deficits may be seen, along with a neuroradiological picture of a basilar meningitis (Figure 59C.4). The CSF shows a mononuclear, or occasionally eosinophilic, pleocytosis, elevated protein, and low glucose. In meningeal disease, 70% of patients have positive complement fixing antibody in the CSF; less than one-half have positive CSF culture results. Rarely, patients have only a positive antibody or culture result at the time of presentation.

In many patients, especially those who are immunocompetent and awake, oral fluconazole (minimum dosage, 400 mg/day) has obviated the need for intrathecal amphotericin B for coccidioidal meningitis (Galgiani et al. 1993; Kauffman 1997). However, therapy is usually prolonged (at least 12 months) and may be required for life, because relapses often occur once the drug is stopped. Immunosuppressed hosts without AIDS usually require fluconazole for life. For those patients who do not respond to fluconazole or whose mental status is impaired at presentation, systemic and intrathecal amphotericin B may be necessary (Sarosi and

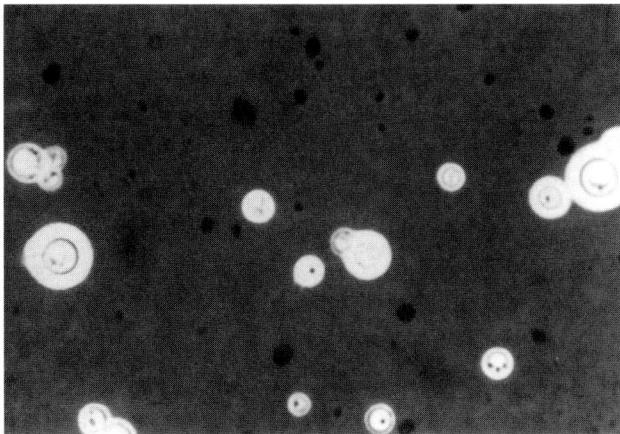

FIGURE 59C.3 An India ink preparation of cerebrospinal fluid revealing numerous cryptococci with wide, optically clear capsules. (Courtesy of R. Kim.)

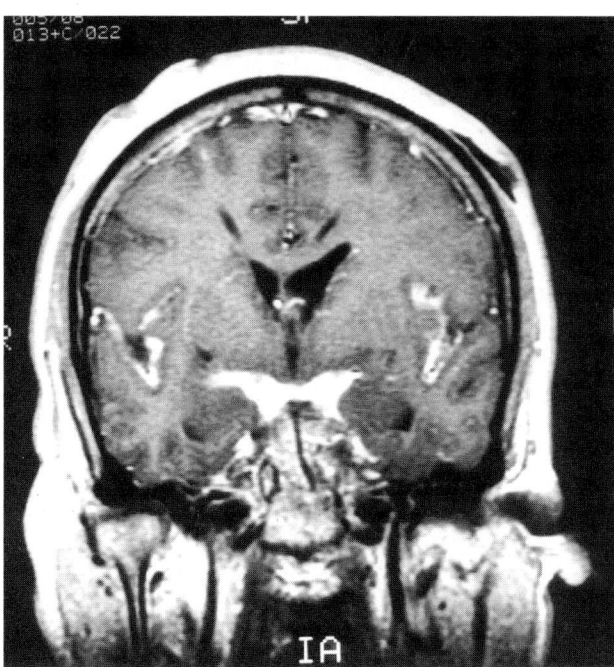

FIGURE 59C.4 Coccidioidomycoctic meningitis. T1 coronal magnetic resonance image with gadolinium showing abnormal enhancement in suprasellar cistern, basal cisterns, sylvian fissures, and along convexity. (Courtesy of J. Healy.)

Davies 1994). With improvement, change to fluconazole (400–800 mg/day) for at least 12 months may be possible. Response to treatment is followed with CSF complement-fixing antibody titers. Because of the predilection of *C. immitis* for the basal meninges, lumbar or cisternal CSF are better indicators of disease activity than ventricular CSF.

Paracoccidioides brasiliensis

Paracoccidioidomycosis is a systemic infection caused by *Paracoccidioides brasiliensis*. The disease is endemic in Central and South America, particularly Brazil. Usually a self-limited pulmonary infection, dissemination in immunosuppressed patients and, occasionally, younger patients produces progressive pulmonary disease, in addition to extrapulmonary involvement of skin, lymph nodes, mucosal surfaces, and the CNS. Cerebral and cerebellar masses have been recognized; yeast-phase organisms are found in biopsy tissue. Treatment, often difficult, includes amphotericin, itraconazole, or sulfonamides.

Histoplasma capsulatum

Histoplasmosis is a systemic fungal infection contracted through inhalation of infectious spores of *H. capsulatum*, originating in soil. *H. capsulatum* has a global distribution and grows well in soil containing bird excreta. Highly endemic areas in the United States include the Ohio, central Mississippi, and St. Lawrence river valleys.

Most primary infections are asymptomatic and many cases are diagnosed retrospectively by skin test conversion or chest roentgenography. Acute pulmonary histoplasmosis is an influenzalike illness that may be accompanied by erythematous skin lesions. The disseminated disease, which may be mistaken for miliary TB, is an acute or chronic febrile illness with diffuse pulmonary infiltrates, abnormal liver function, mucosal ulcerations, and, uncommonly, CNS disease in the form of basilar meningitis, focal cerebritis, or granulomas. Clinical evidence of CNS involvement includes headache and fever; nuchal rigidity is seen in only one-half of cases. Disseminated disease may occur soon after acute exposure or, should immunosuppression develop, long after the patient has left an endemic area. As in coccidioidomycosis, hematogenous dissemination is seen more frequently in immunocompromised individuals, male subjects, and at the very extremes of age.

CSF examination reveals a mixed WBC pleocytosis, elevated total protein, and normal to low glucose. Blood or bone marrow culture results may be positive. Otherwise, diagnosis depends on detection of antibodies by complement fixation. However, the sensitivity and specificity of serological tests are not high, and there is significant cross-reactivity with other fungal or granulomatous diseases. CSF cultures are rarely positive. There is currently a radioimmunoassay and a more investigational enzyme-linked immunosorbent assay for measurement of *Histoplasma* capsular antigen in blood and urine with better specificity (Durkin et al. 1997; Gomez et al. 1997). Antigen detection methods may provide a means of following treatment response. Although itraconazole is highly effective for treatment of histoplasmosis, amphotericin B is indicated for cases of life-threatening and CNS infection (Bradsher 1996). For both immunocompetent and immunosuppressed patients without AIDS, some authors suggest intravenous amphotericin B (500–1,000 mg total dose) until stable, followed by itraconazole (400 mg/day) for 6 months (Sarosi and Davies 1994). *Histoplasma* meningitis is difficult to treat, with cures in only approximately 50% of patients, and frequent relapses.

Blastomyces dermatitidis

Blastomycosis is a systemic disease caused by *Blastomyces dermatitidis*, which grows as a soil saprophyte, and humans contract disease after inhaling the infectious mycelial form. Most cases occur in North America, particularly in the Mississippi, Ohio, and St. Lawrence river basins, the Great Lakes area, and the southeastern United States. Primary infection is a mild, self-limited respiratory illness in immunocompetent individuals. The major clinical forms of blastomycosis are systemic and cutaneous, both of which may follow a pulmonary inception.

In the normal host, CNS disease is rare, affecting less than 5% of individuals with blastomycosis, but affecting up to 40% of patients with AIDS with the infection. CNS disease occurs as either intracranial or spinal abscesses or meningitis, with meningitis often a late and rapidly progressive complication of widely disseminated disease. Osteolytic, often painless, infection of vertebrae may develop and spread to contiguous soft tissue areas. Although endogenous reactivation of residual pulmonary disease has been reported in cell-mediated immunodeficiency patients, blastomycosis is so infrequently encountered as an opportunistic infection that it is not identified as an AIDS-defining infection.

Diagnosis relies on visualization or culture of the organism, which is extremely difficult or, more recently, a sandwich enzyme immunoassay; however, serodiagnosis of blastomycosis remains problematic (Areno et al. 1997). Although itraconazole is highly effective for immunocompetent patients with extraneural blastomycosis in the absence of life-threatening systemic disease, amphotericin B is the treatment of choice in the face of CNS involvement (Sarosi and Davies 1994; Bradsher 1996; Bradsher 1997). Increasing doses of intravenous amphotericin, to a total cumulative dose of 2,000–3,000 mg of intravenous amphotericin, with maximal doses of 1.5 mg/kg per day, are recommended, followed by itraconazole for 6 months in immunosuppressed patients without AIDS (Sarosi and Davies 1994). A protocol for incremental dosing for amphotericin B is presented in the therapeutic agent section below.

Candida albicans

Although many *Candida* species colonize the normal human respiratory, gastrointestinal, and genitourinary tracts, in immunodeficient patients, *Candida* species are important causes of nosocomial infections and agents of disseminated disease in immunodeficient patients. *C. albicans* is the most important pathogenic species with regard to CNS infection. At risk are patients with malignancies, severe disease or debilitation, patients receiving corticosteroids or broad-spectrum antibiotics, transplant recipients, critically ill neonates, and postoperative neurosurgery patients (Nguyen and Yu 1995). Disseminated candidiasis involves one or multiple organs, including the brain parenchyma, meninges, and eye. Cerebral abscesses, small vessel thromboses formed by pseudohyphae, and microinfarcts surrounding areas of vasculitis occur and tend to have a predilection for the middle cerebral artery. Eye and skin infections can provide helpful clues to the diagnosis of candidiasis. Patients with endophthalmitis note blurred vision, eye pain, or scotoma; white, cottonlike exudates are seen in the retina on funduscopic examination.

Nearly all patients with *Candida* meningitis have a CSF pleocytosis, usually lymphocytic, with cell counts of approximately 600 cells/µl. Low glucose and elevated protein may occur in 60%, and the organism may be seen on wet mount or Gram's stain in 40% of patients. Development of simple, reliable serological tests for the diagnosis of *Candida* has proven difficult; diagnosis therefore generally rests on demonstration of the fungus on CSF Gram's stain, wet mount, or culture. Treatment of CNS *Candida* usually includes intravenous or intrathecal amphotericin and flucytosine (Sanchez and Noskin 1996).

Aspergillus fumigatus

Aspergillus species, growing on stored grain or decaying vegetation, are ubiquitous in the environment and are agents of sinus disease, hypersensitivity pneumonitis, and invasive or disseminated infections. *A. fumigatus*, most often associated with human infections, causes CNS disease by direct extension or embolization (Figure 59C.5). In immunosuppressed patients, particularly transplant recipients, cerebral vascular occlusion and strokes follow dissemination of *Aspergillus* from a primary pulmonary process and the posterior circulation is particularly vulnerable. In nonimmunosuppressed patients, strokelike syndromes may result from vasculitis or parenchymal granulomas. Nonimmunosuppressed patients more commonly develop progressive focal neurological disease, with signs and symptoms of brain abscess. Invasive *Aspergillus* sinusitis is one cause of the rhinocerebral syndrome and invasive pulmonary *Aspergillus* may extend to the thoracic vertebrae and epidural space, causing cord compression. Meningitis caused by *Aspergillus* is rare, but has occurred after drug abuse or transsphenoidal surgery.

CSF examination reveals a mixed (but often predominantly neutrophilic) pleocytosis, elevated protein, and normal glucose. There is currently no reliable serodiagnostic marker for aspergillosis infection; diagnosis rests on demonstration of tissue invasion on biopsy (Sanchez and Noskin 1996). Treatment of invasive aspergillosis is by surgical débridement of necrotic tissue in addition to prolonged amphotericin B, usually in doses up to 1.5 mg/kg per day intravenously (Sanchez and Noskin 1996). Of the orally administered agents, itraconazole has the best activity against aspergillosis; once the disease has been stabilized, itraconazole can be administered in dosages of 400–800 mg per day (Sarosi and Davies 1994).

Zygomycetes rhizopus (Mucor)

Zygomycosis is the unifying term for the various diseases caused by saprophytic fungi of the class Zygomycetes. The zygomycoses are sporadic diseases with worldwide distribution and include the order Mucorales, common fungi occurring on decaying vegetation or foods of high sugar content. Invariably, compromised host resistance is present when CNS infection occurs. Diabetes and acidosis are the most frequent predisposing conditions; however, malignancies, high-dose corticosteroids, and renal transplantation also have been described as underlying conditions.

The clinical forms of mucormycosis include pulmonary disease, cutaneous disease, rhino(orbito)cerebral mucormycosis, and cerebral mucormycosis, occurring after open head trauma or intravenous drug use. A vascular invasive fungus, Mucor produces occlusive, ischemic lesions in one or several anatomically related sites. Within the CNS, zygomycosis causes an acute necrotizing tissue reaction and thrombosis of neighboring vessels. Cavernous sinus and internal carotid artery thromboses are common. In either the rhinocerebral syndrome or open head wound cases, a black discharge indicates necrosis of underlying tissue and should suggest the diagnosis of mucormycosis. In the eye, ischemic changes may be indicated by vision loss with optic nerve pallor, corneal ulcer, ocular gangrene, choroidal infarction, and central retinal or ophthalmic artery occlusion.

Like aspergillosis, serodiagnostic tests for mucormycosis remain insensitive (Sanchez and Noskin 1996). Patients are treated by aggressively débriding necrotic tissue and with amphotericin B (Sanchez and Noskin 1996; Sarosi and Davies 1994). Sensory changes in a V_1 distribution only, sparing V_2 and V_3, suggest disease might be confined to the orbit, and there is a chance of surgical cure by radical orbital exenteration for these cases. Overall, mortality from rhinocerebral mucormycosis is greater than 50%.

Other Pathogens

Sporotrichosis, infection by Sporothrix schenkii, causes either superficial or deep infection, and disseminated infections with meningitis in patients with human immunodeficiency virus. Cutaneous lesions appear as either a single, chronic ulcer, or multiple ulcers spread along regional lymphatics. Disseminated lesions affect the meninges, joints, or lungs. Diagnosis is by culture, biopsy, skin test, or antibody

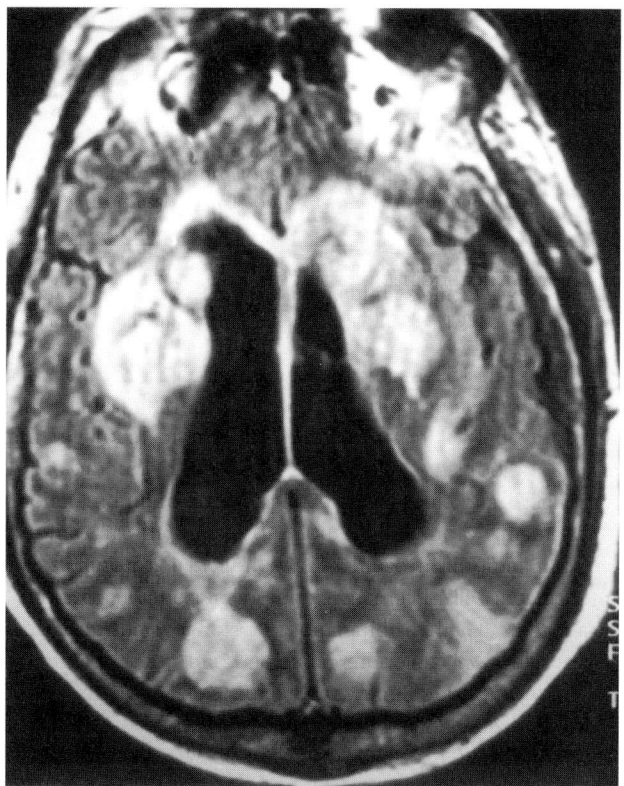

FIGURE 59C.5   Central nervous system *Aspergillus*. Axial magnetic resonance fluid attenuation inversion recovery sequence showing multiple areas of high signal intensity in the basal ganglia, centrum semiovale, and the gray-white junction of parietal and occipital cortices. (Courtesy of J. Healy.)

in the CSF or serum. The cutaneous forms are treated with itraconazole for 2–4 months; meningitic forms with amphotericin B either systemically or intrathecally.

The dematiaceous fungi, or *Phaeohyphomycoses*, common environmental molds with brown pigmented walls, are rare causes of CNS abscesses in immunocompetent hosts. *Cladosporium trichoides* is the most common isolate of this group. Surgical resection is required for cure of superficial infections, plus amphotericin B if intracranial extension occurs.

Pseudallescheria boydii is another uncommon, opportunistic pathogen with poor response to antifungals and high mortality, which characteristically presents as a neutrophilic meningitis or multiple brain abscesses. Factors predisposing to CNS infection include immunosuppression or near drowning with aspiration of contaminated water.

THERAPEUTIC AGENTS

Amphotericin B is the most reliable agent against nearly all of the invasive mycoses; however, the introduction of the triazoles, itraconazole and fluconazole, and newer

Table 59C.1:   Therapy for central nervous system fungal infections

Organism	Immunocompetent host	Immunosuppressed host without acquired immunodeficiency syndrome
Cryptococcus neoformans	Amphotericin B, 0.3–0.5 mg/kg/day, with flucytosine, 150 mg/kg/day (in four divided doses) for 6 wks *or* amphotericin B, 0.3–0.5 mg/kg/day for 10 wks	Amphotericin B, 0.7 mg/kg/day, with flucytosine, 150 mg/kg/day (in four divided doses) for at least 6 wks
Coccidioides immitis	Fluconazole, 400–800 mg/day for 12 mos or longer *or* amphotericin B, 0.3–0.5 mg/kg/day, followed by fluconazole, 400–800 mg/day for at least 12 mos	Amphotericin B, 0.3–0.5 mg/kg/day, followed by fluconazole, 400–800 mg/day for life
Histoplasma capsulatum	Amphotericin B, 500–1,000 mg total until stable, followed by itraconazole, 400 mg/day for 6 mos	Amphotericin B, 1,000 mg total until stable, followed by itraconazole, 400 mg/day for 6 mos
Blastomyces dermatitidis	Amphotericin B, 2,000–3,000 mg total until stable, followed by itraconazole, 400 mg/day for 6 mos	Amphotericin B, 2,000–3,000 mg total until stable, followed by itraconazole, 400 mg/day for 6–12 mos
Candida albicans	Amphotericin B, 0.3–0.5 mg/kg/day, with flucytosine, 150 mg/kg/day (in four divided doses) for 4–6 wks	Amphotericin B, 0.3–0.5 mg/kg/day, with flucytosine, 150 mg/kg/day (in four divided doses) for 4–6 wks
Aspergillus fumigatus	Amphotericin B, 0.7–1.5 mg/kg/day, followed by itraconazole, 400–800 mg/day	Amphotericin B, 1.5 mg/kg/day, followed by itraconazole, 400–800 mg/day
Zygomycetes rhizopus	Amphotericin B, 1.5 mg/kg/day	Amphotericin B, 1.5 mg/kg/day

fungicidal agents has expanded our therapeutic options. Except for coccidiomycosis and perhaps paracoccidiomycosis or *Pseudallescheria boydii* infections, all CNS fungal infections are treated with amphotericin B. New protocols using fluconazole alone for the treatment of coccidioides have been established. Sulfonamides or itraconazole are used for *Paracoccidioides brasiliensis* and itraconazole for *Pseudallescheria boydii*. Miconazole and ketoconazole currently have no role in the primary treatment of serious CNS fungal infections. No universal consensus as to optimal regimen, total dose, or total duration of therapy exists, in part because of the great variability in clinical response, extent of infection, and patients' tolerance of the drugs.

Amphotericin B

Amphotericin B is the treatment of choice for most fungal infections of the CNS, particularly those that are life-threatening (Table 59C.1). It is a polyene that preferentially binds to fungal cytoplasmic membrane sterols, increasing membrane permeability. Because of poor oral and intramuscular absorption, amphotericin B should be given by the intravenous or intrathecal route. It is refrigerated as a powder, reconstituted with sterile water (without a bacteriostatic agent), and administered at a concentration of 0.1 mg/ml of 5% dextrose in water for injection. A colloidal preparation of this drug is also available for intravenous or intrathecal administration. A test dose of 1 mg by slow infusion has been advocated to assess for severe hypotension or anaphylaxis. Otherwise, the usual initial recommended dose, after a minimum of 4 hours, is 0.25 mg/kg per day in a single dose administered slowly over 2–6 hours. If this is well-tolerated,

the daily dose may be increased by increments of 0.25 mg/kg per day to a maximum of 1.5 mg/kg per day. After intravenous administration, the serum half-life is approximately 24–48 hours. The drug is slowly eliminated by the kidneys; however, renal impairment does not appear to significantly change excretion. Thus, the intent of dosage alteration in the setting of renal impairment is to protect the kidneys against further drug-induced toxicity.

Side effects are common, often serious, and treatment limiting with amphotericin. Renal impairment, sometimes irreversible, is the most significant adverse reaction associated with amphotericin, especially if the total dose exceeds 4–5 g. Thus, it is important to monitor renal function carefully throughout treatment. Lipid-containing formulations of amphotericin B, only recently approved, may significantly reduce its nephrotoxicity; however, their comparative efficacy versus conventional amphotericin is not established. During the infusion period, fever, chills, headache, anorexia, nausea, vomiting, malaise, and pain at the infusion site may occur with amphotericin. Premedication with antipyretics, antihistamines, and antiemetics may reduce the severity of these reactions; intravenous meperidine rapidly terminates shaking chills. With repeated administration, thrombophlebitis, normocytic anemia, hypokalemia, and hypomagnesemia, all generally reversible, can be seen. Nephrotoxicity, when it occurs, can sometimes be handled by holding the medication until renal function normalizes or switching to alternate-day dosing. Blood cell counts, electrolytes, and renal and liver function should be monitored. The recommended duration of treatment is 6–8 weeks or 4 weeks after the last positive culture result. When amphotericin is combined with flucytosine (see Flucytosine, later in this chapter), therapy can be shortened to 3–6 weeks.

Intrathecal administration of amphotericin may be necessary in the face of severe illness or immunosuppression, if there is no improvement after 4 weeks, or if disease recurs despite a complete course of intravenous therapy. When amphotericin is given intrathecally by lumbar puncture or through an Ommaya reservoir, a maximum dose of 0.50 mg twice a week is generally used. A test dose of 0.025 mg is given initially. This is followed every second day by doses that are increased in increments of 0.025 mg until a level of 0.50 mg is attained. In addition to blood monitoring, all CSF samples should be examined carefully. The most common adverse reactions to intrathecal administration of amphotericin B include chemical meningitis, cranial nerve palsies, and paresthesias; less frequently, encephalopathy, convulsions, and even paraplegia have been described. Secondary bacterial infections of shunts, shunt occlusions, and hydrocephalus as a result of arachnoid adhesions should be anticipated as possible complications of intrathecal amphotericin treatment.

Flucytosine

Flucytosine is a fluorinated cytosine analogue that appears to be deaminated to the cytotoxic antimetabolite fluorouracil by an enzyme present in fungal, but not human cells. It probably interferes with DNA synthesis. Flucytosine is indicated for serious infections involving *Candida* or *Cryptococcus* in combination with amphotericin. It should not be used as a single agent because of treatment failures as a result of the development of resistant strains. For this reason, it is usually administered in conjunction with amphotericin B and, because of their synergy, allows use of a lower dose of amphotericin. Flucytosine is well absorbed after oral administration, has adequate penetration of the CNS, and is eliminated by the kidneys. Serum half-life of flucytosine is only 3–5 hours; therefore, it is usually given at 6-hour intervals. The recommended oral dosage of flucytosine is 100–150 mg/kg per day, in four divided doses. Serum levels should be monitored to keep the peak concentrations between 50 and 100 µg/ml. Dosage must be reduced in the presence of impaired renal function, and regimens involving reduced dosage at 6-hour dosing intervals have been recommended. Prolonged high serum levels of flucytosine may result in hair loss, bone marrow depression, and abnormal liver function. These reactions are uncommon at normal therapeutic doses and usually reverse following dosage reduction or discontinuation of the drug.

Fluconazole

Fluconazole is a synthetic bistriazole that can be given orally or intravenously and most likely acts by inhibiting sterol synthesis in fungal membranes. It is used to treat coccidioidal meningitis. In addition, in patients with cryptococcal meningitis, fluconazole is often used following induction with amphotericin B and flucytosine. Fluconazole is well absorbed after oral administration and is eliminated by the kidneys, with a serum half-life of 20–50 hours. It is generally well tolerated and has good CNS penetration. The recommended dosage, either orally or intravenously, is 200–400 mg per day. Often, it is administered as 400 mg per day for 3 days followed by 200 mg per day for a period of 10 days to 3 months. Headache, nausea, vomiting, abdominal pain, and diarrhea are the most common adverse effects of fluconazole. More serious, but rare, events include severe hepatic injury and Stevens-Johnson syndrome. Serum creatinine and liver function tests should be monitored at least weekly.

Itraconazole

Itraconazole is a triazole compound that inhibits fungal ergosterol synthesis, thus interfering with membrane function and permeability. It is effective for CNS histoplasmosis and blastomycosis after induction with amphotericin B. Following oral administration, absorption can be quite variable, although it is clearly increased when the drug is taken with food. Peak plasma itraconazole concentrations are achieved in 1.5–4.0 hours. Elimination half-life is approximately 20 hours after a single oral dose of 100 mg and approximately 30 hours after 2–4 weeks of therapy. The recommended oral dosage is 400 mg per day. It is generally well tolerated, although the incidence of side effects increases with duration of therapy. Gastrointestinal disturbances are the most common adverse events; hypokalemia and transient elevation of liver enzymes have been observed also.

REFERENCES

Areno J, Campbell GJ, George R. Diagnosis of blastomycosis. Semin Respir Infect 1997;12:252–262.

Bradsher R. Histoplasmosis and blastomycosis. Clin Infect Dis 1996;22(Suppl. 2):S102–S111.

Bradsher R. Therapy of blastomycosis. Semin Respir Infect 1997; 12:263–267.

DeShazo R, Chapin K, Swain R. Fungal sinusitis. N Engl J Med 1997; 337:254–259.

Durkin M, Connolly P, Wheat L. Comparison of radioimmunoassay and enzyme-linked immunoassay methods for detection of *Histoplasma capsulatum* var. *capsulatum* antigen. Clin Microbiol 1997;35:2252–2255.

Galgiani J, Catanzaro A, Cloud G, et al. Fluconazole therapy for coccidioidal meningitis, The NIAID-Mycoses Study Group. Ann Intern Med 1993;119:28–35.

Gomez B, Figueroa J, Hamilton A, et al. Development of a novel antigen detection test for histoplasmosis. J Clin Microbiol 1997;35:2618–2622.

Kauffman C, Carver RL. Antifungal agents in the 1990s: current status and future developments. Drugs 1997;53:539–549.

Nguyen M, Yu V. Meningitis caused by *Candida* species: an emerging problem in neurosurgical patients. Clin Infect Dis 1995;21:323–327.

Sanchez J, Noskin G. Recent advances in the management of opportunistic fungal infections. Compr Ther 1996;22:703–712.

Sarosi G, Davies S. Therapy for fungal infections. Mayo Clin Proc 1994;11:1111–1117.

Chapter 59
Infections of the Nervous System

D. PARASITIC INFECTIONS
Marylou V. Solbrig

Parasite is from the ancient Greek word, *parasitos*, one who eats at the table of another. The protozoa and helminths, remarkable for their biodiversity and environmental mastery, are important general and nervous system pathogens and chemotherapeutic challenges. Parasitic diseases can be counted among the most common diseases of humans as a result of vector proliferation, habitat change, occupational contact, immunosuppression, and bad luck.

The protozoa, single-celled organisms that can multiply in humans, include several major worldwide pathogens and agents of severe disease in patients with acquired immunodeficiency syndrome. They are agents of acute meningitis or meningoencephalitis (*Naegleria*, African trypanosomes), encephalopathy (the falciparum malaria parasites), subacute or chronic meningitides (*Acanthamoeba*, *Toxoplasma*), space-occupying lesions (*Toxoplasma*, *Entamoeba histolytica*), neuropathy (American trypanosomes, *Leishmania* species), myositis (malarial or *Sarcocystis* parasites), and the most common cause of infection of the retina (*Toxoplasma*).

Helminths, or worms, that cause central nervous system (CNS) disease are problems for humans because of their size, mobility, and challenge to the host immune system. For some, such as the schistosomes, humans are a normal host. Granulomas form around eggs or larval stages, but the worm usually completes its life cycle to the adult stage, which is more or less tolerated. Deposited eggs or larval forms enter the cerebral circulation or embolize from more distant sites to encyst, grow, or antigenically load the CNS. For zoonotic and human parasites less well-adapted to humans, such as another trematode, paragonimiasis, the adult stage may develop but not be well tolerated. Inflammatory reactions develop around both larval and adult forms, with resulting multiorgan inflammatory diseases. For

still others, such as *Gnathostoma* or *Toxocara* parasites, humans are an aberrant host; the parasite life cycle cannot be completed, but larvae remain in the body and elicit a continuing reaction. Similarly, humans are poorly tolerant of parasite life-cycle aberrations. When humans are the wrong host for one stage of the parasite, such as the larval stage, or cysticercal form of *Taenia solium*, the cysticercus also remains in the body, unable to complete its life cycle.

Clinical signs reflect the size and location of the parasite or its migratory path. Some tissue-invasive helminths migrate and enter the CNS through the foramen of the skull or vertebral column, or through connective tissue surrounding nerves or vessels. Exposure history, the presence of peripheral eosinophilia, or elevated IgE levels increase the physician's suspicion of helminth infection.

Ectoparasites attach to host surfaces and cause neurological diseases by toxin release or by the excavation of sinus tracts from a mucosal or skin surface into the CNS.

For most pathogens, definitive diagnosis depends on classic parasitological techniques, aided by serology, antibody or antigen enzyme-linked immunosorbent assay (ELISA) format or nucleic acid detection techniques, neuroimaging, and pathology. A diagnosis of one pathogen does not exclude all others. A host permissive for one may well harbor others, and the course of advanced (parasitic) illness may be punctuated by recurrent or severe concurrent viral or bacterial infections.

Treatment of parasitic diseases, as in all infectious diseases, is rendered difficult by the toxicity of existing chemotherapeutic agents and the emergence of resistant strains. Among the antiparasitic drugs are the most neurotoxic of all antimicrobials (Table 59D.1, Plate 59D.I), which complicate the neurological outcome of many cases.

Table 59D.1: Antiparasitic drugs with significant toxicities

Drug	Indications	Neurotoxicity
Diethylcarbamazine	Loiasis, filariasis	Encephalopathy
Melarsoprol	African trypanosomiasis (*Trypanosoma brucei rhodesiense*)	Arsenical encephalopathy
Nifurtimox	American trypanosomiasis, arsenic-resistant *Trypanosoma brucei gambiense*	Encephalopathy (convulsions, psychosis) neuralgia, paresthesias
Benznidazole	American trypanosomiasis	Neuropathy
Pentavalent antimonials	Leishmaniasis	Myositis, neuropathy
Stilbamidine	Pentavalent antimony-resistant leishmaniasis	Trigeminal neuralgia
Quinine	Falciparum malaria	Cinchonism (tinnitus, headache, vomiting, blurred vision)
Chloroquine	Malaria	Peripheral neuropathy, myopathy, retinopathy (>5 yrs prophylaxis) (see Plate 59D.I)
Clioquinol	Amebic dysentery use in the 1950s and 1960s	Subacute myelo-optic-neuropathy

EOSINOPHILIC MENINGITIS

Eosinophilic meningitis, the presence of eosinophils in the cerebrospinal fluid (CSF), is caused by certain helminth and protozoan parasites as well as other infectious and noninfectious processes. The principal agent is the rat lungworm, *Angiostrongylus cantonensis*, known to produce CSF eosinophilic responses of 10–90% while growing on the surface of the brain and spinal cord and in the subarachnoid spaces. Although few pathogens achieve this intensity of CSF eosinophilia, eosinophilic meningeal reactions also occur with gnathostomiasis, neural larva migrans (*Toxocara* and *Baylisascaris* species), cysticercosis, echinococcosis, paragonimiasis, schistosomiasis, trichinosis, strongyloidiasis, onchocerciasis, loiasis, myiasis, amebic meningoencephalitis, trypanosomiasis, coccidioidomycosis, cryptococcosis and tuberculosis (TB). Noninfectious causes include CNS malignancies (leukemias and lymphomas), drugs (nonsteroidal anti-inflammatory agents and antibiotics), and myelography dye reactions, ventriculoperitoneal shunt implantation or malfunction.

The three major parasitic agents causing eosinophilic meningitis, *A. cantonensis*, *Gnathostoma spinigerum*, and *Baylisascaris procyonis*, are zoonoses, natural parasites of animals, that fail to mature to adulthood to replicate in humans. Although each may cause severe disease, as infections, they are therefore self-limited in the human host. The neurotropism of *A. cantonensis* and *B. procyonis* in the human host is perhaps a recapitulation of their nervous system localizations in their natural hosts (Weller and Liu 1993).

Spinal fluid with high eosinophil levels does not appear turbid, as in purulent meningitis, but has the clumped texture and appearance of "water after it has been used to wash rice." Eosinophils are fragile cells and may require prompt and specialized specimen handling and examination. Eosinophilic spinal fluid, examined for parasites, also may reveal larvae of *A. cantonensis*, procyclic forms of African trypanosomes, trophozoites of the free-living ameba (*Naegleria fowleri* or *Acanthamoeba* species) or *Entamoeba histolytica*, microfilariae of *Onchocerca volvulus* or *Loa loa*, and cysts or immature larvae of *Trichinella spiralis* and establish a definitive diagnosis. The absence of focal brain parenchymal lesions on neuroimaging studies usually favors a diagnosis of *A. cantonensis*, with its tendency for meningeal, subarachnoid, and brain surface localization.

Tissue damage in cases of eosinophilic meningitis or encephalitis is partly by deposition of toxic eosinophil proteins, some of which are thrombogenic. Therapies are often aimed both at treating the specific pathogen and alleviating the general symptoms of disease. When the antiparasitic drug has poor tissue penetration or CNS activity, treatments to eliminate luminal or other accessible infections are used, together with corticosteroids to inhibit eosinophil activation, degranulation, and CNS cytotoxicity.

Parasitic infections of the CNS are summarized in Table 59D.2. Here we discuss the epidemiological and clinical features of parasitic infections of the central and peripheral nervous systems.

DISEASES OF PROTOZOANS

Malaria

Malaria, caused by protozoa of the genus *Plasmodium*, is the most important parasitic disease of humans, with more than 500 million clinical cases each year throughout the world and at least 1 million malaria-related deaths in Africa. One-third of all humanity live in malaria areas and malaria kills one person, often a child under 5, every 12 seconds. Cerebral malaria is an acute, diffuse encephalopathy, with fever occurring in 0.5–1.0% of cases of *P. falciparum*. Unrecognized, it kills within 72 hours.

Ecology and Transmission

Malaria is found throughout Africa, Asia, Central and South America, Oceania, on some Caribbean islands, and, with increasing frequency, as an import in North America and

Table 59D.2: Parasitic infections of the central nervous system

Parasite	Range	Meningo-encephalitis	Encepha-lopathy	Seizures	Mass lesion	Stroke	Spinal cord	Ocular
Protozoans								
Plasmodium falciparum	Africa, South America, Southeast Asia, Pacific Islands, Haiti		+	+				
Naegleria fowleri	Southern United States, Australia, Europe	+						
Acanthamoeba sp.	Europe	+			+			+
Entamoeba histolytica	Tropics worldwide				+			
Trypanosoma brucei rhodesiense	Africa	+						
Trypanosoma brucei gambiense	Africa	+						
Trypanosoma cruzi	Central and South America	+			+	+		
Toxoplasma gondii	Worldwide	+		+	+			+
Helminths								
Cestodes								
Taenia solium	Worldwide	+		+	+		+	+
Echinococcus granulosus	Worldwide			+	+		+	+
Echinococcus multilocularis	Arctic			+	+			
Taenia multiceps	Worldwide				+			+
Spirometra sp.	Worldwide, mainly Asia, Africa	+		+	+	+		
Nematodes								
Trichinella sp.	Worldwide	+	+	+		+		
Angiostrongylus cantonensis	Asia, Africa, Pacific, Caribbean	+		+				+
Gnathostoma spinigerum	Asia, Israel	+		+	+	+	+	+
Onchocerca volvulus	Africa, Central and South America, Yemen							
Loa loa	Africa		+					+
Toxocara sp.	Worldwide	+		+				+
Baylisascaris procyonis	Worldwide	+		+				
Strongyloides stercoralis	Worldwide	+				+		
Ascaris lumbricoides	Worldwide	+		+				
Halicephalobus deletrix	North America	+						
Trematodes								
Schistosome sp.	Africa, Asia, Brazil	+		+	+	+	+	
Paragonimus sp.	Asia, Central and South America	+		+	+	+	+	
Fasciola hepatica	Worldwide	+		+	+	+		

Europe. Natural transmission of all *Plasmodium* species causing human malaria is by the female *Anopheles* mosquito. Laboratory accident, blood transfusion, experimental infection, and zoonotic infection have accounted for additional cases.

Clinical Features

The incubation period is influenced by the species of malaria parasite, the degree of acquired immunity, and the dose inoculated. In nonimmune patients, the incubation period for *P. falciparum* is approximately 12 days, ranging from 6 to 25 days, and prophylactic drugs may extend the incubation period. The prodromal symptoms of lassitude, myalgia,

headache, and chills may occur before an acute attack. Typical attacks sequentially show shaking chills, fever to 105°F, then diaphoresis, with the periodicity of fever determined by the length of the asexual cycle. In *P. falciparum*, fever is every third day. Other signs and symptoms may include backache, arthralgia, abdominal pain, nausea, vomiting, cough, tachypnea, and enlarged liver or spleen. Muscle pain and weakness, even necrosis, may occur because of increased blood viscosity or capillary obstruction.

The time of prodromal, systemic illness to cerebral malaria is from several days to 2 weeks in adults, but as short as 6–12 hours in children. Seizures with persistent unconsciousness is a common presentation, but clinical manifestations also include headache, meningismus, delirium, focal neurological features (aphasia, ataxia, hemiparesis), extrapyramidal signs (chorea, tremor, or rigidity), dysconjugate gaze, retinal hemorrhage (in up to 15% of patients), and papilledema (<1%).

The presence of CNS symptoms relates to the number of *P. falciparum* parasitized erythrocytes sequestered in cerebral vessels, but the pathogenesis of cerebral malaria is incompletely understood. There is evidence of an immune-mediated inflammatory reaction with release of proinflammatory cytokines that produce endothelial damage; increased intracranial pressure and blood-brain barrier permeability are sometimes found. Infected erythrocytes, adherent to vascular endothelium, produce microvascular congestion and tissue hypoxia, whereas hypoglycemia, a frequent complication of cerebral malaria, can produce or augment encephalopathy, depressed consciousness, or focal neurological signs.

Diagnosis

Diagnosis and species determination is by examination of thin blood films and an unspread drop of blood (thick film) stained with Giemsa. Ring-shaped trophozoites are seen within erythrocytes. If initial smear results are negative and falciparum infection is suspected, the smears are repeated at 6- to 8-hour intervals. Cerebral malaria as well as other complications of falciparum malaria are more likely if erythrocyte parasitemia exceeds 5% or if 10% of infected cells contain more than one parasite.

In cerebral malaria, the CSF is usually normal, but may have elevated protein levels (to 200 mg/dl) or mild lymphocytic pleocytosis (10–50 cells/μl). A computed tomographic (CT) scan or magnetic resonance imaging (MRI) can be normal or show slight brain swelling, generally attributed to increased intracerebral blood volume.

The signs and symptoms of malaria (fever, rigors, disturbed consciousness, jaundice, diarrhea, hemorrhage, renal failure, shock, or respiratory distress) are not specific. The differential diagnosis includes yellow fever, other viral hemorrhagic fevers, bacterial meningitis, relapsing fever, enteric infections, leptospirosis, and heat stroke.

Cases of cerebral malaria without confirmatory blood smears may occur; treatment with a broad-spectrum antibiotic, such as tetracycline, can suppress parasitemia and some symptoms. Cerebral malaria also may develop after presumed adequate treatment of malaria. A very ill patient with malaria exposure and a suggestive clinical picture should be treated for presumed cerebral malaria without delay.

Treatment

Because of widespread chloroquine-resistant falciparum malaria in Southeast Asia and sub-Saharan Africa, quinine is used first for the treatment of cerebral malaria in most areas. Quinine dihydrochloride, 7 mg/kg as a dextrose or saline intravenous solution, is infused over 30 minutes, followed by 10 mg/kg over 4 hours. Maintenance is with 10 mg/kg infused over 2–8 hours, and the maximum daily dose of quinine is 1,800 mg. Where intravenous quinine is not available, intravenous quinidine gluconate as a 10 mg/kg loading dose, followed by 0.02 mg/kg per minute, is an alternative, and simultaneous cardiac monitoring is required. Intravenous treatment with either agent is continued for up to 72 hours, or until parasitemia drops to 1%. A change to oral administration is recommended as soon as medically feasible, and treatment is for a total of 7 days (White 1996).

Multidrug-resistant falciparum malaria (chloroquine-, sulfadoxine-pyrimethamine–, mefloquine-, and quinine-resistant) is treated with artemeter (derived from the traditional Chinese medicine *ginghaosu*), 160 mg intramuscularly as a loading dose, followed by 80 mg intramuscularly daily for 4 days, and mefloquine, 750 mg orally on the last day of treatment; or artesunate, a 2 mg/kg intravenous loading dose, followed by 1 mg/kg intravenously at 4 hours and 24 hours, then daily for 6 days (Nakamura et al. 1997). In patients with shock, the unpredictable absorption and distribution of intramuscular medications may limit the effectiveness of artemeter (Murphy et al. 1997).

Antimalarials should terminate acute attacks within 12–96 hours in falciparum infections, and blood smears should be examined during treatment. Recurrence of parasitemia after treatment of falciparum malaria may reflect either treatment failure or a delayed primary attack of vivax malaria.

Hypoglycemia can arise because of increased consumption by parasites, malabsorption, or increased pancreatic secretion of insulin induced by quinine and is treated by rapid infusion of 50% dextrose. Other complications of severe malaria include hemolytic anemia, renal failure, pulmonary edema, lactic acidosis, disseminated intravascular coagulation, shock, gastrointestinal hemorrhage, and gram-negative sepsis. Exchange transfusion is sometimes used for high parasitemia. Correction of lactic acidosis and anemia, anticonvulsant administration, and intracranial pressure monitoring in children are other aspects of patient care. Corticosteroids used with quinine prolong coma and worsen outcome, compared with quinine alone.

Cerebral malaria, potentially completely reversible, proves fatal in 20–50% of cases, especially among young children and nonimmune adults. Untreated cerebral malaria is 100% fatal. Hypoglycemia, lactic acidosis, and prolonged coma or seizures are poor prognostic signs. Concurrent human immunodeficiency virus (HIV) infection has not been related to severity of malaria, but progression or acceleration of HIV infection during malaria infection has been reported.

Uncomplicated chloroquine-resistant falciparum cases are treated with oral quinine sulfate (salt, 10 mg/kg every 8 hours for 7 days) plus pyrimethamine-sulfadoxine or quinine plus tetracycline in regions with known resistance to antifolates. Oral quinine can cause cinchonism with tinnitus, headache, nausea, and visual changes. Mefloquine, an alternative oral agent for treatment and prophylaxis, has been associated with psychotic side effects.

Delayed or late neurological complications, designated the *postmalaria neurological syndromes*, also occur. Patients who recover from cerebral malaria may relapse within 1–2 days into coma. The CSF contains elevated protein levels (200–300 mg/dl) with or without a lymphocytic pleocytosis. Poor, incomplete, or full recovery occurs. Another, more benign, postmalaria neurological syndrome follows uncomplicated malaria with *Plasmodium vivax* or mixed infections. Patients are aparasitemic when they develop psychosis, encephalopathy, seizures, tremor, or cerebellar ataxia, which lasts several days to weeks and is followed by complete recovery (White 1996). Oral mefloquine may be a risk factor for the postmalaria neurological syndrome (Nguyen et al. 1996).

Prevention

Prevention depends heavily on chemoprophylaxis during travel in endemic areas. Recommended medications include chloroquine (300 mg base per week), proguanil (100 or 200 mg/day), or mefloquine (250 mg/week). Country-specific recommendations are available from the Centers for Disease Control and Prevention, Atlanta, GA, or the World Health Organization. Vector eradication programs have been curtailed because of the evolution of mosquito resistance to dichlorodiphenyltrichloroethane (DDT).

Free-Living Amoebae

The free-living amoebae, *Naegleria fowleri, Acanthamoeba* species, and *Balamuthia mandrillaris* (formerly, *Leptomyxid amebae*) are causes of sporadic meningoencephalitis with mortalities that approach 100%. There have been approximately 200 cases of either primary amebic meningoencephalitis (PAM) or granulomatous amebic encephalitis (GAE) worldwide.

Ecology and Transmission

Free-living amebas have been isolated from fresh and frozen water, vegetables, heating and air-conditioning units, cooling towers of electric and nuclear power plants, sewage, medicinal pools, dental treatment units, dialysis units, cell cultures, contact lens solutions, corneal scrapings, skin lesions, and the CNS. *Naegleria* species prefer heated aquatic and soil environments; *Acanthamoeba* are everywhere. Cystic forms, resistant to short periods of drying, may distribute in blown soil. *Naegleria* and *Acanthamoeba* spp. may even harbor pathogenic bacteria, such as *Legionella* and *Vibrio cholera*, protecting the bacteria from chlorine in water supplies.

Naegleria infection results from introduction of contaminated water into the nasal cavity, then direct spread along the olfactory neuroepithelium through the cribriform plate.

Rarely, when there has been no history of water exposure, infection probably occurs by inhalation of dust or soil containing cysts. *Acanthamoeba* or *B. mandrillaris* spread hematogenously from either a pulmonary or cutaneous source to the CNS in immunocompromised or debilitated patients. *B. mandrillaris* in an immunocompetent host is probably also acquired by inhalation (Visvesvara 1993).

Clinical Features

PAM, a fulminant meningoencephalitis of healthy children and young adults, follows exposure to *N. fowleri* in warm water. Most often the patient had been swimming in warm freshwater lakes or ponds. After a 2- to 5-day incubation period (with an extreme of 14 days), there is abrupt headache, fever, pharyngitis, nasal obstruction, meningismus, vomiting, drowsiness, coma, and convulsions. Some patients notice a change in taste or smell before onset of severe disease, and myocarditis has been recognized in some cases. Mortality is high, usually within 1 week of onset of clinical disease.

GAE is a different disease: a subacute or chronic meningitis or meningoencephalitis with focal features. Mental status changes, seizures, hemiparesis, visual disturbances, and ataxia are reported. Inflammatory changes and associated arteritis vary, depending on the immunological status of the host. The duration of CNS disease is from 7 to 120 days, with fatal outcome.

In immunocompetent children with *B. mandrillaris*, vasculitis dominates the clinical syndrome. Progressive and eventually fatal stroke syndromes accompanied by CSF monocytosis were reported in previously healthy children (Griesemer et al. 1994). In immunocompetent adults, *Acanthamoeba* species may cause subacute or chronic keratitis after soft contact lens use or minimal ocular trauma.

Diagnosis

PAM is considered in the differential diagnosis of children and young adults with acute meningoencephalitis or purulent meningitis that fails to respond to antibiotics. In PAM, the CSF is hemorrhagic with elevated pressure. CSF WBCs may be normal early in disease, but soon rise to 400–26,000 WBC/μl, with predominant polymorphonuclear leukocytes, low glucose, and elevated protein. A wet mount of CSF should be examined for amebic trophozoites in any patient with purulent CSF and no bacteria on Gram's stain. Amebic trophozoites may be detected moving in a drop of CSF, or may stain with Wright's or Giemsa's stains in CSF smears. Diffuse contrast enhancement of gray matter and obliteration of basal cisterns is seen on CT scan. The purulent CSF profile helps distinguish PAM from herpes encephalitis.

A diagnosis of GAE is made when amebic trophozoites and cysts are identified in tissue or the CSF, or when cultured. Skin nodules or ulcers should be biopsied and examined for *Acanthamoeba* spp. in patients with suspected GAE. Serological tests using an indirect fluorescent antibody test may be helpful because GAE is a chronic infection. Examination of the CSF reveals a lymphocytic pleocytosis, elevated protein, and normal glucose. Unlike the meningoencephalitis of *N. fowleri*, *Acanthamoeba* spp. and *B. mandrillaris* are not readily demonstrated in the CSF. Abscess, microabscesses, cerebritis, meningitis, or arteritis appear on CT or MRI. The differential diagnosis includes bacterial, fungal, TB abscesses, or granulomatous meningitis caused by syphilis, TB, or fungi. *B. mandrillaris* is included also in the differential diagnosis of progressive or atypical childhood stroke.

Treatment

PAM is treated with systemic and intrathecal amphotericin B. Intravenous amphotericin B is increased as tolerated to 1.0–1.5 mg/kg per day for a 10-day treatment course, with periodic tests of renal, liver, and hematological function. For intrathecal treatment, 0.5 mg is injected three times weekly. Other antiamebic agents such as systemic and intrathecal miconazole (350 mg/m^2 body surface per day intravenously with 10 mg administered intrathecally on alternate days); oral rifampin (10 mg/kg/day for 9 days); and sulfisoxazole, doxycycline, or chloramphenicol also have been used or added. However, PAM is fatal in greater than 95% of cases.

GAE, also treated with tissue amebicides in combination, also has a poor prognosis. If possible, each clinical isolate should be tested for drug sensitivities. The diamidine derivatives, including pentamidine, have the greatest activity against *Acanthamoeba*. In vitro activity also has been demonstrated for ketoconazole, miconazole, neomycin, paromomycin, 5-fluorocytosine, chloroquine, and amphotericin B. Single *Acanthamoeba* or *B. mandrillaris* abscesses should be removed surgically.

Prevention

Where geographic clusters of PAM cases occur, public health officials consider the closure of lakes to swimming. Monoclonal antibody and polymerase chain reaction (PCR)-based reactions may be useful in the future for the analysis of clinical samples and detection of pathogenic species in environmental samples.

Amebiasis (*Entamoeba histolytica*)

Entamoeba histolytica infects approximately 10% of the world's population. A rare secondary manifestation of infection, cerebral amebiasis occurs in an estimated 0.1% of patients.

Ecology and Transmission

Humans are the primary reservoir of infection. Transmission is by ingestion of cysts in contaminated food or water.

Clinical Features

Intestinal infection varies from asymptomatic to inflammatory colitis. Extraintestinal infection occurs with abscesses in the liver, lung, pericardium, or skin. CNS spread is hematogenous, from hepatic or pleuropulmonary amebiasis. Cerebral amebiasis usually presents as fever and rapid deterioration of mental status in a patient with concurrent hepatic abscess. Frontal or basal ganglia abscesses are the most frequent CNS lesions. Rupture or breakdown of a cerebral abscess may cause purulent meningitis.

Diagnosis

Patients with metastatic amebic abscesses and invasive intestinal amebiasis have positive serology. ELISAs are the most sensitive and specific. Indirect fluorescent antibody (IFA), indirect hemagglutination assay, radioimmunoassay, and counterimmunoelectrophoresis tests to detect antiamebic antibody are also available. In CNS cases, stool examinations are unlikely to demonstrate either cysts or trophozoites. The differential diagnosis of hepatic mass with headache or brain abscess includes echinococcosis, fascioliasis, and pyogenic or mycobacterial abscess.

Treatment

Treatment of extraintestinal amebiasis is with intravenous metronidazole, 750 mg three times a day for the first 5–10 days, followed by oral metronidazole for 2–4 weeks. A luminal agent to eradicate cysts and prevent further transmission is used also. Although metronidazole penetrates the CSF and abscess lumen well, cerebral amebiasis has a greater than 90% mortality. Neurosurgery, previously limited to treatment of raised intracranial pressure and impending herniation, has been reported to achieve cures when combined with medical treatment (Shah et al. 1994).

Prevention

Prevention requires adequate sanitation and elimination of cyst carriage.

African Trypanosomiasis

African trypanosomiasis (sleeping sickness, *maladie du sommeil*, somnolencia), caused by flagellated protozoans *Trypanosoma brucei gambiense* in West and Central Africa or by *Trypanosoma brucei rhodesiense* in East and Southeast Africa, is a systemic febrile illness followed weeks, months, or years later by a progressive meningoencephalitis. Untreated, African trypanosomiasis is fatal. At least 20,000–50,000 cases are reported annually, but actual numbers may be ten times that amount.

Ecology and Transmission

Both subspecies are transmitted by bites of tsetse flies. Within the tsetse fly belt (a band across sub-Saharan Africa from 20°N to 20°S latitude), the *T. brucei* species occurs in over 200 endemic loci. Reservoir hosts include pigs and dogs for *T. b. gambiense* and antelope, wild hogs, and cattle for *T. b. rhodesiense*. Laboratory accident, blood transfusion, transplacental spread, and, perhaps, other biting insects, account for additional cases.

Clinical Features

The earliest sign of disease is a hard, painful lesion (chancre or trypanoma) at the site of the insect bite, which develops in 20–50% of patients. The chancre is followed by successive hemolymphatic and meningoencephalitic stages; yet patients with the *T. b. rhodesiense* form may progress rapidly through the disease stages, appearing instead to have a rapid, septicemic disease with CNS symptoms developing within 1 to several weeks. Discreet stages of disease are more clearly defined in the more chronic *T.b. gambiense* cases, with CNS symptoms developing after months or years.

Recognition of disease at the hemolymphatic stage provides the opportunity to treat early and improve clinical outcome. The hemolymphatic phase is characterized by fever, lymphadenopathy, rash, headache, dizziness, tachycardia, debility, sterility, and amenorrhea as the organisms disseminate through the bloodstream and lymphatics. Parasite populations appear at sequential intervals in the blood, with each successive population exposing a different antigen on the surface coat of the flagellates. The systemic phase of trypanosomiasis occurs in recurrent fashion: episodes last from 1–6 days and occur at several-week intervals. At this stage also, minor bumps or soft tissue compressions may produce a deep hyperesthetic pain out of proportion to the degree of injury, known as Kerandel's sign. Posterior cervical lymphadenopathy (Winterbottom's sign) is seen in the Gambian form.

Psychological and behavioral changes are often the first indicators of CNS involvement. In Gambian trypanosomiasis, insomnia, disturbed appetite (bulimia or anorexia), indifference, euphoria, or depression are seen. Progression of the CNS disease is indicated by: more disturbed sleep patterns (daytime somnolence); disruption of other circadian rhythms (such as cortisol and prolactin secretion) (Radomski et al. 1995); altered thermoregulation; pathological reflexes; extrapyramidal signs (rigidity, resting and action tremors, bradykinesia, choreoathetosis, and other dyskinesias); hemiplegia, ataxia, seizures, cranial neuropathies, hyperesthesia, and proprioceptive loss; and, finally, coma. The clinical features of the Rhodesian form are similar, but more acute. All untreated cerebral cases are fatal. For most of the CNS course, parasites are sequestered in choroid or collect around Virchow-Robin spaces, producing a CNS pathology dominated by perivascular inflam-

mation. Actual brain parenchymal penetration by the parasite may only occur in terminal stages of disease.

Diagnosis

Diagnosis is made by demonstrating the parasite in blood, lymph node aspirate, bone marrow, or CSF. Stained blood films, particularly thick films, are first examined, but concentration techniques, such as microhematocrit centrifugation, anion exchange, or buffy-coat preparations of blood, are used to detect low levels of parasitemia. Repeated parasitological examinations over several days increase the likelihood of diagnosis because both acute and chronic infections have fluctuating aparasitemic periods. The field-adapted serological tests, such as the card agglutination trypanosomiasis test using a variant antigen type found in the majority of *T. b. gambiense* isolates, are useful epidemiological tools, but are generally not used for acute diagnosis.

The CSF contains elevated protein and IgM levels, oligoclonal bands, and a pleocytosis, which may contain morular or Mott's cells (modified plasma cells containing large eosinophilic inclusions of IgG). Trypanosomes are sometimes found in centrifuged CSF specimens. A CT scan can show choroid or meningeal enhancement, or parenchymal areas of increased contrast uptake without ring enhancement. Electroencephalography in late stages shows delta-dominated rhythms. African trypanosomiasis is included in the differential diagnosis of irregular fevers, headaches, somnolence and posterior cervical adenopathy, along with malaria, infectious mononucleosis, arboviral encephalitides, leukemia, lymphoma, TB, syphilis, brucellosis, relapsing fever, toxoplasmosis, and onchocerciasis. Tachycardia unrelated to fever, signifying arrhythmias or congestive heart failure, is described in early *T. b. rhodesiense* before CNS involvement.

Treatment

If sleeping sickness is suspected, positive identification of the parasite is necessary before beginning chemotherapy. *T. b. gambiense* in the hemolymphatic phase is treated with intramuscular pentamidine at 3 mg/kg per day for 10 doses. *T. b. rhodesiense* in the hemolymphatic phase is treated with intravenous suramin, given initially as 100–200 mg, then increased as tolerated to 1 g on days 1, 3, 7, 14, and 21. Because suramin can cause renal tubular damage, it is contraindicated in patients with pre-existing renal disease. Because suramin is macrofilaricidal, it is contraindicated also in patients with onchocerciasis. Prolonged or repeat treatments are associated with axonal or demyelinating sensorimotor neuropathies. Neither suramin nor pentamidine penetrate the CNS well enough to treat the meningoencephalitic disease.

Eflornithine (difluoromethylornithine, DFMO), a polyamine synthesis inhibitor, has shown promise as effective treatment for meningoencephalitic disease caused by *T. b. gambiense*, but it is expensive. Regimens in use include a 14-day course of

DFMO, 100 mg/kg intravenously every 6 hours for primary treatment of meningoencephalitic trypanosomiasis; and a 7-day course for treating relapses following use of another agent (Khonde et al. 1997). Elevated CSF IgM levels are one indicator of relapse. Because the response of *T. b. rhodesiense* to DFMO has been variable, patients with rhodesiense CNS disease continue to be treated with organic arsenicals, such as melarsoprol (Iten et al. 1995).

Melarsoprol is used in a series of three to four daily intravenous injections with a maximum of 200–500 mg per injection to a total dose of 3.6 mg/kg. For severe CNS involvement, up to four courses of treatment may be necessary, waiting 7–10 days between series. Arsenical encephalopathy, occurring between the first and fifteenth day of treatment, complicates an estimated 10% of cases and may result in death. Risk of arsenical encephalopathy increases with high CSF WBCs (Pepin et al. 1995) and simultaneous use of thiabendazole to treat helminth infections (Ancelle et al. 1994). Pretreatment with intramuscular pentamidine or suramin, corticosteroids, an antihelminth, nutritional supplementation for debilitated patients, and an anticonvulsant are now recommended.

Arsenical encephalopathy is characterized by sudden loss of consciousness, with or without convulsions, and fever. Arsenical encephalopathy is treated urgently with osmotic diuretic agents (mannitol or glucose), parenteral corticosteroids, and anticonvulsants.

CSF cell and protein contents remain elevated for several months after treatment. Relapse following melarsoprol therapy is signaled by new headache, fever, neurological signs, and worsening CSF profile. *T. b. rhodesiense* relapse is retreated with melarsoprol, and *T. b. gambiense* with eflornithine. MRI, if available, may assist in distinguishing recurrent disease from arsenical reactive encephalitis. Focal, bilateral high-signal areas in white matter without edema on T2-weighted MRI have been reported to signify disease recurrence or incomplete treatment (Sabbah et al. 1997).

Surveillance for 2–3 years after treatment is recommended. The prognosis following treatment of early or second-stage infections is very good. Eradication of infection may be achieved even in 90% of cerebral cases. However, neuropsychiatric sequelae, including irritability, insomnia, and poor impulse control, may occur. The CT scans of treated cases can show cerebral atrophy.

Prevention

Preventive measures include regular medical surveillance of at-risk populations, treatment of early stage disease, fly trapping around active areas, and use of protective, light-colored clothing.

American Trypanosomiasis

American trypanosomiasis (Chagas' disease), infection by the hemoflagellate protozoan *Trypanosoma cruzi*, is a cause of cardiac disease, dysautonomia, or gastrointestinal tract deafferentation (mega disease) years after primary infection; and meningoencephalitis or CNS mass lesions in patients with HIV.

Ecology and Transmission

T. cruzi is a zoonotic infection, transmitted by triatomine cone-nosed bugs to humans and to wild and domestic animals. Infection follows contamination of the skin or mucous membranes by the insect's infected fecal material. The parasite also can be acquired by blood transfusion, organ transplant, or in utero. Chagas' disease is found in Central and South America, with additional cases reported in the Caribbean and the United States.

Clinical Features

Acute Chagas' disease is usually a flulike illness 1 week after inoculation, with fever, malaise, and rarely, meningoencephalitis. An inoculation chagoma, a swollen or indurated area, is seen in fewer than one-half of cases.

Immune response is important in both resistance to and pathogenesis of early and late disease. In endemic areas, early myocarditis, encephalitis, or reactivated Chagas' disease increase clinical suspicion of concurrent HIV disease (Ferreira et al. 1997).

Chronic Chagas' disease develops years or decades after initial infection, with the heart, gastrointestinal tract, and nervous system as the main targets. Cardiac involvement is most common, with syncopal or congestive cardiomyopathy presentations, or embolization of mural thrombi from a left ventricular apical aneurysm. Autoimmune destruction of cardiac autonomic nerves and ganglia produces a dysautonomic syndrome with postural hypotension, dizziness, and arrhythmias, whereas similar injury to the autonomic innervation of the gut produces visceral organ dilatation. Sensory neuropathies are reported also.

Diagnosis

Acute Chagas' disease can be diagnosed by approximately the third week of infection. Parasites are detected in fresh drops of blood or buffy coat, or in (thin or thick) blood smears in more than 90% of patients. Serology converts after 1 month in the sequence of hemagglutination, fluorescence, and complement fixation antibodies and remains positive for life. Chronic Chagas' disease is diagnosed serologically. However, antibodies should be positive on at least two different test results because of the presence of cross-reacting antibodies in patients with syphilis, leishmaniasis, malaria, leprosy, and collagen vascular disorders.

Treatment

Acute and congenital Chagas' disease is treated with benznidazole (7.5 mg/kg/day orally) for 60 days. Side effects include neuropathy and neutropenia after 30 days. Oral nifurtimox for 120 days, starting at 5 mg/kg per day and advancing to final doses of 17 mg/kg per day, is a more toxic alternative, with side effects including hemolytic anemia, peripheral neuritis, and psychosis. Chronic Chagas' disease is treated with allopurinol (8.5 mg/kg/day for 60 days), which has an in vitro antiparasite effect, and itraconazole (6 mg/kg/day for 120 days). Benznidazole, followed by itraconazole and fluconazole may improve the outcome in encephalitis patients with concurrent HIV and *T. cruzi* infections (Ferreira et al. 1997).

Prevention

Prevention focuses on blood donor screening and on measures to interrupt transmission within the home.

Toxoplasmosis

Toxoplasmosis is caused by *Toxoplasma gondii*, an intracellular protozoan infecting humans, other mammals, and birds. Toxoplasmosis is a common ocular infection, accounting for 35% of cases of chorioretinitis in the United States and Europe, a rare cause of myositis or meningoencephalitis in immunocompetent patients, a frequent cause of meningoencephalitis and cerebral mass lesions in immunocompromised patients, and a cause of congenital infection.

Ecology and Transmission

Because of its presence in migratory birds, it has a worldwide range. Cats harboring the intestinal infection are associated with the majority of transmitted disease. Most human infections are acquired by mouth by ingesting oocytes contained in food products or soil, or tissue cysts contained in raw meat. Transmission also occurs across the placenta, by blood transfusion, and by organ transplantation.

Clinical Features

Primary toxoplasmosis in immunocompetent patients presents as a lymphadenopathy syndrome or as a vague mononucleosislike illness 1–2 weeks after cyst ingestion. Rarely, adults with no known underlying disease have developed disseminated toxoplasmosis with CNS meningoencephalitis.

Congenital infection, the result of transplacental spread of infection acquired by the mother during gestation causes chorioretinitis (usually bilateral), strabismus, blindness, epilepsy, encephalitis, psychomotor retardation, microcephaly, intracranial calcification, hydrocephalus (Figure 59D.1), hypotonia, jaundice, hepatosplenomegaly, and pituitary insufficiency. Infants may be born without evidence of infection and symptoms develop later.

Most causes of *Toxoplasma* chorioretinitis are congenital infections. Acquired infections are usually unilateral. A focal, necrotizing retinitis with yellow-white patches is first seen. Healing produces white or darkly pigmented scars (Plate 59D.II). Panuveitis, papillitis, scotoma, defects in central vision, photophobia, glaucoma, microphthalmia, strabismus, and cataracts may be associated.

Recrudescent toxoplasmosis after immunosuppression leads to diffuse or focal encephalitis, cerebral mass lesions, chorioretinitis, myocarditis, myositis, or pneumonitis and is discussed in Chapter 59E.

Diagnosis

A number of antibody detection methods are available, including the Sabin-Feldman dye test, but IgG antibodies are present in many adults. Serological diagnosis of acute or congenital infection depends on finding persistent or increasing IgG titers and a positive IgM titer. Negative IgG levels in immunocompetent individuals with chorioretinitis usually excludes toxoplasmosis. The CSF of patients with encephalitis shows elevated protein and monocytic pleocytosis and may contain *T. gondii* DNA sequences by PCR. Differential diagnosis of the neonatal disease includes human cytomegalovirus, herpes, rubella, syphilis, *Escherichia coli* meningitis, sepsis, and erythroblastosis fetalis. Aicardi's syndrome of female infants, with microcephaly and lacunar retinal lesions resembling congenital toxoplasmosis, is distinguished radiologically by agenesis of the corpus callosum and costovertebral anomalies. Chorioretinitis caused by toxoplasmosis may resemble ocular signs of human cytomegalovirus, syphilis, toxocariasis, TB, herpes, disseminated candidiasis, or retinoblastoma.

Treatment

Asymptomatic infections in children or iatrogenic infections should be treated. Symptomatic patients are treated until disappearance of disease manifestations or there is serological evidence of immunity. Most effective drugs are the antifolates pyrimethamine and the sulfonamides. In adults, pyrimethamine, 75 mg daily for 3 days, then 25 mg daily; sulfadiazine, 500 mg four times a day; and folinic acid are used. Patients with ocular toxoplasmosis are treated for 1 month with pyrimethamine and sulfadiazine. Pregnant women are treated with a sulfonamide until delivery.

Congenital toxoplasmosis is treated for a total of 12 months with sulfadiazine (50 mg/kg twice daily), pyrimethamine (2 mg/kg/day for 2 days, then 1 mg/kg/day for 2–6 months, then 1 mg/kg/day three times a week for an additional 6 months), and folinic acid. Ventricular shunting may be required. Response to therapy is judged by serial serology, radiology, and ophthalmological and CSF examinations.

Prevention

Prevention involves, especially during pregnancy, the use of gloves when handling cat litter boxes or potentially contaminated soil, and thorough cooking of meat.

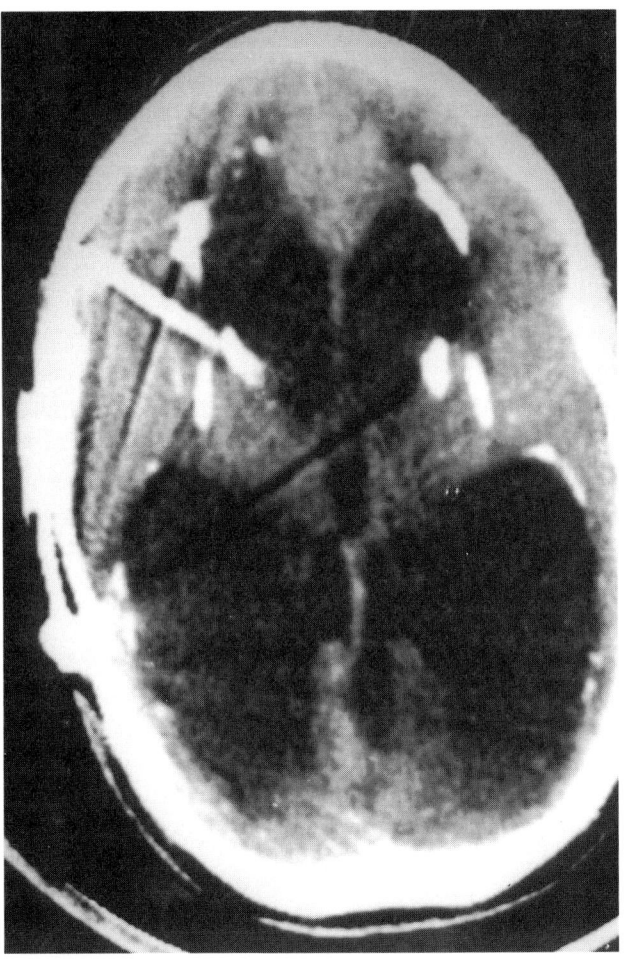

FIGURE 59D.1 Congenital toxoplasmosis. Computed tomographic scan showing periventricular calcifications, obstructive hydrocephalus, and ventricular shunt. (Courtesy of J. Healy.)

Leishmaniasis

Leishmaniasis, infections by protozoans of the genus *Leishmania*, occurs in the tropics of the Americas, parts of Asia, Europe, and Africa north of the equator. Transmission is by sandfly bite. Sensory, motor, cranial, and inflammatory neuropathies of Guillain-Barré type have been reported with visceral disease.

Clinical Features

Cutaneous, mucosal, and visceral forms occur. The cutaneous forms present a spectrum of disease between two polar extremes, with anergy at one end and mutilating hypersensitivity disease at the other. Visceral leishmaniasis, characterized by recurrent fever, hepatosplenomegaly, pancytopenia, hypergammaglobulinemia, and progressive wasting, also has been associated with retinal hemorrhage, uveitis, and peripheral or cranial neuropathies. Burning feet, footdrop, or hearing loss are the most common presentations (Hashim et al. 1995).

Diagnosis

Splenic aspiration is the most sensitive parasitological diagnostic method. Visceral leishmaniasis is an intracellular infection in a patient who has failed to express cellular immunity, but antibodies are readily detected by IFA, ELISA, countercurrent immunoelectrophoresis, and direct agglutination tests. The differential diagnosis includes chronic malaria with tropical splenomegaly, brucellosis, endocarditis, disseminated TB, schistosomiasis, and hematopoietic malignancy. One patient with Guillain-Barré syndrome, relapsing after plasma exchange, was subsequently diagnosed by needle biopsy of the spleen as having early visceral leishmaniasis and successfully treated with one of the pentavalent antimonials.

Treatment

Intravenous or intramuscular doses of 20 mg antimony per kilogram of body weight daily for 3–4 weeks is used in previously untreated patients. Hearing loss or sensory complaints improve during the first 2 weeks of treatment, but motor recovery is slower. Neuropathy is a side effect of sodium stibogluconate. Antimony resistance is reported in India and Sudan, and treatment alternatives are aminosidine, amphotericin B, liposomal amphotericin, or pentamidine. Patients who do not respond to therapy or repeatedly relapse may have HIV coinfection.

Prevention

Control is by treatment and elimination of animal reservoirs of infection, sandfly control, and vaccination, using live *L. major*.

Sarcocystosis

Sarcocystosis, a rare cause of myositis, is caused by accidental infection of humans by ingestion of infectious sporocysts in the feces of an infected carnivore. Muscle pain, swelling, fever, and eosinophilia are features. Corticosteroids can improve the inflammatory reaction, and pyrimethamine-sulfadiazine treats early stages of infection.

DISEASES OF HELMINTHS

Cestodes

Cysticercosis

Human cysticercosis is invasion of tissue by the larval stage (a cysticercus) of the pork tapeworm *T. solium*. A frequent brain autopsy finding in endemic areas, CNS cysticerci are the most common neurological infections in the world.

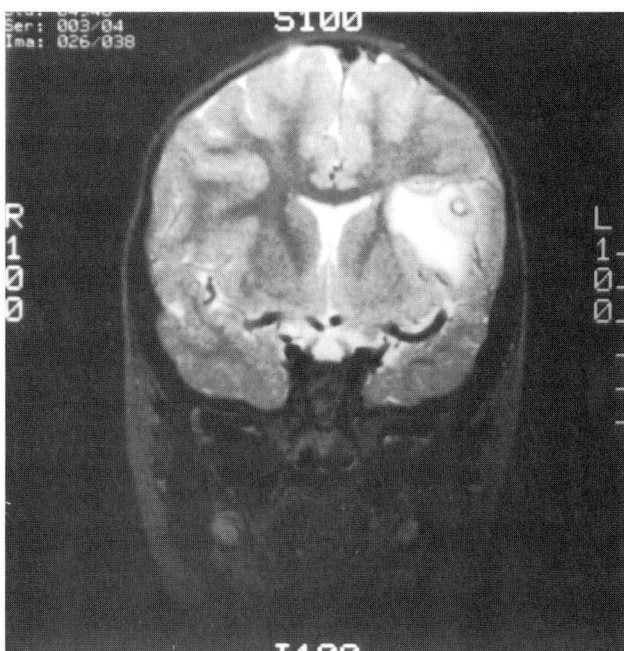

FIGURE 59D.2   Cysticercosis. Coronal T2-weighted magnetic resonance image showing scolex in left temporal lobe with surrounding edema. (Courtesy of J. Healy.)

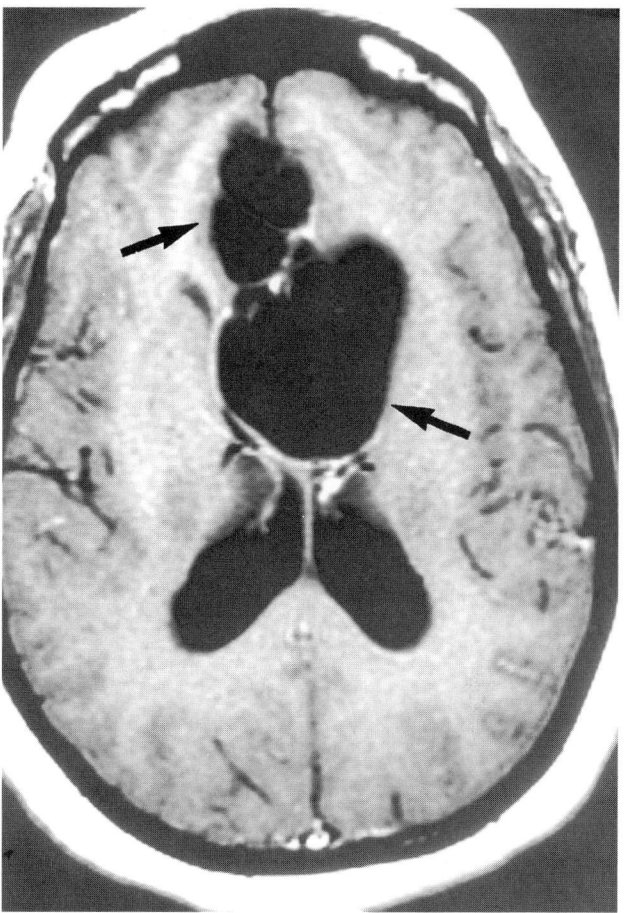

FIGURE 59D.3   Intraventricular cysticercosis. Axial T1 gadolinium magnetic resonance image showing racemose cysts (*arrows*) in pericallosal cistern with signal similar to cerebrospinal fluid and compressing the lateral ventricles. (Courtesy of J. Healy.)

Ecology and Transmission.   Cysticercosis occurs throughout the world in areas where pork production and poor hygiene and sanitation overlap, with a high prevalence in Central and South America, Southeast Asia, and parts of Africa. The tapeworms are acquired by eating undercooked pork containing cysticerci. Human cysticercosis, on the other hand, is a fecal-oral infection, caused by accidental ingestion of eggs excreted in the feces of a human tapeworm carrier. Tapeworm eggs hatch in the gastric tract, develop into invasive larvae, penetrate the bowel wall, and migrate into host tissues, where early larval forms mature to cysticerci. Cysticerci are found most commonly in CNS, muscle, eye, and subcutaneous tissues.

Clinical Features.   Onset of symptoms is from 1–35 years after exposure, with clinical presentations that include child or adult-onset focal or generalized epilepsy, focal neurological deficits, signs of raised intracranial pressure or hydrocephalus, papilledema, cognitive decline or neuropsychological syndromes, acute or chronic meningitis, or myelopathy. A rare presentation is a fulminant encephalitic form progressing to death within 1 week. Clinical features depend on the number and location of cysticerci and whether they are intact or degenerating. Severe meningitis or large cysts at the base of the brain may develop in patients with the racemose (lobulated) form of neurocysticercosis, an aberrant cysticercus that lacks a scolex and continuously grows. Ocular cysts occur in the vitreous or beneath the retina, causing periorbital pain, scotoma, or visual loss in cases with severe inflammation. Cysticerci deposition in muscle causes focal or generalized muscle enlargement.

Diagnosis.   In patients from endemic areas, almost any neurological or psychiatric complaint may be caused by neurocysticercosis. The diagnosis should be considered in patients with seizures, hydrocephalus, a cerebral mass lesion, or meningitis, but there is nothing specific about the neurological presentation. Subcutaneous or muscle cysts may appear as soft tissue calcification on plain films, but a search for peripheral eosinophilia, stool ova, and parasites is usually not helpful. Support for the diagnosis comes from imaging the parasites within the brain (Figure 59D.2) and from serology. MRI is better for visualizing intraventricular or subarachnoid cysts and cysts in the brainstem, cord, eye, or at the base of the brain. The racemose form appears as grapelike clusters of proliferating larval membranes in the subarachnoid spaces (Figure 59D.3) or at the base of the brain and may be associated with meningitis. CT scans are better for demarcating granulomas and calcified lesions. Inactive cysts appear as scattered small calcifications and active larvae as ring-enhancing lesions, with associated edema. The time required for a lesion to progress through these stages varies from 2–10 years, with an average of 5 years. A patient with multiple lesions at different stages is often seen. If the patient has only a granulomatous lesion without coexisting lesions at other stages, the CT and MRI findings are inconclusive and a biopsy may be needed for diagnosis. CSF may show mononuclear or lymphocytic pleocytosis or eosinophils and positive cysticercal titer results.

Immunodiagnostic tests in serum have high false-positive rates or cross-reactivity with echinococcus, schistosomes, or other tapeworms, whereas ELISA tests (using either *T. solium* cysts or cyst fluid as antigens) on CSF are considered more sensitive and specific. Existing serological tests can be used to screen epileptic or other neurological patients, although patients with solitary CNS lesions may be seronegative. In a study from Zimbabwe, serum antibodies detected by ELISA had a positive predictive value of 87% and negative predictive value of 85% for active neurocysticercosis. The differential diagnosis for intraparenchymal cysts on CT or MRI scan includes echinococcosis, paragonimiasis, sparganosis, cryptococcosis, and cystic astrocytomas. The differential diagnosis for extra-axial cysts includes echinococcosis, coenurosis and CNS tumors, and epidermoid, arachnoid, and colloid cysts.

Treatment. Active neurocysticercosis, with parenchymal, subarachnoid, or spinal cysts, is treated with albendazole or praziquantel. Albendazole has the advantages of being cheaper, having activity against the giant subarachnoid cysts, and being without pharmacological interference by corticosteroids. Albendazole, 15 mg/kg per day divided in two oral doses, is given for 8 days, together with dexamethasone, 10 mg intramuscularly per day for the first 4 days. As an alternative, a single day regimen of praziquantel and corticosteroids has been used. Praziquantel is given in three oral doses of 25 mg/kg every 2 hours, followed 5 hours later by dexamethasone, 10 mg intramuscularly, then 10 mg intramuscularly on each of the following 2 days (Sotelo 1997). Dexamethasone is recommended to follow praziquantel by several hours because the simultaneous administration of the two agents reduces plasma levels of praziquantel and decreases uptake of praziquantel into the cysts. Encephalitis and intracranial hypertension are contraindications to commencing antihelminth treatment. Acute inflammatory responses to treatment occur within several hours to days of initiating therapy, are more common if there are many cysts, and are signaled by headache or signs of increased intracranial pressure. Encephalitis, vasculitis, arachnoiditis also are treated with corticosteroids. The efficacy of medical treatment is evaluated by neuroimaging after 2–3 months. In refractory parenchymal cases, both drugs are used. Racemose cisternal forms usually respond poorly to drugs. Hydrocephalus caused by arachnoiditis is treated by ventricular shunt and alternate day prednisone. Hydrocephalus caused by intraventricular cyst(s) is treated by shunt and surgical removal. Spinal cysts also are treated surgically. Inactive neurocysticercosis, as shown by granuloma and calcifications, is treated symptomatically, with antiepileptics, for example.

Prevention. Prevention depends on treatment of *T. solium* carriers, pork inspection, and improved sanitation.

Echinococcosis

Echinococcosis (hydatid disease), infection by larval tapeworms of the genus *Echinococcus*, causes cystic lesions of the liver and lung, brain parenchyma, and intraventricular and subarachnoid spaces.

Ecology and Transmission. Human disease is caused by *Echinococcus granulosus*, *E. multilocularis*, or rarely, *E. vogeli*. *E. granulosus* is distributed widely throughout Europe, Asia, Australia, Africa, northern America, and southern Canada. It includes dog and sheep strains, a sylvatic (wolf) strain, and a dog and horse strain. *E. multilocularis* infects the Arctic fox and foxes and coyotes in North America. *E. vogeli* is found in bush and domestic dogs of the South American tropics. Humans are infected by contact with infected animals or by ingesting food contaminated by tapeworm eggs. Close or playful contact with dogs is an important source of infection. Ingested eggs hatch, release embryos that penetrate the intestinal mucosa, and are hematogenously carried to the liver or other sites, where their cystic development begins.

Clinical Features. Onset of symptoms is 2–20 years from infection, with signs and symptoms of cystic lesions of the liver and lung (abdominal pain, hepatomegaly, or cough), or rupture of the cyst (acute abdomen, dyspnea, hemoptysis, or hypersensitivity reaction). CNS cysts present as seizures or space-occupying lesions: cysts occupy intraparenchymal, intraventricular, subdural, or spinal locations. Other presentations include cord compression caused by hydatid bone disease (hydatid Pott's disease) with vertebral collapse or unilateral proptosis caused by intraorbital cysts.

Diagnosis. CNS cysts often occur with cysts elsewhere in the body. Calcified lesions of plain abdominal films may give the first diagnostic clues; peripheral or CSF eosinophilia may be present. Neuroimaging, demonstrating single or multiple cysts, together with ELISA or indirect hemagglutination assay serology, can often make the diagnosis. *E. granulosus* cysts tend to be solitary well-defined spherical cysts without edema and contrast enhancement, whereas *E. multilocularis* cysts are expansive, complex cysts with multichambered cavities and metastatic potential. Most cysts grow slowly. The differential diagnosis of slowly evolving proptotic eye disease includes gnathostomiasis, sparganosis, ocular larva migrans, cysticercosis, and retro-ocular and periorbital tumors including Burkitt's lymphoma.

Treatment. Surgical resection of the intact hydatid cyst is the treatment of choice. Care is taken to minimize rupture, which carries the risk of anaphylaxis or recurrent disease from dissemination of infectious scolices. Albendazole (15 mg/kg/day for 40 days) or mebendazole (50 mg/day) is recommended before surgery to shrink cysts. Treatment of nonresectable echinococcosis is with albendazole (400 mg twice daily) for at least 3 months. Patients having subtotal cyst resections usually require lifelong therapy. Response to treatment is assessed by repeated neuroimaging studies.

Prevention. In endemic areas, prevention involves personal hygiene with respect to contact with dogs, eliminating contact of pet dogs with sheep offal, or prophylactic treatment of domestic dogs with praziquantel, 5 mg/kg at monthly intervals.

Coenurosis

Coenurosis, infection by a coenurus, the larval form of the dog tapeworm, *Taenia multiceps* or *Taenia serialis*, causes space-occupying cystic lesions in the CNS.

Ecology and Transmission. Dogs and other canids are the definitive hosts. Sheep, goats, rabbits, and various rodents are intermediate hosts. Humans are infected by ingesting tapeworm eggs.

Clinical Features. Patients have signs and symptoms of CNS, ocular, or subcutaneous cysts. Patients may present with headaches modified by posture or paroxysms of headache, dimming vision, or obtundation, all signs of ball valve obstruction of the third ventricle. Commonly located in the subarachnoid spaces and ventricular system, the cysts predispose to obstructive hydrocephalus.

Diagnosis. Cysts in the brain may be spherical or racemose (lobulated). They appear on CT scan as clear cysts at least 2 cm in diameter with no discernible internal structure. Definite diagnosis depends on histological examination.

Treatment. Treatment is surgical.

Prevention. The same measures that are effective for *Echinococcus*, avoidance of infected carnivores and good hygiene, are recommended.

Diphyllobothriasis

Diphyllobothriasis, or fish tapeworm disease, is caused by cestodes of the genus *Diphyllobothrium*. *D. latum*, the most common, absorbs large quantities of vitamin B_{12}, causing megaloblastic anemia or neurological sequelae of vitamin B_{12} deficiency in 2% of infected patients.

Ecology and Transmission. Infection is acquired by ingestion of larvae in flesh, roe, or liver of raw or undercooked fish. *D. latum* is a common cestode in people of Northern Europe.

Clinical Features. Most infections are asymptomatic or cause transient diarrhea, headache, or malaise. Neurological sequelae are more common in elderly patients.

Diagnosis. Diagnosis is based on finding proglottids or eggs in the stool.

Treatment. Treatment is with praziquantel as a single oral dose of 10 mg/kg and vitamin B_{12} supplementation. Niclosamide, in a single oral dose of 2 g, is an alternative.

Sparganosis

Sparganosis, infection by a sparganum, the second stage larva of tapeworm of the genus *Spirometra*, is a rare cause of focal neurological deficits or CNS hemorrhage. Spirometra cestodes resemble *Diphyllobothrium* spp. in their life cycles, with fish serving as intermediate hosts.

Ecology and Transmission. Sparganosis in humans has been reported worldwide, but is most common in East, Southeast Asia, and East Africa. Humans acquire disease by drinking water containing infected *Cyclops*; after eating flesh of infected fish, snakes, or amphibians; or after using the flesh of the these species as a wound poultice.

Clinical Features. Sparganosis usually presents with growing or migratory subcutaneous swellings on the chest or legs or with periorbital swellings. Penetration of larvae into the CNS causes seizures, focal cerebral signs or symptoms, and bland or hemorrhagic infarcts. Changing parasite position, documented on serial head CT or MRI scans, attests to the viability and extreme mobility of this parasite in situ.

Diagnosis. The *Sparganum* is a mobile worm that stimulates an inflammatory response and peripheral eosinophilia as it moves through host tissue. ELISA for detection of antisparganum IgG antibody has been developed, but definitive diagnosis depends on excision and pathological examination of the worm. Cerebral sparganosis may appear as cystic, nodular, hemorrhagic, or calcified lesions on neuroimaging studies. In endemic areas, the combination of irregular or nodular enhancing lesions, small punctate calcifications, and widespread white matter of low density associated with adjacent ventricular dilatation is considered specific for the diagnosis.

Treatment. Treatment is surgical excision, because size (up to 50 cm) and intracranial mobility together predispose to CNS hemorrhage. Spargana are resistant to praziquantel, other antihelminths, and gamma irradiation (Kim et al. 1996).

Prevention. Prevention is achieved by avoiding contaminated foods and water.

Hymenolepis

Hymenolepis is caused by the intestinal tapeworm of humans, *H. nana*, which occurs worldwide, most commonly in areas of poor personal hygiene and poor sanitation. Heavy infections are associated with headache, dizziness, irritability, abdominal pain, anorexia, growth retardation, and seizures. Diagnosis is based on finding embryonated eggs in the stool. An ELISA test is available, but there is cross-reaction with other cestodes. Praziquantel, 25 mg/kg once, treats both adult worms and the cysticercoids in the intestine. Prevention is by improved sanitation.

Nematodes

Trichinosis

Trichinosis (or trichinellosis) infection by the nematodes *Trichinella spiralis* (of omnivores), *T. nativa* (of Arctic bears), or *T. nelsoni* (of scavengers of equatorial Africa) cause myositis and, in severe cases, myocarditis, encephalitis, encephalopathy, or death. *Trichinella* cysts, embalmed along with their human hosts, have been found in Egyptian mummies from 1200 BC.

Ecology and Transmission. Trichinosis is worldwide, acquired by ingestion of undercooked pork in temperate zones, bear or walrus in Arctic zones, and various "bush meats" in the tropics.

Clinical Features. Trichinosis begins as a febrile illness with gastrointestinal symptoms 1–2 days after ingestion. Periorbital edema, myalgia, subconjunctival hemorrhages, and eosinophilia accompany the muscle invasive phase, from 5 days after infection. Pain, swelling, and weakness usually begin in the extraocular muscles and progress to masseter, bulbar, neck, diaphragmatic, intercostal, paraspinal deltoid, and limb muscles. Myocarditis and respiratory failure are seen in severe infections. Larval invasion of the CNS, in approximately 10% of cases, causes meningoencephalitis, presenting as seizures or delirium, CNS hemorrhage, infarction, and major vein thrombosis. An early cardioneurological syndrome, characterized by diffuse encephalopathy or focal neurological deficits, acute myocardial injury, hypereosinophilia, and small multifocal cortical and subcortical ischemic lesions has been recognized (Fourestie et al. 1993). Necrotizing arteritis, resembling polyarteritis nodosa and causing mononeuritis multiplex, has been reported in less fulminant cases.

Diagnosis. Symptomatic patients have blood eosinophilia, elevated serum IgE levels, and elevated muscle enzymes. The definitive test is muscle biopsy, particularly gastrocnemius, deltoid, or pectoralis, at a site of swelling or tenderness. Fresh muscle should be pressed between glass slides and examined microscopically for the presence of larvae, in addition to examinations using standard muscle histopathology techniques. Antibody can be detected between 2 and 4 weeks after infection by bentonite or latex tests, IFA, or ELISA. The differential diagnosis includes infectious and inflammatory causes of myositis, including the eosinophilic-myalgic syndrome linked to tryptophan, other tissue-invasive helminths, and necrotizing vasculitides such as polyarteritis nodosa. Chagas' orbital edema may resemble early trichinosis.

Treatment. In cases of known ingestion of trichinous meat, mebendazole treats the acute gastrointestinal phase. For disseminated infection, treatment is directed toward the larvae and subsequent immune reactions. Oral mebendazole (20 mg/kg every 6 hours), administered for 2 weeks, is active against enteric stages, but inactive against intramuscular cysts. Severe allergic reactions are treated with prednisone, initially at 60 mg per day and tapered over a period of 2–3 weeks. Patients with mild infections recover with bed rest, antipyretics, and analgesics.

Prevention. Prevention is by adequate cooking of pork. Meat storage at –18° to –15°C for 20 days destroys cysts.

Angiostrongyliasis

Angiostrongyliasis, infection by the rat lungworm, *Angiostrongylus cantonensis*, causes a primary eosinophilic meningitis or meningoencephalitis.

Ecology and Transmission. Human disease occurs following the ingestion of snails (including *Pila* snails or the giant African snail, *Achatina fulica*), slugs, undercooked prawns, or crab infected with *A. cantonensis*. Cases have been reported in Asia and the Pacific, Africa, and the Caribbean.

Clinical Features. Headache, nausea, vomiting, and stiff neck follow 1–36 days after ingestion, the time it takes parasites to reach the CNS. Paresthesias, impaired vision, cranial neuropathies (optic neuritis, facial and sixth nerve palsies), generalized weakness, muscle twitching, seizures, pathological reflexes, papilledema, depressed consciousness, and coma may accompany or follow the initial headache. In most cases, the CNS syndrome resolves after several weeks. Worms or larvae also may occur in the vitreous or anterior chamber.

Diagnosis. Diagnosis is based on the CSF findings and compatible clinical history. CSF pressure is elevated, and the fluid contains elevated protein, normal glucose, and WBC counts between 150 and 2,000/µl, 10–90% of which are eosinophils. *A. cantonensis* larvae also may be found in the CSF. The usual absence of focal lesions on neuroimaging studies helps distinguish *A. cantonensis* from gnathostomiasis or neurocysticercosis. ELISA tests of sera and CSF may be positive and worms are occasionally seen on ophthalmoscopic or slit-lamp examination.

Treatment. The spinal tap greatly improves the headache; otherwise, there is no consensus on treatment. Because larvicidal agents may exacerbate CNS disease, and because many cases are self-limited, if the CSF eosinophil counts are decreasing after 1 month, treatment is generally supportive, with analgesics, sedatives, and corticosteroids in severe cases.

Prevention. Prevention is achieved by rodent control and adequate cooking of infected mollusks.

Gnathostomiasis

Gnathostomiasis (Yangtze River edema, Shanghai's rheumatism, Consular disease, nodular eosinophilic panniculitis, woodbury bug), infection by *Gnathostoma* parasites of dogs and cats, causes an eosinophilic meningoencephalitis or radiculomyelitis and invasive masses of the eye.

Ecology and Transmission. Humans are infected after eating undercooked or fermented freshwater fish, reptiles, birds, or other aquatic animals that have ingested microscopic crustaceans containing *Gnathostoma* larvae. Gnathostomiasis has been reported in East Asia, South Asia, and Israel.

Clinical Features. Localized subcutaneous edema or migrating red skin rash, fever, and eosinophilia appear 3 weeks after exposure, but CNS disease may occur without antecedent cutaneous swellings. CNS invasion is signified by a multifocal neurological illness with headache, meningitis, cranial nerve palsies, focal sensory or motor deficits, depressed consciousness, and spinal cord involvement. A painful radiculomyelopathy with segmental, usually, girdle pain and paraparesis is the most characteristic neurological presentation. Gnathostome migration in the soft tissues of the face or in or around the eyes produces cranial neuritis, uveitis, hemorrhage, or retinal detachment; more distal migrations may cause mononeuritis.

Diagnosis. CSF may be hemorrhagic or xanthochromic with eosinophilic pleocytosis. Diagnosis is based on CSF eosinophilia, compatible clinical presentation, and exposure history. CT or MRI scan may show enhancing lesions. Antibody-based diagnostic tests have so far lacked specificity. Where angiostrongyliasis and gnathostomiasis geographically overlap, the diagnosis of gnathostomiasis is favored by a more hemorrhagic spinal fluid and a more diffuse neurological disorder, which includes painful radiculomyelopathy.

Treatment. Albendazole (400–800 mg daily for 21 days) with corticosteroids has been used for treatment, along with surgical removal of the parasite if it migrates to an accessible location.

Prevention. Prevention is best accomplished by thorough cooking of potential sources of infectious larvae.

Onchocerciasis

Onchocerciasis (river blindness, white water disease), infection by the filarial nematode *Onchocerca volvulus*, is an important cause of preventable blindness.

Ecology and Transmission. Onchocerciasis occurs in Central and West Africa, Latin America, and Yemen, where transmission from person to person is by blackflies of the *Simulium* species. Endemic areas are tropical, near rushing rivers or streams that contain vegetation.

Clinical Features. A pruritic or depigmenting dermatitis, onchocercal nodules in subcutaneous sites, and eye lesions are the most frequent manifestations. A punctate keratitis, appearing as snowflakelike opacities, is a tissue reaction to dead microfilariae in the cornea and an early sign of corneal involvement. Heavy microfilarial infection and penetration of the eye causes conjunctivitis, sclerosing keratitis, iridocyclitis with secondary glaucoma, anterior uveitis, chorioretinitis, and optic atrophy, and eye lesions vary widely in endemic geographical areas. The blinding pathologies are the anterior changes (sclerosing keratitis and iritis) and posterior lesions (chorioretinitis and optic atrophy).

Diagnosis. Diagnosis is by examining skin snips for microfilariae or detection of adult worms in excised nodes. Slit-lamp examination may show microfilariae in the cornea or anterior chamber. IFA and ELISA antibody detection techniques currently available may be positive in other nematode infections and cannot distinguish between recent and remote infection. Significant clinical benefit would derive from the development of sensitive and specific immunodiagnostic or PCR-based tests to detect infection before the appearance of microfilariae.

Treatment. Ivermectin (in a single oral dose of 0.4 mg/kg or 150 µg/kg), which kills microfilariae without allergic ocular side effects, is replacing diethylcarbamazine citrate (DEC) as primary therapy. Microfilariae disappear from the skin in approximately 48 hours, but more slowly from the eye. Retreatment may be necessary after 6 months and follow-up skin snips are examined 6–12 months after treatment. Studies indicate that annual ivermectin treatment has reduced the incidence of blindness by 80% in endemic areas. Improved seizure control also has been noted in patients in areas receiving mass treatment with ivermectin. This phenomenon potentially relates either to the drug's microfilarial effect, its simultaneous cure of other helminths, or its pharmacological property of GABAergic enhancement. Ivermectin is contraindicated in young children, in pregnant or lactating women, or in patients with inflamed meninges.

Nodulectomy removes adult worms and is widely used in Central and South America to reduce the incidence of ocular onchocerciasis. The procedure is less successful in African patients, in whom nodules are deeper and more fibrotic. The macrofilaricidal agent, Suramin, is used if total cure is necessary.

Prevention.   Vector control and protective clothing aid prevention.

Loiasis

Loiasis, infection by the filarial nematode, *Loa loa* or African eyeworm, causes episodic localized angioedema or worm migration across the eye, and its treatment provokes encephalopathy or coma.

Ecology and Transmission.   Loiasis occurs in the transitional savanna and rain forests of West and Central Africa. Humans are infected by the bites of mango flies. Larvae develop into adult filariae; gravid females shed microfilariae into the bloodstream. Loiasis is also iatrogenic, transmitted by blood transfusion.

Clinical Findings.   Signs of infection are the "fugitive" or Calabar swellings (after the slave port of Calabar, Nigeria) characterized by itching, erythema, and edema or the migration of the adult worm across the eye in the subconjunctival space, or under the skin.

Diagnosis.   Loiasis is diagnosed by identifying microfilariae in blood films. Peak circulation of microfilariae occurs in the early afternoon, because microfilariae rest in capillaries of the lung and other deep organs at night. Most infected persons have antibodies to filarial antigens on IFA or ELISA tests. Subcutaneous *L. loa* causes relatively mild dermal reactions, which only last a few minutes, whereas the other helminths that migrate under the skin, cutaneous larvae migrans, produce more intense inflammation and multiple tracks. In the eye, *L. loa* is subconjunctival and much larger than *Toxocara*, which has an anterior chamber location.

Treatment.   Treatment is with the microfilaricidal agent DEC (8–10 mg/kg/day in three divided doses) for 21 days. DEC has some activity against adult worms, and several treatments may be necessary to eradicate infection. Ocular inflammation and encephalopathy are significant complications of DEC treatment. Encephalopathy is related to level of microfilaremia, occurring when parasite density exceeds 50,000/ml and may be heralded by retinal hemorrhages. In patients with heavy infections, lower starting doses of DEC (0.5 mg/kg/day) plus corticosteroids, antihistamines, or nonsteroidal anti-inflammatory agents are recommended. Alternatively, a drug with a lower level of microfilaricidal activity, such as mebendazole, may be used

first. Exchange transfusion has been used in cases of high microfilarial load. In regions where loiasis and onchocerciasis overlap, thoughtful consideration of treatment options are indicated, because ivermectin has been shown to provoke the passage of *L. loa* into the CSF in patients with high microfilaremia (Gardon et al. 1997).

Prevention.   Preventive measures include protective clothing and vector control.

Lymphatic Filariasis

Bancroftian filariasis, infection by the parasitic nematodes *Wuchereria bancrofti*, *Brugia malayi*, and *Brugia timori* lasting up to 20 years, is associated with inflammatory neuropathies or compression neuropathies following lymphatic system damage.

Ecology and Transmission.   Spread by mosquitoes in tropical area of both East and West Hemispheres, lymphatic filariasis is widespread in equatorial Africa and Southeastern Asia.

Clinical Features.   The typical presentation is sudden fever, acute groin pain with tender lymph nodes, and a swollen leg. Infection causes lymphadenitis; lymphedema; elephantiasis of the limbs, breasts, or external genitalia; and the tropical pulmonary eosinophilic syndrome. Nerve compression palsies may occur, caused by pressure from enlarged or calcified lymph nodes and dilated pelvic and retroperitoneal lymphatics. Recurrent Guillain-Barré syndrome has been reported after flare-ups of acute filariasis (Bhatia and Misra 1993). Eye involvement, including conjunctivitis, anterior uveitis, or adult worms in the anterior chamber, has been described.

Diagnosis.   Diagnosis is by identifying microfilariae in blood or adult worms or microfilariae in tissue sections. Peak parasitemia is 11 PM to 2 AM and corresponds to the biting and activity habits of their mosquito vectors. IFA and ELISA tests have been developed for antibody detection, whereas IgE and IgG4 antibody tests show greater specificity.

Treatment.   Treatment is with the microfilaricidal agent DEC (6 mg/kg/day in three divided doses for 12 days). DEC is also capable of killing adult *W. bancrofti*, *B. malayi*, and *B. timori*, and DEC treatment is recommended before surgical procedures.

Prevention.   The main means of prevention are chemotherapy of selected communities and mosquito control.

Dracunculiasis

Dracunculiasis, or Guinea worm, is caused by *Dracunculus medinensis*. Parasite-produced ulcers that communicate with the skin surface and surround adult worms through their course, are causes of epidural abscesses and tetanus.

Ecology and Transmission.   Infection, by ingesting water containing *D. medinensis* larvae-infected copepods (water fleas), occurs in West Africa, the Nile Valley, the Arabian Peninsula, India, and Pakistan. The adult females are the longest nematodes to infect humans, reaching lengths of 70–120 cm.

Clinical Features.   The first symptoms usually occur in the days before the worm pierces and emerges from the skin. The dermis swells and a blister develops, most often in the arms or legs. Burning dysesthesias or pruritus accompanies formation of the ulcer. The female worm, having completed a migration through subcutaneous tissues to the surface, emerges through the ulcer in the skin. Worm-induced ulcers may become secondarily infected with any number of environmental, cutaneous, or soil bacteria, including *C. tetani*. *D. medinensis* has been isolated from thickened peripheral nerves, and worms located close to joints may cause arthritis and fixed joint deformities. *D. medinensis* in the region of the eye cause periorbital abscesses or proptosis and in axial locations have caused spinal epidural abscesses.

Diagnosis.   Guinea worm infections are usually not diagnosed during the 8–10 months of their subcutaneous migration. The diagnosis is made at the time the worm emerges. Peripheral eosinophilia is common.

Treatment.   Treatment is by slow extraction of the worm using a small stick. Wound hygiene and tetanus vaccination should be included. Niridazole may reduce inflammation and facilitate extraction.

Prevention.   Prevention is by provision of safe drinking water.

Toxocariasis and Neural Larva Migrans

Larva migrans refers to conditions of protracted migration and persistence of helminth larvae in tissues. Neural larval migrans is a rare cause of seizures or behavior disorders in children. The pathogens most commonly implicated are the roundworms of dogs, *Toxocara canis*; of cats, *Toxocara cati*; and of raccoons, *Baylisascaris procyonis*.

Ecology and Transmission.   Humans contract larva migrans after inadvertent ingestion of infective eggs from material contaminated with the feces of dogs, cats, or raccoons. Young children with histories of pica or geophagia are at risk. Infective larvae hatch from eggs in the small intestine, penetrate the intestinal wall, and migrate.

Clinical Features.   Although most infections are asymptomatic, cutaneous, visceral, neural, and ocular forms of disease are recognized. Cutaneous larva migrans produce slow moving, creeping eruptions with serpiginous tracts, and heavy worm burdens are associated with eosinophilia, fever, and hepatomegaly. Larvae may migrate to any portion of the brain or spinal cord. Encephalitic, epileptic, paretic, or childhood dementing syndromes are the results of CNS traumatic injury, infarcts from vasculitic lesions, inflammation, and eosinophilic granulomas. Entrapment of *T. canis* larvae in the eye results in the retinal inflammatory mass of ocular larva migrans (Plate 59D.III).

Diagnosis.   The diagnosis of neural larva migrans is considered in young children with history of dog or cat exposure, CSF eosinophilia, peripheral eosinophilia, and an encephalitis illness. Suspected *Toxocara* and *Baylisascaris* infections may be confirmed by ELISA or Western blots using larval excretory-secretory antigens. The differential diagnosis includes other migrating helminths or larvae with cutaneous eruption and CNS inflammatory disease: loiasis, gnathostomiasis, strongyloidiasis, and human myiasis by larvae of the horse botfly and cattle grub fly. The granulomatous retinal lesions of ocular larva migrans can appear similar to retinoblastoma, toxoplasmosis, histoplasmosis, optic neuritis, and Coats' disease. Many eye globes containing *Toxocara* spp. have been enucleated because of suspected retinoblastoma.

Treatment.   Corticosteroids are used to reduce the inflammatory complications of neural larva migrans and an antihelminth, such as thiabendazole, 25 mg/kg twice daily for at least 5 days; mebendazole, 100 mg three times daily for 7 days; or albendazole may be added. DEC has also been a first-line drug for *Toxocara* species. Prognosis is poor in CNS infections by the more aggressive *Baylisascaris*. When the larvae are remote from the macula or disk, laser photocoagulation has been used to kill intraretinal larvae (Goldberg et al. 1993).

Prevention.   Human protection is best achieved by sensible hygiene and sanitation practices. Dogs can be periodically tested and treated for *T. cani*.

Strongyloidiasis

Strongyloidiasis, caused by the gastrointestinal nematode *Strongyloides stercoralis*, is associated with severe disseminated infections, including CNS infections, in immunosuppressed and patients with human T-cell leukemia virus I.

Ecology and Transmission.   *Strongyloides* is found in many tropical and subtropical regions of the world. Identified risk groups include (1) residents or emigrants of any developing country, and southern, eastern, and central Europe; (2) residents of the Appalachian region of the United States; and (3) institutionalized individuals. *Strongyloides* infects humans as a result of skin penetration by filariform larvae.

The parasite has the uncommon capacity among human helminth infections of multiplying within the host. Indefinite multiplication in the host is a serious problem for chronically ill or immunosuppressed individuals, and the result is overwhelming autoinfection, called *hyperinfection*.

Clinical Features.   Abdominal pain, distention, jaundice, pulmonary complaints, or gram-negative sepsis are signs of disseminated strongyloidiasis. Because parasites migrating from the gut carry enteric bacteria to various body organs, CNS syndromes include polymicrobial bacterial meningitis as well as eosinophilic meningitis, cerebritis, chronic meningoencephalitis, or cerebral vasculitis with multiple infarcts.

Diagnosis.   The diagnosis of disseminated strongyloidiasis is considered in cases of polymicrobial meningitis caused by gram-negative enteric bacteria. Diagnosis is based on finding larval stages, adult females, or eggs in the stool. *S. stercoralis*–induced antibodies cross-react with other helminths and filariae. Eosinophilia, present in early stage infection, usually disappears with dissemination.

Treatment.   The recommended treatment for immunocompetent patients with uncomplicated infection is oral albendazole, 400 mg once or twice daily for 3 days, thiabendazole, 25 mg/kg twice a day for 3 days, or ivermectin in a single dose of 200 mg/kg. For immunodeficient patients with hyperinfection or dissemination, thiabendazole, 50 mg/kg twice a day, is continued for 2–4 weeks. Other therapies are directed toward the intercurrent bacterial infections or inflammatory conditions.

Prevention.   Precautions are the same as for hookworm: proper sanitation and protective footwear. Disseminated strongyloidiasis can be prevented in some cases by screening stool specimens before immunosuppressive treatments.

Ascariasis

Ascariasis, caused by parasitic roundworms of the genus *Ascaris*, is found in the tropical and subtropical regions of Asia, Africa, Europe, and the Americas. Possibly one in four of the world's population is infected. Infection is acquired from ingestion of eggs in contaminated soil. The main clinical syndromes are abdominal discomfort; small bowel, biliary, or pancreatic ductal obstruction; and eosinophilic pneumonitis. Kwashiorkor and vitamin A deficiency have been associated with ascariasis gastrointestinal infection. Ectopic migration of adult worms from the bowel to the CNS may establish epileptogenic foci or introduce *Bacteroides* or enteroviruses to the CNS. An epidemiological relation between *Ascaris* infection and poliomyelitis has been suggested.

Diagnosis can be made from passage of worms or eggs in stool. Radiological examination of the gastrointestinal tract after an opaque meal often displays the worms. Anti-bodies can be detected by various techniques: complement fixation, precipitin, and immunoelectrophoresis, but cross-reactivity with other helminths is high. Skin test results may be positive because of *Ascaris* hypersensitivity in humans.

Treatment is with a single dose of pyrantel pamoate, 10 mg/kg body weight, albendazole (200 mg for children 2–5 years; 400 mg for older children and adults once), or mebendazole (two 100-mg doses in one day).

Halicephalobiasis

Halicephalobiasis (micronemiasis) is a rare accidental infection of humans and horses caused by invasion of tissues and organs by the saprophytic nematode *Halicephalobus deletrix*. Members of the genus *Halicephalobus* are free-living or saprophytic nematodes distributed throughout the world in decaying humus, soil, and small collections of fresh water. Humans are infected by entry of the worm through skin or broken skin. Three fatal meningoencephalitis cases have been reported from North America. One was a 5-year-old farm boy who accidentally traveled through the blades of a manure spreader and died 24 days later.

Fever, somnolence, and CSF lymphocytic pleocytosis (100–300 cells per µl) are characteristic. In each case, death was attributed to direct parasitic infection of the brain and the diagnosis was made postmortem. *H. deletrix* has not been cultured in vitro. Neither diagnostic reagents nor serological tests are yet available.

Trematodes

Schistosomiasis

Schistosomiasis, infection by the trematode parasites, *S. mansoni*, *S. haematobium*, and *S. japonicum*, ranks as the second most important cause of parasitic death, after malaria. In endemic areas, *S. mansoni* and *S. haematobium* are important causes of spinal cord syndromes. Less frequently, *S. mansoni* or *S. japonicum* cause CNS mass lesions or cerebral vasculitis.

Ecology and Transmission.   *S. mansoni* is found in Africa, Brazil, and the West Indies; *S. haematobium* in Egypt, the Middle East, and Africa; and *S. japonicum* in Asia. Humans are infected by contact with fresh water in which infectious larvae (cercariae) are shed by snails, the intermediate host. Developing worms migrate to portal and hepatic (*S. mansoni* and *S. japonicum*) or pelvic and urinary venous systems (*S. haematobium*).

Clinical Features.   Patients may notice pruritus immediately after exposure and 11–50 days later develop signs and symptoms of acute toxemic schistosomiasis (Katayama's fever), a systemic allergic reaction characterized by fever, myalgia, headache, urticaria, and lymphadenopathy.

S. mansoni infections at this stage also may produce transient meningoencephalitis or a generalized vasculitis.

Chronic infections are established once worms complete their intravascular migrations and settle in the venules of the mesentery, bladder, or ureters, depending on the species. Chronic infections may be associated with hepatosplenomegaly, portal hypertension, hepatic fibrosis, or cystitis or be asymptomatic until a neurological problem develops.

Cauda equina and conus medullaris syndromes, transverse myelitis, cord infarct, and granulomatous cord compression are associated with *S. mansoni* and *S. haematobium*. Ectopic eggs or worms within the spinal canal or cord parenchyma, with the route of infection thought to be via arterial egg embolization or reflux through valveless intervertebral venous plexus of Batsons, cause the inflammatory or ischemic cord injuries. Infections in ectopic locations and the accompanying inflammatory response are linked also to the seizures, focal sensory or motor deficits, and multinodular cerebral masses associated with *S. japonicum* infections and the cerebral vasculitis or mass lesions of chronic *S. mansoni* infections (Case Records 1996).

Additionally, migrating worms may carry *Salmonella* to other body locations to cause recurrent salmonellosis.

Diagnosis.   Schistosomiasis is considered in the differential diagnosis of any painful cauda equina or spinal cord syndrome in residents of endemic areas or travelers with fresh water exposure. A search for stool or urine ova and parasites or peripheral eosinophilia is usually not helpful in spinal cord or CNS cases. CSF eosinophilia may accompany cauda equina syndromes, and CT or MRI may demonstrate lower cord enhancement of granulomas or enlargement. In CNS cases, focal granulomas, developed around embolized eggs, can appear as multiple, nonspecific enhancing nodules with surrounding edema.

Multiple serological techniques may detect antibodies to egg, cercarial, schistosomular, or adult worm antigens and provide a presumptive diagnosis; confirmation is made by finding eggs in feces or urine or by rectal, liver, or bladder biopsy. Direct diagnostic techniques have been greatly aided by two tests. An ELISA using keyhole limpet hemocyanin distinguishes between acute and chronic antibody responses and the circulating anodic antigen test for schistosomal antigens in serum or urine by enzyme immunoassay can be positive before eggs are excreted.

Treatment.   A spinal cord syndrome in patients with exposure history should be treated urgently with praziquantel and corticosteroids (Shakir and Stern 1996). Praziquantel is active against all human schistosome species. A single oral dose of 40 mg/kg treats *S. haematobium* and *S. mansoni*. *S. japonicum* and *S. mekongi* are treated with three doses of 20 mg/kg at 4-hour intervals. Metrifonate and oxamniquine are effective against *S. haematobium* and *S. mansoni*, respectively. Corticosteroids, surgical decompression, or both may be necessary to treat CNS mass lesions or cord compressive lesions, and corticosteroids also have been used for the allergic meningoencephalitis of acute schistosomiasis or CNS inflammatory lesions.

Prevention.   Preventive measures are region-specific and include chemotherapy, molluscicides, modifications of aquatic environments, and anticipatory impact studies of new agriculture programs or human-made water systems.

Paragonimiasis

Paragonimiasis, or Oriental lung fluke, is caused by infection by trematodes of the *Paragonimus* species. The brain is the most common extrapulmonary site of infection, resulting in acute or chronic encephalitic, epileptic, or focal CNS syndromes.

Ecology and Transmission.   *Paragonimus* species are distributed through East and South Asia, the Americas, and West Africa. Humans are infected by the consumption of larval metacercaria in raw or undercooked freshwater crustaceans or water plants. Maturing larvae migrate from the gastrointestinal tract to the lung.

Clinical Features.   Acute infections are characterized by cough, fever, pleural effusions, and hepatosplenomegaly; chronic infections by cough with brown purulent sputum, chest pain, and night sweats. Aberrant migration of young or mature flukes to brain or spinal cord produces an acute or fluctuating meningoencephalitis or myelitis. Host reaction to worms and eggs, by forming cysts, abscesses, or granulomas, clinically manifests as seizures or focal cerebral signs. Migration or embolization may produce CNS hemorrhage or infarction, and chronic forms cause space-occupying lesions, raised intracranial pressure, papilledema, optic atrophy, or mental retardation.

Diagnosis.   Diagnosis is by examination for eggs of samples of blood-stained sputum, by serological (complement fixation or ELISA) and intradermal tests, and chest roentgenography. Eggs may be difficult to isolate from chronic cases. Early stage cerebral paragonimiasis may appear as multiple, ring-enhancing abscesslike cysts with surrounding edema in posterior parts of the brain on CT or MRI. Chronic forms show punctate or nodular areas of calcification, hydrocephalus, or multiple intraparenchymal lesions with adjacent tissue atrophy on CT, rendering the soap bubble appearance of dilated ventricles, multiple dense calcifications and calcified cystic lesions (Kusner and King 1993). CSF examination shows lymphocytic pleocytosis, elevated protein, and eosinophils in approximately 10% of cases. Paragonimiasis is included along with TB, bacterial pneumonias, amebiasis, gnathostomiasis, and melioidosis in the differential diagnosis of new headache or CNS syndrome in patients with pulmonary symptoms and hemoptysis. In endemic areas among children with suspect diets, paragonimiasis is a cause of mental retardation.

Treatment. Oral praziquantel at a dosage of 25 mg/kg three times per day for 3 days is recommended. Niclofolan in a single dose of 2 mg/kg is an alternative. Corticosteroids for inflammatory treatment reactions and surgery for compressive myelopathy or ventricular shunt placement may be indicated also. Other neurosurgical procedures are decided on a case-by-case basis.

Prevention. Adequate cooking of shellfish kills larval metacercaria.

Fascioliasis

Fascioliasis, a common liver fluke infection of cattle, sheep, and other ungulates worldwide, is a rare zoonotic infection of humans. *Fasciola hepatica* causes liver disease, late-stage ascites, and CNS syndromes caused by ectopic migration.

Ecology and Transmission. Where livestock, snails, and humans live in close proximity, human infection occurs after ingesting larval metacercaria in uncooked watercress, water plants, or crustaceans.

Clinical Features. Patients usually present with abdominal or right upper quadrant pain and diarrhea 2–3 months after ingestion. Extrahepatic manifestations include meningitis, cerebral mass lesions, and a single case report of an antiphospholipid syndrome with cerebral arterial thromboses, cardiac mural thrombus, and subungual splinter hemorrhages.

Diagnosis. Diagnosis is by examining stool samples for eggs or by positive serological (ELISA, counterimmunoelectrophoresis, IFA) and intradermal tests.

Treatment. Treatment is with bithionol, 30–50 mg/kg orally on alternate days for 10–15 days. A single oral dose of triclabendazole, 10 mg/kg, after an overnight fast is an alternative, but repeated treatments may be required. Praziquantel is not effective against *F. hepatica*. Dehydroemetine combined with anticoagulation and prednisone improved the case of antiphospholipid syndrome (Frances et al. 1994).

Prevention. Control measures include elimination of the disease in livestock, use of molluscicides, and avoidance of uncooked water plants and contaminated water.

DISEASES OF ECTOPARASITES

Tick paralysis is an ascending flaccid paralysis caused by the following species: *Dermacentor andersoni* (North American wood tick), *D. variabilis* (dog tick), and *Amblyomma maculatum* in North America; *Ornithodoros lahorensis* in the Russian Republic; *Otobius megnini*, *Ixodes rubicundus*, and *Rhipicephalus simus* in South Africa; *Ixodes tancitarus* in

Mexico; and *Amblyomma cyprium aeratipes* in the Philippines. *Ixodes holocyclus* of eastern Australia causes a unique paralysis, becoming more severe 2 days after the tick has been removed, and an antiserum is available. A tick is removed by grasping its head with forceps and pulling from the point of attachment; or by inducing it to release its hold with lighter fluid or chloroform. Fatal tick paralysis has been caused by an unrecognized tick attached to the tympanic membrane. The viral, bacterial, and rickettsial pathogens harbored by ticks and their associated illnesses are discussed in their respective sections.

Myiasis, or infestation by maggots, may occur in comatose or immobile patients. Meningitis may follow dissection of larvae through soft tissue and bone.

REFERENCES

Ancelle T, Barret B, Flachet L, Moren A. Two epidemics of arsenical encephalopathy in the treatment of trypanosomiasis, Uganda, 1992–1993. Bulletin de la Societe de Pathologie Exotique 1994;87:341–346.

Bhatia B, Misra S. Recurrent Guillain-Barré syndrome following acute filariasis. J Neurol Neurosurg Psychiatry 1993;56: 1133–1134.

Blunt SB, Boulton J, Wise R. MRI in schistosomiasis of conus medullaris and lumbar spinal cord. Lancet 1993;341:557.

Case Records of the Massachusetts General Hospital. Weekly clinicopathological exercises. Case 39-1996. A 30-year-old man with a generalized tonic-clonic seizure and a left temporal-lobe mass. N Engl J Med 1996;335:1906–1914.

Ferreira MS, Nishioka S, Silvestre MT, et al. Reactivation of Chagas' disease in patients with AIDS: report of three new cases and review of the literature. Clin Infect Dis 1997; 25:1397–1400.

Fourestie V, Douceron H, Brugieres P, et al. Neurotrichinosis: a cerebrovascular disease associated with myocardial injury and hypereosinophilia. Brain 1993;116:603–616.

Frances C, Piette J-C, Saada V, et al. Multiple subungual splinter hemorrhages in the antiphospholipid syndrome: a report of five cases and review of the literature. Lupus 1994;3:123–128.

Gardon J, Gardon-Wendel N, Demanga Ngangue, et al. Serious reactions after mass treatment of onchocerciasis with ivermectin in an area endemic for *Loa loa* infection. Lancet 1997; 350:18–22.

Goldberg MA, Kazacos KR, Boyce WM, et al. Diffuse unilateral subacute neuroretinitis. Morphometric, serologic, and epidemiologic support for Baylisascaris as a causative agent. Ophthalmology 1993;100:1695–1701.

Griesemer DA, Barton LL, Reese CM, et al. Amebic meningoencephalitis caused by *Balamuthia mandrillaris*. Pediatr Neurol 1994;10:249–254.

Hashim FA, Ahmed AE, el Hassan M, et al. Neurologic changes in visceral leishmaniasis. Am J Trop Med Hyg 1995; 52:149–154.

Iten M, Matovu E, Brun R, Kaminsky R. Innate lack of susceptibility of Ugandan *Trypanosoma brucei rhodesiense* to DL-alpha-difluoromethylornithine (DFMO). Trop Med Parasitol 1995;46: 190–194.

Khonde N, Pepin J, Mpia B. A seven days course of eflornithine for relapsing *Trypanosoma brucei gambiense* sleeping sickness. Trans R Soc Trop Med Hyg 1997;91:212–213.

Kim DG, Paek SH, Chang KH, et al. Cerebral sparganosis: clinical manifestations, treatment and outcome. J Neurosurg 1996;85:1066–1071.

Kusner DJ, King CH. Cerebral paragonimiasis. Semin Neurol 1993;13:201–208.

Murphy SA, Mberu E, Muhia D, et al. The disposition of intramuscular artemeter in children with cerebral malaria: a preliminary study. Trans R Soc Trop Med Hyg 1997;91:331–334.

Nakamura KI, Rabbege JR, Baird JK, et al. Malaria. In DH Connor, FW Chandler, DA Schwartz, et al. (eds), Pathology of Infectious Diseases (Vol. 2). Stamford, CT: Appleton & Lange, 1997;1205–1221.

Nguyen TH, Day NP, Ly VC, et al. Post-malaria neurological syndrome. Lancet 1996;348:917–921.

Pepin J, Milord F, Khonde AN, et al. Risk factors for encephalopathy and mortality during melarsoprol treatment of Trypanosoma brucei gambiense sleeping sickness. Trans R Soc Trop Med Hyg 1995;89:92–97.

Radomski MW, Buguet A, Montmayeur A, et al. Twenty-four-hour plasma cortisol and prolactin in human African trypanosomiasis patients and healthy African controls. Am J Trop Med Hyg 1995;52:281–286.

Sabbah P, Brosset C, Imbert P, et al. Human African trypanosomiasis: MRI. Neuroradiology 1997;39:708–710.

Shah AA, Shaikh H, Karim M. Amoebic brain abscess: a rare but serious complication of Entamoeba histolytica infection. J Neurol Neurosurg Psychiatry 1994;57:240–241.

Shakir RA, Stern GM. Tropical Neurology. In GC Cook (ed), Manson's Tropical Diseases (20th ed). London: Saunders, 1996;193–209.

Sotelo J. Cerebral Cysticercosis. In RT Johnson, JW Griffin (eds), Current Therapy in Neurologic Disease (5th ed). St Louis: Mosby–Year Book, 1997.

Visvesvara GS. Epidemiology of infections with free-living amebas and laboratory diagnosis of microsporidiosis. Mt Sinai J Med 1993;60:283–288.

Weller PF, Liu LX. Eosinophilic meningitis. Semin Neurol 1993;13:161–168.

White NJ. Malaria. In GC Cook (ed), Manson's Tropical Diseases (20th ed). London: Saunders, 1996;1087–1164.

Chapter 59
Infections of the Nervous System

E. NEUROLOGICAL MANIFESTATIONS OF HUMAN IMMUNODEFICIENCY VIRUS INFECTION
Cheryl A. Jay

EPIDEMIOLOGY AND PATHOPHYSIOLOGY

Nearly simultaneous outbreaks of *Pneumocystis carinii* pneumonia (PCP), reported in 1981, among homosexual men and drug abusers in New York and Los Angeles signaled the beginning of the acquired immunodeficiency syndrome (AIDS) epidemic. Cutaneous anergy and CD4 lymphocyte depletion noted in these early patients suggested defective cellular immunity, and outbreaks of other opportunistic infections (OIs) and neoplasms, such as mucosal candidiasis and Kaposi's sarcoma, soon followed. In addition to homosexual men and parenteral drug users, transfusion recipients and their sexual partners were at risk for the newly described syndrome. By 1984, the retrovirus now known as *human immunodeficiency virus* (HIV) had been isolated by groups in France and the United States. HIV binds to cells bearing the CD4 receptor. Helper T-lymphocyte infection eventually depletes these cells, and the resulting profound immunosuppression leads to systemic and neurological OIs and neoplasms. Infected macrophages carry HIV into the nervous system, resulting in dementia in some patients, and probably contributing also to the pathogenesis of HIV-related myelopathy and distal symmetrical polyneuropathy (Tyor et al. 1995).

Nearly two decades into the epidemic, HIV infection and AIDS have exacted a staggering toll. Over 1.1 million AIDS cases had been reported to the World Health Organization through June 1995, from nearly every country in the world. Given underreporting, the World Health Organization estimates the actual figure to be 4.5 million cases. In the United States, more than 500,000 cases had been reported to the Centers for Disease Control and Prevention (CDC) through October 1995 (Gourevitch 1996). AIDS is a leading cause of death in persons aged 25–44 years in the United States and in parts of Africa. Currently, sexual contact, exposure to blood and other infectious body fluids, and vertical transmission from infected mother to infant constitute the principal routes of HIV infection. In the developing world, heterosexual transmission causes most cases. Routine screening of the U.S. blood supply since 1985 has decreased the incidence of transfusion-related HIV infection. Perinatal infection rates of 15–30% decrease substantially with zidovudine monotherapy, highlighting the importance of access to antiretroviral therapy. With highly active antiretroviral therapy (HAART), consisting of several drugs targeting specific enzymes in the HIV replication pathway (Table 59E.1), death rates from AIDS in the United States have decreased.

The high prevalence and striking diversity of neurological disorders complicating AIDS were recognized early. Neurological OIs and malignancies predominated in early case series, but it was also clear that AIDS was associated with distinct syndromes, such as dementia, myelopathy, and painful neuropathy, that appeared to result from HIV itself. Clinically

Table 59E.1: Antiretroviral drugs

Drug	Neurological side effects
Nucleoside reverse transcriptase inhibitors	
Zidovudine*	Myopathy
Didanosine	Neuropathy
Zalcitabine	Neuropathy
Lamivudine	—
Stavudine*	Neuropathy
Non-nucleoside reverse transcriptase inhibitors	
Nevirapine*	—
Delavirdine	—
Protease inhibitors	—
Saquinavir	—
Ritonavir	Circumoral paresthesias
Nelfinavir	—
Indinavir*	—

*Penetrates cerebrospinal fluid

apparent neurological disease develops in approximately one-half of HIV-infected patients. Neuropathological abnormalities are nearly universal in patients dying with AIDS, suggesting subclinical disease, underdiagnosis, or both. Neurological disorders cause significant morbidity and mortality and may be an AIDS-defining illness in previously asymptomatic HIV disease or, occasionally, herald unrecognized HIV infection. Nervous system complications may directly threaten life, as well as impair ability to comply with complex therapeutic regimens necessary to manage HIV disease optimally. As HIV infection advances, the CD4 count decreases and the risk of neurological complications increases. These disorders affect every level of the neuroaxis, and a given patient may carry several neurological diagnoses. Familiarity with the common HIV-related neurological syndromes (Table 59E.2) facilitates their recognition, even in the medically complex patient with several neurological diagnoses.

CLINICAL APPROACH TO THE PATIENT WITH KNOWN HUMAN IMMUNODEFICIENCY VIRUS INFECTION

The high frequency of multiple neurological diagnoses in an individual HIV-infected patient means it is not always possible to adhere strictly to the principle of diagnostic parsimony. Even so, the basic principles of neurological assessment, combining neuroanatomical localization based on symptoms and signs with the overall clinical context, still apply. Practically, determining whether the predominant clinical features suggest focal or global cerebral dysfunction, meningitis, spinal cord disease, peripheral neuropathy, or myopathy is an important initial step in diagnosis. Given the high prevalence of neurological disease in HIV infection, it is reasonable to maintain a high index of suspicion for these disorders, particularly because manifestations may be subtle or overshadowed by systemic illness. The stage of systemic HIV infection influences

both the risk of neurological disease, as well as likely etiologies, and hence CD4 count provides critical information that helps guide the evaluation (Figure 59E.1). In early infection, corresponding to CD4 greater than 500/μl, autoimmune disorders, such as demyelinating neuropathies, may develop. During midstage infection, or CD4 levels of 200–500/μl, primary HIV-related disorders, such as dementia, may become symptomatic, as do some infections such as varicella zoster virus (VZV) radiculitis (shingles). In advanced HIV infection, defined as CD4 count less than 200/μl, the risk of dementia, myelopathy, and painful neuropathy increases further, and patients become vulnerable to major OIs such as cerebral toxoplasmosis, progressive multifocal leukoencephalopathy (PML), and cryptococcal meningitis, as well as to neoplasms such as primary central nervous system lymphoma (PCNSL). HAART can significantly increase CD4 count, and it is uncertain whether the nadir or most recent value better predicts risk for OIs, systemic or neurologic. Plasma viral load, which provides an assessment of HIV replication, helps guide HAART, but its role in assessing and managing HIV-related neurological disorders has yet to be determined.

Another important, frequently overlooked, aspect of the clinical evaluation is medication history. Some antiretroviral agents or antibiotics commonly used to manage HIV infection cause significant neurological side effects (see Table 59E.1). Moreover, prophylaxis for systemic OIs may influence the likelihood of some neurological OIs, or raise concern for nervous system infection with resistant organisms. Particularly in advanced HIV infection, the combined effects of severe, chronic systemic illness and brain disease may render patients particularly susceptible to the cerebral side effects of medications. Knowledge of specific HIV risks is also important. Regardless of HIV status, hemophiliacs remain vulnerable to intracerebral hemorrhage and injection drug users are at risk for developing spinal epidural abscess. Similarly, although it is prudent to associate neurological symptoms or signs in a known seropositive patient with a disorder related to HIV, it is important to realize that these individuals also develop common, unrelated neurological disorders such as migraine or lumbar spondylosis.

Several important principles govern therapy of the HIV-infected patient. Most OIs, including those involving the nervous system, require chronic, suppressive therapy to prevent relapse. Adverse reactions to medications, including standard anticonvulsants and other drugs used to manage neurological disorders, occur commonly in HIV disease. Drug interactions are another concern, particularly given the complexity of modern anti-HIV regimens. Protease inhibitors, for example, interact with many drugs. Medication interactions that decrease antiretroviral efficacy can favor the development of resistant HIV strains.

FOCAL BRAIN DISORDERS

Three disorders account for most HIV-related focal cerebral dysfunction: cerebral toxoplasmosis, PCNSL, and

Table 59E.2: Anatomical and etiological classification of neurological disease in human immunodeficiency virus (HIV) infection

	Autoimmune	Primary HIV	Opportunistic infection	Neoplasm	Medications
Brain	Demyelinating syndromes	HIV-associated dementia*	Toxoplasmosis*, progressive multifocal leukoencephalopathy*; Bacterial: TB, syphilitic gumma; Fungal: Aspergillus, Mucor, Histoplasma; Viral: CMV, VZV	Primary central nervous system lymphoma*	Sensitivity to neuroleptic and other medication side effects
Meninges		Acute aseptic or chronic meningitis; Asymptomatic cerebrospinal fluid abnormalities*	Cryptococcal meningitis; Bacterial: TB, syphilis, Salmonella, pneumococcus, Listeria; Fungal: Histoplasma, Coccidioides, Candida; Parasitic: Acanthamoeba	Lymphomatous meningitis	TMP-SMX, nonsteroidal anti-inflammatory drugs, intravenous immunoglobulin
Spinal cord		Vacuolar myelopathy*	Herpesviruses: VZV, CMV, herpes simplex virus; Others: syphilis, TB	Metastatic lymphoma	
Peripheral nerve Root			CMV polyradiculitis, syphilis, TB	Lymphomatous meningitis	
Nerve	Acute and chronic inflammatory demyelinating polyneuropathies, mononeuritis multiplex	Distal symmetrical polyneuropathy*	CMV mononeuritis multiplex		Nucleosides: didanosine, zalcitabine, stavudine; Dapsone, metronidazole, isoniazid, pyridoxine, vincristine
Muscle	Inflammatory myopathy		Toxoplasma gondii, pyomyositis		Zidovudine, TMP-SMX(?)

CMV = cytomegalovirus; TB = tuberculosis; TMP-SMX = trimethoprim-sulfamethoxazole; VZV = varicella zoster virus.
*Common neurological disorders.

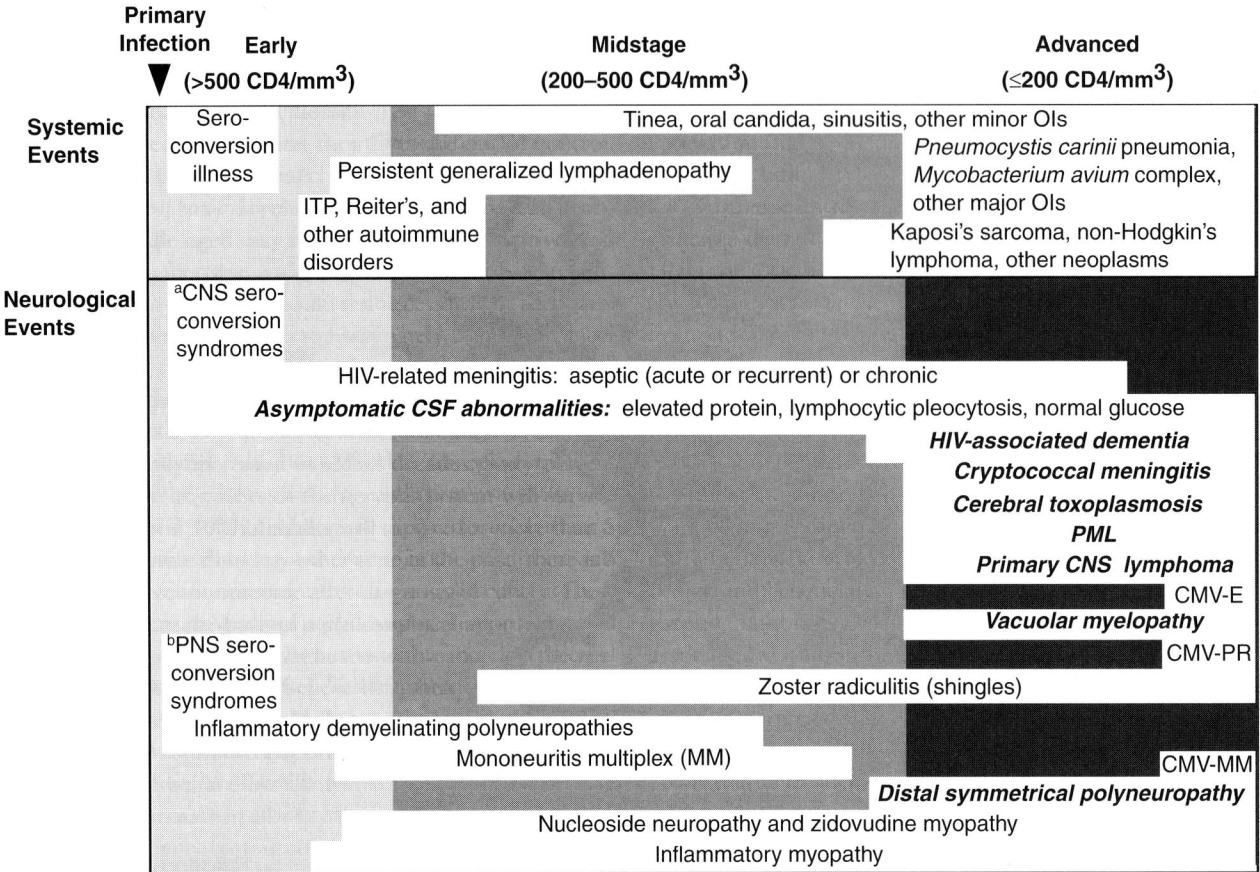

FIGURE 59E.1   Systemic and neurological events in human immunodeficiency virus (HIV) infection. Temporal sequence is approximate and indicates the increasing risk of systemic and neurological complications as HIV infection advances. (CMV-E = cytomegalovirus encephalitis; CMV-PR = CMV polyradiculitis; CNS = central nervous system; CSF = cerbrospinal fluid; ITP = idiopathic thrombocytopenic purpura; OIs = opportunistic infections; PML = progressive multifocal leukoencephalopathy PNS = peripheral nervous system.) [a]Includes, in addition to HIV-related meningitis and asymptomatic cerebrospinal fluid abnormalities, meningoencephalitis, acute demyelinating syndromes, myelopathy. [b]Includes, in addition to acute inflammatory demyelinating polyneuropathies, sensory ganglioneuritis, brachial plexitis, and rhabdomyolysis. Common neurological syndromes are in bold italics.

PML. All are disorders of advanced HIV infection, when CD4 counts decrease below 200/μl. Although they share focal hemispheral or, less commonly, brainstem or cerebellar symptoms as a prominent clinical feature, other aspects of the history, supplemented by neuroimaging studies, response to therapeutic trial, and occasionally brain biopsy, usually allow each to be diagnosed quickly and accurately.

Cerebral Toxoplasmosis

The most common cerebral mass lesion in AIDS, cerebral toxoplasmosis results from reactivation of prior, often minimally symptomatic, infection with the parasite *Toxoplasma gondii*. As such, toxoplasmosis is a syndrome of advanced HIV infection. Prevalence in a given AIDS population varies with the background seropositivity rate (Dal Pan and McArthur 1996), which ranges from approximately 30% in the United Kingdom and United States to 90% in France.

In the United States, 5–10% of patients with AIDS develop toxoplasmosis, consistent with estimates that approximately one-fourth of HIV-infected *Toxoplasma*-seropositive individuals ultimately develop cerebral disease. The typical clinical presentation consists of focal cerebral dysfunction accompanied by fever, headache, and confusion, developing over days to weeks. The absence of headache or fever, however, should not be used to exclude the diagnosis solely on clinical grounds. Systemic PCP prophylaxis with trimethoprim-sulfamethoxazole (TMP-SMX) or dapsone, unlike inhaled pentamidine, confers some protection against toxoplasmosis. In addition to lowering the probability that a given patient with an otherwise compatible clinical syndrome has toxoplasmosis, systemic PCP prophylaxis may eventually decrease the overall incidence and prevalence of toxoplasmosis.

Cranial computed tomography (CT) or magnetic resonance imaging (MRI) reveals ring-enhancing lesions with mass effect, particularly in the basal ganglia and at the gray-white junction (Figure 59E.2). Lesions are multiple in over

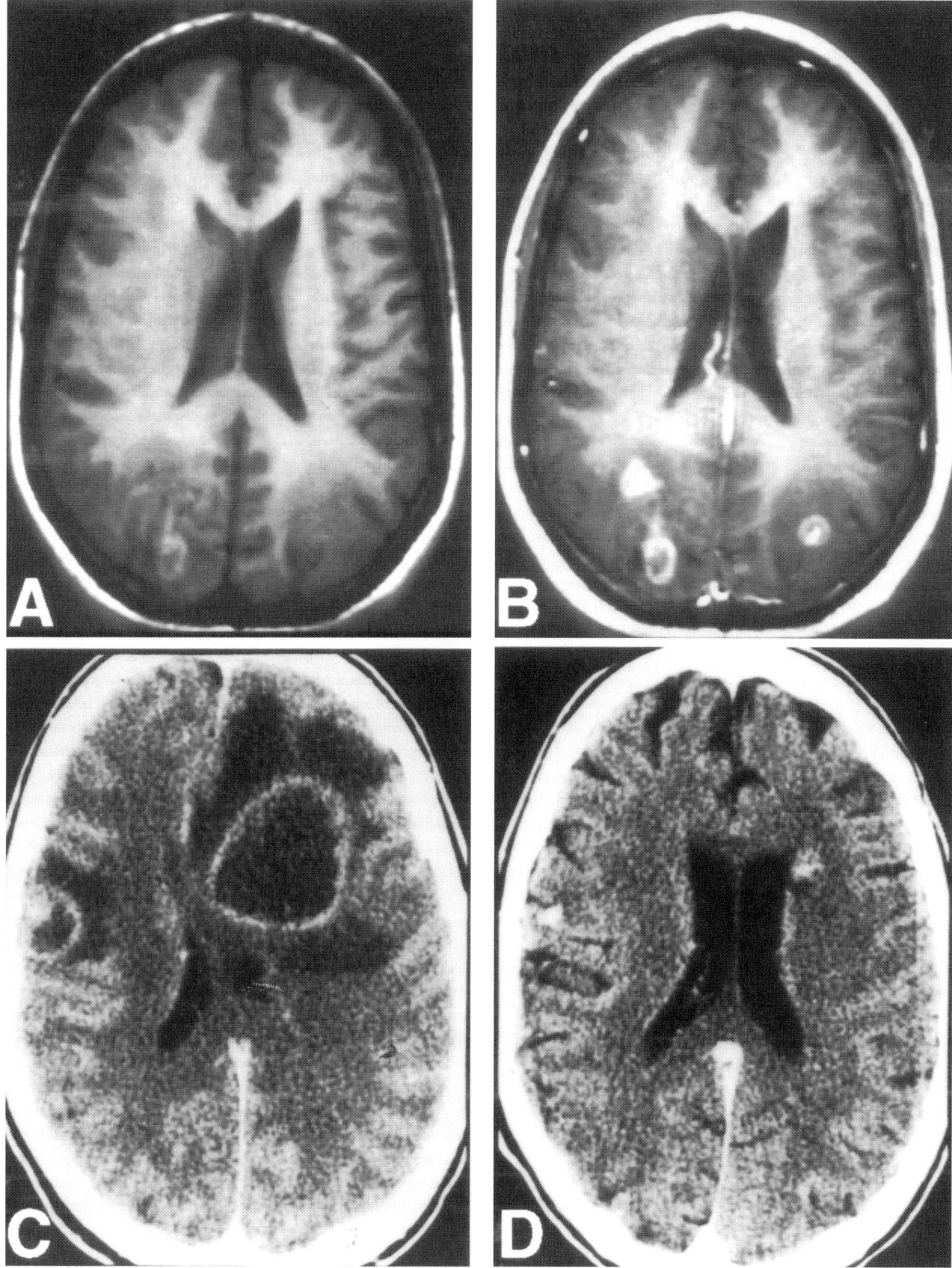

FIGURE 59E.2 Cerebral toxoplasmosis. T1-weighted magnetic resonance images obtained (**A**) before and (**B**) after gadolinium administration reveal multiple ring-enhancing lesions with surrounding edema. (**C**) Contrast-enhanced computed tomographic scan from another patient shows enhancing lesions at presentation. (**D**) Repeat computed tomographic scan after antitoxoplasma therapy reveals residual calcification at sites of original lesions, with resolution of edema. (Courtesy of Dr. Alisa D. Gean.)

70% of cases. MRI detects more lesions than CT, and hence is more sensitive, but it is unusual to miss the diagnosis entirely with contrast-enhanced CT, according to Porter and Sande in 1992. Because these necrotic protozoal abscesses almost always represent reactivated infection, *Toxoplasma* immunoglobulin (IgG) titers are usually, but not invariably, positive. Positive titers are consistent with the diagnosis, but do not establish it unequivocally. Negative titers, however, may increase the likelihood of an alternative diagnosis, such as PCNSL. The diagnosis of toxoplasmosis is typically made when an empiric trial of antitoxoplasma therapy leads to clinical and radiological improvement. First-line acute therapy consists of pyrimethamine (100–200 mg loading dose, followed by 50–75 mg daily, divided thrice daily), sulfadiazine (6–8 g daily, divided four times daily), and folinic acid, 5–10 mg daily, to prevent pyrimethamine-associated hematological toxicity. Medication side effects, such as rash and renal insufficiency, develop in over one-third of patients. In sulfa-intolerant patients, clindamycin, 600 mg three to four times daily, may be substituted. Third-line agents include atovaquone, clarithromycin, and azithromycin. Clinical improvement, accompanied by radiological regression of lesions, as documented by repeat neuroimaging studies after approximately 10–14 days of therapy, confirms the diagnosis. Failure to improve with antitoxoplasma therapy suggests an alternative diagnosis such as PCNSL, and the need for continued evaluation, often including stereotactic brain biopsy. Unless symptomatic increased intracranial pressure (ICP) necessitates their use, corticosteroids are generally avoided, to ensure that resolution can be ascribed to antitoxoplasma therapy alone. Patients whose acute presentation obligates corticosteroids, broad-spectrum antibiotic coverage, or both, may require serial neuroimaging studies over longer periods, as corticosteroids are tapered and other antibiotics are discontinued. Once improvement is documented, lifelong maintenance therapy should be started with sulfadiazine, 500–1,000 mg divided four times daily; pyrimethamine, 25–75 mg daily, and folinic acid, 10 mg daily (USPHS/IDSA Prevention of Opportunistic Infections Working Group 1997). In patients who do not tolerate sulfa drugs, clindamycin (300–450 mg three or four times daily) can be substituted. Practically, poor adherence and intolerance to maintenance therapy pose significant problems. If these obstacles can be overcome, cerebral toxoplasmosis can be compatible with long-term survival. Rarely, toxoplasmosis manifests as acute meningoencephalitis, variably accompanied by muscle involvement. In the even more unusual circumstance in which the diagnosis is made premortem, antitoxoplasma therapy may be lifesaving.

Primary Central Nervous System Lymphoma

In the patient whose neuroimaging studies reveal enhancing cerebral lesions that do not respond to antitoxoplasma therapy, PCNSL is a major diagnostic consideration, and develops in up to 5% of patients with AIDS. Epstein-Barr virus genome is nearly universal in tumor cells of this high-grade B-cell tumor, which complicates advanced HIV infection (Forsyth and DeAngelis 1996). Patients typically present with headache, impaired cognition, and focal cerebral dysfunction evolving over weeks. Compared with toxoplasmosis, the course tends to be less acute and fever less prominent in patients with PCNSL. Neuroimaging studies show one or more lesions with homogeneous enhancement and modest mass effect (Figure 59E.3). Hence both clinical and radiological manifestations of toxoplasmosis and PCNSL overlap significantly. Features favoring the diagnosis of PCNSL include systemic PCP prophylaxis with TMP-SMX or dapsone and good adherence, negative *Toxoplasma* IgG, a solitary lesion by MRI, and failure of lesion(s) to regress with empiric antitoxoplasma therapy. From a neuroimaging perspective, periventricular lesions, particularly in the corpus callosum or subependymal regions, favor a diagnosis of PCNSL over toxoplasmosis.

The optimal timing of diagnostic brain biopsy in patients with AIDS with intracranial mass lesions remains controversial (American Academy of Neurology Quality Standards Subcommittee 1998). The risk of intracerebral hemorrhage following brain biopsy may be higher for patients with AIDS than for individuals without HIV infection. In patients with PCNSL, empiric antitoxoplasma therapy for 10–14 days risks neurological deterioration. Although biopsy remains the gold standard for diagnosing PCNSL, efforts continue to find ways to establish the diagnosis earlier and less invasively. Positive cerebrospinal fluid (CSF) cytology is unusual, but occasionally obviates the need for brain biopsy. Thallium-201 single-positron emission CT may help differentiate PCNSL from toxoplasmosis and is an option at centers experienced in performing and interpreting single-positron emission CT scans. Identification of Epstein-Barr virus nucleic acid in CSF by polymerase chain reaction (PCR) is being studied as a less invasive ancillary test for the diagnosis of PCNSL (Cinque et al. 1997).

Without treatment, mean survival in patients with PCNSL is approximately 1 month. Randomized clinical trial data are lacking, but with whole-brain external beam radiotherapy and corticosteroids, mean survival is 4–6 months. Although newer chemotherapy regimens have improved survival of PCNSL patients without associated HIV infection, most patients with AIDS are too immunocompromised or otherwise systemically ill to tolerate aggressive chemotherapy. As HAART extends survival with advanced HIV infection, PCNSL may become a more common cerebral mass lesion in AIDS, particularly if systemic PCP prophylaxis significantly decreases the incidence and prevalence of toxoplasmosis.

Progressive Multifocal Leukoencephalopathy

PML, a reactivated infection by the JC virus, affects up to 4% of patients with AIDS (Sadler and Nelson 1997b). Sim-

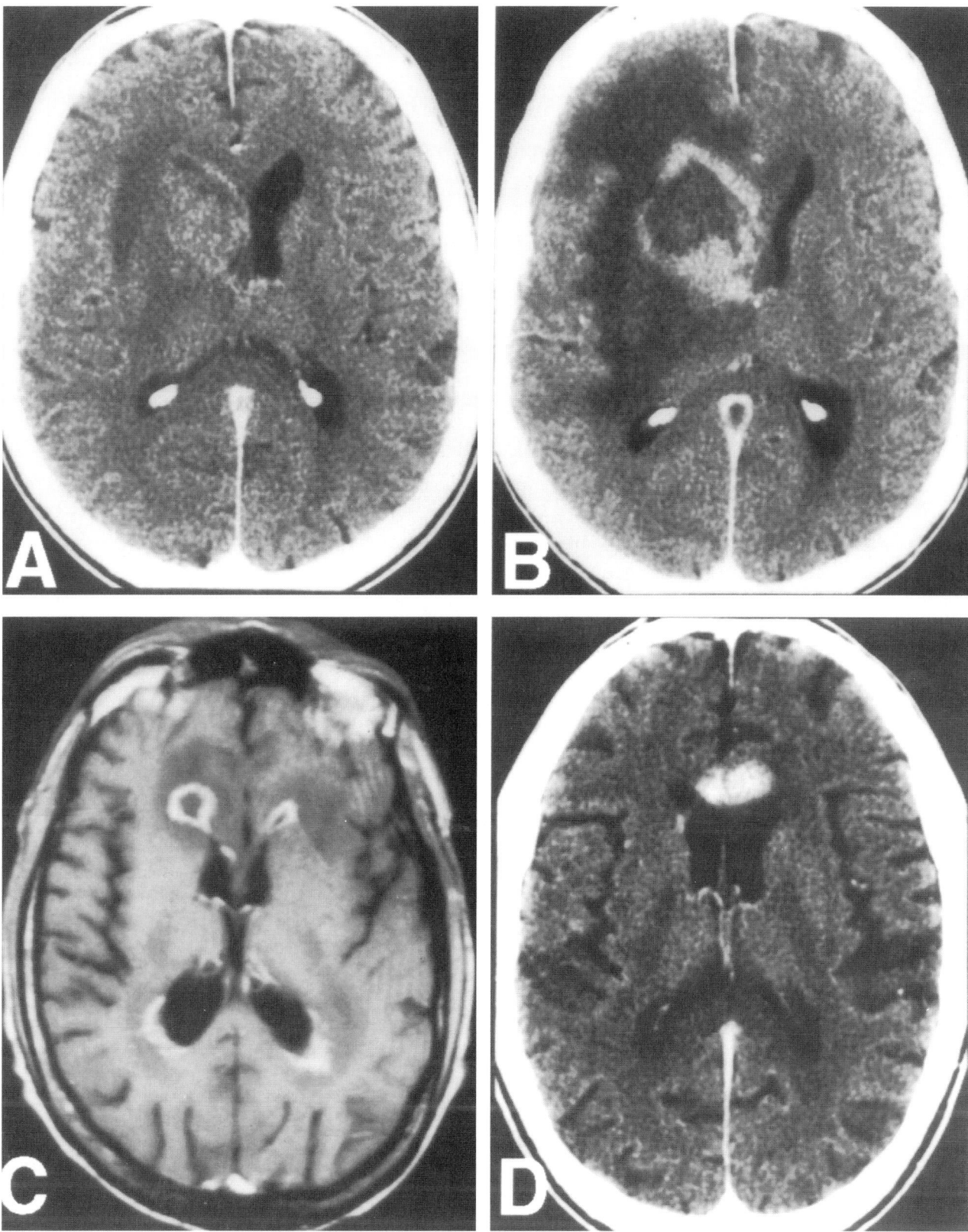

FIGURE 59E.3 Primary central nervous system lymphoma. (A) Contrast-enhanced computed tomographic scan shows a solitary, enhancing lesion adjacent to the right frontal horn with edema and mass effect. (B) Repeat contrast-enhanced computed tomographic scan after empiric antitoxoplasma therapy shows increased lesion size, enhancement, edema, and mass effect, consistent with lymphoma. Images from two additional patients show involvement of subependymal regions on (C) gadolinium-enhanced T1 magnetic resonance imaging and (D) corpus callosum on contrast-enhanced computed tomographic scan. (Courtesy of Dr. Alisa D. Gean.)

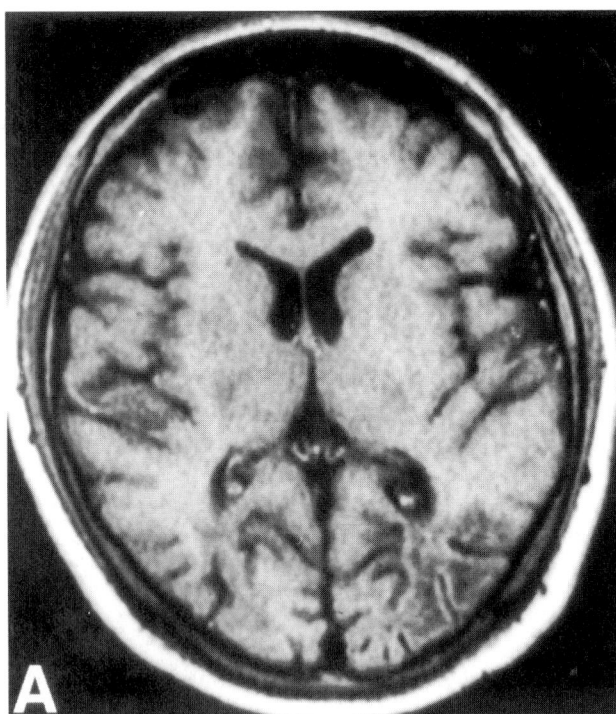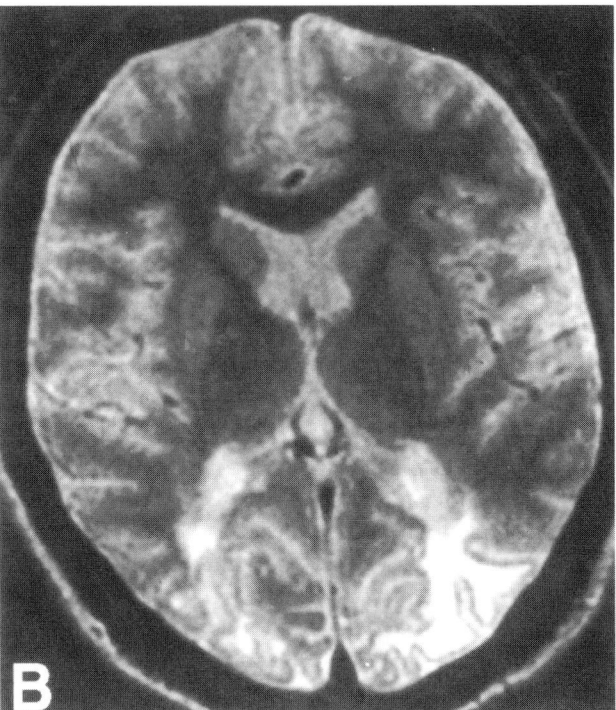

FIGURE 59E.4   Progressive multifocal leukoencephalopathy. **(A)** T1 and **(B)** T2 cranial magnetic resonance images show bilateral lesions in occipital white matter without mass effect.

ilar to PCNSL, PML develops during advanced HIV infection, may be increasing in frequency as systemic management of HIV infection improves, and generally carries a poor prognosis. Clinical manifestations include focal cerebral deficits, usually without headache or fever, typically progressing over months, in a more subacute manner than either toxoplasmosis or PCNSL. Primary infection with JC virus, a human papillomavirus, is nearly universal and often clinically inapparent. With immunosuppression, viral infection reactivates in oligodendroglia, causing demyelination. Neuroimaging studies reveal multiple, well-defined white matter lesions with neither enhancement nor mass effect, findings quite distinct from those of toxoplasmosis or PCNSL, and best appreciated by MRI (Figure 59E.4). Neuroradiological findings in PML can resemble those of HIV-associated dementia, but the strikingly focal symptoms and signs of PML differ significantly from the global cognitive dysfunction that characterizes HIV-associated dementia.

Although definitive diagnosis requires brain biopsy, which reveals bizarre giant astrocytes with pleomorphic hyperchromatic nuclei, altered oligodendrocytes with enlarged nuclei that contain inclusions, and myelin loss, clinical and radiological features usually suffice for making the diagnosis. Routine CSF studies typically show nonspecific changes related to HIV infection. CSF PCR for JC virus DNA appears to be more specific than sensitive for the diagnosis of PML, but eventually may decrease the need for brain biopsy in practice and in clinical trials. Mean sur-

vival is 2–4 months; approximately 8% of patients experience spontaneous remission (Simpson and Berger 1996). Despite anecdotal evidence describing benefit from intrathecal or intravenous cytosine arabinoside therapy, a controlled study showed no benefit. Candidate drugs awaiting controlled clinical study include cidofovir, interferon-α, and the topoisomerase inhibitors camptothecin and topotecan. Even though evidence for efficacy is anecdotal, many clinicians prescribe HAART in hopes that improved immune function will slow progression.

Stroke

Cerebrovascular disease also causes focal brain dysfunction in HIV infection. Ischemic and hemorrhagic stroke have been reported in up to 4% of clinical series and up to 34% of autopsy series (Pinto 1996). Whether HIV infection elevates stroke risk more than other serious, multisystem illnesses remains uncertain. Thrombocytopenia, coagulopathy related to liver disease or disseminated intravascular coagulation, PCNSL, metastatic Kaposi's sarcoma, and, rarely, toxoplasmosis, may be associated with cerebral hemorrhage. Causes of ischemic stroke include bacterial endocarditis, particularly in parenteral drug users, as well as nonbacterial thrombotic endocarditis, vasculitis, and procoagulant states. Granulomatous angiitis of the nervous system has been reported in AIDS. VZV and meningovascular syphilis can cause infectious vasculitis, as can the angioinvasive fungi *Aspergillus* and *Mucor*.

Other Focal Brain Disorders

Numerous other infections have been reported to cause focal cerebral dysfunction in HIV-infected patients. Bacteremia from indwelling catheters needed to manage other aspects of HIV infection or from parenteral drug use predisposes to bacterial brain abscess. Other bacterial causes of focal cerebral dysfunction include *Mycobacterium tuberculosis* abscess, syphilitic gumma, *Bartonella henselae*, and *Nocardia asteroides*. Fungal causes of focal brain disease, in addition to the angioinvasive fungi discussed previously, include cryptococcoma, *Blastomyces dermatitidis*, and *Histoplasma capsulatum* (Minamoto and Rosenberg 1997). Among parasites, relevant diagnostic considerations in patients who have lived in or traveled through endemic areas are cysticercosis and intracerebral Chagas' disease (*Trypanosoma cruzii*). VZV can cause a demyelinating syndrome with lateralizing features, and cytomegalovirus (CMV) has been reported to cause mass lesions (Moulignier et al. 1996). Interestingly, HIV infection does not appear to increase significantly risk for herpes simplex virus encephalitis.

DIFFUSE BRAIN DISORDERS

A broad differential diagnosis applies to the HIV-infected patient in whom impaired cognition or alertness predominates over focal cerebral signs. Organ failure or electrolyte disturbances may cause metabolic encephalopathy. HIV infection may render patients more vulnerable to CNS side effects of neuroleptics and other medications. As HIV infection advances, patients become increasingly vulnerable to other causes of global cerebral dysfunction. For example, when HIV-related focal brain disorders cause multiple lesions, lateralizing symptoms and signs may be less apparent, and the clinical features more consistent with a diffuse encephalopathy. When medication history, screening blood work, and neuroimaging studies do not adequately explain diffuse cerebral dysfunction in a patient with HIV disease, diagnostic considerations include HIV-related dementia, CMV encephalitis syndromes, and various forms of meningitis.

Human Immunodeficiency Virus–Associated Dementia

A disorder unique to AIDS, HIV-associated dementia also has been called the AIDS dementia complex, HIV-1 associated cognitive-motor complex, HIV encephalopathy, subacute encephalitis, and multinucleated giant cell encephalitis. Characteristic cognitive, motor, and behavioral abnormalities define a distinct clinical syndrome consistent with a subcortical dementia. Cognitive features include mental slowing with impaired concentration and memory. Motor involvement manifests as slowed rapid limb movements, gait disorder, spasticity, and hyperreflexia. Prominent behavioral changes include apathy and withdrawal; approximately 10% of patients develop features of organic psychosis. Varying diagnostic criteria and case ascertainment methods have yielded prevalence figures from 7% in a more recent epidemiologic survey to 66% in a retrospective autopsy-based series collected early in the AIDS epidemic (Dal Pan and McArthur 1996). Consistent across many studies is the observation that dementia complicates advanced HIV infection, rarely developing before a diagnosis of AIDS. In the Multicenter AIDS Cohort Study, annual incidence varied from 0.46% among patients with CD4 levels greater than 500/μL to 7.3% at CD4 levels of 100 μl or less (Bacellar et al. 1994). Risk factors for the development of dementia include older age, constitutional symptoms including weight loss, and anemia.

Poor concentration, slowed thinking, apathy, and social withdrawal may overshadow motor manifestations in mild HIV-associated dementia and resemble depression. In more severe dementia, motor signs such as impaired rapid movements, saccadic pursuits, hyperreflexia, and frontal release signs accompany unequivocal memory impairment. Patients with end-stage HIV-associated dementia are mute, quadriparetic, and incontinent. Vacuolar myelopathy (VM) and painful neuropathy frequently coexist with advanced dementia. Lateralizing cerebral signs are distinctly uncommon in HIV-associated dementia and should prompt consideration of alternative or additional neurological diagnoses. Cognitive, behavioral, and motor symptoms and signs typically, but not invariably, progress over months. Approximately 30% of HIV-infected individuals experience mild neurological dysfunction, called *HIV-associated minor cognitive/motor disorder*, that does not clearly predict development of subsequent dementia (McArthur 1997). Whether this relates to true neuropsychological impairment in asymptomatic HIV infection or instead to confounding effects of head trauma, substance abuse, and lack of education remains uncertain.

Neuropathological findings include cerebral atrophy, myelin pallor, chronic perivascular inflammation, multinucleated giant cells derived from HIV-infected macrophages and microglia, microglial nodules, and reactive gliosis. White matter lesions are thought to reflect blood-brain barrier abnormality, rather than frank demyelination. Several lines of evidence implicate HIV in the pathogenesis of dementia. HIV recovery from CSF and intrathecal synthesis of antibodies against HIV suggest the virus crosses the blood-CSF barrier, an event that may occur early and without obvious symptoms. HIV and its antigens and nucleic acids have been identified in brain, principally in cells of monocyte-macrophage lineage. Neurons do not appear to be infected by HIV, although nonproductive infection of astrocytes may occur. Indeed, HIV strains demonstrating

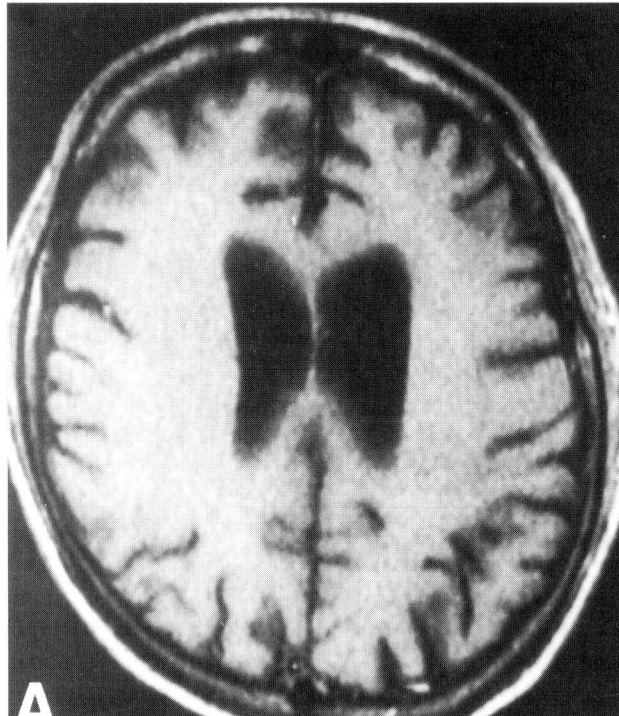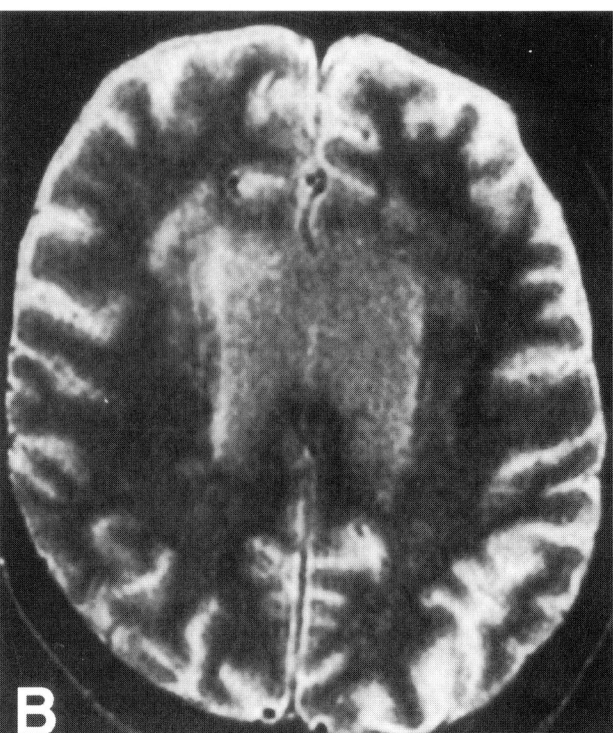

FIGURE 59E.5   Human immunodeficiency virus–associated dementia. Gadolinium-enhanced (**A**) T1 and (**B**) T2 magnetic resonance images, obtained from a patient with acquired immunodeficiency syndrome and progressive cognitive impairment, show marked cerebral atrophy and diffuse white matter abnormalities.

tropism for monocytes and macrophages, as opposed to lymphocytes, are associated with development of dementia, consistent with the hypothesis that infected monocytes and macrophages carry HIV into the brain. Although it is clear that HIV is present in the brain, however, specifics of pathogenesis remain elusive. Clinical and pathological severity do not correlate particularly well. Mild neuropathological features can underlie clinically dramatic dementia, perhaps suggesting neurotoxic pathogenesis. Putative neurotoxins include the viral envelope glycoprotein gp120 and cytokines induced by systemic and cerebral HIV infection. *N*-methyl-D-aspartate receptor activation and calcium influx, resulting from toxins elaborated by interactions of HIV-infected monocytes and macrophages, cytokines, and astrocytes, have been proposed as mechanisms of neuronal injury.

HIV-associated dementia is a clinical diagnosis, with evaluation geared toward excluding other causes of cognitive impairment. Because cognitive and motor slowing are such prominent features of the disorder, screening instruments, such as the Modified Mini-Mental State Examination, that do not incorporate timed tests perform poorly for early detection of HIV-associated dementia. Consideration of medication side effects and depression should accompany screening for thyroid disease, vitamin B_{12} deficiency, and neurosyphilis. As a syndrome of advanced HIV disease, dementia typically develops when patients are also vulnerable to cerebral OIs and neoplasms. Contrast-enhanced cranial CT or MRI help exclude cerebral toxoplasmosis,

PCNSL, and unusual presentations of PML as causes of global cerebral dysfunction. Neuroimaging studies document the cerebral atrophy usually present in more severe cases. MRI may reveal ill-defined, symmetrical, high-signal white matter lesions on T2-weighted images, radiological correlates of myelin pallor observed pathologically, that support the diagnosis of HIV-associated dementia (Figure 59E.5). CSF examination helps rule out neurosyphilis, cryptococcal meningitis, and CMV encephalitis. In dementia, CSF findings include nonspecific changes related to HIV infection: normal glucose, mild protein elevation, and lymphocytic pleocytosis. A variety of conditions, including HIV-related dementia, raise CSF β_2 microglobulin and neopterin levels, and such findings support the diagnosis in the absence of cerebral OI or neoplasm (Price 1996).

Clinical trial and epidemiological data, combined with anecdotal experience, suggest zidovudine helps prevent and ameliorate HIV-associated dementia. Because clinical trials used doses (1,000–2,000 mg daily) exceeding contemporary lower dose regimens (400–500 mg daily), the optimal dose of zidovudine for dementia remains uncertain. Evidence from controlled trials that other antiretroviral drugs modify the course of HIV-associated dementia is lacking. In particular, it remains uncertain whether HAART, which has proven so effective in controlling systemic HIV infection, does the same in the brain, and whether an antiretroviral's ability to penetrate the CSF (see Table 59E.1) predicts efficacy for HIV-associated dementia. In addition to zidovudine, antiretrovirals achieving significant levels in CSF include stavudine, indinavir, and nevirapine. Treatment strategies directed at controlling neurotoxicity thought to be induced by HIV are under investigation (Melton et al. 1997).

Cytomegalovirus Encephalitis and Ventriculoencephalitis

Unusual causes of global cerebral dysfunction in advanced AIDS (CD4 <50/µL), CMV encephalitis and ventriculoencephalitis often cause death within weeks to months (McCutchan 1995). Prior or active disseminated CMV disease, such as retinitis, esophagitis, or colitis, may provide important clues to the neurological diagnosis. CMV encephalitis typically presents as a confusional state evolving over weeks and can resemble HIV-associated dementia. In addition to a course that is more subacute than chronic, focal cerebral signs, hyponatremia, and cranial MRI showing periventricular enhancement are other factors that favor a diagnosis of CMV encephalitis over HIV-associated dementia. CSF abnormalities are typically nonspecific, and CMV PCR is positive in fewer than one-half of cases. Pathological findings include microglial nodules and cytomegalic cells in cortical and subcortical gray matter, thought to be consistent with hematogenous spread of CMV to brain. By contrast, CMV ventriculoencephalitis may reflect dissemination from CSF and presents more acutely than CMV encephalitis, often on a background of CMV retinitis or concurrently with polyradiculitis. Brainstem signs and neuroimaging studies revealing dilatated ventricles also suggest the diagnosis. CSF abnormalities tend to be more striking than CMV encephalitis, revealing elevated protein, polymorphonuclear or lymphocytic pleocytosis, and normal or low glucose. Identifying CMV DNA in CSF by PCR helps confirm the diagnosis. Pathological features include ependymal necrosis and subependymal gliosis with cytomegalic cells, but no microglial nodules. CMV viremia is quite common in late-stage AIDS, and hence detection in this setting by culture, antigen testing, or PCR from blood does not help establish the diagnosis of CMV-related neurological syndromes. Prospective data are needed to confirm the impression that CSF PCR for CMV DNA is specific and reasonably sensitive for these and other CMV-related neurological disorders. Clinical trial data for the efficacy of ganciclovir, foscarnet, cidofovir, or combination therapy for CMV encephalitis and ventriculoencephalitis are lacking, though a trial of empiric therapy is probably appropriate given the poor prognosis.

MENINGITIS

HIV-infected patients are at risk for developing meningitis from a wide array of pathogens, including HIV itself, leptomeningeal spread of systemic lymphoma, and, rarely, medications. The familiar syndrome of fever, headache, and meningismus, with or without altered mentation or cranial neuropathies, observed in immunocompetent patients with meningitis is not always fully expressed in patients with HIV disease. Moreover, HIV infection commonly causes asymptomatic CSF abnormalities that can complicate interpretation of CSF obtained for other diagnostic purposes. As is the case for parenchymal cerebral disorders in HIV infection, the risk of meningitis, particularly from ominous causes, increases as immune function deteriorates.

Human Immunodeficiency Virus–Related Meningitis and Asymptomatic Cerebrospinal Fluid Abnormalities

Diverse forms of meningitis, without other evident cause, may develop during HIV infection. Included among these HIV-related meningitis syndromes is acute aseptic meningitis, which occasionally accompanies or follows the flulike, febrile illness frequently associated with HIV seroconversion. By definition, preserved alertness and cognition accompany headache and other symptoms of meningeal inflammation. CSF shows lymphocytic pleocytosis, elevated protein, and normal glucose. A similar illness with signs and symptoms of parenchymal cerebral dysfunction suggests meningoencephalitis related to HIV, an even rarer seroconversion syndrome. Patients suspected of having these syndromes with an initially negative HIV test result require repeat testing in several months, because HIV antibodies may not be detectable in early infection. HIV-related aseptic meningitis may recur or be accompanied by cranial neuropathies and also occurs during more advanced HIV disease. Chronic meningitis also may develop, sometimes in association with declining CD4 counts (Price 1996). HIV-related meningitis is principally a diagnosis of exclusion, and hence evaluation for other causes of aseptic or chronic meningitis, such as parameningeal infection, other infections (syphilis, tuberculosis, Listeria, fungi, among others), lymphomatous or carcinomatous meningitis, other noninfectious etiologies (sarcoid, Behçet's syndrome, among others) or medications (TMP-SMX, among others) is usually undertaken. The HIV-related meningitis syndromes do not require specific therapy.

Far more common than HIV-related meningitis are asymptomatic CSF abnormalities, which develop throughout the course of HIV infection (Hollander et al. 1994). The typical CSF profile consists of elevated protein (<100 mg/dl) and lymphocytic pleocytosis (<25/µl), with normal glucose. Meningeal exposure to HIV can occur early in systemic infection, as inferred by recovery of HIV from CSF and evidence of intrathecal anti-HIV IgG synthesis. The practical consequence of CSF abnormalities routinely observed in HIV infection is that they can complicate interpretation of CSF obtained to diagnose other neurological disorders.

Cryptococcal Meningitis

Approximately 10% of patients with AIDS develop cryptococcal meningitis, a neurological OI by the encapsulated yeast *Cryptococcus neoformans*. This complication of advanced HIV infection, with CD4 counts less than 200/µl, sometimes presents as headache, fever, stiff neck, and photophobia. However, meningeal symptoms and signs are minimal or absent in over one-half of cases, and the rather broad clinical spectrum includes failure to thrive, personality change, cognitive impairment, cranial neuropathy, or coma. Cranial CT or MRI, typically obtained to exclude focal cerebral disorders, sometimes reveals complications of cryptococcal meningitis, such as hydrocephalus, gelatinous pseudocyst, infarction, or cryptococcoma. More commonly, however, neuroimaging reveals only cerebral atrophy related to advanced HIV infection. The CSF profile ranges from striking protein elevation, lymphocytic pleocytosis, and hypoglycorrhachia to minimal abnormalities that overlap with those attributable to HIV alone. Fungal CSF culture is the gold standard, but the weeks that may pass before a positive result is obtained limit its clinical utility. India ink smear is helpful when positive, but is too insensitive to exclude the diagnosis if negative. Fortunately, CSF cryptococcal antigen (CrAg) testing is a rapid, specific test with a sensitivity exceeding 90%. The rather diverse clinical presentations of cryptococcal meningitis may indicate that CrAg be performed routinely in patients with AIDS undergoing diagnostic CSF examination.

A typical acute regimen for cryptococcal meningitis consists of amphotericin B (0.5–0.7 mg/kg/day) with or without flucytosine (75–150 mg/kg/day) for 2–3 weeks. Renal insufficiency, hypokalemia, and hypomagnesemia may complicate amphotericin B therapy, and the hematological toxicity of flucytosine sometimes precludes its use in patients with AIDS, in whom pancytopenia is common. Patients who are doing well can be switched to fluconazole, 200 mg twice a day for 8–10 weeks (Simpson and Berger 1996), and then placed on maintenance therapy of 200 mg daily to prevent relapse daily (USPHS/IDSA Prevention of Opportunistic Infections Working Group 1997). Although fluconazole therapy may be as effective as amphotericin B for acute therapy of cryptococcal meningitis, delayed CSF clearance of the fungus and a trend toward poorer outcomes among fluconazole-treated patients suggest this approach be reserved for patients with mild disease.

Poor prognostic features at presentation include altered level of consciousness, CSF cell count less than 20 cells/μl, and CSF CrAg greater than 1 to 1,024. Acute mortality approaches 30% and is related to increased ICP at presentation. Medical management with corticosteroids or acetazolamide and CSF drainage with repeated lumbar punctures or ventriculostomy can be used to lower ICP, although none of these interventions has been subjected to clinical trial (Zeind et al. 1996). Optic nerve sheath fenestration has been suggested as an adjunct to these measures when increased ICP threatens vision. Focal cerebral signs accompanying cryptococcal meningitis may suggest stroke from infectious vasculitis or cryptococcoma. Other complications include cranial neuropathies and obstructive or communicating hydrocephalus. Without chronic suppressive therapy, relapse rates exceed 50%. As noted, first-line maintenance therapy is fluconazole, 200 mg daily; second-line agents include weekly amphotericin B or itraconazole. In patients who escape early complications, cryptococcal meningitis is compatible with long-term survival in patients who tolerate and adhere to chronic suppressive therapy.

Neurosyphilis

Diagnosis and management of neurosyphilis in HIV-infected patients pose complex challenges. Syphilis and HIV infection often coexist, as the disorders share risk factors. Moreover, both infections are characterized by diverse neurological syndromes affecting brain, meninges, spinal cord, and nerve roots. CNS invasion in early syphilis appears to occur at similar rates in patients with and without HIV infection (Rolfs et al. 1997). Individuals without HIV infection frequently clear *Treponema pallidum* from CSF even without antibiotic therapy. Whether the same is true in HIV-infected patients is less certain. Meningeal forms characteristic of early neurosyphilis dominate case reports of HIV infection and neurosyphilis, perhaps implicating impaired CSF clearance of *T. pallidum* in HIV-infected patients, even with adequate therapy for early syphilis. Other clinical syndromes described in association with HIV infection include syphilitic eye disease, gumma, and myelopathy.

Several factors complicate the diagnosis of neurosyphilis, particularly asymptomatic forms, in the setting of HIV infection. Individuals coinfected with HIV and *T. pallidum* may demonstrate unusual serological responses. When clinical suspicion for neurosyphilis is high and syphilis serology results are negative, repeat testing to exclude the prozone effect or biopsy, dark-field examination, or immunofluorescence staining of lesions may be necessary (Berger and Levy 1997). Assuming atraumatic lumbar puncture, CSF VDRL is quite specific, but not particularly sensitive, for diagnosing neurosyphilis. Moreover, relying on CSF pleocytosis and protein elevation to make the diagnosis, as is done for HIV-negative individuals, is complicated by the high frequency of these CSF abnormalities caused by HIV infection alone. Treponeme-specific tests in CSF are quite sensitive, but not specific, for neurosyphilis. Hence negative CSF fluorescent treponemal antibody or microhemagglutination–*T. pallidum* excludes the diagnosis of neurosyphilis, but a positive result does not establish the diagnosis. The CDC recommends that HIV-infected patients with late latent syphilis or syphilis of unknown duration undergo CSF examination before therapy, regardless of whether there are associated ophthalmic, vestibular, or neurological symptoms (Centers for Disease Control 1998).

Regardless of HIV status, recommended treatment for neurosyphilis consists of a 10- to 14-day course of either aqueous crystalline penicillin G, 3–4 million units intravenously every 4 hours, or procaine penicillin, 2.4 million units intramuscularly daily, with oral probenecid, 500 mg four times a day. Because alternative agents, such as doxycycline and tetracycline, are of uncertain efficacy in neurosyphilis, desensitization should be considered in patients allergic to penicillin. The CDC recommends CSF examination every 6 months after therapy for all patients with neurosyphilis, regardless of HIV status, until pleocytosis, if initially present, resolves. Whether this is appropriate for patients with HIV infection and neurosyphilis remains uncertain. Treatment failures may occur more commonly in the setting of HIV infection, and neurological status and serum serologies should be carefully monitored as well.

Other Meningitis and Meningoencephalitis Syndromes

Other causes of meningitis complicating HIV infection include neoplasm, rarer infections, and medications. Patients with AIDS are at increased risk for systemic lymphoma, which can cause lymphomatous meningitis. Additional infectious causes of meningitis include bacteria (*Salmonella*, pneumococcus, *M. tuberculosis*, syphilis, *Nocardia*, *Listeria*, *B. henselae*) and fungi (*Histoplasma* and *Coccidioides* in individuals who have lived in endemic regions, *Candida*, *Blastomyces*, *Sporothrix*). Medications are often overlooked as a cause of meningitis; implicated agents in common use for HIV infection include nonsteroidal anti-inflammatory drugs, TMP-SMX, and intravenous immunoglobulin. Causes of meningoencephalitic syndromes include VZV and the parasites *T. gondii*, *T. cruzii*, and *Acanthamoeba* spp.

MYELOPATHY

Vacuolar Myelopathy

VM is the most common cause of spinal cord dysfunction in patients with AIDS, apparent pathologically in 25–55% of AIDS autopsy series (Dal Pan et al. 1994). Affected patients develop gait difficulty, caused by spasticity, leg weakness, and impaired proprioception, often accompanied by sphincter dysfunction, evolving over months. Back pain is not a prominent feature. VM complicates late HIV infection and frequently coexists with dementia and distal symmetrical polyneuropathy. Examination reveals spastic paraparesis with Babinski's signs and hyperreflexia, unless concomitant neuropathy is severe. Sensation in the legs, particularly proprioception and vibratory sense, is usually impaired, although a clear sensory level over the trunk is unusual. The arms are typically spared until VM is advanced. Pathological findings are most striking in the dorsolateral thoracic cord and include vacuolar changes in myelin sheaths with relative preservation of axons. MRI may occasionally reveal cord atrophy, but usually is unremarkable. Despite the clinical and pathological resemblance to combined systems degeneration, vitamin B_{12} levels are typically normal in affected patients. HIV-induced release of neurotoxic cytokines or abnormalities in vitamin B_{12} uti-

lization may contribute to the development of VM; primary HIV infection of the spinal cord seems unlikely. Antiretroviral drugs do not appear to modify the progressive course of VM, and hence therapy is largely supportive and directed toward ensuring safe mobility and managing spasticity and bladder and bowel dysfunction.

Other Myelopathies

Numerous other infectious, neoplastic, and metabolic disorders occasionally cause myelopathy in patients with HIV infection. Compared with VM, these disorders may progress more rapidly, often with associated back or radicular pain. CMV, VZV, and herpes simplex virus may cause myelitis. Helpful diagnostic tests include spinal MRI, which may reveal cord swelling with intramedullary enhancement and T2 signal prolongation, and CSF PCR testing for viral DNA. Because HIV shares risk factors with human T-cell lymphotropic virus I and II, coinfection with these retroviruses also may cause myelopathy in the HIV-infected patient. Other causes of myeloneuropathy complicating HIV infection include neurosyphilis and vitamin B_{12} deficiency. HIV-infected parenteral drug users may develop spinal epidural abscess, a neurosurgical emergency whose clinical manifestations do not appear to be significantly modified by HIV infection (Heary et al. 1994). Rarer infectious causes of myelopathy include *M. tuberculosis* and *T. gondii*. Patients with AIDS are susceptible to systemic lymphoma, which can cause myelopathy from epidural metastases.

NEUROMUSCULAR DISORDERS

Peripheral nervous system complications may be even more prevalent than the various CNS disorders that develop during HIV infection. In the face of significant systemic illness and CNS dysfunction, neuromuscular disorders may be difficult to recognize. Although rarely life-threatening, nerve and muscle disease can interfere with activities of daily living and impair quality of life. As is the case with HIV-related CNS complications, peripheral nervous system dysfunction develops in a relatively stage-specific fashion, caused by primary effects of HIV, consequences of immunological dysfunction, or medication toxicity.

Neuropathies

Of the various peripheral nerve syndromes that complicate HIV infection, the most common is distal sensory polyneuropathy (DSP), also called *HIV-associated neuropathy* or *AIDS neuropathy*. This axonal, predominantly sensory, polyneuropathy develops in approximately one-third of patients with AIDS, becoming more prevalent as the CD4 count decreases (Sadler and Nelson 1997a). Depressed or absent ankle jerks and mild pain, temperature, and vibratory sensory loss in the feet, with or without associated foot paresthesias and numbness, may be the only evidence of the disorder, and probably make up the more common clinical syndrome. Less frequently, severe burning paresthesias develop in the feet, often disrupting sleep in a manner reminiscent of diabetic or alcoholic polyneuropathies. Symmetrical involvement is a characteristic clinical feature, and hands are usually spared until the disorder is advanced. Even though DSP typically spares motor function and proprioception, walking may be impaired because of severe pain. Why advanced HIV infection is so commonly associated with axonal neuropathy remains uncertain. Cytokine upregulation in advanced infection has been proposed, as have dorsal root ganglion toxicity of HIV envelope glycoprotein gp120 and effects of chronic, multisystemic illness. The rather typical clinical features usually obviate the need for electromyography and nerve conduction studies. Exposures to neurotoxins, including ethanol, should be reviewed. Neurotoxic drugs commonly used to manage HIV infection include the nucleoside antiretrovirals didanosine, zalcitabine, and stavudine (see Table 59E.1), in addition to isoniazid, pyridoxine, dapsone, metronidazole, and vincristine. Many clinicians screen for vitamin B_{12} deficiency, and it also may be reasonable to test for diabetes mellitus in selected patients. Goals of treatment include minimizing neurotoxic exposures and managing pain. Tricyclic antidepressants and anticonvulsants ameliorate neuropathic pain, including that caused by DSP. When there is coexisting dementia or other cerebral disease, the anticholinergic effects of amitriptyline may be poorly tolerated. Using very low doses or switching to a less anticholinergic tricyclic antidepressant such as nortriptyline may facilitate tolerance. With regard to anticonvulsants, the high rate of adverse reactions and drug interactions with carbamazepine and phenytoin in patients with AIDS limits their utility for the management of neuropathic pain. The favorable side effect and drug interaction profile of gabapentin may make it a promising agent for managing neuropathic pain in AIDS. Because it is not given systemically, topical capsaicin is an appealing choice, but it can be difficult for patients to use successfully. Other occasionally useful adjuncts include nonsteroidal anti-inflammatory drugs, transcutaneous electrical nerve stimulator units, and acupuncture, but some patients may require chronic narcotic therapy.

Nucleoside neuropathy, a painful neuropathy that closely resembles DSP, is the major dose-limiting toxicity for the antiretroviral agents didanosine, zalcitabine, and stavudine. Two clinical features can help distinguish nucleoside neuropathy from DSP. First, nucleoside neuropathy typically evolves over weeks, in contrast to DSP, which progresses over months or even years. Second, stopping the offending agent eventually leads to regression of nucleoside neuropathy over several months, although an unusual phenomena known as *coasting* may supervene, in which symptoms worsen for several weeks before improving. Although pre-existing DSP increases the risk for nucleoside neuropathy, many patients with DSP tolerate neurotoxic antiretrovirals, particularly if the dose can be kept low. Similarly, many patients who develop nucleoside neuropathy can resume therapy at a lower dose or may tolerate a different neurotoxic drug. Other aspects of the evaluation and treatment are similar to DSP.

Less common than the painful neuropathies related to HIV or nucleoside antiretrovirals are acute and chronic inflammatory demyelinating polyneuropathies (IDPs). These disorders resemble the syndromes seen in individuals without HIV infection with regard to pathogenesis and most clinical features. The precise prevalence is unknown, but case series from the United States and Africa suggest that the IDPs often develop during early HIV infection, sometimes around the time of seroconversion. Before the frank immunosuppression of AIDS, immune dysregulation can cause autoimmune disorders, such as the IDPs, in early HIV infection. Acute IDP, or Guillain-Barré syndrome, typically presents as rapidly progressive ascending weakness with areflexia, variably accompanied by respiratory failure and dysautonomia. The Miller-Fisher variant, in which cranial nerve dysfunction, areflexia, and sensory ataxia are more prominent than limb or respiratory weakness, also has been described during HIV infection. In chronic IDP (CIDP), neuropathic weakness and sensory loss occurs in a more indolent and episodic manner. Cranial nerves may be involved in CIDP, but respiratory failure or autonomic dysfunction are unusual. In both Guillain-Barré syndrome and CIDP, electrophysiological studies reveal slowed conduction, temporal dispersion, and prolonged F waves, indicating demyelination. CSF from seronegative patients with IDP typically reveals only elevated protein, without associated pleocytosis. In contrast, HIV-infected patients with IDP may demonstrate lymphocytic pleocytosis in addition to increased protein. Uncontrolled series suggest that intravenous immunoglobulin, plasmapheresis, and corticosteroids are beneficial. The lower cost of corticosteroids may be offset somewhat by concerns that chronic use may accelerate immunosuppression caused by HIV.

Mononeuritis multiplex, another relatively rare peripheral nerve syndrome of HIV infection, manifests clinically as multifocal, asymmetrical peripheral nerve lesions that may include cranial nerves. When the syndrome develops in early or midstage HIV infection, it is typically self-limited, only rarely requiring immunosuppressive therapy. Mononeuritis multiplex complicating advanced HIV infection, with CD4 count less than 50/µl, may be caused by CMV and responds to intravenous ganciclovir.

Polyradiculitis, another uncommon HIV-related peripheral nerve disorder, results from a variety of infectious agents, usually CMV. Clinical manifestations suggest a cauda equina syndrome, with leg weakness, sphincter dysfunction, sacral and leg paresthesias and sensory loss, and areflexia, typically evolving over several days. When such a syndrome develops in a patient with a CD4 count less than 50/µl, and CSF reveals marked polymorphonuclear pleocytosis, elevated protein, and low to normal glucose, CMV infection of the nerve roots, with subsequent inflammation and necrosis, is the likely cause. CMV PCR or branched DNA assay in CSF is a helpful confirmatory test, but treatment should not be delayed pending these results. Uncontrolled reports indicate that intravenous ganciclovir is beneficial for CMV polyradiculitis, which is fatal without treatment (McCutchan 1995). Polyradiculitis caused by ganciclovir-resistant CMV has been reported and may portend broader use of foscarnet, either alone or with ganciclovir for this disorder. Other causes of polyradiculitis in AIDS include tuberculosis, neurosyphilis, and lymphomatous meningitis.

Myopathies

Among the first of the muscle diseases recognized as a complication of HIV infection was a syndrome resembling polymyositis, now called *HIV-associated inflammatory myopathy*. Patients develop proximal weakness, and less commonly, myalgia, both of which are often ascribed to HIV infection, rather than coexisting primary muscle disease. Creatine kinase is elevated in most cases, and electrophysiological studies often reveal myopathic units and spontaneous activity typical of an inflammatory myopathy. Muscle biopsy reveals fiber size variability, fiber degeneration, and endomysial infiltrates. Cytoplasmic bodies and nemaline rod bodies are other common histological features. HIV does not appear to directly infect muscle fibers, but rather induces them to express major histocompatibility complex I, triggering cell-mediated muscle injury. Even so, inflammatory myopathy is among the few HIV-related neurological disorders that develops at any time during HIV infection. Anecdotal evidence supports the cautious use of corticosteroids for the management of HIV-associated inflammatory myopathy. Given the potential risks of corticosteroid therapy in the setting of HIV infection, treatment should be reserved for management of functionally significant weakness, and not just elevated creatine kinase levels. Inclusion body myositis also has been reported in association with HIV infection (Cupler et al. 1996).

Zidovudine myopathy is a toxic mitochondrial disorder that presents with insidious onset of proximal weakness and myalgia, making it difficult to distinguish clinically from HIV-associated inflammatory myopathy (Grau et al. 1993). Though first described in patients taking zidovudine in doses of 1,000 mg per day or more, zidovudine myopathy also develops on lower dose regimens in current use. Affected patients typically have taken zidovudine for at least 6 months. Creatine kinase may be normal or elevated, and muscle biopsy shows histological features suggesting mitochondrial dysfunction, which may coexist with varying degrees of inflammation. Controversy persists as to whether mitochondrial abnormalities should be attributed to zidovudine or HIV and whether drug holiday or corticosteroids is more likely to ameliorate symptoms and improve strength. Even so, data from in vitro and animal studies, along with ^{31}P muscle magnetic resonance spectroscopy studies in humans, implicate zidovudine as a mitochondrial toxin. Clinical response to drug holiday or reduction in zidovudine dose often obviates the need for muscle biopsy. Whether stavudine or lamivudine are clinically significant myotoxins is uncertain, but clinical experience indicates that didanosine and zalcitabine are not.

Pyomyositis, a focal suppurative bacterial muscle infection, was common in the tropics but rare in developed nations, before the AIDS epidemic (Medina et al. 1995). Clinical features include fever accompanied by local muscle pain and swelling evolving over several weeks. A source of bacteremia may be evident by history or general examination. Typically, the affected area is swollen and indurated, but not fluctuant. Peripheral white count and creatine kinase are usually normal, prompting consideration of cellulitis or deep venous thrombosis as the initial diagnosis. Ultrasound, CT, or MRI of the affected area establishes the diagnosis. Blood cultures may reveal the causative organism, usually *Staphylococcus aureus* or, less commonly, *Salmonella* or other gram-negative bacilli. Empiric intravenous antibiotic therapy should cover these pathogens. Surgical drainage may be required, and a high suspicion maintained for secondary abscesses. Intravenous therapy for 1–2 weeks is usually followed by oral antibiotic therapy for up to 8 weeks.

A variety of other myopathic syndromes have been reported as complications of HIV infection. Rhabdomyolysis may occasionally be associated with seroconversion, or possibly as a consequence of TMP-SMX therapy. HIV infection also has been associated with adult-onset nemaline rod body myopathy. Finally, disseminated infection with *C. neoformans*, *T. gondii*, *M. tuberculosis*, *Mycoplasma avium-intracellulare*, and *Microsporidia* occasionally may involve muscle also.

Other Neuromuscular Disorders

Other neuromuscular disorders reported in association with HIV infection include motor neuron disease and myasthenic syndromes (Lange 1994). Reports of motor neuron disease have been rare, with atypical features, suggesting, perhaps, coincidence rather than true association. Myasthenia gravis has been reported in association with HIV infection. Whether true association or coincidence, myasthenia tends to improve as HIV disease advances, presumably caused by virally mediated immunosuppression.

HUMAN IMMUNODEFICIENCY VIRUS TESTING IN NEUROLOGICAL PRACTICE

Most of the literature pertinent to the neurological consequences of HIV infection address nervous system disorders in patients with known HIV disease. It is important to appreciate, however, that neurological disease may signal previously unrecognized HIV infection. HIV seroconversion often manifests as an acute febrile illness lasting 1–2 weeks, occasionally accompanied by neurological syndromes including headache with or without aseptic meningitis, acute CNS demyelinating disorders, meningoencephalitis, cranial neuropathy, myelopathy, brachial plexitis, sensory ganglioneuritis, Guillain-Barré syndrome, and rhabdomyolysis (Berger and Levy 1997). As described previously, nervous system disorders developing in early, and therefore previously undiagnosed, HIV infection include the IDPs, particularly when accompanied by CSF pleocytosis, mononeuritis multiplex, and inflammatory myopathy. Demyelinating syndromes resembling multiple sclerosis also have been described in early HIV infection. Unexplained dementia, myelopathy, and painful neuropathy may indicate HIV disease, particularly if accompanied by constitutional symptoms. The CDC recommends HIV testing for all patients with syphilis, including neurosyphilis. Obviously, cerebral toxoplasmosis, PCNSL, PML, and cryptococcal meningitis may indicate underlying HIV infection, particularly if no other cause of immunosuppression is apparent.

The aforementioned neurological disorders should prompt inquiry into HIV risks. Counseling by an individual knowledgeable about the interpretation of HIV test results as well as potential associated risks and benefits should be provided before consent for testing is obtained and again when results are provided to the patient. False-negative results may occur in patients who have been recently infected (Gold 1996), and retesting in 3–6 months is appropriate when very early HIV infection is suspected. Unfortunately, patient concerns regarding confidentiality, insurability, discrimination, and social stigma related to HIV status remain justified nearly three decades into the AIDS epidemic. However, diagnosing HIV infection often influences optimal management of the related neurological disorder. Perhaps even more importantly, it provides an opportunity to take advantage of the increasingly effective therapies that improve both quality of life and survival for individuals living with HIV.

REFERENCES

American Academy of Neurology Quality Standards Subcommittee. Evaluation and management of intracranial mass lesions in AIDS. Neurology 1998;50:21–26.

Bacellar H, Muñoz A, Miller EN, et al. Temporal trends in the incidence of HIV-1-related neurological diseases: multicenter AIDS cohort study, 1985–1992. Neurology 1994;44:1892–1900.

Berger JR, Levy RM (eds). AIDS and the Nervous System (2nd ed). Philadelphia: Lippincott–Raven 1997.

Centers for Disease Control and Prevention. 1998 guidelines for treatment of sexually transmitted diseases. MMWR Morb Mortal Wkly Rep 1998;47(RR-1):1–111.

Cinque P, Scarpellini P, Vago L, et al. Diagnosis of central nervous system complications in HIV-infected patients: cerebrospinal fluid analysis by the polymerase chain reaction. AIDS 1997;11:1–17.

Cupler EJ, Leon-Monzon M, Miller J, et al. Inclusion body myositis in HIV-1 and HTLV-1 infected patients. Brain 1996;119:1887–1893.

Dal Pan GJ, Glass JD, McArthur JC. Clinicopathologic correlations of HIV-1-associated vacuolar myelopathy: an autopsy-based case-control study. Neurology 1994;44:2159–2164.

Dal Pan GJ, McArthur JC. Neuroepidemiology of HIV infection. Neurol Clin 1996;14:359–382.

Forsyth PA, DeAngelis LM. Biology and management of AIDS-associated primary CNS lymphomas. Hematol Oncol Clin North Am 1996;19:1125–1134.

Gold JWM. The diagnosis and management of HIV infection. Med Clin North Am 1996;80:1283–1307.

Gourevitch MN. The epidemiology of HIV and AIDS: current trends. Med Clin North Am 1996;80:1223–1238.

Grau J, Masanés F, Pedrol E, et al. Human immunodeficiency virus type 1 infection and myopathy: clinical relevance of zidovudine therapy. Ann Neurol 1993;34:206–211.

Heary RF, Hunt CD, Krieger AJ, Vaid C. HIV status does not affect microbiologic spectrum or neurological outcome of spinal infections. Surg Neurol 1994;42:417–423.

Hollander H, McGuire D, Burack JH. Diagnostic lumbar puncture in HIV-infected patients. Analysis of 138 cases. Am J Med 1994;96:223–228.

Lange DJ. AAEM minimonograph #41: neuromuscular diseases associated with HIV-1 infection. Muscle Nerve 1994;17:16–30.

McArthur JC. NeuroAIDS: diagnosis and management. Hosp Pract 1997;32:73–97.

McCutchan JA. Cytomegalovirus infections of the nervous system in patients with AIDS. Clin Infect Dis 1995;20:747–754.

Medina F, Fuentes M, Jara LJ, et al. Case report: *Salmonella* pyomyositis in patients with the human immunodeficiency virus. Br J Rheumatol 1995;34:568–571.

Melton ST, Kirkwood CK, Ghaemi SN. Pharmacotherapy of HIV dementia. Ann Pharmacotherapy 1997;31:457–473.

Minamoto GY, Rosenberg AS. Fungal infections in patients with acquired immunodeficiency syndrome. Med Clin North Am 1997;81:381–409.

Moulignier A, Mikol J, Gonzalez-Canali G, et al. AIDS-associated cytomegalovirus infection mimicking central nervous system tumors: a diagnostic challenge. Clin Infect Dis 1996;22:626–631.

Pinto AN. AIDS and cerebrovascular disease. Stroke 1996;27:538–543.

Price RW. Neurological complications of HIV infection. Lancet 1996;348:445–452.

Rolfs RT, Joesoef MR, Hendershot EF, et al. A randomized trial of enhanced therapy for early syphilis in patients with and without human immunodeficiency virus infection. N Engl J Med 1997;337:307–314.

Sadler M, Nelson M. Peripheral neuropathy in HIV. Int J STD AIDS 1997a;8:16–22.

Sadler M, Nelson MR. Progressive multifocal leukoencephalopathy in HIV. Int J STD AIDS 1997b;8:351–357.

Simpson DM, Berger JR. Neurological manifestations of HIV infection. Med Clin North Am 1996;80:1363–1394.

Tyor WR, Wesselingh SL, Griffin JW, et al. Unifying hypothesis for the pathogenesis of HIV-associated dementia complex, vacuolar myelopathy, and sensory neuropathy. J Acquir Immune Defic Syndr Hum Retrovirol 1995;9:379–388.

USPHS/IDSA Prevention of Opportunistic Infections Working Group. 1997 USPHS/IDSA guidelines for the prevention of opportunistic infections in persons infected with human immunodeficiency virus: disease-specific recommendations. Clin Infect Dis 1997;25(Suppl.3):S313–335.

Zeind CS, Cleveland KO, Menon M, et al. Cryptococcal meningitis in patients with the acquired immunodeficiency syndrome. Pharmacotherapy 1996;16:547–561.

Chapter 59
Infections of the Nervous System

F. TRANSMISSIBLE SPONGIFORM ENCEPHALOPATHIES
Paul Brown

The Icelandic pathologist Sigurdsson first used the term *slow infection* in 1954 in reference to scrapie, an endemic degenerative brain disease of sheep that two decades earlier had been shown by Cuillé and Chelle in France to be experimentally transmissible to healthy sheep. In 1957, Gajdusek and Zigas described a progressive fatal ataxia among the Foré people of eastern New Guinea, who lived in relative isolation and practiced ritual cannibalism. In 1959, Hadlow, a veterinarian, noted remarkable similarities between the clinical and pathological features of kuru and scrapie, stimulating Gajdusek and Gibbs to extend their ongoing attempts to transmit kuru to small rodents and monkeys to include the long-term surveillance of inoculated chimpanzees. In 1966, they succeeded in transmitting kuru to chimpanzees after incubation periods of 18–24 months, and 2 years later, also transmitted Creutzfeldt-Jakob disease (CJD) after similarly long incubation periods. More recently, two other varieties of human spongiform encephalopathy also have been shown to be experimentally transmissible: Gerstmann-Sträussler-Scheinker syndrome (GSS) and fatal familial insomnia (FFI). The known and speculative interrelationships between these human spongiform encephalopathies and their animal counterparts are shown in Figure 59F.1.

Since the 1970s, advances in cellular and molecular biology have yielded increasingly persuasive evidence that transmissible spongiform encephalopathy (TSE) results, not from invasion by a foreign pathogen, but from the accumulation of an abnormal amyloid form of a host-encoded proteinase-resistant protein (PrP, or "prion") specified by a gene (*PRNP*) on chromosome 20 (Prusiner 1994a). It is a plasma membrane–bound glycoprotein with a molecular weight of 35,000 daltons and several α-helical domains; its normal function is unknown. By an as yet unexplained mechanism, in disease-affected individuals the α-helical domains are flipped into a β-sheet configuration that converts the entire three-dimensional structure into an insoluble β-pleated amyloid macromolecule that is deposited both within neurons and in the extracellular space (sometimes in aggregates that are large enough to be visible histologically as plaques). Of even greater importance, the amyloid protein thus produced, alone or perhaps in association with another unidentified molecule, has the capacity to transmit disease when inoculated into a new host. The protein conversion step has been accomplished in vitro, but it has not yet been possible to show that the converted protein is infectious (Kocisko et al. 1994).

KURU

Kuru is a progressive cerebellar ataxia that was at one time epidemic among the Foré people in the Eastern Highlands of New Guinea. Its description and study played a crucial role in the development of the concept of TSE. An early ambulant phase is characterized by minimal ataxia, postural instability, dysarthria, and generalized shivering tremor. There follows a sedentary period characterized by emotional lability and worsening ataxia and tremor, on which choreoathetotic and other involuntary movements may become superimposed. In the terminal phase the individual develops hyperreflexia, dysarthria, and dysphagia. Motor weakness, sensory impairment, and cranial nerve deficits (apart from strabismus) are rarely seen. Death usually occurs within 12 months of the appearance of neurological symptoms. The disease occurred most often in women and children, a phenomenon explained by the fact

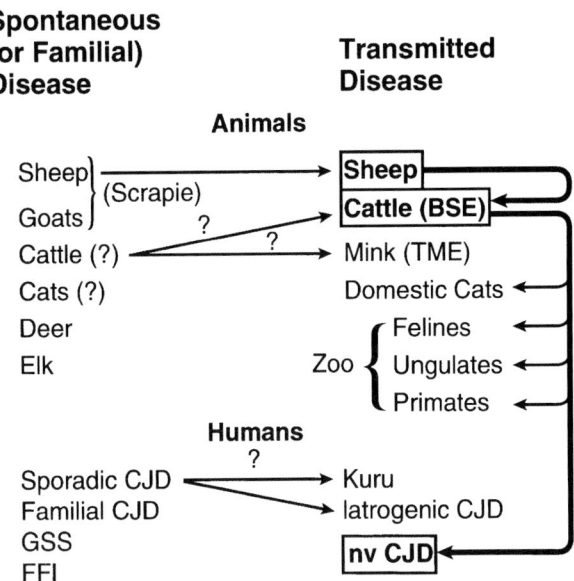

Spontaneous (or Familial) Disease

Transmitted Disease

Animals

Sheep
Goats } (Scrapie)   →   Sheep
Cattle (?)   →   Cattle (BSE)
Cats (?)   →   Mink (TME)
Deer   Domestic Cats
Elk   Zoo { Felines / Ungulates / Primates }

Humans

?
Sporadic CJD   →   Kuru
Familial CJD   →   Iatrogenic CJD
GSS
FFI   →   nv CJD

FIGURE 59F.1 Known and speculative interrelationships among human and animal transmissible spongiform encephalopathies. (BSE = bovine spongiform encephalitis; CJD = Creutzfeldt-Jakob disease; FFI = fatal familial insomnia; GSS = Gerstmann-Sträussler-Scheinker syndrome; nvCJD = new variant CJD; TME = transmissible mink encephalopathy.)

that they, rather than the adult men, prepared the body, and preferentially consumed the nonmuscular tissues, including brain. With the discontinuance of cannibalism, kuru has all but disappeared, although an occasional case is still occurring after longer and longer incubation periods (currently 35–40 years after infection). The neuropathology is similar to that of CJD, but with less spongiform change, more severe cerebellar atrophy, and the presence of kuru-type amyloid plaques in approximately three-fourths of cases.

CREUTZFELDT-JAKOB DISEASE

In 1921, Jakob published four cases of chronic neurological disease that he considered to be similar to a case reported a year earlier by Creutzfeldt. Although only one of these cases meet the current criteria for what has since become known as CJD, Jakob and his students gradually came to appreciate the defining clinical and pathological features of the disease entity, and with the successful use of experimental transmissibility as a basis for the diagnosis during the 1970s and 1980s, the spectrum of disease characteristics was essentially completed (Brown et al. 1994a).

CJD has a worldwide incidence of approximately 0.5–1.0 cases per million per year. Typically, it affects individuals from 50–75 years of age, but cases have occurred both in younger and older individuals; there is slight excess of female subjects. The average time of survival is approximately 7 months, but many patients progress to death in 2 months or less, and a small proportion of cases evolve over

2 or more years. Approximately 90% of CJD cases are sporadic, without any detectable cause, and a familial (inherited) form of the disease, associated with pathogenic mutations in the *PRNP* gene, accounts for most of the remaining 10%. In addition, a small but increasing number of cases of iatrogenic CJD have resulted from cross-contamination through neurosurgical procedures and dura mater grafts, and from therapy with contaminated cadaveric pituitary hormones. Between 1995 and 1999, 40 cases of a new variant of CJD (nvCJD) occurred in Great Britain that are thought to have resulted from the consumption of tissue from cattle infected with bovine spongiform encephalopathy (BSE).

Clinical Features

Prodromal symptoms, experienced by approximately one-fourth of patients, may occur weeks to months preceding the onset of progressive dementia, the hallmark of the illness. These include vegetative symptoms such as asthenia, altered sleep patterns and appetite (bulimia and anorexia), weight loss, and loss of libido. Sometimes, the patient is merely aware of "not feeling right," or has a sense of impending doom.

Whether indefinably fusing with a vague prodromal phase or as the initial manifestation, the onset of recognizable neurological disease usually begins with deficits in concentration, memory, and problem-solving abilities. Family members may notice a change in behavior, including apathy, paranoia, self-neglect, depression, irresponsibility, and inappropriate behavior. They also may comment on episodes of disorientation, hallucinations, and emotional lability. Physical complaints heralding the illness are usually cerebellar or visual in nature, including gait ataxia, clumsiness, dysarthria, diplopia, nystagmus, blurred or distorted vision, altered color perception, field defects, supranuclear palsies, and visual agnosias. Headaches and vertigo are less frequent, and sensory symptoms and abnormal movements are rare. Typically, the onset is gradual, occurring over a period of weeks or even months, but in approximately 15% of patients the onset may occur over a period of a few days or even with strokelike suddenness.

As the illness evolves, increasing impairment of memory and temporospatial orientation occur, eventually progressing to global dementia. Visual symptoms may progress to cortical blindness, and increasingly severe ataxia, in conjunction with pyramidal or extrapyramidal deficits in over one-half of patients, lead to a bedridden state. Abnormal movements, especially myoclonic, but often athetotic or choreiform, are ultimately observed in nearly all patients. Seizures and lower motor neuron signs are less common and usually late in appearance. The clinical course is typically one of more or less continuous progression, with occasional short periods of stability; however, in the small proportion of patients with long clinical courses, the illness may at first evolve rapidly with a subsequently prolonged period of stability, or as a slowly progressive memory deficit followed by a rapid terminal dementia and physical deterioration. The frequency of signs and symptoms at onset, clinical presentation, and in the fully developed illness in a large series of experimentally transmitted cases is shown in Table 59F.1.

Laboratory Diagnostic Aids

Routine examination of the cerebrospinal fluid (CSF) is usually normal, although on occasion the protein may be slightly elevated (almost never higher than 100 mg/dl). An elevation of the immunoglobulin G (IgG) to total CSF protein ratio, sometimes with oligoclonal bands, has been reported to occur in up to 20% of cases. An important new immunoassay that detects a class of 14-3-3 proteinase inhibitor proteins released into the CSF from damaged neurons, although not pathognomonic of CJD, has proved extremely useful in the diagnosis of difficult cases (Hsich et al. 1996). The sensitivity and specificity of the test exceeds 90% (Zerr et al. 1998) and is performed as a service by the Laboratory of CNS Studies, NINDS, National Institutes of Health, Bethesda, MD (Tel. 301-496-4821).

Electroencephalography (EEG) is the most useful routine study in patients with CJD. The typical EEG abnormality in advanced disease consists of one to two cycles per second triphasic sharp waves superimposed on a depressed background (Steinhoff et al. 1996, Figure 59F.2). They are usually asymmetrical in nature, may occur in synchrony with myoclonic jerks, and tend to become slower with the progression of the disease. Less specific but often seen alternative patterns are symmetrical theta and delta waves on an irregularly depressed background, or a burst-suppression slow-wave pattern. With serial tracings, the characteristic triphasic sharp wave pattern is seen in up to 80% of patients at some time during the course of illness.

Computed axial tomographic studies of the brain remain normal in the majority of cases, but may show cerebral atrophy with enlargement of the ventricles and cisterns, widening of the sulci, or cerebellar atrophy. Magnetic resonance imaging also may reveal cerebral atrophy, or a distinctive symmetrical increase in signal intensity in the basal ganglia (Finkenstaedt et al. 1996). Positron emission tomography has been carried out in only a few patients, in whom regional hypometabolism of glucose has shown some correlation with neuropathological lesions found at autopsy.

Diagnosis

The triad of progressive dementia in an older adult associated with cerebellar signs, myoclonus or other abnormal movements, and one to two cycles per second periodic EEG activity, elevated levels of 14-3-3 protein in the CSF, or

Table 59F.1: Clinical characteristics of 209 experimentally transmitted cases of sporadic Creutzfeldt-Jakob disease: percentage of patients with symptoms or signs

Symptoms or signs	At onset	On first examination	During course
Mental deterioration	71	84	100
Memory loss	52	65	100
Behavioral abnormalities	29	38	55
Higher cortical functions	16	36	73
Cerebellar	33	54	70
Visual/oculomotor	19	30	41
Vertigo/dizziness	12	14	19
Headache	11	12	20
Sensory	5	6	11
Involuntary movements	4	19	88
Myoclonus	0.5	9	80
Other (including tremor)	3	10	36
Pyramidal	1.5	16	62
Extrapyramidal	0.5	9	56
Lower motor neuron	0.5	2	11
Seizures	0	2	20
Pseudobulbar	0	0.5	7

both, establishes with high precision a diagnosis of CJD. Alternative diagnoses are most practically grouped according to treatable and untreatable diseases.

Among the treatable diseases that can mimic the clinical presentation of CJD, the physician should first consider the presence of vitamin deficiencies, endocrine metabolic disorders, and drug toxicities. These include thiamine and vitamin B_{12} deficiency, alcoholic and hepatic encephalopathy, hyperparathyroidism, and cyclical antidepressive and lithium toxicity. Infections (including herpes encephalitis and cryptococcal meningoencephalitis) and small occult tumors have also been confused with CJD.

The list of untreatable conditions that can be mistaken for CJD either early or late in the course of illness includes many of the primary brain degenerative diseases: progressive supranuclear palsy, Huntington's disease, Parkinson's disease with dementia, amyotrophic lateral sclerosis with dementia, Pick's disease, and, above all, Alzheimer's disease, from which CJD can sometimes only be distinguished at autopsy.

Biopsy is not recommended unless the differential diagnosis includes a treatable disease; it does the patient no good to learn that he or she has Alzheimer's disease instead of CJD, and patients do not tolerate the procedure well (up to 20% die within 2 weeks of the procedure). In patients with inherited disease, pathogenic mutations in the PRNP gene can be identified by molecular genetic analysis of DNA from peripheral blood leukocytes. The definitive diagnosis of CJD is made by histological examination of brain tissue obtained at autopsy. In addition, immunohistological study of fixed brain tissue sections or Western immunoblot analysis of frozen brain tissue homogenates in virtually every case reveals the presence of pathognomonic PrP.

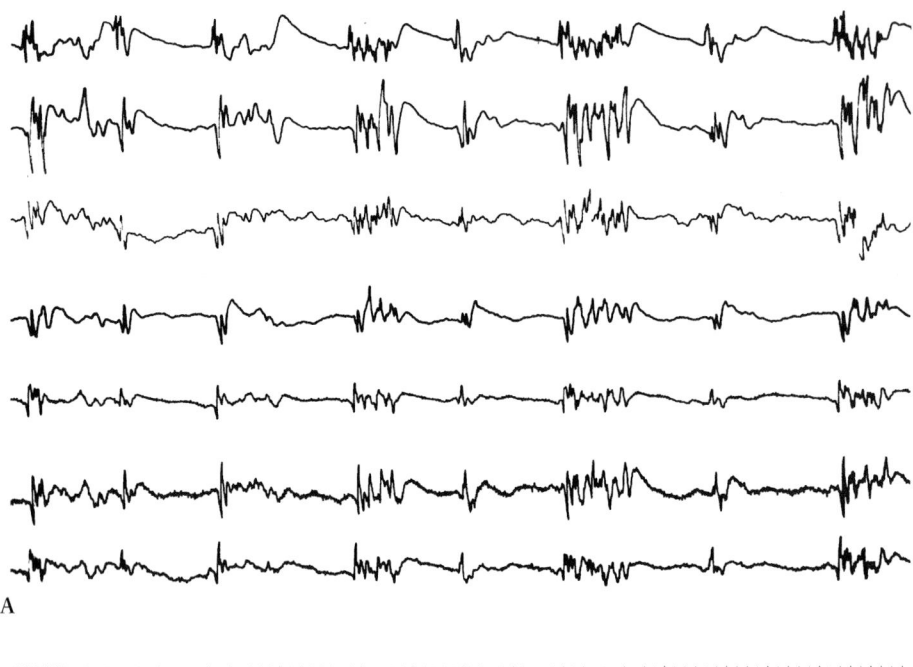

A

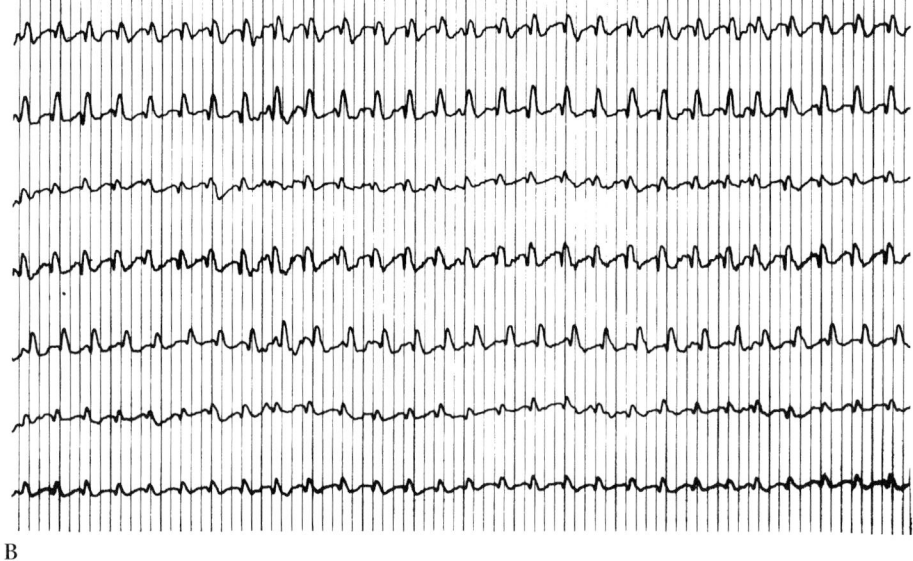

B

FIGURE 59F.2   Electroencephalograms from two patients with Creutzfeldt-Jakob disease. (A) A suggestive but nonspecific burst-suppression pattern. (B) Pathognomonic 1–2 cycles per second triphasic sharp wave pattern.

Pathology

Macroscopically, the brain may appear normal or show varying degrees of atrophy, in part depending on the duration of illness. Historically, a number of subtypes of CJD have been described based on clinicopathological features: corticostriatospinal (Jakob), occipital (Haidenhain), diffuse (Stern and Garcin), ataxic (Brownell-Oppenheimer), and panencephalitic (Tateishi). It has become clear, however, that these subclassifications represent scenes in a continuum of neuropathological pictures and mainly serve the medical tradition of eponyms to honor the physicians who first described them.

Microscopically, the predominant findings are spongiform degeneration, atrophy and loss of nerve cells, and astrocytic gliosis. Spongiform changes, widely but variably distributed from patient to patient, describe small vacuoles in the neuropil that are usually ovoid to round, translucent, and occasionally coalescent (Plate 59F.I). They are usually most prominent in the cerebral cortex, striatum, and molecular layer of the cerebellum. Reactive astrocytic gliosis is a prominent accompanying feature, and neuronal loss may be either mild or severe. An overt inflammatory response is not found, and the reaction of microglia and macrophages is minimal. In approximately 5–10% of cases, amyloid plaques can be seen in the cerebral cortex, cerebellum, or both (Plate 59F.IIA). When present, the plaques usually stain with periodic acid–Schiff reagent, silver, and Congo red, and under denaturing conditions (especially treatment with formic acid, or with

Table 59F.2:   Summary of all known or highly probable cases of iatrogenic Creutzfeldt-Jakob disease

Mode of infection	Number of patients	Agent entry into brain	Mean incubation period (range)	Clinical presentation
Corneal transplant	3	Optic nerve	16, 18, 20 mos	Dementia, cerebellar, or both
Stereotactic electroencepha- lography	2	Intracerebral	16, 20 mos	Dementia, cerebellar, or both
Neurosurgery	4	Intracerebral	20 mos (15–28)	Dementia, visual, cerebellar, or all
Dura mater graft	82	Cerebral surface	6 yrs (1.5–16.0)	Cerebellar, visual, dementia, or all
Gonadotropin	5	Hematogenous	13 yrs (12–16)	Cerebellar
Growth hormone	113	Hematogenous	12 yrs (5–30)	Cerebellar

hydrochloric acid at 121°C), can be stained with antibodies raised against the prion protein.

Iatrogenic Creutzfeldt-Jakob Disease

The first reports of CJD resulting from human-to-human transmission of the disease appeared in the 1970s, involving a contaminated corneal graft and contaminated stereotactic EEG needles. In the first instance, the diagnosis of CJD in the graft donor was not suspected until autopsy, and in the second instance, customary sterilization techniques for the EEG needles were thought to be adequate to inactivate the infectious agent. Retrospective studies in England and France uncovered a handful of other patients who had probably also died as a result of inadequately sterilized neurosurgical instruments.

In 1985, the first case in what has become a tragic outbreak of CJD among recipients of cadaveric human growth hormone was recognized. As of 1999, there have been 113 deaths to date, almost all occurring in France, England, and the United States, with a few new cases occurring each year after incubation periods that have ranged from less than 5 years to more than 30 years. It is likely that the annual number of new cases will soon dwindle to zero, because of the change from cadaveric natural hormone to recombinant hormone that occurred when the first case was discovered in 1985.

Shortly after the human growth hormone story came the recognition of still another cadaveric source of iatrogenic CJD: contaminated dura mater grafts. The first case was reported in 1988, and the total number in 1999 is 82 cases, of which 54 have occurred in Japan. Unlike the random contamination of hormones, however, almost all the infected dura mater grafts were prepared during the early 1980s by a single manufacturer in Germany, who added an effective sterilizing step to the processing protocol in 1987. The U.S. Food and Drug Administration has stipulated a set of rules governing the collection and processing of grafts that should be adequate to prevent any future iatrogenic occurrences from this source.

A summary of all known or highly probable iatrogenic cases is presented in Table 59F.2. The length of incubation period and clinical presentation depends on the route of introduction of the infectious agent (Brown 1996). When introduced directly into the brain (as by EEG needles or surgical instruments), the incubation period is usually measured in months (comparable with the incubation period in intracerebrally inoculated experimental animals), and the clinical presentation is indistinguishable from sporadic CJD. When applied to the surface of the brain (dura mater grafts) the incubation period ranges from a few months to more than a decade, and the clinical presentation may resemble sporadic disease or have a prominent cerebellar or visual onset. When injected by a peripheral route (e.g., pituitary hormones), the average incubation period is 15 years (and may extend as far as 30 years), and the clinical presentation is invariably cerebellar in nature. As a group, iatrogenic cases have clinical evolutions, durations of illness, and neuropathology similar to sporadic CJD.

New Variant Creutzfeldt-Jakob Disease

In 1996, a report of 10 cases of CJD with an unusual clinical presentation, comparatively long duration, and distinctive neuropathology in British adolescents and young adults ended with the electrifying suggestion that they might represent a new disease variant resulting from exposure to BSE, an epidemic disease of cattle that had begun a decade earlier (Will et al. 1996). More recent evidence from the laboratory has strengthened this presumptive connection, in that (1) the deglycosylated protein banding pattern of PrP extracted from nvCJD brain tissue resembles that seen in BSE-infected cattle, but not in sporadic cases of CJD; and (2) nvCJD brain homogenates inoculated into a panel of inbred mouse strains produce an assortment of incubation periods and lesion topographies that resemble those seen after inoculation of BSE, but not sporadic CJD (Hill et al. 1997; Bruce et al. 1997).

Clinically, the most striking peculiarity of nvCJD is the comparative youthfulness of the victims, ranging in age from 16–52 years (average, 28 years), and thus clearly separate from the 50- to 75-year age bracket characteristic of sporadic disease (Zeidler et al. 1997). In addition, the clin-

1428 NEUROLOGICAL DISEASES

Table 59F.3: Mutations of the *PRNP* gene associated with inherited forms of transmissible spongiform encephalopathy

Mutation	Disease phenotype
Octarepeat insertion of 24, 48, 96, 120, 144, 168, 192, or 216 base pairs between codons 51 and 91	CJD, GSS, or atypical dementias
P102L (Pro Leu)	GSS, classical ataxic form
P105L (Pro Leu)	GSS, spastic paraparetic variant
A117V (Ala Val)	GSS, pseudobulbar variant
Y145* (Tyr Stop)	Alzheimer's-like dementia
D178N (Asp Asn)	CJD (129V on mutant allele)
D178N (Asp Asn)	Fatal familial insomnia (129M on mutant allele)
V180I (Val Ile)	CJD
T183A (Thr Ala)	Alzheimer's-like dementia
H187R (His Arg)	GSS, classical ataxic form
F198S (Phe Ser)	GSS with neurofibrillary tangles
E200K (Glu Lys)	CJD
D202N (Asp Asn)	GSS with neurofibrillary tangles
R208H (Arg His)	CJD
V210I (Val Ile)	CJD
Q212P (Gln Pro)	GSS with Lewy bodies
E217R (Glu Arg)	GSS with neurofibrillary tangles
M232R (Met Arg)	CJD

CJD = Creutzfeldt-Jakob disease; GSS = Gerstmann-Sträussler-Scheinker syndrome.

ical presentation seen in most patients has consisted of psychiatric or sensory symptoms, rather than the usual mental and cerebellar onset of sporadic CJD. The illness progresses at a comparatively leisurely pace (average duration, 14 months), during which most of the features of sporadic disease occur (including dementia and myoclonus, but without periodic EEG activity). At autopsy, the defining feature is the widespread occurrence of amyloid plaques surrounded by petals of spongiosis (daisy plaques), together with the usual astrocytosis and neuronal loss seen in sporadic CJD (Plate 59F.IIB).

As of May 1999, there were 40 cases of nvCJD in Great Britain and one in France, a major importer of British beef. New cases continue to appear at the rate of approximately four to five per year, with no evident trend toward increasing, but it will still be another few years before it is known whether these cases represent BSE infection in a small susceptible subset of the British population, or whether they herald a burgeoning nvCJD epidemic of unknown proportions.

FAMILIAL DISEASE AND MOLECULAR GENETICS

The existence of familial forms of TSE has long been recognized; indeed, both familial CJD and GSS were described before 1930. Familial disease has invariably shown an autosomal dominant pattern of inheritance, and in most instances, has been fully penetrant. The discovery of a host gene encoding a protein that is critically involved in the pathogenesis of disease (and perhaps is itself the infectious

agent) opened the door to a search for mutations that could account for familial TSE. Since the late 1980s, the search has been rewarded with the discovery of 24 pathogenic mutations, and although only a few families have had enough informative members to allow formal genetic linkage to be demonstrated, there can be little doubt that each of the mutations does, in fact, cause inherited forms of the disease (Prusiner 1994b). All currently recognized mutations are listed in Table 59F.3.

The mechanism by which these mutations cause disease is unknown. If sporadic CJD results from a spontaneous conversion of the normal to abnormal form of prion protein at a frequency sufficient to produce the observed sporadic incidence of one case per million people per year, it seems plausible to suppose that focal alterations in the character of the normal protein (e.g., ionic charge or hydrogen bonding) brought about by the mutation-directed substitution of one amino acid by another could facilitate the propensity of the protein to assume a β-pleated sheet configuration, such that the one-in-a-million chance conversion would be guaranteed to occur during the lifetime of a person producing the mutated protein. This wholly speculative theory is unburdened by evidence, but nevertheless remains the approved current working hypothesis for the pathogenesis of familial disease.

Knowledge of the molecular genetic basis of TSE has led to a good deal of generalizing about genotype-phenotype correlations, much of which is justified, but susceptible to overinterpretation. Different mutations do in most cases associate with distinctive phenotypes, but it must be emphasized that phenotypic variations between families carrying the same mutation, and even among members of the same family, is the rule rather than the exception, and in virtually all families with several studied members, whether with CJD, GSS, or FFI, at least one member is found to have had an illness similar to sporadic CJD. Generalizations about genotype-phenotype correlation should be read with this fact in mind.

Familial Creutzfeldt-Jakob Disease

The first and still most common mutation to be associated with familial CJD was found as a point mutation at codon 200 of the *PRNP* gene. It is responsible for the exceptionally high incidence of CJD in the Orava region of rural Slovakia, and among Sephardic Jews (including Libyan-born Israelis) living in many different countries of Europe, North Africa, and the Americas. Except for a slightly earlier average age at onset (55 years), the phenotype is indistinguishable from sporadic CJD. Nearby mutations at codons 208 and 210, seen mostly in Italian families, also produce a typical sporadic CJD phenotype. All three mutations are unusual in exhibiting incomplete penetrance: Only approximately one-half of mutation-positive carriers die from CJD.

The second most common mutation associated with familial CJD is found at codon 178. It occurs among families of northern European origin and causes an illness that differs from sporadic CJD in having an earlier onset (usually in the fifth decade), longer duration (1–2 years), and no EEG periodicity.

Other mutations associated with CJD-like syndromes have been described in only one or two families of diverse ethnic origins. These include a point mutation at codon 180 and 183, and several different insert mutations in the octapeptide-repeat region between codons 51 and 91. The point mutations are associated with a typical CJD phenotype, whereas the insert mutations produce mostly atypical syndromes characterized by a markedly earlier age at onset (third and fourth decades) and much longer duration of illness (5–10 years) than any of the other mutations. Japanese authors also have reported a point mutation at codon 232 in a few patients with CJD without known familial disease.

Gerstmann-Sträussler-Scheinker Syndrome

GSS syndrome was first described by Gerstmann and coworkers in 1928 and 1936 as a familial disease with autosomal dominant inheritance. It had been considered an inherited variant of CJD, but its classification as a distinct syndrome has since been validated by molecular genetics, being linked to a different set of mutations than are found in families with the CJD phenotype (Boelläard et al. 1999; Ghetti 1996).

The original family, as well as most of the families discovered later, have a point mutation at codon 102. Onset in the third or fourth decades and a protracted clinical course over several years are common. Patients initially present with cerebellar dysfunction (ataxia or dysarthria), whereas dementia appears later in the course of illness. In some families extrapyramidal or parkinsonian features predominate; others show gaze palsies, deafness, or cortical blindness. Examination frequently reveals loss of deep tendon reflexes in the legs with extensor plantar responses. Myoclonus is comparatively infrequent. The neuropathology of GSS chiefly differs from CJD by the prominence of amyloid plaques, including morphologically distinctive multicentric plaques (Plate 59F.IIC). The classical P102L ataxic form of GSS shows systemic atrophy of the spinocerebellar tracts; other variant features have been associated with different mutations, notably the occurrence of a pseudobulbar syndrome in patients with a mutation at codon 117, and the presence of Alzheimer-type neurofibrillary tangles in families with mutations at codon 198 and codon 217. GSS associated with the H187R point mutation and with insert mutations resembles the classical P102L syndrome.

Fatal Familial Insomnia

Medori and colleagues in 1992 described FFI, which is the most recent TSE. This autosomal dominant disorder presents with intractable progressive insomnia and autonomic systemic disturbances caused by sympathetic overactivity such as hypertension, hyperthermia, hyperhidrosis, and tachycardia. Motor system abnormalities include tremor, ataxia, hyperreflexia, and myoclonus. Frank dementia may or may not develop, but most patients have attention and memory deficits, disorientation, confusion, or complex hallucinations. Endocrine abnormalities consist of loss of circadian rhythm for the secretion of melatonin, prolactin, and growth hormone. Secretion of adrenocorticotropic hormone is decreased, whereas secretion of cortisol is increased. The neuropathology of FFI shows profound selective neuronal loss and astrogliosis in the ventral anterior and medial dorsal nuclei of the thalamus. The inferior olives, and, to a lesser degree, the cerebral cortex show focal areas of spongiosis and gliosis.

The remarkable molecular genetic interest of FFI resides in the fact that the phenotype is associated with the same mutation at codon 178 that produces a CJD-like phenotype in other families. The cause of this unique division of phenotypes linked to the same mutation has been traced to the genotype of polymorphic codon 129: When it encodes methionine on the mutant 178 allele the result is FFI; when it encodes valine on the mutant allele the result is CJD.

THERAPY AND PRECAUTIONS

To date there is neither preventive nor curative treatment for TSE, other than the possibility of eliminating familial disease through an acceptance by mutation-positive family members either to forebear having children, or to request intrauterine fetal mutation screening with a view to therapeutic abortion if the fetus has a positive result (Brown et al. 1994b). Future therapies may be directed toward biochemical interruption of the conversion of normal to abnormal protein or by gene ablation or antisense oligonucleotide therapy to inhibit PRNP gene transcription, as studies in mice have shown that ablation of the PRNP gene has no evident detrimental effect on either the health or life span of genetically altered animals.

Universal precautions should be observed in the general care and management of hospitalized patients. Although the infectious agent of CJD can be found in many organs of the body, it does not appear to be present in any external secretion or excretion, including tears, saliva, perspiration, urine, and feces. It is, however, frequently present in CSF, and rarely present in blood; therefore, gloves should be worn when handling blood or CSF, or when treating oozing wounds or bedsores. As with hepatitis B or acquired immunodeficiency syndrome, the golden rule is to avoid penetrating injuries from potentially contaminated instruments (e.g., spinal tap or venipuncture needles or scalpels). Accidental contamination of intact skin should be treated with the application of fresh undiluted bleach or 1 N sodium hydroxide to the area for approximately a minute, followed by thorough washing with soap and water. Disposable instruments and other materials should be used whenever possible; if retained, instruments can be disinfected by steam autoclaving for 1 hour at 132°C, or by immersion in 1 N sodium hydroxide or undiluted bleach for 1 hour at room temperature.

REFERENCES

Boelläard JW, Brown P, Tateishi J. Gerstmann-Sträussler-Scheinker disease: the dilemma of molecular and clinical correlations. Clin Neuropathol 1999, in press.

Brown P. Environmental causes of human spongiform encephalopathy. In HF Baker, RM Ridley (eds), Prion Diseases. Totowa, NJ: Humana Press, 1996;139–154.

Brown P, Cervenáková L, Goldfarb LG, et al. Molecular genetic testing of a fetus at risk of Gerstmann-Sträussler-Scheinker syndrome. Lancet 1994b;343:379–384.

Brown P, Gibbs CJ Jr, Rodgers-Johnson P, et al. Human spongiform encephalopathy: the National Institutes of Health series of 300 cases of experimentally transmitted disease. Ann Neurol 1994a;35:513–529.

Bruce ME, Will RG, Ironside JW, et al. Transmissions to mice indicate that "new variant" CJD is caused by the BSE agent. Nature 1997;389:498–501.

Finkenstaedt M, Szudra A, Zerr I, et al. MR imaging of Creutzfeldt-Jakob disease. Radiology 1996;199:793–798.

Ghetti B. Prion protein amyloidosis. Brain Pathol 1996;6:127–145.

Hill AF, Desbruslais M, Joiner S, et al. The same prion strain causes vCJD and BSE. Nature 1997;389:448–450.

Hsich G, Kenney K, Gibbs CJ Jr, et al. The 14-3-3 brain protein in cerebrospinal fluid as a marker for transmissible spongiform encephalopathies. N Engl J Med 1996;335:924–930.

Kocisko DA, Come JH, Priola SA, et al. Cell-free formation of protease-resistant prion protein. Nature 1994;370:471–474.

Prusiner SB. Human prion diseases. Ann Neurol 1994a;35:385–395.

Prusiner SB. Inherited prion disease. Proc Natl Acad Sci U S A 1994b;91:4611–4614.

Steinhoff BJ, Racker S, Herrendorf G, et al. Accuracy and reliability of periodic sharp wave complexes in Creutzfeldt-Jakob disease. Arch Neurol 1996;53:162–166.

Will RB, Ironside JW, Zeidler M, et al. A new variant of Creutzfeldt-Jakob disease in the UK. Lancet 1996;347:921–925.

Zeidler M, Stewart GE, Barraclough CR, et al. New variant Creutzfeldt-Jakob disease: neurological features and diagnostic tests. Lancet 1997;350:903–907.

Zerr I, Bodemer M, Gefeller O, et al. Detection of 14-3-3 protein in the cerebrospinal fluid supports the diagnosis of Creutzfeldt-Jakob disease. Ann Neurol 1998;43:32–40.

Chapter 60
Multiple Sclerosis and Other Inflammatory Demyelinating Diseases of the Central Nervous System

Michael J. Olek and David M. Dawson

Diseases affecting central nervous system (CNS) myelin can be classified on the basis of whether a primary biochemical abnormality of myelin exists (dysmyelinating) or whether some other process damages the myelin or oligodendroglial cell (demyelinating). Demyelinating diseases in which normal myelin is disrupted include autoimmune, infectious, toxic and metabolic, and vascular processes (Table 60.1). Dysmyelinating diseases in which a primary abnormality of the formation of myelin exists include several hereditary disorders (see Table 60.1; see Chapter 68). Infectious demyelinating disease (progressive multifocal leukoencephalopathy) is discussed in Chapter 59; toxic and metabolic demyelinating diseases in Chapter 62; and vascular demyelinating disease (Binswanger's disease) is discussed in Chapter 57. The present chapter concentrates on multiple sclerosis and other inflammatory demyelinating diseases of myelin (acute disseminated encephalomyelitis [ADEM] and acute hemorrhagic leukoencephalopathy), as well as other CNS diseases that are presumably immune-mediated (see Table 60.1). The paraneoplastic disorders are discussed in Chapter 58.

MULTIPLE SCLEROSIS

Multiple sclerosis (MS) is the most common disease caused by an inflammatory demyelinating process in the CNS. MS is a leading cause of disability in young adults. In the United States the annual cost, including services, alterations to home and vehicle, medications, purchase of special equipment, and loss of earnings, is $35,000 per patient in 1994 dollars. This translates into a national annual cost of $9.7 billion, and a mean lifetime cost per case of $2.5 million, all in 1994 dollars.

Pathologically, MS is characterized by multifocal areas of demyelination with relative preservation of axons, loss of oligodendrocytes, and astroglial scarring. Certain clinical features are typical of MS, but the disease has a highly variable pace and many atypical forms. Investigative studies are often needed to confirm the diagnosis and exclude other possibilities. Advances in disease monitoring and treatment hold promise of slowing the progression of disability. Our understanding of the basic nature of the disease remains limited, and true control of the disease, and repair of damaged myelin, remain as goals for the future.

Pathophysiology

The symptoms and signs of MS must be the manifestations of the pathological lesions seen in the CNS, namely demyelination with, in general, axonal preservation. However, detailed pathological and magnetic resonance (MR) spectroscopy studies indicate axonal loss of a moderate degree can occur in MS plaques (Trapp et al. 1998). A comparison

Table 60.1:   Diseases of myelin

Autoimmune
   Acute disseminated encephalomyelitis
   Acute hemorrhagic leukoencephalopathy
   Multiple sclerosis
Infectious
   Progressive multifocal leukoencephalopathy
Toxic/metabolic
   Carbon monoxide
   Vitamin B_{12} deficiency
   Mercury intoxication (Minamata disease)
   Alcohol/tobacco amblyopia
   Central pontine myelinolysis
   Marchiafava-Bignami syndrome
   Hypoxia
   Radiation
Vascular
   Binswanger's disease
Hereditary disorders of myelin metabolism
   Adrenoleukodystrophy
   Metachromatic leukodystrophy
   Krabbe's disease
   Alexander's disease
   Canavan–van Bogaert disease
   Pelizaeus-Merzbacher disease
   Phenylketonuria

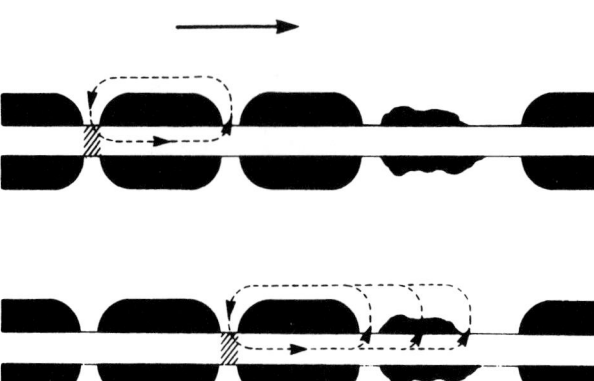

FIGURE 60.1   Schematic diagram of impulse conduction in normal (upper panel) and demyelinated (lower panel) regions of a nerve fiber. The solid arrow indicates the direction of impulse conduction; the shaded area indicates the region occupied by the impulse. Current flow is indicated by the broken arrows. In normally myelinated regions (top), the high-resistance, low-capacitance directs the majority of action current to the next node of Ranvier. In contrast, in demyelinated regions (bottom), action current is short-circuited through the damaged myelin sheath or denuded regions of the axion, and hence further propagation of the action potential is blocked. (Reprinted with permission from SG Waxman. Membranes, myelin, and the pathophysiology of multiple sclerosis. N Engl J Med 1982;306:1529–1533.)

of the physiological properties of normally myelinated axons and of demyelinated axons provides insight into the basis for the symptoms and signs characteristic of MS.

Compacted myelin is the lipid-rich plasma membrane of oligodendrocytes that provides insulation for electric impulses traveling along axons. Myelinated axons propagate nerve impulses rapidly in a saltatory fashion with a high safety factor for transmission (five to seven times above threshold) (Waxman and Ritchie 1993). Current is induced by the opening of voltage-gated Na^+ channels found at the nodes of Ranvier. The resultant Na^+ influx creates a current that then moves toward the next node of Ranvier, as current cannot flow outward in myelinated internodal segments (Figure 60.1). K^+ channel opening terminates current flow and leads to repolarization. Several types of K^+ channels exist in the axon. Fast K^+ channels sensitive to 4-aminopyridine are located in internodal axonal membrane and contribute to repolarization of demyelinated axons. Slow K^+ channels are found at the nodes of Ranvier and have a role in modulating repetitive firing. The Na^+, K^+-adenosinetriphosphatase (ATPase) in the axon membrane restores ionic balance following high-frequency firing.

Demyelination interrupts current flow by removing the insulator of internodal axon current flow. For short segments (one or two internodes) demyelination is not critical because of a high transmission safety factor. However, longer segments of demyelination can result in interruption of current flow, because current must flow by continuous propagation. The low density of internodal Na^+ channels,

at least in the early stages of demyelination, inhibits impulse propagation. If conduction does occur, it is at a much reduced speed (5–10% of normal). The refractory period of demyelinated axons is prolonged, and repetitive volleys may be blocked when encountering an axon segment in a refractory period. Persistent neurological deficits or negative symptoms of MS are caused by regions in which conduction block persists, such as in regions of large plaques, whereas transient worsening of function reflects a drop below the safety threshold for conduction because of physiological changes involving the partially demyelinated axon (Uhthoff's phenomenon, worsening with increased body temperature).

Mechanical stimulation of demyelinated axons can generate action potentials de novo in the axon and may explain Lhermitte's phenomenon, electric shock–like sensations on flexing the neck. Spontaneous action potentials have been recorded from demyelinated axons and, if present in the CNS, could explain paroxysmal positive symptoms of MS such as trigeminal neuralgia, myokymia, and visual phosphenes.

In addition to structural changes, one must consider functional impairment of nerve transmission caused by edema or factors liberated by immunocompetent cells (cytokines, adhesion molecules) in the plaque and periplaque regions that may be toxic to cells or axons. Rapid recovery of function may be caused by resolution of edema, pH changes, and reduction of cellular infiltrates, whereas more delayed recovery may reflect use of alternate axonal pathways or an increase of internodal Na^+ channels.

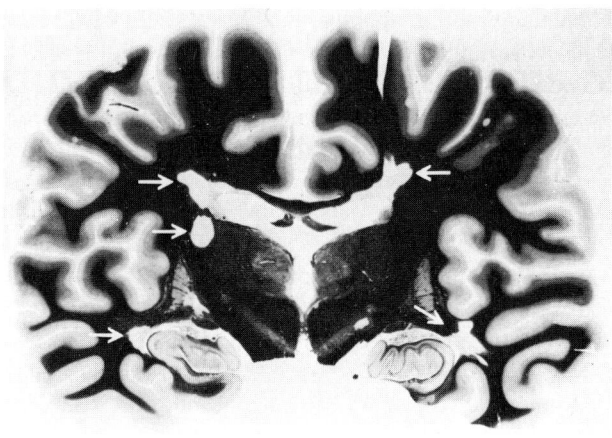

FIGURE 60.2   Coronal section of brain showing large plaques adjacent to lateral ventricles and temporal horns. A plaque is seen also in the left internal capsule (*arrows*) (stain, Heidenhain's myelin). (Courtesy of Dr. S. Carpenter.)

Pathology

The pathological hallmark of MS is the cerebral or spinal plaque, which consists of a discrete region of demyelination with relative preservation of axons, although spectroscopic and pathological studies suggest axonal loss may be an integral part of the demyelinating process.

Gross examination of the brain in MS often reveals variable degrees of atrophy and ventricular dilatation. Plaques may be visible on the surface of the spinal cord on inspection. The cut surface of the brain reveals the plaques, which, when active, appear whitish yellow or pink, with somewhat indistinct borders. Older plaques appear translucent with a blue-gray discoloration and sharply demarcated margins. These plaques often have a hard or rubbery consistency. Individual lesions are generally small (1–2 cm), but may become confluent, generating large plaques. Plaques develop in a perivenular distribution and are seen most frequently in the periventricular white matter, brainstem, and spinal cord (Figures 60.2 and 60.3), a finding confirmed with magnetic resonance imaging (MRI) studies. However, large numbers of small plaques, often detected only by microscopy, are found in cortical regions affecting intracortical myelinated fibers.

One of the earliest features of acute MS lesions is a disruption of the blood-brain barrier (BBB) as detected by MRI studies. The cause for the early disruption of the BBB is unclear, but it appears to be a critical early step in lesion pathogenesis. Histological examination of active plaques reveals perivascular infiltration of lymphocytes (predominantly T cells) and macrophages with occasional plasma cells. Perivascular and interstitial edema may be quite prominent. In the plaque, myelin is disrupted, resulting in myelin debris found in clumps or within lipid-laden macrophages. Macrophages, most prominent in the plaque center, appear to have an integral role in stripping myelin lamellae from axons. Reactive astrocytes are prominent in plaques. Immunohistochemical studies have found increased levels of cytokines in active plaques indicative of ongoing immunoreactivity that may have some role in neural dysfunction.

The fate of oligodendroglia in MS lesions is disputed; consensus opinion is that oligodendroglia number is reduced proportionate to myelin loss in the plaque center, whereas at the plaque edge oligodendroglia are preserved

FIGURE 60.3   Brainstem and spinal cord sections from patient with multiple sclerosis stained with (**A**) Heidenhain's myelin stain; (**B**) Holzer's stain for gliosis; and (**C**) Bodian's stain for axons. Note mirror image of myelin and Holzer's stains in the pons. Also note dramatic demyelination of sacral cord with preserved myelin in nerve roots (**A**, bottom). (Courtesy of Dr. S. Carpenter.)

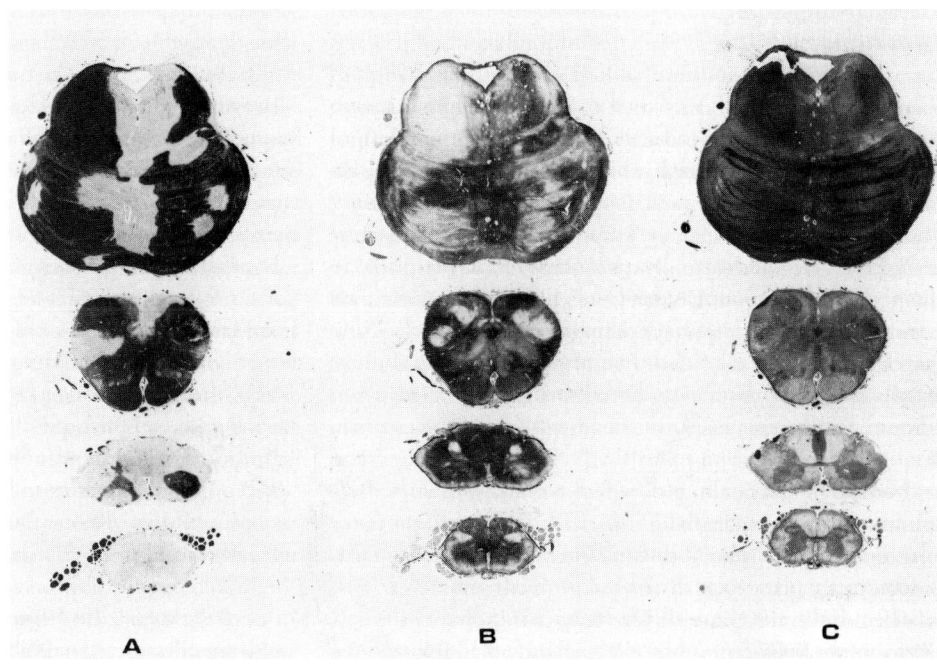

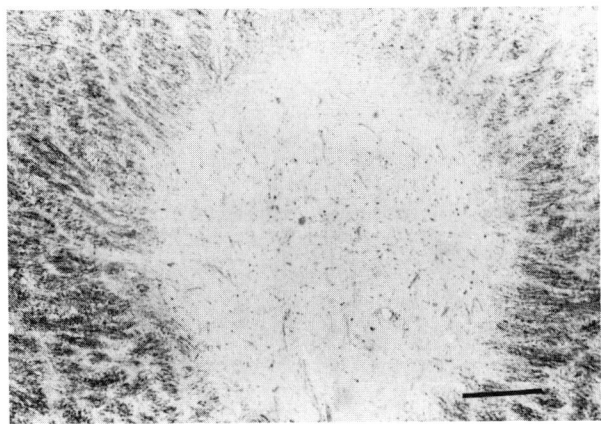

FIGURE 60.4 Punched-out appearance of old multiple sclerosis plaque surrounded by regions with varying amounts of myelin preservation (periodic acid–Schiff Luxol fast blue; bar = 100 μm). (Courtesy of Dr. S. Carpenter.)

or even increased, suggesting an attempt at remyelination. Remyelination has previously been considered improbable in the CNS (as opposed to the peripheral nervous system [PNS]), yet the finding of shadow plaques (areas of thinly myelinated axons) supports the concept of central remyelination (Prineas et al. 1993a). Remyelination may involve either oligodendrocytes that previously produced myelin or maturation of progenitor cells. Such remyelination may explain the clinical finding of slow and delayed recovery from an acute attack, whereas rapid clinical recovery presumably reflects the resolution of edema, inflammation, and removal of toxic factors associated with acute plaques in which myelin destruction is minimal.

Studies of plaques with recurrent demyelination provide insights into a possible mechanism whereby permanent demyelination occurs. Significant numbers of shadow plaques show evidence of recurrent demyelination either overlapping the shadow plaque or within its boundaries (Prineas et al. 1993b). Evidence of recurrence of activity in old plaques may be demonstrated by gadolinium-enhanced MRI. Chronic demyelinated plaques could thus result not from a single severe episode of demyelination, but rather recurrent bouts of demyelination at the same site (Prineas et al. 1993b). This could eventually exceed the ability of oligodendroglia to remyelinate or result in tissue changes that eventually prevent remyelination.

The specific target of the immune-mediated injury in MS remains undetermined. A proportionate loss of oligodendroglia and myelin would imply a primary attack against either oligodendroglia or an antigen present on oligodendroglial cell bodies and myelin. Alternatively, myelin may be the primary target of disease, and the oligodendroglia may survive demyelination, at least in the initial stages of disease.

The active lesions contain T lymphocytes and macrophages in the perivascular regions and parenchyma. Most of the T cells express the α/β T-cell receptor. Both CD4+ and CD8+ T cells are present. An apparent increase in CD8+ cells occurs in the CNS, when compared with the prevalence of this subset in the peripheral blood. CD4+ cells extend from the periphery of active plaques into adjacent white matter, whereas CD8+ cells predominate in the perivascular regions. Some MS lesions also have an accumulation of T cells expressing the γ/δ T-cell receptor, which may mediate cytolysis of CNS cells expressing heat shock proteins.

Among the lymphocytes are cells specifically sensitized to myelin antigens. Reports vary with regard to the extent of restriction and the precise profile of the T-cell receptor repertoire of CNS T cells. T-cell sensitization could occur via direct exposure to myelin antigens within the CNS or within cervical lymph nodes, a site to which CNS antigens are transported, or via exposure to exogenous agents sharing antigenic determinants with myelin. The latter has been termed *molecular mimicry*. Microglial cells, endothelial cells, and possibly astrocytes can be induced to express major histocompatibility complex antigens and function as antigen-presenting cells, thus potentially promoting myelin antigen interaction with immune-mediating cells.

Activated T cells and the microglia-macrophages can contribute to tissue injury via nonantigen-restricted mechanisms. Each of these cell types releases an array of soluble factors that can contribute to tissue injury including oligodendroglia. Cytokines characteristic of T cells include interleukin 2 (IL-2), interferon-γ, and tumor necrosis factor-β (TNF-β) (lymphotoxin). Soluble factors released by macrophages and microglia include TNF-α, leukotrienes, thromboxanes, proteases, and complement components. Many of these immunologically active substances can result in upregulation of adhesion molecules, which can promote or facilitate nonspecific lymphocyte-macrophage migration to the site of immune injury and immune effector-target cell interactions.

B cells and immunoglobulin are also found in MS lesions. To date, no specific myelinotoxic antibody is identified in MS. Antimyelin antibodies are shown, however, to enhance the disease severity in the experimental allergic encephalomyelitis (EAE) model, suggesting that both cellular and humoral mechanisms may be needed for full expression of immune injury.

Chronic, inactive plaques display sharp demarcation from surrounding brain and are hypocellular (Figures 60.4 and 60.5). The plaques show astrocytic proliferation with denuded axons and an absence of oligodendroglia. Axonal shrinkage or loss also may be noted to a variable extent. Microglia and macrophages, occasionally with a foamy appearance, are scattered throughout the lesion. The edge of chronic plaques may still exhibit hypercellularity, suggesting continued disease activity.

Pathological differences are described between classical MS and disorders considered as variants of the disease. Baló's concentric sclerosis is characterized by alternating bands of myelinated and demyelinated fibers in white matter. Clinically, the illness is more fulminant in onset and course than typical MS and has a more inflammatory cerebrospinal fluid (CSF). Transitional forms exist with typical MS. The affected CNS structures in Devic's neuromyelitis optica show more necrosis, cyst formation, and vascular proliferation than is seen in the usual MS case (Mandler et al. 1993).

Etiology

Autoimmunity

Low levels of autoreactive T cells and B cells are present in normal individuals. Presumably they have escaped from clonal depletion during the process of immune development and are now tolerant of their antigens. Autoimmunity develops when these cells lose tolerance and a complex process of immune reactivity in target tissues begins. One potential way in which tolerance can be broken is by means of molecular mimicry between self-antigens and foreign antigens, for example, viral components. Several viral and bacterial peptides share structural similarities with important proteins of myelin, and a few of them are able to activate specific T-cell clones derived from patients with MS. Another way in which tolerance can be broken is by CNS infection, causing tissue damage and releasing antigens into the peripheral circulation where they may encounter corresponding autoreactive T cells.

Myelin basic protein (MBP) has long been considered one of the primary candidates for an autoimmune attack. T cells that respond to MBP are found in the peripheral blood in normal persons and those with MS, possibly at higher levels in patients with MS with active disease. MBP can be an antigen for EAE, the primary animal model of MS. MBP accounts for 30% of the protein of myelin.

Several other proteins characteristic of myelin are also candidates for an autoimmune attack. Proteolipid protein accounts for 50% of myelin protein and is an integral membrane protein of the myelin leaflets. In the PNS P0 protein fulfills this role. Myelin-associated glycoprotein, myelin oligodendrocyte glycoprotein, and cyclic nucleotide phosphodiesterase are proteins that account for a few percent of myelin. Myelin oligodendrocyte glycoprotein and cyclic nucleotide phosphodiesterase are not found in peripheral nerve myelin and are therefore of interest because MS is a disease affecting only central myelin.

Infection

A possible role for viral infection in the causation of MS has been a matter of ongoing debate for decades. The epidemiology of MS (see Epidemiology, later in this chapter) suggests an exogenous or environmental factor of some type. Beyond epidemiology, and much speculation, there is little to support the concept of a role for viral infection. Innumerable efforts to culture a virus from autopsy-derived or biopsy material have yielded no consistent result. Serological data are difficult to interpret because titers may reflect only a nonspecific tendency

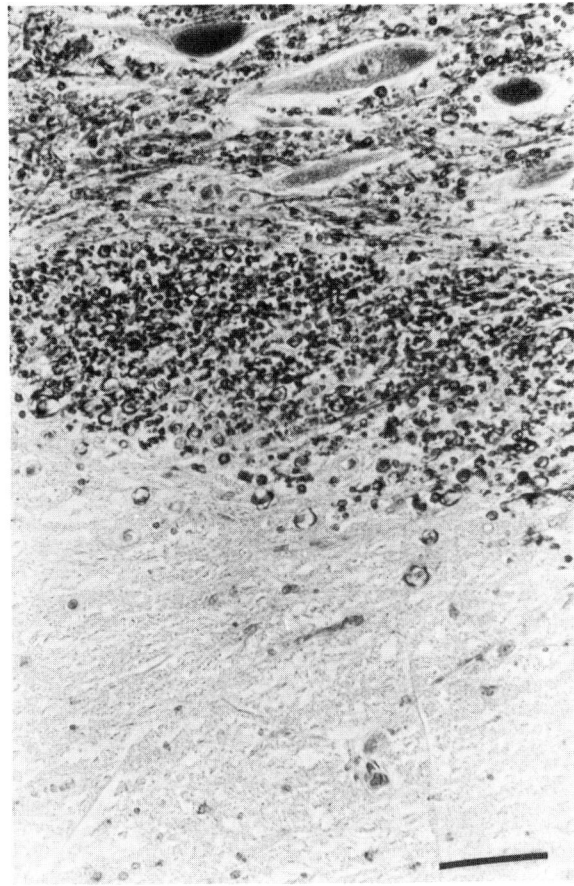

FIGURE 60.5   Plaque edge of old plaque with sharply demarcated zone of demyelination with normal myelin above (periodic acid–Schiff Luxol fast blue; bar = 50 µm). (Courtesy of Dr. S. Carpenter.)

toward increased immune reactivity. Specific efforts to recover a known viral genome (e.g., that of human T-cell lymphotropic virus type 1 [HTLV-1]) have proven negative. Retrovirus infection is unlikely because reverse transcriptase is absent from the CSF, despite the use of sensitive assay techniques.

Human herpes virus 6 may be cultured from 70% of the brains of patients with MS, and an equal number of controls. It may be cultured from nuclei, rather than cytoplasm, of oligodendrocytes in patients with MS. This suggestion of persistent herpes 6 infection is under active investigation; it may suggest an aberrant response to a common and asymptomatic infection.

Epidemiology

The epidemiology (see Chapter 44) and genetics of MS are complex topics. The interested reader is referred to the articles of Sadovnick and Ebers (1993) and Ebers and Sadovnick (1994).

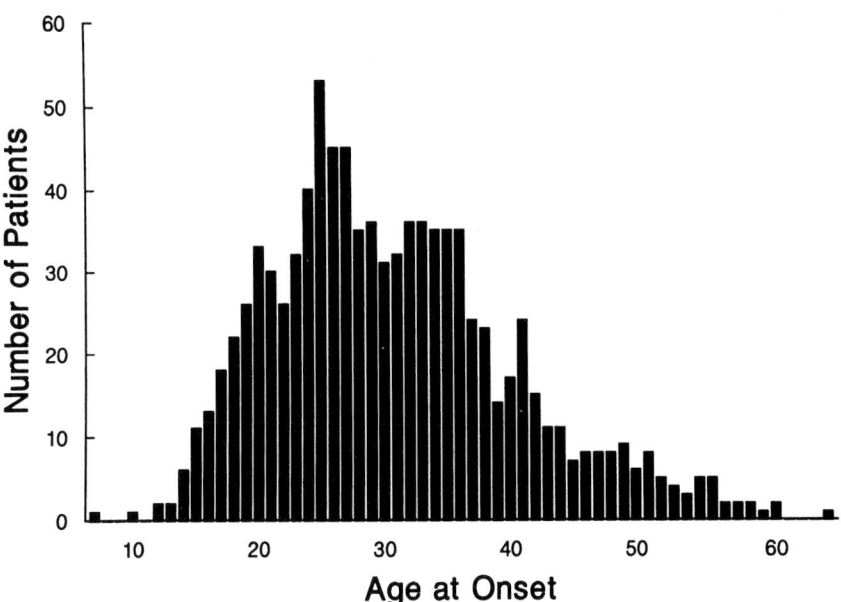

FIGURE 60.6 Age at onset of symptoms of multiple sclerosis in 940 patients followed at the multiple sclerosis clinic of the Montreal Neurologic Institute. Mean age of onset is 30.6 years, median is 27 years, and peak incidence is 25 years.

Age of Onset

Most studies agree that the median age of onset is 23.5 years of age (Figure 60.6). The peak age of onset is approximately 5 years earlier for women than for men. The mean age of onset is 30. Relapsing-remitting MS tends to have an earlier onset, averaging 25–29 years, compared with the relapsing-remitting progressive type with an average of onset of 25–29 years, and a mean age of conversion to progressive MS of 40–44 years. Primary progressive MS has a mean age of onset of 35–39 years. The onset of MS can occur as late as the seventh decade, although rarely.

Sex Distribution

Autoimmune diseases in general and MS in particular affect more women than men. In a summary of 30 incidence and prevalence studies, a cumulative ratio of female to male subjects was 1.77 to 1.00.

Mortality

Mortality caused by MS is difficult to ascertain because of poor data collection and reporting. The U.S. Department of Health and Human Services report of deaths in the year 1992 indicates that 1,900 U.S. citizens died of MS in that year, giving MS a U.S. mortality of 0.7 per 100,000. A breakdown of these numbers shows 1,187 women (89% white, 10% black) died, whereas 713 men (90% white and 9% black) died of MS. The mean age of death of all patients with MS was 58.1 years, compared with a national average of 70.5 for all causes of death. The life expectancy

of patients with MS was therefore calculated to be 82.5% of the normal life span.

In another study, MS mortality figures were calculated for England and Wales for the years 1963–1990. Over this span of years there was a steady and consistent decline in the death rate attributable to MS compared with the overall death rate. Deaths for ages up to age 59 declined from 536 to 360, whereas those above the age of 60 increased from 275 to 440. Patients with MS tended to live longer, and other diseases were more likely to be the cause of death.

Geographic and Racial Distribution

More than 250 prevalence surveys have been carried out, serving as the basis for the delineation of geographic risk for MS that is depicted in Figure 60.7. High-frequency areas of the world, with current prevalence of 60 per 100,000 or more, include all of Europe including Russia, southern Canada, and the northern United States, New Zealand, and the southeastern portion of Australia. In many of these areas the prevalence is more than 100 per 100,000, with the highest reported rate of 300 per 100,000 occurring in the Orkney Islands. In the United States, the prevalence is 0.1%, or a total of 250,000 persons with MS.

Medium frequency areas comprise most of Australia, the southern United States, the Mediterranean basin (other than Italy), the Asian parts of the former Soviet Union, parts of South America, and the white population of South Africa.

Low-risk areas include most of South America, most of Asia, Mexico, and all of Africa. One possible conclusion is that MS is a place-related illness, with a latitude gradient. However, notable exceptions then need to be explained. Japan, situated at the same latitude as areas of high preva-

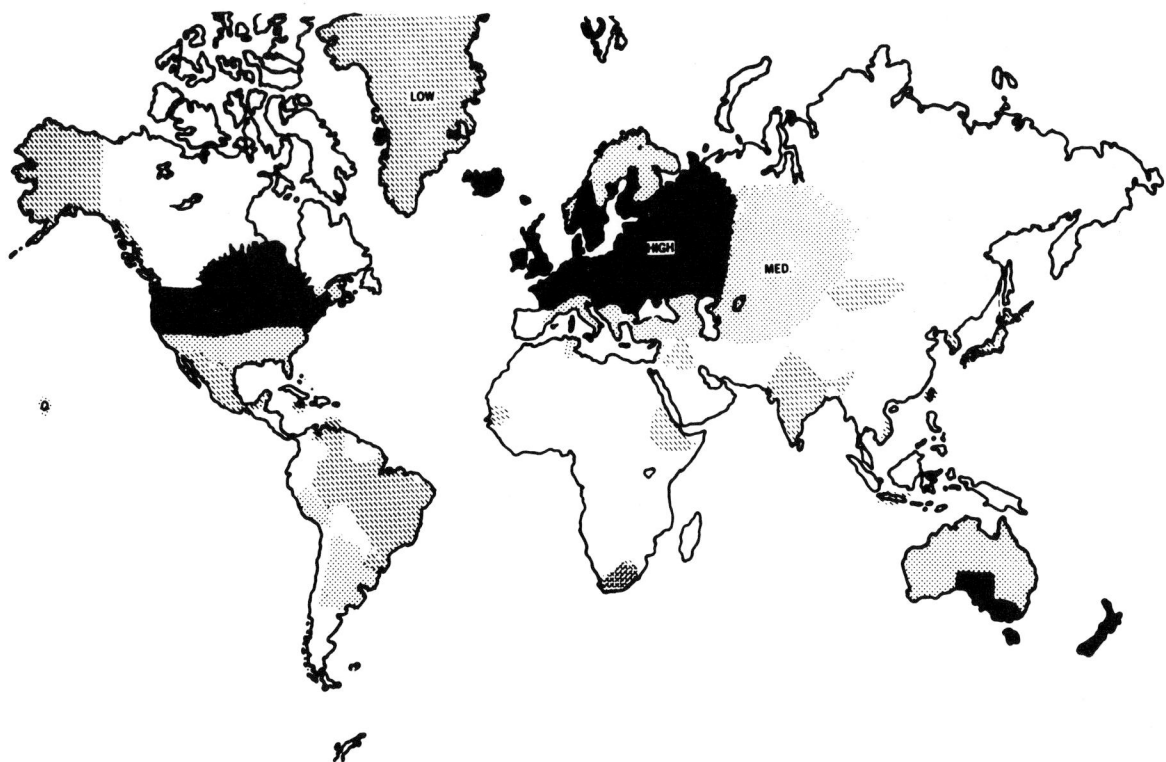

FIGURE 60.7   Worldwide distribution of multiple sclerosis as of 1980. High-frequency areas (>30 per 100,000 population) are indicated in black, medium-frequency areas (5–25 per 100,000) with dots, and low-frequency areas (<5 per 100,000) with diagonal dashes. Open areas are regions without data. South American frequencies are tentative. The low frequency in South Africa is for native South Africans, with medium frequency for persons of European stock native to South Africa. (Reprinted with permission from JF Kurtzke. The geographical distribution of multiple sclerosis—an update with special reference to Europe and the Mediterranean region. Acta Neurol Scand 1980;62:65–80. Copyright 1980 Munskgard International Publishers Ltd., Copenhagen, Denmark.)

lence in Europe, is a low-risk area. Second-generation Japanese in the United States retain their parents' low risk of MS. The white population of South Africa, of medium prevalence of MS, is surrounded by a black population in which the disease is uncommon. Native North Americans, especially of pure Amerindian background, have a very low prevalence, but are surrounded by a white population with a medium or high risk for MS.

It seems plausible that race is a determinant of MS risk, with populations of white extraction, especially from Northern Europe being the most susceptible. People of Asian, African, or Amerindian origin have the lowest risk, whereas other groups are variably intermediate.

Migration data have often been used to support the view that a transmissible agent is involved in the pathogenesis of MS. The data indicate that persons migrating from an area of high risk to an area of low risk after the age of puberty carry their former high risk with them. With migration during childhood the risk seems to be that of the new area to which the person has migrated. The data are not always clear-cut. Japanese in Japan are at low risk for MS. People of Japanese extraction, living in the United States, have a higher risk, although less than their neighbors of Northern European extraction. However, those Japanese who migrate to this country do not seem to acquire the risk of their new area. Comparable data are available for persons moving to Israel from Europe (high risk) compared with those arriving from countries in the Middle East.

Genetic and Racial Distribution

The frequency of familial occurrence of MS has varied from 3–23% in different studies. The studies with the higher percentages are those in which ascertainment was more intense; that is, the more one looks, the more one finds. An overall risk in first-, second-, and third-degree relatives of at least 15% seems a reasonable estimate. The risk is highest for siblings and decreases progressively for children, aunts, uncles, and cousins (Table 60.2). For genetic counseling purposes, it may be stated that the sibling risk is 3–5%, approximately 30–50 times the background risk for this same population. In some studies unaffected family members may have been found to have abnormalities on MRI, implying that the risk may be even higher. The risk applies to blood relatives; only a few studies of adopted children

Table 60.2: Age-adjusted risk of developing multiple sclerosis for relatives of index cases

Relationship to index case	Female index (%)	Male index (%)
Parent	3.0±0.7	2.6±0.9
Sibling	4.0±0.9	3.8±0.7
Child	2.6±1.1	2.5±1.7
Uncle/aunt	1.6±0.3	2.7±0.7
Niece/nephew	1.8±0.7	1.5±0.8
Cousin (first)	2.4±0.4	1.5±0.6

Source: Modified from AD Sadovnick, PA Baird, RH Ward, et al. Multiple sclerosis: updated risks for relatives. Am J Med Genet 1988;29:533–541.

have been done, but they show no increased risk. One unexplained finding is the marked deficiency of transmission from father to son.

Twin studies have shown the familial nature of MS in dramatic fashion. The risk for dizygotic twin pairs is the same as that for siblings, that is, 3–5%. The risk for monozygotic twins is at least 20%, and if the subjects are followed for long periods of time, and if various nonclinical data are included, the risk may reach 38.5%. Because the highest rates for the genetic basis of MS are less than 50%, there must be a contribution by nongenetic factors. There are several candidate genes for MS, including human leukocyte antigen, T-cell receptor, MBP, portions of the immunoglobulin chain, and mitochondrial genes. Three entire genomic scans for MS susceptibility genes have been reported, without an identifiable region of major interest. The data argue for nonmendelian polygenic inheritance.

Clinical Symptoms and Physical Findings

Although the clinical syndrome of MS is classically described as a relapsing-remitting disorder that affects multiple white matter tracts within the CNS, with usual onset in young adults, the disorder displays marked clinical heterogeneity. This variability includes age of onset, mode of initial manifestation, frequency, severity and sequelae of relapses, extent of progression, and cumulative deficit over the course of time. The varied clinical features reflect the multifocal areas of CNS myelin destruction (MS plaques), although discrepancies occur between the extent of clinical and pathological findings.

Cognitive Impairment

Frank dementia is an uncommon feature of MS, occurring in less than 5% of patients, and is usually only encountered in severely affected individuals. However, patients frequently complain of having a poor memory, having a decreased capacity for sustained mental effort, and being distractible. The specificity of such complaints in MS is dif-

ficult to establish. Data from formal neuropsychological studies suggest that cognitive involvement has been underreported in MS. Neuropsychological test results have shown that 34–65% of patients with MS have cognitive impairment. The most frequent abnormalities are with abstract conceptualization, recent memory, attention, and speed of information processing. Total lesion load based on MRI has been found to correlate with impairment on neuropsychological testing.

Cross-sectional studies have shown some degree of affective disturbance in up to two-thirds of patients with MS (Rao et al. 1993). Depression is the most common manifestation and is in part secondary to the burden of having to cope with a chronic, incurable disease. Some data suggest that depression is more common in patients with MS than in others with chronic medical conditions, in whom the lifetime risk of depression was 12.9% in one study. This contrasts with a study of 221 patients with MS, in whom the risk for depression was 34%. It is not known whether this rate of depression in patients with MS reflects a comorbid association with bipolar illness or an effect of frontal or subcortical white matter disease. Euphoria is usually associated with moderate or severe mental impairment. Patients may manifest a dysphoric state with swings from depression to elation.

On occasion, acute cerebral lesions can manifest as a confusional state associated with progressive focal paralysis, changes suggestive of a tumor (Zagzag et al. 1993). Epilepsy is more common in patients with MS than in the general population, with a cited figure of 3%. Convulsions may be either tonic-clonic in nature or partial complex. They generally respond well to anticonvulsants. The prevalence of cortical syndromes such as aphasia, apraxia, and agnosia is low.

Cranial Nerve Dysfunction

Impairment of the Visual Pathways. Optic neuritis (ON) is the most frequent type of involvement of the visual pathways, usually presenting as an acute or subacute unilateral syndrome characterized commonly by pain in the eye accentuated by ocular movements, which is then followed by a variable degree of vision loss (scotoma) affecting mainly central vision. Bilateral ON does occur, but one needs to distinguish whether it is truly simultaneous or sequential. Bilateral simultaneous ON is rare in MS and its occurrence in isolation may suggest another diagnosis such as Leber's hereditary optic atrophy or toxic optic neuropathy (see Chapter 14). In bilateral ON in MS cases, the impairment begins asymmetrically and is usually more severe in one eye. Recurrence is highly variable. In a large ON treatment trial, 15% of placebo-treated patients developed recurrent (ipsilateral or contralateral eye) ON within 6–24 months following the initial bout of ON. Mapping of visual fields reveals a central or cecocentral scotoma (central scotoma involving the physiological blind spot). The finding of a bitemporal hemianopia is rare in MS; if present, it should raise the suspicion of a mass lesion compressing the optic chiasm. Although uncommon, homonymous field defects can be seen in MS caused by involvement of the optic radiations (see Chapters 14 and 41).

Patients with ON have a relative afferent pupillary defect (Marcus Gunn pupil) (see Chapter 41). The afferent pupillary defect is tested by shining a bright light alternately in each eye (the swinging flashlight test), and, in the case of unilateral optic nerve dysfunction, the abnormal pupil paradoxically dilates when the light is shifted from the normal to the affected eye. The interpretation of this sign becomes difficult when the degree of optic nerve impairment is similar in the two eyes. When the acute ON lesion involves the head of the optic nerve, one observes disc edema (papillitis), a finding more commonly seen in children than in adults. More often, the lesion of the optic nerve is retrobulbar, and funduscopic examination is normal in the acute stage. Later the optic disc becomes pale as a result of axonal loss and resultant gliosis. This pallor predominates in the temporal segment of the disc (temporal pallor). After an attack of acute ON, 90% of patients regain normal vision, typically over a period of 2–6 months. Desaturation of bright colors, particularly red, is often reported by recovered patients; some also report a mild nonspecific dimming of vision in the affected eye.

Uhthoff's phenomenon refers to a decrease in visual acuity following an increase in body temperature. This can occur following exercise, a hot bath, or fever. This phenomenon, which reflects subclinical demyelination or preexistent injury to the optic nerve, may occur without a prior history of clinical involvement of the optic nerve. A similar phenomenon can occur at other sites of CNS dysfunction with an increase in body temperature.

Impairment of the Ocular Motor Pathways.   Impairment of individual ocular motor nerves is infrequent in MS. When present, the involved nerves are, in decreasing order of frequency, cranial nerves VI, III, and, rarely, IV. The resulting diplopia usually remits. More frequent findings are those that reflect lesions of vestibulo-ocular connections and internuclear connections. Nystagmus is a common finding in MS (see Chapters 14 and 40). One form of nystagmus particularly characteristic of MS is acquired pendular nystagmus, in which there is rapid, small amplitude pendular oscillations of the eyes in the primary position resembling quivering jelly. Patients frequently complain of oscillopsia (subjective oscillation of objects in the field of vision). This type of nystagmus usually is seen in the presence of marked loss of visual acuity.

Internuclear ophthalmoplegia, defined as abnormal horizontal ocular movements with lost or delayed adduction and horizontal nystagmus of the abducting eye, is secondary to a lesion of the medial longitudinal fasciculus on the side of diminished adduction. Convergence is preserved. When present bilaterally, it is usually coupled with vertical nystagmus on upward gaze. Although most suggestive of MS, a bilateral internuclear ophthalmoplegia can be observed with other intra-axial brainstem lesions, including brainstem glioma, vascular lesions, Arnold-Chiari malformations, and Wernicke's encephalopathy.

Ocular pursuit movements are frequently saccadic rather than smooth. Ocular dysmetria may coexist with other signs of cerebellar dysfunction and other ocular oscillations, such as intrusive saccadic movements (square wave jerks).

Impairment of Other Cranial Nerves.   Impairment of facial sensation, subjective or objective, is a relatively common finding in MS. The occurrence of trigeminal neuralgia in a young adult is frequently an early sign of MS. Facial myokymia, a fine undulating wavelike facial twitching, and hemifacial spasm can be caused by MS, but other causes of a focal brainstem lesion must be excluded. Unilateral facial paresis can occur, but taste sensation is almost never affected. In these syndromes, as with acute oculomotor palsy, the nerve is affected in its course within the neuraxis, rather than peripherally. Vertigo is a reported symptom in 30–50% of patients with MS and is commonly associated with dysfunction of adjacent cranial nerves. Resulting symptoms include hyperacusis or hypoacusis, facial numbness, and diplopia. Complete hearing loss, usually unilateral, is an infrequent complaint. Malfunction of the lower cranial nerves is usually of the upper motor neuron type (pseudobulbar syndrome).

Impairment of the Sensory Pathways

Sensory manifestations are a frequent initial feature of MS and are present in almost every patient at some time during the course of disease. The sensory features can reflect spinothalamic, posterior column, or dorsal root entry zone lesions. The sensory symptoms are commonly described as numbness, tingling, pins and needles, tightness, coldness, or swelling of limbs or trunk. Radicular pains, unilateral or bilateral, can be present, particularly in the low thoracic and abdominal regions. An intensely itching sensation, especially in the cervical dermatomes, usually unilateral, suggests MS.

The most frequent sensory abnormalities on clinical examination are the following: varying degrees of impairment of vibration and joint position sense, decrease of pain and light touch in a distal distribution in the four extremities, and patchy areas of reduced pain and light touch perception in the limbs and trunk. A bilateral sensory level is a more frequent finding than a hemisensory (Brown-Séquard) syndrome. Patients commonly report that the feeling of pinprick is increased or feels like a mild electric shock, or that the stimulus spreads in a ripple fashion from the point at which it is applied. The sensory useless hand is a characteristic but uncommon feature, consisting of an impairment of function secondary to a pronounced alteration of proprioception, without loss of power. A lesion of the relevant root entry zones in the spinal cord is postulated in such cases.

Impairment of Motor Pathways

Corticospinal tract dysfunction is common in MS. Paraparesis, or paraplegia, is a much more common occurrence than is significant weakness in the upper extremities caused by the frequent occurrence of lesions in the descending motor tracts of the spinal cord. With severe spasticity, extensor or flexor spasms of the legs and sometimes the trunk may be provoked by active or passive attempts to rise from a bed or wheelchair. The physical findings include spasticity, usually more marked in the legs than in the arms. The deep tendon reflexes are exaggerated, sustained clonus may be elicited, and extensor plantar responses are observed. All of these manifestations are commonly asymmetrical. Occasionally, deep tendon reflexes may be decreased because of lesions interrupting the reflex arc at a segmental level, and one may observe an inverted reflex wherein one reflex, such as the triceps, is lost and the efferent component is represented by a contraction of a muscle below the lesion, such as the triceps muscle. The Achilles' reflex can be absent in lesions of the sacral segments of the spinal cord with or without concomitant sphincter and sexual problems. Occasionally, reduced reflexes reflect hypotonia resulting from cerebellar pathway lesions. Amyotrophy, when observed, is usually of the disuse type, and most frequently affects the small muscles of the hand; less frequently, lesions of the motor root exit zones may produce muscle denervation caused by axon loss. Secondary entrapment neuropathies are also a cause of muscle atrophy in patients with MS.

A common pattern of disease evolution seen in the spinal form of MS is an ascending pattern of weakness that begins with involvement of the lower extremities and spreads to involve first one upper extremity and then the other. Frequently, there is an associated weakness of the trunk muscles with abnormal posture and involvement of respiratory muscles.

Impairment of Cerebellar Pathways

Cerebellar pathway impairment results in gait imbalance, difficulty in performing coordinated actions with the arms, and slurred speech. Examination reveals the usual features of cerebellar dysfunction, such as dysmetria, decomposition of complex movements, and hypotonia, most often observed in the upper extremities. An intention tremor may be noted in the limbs and head. Walking is impaired by truncal ataxia. Ocular findings of nystagmus, ocular dysmetria, and failure of fixation suppression suggest cerebellar or cerebellovestibular connection dysfunction. Speech can be scanning or explosive in character. In severe cases there is complete astasia (inability to stand), inability to use the arms because of a violent intention tremor, and virtually incomprehensible speech. Cerebellar signs are usually mixed with pyramidal (corticospinal) tract signs.

Impairment of Bladder, Bowel, and Sexual Functions

The extent of sphincter and sexual dysfunction often parallels the degree of motor impairment in the lower extremities. The most common complaint related to urinary bladder dysfunction is urgency, usually the result of uninhibited detrusor contraction, a reflection of a suprasegmental lesion. As the disease progresses, urinary incontinence becomes more frequent. With involvement of sacral segments of the spinal cord, symptoms of bladder hypoactivity may evolve, such as decreased urinary flow, interrupted micturition, and incomplete bladder emptying. An atonic dilatated bladder that empties by overflow results from loss of perception of bladder fullness and is usually associated with urethral as well as anal and genital hypoesthesia, and sensory deficits in the sacral dermatomes. When evaluating bladder incontinence or urgency in patients with MS, one must exclude other causes, particularly in multiparous women. Urinary tract infections are common in MS, especially in women. These infections usually do not cause fever and back pain and may increase the extent of bladder dysfunction.

Constipation is more common than fecal incontinence and can reflect both upper and lower motor neuron impairment in addition to decreased general mobility. Almost all patients with paraplegia require special measures to maintain regular bowel movements.

Sexual dysfunction, although frequently overlooked, is a common occurrence in MS. Approximately 50% of patients become completely sexually inactive secondary to their disease, and an additional 20% become sexually less active. Men experience various degrees of erectile dysfunction, often with rapid loss of erection at attempted intercourse, whereas loss of ejaculation is less common. Most women preserve their orgasmic capabilities, sometimes even in the presence of complete loss of bladder and bowel function. Sexual dysfunction can be the result of multiple problems, including the direct effects of lesions of the motor and sensory pathways within the spinal cord in addition to psychological factors involved with self-image, self-esteem, and fear of rejection from the sexual partner. Mechanical problems created by spasticity, paraparesis, and incontinence further aggravate the problem.

Clinical Features Distinctive of Multiple Sclerosis

Although there are no clinical phenomena that are unique to MS, some are highly characteristic of the disease (Table 60.3). Bilateral internuclear ophthalmoplegia has been mentioned previously. Lhermitte's phenomenon is a transient sensory symptom described as an electric shock radiating down the spine or into the limbs on flexion of the neck. It may be infrequent or occur with the least movement of the head or neck. Although most frequently encountered in MS, this symptom can be seen with other lesions of the cervical cord, including tumors, cervical disc herniation, postradiation myelopathy, and following trauma.

Paroxysmal attacks of motor or sensory phenomena may arise as a manifestation of demyelinating lesions. Within the brainstem, lesions can cause paroxysmal diplopia, facial paresthesia, trigeminal neuralgia, ataxia, and dysarthria. Motor system involvement results in painful tonic contractions of muscles of one or two (homolateral) limbs, trunk, and occasionally the face, but these only rarely occur in all four limbs or the trunk. These paroxysmal attacks usually respond to low doses of carbamazepine and frequently remit after several weeks to months, usually without recurrence.

Heat sensitivity is a well-known occurrence in MS (Uhthoff's phenomenon; see discussion under Impairment of the Visual Pathways, earlier in this chapter); small increases in the body temperature can temporarily worsen current or pre-existing signs and symptoms. This phenomenon is encountered in other neurological diseases, but to a lesser extent, and is presumably the result of conduction block developing in nerves as the body temperature increases. Normally, the nerve conduction safety factor decreases with increasing temperature until a point is reached at which conduction block occurs; this point of conduction block is reached at a much lower temperature in demyelinated nerves.

Fatigue is a characteristic finding in MS, usually described as physical exhaustion that is unrelated to the amount of activity performed. Many patients complain of feeling exhausted on waking, even if they have slept soundly. Fatigue can appear also during the day but may be partially or completely relieved by rest. There is a poor correlation between fatigue and the overall severity of disease or with the presence of any particular symptom or sign. Fatigue is often seen in association with an acute attack and may precede the focal neurological features of the attack and persist long after the attack has subsided.

Diagnostic Criteria

The cornerstone of the diagnosis of MS remains the neurological history and physical examination. To improve the homogeneity of MS patient groups being studied, the Schumacher Committee on Diagnostic Criteria for MS elaborated six items required to diagnose clinically definite MS: objective CNS dysfunction, involvement of white matter structures, two or more sites of CNS involvement, relapsing-remitting or chronic (more than 6 months) progressive course, age 10–50 years at onset, and no better explanation of symptoms as assessed by a competent neurologist. These criteria made no use of laboratory studies. Such stringent criteria would exclude some patients with MS; for example, they were fulfilled in only 95% of a group of patients who came to autopsy study. The criteria have been modified for diagnosis, expanding the age at onset to 59 years and using data derived from laboratory studies, including analysis of the CSF, evoked potentials (EP), and neuroimaging (Table

Table 60.3: Common clinical features of multiple sclerosis

Clinical features suggestive of multiple sclerosis	Clinical features not suggestive of multiple sclerosis
Onset between ages 15 and 50	Onset before age 10 or after 60
Relapses and remissions	Steady progression
Optic neuritis	Early dementia
Lhermitte's sign	Rigidity, sustained dystonia
Internuclear ophthalmoplegia	Cortical deficits such as aphasia,
Fatigue	apraxia, alexia, neglect
Worsening with elevated body temperature	Deficit developing within minutes

60.4). These criteria were developed to ensure that only patients with MS were included in research studies.

There remains the clinical problem, distinct from research criteria, of the patient early in the course who does not meet such diagnostic criteria. The advent of MRI, clearly the most sensitive diagnostic test for MS, has largely alleviated this problem. In the setting of a monophasic neurological illness that is clinically consistent with MS and in the presence of multifocal white matter lesions on MRI consistent with demyelinating plaques, the diagnosis of MS is almost certain. However, rare cases of postinfectious encephalomyelitis and ADEM or vasculitis may present in a similar fashion. In addition, follow-up studies have shown that a significant percentage of patients with MRI lesions detected at onset do not progress to clinically symptomatic MS, at least in 5 years of follow-up. The issue of the monophasic demyelinating disease is discussed in the next section. Such patients may be classed as suspected MS; they may in fact represent particularly benign forms of the disease.

Differential Diagnosis

The differential diagnosis of MS (Table 60.5) is quite limited in the setting of a young adult with two or more clinically distinct episodes of CNS dysfunction with at least partial resolution. Problems arise with atypical presentations, monophasic episodes, or progressive illness. The unusual nature of some sensory symptoms and the difficulty patients experience in describing such symptoms may result in a misdiagnosis of hysteria. The retrospective nature of inquiries also blurs details of prior events, making clear ascertainment of prior attacks difficult in some cases. A monophasic illness with symptoms attributable to one site of the CNS creates a large differential diagnosis that includes neoplasms, vascular events, or infections. Appropriate imaging studies may help clarify the situation, depending on the site of involvement and clinical progression. The most trouble arises with progressive CNS dysfunction, in which great care must be taken to exclude treatable etiologies (compressive spinal cord lesions, arterio-

Table 60.4:   Poser committee diagnostic criteria for multiple sclerosis

Category	Attacks	Clinical evidence	Paraclinical* evidence	Cerebrospinal fluid OCB/IgG
Clinically definite				
CDMS A1	2	2	—	—
CDMS A2	2	1 and	1	—
Laboratory-supported definite				
LSDMS B1	2	1 or	1	+
LSDMS B2	1	2	—	+
LSDMS B3	1	1 and	1	+
Clinically probable				
CPMS C1	2	1	—	—
CPMS C2	1	2	—	—
CPMS C3	1	1 and	1	—
Laboratory-supported probable				
LSPMS D1	2	—	—	+

CDMS = clinically definite multiple sclerosis; CPMS = clinically probable multiple sclerosis; LSDMS = laboratory-supported definite multiple sclerosis; LSDMS B2 and B3 = the two lesions (clinical or clinical and paraclinical) must not both be present at the initial evaluation but must be separated in time by at least 1 month; LSPMS = laboratory-supported probable multiple sclerosis (refers only to cerebrospinal fluid OCB or elevated production of IgG in the cerebrospinal fluid); OCB/IgG = oligoclonal bands/increased IgG; 1, 2 = number of attacks or number of sites of clinical or paraclinical abnormalities; + = presence of OCB or elevated IgG.
*Paraclinical includes neuroimaging, electrophysiological, or urological testing.
Source: Modified from CM Poser, D Paty, LS Scheinberg, et al. New diagnostic criteria for multiple sclerosis. Ann Neurol 1983;13:227–231.

venous malformations, cavernous angiomas, Arnold-Chiari malformation), infectious causes (HTLV-1, human immunodeficiency virus), or hereditary disorders (adult metachromatic leukodystrophy, adrenomyeloleukodystrophy, spinocerebellar disorders).

A common error is to overinterpret multiple hyperintense lesions on MRI as equivalent to MS. Clinical symptoms must be consistent with MS. A few white matter lesions in T2-weighted MRI scans are not infrequent, particularly in the elderly, and do not indicate a diagnosis of MS. CNS vasculitides such as systemic lupus erythematosus (SLE), Sjögren's disease, polyarteritis nodosa, syphilis, retroviral diseases, and Behçet's disease may all produce multifocal lesions with or without a relapsing-remitting course. SLE can present as a recurrent neurological syndrome before the systemic manifestations of this disease declare themselves. Behçet's syndrome is characterized by bucco-genital ulcerations in addition to the multifocal neurological findings. Although rare, ADEM must be considered in the differential diagnosis (see Acute Disseminated Encephalomyelitis, later in this chapter). An MS-like phenotype associated with mitochondrial gene defects has been described; it is of note that when there are multiple MS cases in a family, maternal transmission is more frequent than paternal transmission.

Possibly more important than features characteristic for MS in the differential diagnosis are features that should prompt the clinician to reconsider the diagnosis of MS. Many physicians fail to pursue further diagnostic steps when a patient is labeled as having MS. Features that should alert the clinician to the possibility of other diseases include (1) family history of neurological disease, (2) a well-demarcated spinal level in the absence of disease above the

foramen magnum, (3) prominent back pain that persists, (4) symptoms and signs that can be attributed to one anatomical site, (5) patients who are over 60 years of age or less than 15 years at onset, and (6) progressive disease (see Table 60.3). None of these features excludes the diagnosis

Table 60.5:   Differential diagnosis in multiple sclerosis

Inflammatory diseases
  Granulomatous angiitis
  Systemic lupus erythematosus
  Sjögren's disease
  Behçet's disease
  Polyarteritis nodosa
  Paraneoplastic encephalomyelopathies
  Acute disseminated encephalomyelitis, postinfectious
    encephalomyelitis
Infectious diseases
  Lyme neuroborreliosis
  Human T-cell lymphotropic virus type 1 infection*
  Human immunodeficiency virus infection
  Progressive multifocal leukoencephalopathy*
  Neurosyphilis*
Granulomatous diseases
  Sarcoidosis
  Wegener's granulomatosis
  Lymphomatoid granulomatosis
Diseases of myelin
  Metachromatic leukodystrophy (juvenile and adult)*
  Adrenomyeloleukodystrophy*
Miscellaneous
  Spinocerebellar disorders*
  Arnold-Chiari malformation
  Vitamin B_{12} deficiency*

*Indicates disorders that are predominantly important to differentiate in the setting of progressive disease.

of MS, but in these situations one should seek other etiologies before accepting the diagnosis of MS.

Course

The most characteristic clinical course of MS is the occurrence of relapses (Figure 60.8), which can be defined as the acute or subacute onset of clinical dysfunction that usually reaches its peak from days to several weeks followed by a remission during which the symptoms and signs resolve to a variable extent. The minimum duration for a relapse has been arbitrarily established at 24 hours. Clinical symptoms of shorter duration are less likely to represent what is considered as a true relapse (i.e., new lesion formation or extension of previous lesion size). Worsening of previous clinical dysfunction can occur concurrently with fever, physical activity, or metabolic upset and last for hours to a day or more. Such worsening is thought to reflect conduction block in previously demyelinated axons. Relapses of MS vary markedly with regard to the CNS site involved; the frequency of attacks (the free interval between relapses ranges from weeks to years); the mode of onset (from quite sudden to subacute); and the duration, severity, and quality of remission. The frequency of relapses is highly variable and depends on the population studied and the closeness of observation and recording by patients and physicians. Summaries of many studies provide an average figure of 0.4–0.6 relapses per year. Patients followed closely in clinical trials have higher relapse rates, probably reflecting closer reporting and examinations in such studies. The attack rate in the placebo group in clinical studies ranges from 0.8–1.2 attacks per year. In general, relapses are more frequent during the first years of the disease and tend to wane in later years. A course marked by relapses, interspersed by periods during which the disease seems relatively dormant, is termed relapsing-remitting.

Approximately 15% of patients never experience a second relapse. The exact frequency of such benign MS is unknown, however, because many such individuals never come to medical attention. Autopsy studies found significant numbers of cases with CNS pathology consistent with MS and yet no documented clinical evidence of such disease. Similarly, MRI studies have shown MS-like plaques in T2-weighted scans in patients who have never had a neurological episode. Asymptomatic relatives of patients with MS have MRI lesions consistent with demyelination in up to 15% of these relatives (Sadovnick et al. 1993). The use of MRI may expand the spectrum of MS by detecting milder cases that previously were not included in prognosis studies.

A standardization of terms has been agreed on, to determine the pattern and course of the illness (Lublin and Reingold 1996). Four categories of disease are described:

- Relapsing-remitting MS: Clearly defined relapses with full recovery or with sequelae and residual deficit on

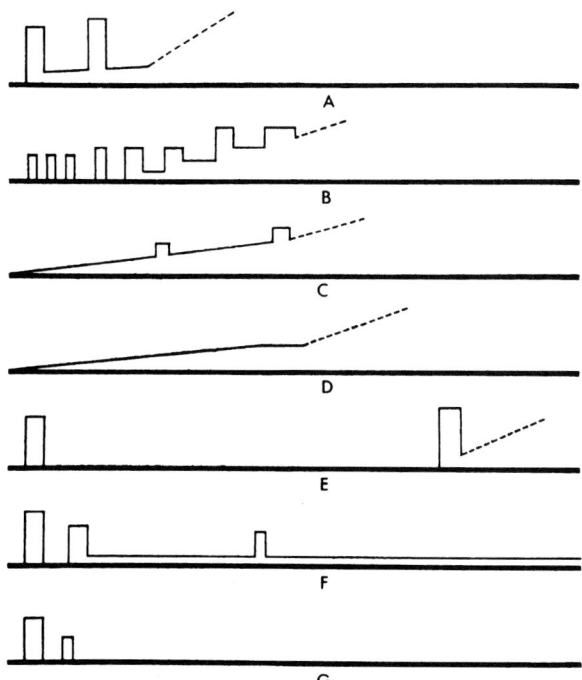

FIGURE 60.8 The course of multiple sclerosis. (**A**) Severe relapses, increasing disability, and early death. (**B**) Many short attacks, tending to increase in duration and severity. (**C**) Slow progression from onset, superimposed relapses, and increasing disability. (**D**) Slow progression from onset without relapses. (**E**) Abrupt onset with good remission followed by long latent phase. (**F**) Relapses of diminishing frequency and severity, slight residual disability only. (**G**) Abrupt onset, few if any relapses after first year, no residual disability. (Reprinted with permission from D McAlpine, A Compston, G Ebers, et al. McAlpine's Multiple Sclerosis [3rd ed]. London: Churchill Livingstone, 1998;32.)

recovery. The periods between disease relapses are characterized by a lack of disease progression.
- Primary-progressive MS: Disease progression from onset with occasional plateaus and temporary minor improvements allowed.
- Secondary-progressive MS: Initial relapsing-remitting disease course followed by progression with or without occasional relapses, minor remissions, and plateaus.
- Progressive-relapsing MS: Progressive disease from onset, with clear acute relapses, with or without full recovery. The periods between relapses are characterized by continuing progression.

Two severity outcomes are also described: (1) Benign MS is disease in which the patient remains fully functional in all neurological systems 15 years after the disease onset; and (2) malignant MS is disease with a rapid progressive course, leading to significant disability in multiple neurological systems or death in a relatively short time after disease onset.

Data from a clinic-based study of 1,100 patients who represented the population of the region found that 66% of patients at onset had relapsing and remitting disease, 15%

had relapsing-progressive, and 19% had progressive disease from the onset. Patients evolved from a relapsing-remitting course to a progressive course; 85% of patients began with a relapsing course, but the proportion continuing as relapsing disease decreased steadily, so that by 9 years from onset, only one-half were still relapsing. Likewise, the probability of reaching 6 on the Kurtzke disability score was 50% 16–17 years after onset. The course of MS with onset after the age of 40 was progressive in over 60% of patients.

The rate of clinical progression of MS is variable. The commonly used index of clinical disability, the Kurtzke disability status score (DSS), or the expanded version called the expanded disability status score (EDSS), uses numbers ranging from 0 for normal examination and function to 10 for death caused by MS. This scale is nonlinear, with great emphasis on ambulation capabilities with scores above 4. Most MS populations have bimodal distributions of EDSS scores, with peaks at values of 1 and 6 (ambulation with unilateral assistance). The time spent by a patient at a given level of disability varies with the score. Thus, for patients with DSS scores of 4 or 5, median time spent at these levels was 1.2 years, whereas for those at DSS 1, median time to stay at that level was 4 years, and at DSS 6, 3 years. These results have powerful implications for the conduct of clinical studies with respect to patient selection, stratification, and duration of follow-up: If many patients of DSS 1 or 6 are included, little movement is seen in a group followed for a year or two. The rate of progression with chronic progressive disease in the placebo groups of three clinical trials ranged from 0.5–0.7 points per year on the DSS scale.

In a cohort of patients followed for 25 years, the following data emerged (Runmaker and Andersen 1993): 80% of the patients had reached the progressive phase by 25 years; 15% of the patients had died; 65% of the patients had reached EDSS 6 (requiring aids for walking); and 50% of the patients reached EDSS 6 within 16 years of onset.

The EDSS, although universally used in clinical trials, has a number of serious limitations. Even with special training and examiner blinding, interrater and intrarater variations in scoring are common. EDSS scores of 4 and higher depend almost entirely on the ability to walk, and developing dementia, vision loss, or weakness of hands may pass undetected by the scoring. An obvious implication of these facts is that other outcome measures should be used as well, and that minor changes in EDSS alone should not be over-interpreted.

Effect of Exogenous Factors on the Course

The role of a variety of exogenous factors either influencing the development of MS or inducing disease exacerbations has been examined using epidemiological techniques. A disproportionately high number of relapses occur in patients with MS who have suffered recently from viral infections, and a high number of infections are followed by acute attacks. Increased interferon-γ and TNF-α produced by cells of the immune system during viral infections may play a role in this increased relapse rate by increasing expression of major histocompatibility complex class II antigens and adhesion molecules on cells of the immune system and CNS, with a resultant increase in the number of activated T cells being attracted to the CNS.

Controversy exists about a link between occurrence of stressful events and exacerbation of MS. Trauma appears not to be implicated in disease induction or relapse, although in the experimental animal model EAE, lesions are most prominent at sites of pre-existent traumatic lesions. Performance of neurological diagnostic procedures such as myelography and lumbar puncture has not been linked with aggravation of the MS disease course, nor has administration of local or general anesthetics. Although data do not strongly establish a link between vaccination and disease exacerbations, some clinicians advise that their patients not receive vaccinations, because experimental studies indicate that an augmentation of immune reactivity can result in recurrence of the disease EAE.

Effect of Pregnancy on the Course

MS is a disease that predominantly affects women and has a maximum incidence during childbearing years. The influence of pregnancy on MS has been repeatedly examined, with evidence that relapses are reduced late in pregnancy and are more frequent than expected in the 3-month post-partum period. However, this is not the finding in all studies. There is general agreement that the overall prognosis is no different in women who have been pregnant, compared with those who have not. Studies of women with MS reveal no increase in stillbirths, ectopic pregnancies, or spontaneous abortions. These data would suggest that pregnancy has no ill effect on MS and that MS has no negative effect on the fetus or the course of pregnancy. In a study of postmenopausal women, there was no difference in disease severity in multiparous or nulliparous women. An important issue in the pregnant woman with MS is to avoid exposing the fetus to toxic drugs (Table 60.6).

Prognosis

Although great individual variability exists with regard to disease prognosis, a variety of factors have been identified as possible prognostic indicators.

- *Sex:* MS appears to follow a more benign course in women than in men.
- *Age at onset:* The average age at onset of MS is 29 years. Onset at an early age is seemingly a favorable factor, whereas onset at a later age carries a less favorable prognosis. As previously stated, the pattern of disease

varies in different age groups, with the relapsing-remitting form being more common in younger patients and the progressive form being more common in the older age group. Data are lacking as to whether prognosis differs as a function of age in patients with similar patterns of disease.

- *Initial disease course:* The relapsing form of the disease is associated with a better prognosis than progressive disease. A high rate of relapses early in the course of illness may correlate with shorter time to reach EDSS 6, as does a short first interval between attacks.
- *Initial complaints:* Among initial symptoms, impairment of sensory pathways or cranial nerve dysfunction, particularly ON, are found in several studies to be favorable prognostic features, whereas pyramidal and particularly brainstem and cerebellar symptoms carry a poor prognosis.

Both benign and fulminant forms of MS are recognized. There is no agreement among workers in the field as to the meaning of these terms. It is the general experience that a patient whose disease has had a benign course for 15 years only rarely develops a more severe course. Patients with mild disease (EDSS score 0–3) 5 years after diagnosis only uncommonly progress to severe disease (EDSS score 6) by 10 years (7.5% of patients) and 15 years (11.5% of patients). The term *malignant MS* is variably used by different workers; some use it to imply a rapid course, others to a clinical course in which there are frequent severe relapses with little recovery. Clues to etiology, susceptibility, and resistance factors must be present in such extremes of the clinical spectrum but they remain elusive at present. Entities such as Devic's disease, Baló's concentric sclerosis, and particularly Marburg's disease are more fulminant variants of MS with early disability and even death.

Risk of Multiple Sclerosis after Monosymptomatic Episodes

Optic Neuritis

The reported risk of later development of MS, based on clinical criteria in patients presenting with ON, is cited to range from 15–75%. A population-based study found that 60% of patients with ON progressed to MS by 40 years after the bout of ON (Rodriguez et al. 1995); the finding of oligoclonal bands (OCBs) in the CSF of such patients has been associated with an increased risk of developing MS. A series of reports indicates that 50–72% of ON patients have cranial MRI appearances consistent with MS and that of those with lesions, there is a 55–70% risk of developing clinically definite MS or laboratory-supported definite MS within 5 years (Morrissey et al. 1993). Patients with iso-

Table 60.6: Safety in pregnancy of drugs used in the treatment of multiple sclerosis

Category B: Animal data showing no harm to the fetus; no human data available
Glatiramer acetate (Copaxone)
Pemoline
Oxybutynin
Fluoxetine (and other selective serotonin reuptake inhibitors)
Desmopressin
Category C: Animal data shows harm to the fetus; no human data available
Corticosteroids
Interferon-β_{1a}
Interferon-β_{1b}
Baclofen
Amantadine
Tizanidine
Carbamazepine
Category D: Known to cause fetal harm when administered to pregnant women
Azathioprine
Cladribine
Cyclophosphamide
Category X: Contraindicated for use during pregnancy
Methotrexate

Source: Modified from DM Damek, EA Shuster. Pregnancy and multiple sclerosis. Mayo Clin Proc 1997;72:977–989.

lated ON and no evidence of disseminated lesions by MRI have a risk of 6–16% of developing MS after 4 years or more of follow-up (Morrissey et al. 1993). The incidence of MRI abnormalities in children with ON is less than that in adults, and this factor, coupled with clinical experience, suggests that the rate of progression to MS in children with isolated ON may well be less than that in adults. Five-year data from the original Optic Neuritis Treatment Trial revealed that the 5-year cumulative probability of developing clinically definite MS was 30% and did not differ by treatment group (oral prednisone, intravenous methylprednisolone, placebo). However, MRI was a strong predictor; the 5-year risk of developing clinically definite MS was 16% in patients with no brain MRI lesions and 51% in patients with three or more lesions.

Myelopathic Syndromes

Acute Myelopathy.   Patients presenting with acute complete transverse myelitis have a cited risk of MS of only 5–10%. However, partial or incomplete myelitis is a much more common clinical entity and bears more relevance to MS. Studies examining the issue of acute partial myelitis as an initial presentation of MS found that 57–72% of such patients had cranial MRI abnormalities consistent with MS. Follow-up from 3–5 years found that 60–90% of these patients developed MS, whereas 10–30% of those with normal MRI developed MS (Morrissey et al. 1993).

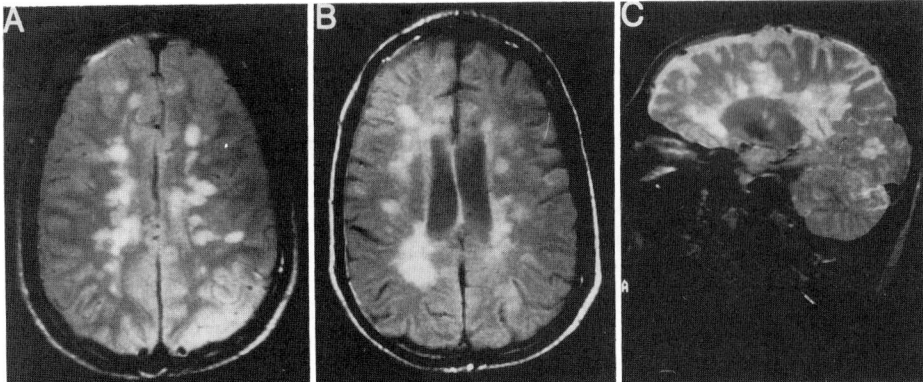

FIGURE 60.9   Magnetic resonance imaging studies in a 29-year-old man. (**A**) Multifocal lesions in the centrum semiovale (proton density image). (**B**) Multiple, at times confluent, white matter lesions abutting the lateral ventricles (proton density image). (**C**) Lesions dis-tributed in a radiating fashion from the corpus callosum. Significant cerebral atrophy with ventriculomegaly and cortical atrophy is also noted (T2-weighted image).

CSF studies suggest that patients with monosymptomatic disease with positive OCBs have a higher risk of evolution to MS than those without OCBs, although CSF results do not help further in prognosis when compared with MRI alone. CSF analysis would be most useful in a situation in which MRI is not available.

Chronic Myelopathy.   In patients with chronic progressive myelopathy, 60–70% have cranial MRI abnormalities con-sistent with MS in the absence of clinical evidence of dis-ease above the level of the spinal cord. What remains unclear is whether the remaining 30% have a disease other than MS or whether MS can manifest as a purely spinal dis-order. Probably both situations apply; improved spinal neu-roimaging should help resolve this issue.

Diagnostic Studies

Although the diagnosis of MS remains clinical, a number of ancillary laboratory tests can aid in the diagnosis of MS. The tests used most often are neuroimaging, particularly MRI, analysis of CSF, and, to a lesser extent, EP studies.

Neuroimaging

Magnetic Resonance Imaging.   MRI has changed signifi-cantly the approach to MS and is now the modality of choice as an aid to the diagnosis. MS plaques are typically found in the periventricular region, corpus callosum, cen-trum semiovale, and to a lesser extent, deep white matter structures and basal ganglia. Features typical of MS plaques have an ovoid appearance; lesions are arranged at right angles to the corpus callosum as if radiating from it. The

plaques appear hyperintense on proton density and T2-weighted studies (Figure 60.9), whereas the plaques appear (if visible at all) hypointense on T1-weighted images.

The earliest studies of cranial MRI in MS rapidly estab-lished that MRI detected many more lesions than did computed tomographic (CT) scanning (Figure 60.10). Fur-thermore, plaques were readily detected in regions that were rarely abnormal on CT, such as the brainstem, cere-bellum, and spinal cord. Most lesions seen on MRI cor-relate with lesions seen on pathology. However, some lesions that are quite extensive on MRI show only small plaques on pathological examination, suggesting that much of the abnormal MRI signal may be a result of increased water content of the brain around such plaques caused by presumed BBB disruption. This would be con-sistent with the finding of reduction of size of plaques in serial studies of MS using MRI.

The major effect of MRI technology has been on diag-nosis. Patients with clinically definite MS have white mat-ter lesions typical of MS in over 90% of cases. One must keep in mind that other CNS diseases (e.g., ischemia, SLE, Behçet's disease, other vasculitides, HTLV-1, sarcoidosis) may have lesions on MRI that appear similar to MS. This is particularly true for ischemic lesions, which make MRI criteria much less reliable for the diagnosis of MS in patients over the age of 50 (Offenbacher et al. 1993). Sev-eral sets of criteria have been proposed for determining if lesions seen on MRI are caused by MS. The criteria take into account the typical sites of MS plaques and also con-sider the relatively frequent finding of scattered hyperin-tense signals on T2-weighted images seen in the more elderly population and thought to be caused by vascular disease. For patients with at least three lesions, lesions abutting the ventricles, lesions in the posterior fossa, and

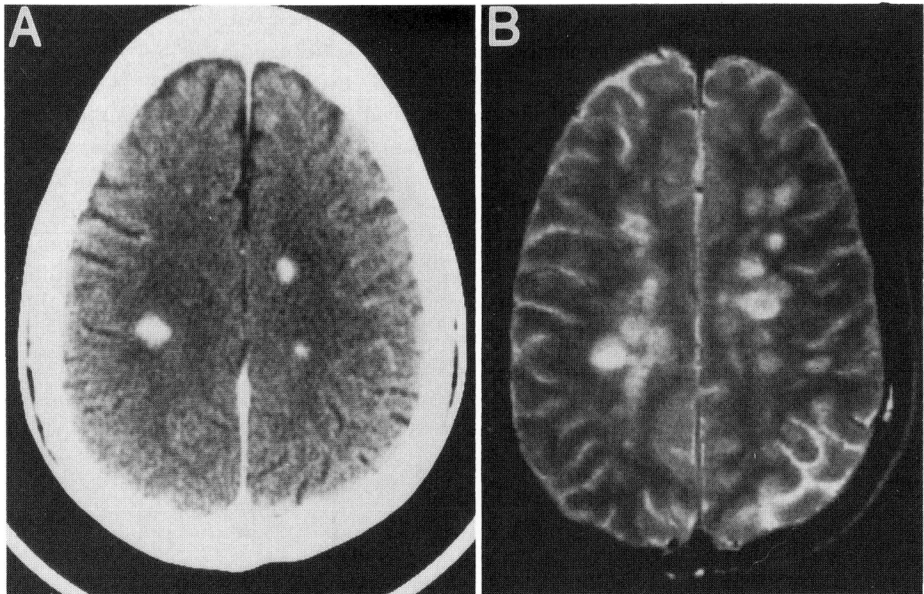

FIGURE 60.10 (A) Computed tomographic scan (same patient as in Figure 60.9, 3 years earlier) with contrast infusion demonstrating three regions of contrast enhancement typical of acute multiple sclerosis plaques. (B) Magnetic resonance imaging performed at the same time and at a comparable anatomical level demonstrating a multiplicity of lesions not detected by computed tomography.

lesions of greater than 5 mm are typical for MS. If at least two of these three criteria were met in an initial group of patients with MS and elderly controls, these criteria had a sensitivity of 88% and specificity of 100%. Testing of a larger, more diverse patient population indicated that these criteria had a sensitivity of 81% and a specificity of 96% (Offenbacher et al. 1993).

MRI scanning is both more sensitive and more specific for predicting evolution to clinically definite MS than other paraclinical measures such as CT scans, CSF, or EP. Two-year follow-up of 200 patients referred for suspected MS showed that 30% (50% of those under age 50) had developed clinically definite MS, of whom 84% had initial MRI scans that were strongly suggestive of MS. Subsequent studies have shown even higher rates of progression to MS (Morrissey et al. 1993) and that total MRI lesion number and load correlated with subsequent development of MS, degree of disability, and lesion load at follow-up (Filippi et al. 1994).

Efforts continue to delineate differences in the MRI appearance of acute or active lesions and chronic lesions. Acute lesions tend to be larger, with somewhat ill-defined margins when acute, and become smaller with sharper margins as resolution occurs. This presumably reflects resolution of edema and inflammation present at the time of acute plaque formation, leaving only residual areas of demyelination, gliosis, and enlarged extracellular space with remission. The MRI appearance of primary progressive MS shows a smaller total disease burden, a greater preponder-

ance of small lesions, fewer gadolinium-enhancing new lesions, and acquisition of fewer lesions per unit time than the secondary progressive form of MS.

Gadolinium-diethylenetriaminepentaacetic acid, a paramagnetic contrast agent that can cross only disrupted BBB, has been used to assess plaque activity. Gadolinium increases signal intensity on T1-weighted images. The accumulation of gadolinium in plaques is associated with new or newly active plaques and has been associated with pathologically confirmed acute inflammation in MS. Gadolinium enhancement usually persists for less than 4 weeks but may persist up to 8 weeks in acute plaques. Gadolinium enhancement diminishes or disappears after treatment with corticosteroids, a therapy thought to restore the integrity of BBB permeability.

Allied to the concept of using MRI data as outcome measures of MS therapeutic studies is the notion of following disease burden, which is the total volume of brain affected by plaques as detected on MRI scans. This can be done by measuring the surface area of all plaques and multiplying by the slice thickness. This is most reliable for thin-slice techniques and preferably with three-dimensional acquisition. A number of studies have examined the ability to detect lesion burden changes over time and have found that it is possible to detect changes that may not be clinically apparent.

The extent of cranial MRI abnormalities (and even pathology) does not necessarily correlate with the degree of clinical disability. Patients with small numbers of lesions may be quite disabled, whereas others may function well despite a large burden of disease as detected by MRI. Several possible explanations exist for this. Lesions may occur in areas that are clinically silent; small lesions in the spinal cord can cause major disability. In the absence of cerebral lesions, MRI may miss lesions that are clinically relevant such as those in cortex, basal ganglia, and brainstem; and large plaques detected by MRI may not have functional correlates but reflect increased tissue water without impairment of neural function.

Several studies have shown that the amount of ongoing MRI activity (new or enlarging lesions, gadolinium-enhancing lesions, or both) exceeds the observed clinical activity by a factor of 2–10. This may reflect not only the factors discussed previously, but also may partly reflect underreporting of minor symptoms and under-recognition of minor signs in patients with MS. It does, however, suggest that MS is a much more dynamic and active disease, both in progressive and relapsing MS, than is clinically apparent and that MRI is essential to studies of therapy in MS.

The utility of cranial MRI in relation to spinal myelopathies is addressed previously in the section on monosymptomatic disease. Spinal MRI is an evolving technology that can detect lesions consistent with demyelination in some but not all patients. In part, this may be caused by technical limitations of spinal MRI, but also may reflect involvement of small tracts in a relatively small anatomical structure. Many of the pathological lesions extend vertically in the affected tract, and such lesions may be best detected by transverse imaging. Newer technology detects lesions in 75% of patients with definite MS (Kidd et al. 1993). The frequency of abnormal signals in normal individuals is only 3%, as the non-MS hyperintense signal seen in older patients on cranial MRI appears not to occur in the spinal cord.

Conventional MRI technology provides excellent images, but makes it difficult to distinguish edema of an acute plaque from gliosis and demyelination of a chronic plaque. Using phosphorus MR spectroscopy, information on phospholipid metabolism can be obtained, whereas proton MR spectroscopy can generate information about other metabolic components, such as N-acetylaspartate (NAA), an exclusively neuronal marker, creatine phosphate (Cr) (energy marker), choline (membrane component), and lactic acid. Brains of patients with chronic MS have a reduced amount of NAA in comparison with choline and Cr; a reduced NAA to Cr ratio is the common means of expressing such a reduction. This reduced ratio implies loss of neurons or axons, which is consistent with pathological studies and appears to parallel disability in MS (Arnold et al. 1994) (Figure 60.11). In acute MS lesions studied by MR spectroscopic imaging, the NAA to Cr ratio may be transiently reduced, whereas the levels of choline and lactic acid may be elevated, perhaps related to myelin membrane disruption and tissue acidosis associated with acute plaque formation. Some investigators have found abnormal lipid peaks on MR spectroscopy, suggesting acute demyelination

(Davie et al. 1994). The use of these metabolic parameters may both lead to a better understanding of the evolution of plaques in vivo and be useful as further adjunct measures of disease progression that antedates clinical disability. A number of new technological advances appear likely to enhance yet further the ability to understand the pathogenesis of the disease process.

Computed Tomography. The current utility of CT scans in the evaluation of patients with MS is largely to exclude other treatable or ominous etiologies as the cause of symptoms. Findings on CT of patients with MS include nonspecific atrophy, hypodense lesions often in a periventricular distribution, and contrast-enhancing lesions presumed to be active plaques with disruption of the BBB (see Figure 60.10). However, the sensitivity of CT scans for plaques is not high, even when using the double-dose contrast technique coupled with delayed scanning. Only 50–60% of scans during an acute relapse demonstrate plaques, and this figure decreases to 40% with an attack in the preceding 3 months and 13% with inactive disease. The CT scan also may only discern a single lesion, which greatly widens the differential diagnosis as compared with multifocal lesions. Plaques in the posterior fossa are poorly visualized, if at all.

Cerebrospinal Fluid

CSF findings alone cannot make or exclude the diagnosis of MS, but they can be useful adjuncts to clinical criteria. CSF abnormalities are an integral part of the laboratory-assisted diagnostic criteria (see Table 60.4). The CSF is grossly normal in MS, being clear, colorless, and under normal pressure. Total leukocyte count is normal in two-thirds of patients, exceeding 15 cells/μl in less than 5% of patients and only rarely exceeding 50 cells/μl (a finding that should raise suspicion of another etiology). The predominant cell type is the lymphocyte, the vast majority of which are T cells.

CSF protein (or albumin) level is normal in the majority of patients with MS. Albumin determinations are preferable because albumin is not synthesized in the CNS and thus gives a better indication of BBB disruption than does total protein, some of which may be synthesized within the CNS (i.e., immunoglobulin). Albumin levels are elevated in 20–30% of patients, although less than 1% of patients have a level twice that of normal (Table 60.7). A common finding in MS is an elevation of CSF immunoglobulin level relative to other protein components, implying intrathecal synthesis. The immunoglobulin increase is predominantly IgG, but the synthesis of IgM and IgA is increased also. The IgG shows an excess of IgG1 and κ light chains. The IgG level may be expressed as a percentage of total protein (normal <11%), as a percentage of albumin (normal <27%), by use of the IgG index (normal value <0.66), or by use of a formula for intra-BBB synthesis of IgG. An abnormality of

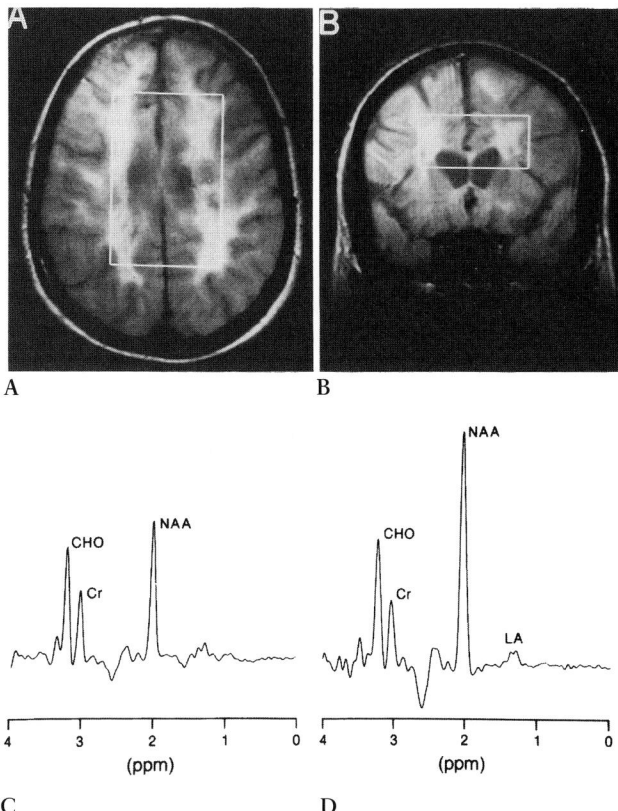

FIGURE 60.11 (A, B) Areas of confluent demyelination in a severely affected progressive multiple sclerosis patient. Outlines show volume of interest selected for spectroscopy study. (C) Spectra obtained with proton spectroscopy in this patient. (D) Spectra of normal brain. Note the reduced height of the N-acetylaspartate (NAA) peak with resultant reduction in the ratio of NAA to creatine (Cr). (CHO = choline; LA = lactic acid.)

CSF IgG production as measured by the IgG index or IgG synthesis rate is found in more than 90% of patients with clinically definite MS, and different formulas appear to have differing sensitivity and specificity. The sensitivity of IgG as a percentage of protein or albumin is slightly lower (see Table 60.7).

Linked to the elevation of IgG is the finding of OCBs in the cathodal region of an electrophoretic analysis of CSF. When normal CSF is electrophoresed, the cathodal region shows only a homogeneous blur of immunoglobulin. In MS and other conditions usually associated with inflammation, electrophoretic analysis reveals a number of discrete bands distinct from the background; these bands represent excess antibody produced by one or more clones of plasma cells (Figure 60.12). In subacute sclerosing panencephalitis, the majority of these OCBs represent antibody directed against the causative agent, measles virus. However, in MS, there is no disease-specific antigen yet identified against which

the majority of bands are directed. The pattern of banding remains relatively consistent in individual patients during the disease course, although bands may be added over time. Occasionally, patients with definite autopsy-proved MS do not have OCBs.

A common method for electrophoresis uses agarose gels, but a more sensitive assay is the use of isoelectric focusing on polyacrylamide gels. OCBs are found in 85–95% of patients with clinically definite MS (see Table 60.7). Up to 8% of CSF samples from non-MS patients show OCBs; most are from cases of chronic CNS infections, viral syndromes, and autoimmune neuropathies. The presence of OCBs in monosymptomatic patients predicts a significantly higher rate of progression to MS than the absence of bands: 25% versus 9% at 3 years' follow-up. However, one must not assume that the presence of OCBs is equivalent to a diagnosis of MS, given the number of false-positive results that can occur and the variability in technique and interpretation in different laboratories.

The presence of myelin components and antimyelin antibodies in CSF and other body fluids has been used to a limited extent as a measure of CNS myelin destruction and presumed demyelinating activity in the CNS (Whitaker et al. 1993).

Evoked Potentials

EPs are the CNS electrical events generated by peripheral stimulation of a sensory organ (see Chapter 37A). The utility of EPs is the detection of a CNS abnormality of function that may be clinically undetectable. In the case of MS, detection of a subclinical lesion in a site remote from the region of clinical dysfunction supports a diagnosis of multifocal disease. The EPs also may help define the anatomical site of the lesion in tracts not easily visualized by imaging (optic nerves, dorsal columns). The three most frequently used EPs are somatosensory (SSEP), visual (VER), and brainstem auditory evoked responses. MRI technology has largely eliminated the utility of EPs, given the much greater anatomical information obtained and the much higher sensitivity of MRI in the diagnosis of MS (Table 60.8).

SSEPs have abnormal results in 65–80% of patients with MS, including approximately one-half of patients with MS who do not have sensory signs or symptoms. Some patients with clinical evidence of posterior column dysfunction may have normal SSEPs. Using pattern shift VERs, abnormalities are detected in over 90% of patients with a history of ON, even when visual acuity has returned to normal. Patients with clinically definite MS have abnormal VERs with a frequency of 85%. The VER is particularly useful in those patients lacking clear clinical evidence of dysfunction above the level of the foramen magnum, such as those with a chronic progressive myelopathy. Ocular or retinal disorders must be excluded before attributing abnormal VERs

Table 60.7: Cerebrospinal fluid abnormalities in multiple sclerosis

	Albumin	IgG/TP	IgG/albumin	IgG index	Oligoclonal banding of Ig
Clinically definite multiple sclerosis	23%	67%	60–73%	70–90%	85–95%
Normal controls	3%	—	3–6%	3%	7%*

IgG/TP = IgG value/total protein.
*Other neurological diseases.

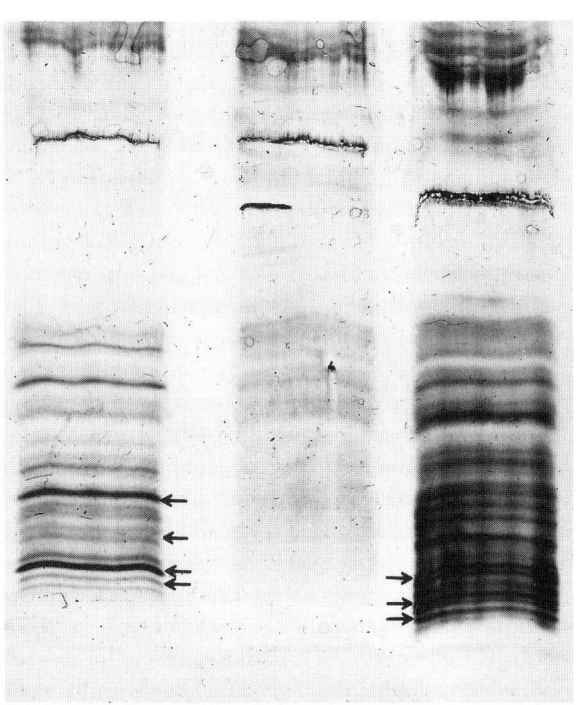

FIGURE 60.12 Isoelectric focusing of cerebrospinal fluid on polyacrylamide gel. Oligoclonal bands are seen (*arrows*) in the cathodal (bottom) region of gel in the left- and right-hand lanes (both multiple sclerosis patients). The center lane is from a patient with headache.

to demyelination in the optic pathways. Brainstem auditory evoked response abnormalities are less frequent in MS than VER or SSEP abnormalities, being present in 50–65% of patients with MS.

Variants of Multiple Sclerosis

MS is a condition with many variable forms, but in most cases the common signs and symptoms described previously are readily apparent, and with proper laboratory confirmation the diagnosis is not difficult. However, there are several inflammatory demyelinating disorders that bear an unknown relationship to MS. They are listed here as variants of MS, rather than as separate illnesses, because it is

often found, after long follow-up, that the disease has reverted to a more standard variety of MS.

Recurrent Optic Neuropathy

There are patients whose entire clinical illness is confined to the optic nerves. They may have sequential affection of one nerve, then the other, or they may have simultaneous bilateral vision loss, a state that is quite uncommon in classic MS. In some instances MRI of the head shows (in addition to lesions of the optic nerves) scattered intracerebral lesions, or a CSF examination shows OCB, attesting to some degree of dissemination of the lesions. Children and preadolescent patients are more likely than adults to have recurrent or simultaneous optic neuropathy. Rarely there is slowly progressive optic neuropathy, similar to that seen with optic nerve sheath tumors, such as meningioma. The distinction from an MS variant can be quite challenging. In bilateral ON, sarcoidosis is commonly a diagnostic consideration.

Devic's Disease (Neuromyelitis Optica)

A combination of bilateral optic neuropathy and cervical myelopathy make up this condition, which most authorities now classify as a variant of MS. Reported cases indicate that the myelopathy tends to be more severe, with less likelihood of recovery, and that the neuropathological features at autopsy are those of a much more severe necrotic lesion of the cord rather than incomplete demyelination. In some patients the optic neuropathy and the myelopathy occur at the same time, in others one or the other component is delayed. The longer the interval, the more like typical MS is the pathology. Because the optic nerve and the cervical spinal cord are two of the locations in the nervous system in which the lesions of MS are typically found, many patients could be classified as having Devic's disease, or syndrome. Little is to be gained by this nomenclature, because Devic's syndrome can be a manifestation of ADEM (see Acute Disseminated Encephalomyelitis, later in this chapter), or rarely of other autoimmune disease, such as SLE. This seems to be especially true of patients with relapsing Devic's syndrome, making up approximately one-half the patients. In a few patients the distinction between an MS variant and SLE (so-called lupoid sclerosis) is essen-

Table 60.8:   Comparison of sensitivity of laboratory testing in multiple sclerosis

	VER	BAER	SSEP	OCB	MRI
Clinically definite multiple sclerosis	80–85%*	50–65%	65–80%	85–95%	90–97%

BAER = brainstem auditory evoked response; MRI = magnetic resonance imaging; OCB = oligoclonal bands; SSEP = somatosensory evoked potentials; VER = visual evoked response.
*Numbers show the percentage of patients with abnormal study results.

tially impossible to make, and some of these are patients with neuromyelitis optica.

Slowly Progressive Myelopathy

A syndrome of slowly progressive spinal cord dysfunction can present a major diagnostic challenge. If there are no sensory signs or symptoms, the entity known as primary lateral sclerosis, one of the group of motor neuron disease, may be the cause. HTLV-1 infection, vitamin B_{12} deficiency, and human immunodeficiency virus infection all can be excluded by appropriate testing. Spinal dural arteriovenous fistula can cause a steadily or stepwise progressive myelopathy, usually in the lower spinal segments. Adrenomyeloneuropathy should be considered.

A number of patients remain who do not fit into these categories, and whose spinal MRI results are repeatedly negative. VERs, CSF OCBs, and MRI of the head show no sign of demyelination elsewhere. No firm diagnosis is possible. Minor clues that MS is present may be furnished by a Lhermitte's sign that has come and gone, or by undue sensitivity to elevated temperature. The degree of compression of the cervical cord by intervertebral disc disease is often an issue in the middle-aged patient, because a majority of persons have some degree of disc disease. There is little doubt that some laminectomies have been carried out for cervical spondylosis where MS was the final correct diagnosis.

Progressive myelopathy caused by MS is part of the primary progressive MS group and carries the poor prognosis typical of that group. The choice of therapy is difficult. Some patients do better for a time with monthly intravenous corticosteroid therapy.

Acute Tumorlike Multiple Sclerosis (Marburg Variant)

Some patients with demyelinating disease present with a large acute lesion of one hemisphere (Figure 60.13) or rarely other locations, such as the spinal cord. Mass effect may occur, with compression of the lateral ventricle and shift across the midline. The clinical abnormalities in such patients are variable: They may be slight even in a patient with a massive lesion, whereas confusion, hemiparesis, or neglect syndrome may be seen in another patient with a lesion that appears no different. Much of the T2 bright lesion volume is often caused by edema and may be rapidly responsive to corticosteroids. (This change with corticosteroids also may occur with glioma or CNS lymphoma and

is therefore not a useful diagnostic criterion.) Biopsy is often required.

In one series of 31 patients, the prognosis was good, most patients recovered well clinically, and their lesion volume rapidly cleared. In 24 of the patients the demyelinating lesion was solitary, whereas in the others one or more satellite nodules existed. Six of the patients were older than 57. In follow-up, 28 of the patients did not develop additional evidence of demyelinating activity during a period of 9 months to 12 years. Other authorities have reported a higher rate of recurrent disease, in particular a conversion to more ordinary types of MS, both clinically and by MRI scan criteria.

Treatment and Management

In prior decades, treatment of this often progressive disease of young adults was judged to be ineffective and many clinicians and patients adopted a nihilistic and pessimistic attitude. The advent of more effective symptomatic therapy, and the widely publicized U.S. Food and Drug Administration (FDA) approval of three agents capable of modifying the disease course have drastically changed that view. There remain many problems, particularly the treatment of progressive MS, yet there are clearly reasons for hope.

Treatment of MS should be directed toward these basic goals:

- Relief or modification of symptoms
- Shortening the duration or limiting the residual effects of an acute relapse
- Preventing progression or slowing its pace
- Supporting family and patient, alleviating social and economic effects, and advocating for the disabled or handicapped

Monitoring Disease Activity

Magnetic Resonance Imaging.   A surrogate marker for disease activity in MS is badly needed. It is now clear from several of the completed interferon therapy trials that there is far more activity in MRI scans of patients than is apparent clinically. Some authors estimate a ratio of new MRI lesions to clinical events as 10 to 1 in patients with active relapsing-remitting MS. New MRI lesions may be measured by change in total T2 visible lesion load, by new or enlarg-

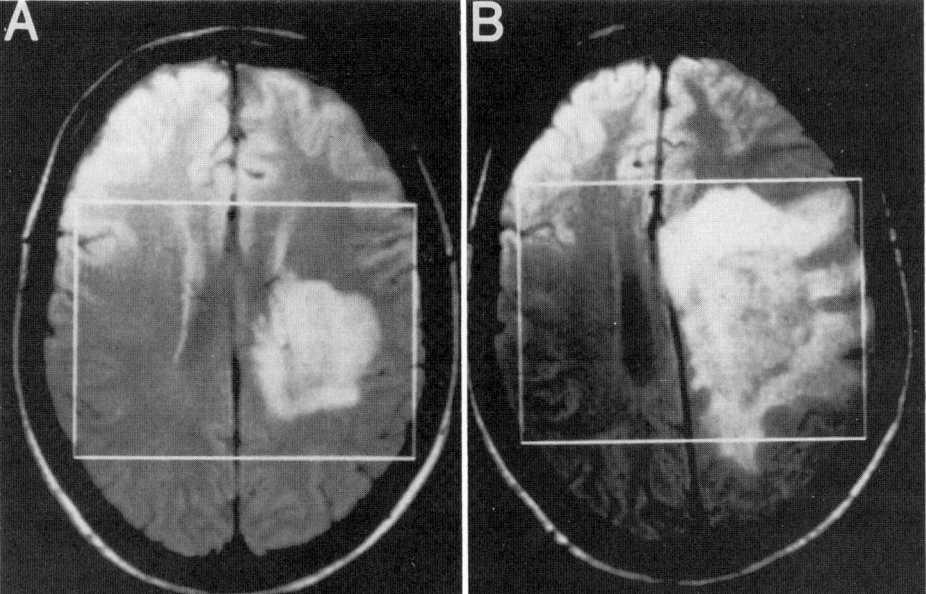

FIGURE 60.13 (A) Magnetic resonance scan showing a large white matter lesion initially without mass effect in a young woman with right hemiplegia developing over 5 days. (B) Marked increase in size of lesion with associated edema and mass effect 1 month later while on corticosteroids and at a time when clinical deficits were improving. Biopsy showed evidence of demyelination.

ing lesions, or by gadolinium enhancement. All three criteria have been used with success in one trial or another.

Several therapies are known to reduce the accumulation of MRI lesions in clinical trials; these include interferon-β_{1a}, interferon-β_{1b}, and mitoxantrone. Unpublished data suggest that cyclophosphamide blocks the appearance of new gadolinium-positive lesions. The MRI data have been strong indicators of clinical effectiveness in clinical trials and are clearly now a cornerstone of therapeutic investigations in MS. Nevertheless, problems exist. In the care of patients who are not enrolled in large-scale trials, MRI plays only a doubtful role in monitoring the progress of treatment. Data from the National Institutes of Health trials of relapsing MS demonstrate that frequent scanning of an individual patient is required to obtain reliable information, possibly as often as once a month. Infrequent scans can miss lesions that have come and gone. In patients with progressive MS, the lesion load in the head MRI scans can remain unchanged while the patient steadily worsens. Often this state of affairs is caused by progressive spinal disease, which cannot be imaged well. A minority of patients with MS, possibly as many as 5%, have no MRI lesions characteristic of MS at all.

Advantages exist in some instances for single or relatively infrequent scans. In the early stages of illness, after a monosymptomatic relapse, many patients wish to know their risk of developing MS, which can often be defined by MRI (see previous sections). In patients under treatment in whom disease activity develops and a change of therapy is contemplated, additional evidence, for or against the change, can sometimes be derived from an MRI scan.

Immunological Data. Thus far, few relevant data exist about levels of cytokines or T-cell subsets as measurements of disease activity. The expression of different T-cell subsets is not relevant. Levels in blood of the inflammatory cytokine IL-12 appear to correlate with activity of relapsing MS and may function as a surrogate marker. Interferon-γ, a cytokine that can itself provoke relapses in patients with MS, may decrease in blood levels when MS is treated successfully. Many investigators are in the process of measuring IL-2, TNF-α, IL-10, and other cytokines (see Chapter 46 for more details).

Clinical Examination. The eventual gold standard of success in MS treatments is the clinical condition of the patient. Every clinical trial includes these data as a primary or secondary outcome. Yet the difficulties of clinical measurement are exemplified by the number of scales and indices that are used. The problems of the EDSS are noted previously. A one-point increase or decrease in the EDSS is often taken as an end point; this may require special training of observers, and even then variability of observations occurs. The Ambulation Index, a direct assessment of walking, is useful in most patients. MRI is increasingly considered as the primary end point.

Relief or Modification of Symptoms

Spasticity. Spasticity slows voluntary movement, impairs balance and gait, and may cause painful flexor or extensor spasms. Partial control is often possible, although recovery of motor power is rare.

Baclofen is a γ-aminobutyric acid agonist that can effectively relieve spasms and has modest effects in improving performance. Daily divided doses of 20–80 mg and occasionally more are used. Too large a dose may produce drowsiness or sufficient hypotonicity as to increase the degree of weakness. Intrathecal baclofen via an implanted pump can be effective against spasticity in suitable patients.

Tizanidine (Zanaflex), a centrally active α_2-noradrenergic agonist, may be used alone or in combination with baclofen because the mechanism of action is different. The medication, available in 4-mg tablets, must be gradually increased starting at 2 mg at bedtime. The side effects are similar to baclofen; however, a blind prospective trial in patients with MS showed that while relieving spasticity it did not affect strength.

Benzodiazepines contribute to the control of spasticity, although sedation and possible drug dependency are limiting factors.

Dantrolene sodium (Dantrium), an agent that acts within muscles on excitation-contraction coupling, is rarely used because of the risk of liver damage. If used, the medication must be titrated from 25 mg daily up to 100 mg three times a day.

4-Aminopyridine and 3,4-diaminopyridine (3,4-DAP) are compounds that block potassium channels in the axolemma, thereby increasing nerve conduction. These compounds may be helpful for a variety of symptoms, especially temperature-related symptoms. A double-blind trial showed improvement in motor strength. The risk of seizure and hepatitis has limited the use of these compounds until further studies are completed.

Botulinum toxin type A (Botox) also has been shown to be effective in selective cases.

Tremor.   One of the most disabling and hard to treat symptoms in MS is tremors. Appendicular tremors are usually seen in action or intention and may limit activities of daily living.

Weighted wrist bracelets and specially adapted utensils are a nonpharmaceutical option.

Isoniazid, 800–1,200 mg per day, with pyridoxine, 100 mg per day, may have marginal success.

Anticonvulsants also have been reported to be helpful with tremor. Primidone (Mysoline), 125–250 mg two to three times per day, is recommended. Dizziness, somnolence, and nausea are the primary side effects. Carbamazepine (Tegretol) in divided doses up to 800 mg per day has been used also. Gabapentin (Neurontin) in daily divided doses up to 3,600 mg has shown some benefit.

Clonazepam (Klonopin), 0.5–2.0 mg one to four times daily, is effective, however the side effects, including ataxia, behavioral changes, confusion, and respiratory depression, must be kept in mind when treating patients.

Propranolol (Inderal), 20–40 mg two to three times daily, is another option. Caution must be taken in patients with concomitant cardiac, circulatory, or respiratory disorders.

Ondansetron (Zofran), 4–8 mg once or twice daily, has been reported effective in case studies of patients with MS. Side effects include diarrhea, headache, and elevated liver enzymes.

Surgical thalamotomy may be used in patients with refractory disease.

Fatigue.   Fatigue is seen in as many as 78% of patients and interferes with daily activities. Fatigue must be separated from depression, medication side effects, or physical exhaustion from gait alterations.

Amantadine (Symmetrel), 100 mg twice a day, has relatively few side effects and is well tolerated by most patients. Caution must be taken in patients with renal insufficiency or seizure disorders. Studies have found an efficacy rate of 40%.

Pemoline (Cylert) is an alternative medication if no response to amantadine is seen. The starting dose is 18.75 mg twice daily and can be increased to a maximum of six tablets per day. The risk of hepatic failure is an obstacle to using this drug as first-line therapy. Some patients also may respond to methylphenidate (Ritalin), 10–60 mg per day in two to three divided doses.

Selective serotonin reuptake inhibitors, in addition to treating the depressive symptoms associated with MS, have been used to treat fatigue. Fluoxetine (Prozac), 10–20 mg once or twice daily, has a side effect profile including nausea, headache, extrapyramidal effects, hypotension, and mania.

Bladder Dysfunction.   Symptomatic bladder dysfunction can be identified at some time during the course of MS in 50–80% of patients. The severity of bladder symptoms is unrelated to the duration of the disease but parallels the severity of other neurological symptoms. Differentiating between bladder spasticity and hypotonia should be evaluated before initiating therapy because different medications are employed for each condition. Common disorders such as urinary tract infections, prostate and bladder cancer, and benign prostatic hypertrophy may mimic symptoms of neurological dysfunction and should be excluded.

Initial steps include fluid management, timed voiding, and bedside commode.

Oxybutynin (Ditropan) is a first-line medication for hyperreflexic bladder without outlet obstruction. Dosage ranges from 2.5–5.0 mg one to three times daily. General precautions and side-effect profiles of the anticholinergics must be observed.

Propantheline (Pro-Banthine), 15 mg three to four times per day, is another anticholinergic option for hyperreflexic bladders without outlet obstruction.

Imipramine (Tofranil), a tricyclic antidepressant, 50–300 mg in divided daily doses, is also helpful, especially with enuresis. Side effects are similar to the anticholinergics. This medication has the dual effect of treating concomitant depression.

Desmopressin is also effective with hyperreflexic bladder without outlet obstruction. Doses of 20–40 µg daily is suggested. Adverse effects include nausea, flushing, and headache.

Tolterodine (Detrol) is a muscarinic receptor antagonist with fewer side effects than anticholinergic medications. This medicine, given at 2 mg twice daily, was shown to reduce bladder frequency and urgency as well as urge incontinence.

Detrusor hyperreflexia with outlet obstruction may respond to Credé's maneuvers, antispasticity medications, or anticholinergics in combination with alpha-sympathetic blocking agents such as terazosin hydrochloride (Hytrin). The maintenance dose is 2–10 mg daily. Adverse effects include tachycardia, dizziness, syncope, headache, and asthenia.

Detrusor areflexia may respond to Credé's maneuvers, alpha-sympathetic blocking agents, or bethanechol chloride (Urecholine). The usual dose is 10–50 mg three to four times a day with a side-effect profile including diarrhea, excessive lacrimation, and flushing of the skin. This medication is also contraindicated in many common medical conditions.

Catheterization may be employed if the previously mentioned measures are ineffective; however, the long-term effects of catheterization must be considered. Squamous metaplasia of the bladder was significantly greater in patients who had been catheterized for more than 10 years (80%) in comparison with those catheterized for less than 10 years (42%) and those without catheters (20%).

Surgical correction, such as augmentation of bladder capacity with an exteriorized loop of bowel, for appropriate patients is another alternative.

Depression.   Prevalence rates for depression in patients with MS range from 14 to 57% as compared with 1.3–3.7% in the general population. The lifetime prevalence of depression in a group of patients with chronic medical disorders was 12.9%. The nature of a chronic debilitating neurological disorder contributes to depressive symptoms and coping problems. Patients taking multiple medications are prone to depression, and the side-effect profile of the interferon-β medications includes depression.

Selective serotonin reuptake inhibitors are the medication of choice for depressive symptoms in patients with MS. In addition to the previously mentioned fluoxetine, any of the other medications in this class may be used.

Amitriptyline (Elavil), 25–100 mg daily (or other tricyclic antidepressants in equivalent dosage), is a second-line choice because of anticholinergic side effects. However, anticholinergic properties may be helpful to patients with symptoms of bladder spasticity or chronic pain, thus avoiding polypharmacy.

Sexual Dysfunction.   Studies suggest that 45–74% of women with MS experience sexual dysfunction. These symptoms have been associated with depression, bowel dysfunction, fatigue, spasticity, and pelvic floor weakness. There was no association between duration of disease, type of disease, recent exacerbations, or disability scores. Erectile dysfunction in men is common, especially in patients with spinal cord involvement. Symptoms also may be caused by medications or psychological issues.

Sildenafil (Viagra) has supplanted traditional approaches to erectile dysfunction in men, which used to include intracavernous papaverine, prostaglandin E, phentolamine, vacuum devices, and penile prostheses. Doses of 25–100 mg 1 hour before sexual intercourse daily are used with minimal side effects, which include headache, flushing, dyspepsia, and musculoskeletal pain. Reports suggest caution in patients with cardiovascular disease. Sildenafil is probably also effective in women.

Cognitive Impairment.   Problems with cognition are increasingly being recognized as an important deficit affecting patients with MS. Studies have found a correlation between dementia and lesion burden on MRI as well as atrophy of the corpus callosum. In a study of patients with chronic progressive MS who underwent MRI scans and a neuropsychological screening battery, those who were impaired according to the neuropsychological screening battery had significantly more cerebral lesions than those who were judged unimpaired. Treatment of cognitive deficits consists of support, improvement of coping strategies, and treatment of depression.

Paroxysmal Symptoms.   A variety of paroxysmal symptoms consist of brief, almost stereotypic, events occurring frequently and often triggered by movement or sensory stimuli. They are likely caused by ephaptic transmission of nerve impulses at sites of previous disease activity. These symptoms include, but are not limited to, trigeminal neuralgia, pain, paresthesia, weakness, tonic seizures, dysarthria and ataxia, pruritus, diplopia, akinesia, and hemifacial spasm and dystonia.

Anticonvulsants, especially carbamazepine and valproate (Depakote), have been used in their usual doses with some benefit. Newer anticonvulsants, such as gabapentin, have been used in small case studies.

Benzodiazepines also have been effective in some patients.

Baclofen, acetazolamide (Diamox), ibuprofen, and bromocriptine are cited as potentially beneficial with these paroxysmal symptoms.

Treatment Strategies

For some patients MS is a disease with one or two acute neurological episodes with no further evidence of disease activity. In others it is a chronic, relapsing, or progressive

Table 60.9: Multiple sclerosis treatment strategies

Disease course/stage	Treatment options
Monosymptomatic (e.g., optic neuritis)	IV methylprednisolone, 1,000 mg for 5 days, without oral taper
Relapsing-remitting, no disease activity for several years, and/or no activity on magnetic resonance imaging	IV corticosteroids if attack does occur
Relapsing-remitting, current disease activity and/or activity on magnetic resonance imaging	IV corticosteroids for attacks, plus (1) interferon-β_{1a} (Avonex), 30 μg IM weekly; or (2) interferon-β_{1b} (Betaseron), 1 ml SC qod; or (3) glatiramer acetate (Copaxone), 20 μg SC daily
Relapsing-remitting, disease activity while on interferon or Copaxone	Add monthly bolus of IV methylprednisolone; consider increasing dose of interferon
Relapsing-remitting, accumulating disability (interferon/Copaxone/corticosteroid nonresponders)	IV monthly cyclophosphamide and pulse therapy
Rapidly progressing disability	IV cyclophosphamide and corticosteroid 8-day induction, followed by pulse maintenance
Very rapidly progressing disability	Plasma exchange
Secondary progressive	IV corticosteroid monthly pulses
	IV cyclophosphamide/corticosteroid monthly pulses
	Methotrexate, oral or SC, 7.5–20 mg/wk, with or without monthly corticosteroid pulses
	Consider addition of interferon-β if not currently taking
Primary progressive	IV corticosteroid monthly pulses
	Methotrexate, oral or SC, 7.5–20 mg/wk, with or without monthly corticosteroid pulses
	Cladribine, IV or SC
	Consider mitoxantrone

disease with an unpredictable clinical course that generally spans 10–20 years during which time neurological disability accumulates. Treatment of MS, as with other branches of medicine, has come to rely on prospective clinical trials. Yet, the variety of patient disabilities and variation in the course of the disease make the choice of treatment for the individual patient difficult. Patients may differ markedly from those who have been treated in clinical trials. Table 60.9 outlines the treatment paradigm used at our institution.

Treatment of Acute Attacks

Acute attacks are typically treated with corticosteroids. Indications for treatment of a relapse include functionally disabling symptoms with objective evidence of neurological impairment such as loss of vision and motor, cerebellar, or both kinds of symptoms. Thus, mild sensory attacks are typically not treated. In the past, adrenocorticotropic hormone and oral prednisone were primarily used. More recently, treatment with short courses of intravenous methylprednisolone, 500–1,000 mg daily for 3–7 days, with or without a short prednisone taper is commonly used. ON may occur anytime during the course of MS or be one of the initial symptoms. A randomized therapeutic trial in ON demonstrated that patients treated with oral prednisone alone were more likely to suffer recurrent episodes of ON as compared with those treated with methylprednisolone followed by oral prednisone (Beck et al. 1993). Furthermore, definite MS developed in 7.5% of

the intravenous methylprednisolone group, 14.7% of the oral prednisone group, and 16.7% of the placebo group over a 2-year period (Beck et al. 1993). These data support the use of high-dose intravenous methylprednisolone for acute MS attacks. High-dose intravenous methylprednisolone appears to be accompanied by relatively few side effects in most patients, although mental changes, unmasking of infections, gastric disturbances, and an increased incidence of fractures have been reported. Baseline and yearly bone density scans are recommended for patients undergoing repeated courses of corticosteroid therapy. Anaphylactoid reactions and arrhythmias are rare, but may also occur. The immunological mechanisms of high-dose corticosteroids include reduction of CD4+ cells, decrease in cytokine release from lymphocytes and cytokines including TNF, interferon-γ, and decreased class II expression (Kupersmith 1994). Corticosteroids have been shown to decrease IgG synthesis in the CNS and reduce CSF antibodies to MBP and OCBs. Intravenous methylprednisolone may decrease the entry of cells into the brain and may affect cytokine patterns also.

Two other trials have focused on oral corticosteroid use. A double-blind, placebo-controlled trial of oral methylprednisolone use in acute attacks involving 51 patients followed over 8 weeks showed a statistically significant beneficial effect of oral corticosteroids. Patients received a total of 3,676 mg of oral methylprednisolone over 15 days with no serious adverse events. A second randomized trial of 80 patients evaluated oral versus intravenous methylprednisolone in acute relapses. The results showed no statistical difference between the treatment groups.

Disease-Modifying Treatments

The first medication approved by the FDA for use in MS was recombinant interferon-β_{1b} (Betaseron) that has been shown in a double-blind, placebo-controlled trial of 372 patients to decrease the frequency of relapses from 1.27 per year to 0.84 per year after 2 years in relapsing-remitting patients receiving 8 mIU every other day. This is a 34% reduction in the relapse rate compared with placebo (IFNB MS Study Group 1993). It did not affect clinical disability in patients followed over the 3-year period, but it did significantly affect accumulation of lesions on the MRI (Paty et al. 1993), suggesting that the underlying disease process was affected. Five-year follow-up data reveals that disease progression was less in the interferon-β_{1b} group (35%) compared with the placebo group (46%) (IFNB MS Study Group 1995). Also seen was a 30% decrease in the annual exacerbation rate in the treated group over 5 years. Although this was not statistically significant, the treatment benefit trend was maintained. The MRI data showed no significant increase in the median MRI lesion burden (3.6%) in the patients receiving interferon-β_{1b}, whereas the patients on placebo had an increase in median MRI lesion burden of 30.2% over 5 years. Betaseron is administered every other day under the skin by self-injection. Side effects include flulike symptoms, depression, and reactions at the injection site, but these tend to diminish with time. Elevated liver enzymes, leukopenia, and anemia were seen, and blood monitoring is suggested every 3 months. Presently, it is not known how interferon-β_{1b} will affect the progression of MS in patients with relapsing-remitting disease or the accumulation of disability over time, although further experience with the drug over the next years will help clarify this issue. Not all patients respond to the drug, and with time all patients have had additional attacks. Also 34% of patients developed neutralizing antibodies that may reduce the clinical efficacy of the drug. The mechanism of action of interferon-β_{1b} is currently unknown.

A second double-blind, placebo-controlled study in 301 patients with relapsing-remitting disease investigated the efficacy of weekly intramuscular injections of 6 million U (30 µg) of interferon-β_{1a} (Avonex), a glycosylated recombinant interferon-β (Jacobs et al. 1996). Over 2 years the annual exacerbation rate was 0.90 in the placebo group and 0.61 in the Avonex group. This is a 29% reduction in the relapse rate compared with placebo. After 2 years the MRI data revealed a lesion volume of 122.4 (mean) in the placebo group compared with 74.1 (mean) in the Avonex group. The number of enhancing lesions on MRI over 2 years was 1.65 (mean) in the placebo group and 0.80 (mean) in the Avonex group. The proportion of patients progressing by the end of 104 weeks of the trial was 34.9% in the placebo group and 21.9% in the Avonex group. Adverse events included mild flulike symptoms and mild anemia. No skin reactions occurred because the injection is deep. Laboratory monitoring is suggested, but not mandatory because no serious liver toxicities occurred. Also, 22% of patients on treatment developed neutralizing antibodies.

Glatiramer acetate/copolymer 1 (Copaxone), a daily subcutaneous injectable synthetic polymer, showed positive effects in a small double-blind trial of relapsing-remitting MS, but not in progressive disease. In a large double-blind trial in relapsing-remitting disease involving 251 randomized patients (Johnson et al. 1995), the patients receiving Copaxone had a 2-year relapse rate of 1.19, compared with 1.68 for patients receiving placebo. There was a 29% reduction in the relapse rate over 2 years for those using Copaxone. Extension data shows that over 140 weeks 41% of patients receiving placebos experienced worsening of their disability by greater than or equal to 1.5 EDSS steps, whereas only 21.6% of Copaxone-treated patients had worsening (Johnson et al. 1998). No MRI data are available at this time. Side effects included local injection site reactions and transient systemic postinjection reactions including chest pain, flushing, dyspnea, palpitations, and anxiety. No laboratory monitoring is necessary. No neutralizing antibodies were detected in the study. This molecule is a random polymer whose initial design was based on the amino acid composition of MBP. The mechanism by which copolymer 1 may work in humans is unknown.

Another factor to consider is that all three medications (Betaseron, Avonex, Copaxone) are contraindicated in pregnancy. With all three agents, when pregnancy occurs, treatment should be discontinued, and if relapses occur during pregnancy they are treated with intravenous corticosteroids. In addition, the safety of symptomatic medications for pregnancy must be kept in mind when managing these patients (see Table 60.6).

A randomized, double-blind, placebo-controlled study of interferon-β_{1a} in higher doses was conducted in Europe (European Study Group 1998). This involved 560 patients with relapsing-remitting disease given subcutaneous interferon-β_{1a} (Rebif). Patients were randomized to placebo, 22 µg, or 44 µg of Rebif three times a week for 2 years. There was a 27% reduction in the relapse rate in the group receiving 66 µg per week and a 33% reduction in the group receiving 132 µg per week. The MRI lesion burden showed a decrease of 1.2% in the group receiving 66 µg per week, a decrease of 3.8% in the group receiving 132 µg per week, and an increase of 10.9% in the group receiving placebo. The side-effect profile was similar to the other interferons. Of note, 23.8% of the group receiving 66 µg per week and 12.5% of the group receiving 132 µg per week were positive for neutralizing antibodies. The presence of neutralizing antibodies did not affect the mean relapse count. This medication is currently approved in Canada and is awaiting FDA approval in the United States.

Much controversy has arisen since the introduction of the three approved medications for MS. Analysis and comparison of these trials has been difficult because each trial used slightly different statistical, clinical, laboratory, and MRI measures. No direct comparison can be made because each drug was tested against placebo and not each other. The neutralizing antibody issue is another point of contention. The current consensus does not recommend the routine testing of neutralizing antibody and does not recommend switching between interferons if neutralizing antibodies are in the high titer range.

Treatment of Progressive Disease

Treatment directed at the progressive phase is the most difficult because the disease may be harder to affect once the progressive stage has been initiated. Immunosuppressive agents such as total lymphoid radiation, cyclosporine, methotrexate, 2-chlorodeoxyadenosine, cyclophosphamide (Cytoxan), mitoxantrone, azathioprine, and interferon-β_{1b} have shown some positive clinical effects in progressive disease. All of these nonspecific immunosuppressive agents suffer from the same basic defect: They may temporarily halt a rapidly progressive downhill course, but it is difficult, or dangerous, to employ them for more than a few months. MS is an illness of decades, not months. Therefore, nonspecific immunosuppression often is a temporary solution, even if effective.

Total lymphoid irradiation has potent immunosuppressive effects, and a double-blind study of lymphoid irradiation reported benefit in patients with progressive MS. The absolute lymphocyte count appeared to be an indicator of therapeutic efficacy, with greater efficacy in patients with lower counts. Many patients began progressing again after initial therapy and a major limitation of the use of total lymphoid radiation is that it may preclude the use of other treatments that affect the immune system at a subsequent time.

Large multicenter trials of cyclosporine indicate that cyclosporine has a beneficial, albeit modest, effect in ameliorating clinical disease progression, but it has not found clinical use because of the narrow benefit-to-risk ratio.

Weekly low-dose oral methotrexate (7.5 mg) was studied in a randomized, double-blind, placebo-controlled trial in 60 patients with chronic progressive disease and has been reported to positively affect measures of upper extremity function in progressive MS. Lower extremity function was not affected (Goodkin et al. 1995).

Cladribine (2-chlorodeoxyadenosine, Leustatin), a potent immunosuppressive agent useful in the treatment of hairy cell leukemia, was reported in preliminary studies to be of benefit in chronic progressive MS.

Cyclophosphamide (Cytoxan) has been in use for treatment of patients with MS, despite conflicting data, since the early 1980s. When used, the drug is now given in monthly bolus injections and maintained over a year or more, usually with intravenous corticosteroids. Effects often can be observed in patients younger than age 40, and especially in those who have been in the progressive phase for less than a year. The drug appears to be ineffective for primary progressive MS. Duration of treatment is limited by the risk of bladder cancer, which appears to increase with time and may depend on total accumulated drug dose.

A trial of mitoxantrone in 42 patients with active MS was published (Edan 1997), in which patients were treated monthly with either intravenous methylprednisolone plus intravenous mitoxantrone or intravenous methylprednisolone alone over 6 months. Although the numbers were small, a statistically significant reduction occurred in the number of relapses and an increase in the number of patients free of attack. Also, 90% of the group receiving intravenous methylprednisolone/intravenous mitoxantrone showed no new enhancing lesions on MRI versus only 31% in the group receiving intravenous methylprednisolone. The risk of cardiotoxicity prevents prolonged usage.

Azathioprine has been studied in both relapsing-remitting and chronic progressive MS since 1971. A meta-analysis of the results of five double-blind and two single-blind, randomized, controlled trials of azathioprine use in MS showed only a small difference in favor of azathioprine after 2 years.

Interferon-β_{1b} was studied in patients with secondary progressive MS in 32 centers in Europe. In this study 358 patients received placebo and 360 patients received interferon-β_{1b} every other day subcutaneously for up to 3 years (European Study Group 1998). In the group receiving interferon-β_{1b} a relative reduction of 21.7% occurred in the proportion of patients with progression. The time to becoming wheelchair-bound was also significantly delayed, equivalent to 12 months ($P < .01$). The mean relapse rate was reduced overall by approximately 30% in the treatment group. In terms of MRI lesion volume, the group receiving placebo showed a mean increase of 8% compared with the group receiving interferon-β_{1b}, which showed a mean decrease of 5%. This study has major implications for the treatment of the largest single category of MS, and the effect on the cost of medical care and the search for other treatments are obvious.

Monthly bolus intravenous corticosteroids, typically 1,000 mg of methylprednisolone, are used at many institutions for treatment of primary or secondary progressive MS. This use remains empiric because no relevant studies have been reported.

Future Directions

A great deal has been learned about the mechanism of oral tolerance, and oral tolerance has been applied successfully to several animal models of autoimmune diseases including animal models of MS (Weiner 1994). The doses and strategy being used in clinical trials is to generate regulatory T

Table 60.10:   Acute disseminated encephalomyelitis and related disorders

Acute disseminated encephalomyelitis
  Uniphasic parainfectious or postvaccination inflammatory
    demyelinating disorder of the central nervous system
Acute hemorrhagic leukoencephalitis
  Hyperacute form of acute disseminated encephalomyelitis,
    usually occurring after upper respiratory infections, with
    more tissue-destructive pathology
Site-restricted forms of uniphasic acute inflammatory
    demyelinating disorders that may occur after viral illness or
    vaccination
  Transverse myelitis
  Optic neuritis
  Cerebellitis
  Brainstem encephalitis
Chronic or recurrent forms of parainfectious or postvaccination
    encephalomyelitis
  Relationship with multiple sclerosis?
Combined peripheral and central nervous system inflammatory
    demyelinating disorders
  Postvaccination: rabies, influenza?
  Postinfectious: measles

cells that suppress inflammation at the target organ. A multicenter trial of bovine myelin in patients with relapsing-remitting disease found that both the treated and placebo groups had a 50% reduction in attack rate over 2 years.

The use of systemic recombinant interferon-α_{2a} and oral interferon-τ are under consideration.

Immune globulin may help a number of autoimmune diseases and has been tried in MS. A randomized, placebo-controlled trial of monthly intravenous immunoglobulin in relapsing-remitting MS involved 150 patients over 2 years (Fazekas 1997). In the group receiving placebo there were 116 relapses compared with 62 in the group receiving intravenous immunoglobulin, and 36% of the group receiving placebo were relapse-free compared with 53% of the group receiving intravenous immunoglobulin, with a significant P value of .03. The challenge in MS therapeutics at this point is to advance beyond the currently available partially effective treatments. Statistically convincing data derived from large randomized clinical trials may not translate into reliable treatments in the clinic.

ACUTE DISSEMINATED ENCEPHALOMYELITIS

History

ADEM is classically described as a uniphasic syndrome, occurring in association with an immunization or vaccination (postvaccination encephalomyelitis) or systemic viral infection (parainfectious encephalomyelitis). This is char-

acterized pathologically by perivascular inflammation, edema, and demyelination within the CNS and clinically by rapid development of focal or multifocal neurological dysfunction. The most precise clinical and pathological observations regarding ADEM are derived from case studies in which epidemiological data have established the link between the specific virus infection or vaccine and the syndrome. In this regard, the syndrome arising after acute measles infection or rabies vaccine administration can be considered the prototype of the illness. Uncertainty remains regarding diagnosis when cases with the clinical features of the syndrome occur with viral infections or vaccine administration not significantly linked with the syndrome by epidemiological criteria.

In addition to the well-defined clinical and pathological entity of ADEM occurring as a parainfectious or postvaccination event (Table 60.10), presumed variants of the disorder also exist. The rarity of these latter entities has impeded attempts to define precisely the relation of each of these entities to either ADEM or MS.

Postvaccination Acute Disseminated Encephalomyelitis

The occurrence of neuroparalytic accidents as a consequence of the Pasteur rabies vaccine prepared from spinal cords of rabbits inoculated with fixed rabies virus was recorded soon after introduction of the treatment. Similar neurological complications were observed as a consequence of the Jenner vaccine used for the prevention of smallpox. Evidence confirmed the postulate that these accidents were not caused by the direct cytopathic effects of the virus but rather to immune-mediated mechanisms directed against specific components of the CNS. In these studies, homogenates of normal rabbit brain were injected repeatedly into monkeys, who after some 6 months, developed an inflammatory encephalomyelitis that resembled the clinical syndromes cited previously. These studies further established the concepts regarding the capacity of immune mechanisms to induce injury to self-tissue (autoimmunity). The model disorder of immune-mediated disease of the CNS, EAE, can be either an acute or a relapsing disorder and can be induced with a number of specific myelin protein antigens, such as MBP and proteolipid protein. The development of animal model diseases, such as Theiler's virus disease, in which an initial viral infection of the CNS can result in a chronic inflammatory demyelinating disorder, and whose severity can be reduced by immunosuppressive therapy, raises further important questions regarding the interaction of viruses and the immune system with regard to inducing encephalomyelitis.

The concern regarding the presence of neural tissue in vaccines as the major factor in predisposing to neuroparalytic accidents has led to attempts to develop vaccines devoid of CNS tissue in the case of rabies and to the discontinuation of routine smallpox vaccination as the virtual eradication of the natural disease was being achieved. The incidence of encephalomyelitis associated with the original Pasteur rabies vaccine prepared in rabbit brain has been estimated at 1 per 3,000–35,000 vaccinations. An incidence rate of 1 per 25,000 vaccinations occurred with duck embryo rabies vaccine, a preparation containing minimal amounts of neural tissue; many of the complications with this vaccine involved the PNS. Introduction of the non-neural, human diploid cell vaccine has virtually eliminated neuroparalytic complications of rabies vaccinations.

Reports have associated ADEM with other vaccines, including pertussis, rubella, diphtheria, and measles. The association of influenza vaccination, particularly the swine flu vaccine, with ADEM has been the subject of medicolegal controversy. In fact, ADEM is not known to be associated with any vaccine currently used in the United States, and the administration of influenza vaccine to people with MS does not induce relapse. ADEM developing after drug administration has been reported with sulfonamides and para-aminosalicylic acid/streptomycin. The aforementioned associations can only be substantiated by strong epidemiological evidence or by the development of a pathognomonic laboratory finding for ADEM, neither of which yet exists.

Measles-Induced Acute Disseminated Encephalomyelitis

The initial recognition of the occurrence of neurological complications in temporal association with measles infection has been attributed to Lucas, who in 1790 described the development of a myelopathy in a 23-year-old woman with onset of measles 8 days previously. Descriptions of cerebral and cerebellar abnormalities appeared in the mid- to late nineteenth century. By 1928, Ford summarized more than 100 cases and delineated subgroups of cases including those with diffuse cerebral features, focal or multifocal cerebral findings, cerebellar dysfunction, and spinal cord abnormalities. The overall experience suggests that neurological sequelae complicate 1 in 400–1,000 cases of measles infection, and that patients do not develop peripheral nerve damage or relapses of disease. The introduction of measles vaccination has greatly reduced the incidence of measles and its neurological complications, but the disease continues to occur in large epidemics in specific geographic areas.

Idiopathic Acute Disseminated Encephalomyelitis

Cases of acute encephalomyelitis occurring in the setting of nonspecific viral illness are difficult to diagnose with certainty and to distinguish from episodes of MS. Cases occurring in children, at an age too young to overlap with MS, are perhaps the most readily delineated. Features deemed characteristic of ADEM include simultaneous

bilateral ON, loss of consciousness, meningismus, loss of deep tendon reflexes and retained abdominal reflexes in the presence of Babinski's reflexes, central body temperature of greater than 100°F, and severe shooting limb pains. Recovery from ADEM is more rapid compared with MS (days versus weeks) and usually more complete. Tentative associations with ADEM have been made with a wide array of viral and bacterial infections: rubella, mumps, herpes zoster, herpes simplex, influenza, Epstein-Barr virus, coxsackievirus, *Borrelia burgdorferi*, *Mycoplasma*, and *Leptospira*.

Clinical Features

The clinical features of ADEM are best described on the basis of observations made of relatively large numbers of cases occurring in association with either specific vaccination programs (rabies vaccine) or viral infection epidemics (measles). An immunogenetic predisposition, as measured by human leukocyte antigen association, is suggested but not established. The clinical features of the postrabies vaccination and parameasles infection syndromes are summarized in Table 60.11. The age group developing ADEM reflects those who are most susceptible to the particular virus infection (e.g., usually children for measles infection) or who require vaccination (e.g., those exposed to rabid animal bites). Postmeasles cases of ADEM are described in infants less than 1 year of age. Postrabies vaccination neurological complications are reported to be rare in children, but in an Indian population receiving either betapropiolactone-inactivated or phenolized rabies vaccine, the age range of affected individuals was 2–67 years. The clinical features of the postvaccination and parainfectious syndromes are strikingly similar, with the exception that the postrabies vaccination complications frequently involve the PNS as well as the CNS, probably reflecting inclusion of PNS tissue in the preparation of specific types of rabies vaccine. Many patients with postrabies immunization illness had only mild clinical features of fever, headache, or myalgia without CSF pleocytosis.

The hallmark clinical feature of the disorder is the development of a focal or multifocal neurological disorder following exposure to virus or receipt of vaccine. In some, but not all, cases, a prodromal phase of several days of fever, malaise, and myalgias occurs. The onset of the CNS disorder is usually rapid (abrupt or up to several hours), with peak dysfunction within several days. Initial features include encephalopathy ranging from lethargy to coma, seizures, and focal and multifocal signs reflecting cerebral (hemiparesis), brainstem (cranial nerve palsies), and spinal cord (paraparesis) involvement. Other reported findings include movement disorders and ataxia. Each of these findings may occur as an isolated feature or in various combinations.

Table 60.11: Clinical and laboratory parameters in patients with acute disseminated encephalomyelitis following postrabies vaccination and measles virus infection

	Rabies vaccination (Betapropiolactone-inactivated)	Measles virus infection
Clinical features		
Age of onset		
Mean	27 yrs	5 yrs
Range	2–67 yrs	1–20 yrs
Interval after first vaccination or onset of infection		
Mean	12 days	5 days
Range	2–60 days	8–20 days
Prodromal illness (3–4 days of fever, malaise, myalgia)	60%	16%
Clinical findings	—	—
Central nervous system	—	—
Encephalopathy (headache, vomiting, altered sensorium)	45% (8%)*	100%
Seizures	5%	47%
Brainstem dysfunction—cranial nerve palsies	18%	5%
Myelopathy	67% (9%)*	58%
Peripheral nervous system	—	—
Radiculopathy	82% (24%)*	0%
Treatment	Corticosteroids	—
	Cyclophosphamide	—
Laboratory findings	—	—
Peripheral blood-MBP reactive T cells and anti-MBP antibodies	+	+
Cerebrospinal fluid	—	—
Cells	—	—
Normal	45%	28%
5–100/µl	41%	72%
>100/µl	14% (some with polymorphonuclear neutrophils)	13% (within first 2 days)
Protein	—	—
>45 mg/dl	60%	44%
>100 mg/dl	21%	10%
Increased MBP content	—	60%
Increased IgG index	—	<10%
Electrophysiological studies	—	—
Electroencephalography: slowing, seizure discharge	43%	—
Visual evoked potentials: abnormal	22%	—
Clinical course	—	—
Death	18%	5–20%
Complete recovery	—	—
Rapid	18%	—
Delayed	68%	5%
Partial recovery	32%	95%

MBP = myelin basic protein.
*Percentage of patients with clinical features as an isolated finding.
Source: Adapted from HS Swamy, SK Shankar, PS Chandra, et al. Neurological complications due to betapropiolactone (BPL)-inactivated antirabies vaccination. J Neurol Sci 1984;63:111–128; T Hemachudha, P Phanuphak, RT Johnson, et al. Neurologic complications of Semple-type rabies vaccine: clinical and immunologic studies. Neurology 1987;37:550–556; RT Johnson, DE Griffin, RL Hirsch, et al. Measles encephalomyelitis—clinical and immunologic studies. N Engl J Med 1984;310:137–141.

Recovery can begin within days, with complete resolution noted on occasion within a few days, but more often over the course of weeks or months. The mortality varies between 10% and 30%, with complete recovery in 50%. Poor prognosis is correlated with severity and abruptness of onset of the clinical syndrome. In the postrabies vaccine case series, a mortality of 18% was recorded. At a mean follow-up of 17 months, 68% of survivors were completely recovered, and 32% were partially recovered, most with minimal deficits. In three patients in the series, a relapse of neurological deficits occurred during the recovery period. No patients were recorded as having relapses after complete recovery had occurred.

Measles virus-associated ADEM may carry a worse prognosis than vaccine-associated disease. In earlier series, the occurrence of acute hemiplegias, which were interpreted as vascular occlusions and akin to the syndrome of acute hemiplegia of childhood, carried a particularly unfavorable prognosis with respect to recovery. Relapses are rare.

Laboratory Features

The hallmark lesions of ADEM are perivascular inflammation and surrounding demyelination within the CNS (Figures 60.14 and 60.15). Vessel necrosis is frequently observed. The demyelinating aspect may be minimal or widespread, with coalescence of the multiple lesions. Some meningeal reaction may be apparent also. Reports of MRI studies, largely from apparent sporadic cases of ADEM, describe multifocal CNS lesions initially indistinguishable from those observed in MS. In ADEM after several weeks, lesions show at least partial resolution without the appearance of new lesions, unlike MS. In some cases lesions can persist. MRI in ADEM, as with MS, is more sensitive than CT scanning, which may in some cases show enhancing lesions. The usual CSF formula is normal pressure, little or no increase in cell count (<100 cells/μl), and a modest increase in protein. Well-documented cases exist with totally normal CSF. Cases with high cell counts, including some polymorphonuclear cells and high protein values, occur and seemingly reflect a more necrotizing disease process. The high counts usually return to normal within a few days. The CSF immunoglobulin content is not usually increased, and OCB patterns are not usually observed. The content of MBP in the CSF may be increased, as it can be in many conditions in which myelin destruction occurs. In many patients with postrabies vaccination and postmeasles ADEM, one can show some systemic blood lymphocyte sensitivity to MBP in vitro. Although technically difficult to assess, CSF lymphocyte sensitivity to MBP may be even more marked than is systemic lymphocyte sensitivity. The occurrence of cases without MBP sensitivity indicates that this assay is insufficiently sensitive to establish or exclude the diagnosis of ADEM.

The diagnosis of ADEM can usually be made with confidence in the setting of a clear-cut antecedent event strongly associated with the disorder, such as measles infection or vaccination. The occurrence of an acute focal or multifocal CNS syndrome subsequent to a more nonspecific viral illness or vaccination in which the epidemiological link with ADEM is weak does create a wider differential diagnosis, particularly depending on the age of the patient and the clinical manifestations of the disease. The following would be included in this differential diagnosis: (1) An initial episode of what will prove to be MS; the presence of CSF-increased IgG levels may favor this diagnosis while follow-up MRI may be needed, because initial MRI scans may appear similar. The occurrence of a nonspecific viral illness before the onset of the clinical neurological syndrome does not distinguish between MS and ADEM, because the incidence of exacerbations of MS is increased following such infections; (2) CNS vasculitis with or without systemic features (such as disseminated intravascular coagulation or serum sickness); (3) multiple cerebral infarcts, particularly embolic from infected cardiac valves; and (4) chronic meningitis or granulomatous disease (sarcoidosis). If the main clinical feature is unifocal, encephalitis, abscess, or tumor needs to be excluded.

Treatment

The current favored therapy for ADEM is corticosteroids, based to some extent on their efficacy in EAE, although no clinical controlled studies have been conducted. Immunosuppressants such as cyclophosphamide have been used in refractory cases, as well as plasmapheresis. Data on the various other immunotherapies described in the section on MS are lacking.

OTHER INFLAMMATORY DEMYELINATING DISEASES OF THE CENTRAL NERVOUS SYSTEM

Acute Hemorrhagic Leukoencephalitis

Acute hemorrhagic leukoencephalitis is a rare entity that represents a hyperacute form of ADEM, in a parallel fashion to the hyperacute forms of EAE. The most frequent antecedent history is that of an upper respiratory infection. Given the nonspecific nature of the antecedent event and the lack of a specific diagnostic clinical laboratory test, the exact incidence and full clinical spectrum of the disorder can only be estimated and are based largely on descriptions of autopsy-proved cases. The clinical manifestations mimic ADEM, but are more abrupt in their development and more severe. They include focal or multifocal signs, seizures, and obtundation. Relapse following initial recovery has been described. Fever is common. The CSF usually demonstrates increased pressure, protein, and both white and red cells. The peripheral white blood cell count also is usually increased. CT scans in suspected clinical cases show an initially normal scan followed by low-density white matter lesions developing within 72 hours of the first symptoms. With improvement, the lesions on CT may largely resolve. MRI may yield additional information on lesion evolution.

The differential diagnosis of this syndrome includes entities that present as rapidly evolving focal cerebral disorders with fever and obtundation. These include brain abscess and encephalitis, particularly caused by herpes simplex, in addition to those syndromes considered in the section on ADEM.

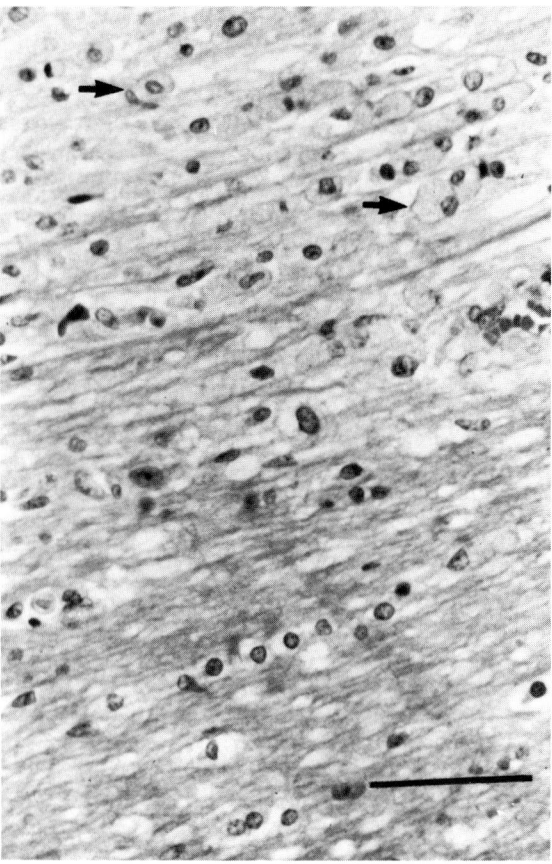

FIGURE 60.14 Lesion of acute disseminated encephalomyelitis showing demyelination and macrophage infiltration (*arrows*) (hematoxylin and eosin; bar = 50 μm). (Courtesy of Dr. S. Carpenter.)

Pathology

This disorder represents a more severe and destructive form of ADEM. The CNS white matter shows necrotizing vasculitis involving venules and capillaries. There are perivascular accumulations of polymorphonuclear cells and red blood cells. The perivascular demyelinating lesions frequently coalesce to form large lesions.

Treatment

Corticosteroids are frequently used in suspected cases, with no firm data yet available regarding efficacy.

Chronic or Recurrent Forms of Postinfectious and Postvaccination Encephalomyelitis

As previously stated, the clinical hallmark of ADEM occurring after measles infection or rabies vaccination is its course. Relapses occurring during the recovery phase could well represent physiological conduction blocks rather than true reactivation of immune-mediated mechanisms. Recurrent encephalomyelitis cases are described, however, particularly in the pediatric age groups. Recurrent cases in adults, if they occur, would be difficult to distinguish from MS. The existence of chronic or recurrent encephalomyelitis cases might be considered as a parallel of the peripheral neuritis syndromes, of which acute nonrelapsing Guillain-Barré syndrome is the prototype, but in which chronic and recurrent cases are reported. The basis of these latter syndromes and their relation to classic Guillain-Barré syndrome remain unre-

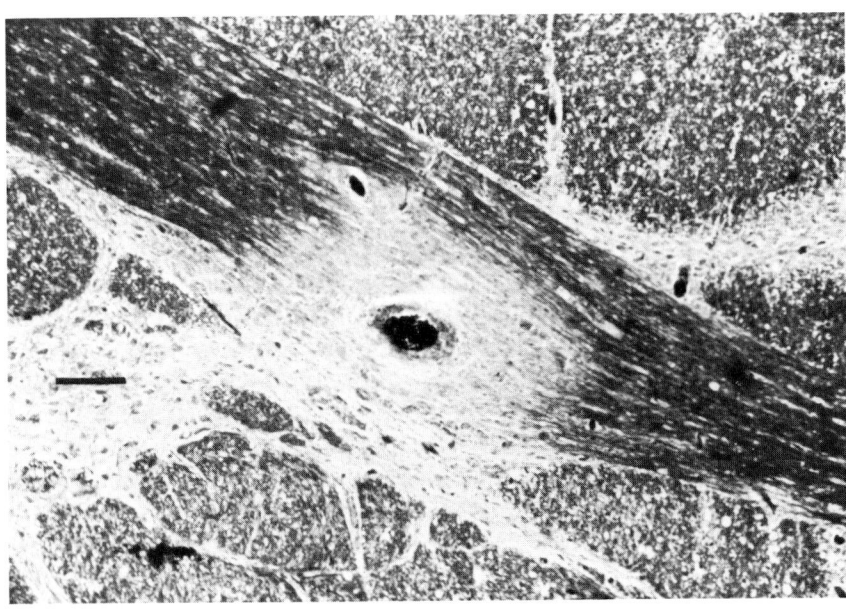

FIGURE 60.15 Perivenular zone of demyelination in brainstem of patient with acute disseminated encephalomyelitis (Heidenhain Woelke stain; bar = 100 μm). (Courtesy of Dr. S. Carpenter.)

solved. The animal models of encephalomyelitis (experimental allergic encephalomyelitis) and peripheral neuritis (experimental allergic neuritis) can both be induced in relapsing form, if one selects animals of critical age and specific genetic background.

Combined Central and Peripheral Demyelinating Disease

The existence of combined central and peripheral demyelinating disease as a postinfectious disorder or as a complication following administration of vaccines not known to contain PNS and CNS tissue remains highly questionable based on available epidemiological evidence. Cases of combined PNS and CNS involvement following swine flu vaccination were reported, but some of these cases had subacute progressive courses. To date, no convincing in vitro immune sensitization to either viral or neural antigens has been shown in such cases. Reports of combined central and peripheral demyelination syndromes do exist in which onion bulb formation in the PNS is demonstrated, indicating recurrent demyelination and remyelination. Some, although not all, of these patients have clinical features consistent with MS. Whether such combined demyelination represents a chance occurrence of two processes or a distinct disease is unresolved.

Site-Restricted Forms of Postinfectious Demyelinating Disorders

Acute and Subacute Transverse Myelitis

Acute and subacute transverse myelitis is defined as the development of isolated spinal cord dysfunction over hours or days in patients in whom no evidence exists of a compressive lesion. In the combined experience of several series reviewing complete transverse myelitis, 37% of patients reported a preceding febrile illness. The initial symptoms are paresthesias, back pain, or leg weakness; 37% of patients had the maximal deficit within 1 day, 45% in 1–10 days, and 18% in more than 10 days. Outcome was rated as good in 42%, fair in 38%, and poor in 20%. The prognosis may be worse in the rapid-onset group of patients. Only approximately 7% of patients develop MS by clinical criteria. Whether these cases represent a homogeneous entity remains speculative and doubtful, particularly because the ages of reported cases range from 4–83 years. In addition, acute transverse myelitis is known to occur on a background of systemic vasculitis, such as SLE and that associated with heroin abuse. One must distinguish complete transverse myelitis from the partial or incomplete syndromes that more frequently predict evolution to MS in 50–90% of patients.

Optic Neuritis

The clinical features of ON are described in the previous section on MS. In ON associated with MS, the majority of clinical episodes are unilateral, although VERs also may indicate involvement of the contralateral eye. Simultaneous bilateral ON is rare in MS, although somewhat more frequent in Devic's disease. The estimated incidence of subsequent development of MS following an initial episode of ON varies widely among different series (from less than 20% to more than 70%). The issue remains whether some cases of isolated ON do represent formes frustes of ADEM. In this regard, cases of ON occurring after childhood exanthems would represent the best example of parainfectious ON. Cases are reported following measles, rubella, mumps, and varicella. Most patients had bilateral optic nerve involvement; additional neurological abnormalities occurred in only a minority of patients. The young age of the patients further suggests that these events are not the initial manifestations of MS. The prognosis for recovery of vision is good in most cases, perhaps less so in postvaricella cases.

Cerebellitis

Acute, isolated ataxia has been observed after many different viral illnesses but most frequently in association with varicella infections. Cerebellar ataxia accounts for 50% of the postvaricella neurological syndromes, which overall occur in 1 in 1,000 cases of childhood varicella. The prognosis for recovery is excellent, although the duration of symptoms varies from a few days up to 3–4 weeks. The fact that most cases remit spontaneously and the etiology (direct invasion versus autoimmune) is unresolved leaves the issue of corticosteroid therapy unsettled.

REFERENCES

Arnold DA, Riess GT, Matthews PM, et al. Use of proton magnetic resonance spectroscopy for monitoring disease progression in multiple sclerosis. Ann Neurol 1994;36:76–82.

Beck RW, Cleary PA, Trobe JD, et al. The effect of corticosteroids for acute optic neuritis on the subsequent development of multiple sclerosis. N Engl J Med 1993;329:1764–1769.

Brønnum-Hansen H, Koch-Henriksen N, Hyllested K. Survival of patients with multiple sclerosis in Denmark. Neurology 1994;44:1901–1907.

Coffey RJ, Cahill D, Steers W, et al. Intrathecal baclofen for intractable spasticity of spinal origin: results of a long-term multicenter study. J Neurosurg 1993;78:226–232.

Davie CA, Hawkins CP, Barker GJ, et al. Serial proton magnetic resonance spectroscopy in acute multiple sclerosis lesions. Brain 1994;117:49–58.

Ebers GC, Sadovnick AD. The role of genetic factors in multiple sclerosis susceptibility. J Neuroimmunol 1994;54:1–17.

Edan G, Miller D, Clanet M, et al. Therapeutic effect of mitoxantrone combined with methylprednisolone in multiple sclerosis: a randomized multicentre study of active disease using MRI and clinical criteria. J Neurol Neurosurg Psychiatry 1997;62:112–118.

European Study Group on Interferon Beta-1b in Secondary Progressive MS. Placebo-controlled multicenter randomised trial of interferon beta-1b in treatment of secondary progressive multiple sclerosis. Lancet 1998;352:1491–1497.

Fazekas F, Deisenhammer F, Strausser-Fuchs S. Randomized placebo-controlled trial of monthly intravenous immunoglobin therapy in relapsing-remitting multiple sclerosis. Austrian Immunoglobin in Multiple Sclerosis Study Group. Lancet 1997;349:586–587.

Filippi M, Horsfield MA, Morrissey SP, et al. Quantitative brain MRI lesion load predicts the course of clinically isolated syndromes suggestive of multiple sclerosis. Neurology 1994;44:635–641.

Gass A, Barker GJ, Kidd D, et al. Correlation of magnetization transfer ratio with clinical disability in multiple sclerosis. Ann Neurol 1994;36:62–67.

Goodkin DE, Rudick RA, Medendorp SV, et al. Low dose (7.5 mg) oral methotrexate reduces the rate of progression in chronic progressive multiple sclerosis. Ann Neurol 1995;37:30–40.

Hillert J, Olerup O. Multiple sclerosis is associated with genes within or close to the HLA-OR-OO subregion on a normal OR15, DQ6, DW2 haplotype. Neurology 1993;43:163–168.

IFNB Multiple Sclerosis Study Group. Interferon beta-1b is effective in relapsing-remitting multiple sclerosis. I. Clinical results of a multicenter, randomized, double-blind, placebo-controlled trial. Neurology 1993;43:655–661.

IFNB Multiple Sclerosis Study Group, University of British Columbia MS/MRI Analysis Group. Interferon beta-1b in the treatment of multiple sclerosis: final outcome of the randomized controlled trial. Neurology 1995;45:1277–1285.

Jacobs L, Cookfair D, Rudick R, et al. Results of a phase III trial of intramuscular recombinant interferon as treatment for multiple sclerosis [abstract]. Ann Neurol 1994;36:259.

Jacobs LD, Cookfair DL, Rudick RA, et al. Intramuscular interferon beta-1a for disease progression in relapsing multiple sclerosis. Ann Neurol 1996;39:285–294.

Johnson KP, Brooks BR, Cohen JA, et al. Copolymer 1 reduces relapse rate and improves disability in relapsing-remitting multiple sclerosis: results of a phase III multicentre double-blind, placebo-controlled trial. Neurology 1995;45:1268–1276.

Johnson KP, Brooks BR, Cohen JA, et al. Extended use of glatiramer acetate (copaxone) is well tolerated and maintains its clinical effect on multiple sclerosis relapse rate and degree of disability. Copolymer 1 Multiple Sclerosis Study Group. Neurology 1998;50:701–708.

Karussis D, Meiner Z, Lehmann D, et al. Treatment of secondary progressive multiple sclerosis with the immunomodulator linomide: results of a double-blind, placebo-controlled study with monthly MRI evaluation [abstract]. Neurology 1995;45(Suppl. 4):A417.

Kepes JJ. Large focal tumor-like demyelinating lesions of the brain: intermediate entity between multiple sclerosis and acute disseminated encephalomyelitis? A study of 31 patients. Ann Neurol 1993;33:18–27.

Kidd D, Thompson A, Thorpe JW, et al. Spinal cord MRI using multi-array coils and fast spin echo. II. Findings in multiple sclerosis. Neurology 1993;43:2632–2637.

Lublin FD, Reingold SC, The National Multiple Sclerosis Society USA Advisory Committee on Clinical Trials of New Agents in Multiple Sclerosis. Defining the clinical course of multiple sclerosis: results of an international survey. Neurology 1996;46:907–911.

Mandler RN, Davis LE, Jeffery DR, Kornfeld M. Devic's neuromyelitis optica: a clinicopathological study of 8 patients. Ann Neurol 1993;34:162–168.

Martin R, Voskuhi R, Flerlage M, et al. Myelin basic protein-specific T-cell responses in identical twins discordant or concordant for multiple sclerosis. Ann Neurol 1993;34:524–535.

Morrissey SP, Miller DH, Kendall BE, et al. The significance of brain magnetic resonance imaging abnormalities at presentation with clinically isolated syndromes suggestive of multiple sclerosis. Brain 1993;116:135–146.

Offenbacher H, Fazekas F, Schmidt R, et al. Assessment of MRI criteria for a diagnosis of MS. Neurology 1993;43:905–909.

Optic Neuritis Study Group. The 5-year risk of MS after optic neuritis: experience of the Optic Neuritis treatment trial. Neurology 1997;49:1404–1413.

Panitch HS, Bever CT. Clinical trials of interferons in multiple sclerosis: what have we learned? J Neuroimmunol 1993;46:155–164.

Paty DW, Li DKB, UBC Study Group, IFNB Multiple Sclerosis Study Group. Interferon beta-1b is effective in relapsing-remitting multiple sclerosis; II. MRI analysis results of a multicenter, randomized, double-blind, placebo-controlled trial. Neurology 1993;43:662–667.

Prineas JW, Barnard RO, Kwon EE, et al. Multiple sclerosis: remyelination of nascent lesions. Ann Neurol 1993a;33:137–151.

Prineas JW, Barnard RO, Revesz T, et al. Multiple sclerosis: pathology of recurrent lesions. Brain 1993b;116:681–693.

PRISMS Study Group. Randomised double-blind placebo controlled study of interferon beta-1a in relapsing/remitting multiple sclerosis. Lancet 1998;352:1498–1504.

Rao SM, Reingold SC, Ron MA, et al. Workshop on neurobehavioural disorders in multiple sclerosis. Arch Neurol 1993;50:658–662.

Rodriguez M, Siva A, Cross SA, et al. Optic neuritis: a population-based study in Olmstead County, Minnesota. Neurology 1995;45:244–250.

Rudick RA, Cohen JA, Weinstock-Guttman B, et al. Management of multiple sclerosis. N Engl J Med 1997;337:1604–1611.

Runmaker B, Andersen O. Prognostic factors in a multiple sclerosis incidence cohort with twenty-five years of follow-up. Brain 1993;116:117–134.

Sadovnick AD, Armstrong H, Rice GPA, et al. A population-based study of multiple sclerosis in twins: update. Ann Neurol 1993;33:281–285.

Sadovnick AD, Ebers GC. Epidemiology in multiple sclerosis: a critical overview. Can J Neurol Sci 1993;20:17–29.

Snipe JC, Romine JS, Koziol JA, et al. Cladribine in treatment of chronic progressive multiple sclerosis. Lancet 1994;344:9–13.

Trapp BD, Peterson J, Ransohoff RM, et al. Axonal transection in the lesions of multiple sclerosis. N Engl J Med 1998;338: 278–285.

Waxman SG, Ritchie JM. Molecular dissection of the myelinated axon. Ann Neurol 1993;33:121–136.

Weiner HL, Friedman A, Miller A. Oral tolerance: immunologic mechanisms and treatment of animal and human organ-specific autoimmune diseases by oral administration of autoantigens. Ann Rev Immunol 1994;12:809–837.

Whitaker JN, Layton BA, Herman PK, et al. Correlation of myelin basic protein-like material in cerebrospinal fluid of multiple sclerosis patients with their response to glucocorticoid treatment. Ann Neurol 1993;33:10–17.

Zagzag D, Miller DC, Kleinman GM, et al. Demyelinating disease versus tumor in surgical neuropathology: clues to a correct pathological diagnosis. Am J Surg Pathol 1993;17: 537–545.

Chapter 61
Anoxic and Ischemic Encephalopathies

Bruce D. Snyder and Robert B. Daroff

Hypoxic and ischemic states may result from a number of conditions, such as cardiac arrest, carbon monoxide intoxication, or septic shock. Corrective action aimed at the underlying disorders must be instituted immediately to ensure survival and minimize residual central nervous system (CNS) damage. Traditionally, hypoxic states have been subdivided into four categories: (1) insufficient cerebral blood flow, (2) reduced oxygen availability, (3) reduced oxygen carriage by the blood, and (4) metabolic interference with the use of available oxygen. Clinically, these mechanisms often coexist, causing an anoxic-ischemic encephalopathy (AIE), and can result in a wide spectrum of CNS dysfunction (Table 61.1).

SYNCOPE AND CONFUSIONAL STATES

Syncopal attacks (see Chapter 2) are brief episodes of global cerebral ischemic anoxia. The brief loss of consciousness is followed by an almost immediate return of full awareness. If the drop in cardiac output is prolonged beyond a few seconds, a few clonic movements or an actual generalized tonic-clonic seizure may occur. Distinguishing a syncopal attack from a primary convulsive disorder can at times be difficult; however, the prompt cessation of ictal activity after circulation is restored and the usually brief or absent postictal state found in syncopal attacks can be helpful.

More prolonged but still brief episodes of global hypoxia may be followed by minutes to hours of confusion (see Chapter 4) and potentially the appearance of a fixed amnestic syndrome resembling Korsakoff's psychosis (see Chapter 63).The predominantly anterograde amnesia may persist for weeks and occasionally is permanent. The presence of persistent anterograde amnesia, with otherwise preserved cognition, presumably reflects the selective vulnerability of hippocampal neurons to anoxic insult.

Certain agents, such as carbon monoxide and cyanide (see Chapter 64), can produce states of histotoxic hypoxia. Cellular mechanisms for carrying and using oxygen are disrupted by these types of poisons. Nervous system damage is virtually identical to lesions resulting from ischemic or anoxic hypoxia.

Prolonged states of marginal cerebral perfusion or reduced oxygen availability (e.g., respiratory failure, high-altitude exposure, or profound hypotension), or both, initially result in mild cognitive deficits that may progress to frank confusion. If such conditions are more severe and prolonged, a typical delirium is seen with fluctuating levels of alertness, hallucinations, and delusions. Sensitivity to given levels of arterial blood pressure, oxygen, and carbon dioxide varies significantly among patients. Delirium in the critically ill patient is, of course, nonspecific, and hypoxia may be one of many factors to consider (see Chapter 4).

Acute mountain sickness (see Chapter 64E) is common among nonacclimatized persons who ascend higher than 6,500 feet. Headache, malaise, anorexia, and nausea occur and are due to the development of mild cerebral edema. Factors that suppress ventilatory drive, such as sedation (e.g., ethanol ingestion), worsen the condition. Symptoms of headache with nausea, vomiting, and especially obtundation require immediate descent and treatment with acetazolamide, corticosteroids, and oxygen. Stroke-prone individuals are at greater risk at high altitudes, and previously asymptomatic intracranial masses may declare themselves.

FOCAL CEREBRAL ISCHEMIA

Prolonged hypotensive episodes associated with delirium or impaired levels of consciousness may result in cerebral infarction. Focal neurological deficits may then coexist with diffuse dysfunction due to generalized neuronal

Table 61.1:   Clinical syndromes of central nervous system hypoxia and ischemia

"Mild" sustained hypoxia
  Cognitive impairment
  Confusional states
  Delirium
Brief anoxic-ischemic events
  Syncope
  Abortive or actual generalized seizure activity
Sustained severe hypoxia
  Coma with residual neurological deficits
    Dementia
    Vegetative state
    Brain death
  Seizure activity
  "Watershed" infarction of cerebrum, cerebellum, spinal cord
  Infarction distal to a pre-existing arterial stenosis or occlusion
  Postanoxic demyelination

Source: Adapted from JJ Caronna, S Finklestein. Neurological syndrome after cardiac arrest. Stroke 1978;9:517–520.

injury. Several mechanisms of infarction (hemodynamic, embolic, and thrombotic) may be involved. Failure of perfusion pressure can result in areas of infarction in the arterial watershed zones, the end-arteriolar territories lying at the boundary of brain areas supplied by a single major intracranial artery, such as the middle cerebral artery. These border-zone areas are last in line for blood supply when cerebral perfusion pressure is reduced. Watershed zones extend high over the cortical convexity to involve the visual cortex, visual association areas, and superior parietal lobules. Further anteriorly, the upward extent of the primary motor and sensory cortices, including interhemispheric structures, may be damaged. Cortical areas surrounding the primary speech areas are within these vulnerable zones, as are sectors of cerebellar cortex, the basal ganglia, and the thoracic spinal cord.

Infarction in watershed areas can result in characteristic clinical signs, including transcortical aphasias, cortical blindness (with varying degrees of anosognosia), bibrachial paresis with possibly some gait dysfunction (man-in-a-barrel syndrome), cerebellar dysmetria, and anterolateral spinal cord infarction (usually midthoracic). Rarely, extensive and selective loss of central spinal cord gray matter can result in a diffuse amyotrophic picture. Although watershed infarctions are generally symmetrical, underlying pre-existing cervical atherosclerotic disease (e.g., unilateral carotid occlusion or high-grade stenosis) may lead to strictly unilateral or predominantly unilateral infarction. In these circumstances, the infarct is in the central area of perfusion of the stenotic vessel; hence, the distribution of the lesions is the inverse of watershed infarcts (see Chapter 57A).

Cardiogenic embolization may complicate myocardial infarction, cardiac arrhythmias, valvular heart disease, or cardiopulmonary arrest (CPA). Resultant cerebral or brainstem infarctions may occur. Hypotensive crises due to sepsis

or hypovolemia can be associated with cerebral venous thrombosis with parasagittal or mesodiencephalic infarction (see Chapter 57A). Parasagittal venous cortical infarctions are generally hemorrhagic and often heralded by prominent focal seizure activity. Thrombosis of the cerebral venous system can propagate to the cerebral venous sinuses, resulting in impaired cerebrospinal fluid (CSF) absorption and the development of hydrocephalus with gradually declining alertness. Thrombotic propagation to the straight sinus and vein of Galen can cause high midbrain infarction with an irreversible comatose state.

POSTANOXIC COMA

The specific duration of anoxia necessary to produce prolonged loss of consciousness and profound cerebral damage is unknown. Individual variation is significant. Factors such as prearrest blood glucose levels, preischemic medications (e.g., aspirin or calcium-channel blockers), and associated hypothermia (as in cold-water drownings and avalanche victims) may be important. Young children are somewhat more resistant to anoxic damage.

After resuscitation, the severely anoxic patient is in deep coma, often transiently without even the most resilient brainstem response, the pupillary light reflex. Survivors regain brainstem functions over the first 1–3 hours but generally require supported ventilation. Initially flaccid, the patient subsequently manifests decerebrate or decorticate posturing. Seizure activity of various kinds appears in almost one of every three patients within the first few days. Axial myoclonus can be so violent that mechanical ventilation is disrupted. The increased cardiovascular strain due to seizure activity may be dangerous to the patient; additionally, hyperthermia and increased cerebral metabolic demand due to seizures may reduce the chances of cerebral recovery. Asynchronous distal limb myoclonus also may be seen. Generalized tonic-clonic seizures occasionally occur and may be due to a variety of toxic or metabolic factors, such as aminophylline or lidocaine intoxication, azotemia, or hyponatremia.

Later, when some degree of cerebral recovery has occurred, partial simple and partial complex seizures may occur. Partial complex status epilepticus should be considered carefully because it can appear to be simply a prolongation of the patient's postanoxic stupor or confusional state. The clinician should consider this diagnosis in patients who plateau in a stuporous state or secondarily decline in level of alertness. Often, the only clinical sign may be gaze deviation with nystagmoid eye movements.

Recovery rates vary among these patients. With time, initial flaccidity is replaced by reflex motor posturing. This, in turn, is succeeded by avoidance movements, reflex grasping, eye opening, and, finally, arousal, as manifested by complex interaction with the environment. As patients emerge from postanoxic coma, several clinical patterns are seen. The patient arousing early (within 24 hours) is frequently agitated and confused for a period of hours to days but ultimately recovers most cognitive functions. The patient's combativeness may necessitate the use of neuroleptics and poses difficulties for nursing care and cardiopulmonary stability. Haloperidol or similar, less sedating, nonanticholinergic dopaminergic blocking agents may provide good control without further clouding the sensorium.

As awareness is regained, the clinician can begin to assess cognitive and sensorimotor deficits. The effects of focal or multifocal infarction become apparent. Patients with more diffuse cortical damage display affective shallowness and lability, inattention, impaired logical flow of thought, hallucinations, and delusions. These gradually clear at varying rates and to varying degrees. Involvement of the basal ganglia, either because of watershed infarction or diffuse neuronal loss (particularly after carbon monoxide intoxication), can result in prominent movement disorders that may be choreoathetoid or even strikingly parkinsonian. Similarly, cerebellar signs, such as limb dysmetria or truncal ataxia, may appear. Most typically, in patients with residual motor dysfunction, combinations of these signs are seen.

Recent memory function seems particularly sensitive to hypoxia. After a significant hypoxic episode, anterograde amnesia with deficits in acquiring and retaining new information may be permanent. Some patients whose coma persists beyond 4 or 5 days slowly become responsive to the environment, if only in a limited fashion. These patients remain cognitively impaired, although recovery proceeds to some extent for up to a year. Structured environments, neuroleptic medication, bladder and bowel programs, and rehabilitative therapy may help optimize functioning.

PERSISTENT VEGETATIVE STATE

An important subgroup of postanoxic comatose patients develops a vegetative state. They begin to open their eyes within a few days but make no apparent contact with the environment. Motor responses continue to be decorticate or decerebrate posturing. Triple-flexion leg withdrawal may be seen, along with spontaneous clonus, flexor or extensor thrusting of the legs, or shivering. Brainstem reflexes recover quickly; sleep-wake cycles appear. With eye opening, other behaviors emerge, such as yawning, bruxism, smiling, crying, sneezing, and blinking when the examiner's hand is thrust toward the eyes. Absolutely no consistent nonreflexive response to stimulation can be established with the patient. These patients do not consistently follow moving people or objects with their gaze. They meet the criteria for being called *vegetative*. If this condition persists for a month after resuscitation, it is considered a persistent vegetative state (PVS) (Ashwal et al. 1995). Pathologically, there is virtually complete forebrain necrosis with preservation of the brainstem. The electroencephalogram (EEG) is severely abnormal. These patients must be distinguished from those with ventral pon-

tine infarctions, who are locked in or de-efferented but have normal cognition with preserved awareness. Other comalike states should be distinguished from PVS (American Neurological Association Committee on Ethical Affairs 1993) as well.

CEREBRAL EDEMA

The mechanisms for the development of cerebral edema in hypoxia are discussed in Chapter 65, but the role of edema in AIE remains uncertain. Patients with AIE do not develop papilledema, although ischemic papillopathy may be observed rarely. Measurements of intracranial pressure (ICP) have been performed rarely, and then with equivocal results. In small reported series, some—but not all—postresuscitation patients have had either elevated ICP or evidence of diffuse cerebral edema on imaging studies. Intracranial hypertension may be more likely to occur after cardiac arrest due to respiratory failure. The effects of prearrest hypercapnia and acidosis are unclear.

Autopsies of patients in coma due to AIE have revealed the presence of gross brain edema and cerebral liquefaction if there had been both a very deep level of coma and prolonged survival (5 days or more). Patients who died within 24 hours of CPA in deep coma do not show cerebral edema or liquefaction, suggesting that brain swelling is a postnecrotic phenomenon in these patients. In the setting of global anoxic ischemia, the presence of high ICP may portend a poor prognosis related to antecedent widespread tissue death. There is no established indication for the use of corticosteroids, osmotic diuretics, hyperventilation, or ventriculostomy.

DELAYED POSTANOXIC DETERIORATION

Occasionally, patients seem to arouse early and begin to recover well from anoxic coma, only to relapse with the appearance of apathy, confusion, gait disturbance, spasticity, incontinence, movement disorders, and dysarthria. Pathologically, there are varying degrees of demyelination in the centrum semiovale, bilateral pallidal necrosis, and patchy cortical necrosis, especially in the hippocampi. With supportive care, these patients may recover but are often left with residual deficits. This unusual disorder is most often seen after carbon monoxide poisoning. Individuals older than 30 years are at greater risk for delayed deterioration. The overall frequency in several series of cases of carbon monoxide intoxication approximates 2.75% (Gottfried et al. 1997). It has been postulated that an oligodendroglial injury results in delayed demyelination, but this remains speculative.

OTHER SEQUELAE

Recovery of cognitive functions generally proceeds rapidly during the first several weeks after anoxic injury and seems to plateau by 3 months. Moderate to severe biparietal deficits (dyscalculia, dyspraxia) occur in one of every three survivors. Almost one-half of patients are left with moderate to severe memory impairment. Problems with planning and organizational skills are common, but speech deficits are infrequent. Depression is another common problem for these patients. It remains unclear whether patients with postanoxic encephalopathy may show some continued cognitive recovery in the first several years after their AIE.

Movement disorders frequently emerge during recovery from severe hypoxic events. Bilateral hemiparesis, pseudobulbar palsy, parkinsonism, tremor, choreoathetosis, and dystonia may appear as the patient awakens from coma or may develop weeks to months later (Govaerts et al. 1998). Features of different disorders may coexist in a given patient. Treatment is often unsatisfactory, and medications that seem to benefit one aspect of a patient's condition may well worsen other problems.

Epilepsy is uncommon in surviving postanoxic patients, although one syndrome deserves mention: Delayed-onset myoclonus can be extremely disabling and may occur in patients who have made good cognitive recoveries from AIE. Intractable stimulus- and action-sensitive, asynchronous, distal limb myoclonus occasionally emerges days to weeks after recovery from anoxic coma. These patients often improve over the course of years after onset of myoclonus (Werhahn et al. 1997). Clonazepam and valproic acid may be therapeutically effective.

PROGNOSIS OF ANOXIC COMA AFTER CARDIOPULMONARY ARREST

Cardiopulmonary arrest is associated with a high rate of morbidity and mortality and is the most common cause of severe anoxic injury. Of patients who survive until hospital admission, in-hospital mortality rates range from 54% to 88%. Of those surviving to hospital discharge, 20% die in 1 year and 40% within 3 years; of the remaining patients, 75% have severe neurological impairment (Mullner et al. 1998), often with severe memory deficits (Mecklinger et al. 1998).

Statistics describing the outcome for patients in anoxic coma have varied somewhat in different clinical series, largely because of patient selection criteria. Some investigators reported series of consecutively resuscitated patients, whereas others have selected those who remain in deep coma for some specified period. The clinician must be aware of the differences in selection criteria when attempting to apply a specific set of published statistics to the patient at hand. The use of sedatives, analgesics, muscle relaxants, and anticonvulsants may weaken the applicability of published statistics to a specific case.

Survival after CPA is closely correlated with the duration of coma. Individuals who are either arousable or fully alert within 12 hours of resuscitation tend to do well neurologically, although they still experience a 25% mortality rate, related primarily to their underlying cardiac disease. In a series of consecutive patients with an overall 40% survival rate, the presence of initial postanoxic unarousability was a negative prognostic sign, with only 28% of that group surviving. The level of consciousness or motor responsiveness to stimulation may fluctuate after resuscitation; a decline within 48 hours is generally associated with a fatal outcome. A declining level of consciousness at any time during hospitalization also is associated with reduced survival rate and poorer outcome. Prognosis in the first few hours of resuscitation remains uncertain. Patients making reflex responses to pain (decorticate or decerebrate posturing) within 1–3 hours of CPA still have a 20–30% possibility of survival with good outcome. Patients who achieve arousal within 72 hours of resuscitation may do well. Such arousal, however, does not guarantee either survival or independent functioning. The clinician should be cautiously optimistic while continuing vigorous life support in such situations. In every series, a few patients achieve full alertness 5–10 days after CPA. The delay may relate to some superimposed or associated metabolic factor, in which case outcome may still be quite good. When no such factor can be identified and reversed, however, the ultimate functional status of the patient seems universally poor.

Cranial nerve reflexes correlate in a highly significant fashion with outcome. The absence of pupillary light reflexes or corneal responses for more than 6 hours after arrest is virtually incompatible with survival. Highly significant correlations exist between the number of brainstem reflex abnormalities and the possibility of survival (Table 61.2). When brainstem reflexes are lost after having been initially present (e.g., the recurrent loss of pupillary reactions), survival is extremely unlikely. It should be noted, however, that, whereas the absence of brainstem reflexes is highly predictive of poor outcome and death, the presence of intact brainstem reflexes is not a clear indicator of good outcome. Guidelines for predicting very good and very poor prognosis appear in Table 61.3.

This sort of prognostic information is used to guide clinician and family in decisions related to life support and the aggressiveness of clinical management. A discussion of the complex ethical issues behind these decisions is beyond the scope of this chapter. Medicolegal considerations are evolving and vary from state to state and country to country. In the United States, the sanctioned termination of life support is currently restricted to situations of brain death. Prognosis for life and function in postanoxic PVS patients is virtually nil; however, there are rare cases of very long survival and eventual recovery of awareness but with profound sensorimotor disability.

Clinical data for the prediction of outcome from anoxic injury in infants and children are not reviewed here (see Kriel et al. 1994), but the combination of magnetic resonance imaging and spectroscopy may provide the best prognostic information (Dubowitz et al. 1998). Outcome assessments in children must be based on more prolonged follow-up, with recognition of the difficulty of judging intellectual capabilities in the developing child. Young mammals seem to be more resistant to anoxic injury than their elders, which suggests that data collected in adult clinical series are not directly applicable to children. After aquatic submersion, immediate resuscitation significantly improves outcome (Kyraicou et al. 1994). Further discussion of the assessment of the critically ill child is presented in Chapter 8.

BRAIN DEATH

Guidelines for determining death in the adult are well established (see Chapter 5). The two principal categories are irreversible cessation of cardiopulmonary function and irreversible cessation of CNS function. In the former group, clinical examination is all that is necessary to determine death. In the latter group, a patient with ongoing circulatory function who is being artificially ventilated presents a more difficult issue. The diagnosis of brain death is based on absence of all cerebral and brainstem functions persisting over a period of observation sufficient to exclude any possibility of recovery. Once a patient has met brain-death criteria, a repeat evaluation 6 hours later is advised (Wijdicks 1995). Twenty-four hours of observation is recommended in states of postanoxic damage. Periods of observation may be reduced if suitable techniques, such as a nuclear medicine cerebral blood flow study, establish beyond a doubt that no blood flow exists to the brain. Electrocerebral silence on EEG is considered a desirable but not necessary confirmatory feature; in any event, EEG recordings to establish cerebral death require a high level of technical and interpretive expertise.

Complicating conditions, such as hypothermia, neuromuscular blockade, severe peripheral neuropathies, lower motor neuron disorders, and comalike states (e.g., locked-in

Table 61.2: Cranial nerve reflex abnormalities and survival after cardiopulmonary arrest

Time after cardio-pulmonary arrest	Number of cranial nerve reflex abnormalities*	Survivors (%)
<3 hrs	0	80
	1	46
	2	29
	3	0
<6 hrs	0	80
	1	37
	2	27
	3	0
<24 hrs	0	81
	1	38
	2	21
	3	0
<24–48 hrs	0	76
	1	21
	2	0
	3	0

*Absent pupillary light reflex, absent corneal responses, absent spontaneous conjugate roving gaze; each count as one abnormal finding.
Source: Adapted from BD Snyder, RJ Gumnit, IE Leppik et al. Neurologic prognosis after cardiopulmonary arrest: IV. Brainstem reflexes. Neurology 1981;31:1092–1097.

syndrome, the presence of sedative or analgesic drugs, or reversible metabolic abnormalities), must all be considered and ruled out before making a diagnosis of brain death.

Guidelines for determining brain death in children must deal specifically with the age group from full-term newborn to the 5-year-old. Features unique to the childhood criteria are primarily the changing periods of recommended observation relative to the patient's age. For children of age 7 days to 2 months, two examinations and two EEGs 48 hours apart are required. For those of age 2 months to 1

Table 61.3: Guidelines that identify patients with poor or good prognosis after cardiopulmonary arrest

Time after cardiac arrest clinical sign	Patients with virtually no chance of regaining independence	Patients with best chance of regaining independence
Initial examination	No pupillary light reflex*	Pupillary light reflexes present; motor response decorticate posturing or decerebrate posturing; spontaneous eye movements conjugately roving or orienting
1 day	1-day motor response no better than decorticate posturing; spontaneous eye movements neither orienting nor conjugate; roving	1-day motor response withdrawal or better; 1-day eye opening to noise or spontaneously
3 days	3-day motor response no better than decorticate posturing	Motor response withdrawal or better; spontaneous eye movements normal
1 wk	Not obeying commands; spontaneous eye movements neither orienting nor conjugate	Obeying commands

*In the absence of some other cause.
Source: Adapted from DE Levy, JJ Caronna, BH Singer et al. Predicting outcome from hypoxic-ischemic coma. JAMA 1985;253:1420–1426.

year, a 24-hour interval is adequate. After 1 year of age, laboratory testing need not be performed, and a 12-hour interval is adequate for most cases.

ELECTRODIAGNOSTIC STUDIES

Electroencephalography

Cardiac arrest results in a stereotyped sequence of EEG changes (see Chapter 37A). In the first 6–9 seconds after a CPA, there is no change in ongoing EEG activities. At 7–9 seconds, there is a transition from normal frequencies to generalized, frontal-dominant 100- to 200-μV delta activity. By 14–18 seconds after CPA, there is generalized voltage attenuation with no recognizable EEG activity. If the cardiac arrest is brief, EEG activities recover in 5–12 seconds after a reverse sequence.

Normothermic individuals incurring a hypoxic-ischemic insult develop varying degrees of cerebral damage. A wide variety of abnormal EEG patterns appear in such individuals, some of which have prognostic significance for neurological outcome. Burst-suppression activity and other periodic generalized phenomena denote severe cerebral dysfunction in the context of AIE (Young et al. 1994).

The term *alpha coma* refers to an EEG pattern comprising widespread alpha-frequency activity that is not reactive to eye opening or other stimulation, recorded from a patient in coma. It occurs in patients after anoxic-ischemic insults and drug intoxication. Because continuous EEG recording has not been widely used in monitoring comatose individuals, the actual incidence and significance of alpha coma is unclear. An alpha coma pattern resolving within 24 hours after CPA denotes a more favorable prognosis than the same pattern detected 24 or more hours after the onset of coma. A persistent alpha coma pattern is usually associated with a fatal outcome.

The absence of detectable EEG activity in individuals studied after CPA is ominous, although one must consider how long after CPA the tracing was taken. Proper interpretation of EEGs demonstrating no detectable cortical activity requires ascertaining conditions capable of causing temporary reversible loss of EEG activity (e.g., sedatives, hypothermia). Occasional patients with no detectable EEG activity for up to 8 hours after resuscitation have subsequently regained consciousness.

There are several detailed systems of grading the conventional EEG in adults to aid in determining prognosis after CPA (Yamashita et al. 1995). EEGs showing normal or near-normal frequency, activity, topography, and reactivity are assigned low grades; those with delta activity, intermittent voltage attenuation, electrocerebral silence, or the patterns mentioned in the preceding paragraphs are assigned higher grades. Patients with grade 1 EEGs (normal or near normal) have a good prognosis for neurological recovery. Patients with grade 4 or 5 EEGs (e.g., alpha coma, intermittent voltage attention, or electrocerebral silence) die, usually without regaining consciousness. Patients with grade 2 or 3 EEGs (mild or moderate abnormalities) experience variable outcomes not accurately predicted by a single post–cardiac arrest EEG. In these patients, sequential EEGs may be of some prognostic assistance.

The labor-intensive nature of prolonged conventional EEG monitoring and interpretation renders widespread clinical application in AIE impractical. One solution to this problem is to transform the conventional EEG data (time-versus-voltage plots) into the frequency domain (frequency-versus-voltage power plots) via microprocessor-based fast Fourier transforms. The data then can be displayed in a succinct graphic format, such as the compressed spectral array. There is a high correlation between the initial and 24-hour postresuscitation compressed spectral array patterns with respect to level of consciousness and ultimate outcome for individuals after CPA.

Evoked Potential Studies

The absence of the early cortical complex (N20-P27) of somatosensory-evoked potentials (SSEPs) in comatose patients (excluding those with brain disease, drug intoxication, major medical abnormalities other than acidosis, or coma of unknown origin) makes it unlikely that the patient will ever regain consciousness. Combining the results of the clinical examination, EEG, and SSEPs improves the sensitivity for predicting prognosis (Chen et al. 1996).

A practical clinical approach to the electrophysiological study of individuals (Figure 61.1) with AIE may begin with a conventional bedside EEG and SSEPs recorded 8–24 hours after resuscitation. If clinically required, additional recordings can be made on days 3 and 7 after resuscitation. Additional recordings allow detection of specific EEG and SSEP patterns that denote a poor neurological prognosis. In addition, the rate and direction of changes in electrocortical activity can be established, with attendant short-term and long-term prognostic implications.

The proper use of these electrophysiological techniques requires technical and interpretive experience and expertise. Minimal technical standards and guidelines are available to assist the clinician (American Electroencephalographic Society 1994). Most of these patients are studied in the intensive care unit, where sources of artifact are legion and often difficult to eliminate. Recognizing artifact is essential.

Other Laboratory Aids in Assessing Prognosis

In addition to the electrophysiological techniques reviewed here, investigators have explored other laboratory techniques for predicting outcome after CPA. Neuroimaging and radionuclide studies have been useful in establishing cerebral nonperfusion and brain death. The concentrations of

FIGURE 61.1 Time course and neurological implications of electroencephalographic (EEG) and evoked potentials in hypoxic ischemic coma.

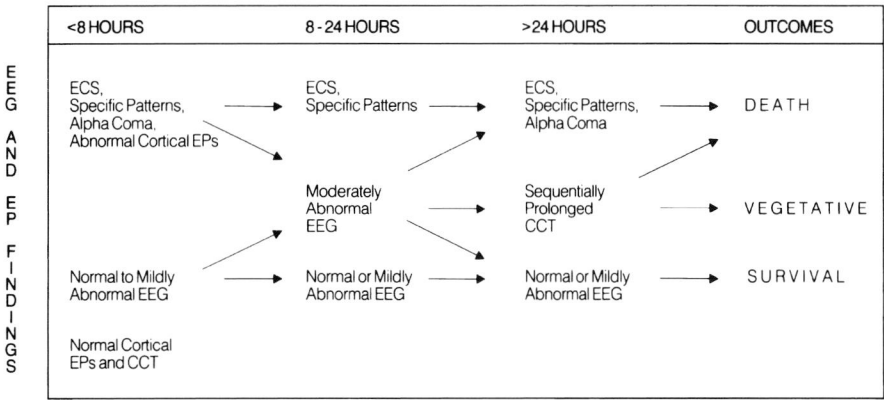

potassium and lactate in the CSF correlate with the severity of CNS insults in clinical series of patients with a variety of disorders. Correlations have not been established, however, for patients with AIE alone. Large elevations of CSF creatine kinase-BB levels are closely correlated with poor outcome but are no more accurate than EEGs and SSEPs in outcome prognostication. Levels of S-100 protein are increased in patients with poor prognosis (Rosen et al. 1998). Magnetic resonance spectroscopy in vivo is also prognostically useful (Berek et al. 1997).

MANAGEMENT OF COMA DUE TO ANOXIC-ISCHEMIC ENCEPHALOPATHY

The patient who is confused, delirious, or comatose during or after an anoxic injury presents difficult diagnostic and treatment issues.

AIE after CPA is a metabolic coma with static or improving course that is often complicated by seizure activity. Diagnostic difficulty is increased because new factors, such as sepsis and drug effects, may come into play during the patient's prolonged illness. Primary intracranial disease can resemble anoxic states and may coexist with them, and care must be taken to rule out other significant factors. Patients presenting with cardiac arrhythmias may have sustained a primary intracranial insult, such as a subarachnoid or intracerebral hemorrhage. The optic fundi should be inspected carefully for papilledema, peripapillary nerve fiber layer hemorrhages, or subhyaloid hemorrhages. Findings such as these or unilateral third cranial nerve palsies should lead to a careful search for other intracranial pathology.

Continued monitoring of the neurological status serves to warn of deteriorating medical status, to establish the neurological prognosis (as outlined earlier), and to identify neurological complications, such as status epilepticus. Computed tomographic brain scan, lumbar puncture, and EEG

techniques may assist in ruling out other diagnoses. Complications of anoxic coma may involve virtually every organ system. Fluid and electrolyte management may be complex. Hyperglycemic hyperosmolar crises may result from combinations of endogenous and exogenous catecholamines, corticosteroids, osmotic diuretics, and glucose infusions, particularly in the diabetic patient. The syndrome of inappropriate secretion of antidiuretic hormone is unusual; diabetes insipidus is extremely rare.

Stress ulceration of the stomach is best prevented by parenteral histamine H_2-receptor blockers, such as ranitidine. Other aspects of routine coma care involve preventing decubitus ulcers, ensuring suitable bladder drainage, and maintaining nutrition.

Currently, there is no known specific treatment that reverses AIE. Rapidly re-establishing circulation and maintaining a normal or somewhat increased systemic arterial pressure for the given individual is essential. Normal arterial blood gas concentrations should be maintained. It is not known if higher levels of arterial oxygen concentration are useful. Hyperthermia and seizure activity increase CNS metabolic activity and should be controlled.

Anticonvulsant therapy is indicated if seizure activity does not respond promptly to the correction of metabolic factors. Axial myoclonus can be very difficult to control. Benzodiazepines (clonazepam or lorazepam) or valproic acid may be effective, but neuromuscular blockade or deep sedation with morphine will more likely be required to prevent disruption of ventilation and interference with nursing care.

As noted previously, current evidence suggests that post-CPA brain swelling is a postnecrotic event. There is no indication for the active treatment of brain edema in this setting. Glucocorticoids and calcium-channel blockers are of no value in treating AIE.

The patient with emerging focal neurological deficits may have sustained one or more cerebral infarctions. Diagnostic considerations must be raised and studies obtained to rule out other intracranial structural lesions when focal deficits are seen. Anticoagulation may be indicated in patients at high risk for recurrent infarction (e.g., those with atrial fibrillation, intracardiac thrombus), but routine anticoagulation after CPA has not been studied for evidence of benefit.

REFERENCES

American Electroencephalographic Society. Guidelines in EEG and evoked potentials 1994. J Clin Neurophysiol 1994;11:37–39, 114–115.

American Neurological Association Committee on Ethical Affairs. Persistent vegetative state. Ann Neurol 1993;33:386–390.

Ashwal S, Cranford RE, Rosenberg JH. Commentary on the practice parameters for the persistent vegetative state. Neurology 1995;45:859–860.

Berek K, Jeschow M, Aichner F. The prognostication of cerebral hypoxia after out-of-hospital cardiac arrest in adults. Eur Neurol 1997;37:135–145.

Chen R, Bolton CF, Young GB. Prediction of outcome in patients with anoxic coma: a clinical and electrophysiologic study. Crit Care Med 1996;24:672–678.

Dubowitz DJ, Bluml S, Arcinue E, Dietrich RB. MR of hypoxic encephalopathy in children after near drowning: correlation with quantitative proton MR spectroscopy and clinical outcome. AJNR Am J Neuroradiol 1998;19:1617–1627.

Gottfried JA, Mayer SA, Shungu DC, et al. Delayed posthypoxic demyelination. Association with arylsulfatase A deficiency and lactic acidosis on proton MR spectroscopy. Neurology 1997; 49:1400–1404.

Govaerts A, Van Zandijcke M, Dehaene I, St-Jan AZ. Posthypoxic midbrain tremor. Mov Disord 1998;13:359–361.

Kriel R, Krach LE, Luxenberg MG, et al. Outcome of severe anoxic ischemic brain injury in children. Pediatr Neurol 1994;10:207–212.

Kyriacou DN, Arcinue EL, Peek C, Kraus JF. Effect of immediate resuscitation on children with submersion injury. Pediatrics 1994;94:137–142.

Mecklinger A, von Cramon Y, Matthes-von Cramon G. Event-related potential evidence for a specific recognition memory deficit in adult survivors of cerebral hypoxia. Brain 1998;121:1919–1935.

Mullner M, Sterz F, Behringer W, et al. The influence of chronic pre-arrest health conditions on mortality and functional neurological recovery in cardiac arrest survivors. Am J Med 1998;104:369–373.

Rosen H, Rosengren L, Herlitz J, Blomstrand C. Increased serum levels of the S-100 protein are associated with hypoxic brain damage after cardiac arrest. Stroke 1998;29:473–477.

Werhahn KJ, Brown P, Thompson PD, Marsden CD. The clinical features and prognosis of chronic posthypoxic myoclonus. Mov Disord 1997;12:216–220.

Wijdicks EFM. Determining brain death in adults. Neurology 1995;45:1003–1011.

Yamashita S, Morinaga T, Ohgo S, et al. Prognostic value of electroencephalogram (EEG) in anoxic encephalopathy after cardiopulmonary resuscitation: relationship among anoxic period, EEG grading and outcome. Intern Med 1995;34:71–76.

Young GB, Blume WT, Campbell VM, et al. Alpha, theta and alpha-theta coma: a clinical outcome study utilizing serial recordings. Electroencephalogr Clin Neurophysiol 1994;91:93–99.

Chapter 62
Toxic and Metabolic Encephalopathies

Alan H. Lockwood

Toxic and metabolic encephalopathies are a group of neurological disorders whose hallmark is an altered mental status. Typically, they are caused by the failure of organs other than the nervous system or the presence of an endogenous or exogenous toxin or drug. Although the brain is isolated from the rest of the body by the blood-brain barrier (BBB), the nervous system often is affected severely by organ failure that leads to the buildup of toxic substances normally removed from the body by the affected organ. This is encountered in patients with hepatic and renal failure. Damage to homeostatic mechanisms affecting the internal milieu of the brain, such as the abnormalities of electrolyte and water metabolism associated with renal failure or the syndrome of inappropriate secretion of antidiuretic hormone (SIADH), also may be seen. In some cases, deficiency of a critical substrate after the catastrophic failure of an organ, such as hypoglycemia caused by fulminating hepatic failure, is the precipitating factor. Frequently, the history and physical examination provide information that defines the affected organ system. In many cases, the cause is evident only after laboratory data are examined.

CLINICAL MANIFESTATIONS

Encephalopathy that develops insidiously may be difficult to detect. The slowness with which abnormalities evolve and replace normal cerebral functions makes it difficult for patients and families to recognize their deficits. When examining patients with diseases of organs that are commonly associated with encephalopathy, neurologists should include encephalopathy in the differential diagnosis.

Mental status abnormalities are always present and may range from subtle abnormalities, detected by neuropsychological testing, to deep coma. The level and content of consciousness reflect involvement of the reticular activating system and the cerebral cortex, respectively. Fundamental deficits may be present in the spheres of selective attention and the ability to process information. These deficits are manifested as disorders of orientation, cognition, memory, affect, perception, judgment, and the ability to concentrate on a specific task. Evidence from studies of patients with cirrhosis (see Hepatic Encephalopathy, later in this chapter) suggests that metabolic encephalopathies are the result of a multifocal cortical disorder rather than uniform involvement of all brain regions. Among patients with coma of unknown etiology, nearly two-thirds ultimately are found to have a metabolic etiology. A complete discussion of coma is found in Chapter 5.

The neuro-ophthalmological examination is extremely important when examining patients with metabolic disorders. The pupillary light reflex and vestibular responses are almost always present, even in patients with deep coma. However, it is common for these reflexes to be blunted. Exceptions include severe hypoxia; ingestion of large amounts of atropine or scopolamine; and deep barbiturate coma, which is usually associated with circulatory collapse and an isoelectric electroencephalogram (EEG). The pupils are usually slightly smaller than normal and may be somewhat irregular. The eyes may be aligned normally in patients with mild encephalopathy. With more severe encephalopathy, dysconjugate roving movements may occur. Other cranial nerve abnormalities may be present but are less useful in constructing a differential diagnosis.

Motor system abnormalities, particularly slight increases in tone, are common. Other signs and symptoms of metabolic disorders may include spasticity with extensor plantar signs (in patients with liver disease), multifocal myoclonus (in patients with uremia), cramps (in patients with electrolyte disorders), Trousseau's sign (in patients with hypocalcemia), tremors, and weakness.

Asterixis, a sudden loss of postural tone, is common. To elicit this sign, the patient should extend the arms and elbows while dorsiflexing the wrists and spreading the fingers. Small lateral movements of the fingers may be the earliest manifestation. More characteristically, there is a sudden flexion of the wrist with rapid resumption of the extended position, the so-called flapping tremor. Asterixis

Table 62.1: Features distinguishing fulminating hepatic failure from chronic hepatic encephalopathy or portal systemic encephalopathy

Feature	Fulminating hepatic failure	Portal systemic encephalopathy
History		
Onset	Usually acute	Varies; may be insidious or subacute
Mental state	Mania may evolve to deep coma	Blunted consciousness progresses to coma
Precipitating factor	Viral infection or hepatotoxin	Gastrointestinal hemorrhage, exogenous protein, drugs, uremia
History of liver disease	No	Usually yes
Symptoms		
Nausea, vomiting	Common	Unusual
Abdominal pain	Common	Unusual
Signs		
Liver	Small, soft, tender	Usually large, firm, no pain
Nutritional state	Normal	Cachectic
Collateral circulation	Absent	Present
Ascites	Absent	May be present
Laboratory tests		
Transaminases	Very high	Normal or slightly high
Coagulopathy	Present	Often present

also may be evident during forced extrusion of the tongue, forced eye closure, or at the knee in prone patients asked to sustain flexion of the knee. Electrophysiological studies have shown the sudden onset of complete electrical silence of muscles that coincides with the lapse of posture. This sign, once thought to be pathognomonic of hepatic encephalopathy, occurs in a variety of conditions, including uremia, other metabolic encephalopathies, and drug intoxication. Occasionally, asterixis is present in patients with structural brain lesions.

Generalized seizures occur in patients with water intoxication, hypoxia, uremia, and hypoglycemia, but only rarely as a manifestation of liver failure. Focal seizures, including epilepsia partialis continua, may be seen in patients with hyperglycemia. Multifocal myoclonic seizures may occur in patients with uremia, after hypoxic brain injury, and in other disorders (see Chapters 25 and 75).

TOXIC ENCEPHALOPATHIES

Hepatic Encephalopathy

Liver disease is the seventh ranked cause of death due to disease. Among the poor, the incidence of cirrhosis may be as much as 10 times higher than the national average and accounts for almost 20% of the excess mortality. As patients with chronic liver disease enter the terminal phases of their illness, encephalopathy becomes an increasingly important cause of morbidity and mortality. However, it is important to stress that mild encephalopathy is common in patients with cirrhosis. This treatable problem is commonly overlooked. The unfortunate term *subclinical encephalopathy* has been used by some to describe a mild form of encephalopathy.

Liver disease causes encephalopathy by two mechanisms: hepatocellular failure and the diversion of toxins from the hepatic portal vein into the systemic circulation. Usually, one mechanism predominates, or both coexist to variable degrees, particularly in patients with cirrhosis in whom shunts are common and encephalopathy waxes and wanes. The term *portal systemic encephalopathy* commonly is applied to patients with cirrhosis with shunts. Patients with fulminant hepatic failure, a disorder occurring in patients with previously normal livers who exhibit neurological signs within 8 weeks of developing liver disease, have pure hepatocellular dysfunction; occasional patients with congenital abnormalities or surgical portacaval shunts have symptoms caused only by the shunt. The features that differentiate patients with fulminant hepatic failure from those with the much more common portal systemic encephalopathy are shown in Table 62.1.

An episode of hepatic encephalopathy may be precipitated by one or more factors, some of which are iatrogenic. In one series, the use of sedatives accounted for almost 25% of all cases. A gastrointestinal (GI) hemorrhage was the next most common event (18%), followed by drug-induced azotemia and other causes of azotemia (15% each). Excessive dietary protein accounted for 10% of episodes; hypokalemia, constipation, infections, and other causes accounted for the remaining cases. As liver disease progresses, patients appear to become more susceptible to the effects of precipitants. This phenomenon has been referred to as *toxin hypersensitivity*. Other data that show older patients are more likely to develop hepatic encephalopathy after the transjugular intrahepatic portosystemic shunts suggest that age-related changes in the brain affect the susceptibility to the agents that cause hepatic encephalopathy.

The diagnosis of hepatic encephalopathy is based on the signs and symptoms of cerebral dysfunction in a setting of hepatic failure. Usually, standard laboratory test results, including serum bilirubin and hepatic enzymes, are abnormal. Products of normal hepatic function, including serum

Table 62.2: Neuropsychiatric abnormalities associated with cirrhosis

	Severity of encephalopathy*		
	Grade 1 (mild)	Grade 2 (moderate)	Grade 3 (severe)
Consciousness	Alert, trivial lack of awareness, short attention span	Slight blunting	Lethargic, somnolent
Behavior	Personality change, fatigue, abnormal sleep pattern	Slight lethargy, disinhibition	Bizarre, paranoia
Affect	Irritable, depressed	Anxious, angry	Blunted
Cognition	Selective visuospatial abnormalities	Impaired	Too impaired to test reliably
Neurological examination	Tremor, asterixis, hyperactive reflexes, Babinski's reflex	Blunted consciousness, slurred speech	Dilation of pupils, nystagmus

*Grade 0: Overtly normal in all spheres. Grade 4: Coma, intact oculocephalic and pupillary light reflexes, no appropriate response to noxious stimuli.

albumin and clotting factors, often are low, leading to prolongation of the prothrombin time. Measurements of the arterial ammonia level may be helpful in diagnosing hepatic encephalopathy. When obtaining blood samples for an ammonia determination, care must be taken to be certain that the sample is of arterial origin (venous ammonia levels may be artificially high, especially after the outpouring of ammonia by muscle made ischemic by applying a tourniquet). The sample should be placed on ice and carried by hand to the laboratory for immediate analysis. Delays can result in ammonia production in the specimen, producing a spuriously elevated result. Normal or minimally elevated blood ammonia values in a comatose patient with long-standing disease should be interpreted with some caution because of the possibility of an altered dose-response relationship between the arterial ammonia concentration and blood flow and oxygen metabolism, discussed elsewhere in this section.

The EEG may be the most useful of the commonly used laboratory diagnostic tests. Bursts of moderate-to-high amplitude (100–300 µV), low-frequency (1.5- to 2.5-Hz) waves are the most characteristic abnormality. There are three stages in the EEG's evolution: a theta stage with diffuse 4- to 7-Hz waves; a triphasic phase with surface-positive maximum deflections; and a delta stage, characterized by random, arrhythmic slowing with little bilateral synchrony.

Neuropsychological tests are an underused and valuable means to diagnose encephalopathy and monitor the response to therapy. Sixty percent or more of all patients with cirrhosis with no overt evidence of encephalopathy exhibit significant abnormalities when given a battery of neuropsychological tests (Table 62.2). Test results of attention, concentration, and visuospatial perception are the most likely to be abnormal. Specific tests that are useful include Trails A and B, the digit symbol, block design subtests of the Wechsler Adult Intelligence Scale (Revised), and the Purdue Pegboard. These abnormalities appear regardless of the cause of the cirrhosis. Patients with alcoholic cirrhosis may have more difficulty with memory deficits than patients with nonalcoholic cirrhosis. Even though these patients appear to be normal, the degree of impairment, particularly in the visual-spatial sphere, may be severe enough to interfere with the safe operation of an automobile or other dangerous equipment, especially if visual-spatial performance is required. Treatment with lactulose lessens the severity of the test score abnormalities in many cases. These data, combined with other studies showing that the quality of life is affected by these abnormalities, suggest that neuropsychological tests should be used more extensively for the routine evaluation of all patients with cirrhosis, particularly those without overt evidence of hepatic encephalopathy.

Event-related potentials may be abnormal in patients with mild encephalopathy. Prolonged latencies and altered waveforms characterize visual event-related potentials. Although there has been less experience with auditory P300 potential recordings, in which the subject is asked to discriminate between a rare and common tone, differences in latencies and waveforms also have been associated with encephalopathy. A combination of visual-evoked potentials, auditory P300s, and selected neuropsychological tests (such as Trails A and B) may be useful in detecting minimal encephalopathy in cirrhotic subjects. It is uncertain whether this less complex approach to detecting minimal encephalopathy will prove to be more reliable and cost-effective than a focused neuropsychological test battery.

Neuroimaging

Magnetic resonance (MR) imaging and spectroscopical studies have revealed new insights into the pathophysiology of hepatic encephalopathy (Lockwood et al. 1997). On T1-weighted images, it is common to find abnormally high signals arising in the pallidum. These are seen as whiter than normal areas in this portion of the brain as shown in Figure 62.1. In addition to these more obvious abnormalities, a systematic analysis of MR images shows that the T1 signal abnormality is quite widespread and found in the limbic, extrapyramidal systems and generally throughout the white matter. A generalized shortening of the T2 signal occurs also. This abnormality is less evident on visual inspection of the images because of the generally short

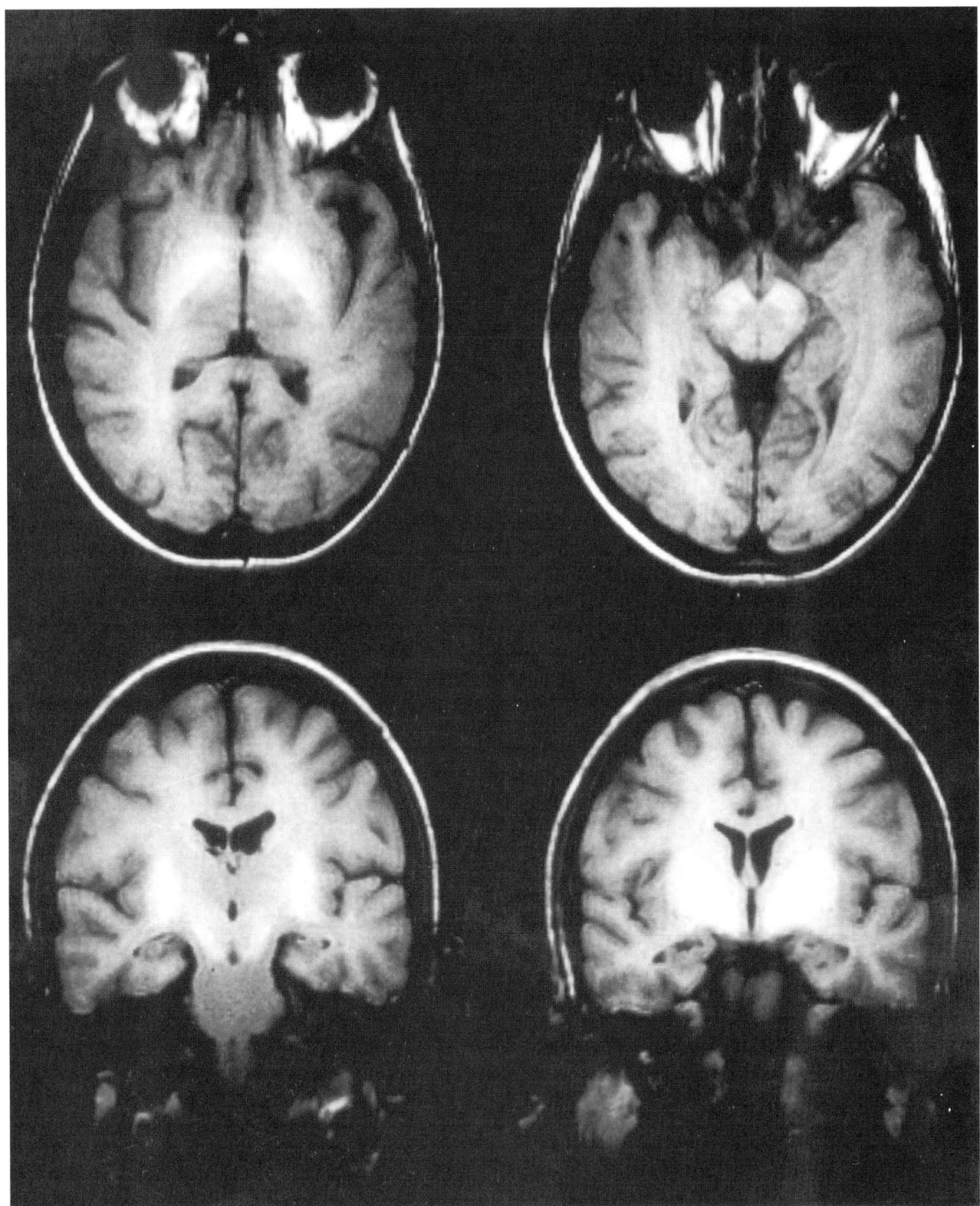

FIGURE 62.1   T1-weighted magnetic resonance images from a patient with cirrhosis of the liver. Note high signal in basal ganglia, cerebral peduncles, and substantia nigra.

duration of T2 signals. These abnormalities have been linked to an increase in the cerebral manganese content. The abnormalities become more prominent with time and regress after successful liver transplantation. The unexpected finding of high T1 signals in the pallidum should suggest the possibility of liver disease.

Proton MR spectroscopical techniques also have been applied to the study of patients with cirrhosis. In the absence of absolute measures that are referable to concentrations, the signal of specific compounds is usually referenced to creatine and expressed as a compound to creatine ratio. There is general agreement among studies that an increase in the intensity of the signal occurs at approximately 2.5 ppm that is attributed to glutamine plus glutamate. With high-field-strength magnets, this peak can be resolved into its components. Results show that the increase is attributable to glutamine, as expected on the basis of animal investigations. Correlations between the glutamine concentration, generally considered to be a reflection of exposure of the brain to ammonia, and the severity of the encephalopathy, have led some to propose that MR spectroscopy may be useful in the diagnosis of hepatic encephalopathy.

Myoinositol and choline signals decrease, whereas N-acetylaspartate resonances (a neuronal marker) are consistently normal. MR spectroscopic studies are difficult and expensive to perform. Because they show no clear advantage over less costly and readily accessible psychometric tests, they are not likely to be used clinically. Neuroimaging studies are not generally required in patients with hepatic encephalopathy. They may be useful in the diagnosis of coexisting brain problems, such as subdural hematomas or other evidence of cerebral trauma, or complications of alcohol abuse and thiamine deficiency, such as midline cerebellar atrophy, or mamillary body atrophy.

Pathophysiology

The pathophysiological basis for the development of hepatic encephalopathy is still not completely known. However, treatment strategies for the disorder are all founded on theoretical pathophysiological mechanisms. A number of hypotheses have been advanced to explain the development of the disorder. Suspected factors include hyperammonemia; altered amino acids and neurotransmitters, especially those related to the γ-aminobutyric acid (GABA)–benzodiazepine complex mercaptans; and short-chain fatty acids. Although none of the current hypotheses is completely capable of explaining the development of hepatic encephalopathy, it is likely that ammonia plays a central role. Because of the complexity of the metabolic derangements that attend liver disease, other factors probably contribute synergistically to the development of this complex disorder.

Cerebral Blood Flow and Glucose Metabolism. Whole-brain measurements of cerebral blood flow (CBF) and metabolism are normal in patients with grade 0–1 hepatic encephalopathy, but reductions occur in more severely affected patients. Positron emission tomography (PET) has been used to study CBF and glucose metabolism in patients with minimal encephalopathy. Although whole-brain values are normal, both blood flow and glucose metabolism patterns are affected significantly. These same studies show that regional values can be used reliably to differentiate patients with liver disease from normal controls. The PET data show clearly that minimal forms of hepatic encephalopathy are caused by the selective impairment of specific neural systems rather than global cerebral dysfunction. This is a novel concept, as more traditional thinking suggests that brain regions are affected more uniformly by the action of toxins. More sophisticated statistical techniques have made it possible to identify specific brain regions in which glucose metabolism is abnormal in patients with grade 0 encephalopathy but in whom neuropsychological tests reveal abnormalities (Lockwood et al. 1993). Reductions occur in the cingulate gyrus (an important element in the attentional system of the brain); increases occur in visual associative cortex. These PET data are in accord with data implicating attentional mechanisms in mildly encephalopathic patients. The increases in metabolism in associative cortex may be compensatory. When compared with normal subjects, patients with cirrhosis and defective attentional systems may have more processing demands placed on visual associative cortex as they seek to adapt to visually novel environments.

Role of Ammonia. A substantial amount of information clearly links the development of encephalopathy to exogenous amounts of ammonia in the blood of patients with liver disease. Patients with encephalopathy have elevated blood ammonia levels that correlate to a degree with the severity of the encephalopathy. Metabolic products formed from ammonia—most notably glutamine and its transamination product, ketoglutaramic acid—also are present in excess cerebrospinal fluid (CSF) in patients with liver disease. Treatment strategies that lower blood ammonia levels are the only ones that are beneficial.

Tracer studies performed with ^{13}N-ammonia have helped clarify the role this toxin has in the pathophysiology of hepatic encephalopathy. Ammonia always is extracted by the brain as arterial blood passes through the cerebral capillaries. When ammonia enters the brain, metabolic trapping reactions convert free ammonia into metabolites (Figure 62.2). The adenosine triphosphate (ATP)-catalyzed glutamine synthetase reaction is the most important of these reactions that occur in small compartments within the brain, with ammonia pool turnover half-times of seconds or less and providing evidence that the glutamine synthetase reaction occurs in astrocytic end-feet that encase brain capillaries. The BBB is approximately 200 times more permeable to uncharged ammonia gas (NH_3) than it is to the ammonium ion (NH_4+); however, because the ionic form is much more abundant than the gas at physiological pH values, substan-

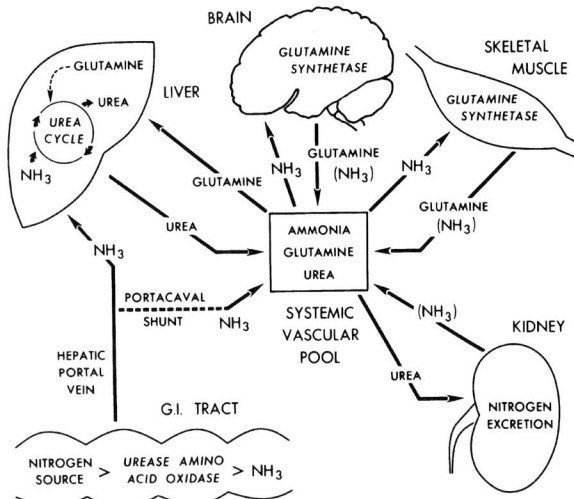

FIGURE 62.2 Human ammonia metabolism. Ammonia and other toxins are formed in the gastrointestinal tract and carried to the liver by the hepatic portal vein, where toxification reactions take place. Portal systemic shunts cause ammonia to bypass the liver and enter the system circulation, where it is transported to the various organs as determined by their blood flow. Ammonia delivered to the brain has deleterious effects on a number of cerebral functions, as described in the text, resulting in altered consciousness or coma. The brain becomes more sensitive to ammonia as time progresses. In addition, ammonia may cause anorexia by stimulating hypothalamic centers, leading to reductions in muscle mass and an impaired ability of muscle to detoxify ammonia. This mechanism is particularly important in patients with extensive portal-systemic shunting, in whom skeletal muscle may become the primary organ of ammonia homeostasis. (G.I. = gastrointestinal.) (Adapted from AH Lockwood, JM McDonald, RE Reiman, et al. The dynamics of ammonia metabolism in man: effects of liver disease and hyperammonemia. J Clin Invest 1979;63:449–460.)

tial amounts of both species appear to cross the BBB in humans. Because of this permeability difference and because ammonia is a weak base, relatively small changes in the pH of blood relative to the brain have a significant effect on the ease with which ammonia is extracted by the brain. As blood becomes more alkalotic, more ammonia is present as the gas and cerebral ammonia extraction increases; however, the role this has in the production of hepatic encephalopathy is not known.

Liver disease itself appears to affect the ease with which ammonia enters the brain. Initial studies of cerebral ammonia metabolism showed that the rate at which ammonia was extracted and trapped as a metabolite increased as the arterial ammonia concentration increased. When blood ammonia doubles, however, more than twice as much ammonia is taken up by the brain. In 1992, Lockwood and colleagues stated that the apparent permeability surface area product of the BBB to ammonia is significantly higher in patients with cirrhosis and encephalopathy than it is in normal controls. An increase in the ammonia permeability surface area product allows additional amounts of ammonia to enter the brain to exert putative harmful effects. This

observation may explain the presence of encephalopathy in patients with near-normal arterial ammonia levels and the development of toxin hypersensitivity. The mechanism that underlies this increase in the permeability surface area product is unknown.

Other Pathophysiological Mechanisms

Abnormalities of Neurotransmission. Since the early 1970s, a variety of hypotheses have suggested that hepatic encephalopathy is caused by disordered neurotransmission. Although early hypotheses related to putative false neurotransmitters were disproved, there is still a substantial effort in this direction.

As a result of the false neurotransmitter hypothesis, it was shown that the ratio of plasma amino acids (valine + leucine + isoleucine) to (phenylalanine + tyrosine) was abnormal in encephalopathic patients, leading to the development of amino acid solutions designed to normalize this ratio that are now commercially available. Although infusion of the solutions normalizes the ratio and patients improve, the results of several controlled clinical trials are inconclusive; it is not clear whether the amino acids or the associated supportive care measures caused the improvement noted.

Substantial effort has been focused on potential abnormalities of the GABA-benzodiazepine complex. Initial attention was directed at GABA itself. Early reports that GABA concentrations were elevated in patients with encephalopathy have been disproved, and attention has shifted toward the presence of benzodiazepines or benzodiazepinelike compounds. A number of anecdotal reports have described dramatic improvements in patients who were refractory to more conventional therapy after they were given flumazenil. Some of the patients in the reports had been given benzodiazepines during the course of their care; however, whether a patient has been given benzodiazepines is not always clearly the case, and very low concentrations of benzodiazepines and their metabolites may be found in blood and CSF of patients with encephalopathy. Typically, these concentrations are substantially lower than concentrations that relieve anxiety and appear to be too low to produce coma. In controlled studies, patients given flumazenil are more likely to improve than those given placebo, but it is not clear that benzodiazepine displacement is the mechanism, because these patients do not have benzodiazepines in their systems. This raises the possibility that any of flumazenil's beneficial actions are unrelated to the displacement of an endogenous benzodiazepine from the receptor site and may be related to some other action of the drug. More recent theories have linked the presence of a increased expression of peripheral types of benzodiazepine receptors to hepatic encephalopathy. These receptors are found on mitochondrial membranes and are implicated in intermediary metabolism and neurosteroid synthesis. Hyperammonemia causes an increase in peripheral types of benzodiazepine receptors and creates a potential for an increase in inhibitory tone in the brain. In addition, there are significant alterations in cerebral serotonin and dopamine metabolism, and a reduction in postsynaptic glutamate receptors of the *N*-methyl-D-aspartate type. Thus, there is a substantial interest in the potential role of neurotransmitters in the pathogenesis of hepatic encephalopathy. As of yet, there is no unifying hypothesis and no rational therapeutic approach based on altering neurotransmission.

Fatty Acids. Short-chain fatty acids affect a variety of metabolic processes, including uncoupling oxidative phosphorylation, altering the mitochondrial respiratory state and state control mechanisms, and inhibiting the urea cycle that may, in turn, lead to hyperammonemia. They work synergistically with ammonia to produce coma in experimental animals.

Medium-chain fatty acid dehydrogenase activity deficiency may lead to the development of a clinical syndrome similar to Reye's syndrome (see Chapter 55B). Indeed, many early cases of Reye's syndrome may have been caused by this metabolic deficiency.

Mercaptans. Mercaptans are thio-alcohols. In this class of compounds, the -OH group is replaced by an -SH group. Methanethiol is the principal mercaptan in humans, is formed by the catabolism of methionine, and occurs in measurable amounts in blood and exhaled air. Injecting or inhaling mercaptans produces coma in animals, and there were early reports of correlations between the concentration of mercaptans in the blood and the severity of encephalopathy in individual patients. An improved methodology for measuring mercaptans has confirmed their presence in elevated amounts in encephalopathic patients, but the correlation between the concentration and the neurological status is poor. Because mercaptans work synergistically with short-chain fatty acids, ammonia, or both to produce coma, synergistic effects may be of importance in humans.

Neuropathology

The Alzheimer type II astrocyte is the neuropathological hallmark of hepatic coma. An account of the original descriptions of this change was provided in translation by Adams and Foley in 1953. In this report, they presented their own findings of this astrocyte change in the cerebral cortex and the lenticular, lateral thalamic, dentate, and red nuclei, offering the tentative proposal that the severity of these changes might be correlated with the length of coma. The cause of the astrocyte change was established by studies that reproduced the clinical and pathological characteristics of hepatic encephalopathy in primates by continuous infusions of ammonia. In studies of rats with portacaval shunts, astrocyte changes become evident after the fifth week. Before coma develops, there is an increase in astrocytic protoplasm and a proliferation of endoplasmic reticulum and mitochondria, suggesting that these are metabolically activated cells. After the production of coma, the more typical signs of the Alzheimer type II change became evident as mitochondrial and nuclear degeneration appeared. Norenberg suggested that hepatic encephalopathy is an astrocytic disease, although oligodendroglial cells are affected as well.

The neuropathological-neurochemical link between astrocytes and the production of hyperammonemic coma is strengthened by immunohistochemical studies that localized glutamine synthetase to astrocytes and their end-feet. Similar findings for glutamate dehydrogenase have been described. Long-standing or recurrent hepatic encephalopathy may lead to the degenerative changes in the brain characteristic of non-Wilsonian hepatocerebral degeneration. Brains of these patients have polymicrocavitary degenerative changes in layers five and six of the cortex, underlying white matter, basal ganglia, and cerebellum. Intranuclear inclusions that are test positive by periodic acid–Schiff also are seen, as are abnormalities in tracts of the spinal cord.

Treatment

Ideally, the management of patients with cirrhosis should involve a cooperative effort between hepatologists, surgeons, neurologists, and psychologists. Diagnostic efforts should be directed toward identifying patients with minimal encephalopathy and monitoring the effects of treatment. Additional effort is required to diagnose and treat precipitating factors, such as infection, electrolyte imbalance, and GI hemorrhage, and to avoid the inappropriate use of drugs, particularly benzodiazepines and sedatives.

The hypothesis that hyperammonemia is a central factor in the pathogenesis of hepatic encephalopathy has led to the most successful and standard treatments of the disorder. Because the majority of the ammonia in the hepatic portal system originates in the colon, the latter has been the principal focus of attention. Treatment of acute encephalopathy should include a number of measures, including careful control of the diet; cleansing the colon with enemas; and administering lactulose, a poorly absorbed antibiotic such as neomycin, or both.

Lactulose. Lactulose is a mainstay for the treatment of both acute and chronic forms of hepatic encephalopathy. It is a synthetic disaccharide metabolized by colonic bacteria to produce acid, causing an osmotic diarrhea.

A widely held but incorrect theory concerning the mechanism of action of lactulose centers on its ability to acidify the colon. Acidification presumably trapped ammonia as the charged and nonabsorbable ammonium ion, thereby preventing ammonia absorption. This theory has been questioned because lactulose treatment does not increase the fecal ammonia concentration or the total amount of ammonia excreted. The effect of lactulose is attributable to its role as a substrate in bacterial metabolism, leading to an assimilation of ammonia by bacteria or reducing deamination of nitrogenous compounds. It is probably the single most important agent in the treatment of acute and chronic encephalopathy. The usual dose of lactulose is 20–30 g three or four times a day or an amount sufficient to produce two or three stools per day. Lactulose also can be given as an enema. Lactitol, another synthetic disaccharide, is also effective. Although it is not yet available in the United States, it may have some advantages over lactulose because it can be prepared in a crystalline form that may make it more acceptable to patients who may object to the taste of lactulose preparations.

Amino Acids. The hypothesis that altered plasma amino acid ratios (discussed earlier), especially the (valine + leucine + isoleucine) to (phenylalanine + tyrosine) ratio, affect brain neurotransmitter pools has led to attempts to treat encephalopathy by normalizing the blood–amino acid profile with branched-chain amino acids. After preliminary open trials suggested a possible therapeutic benefit, a number of controlled trials were undertaken. Although they failed to show a clear beneficial effect, amino acid solutions (oral and parenteral) are still used. Prudence would suggest that they should not be used alone.

Diet. Recent dietary recommendations from hepatologists emphasize the importance of a proper diet containing adequate amounts of protein to permit the recovery of liver function. These replace earlier recommendations of strict limitations of protein content. Dietary measures alone may be sufficient to control chronic portal systemic encephalopathy. Some authors suggest that protein derived from vegetable sources is less likely to produce encephalopathy than animal protein.

Complications and Prognosis

The incidence of hepatic encephalopathy is probably underestimated, mainly because non-neurologists are usually the primary physicians of these patients and may miss early, subtle signs. It is important to establish the diagnosis of hepatic encephalopathy promptly and proceed with vigorous treatment. Although hepatic encephalopathy is potentially completely reversible, prolonged or repeated episodes risk transforming this reversible condition into non-Wilsonian hepatocerebral degeneration, a severe disease with fixed or progressive neurological deficits, including dementia, dysarthria, gait ataxia with intention tremor, and choreoathetosis. Other patients may develop evidence of spinal cord damage, usually manifested by a spastic paraplegia. This complication may be a part of the spectrum of hepatocerebral degeneration. Differentiating correctly between early myelopathy or hepatocerebral degeneration and the motor abnormalities that characterize reversible encephalopathy may not always be possible. Because of the high sensitivity of magnetic resonance imaging, it is possible that this technology will aid in this difficult task. Patients with hepatic encephalopathy may develop toxin hypersensitivity, wherein previously, innocuous levels of toxins caused symptoms. This concept implies that there may be a steadily

increasing risk for developing permanent neurological damage as toxin hypersensitivity evolves.

Severe hepatic coma carries a substantial risk of death. Fulminant hepatic failure is usually the result of massive necrosis of hepatocytes and is defined as a syndrome in which the signs of encephalopathy develop within 8 weeks of the onset of the symptoms of liver disease in a patient with a previously normal liver. This condition has been described as "metabolic chaos," because of coexisting acid–base, renal, electrolyte, cardiac, and hematological abnormalities usually culminating in GI bleeding, ascites, sepsis, and death frequently caused by cerebral edema. In spite of intensive treatment, patients who become comatose have an 80–85% mortality. Improvements in liver transplantation have led to better treatment and improved survival for these patients. Transplantation is associated with its own spectrum of neurological problems (see Chapter 56A).

Uremic Encephalopathy

Neurological disorders in patients with renal failure may present more problems for the neurologist than are found in patients with failure of other organ systems. This is primarily because of the complexity of the clinical status of many of these patients. Many of the disorders that lead to the development of renal failure, such as hypertension, systemic lupus erythematosus, diabetes mellitus, and others, are frequently associated with disorders of nervous system function. Thus, it may be difficult to determine whether new neurological problems are caused by the primary disease or by secondary effects of uremia. Similarly, it is frequently difficult to determine whether neurological problems are the consequence of the progression of renal disease and progressive azotemia or of treating renal failure, such as dialysis and its associated disequilibrium and dementia syndromes, or a complication of transplantation and immunosuppression. With increasing numbers of renal transplants and improved treatment designed to prevent rejection, it is likely that the complexity of these issues will continue to increase. For these reasons, good cooperation and communication between neurologists and the nephrologists and transplant teams who care for these patients are important.

Pathophysiology

Clinically, patients with uremic encephalopathy exhibit many of the signs and symptoms described earlier in this chapter. Perhaps the most notable difference between these patients and those with other forms of metabolic encephalopathy is the frequent coexistence of signs of obtundation (suggesting nervous system depression) and twitching, myoclonus, agitation, and occasionally seizures (suggesting neural excitation). Little is known of the pathophysiology of uremic encephalopathy. As in hepatic encephalopathy, the complexity of the normal kidney's functions makes it likely that failure of the organ leads to a variety of abnormalities that exert synergistic deleterious effects on the brain.

As in other metabolic encephalopathies and other conditions associated with a depression of consciousness, CBF and metabolism are reduced.

Water, Electrolyte, and Acid–Base Balance.   Although derangements in electrolyte, water, and acid–base balance are common in patients with renal failure, they do not appear to contribute substantially to the development of uremic encephalopathy. Disordered water balance is, however, a major factor in the syndrome of dialysis disequilibrium (see Syndromes Related to Dialysis, later in this chapter). Many patients complain of headache, fatigue, and other relatively nonspecific symptoms at the time of dialysis that are attributable to the removal of free water and solutes from the vascular compartment and a lag in re-establishing a new steady-state osmotic equilibrium with the brain. More severe forms of dialysis disequilibrium are now rare. Before the current level of sophistication in equipment, membranes, and schedules for dialysis was developed, severe abnormalities of the EEG, epileptic seizures, coma, and even death occurred as the result of this syndrome.

Calcium and Parathyroid Hormone.   Abnormal calcium metabolism and abnormal control of the parathyroid glands are common in uremic patients, including those receiving dialysis. Experimental studies have shown a doubling of the brain calcium content and serum parathyroid hormone levels within days of the onset of acute renal failure. EEG slowing correlates with elevations in the plasma content of the N-terminal fragment of parathormone. Treatment with 1,25 dihydroxyvitamin D leads to improvements in the EEG and reductions in N-terminal fragment parathyroid hormone concentrations. Brain calcium concentrations may be related to the activity of an ATP-dependent sodium-calcium transporter protein.

Neurotransmitters.   Disorders of plasma amino acids, most notably glutamine, glycine, aromatic and branched-chain amino acids, and potential relationships to GABA, dopamine, and serotonin, have led to speculations that neurotransmitter function may be abnormal in patients with uremic encephalopathy. Others have suggested that brain calcium abnormalities may exert an effect on neurotransmitter release. These hypotheses remain unproven.

Treatment and Its Complications

Dialysis is the primary treatment for uremic encephalopathy. Usually, hemodialysis is chosen, although occasionally peritoneal dialysis is used in its place. After stabilization on dialysis, renal transplantation may be required. Although the details of these treatments are beyond the scope of this text, treatment strategies directed at neurological symptoms associated with uremia and its complications do require management by a neurologist.

Epileptic seizures occur in up to one-third of all uremic patients. In evaluating patients with seizures, it is essential to determine whether the seizure is the result of uremia or the consequence of some other coexisting or causative illness, such as malignant hypertension with encephalopathy, intercurrent infection, dialysis disequilibrium syndrome, or cerebral infarction. Usually, the seizures caused by uncomplicated uremia are generalized, but focal motor seizures and epilepsia partialis continua occur.

Treatment of uremic seizures is complicated by abnormalities of anticonvulsant metabolism and plasma binding encountered in patients with renal failure; phenytoin, a mainstay in seizure treatment, is affected particularly. Regardless of the route of phenytoin administration, uremic patients have lower drug levels than do nonuremic controls, and plasma levels of the metabolite 5-phenyl-5-para-hydroxylphenylhydantoin are higher. The half-life of phenytoin is shortened in uremia and unrelated to the binding of phenytoin to plasma proteins or to the volume of distribution. Plasma protein binding studies of phenytoin in normal and uremic patients show that normal people have approximately 8% unbound, or free, whereas uremic patients have between 8% and 25% in the unbound state. The unbound fraction correlates well with both the blood urea nitrogen and the creatinine concentration in blood, with better correlation with creatinine than blood urea nitrogen. In regulating phenytoin doses in uremic patients, it is critical to use the free drug level rather than the more commonly used total drug level. As a general rule, the free level should be kept between 1 and 2 µg/ml, roughly 10% of the therapeutic level for total phenytoin. Phenytoin toxicity is difficult to manage in uremic patients because the drug is not removed by dialysis.

Phenobarbital is also a useful drug for treating seizures in uremic patients in spite of the fact that it is excreted by the kidneys. Plasma phenobarbital levels are unaffected by uremia and may be used to monitor therapy.

Other abnormalities detected on examination of uremic patients include asterixis, tremor (which may appear before asterixis), and myoclonus. These signs do not require specific therapy and usually clear as the mental status responds to dialysis or transplantation. Tetany and spontaneous carpopedal spasms also may occur.

Treating renal failure by dialysis and transplantation has given rise to a number of neurological syndromes. Because of the large number of patients being treated by these modalities, especially dialysis, it is important to recognize currently described complications and to be alert to the possibility that new syndromes will emerge as treatment modalities evolve.

Although dialysis is clearly an important life-sustaining treatment modality for patients with renal failure, two important neurological syndromes related to this modality are recognized: dialysis disequilibrium syndrome and dialysis dementia syndrome. The former is an acute syndrome that may be seen during or after a single dialysis treatment; the latter is a chronic condition that emerges subacutely or chronically after prolonged treatment by dialysis. The treatment and prophylaxis of these syndromes have become much more successful as our understanding of their pathophysiology has improved.

Dialysis disequilibrium syndrome occurs during or immediately after treatment by either hemodialysis or peritoneal dialysis. Symptoms range from subtle to lethal and include seizures (usually grand mal, although focal seizures may occur), coma, and death. These symptoms were more common before 1970 and are now seen less frequently because of improved dialysis techniques. Other symptoms that may be encountered include disorientation, headache (often associated with nausea, restlessness, or fatigue), muscle cramps, and tremulousness. During the acute syndrome, disorganization and EEG slowing may be seen, and CSF pressure is elevated. EEGs recorded during chronic maintenance hemodialysis show that there is usually some abnormality during the treatment of stable patients, with the most significant abnormalities seen in patients reporting symptoms such as fatigue.

The symptoms of dialysis disequilibrium are probably caused by the development of cerebral edema. Uremic patients have increased serum and brain osmolality because of the accumulation of urea and idiogenic osmoles. When rapid hemodialysis is compared with slow hemodialysis, the water and osmole content of brains of the animals treated by rapid dialysis is found to be greater than in those treated by slow dialysis. Urea concentration in the CSF and the brain exceeds the plasma urea concentration in both treatments. Rapid hemodialysis also is associated with the development of CSF acidosis and a significant osmotic gradient between blood and brain not explained by sodium, potassium, chloride, or urea concentration. These conditions result in the obligatory water retention by the brain relative to blood, which causes the brain to swell. Idiogenic osmoles are probably of critical importance in the development of this syndrome. Presumably under conditions of slower dialysis, the brain has an opportunity to rid itself of idiogenic osmoles and is less susceptible to the development of edema during dialysis. The presence of acidosis in the central nervous system also may be important. Recognizing these mechanisms has led to a reduction in the severity and incidence of this potentially fatal disorder.

Dialysis dementia syndrome is a much rarer and more serious syndrome. It is a subacute syndrome of impaired memory with personality changes, apractic dysarthric speech, myoclonus, seizures (usually multifocal), and an abnormal EEG characterized by slowing with multifocal bursts of more profound slowing and spikes. Aluminum levels in the brains of patients with the syndrome are higher than the levels in controls, in uremic patients not receiving dialysis, and in uremic patients on dialysis but without the syndrome. Epidemiological studies of the relationship of the syndrome to the aluminum content of dialysate fluid have established the latter as the probable source of the aluminum and the most likely cause of most cases of the syndrome. In general, all areas with large numbers of cases of the dialysis dementia syndrome had high aluminum concentrations in dialysis fluid (100–500 pg/liter). Cases occurred most frequently in areas with a high aluminum content in the municipal water supply; removal of aluminum from dialysis baths, preferably by deionization, has markedly reduced the incidence of the syndrome. Although it seems clear that the majority of cases of dialysis dementia can be related to aluminum in the dialysate, there are unexplained sporadic cases occurring in centers with low aluminum levels. In these patients, blood aluminum levels appear to be high, suggesting that GI aluminum absorption may be of occasional importance in the pathogenesis of the disorder.

Treatment of the syndrome has been difficult, and little success has been reported. The most promising form of therapy involves the parenteral administration of deferoxamine. This treatment also appears to have a positive effect on this same group of patients who also have fractures caused by osteomalacia.

METABOLIC DISTURBANCES

Disorders of Glucose Metabolism

Under normal conditions, glucose is the exclusive fuel for the brain. The brain, unlike other organs such as the liver and skeletal muscle, is able to store only trivial quantities of glucose as glycogen. Because brain glucose concentrations are normally low, approximately 25% of the plasma concentration, and the cerebral metabolic rate for glucose is high, the brain is highly vulnerable to interruptions in the supply of glucose. Hyperglycemia is tolerated by the brain better than hypoglycemia, but it, too, produces neurological symptoms, largely because of osmotic effects.

Physiology

Glucose Homeostasis.   After ingesting food, blood glucose levels begin to climb, which, in concert with a number of complex factors, leads to the release of insulin from the pancreas. Insulin has the combined effects of suppressing hepatic glucose production and fostering the storage of glucose, particularly as glycogen in the liver. After carbohydrate absorption is complete, homeostasis is maintained predominantly by hepatic glycogenolysis. Normally, the liver contains sufficient glycogen stores to maintain the blood glucose concentration at 80–90 mg/dl for 24–36 hours. After this time, gluconeogenesis becomes the principal mechanism for maintaining adequate plasma glucose levels. Alanine and glutamine are the amino acids that, along with lactate and pyruvate, are the most important glucose precursors. Initially, most gluconeogenesis takes place in the liver, but with extended starvation, the kidney begins to produce glucose, accounting for roughly one-half of the glucose produced. Approximately one-half of the glucose produced in the postabsorptive state is metabolized by the brain. Because the metabolic processes of glucose homeostasis, including insulin release, glycogen breakdown, and gluconeogenesis, are complex and involve the pancreas, liver, and other organs, it is not surprising that an extensive list of conditions may present as hypoglycemia.

Cerebral Glucose Metabolism. Under normal conditions with a mean CBF of 50 ml/100 g of brain per minute and a glucose concentration of approximately 5 mmol/liter, large amounts of glucose are presented to the brain at all times. Approximately 10% of this total is transported across the BBB by a glucose transporter enzyme that exhibits Michaelis-Menten kinetics. The glucose transporter does not require energy and is capable of transporting other hexoses that may competitively inhibit glucose transport. Defects in glucose transport across the BBB have been encountered in several children with persistently low CSF glucose concentrations, seizures, and developmental delay.

Once in the brain, the majority of the glucose is metabolized by the glycolytic pathway and then by the tricarboxylic acid cycle to generate the ATP needed to maintain brain function. Normally, approximately 85% of the glucose that enters the brain is metabolized in this fashion. The remaining glucose is metabolized by the hexose monophosphate shunt and converted to glycogen. The complete oxidation of 1 mole of glucose requires 6 moles of oxygen and produces 6 moles of carbon dioxide and water. The failure to observe exact stoichiometric relationships experimentally is evidence that glucose carbon skeletons are diverted into the formation of other organic compounds in the brain. After the administration of uniformly labeled glucose, label appears in carbon dioxide in the venous blood in less than 1 minute and eventually appears in a variety of amino acids, proteins, and other compounds.

Measuring cerebral glucose metabolism was revolutionized by the development of the [14C]-2-deoxy-2-D-glucose method. This autoradiographic method for investigating metabolism in animals was followed quickly by the development of an ^{18}F analogue, fluorodeoxyglucose. This compound is also a useful tracer of cerebral glucose metabolism and is well suited to in vivo studies in humans when combined with PET scan data. Fluorodeoxyglucose PET scans of the brain are now an important aspect in the preoperative investigations of patients with intractable seizure disorders.

Clinical Aspects of Hypoglycemia

Diagnosing hypoglycemia on the basis of clinical symptoms is fraught with hazards. Although the majority of symptoms are attributable to nervous system dysfunction, they are extremely varied, nonspecific, and not always present, even when blood glucose levels are very low. In recognition of the close link between the symptoms of hypoglycemia and the brain, some authors use the term *neuroglycopenia* to refer to symptomatic hypoglycemia. There are three syndromes: acute, subacute, and chronic.

The acute syndrome most commonly develops as the result of the action of short-acting insulin preparations or oral antihyperglycemics and begins with vague symptoms of malaise, feeling detached from the environment, restlessness associated with hunger, nervousness that may lead to panic, sweating, and ataxia. Patients may recognize these symptoms. The symptoms respond quickly to oral or parenteral glucose. An EEG during this period may reveal nonspecific abnormalities. Attacks may terminate spontaneously or proceed rapidly to generalized seizures and coma, with the attendant risk of permanent brain injury. These patients may arrive in the emergency department in coma with no history.

The subacute syndrome is the most common form and occurs in the fasting state. Most of the symptoms listed for the acute syndrome are absent. In their place is a slowing of thought processes and a gradual blunting of consciousness with a retention of awareness, although amnesia for the episode is common. The diagnosis may be difficult to establish until the possibility of hypoglycemia is considered or routine testing uncovers the abnormality. Hypothermia is encountered frequently in this form of the disorder, and unexplained low body temperatures always should be followed by a blood glucose measurement.

Chronic hypoglycemia is rare and, if confirmed, suggests a probable insulin-secreting tumor or obsessively good control of a diabetic. Plasma protein C levels are helpful in making this differential diagnosis. This syndrome is characterized by insidious changes in personality, memory, and behavior that may be misconstrued as dementia. Unlike those of the acute and subacute forms of hypoglycemia, these symptoms are not promptly relieved by administering glucose, suggesting the presence of neuronal injury. Clinical improvement after removal of the source of the exogenous insulin is gradual, extending over periods as long as a year.

The symptoms of sweating, tremor, and the sensation of warmth may be attributed to activity of the autonomic nervous system. The inability to concentrate, weakness, and drowsiness are attributable to neuroglycopenia. Hunger, blurred vision, and other symptoms are of uncertain cause.

Diabetics may develop hypoglycemia without being aware of the usual warning symptoms, a condition known as *hypoglycemia unawareness*, which may occur in a complete or partial form in up to 17% of all episodes in patients with type I diabetes (MacLeod et al. 1993). The underlying mechanisms appear to be related to the occurrence of prior episodes of hypoglycemia, altered neuroendocrine responses that regulate blood glucose levels, and central nervous system dysfunction that may interfere with symptom detection and analysis (Lingenfelser et al. 1993).

There are special problems associated with detecting hypoglycemia in neonates and children that center on the various nonspecific symptoms (e.g., pallor, irritability, and

Table 62.3:   Causes of hypoglycemia

Postprandial hypoglycemia (reactive)
   Postoperative rapid gastric emptying (alimentary hyperinsulinism)
   Fructose intolerance
   Galactosemia
   Leucine intolerance
   Idiopathic
Fasting hypoglycemia
   Overuse of glucose
      Elevated insulin levels
         Exogenous insulin (therapeutic, factitious)
         Oral hypoglycemic (therapeutic, factitious)
         Islet cell disorders (adenoma, nesidioblastosis, cancer)
         Excessive islet cell function (prediabetes, obesity)
         Antibodies to endogenous insulin
      Normal to low insulin levels
         Ketotic hypoglycemia
         Hypermetabolic state (sepsis)
         Rare extrapancreatic tumors
         Carnitine deficiency
         Antibodies to endogenous insulin
   Underproduction of glucose
      Hormone deficiencies (growth hormone, glucagon,
         hypoadrenalism)
      Enzyme disorders
         Glycogen metabolism (glycogen phosphorylase, glycogen
           synthetase)
         Hexose metabolism (glucose-6-phosphatase, fructose-
           1,6-biphosphatase)
         Glycolysis, Krebs' cycle (phosphoenolpyruvate carboxy-
           kinase, pyruvate carboxylase, malate dehydrogenase)
      Alcohol and probably other drugs
      Liver disease (cirrhosis, fulminant hepatic failure)
      Severe malnutrition

feeding difficulties) and on the variable sensitivities of individual children to a given plasma glucose concentration. As with adults, the diagnosis is most likely to be made when the physician consciously keeps his or her index of suspicion high and when glucose measurement is done routinely when there is any doubt about a diagnosis. The risk of missing the diagnosis and having irreversible neuronal injury develop in the patient justifies liberal use of screening measures and, in some cases, presumptive treatment with parenteral glucose.

Because of the complexity of glucose homeostasis, the causes of hypoglycemia are many and varied, and a detailed discussion is beyond the scope of this chapter. In general, most authors present a physiological classification as shown in Table 62.3.

Drugs are frequently cited as an important cause of hypoglycemia. In some cases the effect of a drug may be potentiated by a restriction of food intake. Age-varying causes have been found and should aid in the diagnosis of the disorder. In the newborn period, administration of sulfonylureas to the mother dominated as a cause of hypoglycemia. From 0–2 years, salicylate ingestion dominates. Surprisingly, alcohol predominated as a cause in the 2- to 7-year age group. Alcohol-

containing cough syrups and alcoholic beverages were responsible. Sulfonylureas again dominate in the 11- to 30-year and 50 and older age groups. Alcohol predominated between the ages of 30 and 50 years. Significant numbers of patients in most age groups were encountered in whom beta blockade with propranolol was a factor in masking the symptoms of developing hypoglycemia. The use of beta blockers in patients receiving insulin or oral hypoglycemic agents, therefore, should be avoided. A number of risk factors have been recognized that predispose to the development of hypoglycemia. These include (in addition to diabetes) decreased caloric intake (usually related to severity of some illness or disruption of dietary routines), uremia, liver disease, infection, shock, pregnancy, neoplasia, and burns.

A substantial morbidity is associated with hypoglycemia. A study of 600 diabetics showed that the frequency of severe hypoglycemia was 1.60 episodes per patient per year and that it occurred twice as often in patients with the type I form of the disorder (MacLeod et al. 1993). Among patients with severe episodes of hypoglycemia, injuries and convulsions occurred at rates of 0.04 and 0.02 episodes per patient per year. Five patients had automobile accidents caused by hypoglycemia. Patients with episodes of severe hypoglycemia were more likely to have had prior severe episodes, were on insulin longer, and had lower mean glycated hemoglobin concentrations. A southern California medical examiner found 123 deaths caused by hypoglycemia in a series of 54,850 autopsies. The risk of death is highest in patients with the most severe hypoglycemia and the largest number of risk factors. Among hospitalized patients, whites have the lowest mortality (approximately 6%), whereas black and Hispanic patients have mortalities of 30% and 46%, respectively.

Hypoglycemia is a medical emergency, and all patients suspected of being hypoglycemic, including all patients with coma of unknown cause, should be treated with parenteral glucose after adequate blood samples are obtained for laboratory testing. It is prudent to draw extra blood so that insulin and C peptide levels can be measured if indicated by the patient's subsequent course. Measuring insulin and C peptide levels is particularly important in patients with obscure histories and in whom factitious hypoglycemia may be present. The total amount of glucose administered may be of little consequence if the patient is found to have a normal or elevated plasma glucose concentration. Evidence suggests, however, that exogenous glucose may be harmful to the brain during hypoxia or ischemia, and caution must be exercised in administering glucose to this group of patients.

Clinical Aspects of Hyperglycemia

Although there are many causes of hyperglycemia, diabetic ketoacidosis (DKA), nonketotic hyperosmolar coma, and iatrogenic factors, such as parenteral hyperalimentation, are the most important. DKA is a relatively common disorder affecting type I diabetics. It is frequently precipitated by an infectious process in a patient who has been otherwise stable, develops over several days, and is heralded by polyuria and polydipsia caused by the osmotic diuresis produced by glucosuria. These symptoms are followed by anorexia, nausea, disorientation, and coma. On physical examination, sustained hyperventilation is common, especially in patients with severe acidosis. The diagnosis is frequently suspected on the basis of clinical findings, but laboratory data, including the plasma glucose, arterial blood gases, electrolytes, and an appropriate test for ketone bodies, are essential for confirming the diagnosis and management.

Nonketotic hyperosmolar coma, by contrast, is a feature of type II diabetes and is thus encountered in older patients, commonly as the first manifestation of the disease. This syndrome evolves more slowly than DKA, and the period of polyuria is more prolonged, leading to much more severe dehydration. Because glucose is a less effective dipsogen than other solutes, water-seeking behavior is not as strong in this group of patients as it is in patients with hypernatremic hyperosmolality, thus promoting the development of dehydration. Suppressed water-seeking behavior, combined with the inhibitory effect of hypertonicity on insulin release, can lead to severe dehydration and hyperglycemia that can be in excess of 2,000 mg/dl. The disorder's signs and symptoms are those of hyperosmolality, hypovolemia, and cerebral dysfunction, with epileptic seizures occurring in some individuals. Precipitating factors include infection, gastroenteritis, pancreatitis, and, occasionally, treatment with glucocorticoids or phenytoin. Because many total parenteral nutrition protocols use solutions with high glucose contents, hyperglycemia is a potential complication of their use.

DKA is an insulin-deficient state, and administering insulin is the cornerstone of therapy. In the absence of insulin, peripheral glucose uptake and glycogen formation are reduced, and glycogenolysis and lipolysis are accelerated, leading to the formation of acidic ketone bodies and hyperglycemia. When plasma glucose levels exceed the renal threshold (usually approximately 180 mg/dl), glucosuria and a forced osmotic diuresis ensue. The treatment of DKA is designed to reverse these pathophysiological abnormalities and consists of administering insulin to enhance glucose uptake, enhance glycogen formation by noncerebral tissues, and reduce the rate of ketone body formation that occurs during low-insulin, high-glucagon states that promotes the entry of fatty acids into mitochondria, where they are converted to ketones. Replacing fluid and electrolytes also is required, as is treatment of precipitating factors. It is important to remember that overly vigorous treatment with rapid restoration of plasma osmolality to normal levels can lead to the development of cerebral edema (see Complications of Treatment, later in this chapter).

Neurologists may become involved in the diagnosis and management of patients with nonketotic hyperosmolar coma when a patient has no prior history of diabetes and is brought to the emergency department with unexplained coma or seizures. Because hyperosmolality and the associated hypovolemia are usually much more severe in this con-

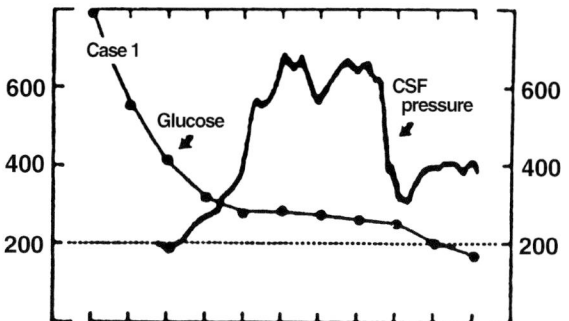

FIGURE 62.3   Blood glucose and intracranial pressure during treatment of diabetic ketoacidosis. The untreated hyperosmolar state leads to the intracerebral accumulation of idiogenic osmoles. As blood glucose and osmolality levels decrease during treatment, free water enters the brain more rapidly than idiogenic osmoles are shed, leading to an increase in intracranial pressure from the swollen brain. This mechanism presumably operates in all cases in which hyperosmolality is corrected rapidly. (CSF = cerebrospinal fluid.) (Reprinted with permission from RS Clements Jr, SA Blumenthal, AD Morrison, et al. Increased cerebrospinal fluid pressure during treatment of diabetic ketoses. Lancet 1971;2:671–675.)

dition than in DKA, maintaining an adequate blood pressure and cardiac output are the first priorities in treatment. One or 2 liters of normal saline should be given rapidly to restore blood volume and to begin to reduce plasma osmolality. Additional fluid and insulin therapy then can be initiated as indicated by laboratory and clinical data. These patients may require intensive monitoring with arterial and Swan-Ganz catheters to monitor the circulatory system status and avoid inducing a volume overload; at the same time, adequate amounts of fluid should be given to restore osmolality to normal levels. The exact mechanisms leading to the development of the syndrome, particularly the absence of ketosis, are not fully explained.

Complications of Treatment.   Although treatment of DKA has improved, the syndrome's mortality is still appreciable. The majority of patients who succumb die in cardiovascular collapse or from complications of the precipitating factor. A small number of patients die unexpectedly when laboratory and clinical indicators all show initial improvement.

Clinically, patients with DKA who die experience rapid neurological then cardiovascular deterioration. Postmortem examinations of the brains show lesions similar to those seen in acute asphyxia, including capillary dilation with perivascular and pericellular edema. Death is heralded by a rapid evolution of signs and symptoms indicating an increase in intracranial pressure. Approximately one-half die during the initial episode of DKA. The rate and degree to which the plasma glucose level is lowered is not a major risk factor for death.

Some degree of cerebral edema attends the treatment of most patients with DKA, occasionally to the high level of 600 mm CSF pressure, as shown in Figure 62.3.

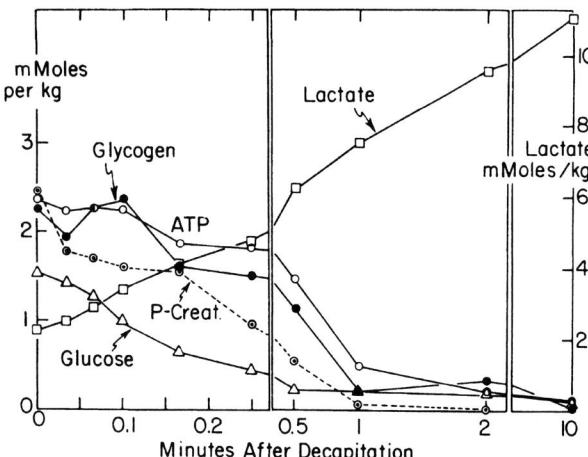

FIGURE 62.4 Neurochemical consequences of decapitation. Experimental animals were decapitated and then frozen at various times thereafter. Brains were assayed for metabolites, as shown in the figure. As can be seen, high-energy phosphates are depleted rapidly. Glucose and glycogen also are consumed, generating lactate, as metabolism changes from the normal aerobic condition to an anaerobic state. The changes shown in this figure are analogous to those following acute hypoxia or cerebral infarction. (ATP = adenosine triphosphate; P-Creat = phosphocreatine.) (Reprinted with permission from OH Lowry, JV Pasonneau. The relationships between substrates and enzymes of glycolysis in brain. J Biol Chem 1964;239:31–42.)

The data suggest that at least mild, clinically silent cerebral swelling may be much more common than is realized in cases of DKA. Rare, unknown factors appear to trigger a malignant increase in intracranial pressure in a small number of patients, producing a syndrome characterized by rapid neurological deterioration and death caused by neurological and circulatory collapse. Published experience suggests that if this diagnosis is made, prompt, aggressive treatment of cerebral edema is indicated, preferably using intracranial pressure monitoring as a guide to therapy. Nevertheless, there is still a high mortality.

Glucose and Cardiopulmonary Resuscitation. A number of studies suggest that hyperglycemia is associated with an increase in the severity of complications of cerebral ischemia and hypoxia. The presumption is that blood, and hence brain, glucose levels are higher in hyperglycemic individuals and that this glucose produces more lactate during the hypoxic-ischemic insult. This sequence is shown in Figure 62.4, in which the metabolic consequences of decapitation in animals are shown. Glucose is metabolized anaerobically to lactate, which, with the hydrolysis of ATP, causes acidosis. A large number of experimental studies suggest that cerebral acidosis is an important determinant of brain injury, including acidosis associated with lactate production during ischemia. The results of these studies have been extended to humans, in whom a less favorable outcome was suggested for stroke patients with diabetes and hyperglycemia compared with euglycemic diabetic stroke patients.

A number of animal studies have shown that the risk of neurological injury during resuscitation from cardiopulmonary arrest increases if exogenous glucose is administered. This issue has been investigated in humans by Longstreth et al. (1993), who randomly administered 5% dextrose in water or half-normal saline while treating out-of-hospital cardiopulmonary arrest. These treatments did not produce significant differences among three measures of outcome: awakening, survival to admission to the hospital, or discharge from the hospital. Because patients with ventricular fibrillation or asystole with high blood glucose levels at the time of admission to the hospital were less likely to awaken than patients with lower blood glucose levels, however, they concluded that it is appropriate to restrict the amount of glucose administered during cardiopulmonary resuscitation.

Disorders of Water and Electrolyte Metabolism

Patients with abnormalities of water and electrolyte metabolism frequently exhibit signs and symptoms of cerebral dysfunction. Typically, these patients have altered states of consciousness or epileptic seizures that herald the onset of the abnormality. The vulnerability of the nervous system to abnormalities of water and electrolyte balance arises from changes in brain volume, especially the brain swelling that may be associated with water intoxication; the abnormalities are symptomatic almost immediately because the brain is enclosed by the rigid skull. The role played by electrolytes is also important in maintaining transmembrane potentials, neurotransmission, and a variety of metabolic reactions, such as those involving the role of calcium and calmodulin. Although most clinicians are aware of the importance of water and electrolyte disturbances as a cause of brain dysfunction, the importance of the brain in the control of water and electrolytes is less well appreciated.

Disordered Osmolality

Osmotic Homeostasis. The serum, and hence whole-body osmolality, are regulated by complex neuroendocrine and renal interactions that control thirst and water and electrolyte balance. When serum osmolality increases, the brain loses volume; when osmolality falls, the brain swells. Events related to water loss are illustrated in Figure 62.5. The brain has little protection in terms of volume changes when an osmotic stress is acute. Examples of acute osmotic stress may be found in patients with heat stroke, inadvertent solute ingestion (particularly in infants), massive ingestion of water (which may be psychogenic), hemodialysis, and diabetics with nonketotic coma. When osmotic stress is applied more slowly over a longer period of time, the predicted volume changes are smaller than would be expected. The mechanisms that underlie these protective adaptations are not known completely but involve the gain of amino acids in the

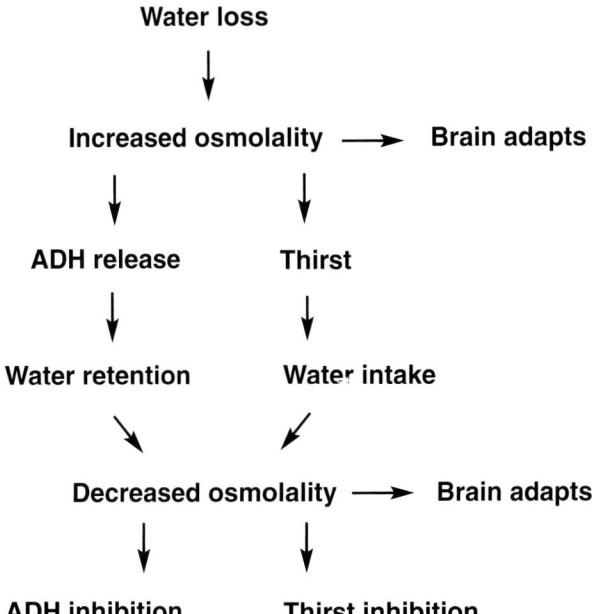

Water loss

↓

Increased osmolality → **Brain adapts**

↓   ↓

ADH release   **Thirst**

↓   ↓

Water retention   **Water intake**

↘   ↙

Decreased osmolality → **Brain adapts**

↓   ↓

ADH inhibition   **Thirst inhibition**

FIGURE 62.5   Water balance and the brain. A reduction in water (or an increase in water loss or solute gain) stimulates thirst and vasopressin release, leading to increased water conservation and intake, which in turn reduces vasopressin levels and ends thirst. Excessive water intake or excessive water loss leads to hypo-osmolality or hyperosmolality and the loss or gain of osmotically active particles in the brain, respectively. Excessively rapid treatment of these conditions may lead to the development of neurological symptoms. (ADH = antidiuretic hormone.)

Table 62.4:   Causes of hyponatremia

Combined water and sodium depletion (hypovolemia)
   Renal loss
      Primary renal disease
      Osmotic diuresis (glucose, mannitol)
      Adrenal insufficiency
   Nonrenal loss
      Gastrointestinal (diarrhea, suction, vomiting)
      Transcutaneous (sweating, burns)
      Sequestration (ascites, peritonitis)
Hyponatremia without water loss
   Edema with water and sodium retention
   Dilutional (iatrogenic, psychogenic)
   Sick cell syndrome
   Hyperosmotic (hyperglycemia or mannitol administration)
   Syndrome of inappropriate antidiuretic hormone secretion
      (see Table 62.5)
   Artifact (laboratory error, hyperlipemia)

case of the hyperosmolar state and the loss of potassium in the hypo-osmolar state. Experimental studies have failed to identify all of the osmotically active particles that must exist in the brain after a given osmotic stress is applied. These unidentified molecules are called *idiogenic osmoles.*

Hypo-osmolality and Hyponatremia.   Hypo-osmolality almost always is associated with hyponatremia, and the diagnosis usually is made by laboratory testing. Conditions associated with hyponatremia are shown in Table 62.4. When hyponatremia is encountered, a measurement of serum osmolality should be performed to differentiate true from pseudo hypo-osmolality, which may be encountered in patients with lipemic serum or in neurological patients treated with mannitol.

A large and diverse group of neurological conditions is associated with hyponatremia as a result of SIADH, as shown in Table 62.5. SIADH is characterized by hyponatremia in the face of normal or increased blood volume, normal renal function, and the absence of factors that normally operate to produce antidiuretic hormone release. The syndrome may be relatively asymptomatic, in which case, water restriction is the treatment of choice. In more severe cases, hypertonic saline combined with a diuretic may be required. Overly zealous treatment may produce central

pontine myelinolysis (see Therapy, later in this chapter). Chronic syndromes have been treated successfully with a variety of drugs, including the tetracycline demeclocycline, which interferes with the action of antidiuretic hormone on the renal tubules.

Great care must be taken when considering the diagnosis of SIADH in patients with subarachnoid hemorrhage. Patients with subarachnoid hemorrhage, hyponatremia, and reduced blood volume may not have true SIADH. In these patients fluid restriction may lead to further volume reduction and cerebral infarcts during the period of the highest risk for vasospasm. The mechanisms underlying this phenomenon are not clear but may be related to the complexity of the peptidergic neurotransmitter systems in the vicinity of the third ventricle and to the possibility that they are damaged by the ruptured aneurysm. Damage is especially likely with an aneurysm on the anterior communicating artery. Hyponatremia occurs in approximately 1% of patients with recent surgical procedures. Because the symptoms are frequently mild or attributed to the surgery itself, this diagnosis may be missed. Typically, these patients seem to do well in the immediate postoperative period and then develop symptoms and signs of encephalopathy. Men and postmenopausal women are less likely to develop postoperative hyponatremia than women who are still menstruating. Complications, such as respiratory arrest, are particularly likely to occur in menstruating women and occur at higher serum sodium concentrations than in men or menopausal women. Thus, it is important to be particularly vigilant when evaluating younger women with postoperative encephalopathy.

Therapy.   The treatment of hyponatremia always has been controversial and has become more so since the link between hyponatremia and the subsequent development of central pontine myelinolysis was recognized and experimental replication of the syndrome achieved. Harris et al. (1993) reviewed this problem. They were not able to iden-

Table 62.5: Causes of the syndrome of inappropriate secretion of antidiuretic hormone

Malignant neoplasms
   Small cell carcinoma of lung
   Pancreas
   Thymoma
   Mesothelioma
   Lymphoma (lymphosarcoma, reticulum cell sarcoma,
      Hodgkin's disease)
   Bladder, ureter, prostate
   Duodenum
   Ewing's sarcoma
Central nervous system disorders
   Infections (meningitis, encephalitis, abscess, Rocky Mountain
      spotted fever)
   Trauma
   Subarachnoid hemorrhage
   Infarction
   Guillain-Barré syndrome
   Acute intermittent porphyria
   Hydrocephalus
   Neonatal hypoxia
   Shy-Drager syndrome
   Delirium tremens
   Systemic lupus erythematosus
Drugs
   Vasopressin
   Oxytocin
   Vinca alkaloids
   Thiazides
   Chlorpropamide
   Phenothiazines
   Carbamazepine
   Clofibrate
   Nicotine
   Monoamine oxidase inhibitors
   Tricyclic antidepressants
   Cyclophosphamide
   Narcotics
Pulmonary diseases
   Tuberculosis
   Other pneumonias
   Abscess or cavity
   Empyema
   Cystic fibrosis
   Obstructive airway disease
   Pneumothorax
   Asthma
   Positive pressure ventilation
Miscellaneous causes
   Hypothyroidism
   Acute psychosis
   Postoperative state
   Idiopathic

tify the rate at which serum sodium was corrected, the absolute magnitude of the correction, or the type of solution infused as a factor that predisposed to the development of central pontine myelinolysis. They noted that there are undoubtedly thousands of patients with symptomatic hyponatremia who have been treated successfully using a large number of protocols but who have not been reported. This makes it impossible to estimate the risk of central pontine myelinolysis associated with any given treatment regimen. However, because they were unable to identify any cases of central pontine myelinolysis among the 185 published examples of symptomatic hyponatremia (published since 1954) in which patients were allowed to "self-correct" during a period of water restriction (as opposed to the infusion of saline solutions of varied concentrations), they suggested that the preferred therapy of hyponatremia might be water restriction and discontinuing diuretics. Fraser and Arieff (1997) recommend the use of hypertonic sodium chloride for the treatment of symptomatic hyponatremia. Infusions should be adjusted to increase the plasma sodium concentration at a rate of 1 mmol/liter per hour. Complicating factors such as evidence for cerebral edema or seizures require more rapid correction of the deficit. A rate of 4–5 mmol/liter per hour was suggested. Hypertonic saline therapy may be discontinued when patients become asymptomatic, when the serum sodium reaches 120–125 mmol/liter, or when the plasma sodium has increased by a total of 20 mmol/liter. Protection of the airway and ventilator support may be required. Diuretics acting at the loop of Henle, such as furosemide, may be required. It is important to monitor electrolytes at frequent intervals (every 2 hours) and to avoid the administration of excessive amounts of sodium and the production of hypernatremia.

Hyperosmolality. Hyperosmolality is less common than hypo-osmolality but may present with similar symptoms or evidence of intracranial bleeding caused by the tearing of veins that bridge the space between the brain and dural sinuses. Usually, hyperosmolality is diagnosed by laboratory findings of an elevated serum sodium or, perhaps more commonly, hyperglycemia in diabetics. The syndrome frequently is caused by dehydration, especially in hot climates; by uncontrolled diabetes with or without ketosis; and, less frequently, by central lesions that reset the osmotically sensitive regions of the brain. As with hypo-osmolality, cautious correction of the defect is important. The following formula can be used to estimate the water deficit:

Deficit in liters = 0.6 (body weight in kg) × (1–140/plasma Na)

Thus, a 70-kg patient with a serum sodium of 150 mEq/liter would have a deficit of 2.8 liters. Replacement should be given orally, if possible. The first half of the deficit can be given rapidly, but the second half must be given with much more caution to avoid producing iatrogenic brain swelling as the whole-body osmotic pressure decreases.

Chronic hyperosmolality is associated with relative brain volume preservation as a result of the production of idiogenic osmoles, as described earlier. Administering free water at a rate that exceeds the rate at which the brain is able to rid itself of idiogenic osmoles is associated with the development of paradoxical brain edema that occurs at a time when serum glucose and electrolyte concentrations are normalized. This is illustrated by the data in Figure 62.3, in which the CSF pressure was measured continuously as hyperglycemia caused by diabetes mellitus was corrected. The increase in intracranial pressure is undoubtedly caused by adapted brain cells imbibing free water as serum osmolality decreases in response to therapy. If patients undergoing treatment for hyperosmolar states develop new neurological signs, including altered consciousness and seizures, the diagnosis of brain swelling should be considered. Mannitol treatment to restore osmolality to the prior elevated level may be required to prevent death caused by brain swelling.

Disorders of Calcium

Hypercalcemia and hypocalcemia both have diverse causes associated with disordered parathyroid gland function and a variety of other conditions. Under normal circumstances, approximately one-half of the total serum calcium is bound to proteins, mainly albumin, and one-half is in the ionized form, the only form in which it is active. When there is doubt about the ionized calcium concentration, as in patients with hypoalbuminemia, direct measurement of ionized calcium with ion-sensitive electrodes may be advisable.

Hypercalcemia is associated with hyperparathyroidism; granulomatous diseases, especially sarcoidosis; treatment with drugs including thiazide diuretics; vitamin D; calcium itself; tumors that have metastasized to bone; and thyroid disease. Many cases are idiopathic. The symptoms and signs of hypercalcemia may be protean. Severe hypercalcemia affects the brain directly, causing coma in extreme cases. In this group of patients, metastatic tumors are common, especially multiple myeloma and tumors of the breast and lung. Cancer patients seem to be particularly vulnerable to developing hypercalcemia after a change in therapy. Less severe hypercalcemia may cause altered consciousness with a pseudodementia syndrome and weakness. GI, renal, and cardiovascular abnormalities also may be present.

Severe hypercalcemia is life threatening. Initial treatment consists of a forced diuresis using saline and diuretics. Because the volumes of saline that are required may be large, a central venous or Swan-Ganz catheter may be needed to monitor therapy. Under these circumstances, in elderly patients or in those with cardiovascular or renal disease, treatment should be undertaken in collaboration with an internist. Once the initial phase of treatment is accomplished, further management is determined by the cause of the hypercalcemia.

Hypocalcemia usually is associated with hypoparathyroidism. The neurological symptoms are caused by the enhanced excitability of the nervous system. Symptoms include paresthesias around the mouth and fingers, cramps caused by tetanic muscle contraction, and in more extreme cases, epileptic seizures. In more chronic hypocalcemia, headache caused by increased intracranial pressure may occur, and extrapyramidal signs and symptoms such as

chorea or parkinsonism may be encountered. These patients may have calcification of the basal ganglia, evident on computed tomographic scans of the brain. The physical examination should include attempts to elicit Chvostek's and Trousseau's signs. Cataracts and papilledema may be seen.

Severe hypocalcemia should be treated with infusions of calcium to treat or prevent epileptic seizures or laryngeal spasms, both of which are life-threatening but unusual complications. Chronic therapy usually involves administering calcium and vitamin D. Care must be taken to avoid hypercalcemia and hypercalciuria. Consultation with an endocrinologist is prudent, but continued neurological care may be necessary, especially in patients with extrapyramidal syndromes, who may require specific treatment.

Disorders of Magnesium

Hypermagnesemia is an unusual condition because of the ease with which normal kidneys act to preserve magnesium homeostasis. The most frequent cause of hypermagnesemia is infusions given to treat symptoms of eclampsia, in which its effect to lower blood pressure and inhibit the nervous system is desirable. Care must be observed in administering magnesium to patients with renal failure because of any cause. This group of patients is the most vulnerable and the most likely to develop hypermagnesemia because the kidneys' homeostatic function is impaired. Hypocalcemia potentiates the effects of excess magnesium. Severe hypermagnesemia is life threatening, and concentrations in excess of 10 mEq/liter must be treated. Usually, discontinuing magnesium preparations suffices. When cardiac arrhythmias are present or circulatory collapse is possible, calcium must be infused, especially when hypocalcemia is present.

Isolated hypomagnesemia is unusual. Magnesium deficiency usually occurs in patients with deficiencies of other electrolytes. Hypomagnesemia may result from a diet deficient in magnesium, including prolonged parenteral alimentation with insufficient or no magnesium replacement, malabsorption, and alcoholism. Excess magnesium loss from the GI tract or the kidneys also can lead to calcium deficiency. Magnesium deficiency is usually part of a complex electrolyte imbalance, and accurate diagnosis and management of all aspects of the state are necessary to ensure recovery.

Pure magnesium deficiency has been produced experimentally and is expressed primarily through secondary reductions in serum calcium levels in spite of adequate dietary calcium intake. Ultimately, anorexia, nausea, a positive Trousseau's sign, weakness, lethargy, and tremor develop but are rapidly abolished by magnesium repletion. Balance studies indicate that magnesium deficiency causes a positive sodium and calcium balance and a negative potassium balance. Magnesium is necessary for proper mobilization and homeostasis of calcium and the intracellular retention of potassium. Some of the effects of magnesium depletion are secondary to abnormalities of potassium and calcium metabolism.

Table 62.6:   Characteristics of drug overdose

1. Toxicity predicted by drug level—specific therapy determined by toxicology
   Acetaminophen, digoxin, ethylene glycol (not detected by most systems), lithium, salicylates, theophylline
2. Toxicity parallels drug level—supportive care required
   Barbiturates, ethanol, phenytoin
3. Toxicology confirms only clinical impression—clinical decisions determined by direct patient evaluation
   Cyanide, narcotics, organophosphates, tricyclic antidepressants
4. Toxicity correlates poorly with drug level—clinical decisions determined by direct patient evaluation
   Amphetamines, benzodiazepines, cocaine, hallucinogens, neuroleptics, phencyclidine, phenylpropanolamine

Source: Based on report of JD Mahoney, PL Gross, TA Stern, et al. Quantitative serum toxic screening in the management of suspected drug overdose. Am J Emerg Med 1990;8:16–22.

Disorders of Manganese

Manganese poisoning occurs primarily in manganese ore miners and causes parkinsonism. As presented in the section on hepatic encephalopathy, there is increasing evidence that accumulation of this metal in the brain causes the T1 magnetic resonance imaging hyperintensities and may be associated with disorders of dopaminergic neurotransmission.

DRUG OVERDOSE AND TOXIC EXPOSURES

The tentative diagnosis of intentional or accidental drug overdose must be considered during the course of the evaluation of almost all emergency department patients with altered behavior (see Chapter 64). Most overdoses are attributable to drugs in one of six groups that account for more than 80% of all positive laboratory results. They are, in order of decreasing frequency, ethanol, benzodiazepines, salicylates, acetaminophen, barbiturates, and tricyclic antidepressants. Table 62.6 classifies drugs into four groups based on the usefulness of toxicological information and the relationships between drug levels and symptomatology. Regional poison control centers usually are staffed by well-informed, helpful personnel and should be consulted if further information is needed or there is uncertainty about the contents of specific products. Reported patterns of drug overdoses vary among communities and with time. Illicit drug availability varies substantially by region and evolves constantly. So-called designer drugs are unpredictable. As benzodiazepine use has increased and replaced barbiturates used as sleeping pills, barbiturate intoxications have declined. The prevalence of overdose varies as a function of the number of prescriptions written.

Miscellaneous Disorders

Neurologists may be asked to evaluate patients with vague complaints such as headache, poor concentration and memory, and other symptoms to determine whether toxin exposure is a contributing factor. These requests may occur during the course of ordinary patient care, litigation, or more systematic population-based investigations. In some instances, the doctor-patient relationship is clouded by political or legal ramifications of the questions asked and the possible answers. Current concerns about Gulf War syndrome typify this dilemma (Lockwood 1997). Many veterans of the Persian Gulf conflict contend that a variety of problems ranging from the complaints outlined previously to more definitive problems, such as amyotrophic lateral sclerosis, a variety of cancers, birth defects among their children, and others, are the consequence of exposure to chemicals, including insecticides, pyridostigmine bromide, and nerve agents. This anxiety was heightened by the revelation in the summer of 1997 that the destruction of a munitions depot in Khamisiyah, Iraq, in March 1991 released a cloud of sarin that exposed almost 100,000 troops to this nerve agent. Even though there were no documented acute effects of sarin on the exposed combatants, suspicion and distrust of the federal authorities charged with evaluating the Gulf War veterans were heightened by the charges of cover-up that were inevitable because of the delay in acknowledging the exposure. In spite of investigations that have failed to show excess mortality in Gulf War veterans, increases in birth defects in their children, or more frequent hospitalizations, this issue is far from settled. The findings of a Presidential Advisory Council and an independently chartered committee appointed by the National Academy of Sciences Institute of Medicine also have failed to satisfy those who believe that Gulf War syndrome is a real entity.

A similar and parallel situation has arisen among some who complain that pesticide exposure has affected their health. Because many pesticides are organophosphate cholinesterase inhibitors (OPCI, differing from nerve agents in potency), links between exposure and a variety of complaints have been claimed or sought. Worldwide, OPCIs are a common cause of death in agricultural workers, particularly in undeveloped nations. In Western countries, death is uncommon, but accidental or intentional exposure may occur (ingestion by children, overdose by adults, and so forth). OPCIs may cause peripheral neuropathy, as described in Chapter 64. Comparisons among control populations and OPCI-exposed subjects have shown differences in performance on certain neuropsychological tests, buttressing claims of disability and distress among exposed individuals. Again, in this area, emotions, politics, and other considerations may dominate. As a result of these concerns, the National Research Council on Pesticide Residues in the Diets of Infants and Children was established. This group concluded that some children may indeed be exposed to more than a reference dose of some pesticides. Among their recommendations, the panel urged abolition of "pesticide tolerances" defined by the pesticide industry on the basis of agricultural practices and replacement by considerations based on health.

For both of these examples, there is a uniform recognition that there is a cohort of patients who have real complaints and real illnesses. They deserve treatment independent of other issues related to unresolved classification and etiology issues. The clinical neuroscience community faces a major challenge in the development of regulations that govern exposure to potential toxins that are within the limits of science while providing adequate protection for the public and social accountability.

REFERENCES

Fraser CL, Arieff AI. Epidemiology, pathophysiology, and management of hyponatremic encephalopathy. Am J Med 1997;102:67–77.

Harris CP, Townsend JJ, Baringer JR. Symptomatic hyponatremia: can myelinolysis be prevented by treatment? J Neurol Neurosurg Psychiatry 1993;56:626–632.

Kulisevsky J, Pujol J, Balanzo C, et al. Pallidal hyperintensity on magnetic resonance imaging in cirrhotic patients: clinical correlations. Hepatology 1992;16:1382–1388.

Lingenfelser T, Renn W, Sommerwerck U, et al. Comprised hormonal counterregulation, symptom awareness, and neurophysiological function after recurrent short-term episodes of insulin-induced hypoglycemia in IDDM patients. Diabetes 1993;42:610–618.

Lockwood AH. Exposure to environmental toxins. Curr Opin Neurol 1997;10:507–511.

Lockwood AH, Murphy BW, Donnelly KZ, et al. Positron-emission tomographic localization of abnormalities of brain glucose metabolism in patients with minimal hepatic encephalopathy. Hepatology 1993;18:1061–1068.

Lockwood AH, Weissenborn, Butterworth RF. An image of the brain in patients with liver disease. Curr Opin Neurol 1997;10:525–533.

Longstreth WT Jr, Copass MK, Dennis LK, et al. Intravenous glucose after out-of-hospital cardiopulmonary arrest: a community-based randomized trial. Neurology 1993;43:2534–2541.

MacLeod KM, Hepburn DA, Frier BM. Frequency and morbidity of severe hypoglycemia in insulin-treated diabetic patients. Diabetic Med 1993;10:238–245.

Chapter 63
Deficiency Diseases of the Nervous System

Yuen T. So and Roger P. Simon

Undernutrition causes a wide spectrum of neurological disorders, ranging from isolated optic neuropathy to diffuse damage of the peripheral and central nervous systems. Of the more than 40 nutrients recognized today, vitamins are the most significant to neurologists. Although deficiency of almost any of the vitamins has been reported to produce neurological symptoms of some kind, the B vitamins (thiamine, pyridoxine, nicotinic acid, and vitamin B$_{12}$), vitamin E, and perhaps folic acid are the most important.

Nutritional deficiency is still a serious worldwide problem despite great advances since the turn of the twentieth century. Kwashiorkor and marasmus are endemic in many underdeveloped countries. The problem in Western countries is usually the result of dietary insufficiency from chronic alcoholism or malabsorption states from gastrointestinal (GI) diseases (Table 63.1). Drugs such as isoniazid and hydralazine also interfere by altering vitamin metabolism.

Most causes of nutritional deficiency, whether dietary or malabsorptive, do not selectively deplete a single vitamin. This is especially true among the malnourished populations in underdeveloped countries, where the diet may lack more than one vitamin and overlapping neurological syndromes

are the result. One exception is pernicious anemia, in which malabsorption is restricted to vitamin B$_{12}$.

Individual vitamin requirements are influenced by many factors. The daily need for both thiamine and nicotinic acid, important compounds in energy metabolism, increases proportionally with increasing caloric intake and energy need (e.g., symptoms of thiamine deficiency often occur in at-risk patients during periods of vigorous exercise and high carbohydrate intake). Other factors, such as growth, infection, and pregnancy, are known to worsen deficiency states, although the precise relationship is inadequately understood. Vitamin requirement is genetically determined in some cases, as in some infants dependent on unusually large doses of pyridoxine to prevent seizures. Low serum levels of vitamins in many individuals do not necessarily correlate with the occurrence of symptoms. As always, laboratory data should be interpreted in light of clinical findings.

The most frequent neurological deficits fall into several categories (Table 63.2). Peripheral neuropathy, the most common, occurs with the deficiency of many vitamins. Cerebral dysfunction, ranging from mental dullness to acute encephalopathy, may occur with deficiency of vita-

Table 63.1:   Causes of nutritional deficiencies and associated neurological syndromes

Underlying causes	Deficient nutrients	Neurological syndromes
Dietary deficiency	Protein and calories	Kwashiorkor and marasmus
	Thiamine	Beriberi, Wernicke-Korsakoff syndrome
	Nicotinic acid	Pellagra
	Pyridoxine	Encephalopathy, seizures, neuropathy
	Folate	Myelopathy, neuropathy, dementia
	Iodine	Cretinism
	Vitamin D	Myopathy
Alcoholism	Thiamine	Wernicke-Korsakoff syndrome
	Multifactorial	Neuropathy, cerebellar degeneration, Marchiafava-Bignami disease, amblyopia, and others
Malabsorption	Vitamin B_{12}	Combined system degeneration
	Vitamin E	Myelopathy, spinocerebellar degeneration
	Vitamin D	Myopathy
	Folate	Myelopathy, neuropathy, dementia
Congenital defect of absorption	Vitamin E	Bassen-Kornzweig syndrome
	Folate	Mental retardation, seizures
	Tryptophan and other amino acids	Hartnup disease
Drug antagonism—isoniazid	Pyridoxine	Neuropathy and seizures

min B_{12} or in Wernicke-Korsakoff syndrome. Myelopathy usually suggests a deficiency of vitamin B_{12}, although vitamin E and folate have been implicated in rare instances.

VITAMIN B_{12} DEFICIENCY

Vitamin B_{12}, cyanocobalamin, is one of several cobalamins having biological activity in the body. Cobalamins are abundant in meat, fish, and most animal by-products. Although vegetables are generally devoid of the vitamin, strict vegetarians almost never develop a clinical deficiency, because only 5 μg of vitamin B_{12} is needed per day and an adequate amount is available in legumes. Intrinsic factor, a binding protein secreted by gastric parietal cells, is needed for intestinal absorption of vitamin B_{12}; malabsorption caused by inadequate availability of intrinsic factor is probably the most common cause of vitamin B_{12} deficiency. Vitamin B_{12} deficiency is one of a few nutritional diseases encountered regularly by neurologists in North America.

Table 63.2:   Neurological manifestations in deficiency diseases

Neurological manifestations	Associated nutritional deficiencies
Dementia, encephalopathy	Vitamin B_{12}, nicotinic acid, thiamine, folate
Seizures	Pyridoxine
Myelopathy	Vitamin B_{12}, vitamin E, folate
Myopathy	Vitamin D, vitamin E
Peripheral neuropathy	Thiamine, vitamin B_{12}, vitamin E, pyridoxine, folate
Optic neuropathy	Vitamin B_{12}, thiamine, folate, and probably others

Clinical Features

The onset of symptoms is insidious, with paresthesias in the hands or feet in the majority of patients. Weakness and unsteadiness of gait are the next most frequent complaints. Lhermitte's sign may be present. Cerebral symptoms, such as mental slowing, depression, confusion, delusions, and hallucinations, are quite common, and occasionally patients present with only cognitive or psychiatric symptoms. Many patients also complain of dyspepsia, flatulence, altered bowel habits, or other GI symptoms.

On examination, most patients show signs of both peripheral nerve and spinal cord involvement, although either can be affected first in the early stage of the disorder. Loss of vibration or joint position sense in the legs is the most consistent abnormality. If impaired position sense is severe, Romberg's sign may be present. Tendon reflexes often are decreased or absent in the legs, although the effect on reflexes is quite variable. Motor impairment, if present, results from pyramidal tract dysfunction and is most severe in the legs, ranging from mild clumsiness and hyperreflexia to spastic paraplegia and extensor plantar responses. Visual impairment occasionally is encountered and may antedate other manifestations of vitamin deficiency; ophthalmological examination reveals bilateral visual loss, optic atrophy, and centrocecal scotomata. Brainstem or cerebellar signs or even reversible coma may occur.

Laboratory Studies

The classic picture of macrocytic anemia is seen inconsistently. Erythrocyte or bone marrow macrocytosis or hypersegmentation of polymorphonuclear cells may be present without anemia. Occasionally, hematological abnormalities may be completely absent at the time of neurological presentation. Achlorhydria is present in many patients with pernicious anemia, but measuring gastric pH is no longer diagnostically useful since the widespread availability of serum assay of vitamin B_{12}.

Serum cobalamin may be measured either with a radioassay or a chemiluminescence assay. The later is becoming increasingly popular, but it yields a higher normal reference range (250–1,100 pg/ml as compared with 170–900 pg/ml for radioassay). A normal serum cobalamin level does not exclude a deficiency state (Savage et al. 1994). Serum measurement of vitamin B_{12} is complicated by most of the cobalamins present in serum being bound to several transport proteins (transcobalamins I, II, and III). The cobalamin bound to transcobalamin II is the most important physiological fraction, but it accounts for only 10–30% of the serum level measured by standard laboratory methods. Serum levels are influenced by conditions that may affect transcobalamin concentrations. Myeloproliferative and hepatic disorders may raise the concentration of transcobalamin I and III, and cause a falsely normal serum level. A misleadingly high serum level also may result from the presence of an abnormal cobalamin-binding protein. In contrast, pregnancy may give low measurements in the absence of deficiency, and low values may be encountered in patients without macrocytosis or clinical disease.

Homocysteine and methylmalonic acid, precursors of vitamin B_{12}–dependent pathways, are elevated in more than 90% of patients with cobalamin deficiency. Assay of these metabolites is appropriate in patients with suspected clinical disease. In 1992, Pennypacker and colleagues suggested it is especially useful in those with low normal serum vitamin B_{12} levels in the range of 200–350 pg/ml and in those with neurological deficits secondary to nitrous oxide abuse (see Pathogenesis and Etiology, later in this chapter).

Abnormally low serum vitamin B_{12} or elevated metabolite levels provide confirmatory evidence of deficiency in the presence of an appropriate neurological picture. Further evaluation should include measurement of antibodies against parietal cell and against intrinsic factor, either of which may be elevated in 60–90% of patients. A dietary history is helpful occasionally, though inadequate dietary intake is seldom a sole cause of cobalamin deficiency. Schilling's test should be considered to further document the underlying cause of malabsorption. If uncertainty persists, a therapeutic trial of vitamin B_{12} may be useful.

There may be other laboratory abnormalities but they are seldom helpful in establishing the diagnosis. Nonspecific electroencephalographic abnormalities may be present and follow-up electroencephalography in selected cases can provide one of the earliest objective responses to vitamin B_{12} therapy. Visual and somatosensory responses are frequently abnormal; nerve conduction studies show small or absent sural nerve sensory potentials in approximately 80% of patients, providing evidence for an axonal polyneuropathy.

Physiology

Dietary vitamin B_{12} binds readily to intrinsic factor, and the complex is transported to the ileum, where it is absorbed into the circulation via specific receptors on ileal mucosal cells. Once absorbed, vitamin B_{12} binds to transcobalamins for transport to tissues. As much as 90% of total body vitamin B_{12} (1–10 mg) is stored in the liver. Even when vitamin absorption is severely impaired, many years are needed to deplete the body store. A clinical relapse in pernicious anemia after interrupting vitamin B_{12} therapy takes an average of 5 years to be recognized.

Biochemistry

Two biochemical reactions depend on vitamin B_{12}. The one that has received the most attention is a folate-dependent reaction in which the methyl group of methyltetrahydrofolate is transferred to homocysteine to yield methionine. The homocysteine-to-methionine reaction depends on the enzyme methionine synthase, which has cobalamin as a cofactor. Reduced cofactor activity from cobalamin deficiency eventually leads to impaired DNA synthesis, although the precise mechanism is not settled (Tefferi and Pruthi 1994). The other cobalamin-dependent reaction, conversion of methylmalonyl coenzyme A to succinyl coenzyme A, is of unclear significance in the nervous system complications of vitamin B_{12} deficiency.

Pathology

The term *subacute combined degeneration of the spinal cord* describes the pathological process seen in vitamin B_{12} deficiency. Microscopically, spongy changes and foci of myelin and axon destruction are seen in the white matter of the spinal cord. The most severely affected regions are the posterior columns at the cervical and upper thoracic levels (Figure 63.1); pathological changes also are seen commonly in the lateral columns, whereas the anterior columns are involved in only a small number of the advanced cases. The pathological findings of the peripheral nervous system are those of axonal degeneration, but in some cases there is evidence of demyelination. Involvement of the optic nerve and cerebral white matter also occurs.

Pathogenesis and Etiology

Pernicious anemia caused by defective intrinsic factor production by parietal cells probably accounts for most cases of vitamin B_{12} deficiency. Many of these patients have circulating antibodies to parietal cells or lymphocytic infiltrations of the gastric mucosa, suggesting an underlying autoimmune disorder. Another cause of intrinsic factor defi-

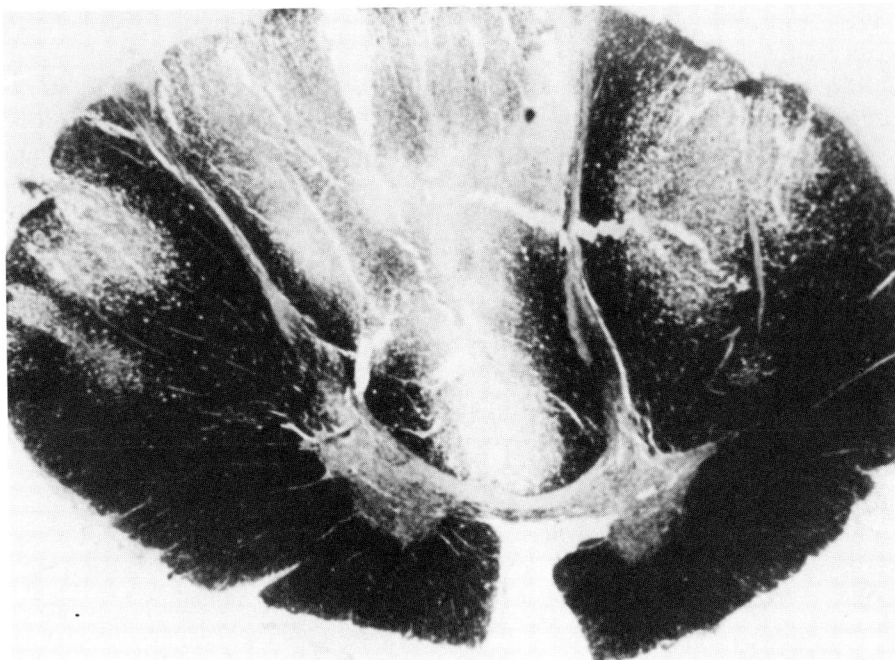

FIGURE 63.1 Subacute combined degeneration of the spinal cord in vitamin B_{12} deficiency. Demyelination and loss of axons are more widespread in posterior than in lateral columns. (Weigert's stain.) (Courtesy of Dr. Michael F. Gonzales.)

ciency is gastrectomy, although it rarely leads to symptomatic deficiency in isolation. Other cases of malabsorption are surgical resection of the terminal ileum and blind loop syndrome. Drugs such as colchicine also cause megaloblastic anemia, presumably via interference with the intestinal absorption of the vitamin. Rare cases of dietary insufficiency occur in strict vegetarians (vegans) without evidence of vitamin B_{12} malabsorption. Low serum level of vitamin B_{12} also occurs in approximately 20–30% of patients with acquired immunodeficiency syndrome (AIDS). Even in AIDS patients with a low cobalamin level, serum homocysteine and methylmalonic acid levels are often within the normal range (Paltiel et al. 1995). Whether the cobalamin abnormalities in AIDS are merely laboratory phenomena or important contributors to the neurological complications of AIDS awaits clarification.

After heavy abuse of nitrous oxide, subjects may develop a clinical syndrome of myeloneuropathy indistinguishable from that of vitamin B_{12} deficiency. Symptoms include numbness, paresthesia, Lhermitte's sign, gait ataxia, and leg weakness. Subjects improve slowly when nitrous oxide is stopped but the myelopathy may never completely recover. Serum vitamin B_{12} level and Schilling's test result are almost always normal, and hematological derangements are usually inconspicuous. The mechanism appears to be an interference with the vitamin B_{12}-dependent conversion of homocysteine to methionine. The other pathway, conversion of methylmalonyl coenzyme A to succinyl coenzyme A, is unaffected by nitrous oxide. Prolonged exposure to nitrous oxide is necessary to produce neurological symptoms in normal individuals. By contrast, patients who are already vitamin B_{12} deficient may experience neurological

deficits after brief exposures to nitrous oxide during general anesthesia. Symptoms typically appeared 2–6 weeks after surgery and resolved quickly with vitamin B_{12} treatment (Green and Kinsella 1995).

Course and Prognosis

With proper treatment, at least partial improvement can be expected in most instances. Most of the symptomatic improvement occurs during the first 6 months of therapy, although it may not be complete for a year or more. The need for early diagnosis and treatment is underscored by the remission of symptoms being correlated inversely with the time lapse between onset of symptoms and initiation of therapy. Recently acquired manifestations are much more likely to reverse than those that are long-standing.

Treatment and Management

Any patient with clinically overt vitamin B_{12} deficiency should be treated with parenteral vitamin therapy aimed at replenishing the total body pool. The usual regimen uses intramuscular injections of 100 mg daily or 1,000 mg twice weekly for 2 weeks. This is followed by weekly injections of 1,000 mg for another 2–3 months. If Schilling's test demonstrates malabsorption of vitamin B_{12}, the patient should be placed on lifelong maintenance therapy, usually in the form of monthly 1,000-mg injections. Oral preparations of intrinsic factor are available but unfortunately are not reliable for clinical use. Antibodies to intrinsic factor may nullify its effectiveness in the intestinal lumen, and many patients eventually become refractory to intrinsic factor therapy. The parenteral dose of vitamin B_{12} recommended here provides quantities considerably higher than the usual body requirement. Although there is no evidence that overdosing can speed neurological recovery, adverse reactions to high doses of vitamin B_{12} are unknown.

FOLATE DEFICIENCY

Theoretically, folate deficiency can produce neurological deficits identical to those seen in vitamin B_{12} deficiency. Methyltetrahydrofolate, a folic acid derivative, is central to the vitamin B_{12}-dependent reaction that converts homocysteine to methionine. However, the importance of folate in neurological diseases continues to be debated. A low serum folate level is commonly encountered in elderly patients, many of whom are asymptomatic. Folate generally is present in the brain at concentrations several times higher than that in serum, and it is uncertain how a low serum level correlates with deficiency in neural tissues. Human folate deficiency often coexists with diseases such as alcoholism and generalized malabsorption, both of which can produce neurological complications. It is difficult to prove a causal relationship even if clinical improvement occurs at the same time as therapy; concurrently administered treatments, such as increased attention to diet, psychosocial support, and physical therapy, conceivably may account for many of the so-called folate-responsive cases. Supplemental vitamins also may be inadvertently given, for example, an injection of cobalamin during Schilling's test is sufficient to reverse transiently the symptoms of vitamin B_{12} deficiency.

Clinical Features

The vast majority of patients with folate deficiency have only hematological abnormalities without neurological changes. Of the neurological syndromes attributable to folate deficiency, the most carefully documented resembles, in all practical aspects, the subacute combined degeneration of pernicious anemia. Presenting symptoms are weakness and gait unsteadiness. Patients have megaloblastic anemia, impaired position and vibration sense, pyramidal signs, and, possibly, dementia. A causal relationship between folate deficiency and peripheral neuropathy is difficult to establish.

Chronic alcoholism is probably the most important cause of folate deficiency. Folate deficiency is also a common complication of diseases of the small intestine. Other populations at risk are pregnant women and patients receiving anticonvulsant drugs that interfere with folate metabolism. Patients with Crohn's disease and ulcerative colitis often have low serum folate levels and occasionally megaloblastic hematological changes. Probably only a small proportion of patients with low serum folate develop nervous system manifestations.

Laboratory Studies

Assays of serum erythrocyte folate level are readily available. Erythrocyte folate is less affected by short-term fluctuation in intake but may be falsely low in patients with vitamin B_{12} deficiency. The hematological picture of the megaloblastic anemia is identical to that seen in pernicious anemia.

Physiology and Biochemistry

Folic acid refers to a group of pteridine compounds necessary for a number of one-carbon transfer reactions in the body. Its major function is probably in the biosynthesis of purines and other biological macromolecules.

Treatment and Management

Although there may be doubts about the importance of folate deficiency in neurological diseases, its pathogenic role in megaloblastic anemia is undeniable. Moreover, it is an easily treatable condition. The initial dose is usually 1 mg of folate several times per day, followed by a maintenance dose of 1 mg per day. For acutely ill patients, parenteral doses of 1–5 mg may be given. Even with oral doses as high as 15 mg per day, there is no substantiated report of toxicity. It is important to keep in mind that large doses of folate can correct the megaloblastic anemia of vitamin B_{12} deficiency without altering the neurological abnormalities. A hematological response to folate, therefore, does not preclude the diagnosis of pernicious anemia.

VITAMIN E DEFICIENCY

Clinical Features

Like other fat-soluble vitamins, vitamin E normally is stored to a massive degree in the body. Clinical symptoms, therefore, do not begin until many years of malabsorption have depleted the vitamin reserves. In adults, this usually takes 15–20 years, but an onset as early as 2–3 years of age occurs in children, presumably because of their small vitamin reserves.

The presenting symptoms are usually weakness or gait unsteadiness. Neurological examination reveals a syndrome of spinocerebellar degeneration, often accompanied by a varying degree of peripheral nerve involvement. Some patients are diagnosed erroneously with Friedreich's ataxia. The most consistent abnormalities are limb ataxia, areflexia, and severe loss of vibration and position sense. Cutaneous sensation usually is spared or affected to a lesser degree. Approximately one-half of the patients have nystagmus, ptosis, or partial external ophthalmoplegia. Mild

Table 63.3:   Causes of vitamin E deficiency

Gastrointestinal diseases
   Biliary atresia, chronic cholestasis
   Intestinal resection
   Crohn's disease
   Pancreatic insufficiency (e.g., cystic fibrosis)
   Blind loop syndrome and bacterial overgrowth
   Bowel irradiation
   Other causes of steatorrhea
   Celiac disease
Hereditary diseases
   Abetalipoproteinemia
   α-Tocopherol transfer protein mutation

to moderate proximal weakness is common, although weakness can be diffuse or predominantly distal. Babinski's sign is present in fewer than one-half of the reported cases.

Laboratory Studies

The diagnosis is not difficult when the appropriate neurological syndrome and a low serum vitamin E level are both present. Serum level always should be interpreted in light of the clinical findings. Many patients with low levels do not have demonstrable neurological deficits. Moreover, plasma vitamin E is largely incorporated into chylomicrons and is, therefore, highly dependent on the concentrations of total plasma lipids, cholesterol, and very-low-density lipoproteins.

Other laboratory abnormalities, despite their nonspecific nature, help to clarify the diagnosis. Stool fat is increased in many patients, and serum carotene concentration is often abnormally low, both reflecting a generalized state of fat malabsorption. Cerebrospinal fluid should be normal. Nerve conduction studies usually reveal a mild axonal neuropathy, with diminished or absent sural nerve action potentials and normal or slightly slow motor nerve conduction. Somatosensory and visual evoked responses are frequently abnormal. Whether a vitamin E deficiency myopathy exists in humans as it does in animals is not settled.

Physiology and Biochemistry

Vitamin E has been known for some time to be an excellent scavenger of free radical groups in the body. By reacting with free radicals and perhaps with other oxidative intermediates, vitamin E functions as an effective antioxidant capable of stabilizing polyunsaturated membrane lipids. It is, therefore, potentially important in maintaining the integrity of cellular membranes. Whether this action bears any relationship to the development of neurological deficits in the deficiency state is uncertain.

Pathology

Few cases of proven vitamin E deficiency have come to autopsy. Degeneration of large myelinated fibers may be present in the peripheral nerves, posterior columns, and sensory roots. Accumulations of lipopigments are seen in both neurons and endothelial cells, especially prominent in the spinal cord and the cerebellum.

Pathogenesis and Etiology

Like other fat-soluble compounds, vitamin E depends on the presence of pancreatic esterases and bile salts for its solubilization and absorption in the intestinal lumen. Neurological symptoms of deficiency occur most commonly in patients with significant fat malabsorption (Table 63.3). A reduced bile salt pool may be caused either by reduced hepatic excretion, as in congenital cholestasis, or by interruption of the enterohepatic reabsorption of bile, as in patients with extensive small bowel resection. Another setting for malabsorption is cystic fibrosis.

A rare familial form of fat malabsorption is abetalipoproteinemia (Bassen-Kornzweig syndrome), a disorder in which impaired chylomicron and lipoprotein synthesis is at least partly responsible for the impaired fat absorption (Kayden 1993). In addition to a neurological syndrome strikingly similar to that seen in other vitamin E–deficient states, spiky red blood cells (acanthocytes) and retinal pigment changes are characteristic. Vitamin E therapy may halt or even reverse the progression of neurological impairment in these patients.

Isolated vitamin E deficiency occurs in patients without any GI disease or generalized fat malabsorption. This syndrome may be inherited in an autosomal recessive manner. The defect appears to be impaired incorporation of the vitamin into hepatic lipoproteins that are necessary for delivery to tissues. Different mutations in the α-tocopherol transfer protein gene on chromosome 8q13 may occur in some patients (Cavalier et al. 1998).

Treatment and Management

The recommended daily requirement of vitamin E in normal adults is 10 mg (equivalent to 10 IU) of d,l-alpha-tocopherol acetate, a commonly available form of the vitamin. In the deficiency state, a wide range of doses has been used, ranging from 200 mg per day to 100 mg per kg per day. Although there is little consensus on the optimal therapeutic dosage, there is also no evidence of toxicity from overdose. A reasonable approach is to begin therapy with an oral preparation of water-miscible tocopherol at a dose of 200–600 mg per day. The clinical picture and serum level should be followed; if no improvement occurs, higher oral dosages or even parenteral administration should be tried. Supplementation of bile salts may be of value in some patients.

PELLAGRA (NICOTINIC ACID DEFICIENCY)

Nicotinic acid (*niacin*, another term for nicotinic acid, was introduced to avoid confusion with the alkaloid nicotine) is converted in the body to two important coenzymes in carbohydrate metabolism: nicotinamide adenine dinucleotide and nicotinamide adenine dinucleotide phosphate. Dietary deficiency of nicotinic acid produces the syndrome in humans known as *pellagra* (from the Italian *pelle agra*, meaning *rough skin*). Pellagra occurs in populations whose diet consists chiefly of corn. Corn lacks nicotinic acid as well as tryptophan, a precursor that can be converted in the body to nicotinic acid. In many underdeveloped countries, pellagra is still a common health problem. Even in the United States, pellagra was endemic until approximately 1940 in the South and in alcoholic populations. It has now largely disappeared, credited to the widespread consumption of bread enriched with niacin.

Clinical Features

Pellagra classically affects three organ systems in the body: the GI tract, skin, and nervous system (hence the mnemonic of the three Ds: diarrhea, dermatitis, and dementia). The chief GI symptoms are anorexia, diarrhea, stomatitis, and abdominal discomfort. Skin changes range from erythema to a reddish-brown hyperkeratotic rash distributed over much of the body, with the face, chest, and dorsal surfaces of the hands and feet being most frequently involved.

The neurological syndrome of pellagra is not well defined. Reported cases, especially of patients with alcoholic pellagra, frequently are confounded by other coexisting central nervous system disorders. The primary early symptoms are neuropsychiatric (e.g., irritability, apathy, depressed mood, inattentiveness, memory loss) and may progress to stupor or coma. In addition to the confusional state, spasticity, Babinski's sign, gegenhalten, and startle myoclonus may be prominent on neurological examination.

Nonendemic pellagra occurs rarely in patients with alcoholism or malabsorption secondary to GI disease. The diagnosis of nonendemic pellagra can be made only on clinical grounds because there is no available blood niacin level determination, and diagnosis is frequently difficult because diarrhea and dermatological changes may be absent. Unexplained progressive encephalopathy in alcoholic patients not responsive to thiamine therapy (see Wernicke-Korsakoff Syndrome, later in this chapter) should raise the possibility of pellagra.

Treatment and Management

The recommended daily allowance for nicotinic acid is 6.6 mg/1,000 kcal dietary intake. Oral nicotinic acid in doses of 50 mg several times a day is usually sufficient to treat symptomatic patients. Alternatively, parenteral doses of 25 mg can be given two to three times a day. Nicotinamide has similar therapeutic efficacy in pellagra, but it does not have the vasodilatory and cholesterol-lowering activities of niacin.

VITAMIN B$_6$ (PYRIDOXINE) DEFICIENCY

Although the term *pyridoxine* often is used synonymously with vitamin B$_6$, two other closely related compounds—pyridoxal and pyridoxamine—also exist in nature, and both possess biological activities similar to pyridoxine. All three compounds are readily converted to pyridoxal phosphate, the coenzyme form important for the metabolism of many amino acids.

History

The original recognition of one of the complications of pyridoxine deficiency provides a useful lesson in nutrition. In the early 1950s, physicians in the United States encountered cases of an unusual seizure disorder affecting infants at the age of several weeks to a few months. The seizures were difficult to control with the usual anticonvulsant therapy. In contrast, the response was often dramatic when vitamin B$_6$ was given. As more patients were identified, it became clear that the symptomatic infants had been fed a commercially prepared liquid formula that contained only 60 mg/liter of vitamin B$_6$, or approximately one-third the amount found in other infant formulas. The underlying cause eventually was traced to a manufacturing process that apparently reduced the formula's pyridoxine content.

Clinical Features

Even with better awareness of the problem, sporadic cases of infantile seizures from dietary vitamin B$_6$ deficiency still occur, most commonly as a result of breast-feeding by malnourished mothers from poor socioeconomic backgrounds or in underdeveloped countries. The typical patients have a normal birth history and are entirely healthy until the development of hyperirritability and an exaggerated auditory startle. Recurrent convulsions often occur abruptly, as may status epilepticus. Once the dietary insufficiency is corrected, patients become free of seizures and develop normally.

Another form of pyridoxine-responsive seizure occurs in infants who develop symptoms despite a normal supply of pyridoxine from the diet and appear to have a congenital dependency on pyridoxine. In contrast to patients with dietary deficiency, these children manifest seizures earlier in life (within days of birth) and require much larger doses of pyridoxine (5–100 mg) to control their convulsions. Long-term administration of large amounts of pyridoxine is needed, generally in the range of 10 mg per day. Even after several years of successful treatment, seizures often reappear within days of pyridoxine withdrawal.

Whereas children with the classic pyridoxine-dependency syndrome manifest seizures in the neonatal period, cases may present later in infancy. Whether these infants have the same metabolic disease is uncertain. In any case, pyridoxine dependency should be considered in infants with undiagnosed seizures, especially in those with a poor response to anticonvulsants.

Adults in general are much more tolerant of vitamin B_6 deficiency. Not only are most adult diets adequate in pyridoxine and related compounds, symptoms are rare even when there is demonstrable vitamin deficiency. Isoniazid and a few other drugs, such as hydralazine and penicillamine, are probably responsible for most adult cases. This is especially a problem in slow inactivators of isoniazid, among whom as many as 50% may develop peripheral neuropathy when treated with the drug. Sensory symptoms generally appear first, consisting of numbness, tingling, and occasionally burning pain in the distal portions of the feet. If the drug is continued, symptoms may spread proximally to the knees and hands. Burning pain is disabling in some instances. On examination, there is distal weakness, depressed tendon reflexes, and impaired distal sensation.

Use of high doses of pyridoxine (1,000 mg per day or more) for several months causes a sensory neuropathy in a dose-dependent manner, according to Berger and colleagues' reporting in 1992. Reported patients ingesting such a high dose for a prolonged period had a syndrome of sensory ataxia, with impaired cutaneous and deep sensation, areflexia, and Romberg's sign. Many years of taking doses as low as 200 mg per day may also cause a mild, predominantly sensory polyneuropathy. Hence, in therapeutic use of pyridoxine, it seems prudent to limit dosage to 100 mg per day or less.

Treatment and Management

Treatment of pyridoxine-related seizures in infants was discussed earlier. The neurotoxicity of isoniazid and hydralazine is dose dependent. Even with high doses of isoniazid, pyridoxine supplements of 50 mg per day can prevent the development of neuropathy in nearly all patients.

BERIBERI (THIAMINE DEFICIENCY POLYNEUROPATHY)

Beriberi literally means extreme weakness. It affects the heart and peripheral nerves, producing congestive cardiomyopathy, sensorimotor polyneuropathy, or both. The classical wet and dry forms refer to the presence or absence of edema.

Clinical Features

The neuropathy generally progresses over several weeks or months. Affected patients characteristically complain of paresthesias or pain of the lower extremities. Walking may become difficult. Distal muscle weakness appears as the neuropathy worsens. Muscle tenderness and cramps, especially of the calves, are prominent in some cases. When cardiac dysfunction is present, patients also experience tachycardia, palpitations, dyspnea, fatigue, and peripheral edema at the ankles.

The most common neurological finding is a stocking-glove distribution of cutaneous sensory loss. Weakness, when present, occurs first in the finger and wrist extensors and the dorsiflexors of the ankle. Deep tendon reflexes of the ankles are lost in the majority of patients. Cranial nerve deficits are unusual, although there may be laryngeal nerve paralysis producing hoarseness and weakness of voice. A subacute optic neuropathy may be present and may occur rarely in thiamine-deficient patients given a ketogenic diet to control epilepsy.

Laboratory Studies

Diagnosis of beriberi is based primarily on recognizing the appropriate clinical features in a background of significant nutritional deficiency. Thiamine levels in serum and urine may be decreased in patients with beriberi. The assay, however, is of limited usefulness, because the level does not reliably reflect tissue concentrations. Erythrocyte transketolase activity level is dependent on thiamine and provides a better assay of functional status. Pyruvate accumulates during thiamine deficiency, and elevated serum level provides additional confirmation. A blood sample should be drawn before initiation of treatment because these laboratory abnormalities normalize quickly.

Electrodiagnostic studies show an axonal neuropathy with reduced amplitude of sensory or motor responses, normal or mildly reduced conduction velocity, and neurogenic changes on electromyography. Lumbar puncture sometimes shows a mildly elevated opening pressure, a finding probably related to the presence of congestive heart failure. Cerebrospinal fluid examination is otherwise unremarkable. If cardiac impairment is present, electrocardiographic abnormalities or cardiac enlargement on chest roentgenography may occur.

Physiology and Biochemistry

Thiamine is the precursor for the coenzyme thiamine pyrophosphate, which catalyzes the oxidative decarboxylation of pyruvate and alpha-ketoglutarate, with the eventual production of coenzyme A. Thiamine pyrophosphate also serves as a cofactor for the transketolase reaction in the hexose monophosphate shunt. A corollary of the biochemistry is the dependence of the thiamine requirement on the body's metabolic rate, with the requirement being greatest during periods of high metabolic demand or high glucose intake. This explains the clinical observation that symptoms of thiamine deficiency frequently occur during periods of refeeding or intravenous administration of glucose.

Pathology

Ultrastructural and morphometric analysis of sural nerve biopsy reveals axonal loss of wallerian type. Segmental demyelination is infrequent and probably secondary to axonal degeneration.

Epidemiology

Beriberi is rare in most industrialized nations. Even in Japan, where beriberi once accounted for over 20,000 deaths a year, the disease has all but disappeared. An exceptional outbreak in the 1970s occurred primarily in young people with a history of an unbalanced diet high in instant food, unfortified rice, and other carbohydrates and deficient in protein and vegetables. The symptoms typically appeared acutely or subacutely after a period of strenuous athletic training or heavy work. Exercise presumably precipitated the condition by raising the metabolic requirement for thiamine. Other causes of increased metabolic demands such as pregnancy, malignancy, and systemic infection may rarely precipitate symptoms, especially in people with marginal nutritional status. In developed countries, many cases are probably related to alcoholism, but it is often difficult to distinguish beriberi from alcoholic neuropathy.

Course and Prognosis

Gradual return of sensory and motor function can be expected after thiamine replenishment. Mildly affected patients experience considerable improvement after a few weeks of treatment; in severe cases, improvement may take many months and may be incomplete.

Treatment and Management

The major goal is to initiate a balanced diet with supplements of thiamine and other vitamins. Thiamine is water soluble and usually supplied as thiamine hydrochloride, either in crystalline form or as a 100-mg/ml solution. The minimum daily requirement is 0.3 mg/1,000 kcal dietary intake in normal subjects, but the requirement is higher during pregnancy and old age. For therapeutic purposes, 50–100 mg per day generally is used. The parenteral form of thiamine should be considered whenever there is doubt about adequate GI absorption.

Infantile Beriberi

An acute syndrome of thiamine deficiency in infants occurs in the rice-eating populations of Asia, most frequently in breast-fed infants less than 1 year of age; thiamine is often deficient in breast milk from mothers who eat primarily polished rice. Although the disorder is called *infantile beriberi*, it bears little resemblance to the adult form. Acute cardiac symptoms are common, often preceded by a prodrome of anorexia, vomiting, deficient weight gain, and restlessness. Dyspnea, cyanosis, and signs of heart failure follow and can lead rapidly to death. Arytenoid edema and recurrent laryngeal neuropathy give rise to hoarseness, dysphonia, and eventually aphonia. Early warning signs of coughing and choking may be mistaken for respiratory tract infections. Central nervous system manifestations include drowsiness, ophthalmoplegia, and convulsions. These symptoms often begin abruptly and carry a grave prognosis. Parenteral administration of 5–20 mg of thiamine can be lifesaving and should never be delayed.

WERNICKE-KORSAKOFF SYNDROME

Wernicke's Encephalopathy

History

Even though there were earlier descriptions of patients who probably had this form of encephalopathy, Carl Wernicke generally is credited with initially recognizing the disease. In 1881, he described an acute syndrome of mental confusion, ophthalmoplegia, and gait ataxia in three patients, two of whom were alcoholics. At autopsy, multiple small hemorrhages were seen affecting the periventricular gray matter, primarily around the aqueduct and the third and fourth ventricles.

Clinical Features

Although the most common clinical setting for Wernicke's encephalopathy is chronic alcoholism, a large number of cases occurs in other conditions, with the only prerequisite being a poor nutritional state, either from inadequate intake, malabsorption, or increased metabolic requirement (Table 63.4). Wernicke's encephalopathy may be precipitated acutely in at-risk patients by intravenous glucose administration or carbohydrate loading.

Wernicke's original description of the clinical triad of confusion, ophthalmoplegia, and ataxia is still diagnostically useful. Patients with classic Wernicke's encephalopa-

Table 63.4: Associated conditions in nonalcoholic patients with Wernicke's encephalopathy

Hyperemesis of pregnancy
Systemic malignancy
Gastrointestinal surgery
Hemodialysis or peritoneal dialysis
Prolonged intravenous feeding
Refeeding after prolonged fasting or starvation
Anorexia nervosa
Acquired immunodeficiency syndrome

thy experience a confusional state developing over days or weeks, with inattention, apathy, disorientation, and memory loss. Stupor or coma is rare. Most patients have horizontal nystagmus on lateral gaze, and many also have vertical nystagmus on upgaze. Ophthalmoplegia, when present, commonly involves both lateral recti, either in isolation or together with palsies of other extraocular muscles. Sluggish reaction to light, light-near dissociation, or other pupillary abnormalities sometimes are seen. Truncal ataxia is common, but limb ataxia is not, findings similar to those seen in alcoholic cerebellar degeneration.

Other frequent findings include hypothermia and postural hypotension, reflecting involvement of hypothalamic and brainstem autonomic pathways. Signs of nutritional deficiency and complications of alcoholism are common as are peripheral neuropathy, tongue redness, skin changes, and liver abnormalities. Many patients also show signs of acute alcohol withdrawal, with tremor, delirium, and tachycardia.

Laboratory Studies

Wernicke's encephalopathy remains a clinical diagnosis, as there is no distinctive laboratory abnormality. High-resolution magnetic resonance imaging may show shrunken mamillary bodies later in the disease or after repeated attacks. The cerebrospinal fluid is either normal or shows a mild elevation in protein content. Serum thiamine level and erythrocyte transketolase activity may be depressed, and there also may be an elevation of serum pyruvate, but the predictive values of these test results are unclear. Treatment should not be withheld while the clinician waits for laboratory results.

Physiology

The clinical findings reflect the localization of pathological abnormalities in this disease, namely, the prominent involvement of periventricular structures at the level of the third and fourth ventricles. Lesions of the nuclei of the III, VI, and vestibular nerves are responsible for the eye findings, and the truncal ataxia is probably caused by the vestibular dysfunction and involvement of the superior cerebellar vermis.

Biochemistry

Biochemistry is discussed in the section on beriberi.

Pathology

The pathological process depends on the age of the lesions. Macroscopically, varying degrees of congestion, petechial hemorrhages, shrinkage, and discoloration may be present (Figure 63.2). Chronic lesions are characterized by foci of glial proliferation and myelin pallor primarily affecting the aforementioned locations. In acute lesions, dilatation and hyperplasia of small blood vessels occur, with punctate hemorrhages in the subependymal gray matter.

Epidemiology

The frequency of Wernicke's encephalopathy as estimated from various autopsy studies is approximately 0.8–2.8%, a figure far greater than that expected from clinical studies. Only 20% of the cases in one series were diagnosed during life. This is disturbing because Wernicke's encephalopathy is readily preventable and treatable. One reason for this underrecognition is that some patients do not have the classic triad of ataxia, ophthalmoparesis, and encephalopathy. The misdiagnosis also may be caused by the overemphasis on chronic alcoholism as a cause. Wernicke's encephalopathy occurring under other settings may be mistaken for encephalopathy of uremia, dialysis, sepsis, or other systemic diseases.

Course and Prognosis

If left untreated, Wernicke's encephalopathy is progressive; the mortality, even with thiamine treatment, is 10–20%. The majority of ocular signs resolve rapidly within hours of treatment, although a fine horizontal nystagmus persists indefinitely in approximately 60% of patients. Apathy and lethargy improve over days or weeks. The gait disturbance resolves much more slowly, and in one-third or more of cases, gait may be abnormal even months after treatment. As the global confusional state recedes, many patients are left with a disorder of impaired memory and learning, that is, Korsakoff's syndrome.

Treatment and Management

To avoid precipitating acute worsening of symptoms, any patient suspected of Wernicke's encephalopathy should be given thiamine before administration of glucose. Thiamine is the only treatment known to alter the outcome of this disorder. The need to administer thiamine in patients with unexplained stupor or coma should be emphasized. Thiamine always should be given parenterally in the acute stage because intestinal absorption is unreliable in debilitated and alcoholic patients. Doses of 50–100 mg can be

FIGURE 63.2   Acute Wernicke's disease. Hemorrhagic areas are seen adjacent to the fourth ventricle and aqueduct in the (from right to left) medulla, pons, and midbrain. (Courtesy of Dr. Michael F. Gonzales.)

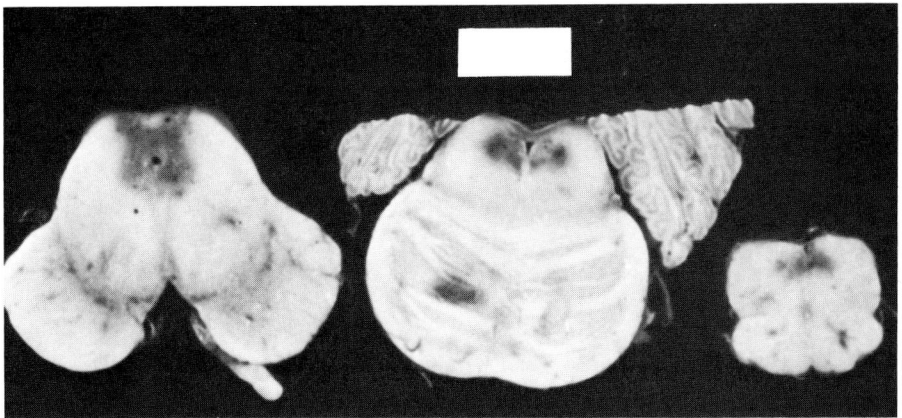

given safely via the intravenous route and should be continued daily throughout the acute period.

Korsakoff's Syndrome

Korsakoff's syndrome refers to a cognitive disturbance in which memory is impaired out of proportion to other cognitive functions. Its anatomical basis lies in the diencephalon and the temporal lobes. Injury to these regions (e.g., infarction in, or trauma to, bilateral inferomedial temporal lobes, temporal lobe epilepsy, third ventricular or thalamic tumors, or herpes simplex encephalitis) potentially can produce a syndrome indistinguishable from the amnesia syndrome seen in alcoholic patients. Like Wernicke's encephalopathy, Korsakoff's syndrome is best defined in chronic alcoholism. Korsakoff's syndrome and Wernicke's encephalopathy do not represent separate diseases but are different stages of one disease process (Wernicke-Korsakoff syndrome). Korsakoff's syndrome typically follows Wernicke's encephalopathy, emerging as ocular symptoms and encephalopathy subside.

History

Shortly after Wernicke's original treatise, Korsakoff, a Russian psychiatrist, described this amnesia syndrome in 20 alcoholic men. At the time, however, neither Wernicke nor Korsakoff recognized the relationship between the encephalopathy and impaired memory. Some of Korsakoff's patients had nystagmus and ophthalmoplegia, and several of Wernicke's original patients had amnestic psychosis. The clinical connection and the pathological similarity between the two conditions were not appreciated until 10 years later by other investigators.

Clinical Features

The memory impairment is characterized by the presence of both anterograde and retrograde amnesia. Affected patients have severe difficulty establishing a new memory, always coupled with a limited ability to recall events that antedate the onset of illness by several years. Most patients are disoriented as to place and time. Alertness, attention, social behavior, and most other aspects of cognitive functions are relatively preserved. Confabulation can be a prominent feature, especially in the early stages, although it may be absent in some patients.

Pathology

The histopathological changes in patients with Korsakoff's syndrome are similar to those in patients with predominantly Wernicke's encephalopathy. Patients with Korsakoff's syndrome have, in addition, involvement of the dorsal medial nucleus of the thalamus. Although present data do not allow confident identification of the anatomical lesion responsible for amnesia, Victor (1993) suggested that the memory disturbances are caused by these thalamic lesions.

Course and Prognosis

Despite treatment with thiamine, improvement in memory function is slow and usually incomplete, and those who improve usually do so after a 1-month delay or longer. Occasionally, patients may not achieve maximal improvement for more than a year.

Treatment and Management

Except for the initial thiamine administration, treatment usually is limited to social support. Many patients require at least some form of supervision, either at home or in a chronic care facility.

OTHER NUTRITIONAL DISEASES ASSOCIATED WITH ALCOHOLISM

The neurological consequences of alcohol abuse have been recognized for centuries, but little is known about their

1506 NEUROLOGICAL DISEASES

Table 63.5: Neurological complications associated with alcohol abuse

Nutritional deficiency
   Wernicke's encephalopathy
   Korsakoff's syndrome
   Pellagra
Partly nutritional in origin
   Alcoholic polyneuropathy
   Amblyopia
Direct toxic effects of alcohol
   Acute intoxication
   Delirium tremens
   Fetal alcohol syndrome
Abnormalities of serum electrolytes and osmolality
   Central pontine myelinolysis
Withdrawal
   Tremor
   Delirium tremens
Diseases of uncertain pathogenesis
   Cerebellar degeneration
   Marchiafava-Bignami disease
   Alcoholic myopathy
   Alcoholic dementia

pathogenesis. A nutritional cause is often invoked (Table 63.5); however, with the exception of Wernicke-Korsakoff syndrome, in which thiamine deficiency is the accepted cause, no single nutritional factor has been defined conclusively. Many investigators instead have proposed a direct neurotoxicity of alcohol, but this is a subject of much debate.

One fact is clear: Dietary deficiency is prevalent in the majority of alcoholic patients. Alcohol contains so-called empty calories because it does not provide significant amounts of protein and vitamins. A gram of pure ethanol contains 7 calories. A person who drinks a pint of 86-proof liquor daily consumes well over 1,000 calories a day, approximately one-half of the daily caloric requirement, and the alcohol consumption inevitably results in reduced intake of other foods. The problem is compounded further by malabsorption and abnormal metabolism of vitamins, both of which are common in alcoholics.

Alcoholic Neuropathy

Neuropathy is the most frequent neurological complication of alcoholism. Depending on the method of ascertainment, it may be diagnosed in 10–75% of alcoholic patients. Most affected patients are between 40 and 60 years of age, and in essentially all cases, there is a history of chronic and heavy alcohol intake.

Clinical Features

Alcoholic neuropathy is a mixed sensory and motor disorder. The onset of symptoms is usually insidious, beginning in the feet and progressing proximally and symmetrically. Paresthesia is the most common presenting complaint. A significant portion of patients also complains of pain, either an aching discomfort in the calves or a burning sensation over the soles. Dysesthesias at times become so severe that a light touch or gentle rubbing over the skin is interpreted as intensely unpleasant. Interestingly, pain is more often a problem in those with milder neuropathy.

On examination, signs of a distal symmetrical polyneuropathy are invariably present. Both deep and superficial sensation are affected approximately to the same degree. Ankle tendon reflexes and sometimes knee reflexes are absent. Weakness and wasting are limited to the distal feet in mild cases but can involve the distal upper extremities in more severe cases. Rarely, there may be vagus–recurrent laryngeal nerve involvement, with prominent hoarseness and weakness of voice.

Other manifestations of chronic alcoholism are often evident. Liver cirrhosis, hepatic encephalopathy, Wernicke-Korsakoff syndrome, alcoholic cerebellar degeneration, and alcohol withdrawal symptoms all occur frequently at the time of evaluation. Also sometimes encountered are trophic skin changes in the form of hyperpigmentation, edema, ulcers, and cellulitis in the distal part of the feet. There may be radiological suggestions of a distal neuropathic arthropathy (Charcot's forefeet, acrodystrophic neuropathy), with phalangeal atrophy, bony resorption, and subluxation of small joints in the feet. Repeated trauma and infections to insensitive parts of the feet are probably responsible. This syndrome is particularly prevalent in the south of France and Spain, where the term *Thévenard's syndrome* is applied.

Laboratory Studies and Pathology

Both electrophysiological and histological studies have confirmed that alcoholic neuropathy is predominantly axonal. Nerve conduction studies show severely reduced sensory nerve amplitudes with normal or mildly reduced conduction velocities. Electromyography may reveal signs of denervation and reinnervation in distal muscles of the lower extremities. Axonal degeneration of both myelinated and unmyelinated fibers is present on sural nerve biopsy. In approximately one-fourth of patients, autonomic dysfunction may be demonstrated by abnormalities in heart rate variation to deep breathing, Valsalva's maneuver, and postural change (Monforte et al. 1995).

Pathogenesis

Both alcohol neurotoxicity and thiamine deficiency may play major roles in the pathogenesis of alcoholic neuropathy. Some have argued that alcoholic neuropathy is clinically and pathologically identical to beriberi and that a nutritional deficiency of thiamine is responsible. One difficulty with this view is that many patients with alcoholic neuropathy have no evidence of nutritional deficiency. Others have suggested that alcohol is directly toxic to peripheral nerves but attempts to reproduce neuropathy in animal models have been disappointing. There are also reports that a balanced diet and supplemental vitamins produce improvement in neuropathy in those patients who continued to drink heavily.

Treatment and Management

It seems prudent to treat most affected patients with supplemental multivitamins and a balanced diet. Most patients probably do not respond to vitamin supplements alone, and abstinence from alcohol is paramount for treatment success. Even under ideal conditions, recovery is often slow and incomplete.

Tobacco-Alcohol or Nutritional Amblyopia

This is a syndrome of vision loss caused by a selective lesion of the optic nerves. In Western countries, most affected patients are chronic and severe alcoholics, often with a history of poor dietary intake or marked weight loss. Vision loss occurs insidiously and painlessly, progressing in both eyes over a period of several weeks. The most common deficits are impaired visual acuity and the presence of central or centrocecal scotomata. Even in severely affected subjects, the optic discs may show only mild pallor.

Although it is commonly called tobacco-alcohol amblyopia, neither agent has been proved to be directly responsible for the vision loss. The underlying cause is probably a nutritional deficiency. The disease is essentially identical to the amblyopia seen in prisoners of war and malnourished individuals who have no access to either alcohol or tobacco. Moreover, treatment with a combination of an adequate diet and B vitamins, despite the continuation of drinking and smoking, results in visual recovery. Dietary deficiencies of vitamin B_{12}, thiamine, folate, and riboflavin, all of which have been linked to optic neuropathy, may individually, or together, be responsible.

Marchiafava-Bignami Disease

In 1903, Marchiafava and Bignami, two Italian pathologists, described a curious syndrome of selective demyelination of the corpus callosum in alcoholic Italians who indulged in large quantities of red wine. The disease seems to affect severe and chronic alcoholics in their middle or late adult life, with a peak incidence between 40 and 60 years of age. It is not restricted to Italians and consumption of red wine is not an invariable feature. Because of the background history of alcohol abuse, a nutritional cause has been invoked, but no nutritional factor has been identified. A toxic cause, such as direct toxicity of ethanol or other constituents, seems equally plausible.

A clinical diagnosis is often difficult, because neurological presentations vary considerably. Many patients present in terminal coma, which often precludes a premortem diagnosis. Mental and motor slowing, other personality and behavior changes, incontinence, dysarthria, seizures, and hemiparesis occur to a varying extent. The most common picture on neurological evaluation is probably that of a frontal lobe or dementing syndrome. Sucking, grasping, and gegenhalten may be prominent. These symptoms have a tendency to remit, and many patients survive and later die of an unrelated cause.

Pathologically, selective involvement of the central portion of the corpus callosum occurs; the dorsal and ventral portions are spared or affected to a much lesser degree. There also may be symmetrical involvement of other white matter tracts. Magnetic resonance imaging is valuable for premortem visualization of these white matter lesions and provides a means of in vivo diagnosis.

Treatment should be directed at nutritional support and rehabilitation from alcoholism. In those patients who recovered, it is not clear whether improvement was a result of vitamin supplementation or merely a reflection of the disease's natural history.

Alcoholic Cerebellar Degeneration

Although the prevalence of this disorder is not known, alcoholic cerebellar degeneration is likely the most common of the acquired degenerations of the cerebellum. Men are affected more frequently than women, and the incidence peaks in the middle decades of life. Alcohol abuse is long-standing in all patients, and alcohol polyneuropathy accompanies most patients. The clinical syndrome is remarkably stereotyped. The usual presentation is a progressive unsteadiness in walking, evolving over weeks or months. Less commonly, a mild gait difficulty may be present for some time, only to worsen acutely during binge drinking or an intercurrent illness. On examination, the most striking finding is truncal ataxia, readily demonstrated by a wide-based gait and difficulty with tandem walking. Limb ataxia, if present, is much milder than truncal ataxia and more severe in the legs than in the arms. In contrast to Wernicke's encephalopathy, nystagmus and ocular dysmetria are uncommon. Dysarthria, tremor, and hypotonia are rare findings. With abstinence from alcohol and nutritional supplements, improvement in cerebellar symptoms occurs slowly but is often incomplete.

The pathological changes consist of selective atrophy of the anterior and superior parts of the cerebellar vermis, with the cerebellar hemispheres involved to a much lesser extent. Computed tomography or magnetic resonance imaging is useful in demonstrating the atrophy during life. Histologically, cell loss involves all neuronal types in the cerebellum, although Purkinje's cells are the most severely affected. A mild secondary loss of neurons is common in the deep cerebellar nuclei and the inferior olivary nuclei. In some patients, concomitant pathological changes of Wernicke's encephalopathy may be present.

MISCELLANEOUS DEFICIENCY DISEASES

Strachan's Syndrome and Related Disorders

In 1887, Strachan, a medical officer in the West Indies, described a syndrome of severe painful polyneuropathy, sensory ataxia, vision loss, and mucocutaneous excoriations. Although it was originally known as *Jamaican neuritis*, hundreds of cases were quickly recognized around the world. More recent cases are seen primarily in underdeveloped countries and in prisoners of war. Most investigators agree that nutritional deficiency plays a leading role in the pathogenesis of this disorder, but specific vitamins have not been implicated. The majority of patients undoubtedly had deficiencies of multiple vitamins, especially that of thiamine.

Although the clinical picture varies from patient to patient, the essential features are (1) a polyneuropathy that is often sufficiently severe to produce sensory ataxia; (2) amblyopia with optic atrophy; (3) tinnitus, hearing loss, and sometimes vertigo; and (4) a varying combination of stomatoglossitis, genital soreness and excoriation, and corneal degeneration. Gait ataxia and loss of sensation to vibration and joint position are prominent findings.

In the absence of a distinctive cause, there seems to be little value in distinguishing Strachan's syndrome from nutritional amblyopia and polyneuropathy. As in other deficiency diseases, treatment is directed toward establishing adequate diet and replenishing vitamins. Some degree of improvement can be expected, especially in the polyneuropathy.

A relatively recent outbreak of optic neuropathy in Cuba provides further insight into the etiology of nutritional optic and peripheral neuropathy (Roman 1994). The Cuban outbreak occurred in 1992–1993, coinciding with a period of food shortage and rationing. Clinical manifestations included a varying combination of retrobulbar optic neuropathy, peripheral neuropathy, sensorineural deafness, spasticity, position and vibration sense loss, dysphonia, and dysphagia. Increased risk was associated with poor dietary intake, smoking, heavy alcohol drinking, weight loss, and excessive sugar consumption. No toxic etiological agent was identified. Supplementation of multivitamins to the entire Cuban population coincided with abatement of the epidemic. A dependence on cane sugar, relative deficiency of meat and vegetables, and hence, B-vitamins deficiency, seemed responsible for the outbreak.

Vitamin A

Dietary deficiency of vitamin A is uncommon in Europe and the United States. Deficiency may occur rarely in fat malabsorption syndromes, such as sprue, biliary atresia, and cystic fibrosis. A few cases occurred in infants put on nondairy formula free of vitamin A.

The earliest sign of deficiency is reduced ability to see in dim light. Retinol, an aldehyde form of vitamin A, binds with the protein opsin to form rhodopsin, which is responsible for vision at low light level. Xerosis, or keratinization, of the conjunctiva and cornea often accompanies night blindness. Some patients have the characteristic Bitot's spots, which are white, foamlike spots appearing at the side of the cornea. These eye findings are caused by metaplasia of epithelial cells and, if severe, can lead to permanent blindness. Rarely, infants may manifest a syndrome of raised intracranial pressure, bulging fontanelles, and lethargy.

Patients with signs of vitamin A toxicity are more likely to see a neurologist than are those with a deficiency of the vitamin. The classic syndrome of toxicity is that of pseudotumor cerebri with headache and papilledema. The skin is often dry and pruritic, and patients may complain of generalized joint or bone pain. Especially in children, joint swelling and hyperostoses are often evident on roentgenography. Chronic daily consumption of more than 25,000 IU may produce toxicity, although most reported patients consumed much higher doses over a shorter period of time. Unusual foods, such as polar bear liver and halibut liver, contain high concentrations of vitamin A and have caused acute toxicity. Serum retinol level is useful in the diagnosis. The generally accepted lower limit of normal is 20 mg/dl, whereas concentrations in excess of 100 mg/dl are suggestive of toxicity.

Vitamin D

A syndrome of pain and proximal weakness has long been recognized in association with osteomalacia caused by a diversity of causes, including hyperparathyroidism, hypophosphatemia, anticonvulsant use, malabsorption, and dietary deficiency. Although the pathogenesis of the disorder remains obscure, many patients recover partially or completely with vitamin D treatment.

The best documentation of this disorder is provided by studies of undernourished patients in India who probably have dietary deficiency of vitamin D. Proximal weakness, particularly in the pelvic girdle, is the most prominent finding on examination as is a waddling gait. Neck muscles also may be weak, but bulbar and ocular weakness are not present. Tendon reflexes and sensation are normal. Aside from the manifestations of myopathy, accompanying clinical features include a long history of multiple bone fractures, vertebral collapse, and disabling bone pain. Bone pain mainly affects the pelvic girdle; the muscles are usually not painful. The pain may make the actual degree of weakness difficult to assess. When vitamin D therapy is instituted, the pain disappears quickly and true muscular weakness is unmasked.

Serum creatine kinase level is usually normal or mildly elevated. Nonspecific type II muscle fiber atrophy is seen on biopsy. Electromyography typically shows short-duration, low-amplitude, and polyphasic motor unit potentials without spontaneous activities, features similar to those of other metabolic myopathies. Other laboratory abnormalities of deranged bone metabolism are present. Osteomalacia is evident by roentgenography. Serum alkaline phosphatase almost always is elevated, and serum calcium and phosphorus may be normal or mildly decreased. These laboratory studies return to normal after a short period of vitamin D therapy. Muscle weakness, however, recovers much more slowly over a period of several months.

Vitamin D deficiency and compensatory increase of parathyroid hormone are common in hospitalized or immobilized patients (Thomas et al. 1998). Some of the contributing factors include insufficient exposure to sunlight, anticonvulsant drug therapy, renal dialysis, and Parkinson's disease. The deficiency poses a risk for bone loss and fracture. Its effect on neuromuscular function in this population is uncertain.

Protein-Calorie Malnutrition

Millions of infants and children in underdeveloped countries suffer from varying degrees of protein and calorie deficiencies and manifest two interrelated syndromes, marasmus and kwashiorkor. Marasmus is primarily a result of caloric insufficiency and characterized by extreme emaciation and growth failure in early infancy. These infants usually have never been breast-fed or were weaned before the age of 1 year. Kwashiorkor is seen most commonly in children weaned between 2 and 3 years of age, and its primary underlying cause is protein deficiency. The signs of kwashiorkor are edema, ascites, hepatomegaly, sparse hair, and skin depigmentation.

The earliest and most consistent neurological signs in these children are apathy to the environment and extreme irritability. In addition, weakness, generalized muscle wasting, hypotonia, and hyporeflexia frequently occur. Cognitive deficits may be permanent despite improved nutrition after the initial treatment. It is difficult to separate the effects of malnutrition from those of socioeconomic deprivation, but comparison studies in siblings show persistent impairment of intelligence attributable to malnutrition. Computed tomography of the brain shows subtle cerebral atrophy in 25% of patients. Autopsy studies further document that the brain tends to be smaller and neuronal development less mature in these patients.

A mild encephalopathy, usually no more than transient drowsiness, sometimes occurs during the first week of dietary treatment. Occasionally, children develop asterixis or coma or even die as a result of their treatment. Other children manifest a transient syndrome of rigidity, coarse tremors, myoclonus, and exaggerated tendon reflexes during the first few weeks of recovery from malnutrition. Little is known about the pathogenesis of these cases.

REFERENCES

Cavalier L, Ouahchi K, Kayden HJ, et al. Ataxia with isolated vitamin E deficiency: heterogeneity of mutations and phenotypic variability in a large number of families. Am J Hum Genet 1998;62:301–310.

Green R, Kinsella LJ. Current concepts in the diagnosis of cobalamin deficiency. Neurology 1995;45:1435–1440.

Kayden HJ. The neurologic syndrome of vitamin E deficiency: a significant cause of ataxia. Neurology 1993;43:2167–2169.

Monforte R, Estruch R, Valls-Sole J, et al. Autonomic and peripheral neuropathies in patients with chronic alcoholism. A dose-related toxic effect of alcohol. Arch Neurol 1995;52:45–51.

Paltiel O, Falutz J, Veilleux M, et al. Clinical correlates of subnormal vitamin B_{12} levels in patients infected with the human immunodeficiency virus. Am J Hematol 1995;49:318–322.

Roman GC. An epidemic in Cuba of optic neuropathy, sensorineural deafness, peripheral sensory neuropathy and dorsolateral myeloneuropathy. J Neurol Sci 1994;127:11–28.

Savage DG, Lindenbaum J, Stabler SP, et al. Sensitivity of serum methylmalonic acid and total homocysteine determinations for diagnosing cobalamin and folate deficiencies. Am J Med 1994;96:239–246.

Tefferi A, Pruthi RK. The biochemical basis of cobalamin deficiency. Mayo Clin Proc 1994;69:181–186.

Thomas MK, Lloyd-Jones DM, Thadhani RI, et al. Hypovitaminosis D in medical inpatients. N Engl J Med 1998;338:777–783.

Victor M. Persistent altered mentation due to ethanol. Neurol Clin 1993;11:639–661.

Chapter 64
Effects of Toxins and Physical Agents on the Nervous System

A. EFFECTS OF OCCUPATIONAL TOXINS ON THE NERVOUS SYSTEM
Michael J. Aminoff

Neurotoxic disorders, especially those with an iatrogenic basis, are well recognized. Hence, any unexplained symptom may be thought to be caused by a neurotoxin and may be the subject of potential litigation. Nevertheless, neurotoxic disorders are occurring increasingly as a result of occupational or environmental exposure to chemical agents and often go unrecognized.

RECOGNITION OF NEUROTOXIC DISORDERS

Exposure to neurotoxins may lead to dysfunction of any part of the central, peripheral, or autonomic nervous systems and the neuromuscular apparatus. Neurotoxic disorders are recognized readily if a close temporal relationship exists between the clinical onset and prior exposure to a chemical agent, especially one known to be neurotoxic. Known neurotoxins produce stereotyped or characteristic neurological disturbances that generally cease to progress soon after exposure is discontinued and ultimately improve to a variable extent. Recognition of a neurotoxic disorder is more difficult when exposure is chronic or symptoms are nonspecific. Diagnosis may be clouded by concerns about possible litigation, and the problem is compounded when

the exposure history is unclear. Patients often attribute symptoms to chemical exposure when no other cause can be found. Such patients have often been exposed to several chemical agents or are known to abuse alcohol or other drugs, thereby further confounding the issue.

Single case reports that an agent is neurotoxic are unreliable, especially when the neurological symptoms are frequent in the general population. Epidemiological studies may be helpful in establishing a neurotoxic basis for symptoms. However, many of the published studies are inadequate because of methodological problems such as the selection of appropriate control subjects. Recognition of a neurotoxic basis for neurobehavioral disorders, for example, requires matching of exposed subjects and unexposed controls, not only for age, gender, and race, but also for premorbid cognitive ability, educational, social, and cultural background, and alcohol, recreational drug, and medication use. Laboratory test results are often unhelpful in confirming that the neurological syndrome is caused by a specific agent, either because the putative neurotoxin cannot be measured in body tissues or because the interval since exposure makes such measurements meaningless.

Dysfunction of any part of the central, peripheral, or autonomic nervous systems and of the neuromuscular apparatus may result from exposure to neurotoxins, depending on the responsible agent. The pathophysiological basis of the clinical disorder is often unknown. In considering the possibility of a neurotoxic disorder, it is important to obtain a detailed account of all chemicals to which exposure has occurred, including details of the duration and severity of exposure, whether any protective measures were taken, and the context in which exposure occurred. Then, it must be determined whether any of these chemicals are known to be neurotoxic and whether symptoms are compatible with the known toxicity of the suspected compound. Many neurotoxins can produce clinical disorders that resemble metabolic, nutritional, or degenerative disorders, and it is therefore important to consider these and any other relevant disease processes in the differential diagnosis. Neurotoxins cause diffuse rather than focal or lateralized neurological dysfunction. In recognizing new neurotoxic disorders, a clustering of cases is often important, but this may not be evident until patients are referred for specialist evaluation.

The neurological disorder is typically monophasic. Although progression may occur for several weeks after exposure has been discontinued ("coasting"), it is eventually arrested and improvement may then follow, depending on the severity of the original disorder. Prolonged or progressive deterioration long after exposure has been discontinued, or the development of neurological symptoms months to years after exposure, suggest that a neurotoxic disorder is not responsible.

In this section, we review the neurotoxicity of occupational and environmental agents, in alphabetical order.

ORGANIC CHEMICALS

Acrylamide

Acrylamide polymers are used as flocculators and are constituents of certain adhesives and products such as cardboard or molded parts. They also are used as grouting agents for mines and tunnels, a solution of the monomer being pumped into the ground where polymerization is allowed to occur. The monomer is neurotoxic, and exposure may occur during its manufacture or in the polymerization process. Most cases of acrylamide toxicity occur by inhalation or cutaneous absorption. The acrylamide is distributed widely throughout the body and is excreted primarily through the kidney. The mechanism responsible for its neurotoxicity is unknown. Studies in animals have shown early abnormalities in axonal transport, and this may account for the histopathological changes discussed here.

Clinical manifestations of acrylamide toxicity depend on the severity of exposure. Acute high-dose exposure results in confusion, hallucinations, reduced attention span, drowsiness, and other encephalopathic changes. A peripheral neuropathy of variable severity may occur after acute high-dose or after prolonged low-level exposure. The neuropathy is a length-dependent axonopathy involving both sensory and motor fibers. It is accompanied by hyperhidrosis and dermatitis that may develop before the neuropathy is evident clinically in those with repeated skin exposure. Ataxia from cerebellar dysfunction also occurs and relates to degeneration of afferent and efferent cerebellar fibers and Purkinje's cells. Neurological examination reveals distal sensorimotor deficits and early loss of all tendon reflexes, rather than simply the Achilles' reflex, which is usually affected first in most length-dependent neuropathies. Autonomic abnormalities other than hyperhidrosis are uncommon. Gait and limb ataxia are usually greater than can be accounted for by the sensory loss. With discontinuation of exposure, the neuropathy coasts, arrests, and may then slowly reverse, but residual neurological deficits are common. These consist particularly of spasticity and cerebellar ataxia; the peripheral neuropathy usually remits, because regeneration occurs in the peripheral nervous system. No specific treatment exists.

Electrodiagnostic studies provide evidence of an axonal sensorimotor polyneuropathy. Workers at risk of developing the disorder may be monitored electrophysiologically by recording sensory nerve action potentials, which are attenuated early in the course of the disorder, or by measuring the vibration threshold (Calleman et al. 1994). Histopathological studies show the accumulation of neurofilaments in axons, especially distally, and distal degeneration of peripheral and central axons. The large myelinated axons are involved first. The affected central pathways include the ascending sensory fibers in the posterior columns, the spinocerebellar tracts, and the descending corticospinal pathways. Involvement of postganglionic sympathetic efferent nerve fibers accounts for the sudomotor dysfunction. Measurement of hemoglobin-acrylamide adducts may be useful in predicting the development of peripheral neuropathy (Calleman et al. 1994).

Allyl Chloride

Allyl chloride is used for manufacturing epoxy resins, certain insecticides, and polyacrylonitride. Exposure leads to a mixed sensorimotor distal axonopathy. Cessation of exposure is followed by recovery of variable degree. Intraaxonal accumulation of neurofilaments occurs multifocally before axonal degeneration in animals exposed to this compound. Similar changes may occur also in the posterolateral columns of the spinal cord.

Carbon Disulfide

Carbon disulfide is used as a solvent or soil fumigant, in perfume production, in certain varnishes and insecticides, in the cold vulcanization of rubber, and for manufacturing viscose rayon and cellophane films. Toxicity is primarily from inhalation or ingestion, but also may occur transdermally. The pathogenetic mechanism is uncertain, but may involve a chelating effect of carbon disulfide metabolites, direct inhibition of certain enzymes, or the release of free radicals following cleavage of the carbon-sulfur bond. Most reported cases have been from Europe and Japan.

Acute inhalation of concentrations exceeding 300–400 ppm leads to an encephalopathy with symptoms that vary from mild behavioral disturbances to drowsiness and, ultimately, to respiratory failure. Behavioral disturbances may include explosive behavior, mood swings, mania or depression, confusion, and other psychiatric disturbances (Huang et al. 1996). Long-term exposure to concentrations between 40 and 50 ppm may produce similar disturbances. Minor affective or cognitive disturbances may be revealed only by neuropsychological testing.

Long-term exposure to carbon disulfide may lead also to extrapyramidal or pyramidal deficits, absent pupillary and corneal reflexes, optic neuropathy, and a characteristic retinopathy. A clinical or subclinical polyneuropathy (Chu et al. 1995) develops after exposure to levels of 100–150 ppm for several months or to lesser levels for longer periods and is characterized histologically by focal axonal swellings and neurofilamentary accumulations.

No specific treatment exists other than the avoidance of further exposure. Recovery from the peripheral neuropathy generally follows the discontinuation of exposure, but some central deficits may persist.

Carbon Monoxide

Occupational or environmental exposure to carbon monoxide occurs mainly in miners, gas workers, and garage employees. The neurotoxic effects of carbon monoxide relate to intracellular hypoxia. Carbon monoxide binds to hemoglobin with high affinity to form carboxyhemoglobin; it also limits the dissociation of oxyhemoglobin and binds to various enzymes. Acute toxicity leads to disturbances of consciousness and a variety of other behavioral changes. Motor abnormalities include the development of pyramidal and extrapyramidal deficits. Seizures may occur, and focal cortical deficits sometimes develop. Treatment involves prevention of further exposure to carbon monoxide and administration of pure or hyperbaric oxygen. Neurological deterioration may occur several weeks after partial or apparently full recovery from the acute effects of carbon monoxide exposure, with recurrence of motor and behavioral abnormalities. The degree of recovery from this delayed deterioration is limited, and some patients lapse into a persistent vegetative state.

Pathological examination shows hypoxic and ischemic damage in the cerebral cortex, as well as in the hippocampus, cerebellar cortex, and basal ganglia. Lesions are also present diffusely in the cerebral white matter. The delayed deterioration has been related to a diffuse subcortical leukoencephalopathy, but its pathogenesis is uncertain.

Ethylene Oxide

Ethylene oxide is used to sterilize heat-sensitive medical equipment and as an alkylating agent in industrial chemical synthesis. A by-product, ethylene chlorohydrin, is highly toxic. Protective ventilatory apparatus is required to prevent occupational exposure, for example, among operators of sterilization equipment. Acute exposure to high levels produces headache, nausea, and a severe, reversible encephalopathy. Long-term exposure to ethylene oxide or ethylene chlorohydrin may lead to a peripheral sensorimotor axonopathy and mild cognitive changes, such as have been reported in operating-room nurses and sterilizer workers (Brashear et al. 1996). Recovery generally follows cessation of exposure. Neuropathy may be produced in rats by exposure to ethylene oxide, and the residual ethylene oxide in sterilized dialysis tubing may contribute to the polyneuropathy occurring in patients undergoing chronic hemodialysis.

Hexacarbon Solvents

The hexacarbon solvents n-hexane and methyl n-butyl ketone are both metabolized to 2,5-hexanedione, which is responsible in large part for their neurotoxicity. This neurotoxicity is potentiated by methyl ethyl ketone, which is used in paints, lacquers, printer's ink, and certain glues. n-Hexane is used as a solvent in paints, lacquers, and printing inks and is used especially in the rubber industry and in certain glues. Workers involved in manufacturing footwear, laminating processes, and cabinetry, especially in confined, unventilated spaces, may be exposed to excessive concentrations. Methyl n-butyl ketone is used in the manufacture of vinyl and acrylic coatings and adhesives and in the printing industry. Exposure to either of these chemicals by inhalation or skin contact leads to a progressive, distal, sensorimotor axonal polyneuropathy. Optic neuropathy or maculopathy, and facial numbness also have followed n-Hexane exposure. The neuropathy is related to a disturbance of axonal transport, and histopathological studies reveal giant multifocal axonal swelling and accumulation of axonal neurofilaments, with distal degeneration in peripheral and central axons. Myelin retraction and focal demyelination are found at the giant axonal swellings.

Acute inhalation exposure may produce feelings of euphoria, associated with hallucinations, headache, unsteadiness, and mild narcosis. This has led to the inhalation of certain glues for recreational purposes, which causes pleasurable feelings of euphoria in the short term but may lead to a progressive, predominantly motor neuropathy and symptoms of dysautonomia after high-dose exposure, and a more insidious sensorimotor polyneuropathy following chronic usage.

Electrophysiologically, increased distal motor latency and marked slowing of maximal motor conduction velocity occur, as well as small or absent sensory nerve action potentials and electromyographical signs of denervation in affected muscles. The conduction slowing relates to demyelinative changes and is unusual in other toxic neuropathies. A reduction in size of sensory nerve action potentials may occur in the absence of clinical or other electrophysiological evidence of nerve involvement (Pastore et al. 1994). Central involvement may result in abnormalities of sensory evoked potentials. The cerebrospinal fluid is usually normal, but a mildly elevated protein concentration is sometimes found. Despite cessation of exposure, progression of the neurological deficit may continue for several weeks or months (coasting) before the downhill course is arrested and recovery begins. Severe involvement is followed by incomplete recovery of the peripheral neuropathy. When the polyneuropathy does resolve, previously masked signs of central dysfunction, such as spasticity, may become evident.

Methyl Bromide

Methyl bromide has been used as a refrigerant, insecticide, fumigant, and fire extinguisher. Its high volatility may lead to concentrations in work areas that are sufficient to result in neurotoxicity from inhalation. Following acute high-level exposure, an interval of several hours or more may elapse before the onset of symptoms. Because methyl bromide is odorless and colorless, subjects may not even be aware that exposure has occurred. Hence, chloropicrin, a conjunctival and mucosal irritant, is commonly added to provide warning of inhalation exposure. Acute methyl bromide intoxication leads to an encephalopathy with convulsions, delirium, hyperpyrexia, coma, pulmonary edema, and death (Deschamps and Turpin 1996). Acute exposure to lower concentrations may result in conspicuous mental changes including confusion, psychosis, or affective disturbances and to headache, nausea, dysarthria, tremulousness, myoclonus, ataxia, visual disturbances, and seizures.

Long-term, low-level exposure may lead to a polyneuropathy in the absence of systemic symptoms. Distal paresthesias are followed by sensory and motor deficits, loss of tendon reflexes, and an ataxic gait. Visual disturbances, optic atrophy, and upper motor neuron deficits may occur also (De Haro et al. 1997). Calf tenderness is sometimes conspicuous. The cerebrospinal fluid is unremarkable, whereas electrodiagnostic study results reveal both sensory and motor involvement. Gradual improvement occurs with cessation of exposure.

Treatment is symptomatic and supportive. Chelating agents have been used in the past, but are of uncertain utility.

Organochlorine Pesticides

The organochlorine pesticides include aldrin, dieldrin, and lindane, as well as the once popular insecticide dichlorodiphenyl-trichlorethylene, commonly called *DDT*. Tremor and convulsions may follow acute, high-level exposure, but the effects of chronic, low-level exposure are uncertain. Chlordecone, which belongs to this group, may produce a neurological disorder characterized by "nervousness," tremor, clumsiness of the hands, gait ataxia, and opsoclonus. Minor cognitive changes and benign intracranial hypertension may occur sometimes. The pathophysiology of the disorder has not been established.

Organophosphates

Organophosphates are used mainly as pesticides and herbicides, but also as petroleum additives, lubricants, antioxidants, flame retardants, and plastic modifiers. Most cases of organophosphate toxicity result from exposure in an agricultural setting, not only among those mixing or spraying the pesticide or herbicide, but also among workers returning prematurely to sprayed fields. Absorption may occur through the skin, by inhalation, or through the gastrointestinal tract. Organophosphates inhibit acetylcholinesterase by phosphorylation, with resultant acute cholinergic toxicity. This has both central and neuromuscular manifestations. Symptoms include nausea, salivation, lacrimation, headache, weakness, and bronchospasm in mild instances, and bradycardia, tremor, chest pain, diarrhea, pulmonary edema, cyanosis, convulsions, and even coma in more severe cases. Death may result from respiratory or heart failure. Treatment involves intravenous administration of pralidoxime (1 g) together with atropine (1 mg) subcutaneously every 30 minutes until sweating and salivation are controlled. Pralidoxime accelerates reactivation of the inhibited acetylcholinesterase, and atropine is effective in counteracting muscarinic effects, although it has no effect on the nicotinic effects such as weakness or respiratory depression. It is important to ensure adequate ventilatory support before atropine is given. The dose of pralidoxime can be repeated if no obvious benefit occurs, but in refractory cases it may need to be given by intravenous infusion, the dose being titrated against clinical response. Functional recovery may take approximately 1 week, although acetylcholinesterase levels take longer to reach normal levels.

Carbamate insecticides also inhibit cholinesterases, but have a shorter duration of action than organophosphate compounds. The symptoms of toxicity are similar to those described for organophosphates, but are generally milder. Treatment with atropine is usually sufficient.

Certain organophosphates cause a delayed polyneuropathy, which occurs approximately 2–3 weeks after acute exposure. In the past, contamination of illicit alcohol with triorthocresyl phosphate ("Jake") led to large numbers of such cases (Woolf 1995). Paresthesias in the feet and cramps in the calf muscles are followed by progressive weakness that typically begins distally in the limbs and then spreads to involve more proximal muscles. The maximal deficit usually develops within 2 weeks. Quadriplegia occurs in severe cases. Although sensory complaints are typically inconspicuous, clinical examination shows sensory deficits. The Achilles' reflex is typically lost, and other tendon reflexes may be depressed also; however, in some instances evidence of central involvement is manifest by brisk tendon reflexes. Cranial nerve function is spared typically. With time, there may be improvement in the peripheral neuropathy, but upper motor neuron involvement then becomes unmasked and often determines the prognosis for functional recovery. There is no specific treatment to arrest progression or hasten recovery. Electrodiagnostic studies reveal an axonopathy, with partial denervation of affected muscles, small compound muscle action potentials, but normal or only minimally reduced maximal motor conduction velocity.

The delayed syndrome follows exposure only to certain organophosphates such as triorthocresyl phosphate, leptophos, trichlorfon, and mipafox. The neurological disturbance relates to phosphorylation and inhibition of an enzyme called neuropathy target esterase (NTE), which is present in essentially all neurons and has an uncertain role in the nervous system (Glynn et al. 1998). In addition, *aging* of the inhibited NTE (loss of a group attached to the phosphorus, leaving a negatively charged phosphoryl group attached to the protein) must occur for the neuropathy to develop. The precise cause of the neuropathy is uncertain, however (Lotti 1995). No specific treatment exists to prevent occurrence of the neuropathy following exposure, but measurement of lymphocyte NTE has been used to monitor occupational exposure and predict the occurrence of neuropathy. Moreover, the ability of an organophosphate to inhibit NTE in the hen may predict its neurotoxicity in humans.

Three other syndromes related to organophosphates require brief comment. The intermediate syndrome occurs in the interval between the acute cholinergic crisis and the development of delayed neuropathy, typically becoming manifest within 4 days of exposure and resolving in 2–3 weeks. It reflects excessive cholinergic stimulation of nicotinic receptors and is characterized clinically by respiratory, bulbar, and proximal limb weakness (Sedgwick and Senanayake 1997). It relates to the severity of poisoning and to prolonged inhibition of acetylcholinesterase activity, but not to the development of delayed neuropathy (De Bleecker 1995). The syndrome of dippers' flu refers to the development of transient symptoms such as headache, rhinitis, pharyngitis, myalgia, and other flulike symptoms in farmers exposed to organophosphate sheep dips. Whether they relate to mild organophosphate toxicity is uncertain. Similarly uncertain is whether chronic effects (persisting behavioral and neurological dysfunction) may follow acute exposure to organophosphates. The occurrence of chronic symptoms in the absence of any episode of acute toxicity is unlikely. Evaluation of reports is hampered by incomplete documentation and because exposure has often occurred to a variety of agents. Carefully controlled studies may clarify this issue in the future.

Pyrethroids

Pyrethroids are synthetic insecticides. Occupational exposure has led to paresthesias that have been attributed to repetitive activity in sensory fibers as a result of abnormal prolongation of the sodium current during membrane excitation. Treatment is purely supportive.

Solvent Mixtures

In the 1970s, a number of reports from Scandinavia suggested that house painters, in particular, developed a disturbance of cognitive function that related to exposure to mixtures of organic solvents. However, further studies (including cases previously diagnosed with the disorder) have failed to validate the earlier reports, which in many instances were methodologically flawed. In consequence, the existence of so-called painter's encephalopathy in those exposed to low levels of organic solvents for a prolonged period remains uncertain.

Styrene

Styrene is used for manufacturing reinforced plastic and certain resins. Occupational exposure occurs by the dermal or inhalation routes and is typically associated with exposure to a variety of other chemicals, thereby making it difficult to define the syndrome that occurs from styrene exposure itself. Acute exposure to high concentrations of styrene has led to cognitive, behavioral, and attentional disturbances. Less clear are the consequences of exposure to chronic low levels of styrene. Abnormalities in psychomotor performance have been reported, but one analysis of the literature suggests that there is little compelling evidence of persisting neurological sequelae in this circumstance (Rebert and Hall 1994).

Toluene

Toluene is used in a variety of occupational settings. It is a solvent for paints and glues and is used to synthesize benzene, nitrotoluene, and other compounds. Exposure occurs among workers laying linoleum or spraying paint, and in the printing industry, particularly in poorly ventilated locations. Chronic high exposure may lead to cognitive disturbances and to central neurological deficits with upper motor neuron, cerebellar, brainstem, and cranial nerve findings, and tremor. An optic neuropathy may occur, as may ocular dysmetria and opsoclonus. Disturbances of memory and attention characterize the cognitive abnormalities. There may be a flat affect. Magnetic resonance imaging shows cerebral atrophy and diffuse abnormalities of the cerebral white matter (Caldemeyer et al. 1996); symmetrical lesions may be present in the basal ganglia and thalamus, and the cingulate gyri. Lower levels of exposure lead to minor neurobehavioral disturbances.

Trichloroethylene

Trichloroethylene is an industrial solvent and degreaser that is used in dry cleaning and the manufacture of rubber. It also has anesthetic properties. Recreational abuse has occurred because it may induce feelings of euphoria. Acute low-level exposure may lead to headache and nausea, but claims that an encephalopathy follows chronic low-level exposure are unsubstantiated. Higher levels of exposure lead to dysfunction of the trigeminal nerve, with progressive impairment of sensation that starts in the snout area and then spreads outward. With increasing exposure, facial and buccal numbness is followed by weakness of the muscles of mastication and facial expression. Ptosis, extraocular palsies, vocal cord paralysis, and dysphagia may occur also, as may an encephalopathy (Szlatenyi and Wang 1996), but there is uncertainty whether a peripheral neuropathy occurs in the limbs. The clinical deficit relates to neuronal loss in the cranial nerve nuclei and degeneration in related tracts. With discontinuation of exposure, the clinical deficit generally resolves, sometimes over 1–2 years, but occasional patients are left with residual facial numbness or dysphagia.

Vacor

Vacor, a rodenticide, has led to severe autonomic dysfunction accompanied by a usually milder sensorimotor axonopathy following its ingestion. The mechanism by which this develops is unclear, but it may relate to an impairment of fast anterograde axonal transport. Acute diabetes mellitus also results from necrosis of the beta cells of the pancreas.

METALS

Aluminum

Aluminum exposure is responsible for dialysis encephalopathy, which is characterized by speech disturbances, cognitive decline, seizures, and myoclonus.

Arsenic

Arsenic poisoning usually results from ingestion of the trivalent arsenite in murder or suicide attempts or following consumption of contaminated well water. Traditional Chinese medicinal herbal preparations may contain arsenic sulfide and mercury and are a source of chronic poisoning. Uncommon sources of accidental exposure include the burning of preservative-impregnated wood and storing food in antique copper kettles. Exposure to inorganic arsenic occurs in workers involved in the smelting of copper and lead ores.

With acute or subacute exposure, nausea, vomiting, abdominal pain, diarrhea, hypotension, tachycardia, and vasomotor collapse occur and may lead to death. Obtundation is common and an acute confusional state may develop. Arsenical neuropathy takes the form of a distal axonopathy, although a demyelinating neuropathy is found soon after acute exposure (Greenberg 1996). The neuropathy usually develops within 2–3 weeks of acute or subacute exposure, although the latent period may be as long as 1–2 months. Symptoms may worsen over a few weeks despite lack of further exposure, but eventually stabilize. With low-dose chronic exposure, the latent period is more difficult to determine. In either circumstance, systemic symptoms are also conspicuous. With chronic exposure, similar but less severe gastrointestinal disturbances develop, as may skin changes such as melanosis, keratoses, and malignancies. Mees' lines are white transverse striations of the nails (striate leukonychiae) that appear 3–6 weeks after exposure (Figure 64A.1). As a nonspecific manifestation of nail matrix injury, Mees' lines can be seen in a number of other conditions including thallium poisoning, chemotherapy, and a variety of systemic disorders.

The neuropathy involves both large- and small-diameter fibers. Initial symptoms are typically of distal, painful dysesthesias and are followed by distal weakness. Proprioceptive loss may be severe, leading to marked ataxia. The severity of weakness depends on the extent of exposure. The respiratory muscles are sometimes affected, and the disorder may simulate the Guillain-Barré syndrome both clinically and electrophysiologically. Electrodiagnostic studies may initially suggest a demyelinating polyradiculoneuropathy, but the changes of an axonal neuropathy subsequently develop. Arsenic levels in hair, nail clippings, or urine may be increased, especially in cases of chronic exposure.

Detection of arsenic in urine is diagnostically useful within 6 weeks of a single large dose exposure, or during ongoing low level exposure. Inorganic arsenic values over 25 µg per 24 hours are abnormal. Methods are available in reference laboratories to distinguish between inorganic (toxic) and organic (seafood-derived) arsenical compounds. Arsenic bound to keratin can be detected in hair or nails months to years after exposure. Pubic hair is preferable to scalp hair for examination because it is less liable to environmental contamination. Levels exceeding 10 µg/g of tissue are abnormal. Other abnormal laboratory features include aplastic anemia with pancytopenia, and moderate cerebrospinal fluid protein elevation. Nerve conduction studies in chronic arsenic neuropathy reflect the changes of distal axonopathy with low-amplitude or unelicitable sensory and motor evoked responses and preserved conduction velocities. Electromyography typically shows denervation in distal extremity muscles. In the subacute stages, however, some electrophysiological features, such as partial motor

FIGURE 64A.1   Mees' lines in arsenic neuropathy.

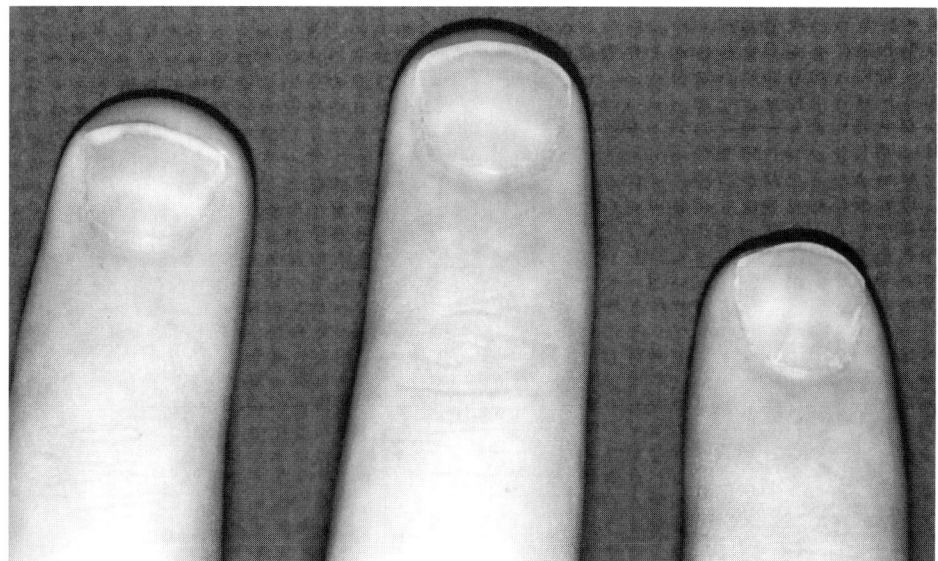

conduction block, absent F responses, and slowing of motor conduction velocities are suggestive of demyelinating polyradiculoneuropathy. Progressive slowing of motor conduction velocities sufficient to invoke consideration of segmental demyelination has been reported in the first 3 months after massive exposure. Biopsies of peripheral nerves show axonal degeneration in chronic cases. Arsenite compounds react with protein sulfhydryl groups, interfere with formation of coenzyme A and several steps in glycolysis, and are potent uncouplers of oxidative phosphorylation. These biochemical reactions are responsible for the impaired neuronal energy metabolism, which in turn results in distal axonal degeneration.

Chelation therapy with either water-soluble derivatives of dimercaprol (DMSA or DMPS) or penicillamine is effective in controlling the systemic effects of acute arsenic poisoning and may prevent the development of neuropathy provided that it is started within hours of ingestion (Graeme and Pollack 1998). There is little evidence that chelation in the later stages of arsenic neuropathy promotes clinical recovery. The neuropathy itself often improves gradually over the course of many months, but depending on the severity of the deficit when exposure is discontinued, a substantial residual neurological deficit is common.

Lead

Occupational exposure to lead occurs in workers in smelting factories and metal foundries, and those involved in demolition, ship breaking, manufacturing batteries or paint pigments, and the construction or repair of storage tanks. Occupational exposure also occurs in the manufacture of ammunition, bearings, pipes, solder, and cables. Nonindustrial sources of lead poisoning are home-distilled whiskey, Asian folk remedies, earthenware pottery, indoor firing ranges, and retained bullets. Lead neuropathy reached epidemic proportions at the end of the nineteenth century because of uncontrolled occupational exposure, but now is rare because of strict industrial regulations. Exposure also may result from paint ingestion in children with pica and the consumption of illicit spirits by adults. Absorption is commonly by ingestion or inhalation, but occasionally occurs through the skin.

The toxic effects of inorganic lead salts on the nervous system differ with age, producing acute encephalopathy in children and polyneuropathy in adults. Children typically develop an acute gastrointestinal illness followed by behavioral changes, confusion, drowsiness, reduced alertness, focal or generalized seizures, and (in severe cases) coma with intracranial hypertension. At autopsy, the brain is swollen, with vascular congestion, perivascular exudates, edema of the white matter, and scattered areas of neuronal loss and gliosis. In adults, an encephalopathy is less common, but behavioral and cognitive changes are sometimes noted. In adults, lead produces a predominantly motor neuropathy, sometimes accompanied by gastrointestinal disturbances and a microcytic, hypochromic anemia. The neuropathy is manifest primarily by a bilateral wrist drop, sometimes accompanied by bilateral footdrop, or by more generalized weakness that may be associated with distal atrophy and fasciculations. Sensory complaints are usually minor and overshadowed by the motor deficit. The tendon reflexes may be diminished or absent. Older reports describe a painless motor neuropathy with few or no sensory abnormalities and distinct patterns of weakness affecting wrist extensors and finger extensors and intrinsic hand muscles. Preserved reflexes, fasciculations, and profound muscle atrophy may simulate amyotrophic lateral sclerosis. A rare sign of lead exposure is a blue line at the gingival margin in patients with poor oral hygiene. Hypochromic microcytic anemia with basophilic stippling of the red cells, hyperuricemia, and azotemia should stimulate a search for lead exposure.

Lead intoxication is confirmed by elevated blood and urine lead levels. Blood levels exceeding 70 µg/100 ml are considered harmful but even levels greater than 40 µg/100 ml have been correlated with minor nerve conduction abnormalities. Lead inhibits erythrocyte δ-aminolevulinic acid dehydratase and other enzymatic steps in the biosynthetic pathway of porphyrins. Consequently, increased red cell protoporphyrin levels emerge together with increased urinary excretion of δ-aminolevulinic acid and coproporphyrin. Excess body lead burden, confirming past exposure, can be documented by increased urinary lead excretion after a provocative chelation challenge with calcium ethylenediaminetetraacetic acid. Only a few electrophysiological studies have been reported in patients with overt lead neuropathy. These investigations indicate a distal axonopathy affecting both motor and sensory fibers. These observations corroborate changes of axonal degeneration seen in human nerve biopsies. Contrary to the findings in humans, lead produces segmental demyelination in animals. Lead is known to cause early mitochondrial changes in cell culture systems, but the biochemical mechanisms leading to neurotoxicity remain unknown.

Lead encephalopathy is managed supportively, but corticosteroids are given to treat cerebral edema, and chelating agents (dimercaprol or 2,3-dimercaptopropane sulfonate) are prescribed also. No specific treatment exists for lead neuropathy other than avoidance of further exposure to lead. Chelation therapy does not hasten recovery.

Manganese

Manganese miners may develop neurotoxicity following inhalation for prolonged periods (months or years) of dust containing manganese. Headache, behavioral changes, and cognitive disturbances ("manganese madness") are followed by development of an extrapyramidal syndrome, with bradykinesia, rigidity, tremor, and dystonic posturing. Neuronal loss occurs in the globus pallidus and substantia nigra pars reticularis, as well as in the subthalamic nucleus and striatum. There is little response to L-dopa of the extrapyramidal syndrome, which may progress over several years (Huang et al. 1998).

Mercury

The toxic effects of elemental mercury (mercury vapor), inorganic salts and short-chain alkyl-mercury compounds predominantly involve the central nervous system and dorsal root ganglion sensory neurons. Inorganic mercury toxicity may result from inhalation during industrial exposure, as in battery factories, mercury processing plants, and electronic applications factories. In the past, exposure occurred particularly in the hat-making industry. No evidence exists that the mercury contained in dental amalgam imposes any significant health hazard. Clinical consequences of exposure include cutaneous erythema, hyperhidrosis, anemia, proteinuria, glycosuria, personality changes, intention tremor ("hatter's shakes"), and muscle weakness. The personality changes ("mad as a hatter") consist of irritability, euphoria, anxiety, emotional lability, insomnia, and disturbances of attention, with drowsiness, confusion, and, ultimately, stupor. A variety of other central neurological deficits may occur, but are more conspicuous in patients with organic mercury poisoning.

The effects of methyl mercury (organic mercury) poisoning have come to be widely recognized since the outbreak that occurred in Minamata Bay (Japan) in the 1950s, when industrial waste discharged into the bay led to contamination of fish that were then consumed by humans. Outbreaks have occurred also following the use of methyl mercury as a fungicide, because intoxication occurs if treated seed, intended for planting, is eaten instead. Methyl- and ethyl-mercury compounds have been used as fungicides in agriculture and in the paper industry. Methyl mercury and elemental mercury are potent neurotoxins causing neuronal degeneration in the cerebellar granular layer, calcarine cortex, and dorsal root ganglion neurons.

The characteristic features of chronic methyl mercury poisoning are sensory disturbances, constriction of visual fields, progressive ataxia, tremor, and cognitive impairment. Electrophysiological studies have shown that these symptoms relate to central dysfunction. Sensory disturbances result from dysfunction of sensory cortex rather than peripheral nerves, and the visual complaints also relate to cortical involvement. Pathological studies reveal neuronal loss in the cerebral cortex, including the parietal and occipital regions, as well as in the cerebellum. A few cases presenting with peripheral neuropathy or a predominantly motor neuronopathy resembling amyotrophic lateral sclerosis have been described in association with intense exposure to elemental mercury vapors.

The diagnosis of elemental or inorganic mercury intoxication usually can be confirmed by assaying mercury in urine. Monitoring blood levels is recommended for suspected organic mercury poisoning.

Chelating agents increase urinary excretion of mercury, but insufficient evidence exists to substantiate the claim that chelation increases the rate or extent of recovery.

Tellurium

Tellurium is used in the manufacture of various alloys, the coloring of glass, ceramics and metalware, the production of rubber, and the manufacture of thermoelectric devices. Inhalation of volatile tellurium compounds may lead to headache, drowsiness, a metallic taste, hypohidrosis, skin rashes and discoloration, and a curious odor resembling garlic in the breath. Recovery generally occurs spontaneously.

Thallium

Thallium salts cause severe neuropathy and central nervous system degeneration that has led to their discontinued use as rodenticides and depilatories. Most intoxications result from accidental ingestion, attempted suicide, or homicide.

After consumption of massive doses, vomiting, diarrhea, or both, occur within hours. Neuropathic symptoms, heralded by limb pain and severe distal paresthesia, are followed by progressive limb weakness within 7 days. Cranial nerves, including optic nerves, may be involved. Ptosis is common. In severe cases, ataxia, chorea, confusion, and coma, as well as ventilatory and cardiac failure may ensue. Alopecia, which appears 2–4 weeks after exposure, provides only retrospective evidence of acute intoxication. A chronic progressive, mainly sensory, neuropathy develops in patients with chronic, low-level exposure. In this form, hair loss is a helpful clue.

Electrocardiographic findings of sinus tachycardia, U waves, and T-wave changes, of the type seen in potassium depletion, are related to the interaction of thallium and potassium ions. Electrophysiological findings are characteristic of distal axonal degeneration. Autopsy study results confirm a distal axonopathy of peripheral and cranial nerves. Studies in animals show accumulation of swollen mitochondria in distal axons before wallerian degeneration of nerve fibers. The diagnosis is confirmed by the demonstration of thallium in urine or bodily tissues. High levels are found in central nervous system gray matter and myocardium. The toxic effects of thallium may be related to binding of sulfhydryl groups or displacement of potassium ions from biological membrane systems.

With acute ingestion, gastric lavage and cathartics are given to remove unabsorbed thallium from the gastrointestinal tract. Oral potassium ferric ferrocyanide (Prussian blue), which blocks intestinal absorption, together with intravenous potassium chloride, forced diuresis, and hemodialysis have been used successfully in acute thallium intoxication.

Tin

Although ingested inorganic tin usually produces little or no systemic and neurological complications, organic tin compounds, which are used in various industrial processes, have definite neurotoxicity. Intoxication with trimethyl tin leads to multifocal central dysfunction, with conspicuous behavioral disturbances, emotional lability, confusion, disorientation, cognitive disturbances, sleep dysfunction, headaches, and visual disturbances. Triethyl tin may lead to severe cerebral edema, with headache, papilledema, and behavioral abnormalities that generally resolve some weeks after discontinuation of exposure.

REFERENCES

Brashear A, Univerzagt FW, Farber MO, et al. Ethylene oxide neurotoxicity: a cluster of 12 nurses with peripheral and central nervous system toxicity. Neurology 1996;46:992–998.

Caldemeyer KS, Armstrong SW, George KK, et al. The spectrum of neuroimaging abnormalities in solvent abuse and their clinical correlation. J Neuroimaging 1996;6:167–173.

Calleman CJ, Wu Y, He F, et al. Relationships between biomarkers of exposure and neurological effects in a group of workers exposed to acrylamide. Toxicol Appl Pharmacol 1994;126:361–371.

Chu CC, Huang CC, Chen RS, Shih TS. Polyneuropathy induced by carbon disulphide in viscose rayon workers. Occup Environ Med 1995;52:404–407.

De Bleecker JL. The intermediate syndrome in organophosphate poisoning: an overview of experimental and clinical observations. J Toxicol 1995;33:683–686.

De Haro L, Gastaut JL, Jouglard J, Renacco E. Central and peripheral neurotoxic effects of chronic methyl bromide intoxication. J Toxicol 1997;35:29–34.

Deschamps FJ, Turpin JC. Methyl bromide intoxication during grain store fumigation. Occup Med 1996;46:89–90.

Glynn P, Holton JL, Nolan CC, et al. Neuropathy target esterase: immunolocalization to neuronal cell bodies and axons. Neuroscience 1998;83:295–302.

Graeme KA, Pollack CV Jr. Heavy metal toxicity, part I: arsenic and mercury. J Emerg Med 1998;16:45–56.

Greenberg SA. Acute demyelinating neuropathy with arsenic ingestion. Muscle Nerve 1996;19:1611–1613.

Huang CC, Chu CC, Chen RS, et al. Chronic carbon disulfide encephalopathy. Eur Neurol 1996;36:364–368.

Huang CC, Chu NS, Lu CS, et al. Long-term progression in chronic manganism: ten years of follow-up. Neurology 1998;40:698–700.

Lotti M. Mechanisms of toxicity and risk assessment. Toxicol Lett 1995;77:9–14.

Pastore C, Marhuenda D, Marti J, Cardona A. Early diagnosis of n-hexane-caused neuropathy. Muscle Nerve 1994;17:981–986.

Rebert CS, Hall TA. The neuroepidemiology of styrene: a critical review of representative literature. Crit Rev Toxicol 1994;24:S57–S106.

Sedgwick EM, Senanayake N. Pathophysiology of the intermediate syndrome of organophosphate poisoning. J Neurol Neurosurg Psychiatry 1997;62:201–202.

Szlatenyi CS, Wang RY. Encephalopathy and cranial nerve palsies caused by intentional trichloroethylene inhalation. Am J Emerg Med 1996;14:464–466.

Windebank AJ. Metal Neuropathy. In PJ Dyck, PK Thomas, JW Griffin, et al. (eds), Peripheral Neuropathy (3rd ed). Philadelphia: Saunders, 1993;1549–1570.

Woolf AD. Ginger Jake and the blues: a tragic song of poisoning. Vet Hum Toxicol 1995;37:252–254.

Chapter 64
Effects of Toxins and Physical Agents on the Nervous System

B. EFFECTS OF DRUG ABUSE ON THE NERVOUS SYSTEM
Yuen T. So

Drug abuse occurs in several different forms. A drug such as heroin or cocaine may be abused simply because it is illegal or obtained illegally. Legal prescription drugs, such as the opioid analgesics and benzodiazepines, also may be abused if taken in excessive amounts or used solely for recreational purposes. *Drug dependence* refers to either a psychological dependence or a physical dependence. In the former, drug craving or drug-seeking behavior emerges when the drug is not available. Physical dependence, on the other hand, implies the appearance of physiological symptoms and signs during drug withdrawal. *Drug tolerance* is generally defined as a diminished response to the same dosage of a drug and may reflect either increased metabolism of the drug or reduced physiological response to the drug at its normal cellular target.

The medical and social importance of drug abuse is enormous. In the United States, approximately one-third of the teenage or older population is said to have used marijuana, and 10% or more have used cocaine, heroin, or other hallucinogens. In the clinical evaluation of patients, a high level of suspicion is necessary, as a confirmatory history may be absent. Multiple agents are often abused concurrently, a fact that is important to bear in mind in the emergency assessment of patients with overdose. Chronic abuse of illicit drugs also coexists frequently with overuse of legal drugs, such as alcohol, tobacco, and prescription medications.

All the substances of abuse have potent acute and chronic effects on the nervous system. It is helpful to divide the neurological consequences of drug abuse into three broad categories according to the mechanism of action (Table 64B.1). First, acute intoxication or overdose often leads to delirium, stupor, or coma, sometimes accompanied by myoclonus, seizures, or serious systemic consequences such as respiratory depression and cardiovascular collapse. Second, chronic use of most of these agents often leads to drug tolerance or dependence. With abrupt abstinence of a habitually used drug, a patient may present for emergency care with an acute withdrawal syndrome. Third, drug abuse may affect the nervous system indirectly, via infectious and embolic consequences of intravenous drug use, hypersensitivity or immunological mechanisms, or some other manner that is not yet understood.

Urine screening of drugs of abuse is widely used in the diagnostic evaluation of patients (Table 64B.2). Positive results may be confirmed by an alternative method such as gas chromatography and mass spectroscopy. The urine test provides only qualitative information of recent drug use. Because urinary levels are dependent on time and clearance, they often do not correlate with toxic symptoms.

The first part of the following discussion reviews the pharmacological effects of commonly abused drugs. The primary concerns are the acute pharmacological effects and the withdrawal syndromes associated with long-term use. The second part of the chapter discusses the indirect effects of drug abuse on the nervous system.

PHARMACOLOGICAL EFFECTS

Opioid Analgesics

The name *opium* came from the Greek word for *juice*, as it was derived from the juice of the poppy. Its medicinal uses were discovered as early as the third century BC. Opium contains more than 20 alkaloids. Morphine was the first to be isolated in 1806 and was named after Morpheus, the Greek god of dreams. Other alkaloids such as codeine were discov-

Table 64B.1:   Neurological complications of drug abuse

Acute intoxication and overdose
Drug withdrawal syndrome
Indirect complications of drug abuse
    Infectious endocarditis
        Cerebral or spinal cord abscess
        Meningitis or encephalitis
        Myelopathy
    Strokes
        Postanoxic encephalopathy
        Hemorrhage
        Cerebral or spinal cord infarct
    Brachial plexitis
    Nerve compression
    Rhabdomyolysis

Table 64B.2:   Common drugs of abuse: maximum time interval after last drug use when drugs and their metabolites are still detectable by enzyme immunoassay of urine

Drug	Maximum detection time after last use
Amphetamine	48 hrs
Cocaine	48 hrs
Benzodiazepines*	5–7 days
Barbiturates, long-acting	7 days
Barbiturates, short- or intermediate-acting	1–2 days
Heroin*	4–5 days
Methadone	3 days
Morphine	48 hrs
Phencyclidine*	2 wks
Propoxyphene	48 hrs

*Maximum detection times given for chronic users. Single dose in nonhabitual users is cleared considerably more rapidly.

ered soon afterward. By the middle of the nineteenth century, the use of these compounds was widespread in medicine.

Pharmacology

Opiates refer only to those drugs derived from opium and include the naturally occurring alkaloids as well as semisynthetic derivatives. Endorphins are endogenous opioid peptides, and encompass the enkephalins, dynorphins, and β-endorphins. The term *opioid* is more inclusive and is used for all agonists and antagonists with morphinelike activities, as well as the naturally occurring and synthetic opioid peptides. These compounds act on the three opioid receptor subtypes, μ, δ, and κ, and have a wide spectrum of activities as analgesics, psychotomimetics, miotics, and suppressants of respiration, cough, and gastric motility.

Development of drug tolerance and dependence is an unavoidable physiological consequence of repeated use of opioids. For example, when used in prolonged treatment of pain, increasingly higher doses of opioids are often required to maintain the same degree of pain control. The pharmacological basis of this phenomenon is poorly understood. At least in animal models, competitive and noncompetitive N-methyl-D-aspartate (NMDA) antagonists, or inhibition of nitric oxide synthase may block the phenomenon of tolerance. Neither tolerance nor dependence reliably predicts drug abuse; thus, the fear that tolerance may develop should not interfere with the appropriate use of opioids.

Drug Abuse

Abuse of opioid analgesics presents in two primary forms. A prescription opioid analgesic may be taken excessively, or a legal drug may be obtained or sold illegally. A typical patient may seek multiple physicians for prescription, present with exaggerated complaints, or engage in other drug-seeking behavior. A second group of drug abusers are the so-called street addicts, typified by the use of the illegal drug heroin. Heroin crosses the blood-brain barrier rapidly. Its effect on the brain is identical to that of morphine. Three milligrams of heroin is roughly equivalent to 10 mg of morphine. Heroin may be snorted (sniffed up the nose), smoked, injected subcutaneously ("skin-popping"), or administered intravenously ("mainlining"). Heroin is sold in the streets in varying degree of purity, and it is sometimes combined with cocaine ("speedball").

Acute Effects

Aside from the analgesic effects, morphine or heroin acutely produce a sense of rush, accompanied by either euphoria or dysphoria. Hallucinations may occur also. Other effects include pruritus, dry mouth, nausea and vomiting, constipation, and urinary retention. Examination may show marked pupillary constriction, such that it may be difficult to discern the light reflex. Overdose of heroin leads to coma, respiratory suppression, and pinpoint pupils. Hypotension and hypothermia may also occur, but seizures are rare.

Acute treatment of severe opioid overdose should include close monitoring of vital signs and provision of blood pressure and respiratory support if necessary. Naloxone is a safe and effective opioid antagonist and should be used immediately in any suspected opioid overdose. Naloxone also provides useful diagnostic information, because it induces immediate reversal of both coma and respiratory depression in a patient with opioid overdose. For treatment of respiratory depression, 2 mg of naloxone may be given parenterally, and the dose repeated as needed up to 10–20 mg. Because the half-life of naloxone (1–4 hours) is shorter than most opioid agonists, it should be given in repeat boluses and the patient should be monitored closely through the at-risk period. With careful titration of the dose, it should be possible to reverse respiratory depression without precipitating acute opioid withdrawal.

Drug Dependence and Withdrawal

With development of drug dependence, symptoms and signs of withdrawal appear hours after the last opioid use. Drug craving appears first, followed by restlessness and irritability. Autonomic symptoms such as sweating, lacrimation, and rhinorrhea then emerge. Still later, piloerection, aching, nausea, abdominal cramps, diarrhea, and coughing develop. The time of the appearance of withdrawal symptoms depends on the duration of action of the drugs. With morphine and heroin, withdrawal symptoms appear in 6–9 hours of the last dose, peak at 24–72 hours, and last approximately 10 days. With methadone, symptoms appear in approximately 12–24 hours, peak at 6 days, and last approximately 3 weeks.

Most of the time, opioid withdrawal in adults, although unpleasant, is not in itself life-threatening. In contrast to adults, opioid withdrawal in neonates is sometimes accompanied by myoclonus, seizures, or even status epilepticus. This occurs typically in newborns of opioid-dependent mothers. Naloxone used during the treatment of respiratory depression sometimes precipitates withdrawal reactions. Acute administration of paregoric or methadone is an effective treatment. Phenobarbital may be used if there has been prenatal exposure to other drugs such as barbiturates and alcohol.

Oral methadone, a long-acting opiate, is used to relieve opioid withdrawal symptoms. A dose of 20 mg once or twice a day is sufficient in opioid-dependent patients. The dose is then gradually reduced, with the hope of eventually achieving detoxification. Clonidine, an α_2-adrenergic agonist, suppresses the autonomic disturbances of opioid withdrawal and is useful when combined with methadone.

Sedatives and Hypnotics

Sedatives and hypnotics as a group have calming effects and are capable of inducing sleep when taken in sufficient dosages. The group includes the benzodiazepines, barbiturates, and various less commonly used agents. Like opioid analgesics, abuse manifestations include excessive use of prescription drugs, recreational use, drug overdose, drug dependence, and withdrawal symptoms. The benzodiazepines are among the most frequently prescribed medications in Western countries. Approximately 2% of the adult population takes these agents on a daily basis, of whom approximately one-fifth use them regularly for 12 months or longer. The benzodiazepines account for over one-half of the overdoses in the United States. Both benzodiazepines and barbiturates are often used in conjunction with heroin by opioid abusers. Alcoholics also sometimes use them to alleviate symptoms of alcohol withdrawal. Overdose with these agents is common.

Benzodiazepines

Benzodiazepines constitute a large group of prescription drugs promoted either as sleeping aids or tranquilizers. They all share similar effects on the central nervous system, and the differences among individual drugs are largely those of dosage and duration of action. The benzodiazepines with rapid onset of action, such as diazepam, are among the most likely to be abused. Benzodiazepines also are abused frequently in conjunction with other drugs, most notably alcohol.

Acutely, the recipient experiences varying degrees of lassitude, drowsiness, confusion, amnesia, euphoria, and impairment of other psychomotor functions. Even in conventional dosages, these neurological effects are potentially dangerous, especially in the elderly. Falls, for example, may result from drowsiness and motor incoordination. Sufficiently severe overdose leads to coma, but benzodiazepines are less likely to cause respiratory or cardiovascular depression than barbiturates and opioids. Thus, benzodiazepine overdose is rarely fatal, unless other drugs are used concurrently. Still, initial treatment of comatose patients should be directed to immediate assessment and management of cardiovascular and respiratory functions. Flumazenil is a specific antagonist for benzodiazepines. It reverses rapidly the stupor or coma of the overdose, although its usefulness is limited by its short duration of action, lasting only 30–60 minutes. A dose of 0.2–5.0 mg given intravenously over 2–10 minutes is sufficient to reverse benzodiazepine overdose. A lack of response is strong evidence that another drug is involved.

Chronic use of benzodiazepines may lead to tolerance and physical dependence. Withdrawal symptoms typically occur within 24 hours of cessation of use of a short-acting benzodiazepine, and approximately 3–7 days after stopping a long-acting agent. Withdrawal symptoms include irritability, increased sensitivity to light and sound, sweating, tremor, tachycardia, headache, and sleep disturbances. In more severe withdrawal states, delirium, hallucinations, and seizures may occur. Withdrawal symptoms may last several weeks. Reinstituting the benzodiazepine, followed by gradual tapering of the dosage is usually sufficient to treat these withdrawal symptoms.

Barbiturates

Like benzodiazepines, abuse of barbiturates is often linked with use of other agents. The acute symptoms are similar to those of alcohol and include euphoria, sedation, slurred speech, and gait ataxia. Severe enough intoxication leads to coma. Hypotension and hypothermia often accompany coma. There are frequently signs of abnormal respiration. Breathing may be slow or rapid and shallow. Cheyne-Stokes breathing, respiratory depression, and eventually apnea occur with sufficient intoxication. Treatment is primarily supportive. The lethal dose varies, but as a general rule of thumb intoxication with more than 10 times the hypnotic dose is likely to be dangerous. Treatment is primarily supportive. Gastric lavage may be useful within 24 hours, because barbiturates may reduce gastric motility. Hemodialysis or hemoperfusion is rarely necessary.

Withdrawal symptoms are similar to those seen with alcohol withdrawal. Insomnia, irritability, tremor, tachycardia, nausea, and vomiting are common. With short-acting barbiturates, symptoms usually begin within 36 hours, and the long-acting barbiturates are associated with a longer delay of several days. In severe cases, delirium tremens and seizures may occur. Treatment of withdrawal is simply reinstitution of the barbiturates, followed by gradual tapering.

Other Sedatives and Hypnotics

Other sedatives and hypnotics are abused much less frequently than barbiturates and benzodiazepines. Methaqualone was popular in the 1970s. Overdose is characterized by delirium, myoclonus, and seizures, sometimes followed by coma and acute congestive heart failure. Glutethimide overdose leads to coma, hypotension, and less frequently, respiratory depression. Abuse of this agent is recognized by its anticholinergic effects that produce dilated unreactive pupils. Other infrequently abused drugs include paraldehyde, chloral hydrate, meprobamate, and ethchlorvynol. Ethchlorvynol overdose is characterized by its long duration of action that may last many days. Treatment includes diuresis, peritoneal or hemodialysis, or hemoperfusion with activated charcoal or resin.

Psychomotor Stimulants

This group of drugs all share sympathomimetic effects on the central nervous system. The main difference is in the duration of action. Cocaine is the most commonly abused. It may be administered intranasally or parenterally, or may be smoked ("crack"). Amphetamine, dextroamphetamine, methamphetamine, and methylphenidate also have significant abuse potential. Another drug of abuse is 3,4-methylenedioxymethamphetamine (MDMA). It is popularly known as *ecstasy*, as it has hallucinogenic effects in addition to its stimulant properties. Other agents such as fenfluramine, phentermine, ephedrine, and phenylpropanolamine have less liability for abuse.

Acute Effects

In moderate doses, these stimulants produce mood elevation, increased alertness, reduced fatigue, decreased appetite, and sometimes enhanced performance in various tasks. Other symptoms may include agitation, palpitation, dysphoria, and headaches. Pupillary dilation, tachycardia, and hypertension are common. There are considerable individual differences in the psychic effects of these stimulants. Some patients develop paranoia, delusions, hallucinations, and violence. Other patients may be depressed or lethargic. Movement disorders such as tics, chorea, and dystonia are sometimes seen (Cardoso and Jankovic 1993). Some patients may present with myoclonus or seizures. Most of these seizures are generalized and self-limiting, although status epilepticus is an uncommon but recognized complication of overdose.

Of the abused stimulants, cocaine is the most likely to cause seizures. Seizures are generally more likely when cocaine is smoked (crack cocaine) or given intravenously. Cocaine also may induce seizures in people with a history of epilepsy (Koppel et al. 1996). The estimate of seizure frequency varies widely from approximately 1–10%, depending on the study population. Typically, seizures occur within 1–2 hours of cocaine use. Other drugs, such as amphetamines, methylphenidate, ephedrine, and phenylpropanolamine also may cause seizures.

Treatment of overdose should include supportive measures such as oxygen, cardiac monitoring, cooling for hyperthermia, antihypertensives, and blood pressure and ventilatory support as necessary. Sedatives may be used judiciously to treat agitation. Seizures are managed with benzodiazepines and phenytoin. Forced diuresis and urine acidification promote drug excretion, but should be avoided if myoglobinuria is present.

Drug Dependence and Withdrawal

After repeated usage of cocaine or amphetamines, tolerance develops to the euphoric and anorexic effects of these agents. The reverse seems to apply to the epileptogenic effect, as repeated use of cocaine may lower seizure threshold. Acute abstinence after chronic use manifests primarily as fatigue and depression. The withdrawal syndrome is seldom life-threatening, with the exception of those patients who encounter suicidal ideations. Treatment with imipramine or other antidepressant drugs may be helpful.

Other Substances of Abuse

Marijuana

Tetrahydrocannabinol is the primary active ingredient of marijuana. Tetrahydrocannabinol has effects on mood, memory, judgment, and sense of time. Often, a sense of relaxation, euphoria, and depersonalization occurs. There may be a subjective slowing of time. Variable amounts of anxiety, paranoia, sedation, or sleepiness may occur also. High doses of tetrahydrocannabinol produce hallucinations, paranoia, or a frank panic reaction. Treatment of such cases generally requires only calm reassurance. Tolerance does develop with chronic usage. Irritability, restlessness, and insomnia are typical after abrupt discontinuation.

Phencyclidine and Ketamine

These drugs were developed as anesthetics. At progressively increasing dosages, analgesia, anesthesia, stupor, and coma develop. At moderate doses, they produce variable degrees of euphoria, dysphoria, relaxation, paranoia, and hallucinations. Psychosis, agitation, bizarre behavior, and catatonia are common. This may be accompanied by physical signs of fever, hypertension, sweating, miosis, and horizontal as well as vertical nystagmus. Treatment is largely supportive. Violent behavior may require restraint. Rhabdomyolysis is common with overdose, and myoglobinuria should be looked for and treated.

Anticholinergics

The recreational use of these agents includes abuse of prescription drugs as well as use of plants that contain the belladonna alkaloids, atropine, and scopolamine. These agents are abused for their pharmacological properties of causing delirium and hallucinations. The psychoactive effects are accompanied by mydriasis, dry and flushed skin, tachycardia, urinary retention, and fever. Severe overdose may lead to myoclonus, seizures, coma, and death. Acute treatment employs intramuscular or intravenous injection of 1 mg of physostigmine. This is followed by titrating doses of 0.5–2.0 mg of physostigmine every 30 minutes to 2 hours.

Inhalants

This includes a wide range of volatile compounds, including various hydrocarbons, nitrites, and nitrous oxide. Many of these chemicals are present in common household and industrial products. Despite the diversity of agents being abused, the acute effects are remarkably similar. At low to moderate doses, these chemicals induce a sense of euphoria, relaxation, incoordination, and slurred speech. For most practical purposes, the effects resemble alcohol intoxication. Higher doses produce psychosis, hallucinations, and seizures. The duration of action is typically only 15–30 minutes, but the effects may be sustained by continual use. Various complications such as cardiac arrhythmia, suffocation from the use of plastic bags, vomiting and aspirations and, rarely, sudden death have been reported.

Aside from the acute neuropsychological effects, different systemic and neurological complications may result from chronic abuse of individual agents. Lead intoxication may result from sniffing gasoline. A peripheral neuropathy with disabling weakness and slow nerve conduction velocities may result from the use of n-hexane. Nitrous oxide abuse leads to a syndrome of subacute combined degeneration similar to that seen in vitamin B_{12} deficiency. Cerebral and cerebellar dysfunctions are seen after chronic toluene abuse. Mild cognitive dysfunction has been associated with chronic exposures to many volatile hydrocarbons. Systemic complications include renal, hepatic, and bone marrow

Table 64B.3: Probable mechanisms of strokes associated with drug abuse

Intravenous drug abuse
Endocarditis, infectious or marantic
Embolization of foreign materials
Right-to-left shunt in pulmonary vasculature
Mycotic aneurysm
Direct effects of drugs
Vascular injury: hypertensive changes, arterial dissection
Acute severe hypertension
Vasoconstriction or vasospasm
Impaired autoregulation
Indirect effects of drugs
Vasculitis
Pre-existing vascular malformation or aneurysm
Cardiomyopathy and arrhythmia
Antiphospholipid antibodies
Nephropathy and secondary hypertension
Hypotension or hypoxia from overdose
Acquired immunodeficiency syndrome or related to human immunodeficiency virus

abnormalities after exposure to benzene, and methemoglobinemia after use of alkyl nitrite.

Hallucinogens

The hallucinogens as a group cause alteration of mood, perception, and thought processes, without significantly changing alertness, memory, and orientation. The synthetic ergot D-lysergic acid diethylamide (usually referred to as *LSD*) is the best example and is still popular among drug abusers. In addition, a wide range of plants and mushrooms are known to be hallucinogenic. Acute ingestion leads to rapid onset of dizziness, blurred vision, nausea, and weakness. This is followed by hallucinations that are often visual and complex. There may be depersonalization and a distortion of time. Sometimes the experience is terrifying (the so-called bad trips), resulting in injuries to self or others. Physical signs include fever, tachycardia, hypertension, mydriasis, seizures, and coma.

INDIRECT NEUROLOGICAL COMPLICATIONS

Stroke

Drug abuse of almost any form increases the risk of strokes. In retrospective studies of young stroke patients between 15 and 44 years of age, drug abusers accounted for 12–31% (Sloan et al. 1998). Drug abuse was the most important risk factor for those younger than 35 years of age. The relative risk of stroke was 6.5 after controlling for other stroke risk factors. The possible mechanisms are diverse (Table 64B.3) and are dependent on the route of drug administration and the chemical agents involved. The risk increase does not take into consideration the abuse of alcohol and tobacco, both of which, though legal, also increase the stroke risk.

Aside from the usual workup of stroke, the evaluation of patients with drug-related strokes should include a careful search for endocarditis or other source of embolization, a full cardiac evaluation, erythrocyte sedimentation rate, and antiphospholipid antibody assay. Cerebral angiography is often necessary, especially when vasculitis, aneurysms, or vascular malformations are suspected (Brust 1993; Kokkinos and Levine 1993).

Embolism

The sources of embolism include valvular disease secondary to infective or marantic endocarditis, mural thrombi of cardiomyopathy, right-to-left shunt, aortic or other arterial dissection, and foreign materials injected during intravenous drug abuse. Strokes occur in approximately 20% of cases of infective endocarditis. Prompt initiation of antibiotic therapy markedly reduces the risk of stroke. Thus, early recognition is important. Mycotic aneurysm complicates 1–3% of endocarditis and is an important cause of intracerebral hemorrhage. Angiography should be considered when mycotic aneurysm is suspected, although the role and timing of surgery are controversial.

Emboli of foreign material are possible when intravenous injections are prepared by crushing or dissolving drug tablets. Examples are methylphenidate, meperidine, and pentazocine. Embolic materials also may include insoluble fillers such as talc. These foreign particles become lodged in the lung after an intravenous injection and cause pulmonary hypertension and arteriovenous fistulae, providing a path to the cerebrovascular circulation.

Vasculitis and Other Vasculopathies

Vasospasm is associated with many drugs of abuse, most notably the psychostimulants such as cocaine, amphetamines, methylphenidate, and phenylpropanolamine. For poorly understood reasons, some drugs of abuse also lead to the development of vasculitis. This has been best documented in some patients with amphetamine abuse and less convincingly in a few patients who abused phenylpropanolamine, cocaine, or heroin. The diagnosis of vasculitis without histological verification is difficult, as the classic angiographic findings of segmental narrowing and beading of intracerebral arteries do not distinguish among vasculitis, vasospasm, arteriosclerosis, and other vasculopathies. Abstinence should be the first step in treatment of patients suspected to have vasculitis. The role of immunosuppressive therapy is undefined. It is not clear if the clinical course and response to treatment of drug-induced vasculitis are different from other vasculitis of the nervous system.

Hypotension and Anoxia

Anoxic brain injury often follows drug overdose, most notably those caused by heroin and other opiates. An autopsy series of heroin addicts observed that 2% had ischemic injury to the globus pallidus. Delayed postanoxic encephalopathy also rarely occurs. The clinical manifestations are similar to those described after prolonged cardiac arrest, respiratory failure, and carbon monoxide poisoning.

Cocaine

Cocaine is without question the most important cause of drug-related stroke and accounts for approximately 50% of all the cases. There are reports of transient ischemic attacks or ischemic infarctions of almost any area of the brain or spinal cord. Intraparenchymal or subarachnoid hemorrhage is another common mode of presentation (Aggarwal et al. 1996). Neurological symptoms typically develop within hours of cocaine use, although rarely symptoms may progress gradually for up to a week. Seizures sometimes accompany the strokes.

The pathophysiological mechanisms of cocaine-induced stroke are varied. Acute hypertension, vasospasm, and vasoconstriction probably play an important role (Kaufman et al. 1998). Pre-existing vascular pathology may be a key factor in some patients. Among those who present with intracranial hemorrhages, approximately one-half have underlying cerebral aneurysms or vascular malformations. Endocarditis, myocardial infarction, cardiac arrhythmias, aortic dissection, and anticardiolipin antibodies are other observed associations.

Myelopathy

An acute myelopathy may develop rarely after drug abuse. The association is best documented in heroin abuse and rarely in cocaine use. For the most part, the syndrome resembles an anterior spinal artery syndrome. Paraparesis, urinary retention, and a segmental sensory level appear acutely. On examination, posterior column function is often relatively spared. Myelography, magnetic resonance imaging, and cerebrospinal fluid are usually normal, although mild elevation of cerebrospinal fluid protein may be present. There are several possible causes. Watershed infarct secondary to hypotension may be responsible in some patients. Embolic infarct from injected particulate material may account for other cases, as may hypersensitivity or vasculitis.

Rhabdomyolysis and Myopathy

It is unclear whether any of the commonly abused drugs are directly toxic to muscles. Evidence of muscle abnormality ranges from asymptomatic elevation of serum creatine kinase to frank myoglobinuria and renal failure. The observations are made most commonly in the abuse of heroin, cocaine, amphetamine, MDMA (ecstasy), and phencyclidine. The patients were typically severely intoxicated. Possible mechanisms include trauma, crush injury, hypotension, hypertension, fever, seizures, and excessive muscular activities.

Repeated intramuscular injections of meperidine, pentazocine, or heroin sometimes lead to focal fibrosis and weakness of the injected muscles. Contractures develop slowly. The affected muscles have a woody and firm quality. Weakness is mild and is limited to the injected muscles. Electromyographical examination of affected areas demonstrates reduced insertional activity (suggesting extensive fibrotic replacement of the muscle), short duration, and small amplitude motor unit action potentials (Louis et al. 1994).

Neuropathy and Plexopathy

Compressive or stretch injuries to peripheral nerves and plexuses may result from drug abuse of any kind. Focal neuropathies may develop also as a result of compartment syndrome and secondary nerve ischemia. The most commonly affected sites are the brachial plexus, the radial nerve at the upper arm, ulnar nerve at the elbow, sciatic nerve in the gluteal region, and peroneal nerve at the fibular head. Some cases of idiopathic brachial or lumbosacral plexitis have been attributed to heroin use. A potential though unproven cause is a hypersensitivity reaction to heroin or the accompanying adulterant.

Many drug abusers have physical signs of a distal sensory or sensorimotor polyneuropathy, but it difficult to establish a causal relationship with the abused drugs, as confounding factors such as alcohol abuse and systemic diseases are frequently present. An exceptional example is in the chronic use of hydrocarbon inhalants (Smith and Albers 1997). The neuropathy is similar to that observed during industrial outbreaks caused by exposure to n-hexane or methyl n-butyl ketone. Distal paresthesias and numbness appear first, followed by development of distal weakness. Weakness worsens with continuing abuse and may progress to involve proximal muscles of both upper and lower limbs.

REFERENCES

Aggarwal SK, Williams V, Levine SR, et al. Cocaine-associated intracranial hemorrhage: absence of vasculitis in 14 cases. Neurology 1996;46:1741–1743.

Brust JC. Clinical, radiological, and pathological aspects of cerebrovascular disease associated with drug abuse. Stroke 1993;24:I129–I133; discussion I134–I135.

Cardoso FE, Jankovic J. Cocaine-related movement disorders. Mov Disord 1993;8:175–178.

Kaufman MJ, Levin JM, Ross MH, et al. Cocaine-induced cerebral vasoconstriction detected in humans with magnetic resonance angiography. JAMA 1998;279:376–380.

Kokkinos J, Levine SR. Stroke. Neurol Clin 1993;11:577–590.

Koppel BS, Damkoff L, Daras M. Relation of cocaine use to seizures and epilepsy. Epilepsia 1996;37:875–878.

Louis ED, Bodner RA, Challenor YB, et al. Focal myopathy induced by chronic intramuscular heroin injection. Muscle Nerve 1994;17:550–552.

Sloan MA, Kittner SJ, Feeser BR, et al. Illicit drug-associated ischemic stroke in the Baltimore-Washington Young Stroke Study. Neurology 1998;50:1688–1693.

Smith AG, Albers JW. n-Hexane neuropathy due to rubber cement sniffing. Muscle Nerve 1997;20:1445–1450.

Chapter 64
Effects of Toxins and Physical Agents on the Nervous System

C. NEUROTOXINS OF ANIMALS AND PLANTS
Yuen T. So

Naturally occurring neurotoxins of animals and plants are of great scientific interest. Many of them are important tools used by investigators to probe the workings of the nervous system. One of the oldest and best-known examples is curare, a plant toxin that was used in Claude Bernard's classical experiments on neuromuscular transmission over 100 years ago. Another example, α-bungarotoxin, was isolated from the venom of the banded krait *Bungarus multicinctus*. α-Bungarotoxin is a competitive blocker of the acetylcholine receptor and has proven to be invaluable in the studies of the neuromuscular junction and myasthenia gravis.

NEUROTOXINS OF ANIMALS

The neurotoxins of animals serve several essential functions in nature. Venoms from reptiles and arthropods may be useful to defend against predators or to immobilize prey. Some venom may contain enzymes that aid in the digestion of consumed food. Many of these agents are among the most potent neurotoxins known to humans (Table 64C.1). Despite their biological potency, mortality caused by these agents is uncommon. The rarity is in part a result of the healthy respect most people have for snakes, spiders, and scorpions. Moreover, most bites result in a relatively small amount of envenomation that is well below lethal dosage.

Snake

The majority of the venomous snakebites in the United States are inflicted by the pit vipers (Crotalidae), a group that includes rattlesnakes, copperheads, and water moccasins. Coral snakes (Elapidae) account for most of the remainder. Important venomous snakes in other parts of the world include other Elapidae (cobras, mambas, kraits, and Australian elapid snakes), Hydrophiidae (sea snakes), and Viperinae (old world vipers or Russell's viper). Not all bites by venomous snakes result in envenomation because approximately 20% of bites are dry. Even with envenomation, signs and symptoms may vary. Morbidity and mortality depend on the venom composition of the local snakes and the availability and sophistication of emergency medical care. In the United States, death occurs in much less than 1% of all incidents. By contrast, over 10,000 deaths are reported yearly from the Nigerian savannas and approximately 23,000 from West Africa.

Snake venoms are composed of a complex mixture of peptides with activities on the neuromuscular junction, platelets, endothelial cells, and the coagulation cascade (see Table 64C.1) (Markland 1997). Some of the toxins also may be directly myotoxic, and rhabdomyolysis is sometimes seen after envenomation. Considerable species and geographic variations occur in the spectrum of biological activities. For example, snakebites may cause primarily neuromuscular paralysis in one region, whereas bites by the same species in another region may cause mainly coagulopathy and hemorrhage. In general, when weakness is present, the pattern of involvement bears resemblance to myasthenia gravis, with predilection of the neck flexors, ocular, bulbar, and proximal limb muscles. Respiratory paralysis, if severe enough and left untreated, may lead to death.

At the time of patient presentation, fear and panic are common symptoms and the accompanying autonomic reac-

Table 64C.1:   Neurotoxins of snakes and arthropods

Source	Toxin	Physiological action
Snake venom	α-Bungarotoxin, cobrotoxin	Postsynaptic, competitive blockade of acetylcholine receptor
Snake venom	β-Bungarotoxin, crotoxin, notexin, taipoxin	Presynaptic inhibition of acetylcholine release
Black widow spider (*Latrodectus mactans*)	α-Latrotoxin	Presynaptic facilitation of acetylcholine release, followed by depletion of acetylcholine
Scorpion (*Tityus serrulatus*)	Tityustoxin	Presynaptic facilitation of acetylcholine release, and postsynaptic inhibition of Na$^+$ inactivation
Scorpion (*Centruroides*)	At least two groups of toxins	Presynaptic membrane depolarization
Tick (*Ixodes holocyclus*)	Holocyclotoxin	Presynaptic inhibition of acetylcholine release

tions should not be mistaken for systemic symptoms of envenomation. The cardinal signs of pit viper envenomation are pain, swelling, and erythema in tissues adjacent to the bite sites. These usually appear within 30 minutes and spread proximally as the venom spreads. More serious systemic symptoms appear over the ensuing 12–24 hours and consist of a variable combination of perioral or limb paresthesias, muscle fasciculations, weakness, hypotension, and shock. In contrast to pit viper envenomation, little pain or swelling accompanies coral snake bites. After a delay of 1–5 hours, ptosis, dysphagia, diffuse weakness, and respiratory suppression may develop, and deep tendon reflexes are lost. The bitten patient should be transferred to the nearest medical facility. Treatment includes calming and supportive measures. Even in the absence of life-threatening symptoms, a patient should be monitored for at least 6 hours if bitten by pit vipers and 12 hours if bitten by coral snakes. Antivenin should be administered as soon as it is certain that significant envenomation has occurred. Precaution should always be taken for anaphylactic reactions to the antivenin. Initial laboratory evaluation should include complete blood cell and platelet counts, coagulation parameters, fibrinogen, serum creatine kinase, and urine analysis. In patients with significant weakness, nerve conduction studies and repetitive nerve stimulation testing may reveal a pattern of either postsynaptic or presynaptic blockade. The observed changes consist of reduced amplitude of the compound muscle action potentials, decremental response to low-frequency repetitive stimulation, and postexercise and post-tetanic facilitation.

Spider

Of the commonly encountered spiders, few produce significant symptoms in humans. The widow spider (*Latrodectus* sp.) is the most important worldwide in terms of morbidity. The black widow spider (*Latrodectus mactans*) venom contains α-latrotoxin, a neurotoxin capable of inducing neurotransmitter release from presynaptic cholinergic, noradrenergic, and aminergic nerve endings. Although the toxin is far more potent than rattlesnake venoms, most bites do not cause many symptoms because only a small amount of venom is injected. Sometimes, an erythematous ring surrounding a paler center (target lesion) develops around the

site of spider bite. Rarely, often within 30–60 minutes of spider bites, intense pain and involuntary muscle spasms may appear dramatically in abdominal muscles and spread to limb muscles. Muscle weakness often follows. The condition may be mistaken for acute signs in the abdomen. Respiratory arrest sometimes results from respiratory muscle involvement. Other associated symptoms include priapism, salivation, sweating, bronchospasm, and bronchorrhea. Hypertension is a nearly universal finding in affected patients (Woestham et al. 1996). Serum creatine kinase may be elevated. Treatment begins with careful monitoring of respiration and vital signs, with intensive care support if necessary. Antivenin shortens the duration of symptoms if administered early, but should be reserved primarily for severe disease. Muscle spasms may be treated with slow infusion of calcium gluconate or methocarbamol. Benzodiazepines and opioids are useful for the control of anxiety and pain.

Scorpion

Although only a few of the approximately 1,400 scorpion species are of neurological importance, bites by poisonous scorpions are generally more dangerous than spider bites. Scorpion envenomation is a public health problem in warm climates. In Mexico alone, there are 100,000–200,000 scorpion bites annually, resulting in 400–1,000 fatalities. Small children in particular are prone to developing neurological symptoms. As many as 80% of the bites are symptomatic in this population. *Buthotus tamulus* of India, *Leiurus quinquestriatus* of North Africa and Near East, *Tityus serrulatus* of Brazil, and *Centruroides suffusus* of Mexico are among the most toxic. The bark scorpion (*Centruroides exilicauda*) is found in southwestern United States. Other species of medical importance include *Androctonus*, *Buthus*, *Parabuthus*, and *Nebo*. The venoms of these scorpions contain a wide range of polypeptides that have a net excitatory effect on autonomic and skeletal neuromuscular systems (see Table 64C.1).

Presenting symptoms are highly variable, from local pain to a general state of intoxication. Paresthesias are common and are usually experienced around the site of bite, but also may be felt diffusely. Autonomic symptoms may include hypertension, tachycardia or bradycardia, diaphoresis, salivation, lacrimation, hyperthermia, and mydriasis. Muscle fasciculations and spasms, dysphagia, and nystagmus are sometimes seen (Gateau et al. 1994). With severe envenomation, encephalopathy, paresis, or seizure may result from direct central nervous system toxicity. Treatment is often limited to symptomatic control. Severe cases should be monitored and treated in an intensive care setting. Scorpion antivenin is the only specific treatment and appears to be relatively safe and effective.

Tick Paralysis

Two types of ticks are of medical importance, Argasidae (soft tick) and Ixodidae (hard tick). Both may harbor infectious organisms, but only ixodid ticks cause paralysis. The ixodid ticks have a hard body plate and attach to the host for a prolonged period for feeding. Forty-six species cause weakness. *Ixodes holocyclus* is responsible for most cases in Australia, and *Dermacentor andersoni* and *Dermacentor variabilis* in North America. *Ixodes holocyclus* contains the neurotoxin, holocyclotoxin, that interferes with the presynaptic release of acetylcholine at the neuromuscular junction. The toxins of the North American ticks have not been characterized.

The hallmark of tick paralysis is an acute flaccid paresis that is nearly impossible to distinguish from Guillain-Barré syndrome. Most cases have been in small children between 1 and 5 years of age. Gait ataxia appears a few days after a tick attaches to the body. Ascending paralysis then develops over 1–2 days, generally more rapidly than in Guillain-Barré syndrome. In addition to limb weakness, weakness of the neck, bulbar, extraocular, and respiratory muscles may be prominent. Some degree of paresthesias is common, but there is no objective sensory loss. The physical examination should include a meticulous search for the tick, especially in the scalp, pubis, and skin areas covered by hair.

Nerve conduction study results may be normal or may show mild slowing of motor nerve conduction velocities. The amplitude of the compound muscle action potentials is often decreased, sometimes to a marked degree. High rates of repetitive stimulation may show a normal result or an abnormal incremental response. There may be important differences in pathophysiology between the North American and Australian cases of tick paralysis. Removal of the North American tick often leads to rapid and dramatic recovery within a few hours. By contrast, removal of *Ixodes holocyclus* is often followed by worsening of paralysis over 24–48 hours before improvement begins (Grattan-Smith et al. 1997).

NEUROTOXINS OF PLANTS AND MUSHROOMS

Pharmacologically active agents are present in thousands of plants and mushrooms species. Although fatal poisoning is relatively rare, many of the commonly encountered species are capable of inducing serious neurological symptoms. In 1993 in the United States, 94,725 cases of plant poisoning and 7,976 cases of mushroom poisoning were reported by poison centers (Litovitz et al. 1994). Clinically significant toxicity occurs under several circumstances. Approximately 75% of the poison center cases occur in children under the age of 6 years. Most of them are a result of accidental ingestion. Adult poisoning may occur when toxic plants or mushrooms are mistaken for edible species. Undoubtedly, an underreported category is the intentional consumption among some adolescents and young adults who choose to seek their highs from botanical sources.

Common names of plants are entirely inadequate in the identification of plants; botanical names should be used whenever possible. Identification is neither easy nor accurate, even with the aid of current computer software (Lawrence 1998). Naming the plant or mushroom involved in a botanical exposure should be left to a trained botanist or mycologist. Even without a definitive identification, the history of exposure and the recognition of an appropriate syndrome are often sufficient to establish a tentative diagnosis. The best treatment is usually empiric, including gastric lavage or catharsis, supportive measures, and control of symptoms. With the exception of the anticholinergic poisoning, there is no antidote.

A few of the important neurological syndromes are discussed in this chapter. A comprehensive review of the botanical toxins is impossible. Table 64C.2 lists several major categories and the commonly associated plants in each category. Omitted are plants that do not have direct toxicity on the nervous system, such as those containing cardiac glycosides, oxalates, taxines, andromedotoxin, colchicine, and phytotoxins. Secondary neurological disturbances may result from these toxins because some of them can cause severe fluid and electrolyte abnormalities or cardiovascular dysfunctions.

Jimson Weed (*Datura stramonium*)

Jimson weed, originally named Jamestown weed, when grown by early settlers in Jamestown, VA, from seeds brought from England, was used to treat asthma. The chief active ingredient is the alkaloid hyoscyamine, with lesser amounts of atropine and scopolamine. It is found throughout the United States. Intoxication is not uncommon, especially among young recreational users in rural areas. Symptoms of anticholinergic toxicity appear within 30–60 minutes after ingestion, and often continue for 24–48 hours because of delayed gastric motility (Centers for Disease Control 1995). Symptoms include blurred vision, delirium, hallucinations, seizures, and coma. They are accompanied by autonomic disturbances such as mydriasis, tachycardia, thirst, dry mouth, and hyperpyrexia. Treatment include gastric lavage, induction of emesis, supportive measures, and symptomatic treatments. Physostigmine is reserved for severe or life-threatening cases.

Peyote (*Lophophora williamsii*)

Peyote is a small cactus native to the southwestern United States and Mexico, but it can be cultivated anywhere. The

Table 64C.2:   Neurotoxicity of plants

Principal toxins	Plants	Clinical features
Tropane (belladonna) alkaloids	Jimson weed (*Datura stramonium*) Deadly nightshade (*Atropa belladonna*) Matrimony vine (*Lycium halimifolium*) Henbane (*Hyoscyamus niger*) Jasmine (*Cestrum* sp.)	Mydriasis, tachycardia, dry mouth, hyperpyrexia, blurred vision, delirium, hallucinations, seizures, coma
Solanine alkaloids	Woody nightshade (*Solanum dulcamara*) Black nightshade (*Solanum nigrum*) Jerusalem cherry (*Solanum pseudocapsicum*) Leaves and roots of common potato (*Solanum tuberosum*) Wild tomato (*Solanum gracile*)	Mydriasis, tachycardia, dry mouth, hyperpyrexia, blurred vision, delirium, hallucinations, seizures, coma
Nicotinelike alkaloids	Tobacco (*Nicotiana* sp.) Golden chain (*Laburnum anagyroides*) Poison hemlock (*Conium maculatum*)	Variable sympathetic and parasympathetic hyper-activities, seizures, hypotension
Cicutoxin	Water hemlock (*Cicuta* sp.) Chinaberry (*Melia azedarach*)	Diarrhea, abdominal pain, salivation, seizures, coma
Miscellaneous hallucinogens	Morning glory (*Ipomoea tricolor*) Peyote (*Lophophora williamsii*) Juniper (*Juniper macropoda*) African yohimbe (*Corynanthe yohimbe*) Catnip (*Nepeta cataria*) Nutmeg (*Myristica fragrans*) Periwinkle (*Catharanthus roseus*)	Delirium, hallucinations
Excitatory amino acids	Chickling pea and others (*Lathyrus* sp.) Cycad (*Cycas circinalis*)	Neurodegenerative diseases

principal agent is mescaline, which has actions similar to those of the hallucinogenic indoles. A peyote button, the top portion of the cactus, contains approximately 45 mg of mescaline. Approximately six to nine buttons (5 mg/kg) are sufficient to be hallucinogenic. Dizziness, drowsiness, ataxia, paresthesias, sympathomimetic symptoms, nausea, or vomiting are frequent accompanying clinical features. Ingestions are rarely life-threatening.

Morning Glory (*Ipomoea tricolor*)

The active agents in morning glory are various amides of lysergic acid. The seeds are consumed for purposes of abuse. The neuropsychological effects are similar to those of lysergic acid diethylamide and consist of hallucinations, anxiety, mood changes, depersonalization, and drowsiness. Acute clinical effects also include mydriasis, nausea, vomiting, and diarrhea.

Water Hemlock (*Cicuta* sp.)

Water hemlock is a highly toxic plant found primarily in wet, swampy areas and is sometimes mistakenly ingested as wild parsnips. Symptoms consist of initial muscarinic effects (abdominal pain, salivation, and diarrhea), followed by generalized convulsions, obtundation, and coma. Seizures may be treated with benzodiazepines.

Lathyrism

Various *Lathyrus* species including the grass or chickling pea (*L. sativus*), *L. clymenum* (Spanish vetch), and *L. cicera* (flat-podded pea) are responsible for lathyrism (Spencer 1995). These hardy plants are an important part of the diet of people in the India continent, Africa, China, and some parts of Europe. Epidemics of lathyrism often coincide with periods of famine or war, probably a result of excessive dietary dependency on these legumes. The disease, known since antiquity, is still endemic in many underdeveloped countries, where astounding prevalence rates as high as 66% have been reported during famines. The putative toxin is beta-N-oxalylamino-L-alanine, an excitatory amino acid that is capable of inducing lathyrism in primate animal models.

Clinically, the affected patients present with subacute or insidious onset of spastic paraparesis, Babinski's sign, and gait instability. Muscle aching and subjective paresthesias may be present, but the sensory examination is largely normal. Cognition and cerebellar functions are spared. Partial recovery after discontinuation of *Lathyrus* intake is possible. Of interest are reports of late deterioration many years

Table 64C.3: Poisonous mushrooms

Principal toxins	Mushrooms	Mode of action	Time of onset/clinical features
Cyclic polypeptides (especially amatoxins)	*Amanita phalloides, A. virosa, A. bisporigera*, and others	Inhibition of mRNA synthesis, hepatotoxin and nephrotoxin	6–24 hrs: gastrointestinal symptoms; 3–5 days: hepatotoxicity and renal failure
Monomethylhydrazines (gyromitrin)	*Gyromitra* genus ("false morels")	Competitive inhibition of pyridoxine	6–12 hrs: gastrointestinal symptoms, hemolysis, seizures that respond to pyridoxine
Coprine	*Coprinus atramentarius*	Inhibition of acetaldehyde dehydrogenase (disulfiramlike)	20–120 mins: flushing, palpitations, and headache only after alcohol ingestion
Muscarine	*Clitocybe* and *Inocybe* genera	Cholinergic agonist	15–120 mins: cholinergic hyperactivity
Muscimol, ibotenic acid	*Amanita muscaria, A. gemmata, A. pantherina, A. cothurnata*	Anticholinergic and γ-aminobutyric acid antagonist	30–120 mins: euphoria, ataxia, mydriasis, delirium, seizures, and coma
Indoles (psilocybin)	*Psilocybe, Panaeolus, Gymnophilus* genera	Actions resemble lysergic acid diethylamide	30–60 mins: euphoria, hallucinations, mydriasis, tachycardia, seizures

later without further exposure; whether this is attributable to aging or other causes is unclear.

Moldy Sugarcane Poisoning

Moldy sugarcane poisoning was first recognized in 1972, and all the cases so far occurred only in China. Proliferation of the fungus *Arthrinium* sp. in sugarcanes stored under suboptimal conditions leads to production of 3-nitropropionic acid. The neurological syndrome consists of acute onset of headache, lethargy, seizures, and coma, followed weeks later by delayed choreoathetosis, torsion spasms, and limb dystonia (He et al. 1995). Brain computed tomography may show bilateral lucencies in the basal ganglia. The pathogenetic mechanism is unknown, although 3-nitropropionic acid appears to interfere with energy metabolism via inhibition of succinic dehydrogenase.

Mushroom Poisoning

Of the more than 5,000 varieties of mushrooms, approximately 100 are known to be toxic. Ingestion by children comprises the majority of cases reported to poison centers. These exposures are generally not serious, because usually only small amounts are ingested and most lawn mushrooms are harmless. Adults more frequently consume mushrooms in larger quantities and more likely develop toxic symptoms. Aside from accidental ingestion, genera such as *Psilocybe, Panaeolus, Amanita muscaria*, and *Amanita pantherina* are popular among drug abusers for their psychoactive effects. Many are used also in tribal ceremonies as an intoxicant.

The classification system most commonly adopted by clinicians divides the poisonous mushrooms into seven groups according to the clinical symptomatology. Six of the seven groups are associated with significant neurological morbidity and are listed in Table 64C.3. The most lethal mushrooms almost all belong to the *Amanita* genus and contain various cyclic polypeptides (phallotoxins and amatoxins). Amatoxins are the main toxins responsible for human disease. They have potent hepatotoxicity and nephrotoxicity. In severely toxic individuals, gastrointestinal symptoms appear initially, followed by fulminant hepatic and renal failure 3–5 days later (see Table 64C.3). Seizures, encephalopathy, and coma often accompany the organ failure. With the exception of poisoning by some monomethylhydrazine-containing genera, toxicities from other groups listed in Table 64C.3 are rarely life-threatening. Nevertheless, neurological symptoms are frequent after ingestion of these mushrooms and provide important clues to diagnosis and treatment.

Although attempts should be made to identify the mushrooms involved, accurate identification is a formidable task. Poisonous species often closely resemble the edible varieties. The specimen also may be distorted during transport or after cooking. The task of taxonomy is best left to a professional mycologist. Even in the absence of a positive identification, the nature of the symptoms and the time of onset of symptoms after ingestion are valuable guides to diagnosis and patient management. Supportive care is the mainstay of treatment. It is further supplemented by specific treatments such as infusion of pyridoxine (gyromitrin poisoning), atropine (muscarine poisoning), or physostigmine (ibotenic acid and muscimol poisoning).

REFERENCES

Bogmolski-Yaholom V, Amitai Y, Stalnikowicz R. Paresthesia in envenomation by the scorpion *Leiurus quinquestriatus*. J Toxicol Clin Toxicol 1995;33:79–82.

Bryson PD. Comprehensive Review in Toxicology for Emergency Clinicians. Washington, DC: Taylor & Francis, 1996.

Centers for Disease Control. Jimson Weed poisoning—Texas, New York, and California, 1994. MMWR Morb Mortal Wkly Rep 1995;44:41–44.

Connolly S, Trevett AJ, Nwokolo NC, et al. Neuromuscular effects of Papuan Taipan snake venom. Ann Neurol 1995;38: 919–920.

Gateau T, Bloom M, Clark R. Response to specific *Centruroides sculpturatus* antivenom in 151 cases of scorpion stings. J Toxicol Clin Toxicol 1994;32:165–171.

Grattan-Smith PJ, Morris JG, Johnston HM, et al. Clinical and neurophysiological features of tick paralysis. Brain 1997;120: 1975–1987.

He F, Zhang S, Qian F, et al. Delayed dystonia with striatal CT lucencies induced by mycotoxin (3-nitropropionic acid). Neurology 1995;45:2178–2183.

Lawrence RA. Poison centers and plants: more pollyanna data? J Toxicol Clin Toxicol 1998;36:225–226.

Litovitz TL, Clark LR, Soloway RA. 1993 annual report of the American Association of Poison Control Centers Toxic Exposure Surveillance System. Am J Emerg Med 1994;12:546–584.

Markland FS Jr. Snake venoms. Drugs 1997;54:1–10.

Spencer PS. Lathyrism. In FA de Wolff (ed), Handbook of Clinical Neurology: Intoxications of the Nervous System. Amsterdam: Elsevier, 1995;1–20.

Woestman R, Perkin R, Van Stralen D. The black widow: is she deadly to children? Pediatr Emerg Care 1996;12:360–364.

Chapter 64
Effects of Toxins and Physical Agents on the Nervous System

D. MARINE TOXINS
Yuen T. So

Marine toxins comprise a group of extremely potent neurotoxins that can cause a wide range of diseases in humans, fish, shore birds, and other animals. With the notable exception of tetrodotoxin in pufferfish, most marine toxins originate from diatoms and dinoflagellates, which are single-cell algae either free floating or attached to solid surfaces. During periods of intense proliferation of these algae, high concentrations of toxins accumulate in fish or mollusks (shellfish), which then act as transvectors of diseases (Table 64D.1). Typically, the toxins do not adversely affect the transvectors. Human diseases follow ingestion of these contaminated fish or shellfish.

Descriptions of unmistakable cases of marine food poisoning have been available since ancient times. Well-known examples include reports of probable ciguatera in the journals of the Captain Cook expedition in 1774 and the mutiny on H.M.S. *Bounty* in 1789, as well as George Vancouver's recognition of paralytic shellfish poisoning in the Pacific Northwest toward the end of the eighteenth century.

The proliferation of diatoms and dinoflagellates depends on poorly understood interactions of a number of environmental and seasonal factors. Outbreaks of shellfish poisoning are associated with the so-called red tides, which refer to periods of bloom of planktons and the subsequent reddish-brown discoloration of the water. Red tides have great economic effect on coastal communities dependent on tourism and fisheries, because blooms can cause massive fish kills and wipe out entire fish farms within hours. Not all red tides are toxic, and shellfish contaminations do not necessarily follow red tides. Moreover, ciguatera or reef fish poisoning, a common form of fish poisoning, is not associated with red tides or any other reliable forewarning.

The marine toxins are generally colorless, tasteless, and odorless and do not alter the flavor of the fish and shellfish. The toxins are also heat and acid stable. Normal food screening and preparation procedures therefore do not prevent intoxication from contaminated seafood. These characteristics pose difficulty in formulation of public health strategies in prevention. Physicians who treat any suspected cases should report to public health agencies, as any index case may be the beginning of an outbreak. Whenever possible, the contaminated food should be retrieved and tested. Diagnosis is dependent on the history of ingestion and the recognition of the appropriate clinical features.

CIGUATERA

Ciguatera is a marine food poisoning endemic in the tropics. The ciguatera toxins are produced by dinoflagellates that thrive in the tropical or subtropical coral reef ecosystem, extending roughly between latitudes 35 degrees north and 35 degrees south. The dinoflagellates are consumed by small fish that in turn are eaten by large carnivores. The toxins therefore accumulate in the marine food chain without noticeable ill effects to the fish. Larger and older fish such as barracuda, grouper, red snapper, and amberjack are in general more toxic, but practically almost any reef fish may cause ciguatera. Although only reef fish are contaminated, outbreaks potentially can occur in residents of temperate areas after return from travel or consumption of imported fish.

Accurate disease incidence is not available because of the unavoidable underrecognition and underreporting. One estimate put an annual number of cases at 10,000–50,000

Table 64D.1:   Fish and shellfish poisoning

Syndrome	Toxin source	Transvector	Principal toxins	Pathophysiology
Ciguatera	Dinoflagellate	Fish	Ciguatoxin, maitotoxin, scaritoxin	Activation of Na^+ and Ca^{2+} channels
Pufferfish (*fugu*)	Bacteria(?)	Fish	Tetrodotoxin	Blockade of Na^+ channels
Scombroid	Bacteria(?)	Fish rich in dark meat	Histamine	Physiological effects of histamine(?)
Paralytic shellfish poisoning	Dinoflagellate (red tide)	Shellfish	Saxitoxin	Blockade of Na^+ channels
Neurotoxic shellfish poisoning	Dinoflagellate (red tide)	Shellfish	Brevetoxin	Activation of Na^+ channels
Amnestic shellfish poisoning	Diatom (red tide)	Shellfish	Domoic acid	Activation of glutamate receptors
Diarrheal shellfish poisoning	Dinoflagellate (red tide)	Shellfish	Okadaic acid	Inhibition of phosphory-lase phosphatase

among people in the endemic areas. A telephone survey estimated that 7% of Puerto Rico residents might have suffered at least one episode of ciguatera in their lifetime. In the United States, almost all cases are encountered in the Caribbean, Hawaii, and Florida. Even in Canada, there are an estimated 1,000 cases per year from tourism and imported fish.

A number of toxins, ciguatoxin, maitotoxin, scaritoxin, and possibly palytoxin and okadaic acid, are responsible for ciguatera. The viscera, especially the liver and gonads, contain the highest concentration of toxins, and the flesh tends to have the lowest concentration. Ciguatoxin is the best known of the toxins. It is lipid soluble and acts on the voltage-gated sodium channels in neurons and cardiac and skeletal muscles, leading to increased sodium permeability and membrane depolarization. Maitotoxin increases calcium ion influx through excitable membranes via its action on the voltage-dependent calcium channels.

Clinical Features

Gastrointestinal symptoms are usually the first to appear. Abdominal pain, nausea, vomiting, and diarrhea may occur within hours of ingestion of the fish. In more severely affected cases, neurological symptoms soon follow and typically dominate the clinical picture (Lange 1994; Swift and Swift 1993). Almost all patients develop paresthesias involving the limbs, oral cavity, pharynx, trunk, and, most disagreeably, the genitalia and perineum. Particularly characteristic is paradoxical dysesthesia or temperature reversal that is present in approximately 80% of the patients. This is a peculiar form of altered sensation characteristically triggered by cold stimuli (Cameron and Capra 1993). Patients perceive cold as burning, tingling, or unbearably hot. A small proportion of patients also may perceive warm objects as cold. Headache, arthralgia, myalgia, and asthenia are common. Ataxia and clinically significant weakness are uncommon. Rare cases of polymyositis have been reported.

Acute but transient cardiovascular abnormalities are sometimes seen. These may include bradycardia, heart block, hypotension, and, rarely, circulatory collapse. Most neurological symptoms typically remit in approximately 1 week, although some degree of paresthesias, asthenia, and headache may persist for months.

Diagnosis

Many attempts have been made to detect ciguatera toxins using bioassay and immunoassay techniques, although none is sufficiently reliable and convenient to be of use in patient management. Diagnosis is largely based on the characteristic gastrointestinal, neurological, and cardiovascular disturbances that develop within hours of eating reef fish. Clustering of cases in people who consumed the same fish help to confirm the diagnosis. However, there is great variation in individual susceptibility, even when two persons eat a similar amount of fish. Nerve conduction studies may show slowing of both sensory and motor nerve conduction velocities, and prolongation of the absolute refractory, relative refractory, and supernormal periods. These findings are consistent with prolonged opening of sodium channels in the nerve membranes.

Treatment

The mainstay of treatment is supportive care, which may include fluid supplementation, control of bradycardia, and symptomatic treatment of anxiety, headache, and pain. Calcium gluconate, anticonvulsants, and corticosteroids have been tried with varying results. Intravenous mannitol has emerged as a specific treatment of acute ciguatera (20% mannitol, 0.5–1.0 g/kg at 500 ml/hour), even though its mechanism of action is unclear. Neurological improvement can be dramatic, especially if mannitol is given within 24–48 hours of symptom onset. Fluid and electrolyte status should be assessed and corrected if necessary before mannitol is given, as mannitol itself may induce severe dehydration and electrolyte derangements. The chronic symptoms of ciguatera are difficult to treat. Amitriptyline or other tricyclic antidepressants may provide partial relief.

OTHER FISH POISONING

Tetrodotoxin (Pufferfish) Poisoning

Tetrodotoxin is the causative agent in pufferfish poisoning, found in fish of the order Tetraodontiformes, which has a worldwide distribution in both fresh and saltwater. Over 100 species are known variously as pufferfish, tambores, porcupine fish, jugfish, blowfish, and others. Other sources include ocean sunfish, blue-ringed octopus, and some newts and salamanders. The source of tetrodotoxin appears to be marine bacteria that colonize the gut and skin of Tetraodontiformes. Persistent levels of toxin are produced by the bacteria and sequestered in the body. Concentrations are especially high in the skin and viscera and relatively low in the muscles. *Fugu* refers to a special preparation of pufferfish in Japan that is considered a delicacy. Specially trained *fugu* chefs fillet the fish in such a way to avoid contamination by the viscera. Despite these precautions, *fugu* poisoning accounts for approximately 50% of the fatal food poisonings in Japan.

Tetrodotoxin selectively blocks the sodium channels in excitable membranes and hence interferes with the inward flow of sodium current during an action potential. The toxin has a wide range of physiological effects in humans. It blocks impulse conduction in somatic and autonomic nerve fibers, reduces the excitability of skeletal and cardiac muscles, and has profound effects on vasomotor tone. The clinical symptoms of tetrodotoxin poisoning are similar to those of paralytic shellfish poisoning, which is caused by saxitoxin, another sodium-channel blocker (see Paralytic Shellfish Poisoning, later in this chapter). Paresthesias appear within minutes of ingestion. Gastrointestinal symptoms such as nausea, vomiting, and diarrhea are common. Progressive weakness of limb muscles appears in moderately severe cases. Dysphonia, dysphagia, respiratory insufficiency, and profound hypotension develop in even more severe cases. Fatality rates are close to 50% and are related to the respiratory insufficiency and hypotension. Treatment is largely supportive. The diagnosis may be confirmed with the mouse bioassay.

Scombroid

Scombroid is among the most common causes of fish toxicity. The syndrome is distinctive and closely resembles an acute allergic reaction. Clinical features include throbbing headache, skin flushing, and gastrointestinal disturbances.

The pathophysiology is incompletely understood, but is believed to be, at least in part, caused by bacterial transformation of histidine to histamine in inadequately refrigerated fish.

SHELLFISH POISONING

Food poisoning caused by shellfish is more likely to be caused by infectious agents than toxins. Nevertheless, the toxic illnesses are of clinical and scientific importance to neurologists. Depending on the toxins involved, at least four syndromes may result from consumption of shellfish contaminated by toxins: paralytic shellfish poisoning, neurotoxic shellfish poisoning, amnestic shellfish poisoning or domoic acid intoxication, and diarrheal shellfish poisoning. Outbreaks tend to be most frequent during the summer months, especially during periods of red tides. However, toxic contamination may occur in any month of the year or in the absence of red tide.

Paralytic Shellfish Poisoning

Paralytic shellfish poisoning is of worldwide importance, with red tides and poisoning cases reported with increasing frequency throughout the world. Saxitoxin and at least 11 other toxins with similar actions are responsible for the neurological symptoms. Dinoflagellates belonging to the species *Alexandrium* are the primary source of toxins. Saxitoxin, the first and best characterized, is a heat-stable toxin that is readily absorbed through the gastrointestinal tract. It acts primarily on the peripheral nervous system, where it binds reversibly to a receptor on excitable membranes and blocks the permeability of the sodium channels. Its action is hence similar to tetrodotoxin. In comparison with tetrodotoxin, saxitoxin has a greater potency to cause skeletal muscle weakness, but has a lesser propensity to induce hypotension and a shorter duration of action.

Symptoms typically appear within 5–30 minutes of ingestion of the contaminated shellfish. Paresthesias develop in almost all patients and initially involve the perioral areas, oral cavity, face, and neck (Gessner and Middaugh 1995). These symptoms spread to the limbs and trunk in severe cases. Some patients complain of an unusual floating sensation in the head. Brainstem symptoms and signs are sometimes present. These include dysarthria, dysphagia, ophthalmoplegia, nystagmus, dilated pupils, and blurred vision. Other neurological symptoms include headache, gait ataxia, and limb incoordination. Despite the name of this syndrome, muscle paralysis does not develop in every patient. If present, weakness may involve muscles of the face, jaw, swallowing, respiration, and the upper and lower limbs. In severe cases, respiratory paralysis appears within 2–12 hours of ingestion. Spontaneous recovery begins to appear after 12 hours and usually is complete within a few days. There is no antidote for the toxins. Treatment is therefore primarily supportive, with special attention to bulbar and respiratory functions. Access to emergency care is a critical determinant of outcome. The overall mortality is as high as 10% in areas without sophisticated medical care, and the illness is more likely to be fatal in children.

Initial diagnosis is largely dependent on the recognition of the history and clinical features. An enzyme-linked immunosorbent assay is available for saxitoxin, but its utility is limited by the variability of toxin constituents in each outbreak. If the contaminated shellfish is available, a useful test is the mouse bioassay. A mouse unit is defined as the minimum amount necessary to induce death of a mouse in 15 minutes. The lethal dose for human is approximately 5,000–20,000 mouse units. The mouse assay also is widely employed to monitor commercial shellfish production in many parts of the world. Nerve conduction studies may show reduced amplitude of the sensory and motor responses, prolonged motor and sensory latencies, and slow nerve conduction velocities. Unlike acute demyelinating neuropathies in which electrophysiological abnormalities lag behind clinical findings, the electrophysiological abnormalities in paralytic shellfish poisoning are most prominent at symptom onset and resolve over a few days as clinical symptoms resolve.

Neurotoxic Shellfish Poisoning

The causative toxins are produced by the dinoflagellate *Ptychodiscus brevis*, which is found primarily in the Gulf of Mexico and the Caribbean sea. Another dinoflagellate similar to *P. brevis* is responsible for diseases in Spain. The toxins are named brevotoxins. They cause depolarization of excitable membranes of peripheral nerves and muscles by inducing an increase in the permeability of the sodium channel.

Clinical presentation is characterized by the simultaneous onset of gastrointestinal and neurological symptoms within a few hours of ingestion. Nausea, diarrhea, and paresthesias are common. Some patients may complain of a choking sensation or throat tightness. They also may report temperature reversal similar to that seen in ciguatera. The neurological symptoms are milder than those of paralytic shellfish poisoning. Brevotoxins are probably more toxic to wildlife than humans, as red tides from blooms of *P. brevis* are typically associated with massive fish and bird kills.

A separate respiratory syndrome, attributed to inhalation of aerosolized brevotoxin by people walking along the seashore, consists of conjunctival irritation, rhinorrhea, cough, and bronchoconstriction.

Amnestic Shellfish Poisoning

In November 1987, over 100 Canadians were stricken by a novel illness after eating mussels harvested off the Prince Edward Island coast. Gastrointestinal symptoms and cognitive dysfunction characterize the syndrome. The toxin was later identified as domoic acid, an amino acid analogue of kainic acid and glutamic acid. A pennate diatom, *Nitzschia pungens*, was the probable source of domoic acid. Very high concentrations of the excitotoxin were found in uneaten mussels and mussels sampled from three river estuaries in Prince Edward Island. One postulate suggested that fertilizer runoff may have contributed to the bloom of the diatom. Since the initial epidemic, domoic acid has been found in species of another phytoplankton *Pseudonitzschia*, and in edible marine species along the Pacific Coast and Gulf of Mexico.

Domoic acid acts as an excitatory neurotransmitter in animal models and is approximately three times more potent than kainic acid and over 30 times more than glutamic acid. Human neurological disease results from its excitotoxic effects, especially on the limbic system. Symptoms usually appear within a few hours of ingestion (median, 5.5 hours). Almost all patients have diarrhea, vomiting, or abdominal cramps, although the severity varies considerably. Roughly one-half of all patients have headache, and approximately 25% present with memory loss. In those with neurological dysfunction, the findings are quite varied. They include disorientation, mutism, seizures, myoclonus, and altered state of consciousness ranging from somnolence to coma. Reflexes may be depressed or hyperactive. Some patients may have Babinski's signs. Two patients had a unique alternating hemiparesis and complete external ophthalmoplegia.

Gradual improvement occurs spontaneously over 3 months. Those with residual deficits often have severe anterograde amnesia with relative preservation of intellect and other higher cortical functions. Some patients develop temporal lobe epilepsy. There also may be coexisting distal limb weakness and atrophy, and electromyography suggests a picture of either a motor neuronopathy or a sensory motor axonopathy. In a few patients who died, autopsy revealed astrocytosis and selective neuronal loss in the amygdala and hippocampus (Cendes et al. 1995). These lesions are reminiscent of those seen in the rat model of kainate-induced seizures.

Treatment is primarily symptomatic. Previous experience suggests that diazepam and phenobarbital, but not phenytoin, are the drugs of choice in the control of seizures. Diagnosis may be established with the use of the same mouse bioassay as in paralytic shellfish poisoning. A surveillance program now exists in Canada to monitor the commercial shellfish operations.

Diarrheal Shellfish Poisoning

Diarrheal shellfish poisoning is a self-limiting gastrointestinal illness without clinical evidence of neurotoxicity. Diarrhea, nausea, and vomiting are almost universal symptoms. Symptoms begin 30 minutes to a few hours after ingestion, and complete recovery is expected within 3 days.

REFERENCES

Cameron J, Capra MF. The basis of the paradoxical disturbance of temperature perception in ciguatera poisoning. J Toxicol Clin Toxicol 1993;31:571–579.

Cendes F, Andermann F, Carpenter S, et al. Temporal lobe epilepsy caused by domoic acid intoxication: evidence for glutamate receptor-mediated exitotoxicity in humans. Ann Neurol 1995;37:123–126.

Gessner BD, Middaugh JP. Paralytic shellfish poisoning in Alaska: a 20-year retrospective analysis. Am J Epidemiol 1995;141:766–770.

Lange WR. Ciguatera fish poisoning. Am Fam Physician 1994;50:579–584.

Swift AE, Swift TR. Ciguatera. J Toxicol Clin Toxicol 1993;31:1–29.

Chapter 64
Effects of Toxins and Physical Agents on the Nervous System

E. EFFECT OF PHYSICAL AGENTS ON THE NERVOUS SYSTEM
Michael J. Aminoff

The nervous system may be damaged by physical agents such as ionizing and nonionizing radiation, electricity, extreme heat or cold, and vibration. The extent of damage depends on the intensity and duration of exposure.

IONIZING RADIATION

Electromagnetic and particulate radiation may lead to cell damage and death. Radiation therapy affects the nervous system by causing damage to exposed regions or to blood vessels supplying neural structures. It may also produce tumors that lead to neurological deficits. Neurological injury is proportional to both the total dose and daily fraction of radiation that were received.

Encephalopathy

Radiation encephalopathy is best considered according to its time of onset after exposure. Acute radiation encephalopathy occurs within a few days of exposure and is characterized by headache, nausea, and a change in mental status that may be related to increased intracranial pressure from breakdown of the blood-brain barrier. Treatment with high-dose corticosteroids usually provides relief.

Early delayed radiation encephalopathy is probably caused by demyelination and occurs between 2 weeks and 3 or 4 months after irradiation. Headache and drowsiness are features, as is an enhancement of previous focal deficits. Symptoms resolve after several weeks without specific treatment. A brainstem encephalopathy also may develop and is manifest by ataxia, nystagmus, diplopia, and dysarthria. Spontaneous recovery over a few weeks is usual, but the disorder sometimes progresses to obtundation, coma, or death.

Delayed radiation encephalopathy occurs several months or longer after cranial irradiation. It may be characterized by diffuse cerebral injury (atrophy) or focal neurological deficits with signs of increased intracranial pressure. The disorder may result from focal cerebral necrosis caused by direct radiation damage or by vascular changes. Immunological mechanisms also may be involved. Occasionally, patients develop a progressive disabling disorder, with cognitive and affective disturbances and a disorder of gait, approximately 6–18 months after whole-brain irradiation. Pathological examination in some instances has shown demyelinating lesions.

Myelopathy

A myelopathy also may result from irradiation. Transient radiation myelopathy usually occurs within the first year or so after incidental cord irradiation in patients with lymphoma and other neoplasms. Paresthesias and Lhermitte's phenomenon characterize the syndrome, which is self-limiting and probably relates to demyelination of the posterior columns. A delayed severe radiation myelopathy may occur approximately 1 year after completion of radiotherapy. Patients present with a focal neurological deficit that progresses over weeks or months to paraplegia or quadriplegia. This may simulate a compressive myelopathy or paraneoplastic subacute necrotizing myelopathy, but the results of magnetic resonance imaging (MRI) are usually normal. The cerebrospinal fluid is usually normal, although the protein concentration is sometimes elevated. Corticosteroids may lead to temporary improvement, but no specific treatment exists. The disorder is caused by necrosis and atrophy of the cord, with an associated vasculopathy. Occasional patients develop sudden back pain and leg weakness several years after irradiation, and MRI reveals hematomyelia; symptoms usually improve with time. In some instances, inadvertent spinal involvement, usually by pelvic irradiation, leads to a selective, focal degeneration of lower motor neurons. The neurological deficit may progress over several months but eventually stabilizes, leaving a flaccid, asymmetrical paraparesis. Recovery does not occur.

Plexopathy

A radiation-induced plexopathy may rarely occur soon after treatment and must be distinguished from direct neoplastic involvement of the plexuses. Paresthesias, weakness, and atrophy typify the disorder, which tends to resolve gradually over several months. It occurs most commonly after treatment for breast cancer. A plexopathy also may develop later (1–2 years) after irradiation of the brachial or lumbosacral plexuses. In this regard, doses of radiation exceeding 6,000 cGy, involvement of the upper part of the brachial plexuses, lack of pain, lymphedema, induration of the supraclavicular fossa, and the presence of myokymic discharges on electromyography all favor a radiation-induced plexopathy.

NONIONIZING RADIATION

Nonionizing radiation that strikes matter is transformed to heat, which may lead to tissue damage. Ultraviolet radiation is produced by the sun, incandescent and fluorescent light sources, welding torches, electrical arc furnaces, and germicidal lamps. Ultraviolet radiation is absorbed primarily by proteins and nucleic acids. Susceptibility to it is increased by certain drugs, such as chlorpromazine and tolbutamide, and by certain plants, such as figs, lemon and lime rinds, celery, and parsnips, which contain furocoumarins and psoralens. Short-term exposure to ultraviolet light can damage the retina and optic nerve fibers. A severe central scotoma may result from macular injury. Prevention requires the use of goggles and face masks in work environments where exposure to high-intensity ultraviolet radiation is likely to occur.

Exposures to laser radiation can induce ocular damage. This is problematic especially when the wavelength of the laser beam is not in the visible portion of the electromagnetic spectrum, because exposure may then be inapparent.

Concern has been raised that occupational or environmental exposure to high-voltage electrical power lines may lead to neurological damage from exposure to high-intensity electromagnetic fields. However, the effects of such exposure are uncertain and require further study.

High-intensity noise may lead in the acute setting to pain in the ear, tinnitus, vertigo, and hearing impairment. Chronic exposure to high-intensity noise of any frequency leads to focal cochlear damage and impaired hearing.

ELECTRICAL CURRENT AND LIGHTNING

Electrical injuries (whether from manufactured or naturally occurring sources) are common. Their severity depends on the strength and duration of the current and the path in which it flows. Electricity travels along the shortest path to ground. Its passage through humans can often be determined by identifying entry and exit burn wounds. When its path involves the nervous system, direct neurological damage is likely among survivors. With the passage of current through tissues, heat is produced that is responsible, at least in part, for any damage, but nonthermal mechanisms may contribute also (Winkelman 1995). In addition, neurological damage may result from circulatory arrest and trauma related to falling or a shock pressure wave.

A large current that passes through the head leads to immediate unconsciousness, sometimes associated with ventricular fibrillation and respiratory arrest. Confusion, disorientation, seizures, and transient focal deficits are common in survivors (Cherington et al. 1993), but recovery generally occurs within a few days. Some survivors develop a cerebral infarct after several days or weeks, attributed to thrombotic occlusion of cerebral blood vessels. Residual memory and other cognitive disturbances are also common. Weaker current leads only to headache or other mild symptoms for a brief period.

When the path of the current involves the spinal cord, a transverse myelopathy may occur immediately or after up to 7 days or so, and may progress for several days. The disorder eventually stabilizes, after which partial or full recovery occurs in many instances. Upper and lower motor neuron deficits and sensory disturbances are common, but the sphincters are often spared. Unlike traumatic myelopathy, pain is not a feature. Autopsy studies show demyelination of long tracts, loss of anterior horn cells, and areas of necrosis in the cord.

Segmental muscle atrophy may occur also within a few days or weeks of electrical injury of the cord. Whether this relates to focal neuronal damage or has an ischemic basis is uncertain. The current pathway is typically across the cervical cord, and the muscle atrophy in the arms then may be accompanied by an upper motor neuron deficit in the legs. Sensory disturbances (in upper or lower limbs) and sphincter dysfunction also occur. Occasional reports have suggested the occurrence of a progressive disorder simulating amyotrophic lateral sclerosis after electrical injury.

Peripheral or cranial nerve injury in the region of an electrical burn is often reversible, except when high-tension current is responsible, in which case thermal coagulation necrosis is likely. Care must be taken to distinguish such neuropathies from compartment or entrapment neuropathies, which are suggested by severe pain and a delay between injury and development of the neuropathy. Compartment syndromes develop because of muscle swelling and necrosis, and entrapment syndromes because of swelling of tissues in confined anatomical spaces.

Occasional patients have developed hemorrhagic or thrombotic stroke after electrical injuries, for uncertain reasons. Venous sinus thrombosis has also been described (Patel and Lo 1993). Suggested mechanisms include coagulation necrosis of part of the vascular wall with aneurysmal distention and rupture, or intramural thrombosis. Intense vasospasm, acute hypertension, intramural dissections, or transient circulatory arrest may contribute.

VIBRATION

Exposure to vibrating tools such as pneumatic drills has been associated with both focal peripheral nerve injuries, such as carpal tunnel syndrome, and vascular abnormalities, such as Raynaud's phenomenon. The mechanism of production is uncertain but presumably reflects focal damage to nerve fibers.

HYPERTHERMIA

Exposure to high external temperatures may lead to heat stress disorders. Heat stroke, the most severe, sometimes has an exertional basis, and disturbances of thermoregulatory sweating may be contributory. Classic heat stroke occurs especially in older persons with chronic disorders such as diabetes or obesity and in hypermetabolic states such as thyrotoxicosis. Anticholinergic or diuretic drugs, or dehydration, predispose to heat stroke because they impair sweating and thereby limit heat dissipation.

Hyperthermia leads to thirst, fatigue, nausea, weakness, muscle cramps, and eventually to confusion, delirium, obtundation, or coma, but coma can develop without any prodrome. Seizures are frequent, focal neurological deficits are sometimes present, and papilledema may occur. With recovery, symptoms and signs generally clear completely, but cognitive changes or focal neurological deficits may persist. Cataracts have been attributed to dehydration. Cardiac output is reduced, pulmonary edema may occur, and adult respiratory distress syndrome is sometimes conspicuous.

Other systemic manifestations include a respiratory alkalosis and often a metabolic acidosis, hypokalemia or hyperkalemia, hypoglycemia, other electrolyte disturbances, and various coagulopathies. Rhabdomyolysis is common, and acute renal failure may occur in exertional heat stroke.

The prognosis depends on the severity of hyperthermia and its duration before initiation of treatment. With proper management, the mortality rate is probably about 5%. Treatment involves control of the body temperature by cooling, rehydration of the patient, correction of the underlying cause of the hyperthermia, and prevention of complications. When excessive muscle activity is responsible, neuromuscular blockade may be necessary. In the malignant hyperthermia syndrome, the responsible anesthetic agent is discontinued, oxygenation is ensured, and intravenous dantrolene is administered. Thyrotoxic crisis is treated with thyroid-blocking drugs. Patients with pheochromocytoma are treated with α-adrenergic antagonists.

Cooling is achieved by evaporation or by direct external cooling, as by immersion of the patient in cold water. The skin should be massaged vigorously to counteract the cutaneous vasoconstriction that results from external cooling and that impedes heat removal from the core. Antipyretic agents are unhelpful. Hypotension is treated by fluid administration rather than vasoconstrictor agents, which should be avoided if possible. High doses of mannitol and use of diuretics may be required to promote urinary output. Electrolyte and glucose abnormalities also may require treatment.

HYPOTHERMIA

A core temperature below 35°C may occur in very young or elderly persons and with environmental exposure, coma, certain endocrinopathies, malnutrition, severe dermatological disorders (because of excessive heat loss and inability to regulate cutaneous vasoconstriction), and alcoholism. Alcohol promotes heat loss by vasodilation and may lead to coma directly or from trauma, with resultant environmental exposure. Hypothermia also occurs in persons exposed to low temperatures in the working environment, such as divers, skiers, and cold-room workers.

The usual compensatory mechanism for cooling is shivering, but this fails at temperatures below approximately 30°C. As the temperature declines, respiratory requirements diminish, cardiac output falls, and significant hypotension and cardiac arrhythmias ultimately develop. Neurologically, there is increasing confusion, psychomotor retardation, and obtundation until consciousness is eventually lost. The tendon reflexes are reduced and muscle tone increases, but extensor plantar responses are not usually found. The electroencephalogram slows and ultimately shows a burst-suppression pattern or becomes isoelectric with increasing hypothermia. At core temperatures below 32°C, the appearance of brain death may be simulated clinically and electroencephalographically, but complete recovery may follow appropriate treatment. Management involves slow rewarming of patients and the prevention of complications such as aspiration pneumonia and metabolic acidosis. Hypotension may occur from dehydration but can be managed usually by fluid replacement. Plasma electrolyte concentrations must be monitored closely, especially because of the risk of developing cardiac arrhythmias. With recovery, there are usually no long-term sequelae.

Nerve damage may occur as a consequence of the tissues becoming frozen by the cold (frostbite). This involves the extremities and is usually irreversible.

BURNS

Following common usage, the term *thermal burn* refers to a burn caused by direct contact with heat or flames. Patients with severe burns may have associated disorders such as anoxic encephalopathy from carbon monoxide poisoning, head injury, or respiratory dysfunction from smoke inhalation. Central neurological disorders otherwise occur later during hospitalization and are secondary to various systemic complications. Thus, metabolic encephalopathies may relate to anoxia, liver or kidney failure, and hyponatremia, and central pontine myelinolysis may occur also. Infections (meningitis or cerebral microabscesses) are common, especially in the second or third week after the burn. Vascular complications including multiple strokes may result from septic infarction, disseminated intravascular coagulation, venous thrombosis, hypotension, or intracranial hemorrhage. Imaging studies are therefore important in clarifying the underlying disorder.

Peripheral complications of burns are also important. Nerves may be damaged directly by heat, leading to coagulation necrosis from which recovery is unlikely. A compartment syndrome may arise from massive swelling of tissues and mandates urgent decompressive surgery. In other instances, neuropathies result from compression, angulation, or stretch as a result of incorrectly applied dressings or improper positioning of the patient. A critical illness polyneuropathy is now well recognized in patients with multiorgan failure and sepsis, including patients with burns, and is discussed in Chapter 80.

REFERENCES

Cherington M, Yarnell P, Hallmark D. MRI in lightning encephalopathy. Neurology 1993;43:1437–1438.

Delattre J-Y, Posner JB. Neurological Complications of Chemotherapy and Radiation Therapy. In MJ Aminoff (ed), Neurology and General Medicine (2nd ed). New York: Churchill Livingstone, 1995;421–445.

Patel A, Lo R. Electric injury with cerebral venous thrombosis: case report and review of the literature. Stroke 1993;24:903–905.

Winkelman MD. Neurological Complications of Thermal and Electrical Burns. In MJ Aminoff (ed), Neurology and General Medicine (2nd ed). New York: Churchill Livingstone, 1995;915–929.

Chapter 65
Brain Edema and Disorders of Cerebrospinal Fluid Circulation

Gary A. Rosenberg

The brain and spinal cord are subject to different physical processes than other organs in the body because they lie within the rigid bony compartments of the skull and spinal canal. These physical processes depend on the fact that the brain is surrounded by and encloses a large volume of cerebrospinal fluid (CSF). The character of the CSF, with its constituents, pressure, and flow, are of great importance to the function of the central nervous system (CNS). Increased intracranial pressure results from increased tissue within the rigid bony box of the skull (space-occupying lesions, such as tumor, abscess, and hematoma), increased fluid (cerebral edema of several types), and impaired flow of CSF (hydrocephalus).

Brain edema is a serious complication of many neurological conditions. Damaged cells swell, injured blood vessels leak, and blocked absorption pathways force fluid to enter brain tissues. Each of these mechanisms results in a potential increase in intracranial volume. Compensation for the potential increase occurs by displacement of CSF and venous blood from the skull. Further volume increases cause brain tissue to shift. Herniation of brain leads to a life-threatening situation, requiring rapid assessment of the cause and urgent treatment.

Brain cells are surrounded by an interstitial fluid (ISF) that is contiguous with the CSF. The CSF and ISF act as one fluid. Therefore, a lumbar puncture to withdraw CSF provides insight into brain cell function that is critical in diagnosis and management of patients. The analysis of CSF gives important information on bleeding, inflammation, and infection in the brain that is not available by other methods. Proper use of the information obtained by lumbar puncture, which is central to neurological diagnosis, requires an understanding of normal CSF and ISF physiology.

The recognition that the total volume of fluid and tissue contained in the rigid skull is constant is called the *Monro-Kellie doctrine*, which was formulated in the eighteenth century. Changes in volume of either blood, CSF, or brain compartments produce compensatory changes in the others, with a resultant increase in CSF pressure (Figure 65.1). Hydrocephalus causes an interstitial edema with enlargement of the CSF space. Masses, such as tumors or abscesses, cause an enlargement of the tissue space. Opening of the blood-brain barrier (BBB) due to disruption of the blood vessel wall leads to vasogenic edema with extravasation of fluid into the brain tissue. Damage to cells leads to cytotoxic edema with narrowing of the extracellular space. Finally, an increase in blood volume, as seen in hypercapnia and hypoxia, increases the intracranial pressure (Table 65.1). Raised intracranial pressure can be diagnosed by neuroimaging when it is due to brain edema from a wide range of brain disorders or to hydrocephalus. Isolated increases in CSF pressure with normal imaging suggest idiopathic intracranial hypertension (IIH) syndrome, which is diagnosed by lumbar puncture. The many surfaces where brain tissue is exposed to the systemic circulation have evolved unique structural, metabolic, and enzymatic mechanisms to preserve the neuronal microenvironment. Fluid and electrolyte balance and immunological protection are lost in the presence of ischemia, inflammation, infection, and tumors.

BLOOD-BRAIN INTERFACES

Cerebral Blood Vessels

Brain cells are separated from the general circulation by a complex series of interfaces that form the BBB. The large

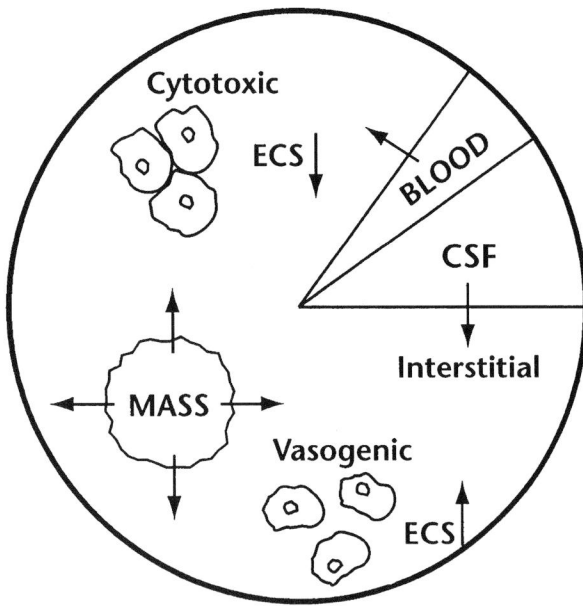

FIGURE 65.1   The rigid skull inhibits expansion of any brain compartments. An increase in blood or cerebrospinal fluid (CSF) volume directly affects CSF pressure. Masses, such as tumors, abscesses, or hematomas, increase brain tissue volume, thereby raising CSF pressure. Cell swelling causes loss of extracellular space (ECS) and cytotoxic edema. Blood-brain barrier damage increases extracellular space, particularly in the white matter with vasogenic edema.

Table 65.1:   Causes of increased intracranial pressure (ICP)

Site of increased ICP	Diseases
Increased tissue volume	Tumor, abscess
Increased blood volume	Hypercapnia, hypoxia, venous sinus occlusion
Cytotoxic edema	Ischemia, trauma, toxins, metabolic diseases
Vasogenic edema	Infections, brain tumors, hyperosmolar states, inflammation
Interstitial edema	Hydrocephalus with transependymal flow

via terminal capillaries and venules or into CSF for eventual absorption through the arachnoid granulations. Drainage of ISF into the cervical lymphatics has been shown in rats and rabbits and most likely occurs in humans (Knopf et al. 1995).

Normally, brain extracellular space comprises 15–20% of the total brain volume. Complex carbohydrates are found in the extracellular space, including hyaluronic acid, chondroitin sulfate, and heparan sulfate. Hyaluronic acid forms large water domains. Other glycosaminoglycans act as charge barriers and binding sites. Around the cerebral capillaries the extracellular matrix forms a layer of basal lamina. Type IV collagen, fibronectin, heparan sulfate, laminin, and entactin make up the various layers of the basal lamina. Entactin connects type IV collagen and laminin to add a structural element to the capillary. Fibronectin from the cells joins the basal lamina to the endothelium. Basal lamina overlays epithelial cells, including the endothelium, and surrounds pericytes and smooth muscles. Basement membranes in general provide structure through type IV collagen, charge barriers by heparan sulfate, and binding sites on the laminin and fibronectin molecules, but the role of the basal lamina in brain blood vessels is unclear.

During development, cerebral blood vessels get the characteristics that distinguish them from systemic capillaries. During embryonic life, vessels destined to form the BBB show increased expression of the cell surface protein, HT7. When quail embryonic brains are grafted into the coelomic cavity of chick embryos, chicken blood vessels growing into the grafted brain express HT7 protein, which is specific for chicken and not expressed in quail (Risau 1995). Systemic blood vessels in the chick embryo at stages 17–20 can form a BBB when implanted into developing brain. The proximity

surface areas of the capillary endothelial cells form the major interface. Choroid plexuses and arachnoid granulations also have barrier surfaces that regulate the exchange of substrates between brain and blood (Table 65.2). At each of the BBB interfaces, bulk transport is restricted by high-resistance junctions (zona occludens) between cells, which make the surface into an epitheliumlike structure (Bradbury 1993). Non–lipid-soluble substances, charged substances, or large molecules are impeded by the epithelial sheets, whereas lipid-soluble substances, such as water and anesthetic gases, pass easily through the cells.

Once substances cross the BBB, they may reach all brain regions through the ISF. Lymphatics are absent in brain, and ISF functions as a lymph fluid. Circulation of ISF begins with its formation at the capillaries. Flowing around cells, ISF brings nutrients, such as glucose and oxygen, to neurons and astrocytes and removes the products of metabolism. ISF is absorbed either into the blood

Table 65.2:   Characteristic features of the blood-brain interfaces

Interface	Tight-junction location	Functional aspects
Blood-CSF	Choroid plexus cell	Active secretion of CSF via ATPase and carbonic anhydrase
CSF-blood	Arachnoid membrane	Arachnoid granulations absorb CSF by one-way valve mechanism
Blood-brain	Capillary endothelial cell	Active transport of ISF via ATPase; increased mitochondria and glucose transporters in the capillary

ATPase = adenosine triphosphatase; CSF = cerebrospinal fluid; ISF = interstitial fluid.

of the astrocytic processes to the capillary cells suggests that the astrocytes provide essential substances to the capillary.

Tight junctions between the endothelial cells create a high electrical resistance that limits transport of non–lipid-soluble substances (Table 65.3). Essential nutrients, such as glucose and amino acids, are selectively transported by carrier molecules that shuttle between the blood and brain sides of the capillaries. Glucose transporters are densely distributed in the capillaries. At low levels of blood glucose, the carriers function at high capacity, but at higher levels, they become saturated. Once they are saturated, any increase in uptake occurs by diffusion. Several isoforms of the glucose transporter molecule have been isolated and cloned (Vannucci et al. 1997). High concentration of one isoform, GLUT1, is found on cerebral blood vessels. GLUT3 is found on neurons and GLUT5 in microglia. GLUT2 is found predominantly in the liver, intestine, kidney, and pancreas. Impairment of glucose transport due to lack of transporters has been described. People with Alzheimer's disease have low levels of the glucose transporter on cerebral capillaries.

Amino acid carrier molecules are also found on cerebral capillaries. Substances that compete with essential amino acids for the carriers block their uptake and lead to deficiency states. For example, high-protein meals provide amino acids that compete for the carriers that transport L-dopa, which may interfere with L-dopa uptake in the treatment of Parkinson's disease. Serotonin uptake is decreased in patients with phenylketonuria.

Steady-state levels of brain electrolytes are preserved by transport mechanisms at the BBB. Potassium is maintained at a constant level in the CSF and brain by the BBB. This prevents fluctuations of electrolyte levels in the blood from influencing brain levels. Calcium is similarly regulated. Glutamate, which is an excitotoxin, is excluded from the brain. High lipid solubility is needed for rapid entry into the brain. Gases, such as carbon dioxide and oxygen, are rapidly exchanged across the capillary. Anesthetic gases are effective because of their rapid entry into the brain. Water rapidly crosses the capillary wall, with only slight impedance found at faster blood flow rates.

Drugs acting on the CNS need to cross the BBB. Early antibiotics, such as penicillin, had to be given in very high doses because they penetrated the nervous system poorly. Newer antibiotics, however, penetrate more readily, making them better agents for treatment of brain infections. Chemotherapy of brain tumors has been hampered by the agents' poor lipid solubility. Heroin is more readily taken up by the brain than morphine because of its increased lipid solubility. Nicotine and alcohol are readily transported into brain, resulting in their addictive potential.

Paradoxical clinical situations arise because of the limitations to transport across the BBB, causing different rates for equilibration of various substances between blood and brain. For example, patients with metabolic acidosis deplete bicarbonate from the brain. A compensatory respiratory alkalosis lowers carbon dioxide. Correction of the metabolic acidosis with bicarbonate raises serum levels before those in the brain. As serum pH rises, normal respirations are restored and carbon dioxide levels return to normal in both brain and blood. This causes a paradoxical fall in brain pH because the low brain bicarbonate levels do not compensate for the increased acidity due to the rise in carbon dioxide. Although treatment is necessary to correct the metabolic acidosis, patients may temporarily worsen as the treatment progresses due to brain acidosis (Figure 65.2).

Table 65.3: Unique features of cerebral capillaries

Tight junctions create high electrical resistance
Adenosine triphosphatase pumps on abluminal surfaces form interstitial fluid
Increased numbers of mitochondria for high energy needs
Glucose transporters and amino acid carriers
Basal lamina, pericytes, and astrocytes

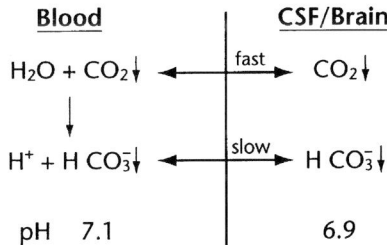

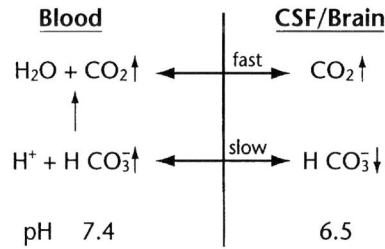

Metabolic Acidosis
(Respiratory Alkalosis)

Blood		CSF/Brain
$H_2O + CO_2\downarrow$	←—fast—→	$CO_2\downarrow$
$H^+ + H CO_3^-\downarrow$	←—slow—→	$H CO_3^-\downarrow$
pH 7.1		6.9

Acidosis Corrected
(Bicarbonate Infusion)

Blood		CSF/Brain
$H_2O + CO_2\uparrow$	←—fast—→	$CO_2\uparrow$
$H^+ + H CO_3^-\uparrow$	←—slow—→	$H CO_3^-\downarrow$
pH 7.4		6.5

FIGURE 65.2 Illustration of the effects of metabolic acidosis with respiratory alkalosis on pH of blood and cerebrospinal fluid (CSF) and brain. Uncompensated, the blood bicarbonate and CO_2 are both low and are mirrored by the levels in CSF and brain. Treatment with bicarbonate restores normal respiration, increasing CO_2 levels in both compartments, but bicarbonate crosses the blood-brain barrier too slowly to compensate for the excess protons. CSF and brain pH paradoxically fall.

Choroid Plexuses and Production of Cerebrospinal Fluid

Choroid plexuses form an important interface between CSF and blood. These secretory structures are in the cerebral ventricles. Tight junctions at the apical surface of choroid plexus ependymal cells form the barrier between blood and CSF. Capillaries beneath the choroidal cells are fenestrated, and they permit substances to pass into the stroma that separates the blood vessels from the choroid plexus epithelial cells. Microvilli line the outer surface and contribute to the secretory function. The presence in the epithelial cells of many mitochondria, Golgi complexes, and endoplasmic reticulum suggests a high level of metabolic activity. The choroid plexus is the main producer of CSF, with the capillaries contributing at varying levels in different species. Production of CSF is constant across species when volume of fluid formed is divided by the weight of the choroid plexus. In humans, the rate of CSF production is 0.35 ml per minute. CSF production occurs at both choroidal and extrachoroidal sites. Estimates of the proportion of CSF from each site vary, depending on the species and the method of measurement. Choroidal production accounts for 60–70% of total CSF production in the cat, but it may be lower in the monkey, where extrachoroidal sources are important. No measurements of the relative proportion of CSF produced at each source have been made in humans.

Higher levels of sodium, chloride, and magnesium and lower levels of potassium, calcium, bicarbonate, and glucose are found in CSF than are expected from a plasma ultrafiltrate, which suggests that the CSF is actively secreted. An adenosine triphosphatase (ATPase) pump on the apical surface of the choroidal cells secretes sodium-rich CSF that draws osmotic water into the ventricles. Carbonic anhydrase converts carbon dioxide and water into bicarbonate, which is removed along with chloride to balance the sodium charge.

Production of CSF is difficult to decrease. Acetazolamide, which inhibits carbonic anhydrase, reduces CSF production, as do hypothermia, hypocarbia, hypoxia, and hyperosmolality. Osmotic agents, such as mannitol and glycerol, increase serum osmolality, lowering CSF production temporarily by about 50%. However, none of these measures is effective in the long-term reduction of CSF production.

Capillaries, which have ATPase on the abluminal surface, are a source of extrachoroidal ISF production. Gray matter has a dense neuropil that restricts water flow, whereas white matter is more regularly arranged, making it a natural conduit for normal flow of ISF and for movement of edema in pathological conditions. Under the pressure gradient maintained by capillary ISF production, bulk flow of fluid occurs in the white matter. Diffusion of water and entrained solutes takes place in gray matter. Magnetic resonance imaging detects the diffusion of water. Images made of water diffusion patterns show abnormal patterns of water movement in pathological states. For example, in a region of ischemic infarct, the swollen cells initially restrict the normal diffusion of water. In the region of a stroke, the diffusion-weighted image is positive very early after the insult. Because of the complex dynamic nature of the diffusion changes, the use of diffusion images is still experimental (Baird and Warach 1998).

Ependymal and Pial Surfaces

Lining the cerebral ventricles is a layer of ependymal cells with cilia. Pial cells line the surface of the brain, forming a limiting glial membrane. Gap junctions (zona adherens) are found between the ependymal cells that line the cerebral ventricles and the pial cells of the cortex. Fluid, electrolytes, and large protein molecules can cross gap junctions, thereby allowing exchange between the CSF and ISF. Intrathecal administration of antibiotics and chemotherapeutic agents has been used to bypass the BBB. After injection into the CSF space, large proteins penetrate the perivascular spaces of Virchow-Robin. These perivascular routes may be important in spread of infection into the brain from the subarachnoid space. Virchow-Robin spaces provide a conduit for substances in the subarachnoid space to enter brain.

Arachnoid Granulations and Absorption of Cerebrospinal Fluid

Arachnoid granulations (pacchionian granulations) are the major sites for the drainage of CSF into the blood. They protrude through the dura into the superior sagittal sinus and act as one-way valves. As CSF pressure increases, more fluid is absorbed. When CSF pressure falls below a threshold value, the absorption of CSF ceases (Figure 65.3). In this way, the CSF pressure is maintained at a constant level, with the rate of CSF production as one determining factor.

Although channels are seen in the arachnoid granulations, actual valves are absent. The tissue appears to collapse around the channel as the pressure falls, and the channels enlarge as the pressure rises. Resistance to the outflow across the arachnoid granulations leads to elevation of the CSF pressure. Substances can clog outflow channels and increase resistance to CSF absorption. Blood cells are trapped in the arachnoid villi, and subarachnoid hemorrhage causes a transient increase in CSF pressure and can occasionally lead to hydrocephalus. Similarly, white blood cells from meningitis can increase CSF pressure.

Lymphatic Drainage of Interstitial Fluid

Brain tissue lacks a lymphatic drainage system, and ISF acts as the lymphatics do in other tissues. Substances of high molecular weight injected into various sites in the brain drain into the cervical lymphatics. Drainage occurs along certain cranial nerves and spinal nerve roots to the lymphatics. One such route is along the olfactory tracts, across the cribriform plate, and into the cervical lymph nodes. Although these drainage pathways are estimated to remove about 30% of ISF in small mammals, the significance in humans is less certain. Small molecules are removed across the blood vessels rather than by the slower route of drainage into the lymph nodes of the neck. Under pathological conditions, protein moieties from brain may reach the cervical lymphatics by this route, where they can cause an immunological response. This has been proposed as a possible mechanism for the development of antibodies against brain antigens (Knopf et al. 1995).

Cerebrospinal Fluid Pressure

For more than 100 years, lumbar puncture has been used to measure CSF pressure, obtain CSF for diagnosis, and inject drugs. The method of measuring pressure and removing fluid was first reported by Quincke in 1891. With the patient in the lateral recumbent position, the spinal needle is introduced into the subarachnoid space and pressure is measured with a manometer. An opening pressure should be recorded. Normal CSF pressure is 80–180 mm H_2O. Three components contribute to the measured pressure: blood, CSF, and brain tissue. Enlargement of any of these causes an increase in CSF pressure.

Small fluctuations from the cardiac pulse and larger fluctuations from respirations take place in the fluid in the manometer. Because veins are thin-walled structures, venous pulsations cause fluctuations in CSF pressure. Arteries with thick elastic walls dampen the pulsations from arterial pressures. Therefore, an increase in CSF outflow pressure at the sagittal sinuses, as occurs when pressure within the thoracic cavity increases, results in an increase in the CSF pressure. Deep respirations cause wide fluctuations in the CSF pressure, whereas changes in arterial pressure are barely visible.

As intracranial pressure rises, tissue compliance falls and reserve capacity of the intracranial contents is lost. At that point, small changes in fluid volume may lead to large increases in intracranial pressure. Patients with increased intracranial pressure have been continuously monitored with catheters placed into the cerebral ventricles or with bolts placed on the dura. Pathological elevations in intracranial pressure cause Lundberg or plateau waves that increase in steps to 50 mm Hg, where they persist for up to 20 minutes before returning to baseline. Less significant waves of 1–2 per minute with lower amplitude are thought to be related to respiration. Head-injured patients with severely reduced levels of consciousness often undergo intracranial pressure monitoring to gauge response to treatment.

BRAIN EDEMA

Molecular Cascade in Injury

Cerebral edema occurs in many neurological diseases. Excess fluid can accumulate in the intracellular or extracellular spaces. Cytotoxic edema is cellular swelling, vasogenic

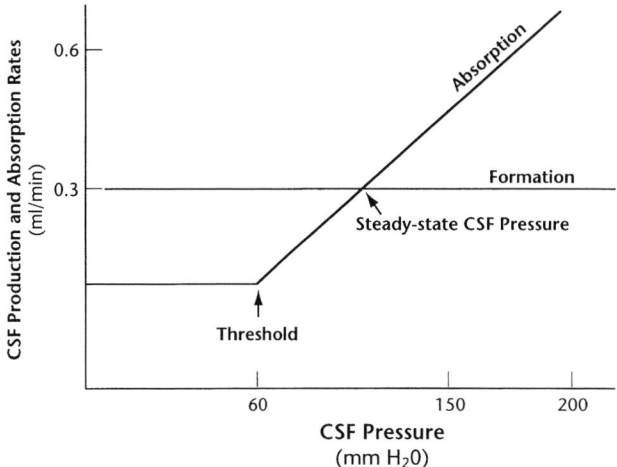

FIGURE 65.3 Schematic drawing of the relationship of cerebrospinal fluid (CSF) formation and absorption to pressure. CSF is formed at a constant rate of 0.35 ml per minute. Absorption begins above a threshold value that varies from person to person. Once CSF absorption begins, it is linear, as seen in a one-way valve. When formation rate equals absorption rate, the steady-state CSF pressure is determined. (Modified with permission from RW Cutler, L Page, J Galicich, GV Watters. Formation and absorption of cerebrospinal fluid in man. Brain 1968;91:707–720.)

edema is blood vessel leakage, and interstitial edema is transependymal flow in hydrocephalus. Rarely is the separation into distinct categories possible; there is often overlap between the various types of edema.

Vasogenic edema expands the extracellular space in the white matter. Cytotoxic edema, which results from pathological processes that damage cell membranes, constricts the extracellular spaces. Cellular and blood vessel damage follows activation of an injury cascade. The cascade begins with glutamate release into the extracellular space. This occurs during a hypoxic, ischemic, or traumatic injury and causes cytotoxic damage. Calcium and sodium entry channels on cell membranes are opened by glutamate stimulation. Membrane ATPase pumps extrude one calcium ion in exchange for three sodium ions. Sodium builds up within the cell, creating an osmotic gradient and increasing cell volume by the entry of water. While the cell membrane is intact, the increase in water causes dysfunction but not necessarily permanent damage. Finally, hypoxia depletes the cell's energy stores, disabling the sodium-potassium ATPase pumps and reducing calcium exchange. Calcium then accumulates inside the cell, activating intracellular cytotoxic processes. An inflammatory response is initiated by the formation of immediate early genes, such as *c-fos* and *c-jun*, and cytokines, chemokines, and other intermediary substances (Ginsberg and Pulsinelli 1994). Microglial cells are activated and release free radicals and proteases, which contribute to the attack on cell membranes and capillaries. Once the membranes are disrupted, recovery of the cell is impossible. In the molecular cascade of injury that accompanies hypoxic, ischemic, and

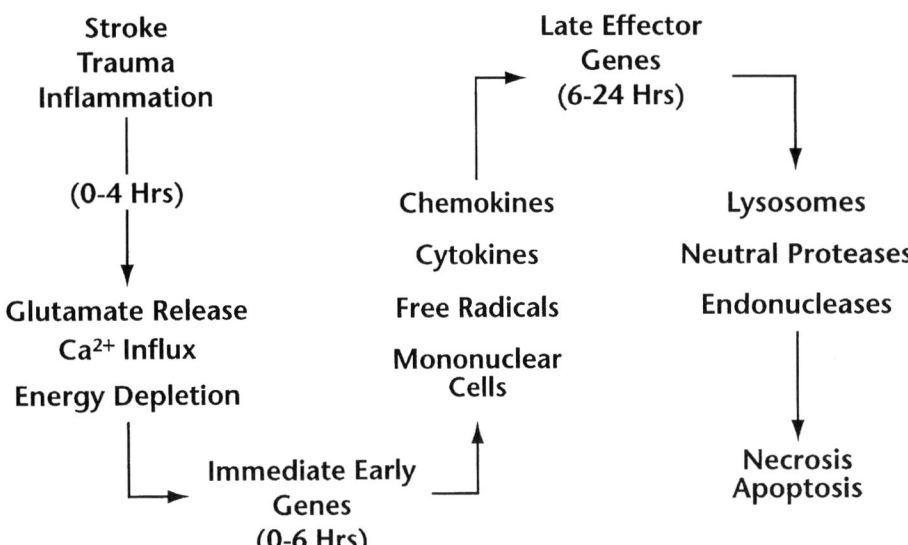

FIGURE 65.4   Mechanisms of ischemic-hypoxic injury leading to cell swelling and death. The chart shows the time course of the early events involving glutamate release, immediate early gene production, and energy failure. This leads to changes in electrolytes and initiation of the inflammatory response. Cytokines continue the damage that results in opening of the blood-brain barrier. Chemokines attract white blood cells to the injury site, where they release free radicals and proteases and enhance the injury. Finally, the proteases attack structural components, leading to membrane damage and cell death.

traumatic injuries, the goal must be to initiate treatment before the point at which the cells swell and the membranes are irreversibly damaged.

Free radicals are toxic to cells. Reactive oxygen species, such as superoxide ion, hydrogen peroxide, and hydroxyl ion, are produced by the arachidonic acid cascade. Release of fatty acids, such as arachidonic acid, provides a supply of damaging molecules (Gobbel et al. 1997). Superoxide dismutase-1 and catalase are the major enzymes that catalyze the breakdown of reactive oxygen species. Other defenses include glutathione, ascorbic acid, vitamin E, and iron chelators, such as the 21-amino steroids. Transgenic mice that overexpress the superoxide dismutase-1 gene have smaller ischemic lesions than controls.

Nitric oxide (NO) is also a source of free radicals. NO synthetase (NOS) has three forms: neuronal NOS (nNOS), endothelial NOS (eNOS), and inducible or immunological NOS (iNOS). Macrophages and activated microglial cells form NO through the action of iNOS in response to ischemia, injury, and inflammatory stimuli. NO acts both as a normal vasodilator of blood vessels, by release of cyclic guanosine monophosphate in smooth muscle, and as a toxic compound in pathological conditions. Peroxynitrite anions ($ONOO^-$) are formed from the reaction of NO with superoxide anions. Manipulation of the NOS gene has helped reveal the action of the enzyme. The free radical nNOS produces toxic free radicals early in ischemic injury. Deletion of the nNOS gene in transgenic mice results in smaller infarcts from middle cerebral artery occlusion (Huang et al. 1994). On the other hand, eNOS causes vasodilatation and increases cerebral blood flow. Removing the eNOS genes leads to increased infarct size. Inflammation induces iNOS, which reaches a maximum at 24 hours (Iadecola 1997).

Vasogenic Edema and the Neuroinflammatory Response

Capillary injury results in opening of the BBB, with leakage of protein and fluids into brain tissue. Vasogenic edema moves through the white matter. Opening of the BBB could occur by loosening of tight junctions, development of pinocytotic vesicles in the endothelial cell, or an alteration in the substrates surrounding the capillaries. Opening of tight junctions between cells has been observed after the infusion of hyperosmotic solutions. There is little evidence to support enhanced pinocytosis. Potentially toxic substances that may injure the capillary and the extracellular matrix include free radicals, cytokines, and proteases. Free radicals from oxygen and nitrogen can increase the permeability of the capillary. Cytokines have also been shown to have toxic effects on blood vessels, particularly tumor necrosis factor-α (TNF-α). Several proteases damage the capillary.

Late effector genes are activated by the immediate early genes, c-fos and c-jun, and by cytokines. Proteases are produced that can attack substrates in the capillary and in the extracellular matrix around it. Neutrophils and macrophages enter the injury site through the blood vessel in response to a variety of injuries (Perry et al. 1993). Proteases in the white blood cells, such as the matrix metalloproteinases, are released by the invading cells. The enzymes enable the white blood cells to penetrate the capillary wall. Neutrophils release free radicals in the respiratory burst. Elastases and cathepsin are also released by neutrophils (Figure 65.4).

Cerebral capillaries are surrounded by astrocytic foot processes attached by integrins to the basal lamina (Wagner et al. 1997). Beneath and next to the astrocytes are pericytes and perivascular microglial cells. Neutral proteases, such as serine proteases and matrix metalloproteinases, attack the extracellular matrix around capillaries. Brain cells make proteases. Astrocytes constitutively secrete the matrix metalloproteinase, gelatinase A or 72-kD type IV collagenase (Gottschall and Deb 1996). Microglia secrete the inflammatory matrix metalloproteinase gelatinase B or 92-kD type IV collagenase (Colton et al. 1993). Proteases are secreted in latent forms and require activation. Free radicals and other proteases have been implicated in the activation of the gelatinases, but the in vivo mechanism is uncertain. Other proteases that may be released during the inflammatory process include elastases, plasmin, and cathepsin. Elastases are released from microglia cells and from invading neutrophils. Plasmin is generated in glia cells by plasminogen activators.

When an activated form of the 72-kD type IV collagenase is injected intracerebrally into rat brain, the BBB is opened. This reaction can be blocked by the tissue inhibitor of metalloproteinases-2 and by synthetic metalloproteinase inhibitors. Direct injection of TNF-α into brain results in the production of the proinflammatory gelatinase B, but only after a 24-hour delay, which correlates with the opening of the BBB (Rosenberg et al. 1995). During an ischemic injury produced by permanent occlusion of the middle cerebral artery, increased levels of gelatinase B are found around 24 hours after the occlusion. Gelatinase A increases approximately 5 days later, when the urokinase-type plasminogen activator is also elevated (Rosenberg et al. 1996). Because both gelatinases and plasminogen activators are important in angiogenesis, the delayed increase in gelatinase A may be occurring in the recovery phase when new blood vessel growth is seen. Because of the highly disruptive properties of these hydrolytic enzymes, they are tightly regulated by tissue inhibitors of metalloproteinases and plasminogen activator inhibitors. Hemorrhagic transformation occurs commonly after a stroke, particularly when ischemic tissue is reperfused (del Zoppo 1994; Hornig et al. 1993). Proteolytic enzymes active in vessel regrowth and extracellular matrix remodeling may be involved.

Infection, Ischemia, and Inflammation

Bacterial meningitis initiates an inflammatory response in the meninges caused by the invading organisms and by the secondary release of cytokines and chemokines. The secondary, inflammatory response may aggravate the infection. Reducing the inflammation with corticosteroids has been shown in children to reduce the incidence of permanent hearing loss and other complications. It is recommended that children be given corticosteroids along with appropriate antibiotics. The goal is to reduce the secondary, inflammatory response that occurs as the bacteria die and release toxic lipopolysaccharide. Cytokines, including TNF-α and interleukin-6, are elevated in the CSF of patients with bacterial meningitis and contribute to the secondary tissue damage. The use of corticosteroids in adults with bacterial meningitis remains to be tested.

Diagnosis of infections of the CNS has been aided by polymerase chain reaction (PCR) to detect messenger RNA from infectious agents. Herpes simplex encephalitis can be rapidly diagnosed by PCR (Elger et al. 1997). Patients with acquired immunodeficiency syndrome frequently have opportunistic CNS infections. Use of PCR assays helps to separate various causes, including toxoplasmosis, Epstein-Barr virus, and JC virus (Antinori et al. 1997).

Cytotoxic Brain Edema

Cytotoxic edema is induced by stroke, trauma, and toxins. After a stroke, brain water increases rapidly due to energy failure and loss of ATP. Cytotoxic edema worsens for 24–48 hours, during which period there is a danger of brain herniation. Capillary injury also takes place as part of the inflammatory phase. Vasogenic edema develops as a result of opening of the BBB. Reperfusion of brain after an ischemic insult increases brain edema. In animal studies of reperfusion injury after a stroke, there is a biphasic opening of the BBB (Belayev et al. 1996). The first opening occurs several hours after reperfusion. This could be due to hyperemia, a rapid proteolytic response, or free radicals. The barrier then closes for an extended period before a second opening of the BBB occurs around the second day. This delayed opening is associated with activation of microglia and influx of inflammatory cells; multiple proteolytic enzymes and free radicals are active at that time. When oxygen is reintroduced into the tissue by reperfusion, brain edema occurs more rapidly, with a greater increase in water content (Yang et al. 1994). The effect of reperfusion on the capillary depends on multiple factors, including the time of occlusion and of reperfusion.

Intracerebral hemorrhage causes brain edema, both around the hemorrhagic mass and in distant regions. Besides the cytotoxic edema at the site of injury, vasogenic edema can spread to other regions when the mass lesion is large. Hemorrhagic transformation after a stroke occurs in approximately 40% of patients, but only a small proportion progress to develop clinical symptoms from the mass lesion (Brott et al. 1997). When intracerebral hematoma develops rapidly, the edema reaches maximum levels around 24–48 hours after the bleed.

In acute hepatic failure, cerebral edema may cause death. Patients with cerebral edema are often young and have an acute cause of liver failure. Often these patients have overdosed on a drug that is toxic to the liver or have infectious hepatitis. Long-standing liver disease with cirrhosis and hepatic encephalopathy shows changes of astrocytes in the brain, but it is generally not complicated by cerebral edema. Reye's syndrome, which is seen primarily in children after an influenza infection, particularly when they are treated with aspirin, has a high incidence of brain swelling. Since the realization of the association of aspirin with the syndrome, the number of cases of postinfluenza hepatic encephalopathy has dramatically declined. The mechanisms involved in the production of cerebral edema with acute hepatic disease are poorly understood.

A posterior edema syndrome is associated with hypertensive encephalopathy (Hinchey et al. 1996). Rapid elevations in blood pressure can occur with kidney disease and in eclampsia. The changes are transient unless hemorrhage or infarction occurs. Rapid reduction in blood pressure is necessary. The reason for the predilection for the posterior circulation in this syndrome is uncertain. Petechial bleeding into the occipital lobe can cause blindness. Eclamptic patients may have visual disturbances as the only neurological manifestation.

Edema may occur secondary to changes in osmolality. Patients treated for diabetic ketoacidosis, with rapid reduction of plasma glucose and sodium, are at risk for edema secondary to water shifts into the brain (Hale et al. 1997). Long-standing hyperosmolality leads to solute accumulation in brain to compensate for the hyperosmolar plasma levels. These idiogenic osmoles are thought to include taurine and other amino acids. Once formed, they are slowly removed from the brain. When blood osmolality is reduced, water follows the osmotic gradient, resulting in cerebral edema. Rapid reduction of serum hyperosmolality, as in diabetic ketoacidosis, should be avoided to prevent brain edema due to the residual idiogenic osmoles. Dialysis disequilibrium may also be due to an osmotic imbalance that results from urea buildup in brain tissue (Silver et al. 1996). Rapid correction of chronic serum hyponatremia can cause a different syndrome, central pontine myelinolysis, which may also be due to osmotic imbalance.

Treatment of Brain Edema

Treatment of brain edema has not kept up with the advances in understanding of the mechanisms producing the edema. Blood volume can be reduced with hyperventilation, which lowers carbon dioxide. However, it also can be detrimental because it constricts blood vessels, causing a worsening of the ischemia. Intraventricular drainage lowers the CSF volume. This is used in some patients with head injuries. Agents that reduce the production of CSF, such as acetazolamide or diuretics, may be used. Osmotic treatment with mannitol reduces brain volume and CSF production and improves blood flow. Corticosteroids lower intracranial pressure primarily in vasogenic edema because of their beneficial effect on the blood vessel. They have been less effective in cytotoxic edema, however, and are not recommended in the treatment of edema secondary to stroke or hemorrhage. In fact, systemic complications of corticosteroids can worsen the patient's condition. Edema surrounding brain tumors, particularly metastatic brain tumors, responds dramatically to treatment with high doses of dexamethasone. The corticosteroid closes the BBB rapidly. Hence, it is important to obtain contrast-enhanced magnetic resonance imaging (MRI) or computed tomographic (CT) scans before treatment with corticosteroids; otherwise, enhancement of the lesion may be missed.

Osmotherapy with mannitol infusions over several days lowers intracranial pressure. Low doses of mannitol (0.25–1.0 g/kg) are effective, although they raise the serum osmolality only slightly. It is unlikely that the major effect is an osmotic shrinkage of tissue. Mannitol reduces CSF and ISF secretion by 50%, which may contribute to its action. Prolonged administration of mannitol results in an electrolyte imbalance that may override its benefit and that must be carefully monitored. Some investigators have proposed that mannitol hyperosmolality alters the rheological properties of blood, whereas others have noted an antioxidant effect.

Opening of the BBB is frequently seen on MRI with gadolinium contrast in patients with multiple sclerosis. The opening of the BBB is associated with elevated levels of the proinflammatory cytokine, TNF-α. Inflammatory lesions, such as those that occur in acute attacks of multiple sclerosis, respond well to high-dose methylprednisolone. Dramatic reduction in enhancement on MRI may be seen after treatment. However, the effect is lost after several months. Corticosteroids are recommended for the treatment of acute spinal injuries, but the role of corticosteroids in head trauma is uncertain.

IDIOPATHIC INTRACRANIAL HYPERTENSION

Before the advent of CT scanners, the complaint of headache and the finding of papilledema raised the suspicion of hydrocephalus or tumor. When pneumoencephalograms showed normal-sized ventricles without evidence of a brain tumor, and a subsequent ventricular or lumbar puncture showed raised CSF pressure, the syndrome was called *pseudotumor cerebri*. Another early name was *otitic hydrocephalus*, which referred to the association of middle ear infections with papilledema, headaches, and increased intracranial pressure, particularly in children. Another name for the syndrome was *benign intracranial hypertension*, but for the occasional patients who lost vision from the increased intracranial pressure, the syndrome was not benign. The best term is IIH, but *pseudotumor cerebri* is also commonly used.

Clinical Features

Patients with IIH have headaches that are diffuse, worse at night, and often wake them from sleep. Headache is aggravated by sudden movements, such as coughing. Headaches may be present for several months before a diagnosis is made. Some patients complain of dizziness. Transient loss of vision (transient obscuration) can occur with change of position. Visual fields may show an enlarged blind spot. Prolonged papilledema may lead to sector scotomas and, rarely, vision loss. Damage to one or both sixth cranial nerves can occur as an effect of shifts of cerebral tissue; because the sixth cranial nerve is remote from the site of the process producing intracranial hypertension, the cranial neuropathy is termed a *false localizing sign*.

Diagnosis requires ruling out other causes of increased intracranial pressure. All patients require a CT or MRI scan to look for hydrocephalus and mass lesions. Lumbar puncture is also needed, but only after the imaging studies have ruled out a space-occupying lesion as the cause of the papilledema. Characteristic findings in the CSF include normal or low protein, normal glucose, no cells, and elevated CSF pressure. The upper limit for normal CSF pressure is above 180 mm H_2O, but borderline readings are difficult to interpret. Measurement of CSF pressure should be done with legs extended and neck unflexed. Movements of the fluid column with respiration should be seen to confirm proper placement of the needle.

IIH occurs more frequently in women than in men. Obesity and menstrual irregularities, with excessive premenstrual weight gain, are often present. Headache, often worse in the morning, is the main complaint. Because many illnesses are associated with IIH, a search for an underlying cause is essential before the diagnosis is made by exclusion. MRI has rekindled interest in conditions that cause occlusions of the venous sinuses. When the sinuses draining blood from the brain are obstructed, absorption of CSF is reduced, causing the pressure of the CSF to increase. MR venography is available in many centers and is better for showing the thrombosed sinuses than conventional MRI.

Several etiologies have been proposed for the increased intracranial pressure. Elevated venous pressure is frequently found in IIH. Pressure increases are seen due to dural sinus outflow obstruction or increased right-sided heart pressure (Karahalios et al. 1996). Venography is helpful and can be done by MR venography or, if that is negative, by conventional angiographic venography. Obesity is often found in women with IIH. Endocrine abnormalities have been extensively investigated in both obese and nonobese subjects, but none has been identified. Drugs associated with the syndrome include tetracycline-type antibiotics, nalidixic acid, nitrofurantoin, sulfonamides, and trimethoprim-sulfamethoxazole (Table 65.4). Withdrawal of corticosteroids can cause an increase in intracranial pressure. Large doses of vitamin A, which are used in the treatment of various skin conditions, may cause the syndrome. Hypercapnia leads to retention of carbon dioxide and increase in blood volume. Sleep apnea and lung diseases may cause headaches and papilledema due to this mechanism. Less frequent causes include Guillain-Barré syndrome, in which IIH may be due to an increase in CSF protein or an inflammatory response. Uremic patients have an increased incidence of papilledema with IIH. Renal failure patients have increased levels of vitamin A, use corticosteroids, and take cyclosporine, which have all been linked to IIH.

Cerebral edema was seen in one patient with early IIH, who had a brain biopsy at the time of subtemporal decom-

Table 65.4: Drugs frequently associated with idiopathic intracranial hypertension

Minocycline
Isotretinoin
Nalidixic acid
Tetracycline
Trimethoprim-sulfamethoxazole
Cimetidine
Prednisolone
Methylprednisolone
Tamoxifen
Beclomethasone

Source: HS Schutta, JJ Corbett. Intracranial Hypertension Syndromes. In RJ Joynt, RC Griggs (eds), Clinical Neurology (12th ed). Philadelphia: Lippincott, 1997;1–57.

pression. However, two IIH patients who came to post-mortem examination had no histologic evidence of cerebral edema (Wall et al. 1995). Blood volume is increased and cerebral blood flow decreased. CSF circulation is impaired. Diseases that chronically raise cerebral venous pressure often produce increased intracranial pressure without increased ventricular size. The primary sites of obstruction may be the superior vena cava, jugular veins, or large cerebral veins. Increased superior sagittal sinus or transverse sinus pressure has been reported in IIH (Karahalios et al. 1996; King et al. 1995). Many investigators favor an elevation of dural venous sinus pressure as a reasonable mechanism.

Treatment

Treatment involves reducing intracranial pressure. Acetazolamide is an inhibitor of carbonic anhydrase that lowers CSF production and pressure. It is given in a starting dose of 250 mg twice daily, increasing to 1 g per day. Electrolytes must be monitored to look for metabolic acidosis. Distal paresthesias are reported to occur in up to 25% of patients. The hyperosmolar agent, glycerol (0.25–1.00 g/kg/dose two or three times daily), and the diuretic, furosemide (20–60 mg daily), lower intracranial pressure. Corticosteroids have been used, but pressure may increase when they are tapered. Drug effects are often transient, and when the syndrome does not resolve spontaneously, other treatments are needed. Although the relationship of obesity to IIH is uncertain, loss of weight can lead to resolution of the syndrome.

Visual fields should be measured and the size of the blind spot plotted. When the papilledema spreads into the region of the macula, visual acuity falls, and in extreme cases, blindness may occur. Although most patients with IIH retain normal vision, a small percentage of patients develop impairment of vision. When vision is threatened, and drugs and lumbar punctures do not lower the CSF pressure, surgical intervention is necessary. Lumboperitoneal shunting has a reportedly high success rate (Eggenberger et al. 1996). However, shunt malfunction is common in lumboperitoneal shunts. Fenestration of the optic nerve sheath to drain CSF into the orbital region reduces the intracranial pressure, and some consider it the treatment method of choice in medically refractory patients (Spoor and McHenry 1993).

HYDROCEPHALUS

Hydrocephalus is defined as enlargement of the ventricles of the brain with an abnormal increase in the amount of CSF relative to brain tissue. Hydrocephalus can be divided into *noncommunicating (obstructive) hydrocephalus* and *communicating hydrocephalus.*

Enlargement of the cerebral ventricles in children younger than 2 years old causes enlargement of the head size because the skull sutures are still open. In the elderly, the onset of symptoms may be gradual, beginning with problems of gait and intellect, which can suggest many different diagnoses. When the CSF outflow tracts are obstructed, as occurs with cerebellar masses that obstruct the exit foramina of the fourth ventricle (foramina of Luschka and Magendie), a noncommunicating type of hydrocephalus results. *Communicating hydrocephalus* refers to enlargement of the ventricles with preserved flow of CSF between the ventricle and the subarachnoid space. Obstruction of CSF circulation may result in increased CSF pressure as ventricles enlarge. Tissue loss results in compensatory ventricular enlargement without obstruction, which is called *hydrocephalus ex vacuo* to distinguish it from excess fluid due to obstruction of CSF outflow, with consequent compression of brain tissue.

Acute hydrocephalus develops rapidly, reaching 80% of maximal ventricular enlargement within 6 hours. A slower phase of enlargement follows the initial rapid expansion, and ventricular enlargement plus continual production of CSF causes cerebral edema in the periventricular white matter.

When the hydrocephalus stabilizes and enters a chronic phase, the CSF pressure may decrease, resulting in a normal pressure recording on random measurements. Atrophy may occur in the chronically hydrocephalic white matter. When the rate of ventricular enlargement stabilizes in patients with incomplete ventricular obstruction, CSF production is balanced by absorption at alternate sites. Arrested hydrocephalus occurs more commonly in communicating hydrocephalus, which tends to produce an incomplete block to CSF circulation. Occasionally, patients with arrested hydrocephalus can undergo decompensation.

Hydrocephalus in Children

Hydrocephalus in children is often due to a structural abnormality, such as Arnold-Chiari malformation with or without meningocele, congenital aqueductal stenosis, aqueductal stenosis due to intrauterine infection or other congenital causes, such as anoxic injury, intraventricular hemorrhage, and obstruction of the CSF pathways after bacterial meningitis. Before the age of 2 years, when the cranial sutures are open, the diagnosis of hydrocephalus is suspected when serial measurements of head circumference fall above the normal developmental curves. Bulging of the anterior fontanelle may be seen, along with thinning of the skull and separation of the sutures. If the diagnosis is delayed, abnormal eye movements and optic atrophy may develop. Spasticity of the lower limbs may be observed at any stage. Acute enlargement of the ventricles is associated with nausea and vomiting.

During the neonatal and early childhood period, irritability is the most common symptom of hydrocephalus. The child feeds poorly, appears fretful, and may be lethargic. In the older child, headache may be a complaint. Vomiting due to increased intracranial pressure may be present in the morning. Remote effects of the increased pressure may affect the sixth cranial nerves on one or both sides, leading to the complaint of diplopia. The enlarged ventricles affect gait. A wide-based ataxic gait may be present due to the stretching of the white matter tracts from the frontal leg regions around the ventricles.

Premature infants weighing less than 1,500 g at birth have a high risk of intraventricular hemorrhage, and approximately 25% of these infants develop progressive ventricular enlargement, as shown by CT or ultrasound scans (Roland and Hill 1997). Ventricular size in the neonate may be followed at the bedside with B-mode ultrasound through the open fontanelle. Long-term follow-up studies of children with intraventricular hemorrhage due to prematurity show that 5% require shunting for hydrocephalus. The survivors of a large intracerebral bleed often have multiple disabilities.

Before the widespread availability of antibiotics and vaccinations, meningitis was a frequent cause of hydrocephalus in children. Often, there was concurrent cerebral infarction, resulting in brain atrophy with ventricular enlargement. Separation of the atrophy from the obstructive hydrocephalus may be difficult. Once the sutures are closed, which generally occurs by the age of 3 years, hydrocephalus causes signs of increased intracranial pressure rather than head enlargement. Meningitis, aqueductal stenosis, Arnold-Chiari malformations, and mass lesions may be the cause of hydrocephalus in these young children. When the aqueduct of Sylvius is closed by a mass, pressure on the brainstem and ventricular enlargement cause acute symptoms that require urgent diagnosis and treatment. Tumors originating from the cerebellum and from the brainstem produce acute symptomatology, including headaches with vomiting, diplopia, visual blurring, and ataxia.

Examination shows papilledema, possible sixth cranial nerve palsy, and spasticity of the lower limbs. When the

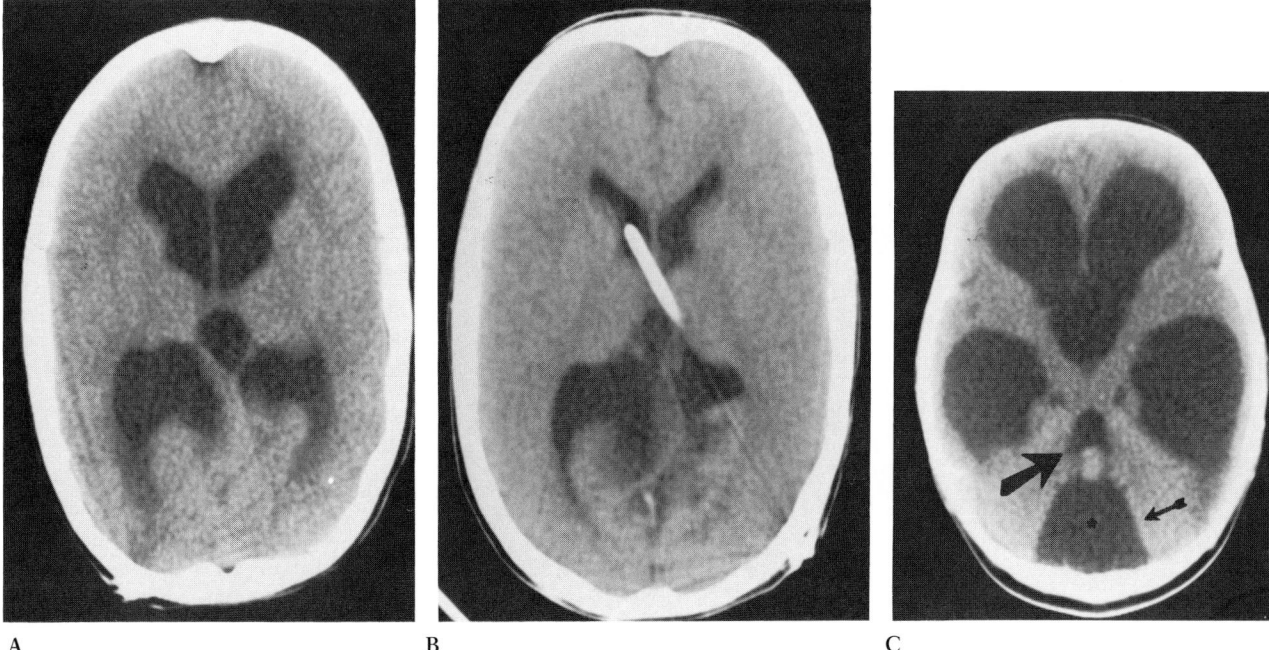

A   B   C

FIGURE 65.5 **(A)** Computed tomographic (CT) scan before shunting demonstrates ventriculomegaly and asymmetrical dilatation of the ventricles. **(B)** A repeat CT scan 2.5 weeks after placement of a shunt, which decompressed the ventricles but crossed the midline. **(C)** A CT scan oriented to show the entire ventricular system. Dilatated fourth ventricle (*large arrow*) is seen in front of an enlarged or mega cisterna magna (*small arrow*).

hydrocephalus is more long-standing, endocrine dysfunction may occur, involving short stature, menstrual irregularities, and diabetes insipidus. Excessively rapid growth of the head is the hallmark of hydrocephalus in the child before closure of the sutures. Charts are available to plot head growth and to compare it with the standardized curves for normals. Bulging of the anterior fontanelle is found even with the child relaxed and upright. After 1 year, the firmness of the fontanelle cannot be used because the sutures have closed. Other findings include the "cracked-pot" sound on percussion of the skull, engorged scalp veins, and abnormalities of eye movements. As spasticity develops, the deep tendon reflexes increase.

Treatment involves shunting CSF from the ventricles to drain fluid into another body cavity (Figure 65.5). In very young children, the shunt is often placed in the right heart (ventriculoatrial shunt) or the peritoneal cavity. As the child grows, the shunt requires frequent revision to keep the end in the correct place. In the older child, a ventriculoperitoneal shunt is generally used. Complications of shunt placement include ventriculitis and subdural hematomas.

Adult-Onset Hydrocephalus

In the adult, symptoms of hydrocephalus include headaches, papilledema, diplopia, and mental status changes. Sudden death may occur with severe increases in pressure. Rarely, hydrocephalus causes an akinetic mutism due to pressure on the structures around the third ventricle. Other symptoms include temporal lobe seizures, CSF rhinorrhea, endocrine dysfunction (e.g., amenorrhea, polydipsia, and polyuria), and obesity, which suggests third-ventricle dysfunction. Gait disturbances are reported in patients with aqueductal stenosis, but hyperreflexia with Babinski's sign is infrequent.

Adult-onset hydrocephalus has similar causes to those in children, but the frequencies differ. As in children, acute obstruction of the ventricles results in rapidly progressive hydrocephalus with symptoms of raised intracranial pressure, which is usually due to tumors or hematomas of the posterior fossa. Adults are more likely than children to present with an acute blockage of CSF flow by intraventricular masses, such as a colloid cyst of the third ventricle or an ependymoma of the fourth ventricle. These tumors cause sudden headaches, ataxia, and loss of consciousness with symptoms that may be intermittent due to the ball-valve effect of the masses. Diagnosis can be made by CT or MRI, which reveals the structural lesion in the ventricular system.

Cerebellar hemorrhage or, less commonly, cerebellar infarction with edema, cause an acute hydrocephalus by compression of the brainstem, blocking the sylvian aqueduct and the outflow of CSF from the fourth ventricle (Figure 65.6). Patients with cerebellar hemorrhage usually have a history of hypertension. The acute onset of headache is

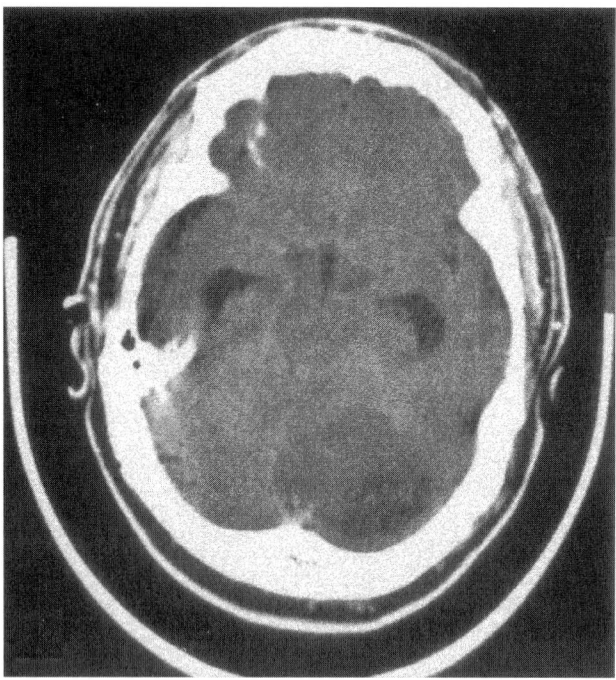
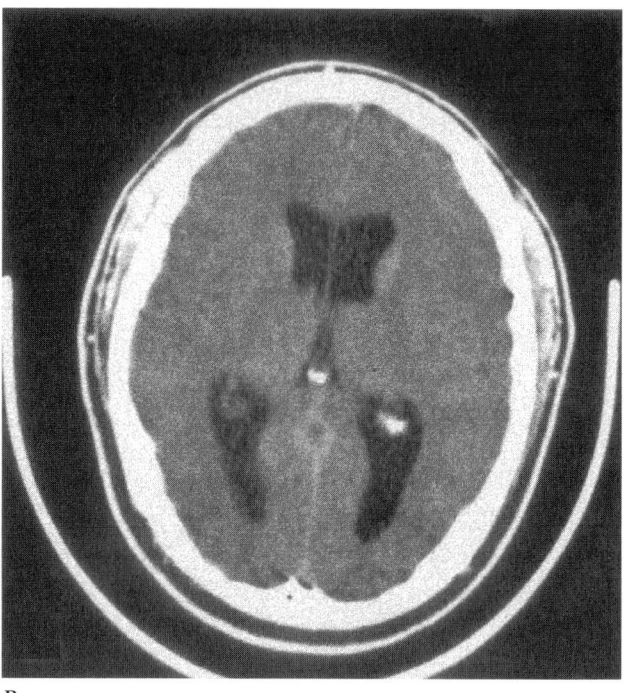

A

B

FIGURE 65.6 Cerebellar infarction causing compression of the fourth ventricle and hydrocephalus. (A) Large cerebellar infarction seen in the posterior region (bottom) of computed tomographic (CT) scan. Note the enlargement of the temporal poles of the lateral ventricles. (B) Acute hydrocephalus causing enlargement of the ventricles in a higher tomographic section of the CT scan.

often followed by increasing drowsiness and difficulty walking. Hemiparesis and brainstem findings evolve after the ataxia, providing a clue that the origin of the problem is in the posterior fossa. The expanding mass in the posterior fossa demands urgent neurosurgical attention, with placement of a ventricular catheter to decompress the lateral and third ventricles, followed by posterior fossa craniectomy to remove the mass effect and pressure on the brainstem.

Chronic hydrocephalus in the adult can produce symptoms of gait disturbance, incontinence, and memory loss, with or without symptoms and signs of raised intracranial pressure, including headache, papilledema, and false localizing signs. Causes of chronic hydrocephalus include subarachnoid hemorrhage, chronic meningeal infections, slow-growing tumors blocking the CSF pathways, and decompensated arrested hydrocephalus. However, about one-third of cases have no obvious cause and are classified as idiopathic.

Treatment of hydrocephalus involves an operation to insert a tube to shunt CSF from the ventricles to another body cavity, such as peritoneum (ventriculoperitoneal shunt). Ventriculoatrial shunts are mainly used for children because they have a higher complication rate than do shunts into the peritoneal cavity. Occasionally, the shunt is placed in the lumbar region with drainage into the abdominal cavity. Generally, the drainage tubes connect the enlarged ventricles with the peritoneal cavity. Hydrocephalic ventricles can be taped without difficulty due to the increase in their size. Shunts may dysfunction after long intervals, causing abrupt decompensation. Symptoms of acute increased intracranial pressure from a shunt malfunction resemble those seen with onset of the hydrocephalic process.

Adult-onset hydrocephalus that is communicating may be due to a tumor in the basal cisterns, subarachnoid bleeding, or infection or inflammation of the meninges, but only a small percentage of these patients require insertion of a shunt. Syphilis, tuberculosis, and fungal infections can cause a chronic obstruction of the subarachnoid pathways, with consequent hydrocephalus. Cultures of the CSF are indicated in the elderly patient with enlarged ventricles, and searching for other sources of infection in lungs and other organs may be helpful in establishing the type of infection.

Normal-Pressure Hydrocephalus

Normal-pressure hydrocephalus (NPH) is a term used to describe chronic, communicating adult-onset hydrocephalus. Typically, patients with NPH have the triad of mental impairment, gait disturbance, and incontinence. Enlarged ventricles are seen on CT or MRI. By definition, lumbar puncture generally reveals a normal CSF pressure. *Normal pressure* is an unfortunate term because patients who have undergone long-term monitoring with this syndrome have intermittently elevated pressures, often during the night.

NPH can develop secondary to trauma, infection, or subarachnoid hemorrhage, but in about one-third, no etiology is found. The presenting symptoms may be related to gait or to mental function. When gait is the presenting factor, the prognosis for treatment is better. NPH causes an apraxic gait, which is an inability to lift the legs as if they were stuck to the floor. The motor strength is intact, reflexes are usually normal, and Babinski's sign is absent. Patients may be misdiagnosed as having Parkinson's disease because the gait disorder is similar in the two syndromes, suggesting that the etiology of the problem in the hydrocephalic patient lies in the basal ganglia. Because many of these patients also have hypertension, and some have small or large strokes, such patients may have other neurological findings, including spasticity and hyperreflexia with Babinski's signs. The combination of cerebrovascular disease and hydrocephalus is a poor prognostic sign for treatment with shunts (Caruso et al. 1997).

NPH leads to a reduction in intellect, which at times may be subtle. The dementia involves slowing of verbal and motor responses with preservation of cortical functions, such as language and spatial resolution. Neuropsychological testing quantitates the decline in intellect and the degree of dementia. Patients are apathetic and may appear depressed. Incontinence of urine may occur early in the course, particularly in patients with prominent gait disturbance. In the early stages of the illness, presumably as the ventricles are undergoing enlargement, patients can experience drop attacks or brief loss of consciousness. Headache and papilledema are not a part of the syndrome.

Diagnosis of adult-onset NPH and selection of patients for placement of a ventriculoperitoneal shunt has been difficult. Many of these patients have hypertensive vascular disease with lacunar infarcts. Features of Parkinson's disease were noted in earlier reports of the syndrome, and it is now recommended that all patients with Parkinson's disease have scans to rule out hydrocephalus. CT and MRI have aided in separating Parkinson's disease, lacunar state, and NPH, although NPH may occasionally coexist with these diseases. Patients diagnosed with vascular diseases, such as lacunar state or subcortical arteriosclerotic encephalopathy (Binswanger's disease), along with the hydrocephalus respond poorly to shunting, and if there is a positive response, it may be transient as the underlying disease progresses. Selection of patients for shunting requires a combination of clinical findings and diagnostic test results, because no test can totally predict whether a patient will likely benefit from an operation.

There may be a correlation between improvement in gait after removal of CSF and improvement after shunting. Cisternography is a useful procedure that involves the injection of a radiolabeled tracer into the CSF with monitoring of its absorption for 3 days. Normally, the labeled material fails to enter the ventricles, moving over the convexity of the brain and leaving the CSF space within 12–24 hours. In patients with large ventricles due to atrophy, there may be a delay in circulation time, with some isotope being seen in the ventricles during the first 24 hours. Communicating hydrocephalus with abnormal CSF circulation shows persistent ventricular filling for more than 48 hours. In patients with NPH, there is reflux of the tracer into the cerebral ventricles by 24 hours and retention in the ventricles for 48–72 hours. This suggests that transependymal absorption is occurring and that periventricular white matter has become an alternate route of CSF absorption. Unfortunately, a positive cisternogram is seen in some patients with hypertensive cerebrovascular disease and Binswanger's encephalopathy.

CT and MRI in NPH show that the temporal horns of the lateral ventricles are enlarged and that cortical atrophy is less than anticipated for age. This is in contrast to patients with hydrocephalus ex vacuo due to a degenerative disease, such as Alzheimer's disease, in which there is atrophy of the cerebral gyri and enlargement of the ventricles. Another useful finding on proton density MRI is the presence of presumed transependymal fluid in the frontal and occipital periventricular regions (Figure 65.7). Quantitative cisternography using single-photon emission CT has been successfully used to predict the results of a shunt (Larsson et al. 1994). Other proposed diagnostic methods, including measuring rate of absorption of CSF by infusion of saline or artificial CSF into the thecal sac, clinical improvement after CSF removal, or the prolonged monitoring of intracranial pressure, have been used with some success to select patients for surgery (Chen et al. 1994; Raftopoulos et al. 1994; Sand et al. 1994). Decreased cerebral blood flow has been reported in NPH (Kristensen et al. 1996); regional cerebral blood flow is reduced in both cortical and subcortical regions. Patients who show clinical improvement with shunting have a concomitant increase in cerebral blood flow (Waldemar et al. 1993). Removal of CSF may result in an increase in cerebral blood flow in patients in whom NPH is likely to respond to shunt therapy.

The number of patients undergoing shunt operations at most centers has fallen as the initial enthusiasm, which resulted in many shunts and a low success rate, has waned. None of the currently available tests by themselves identify the patients that will benefit from shunting. Most helpful is a combination of clinical signs and judiciously chosen laboratory tests.

Success rates vary between investigators, with some reports describing improvement in approximately 80% of treated patients and others reporting lower rates. In one study, 166 patients receiving shunts for presumed NPH found that 36% had a poor response and 28% had major complications, including a high rate of infection and subdural hematomas after shunt placement. Clearly, more information is needed to aid in the management of patients with this uncommon but treatable syndrome.

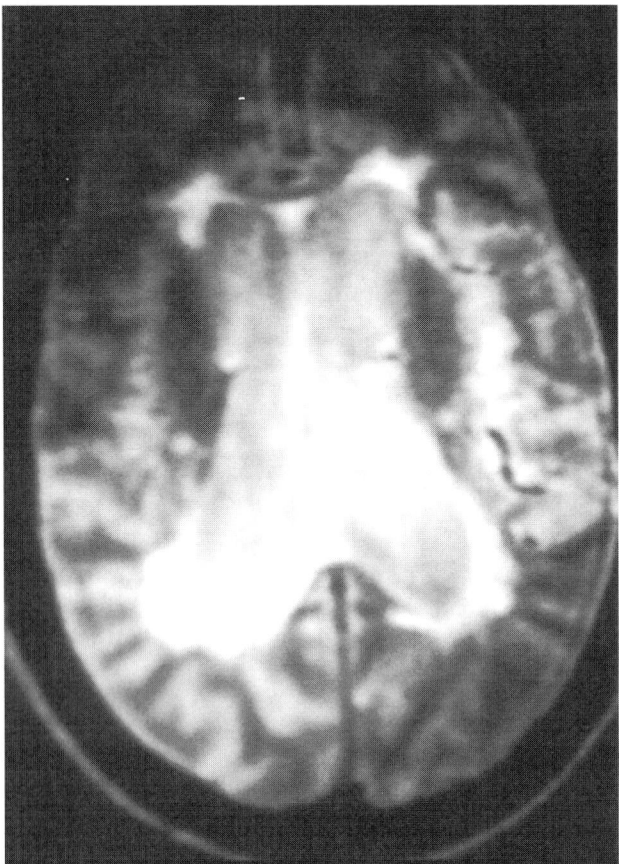

FIGURE 65.7 Magnetic resonance image of a patient with adult-onset hydrocephalus. This intermediate-weighted image (proton density) shows cerebrospinal fluid as gray and water in the periventricular tissue as white. The white area around the ventricle is interstitial edema from transependymal flow of cerebrospinal fluid into brain.

REFERENCES

Antinori A, Ammassari A, De Luca A, et al. Diagnosis of AIDS-related focal brain lesions: a decision-making analysis based on clinical and neuroradiologic characteristics combined with polymerase chain reaction assays in CSF. Neurology 1997;48:687–694.

Baird AE, Warach S. Magnetic resonance imaging of acute stroke. J Cereb Blood Flow Metab 1998;18:583–609.

Belayev L, Busto R, Zhao W, Ginsberg MD. Quantitative evaluation of blood-brain barrier permeability following middle cerebral artery occlusion in rats. Brain Res 1996;739:88–96.

Bradbury MW. The blood-brain barrier. Exp Physiol 1993;78: 453–472.

Brott T, Broderick J, Kothari R, et al. Early hemorrhage growth in patients with intracerebral hemorrhage. Stroke 1997;28:1–5.

Caruso R, Cervoni L, Vitale AM, Salvati M. Idiopathic normal-pressure hydrocephalus in adults: result of shunting correlated with clinical findings in 18 patients and review of the literature. Neurosurg Rev 1997;20:104–107.

Chen IH, Huang CI, Liu HC, Chen KK. Effectiveness of shunting in patients with normal pressure hydrocephalus predicted by temporary, controlled-resistance, continuous lumbar drainage: a pilot study. J Neurol Neurosurg Psychiatry 1994;57:1430–1432.

Colton CA, Keri JE, Chen WT, Monsky WL. Protease production by cultured microglia: substrate gel analysis and immobilized matrix degradation. J Neurosci Res 1993;35:297–304.

del Zoppo GJ. Microvascular changes during cerebral ischemia and reperfusion. Cerebrovasc Brain Metab Rev 1994;6: 47–96.

Eggenberger ER, Miller NR, Vitale S. Lumboperitoneal shunt for the treatment of pseudotumor cerebri. Neurology 1996;46: 1524–1530.

Elger B, Laux V, Schwarz M. Magnetic resonance imaging studies on the effect of the fibrinogen-lowering agent ancrod on cerebral lesions in two rat models of acute stroke. Arzneimittelforschung 1997;47:895–899.

Ginsberg MD, Pulsinelli WA. The ischemic penumbra, injury thresholds, and the therapeutic window for acute stroke (editorial comment). Ann Neurol 1994;36:553–554.

Gobbel GT, Chan TY, Chan PH. Nitric oxide- and superoxide-mediated toxicity in cerebral endothelial cells. J Pharmacol Exp Ther 1997;282:1600–1607.

Gottschall PE, Deb S. Regulation of matrix metalloproteinase expressions in astrocytes, microglia and neurons. Neuroimmunomodulation 1996;3:69–75.

Hale PM, Rezvani I, Braunstein AW, et al. Factors predicting cerebral edema in young children with diabetic ketoacidosis and new onset type I diabetes. Acta Paediatr 1997;86:626–631.

Hinchey J, Chaves C, Appignani B, et al. A reversible posterior leukoencephalopathy syndrome. N Engl J Med 1996;334: 494–500.

Hornig CR, Bauer T, Simon C, et al. Hemorrhagic transformation in cardioembolic cerebral infarction. Stroke 1993;24:465–468.

Huang Z, Huang PL, Panahian N, et al. Effects of cerebral ischemia in mice deficient in neuronal nitric oxide synthase. Science 1994;265:1883–1885.

Iadecola C. Bright and dark sides of nitric oxide in ischemic brain injury. Trends Neurosci 1997;20:132–139.

Karahalios DG, Rekate HL, Khayata MH, Apostolides PJ. Elevated intracranial venous pressure as a universal mechanism in pseudotumor cerebri of varying etiologies. Neurology 1996;46:198–202.

King JO, Mitchell PJ, Thomson KR, Tress BM. Cerebral venography and manometry in idiopathic intracranial hypertension. Neurology 1995;45:2224–2228.

Knopf PM, Cserr HF, Nolan SC, et al. Physiology and immunology of lymphatic drainage of interstitial and cerebrospinal fluid from the brain. Neuropathol Appl Neurobiol 1995;21: 175–180.

Kristensen B, Malm J, Fagerland M, et al. Regional cerebral blood flow, white matter abnormalities, and cerebrospinal fluid hydrodynamics in patients with idiopathic adult hydrocephalus syndrome. J Neurol Neurosurg Psychiatry 1996;60: 282–288.

Larsson A, Arlig A, Bergh AC, et al. Quantitative SPECT cisternography in normal pressure hydrocephalus. Acta Neurol Scand 1994;90:190–196.

Perry VH, Andersson PB, Gordon S. Macrophages and inflammation in the central nervous system. Trends Neurosci 1993;16: 268–273.

Raftopoulos C, Deleval J, Chaskis C, et al. Cognitive recovery in idiopathic normal pressure hydrocephalus: a prospective study. Neurosurgery 1994;35:397–404.

Risau W. Differentiation of endothelium). FASEB J 1995;9: 926–933.

Roland EH, Hill A. Intraventricular hemorrhage and posthemorrhagic hydrocephalus. Current and potential future interventions. Clin Perinatol 1997;24:589–605.

Rosenberg GA, Estrada EY, Dencoff JE, Stetler-Stevenson WG. Tumor necrosis factor-alpha–induced gelatinase B causes delayed opening of the blood-brain barrier: an expanded therapeutic window. Brain Res 1995;703:151–155.

Rosenberg GA, Navratil M, Barone F, Feuerstein G. Proteolytic cascade enzymes increase in focal cerebral ischemia in rat. J Cereb Blood Flow Metab 1996;16:360–366.

Sand T, Bovim G, Grimse R, et al. Idiopathic normal pressure hydrocephalus: the CSF tap-test may predict the clinical response to shunting. Acta Neurol Scand 1994;89:311–316.

Silver SM, Sterns RH, Halperin ML. Brain swelling after dialysis: old urea or new osmoles? Am J Kidney Dis 1996;28:1–13.

Spoor TC, McHenry JG. Long-term effectiveness of optic nerve sheath decompression for pseudotumor cerebri. Arch Ophthalmol 1993;111:632–635.

Vannucci SJ, Maher F, Simpson IA. Glucose transporter proteins in brain: delivery of glucose to neurons and glia. Glia 1997;21:2–21.

Wagner S, Tagaya M, Koziol JA, et al. Rapid disruption of an astrocyte interaction with the extracellular matrix mediated by integrin alpha-6-beta-4 during focal cerebral ischemia/reperfusion. Stroke 1997;28:858–865.

Waldemar G, Schmidt JF, Delecluse F, et al. High resolution SPECT with [99mTc]-d,l-HMPAO in normal pressure hydrocephalus before and after shunt operation. J Neurol Neurosurg Psychiatry 1993;56:655–664.

Wall M, Dollar JD, Sadun AA, Kardon R. Idiopathic intracranial hypertension. Lack of histologic evidence for cerebral edema. Arch Neurol 1995;52:141–145.

Yang GY, Betz AL. Reperfusion-induced injury to the blood-brain barrier after middle cerebral artery occlusion in rats. Stroke 1994;25:1658–1664.

Chapter 66
Developmental Disorders of the Nervous System

Harvey B. Sarnat and Laura Flores

EMBRYOLOGY OF THE NERVOUS SYSTEM

Congenital malformations of the nervous system are best understood in the context of embryology. The scope of modern embryology encompasses classic descriptive morphogenesis as well as the molecular genetic programming of development. *Maturation* refers both to *growth,* a measurement of physical characteristics over time, and *development,* the acquisition of metabolic functions, reflexes, sensory awareness, motor skills, language, and intellect. Molecular development is the maturation of cellular function. In the case of neurons, it includes the development of an energy production system to actively maintain a resting membrane potential, the synthesis of secretory molecules as neurotransmitters, and the formation of membrane receptors. Membrane receptors respond to various transmitters at synapses, to a variety of trophic and adhesion molecules and, during development, substances that attract or repel growing axons in their intermediate and final trajectories. The role of homeobox genes in the differentiation of neural structures is an aspect of development recognized relatively recently. Molecular genetic data are rapidly becoming available because of intense interest in this key to understanding neuroembryology in general and neural induction in particular (Bronner-Fraser and Fraser 1997; Sarnat and Menkes 1999). Other aspects of current investigative interest include the roles of neurotrophic factors, hormones, ion channels, and neurotransmitter systems in fetal brain development.

Maturation progresses in a predictable sequence with precise timing. Insults that adversely affect maturation influence events occurring at a particular time. Some insults are brief (e.g., a single exposure to a toxin), whereas others act over many weeks or throughout gestation, such as some congenital infections, diabetes mellitus, and genetic or chromosomal defects.

The anatomical and physiological correlates of neurological maturation reflect the growth and development of the individual neuron and its synaptic relations with other neurons. The mature neuron is a secretory cell with an electrically polarized membrane. Although many cells are secretory, and others, such as muscle cells, possess excitable membranes, only neurons embrace both functions. The precursors of neurons are neither secretory nor excitable. The cytological maturation of neurons is an aspect of ontogenesis that is as important as their spatial relations with other cells for future function and also for the pathogenesis of some functional neurological disorders of infancy, such as neonatal seizures (Sarnat et al. 1998; Sarnat and Born 1999).

The events of neural maturation after initial induction and formation of the neural tube are each predictive of specific types of malformation of the brain and of later abnormal neurological function. These are (1) mitotic proliferation of neuroblasts, (2) programmed death of excess neuroblasts, (3) neuroblast migration, (4) growth of axons and dendrites, (5) electrical polarity of the cell membrane, (6) synaptogenesis, (7) biosynthesis of neurotransmitters, and (8) myelination of axons.

Malformations of the nervous system are unique. No two individual cases are identical, even if they can both be categorized as similar, such as alobar holoprosencephaly, agenesis of the corpus callosum, or type 2 lissencephaly (Norman et al. 1995). Functional expression of anatomically similar cases also may vary widely. For example, two cases of holoprosencephaly with nearly identical imaging findings and similar histological patterns of cortical architecture and subcortical heterotopia at autopsy may differ in that one infant may have epilepsy refractory to pharmacological control, whereas the other may have no clinical seizures at all. The difference may be at the level of synaptic organization and the relative maturation of afferent input and neuronal maturation (Sarnat and Born 1999).

Neural Maturation

Mitotic Proliferation of Neuroblasts (Neuronogenesis)

The neuroblast is histologically indistinguishable from other stem cells, but it is identified by its location in the primitive neural plate. After formation of the neural tube, neurons and glial cells are generated by proliferation of neuroepithelial cells in the ventricular zone with mitoses at the ventricular surface. The rate of division is greatest during the early first trimester in the spinal cord and brainstem and during the late first and early second trimester in the forebrain. Within the ventricular zone of the human fetal telencephalon, 33 mitotic cycles provide the total number of neurons required for the mature cerebral cortex. Most mitotic activity in the neuroepithelium occurs at the ventricular surface, and the orientation of the mitotic spindle determines the subsequent immediate fate of the daughter cells. If the cleavage plane is perpendicular to the ventricular surface, the two daughter cells become equal neuroepithelial cells preparing for further mitosis. If, however, the cleavage is parallel to the ventricular surface, the two daughter cells are unequal (asymmetrical cleavage). In that case, the one at the ventricular surface becomes another neuroepithelial cell, whereas the one away from the ventricular surface separates from its ventricular attachment and becomes a postmitotic neuroblast ready to migrate to the cortical plate. Furthermore, the products of two genes that determine cell fate, called *numb* and *null*, are on different sides of the neuroepithelial cell. Therefore, with symmetrical cleavages, both daughter cells receive the same amount of each, but with asymmetrical cleavage, the cells receive unequal ratios of each, which also influences their subsequent development (Chenn and McConnell 1995; Mione et al. 1997; Zhong et al. 1996).

Active mitoses cease well before the time of birth in most parts of the human nervous system, but a few sites retain a potential for postnatal mitoses of neuroblasts. One recognized site is the periventricular region of the cerebral hemispheres (Kendler and Golden 1996). The best-documented site is the external granular layer of the cerebellar cortex, where mitoses persist until 1 year of age. Postnatal regeneration of these neurons after most are destroyed by irradiation or cytotoxic drugs is demonstrated in animals and may occur in humans as well. Primary olfactory receptor neurons also retain a potential for regeneration. In fact, if a constant turnover of these neurons did not occur throughout life, the individual would become anosmic after a few upper respiratory infections, which transiently denude the intranasal epithelium.

Disorders of Neuronogenesis

Destructive processes may destroy so many neuroblasts that regeneration of the full complement of cells is impossible. This happens when the insult persists for a long time or is repetitive, destroying each subsequent generation of dividing cells. Inadequate mitotic proliferation of neuroblasts results in hypoplasia of the brain (Figure 66.1). Such brains are small and grossly malformed because neuroblast migration is affected directly or by destruction of the glial cells with radial processes that guide migrating nerve cells. The entire brain may be affected, or portions may be selectively involved. Cerebellar hypoplasia is often a selective interference with proliferation of the external granular layer. In some cases, cerebral hypoplasia and microcephaly are the result of precocious development of the ependyma before all mitotic cycles of the neuroepithelium are complete because ependymal differentiation arrests mitotic activity at the ventricular surface. The mutation of a gene that programs neuronogenesis may be another explanation for generating insufficient neuroepithelial cells, although this pathogenesis remains hypothetical in humans.

Programmed Cell Death (Apoptosis)

Excessive neuroblasts are formed in every part of the nervous system by normal mitotic proliferation. This abundance is reduced by a programmed process of cell death until the definitive number of immature neurons is achieved. The factors that arrest the process of programmed cell death in the fetus are multiple and are in part genetically determined. Cells that do not match with targets are more vulnerable to degeneration than are those that achieve synaptic contact with other cells. Endocrine hormones and neuropeptides modulate apoptosis. Some homeotic genes, such as c-*fos*, are important in the regulation of programmed cell death in the nervous system, and other suppressor genes stop the expression of apoptotic genes.

Two phases of apoptosis are distinguished. One involves yet undifferentiated neuroepithelial cells or neuroblasts with incomplete differentiation; another phase involves fully differentiated neurons of the fetal brain.

Disorders of Programmed Cell Death

Spinal muscular atrophy (see Chapter 78) is an example of a human disease caused by programmed cell death not stopping at the proper time. In this disorder, continued loss of spinal motor neurons after all surplus embryonic neuroblasts are deleted is expressed as a progressive denervating process. Genetic factors are crucial in determining the arrest of cell death, which accounts for the hereditary character of spinal muscular atrophy. The *SMN* defective gene at the 5q13.1 locus has now been isolated and is normally responsible for arresting apoptosis in motor neuroblasts.

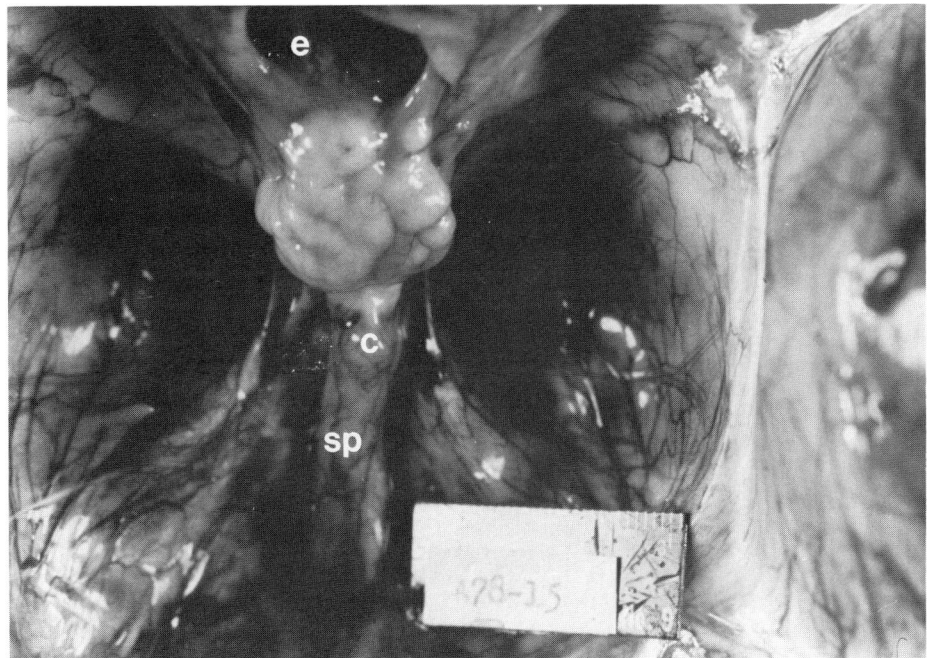

FIGURE 66.1   Severe cerebral hypoplasia. The brain of this term neonate weighed only 12.6 g (normal mean is 350 g), although the cranium was closed and mainly filled with fluid. The dysplastic architecture of the telencephalon, including dysplastic cerebellar tissue, extended into a frontal encephalocele (e) and was not that of a neural tube defect or fetal infarction. The spinal cord (sp) is well formed except for the absence of descending tracts. The cerebellum (c) is small but normally laminated. This brain probably represents lack of neuronal proliferation. Note the well-formed fossae at the base of the skull, despite the absence of cerebral development. (Reproduced with permission from HB Sarnat, DE de Mello, JD Blair, et al. Heterotopic growth of dysplastic cerebellum in frontal encephalocele in an infant of a diabetic mother. Can J Neurol Sci 1982;9:31–35.)

Other neurodegenerative diseases of fetal life and infancy are more widespread within the central nervous system (CNS) rather than limited to one type of neuron, such as the motor neuron. They also are characterized by progressive neuronal loss that is apoptotic rather than necrotic in character: There is no inflammatory or glial reaction and the features of the DNA degradation differ from ischemic necrosis. An example is pontocerebellar hypoplasia, a group of progressive degenerative diseases that begin prenatally and continue postnatally. Despite the name, they involve much more than the cerebellar system. These diseases are associated with extensive cerebral cortical and basal ganglionic abnormalities, even in motor neurons, which causes a clinical presentation at birth resembling spinal muscular atrophy (Barth 1993). This autosomal recessive group of diseases, all genetically distinct from olivopontocerebellar atrophy, exemplifies a semantic difficulty: If an atrophic process begins before development is complete, it results in both hypoplasia and superimposed atrophy.

In the CNS, glial cells also undergo programmed cell death. Glial necrosis is intimately linked to the interhemispheric passage of commissural fibers in the corpus callosum. In a murine model of callosal agenesis, glial cells that do not degenerate act as a barrier to crossing axons and prevent the corpus callosum from forming.

Neuroblast Migration

No neurons of the mature human brain occupy the site in which they were generated from the neuroepithelium. They migrate to their mature site to establish the proper synaptic connections with appropriate neighboring neurons and to send their axons in short or long trajectories to targets. The subependymal germinal matrix (Figure 66.2) is the subventricular zone of the embryonic concentric layers and consists of postmitotic, premigratory neuroblasts and glioblasts. In general, the movement of maturing nerve cells is centrifugal, radiating toward the surface of the brain. The cerebellar cortex is exceptional in that external granule cells first spread over the surface of the cerebellum and then migrate into the folia. Migration of neuroblasts begins at about 6 weeks' gestation in the human cerebrum and is not completed until at least 34 weeks of fetal life, although the majority of germinal matrix cells after midgestation are glioblasts. Glioblasts continue to migrate until early in the postnatal period. Within the brainstem, neuronal migration is complete by 2 months' gestation. Cerebellar external granule cells continue migrating throughout the first year of life.

Neuroblast migration permits a three-dimensional spatial relation to develop between neurons, which facilitates the formation of complex synaptic circuits. The timing and

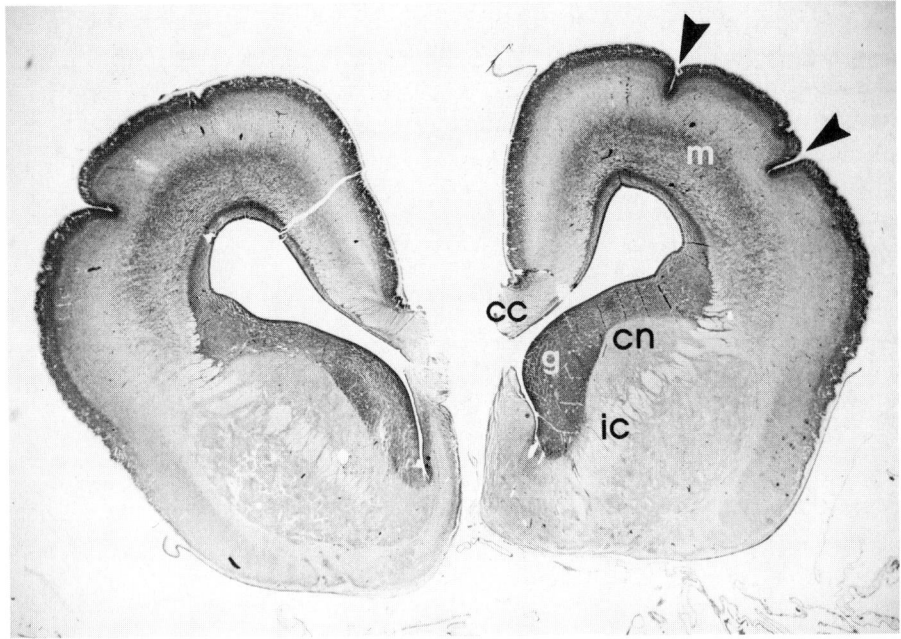

FIGURE 66.2 Coronal section of forebrain of 16-week normal fetus, showing extensive subependymal germinal matrix (g) of neuroblasts and glial precursors that have not yet migrated. The surface of the brain is just beginning to develop sulci (*arrowheads*). Migrating neuroblasts (m) are seen in the subcortical white matter. The corpus callosum (cc) is artifactually ruptured and the two hemispheres should be closely approximated. (cn = caudate nucleus; ic = anterior limb of internal capsule.) (Hematoxylin-eosin stain.)

sequence of successive waves of migrating neuroblasts are precise. In the cerebral cortex, immature nerve cells reach the pial surface and then form deeper layers as more recent arrivals replace their position at the surface. Neurons forming the most superficial layers of neocortex are thus the last to have migrated, although in the three-layered hippocampus, the most superficial neurons represent the earliest migratory wave.

The laminated arrangement of the mammalian cerebral cortex requires a large cortical surface area to accommodate increasing numbers of migrating neuroblasts and glioblasts. Convolutions provide this large surface area without incurring a concomitant increase in cerebral volume. The formation of gyri and sulci is thus a direct result of migration (Figure 66.3). Most gyri form in the second half of gestation, which is a period of predominant gliogenesis and glial cell migration. Therefore, the proliferation of glia in the cortex and subcortical white matter may be more important than neuroblast migrations in the formation of convolutions, but the growth of dendrites and synaptogenesis also may influence gyration by contributing mass to the neuropil. The timing and sequence of gyral formation in the human brain are as predictable as other aspects of cerebral maturation. The gestational age of a premature infant may be determined to within a 2-week period or less from the convolutional pattern of the brain at autopsy.

The Major Mechanism of Neuroblast Migration: Radial Glial Fiber Guides. The genetically determined programming of neuroblast migration begins when cells are still undifferentiated neuroepithelial cells and even before all their mitotic cycles are complete. Neuroepithelial cells express the gene products of *LIS1*, as do ependymal cells

and Cajal-Retzius cells of the molecular layer of cerebral cortex. This gene is defective in type 1 lissencephaly (Miller-Dieker syndrome), a severe disorder of neuroblast migration (Clark et al. 1997; Dobyns et al. 1993). How it functions in migration is not fully understood. Most neurons of the forebrain are guided to their predetermined site from the germinal matrix (embryonic subventricular zone) by long, radiating fibers of specialized fetal astrocytes (Figure 66.4). The entire wall of the fetal cerebral hemisphere is spanned by the elongated processes of these glial cells, whose cell bodies are in the periventricular region and terminate as end-feet on the limiting pial membrane at the surface of the brain (see Figure 66.4). Radial glial cells are the first astroglial cells of the human nervous system to be distinguished, as early as 6 weeks' gestation. On completion of neuroblast and glioblast migration, their radial fiber retracts and the cell is converted into a mature fibrillary astrocyte of the subcortical white matter; some are still present at birth. Mature astrocytes are present throughout the CNS by 15 weeks' gestation, and gliogenesis continues throughout fetal and postnatal life. Several types of glial cells are recognized between 20 and 36 weeks' gestation.

The mechanical process of neuroblasts gliding along a radial glial fiber is facilitated by a number of specialized proteins, such as astrotactin, that are secreted by the neuroblast itself (Zheng et al. 1996). The glial cell (e.g., L1 neural cell adhesion molecules [Jouet and Kenwrick 1995]), and other adhesion molecules (Herman et al. 1993) also facilitate gliding. Ependymal cells may do the same through their radiating processes, which resemble those of the radial glial cell but do not extend beyond the germinal matrix and molecules in the extracellular matrix. Some adhesion molecules are present in the extracellular

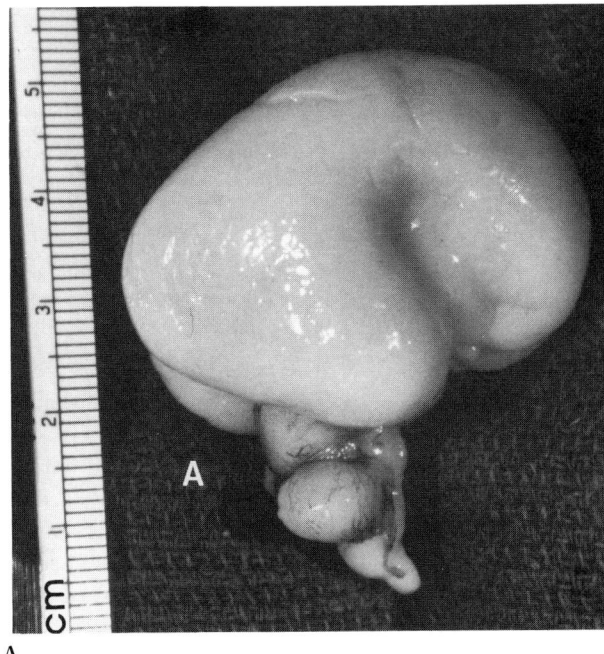

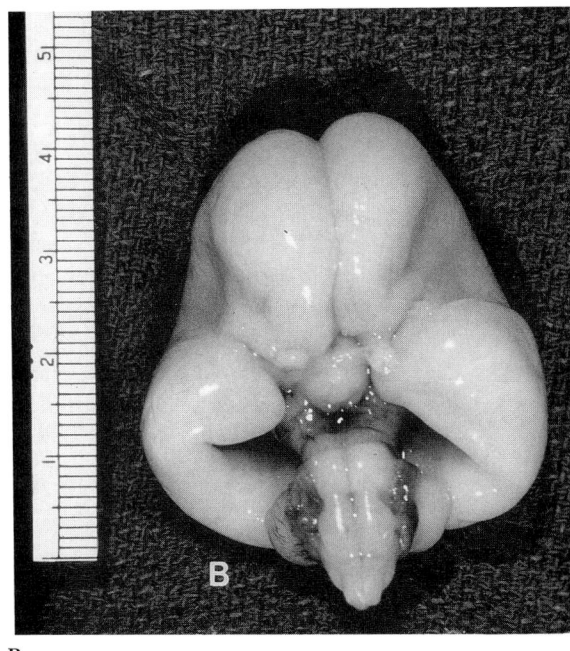

A   **B**

FIGURE 66.3 Lateral (**A**) and ventral (**B**) views of a normal brain of a 16-week fetus. The primary sulci, such as the sylvian fissure, calcarine fissure, and central sulcus, are forming, but secondary and tertiary sulci and gyri are not yet developed, and the surface of the brain is smooth.

FIGURE 66.4 Radial glial fibers extending from subependymal region (*right*) toward cerebral cortex (*left*), guiding migrating neuroblasts in a 16-week fetus. (Glial fibrillary acidic protein reaction; bar = 10 μm.)

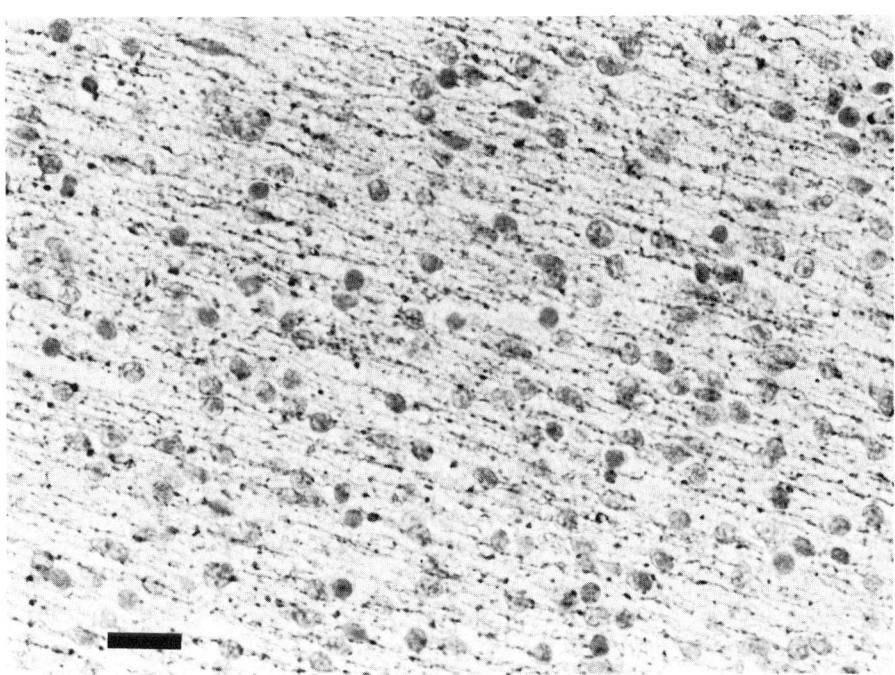

matrix (Thomas et al. 1996). These molecules serve as lubricants, as adhesion molecules between the membranes of the neuroblast and the radial glial fiber, and as nutritive and growth factors. They stimulate cell movement by a mechanism still poorly understood. Deficient molecules lead to defective migration. For example, the L1 adhesion molecule is the defective genetic program in X-linked hydrocephalus accompanied by polymicrogyria and pachygyria (Jouet and Kenwrick 1995).

The process of transformation of radial glial cells into astrocytes and ependymal cells begins during the first half of gestation and is completed postnatally. During midgestation, when neuronal migration is at a peak, many radial glial cells remain attached to the ventricular and pial surfaces, increasing in length and curving with the expansion and convolution of the cerebral wall. From 28 weeks' gestation to 6 years of age, astrocytes of the frontal lobe shift from the periventricular to the subcortical region. The centrifugal movement of this band of normal gliosis marks the end of neuronal migration in the cerebral mantle. Ependyma does not completely line the lateral ventricles until 22 weeks' gestation.

In addition to the radial migration to the cerebral cortex, tangential migration also occurs, but the number of neuroblasts is far smaller (O'Rourke et al. 1995; Rakic 1995). These migrations perpendicular to the radial fibers probably use axons rather than glial processes as guides for migratory neuroblasts, which explains why all cells in a given region of cortex are not from the same clone or vertical column. Tangential migrations occur in the brainstem and olfactory bulb as well as in the cerebrum. The subpial region is another site of neuroblast migration that does not use radial glial cells.

Disorders of Neuroblast Migration. Nearly all malformations of the brain are a direct result of faulty neuroblast migration or at least involve a secondary impairment of migration. Imperfect cortical lamination, abnormal gyral development, subcortical heterotopia, and other focal dysplasias are related to some factor that interferes with neuronal migration, whether vascular, traumatic, metabolic, or infectious. The most severe migrational defects occur in early gestation, often associated with events in the gross formation of the neural tube and cerebral vesicles. Heterotopia of brainstem nuclei also occurs. Later defects of migration are expressed as disorders of cortical lamination or gyration, such as lissencephaly, pachygyria, and cerebellar dysplasias. These insults of the third trimester of gestation cause more subtle or focal abnormalities of cerebral architecture.

Lissencephaly is a condition of a smooth cerebral cortex without convolutions. At midgestation, the brain is essentially smooth; only the interhemispheric, sylvian, and calcarine fissures are formed. Gyri and sulci develop between 20 and 36 weeks' gestation, and the mature pattern of gyration is evident at term, although some parts of the cerebral cortex, such as the frontal lobes, are still relatively small. In lissencephaly type 1 (Miller-Dieker syndrome), the cerebral cortex remains smooth (Figure 66.5) or has a shallow "cobblestone" appearance not evident on imaging. The histopathological pattern is that of a four-layer cortex in which the outermost layer (1) is the molecular layer, as in normal six-layered neocortex. Layer 2 corresponds to layers 2 through 6 of normal neocortex, layer 3 is cell-sparse as a persistent fetal subplate zone, and layer 4 consists of incompletely migrated neurons in the subcortical intermediate zone. In lissencephaly type 2 (Walker-Warburg syndrome), poorly laminated cortex with disorganized and disoriented neurons is seen histologically, and the gross appearance of the cerebrum is one of a smooth brain or a few poorly formed sulci (Figure 66.6). The cerebral mantle may be thin, suggesting a disturbance of cell proliferation as well as of neuroblast migration. Malformations of the

brainstem and cerebellum often are present as well (see Figure 66.6). Lissencephaly of type 1 and type 2 (Walker-Warburg syndrome, Fukuyama type muscular dystrophy, muscle-eye-brain syndrome of Santavuori) are genetic diseases, but lissencephaly also may occur secondary to nongenetic disturbances of neuroepithelial proliferation or neuroblast migration, including destructive encephaloclastic processes, such as congenital infections during fetal life.

Other abnormal patterns of gross gyration of the cerebral cortex also occur secondary to neuroblast migratory disorders (Norman et al. 1995). *Pachygyria* signifies abnormally large, poorly formed gyri and may be present in some regions of cerebral cortex with lissencephaly in other regions (see Figure 66.6). *Polymicrogyria* refers to excessively numerous and abnormally small gyri that similarly may coexist with pachygyria; it does not necessarily denote a primary migratory disorder of genetic origin. Small, poorly formed gyri may occur in zones of fetal ischemia, and they regularly surround porencephalic cysts due to middle cerebral artery occlusion in fetal life. Schizencephaly is a unilateral or bilateral deep cleft in the general position of the sylvian fissure but is not a sylvian fissure: This cleft is the full thickness of the hemispheric wall, and no cerebral tissue remains between the meninges and the lateral ventricle (the pial-ependymal seam). If the cerebral cortical walls on either side of the deep cleft are in contact, the condition is called *closed lips*, and if a wide subarachnoid space separates the two walls, it is known as *open lips*, but these two variants do not provide a clue to pathogenesis. Schizencephaly occurs both as a genetic trait (the defective gene is *EMX2*) and sporadically; in some cases, it is a form of porencephaly due to fetal cerebral infarction.

In the cerebral hemisphere, most germinal matrix cells become neurons during the first half of gestation, and most form glia during the second half of gestation. Nonetheless, a small number of germinal matrix cells are neuronal precursors, migrating into the cerebral cortex in late gestation. Because the migration of the external granular layer in the cerebellar cortex is not completed until 1 year of age, a potential for acquired insults to interfere with late migrations persists throughout the perinatal period. Anatomical lesions, such as periventricular leukomalacia, intracerebral hemorrhages and abscesses, hydrocephalus, and traumatic injuries, may disrupt the delicate radial glial guide fibers and prevent normal migration, even though the migrating cell itself may escape the focal destructive lesion.

Damaged radial glial cells tend to retract their processes from the pial surface. The migrating neuron travels only as far as its retracted glial fibers carry it. If this fiber is retracted into the subcortical white matter, the neuroblast stops there and matures, becoming an isolated heterotopic nodule composed of several nerve cells that were migrating at the same time in the same place. In these nodules, neurons of various cortical types differentiate without laminar organization and with haphazard orientations of their processes, but a few extrinsic axons may prevent total synaptic isolation of the nodule.

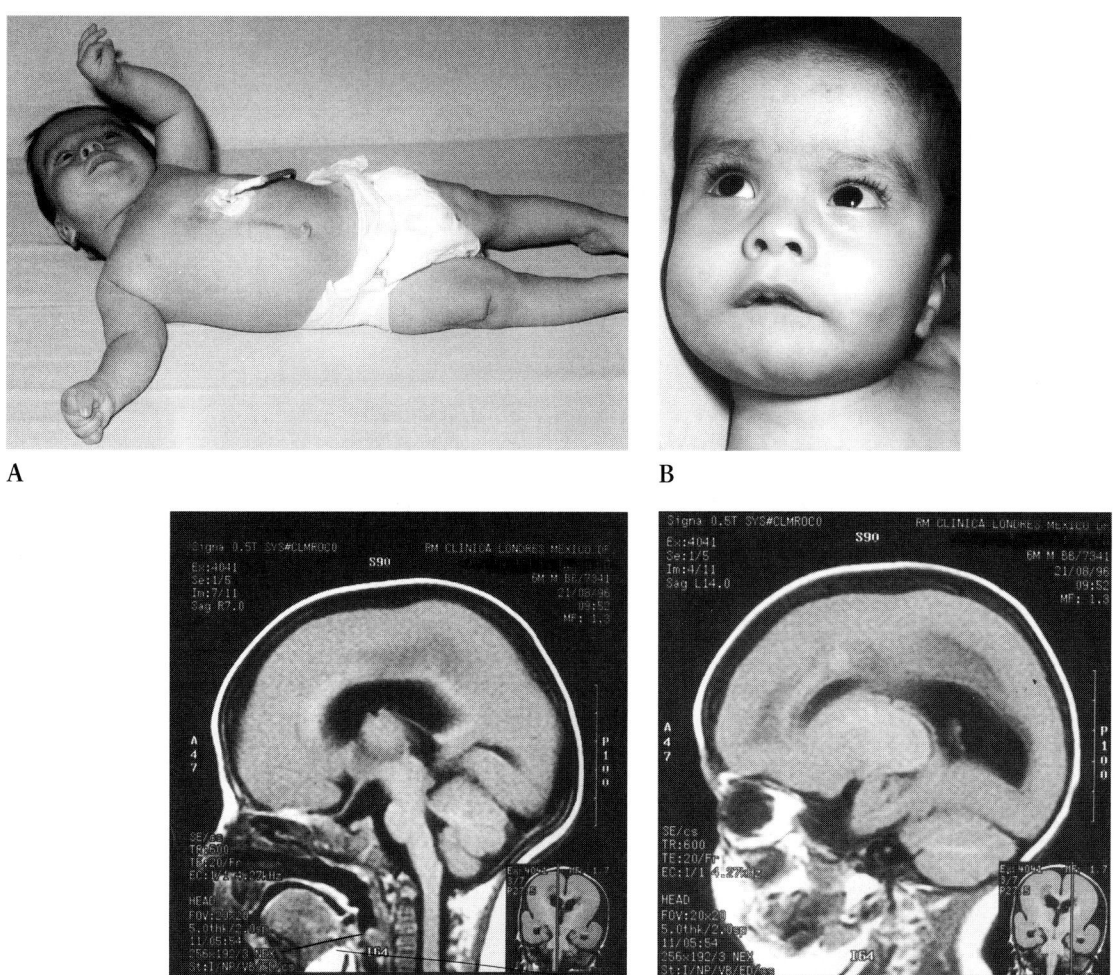

A   B

C   D

FIGURE 66.5 (**A**) This 7-month-old boy has Miller-Dieker syndrome. He has unusual postures of the extremities and opisthotonus, which are not seen in all patients with this genetic disorder. Note the gastrostomy that he required. (**B**) He has the typical facies of this genetic syndrome, with a high brow, upturned nares, and long philtrum (upper lip). His gaze is dysconjugate, but there is no paresis of extraocular muscles. (**C**) Sagittal and (**D**) parasagittal views of T1-weighted magnetic resonance images, showing type 1 lissencephaly with only mild ventriculomegaly. The cerebellum and brainstem, including the basis pontis, are grossly well formed. The corpus callosum is very thin. Extra-axial (i.e., subarachnoid) spaces are wide over the convexities of the cerebral hemispheres and in the cisterns surrounding the brainstem.

Interference with the glial guide fibers in the cerebral cortex itself results in neurons either not reaching the pial surface or not being able to reverse direction and then descending to a deeper layer. The consequence is imperfect cortical lamination, which interferes with the development of synaptic circuits. These disturbances of late neuroblast migration do not produce the gross malformations of early gestation and may not be detected by imaging techniques. They may account for many neurological sequelae after the perinatal period, including seizures, perceptual disorders, impaired coordination of gross or fine motor function, learning disabilities, and mental retardation.

In sum, disorders of neuroblast migration may be due either to defective genetic programming or may be acquired secondary to lesions in the fetal brain that destroy or interrupt radial glial fibers. Cells may not migrate at all and become mature neurons in the periventricular region, as occurs in X-linked periventricular nodular heterotopia (Eksioglu et al. 1996) and in some cases of congenital cytomegalovirus infection. Cells may become arrested along their course as heterotopic neurons in deep subcortical white matter, as occurs in many genetic syndromes of lissencephaly-pachygyria and in many metabolic diseases, including cerebrohepatorenal syndrome of Zellweger and in many aminoacidurias and organic acidurias. The same aberration may occur in acquired insults to the radial glial cell during ontogenesis (Norman et al. 1995). Cells may overmigrate, beyond the limits of the pial membrane into the meninges as ectopic neurons, either singly or in clusters known as *marginal glioneuronal heterotopia* or *brain warts*. Rarely, herniation of the germinal matrix into the lateral ventricle may

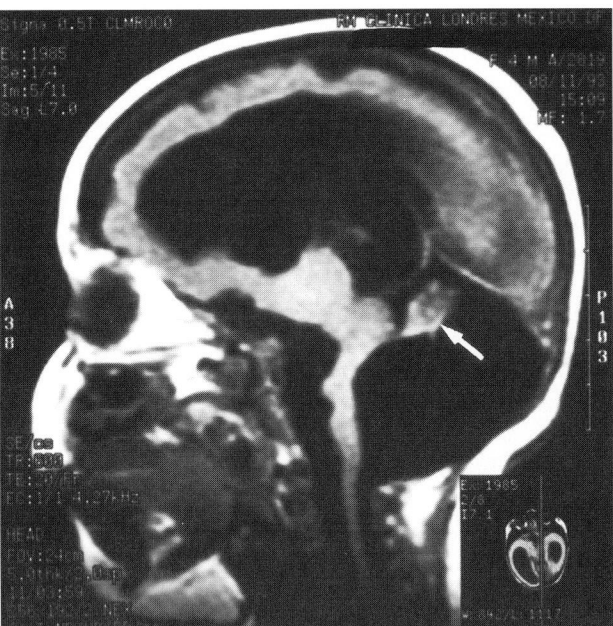

FIGURE 66.6 Sagittal T1-weighted magnetic resonance image of a 10-month-old girl with lissencephaly type 2 and Dandy-Walker malformation. The cerebral mantle is thin, and the lateral ventricle is greatly enlarged. A few abnormal shallow fissures at the cerebral surface may indicate abortive gyration or pachygyria. The cerebellum is severely hypoplastic (*arrow* indicates anterior vermis), and the posterior fossa contains a large, fluid-filled cyst. The brainstem also is hypoplastic, and the basis pontis is nearly absent. A differential diagnosis of this image is pontocerebellar hypoplasia, but the high position of the torcula indicates a Dandy-Walker malformation.

occur through gaps in the ependyma; those cells mature as neurons, forming a non-neoplastic intraventricular mass that may or may not obstruct cerebrospinal fluid (CSF) flow (Flores et al. 1998). Whether disoriented radial glial fibers actually guide neuroblasts to an intraventricular site or are physically pushed into a direction of less resistance is uncertain.

Growth of Axons and Dendrites

During the course of neuroblast migration, neurons remain largely undifferentiated cells, and the embryonic cerebral cortex at midgestation consists of vertical columns of tightly packed cells between radial blood vessels and extensive extracellular spaces. Cytodifferentiation begins with a proliferation of organelles, mainly endoplasmic reticulum and mitochondria in the cytoplasm, and clumping of condensed nuclear chromatin at the inner margin of the nuclear membrane. Rough endoplasmic reticulum becomes swollen, and ribosomes proliferate.

The outgrowth of the axon always precedes the development of dendrites, and the axon forms connections before the differentiation of dendrites begins. The projection of the axon toward its destination was first recognized by Ramón

y Cajal, who named this growing process the *cone d'accroissement* (growth cone). The tropic factors that guide the growth cone to its specific terminal synapse, whether chemical, endocrine, or electrotaxic, have been a focus of controversy for many years. However, it is now well demonstrated that growth cones are guided during their long trajectories by diffusible molecules secreted along their pathway by the processes of fetal ependymal cells and perhaps some glial cells. Some molecules, such as brain-derived neurotrophic growth factor and S-100 protein, attract growing axons, whereas others, such as the glycosaminoglycan *keratan sulfate* (not to be confused with the protein *keratin*), strongly repel them and thus prevent aberrant decussations and other deviations. Matrix proteins, such as laminin and fibronectin, also provide a substrate for axonal guidance. Cell-to-cell attractions operate as the axon approaches its final target. Despite the long delay between the migration of an immature nerve cell and the beginning of dendritic growth, the branching of dendrites eventually accounts for more than 90% of the synaptic surface of the mature neuron. The pattern of dendritic ramification is specific for each type of neuron. Spines form on the dendrites as short protrusions with expanded tips, providing sites of synaptic membrane differentiation.

The Golgi method of impregnation of neurons and their processes with heavy metals, such as silver or mercury, has been used for more than a century and continues to be one of the most useful methods for demonstrating dendritic arborizations. Among the many contributions of this technique to the study of the nervous system, beginning with the elegant pioneering work of Ramón y Cajal, none has surpassed its demonstration of the sequence of normal dendritic branching in the human fetus. Newer immunocytochemical techniques for demonstrating dendrites also are now available, such as microtubule-associated protein 2. These techniques may be applied to human tissue resected surgically, as in the surgical treatment of epilepsy, and the tissue secured at autopsy.

Disorders of Neurite Growth

If a neuron becomes disoriented during migration and faces the wrong direction in its final site, its axon is capable of reorienting itself as much as 180 degrees after emerging from the neuronal cell body. Dendrites, by contrast, conform strictly to the orientation of the cell body and do not change their axis. The dendritic tree becomes stunted if axodendritic synapses are not established.

Because so much dendritic differentiation and growth occurs during the last third of gestation and the first months of the postnatal period, the preterm infant is particularly vulnerable to noxious influences that interfere with maturation of dendrites. Extraordinarily long dendrites of dentate granule cells and prominent basal dendrites of pyramidal cells have been described in term infants on life-support systems. Retardation of neuronal maturation in terms of dendrite development and spine morphology has been described in premature infants, compared with term infants of the same conceptional age, possibly as a result of asphyxia. Infants with fetal alcohol syndrome also have a reduced number and abnormal geometry of dendritic spines of cortical neurons.

Traditional histological examination of the brains of mentally retarded children often shows remarkably few alterations to account for a profound intellectual deficit. The study of dendritic morphology by the Golgi technique has revealed striking abnormalities in some of these cases. The alterations are best documented in chromosomal diseases, such as trisomy 13 and Down syndrome. Long, thin, tortuous dendritic spines and the absence of small, stubby spines are a common finding. Children with unclassified mental retardation but normal chromosome numbers and morphology also show defects in the number, length, and spatial arrangement of dendrites and synapses.

Abnormalities of cerebellar Purkinje's cell dendrites occur in cerebellar dysplasias and hypoplasias. They consist of cactuslike thickenings and loss of branchlet spines. Abnormal development of the dendritic tree is also a common finding in many metabolic encephalopathies, including Krabbe's disease and other leukodystrophies, Menkes' kinky hair disease, gangliosidoses, ceroid lipofuscinosis, and Sanfilippo's syndrome. Among genetically determined cerebral dysgeneses, aberrations in the structure and number of dendrites and spines are reported in cerebrohepatorenal (Zellweger) syndrome and in tuberous sclerosis.

Electrical Polarity of the Cell Membrane

The development of membrane excitability is one of the important markers of neuronal maturation, but little is known about the exact timing and duration of this development. Membrane polarity is established before synaptogenesis and before the synthesis of neurotransmitters begins. Because the maintenance of a resting membrane potential requires considerable energy expenditure to fuel the sodium-potassium pump, the undifferentiated neuroblast would be incapable of maintaining such a dynamic condition as a resting membrane potential. The development of ion channels within the neural membrane is another important factor in the maturation of excitable membranes and the maintenance of resting membrane potentials.

Disorders of Membrane Polarity

Epileptic phenomena are largely due to inappropriate membrane depolarizations. They represent a complex interaction of excitatory and inhibitory synapses that modulate the resting membrane potential, metabolic alterations, and many unknown factors that also contribute to the discharge threshold of neural membranes. Cerebral malformations are often associated with seizures because of abnormal synaptic circuitry, and the role of abnormal resting membrane potentials in development is largely speculative at this time. Electrolyte imbalances in the serum certainly influence the depolarization threshold, and hypothalamic disturbances may alter endocrine function and electrolyte balance.

Synaptogenesis

Synapse formation follows the development of dendritic spines and the polarization of the cell membrane. The relation of synaptogenesis to neuroblast migration differs in different parts of the nervous system. In the cerebral cortex, synaptogenesis always follows neuroblast migration. In the cerebellar cortex, however, the external granule cells develop axonal processes that become the long parallel fibers of the molecular layer and make synaptic contact with Purkinje's cell dendrites before migrating through the molecular and Purkinje's cell layer to their mature internal position within the folium.

Afferent nerve fibers reach the neocortex early, before lamination occurs in the cortical plate. The first synapses are axodendritic and occur both external to and beneath the cortical plate in the future layers I and VI, which contain the first neurons that have migrated.

An excessive number of synapses form on each neuron, with subsequent elimination of those that are not required. Outside the CNS, muscle fibers also begin their relation with the nervous system by receiving multiple sources of innervation, later retaining only one. Transitory synapses also form at sites on neurons where they are not found in the mature condition. The spinal motor neurons of newborn kittens display prominent synapses on their initial axonal segment, where they are never found in adult cats. Somatic spines are an important synaptic site on the embryonic Purkinje's cell, but these spines and their synapses disappear as the dendritic tree develops.

A structure-function correlation may be made in the developing visual cortex. In preterm infants of 24–25 weeks' gestation, the visual evoked potentials (VEPs) recorded at the occiput exhibit an initial long-latency negativity, but by 28 weeks' gestation, a small positive wave precedes this negativity. The change in this initial component of the VEP corresponds to dendritic arborization, and the formation of dendritic spines that occurs at that time.

The electroencephalogram (EEG) of the premature infant follows a predictable and time-linked progression in maturation that has been extensively studied. The EEG reflects synaptogenesis more closely than any other feature of cerebral maturation and thereby provides a noninvasive and clinically useful measure of neurological maturation in the preterm infant. Fetal EEG may even detect neurological disease and seizures in utero.

Disorders of Synaptogenesis

Because the formation of dendritic spines and the formation of synapses are so closely related, the same spectrum of diseases already discussed is equally appropriate for consideration in this section. The rate of maturation of the EEG is often slow in preterm infants, who are generally unwell, even if they do not have specific neurological disease, which may reflect an impairment of synapse formation. Chronic hypoxemia particularly delays neurological maturation.

Biosynthesis of Neurotransmitters

The synthesis of neurotransmitters and neuromodulating chemicals is based on the secretory character of the neuron, without which synaptic transmission is impossible. Several types of substances serve as transmitters: (1) acetylcholine (ACh); (2) monoamines, including dopamine, norepinephrine, epinephrine, and serotonin; (3) neuropeptides, including substance P, somatostatin, and opioid-containing peptide chains, such as the enkephalins; and (4) simple amino acids, including glutamic acid, aspartic acid, γ-aminobutyric acid (GABA), and glycine. Some transmitters are characteristically inhibitory (such as glycine, GABA, and ACh in the CNS). Each neuronal type produces a characteristic transmitter (motor neurons produce ACh, cerebellar Purkinje's cells produce GABA, and granule cells produce glutamic acid in the adult). Neuropeptides may coexist with other types of transmitters in some neurons.

In some parts of the brain, transitory fetal transmitters may appear during development and then disappear. Substance P and somatostatin are present in the fetal cerebellum at midgestation, but these neuropeptides are never found in the mature cerebellum. In the cerebral cortex of the frontal lobe, there is laminar distribution of cholinergic muscarinic receptors of the mature brain that is the inverse of the pattern in the fetus. The functions of these transitory transmitter systems are unknown. Some serve as trophic molecules rather than transmitters in early development. Even amino acid transmitters, such as GABA, may serve mainly a trophic function at an early stage in development. In situ hybridization and new immunocytochemical techniques demonstrate neurotransmitters in neurons of the developing brain of experimental animals and may be applied to human tissue under some circumstances (Dupuy and Houser 1997).

Disorders of Neurotransmitter Synthesis

Ischemic and hypoxic insults impair RNA transcription and result in arrest of the synthesis of secretory products. Many of the clinical neurological deficits observed in neonates who underwent birth asphyxia are probably the result of neurotransmitter depletion and functional synaptic block. Some amino acid neurotransmitters, by contrast, are neurotoxic when released in large quantities. The excitatory amino acids glutamic acid and aspartic acid induce transsynaptic degeneration when released in this way, as might occur with hypoxic stresses, and may be a major source of irreversible brain damage in asphyxiated neonates.

Developmental disorders due to inborn errors of metabolism that block the chemical pathway of transmitter synthesis may hypothetically occur but are probably incompatible with survival if they interfere with the synthesis of a major transmitter, such as ACh, monoamines, or an essential peptide. Defects in the metabolic pathways of particular amino acids are known, and many of these are associated with mental retardation, epilepsy, spastic diplegia, and other chronic neurological handicaps. Phenylketonuria (a disorder of phenylalanine metabolism) and maple syrup urine disease (a disorder of the metabolism of the branched-chain amino acids leucine, isoleucine, and valine) are well-documented examples. However, it is not certain whether absence of the product of the deficient enzyme or toxicity of high levels of precursors upstream from the enzyme deficiency is the principal insult to the nervous system.

Myelination

Myelin insulates individual axons and provides greatly increased speed of conduction. It is not essential in all nerves, and many autonomic fibers of the peripheral nervous system remain unmyelinated throughout life. Conduction velocity in central pathways is important in coordinating time-related impulses from different centers that converge on a distant target and in ensuring that action potentials are not lost by synaptic block. The nervous system functions on the basis of temporal summation of impulses to relay messages across synapses.

Myelination of pathways in the CNS occurs in a predictable spatial and temporal sequence. Some tracts myelinate as early as 14 weeks' gestation and complete their myelination cycle in a few weeks. Examples include the spinal roots, medial longitudinal fasciculus, dorsal columns of the spinal cord, and most cranial nerves. Between 22 and 24 weeks' gestation, myelination progresses in the olivary and cerebellar connections, the ansa lenticularis of the globus pallidus, the sensory trigeminal nerve, the auditory pathways, and the acoustic nerve as well as the trapezoid body, lateral lemniscus, and brachium of the inferior colliculus. By contrast, the optic nerve and the geniculocalcarine tract (i.e., optic radiations) do not begin to acquire myelin until near term.

Some pathways are late in myelinating and have myelination cycles that are measured in years. The corpus callosum begins myelinating at 4 months postnatally and is not complete until midadolescence. Some ipsilateral association fibers connecting the frontal with the temporal and parietal lobes do not achieve full myelination until about 32 years of age.

Myelination can now be accurately measured in specific central pathways of the living patient by using T2-weighted magnetic resonance imaging sequences, but the time at which myelination can be detected is somewhat later than with traditional myelin stains of brain tissue sections, such as Luxol fast blue. Newer neuropathological methods, using gallo-cyanin and immunoreactivity to myelin basic protein, may detect myelination even earlier than the traditional strains. Electron microscopy remains the most sensitive method of demonstrating the earliest myelination in tissue sections.

Disorders of Myelination

Many metabolic diseases impede the rate of myelination. Hypothyroidism is a classic example. Menkes' kinky hair disease, a disorder of copper absorption and metabolism, is another example. Many aminoacidurias, including phenylketonuria, are also associated with delayed myelination. Cerebrohepatorenal (Zellweger) syndrome is well documented with neuropathological findings that include disorders of neuroblast migration and of myelination. Some leukodystrophies, such as Krabbe's disease and perinatal sudanophilic leukodystrophy, are already expressed in fetal life with defective myelination.

Chronic hypoxia in premature infants is probably the most common cause of delayed myelination and contributes to the delay found in clinical neurological maturation. Myelination depends on fatty acids that must be supplied by the maternal and infant diet; nutritional deficiencies during gestation or in postnatal life may result in delayed myelination and are clinically expressed as developmental delay. Unlike disorders of neuronal migration, delay in myelination is not necessarily irreversible if the insult is removed; myelination may catch up to reach the appropriate level of maturity.

Transitory Cells of the Fetal Brain

Three types of cells are found in the human fetal brain but later disappear and are absent or perhaps unrecognized in the adult brain. These three neuroepithelial cell types are the primitive germinal matrix cell, which differentiates into neurons and glia, the Cajal-Retzius neuron, and the subpial granule (glial) cell of the cerebral cortex.

Cajal-Retzius cells are large, mature, stellate neurons in the marginal (outermost) zone of the fetal cerebral cortex. They are the first cells to appear at the surface of the embryonic cerebrum. Unlike other neurons that reach the surface, Cajal-Retzius cells do not reverse direction to enter deeper layers of the cortex as more migrating neurons arrive at the surface. The first afferent processes to enter the marginal layer are dendrites of pyramidal cells of layer VI, neurons also included in the first wave of neuronal migration. Synapses formed between Cajal-Retzius cells and pyramidal cells of layer VI form the first intrinsic cortical circuits (Marín-Padilla 1998).

Cajal-Retzius cells contain acetylcholinesterase and oxidative enzymes and secrete GABA and presumably ACh as neurotransmitters. Their long axons extend parallel to the surface of the brain, plunging short branches into layer II (Figure 66.7). The Cajal-Retzius neurons disappear

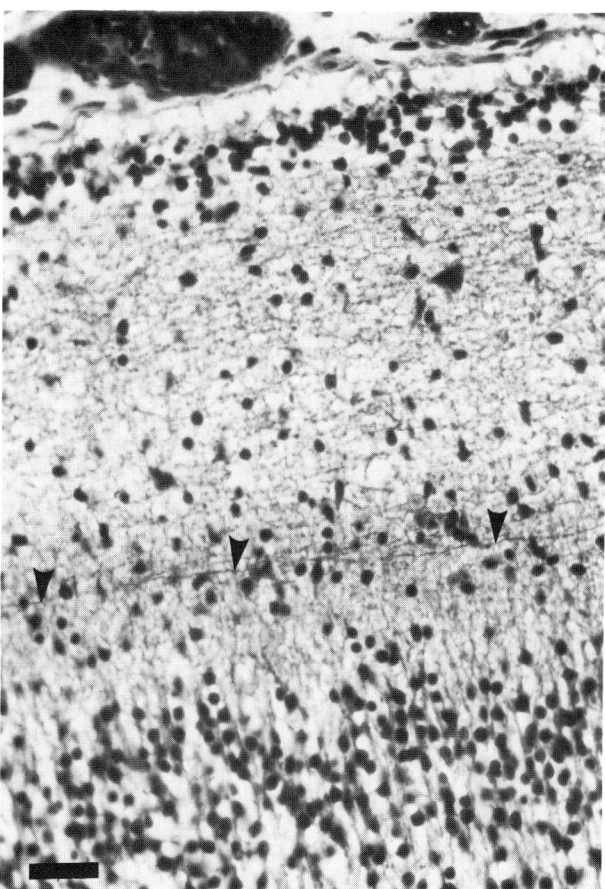

FIGURE 66.7   Silver stain of molecular layer of motor cortex in a 20-week fetus. The long fibers (*arrowheads*) extending parallel to the surface of the brain are axons of Cajal-Retzius neurons. They disappear with further cerebral maturation. (Bielschowsky's stain. Bar = 10 μm.)

shortly after birth, undergoing programmed cell death; a few horizontal cells of Cajal persist in layer I of the adult cerebral cortex, but these may account for only a small percentage of fetal Cajal-Retzius cells. However, a few clusters of Cajal-Retzius cells may persist in the entorhinal cortex of adults. Cajal-Retzius neurons strongly express the transcription product of the *LIS1* gene, which is defective in X-linked hydrocephalus associated with polymicrogyria and defective neuroblast migration. Hence, it is now believed that these fetal neurons play a role in neuroblast migration, although their precise function is not known (Clark et al. 1997). No other specific diseases involving Cajal-Retzius neurons are yet described.

The fetal cerebral cortex has a subpial or external granular layer that histologically resembles that of the cerebellum but are of quite a different character. Cells of the cerebral cortex rise in columns from the germinal matrix of the hippocampus to form a thin layer on the surface of the archicortex at 12 weeks' gestation. They rapidly spread over the neocortex in a predictable sequence to cover the entire convexity by the sixteenth to eighteenth week, with

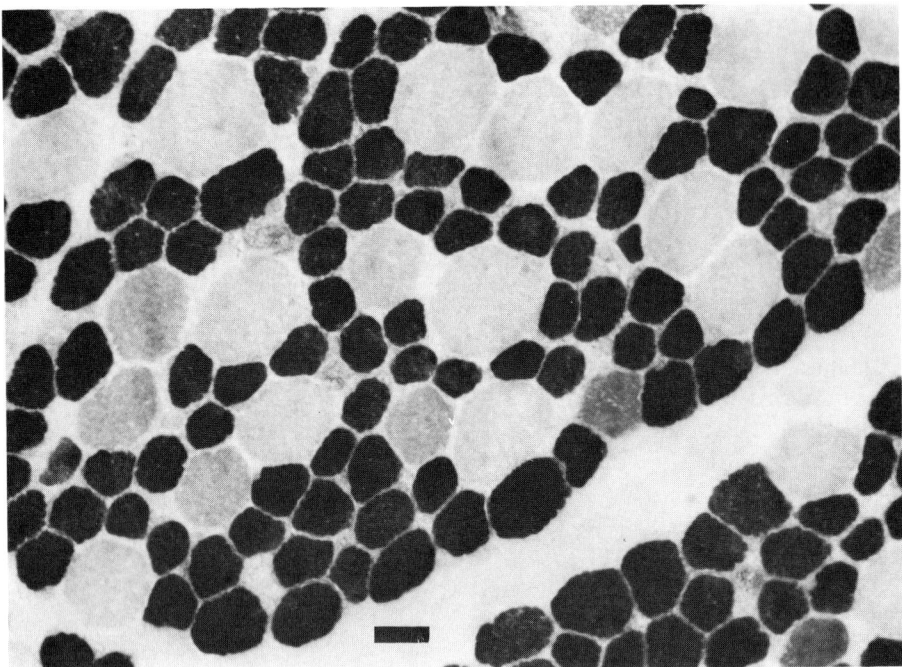

FIGURE 66.8 Histochemical type 2 myofiber numerical predominance and relative smallness of type 2 fibers. Type 1 fibers are stained lightly; type 2 fibers are dark. The small type 2 fibers do not show the angular contour characteristic of denervated muscle fibers or of those atrophic secondary to disuse. This muscle biopsy was taken from a 3-year-old boy with generalized hypotonia and cerebellar hypoplasia. (Myosin ATPase stain preincubated at pH 10.4. Bar = 15 μm.)

the layer reaching the greatest thickness by 22 weeks' gestation. Subsequent involution of the external granular layer results from migration of these cells into the cerebral cortex, where they can no longer be distinguished. Only remnants of this once-prominent layer persist at term, confined to the inferior temporal and orbital surfaces. These surfaces are the last sites from which they finally disappear from the neocortex, although a few may persist over the paleocortex even into adult life. Their fate within the cerebral cortex is unknown, but it is speculated that they mature into glial cells because they lack ultrastructural features of neurons, and they stain immunocytochemically for glial fibrillary acidic protein but not for vimentin.

The subpial granular layer of the cerebral hemispheres is partially or totally absent in most cases of holoprosencephaly, even at the gestational period when it is expected to be most prominent; this absence may contribute to the marginal glioneural heterotopia found in the meningeal spaces and superficial cortical layers. The layer of the subpial granule cells may serve as a barrier to reverse the direction of migration in neuroblasts reaching the surface. In the Fukuyama type of congenital muscular dystrophy associated with cerebral cortical dysplasia, a heterotopic layer of stellate glial cells forms at the surface of the cerebral cortex, into which migrating neurons accumulate as they reach the surface rather than reversing direction and entering deeper layers of the cortex.

Suprasegmental Influences on Muscle Maturation

The effects of denervation of fetal muscle are well defined morphologically and histochemically and differ in several ways from findings in mature muscle after denervation. These differences form the basis of the diagnoses of spinal muscular atrophy and perinatal neuropathy by muscle biopsy. The histochemical changes seen in striated muscle of infants with cerebral dysgenesis are not as well understood but are being better documented.

The motor unit is capable of developing normally in the absence of suprasegmental modification, as in infants with severe hypoplasias of the brain (see Figure 66.1). Malformations of the brainstem and cerebellar hypoplasia in particular are associated with a variety of aberrations in histochemical differentiation. These aberrations include (1) delayed maturation; (2) more than 80% predominance of type 1 or type 2 myofibers, with or without uniform hypoplasia of one or the other type (Figure 66.8); and (3) classic congenital muscle fiber-type disproportion. Malformations limited to the cerebral cortex do not cause fiber-type predominance. Muscle biopsy of children with cerebral palsy from birth asphyxia or other perinatal insults shows only nonspecific type 2 muscle fiber atrophy, with preservation of the normal rations of fiber types, similar to the changes that follow disuse or immobilization of muscle.

It is speculated that many of the small bulbospinal "subcorticospinal" tracts (i.e., vestibulospinal, reticulospinal, olivospinal, tectospinal, and rubrospinal) are more important than are the larger corticospinal tract during the stage of histochemical differentiation of muscle between 20 and 28 weeks' gestation. These small descending pathways are generally well myelinated and functional at that time, whereas the corticospinal tract does not even begin its myelination cycle or proliferation of axonal terminals until after muscle development is complete.

Etiology

The causes of cerebral malformations generally fall into one of two categories. The first category is genetic and chromosomal disease in which there is defective programming of cerebral development. This genetic category also includes many inborn metabolic diseases, in which cerebral dysgenesis may be due to biochemical insults during development rather than, or in addition to, primary errors in molecular genetic codes for neural programming. The second category includes all induced malformations in which a teratogenic influence acts at a particular time in ontogenesis; the malformation depends on the timing of the insult in relation to brain development at that moment. The timing may be brief, as with a single exposure to a toxic drug, a dose of radiation, or a traumatic injury of the fetal brain. It may be repeated two or more times or may be prolonged and involve the fetus at several stages of development. Examples of the latter include certain congenital infections, such as toxoplasmosis and cytomegalovirus disease, which may be active throughout most of gestation, even into the postnatal period. Genetic factors are the most frequent causes of malformations during the first half of gestation; environmental factors are more important in late gestation and may cause disturbances of late neuroblast migrations, particularly in premature infants. In some cases, no definite inductive factor is identified despite intensive clinical investigations during life and meticulous postmortem studies.

Ischemic Encephalopathy in the Fetus

Among the environmental factors that may interfere with the developmental process in utero or postnatally, either briefly or more chronically, none is more important as a cause of morbidity than ischemic or hypoxic encephalopathy. Circulatory insufficiency or hypoxemia may interfere with migrations by causing infarction, which interrupts glial guide fibers.

Ischemia also affects the fetal cerebrum by producing watershed infarcts between zones of arterial supply because of poorer collateral circulation compared with the mature brain. Thin-walled vessels radiate perpendicular to the surface of the brain. The precursors of these radial vessels originate from leptomeningeal arteries and are evident at 15 weeks' gestation in the human embryo; horizontal branches appear in deep cortical layers at 20 weeks' gestation and increase to supply the superficial cortex by 27 weeks' gestation. The capillary network of the cortex proliferates mainly in the postnatal period, as radial arterioles decrease in number. Severe ischemia of the immature brain may result in cuffs of surviving nerve cells surrounding the radial arterioles, with vertical columns of necrotic tissue between these zones related to immaturity of the vascular bed. Alternating radial zones of viable cerebral tissue and infarcted tissue thus occur in the cerebral cortex. Infarcts not only destroy maturing nerve cells that have already completed their migration but also interfere with continuing and future migrations into those regions. The zones of infarction eventually become gliotic, and the geometric architecture of the cortex is disrupted.

The existence of fetal watershed zones of the cortical vascular bed is important in the pathogenesis of ulegyria, an atrophy of gyri that grossly resembles polymicrogyria. Focal areas of cortical atrophy and gliotic scarring after perinatal ischemic or hypoxic encephalopathy have been known for many years. The four-layered cortex of polymicrogyria is traditionally considered quite a different lesion than ulegyria, resulting from a primary disturbance of neuroblast migration. Some authors question this interpretation, however, and provide evidence of postmigratory laminar necrosis of the cortex. Polymicrogyria is frequently distributed in vascular territories of fetal brain and often forms a rim surrounding a porencephalic cyst in the territory of the middle cerebral artery. Multicystic encephalomalacia and hydranencephaly are end-stage sequelae of massive cerebral infarction in the developing brain. Watershed zones also exist in the brainstem, between the territories supplied by paramedian penetrating, short circumferential, and long circumferential arteries, which all originate from the basilar artery. Transient hypoperfusion in the basilar artery in fetal life may produce watershed infarcts in the tegmentum of the pons and medullar oblongata. This is a probable pathogenesis of Möbius' syndrome and probably also of "failure of central respiratory drive" in neonates with hypoventilation not due to pulmonary or neuromuscular disorders. The cause is involvement of the tractus solitarius, which receives afferents from chemoreceptors, such as the carotid body, and provides efferent axons to motor neurons that innervate the diaphragm and intercostal muscles.

CLINICAL EXPRESSION OF MALFORMATIONS OF THE NERVOUS SYSTEM

Table 66.1 summarizes the clinical features of major malformations of the brain.

Disorders of Neurulation (1–4 Weeks' Gestation)

Incomplete or defective formation of the neural tube from the neural placode is the most common type of malformation of the human CNS. Anencephaly has an incidence of 1 per 1,000 live births, although affected fetuses rarely survive. Meningomyelocele is almost as frequent, with geographical and ethnic differences among various populations in the world. Nonetheless, it is a medical problem and human tragedy of much greater proportions because the majority of infants affected with defects of the posterior neural tube survive with major neurological handicaps. The

Table 66.1: Summary of clinical features of major malformations of the brain

	Microcephaly	Encephalocele	Dysmorphic facies	Hydrocephalus	Seizures	Vision impairment	Mental retardation	Hypotonia	Spasticity	Ataxia	Myopathy	Endocrinopathy
Holoprosencephaly, alobar, semilobar	+++	++	+++	+	++	+	++++	+++	+	++	0	++
Holoprosencephaly, lobar	+	0	+	++	++	0	+++	++	+	+	0	+
Septo-optic dysplasia	+	0	+	+	++	+++	+++	++	+	+	0	+++
Callosal agenesis, complete or partial	0	0	++	+	+++	+	+++	+	+	0	0	+
Callosal agenesis, Aicardi's syndrome	++	0	++	0	++++	+	++++	+++	+	+	0	0
Callosal agenesis lipoma	0	0	+	+	++++	0	+	++	0	0	0	0
Colpocephaly, primary	++	0	++	+	++	++	++	++	+	0	0	0
Lissencephaly or pachygyria (Miller-Dieker)	+	0	++++	0	+++	+	++++	+++	+	++	0	+
Lissencephaly or pachygyria (Walker-Warburg)	+++	++	++++	++	+++	+++	++++	+++	++	++	++++	++
Pachygyria (Fukuyama)	+++	0	++	0	+++	+	++++	++++	0	++	++++	+
Cerebrohepatorenal disease (Zellweger)	++	0	++++	+	++++	++	++++	++++	0	0	++	+
Tuberous sclerosis (Bourneville's disease)	+	0	++++	++	++++	+	++++	++	++	+	0	+
Hemimegalencephaly	+	0	++	+	+++	+	+++	+	0	0	0	+
Chiari malformations	+	+	0	++++	+	0	++++	0	+++	+	0	0
Dandy-Walker malformation	0	+	0	+++	+	0	+++	+++	++	+++	0	0
Aqueductal stenosis or atresia	0	0	+	++++	+	0	++	+	++	+	0	0
Cerebellar hypoplasias	0	0	0	0	+	0	++	++++	0	++++	0	0

0 = <5% of patients; + = 5–25%; ++ = 26–50%; +++ = 51–75%; ++++ = >75% of patients involved.

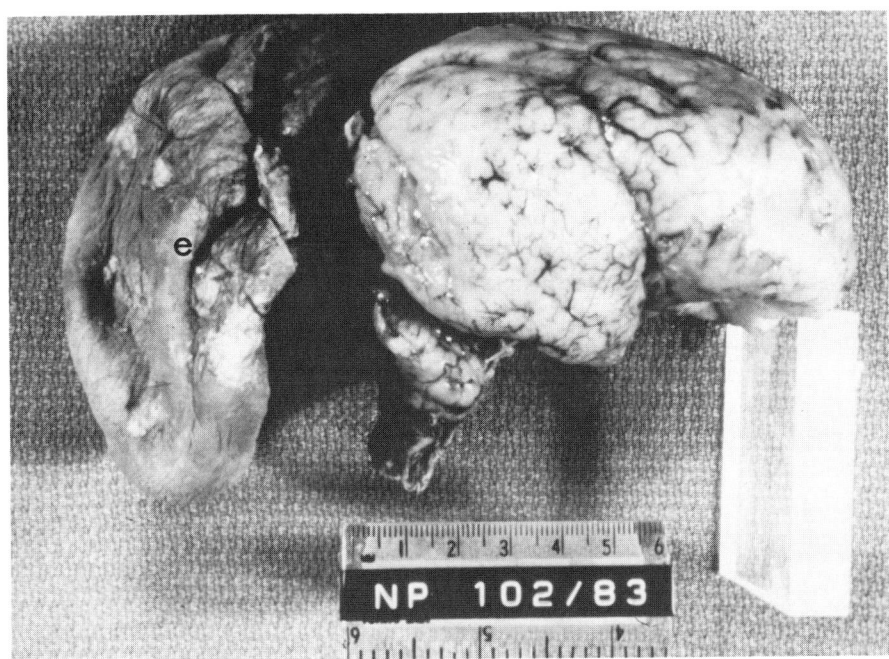

FIGURE 66.9 Lateral view of the brain of a term neonate with Meckel-Gruber syndrome. This dysplasia is a large occipital encephalocele (e) and lissencephaly. The brain is smooth and shows only a sylvian fissure and a few shallow abnormal sulci near the vertex. The encephalocele contains disorganized neural tissue, angiomatous malformations, focal hemorrhages, and zones of infarction.

causes of these disorders of the first month of gestation are usually not evident, despite intensive epidemiological, genetic, dietary, and toxicological surveys.

Anencephaly (Aprosencephaly with Open Cranium)

Anencephaly is a failure of the anterior neuropore to close at 24 days' gestation or perhaps to remain closed. The lamina terminalis does not form, and its derivatives, including most forebrain structures, do not develop. Structures derived from the ventral part of the lamina terminalis, the basal telencephalic nuclei, may form imperfectly. Because the deficient forebrain neuroectoderm does not induce the overlying mesoderm to develop, the cranium, meninges, and scalp also do not close in the sagittal midline, and the remaining brain tissue is exposed throughout gestation to the surrounding amniotic fluid. The original induction failure, however, is probably that of mesodermal tissue on neuroectoderm, due to a defective rostral end of the notochord.

The small nodule of residual telencephalic tissue is called the area cerebrovasculosa and consists of haphazardly oriented mature and immature neurons, glial cells, and nerve fibers. This neural matrix is perfused by an extensive proliferation of small, thin-walled vascular channels, so concentrated in places as to resemble a cavernous hemangioma. This abnormal vasculature, particularly prominent at the surface of the telencephalic nodule, is probably the result of a necrotizing and resorptive process.

The diagnosis of anencephaly can be made prenatally by examination of amniotic fluid for elevated α-fetoprotein and is confirmed by sonographic imaging as early as 12 weeks' gestation.

Encephalocele (Exencephaly)

Encephaloceles are less extreme midline cranial defects than those found in atelencephaly. Most are parietal or occipital (Figure 66.9) and contain supratentorial tissue, cerebellar tissue, or both. Frontal encephaloceles are less common in North America and Europe but are the most frequent variety in Thailand and surrounding countries. They nearly always include olfactory tissue.

The cerebral tissue in the encephalocele sac is usually extremely hamartomatous without recognized architecture. It may include heterotopia from an unexpected site, such as cerebellar tissue in a frontal encephalocele. Zones of infarction, hemorrhage, calcifications, and extensive proliferations of thin-walled vascular channels are common, approaching the disorganized tissue of the area cerebrovasculosa of atelencephaly. The remaining intracranial brain is often dysplastic as well. The ventricular system may be partially herniated into the encephalocele sac, at which point hydrocephalus ensues.

Encephaloceles may be completely covered with skin, or thin, distorted meningeal membranes may be exposed. Leaking CSF rapidly becomes infected. Some encephaloceles, particularly those of the occipital midline, may become so large that they exceed the size of the infant's head. Nasopharyngeal encephaloceles are rare but may be a source of meningitis from CSF leak through the nose. Malformations of the visceral organs often coexist with encephaloceles, and other congenital anomalies of the eyes and face, cleft palate, and polydactyly also are common. The entire brain may be severely hypoplastic (see Figure 66.1).

Clinical neurological handicaps may be severe because even if the herniated tissue within the encephalocele is small and easily excised, concomitant intracranial malformations of the brain often result in epilepsy, mental retardation, motor impairment, and often cortical blindness in the case of occipital encephaloceles. The treatment of choice of small encephaloceles is surgical excision and closure of overlying cutaneous defects. Seizures and hydrocephalus are common but treatable complications. Infants with large encephaloceles usually do not survive the neonatal period, and surgical treatment may be deferred.

Meningomyelocele (Spinal Dysraphism, Rachischisis, Spina Bifida Cystica)

Spinal dysraphism involving the caudal end of the neural tube results from the posterior neuropore not closing at 26 days postnatal. The hypothesis that meningomyelocele and atelencephaly are due to increased pressure and volume of fluid within the primordial ventricular system of the developing neural tube, which causes rupture at one end and prevents reclosure, has not been widely embraced. This is true because the choroid plexuses are not yet formed at the time of neural tube closure and embryological evidence of hydrocephalus at that stage in experimental animals is lacking. Although many theories have been proposed, and several teratogenic drugs, hypervitaminosis A, and genetic models are able to produce neural tube defects and hydrocephalus in experimental animals, none explains the pathogenesis of faulty neurulation in humans.

The spina bifida syndromes are classified on one of two bases: the bony vertebral deformity or the neurological lesion and associated clinical deficit. The latter can cause a range of problems, including no deficit in the case of spina bifida occulta without herniation of tissue or mild spina bifida cystica with herniation of meninges alone. Deficits resulting from herniation of nerve roots and consequent motor, sensory, and autonomic neuropathy (meningomyelocele) also occur, as do extensive defects that also involve the parenchyma of the spinal cord (myelodysplasia). Most lesions are lumbosacral in location, but meningomyelocele also may occur in the thoracic or even the cervical region, usually as an extension rostrally of lumbosacral lesions. The level of involvement determines much of the clinical deficit. Type II Chiari malformation is consistently present, and aqueductal stenosis coexists in 50%. Hydrocephalus is a common complication, involving most patients with meningomyelocele and causing neurological deficit.

The treatment of meningomyelocele is controversial and enters the arena of medical ethics. Small defects are easily closed surgically in the neonatal period, but large defects that cause complete paraplegia and flaccid neurogenic bladder, often accompanied by hydronephrosis, severe hydrocephalus, and other cerebral malformations, are associated with poor quality of life. A decision not to treat such infants or not to prolong survival poses a moral question to be addressed by the physicians in consultation with parents, hospital ethics committees, and other individuals whom the parents may identify.

The most important immediate complications of large meningomyeloceles are hydrocephalus and infection from leaking CSF. Long-term complications include chronic urinary tract infections, decubiti, hydrocephalus, paraplegia, and other neurological deficits. Mental retardation is common but may be mild.

Midline Malformations of the Forebrain (4–8 Weeks' Gestation)

A series of developmental malformations of the prosencephalon are embryologically related to the lamina terminalis not differentiating into telencephalic structures. The lamina terminalis is the rostral membrane of the primitive neural tube that forms with closure of the anterior neuropore. Disorders of the lamina terminalis are expressed mainly as midline defects, not only because of its location in the midline but also because lateral growth of the cerebral hemispheres is affected due to deficient or abnormal cellular migration centrifugally to form the cerebral cortex. The series of midline prosencephalic malformations is related to the embryological time of the beginning of each and includes alobar, semilobar, and lobar holoprosencephaly, arhinencephaly, septo-optic dysplasia, colpocephaly, and agenesis of the corpus callosum.

The lamina terminalis itself, after differentiating the forebrain structures, becomes the anterior wall of the third ventricle in the mature brain, extending between the optic chiasm ventrally and the rostrum of the corpus callosum dorsally. Some authors contend that a defective cephalic notochord induces midline forebrain defects. The complex embryological relationships of neuroectoderm and mesoderm in early ontogenesis are incompletely understood.

Holoprosencephaly

This malformation in which the two cerebral hemispheres are fused in the midline is traditionally attributed to lack of cleavage in the midsagittal plane of the embryonic cerebral vesicle at 33 days. Recent molecular genetic data implicates the strong ventralizing gene, Sonic hedgehog (Shh); the lack of expression of this gene in the prechordal mesoderm ventral to the rostral end of the neural tube results in no neural induction (Roessler et al. 1996). Abnormal Shh expression also may be altered in metabolic diseases with impaired cholesterol synthesis and high serum levels of the cholesterol precursor molecule 7-dehydrocholesterol, as in the Smith-Lemli-Opitz syndrome, which has a high association with holoprosencephaly (Kelley et al. 1996). Holoprosencephaly may result from many genetic defects, and several genes or their transcription products may cause this malformation. An autosomal dominant form maps to the 7p36.2 locus. A defect at the same locus that affects *Shh* at the posterior, rather than the anterior, end of the neural tube results in sacral agenesis (Lynch et al. 1995). A defect in the *Zic-2* gene is associated with 13q deletions, and holoprosencephaly is frequent in infants with trisomy 13 (Brown et al. 1998). The most common association of holoprosencephaly, after chromosomal defects, is with maternal diabetes mellitus; sacral agenesis is another common malformation in infants of diabetic mothers. Both involve downregulation of *Shh*.

Olfactory bulbs and tubercles differentiate a few days after forebrain cleavage, but olfactory agenesis almost always accompanies all but the mildest forms of holoprosencephaly; therefore, the term *arhinencephaly* has often been used interchangeably (and incorrectly). Callosal agenesis also is a uniform feature except in the mildest forms, and the cerebral mantle is grossly disorganized, with multiple heterotopia, poorly laminated cortical gray matter, and ectopic neurons and glial cells in the overlying meninges. Extensions of germinal matrix into the lateral ventricles through gaps in the ependyma are common. Thus, although holoprosencephaly can be dated to about 33 days' gestation at onset, the pathological process extends throughout most of fetal life.

The variants of holoprosencephaly have been classified into three types, reflecting different degrees of abnormal cerebral architecture. Alobar holoprosencephaly is characterized by a brain with a single midline telencephalic ventricle, rather than paired lateral ventricles, and continuity of the cerebral cortex across the midline frontally. The roof of the monoventricle often balloons into a dorsal cyst that may assume a variety of configurations. The corpus striatum and thalamus of the two sides are fused, and the third ventricle may be absent, leaving rudiments of ependymal rosettes in its place. In semilobar holoprosencephaly, an incomplete interhemispheric fissure is formed at least posteriorly, and the occipital lobes, including the occipital horns of the ventricular system, may approach a normal configuration, despite fusion of the frontal lobes across the midline. Lobar holoprosencephaly is the least severe form; the hemispheres are well formed but are in continuity through a band of cortex at the frontal pole or the orbital surface, and the indusium griseum and cingulate gyri overlying the corpus callosum are in continuity. The corpus callosum is incompletely formed but not totally absent, as in alobar and semilobar holoprosencephaly. In the more severe forms of holoprosencephaly, the optic nerves are hypoplastic or fused in and associated with a single median eye. Midline cerebellar defects, absent pyramidal tracts, and malformed brainstem structures accompany the more severe forms of this malformation. The degree of disorganization of the intrinsic architecture of the cerebral cortex and subcortical heterotopia corresponds to the severity of gross hemispheric fusion. Meningeal heterotopia or marginal glioneuronal nodules commonly result from overmigration, perhaps associated with absence of the transitory external granular layer of the fetal brain in holoprosencephaly.

Holoprosencephaly often is diagnosed at the time of delivery because 93% of patients exhibit midline facial dysplasias ranging from hypotelorism to midline facial aplasias with fusion of the eyes into a cyclops appearance, malformation and displacement of the proboscis or nose, and other grotesque abnormalities. About one-third of holoprosencephalic infants have a variety of non-neurological malformations of the viscera and the musculoskeletal system.

Holoprosencephaly is commonly associated with trisomy 13 or other chromosomal abnormalities. In other cases, autosomal dominant or autosomal recessive inheritance has been documented, and the malformation is not uncommon in infants of diabetic mothers. Most commonly, however, holoprosencephaly is sporadic and no genetic factors are apparent.

The various forms of holoprosencephaly are well demonstrated by most imaging techniques (Figure 66.10). The anterior cerebral artery is usually a single azygous vessel coursing just beneath the inner table of the skull, a pathognomonic finding. The sagittal sinuses are deformed or replaced by a network of large abnormal veins that resembles the early embryonic pattern of venous drainage.

The EEG in holoprosencephaly shows multifocal spikes that often evolve into hypsarrhythmia. In the neonatal period, the waking EEG is characterized by almost continuous high-voltage alpha-theta monorhythmic activity, becoming discontinuous in sleep. VEPs also are abnormal or altogether absent.

The clinical course of holoprosencephaly is characterized by severe developmental delay and mental retardation and by a mixed pattern of seizures that often are refractory to anticonvulsant medications. Some patients develop hydrocephalus and require shunting, but this condition is more common in the less severe forms of the malformation. Endocrine dysfunction may be present, associated with hypothalamic or pituitary involvement, and vasopressor-sensitive diabetes insipidus may occur. Treatment is directed toward the complications of seizures, hydrocephalus, and endocrine disturbances.

Arhinencephaly

Absence of olfactory bulbs, tracts, and tubercles commonly accompanies more extensive malformations, such as holoprosencephaly and septo-optic dysplasia, but may occur with callosal agenesis or as an isolated cerebral anomaly. Kallmann's syndrome is an X-linked or autosomal dominant condition limited to males, in which anosmia secondary to arhinencephaly without other forebrain malformations is associated with lack of secretion of gonadotropic hormones. Olfactory reflexes may be elicited in the neonate consistently after 32 weeks' gestation and provide a useful supplement to the neurological examination of newborns suspected of cerebral dysgenesis.

Septo-Optic Dysplasia

The association of a rudimentary or absent septum pellucidum with hypoplasia of the optic nerves and chiasm was

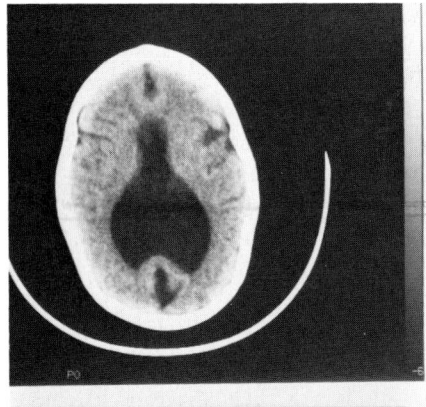
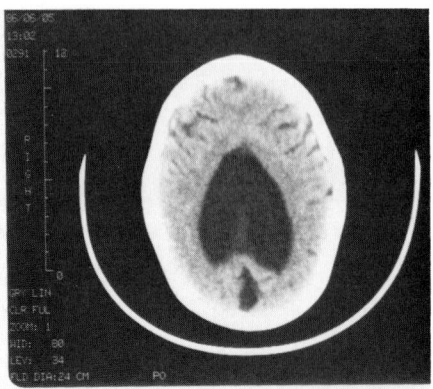
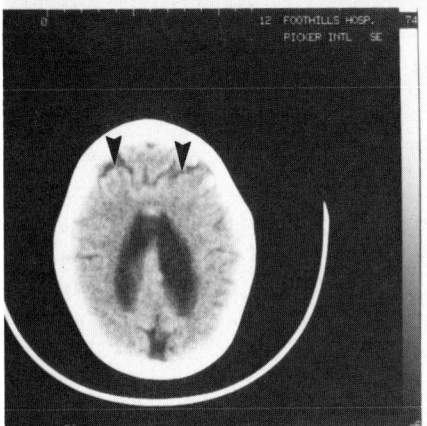
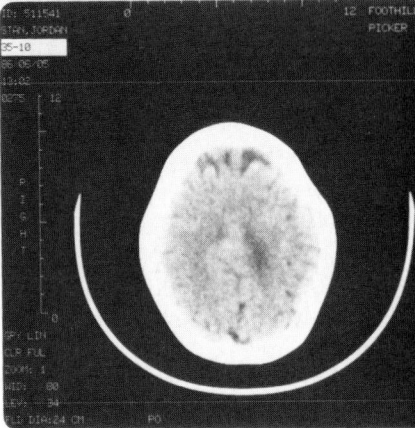

FIGURE 66.10   Unenhanced computed tomographic scan of a 6-year-old boy with semilobar holoprosencephaly. The lateral ventricles are fused, particularly frontally, but show some division into two occipital horns. A deep abnormal sulcus is seen across the fused frontal lobes (*arrowheads*). This is one of several radiological variants of holoprosencephaly.

first recognized by De Mosier in 1956. Underdevelopment of the corpus callosum and anterior commissure and detachment of the fornix from the ventral surface of the corpus callosum are additional features. Patients with this combination of anomalies overlap others with semilobar holoprosencephaly, and some children with septo-optic dysplasia also have arhinencephaly.

Disturbances of the hypothalamic-pituitary axis often occur in septo-optic dysplasia, ranging from isolated growth hormone deficiency to panhypopituitarism and deficient secretion of antidiuretic hormone. Hypothalamic hamartomas, gliosis, and the absence of some hypothalamic nuclei may be associated with a histologically normal pituitary. Absence of the neurohypophysis is demonstrated at autopsy in some cases.

Midline cerebellar defects and hydrocephalus occur inconsistently in septo-optic dysplasia. One cerebellar lesion, called *rhombencephalosynapsis*, is aplasia of the vermis and midline fusion of the cerebellar hemispheres and of the dentate nuclei.

Clinical manifestations relate mainly to the endocrine deficiencies and vision impairment. Ataxia may be compensated if the cerebellar vermis is mildly involved. Seizures are uncommon. Intellectual development usually is normal. Hypertelorism is not a constant finding. Chromosomes are invariably normal. Familial cases are not reported. There is, however, a high incidence of teenage pregnancy and drug abuse in early gestation in mothers of affected infants. Septo-optic dysplasia has been described in an infant of a diabetic mother.

Agenesis of the Corpus Callosum

A commissural plate differentiates within the lamina terminalis at day 39 of embryonic life. The plate acts as a bridge for axonal passage and provides a preformed glial pathway to guide decussating growth cones of commissural axons. The interhemispheric projection of the first axons is preceded by microcystic degeneration in the commissural plate and physiological death of astrocytes. The earliest callosal axons appear at 74 days in the human embryo, the genu and the splenium are recognized at 84 days, and the adult morphology is achieved by 115 days.

The pathogenesis of callosal agenesis is related to two aspects of the commissural plate. If this plate is not available to guide axons across, the corpus callosum does not develop. However, failure of physiological degeneration of a portion of the plate results in a glial barrier to axonal passage, and primordial callosal fibers are deflected posteriorly to some other destination within their hemisphere of origin (bundle of Probst) or disappear.

Agenesis of the corpus callosum is a common malformation, having a 2.3.% prevalence in computed tomographic

(CT) scans in North America and 7–9% prevalence in Japan. Most cases are isolated malformations, but callosal agenesis is an additional feature of many other prosencephalic dysplasias; it also occurs with aplasia of the cerebellar vermis and anomalous pyramidal tract. Simple callosal agenesis may involve the entire commissure or may be partial, usually affecting only the posterior fibers. Hypoplasia or partial agenesis of the commissure is much more common than total agenesis (Bodensteiner et al. 1994). In callosal agenesis, the anterior and hippocampal commissures are always well formed or large.

In the absence of a corpus callosum, the lateral ventricles are displaced laterally and the third ventricle rises between them (Figure 66.11). The ventricles also are often mildly dilated, but intraventricular pressure is normal. The anomaly may be demonstrated by most imaging techniques. The varying degrees of partial callosal agenesis produce several radiographic variants.

Clinical symptoms of callosal agenesis may be minimal and unrecognized in children of normal intelligence, although detailed neurological examination discloses deficits in the interhemispheric transfer of perceptual information for verbal expression. Mental retardation or learning disabilities are found in some cases. Epilepsy is common, particularly in patients who are diagnosed early in life. Seizures may relate more to minor focal cortical dysplasias than to the callosal agenesis itself. Hypertelorism is present in many but not all cases and often is associated with exotropia and inability to converge.

The EEG characteristically shows interhemispheric asynchrony or poor organization, with or without multifocal spikes, but is not specific enough to establish the diagnosis. Asynchronous sleep spindles after 18 months of age are a good clue.

Several hereditary forms of callosal agenesis are described besides its occurrence as an additional anomaly in some cases of tuberous sclerosis and various genetic syndromes. An autosomal recessive syndrome of callosal agenesis, mental deficiency, and peripheral neuropathy is known as Andermann's syndrome. Aicardi's syndrome consists of agenesis of the corpus callosum, chorioretinal lacunae, vertebral anomalies, mental retardation, and myoclonic epilepsy. This disorder is found almost exclusively in girls and is thought to be X-linked dominant (chromosomal locus is Xp22) and generally lethal in the male fetus. The EEG shows a typical asymmetrical and asynchronous burst-suppression pattern. Neuropathological findings in Aicardi's syndrome include a variety of minor dysplasias in addition to agenesis of the corpus callosum and anterior commissure and nonlaminated polymicrogyric cortex with abnormally oriented neurons. Callosal agenesis is a common component in many chromosomal disorders, particularly trisomies 8, 11, and 13. Lipoma replacing part of the corpus callosum is associated with a high incidence of epilepsy.

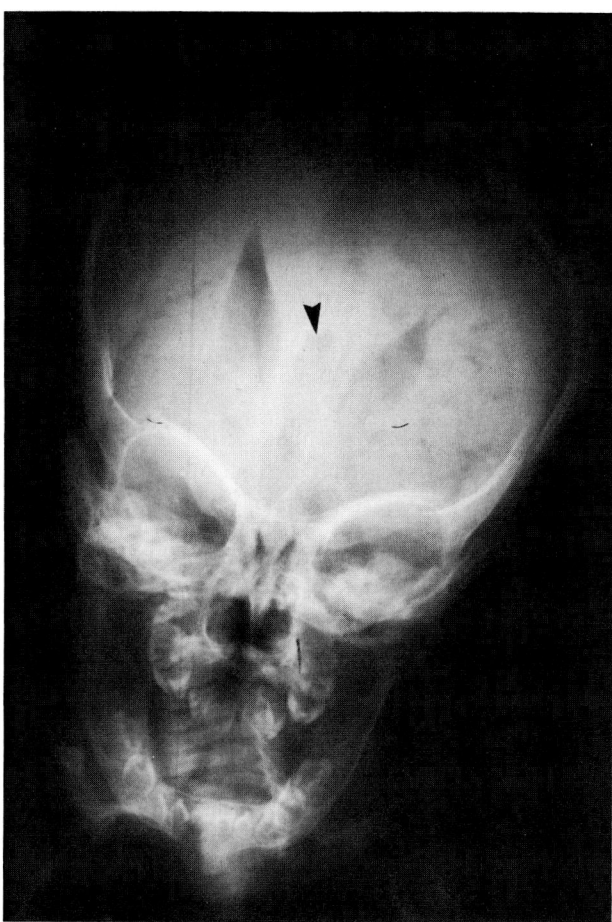

FIGURE 66.11 Pneumoencephalogram of a 6-month-old infant with agenesis of the corpus callosum. The lateral ventricles are widely separated by the bundle of Probst in the dorsomedial part of each hemisphere, and the third ventricle (*arrowhead*) rises between them. The septum pellucidum is absent.

Colpocephaly

Colpocephaly is a selectively much greater dilatation of the occipital horns than of the frontal or temporal horns of the lateral ventricles, not due to increased intraventricular pressure but rather due to loss of surrounding tissue, particularly white matter. Three conditions may cause colpocephaly:

1. It may appear as a primary malformation, histologically associated with poorly laminated striate cortex, subcortical heterotopia, and defective ependyma lining the occipital horns.
2. It is common in many cases of agenesis of the corpus callosum because of absence of the splenium.
3. It may be the acquired result of periventricular leukomalacia, especially in premature infants, because of loss of periventricular white matter in the posterior half of the cerebral hemispheres.

Clinical findings are usually those of mental retardation, spastic diplegia, epilepsy, and vision loss, but it does not always cause complete blindness. Most cases have been demonstrated by CT in the neonatal period or early infancy. The focal ventriculomegaly is not generally associated with increased intracranial pressure, but a few cases have been treated by shunting because of enlarging head size. Isotope cisternography shows normal CSF dynamics in most cases.

The EEG in colpocephaly ranges from normal in mild cases to near-hypsarrhythmia in infants who develop myoclonic epilepsy. Bilateral posterior slowing of low voltage with occipital spikes is common.

Colpocephaly also develops late in fetal life because of infarction and cystic degeneration of the deep white matter of the posterior third of the cerebral hemispheres rather than as a developmental disorder of neuronal migration.

Disorders of Early Neuronal Migration (8–20 Weeks' Gestation)

Lissencephaly (Agyria)

Lissencephaly is a failure of development of convolutions in the cerebral cortex because of defective neuronal migration. The cortex remains smooth, as in the embryonic brain (see Figure 66.9). The migrations of the cerebellum and the brainstem also are usually involved, but the embryonic corpus gangliothalamicus pathway is not disturbed, so the thalamus and basal ganglia are well formed. Structural and metabolic abnormalities of the fetal ependyma may be important factors in disturbing the normal development of radial glial cells (Sarnat 1992).

The cytoarchitecture of the neocortex in lissencephaly takes one of two forms. In the first, a four-layered sequence develops. The outermost layer is a widened molecular zone; layer 2 contains neurons corresponding to those of normal laminae III, V, and VI; layer 3 is cell-sparse; and layer 4 contains heterotopic neurons that have migrated incompletely. Decreased brain size leads to microcephaly, with widened ventricles representing a fetal stage rather than pressure hydrocephalus and an uncovered sylvian fossa representing a lack of operculation. The second form of cortical architectural abnormality in lissencephaly is disorganized clusters of neurons with haphazard orientation, forming no definite layers or predictable pattern. Type 2 lissencephaly is associated with several closely related genetic syndromes: Walker-Warburg syndrome, Fukuyama type muscular dystrophy, muscle-eye-brain syndrome of Santavuori, and Meckel-Gruber syndrome.

Occasionally, lissencephalic brains have deep or shallow symmetrical clefts with open or closed lips. This configuration has been termed *schizencephaly*. Schizencephaly is associated with defective expression of the gene *EMX2* (Granata et al. 1997). Encephalocele may be associated with some cases of lissencephaly (see Figure 66.9).

Miller-Dieker Syndrome

Miller-Dieker syndrome is a familial lissencephaly characterized clinically by microcephaly and a peculiar facies that includes micrognathia, high forehead, thin upper lip, short nose with anteverted nares, and low-set ears. Neurologically, the children are developmentally delayed in infancy and mentally retarded, lack normal responsiveness to stimuli, initially exhibit muscular hypotonia that later evolves into spasticity and opisthotonos, and develop intractable seizures. Death before 1 year of age is common. The EEG often shows focal or multifocal spike-wave discharges that later become bisynchronous bursts of diffuse paroxysmal activity and extremely high-voltage diffuse rhythmic theta and beta activity.

At autopsy, the original cases showed lack of gyral development in the cerebral cortex, but later patients were found with the typical craniofacial features and clinical course but with gyral development, although the convolutions were abnormal and pachygyria predominated. The term *Miller-Dieker syndrome* was proposed to distinguish this syndrome from other cases of lissencephaly without the clinical and dysmorphic facial features. A microdeletion at the chromosome 17p13.3 locus is demonstrated by high-resolution studies in most patients with Miller-Dieker syndrome, and family members of the original patients also show the defect (Chong et al. 1997). The responsible gene is *LIS1*. Histological examination of the brain in Miller-Dieker syndrome confirms the presence of a severe disorder of neuroblast migration, as in other cases of lissencephaly.

Subcortical Laminar Heterotopia (Band Heterotopia, Double Cortex) and Bilateral Periventricular Nodular Heterotopia

Subcortical laminar heterotopia and bilateral periventricular nodular heterotopia both result from X-linked recessive traits that occur almost exclusively in females. Both disorders present clinically as severe seizure disorders in childhood, although they are often associated also with mental retardation and other neurological deficits. In subcortical laminar heterotopia, a band of gray matter heterotopia within the subcortical white matter lies parallel to the overlying cerebral cortex but separated from it by white matter. Histologically, it is not laminated, as is the normal cortex and consists of disoriented neurons and glial cells and fibers with poorly organized architecture. The few male fetuses that have not spontaneously aborted have been born with lissencephaly in addition and even more severe neurological deficits (Pinard et al. 1994). The defective gene and its transcription product in subcortical laminar heterotopia have been identified and are called *doublecortin* (Gleeson et al. 1999). In bilateral periventricular nodular heterotopia, islands of neurons and glial cells occur in the subependymal regions around the lateral ventricles and appear to be neuroepithelial cells that have matured in their site of origin without migrating (Eksioglu et al. 1996). Both conditions are best demonstrated by magnetic resonance imaging, but also are detected by CT.

Disturbances of Late Neuroblast Migration (after 20 Weeks' Gestation)

Although major neuronal migrations in the developing human brain occur in the first half of gestation, late migrations of immature nerve cells continue. A few neuronal precursors continue to migrate to the cerebral cortex after 20 weeks' gestation. Perinatal disorders of cerebral perfusion, small intraparenchymal hemorrhages in premature infants, intracranial infections, and hydrocephalus are examples of common perinatal complications that may interfere with the late neuronal migrations, either by destroying migrating neuroblasts or by disrupting their radial glial fiber guides. Reactive gliosis is detected as early as 20 weeks' gestation in the fetal brain, and proliferation of astrocytes is already evident 4 days after an insult. Neurons may be blocked from traversing a gliotic plaque.

Disorders of Cerebellar Development (32 Days' Gestation to 1 Year Postnatally)

The cerebellum has the longest period of embryological development of any major structure of the brain. Neuroblast differentiation in the cerebellar plates (rhombic lips of His) of the dorsolateral future medulla oblongata and lateral recesses of the future fourth ventricle are recognized at 32 days. Neuroblast migration from the external granular layer is not complete until 1 year postnatally. As a result of this extended ontogenesis, the cerebellum is vulnerable to teratogenic insults longer than are most parts of the nervous system. Malformations of the cerebellum may be focal, confined to the cerebellum, or associated with other brainstem or cerebral dysplasias. The cerebellar cortex is especially susceptible to toxic effects of many drugs, chemicals, viral infections, and ischemic-hypoxic insults.

Selective hypoplasia or aplasia of the vermis, with intact lateral hemispheres, occurs in some genetic disorders, in association with other midline defects involving the forebrain, as in some cases of holoprosencephaly and of callosal agenesis. A specific autosomal recessive disease, Joubert's syndrome, is characterized clinically by episodic hyperpnea, abnormal eye movements, ataxia, and mental retardation and has a variable but often progressively worsening course, with improvement in some cases.

The Dandy-Walker malformation consists of a ballooning of the posterior half of the fourth ventricle, often but not always associated with non-opening of the foramen of Magendie to open. In addition, the posterior cerebellar vermis is aplastic, and there may be heterotopia of the inferior olivary nuclei, pachygyria of the cerebral cortex, and other cerebral and sometimes visceral anomalies. Hydrocephalus from obstruction almost always develops, but if it is treated promptly, the prognosis may be good. Neurological handicaps, such as spastic diplegia and mental retardation, probably relate more to the associated malformations of the brain than to the hydrocephalus.

The Chiari malformation is a herniation of the tonsils and posterior vermis of the cerebellum through the foramen magnum, compressing the spinomedullary junction. This simple form is termed *Chiari type I malformation*. Type II involves an additional downward displacement of a distorted lower medulla and dysplasia of medullary nuclei and is a constant feature of lumbosacral meningomyelocele. Chiari type III malformation is actually a cervical spina bifida with cerebellar encephalocele. Hydrocephalus is commonly associated with Chiari malformations of all types. The pathogenesis has been a matter of controversy for many years and is still not fully resolved, although it is clear that Chiari malformations are not the result of a tethered spinal cord with traction as the vertebral column grows. A small posterior fossa may be the primary defect, with insufficient room for the growth of neural structures.

Selective agenesis of the cerebellar hemispheres is much less common than aplasia of the vermis alone. Other components of the cerebellar system, such as the dentate and inferior olivary nuclei, may also be dysplastic. The lateral hemispheres and the inferior olivary and pontine nuclei more commonly are selectively involved in certain degenerative diseases of genetic origin, such as olivopontocerebellar atrophy and other spinocerebellar degenerations.

Global cerebellar hypoplasia has diverse causes, which include chromosomal and genetically determined diseases, Tay-Sachs disease, Menkes' kinky hair disease, some cases of spinal muscular atrophy, and sporadic cases of unknown cause. Histologically, there may be a selective depletion of granule cells or a loss of Purkinje's cells and other neuronal elements in addition to granule cells (Figure 66.12). In selective granule cell depletion, the axons and dendrites of Purkinje's cells are deformed.

Clinically, the most constant features of cerebellar hypoplasia in infancy are developmental delay and generalized muscular hypotonia. Truncal titubation and ataxia become evident after several months, and nystagmus and intention tremor may appear in severe cases. Tendon stretch reflexes usually are diminished but may be hyperactive if corticospinal tract deficit also is present because of cerebral involvement.

Focal dysplasias and hamartomas of the cerebellar cortex (Figure 66.13) are often incidental findings at autopsy and are often clinically asymptomatic. More extensive lesions present abnormal cerebellar findings clinically. These small focal malformations are a disorder of neuronal migration that may be programmed as genetic

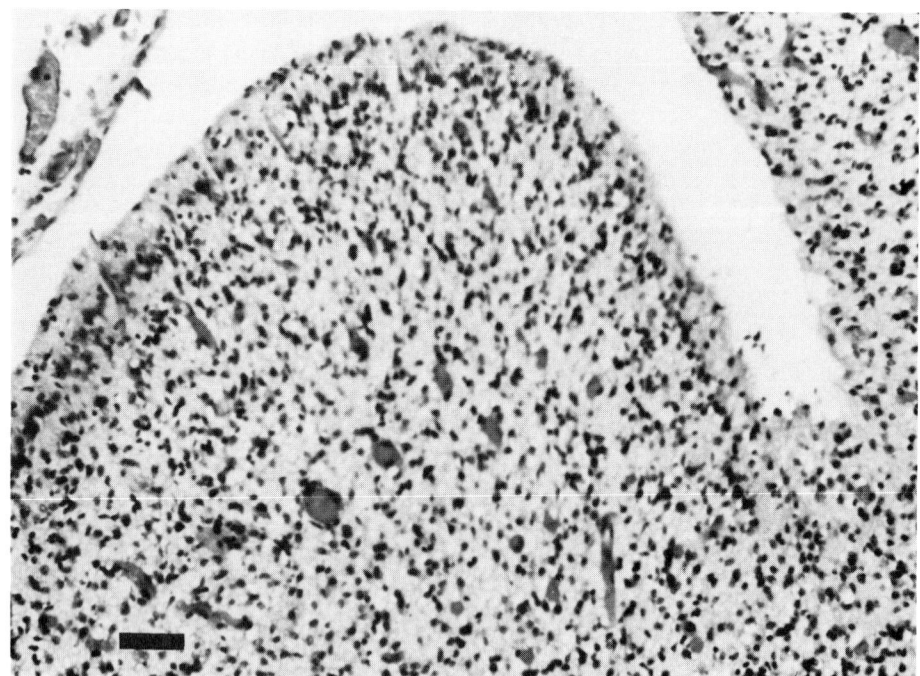

FIGURE 66.12 Cerebellar cortex of infant with cerebellar hypoplasia shows extensive gliosis and loss of all neuronal elements. This histological appearance resembles that of cerebellar sclerosis secondary to acquired injury, but in the latter condition there are usually a few neurons still surviving. Some cases of cerebellar hypoplasia show selective loss of granule cells and preservation of Purkinje's cells. (Hematoxylin-eosin stain. Bar = 100 µm.)

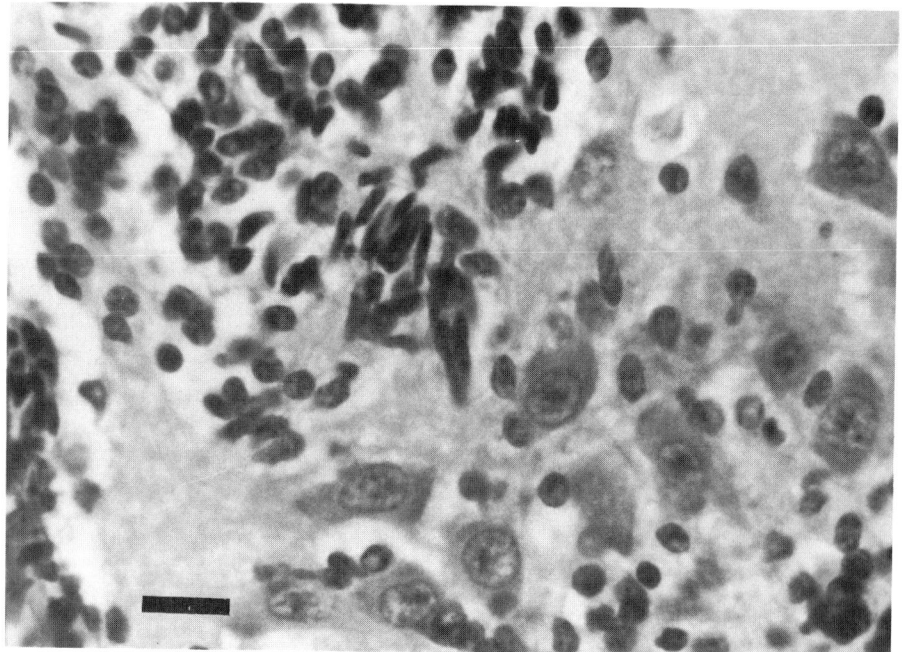

FIGURE 66.13 Focal dysplasia of cerebellar cortex. The normal laminar architecture is disrupted, and granule and Purkinje's cells show a haphazard orientation and array. Some granule cells are spindle shaped, resembling the shape assumed during transit from the external granular layer in normal development. This dysplasia is due to faulty neuronal migration and probably occurred at midgestation. (Hematoxylin-eosin stain. Bar = 15 µm.)

defects or, more commonly, acquired from brief insults during the long period of cerebellar development. Focal ischemic insults and exposure to cytotoxic drugs or viruses are among the more common causes. The granule cells of the cerebellar cortex retain a regenerative capacity lost early in gestation by most other neurons, but the regenerative pattern of lamination in the cerebellar cortex may be imperfect.

REFERENCES

Barth PG. Pontocerebellar hypoplasias. An overview of a group of inherited neurodegenerative disorders with fetal onset. Brain Dev 1993;15:411–422.

Bodensteiner JB, Schaefer GB, Breeding L, Cowan L. Hypoplasia of the corpus callosum: a study of 445 consecutive MRI scans. J Child Neurol 1994;9:47–49.

Bronner-Fraser M, Fraser SE. Differentiation of the vertebrate neural tube. Curr Opin Cell Biol 1997;9:885–891.

Brown SA, Warburton D, Brown LY, et al. Holoprosencephaly due to mutations in *Zic2*, a homologue of *Drosophila* odd-paired. Nat Genet 1998;20:180–183.

Chenn A, McConnell SK. Cleavage orientation and the asymmetrical inheritance of notch 1 immunoreactivity in mammalian neurogenesis. Cell 1995;82:631–641.

Chong SS, Pack SD, Roschke AV, et al. A revision of the lissencephaly and Miller-Dieker syndrome critical regions in chromosome 17p13.3. Hum Mol Genet 1997;6:147–155.

Clark DC, Mizuguchi M, Antalffy B, et al. Predominant localization of the *LIS* family of gene products to Cajal-Retzius cells and ventricular neuroepithelium in the developing human cortex. J Neuropathol Exp Neurol 1997;56:1044–1052.

Dobyns WB, Reiner O, Carrozzo R, Ledbetter DH. Lissencephaly: a human brain malformation associated with deletion of the *LIS1* gene located at chromosome 17p13. JAMA 1993;270:2838–2842.

Dupuy S, Houser CR. Developmental changes in GABA neurons of the rat dentate gyrus: an in situ hybridization and birthdating study. J Comp Neurol 1997;389:402–418.

Eksioglu YZ, Scheffere IE, Cardenas P, et al. Periventricular heterotopia: an X-linked dominant epilepsy locus causing aberrant cerebral cortical development. Neuron 1996;16:77–87.

Flores L, Marhx A, Ramírez-Mayans J. Intraventricular masses: a result of ependymal gaps or failure of apoptosis? VIII International Congress of Pediatric Neurology, Ljubljana, Slovenia, September 13–18, 1998.

Gleeson JG, Minnerath SH, Fox JW, et al. Characterization of mutations in the gene *doublecortin* in patients with double cortex syndrome. Ann Neurol 1999;45:146–153.

Granata T, Farina L, Faiella A, et al. Familial schizencephaly associated with *EMX2* mutation. Neurology 1997;48:1403–1406.

Herman J-P, Victor JC, Sanes JR. Developmentally regulated and spatially restricted antigens of radial glial cells. Dev Dyn 1993;197:307–318.

Jouet M, Kenwrick S. Gene analysis of L1 neural cell adhesion molecule in prenatal diagnosis of hydrocephalus. Lancet 1995;345:161–162.

Kelley RL, Roessler E, Hennekam RC, et al. Holoprosencephaly in RSH/Smith-Lemli-Opitz syndrome: Does abnormal cholesterol metabolism affect the function of *Sonic hedgehog*? Am J Med Genet 1996;66:78–84.

Kendler A, Golden JA. Progenitor cell proliferation outside the ventricular and subventricular zones during human brain development. J Neuropathol Exp Neurol 1996;55:1253–1258.

Lynch SA, Bond PM, Copp AJ, et al. A gene for autosomal dominant sacral agenesis maps to the holoprosencephaly region at 7q36. Nat Genet 1995;11:93–95.

Marín-Padilla M. Cajal-Retzius cells and the development of the neocortex. Trends Neurosci 1998;21:64–71.

Mione MC, Cavanagh JFR, Harris B, Parnavelas JG. Cell fate specification and symmetrical/asymmetrical divisions in the developing cerebral cortex. J Neurosci 1997;17:2018–2029.

Norman MG, McGillivray B, Kalousek DK, et al. Congenital Malformations of the Brain. Pathological, Embryological, Radiological and Genetic Aspects. New York: Oxford University Press, 1995.

O'Rourke NA, Sullivan DP, Kaznowski CE, et al. Tangential migration of neurons in the developing cerebral cortex. Development 1995;121:2165–2176.

Pinard J-M, Motte J, Chiron C, et al. Subcortical laminar heterotopia and lissencephaly in two families: a single X-linked dominant gene. J Neurol Neurosurg Psychiatry 1994;57:914–920.

Rakic P. Radial versus tangential migration of neuronal clones in the developing cerebral cortex. Proc Natl Acad Sci USA 1995;92:11323–11327.

Roessler E, Belloni E, Gaudenz K, et al. Mutations in the human *Sonic hedgehog* gene cause holoprosencephaly. Nat Genet 1996;14:357–360.

Sarnat HB, Born DE. Synaptophysin immunocytochemistry with thermal intensification: a marker of terminal axonal maturation in the human fetal nervous system. Brain Dev 1999;21:41–50.

Sarnat HB, Menkes JH. The new neuroembryology: how to construct a neural tube. J Child Neurol 1999;14:in press.

Sarnat HB, Nochlin D, Born DE. Neuronal nuclear antigen (NeuN): a marker of neuronal maturation in the early human fetal nervous system. Brain Dev 1998;20:88–94.

Thomas LB, Gates MA, Steindler DA. Young neurons from the adult subependymal zone proliferate and migrate along an astrocyte, extracellular matrix-rich pathway. Glia 1996;17: 1–14.

Zheng C, Heintz N, Hatten ME. CNS gene encoding astrotactin, which supports neuronal migration along glial fibers. Science 1996;272:417–419.

Zhong W, Feder JN, Jiang M-M, et al. Asymmetric localization of mammalian numb homolog during mouse cortical neurogenesis. Neuron 1996;17:43–53.

Chapter 67
Developmental Disabilities

Ruth Nass

CEREBRAL PALSY

Diagnosis

Cerebral palsy (CP) is a static encephalopathy of prenatal or perinatal origin that affects motor tone and function, resulting in spasticity, hypotonia, ataxia, and dyskinesias. The diagnosis is based on a history of delayed motor milestones and on clinical examination. CP occurs in approximately 2 per 1,000 children. The likelihood that intellectual impairment and seizures are associated is directly proportional to the severity of motor impairment. The cause of CP is not always known. Documented causes include brain malformations, prematurity, low birth weight, infection (congenital infections and neonatal meningitis), genetic and metabolic disorders, and neonatal hypoxic ischemic encephalopathy. The National Perinatal Collaborative Project monitored more than 50,000 pregnancies and followed the children born of these pregnancies until age 7 years; 200 of these children developed CP. The most important predictors of CP were maternal mental retardation (MR), birth weight less than 2,000 g, a malformation of any organ system, and breech presentation at delivery. Commonly used signs of presumed perinatal asphyxia, such as an abnormal fetal heart rate, presence of meconium, and low Apgar score, did not improve the predictability of CP and were relatively common in ultimately healthy infants. Infants requiring resuscitation are no more likely to develop CP than were those who breathed spontaneously, unless the infant continued to have neurological problems (e.g., lethargy, hypotonia, poor suck, or seizures) in the newborn nursery. Indeed, most infants with low Apgar scores and neonatal problems do not ultimately develop CP. Most congenital infarctions are prenatal, not perinatal, in origin. A relationship exists between ultrasound abnormalities in preterm infants and disabling and nondisabling CP. Those with nondisabling CP are mostly males with uneventful perinatal courses. This suggests a prenatal origin for their CP, which may have been the precipitant of the preterm labor (rather than the result of prematurity). A vanishing twin is often associated with CP in the survivor.

Low-birth-weight or preterm infants comprise more than 50% of the cases of CP. In a population-based study (Hagberg et al. 1996), birth-weight-specific prevalences were 57 per 1,000 for birth weights less than 1,000 g, 68 per 1,000 for 1,000–1,499 g, 14 per 1,000 for weights 1,500–2,499 g, and 1.4 per 1,000 for 2,500 g or heavier. The etiology was prenatal in 8%, perinatal in 54%, and unclassifiable in 38% of preterm and, respectively, in 33%, 28%, and 39% of term children. Hemiplegic, diplegic, and quadriplegic syndromes accounted for 22%, 66%, and 7% of preterm and 44%, 29%, and 10% of term children. An increase in the severity of functional disability, indicated by the proportion of children with severe learning, manual, and ambulation dysfunction, may be occurring.

Evaluation and Etiology

Magnetic resonance imaging studies show that term infants with CP often have brain malformations, whereas preterm infants with CP usually have periventricular leukomalacia. Periventricular leukomalacia is associated with more severe disability in term infants than in preterm infants, and infratentorial pathology is seen in one-fourth of those with ataxic CP (see Chapter 84).

Although most genetic disorders with a phenotype suggesting CP ultimately cause progressive disability, some appear to be static for years. Atypical features of CP and a history of other affected family members should flag some patients for further evaluation. Ataxic CP is most often genetic (see Chapter 68). Dopamine-responsive dystonia may mimic CP and is treatable. Other genetic or metabolic disorders mimicking CP include metachromatic leukodystrophy, Krabbe's disease (spastic diplegia CP), Lesch-Nyhan syndrome, glutaric aciduria 1 (dyskinetic CP), ataxia telangiectasia, Leigh disease, and subacute sclerosing panencephalitis (ataxic CP).

Treatment

Prevention of CP has focused on prevention of prematurity, treatment of the preterm infant during the perinatal period, and development of neuroprotective agents (see Chapter 84). Magnesium sulfate prevents CP in the very-low-birthweight preterm infant, and indomethacin may prevent CP caused by intraventricular hemorrhage. Cesarean section and rapid initiation of supportive care may decrease the frequency of CP in the preterm newborn, because most intraventricular hemorrhage occurs within the first 6 hours after birth and possibly during labor and delivery.

Rehabilitative therapy influences outcome. The main goals of treatment are to improve the child's motor function and to modify the environment to improve mobility. Orthopedic surgery is sometimes required. Dorsal rhizotomy has been used to decrease spasticity and improve gait or make wheelchair-bound patients more comfortable. Botulinum toxin also has a role in the treatment of spasticity. Life expectancy is limited in those who are immobile or profoundly retarded and who require special feeding (Strauss et al. 1998). Otherwise, children with CP may live well into adult life.

MENTAL RETARDATION

Diagnosis

Total MR prevalence in industrialized countries is 1–3%. Prevalence of mild MR (IQ of 55–70) in children is approximately 2%. Psychometrically defined moderate MR is an IQ of 40–55; severe MR is an IQ of 25–40; and profound MR is an IQ of less than 25.

Evaluation and Etiology

The higher rates of mild MR in lower socioeconomic classes may be due to poor living conditions, migration, cultural differences, poor intellectual stimulation, and less resistance to labeling children as mentally retarded. Maternal MR has an adverse effect on the intellectual, academic, and behavioral status of school-aged children significantly greater than poverty alone. Etiological factors, such as endemic diseases, nutritional deficiencies, intoxication, suboptimal perinatal care, and parental exposure to chemical agents and radiation, may also affect prevalence of MR. Maternal smoking during pregnancy is associated with more than a 50% increase in the prevalence of idiopathic MR.

Several lines of evidence suggest that genes coding for intellectual function may be on the X chromosome: (1) the excess of males with MR (overall 20%; moderate handicap 30%), (2) the wider variability in the distribution of IQ in males than in females, and (3) the segregation of nonspecific MR in an X-linked pattern in many families. More than 150 MR syndromes are inherited in an X-linked fashion. Fragile X syndrome is associated with triplet repeats. Increasing numbers of triplet repeats explain generational anticipation in fragile X syndrome; the number of triplet repeats correlates with degree of cognitive deficit. Although chromosome studies generally detect males with fragile X syndrome, DNA studies may be required to detect manifesting female heterozygotes. The prevalence of nonspecific X-linked MR (2.5 per 10,000) is three times that of fragile X syndrome in the moderately handicapped and may be greater in those with mild MR. However, diagnosis is complicated by the fact that affected males with X-linked MR have no phenotypic, neurological, or biochemical features in common other than MR. Consistent with a genetic basis, the risk of recurrence of mild MR is estimated to be 5–35% and of severe MR, 3–10% (Hodgson 1998).

Brain imaging and studies of metabolic function in a child with MR are often unrevealing. Some recognizable syndromes are associated with MR, particularly in those who are severely retarded, of whom approximately one-third have an identifiable syndrome.

Treatment

Treatment focuses on finding the appropriate educational setting and vocational training for the mildly and moderately retarded and determining home or institutional placement for the severely and profoundly retarded.

PERVASIVE DEVELOPMENTAL DISORDER AND AUTISTIC SPECTRUM DISORDERS

Diagnosis

The diagnosis of autistic spectrum disorders (ASDs) and pervasive developmental disorders (PDDs) requires the

Table 67.1: Asperger's disorder diagnostic criteria

A. Qualitative impairment in social interaction, manifested by at least two of the following:
1. Impairment in use of nonverbal behaviors to regulate social interaction
2. Failure to develop peer relationships
3. Lack of spontaneous seeking to share enjoyments and interests
4. Lack of social or emotional reciprocity

B. Restricted repetitive and stereotyped behavior, interests, and activities, manifested by at least one of the following:
1. Encompassing preoccupation
2. Inflexible adherence to nonfunctional routines
3. Stereotyped and repetitive motor mannerisms
4. Persistent preoccupation with parts of objects

C. Disturbance causes significant impairment in functioning
D. No clinically significant language delay
E. No clinically significant cognitive deficit
F. Criteria not met for diagnosis of another pervasive developmental disorder or schizophrenia

Source: Modified from Diagnostic and Statistical Manual of Mental Disorders, 4th ed. Washington, DC: American Psychiatric Association, 1994.

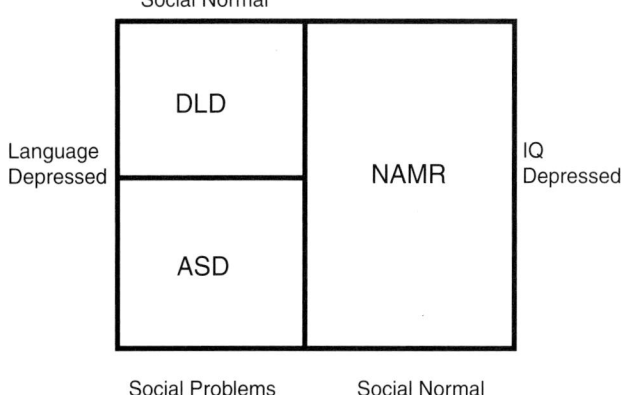

FIGURE 67.1 Developmental language disorders (DLDs) versus autistic spectrum disorders (ASDs) versus nonautistic mental retardation (NAMR). DLDs and ASDs are distinguished by the presence or absence of social disabilities. NAMR is distinguished from DLDs and ASDs by IQ and by language and social normalcy.

early onset of impaired sociability, impaired verbal and nonverbal communication, and restricted activities and interests (Rapin 1997). Autism and Asperger's disorder (AD) (Table 67.1), which probably represents the high-functioning end of the ASD/PDD spectrum, have a reported frequency of 0.4–70.0 per 10,000 children. The symptoms of PDD, like other developmental disorders, often change with age. Approximately one-third of autistic children regress between the ages of 1 and 3 years. Conversely, some toddlers and preschoolers with typical symptoms of autism may not appear autistic by school age. They may seem a bit odd and have peculiarities of language prosody and pragmatics (i.e., *how*, rather than *what*, they communicate). Social skills may be tenuous. Nonverbal learning disabilities (LDs) or attention-deficit hyperactivity disorder (ADHD) may become the school-age diagnosis. Most, however, retain the typical features of autism. The natural history of AD is less well understood. The diagnosis is often delayed until late childhood, adolescence, or even adulthood because by definition early language development must be normal. Nonverbal LDs or ADHD may be the apparent presenting complaint. The characteristic overfocus in a particular, or sometimes peculiar, interest area may escalate over time, but may be the key to a special form of adult success.

Outcome studies suggest that, although overall improvement occurs in approximately 40% during adolescence, deterioration in adolescence may occur in as many as one-third of patients with ASD/PDD. A small minority of patients, usually the higher-functioning group, improve significantly during adolescence, growing to adulthood with no more than the usual social issues. Approximately two-thirds of adults with autism show poor social adjustment

(limited independence in social relations), and one-half require institutionalization. Nonretarded autistic people tend to improve more than do those who are retarded. Higher-functioning people with autism and AD have the best outcome. Although fair-to-good outcomes are reported in 15–30%, only 5–15% become competitively employed, lead independent lives, marry, and raise families. Psychiatric problems are common even in this group. Probably, some odd adults go undiagnosed in childhood and adolescence, thus increasing the proportion of children with ASD/PDD who ultimately function in the mainstream. A small proportion of all those with childhood autism become highly original, emotionally intact adults.

Specific Clinical Features

Intelligence and Cognition

Language and social deficits, but not IQ, define ASD/PDD. Thus, children with ASD/PDD spectrum disorders may function in the inferior, average, or superior range of intellectual ability (Figure 67.1). The majority (70–85%), however, are mentally retarded. A core feature of autism is believed to be an inability to grasp other people's thoughts because of the autistic's own egocentricity, resulting in false beliefs. A theory that individuals with autistic features lack empathy has also been proposed.

Language

Abnormal language is a major symptom of autism. When autistic children have language, it is generally parrotlike

Table 67.2:   Play rating scale

Level 1: No appropriate or functional use of toys or play materials. No symbolic play. Activities restricted to repetitive stereotypic pursuits and indiscriminate sensory use of objects (mouthing, rubbing, etc.) even when directed by an adult.

Level 2: Objects used functionally (drinks from cup), but toy play consists primarily of repetitive stereotypic pursuits (e.g., opening and closing doors) except when directed by an adult. Some capacity to imitate action naming (brushing a doll's hair) with adult support. Beyond this, there is no symbolic play.

Level 3: Objects used functionally, but the range of toys is limited. Prefer cognitive activities (e.g., puzzles) but when left to their own devices, these children tend to use even these activities perseveratively. Activities are primarily repetitive and stereotypical, unless directed by an adult. May learn to engage in simple symbolic play (e.g., doll-house scene).

Level 4: Objects used functionally and a variety of toys used appropriately. These children enjoy running, catching, and tickling games with adults or children. Activities are partly rigid or repetitive and partly constructive, even without adult support. With adult structuring, able to use dolls and people, make puppets talk, and engage in brief sequences of symbolic play (e.g., the boy doll won't eat, mommy doll gets mad, knocks the boy doll down).

Level 5: Objects used functionally. May be extraordinarily competent and knowledgeable in activities involving their circumscribed areas of interest (e.g., board games, computers, electronic games, or high-level word and number tasks). They may engage in these intellectual activities with pleasure and may even appear to use them as a form of play. Activities are partly rigid or repetitive and partly constructive, even without adult support. Use dolls as people, make puppets talk, use an object as if it were a different object (block as phone receiver), act out simple sequences, and with adult help, engage in simple role-taking games.

Source: Modified with permission from L Waterhouse, R Morris, D Allen, et al. Diagnosis and classification in autism. J Autism Dev Dis 1996;26:59–86.

and echolalic; repetitive, stereotyped phrases are uttered without conversational give-and-take. Comprehension of language is impaired or literal. Because they lack interest in communication, young autistic children typically ignore verbal instruction, often leading to the erroneous suspicion of deafness. Several developmental language disorders are found in preschool autistic children: verbal auditory agnosia, phonological syntactic syndrome, semantic pragmatic syndrome, and lexical syntactic syndrome (see Chapter 12B).

The status of language skills at age 5–6 years is the key to long-term prognosis. Those with conversational language do significantly better than those having no or rudimentary language. IQ score at the time of diagnosis is also an important predictor of long-term outcome in autism, especially for those with IQs less than 50, who fare less well.

Abnormalities of play fall within the clinical category of language dysfunction. Atypical play patterns found in autistic children are listed in Table 67.2.

Social Skills

Social dysfunction is a hallmark of autism; several classification schema have been described (Waterhouse et al. 1996). Three groups are identified.

1. The aloof group is most similar to the popular notion of autism. Signs of abnormal attachment are apparent early on. These children do not follow their parents around, do not run to greet them, and do not seek comfort when in pain. They tend to be low functioning in verbal skills and nonverbal communication and exhibit little symbolic play.

2. The passive group is somewhat higher functioning than the aloof group. These children do not make social approaches, but they accept such approaches when made by others. They are capable of some pretend play and join in games, but they take a passive role (e.g., the baby in the game of mothers and fathers).

3. Children in the interactive-but-odd group make spontaneous social approaches to others, but they do so in a peculiar, naive, and one-sided fashion. They tend to talk at other people; their approach may be so persistent as to become unwelcome. Their language lacks pragmatic constraints. Questions are used, for example, as conversational openers without preceding social graces. These children are capable of pretend symbolic play, but it is often extremely repetitive.

An alternative subtyping system defines autism as a spectrum disorder. In this system, four types of sociability deficits are the universal variable, and various language and play deficits are additional subtyping factors. The socially unavailable pattern includes the most severely impaired children, who make no interpersonal contacts. The socially remote category includes children who engage in solitary activity; the child may be interested in activities of another person but not in the person. If someone attempts to intrude, these children ignore, move away, or vocally protest. The inappropriately interactive category includes children who are easier to engage but who have difficulty initiating or maintaining social interactions. The pseudosocial category includes the most verbal children, who can be engaged, although their attempts at social interaction are immature, inadequate, or bizarre (Figure 67.2).

Restricted Range of Behaviors, Interests, and Activities

A restricted range of behaviors, interests, and activities is a necessary feature of autism. In lower-functioning children, these tend to consist of repetitive and stereotyped patterns of behaviors such as twirling, rocking, flapping, toe walking, banging, licking, and covering and uncovering ears or more complex behaviors, such as turning water on and off or opening and closing a door. The so-called idiot savant also exemplifies a restricted repertoire, as do calculating prodigies and hyperlexic children. The possible links with

FIGURE 67.2 Autistic spectrum disorders (ASDs): play, language, and social patterns. (DLD = developmental language disorder; VAA = verbal auditory agnosia.) (Reprinted with permission from D Allen. Autistic spectrum disorder. J Child Neurol 1988:3: 548–556.)

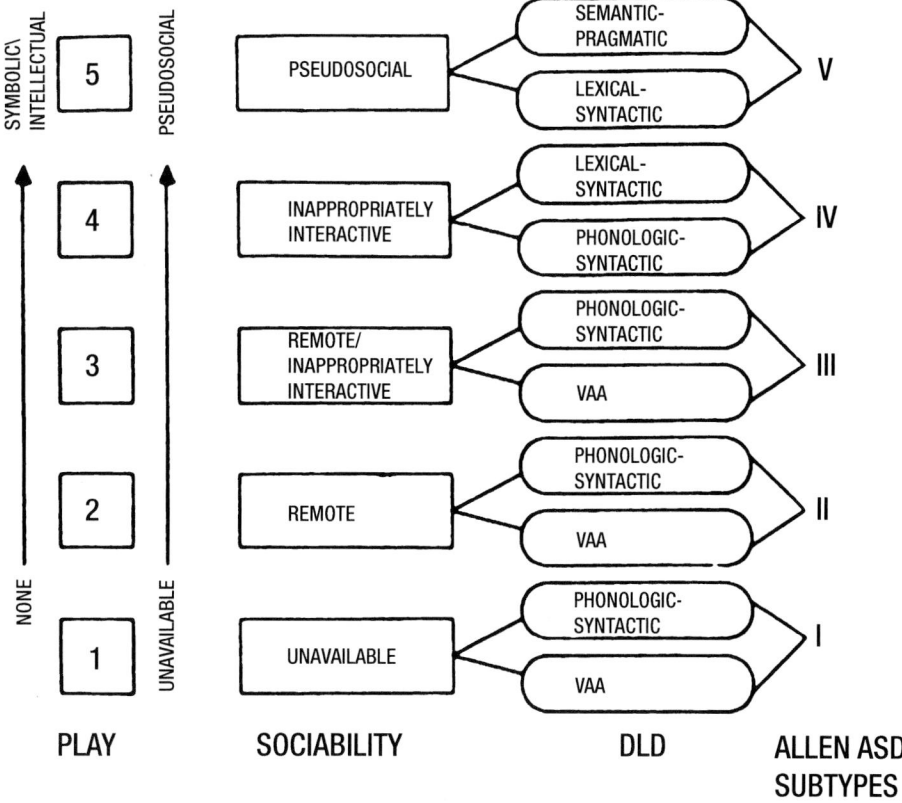

tic disorders and obsessive-compulsive disorders are apparent here. In the higher-functioning autistic child and the child with Asperger's disorder, the restricted range of behaviors, interests, and activities is considerably more complex. Some individuals with exceptional artistic and musical talents may meet other criteria for a diagnosis of an ASD. Some of these children may grow up to be single-minded, peculiar, nonsocial chess or mathematical geniuses. Many of these children have great difficulties with transitions. Not only do they often not focus, but they also become overfocused.

Evaluation and Etiology

The standard neurological examination is generally not abnormal. Careful attention should be paid to the examination of the skin because tuberous sclerosis is probably the most common definable cause of autism. Hearing impairment should be excluded by formal audiologic assessment. An electroencephalogram (EEG), including a sleep record or video-EEG monitoring, is appropriate to exclude subclinical seizures, especially when language comprehension is impaired. Mild-to-severe epilepsy, partial and generalized, occurs in up to one-third of patients with autism by early adulthood. Infancy and peripuberty are particularly vulnerable periods. Those who are retarded are at higher risk,

but epilepsy occurs in high-functioning children as well. Girls may be at greater risk than boys are. Epileptiform EEGs and early epilepsy occur more frequently in children who undergo an early regression (Tuchman and Rapin 1997). The onset of seizures may play a role in adolescent deterioration in some patients.

Imaging of the brain is rarely productive except for research purposes. Structural abnormalities reported in autism include increased brain volume (males), increased ventricular volume, increased white matter volume, and thin splenium of corpus callosum. Also found are decreased axons, hypoplastic cerebellum (vermian lobules VI and VII), 10% hyperplastic cerebellum, hypoplastic parietal lobes, cytoarchitectonic abnormalities in cingulate gyrus, reduced neuronal size, and increased density in hippocampus and amygdala. Although it is inconsistent, most imaging of metabolism in autism reveals hypometabolism in frontal regions and to a lesser extent temporally.

Fragile X chromosome studies should be done if family history or physical features are suggestive (see Mental Retardation, earlier in this chapter). Other metabolic workup depends on clinical suspicions. Some specific causes of ASD/PDD have been identified. ASD/PDD have been found in approximately 20% of children presenting with MR and 10% of children with CP. The high concordance in monozygotic twins and the presence of multiple siblings affected in the same family suggest a genetic component.

Table 67.3:   Medications for autism

Hyperactivity and inattention	Methylphenidate (Ritalin), dextroamphetamine (Dexedrine, Adderal), clonidine (Catapres)
Obsessive-compulsive behaviors	Clomipramine (Anafranil), fluoxetine (Prozac), sertraline (Zoloft), paroxetine (Paxil), fluvoxamine (Luvox), risperidone (Risperdal)
Aggressive behaviors	Carbamazepine (Tegretol), divalproex sodium (Depakote), clonidine, propranolol (Inderal), buspirone (BuSpar), lithium
Self-mutilation	Naloxone (Narcan), propranolol, fluoxetine, clomipramine, lithium
Psychosis	Neuroleptics—haloperidol decanoate (Haldol), risperidone (Risperdal), Thorazine
Others	Adrenocorticotropic hormone and analogues, prednisone, B-complex vitamins

Source: Modified with permission from J Gilman, R Tuchman. Autism and associated behavioral disorders: pharmacologic intervention. Ann Psychopharmacol 1995;29:47–56.

Treatment

Preschool children with ASD/PDD should receive special education in a therapeutic nursery or in a home-based behavioral modification program. Medications that have proved helpful in some cases are listed in Table 67.3.

LEARNING DISABILITIES

LDs occur in approximately 10% of school-aged children and can affect one or several cognitive skills. In addition to developmental language disorders, which are discussed separately (see Chapter 12B), common LDs involve reading (dyslexia), disorders of motor function (dysgraphia, dyspraxia, clumsiness), and the gamut of nonverbal LDs (dyscalculia, visuospatial dysfunction, socioemotional disabilities, and ADHD).

DYSLEXIA

Diagnosis

Developmental dyslexia (Shaywitz 1998), an unexpected difficulty in learning to read, is defined by both exclusive and inclusive criteria. As with other LDs, the dyslexic child may have no major neurological abnormalities, although mild abnormalities (soft signs) may be detected on examination (Table 67.4). Major sensory functions must be normal, but disturbances of cortical visual functioning are presently being explored in relation to reading disability. Some have speculated that in dyslexia, visual processing by a "slow" lateral geniculate magnocellular system (important for monitoring motion, stereopsis, spatial localization, depth, and figure-ground perception) does not appropriately modify the information received from the parvocellular system (crucial for color perception, object recognition, and high-resolution form perception). Normal intelligence is a requirement for a traditional diagnosis. The dyslexic child must have been in a social and educational environment conducive to learning to read. Studies of inner-city elementary schoolchildren show that enrichment programs can help some nonreaders become readers.

With respect to inclusive criteria, reading two grades behind actual or expected grade level is generally required for a diagnosis of dyslexia by educational authorities. The "two-grades-behind" criterion does not take into account that different reading tests yield different reading levels and may be more or less reliable measures and predictors of reading ability at different ages and grade levels because of the complex dynamics of reading acquisition. The age of the child affects the inclusive criteria. Because we do not expect children to read until first grade, the strict definition makes a diagnosis of dyslexia impossible before the third grade. Yet a history of language delay is often predictive of dyslexia, and strict adherence to definition should not preempt consideration of early intervention. In addition, a 2-year discrepancy reflects a greater disability for the younger than for the older child. Whether intelligence should be factored into the diagnosis of reading disability is debated. Spelling difficulties may be a mild form of dyslexia that persists into adulthood or that are present in good readers in dyslexic families (Nass 1998).

Evaluation and Etiology

The assessment of reading itself is the pivot point of an evaluation. Phonological awareness or lack thereof is cur-

Table 67.4:   Common soft signs associated with developmental dyslexia and motor skill disorders

Cranial nerves	Head turns with eyes
	Mouth opens when eyes open
	Difficulty with grimace
Motor	Excess upper extremity posturing on stressed gait
	Excess overflow during finger tapping
	Unsustained one-foot stand
	Difficulty with hopping
	Excess choreiform movements with arms extended
Cerebellar	Dysrhythmic rapid alternating movements
	Excess overflow during rapid alternating movements
	Ballistic finger-nose-finger test
	Difficulty with tandem sequence
Sensory	Extinction of double simultaneous stimuli

rently considered crucial to reading. Few children do not read because of visual perceptual difficulties. The standard neurological examination is generally not abnormal. Routine imaging is rarely abnormal and generally unnecessary, except perhaps in children with atypical features (Table 67.5). Specialized imaging has been more revealing. Approximately two-thirds of normal adult brains show an asymmetry favoring the left planum temporale and left posterior region. By contrast, only 10–50% of dyslexics show a left greater than right posterior asymmetry. Studies assessing structure-function correlations demonstrate that, within the dyslexia group, those with atypical asymmetry patterns tend to have more severe language or reading deficits. The corpus callosum has been implicated in dyslexia because of its role in interhemispheric information transfer. Theoretically, the splenium is the critical region because it contains axons linking the planum temporale and angular gyrus. Some imaging studies do find structural differences in the corpus callosum in normal versus dyslexic readers. Dynamic imaging studies suggest that dyslexics use different pathways for reading than normal readers; posterior regions are underactivated and anterior regions overactivated (Skudlarski et al. 1988). Testing with measures that assess phonological functioning appears to maximize the ability to differentiate dyslexic from normal readers.

Treatment

Numerous techniques for reading remediation have been developed. Controversy persists about whether to remediate to the child's strength or weakness (phonics versus sight vocabulary). Generally, if one technique is unsuccessful, another should be tried, regardless of the theoretical backdrop. Remediation techniques (e.g., reduce contrast, use diffuse colored lights or lenses), which variably inhibit magnocellular and parvocellular systems, have no proved efficacy.

DEVELOPMENTAL DISORDERS OF MOTOR FUNCTION

Diagnosis

Motor skill disorders consist of several discrete, variably co-occurring types: clumsiness, apraxia, dysgraphia, adventitious movements, and anomalous dominance or handedness. Clumsiness is defined as a slowness and inefficiency in performing elemental fine motor and sometimes gross motor movements. Clumsiness is more common in the LD than in the non-LD population, hence the antiquated designation *minimal brain dysfunction* for those with LD. Children with developmental dyspraxia have difficulty with motor learning and motor execution, with or with-

Table 67.5:   Atypical features in dyslexia

Female gender
Left-handed without family history
Strongly left-handed, early declaration
Dyslexic without family history
No history of developmental language problems
Large discrepancy between verbal and spatial skills
Neurological abnormalities or seizures

out clumsiness, and alone or in combination with other LDs. Ideomotor and ideational apraxia occur in children. Dysgraphia (difficulty with writing) can be a manifestation of clumsiness or dyspraxia (part of a generalized deficit or a material-specific deficit) or occur secondary to dyslexia as a higher-order cognitive disorder. Adventitious movements, which can occur normally on a developmental basis, include synkinesis, chorea, tremor, and tics; hence the designation *developmental soft signs* to describe their persistence beyond the age when they normally cease to occur (see Table 67.4). With regard to handedness (manual dominance), most ultimately right-handed children declare after 1 year of age and before age 5 years. Strong left dominance, especially when established before age 1 year, should raise concerns that handedness is pathological (reflects left hemisphere dysfunction). Many infants appear to be transiently left-handed, and the percentage of right-handers (and probably the strength of handedness) increases through age 5 years, reaching more than 90%. Most right-handers are strongly right-handed, whereas most left-handers are ambidextrous. Although there is an increased frequency of LD among left-handers, the dexterity of left-handers equals that of right-handers.

Evaluation and Etiology

A three-tier assessment of motor skills is proposed: (1) history of gross and fine motor milestones; (2) informal examination for adventitious movements, finger tapping, hand turning and toe tapping, sequential motor acts to imitation, pantomime with and without objects and writing and drawing; and (3) formal standardized testing. Synkinesia is best elicited by finger tapping, finger sequencing, and stressed gait testing. Choreiform movements are best elicited by having the child stand with eyes closed and pronated arms extended with fingers spread.

Treatment

Children with significant disorders of motor control may benefit from process-oriented occupational therapy. Computers can facilitate output for those with poor graphomotor skills.

NONVERBAL LEARNING DISABILITIES

Diagnosis

Children with nonverbal LDs (NVLDs) may have (1) emotional and interpersonal difficulties (overlapping with ASD/PDD children); (2) paralinguistic communication problems involving prosody and pragmatics (see Chapter 12B); (3) impaired visuospatial and visuomotor skills (overlapping with children with motor skills disorders), with verbal IQ better than performance IQ; (4) dyscalculia; (5) neurological signs on the left side of the body; (6) ADHD; and (7) marked slowness of performance. Deficits in visual-perceptual-organizational psychomotor coordination and complex tactile-perceptual skills appear to be most representative (in the sense of most discriminative) in NVLD syndrome compared with normal children and to those with other types of LDs.

Evaluation and Etiology

The neuropathological sign most often associated with NVLDs is white matter abnormalities that result in cerebral disconnection.

Treatment

Treatments suggested for those with NVLD include the following:

Observe the child closely in novel or complex situations.
Teach the child in a systematic, step-by-step way.
Encourage detailed descriptions of important events.
Teach appropriate strategies for troublesome, frequently occurring situations.
Encourage the generalization of learned strategies.
Teach the child to use his or her verbal skills appropriately.
Teach the child to make better use of his or her visual-perceptual-organizational skills.
Teach the child to interpret visual information when there is competing auditory information.
Teach the child appropriate nonverbal behavior to facilitate structured peer interactions.
Promote, encourage, and monitor systematic exploratory activities.
Teach the older child how to use available aids in reaching a specific goal to help the child gain insight into easy and troublesome situations.

DYSCALCULIA

Diagnosis

The prevalence of dyscalculia in general is approximately 6% (similar to that of dyslexia and ADHD). Both genders are affected equally. A developmental Gerstmann's syndrome (right-left disorientation, finger agnosia, dysgraphia, and dyscalculia) is said to occur in as many as 2% of school-aged children. Dyscalculia is also seen in children with NVLD. The mean IQ of children with dyscalculia is generally normal; one-fourth show symptoms of ADHD, and approximately one-fifth show symptoms of dyslexia. In one cohort, almost one-half had first-degree relatives with LDs.

Evaluation and Etiology

To study the link between arithmetic dysfunction and brain laterality, subjects were tested on a standardized arithmetic battery and underwent a neurological and neuropsychological evaluation. A diagnosis of left hemisphere dysfunction in 13 subjects was based on right-sided soft neurological signs, performance IQ greater than verbal IQ, dyslexia, and intact visuospatial functions. Criteria for right hemisphere dysfunction in 12 subjects were left body signs, verbal IQ greater than performance IQ, impaired visuospatial functions, and normal language skills. Both groups scored more than 2 standard deviations below the mean adjusted score on the arithmetic battery, but the left hemisphere dysfunction group was significantly worse in addition, subtraction, complex multiplication, and division and made more visuospatial errors.

Treatment

Math remediation is appropriate for the child with isolated difficulties or with math difficulties in combination with other learning difficulties.

ATTENTION-DEFICIT HYPERACTIVITY DISORDER

Diagnosis

The reported prevalence of ADHD in school-aged children ranges from 1% to 20%. This wide range reflects the lack of a biological marker for the disorder. The variation in prevalence is secondary to differing technique of ascertainment: parent, child, or teacher perspective; which diagnostic questionnaire was used; age at ascertainment (standards are most clear-cut for the elementary school–aged child); and even country of study (e.g., there is more ADHD in the United States than in the United Kingdom). Although complete recovery from ADHD used to be expected, it now appears that ADHD persists in 60–70% of adults who were so diagnosed in childhood (Table 67.6). Significant social-emotional difficulties in adulthood occur in 40–50%. Serious psychiatric or antisocial disabilities occur in 10%. Assuming a prevalence of childhood ADHD of 6–10% and using one-third of 6% as a minimum figure and two-thirds of 10% as a

Table 67.6: Criteria for diagnosis of attention-deficit hyperactivity disorder (ADHD)

ADHD with hyperactivity, impulsiveness
Fidgets with hands or feet
Leaves seat in classroom
Runs about or climbs excessively
Has difficulty playing quietly
Often on the go
Talks excessively
Blurts out answers
Difficulty awaiting turn
Interrupts others
ADHD with inattention, distractibility
Has difficulty sustaining attention
Does not give close attention to details
Does not seem to listen
Does not follow through
Has difficulty organizing tasks
Avoids engaging in tasks requiring sustained mental effort
Easily distracted
Forgetful in daily activities

Source: Modified with permission from Diagnostic and Statistical Manual of Mental Disorders, 4th ed. Washington, DC: American Psychiatric Association, 1994.

maximum figure, the prevalence of ADHD in adults may be 2–7%. ADHD can also be diagnosed in the toddler. It may be as much as 4–8 times more common in males. When affected, females have less hyperactivity and more severe general cognitive deficits, which suggests that females manifesting ADHD may do so on account of a greater genetic load.

Clinical Features

Practically speaking, ADHD is defined by inappropriate inattention, impulsivity, distractibility, and hyperactivity for chronological and mental age. Table 67.6 delineates the *Diagnostic and Statistical Manual of Mental Disorders*, 4th edition, criteria for diagnosis, the current gold standard. The preschooler with ADHD may be differently diagnosed (Table 67.7). The physical examination of the ADHD child is generally normal, albeit with soft signs (Table 67.8). Especially common features on the neurological examination are synkinesis and choreiform movements when arms are extended. The neuropsychological profile reveals normal IQ but low scores on the Wechsler IQ subtests that demand attention or rapid processing: digit span, coding, arithmetic, and symbol search. Measures of executive-frontal lobe functioning, tapping the ability to initiate, inhibit, sustain, and shift attention, are often compromised.

Evaluation and Etiology

Although many causes of ADHD exist, it is most frequently genetic. Approximately one-fourth of the first-degree relatives of a child proband with ADHD also have or have had

Table 67.7: Signs of preschool attention-deficit hyperactivity disorder

High activity
Poor persistence
Group instruction problems
Poor behavior modulation
Poor social interactions
Excessive aggression
Silliness
Bossiness
Impulsiveness
"Immature," not on task
Inappropriate behavior
Unproductive

ADHD, generally the father or maternal uncle. As many as 10% of ADHD children probably carry the Tourette gene but may not have tics. Girls with the Tourette gene more often have obsessive-compulsive disorder, whereas boys have ADHD and tics. Metabolic studies suggest dysfunction of frontal lobes and the right-sided prefrontal-striatal systems, whereas imaging studies suggest atypical asymmetry patterns in the basal ganglia. Dopaminergic dysfunction appears to be the biochemical basis of ADHD.

Treatment

Medication, in particular stimulants, is the mainstay of treatment (Table 67.9). Attention must also be given to par-

Table 67.8: Natural history of soft signs

Neurological system affected	Soft sign	Age of appearance or disappearance (yrs)
Cranial nerves	Head does not move with eyes	6–7
	Sticks tongue out for 10 secs	6–7
Motor	Toe-heel walk	3
	Heel walk without associated movements	5
	Hop 10 times	5
	Hops indefinitely	7
	One-foot stand for 30 secs	7
	No longer drifts up and down with pronated and supinated arms	3–4
	Rigid tripod	5
	Dynamic tripod	7–8
	Choreiform movements	7–10
	Athetoid movements	2–4
Cerebellar	Tandem	6
	No overflow during rapid alternating movements	7–8
Sensory	Stereoagnosis, graphesthesia	6
	No longer extinguishes on double simultaneous stimulation	8

Table 67.9: Treatment of attention-deficit hyperactivity disorder

Stimulants	Methylphenidate (Ritalin), dextroamphetamine (Dexedrine, Adderal), pemoline (Cylert)
Alpha agonists	Clonidine (Catapres), guanfacine (Tenex)
Antidepressants	Selective serotonin reuptake inhibitors; tricyclic antidepressants; bupropion (Wellbutrin); trazodone, venlafaxine (Effexor); monoamine oxidase, selegiline (Deprenyl)
Antimanic	Lithium
Mood stabilizers	Carbamazepine (Tegretol), divalproex sodium (Depakote)
Beta blockers	Propranolol (Inderal), atenolol (Tenormin)
Antianxiolytic	Buspirone (BuSpar); clonazepam (Klonopin)
Neuroleptics	Haloperidol decanoate (Haldol); risperidone (Risperdal); phenothiazines

ent skills training, educational supplementation, cognitive behavioral therapy, social skills training, and behavioral modification. (Behavioral modification requires setting goals, defining progress, and determining the incentives.) Approximately 60–75% of children respond to stimulants. In 5–10%, side effects limit treatment (failure to thrive, rebound or afternoon depression, tics). A placebo response probably occurs in approximately 20%. Treatment is often affected by comorbid issues. Many of the medications now used alone or in conjunction with stimulants may mitigate comorbid depression or manic mood disorders (Milberger et al. 1995).

REFERENCES

Hagberg B, Hagberg G, Olow I, van Wendt L. The changing panorama of cerebral palsy in Sweden. VII. Prevalence and origin in the birth year period 1987–90. Acta Paediatr 1996;85:954–960.

Hodgson S. The genetics of learning disabilities/mental retardation. Dev Med Child Neurol 1998;40:137–141.

Milberger S, Biederman J, Faraone SV, et al. Attention deficit hyperactivity disorder and comorbid disorders: issues of overlapping symptoms. Am J Psychiatry 1995;152:1793–1799.

Nass R. Over and Under-Diagnosis, Over and Under-Sophistication, Over and Under-Treatment. In B Shapiro, P Accardo, A Capute (eds), Specific Reading Disability: A View of the Spectrum. Timonium, MD: York, 1998.

Rapin I. Autism. New Engl J Med 1997;337:97–104.

Shaywitz SE. Dyslexia. N Engl J Med 1998;338:307–312.

Skudlarski P, Fletcher J, Katz L, et al. Functional imaging in dyslexia. Proc Natl Acad Sci USA 1998;95:2636–2641.

Strauss DJ, Shavelle RM, Anderson TW. Life expectancy of children with cerebral palsy. Pediatr Neurol 1998;18:143–149.

Tuchman RF, Rapin I. Regression in pervasive developmental disorders: seizures and epileptiform electroencephalogram correlates. Pediatrics 1997;99:560–566.

Waterhouse L, Morris R, Allen D, et al. Diagnosis and classification in autism. J Autism Dev Disord 1996;26:59–86.

Chapter 68
Inborn Errors of Metabolism of the Nervous System

Section Editor
Owen B. Evans

Owen B. Evans, Colette C. Parker, Richard H. Haas, Sakkubai Naidu, Hugo W. Moser, and Hans-Georg O. Bock

Inborn errors of metabolism are inherited diseases that cause abnormalities in the production, synthesis, or catabolism of the cell's metabolic substrates, proteins, or structural constituents. Most inborn errors of metabolism are inherited as autosomal recessive or X-linked traits and are the result of an enzyme defect. Clinical disease usually is caused by the accumulation or deficiency of some metabolites. Some autosomal dominant and X-linked disorders are caused by relative enzyme deficiencies; others are caused by defective structural proteins. Many of these diseases cause neurological impairment.

Although individual metabolic diseases are relatively rare, collectively their prevalence is such that most physicians encounter affected patients. Most of these diseases are diagnosed by relatively simple laboratory tests, even in the neonate. Knowledge of these diseases and an accurate diagnosis are necessary for genetic counseling, heterozygote detection, and prenatal diagnosis. Many of these diseases are treatable.

Metabolic diseases of the nervous system have four major presentations: (1) acute neonatal encephalopathy; (2) recurrent metabolic encephalopathy; (3) mental retardation of unknown cause; and (4) progressive neurological signs, such as dementia, motor impairment, and seizures. Genetic variation is an important feature of these disorders. Variation in

the nature or severity of disease may occur in patients with identical mutant genes. This is especially true for dominantly inherited diseases in which some family members, known to carry the mutant gene, appear unaffected. Diseases transmitted by mitochondrial deoxyribonucleic acid (mDNA) vary considerably in clinical severity, target organ involvement, and age at onset. Although most metabolic diseases have their onset during childhood, many first develop clinical features after the first decade. Some diseases result in early death, but many children survive well into adulthood, and their diseases often go undiagnosed.

The authoritative text on inborn errors of metabolism is almost 5,000 pages in three volumes (Scriver et al. 1995). Each year, additional diseases are discovered or an old disease is reclassified based on the determination of the enzymatic defect. Any review on the subject is outdated by the time of publication. In addition, developments in molecular genetics are rapidly improving our understanding of these diseases, yielding new methods for detection, diagnosis, and treatment. The most up-to-date source of information on all genetic diseases is Online Mendelian Inheritance in Man. This chapter reviews current knowledge of major metabolic disorders without attempting to define the many minor variants.

The inborn errors of metabolism affecting the nervous system can be divided into (1) metabolic encephalopathies that

Table 68.1:   Common laboratory abnormalities of the inborn errors of metabolism

Disorder or enzyme deficiency	Hypoglycemia	Hyperammonemia	Metabolic acidosis	Renal tubular acidosis	Ketosis
Amino acids					
Phenylketonuria	–	–	–	–	–
Tyrosinemia	+	+	–	–	+
Maple syrup urine disease	+	–	+	–	+
Lysine intolerance	–	+	–	–	–
Organic acidosis					
Branched-chain ketoacid disorders	+/–	+/–	+	–	+
Glutaric acidemia	+	+/–	+	–	+
5-Oxoprolinemia	–	–	+	–	–
Propionic acidemia	+/–	+	+	–	+
Methylmalonic acidemia	+/–	+	+	–	+
Multiple carboxylase deficiency	+/–	+	+	–	+
Carnitine deficiency	+	+	+	–	–
Pyruvate metabolism					
Pyruvate dehydrogenase deficiency	–	–	+	–	–
Pyruvate carboxylase deficiency	+	+/–	+	–	+
Mitochondrial disorders	+/–	–	+	+/–	+/–
Galactosemia sugar metabolism	+/–	–	+	+	–
Hereditary fructose intolerance	+	–	+	+	–
Fructose-1,6-diphosphatase	+	–	+	–	+
Glycogen storage diseases I, III	+	–	+	–	+/–

+ = usually present; – = usually absent; +/– = variable.

impair neuronal function because of excessive production of toxic intermediary metabolites, (2) lysosomal storage diseases that cause cell injury because of excessive accumulation of material within cells, (3) diseases of the mitochondria and oxidative metabolism, and (4) peroxisomal disorders.

METABOLIC ENCEPHALOPATHIES

Metabolic encephalopathies are caused by enzyme deficiencies that block metabolic pathways. The results are (1) an impairment of subsequent substrate production, (2) excessive production of intermediary metabolites proximal to the metabolic blockage, and (3) excessive production of metabolites of alternative pathways. The injury to the nervous system is caused by a direct toxic effect of the accumulated metabolites; deficiency of essential substrates; or a disturbance of the internal milieu caused by severe acidosis, hyperammonemia, hypoglycemia, or other metabolic derangement. These secondary metabolic disorders are valuable clues for the rapid detection of many metabolic diseases (Table 68.1).

The initial symptoms are often that of a newborn encephalopathy with altered consciousness and seizures. Typically, the onset begins after dietary exposure to an unmetabolizable substrate. Unlike syndromes associated with chromosomal abnormalities, these infants need not have distinctive dysmorphic features, but some have unusual facies or cerebral malformations, or both. Another common presentation is episodic encephalopathy, with vomiting,

altered consciousness, or ataxia. Less common is a chronic progressive or chronic static course. These disorders differ from the lysosomal storage diseases in that they lack distinctive neurological or physical features that help in clinical diagnosis. Some patients have an unusual odor (Table 68.2).

A diagnosis of metabolic disease caused by an inborn error of metabolism requires a high index of suspicion. Initial tests should include screening of arterial blood gases, blood ammonia, lactate, glucose, and electrolytes for calibration of the anion gap. These studies offer clues to the underlying primary defect (see Table 68.1) and direct subsequent diagnostic evaluation, such as quantitative plasma amino acid analysis, urine organic acid and sugar analysis, enzyme assays, and DNA analysis. More important, these screening tests allow for refinement of the therapy for severe metabolic disturbances. The importance of early diagnosis cannot be overemphasized because rapid initiation of appropriate therapy often can avert a poor neurological outcome and death.

Disorders of Phenylalanine Metabolism

Disorders of phenylalanine metabolism cause accumulation of phenylalanine, phenylpyruvate, and its metabolites. The normal phenylalanine plasma concentration is 1.0–2.0 mg/dl. Neonatal screening programs detect children with hyperphenylalaninemia (Table 68.3). Two-thirds of such children have classic phenylketonuria (PKU) caused by phenylalanine hydroxylase deficiency, and most

Table 68.2: Unusual odors of metabolic diseases

Odor	Disease or enzyme deficiency
Sweaty feet	Glutaric acidemia type II
	Isovaleric acidemia
Tomcat urine	3-Methylcrotonyl-CoA carboxylase
	Multiple carboxylase deficiency
Maple syrup	Maple syrup urine disease
Musty	Phenylketonuria
Rotten cabbage	Tyrosinemia
	Methionine malabsorption
Rotten fish	Trimethylaminuria
Fermentation	Methionine malabsorption

CoA = coenzyme A.

of the remainder have benign non-PKU hyperphenylalaninemia. Approximately 2% of patients with hyperphenylalaninemia have a defect in the generation or recycling of tetrahydrobiopterin, a necessary cofactor for the phenylalanine hydroxylase reaction. An early, precise diagnosis is important because early dietary restriction of phenylalanine prevents the severe complications of classic PKU. Dietary restriction normalizes the plasma phenylalanine in patients with the cofactor deficiency, but does not prevent neurological deterioration unless other therapies are instituted.

Phenylketonuria

Pathophysiology. PKU is the result of impaired conversion of phenylalanine to tyrosine. The deficient enzyme is phenylalanine hydroxylase, for which the gene is located at 12q.24.1. It is an hepatic enzyme and requires tetrahydrobiopterin as a cofactor (Figure 68.1). With deficient enzyme activity, phenylalanine accumulates and is transaminated to phenylpyruvate, which in turn is converted to phenyllactate and phenylacetate. These latter metabolites are the phenylketones that are excreted in the urine.

Classic PKU is an autosomal recessive disorder caused by the almost complete absence of phenylalanine hydroxylase.

Multiple mutant alleles for the phenylalanine hydroxylase enzyme exist. Different combinations of these alleles are responsible for the clinical heterogeneity of classic PKU (Svensson et al. 1993). The incidence of PKU is approximately 1 in 15,000 live births in the United States.

The major impact of PKU is on the developing central nervous system (CNS). The neurological signs of the disease are caused by the toxicity of high concentrations of phenylalanine. The hyperphenylalaninemia adversely affects myelination and cognitive development. Dysmyelination is present even in patients who are treated early and managed carefully (Scriver et al. 1995). Possible pathogenic mechanisms are impaired amino acid transport across the blood-brain barrier, defective proteolipid synthesis, and altered neurotransmitter metabolism.

All 50 states have mandatory screening for PKU, which measures the accumulation of phenylalanine in the blood. For the test to be accurate, the infant should be on protein feedings for at least 24 hours. The two most commonly used screening tests are Guthrie's test (a bacterial inhibition assay) and fluorometric determinations of phenylalanine. False-positive and false-negative results are possible. Infants with positive screening test results must have quantitative measurements of phenylalanine. Tyrosine, urine pterins, and dihydropteridine reductase also must be measured in any child with a positive screening test result, because disorders of tyrosine and pterin metabolism also cause elevations of phenylalanine concentrations. A differential diagnosis for a positive neonatal phenylalanine screening test result is listed in Table 68.3.

Clinical Features. Untreated children with classic PKU are normal at birth and present at 2 months or later with early nonspecific signs of developmental delay. Some have persistent vomiting. After the first year of life, neurological deterioration is the primary clinical feature; most untreated children have an IQ of less than 50. Approximately 2% of patients with PKU have normal intelligence without receiving nutritional therapy. Agitated or aggressive behavior, tremor or other movement disorders, hyper-

Table 68.3: Differential diagnosis of hyperphenylalaninemia in the newborn

Disorder	Etiology	Phenylalanine	Tyrosine (mg/dl)
Phenylketonuria			
Classic phenylketonuria	Phenylalanine hydroxylase <1% residual activity	>20 mg/dl	<5
Benign variants	Phenylalanine hydroxylase 2–35% residual activity	4–20 mg/dl	<5
Malignant variants	Dihydropteridine reductase deficiency	Variable, may be >20 mg/dl	<5
	6-Pyruvoyltetrahydrobiopterin synthetase deficiency	Variable, may be >20 mg/dl	<5
	Guanosine triphosphate cyclohydrolase deficiency	Variable, may be >20 mg/dl	<5
Tyrosinemia			
Tyrosinosis I	Fumarylacetoacetate hydrolase deficiency	Elevated in acute stage	3–12
Tyrosinosis II	Tyrosine aminotransferase deficiency	Normal	15–50
Transitory neonatal tyrosinemia	Unknown	Less than tyrosine level	3–30

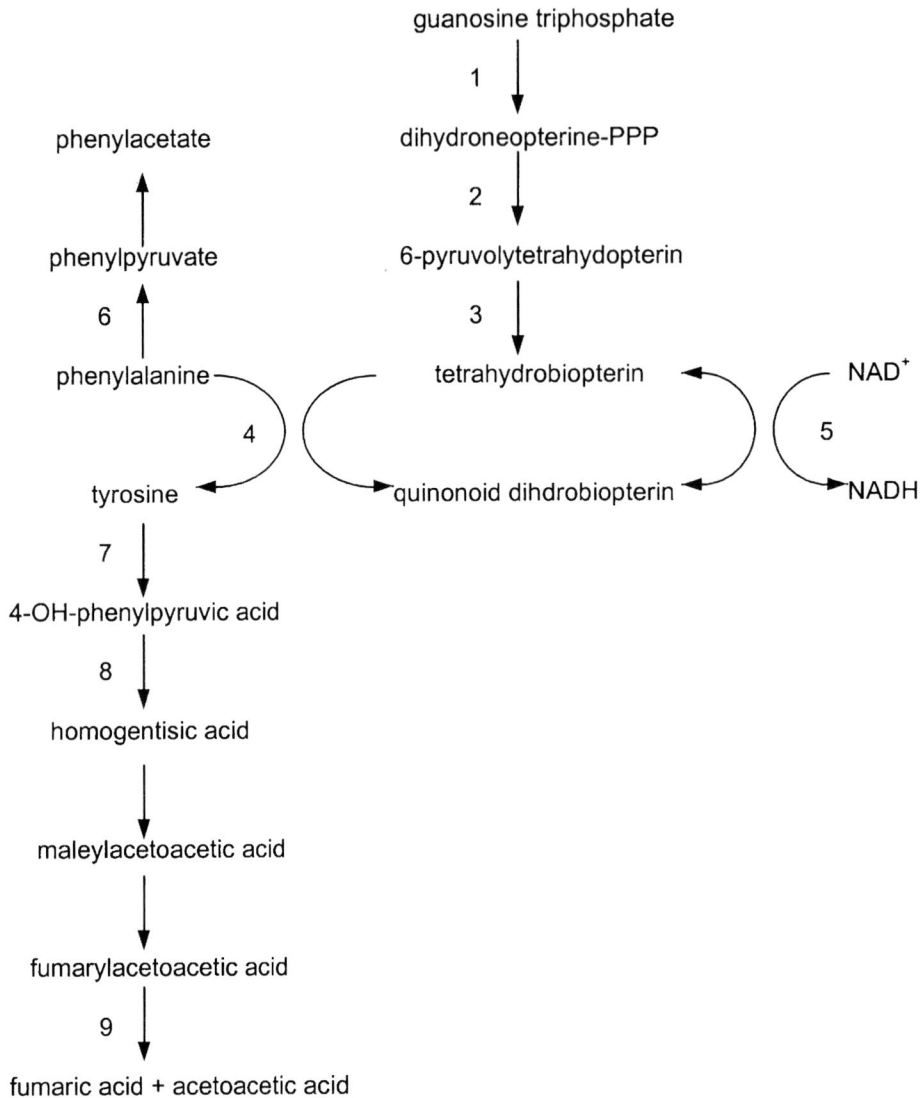

FIGURE 68.1 Phenylalanine and tyrosine metabolism. (1) Guanosine triphosphate cyclohydrolase. (2) 6-Pyruvoyltetrahydrobiopterin synthetase. (3) Sepiapterin reductase. (4) Phenylalanine hydroxylase. (5) Dihydropteridine reductase. (6) Phenylalanine transaminase. (7) Tyrosine transaminase. (8) 4-Hydroxyphenylpyruvic acid dioxygenase. (9) Fumarylacetoacetic acid hydrolase. (NAD = nicotinamide adenine dinucleotide; NADH = NAD reduced; PPP = triphosphate.)

tonia or spasticity, and hyperactivity are present to a greater or lesser degree in every child. Some infants have infantile spasms, and generalized tonic-clonic seizures may occur later in childhood. The skin is usually dry or eczematoid, and the child may have a musty odor caused by the excreted phenylacetate. Small stature, microcephaly, and hypopigmentation (blond hair, blue eyes) are common.

Diagnosis. Untreated PKU should be considered in children with mental retardation. The urine ferric chloride assay is not an adequate test; the diagnosis is made on the basis of the quantitative measurement of phenylalanine and

tyrosine in the blood. A phenylalanine concentration of greater than 20 mg/dl with a normal or reduced tyrosine concentration and urinary excretion of phenylketones is diagnostic of classic PKU. Inability to tolerate a phenylalanine challenge and normal tetrahydrobiopterin concentrations and metabolism differentiate classic PKU from the PKU variants. Prenatal diagnosis is possible.

Treatment. The treatment for classic PKU is the selective restriction of dietary phenylalanine so that plasma phenylalanine concentrations are maintained in the near normal range (4–6 mg/dl). Initiation of dietary therapy by 3 weeks of age prevents severe, irreversible brain damage. Dietary therapy is complicated. Frequent clinical, biochemical, and nutritional evaluations are necessary. Careful, timely adjustment of the dietary intake is required. Nutritional management demands a drastic restriction of all natural protein intake and uses an appropriate mixture of special dietary and natural, low-protein food products. The goal is to provide a complete diet that fulfills the phenylalanine requirements for normal growth and development while avoiding all significant nutrient deficiencies. Aspartame, a synthetic sweetener that is converted to phenylalanine, should be avoided by patients with PKU. Inappropriate nutritional management can result in mental retardation, growth failure, or death. The management is best undertaken and administered by physicians and nutritionists with experience in treating patients with hyperphenylalaninemia. Although treated patients can have normal intelligence, some have behavioral problems, learning disabilities, and attention deficits. Despite these disabilities, most PKU-treated adults generally function well.

When to terminate the diet remains an unresolved question. Children with classic PKU may develop intellectual and behavioral deterioration after dietary relaxation. This is true especially if the off-diet blood phenylalanine level is greater than 18 mg/dl. The mechanism for this late decline is unknown, but may be related to the effects that high phenylalanine concentration has on neurotransmitter concentration and metabolism. Cognitive impairment is at least partially reversible after reinstituting the diet. Continuation of a moderate degree of dietary protein restriction may result in better school performance, behavior, and attention. The ultimate prognosis for intelligence is related directly to how early nutritional management is initiated, the degree of dietary compliance, and how long nutritional management is maintained. It generally is recommended that nutritional management be continued at least through adolescence and preferably indefinitely.

Maternal Hyperphenylalaninemia

Infants born to mothers who have hyperphenylalaninemia are at increased risk for microcephaly, mental retardation, and congenital malformations despite the fact that the infant's enzyme activity is half of normal. Damage to the fetus is related directly to the mother's phenylalanine blood concentration. Strict maintenance of maternal phenylalanine blood concentrations near 4–6 mg/dl before conception and during pregnancy can prevent many of the complications. Hyperphenylalaninemic women are encouraged to maintain nutritional therapy at least through their childbearing years.

Phenylketonuria Variants

Benign Hyperphenylalaninemia. The non-PKU benign hyperphenylalaninemic variants are caused by partial phenylalanine hydroxylase deficiency (residual activity

2–35% of control) and transitory hydroxylase deficiency (see Table 68.3). These patients are detected on neonatal screening and have blood phenylalanine concentrations of less than 20 mg/dl and normal tyrosine levels. The outcome is usually good, even without initiation of a phenylalanine-restricted diet. The dietary phenylalanine should be restricted when phenylalanine exceeds a concentration of 12 mg/dl in the blood. Children with transitory phenylalanine hydroxylase deficiency later are less sensitive to dietary phenylalanine intake, whereas children with classic PKU always have phenylalaninemia of greater than 20 mg/dl on unrestricted protein intake.

Malignant Hyperphenylalaninemia. The malignant hyperphenylalaninemia variants are caused by disorders known as the pterin defects and are responsible for 1–3% of cases of hyperphenylalaninemia. They are caused by disorders in the metabolism of tetrahydrobiopterin, a cofactor for phenylalanine hydroxylase, tyrosine hydroxylase, and tryptophan hydroxylase (see Figure 68.1). The disorders are dihydropteridine reductase (DHPR) deficiency, 6-pyruvoyltetrahydropterin synthase (6-PTS) deficiency, and guanosine triphosphate cyclohydrolase I deficiency. Their initial features can resemble classic PKU, mild hyperphenylalaninemia, or show hypotonia and inactivity in the neonatal period. Progression to mental retardation, seizures, myoclonus, and motor impairment occurs even after initiation of a phenylalanine-restricted diet. A less severe form of guanosine triphosphate cyclohydrolase I deficiency has been reported in an adult who had a slowly progressive course since childhood. Severe disturbances in neurotransmitter metabolism are thought to play a major role in the pathogenesis.

Early detection and differentiation from classic PKU are essential. Finding a marked increase in the urine ratio of neopterin to biopterin suggests a defect in 6-PTS, whereas a low tetrahydrobiopterin concentration is more consistent with DHPR deficiency. Administration of tetrahydrobiopterin consistently lowers blood phenylalanine concentrations in these patients. DHPR should be assayed. The other enzymes can be measured as indicated.

Therapy with tetrahydrobiopterin for the 6-PTS deficiency and with folinic acid for the DHPR deficiency, together with dietary phenylalanine restriction and the administration of L-dopa, carbidopa, and 5-hydroxytryptophan has been effective in some of these patients.

Disorders of Tyrosine Metabolism

Hereditary Tyrosinemia

Pathophysiology. Tyrosinemia type I, or hepatorenal tyrosinemia, is transmitted by autosomal recessive inheritance. It is characterized by a defect in fumarylacetoacetate hydrolase. The disease is characterized by severe hepatocellular destruction and a renal tubular Fanconi's syndrome (Mitchell et al. 1995). The accumulation of succinylacetone inhibits δ-aminolevulinic acid dehydratase and causes episodic features of acute intermittent porphyria.

Clinical Features. The clinical presentation and course vary. The acute early infantile form is characterized by vomiting, diarrhea, failure to thrive, bleeding, jaundice, and hepatomegaly. It progresses rapidly to overwhelming liver failure, coma, and death. A cabbagelike odor may be noted. Children with the more chronic form of hereditary tyrosinemia type I have a later onset of hepatic disease and Fanconi's syndrome, with glycosuria, proteinuria, generalized aminoaciduria, and hypophosphatemic rickets. Severe, chronic liver disease, with hepatic cirrhosis and portal hypertension, progresses to hepatic failure and death, usually within the first two decades. The episodic porphyric complication is a significant source of morbidity and mortality for these patients. Hypoglycemia and hypertensive crisis can be additional problems. Many children with the chronic form of the disease develop hepatocarcinoma.

Diagnosis. Hereditary tyrosinemia type I should be suspected in neonates with acute metabolic encephalopathy and liver failure, and in older children with chronic liver and renal disease. The blood concentration of α-fetoprotein is increased markedly. Plasma concentrations of tyrosine are in the 3–12 mg/dl range (normal is <1 mg/dl). Plasma methionine frequently is increased, whereas plasma phenylalanine concentrations are usually not elevated. Tyrosine, tyrosine metabolites, other amino acids, and δ-aminolevulinic acid are elevated in the urine. The finding of elevated concentrations of succinylacetone in blood or urine in this setting is virtually diagnostic. Enzyme assay documents fumarylacetoacetate hydrolase deficiency. Other enzyme deficiencies reported in patients with this disorder probably represent secondary events. Prenatal diagnosis is possible.

Treatment. The use of phenylalanine- and tyrosine-restricted diet is beneficial but does not stop the progression of the hepatic and renal disease. Liver transplantation provides effective treatment, but is associated with substantial risk for morbidity and mortality. In addition, renal function and some metabolic parameters do not normalize completely. An alternative therapy currently under evaluation in patients with hereditary tyrosinemia type I is the use of 2-(2-nitro-4-trifluoromethylbenzoyl)-1,3-cyclohexanedione, an inhibitor of 4-hydroxyphenylpyruvate dioxygenase according to Lindstedt and colleagues in 1992.

Other Disorders of Tyrosine Metabolism

Tyrosinemia type II, also called *oculocutaneous tyrosinemia* or *Richner-Hanhart syndrome*, is mainly a dermatological disorder caused by a deficiency of hepatic cytosolic tyrosine aminotransferase. Plasma and urine tyrosine concentrations are elevated, but other amino acids and routine laboratory study results are normal. Because tyrosine has limited solubility, it crystallizes within tissues and initiates an inflammatory response. This causes corneal, palmar, and plantar erosions and plaques with secondary hyperkeratosis, which are apparent in infancy. Neurological involvement is inconstant and includes developmental delay, mild to moderate mental retardation, self-mutilating behavior, impaired coordination, and language defects. The disorder is transmitted as an autosomal recessive trait. Treatment with a low-phenylalanine and low-tyrosine diet is therapeutic.

Transient neonatal tyrosinemia is a benign disorder found on routine neonatal screening for hyperphenylalaninemia. It occurs more commonly in premature infants on high-protein diets. Delayed maturation of the hepatic enzyme 4-hydroxyphenylpyruvate dioxygenase is the likely cause. There have been rare reports of mental retardation in children who had neonatal tyrosinemia. Dietary protein restriction to less than 3 g/kg per day and supplementation with ascorbic acid (50–200 mg/day) effectively lowers blood tyrosine and phenylalanine concentrations.

Elevations of blood tyrosine and other tyrosine metabolites occur in people with defective metabolism of 4-hydroxyphenylpyruvate caused by 4-hydroxyphenylpyruvic acid dioxygenase deficiency. These individuals may be normal or present early in life with failure to thrive, microcephaly, chronic metabolic acidosis, and unusual body odor ("swimming pool" odor). The neurological signs are variable and include mental retardation, seizures, ataxia, and a myasthenic syndrome. The acidosis and neurological signs are exacerbated by high protein intake. A diet restricted in phenylalanine and tyrosine may be beneficial, as may be ascorbate supplementation. This appears to be transmitted as an autosomal dominant trait.

Chédiak-Higashi disease is a rare autosomal recessive inherited disorder characterized by tyrosinase-positive oculocutaneous albinism, nystagmus, cerebellar and long-tract signs, mental retardation, and a progressive polyneuropathy. There is neutrophil dysfunction, with decreased bactericidal killing, whereas phagocytosis is preserved. In addition to the neutrophil dysfunction, there is neutropenia, with increased susceptibility to infections, anemia, abnormal platelet function, bleeding, and eventual lymphoreticular malignancy. Death usually occurs before age 10 years, although cases of milder disease have been reported. Giant cytoplasmic inclusions in neutrophils and neurons are characteristic. The absence of an obvious oculocutaneous defect or an apparent predisposition to infections does not preclude this diagnosis. Bone marrow transplantation may be beneficial.

Disorders of Sulfur Amino Acid Metabolites

Homocystinuria

Pathophysiology. Type I (classic) homocystinuria is the major disorder of the sulfur-containing amino acids affecting the nervous system. Homocysteine is catabolized by the remethylation cycle to methionine or the transsulfuration pathway to cystathione (Figure 68.2). A deficiency of cystathionine synthase in the transsulfuration pathway causes homocystinuria with accumulation of several sulfur-containing metabolites, including homocysteine and homocystine, homocysteine-cysteine mixed disulfide, and methionine in the blood, urine, and cerebrospinal fluid (CSF). It is transmitted as an autosomal recessive trait; the incidence of the disease in the United States is 0.5–1.0 in 100,000. Approximately 40% of patients with classic homocystinuria respond to pyridoxine. Other disorders of sulfur amino acid metabolism are summarized in Table 68.4.

High plasma homocysteine concentrations adversely affect collagen metabolism and are responsible for alterations in the blood vessel walls. Intimal thickening and fibrosis cause arterial and venous thromboembolic disease. This is the main cause of neurological complications. Blood coagulation and platelet survival time also may be abnormal.

Clinical Features. Children with classic homocystinuria are normal at birth. Most of the neurological features are the result of cerebral thromboembolic disease, which also occurs in young adult heterozygotes. Homozygotes for homocystinuria are at high risk to have one or more major thrombotic events of the cerebral or other arteries beginning in early childhood. There also is an increased risk for stroke following surgery. Approximately 50% have mental retardation, and psychiatric and extrapyramidal signs are common. Cerebral vascular disease causes hemiplegia, ataxia, dystonia, aphasia, and pseudobulbar palsy. Seizures are present in approximately 20% of patients. Central retinal artery occlusion can cause optic atrophy.

The non-neurological manifestations become apparent later in childhood and include a marfanoid habitus, with arachnodactyly, in approximately one-half of the patients. Other features are pectal and foot deformities, genu valgum, osteoporosis, fractures, biconcavity of the vertebrae ("codfish" vertebrae), kyphoscoliosis, widened condyles, and metaphyseal spicules. Children may have blond, sparse, brittle hair. Many also have erythematous skin lesions on the cheeks and livedo reticularis elsewhere. Eye abnormali-

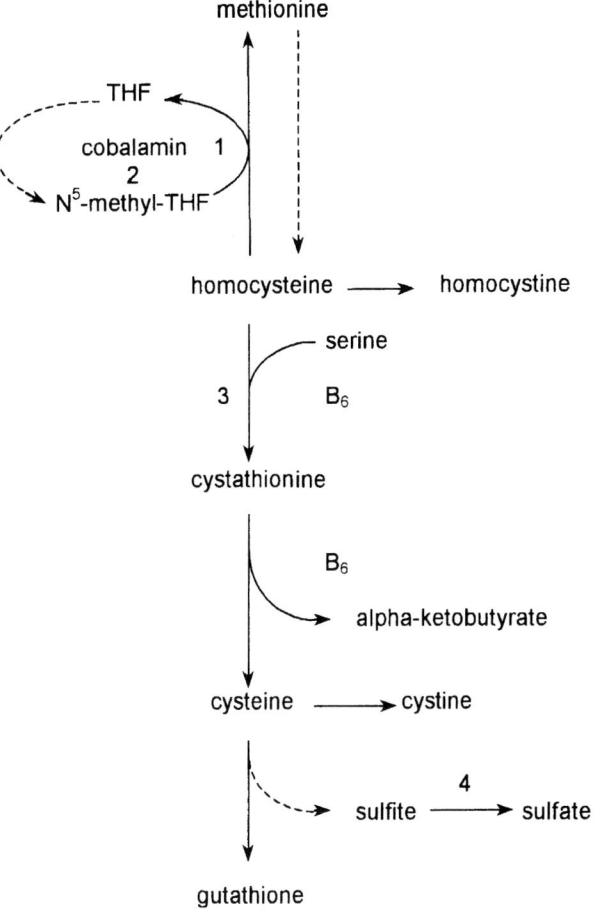

FIGURE 68.2 Sulfur amino acid metabolism. (1) *N*-5-methyl-tetrahydrofolate-homocysteine methyltransferase. (2) Formation of methylcobalamin from B_{12}. (3) Cystathionine synthase. (4) Sulfite oxidase. (THF = tetrahydrofolate.)

ties are characteristic. Typically, myopia is followed by a usually downward dislocation of the lens (*ectopia lentis*) (Figure 68.3). Glaucoma often is produced by the dislocated lens. Iridodonesis, a quivering of the iris, occurs from a lack of support of the iris. Astigmatism, cataracts, and degeneration or detachment of the retina are other possible complications.

Table 68.4: Disorders of sulfur amino acid metabolism

Disorder	Clinical features	Laboratory features
Homocystinuria I (cystathionine synthase deficiency)	Strokes, mental retardation, ectopia lentis, marfanoid habitus	Hypermethioninemia, homocystinuria, methioninuria
Homocystinuria II (defect in methylcobalamin synthesis)	Features of homocystinuria I, episodic metabolic acidosis	Homocystinuria, methylmalonic acidemia and aciduria
Homocystinuria III (defect in tetrahydrofolate metabolism)	Neonatal seizures, apnea, and coma, or later onset mental retardation, seizures, and psychiatric disturbances	Homocystinuria
Sulfite oxidase deficiency	Ectopia lentis, psychomotor retardation, ataxia, seizures	No organic sulfaturia
Oasthouse disease (methionine malabsorption)	Psychomotor retardation, fine white hair, seizures, extensor spasms, unusual odor	Increased urine excretion of α-hydroxy butyric acid; intestinal malabsorption of methionine

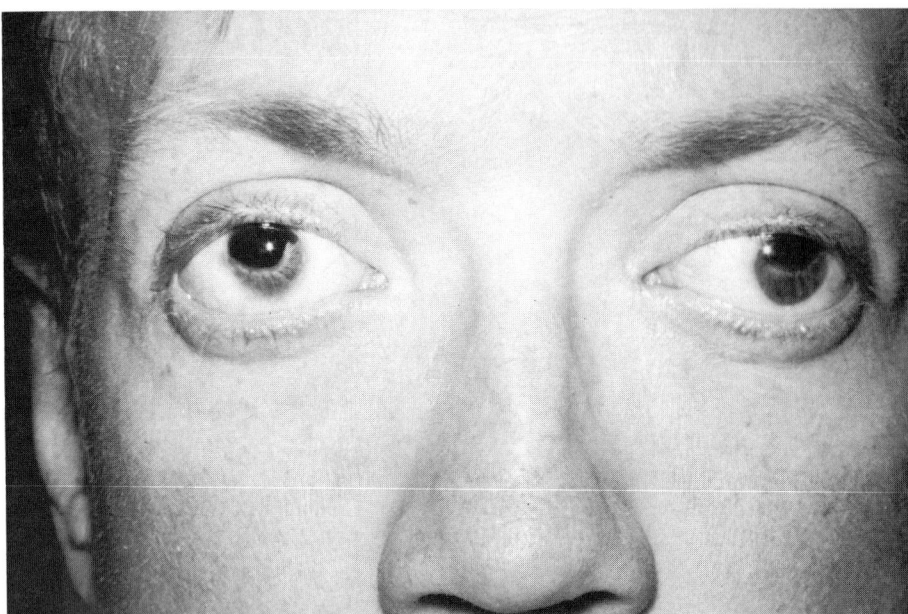

FIGURE 68.3 Ectopia lentis and iridectomy in a patient with homocystinuria.

Mild homocystinemia has been identified as an independent risk factor for atherosclerotic cardiovascular disease that causes premature coronary artery disease, stroke, and other vascular thromboses in early adulthood (Welch and Loscalzo 1998).

Diagnosis. The disease should be suspected in any child with stroke, atraumatically dislocated lenses, or mental retardation. The differential diagnosis is relatively short. Homocystinuria may be confused with Marfan's syndrome because of lens dislocation and dysmorphic features; however, the two disorders are distinguished easily by inheritance pattern, clinical course, and biochemical analysis. Mental retardation is not a typical feature of Marfan's syndrome. Quantitative analyses of blood and urine show the marked elevation of homocystine and methionine. False-negative results can occur if the patient is receiving supplementary pyridoxine. The enzyme can be measured in fibroblasts, amniocytes, and cultured cells from chorionic villi. Other disorders of sulfur amino acid metabolism are summarized in Table 68.4.

Treatment. Therapy is directed at reducing the plasma homocystine concentration. Low doses of pyridoxine (25 mg/day) may correct the biochemical abnormalities in some pyridoxine-responsive patients, but large doses of pyridoxine (250–1,000 mg/day) are required in most. A methionine-restricted diet that is supplemented with cystine benefits some patients but is not palatable, and long-term nutritional management using such restricted diets is difficult to achieve. Betaine, a methyl donor that recycles homocysteine to methionine, is recommended at a dose of 6–9 g per day for those who do not respond to pyridoxine and

do not tolerate a methionine-restricted diet. Even imperfect metabolic control seems to decrease markedly the risk for thromboembolic and other complications. Folate (5 mg/day) is recommended because of a deficiency that may occur with this disease. Aspirin and dipyridamole may help prevent thromboembolic disease. Because of an increased risk of stroke, the total homocysteine blood levels should be reduced as low as possible before any surgery. Intravenous hydration before and after surgery, the use of elastic stockings, and early postoperative physiotherapy also have been recommended to try to minimize the risk of thromboembolic events in such patients.

Disorders of Branched-Chain Amino Acid Metabolism

Maple Syrup Urine Disease

Maple syrup urine disease (MSUD) gets its name from the distinctive odor associated with patients who have this disease. It is one of several disorders of catabolism of branched-chain amino acids (BCAAs) and is transmitted by autosomal recessive inheritance. The incidence of MSUD in the United States is approximately 1 in 200,000.

Pathophysiology. The first step in the catabolism of the three BCAAs—leucine, isoleucine, and valine—is transamination to their respective branched-chain ketoacids (BCKAs) (Figure 68.4). A common BCKA dehydrogenase enzyme complex converts the BCKAs to the respective acyl–coenzyme A (CoA) metabolites. MSUD is caused by a deficiency of mitochondrial BCKA dehydrogenase. This enzyme complex is

FIGURE 68.4   Branched-chain amino acid and ketoacid metabolism. (1) Branched-chain amino acid transaminase. (2) Branched-chain ketoacid dehydrogenase. (3) 2-Methylbranched-chain acyl–coenzyme A (CoA) dehydrogenase. (4) Isovaleryl-CoA dehydrogenase. (5) 3-Methylcrotonyl-CoA carboxylase. (6) 3-Hydroxy-3-methylglutaryl-CoA lyase. (7) β-ketothiolase (mitochondrial acetoacetyl-CoA thiolase).

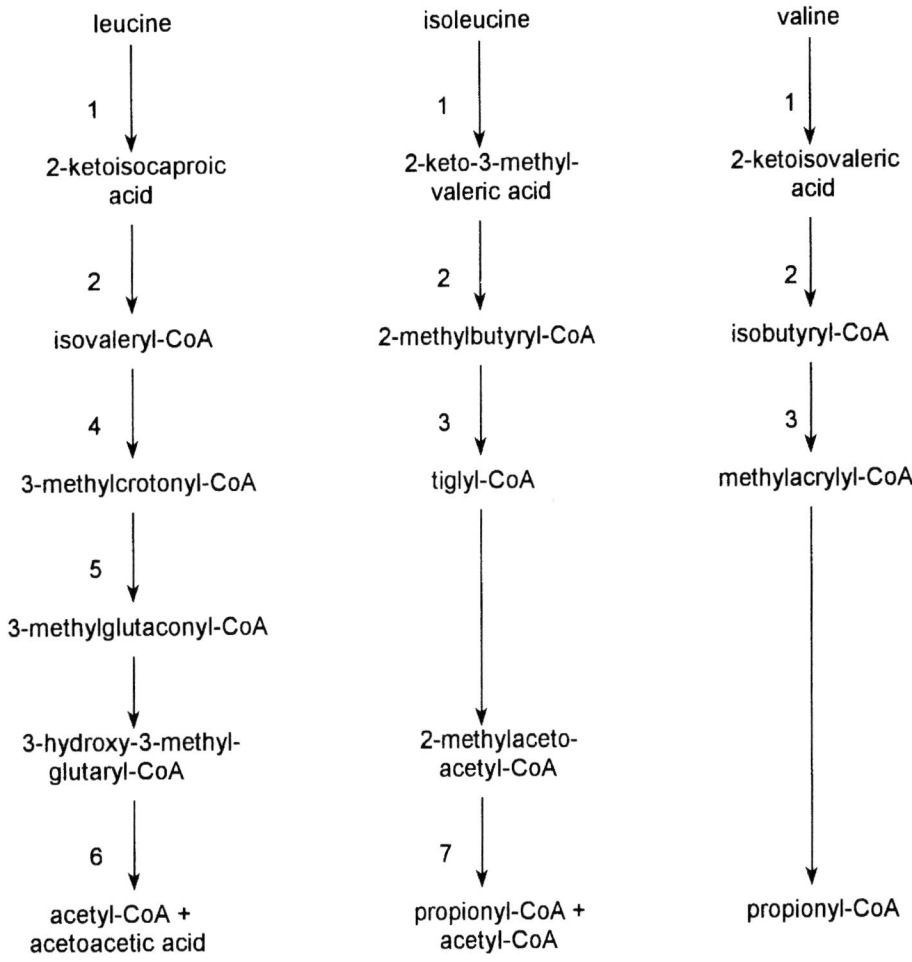

composed of six subunits and is similar to the pyruvate and alpha-ketoglutarate dehydrogenase enzyme complexes. The major abnormality in MSUD is a deficiency of the E1 subunit of BCKA dehydrogenase, but other components of the complex can be affected.

In classic MSUD, the brain has decreased myelination, heterotopias, and spongy degeneration with gliosis. The white matter abnormalities can be visualized on neuroimaging studies. Cerebral edema and encephalopathy accompany the accumulation of BCAAs and BCKAs in untreated patients during periods of metabolic stress.

Clinical Features.   Several clinical subtypes of MSUD are classified according to the nature and severity of the enzyme deficiency. Classic MSUD may present as neonatal apnea and death or as a fulminant encephalopathy after the initiation of protein feedings during the first week postpartum. Feeding difficulty, vomiting, seizures, and lethargy progressing to coma are typical. Large quantities of BCAAs and BCKAs are excreted in the urine, causing the characteristic urine odor. Alloisoleucine, an uncommon isomer of isoleucine, is present in plasma. Other metabolic features in some infants include ketoacidosis and hypoglycemia.

Untreated infants usually die, and survivors have impaired neurological function and mental retardation in proportion to the severity of the neonatal course.

Patients with the most severe type of MSUD have less than 2% of the BCKA dehydrogenase activity of controls. Those with greater residual BCKA dehydrogenase activity have milder variants of MSUD: the intermediate form, the intermittent form, and the thiamine-responsive variant.

Patients with the intermediate type of MSUD present with similar neurological manifestations, but the onset is somewhat later in infancy, again in association with a febrile illness or other catabolic state or when the protein intake becomes excessive. In the absence of vigorous early therapeutic intervention, moderate mental retardation results. Ataxia and failure to thrive are common. BCAA and BCKA concentrations always are elevated, though not as high as in the classic disease. The ketoacidosis is usually milder as well.

Children with the intermittent variant of MSUD have no neonatal complications. The onset is in early childhood, characterized by episodic encephalopathy, ataxia, and ketoacidosis. During attacks, there is excessive excretion of BCAAs and BCKAs in the urine. Permanent neurological damage and even death can occur during intervals of excessive protein

Table 68.5:   Disorders of branched-chain amino acid metabolism

Enzyme deficiency	Clinical signs
BCKA dehydrogenase	
Classic MSUD	Fulminant neonatal encephalopathy, ketoacidosis
Intermediate MSUD	Mild to moderate mental retardation, intermittent ketoacidosis, ataxia, encephalopathy
Intermittent MSUD	Intermittent ketoacidosis, ataxia, encephalopathy
Thiamine-responsive branched-chain ketoaciduria	Mild to moderate mental retardation, intermittent ketoacidosis, ataxia, encephalopathy
BCKA dihydrolipoyl transacylase	Fulminant neonatal encephalopathy
BCKA dihydrolipoyl dehydrogenase	Progressive encephalopathy, severe ketoacidosis
Valine transaminase	Mental retardation, failure to thrive
Isoleucine and leucine transaminase	Mental retardation, failure to thrive, retinal degeneration, deafness

BCKA = branched-chain ketoacid; MSUD = maple syrup urine disease.

intake or catabolic stress, such as during surgery or during a febrile illness. Between attacks, BCAA and BCKA concentrations and the neurological examination may be normal.

Thiamine is a necessary cofactor of BCKA dehydrogenase. The thiamine-responsive variant of MSUD presents primarily with moderate retardation. Elevated BCKAs and BCAAs are present in blood and urine.

Dihydrolipoyl dehydrogenase (E3) deficiency is a variant of MSUD that also causes lactic acidosis. E3 is common to the BCKA, pyruvate, and α-ketoglutarate dehydrogenase complexes. BCAAs are elevated moderately, but patients have lactic acidosis, hyperpyruvicemia, hyperalaninemia, and clinical and pathological features similar to Leigh disease (Chuang and Shih 1995).

Diagnosis.   The diagnosis of MSUD requires clinical suspicion of a metabolic disease in a child with severe neonatal encephalopathy, unexplained mental retardation, psychomotor regression, episodic encephalopathy or ataxia, or unexplained metabolic acidosis or ketonuria. Aside from the unusual odor that may be present, there are no distinguishing physical or neurological features that help with the diagnosis. A presumptive diagnosis can be made by demonstrating the presence of BCAAs in the urine by a ferric chloride test or the 2,4-dinitrophenylhydrazine test. Quantitative measurement of blood and urine BCAAs, including alloisoleucine, and BCKAs is diagnostic. Analysis of urine organic acids by gas chromatography and mass spectroscopy confirms the diagnosis. Quantitation of enzyme activity provides a definitive diagnosis and delineates the most appropriate therapy. Enzyme analysis is possible in leukocytes, cultured fibroblasts, cultured amniotic fluid cells, and chorionic villi. The enzymatic variants and the differential diagnosis of MSUD are summarized in Table 68.5.

Treatment.   During an acute episode, all natural protein intake must be discontinued immediately, and dehydration, electrolyte imbalance, and metabolic acidosis must be corrected. The provision of intravenous glucose, lipids, and BCAA-free amino acids promotes an anabolic state and is beneficial. Cerebral edema and seizures must be controlled. Hemodialysis may be necessary to correct the life-threatening metabolic acidosis. A trial of thiamine at a dose of 10–20 mg/kg per day should be conducted and to document a thiamine-responsive MSUD variant. Long-term therapy of classic and intermediate MSUD consists of the dietary restriction of natural food protein, the use of elemental nutrition products containing few or no BCAAs, and careful monitoring of growth and urine ketones. Children with residual dehydrogenase activity of 5% or greater are more likely to respond to therapy. Children diagnosed early and treated rigorously have a much better prognosis than do those diagnosed after 14 days of age or who do not adhere to therapy. Excessive restriction of dietary BCAA can cause extensive dermatological problems (Northrup et al. 1993).

Hyperglycinemia

There are two major causes for hyperglycinemia. One is an autosomal recessive inherited primary defect of glycine metabolism, glycine encephalopathy (nonketotic hyperglycinemia). The second is a group of inborn errors of metabolism that causes ketotic hyperglycinemia with severe ketoacidosis and includes propionic acidemia, methylmalonic acidemia, isovaleric acidemia, and β-ketothiolase deficiency. These latter disorders are discussed in the section on organic acidemias. Valproic acid also causes hyperglycinemia.

Glycine Encephalopathy (Nonketotic Hyperglycinemia)

Pathophysiology.   Glycine encephalopathy is caused by a defect in the metabolic pathway converting glycine to serine, the glycine cleavage system (GCS) (Tada and Kure 1993). The system is a mitochondrial enzyme complex of four proteins and requires pyridoxine, tetrahydrofolate, and lipoic acid. Serine synthesis is compromised. More important, however, glycine is increased markedly in the blood, urine, CSF, and tissue. It is hypothesized that the high glycine concentration causes excessive activation of excita-

Table 68.6:   Disorders of histidine and diaminopeptides

Disorder	Clinical features	Laboratory features
Carnosinase deficiency	Infantile encephalopathy, mixed seizures, spasticity, mental retardation	Increased carnosine in blood and urine
Imidazole aciduria	Cerebromacular degeneration	Increased urine imidazoles (metabolites of histidine)
Homocarnosinase deficiency	Spastic paraparesis and mental retardation	Increased homocarnosine in CSF
β-Alaninemia (β-alanine transaminase deficiency)	Neonatal encephalopathy, persistent seizures	Increased urine and CSF β-alanine and γ-aminobutyric acid Increased urine taurine and β-aminoisobutyric acid
Formiminoglutamic acid transferase deficiency (folic acid metabolism)	Mental retardation, behavioral disorders, anemia	Increased urine formiminoglutamic acid Normal to high folate
Prolidase deficiency	Chronic dermatitis and ulcerations of the extremities, variable mental retardation, ptosis, optic atrophy, deafness	Glycoprolinuria, iminopeptiduria

CSF = cerebrospinal fluid.

tory amino acid receptors, such as the N-methyl-D-aspartate receptors in the brain. This causes seizures and intracellular calcium accumulation with secondary calcium-activated endonuclease-mediated DNA fragmentation and neuronal death. Unlike the case of patients with ketotic hyperglycinemia, organic acids do not accumulate, and no ketoacidosis, hypoglycemia, hyperammonemia, or lactic acidosis occurs.

Clinical Features.   The most frequent clinical presentation of this heterogeneous disorder is severe neonatal encephalopathy. Patients have no detectable GCS activity. The onset begins shortly after protein feedings are initiated. The clinical course progresses rapidly, with poor feeding, lethargy, hypotonia, myoclonic seizures, and apnea. Hiccups is a common feature and should suggest the diagnosis. Routine blood laboratory studies (blood gases, ammonia, lactate, electrolytes, glucose, cultures) typically are normal. Neonatal death is usual.

Milder cases with greater residual enzyme activity present at a later age with a less severe clinical course. Developmental delay, myoclonic seizures, hiccups, and moderate mental retardation characterize this group. Imaging studies often document atrophy, abnormal myelination, and abnormal or absent corpus callosum.

Diagnosis.   Nonketotic hyperglycinemia is in the differential diagnosis of neonates with progressive encephalopathy and seizures and of older children with intractable seizures, spasticity, and mental retardation. Markedly elevated concentrations of glycine in blood, urine, and CSF in the absence of ketoacidosis or other metabolic disturbances is virtually diagnostic. Enzyme assay of GCS activity in fibroblasts or by DNA analysis is necessary for confirmation.

Treatment.   Acute measures to lower the glycine concentration, such as high-dose benzoate therapy, hemodialysis, peritoneal dialysis, or exchange transfusion, can be life-saving, but survivors have spastic cerebral palsy with severe mental retardation and often intractable seizures with myoclonus.

N-methyl-D-aspartate receptor antagonists, such as dextromethorphan, and the use of benzoate to lower glycine concentrations may be beneficial (Hamosh et al. 1998), but further clinical trials are needed. Diazepam may control seizures. No therapy is proven to be effective. Genetic counseling is indicated and prenatal diagnosis by enzyme assay of GCS activity in chorionic villi or DNA analysis is possible.

Disorders of Histidine Metabolism

Histidinemia is a relatively common, probably benign, disorder that was first detected because imidazolepyruvic acid in the urine causes a positive ferric chloride reaction. This occurred in a number of children with mental retardation, speech disorders, seizures, ataxia, tremor, attention deficit disorder, and a variety of other neurological problems. These patients had a deficiency of histidase. Subsequently, it was shown that many normal people have histidase deficiency with histidinemia and that the association with neurological problems probably was fortuitous, and possibly the result of bias of ascertainment. Treatment with a histidine-restricted diet can normalize the biochemical findings but is not necessary. The clinical significance of histidinemia continues to be controversial. Some reports of clinical improvement in neurological status that occurs in association with dietary manipulation have suggested that a small percentage of histidinemic patients with clinical problems might benefit from reduced histidine intake in the diet. Proprietary formulas for such therapy are available. Histidine is involved in several rare metabolic pathways of diaminopeptides, which are summarized in Table 68.6.

Disorders of Tryptophan Metabolism

Hartnup disease is a relatively common and usually benign inborn error of amino acid transport that causes a neutral aminoaciduria, a photosensitive dermatitis, and

Table 68.7: Disorders of typtophan metabolism

Disorder	Clinical features	Laboratory features
Hartnup disease (defect in neutral amino acid transport)	Pellagralike rash, intermittent personality changes, depression, psychosis, headache, ataxia	Tryptophanuria, neutral aminoaciduria
Tryptophanaemia (defect in synthesis of formylkynurenine from tryptophan)	Mental retardation, pellagralike rash, ataxia	Tryptophanemia, tryptophanuria
Hydroxykynureninuria (kynurinase deficiency)	Mental retardation, migrainelike headaches	Hydroxykynureninuria

neurological dysfunction. Screening programs estimate that the incidence in the United States of this autosomal recessive disease is similar to that of PKU. Intestinal absorption and renal reabsorption of the neutral monoamino-monocarboxylic amino acids, especially tryptophan, is impaired. As a result, the tryptophan concentration in the blood is lower than normal. Tryptophan is a precursor for nicotinic acid. The clinical features include a red, blistering, eczematoid or pellagralike rash and intermittent neurological signs, including personality changes, depression, psychosis, headache, and cerebellar ataxia. Although the aminoaciduria and indole excretion (tryptophan metabolites) are constant, not all patients are symptomatic. The signs and symptoms of the disease typically present in early to late childhood, but do not usually develop with an adequate protein diet. Nicotinamide (25–300 mg/day) supplementation may reverse the skin and neurological complications. The other rare disorders of tryptophan metabolism are summarized in Table 68.7.

Lowe's Syndrome

Lowe's syndrome, or oculocerebrorenal syndrome, is a complex neurodegenerative disease in which there is a generalized renal tubular dysfunction of the Fanconi type, with reduced ammonia production, renal tubular acidosis, phosphaturia, albuminuria, and a generalized aminoaciduria. It is inherited as an X-linked recessive trait. The gene defect causes deficient Golgi-associated phosphatidylinositol-4,5-bisphosphate-5-phosphatase resulting in abnormal function of the Golgi apparatus (Hayashi et al. 1995). The clinical features emerge in infancy, with cataracts, glaucoma, hypotonia, mental retardation, renal rickets, and growth failure in affected male subjects. The growth and bone abnormalities are caused by renal tubular acidosis. Serum concentrations of muscle enzymes are elevated. Female heterozygotes frequently have fine "snowflake" lenticular opacities. Specific treatment is not available. Alkalinization therapy and vitamin D, calcium, phosphate, carnitine, and potassium supplements may be useful. Prenatal diagnosis is possible.

Canavan's Disease

Canavan's disease is caused by a deficiency of the enzyme aspartoacylase that causes the accumulation of the N-acetyl-aspartic acid in the brain (Matalon et al. 1993). It is concentrated especially in the white matter and also excreted in massive amounts in the urine. Patients with Canavan's disease also have elevated concentrations of N-acetylaspartic acid in the blood and CSF.

The clinical presentation of Canavan's disease is one of a progressive encephalopathy beginning with hypotonia early in the first year of life. One of the hallmarks is progressive macrocephaly. Infants become hyperreflexic and hypertonic, have swallowing difficulties with reflux, and eventually develop optic atrophy and seizures. The clinical course may vary considerably from patient to patient. The disease is inherited as an autosomal recessive trait.

Patients with Canavan's disease show demyelination with neuroimaging studies and the excessive concentrations of N-acetylaspartic acid in blood and urine are virtually diagnostic. Pathology specimens show characteristic spongiform degeneration of white matter. The disease resembles Alexander's disease, which also presents with progressive macrocephaly and demyelination; however, the latter disease has a somewhat later onset and slower course. Treatment is not available.

Disorders of Lysine Homeostasis

Lysine, arginine, and ornithine are dibasic amino acids that share a common cellular transport mechanism in renal tubules and intestinal mucosa. Hyperlysinemia and hyperlysinuria can occur in patients with decompensated organic acidemias (see Organic Acidemias, later in this chapter), sometimes in association with hyperammonemia.

Lysinuric Protein Intolerance

This disorder is transmitted as an autosomal recessive trait. Affected individuals have defective transmembrane transport of lysine, arginine, and ornithine, resulting in decreased intestinal absorption and reduced renal tubular reabsorption of these three amino acids. Dibasic aminoaciduria and low plasma concentrations of these amino acids occur that leads to urea cycle dysfunction because ornithine is the substrate for ornithine transcarbamylase. Hyperammonemia (often postprandial only) and orotic aciduria are secondary consequences. Clinical features include feeding difficulties, growth failure, osteoporosis, hepatomegaly, bone marrow depression, obvious aversion to dietary protein, episodic emesis, episodic encephalopathy, developmental delay, hypotonia, mental retardation, psychoses, and seizures. Treatment consists of citrulline supplementation. Monitoring the urine orotic acid and the postprandial blood ammonia levels facilitates nutritional management by documenting the patient's level of protein tolerance. Hyperammonemic crises are treated by intravenous infusion of arginine, discontinuance of dietary protein, intravenous hydration with glucose- and lipid-containing solutions to promote anabolism, and use of benzoate/phenylacetate if indicated.

Familial Hyperlysinemia

Hyperlysinemia with hyperlysinuria has been documented in patients with mental retardation, poor growth, and various other neurological abnormalities in association with a deficiency of alpha-aminoadipic semialdehyde synthase activity (familial hyperlysinemia). Saccharopinuria, hyperdibasic aminoaciduria, and elevated plasma pipecolic acid can occur. Similar biochemical findings in asymptomatic relatives and the absence of the disease in synthase-deficient individuals detected in general population screening suggest that familial hyperlysinemia probably is a benign biochemical variant. Occasional anecdotal reports describe clinical improvement with a lysine-restricted diet, however.

Organic Acidemias

Accumulation of organic acids occurs with impaired catabolism of carbohydrates, lipids, and amino acids (Garcia et al. 1996). Disorders of carbohydrates and lipids are discussed elsewhere in this chapter. Most of the disorders of amino acids are caused by defects in the metabolism of BCKAs, propionic acid, or methylmalonic acid. The common clinical feature of all organic acidemias is either overwhelming neonatal encephalopathy or intermittent encephalopathy, with vomiting, hypotonia, coma, and acidosis. The similar clinical features of organic acidemias, carnitine deficiency, Reye's syndrome, and valproate-induced hepatoencephalopathy suggest a shared pathophysiology that involves carnitine metabolism.

Carnitine Deficiency

Pathophysiology.   Carnitine is synthesized from lysine and methionine by the liver and kidney, but 75% of the total daily requirement is obtained from dietary sources, particularly meat. Ninety percent of total carnitine is in muscle. The carnitine cycle is necessary to transport a number of metabolites across the mitochondrial membrane (Figure 68.5). Carnitine transporter enzyme maintains the intracellular pool of carnitine. Carnitine acyltransferase at the outer mitochondrial membrane converts acyl-CoA esters to acylcarnitine analogues, which is necessary for some metabolites to be transported across the inner mitochondrial membrane. Carnitine/acylcarnitine translocase mediates the mitochondrial transmembrane transfer of acylcarnitine in exchange for free carnitine. The cycle is completed by carnitine acyltransferase on the inner mitochondrial membrane that reconstitutes the acyl-CoA esters and free carnitine. Carnitine is necessary for the transport of long-chain fatty acids across the inner mitochondrial membrane for beta-oxidation, modulation of the acyl-CoA to free CoA ratio inside mitochondria, and shuttling acyl-CoA compounds from peroxisomes into mitochondria. Acylcarnitine is less toxic to mitochondrial enzymes than are acyl-CoA compounds. Acyl-CoA esters inhibit several mitochondrial enzymes, especially those of the urea cycle and pyruvate metabolism. This results in lactic acidosis, hypoglycemia, and hyperammonemia. The acylcarnitine esters are excreted in the urine as a detoxification mechanism.

Carnitine deficiency is either primary or secondary. Primary carnitine deficiency results from deficient transporter enzyme. The resulting deficiency of intracellular carnitine in muscle causes myopathy, and in all other tissues, systemic disease. Secondary carnitine deficiency is a feature of mitochondrial fatty acid oxidation disorders and of several inborn errors of metabolism that cause organic acidosis and excessive production of acyl-CoA compounds. Secondary carnitine deficiency develops when free carnitine is trapped by the formation of acylcarnitine esters that are subsequently lost in the urine. The loss of carnitine further reduces the capacity to buffer toxic acyl-CoA esters and results in further metabolic decompensation. In both primary and secondary carnitine deficiency, the acylcarnitine to free carnitine ratio (normally <0.25) is increased markedly. A similar metabolic profile occurs in patients with Reye's syndrome and valproate-induced hepatic encephalopathy. Dietary deficiencies, impaired liver function, and renal tubular disease contribute to carnitine deficiency.

Clinical Features.   Carnitine transporter deficiency can present in infancy as repeated episodes of acute encephalopathy, lactic acidosis, hyperammonemia, hypoglycemia, and hepatic injury with variable skeletal and cardiac myopathy (Stanley 1995). Serum concentrations of liver enzymes are elevated, but the bilirubin concentration is normal. Metabolic stress, such as infection or starvation, precipitates acute deterioration. Alternatively, carnitine transporter deficiency can present later as a progressive cardiomyopathy and myopathy.

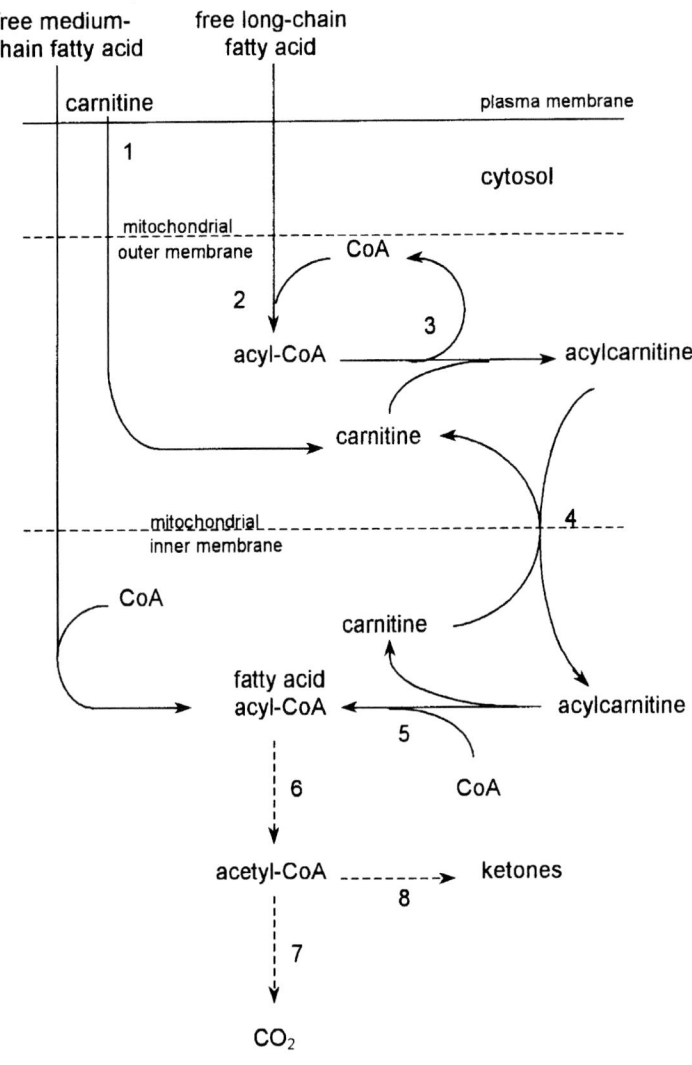

FIGURE 68.5 Carnitine and fatty acid metabolism. (1) Carnitine transporter enzyme. (2) Acyl–coenzyme A (CoA) synthetase. (3) Carnitine palmitoyltransferase I. (4) Carnitine-acylcarnitine translocase. (5) Carnitine palmitoyltransferase II. (6) Beta-oxidation spiral of fatty acids including fatty acid acyl-CoA dehydrogenases: short-chain, medium-chain, long-chain, very-long-chain, and the trifunctional protein-bearing long-chain 2-enol-CoA hydratase. (7) Tricarboxylic acid cycle. (8) HMG-CoA pathway.

Episodic encephalopathy was thought to be typical of *systemic* carnitine deficiency because carnitine is deficient in both blood and muscle, but it also occurs in children with secondary carnitine deficiency associated with organic acidemias or with the mitochondrial fatty acid oxidation deficiencies. *Muscle* carnitine deficiency originally was described as a progressive myopathy, with the pathological features of lipid storage and deficient carnitine concentrations in skeletal muscle. It also was implicated in infantile hypotonia and exercise intolerance. The overlap of clinical features in muscle and systemic carnitine deficiency suggests that they are a spectrum of the same underlying carnitine transporter deficiency. Members of the same family can present with either syndrome.

Diagnosis.   Total, free, and esterified carnitine plasma measurements should be obtained to evaluate a patient suspected of carnitine deficiency. Total plasma carnitine is the sum of free carnitine and acylcarnitine esters and is normally greater than 30 μmol/liter. A free carnitine concentration of less than 20 μmol/liter is abnormal. Acylcarnitine esters normally make up less than 25% of the total; a ratio of esterified to free carnitine greater than 0.4 is abnormal. Patients with carnitine transporter deficiency have a marked decrease in plasma carnitine (<5–10 μmol/liter) and muscle carnitine. Patients with primary muscle carnitine deficiency have normal plasma carnitine but low muscle carnitine concentrations. Patients with secondary carnitine deficiency have moderately decreased serum carnitine concentrations, but the ratio of acylcarnitine to free carnitine is greater than 0.4. The tissue carnitine concentrations are variable in these patients. The excretion of dicarboxylic acids is increased, indicating an impairment of long chain fatty acid beta-oxidation and a shift to omega oxidation in peroxisomes. Ketogenesis during fasting is impaired.

Treatment.   Carnitine deficiency, whether primary or secondary, muscular or systemic, often responds to dietary carnitine supplements. The dosage of L-carnitine is 100–200 mg/kg per day orally or 60 mg/kg per day intravenously.

Table 68.8: Disorders of branched-chain ketoacid metabolism

Disorder and enzyme deficiency	Distinctive features	Clinical syndromes
Isovaleric acidemia (isovaleryl-CoA dehydrogenase)	Sweaty socks odor	Neonatal encephalopathy
	Ketoacidosis	Chronic, mental retardation
3-Methylcrotonyl-CoA carboxylase	Tomcat urine odor	Infantile hypotonia
	Ketoacidosis	Intermittent encephalopathy
3-Hydroxy-3-methyl-glutaryl-CoA lyase	Acidosis	Intermittent encephalopathy and cardiomyopathy
β-Ketothiolase	Ketoacidosis	Intermittent encephalopathy
Glutaric acidemia II (multiple acyl-CoA dehydrogenase)	Sweaty socks odor	Neonatal encephalopathy
		Intermittent encephalopathy
		Late-onset lipid storage
		Myopathy and cardiomyopathy

CoA = coenzyme A.

Disorders of Branched-Chain Ketoacid Metabolism

Clinical Features. Disorders of BCKA metabolism are biochemically located between MSUD and the propionic and methylmalonic acidemias and share similar pathophysiological and clinical features to MSUD and other organic acidemias (see Figure 68.4). Although neonatal, intermittent, or both encephalopathies and an unusual odor are the major clinical features, the clinical spectrum is broad (Sweetman and Williams 1995). Table 68.8 outlines the more common BCKA diseases. Newborns with severe deficiencies have severe ketoacidosis with a fulminant, fatal encephalopathy. Infants and children with partial deficiency have either a chronic or intermittent course. Associated metabolic abnormalities are mild lactic acidosis and hyperammonemia. Thrombocytopenia, leukopenia, and anemia may occur during acute metabolic crisis and survivors are retarded frequently as a result. Also, children with unexplained pancreatitis should be evaluated for BCKA disorders.

Diagnosis. The diagnosis is suggested by the clinical features of acute or intermittent encephalopathy accompanied by ketoacidosis and a "sweaty socks" or "tomcat urine" odor. Analysis of urine organic acids shows increased concentrations of metabolites that suggest the specific diagnosis. Definitive diagnosis requires measuring the enzyme activity in leukocytes or cultured fibroblasts or gene identification.

Treatment. Protein restriction and carnitine administration are the mainstays of treatment. Acylcarnitine is formed and excreted in the urine to eliminate toxic metabolites. Carnitine also increases protein tolerance and provides some protection from encephalopathy during acute illnesses. Glucose infusion during acute attacks reduces protein catabolism.

Glycine enhances the formation of isovalerylglycine, a compound that is excreted readily in the urine. Glycine is recommended in the treatment of isovaleric acidemia, although carnitine supplementation alone is satisfactory in some patients (Fries et al. 1996).

Multiple Carboxylase Deficiency

Pathophysiology. Biotin is a cofactor for several carboxylating systems that incorporate carbon dioxide (CO_2) into intermediary metabolites. The enzymes requiring biotin are propionyl-CoA carboxylase, pyruvate carboxylase (PC), and 3-methylcrotonyl-CoA carboxylase. Deficiencies of each of these enzymes cause an organic acidemia. Acetyl-CoA carboxylase is required for fatty acid synthesis. The inactive apoenzymes are activated by attaching biotin covalently to a lysine E-amino group of the apocarboxylase by holocarboxylase synthetase. Deficient holocarboxylase synthetase affects all enzymes requiring the biotin cofactor. Biotin is recaptured through protein catabolism of the carboxylase enzymes to lysyl-biotin compounds. Biotinidase is required to free biotin for reuse with the apocarboxylases according to Wolf and Heard in 1991. Multiple carboxylase deficiency can be caused by holocarboxylase synthetase deficiency, biotinidase deficiency, defective gastrointestinal absorption of biotin, defective renal reabsorption of biotin, or nutritional causes for biotin deficiency. A complex, but distinctive pattern of abnormal organic acids accumulates in the blood and urine because of the several enzyme deficiencies.

Clinical Features. The usual syndrome is developmental regression and recurrent episodes of metabolic ketoacidosis, hyperammonemia, and vomiting. Many children develop an erythematous skin rash, stomatitis, glossitis, conjunctivitis, candidiasis, alopecia, and a tomcat urine odor. Immunodeficiency with a dysfunction of T and B lymphocytes can occur.

Less common neurological features are seizures, optic atrophy, hypotonia, ataxia, and high-frequency hearing loss. Biotinidase deficiency has a later onset and is less severe; however, considerable overlap exists with the features of holocarboxylase synthetase deficiency.

Diagnosis. The clinical features vary; not all children with neurological dysfunction have cutaneous manifestations or organic aciduria. The diagnosis is confirmed by measuring

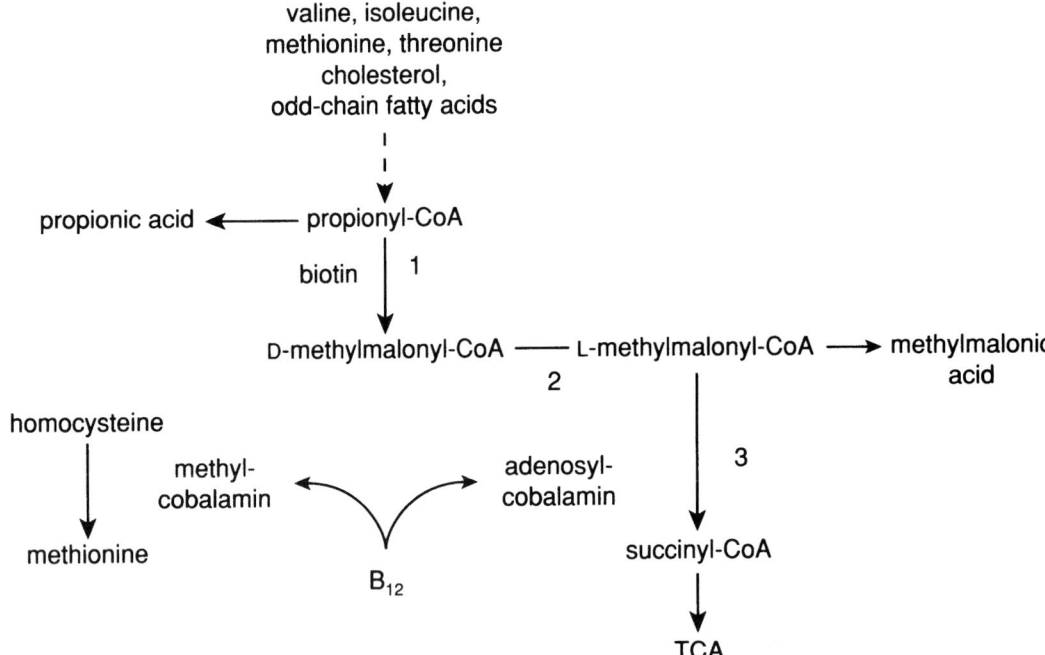

FIGURE 68.6   Propionic acid and methylmalonic acid metabolism. (1) Propionyl–coenzyme A (CoA) carboxylase. (2) Methylmalonyl-CoA racemase. (3) Methylmalonyl-CoA mutase. (TCA = tricarboxylic acid cycle.)

biotin levels in the blood and the biotinidase and holocarboxylase synthetase enzyme activities in leukocytes.

Treatment.   A therapeutic trial of biotin, 10 mg per day, should be considered in any child with compatible clinical features. All forms of holocarboxylase deficiency respond to biotin therapy.

Propionic Acidemia

Pathophysiology.   Propionic acidemia, one of the more frequently encountered organic acidemias, is an autosomal recessively inherited disorder caused by deficiency of the biotin-dependent enzyme propionyl-CoA carboxylase, which converts propionyl-CoA to methylmalonyl-CoA (Figure 68.6). Propionyl-CoA is an intermediary metabolite in the catabolism of BCAAs and BCKAs, odd-chain fatty acids, threonine, methionine, heme, and the 3-carbon side chains of cholesterol. Because propionyl-CoA requires biotin as a cofactor, disorders of biotin also cause propionic acidemia. The urinary excretion of propionylcarnitine causes a secondary carnitine deficiency.

Clinical Features.   Three clinical syndromes are associated with propionic acidemia. The most common is a catastrophic metabolic acidosis of the newborn characterized by encephalopathy and death. This syndrome may be confused with neonatal sepsis or intraventricular hemorrhage; thus, some cases are never diagnosed. The second syndrome has an infantile onset and is characterized by episodic

ketoacidosis, encephalopathy, vomiting, and dehydration. The third presentation is a later onset, mildly progressive disease associated with mental retardation or dementia and movement disorders, especially chorea and dystonia (Fenton and Rosenberg 1995).

Severe acidosis, ketotic hyperglycinemia, and hyperammonemia are the major biochemical features. Other laboratory findings include mild lactic acidosis, hypoglycemia, neutropenia, and thrombocytopenia.

Diagnosis.   The clinical features are not sufficiently distinctive to be diagnostic. The diagnosis should be suspected in the infant or older child with hyperglycinemia, ketoacidosis, and encephalopathy. Measuring blood and urine concentrations of organic and amino acids shows a characteristic biochemical profile. Typical findings include high concentrations of propionic acid, 3-hydroxypropionate, methylcitrate, 3-hydroxyvaleric acid, and propionylglycine and many other intermediary metabolites. The definitive diagnosis is made by measuring the enzyme activity in fibroblasts.

Treatment.   The treatment of all organic acidurias is similar. The overwhelming neonatal form may require peritoneal dialysis or venovenous hemoperfusion. Some may respond to intravenous fluids and therapy for acid–base and electrolyte abnormalities. Management usually requires an intensive care setting. Immediate withdrawal of dietary protein and carnitine supplementation should be initiated as soon as the diagnosis is suspected. Carnitine supplementation increases the tolerance to protein intake and the catabolic stress of illness. Excessive catabolism during time of stress must be reversed rapidly. Parenteral nutrition may be successful in preventing catastrophic injury associated with long-term stress. Patients with multiple carboxylase deficiency respond to biotin supplementation, as discussed earlier. Chronic management relies on L-carnitine therapy and attention to diet using medical specialty formulas that are supplemented with low-protein natural foods.

Methylmalonic Acidemia

Pathophysiology. Methylmalonic acidemia is a heterogeneous group of genetically distinct disorders caused by deficiency of methylmalonyl-CoA mutase activity. This enzyme catalyzes the conversion of L-methylmalonyl-CoA to D-succinyl-CoA and is a major step in the catabolism of the BCAAs, BCKAs, and fatty acids as well as several other metabolic pathways (see Figure 68.6). Methylmalonyl-CoA mutase requires vitamin B_{12} in the form of adenosylcobalamin as a cofactor. Deficiency of the enzyme causes the accumulation of methylmalonyl-CoA, which is hydrolyzed to methylmalonic acid.

Seven genetically distinct classes of methylmalonic acidemia have been identified (Fenton and Rosenberg 1995). Two are caused by deficiencies of the mutase enzyme: One is a complete loss of affinity of the apomutase locus for adenosylcobalamin (mut^O), and the other is a partial deficiency (mut$^-$). The other five are caused by disorders of cobalamin metabolism: mitochondrial cobalamin reductase deficiency (cblA); cobalamin adenosyltransferase deficiency (cblB); cytosolic cobalamin metabolism (cblC and cblD); and lysosomal cobalamin efflux (cblF). cblA and cblB impair the formation of adenosylcobalamin alone. Adenosylcobalamin is necessary only for the methylmalonyl-CoA mutase reaction. cblC, cblD, and cblF interrupt the formation of both adenosylcobalamin and methylcobalamin. cblC complementation defect is the most common inborn error of cobalamin metabolism. Methylcobalamin is a vitamin B_{12} derivative necessary for the remethylation of homocysteine to methionine. Affected individuals have clinical features of homocystinuria and methylmalonic acidosis. Mild methylmalonic aciduria also may occur in acquired cobalamin deficiency.

Clinical Features. The typical onset is a catastrophic encephalopathy after introducing protein feedings. An alternative syndrome presents with episodic attacks of vomiting, dehydration, seizures, hypotonia, and progressive encephalopathy at the time of intercurrent illness. The clinical course may be one of failure to thrive, poor feeding, developmental delay, mental retardation, and abnormal behavior. Thrombocytopenia, anemia, and neutropenia during metabolic crisis can be clinically significant. Frequent infections, T-cell dysfunction, and candidiasis occur when metabolic control is poor.

The biochemical features include severe ketoacidosis, hypoglycemia, hyperammonemia, lactic acidosis, and sec-

ondary carnitine deficiency. The blood and urine glycine concentration is increased, making this one of the ketotic hyperglycinemias. Urine organic acid analysis shows high concentrations of methylmalonic acid and lower concentrations of 3-hydroxypropionate, methylcitrate, and other metabolites of propionyl-CoA.

Patients with the complete mutase deficiency have the poorest prognosis and frequently die during an acute episode. Children with partial mutase deficiency or cblB mutations do somewhat better but are still at high risk for early death. Patients with the cblA type show the greatest response to cobalamin therapy and have the best prognosis of the complementation group of disorders. Patients with combined methylmalonic acidemia and homocystinuria (cblC, cblD, and cblF types) may have neonatal or chronic neurological disease and often have the hematological complications and less severe methylmalonic acidemia. Hyperglycinemia and hyperammonemia are not characteristic findings for these types.

Diagnosis. Methylmalonic acidemia should be suspected in any child with neonatal or episodic encephalopathy associated with ketoacidosis, lactic acidosis, and hyperammonemia. Quantitative analysis of blood and urine organic acids suggests the diagnosis. Definitive diagnosis requires enzyme analysis of cultured fibroblasts or gene identification.

Treatment. Metabolic acidosis, hypoglycemia, and hyperammonemia must be treated aggressively during episodes of metabolic decompensation. Episodes of ketoacidosis and hyperammonemia are best managed by venovenous hemofiltration or peritoneal dialysis. Protein intake should be eliminated initially and the catabolic state reversed as rapidly as possible with glucose infusions. The biochemical and clinical response to intramuscular hydroxocobalamin (1.0–2.0 mg/day) can be dramatic, and all children suspected of having methylmalonic aciduria should be given a trial (Anderson and Shapira 1998). L-Carnitine supplementation is indicated for both acute and chronic management. Parenteral nutrition may be necessary for protracted metabolic stress. Chronic management includes strict dietary protein control and L-carnitine and hydroxocobalamin supplementation. Betaine supplementation is being investigated for use in those with homocystinuria.

Prenatal treatment of the mother with cobalamin can be beneficial for infants at risk. Although metronidazole therapy to reduce the gut flora and potential sources of offending metabolites has been advocated in the treatment of many organic acidurias, the results have been inconclusive (Burns et al. 1996).

Glutaric Acidemia

Pathophysiology. Glutaric acidemia type I is an autosomal recessive disorder caused by a deficiency of glutaryl-

Table 68.9: Disorders of the γ-glutamyl cycle and glutamic acid metabolism

Disease and/or enzyme deficiency	Neurological signs	Other findings
γ-Glutamylcysteine synthetase	Myoclonic seizures, spinocerebellar degeneration, polyneuropathy	Hemolytic anemia, aminoaciduria, glutathione deficiency
5-Oxoprolinase	Benign disease? (possible mental retardation and other signs)	5-Oxoprolinuria (pyroglutamic aciduria)
Glutathione synthetase	Neonatal metabolic acidosis and encephalopathy, progressive ataxia	Hemolytic anemia, jaundice, 5-oxoprolinuria, acidosis
γ-Glutamyl transpeptidase	Mental retardation	Glutathionuria
Glutamic acid decarboxylase	Poorly controlled seizures	Vitamin B_6-responsive seizures
Succinic semialdehyde dehydrogenase	Hypotonia, ataxia, mental retardation; signs improve with age	4-Hydroxybutyric aciduria, dicarboxylic aciduria

CoA dehydrogenase. Patients with type I disease accumulate and excrete large amounts of glutaric acid, which is an intermediary metabolite of tryptophan, lysine, and hydroxylysinecatabolism. Glutaric acidemia type II is caused by a defect in electron transfer from several flavin-dependent acyl-CoA dehydrogenases into the respiratory chain.

Clinical Features.   Children usually present between 3 and 12 months of age with rapid onset of dystonia, choreoathetosis, or other abnormal movements. Subsequently, the course is relatively progressive, but some patients have intermittent encephalopathy. A few patients present later in childhood with a slowly progressive extrapyramidal syndrome. There may be a marked clinical heterogeneity. Minimal to severe disease can occur within the same family.

Diagnosis.   Glutaryl-CoA dehydrogenase should be suspected in any child with a metabolic encephalopathy, especially those with extrapyramidal signs. Neuroimaging studies show marked cerebral and striatal atrophy. The temporal lobes are especially affected. The CSF spaces are enlarged and infants often have macrocephaly at birth. Glutaric acid and 3-hydroxyglutaric acid are elevated in the urine. Increased excretion of the latter compound is pathognomonic for the disease. A definitive diagnosis can be made by enzymatic analysis of cultured fibroblasts or gene identification.

Treatment.   Treatment for acute metabolic encephalopathy includes fluids, correction of acidosis, glucose, and insulin. Early diagnosis and treatment with diets low in lysine and tryptophan can result in normal development. Treatment with L-carnitine and riboflavin is also beneficial. Because γ-aminobutyric brain concentrations are low in patients with glutaric acidemia, agents that increase γ-aminobutyric concentrations, such as baclofen, valproic acid, and vigabatrin, have been used with variable results.

Disorders of the γ-Glutamyl Cycle and Glutamic Acid Metabolism

The γ-glutamyl cycle is a general mechanism for transporting amino acids across cell membranes and is associated intimately with glutathione metabolism. Amino acids react with glutathione to form a γ-glutamyl amino acid that is transported across the cell membrane and then hydrolyzed in the intracellular space, liberating the amino acid and pyroglutamic acid. Reconstitution of glutathione from glutamic acid, cysteine, and glycine completes the cycle. The several diseases associated with defects within the γ-glutamyl cycle are summarized in Table 68.9. Two additional disorders associated with the catabolism of glutamic acid to succinic acid and hydroxybutyric acid are summarized in the table. These diseases are rare and transmitted as autosomal recessive traits. Pyridoxine-dependent seizures respond to pharmacological doses of pyridoxine. Although previously considered the result of abnormal interaction between glutamic acid decarboxylase and its cofactor, recent biochemical and molecular analyses suggest that these patients do not have that enzyme deficiency.

Patients with glutathione synthetase deficiency are at risk for cellular injury from the accumulation of reactive oxygen intermediates. Ascorbate or N-acetylcysteine has antioxidative properties and may be therapeutic in these patients (Jain et al. 1994). No specific therapy exists for these diseases.

L-2-Hydroxyglutaric Acidemia

L-2-Hydroxyglutaric acidemia is an inherited neurometabolic disease transmitted by autosomal recessive inheritance. The disease is characterized by developmental regression in childhood (ages 1–10 years), sometimes associated with growth deficiency and macrocephaly. Neurological features are ataxia, dysmetria, dysarthria, spasticity, and dystonia. Mental retardation is invariable. Generalized febrile and nonfebrile seizures are common.

Screening urinary gas chromatography shows increased excretion of L-2-hydroxyglutaric acid. L-2-hydroxyglutaric acid concentrations also are increased in the CSF and to a lesser extent in the plasma, resulting in an elevated CSF to plasma ratio. Plasma and CSF concentrations of lysine also may be increased. Magnetic resonance imaging (MRI) shows subcortical white matter changes, cerebellar atrophy, and signal changes in the lenticular nuclei. Survival into adulthood is possible. Specific therapy is not available.

Disorders of Sugar Metabolism

Galactosemia

Pathophysiology.   Classic galactosemia is an autosomal recessive inherited disease caused by a deficiency of the enzyme galactose-1-phosphate uridyltransferase (GPUT), which catalyzes the reaction of galactose-1-phosphate to uridyl diphosphogalactose (Figure 68.7). Ingestion of lactose- or galactose-containing foods causes galactosemia and galactosuria as well as accumulation of galactose-1-phosphate and galactitol, the alcohol of galactose. Galactitol is responsible for the development of cataracts. The basis for the neurotoxicity, hepatotoxicity, and other clinical features is less understood but probably relates to the accumulation of galactose-1-phosphate.

Clinical Features.   Infants become symptomatic during the early neonatal interval after dietary exposure to galactose, although occasionally congenital signs of the disease may exist. The classic clinical features are poor feeding, lethargy, failure to thrive, vomiting, and cataracts. Cataracts can occur in the newborn, even if the mother was on a galactose-restricted diet. Untreated infants develop progressive liver disease with hyperbilirubinemia, coagulopathy, and hepatosplenomegaly. Hypoglycemia can occur. Cirrhosis and renal tubular disease with proteinuria, glycosuria, generalized aminoaciduria, and renal tubular acidosis occur unless therapy is begun. *Escherichia coli* sepsis is a common complication of the disease. Death may result from infection, liver failure, or general inanition. Untreated children develop mild to moderate mental retardation, speech defects, learning disabilities, and chronic liver disease. Children with partial deficiency can have a later onset and a milder course. Pseudotumor cerebri has been associated with galactosemia in rare cases. Hypergonadotropic ovarian failure develops in female subjects, resulting in abnormal secondary sexual development, infertility, amenorrhea, and osteoporosis in spite of good compliance with a galactose-restricted diet.

Diagnosis.   The diagnosis should be suspected in any neonate with failure to thrive, emesis, lethargy, cataracts, and liver disease and in older children with cataracts, mental retardation, and chronic liver disease. Patients ingesting galactose have detectable reducing substances in the urine, but the glucose oxidase test result is negative. A negative test result for urine-reducing substances does not exclude galactosemia if galactose has been restricted from the diet or if urine is dilute. A positive test result for urine-reducing substances is not specific for galactose. A qualitative, fluorescent blood enzyme spot test for GPUT provides a rapid, sensitive method to detect enzyme activity and does not require elevated plasma galactose for diagnosis. A neonate or infant who has been transfused may have GPUT activity, however, because of the donor blood cells. Quantitative enzyme assay is necessary to confirm the diagnosis. A galactose-restricted diet should be initiated before final confirmation of the diagnosis.

Treatment.   Treatment for galactosemia requires the treatment of acute metabolic and infectious complications and the elimination of all galactose-containing foods from the diet. Soy formulas and Nutramigen (Mead Johnson) are free of galactose and can be substituted for other proprietary formulas or breast milk. It is important to begin therapy as soon as the diagnosis is suspected. Most of the systemic complications reverse within several days of the diet's initiation, but mental retardation does not improve. Even if treatment with excellent compliance is started immediately after birth, most children experience late-onset galactose toxicity with clinical complications, including hypergonadotropic hypogonadism with ovarian failure, delayed growth, cognitive deficits, psychological problems, tremor, ataxia, or other neurological deficits (Waggoner and Buist 1993). The causes for late complications on a restricted diet are unknown but may be related to cryptic ingestion of galactose and endogenous production of galactose. Cataracts can worsen if the diet is relaxed. Pregnant patients with galactosemia should adhere to a strict diet free of galactose and lactose to reduce passive injury to the fetus.

Variants of Galactosemia

Several genetically distinct variants exist that have a partial deficiency of the transferase enzyme and a milder course. A common galactosemic variant detected in population screening studies is the compound heterozygote, with one classic galactosemia gene and one Duarte galactosemia gene. These patients have approximately 25% of normal GPUT activity and can have galactose intolerance. Approximately 10% of the population are heterozygotes for the normal and Duarte gene. The homozygote for the Duarte gene has approximately 50% of normal enzyme activity but has no clinical symptoms.

Galactokinase catalyzes the reaction of galactose to galactose-1-phosphate (see Figure 68.7). Galactokinase deficiency causes galactose and galactitol accumulation. The sole clinical manifestation is cataracts, which can appear at any age in either the heterozygote or the homozygote. Treatment is similar to that for galactosemia.

Uridyl-diphosphogalactose-4-epimerase deficiency is an autosomal recessive disorder that also causes galactosemia and galactosuria. A benign form and a severe form have been described. The severe form is characterized by a generalized deficiency of this epimerase activity in contrast to the much more common benign form, which has hepatic epimerase activity but deficient erythrocyte and leukocyte epimerase activity. The severe epimerase deficiency phenotype is similar to that of classic galactosemia because of transferase deficiency. These patients have developmental delay, neurosensory deafness, and variable intellectual disability. Individuals with the benign form have no clinical problems, although long-term evaluation studies are not complete.

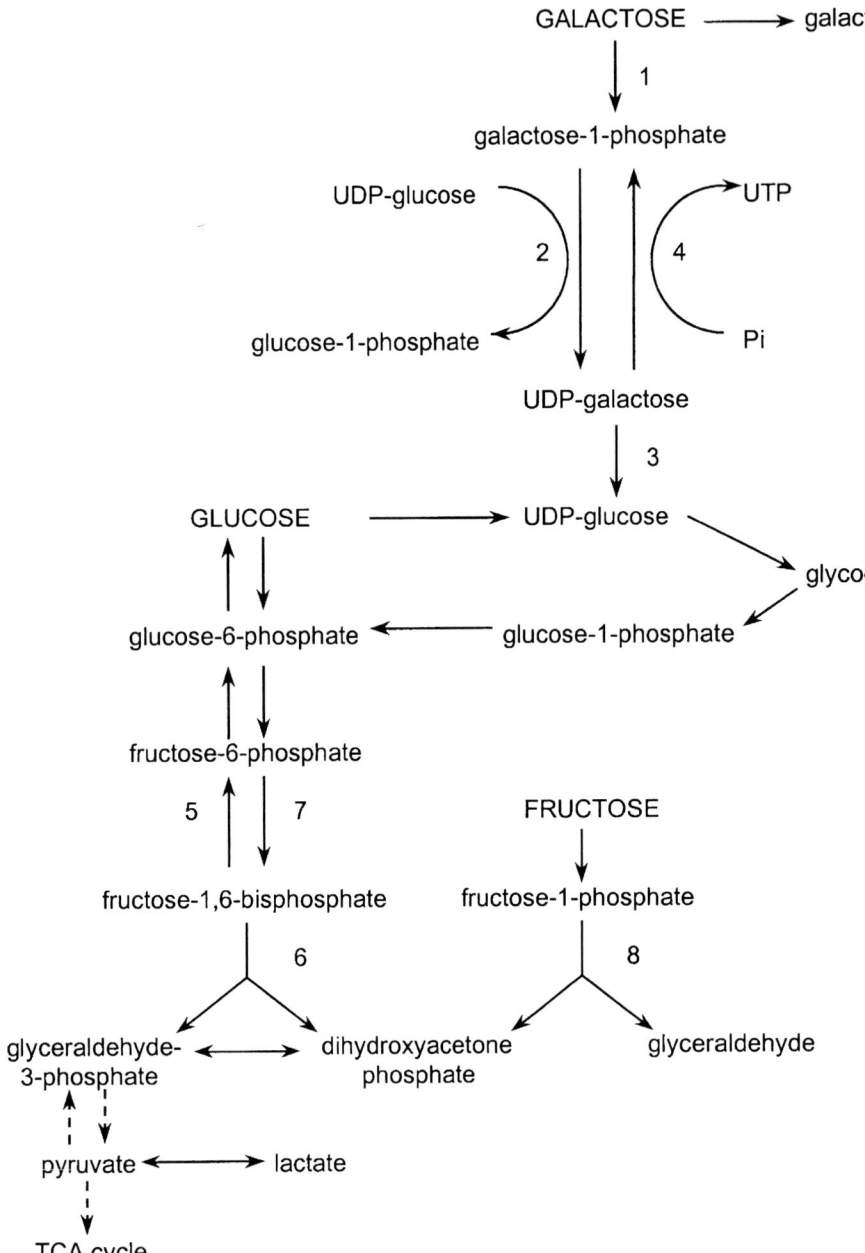

FIGURE 68.7   Fructose and galactose metabolism. (1) Galactokinase. (2) Galactose-1-phosphate uridyl transferase. (3) UDP-galactose epimerase. (4) Hexose-1-phosphate uridyltransferase. (5) Fructose bisphosphatase. (6) Fructose bisphosphatase aldolase. (7) Phosphofructokinase. (8) Fructoaldolase. (Pi = inorganic phoshate; TCA = tricarboxylic acid cycle; UDP = uridine diphosphate; UTP = uridine triphosphate.)

Disorders of Fructose Metabolism

The several disorders of fructose metabolism are not associated with chronic neurological signs, although they often cause seizures and altered consciousness associated with an acute encephalopathy, hypoglycemia, and metabolic acidosis. The clinical features are summarized in Table 68.10. In patients with fructose metabolism disorders, urine test results for reducing substances are positive; however, the glucose oxidase test result is negative. Qualitative chromatography is necessary to identify urine fructose. The hepatic enzymes fructose bisphosphate aldolase and fructose bisphosphatase can be measured for a specific diagnosis. Treatment includes symptomatic support and the removal of fructose and substances that can be converted to fructose (sucrose and sorbitol) from the diet.

Other Metabolic Disorders

Hyperammonemia

Pathophysiology.   Ammonia is derived from protein catabolism and as a metabolic product of bacteria in the

Table 68.10:   Disorders of fructose metabolism

Disease	Enzyme defect	Clinical features
Hereditary fructosuria	Fructokinase	Asymptomatic
Hereditary fructose intolerance	Fructose bisphosphate aldolase	Severe hypoglycemia, vomiting, failure to thrive, liver disease, renal tubular disease, aversion to fruits, lethargy, seizures
Fructose-1,6-bisphosphatase deficiency	Fructose bisphosphatase	Fasting hypoglycemia, keto and lactic acidosis, apnea, hyperventilation, encephalopathy, seizures

gastrointestinal tract. Figure 68.8 outlines the metabolic pathways for the elimination of ammonia by its conversion to urea. Hyperammonemia causes progressive brain disease and, if untreated, results in permanent brain injury. The mechanisms of hyperammonemic coma and brain injury are unknown, but may result from the accumulation of ammonia and amino acids, neurotransmitter alterations, and excitotoxic injury (Batshaw 1994). Astrocytes are rich in glutamine synthetase, and hyperammonemia causes excessive accumulation of glutamine in the brain. This has been implicated as a cause of cerebral edema in patients with hyperammonemia. Plasma and CSF glutamine concentrations anticipate and parallel concentrations of ammonia.

Hyperammonemia has many causes (see Table 68.1). Acquired hyperammonemia usually is caused by extensive

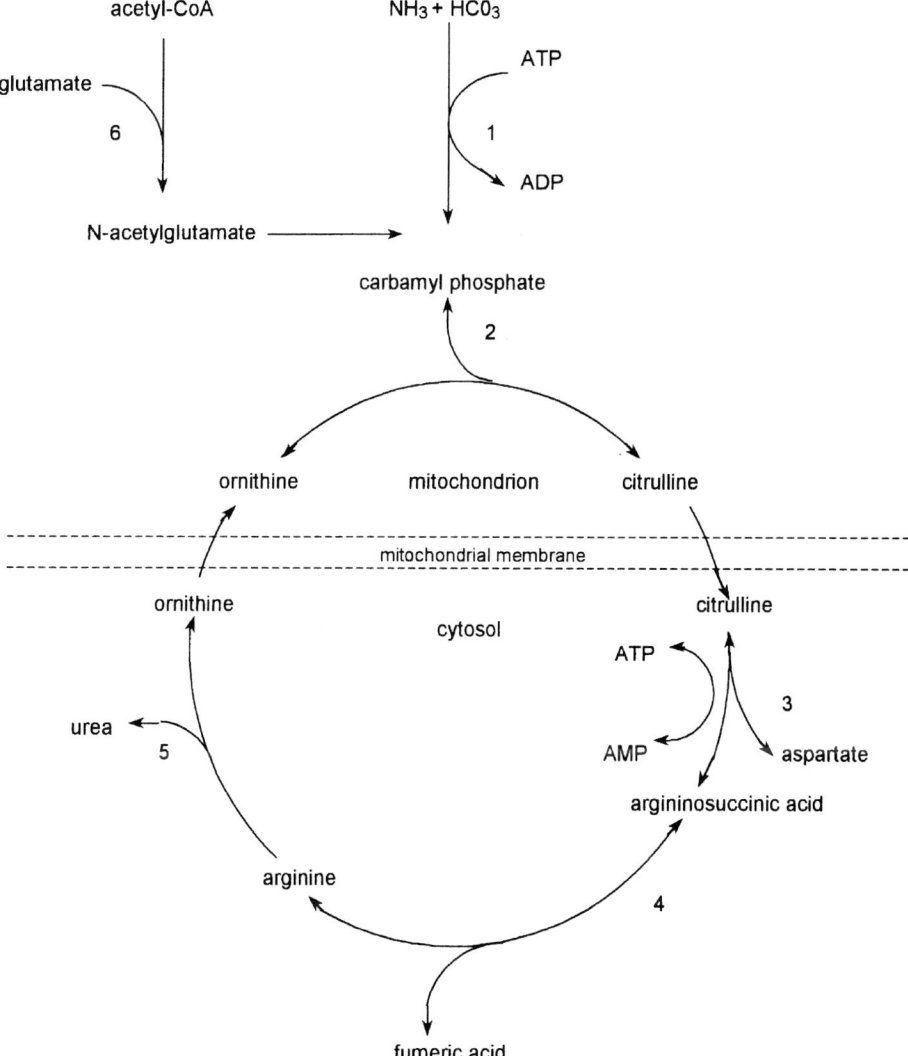

FIGURE 68.8   The urea cycle. (1) Carbamyl phosphate synthetase. (2) Ornithine transcarbamylase. (3) Argininosuccinate synthetase. (4) Argininosuccinate lysase. (5) Arginase. (6) N-Acetylglutamate synthetase. (ADP = adenosine disphosphate; AMP = adenosine monophosphate; ATP = adenosine triphosphate; CoA = coenzyme A.)

Table 68.11:   Urea cycle and related diseases

Enzyme deficiency	Genetics	Clinical features	Laboratory features
Ornithine transcarbamylase	XLD	Males: neonatal encephalopathy, respiratory alkalosis, death or mental retardation Variant: episodic headache, ataxia, lethargy Females: normal or intermittent headaches, vomiting, ophthalmoplegia	Hyperammonemia, orotic aciduria, low plasma citrulline
Argininosuccinate lyase	AR	Neonatal encephalopathy or later onset mental retardation, seizures, trichorrhexis nodosa, episodic vomiting, hepatomegaly, ataxia	Hyperammonemia, arginino-succinate aciduria citrullinuria, orotic aciduria
Argininosuccinate synthetase	AR	Neonatal encephalopathy or chronic ataxia, seizures, recurrent vomiting, trichorrhexis nodosa	Hyperammonemia, citrullinemia, citrullinuria, orotic aciduria
Carbamyl phosphate synthetase I	AR	Neonatal encephalopathy or intermittent vomiting, lethargy with unusual eye movements	Hyperammonemia, low plasma citrulline
Arginase	AR	Mental retardation, microcephaly, seizures, spastic diplegia, recurrent vomiting	Hyperammonemia; hyperargininemia, arginine, cystine, ornithine, and lysine may be increased in urine
N-Acetyl glutamate synthetase	AR	Neonatal encephalopathy	Hyperammonemia, hyperornithinemia
Hyperammonemia, hyperornithinemia, and homocitrullinemia syndrome	AR	Neonatal encephalopathy, myoclonic seizures, ataxia, mental retardation, failure to thrive	Hyperammonemia, hyperornithinemia, homocitrullinemia
Ornithine-ketoacid aminotransferase	AR	Gyrate atrophy of the choroid and retina	None

AR = autosomal recessive; XLD = X-linked dominant.

liver injury. Inborn errors of metabolism of the urea cycle and related diseases are the most common causes of severe hyperammonemia (Table 68.11). Several other metabolic diseases cause hyperammonemia by a secondary effect on urea metabolism. These disorders usually have other metabolic disturbances, such as hypoglycemia, organic acidemia, or lactic acidosis, and are discussed elsewhere in this chapter.

Clinical Features.   The clinical features of hyperammonemia are similar regardless of underlying cause. Infants show lethargy, poor feeding, and vomiting at blood concentrations of 100–150 µmol/liter; hyperventilation, involuntary movements such as asterixis, and further decline in consciousness at blood concentrations of 40–400 µmol/liter; coma at blood concentrations of 400 µmol/liter; and increased intracranial pressure at blood concentrations of 500 µmol/liter.

Several clinical presentations of hyperammonemia are recognized. The first is an acute fulminating neonatal encephalopathy characterized by lethargy, hypotonia, poor feeding, and vomiting. The onset is soon after first exposure to protein feedings. The second is a Reye's-like syndrome with onset in childhood that is precipitated by stress, such as infection or a high protein intake. Children also may present a more indolent course, with ataxia, hyperactivity, anorexia, and behavioral disturbances, including self-injury. The third is a chronic or intermittent syndrome with onset from childhood to young adult life that often mimics more common neurological diseases. It is characterized by intermittent, migrainelike headaches, cyclic vomiting, confusion, hallucinations, visual disturbances, and ataxia. A less common presentation is one of progressive spasticity, mental retardation, seizures, growth retardation, and recurrent vomiting. This clinical pattern is particular to arginase deficiency.

Diagnosis.   The blood concentration of ammonia should be measured in every child with an acute or intermittent encephalopathy and in children with mental retardation or intractable seizures of unknown cause. Hyperammonemia almost always is provoked by an oral protein load in children with urea cycle defects. Further evaluation of hyperammonemia should include analyses of plasma amino acids, lactate, and pyruvate and urine measurements for organic and amino acids.

Patients with organic acidemias associated with hyperammonemia usually have ketoacidosis, hyperglycinemia, and a characteristic organic acidemia and aciduria. Lactic acidosis is never caused by a urea cycle defect and, when associated with hyperammonemia, indicates an organic acidemia or a disorder of pyruvate metabolism. Specific urea cycle defects can be distinguished by measuring the blood concentrations of citrulline, argininosuccinate, arginine, and orotic acid. Acquired liver diseases that cause hyperammonemia, with the exception of Reye's syndrome, usually show hyperbilirubinemia, elevated concentrations of liver enzymes, and other findings of liver failure.

The clinical approach to hyperammonemia is outlined in Figure 68.9. A specific diagnosis can be confirmed with

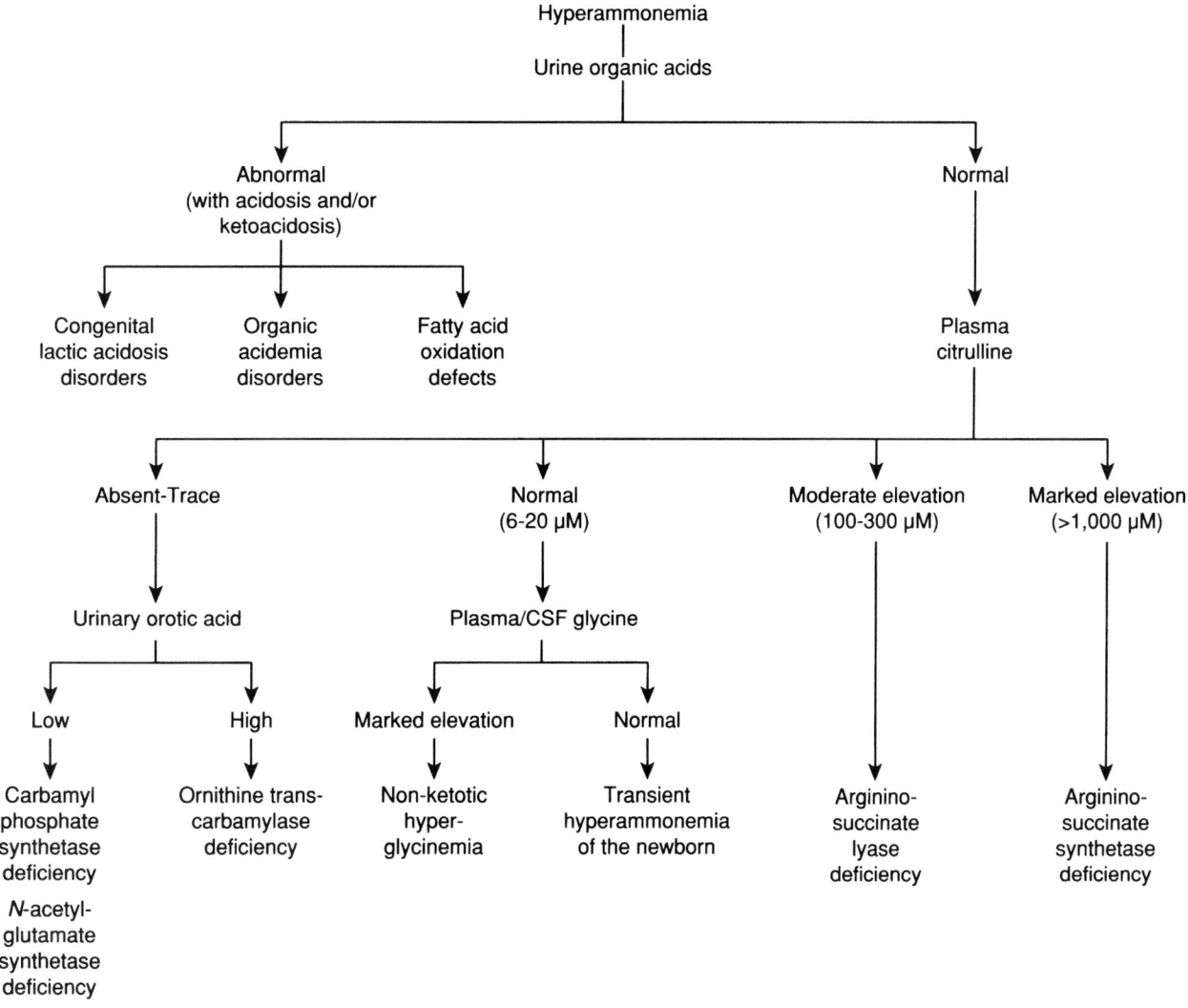

FIGURE 68.9 Algorithm for neonatal hyperammonemia. (CSF = cerebrospinal fluid.) (Modified with permission from ML Bradshaw. Inborn errors of urea synthesis. Ann Neurol 1994;35:133–141.)

enzyme analysis in fibroblasts, red blood cells, or liver tissue. Prenatal diagnosis is possible by DNA analysis or enzyme analysis of cultured cells obtained by amniocentesis.

Treatment.   Blood ammonia concentrations must be lowered quickly in patients with hyperammonemic encephalopathy or coma. Ammonia blood concentrations greater than 200 μmol/liter in a newborn always increase, and immediate hemodialysis is needed. Peritoneal dialysis and continuous arteriovenous hemofiltration are alternative but less efficient methods. Several measures are recommended, pending the specific diagnosis, that dispose of waste nitrogen atoms through alternative metabolic pathways (Table 68.12). When the diagnosis is established prenatally, specific therapy should be instituted within 2 hours of birth. Early treatment is critical because the severity of mental retardation and other permanent neurological disturbances correlates directly with the

time in hyperammonemic coma rather than with the underlying defect. Early, specific interventions may reduce the morbidity considerably.

Chronic therapy is tailored to the specific cause and is usually best managed by experienced physicians. Therapy must balance the need for adequate protein, arginine, and energy to promote growth against the adverse effects of hyperammonemia and hyperglutaninemia (Brusilow and Maestri 1996). Monitoring growth and plasma concentrations of glutamine and ammonia are important for optimal therapy. In patients with urea cycle defects, except for arginase deficiency, arginine becomes an essential amino acid, and restriction of this amino acid results in nitrogen accumulation and other problems. Patients with deficiencies of argininosuccinate synthetase or argininosuccinase benefit from arginine supplementation, which stimulates production of citrulline and argininosuccinic acid for elim-

Table 68.12:   Therapy for hyperammonemia

Therapy for severe neonatal hyperammonemia of unknown cause
   Hemodialysis for ammonia >200 µmol/liter
   No nitrogen intake until diagnosis established
   10% dextrose and intralipid infusion, protein-free enteric
      formula as soon as tolerated
   Biotin, 10 mg/day
   Vitamin B$_{12}$, 1 mg/day
   L-Carnitine, 40 mg/kg/day IV or 100–200 mg/kg/day PO
   Sodium benzoate, 0.25 g/kg initially; then 0.25–0.50 g/kg/day
      constant infusion, decreasing to the lower dose if ammonia
      levels decrease
   Arginine hydrochloride, 0.2–0.6 g/kg initially; then 0.2–0.6
      g/kg/day constant infusion with the higher dose for
      citrullinemia or argininosuccinic acidemia
   Sodium phenylacetate, 0.25 g/kg initially; then 0.25–0.5
      g/kg/day constant infusion decreasing to the lower dose
      if ammonia levels decrease
Maintenance therapy for urea cycle disorders (varies according
   to specific diagnosis)
   Protein-restricted diet (protein, 0.75 g/kg/day)
   Essential amino acids plus arginine, 0.75 g/kg/day
   Sodium benzoate, 0.25–0.50 g/kg/day
   Sodium phenylbutyrate, 0.4–0.6 g/kg/day
   L-Arginine (free base), 0.4–0.7 g/kg/day

ination as waste nitrogen. Patients with carbamyl phosphate synthetase or ornithine transcarbamylase deficiency can use benzoate, phenylacetate, and phenylbutyrate to produce other nitrogenous products that are excreted by the kidneys, thereby reducing ammonia production. Liver transplantation is an alternative approach that offers a potential cure for some diseases.

Disorders of Purine Metabolism

Lesch-Nyhan Disease

Pathophysiology.   Lesch-Nyhan disease is the most common neurological disorder of purine metabolism. It is caused by deficiency of hypoxanthine-guanine phosphoribosyl transferase (HGPRT) (Figure 68.10). HGPRT requires 5-phosphoribosyl-1-pyrophosphate as a substrate. The absence of HGPRT causes an excessive accumulation of 5-phosphoribosyl-1-pyrophosphate, which stimulates the rate-limiting step in purine metabolism. In addition, the products of HGPRT activity normally cause feedback inhibition of purine metabolism. As a result, patients with HGPRT deficiency have increased de novo purine synthesis, resulting in markedly elevated uric acid concentrations in the blood and urine. Xanthine and hypoxanthine are excreted in excessive amounts in the urine. Some of the clinical features are caused by the poor solubility of xanthine and hypoxanthine in body fluids.

The pathophysiology of cerebral impairment is not established. HGPRT activity is especially high in the basal ganglia, and its deficiency may impair dopamine synthesis. There is significant heterogeneity at the clinical, biochemical, and molecular genetic levels. Lesch-Nyhan disease is transmitted as an X-linked recessive trait. Male subjects are affected, and female carriers with partial deficiencies can develop hyperuricemia or gout.

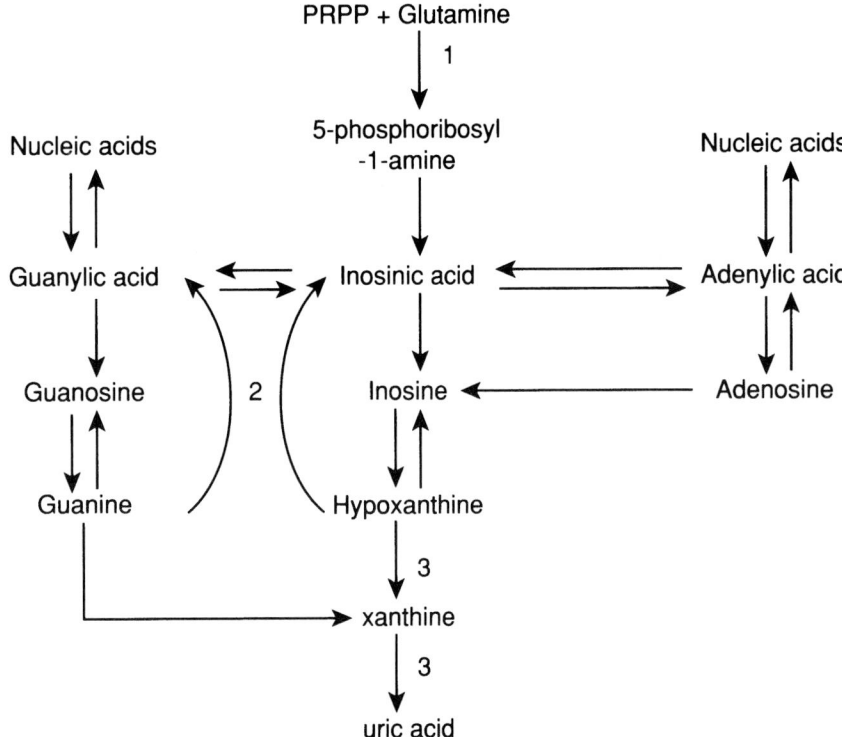

FIGURE 68.10   Purine and uric acid metabolism. (1) PRPP-glutamine aminotransferase. (2) Hypoxanthine-guanine phosphoribosyl transferase. (3) Xanthine oxidase. (PRPP = 5-phosphoribosyl-1-pyrophosphate.)

FIGURE 68.11 Self-mutilation in a patient with Lesch-Nyhan disease.

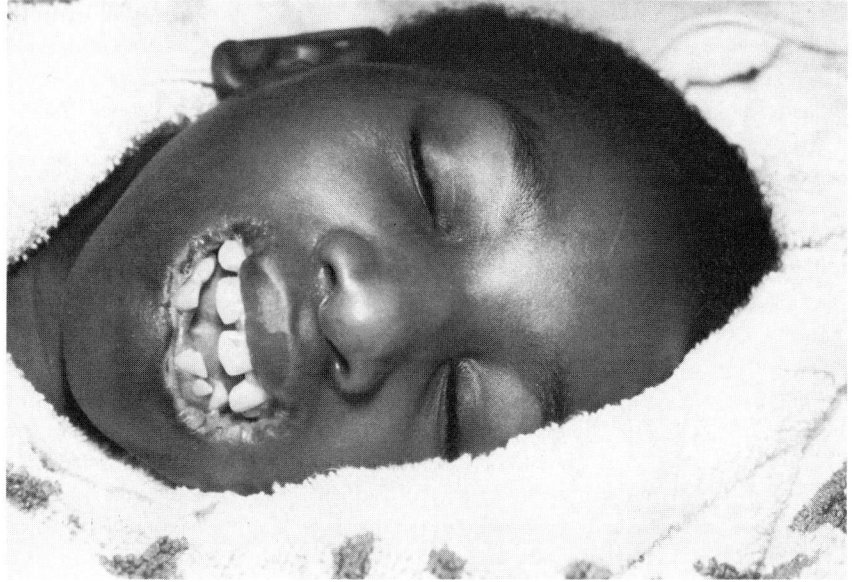

Clinical Features. The clinical features are variable degrees of mental retardation, extrapyramidal movement disorders, self-mutilation, and gout. Infants may have crystalluria, hematuria, or yellow-orange sand in their diapers. Neurological features during the first year are hypotonia that progresses to mild spasticity and psychomotor retardation. The onset of choreoathetosis is in the second and third years. Most children never learn to walk, and approximately one-half have seizures. Variable degrees of self-mutilation develop at 4–8 years of age. Unlike patients with other conditions characterized by self-injury (e.g., mental retardation), children with Lesch-Nyhan disease usually suffer actual tissue loss (Figure 68.11). They are not pain insensitive and appreciate being restrained from hurting themselves. Aggressive behavior and language also may be present. The complete neurological syndrome of spasticity, choreoathetosis, opisthotonos, facial dystonia, impaired communication and feeding, and mild to moderate mental retardation is established by age 10.

The accumulation of uric acid crystals causes arthritis, urate tophi, and renal stones. In untreated patients, death results from renal failure as a complication of nephrolithiasis or from secondary infections.

Partial deficiencies of HGPRT cause several possible milder syndromes. Some patients have only hyperuricemia; others have neurological dysfunction without mental retardation or self-mutilating behavior. The syndrome in one kindred with variant enzyme kinetics was characterized by mild retardation, slowly progressive mild spasticity, and dysmorphic features.

Diagnosis. The diagnosis is suggested by the clinical features and X-linked inheritance and confirmed by elevated blood concentrations of uric acid. A laboratory screening test is the measurement of the urinary uric acid to creatinine ratio. Children with the disease have a ratio greater than 2 to 1. Definitive diagnosis requires measuring HGPRT activity in white blood cells, fibroblasts, or amniocytes.

Treatment. Treatment is directed at preventing complications of hyperuricemia. The course of neurological deterioration cannot be altered. Allopurinol, a xanthine oxidase inhibitor, lowers blood uric acid concentrations and prevents renal and joint disease. A high liquid intake also helps prevent the formation of xanthine stones. Annual renal ultrasonography is recommended. Physical restraints and dental extractions may be necessary to prevent self-mutilation, although some boys respond to behavior modification.

Other Disorders of Purine Metabolism. Xanthinuria is an autosomal recessive disorder of purine metabolism caused by xanthine oxidase deficiency. The deficiency is asymptomatic in most patients. Some have xanthine urinary calculi. Myopathy from deposits of xanthine crystals in muscle is a rare complication.

A rare disorder of purine metabolism is caused by a defect in a molybdenum-containing cofactor necessary for both xanthine oxidase and sulfite oxidase. The onset begins shortly after birth. Clinical features are developmental delay, seizures, cerebral atrophy, and lens dislocation. Death occurs during infancy.

Adenylosuccinase deficiency is a rare disorder that causes variable signs of mental retardation, seizures, autism, growth retardation, and myopathy.

Disorders of Pyrimidine Metabolism

Hereditary orotic aciduria is caused by a deficiency of orotate phosphoribosyltransferase and orotidine-5'-phosphate decarboxylase, which are dual components of uridine-5'-monophosphate synthase. The clinical features are delayed development, megaloblastic anemia, leukopenia, and crystalluria. Strabismus and fine, dry hair are common. Some children have splenomegaly. The diagnosis is difficult on clinical grounds alone. Orotic acid excretion is 1,000 times greater than normal; the enzymes can be measured for definitive diagnosis. An early diagnosis is important because dietary supplementation with uridine, 100 mg/kg per day, corrects the hematological abnormalities and prevents the developmental problems.

The list of disorders that affects the catabolism of the pyrimidines thymine and uracil continues to grow (Van Gennip et al. 1997). Uracil is metabolized in a series of steps to carbomoyl-β-alanine, which is then converted to the neurotransmitter β-alanine by a transaminase. Thymine catabolism has similar steps to carbomoyl-β-aminobutyric acid. Defects proximal to the transaminase cause accumulation uracil and thymine and decreased concentrations of β-alanine. Transaminase deficiency causes increased concentrations of β-alanine. The clinical features are not specific for diagnosis. Patients may have seizures, mental retardation, growth retardation, and microcephaly. Patients with partial deficiency can have severe neurological complications from treatment with the antimetabolite 5-fluorouracil because the drug is metabolized by the same system.

Xeroderma Pigmentosum.   Xeroderma pigmentosum is caused by a defect in DNA repair; seven genetically distinct forms are recognized, of which four have neurological complications (De Sanctis-Cacchione syndrome). Affected individuals are sensitive to ultraviolet (UV) light. Under normal physiological conditions, UV light causes cyclobutane-pyrimidine dimers to form from adjacent pyrimidines in DNA. Normally, such dimers are excised, the gaps filled by DNA polymerase, and the DNA ends rejoined by a ligase. In xeroderma pigmentosum, however, excision of dimers is impaired in most cases; postreplication repair is defective in others.

Defective DNA repair causes severe sensitivity to sun exposure, with chronic exposure causing skin cancer. The neurological features are progressive mental deterioration, microcephaly, choreoathetosis, ataxia, deafness, pyramidal and extrapyramidal signs, and growth failure. Polyneuropathy is almost a constant feature after 10 years of age.

The diagnosis can be made by the typical skin features and neurological signs. Cultured fibroblasts show a high rate of UV-induced mutagenesis. The only treatment is avoiding sun exposure.

Cockayne's Syndrome.   Cockayne's syndrome has similar pathophysiological and clinical features to xeroderma pig-

mentosum. Affected individuals have excessive sensitivity to sun exposure, mental retardation, spasticity, and deafness.

Porphyrias

Pathophysiology.   Porphyrins play an important role in intermediary metabolism by forming metalloporphyrin complexes, which are found in hemoglobin, myoglobin, cytochromes, peroxidases, oxidases, and catalases. The porphyrias are a group of disorders with defects in heme biosynthesis that result in cutaneous signs, neuropsychiatric signs, or both (Kappas et al. 1995). Heme causes feedback inhibition of δ-aminolevulinic acid synthetase, the first enzyme in the heme synthetic pathway. This enzyme is induced by several drugs. Increased production of aminolevulinic acid (ALA) is associated with attacks of porphyria. Cutaneous manifestations of porphyria correlate with the accumulation of porphyrin intermediates (uroporphyrin, coproporphyrin, and protoporphyrin); the neuropsychiatric features correlate with the accumulation of the porphyrin precursors ALA and porphobilinogen (PBG).

Seven enzyme defects cause porphyria; three defects cause only cutaneous disease. The hepatic porphyrias (acute intermittent porphyria, hereditary coproporphyria, and variegate porphyria) are transmitted by autosomal dominant inheritance and characterized by neurological and psychiatric disturbances. Acute intermittent porphyria is not associated with skin photosensitivity (Table 68.13).

Acute intermittent porphyria is the most common dominantly inherited disease of porphyrin metabolism. It is caused by a partial deficiency of PBG deaminase, the third step in heme synthesis. Excessive amounts of ALA and PBG are generated during attacks and are detected easily in the urine. Despite the gene defect's autosomal dominant inheritance, approximately 90% of those with the gene defect have a latent disease and do not have clinical expression. Drugs, hormones, nutrition, and other exogenous factors determine disease expression in acute intermittent porphyria heterozygotes. Onset of symptoms is unusual in childhood, and the gender ratio is approximately equal before puberty. After puberty, it is twice as common in girls as in boys.

Clinical Features.   The most common clinical feature of acute intermittent porphyria is an acute attack of severe abdominal pain, often associated with vomiting and constipation or with diarrhea. The pain usually precedes other clinical features and is described as colicky but may be steady. Other common features are tachycardia, hypertension, and fever, which are thought to be caused by an autonomic polyneuropathy. Less frequent manifestations of autonomic dysfunction in acute intermittent porphyria are urinary retention, hypotension, and diaphoresis.

Peripheral neuropathy, mainly motor, occurs in approximately 50% of attacks. Rare cases have a mononeuropathy multiplex. The neuropathy can progress to complete paralysis over several weeks and is clinically indistinguish-

Table 68.13: Clinical and biochemical features of the hepatic porphyrias

Disease	Enzyme deficiency	Inheritance	Skin sensitivity	Neurological signs	Porphyrins	
					Urine	Stool
Acute intermittent porphyria	Porphobilinogendeaminase	AD	−	+	ALA PBG	−
Hereditary coproporphyria	Coproporphyrinogen oxidase	AD	+	+	ALA PBG COPRO	COPRO
Variegate porphyria	Protoporphyrinogen oxidase	AD	+	+	ALA PBG COPRO	COPRO PROTO
Aminolevulinic dehydratase deficiency porphyria	Aminolevulinic dehydratase	AR	−	+	ALA	−

AD = autosomal dominant; ALA = delta aminolevulinic acid; AR = autosomal recessive; COPRO = coproporphyrin; PBG = porphobilinogen; PROTO = protoporphyrin; + = usually present; − = usually absent.
Source: Adapted with permission from A Kappas, S Sassa, RA Gallbraith, et al. The Porphyrias. In JB Stanburg, JB Wyngaarden, DS Fredrickson, et al. (eds), The Metabolic Basis of Inherited Disease (6th ed). New York: McGraw-Hill, 1989;1305–1365.

able from Guillain-Barré syndrome, except that the neuropathy of acute intermittent porphyria is axonal rather than demyelinating. The weakness usually resolves in days to months after an attack, but resolution may be incomplete following a severe or prolonged attack. The CNS features of acute intermittent porphyria are mainly psychiatric, including episodes of depression, dementia, acute paranoia, schizophrenia, delirium, or agitation. The psychiatric symptoms resolve between attacks in adults, but children can have irreversible cognitive and behavioral disturbances. Nonpsychiatric features are aphasia and apraxias. Seizures occur in 15% of adults and 30% of children.

Several drugs, especially barbiturates, can precipitate acute attacks in acute intermittent porphyria. The list of prohibited drugs includes sulfonamides, griseofulvin, meprobamate, phenytoin, valproate, corticosteroids, succinamides, and many others (Kappas et al. 1995). Other contributing factors in precipitating attacks are starvation, infection, and fever.

Hereditary coproporphyria and variegate porphyria have neurological and cutaneous manifestations (see Table 68.13). The skin is photosensitive, and blistering occurs with excessive sun exposure or mild trauma and leads to moderate scarring. The neurological manifestations are the same as in acute intermittent porphyria.

Diagnosis.   Acute intermittent porphyria should be suspected in every patient with acute or episodic neurological or psychiatric disturbances, especially when the family history is compatible with similar illness. The amount of ALA and PBG excreted increases during attacks, but may be normal in between attacks. Other laboratory abnormalities include hypercholesterolemia, hyperlipidemia, glucose intolerance, and an elevated concentration of CSF protein. Definitive diagnosis requires measuring PBG deaminase

activity in erythrocytes. Screening for the porphyrias is accomplished by measuring stool porphyrins and urinary ALA and PBG concentrations.

Treatment.   Therapy is mainly preventive, with avoidance of low-calorie diets and drugs that are known to induce attacks. Glucose infusions and hematin, substances that inhibit ALA synthetase, are administered during an attack. Seizure management is difficult because several commonly used anticonvulsant drugs may increase the severity of an acute attack. Gabapentin is not metabolized in the liver and may be the drug of choice for managing epilepsy in patients with acute intermittent porphyria (Tatum and Zachariah 1996). Prophylactic hematin therapy has been used to prevent attacks, but its use may be limited because of thrombotic complications. Haem-arginate may be a safer alternative. Cimetidine also has been used as prophylactic therapy (Rogers 1997).

Lipoprotein Deficiencies

Abetalipoproteinemia and Hypobetalipoproteinemia

Pathophysiology.   Lipoproteins are necessary for the transport of certain lipids in the blood. Abetalipoproteinemia (Bassen-Kornzweig syndrome) is an autosomal recessive inherited disease in which apolipoprotein B is completely absent, resulting in very low plasma concentrations of cholesterol and triglyceride. The blood contains no chylomicrons, very low-density lipoproteins, or low-density lipoproteins. More important, the blood concentrations of vitamin E and other fat-soluble vitamins are very low. The neuropathological features are demyelination of peripheral nerves and neuronal degeneration of the cerebellum and spinal neurons. Vitamin E deficiency without fat malabsorption causes a spinocerebellar disease similar to Friedreich's ataxia.

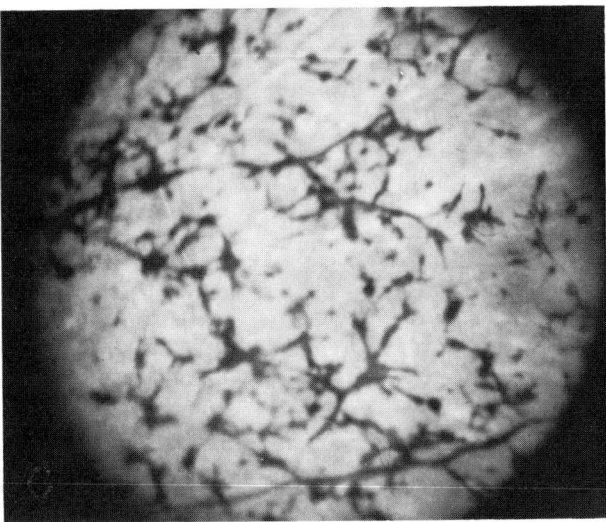

FIGURE 68.12 Retinitis pigmentosa. (Reprinted with permission from OB Evans. Manual of Child Neurology. New York: Churchill Livingstone, 1987;213.)

Clinical Features. The main clinical features are fat malabsorption, retinitis pigmentosa (Figure 68.12), progressive ataxia, polyneuropathy, and acanthocytosis. The lack of beta-lipoproteins causes a malabsorption syndrome in infants, with chronic steatorrhea, poor feeding, and failure to thrive. Retinal degeneration and neurological signs begin in the first decade. Impaired night vision is an early feature. Areflexia, ataxia, nystagmus, and ophthalmoplegia become increasingly more severe during the second and third decades. Pes cavus and scoliosis are associated with the ataxia, adding to the similarity to Friedreich's ataxia.

Hypobetalipoproteinemia has similar but much less severe clinical features. It is transmitted as an autosomal dominant trait.

Diagnosis. The diagnosis should be considered in patients with unexplained progressive ataxia. Laboratory confirmation is made by plasma lipoprotein electrophoresis, measurement of blood cholesterol and triglycerides, and evaluation of red cell morphology. In patients with abetalipoproteinemia or hypobetalipoproteinemia, plasma vitamin E and iron concentrations are decreased.

Treatment. Many of the complications of abetalipoproteinemia and hypobetalipoproteinemia can be prevented by administering 1,000–10,000 mg per day of DL-alpha-tocopherol. Vitamins A and K also should be supplemented (Kane and Havel 1995).

Tangier Disease

Pathophysiology. Tangier disease is a rare disorder characterized by large, orange tonsils and polyneuropathy. It is transmitted by autosomal recessive inheritance. The tonsils and other tissues are laden with cholesterol esters.

The blood cholesterol concentration is decreased, and the triglyceride concentration is normal or increased. High-density lipoproteins are deficient, and electrophoresis shows no alpha lipoprotein mobility and an indistinct pre-beta band.

Clinical Features. The initial symptoms of Tangier disease are recurrent or progressive sensorimotor neuropathy in childhood. Neurological signs include distal weakness, decreased pain and temperature sensation with relative preservation of position and vibratory sensation, and hyporeflexia. Electrodiagnostic studies are compatible with an axonal neuropathy (see Chapter 37B). Less common features are ptosis, ophthalmoplegia, and hepatosplenomegaly.

Diagnosis. Tangier disease should be suspected in any child with neuropathy and enlarged tonsils. The blood lipid profile is diagnostic.

Treatment. Treatment is not available.

Disorders of Copper Metabolism

Dietary copper is absorbed in the gut and transported to the liver. Copper is disbursed to other tissues bound to ceruloplasmin in the blood and binds to metallothionein within the cell. Excess copper is excreted in the bile. Copper is a necessary component of a number of metalloenzymes including cytochrome oxidase (electron transfer), superoxide dismutase (free radical detoxification), trosine and dopamine β-hydroxylase (melanin and catecholamine synthesis), and lysyloxidase (cross linkages in collagen and elastin). Excessive copper is toxic and its metabolism is carefully controlled. Two diseases are related to abnormal copper metabolism. Wilson's disease is caused by an inability to excrete excess copper and Menkes' disease is caused by an inability to absorb copper (DiDonato and Sarkar 1997). A related disease, aceruloplasminemia, is caused by an absence of ceruloplasmin, has similar clinical features to Wilson's disease, normal copper metabolism, and iron storage in the brain.

Hepatolenticular Degeneration (Wilson's Disease)

Pathophysiology. Wilson's disease is transmitted by autosomal recessive inheritance and is characterized by impaired copper excretion in the bile. The responsible gene has been mapped to chromosome 13q14.3. It codes for a membrane-bound, copper binding, ATPase protein that probably acts as a copper pump to transfer copper into bile. The pleiotropic effects of the 25 known mutant gene defects are secondary to excessive accumulation of copper in the liver, brain, cornea, kidneys, and other tissues of untreated patients. The copper concentration in the tissues may be 20–30 times greater than normal. The serum ceruloplasmin concentration is low, and excessive copper exists in the plasma and urine.

In the initial asymptomatic stage, copper accumulates in the hepatic cytosol. After the cytosols are saturated, copper accumulates in hepatic lysosomes and spills into the circulation. Rapid redistribution can cause fulminant hepatic injury or hemolysis. Continued release of copper into the blood causes the gradual development of chronic neurological, hepatic, and renal disease and may cause osteoporosis, arthropathy, and cardiomyopathy.

Nodular cirrhosis of the liver begins during early childhood. The main neuropathological finding is cavitary necrosis of the putamen and caudate nuclei, with neuronal loss, axonal degeneration, and protoplasmic astrocytosis. Cortical atrophy is common, and MRI correlates well with the postmortem findings.

Clinical Features. The onset of symptoms is unusual before age 6 years or after age 40 years. One-half of patients are symptomatic by age 15 years; the mean age of onset for neurological symptoms is age 21 years. One-third of the patients present with liver disease, one-third with neurologic features, and one-third with psychiatric features (Brewer 1995). Liver disease and hemolytic anemia are the typical initial symptoms in children; one-half of affected individuals have liver disease at onset. The liver disease is characterized by an acute hepatitis that either resolves spontaneously or progresses to eventual death from hepatic and renal failure. Less common are asymptomatic hepatomegaly, chronic active hepatitis, or cirrhosis. Other systemic manifestations in children are anorexia, nausea, vomiting, weight loss, fluid retention, splenomegaly, and easy bruising or other bleeding problems. Neutropenia and thrombocytopenia may complicate the hemolytic anemia.

The major neurologic features are dysarthria, poor coordination, tremor, gait and postural abnormalities, and invariably, dystonia. Sensory symptoms are notably absent and chorea is rare. The psychiatric manifestations are insidious and include depression, personality change, and emotional lability. Most patients have impaired work or school performance.

Diagnosis. Wilson's disease should be considered in every child with unexplained liver disease or hemolytic anemia. The diagnosis should be considered in older children and adults who have unexplained extrapyramidal dysfunction, dysarthria, and personality change or depression. A careful family history often discloses consanguinity or a sibling with similar features. No laboratory test is definitive. The most common diagnostic abnormality is the presence of a Kayser-Fleischer ring in the cornea caused by copper accumulation in Descemet's membrane (Figure 68.13). It is present in all patients with neurological disease and in 85% of children with only hepatic disease.

Other findings are increased urinary copper excretion (>100 μg/24 hours) and low plasma ceruloplasmin concentrations (<15 mg/dl). Approximately 10% of patients with Wilson's disease have ceruloplasmin levels that overlap the range for both heterozygotes and control patients. Aceruloplasminemia is a rare disorder with clinical features similar to Wilson's disease; however, the pathophysiology is related to iron deposition in the basal ganglia rather than copper. Nonceruloplasmin copper is consistently elevated

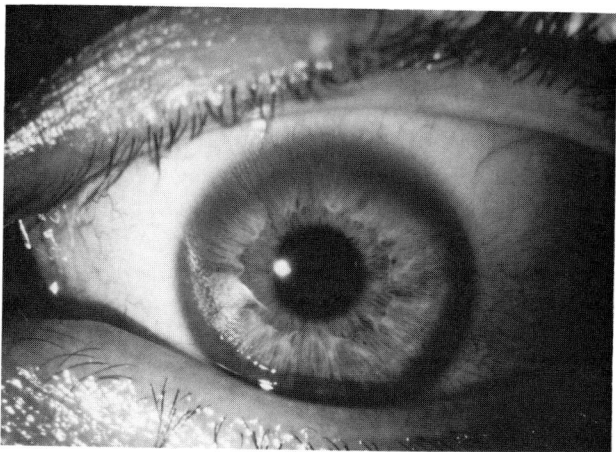

FIGURE 68.13 Kayser-Fleischer ring in a patient with Wilson's disease. (Courtesy of Dr. John Milam.)

in Wilson's disease and in other diseases causing cholestasis. Liver copper concentrations of more than 250 μg/g dry weight of the liver are diagnostic for Wilson's disease. Urinary copper excretion is not diagnostic but is useful to monitor therapy. Normal adult copper excretion is less than 70 μg per day. Radiocopper incorporation into ceruloplasmin is useful when other test results are equivocal. Normally, ^{64}Cu is cleared rapidly from the blood by the liver, but a secondary increase in the plasma concentration occurs within 48 hours as newly synthesized ceruloplasmin binds the radiocopper. This secondary increase is absent in patients with Wilson's disease.

MRI shows cortical atrophy, ventricular dilatation, and lytic lesions in the basal ganglia. In general, asymptomatic patients with normal neurological examinations have normal imaging study results. Therapy often improves the cortical atrophy and especially the basal ganglia lytic lesions.

Treatment. D-Penicillamine is useful for mild disease, even in those who are asymptomatic. The average dose is 0.5 g per day for children less than 10 years of age and 1.0–2.0 g per day for those older than age 10 years. It should be given four times a day before meals. Higher dosages are given briefly for acutely ill patients, and then lowered by 50% for maintenance after the clinical features stabilize and urinary copper excretion diminishes. Both the systemic and neurological complications improve after a delay of several months. Unfortunately, some patients become transiently worse when treatment is initiated. This can be avoided by gradually increasing the dose in combination with a low-copper diet (<1 mg/day) to prevent sudden, excessive mobilization of copper. Among patients with established disease, 50% show significant improvement, 15% remain stable, and the remainder have an initial deterioration. Approximately one-half of those who deteriorate do not recover to their pretreatment state. The liver disease in children improves considerably. If there are also neurological complications, however, only 25% show improved liver function with therapy; 25% deteriorate despite therapy. Early detection and uninterrupted therapy throughout life improves the outcome. Sudden discontinuation of penicillamine causes a rapid clinical deterioration. The side effects associated with D-penicillamine are myelosuppression, lupuslike reactions, glomerulonephritis, anaphylaxis, pyridoxine-responsive anemia, and a myasthenia gravis syndrome. Many patients also develop a rash. The diet should be supplemented with 25 mg per day of pyridoxine.

Patients who cannot tolerate penicillamine can be treated with trientine, 500 mg three times a day before meals. If neither drug is tolerated, elemental zinc, 50 mg three times a day, may be beneficial. Zinc competes for copper absorption in the intestine and stimulates the production of the metallobinding protein metallothionein in the liver, thus binding excess dietary copper. Tetrathiomolybdate is an effective chelator of copper and is less likely to cause neurological deterioration than D-penicillamine (Brewer 1995). When the drug becomes widely available, the initial use of tetrathiomolybdate followed by chronic zinc therapy may be the best strategy for the chronic treatment of Wilson's disease. Liver transplantation is curative.

Menkes' Syndrome

Pathophysiology. Menkes' syndrome (trichopoliodystrophy, or kinky hair syndrome) is an X-linked recessive disorder of copper metabolism. The gene defect at chromosome Xq13.3 impairs placental and intestinal copper transport (DiDonato and Sarkar 1997). Affected male subjects have increased binding and defective release of copper by intestinal mucosa, kidney, and cultured fibroblasts. This causes impaired copper absorption by the intestine. The copper concentration is low in the brain, liver, and plasma, as is the ceruloplasmin level. Copper is a component of many metalloenzymes. Copper deficiency has widespread effects on the nervous system and other tissues, especially connective tissue. Impaired elastin and collagen cross linking by the copper-requiring enzyme lysyl oxidase causes a vasculopathy. Complex IV of the electron transport chain also is affected. Pathologically, there is neuronal degeneration and gliosis. The Purkinje's cells are affected especially, and many show an unusual proliferation of the dendrites.

Clinical Features. Affected infants have hypothermia, failure to thrive, hypotonia, and seizures. Neurological deterioration is rapid, with death early in childhood. The face has a depressed nasal bridge and a cherubic appearance. The hair is colorless and quite friable, with pili torti (twisting) and trichorrhexis nodosa (fragmentation) or monilethrix (periodic narrowing). Systemic manifestations include osteoporosis with diaphyseal fractures, intestinal diverticulae, and markedly tortuous arteries in the brain and other organs.

Milder variants of Menkes' syndrome are characterized by mild mental retardation associated with ataxia and extrapyramidal signs and the occipital horn exostosis syndrome.

Diagnosis. The diagnosis should be suspected in any male child who has early neurological regression associated with the typical hair features. Low plasma concentrations of ceruloplasmin and copper suggest the diagnosis. Gene detection confirms the diagnosis.

Treatment. Copper supplementation with copper histinate may prolong survival. Prenatal diagnosis is possible.

Disorders of Oxidative Metabolism and Mitochondria

Mitochondria are subcellular organelles that have a symbiotic relationship with the cell. A major function of mitochondria is oxidative metabolism. Most structural components of the mitochondria are encoded on nuclear DNA, transported across the mitochondrial membranes, and assembled in mitochondria. Approximately 3% of mitochondrial proteins are encoded by maternally inherited mitochondrial DNA (mtDNA). mtDNA encodes 13 proteins in the respiratory chain, 2 rRNAs, and 22 tRNAs. Several intermediary metabolic pathways converge in mitochondria for the use of carbon skeletons derived from carbohydrates, fatty acids, amino acids, and ketone body metabolism. The combination of acetyl-CoA and oxaloacetate forms citric acid, which is metabolized in the citric acid cycle to produce reducing equivalents (reduced nicotinamide adenine dinucleotide [NADH$^+$H] and reduced flavinadenine dinucleotide [FADH$_2$]) and CO_2. The reducing equivalents are transferred to molecular oxygen in the respiratory chain to produce water. The energy released by electron transport is used by complex V to make adenosine triphosphate (ATP) from adenosine diphosphate. Reactive oxygen species, unavoidable by-products of electron transport, cause cellular protein and DNA damage that accumulates over the life of postmitotic cells and occurs at an accelerated rate in mitochondrial diseases.

The organs and tissues most dependent on mitochondrial energy production include brain, peripheral nerve, heart, skeletal muscle, endocrine glands, kidney, retina, and bone marrow. These are the predominant organ systems, and tissues involved in mitochondrial disease becoming quickly symptomatic when oxidative metabolism is impaired. Mitochondrial diseases are multisystem disorders with variable phenotypes and symptoms overlapping those of common diseases. Asymptomatic or mildly affected individuals often are misdiagnosed, and the onset of significant symptoms may not occur until adulthood. Patients with mitochondrial disease often are diagnosed with cerebral palsy, epilepsy, learning disabilities, autism, neuromuscular disease, and other common neurological disorders. Often patients present with symptoms remote from the nervous system such as symptoms of cardiomyopathy, diabetes mellitus, disorders of gut motility, renal or hepatic disease, or anemia. The biochemical signature of impaired oxidative metabolism is acidosis, especially lactic acidosis. Hypoglycemia and hyperammonemia also may be seen, particularly in younger individuals. Impaired metabolic oxidation of glucose and fatty acids are discussed in this section.

Lactic Acidosis

Pathophysiology.   Lactic acid, the normal end product of anaerobic glucose metabolism, accumulates when production exceeds use. Physiological states, such as anaerobic exercise, produce an oxygen debt in fast-twitch (glycolytic) muscle fibers that causes a transitory lactic acidosis. Pathological lactic acidosis occurs during anoxia-ischemia and in metabolic failure from liver disease or diabetes mellitus. These conditions must be excluded before evaluating children for inborn errors of metabolism. Inborn errors of metabolism that cause lactic acidosis may result from oxidative metabolic defects (primary) or defects in other metabolic pathways (secondary) that impair mitochondrial metabolism. Lactic acid elevation as an artifact of sample collection or handling is a common problem.

Intact oxidative metabolism is critical for normal CNS function. Both primary and secondary lactic acidosis impair cerebral function because of in situ mitochondrial oxidative failure and the neurotoxic effects of excess lactic acid. The high metabolic activity of the basal ganglia makes them especially vulnerable to oxidative defects. Putaminal necrosis is a frequent early feature of Leigh disease and is common in mitochondrial encephalomyopathies. Basal ganglia disease is often a feature of complex I deficiency, which is found in 25% of cases of Leigh disease. In 1992, Shoffner and colleagues reported that dystonia was the initial feature in two families with a novel mtDNA mutation in the ND6 gene of complex I. Some adult-onset neurodegenerative diseases might have a mitochondrial pathogenesis. Decreased tissue concentrations of mitochondrial complex I activity are found in patients with Parkinson's disease (Haas et al. 1995) and Huntington's disease. mtDNA mutations at higher than control frequency have been reported in Alzheimer's disease and Parkinson's disease (Shoffner et al. 1993).

Figure 68.14 provides an overview of oxidative metabolism and indicates the sites of the enzyme defects commonly responsible for Leigh disease. Lactic acid is the end product of pyruvate metabolism and acts as a reservoir for excess pyruvate. Under physiological conditions, lactic dehydrogenase is a reversible enzyme that converts lactate back to pyruvate, which is then further metabolized through the citric acid cycle. The oxidation of lactate to pyruvate produces 1 mole of NADH, an important substrate in the electron transport chain. The blood lactate to pyruvate ratio reflects the NADH to nicotinamide-adenine dinucleotide ratio, or redox state, and is useful in the diagnosis of primary lactic acidosis. Defects of enzymes close to pyruvate in the metabolic pathway usually produce ratios of less than 20, whereas electron trans-

port chain defects that cause NADH accumulation have ratios greater than 20.

Clinical Features.   Disorders of mitochondrial oxidative metabolism that cause lactic acidosis are clinically and biochemically heterogeneous. Leigh disease can be caused by several biochemical defects: pyruvate dehydrogenase (PDH) deficiency, PC deficiency, and defects in the electron transport system. On the other hand, a single enzymatic defect, such as cytochrome oxidase (COX) deficiency, has several clinical phenotypes because the mitochondria themselves and the severity of a mitochondrial defect can vary from organ to organ. An apparently single enzyme defect such as COX deficiency, may result from defects in nuclear or mitochondrial encoded subunits. In addition, different tissue isoforms lead to great variability in phenotypic expression. Mitochondrial encoded tRNA defects may compromise COX subunit translation, leading to COX deficiency. This phenomenon leads to the early confusing reports of multiple electron transport enzyme deficiencies in diseases later shown to be caused by mitochondrial tRNA point mutations. Variability of clinical phenotype is particularly a feature of mtDNA disorders. This arises in large part from heteroplasmy (a mixture of mutant and wild-type mtDNA), which differs from mitochondrion to mitochondrion, cell to cell, and tissue to tissue.

The most common clinical features of primary lactic acidosis are neurological: (1) severe infantile or neonatal lactic acidemia with encephalopathy; (2) subacute necrotizing encephalomyelopathy (Leigh disease); (3) psychomotor delay with static or progressive CNS disease; (4) mitochondrial encephalomyopathy; (5) mitochondrial myopathy; and (6) intermittent ataxia with a progressive spinocerebellar degeneration. In all presentations, involvement of organs other than the CNS is common and should be sought. Cardiomyopathy is particularly common.

Diagnosis.   The first step in diagnosing lactic acidosis is to confirm the blood lactate and pyruvate concentrations. Spurious elevation of blood lactate concentration is caused either by ischemia from the tourniquet used to collect blood or from the normal anaerobic metabolism of red blood cells that occurs when blood lactic dehydrogenase is inhibited inadequately because of inadequate mixing with perchlorate or fluoride. Fasting samples are needed to measure pyruvate because its concentration normally is elevated within 2 hours of a meal. Reliable measurements require a free-flowing venous sample collected without or with brief application of a tourniquet (<20 seconds). Accurate sampling may require an indwelling intravenous catheter. The blood must be mixed well in the collection tube and placed on ice for transport to a laboratory experienced in the measurement of lactate and pyruvate.

Arterial samples are less prone to artifact, but prolonged crying raises arterial lactate. CSF lactate and pyruvate concentrations may be elevated in patients with lactic acidosis

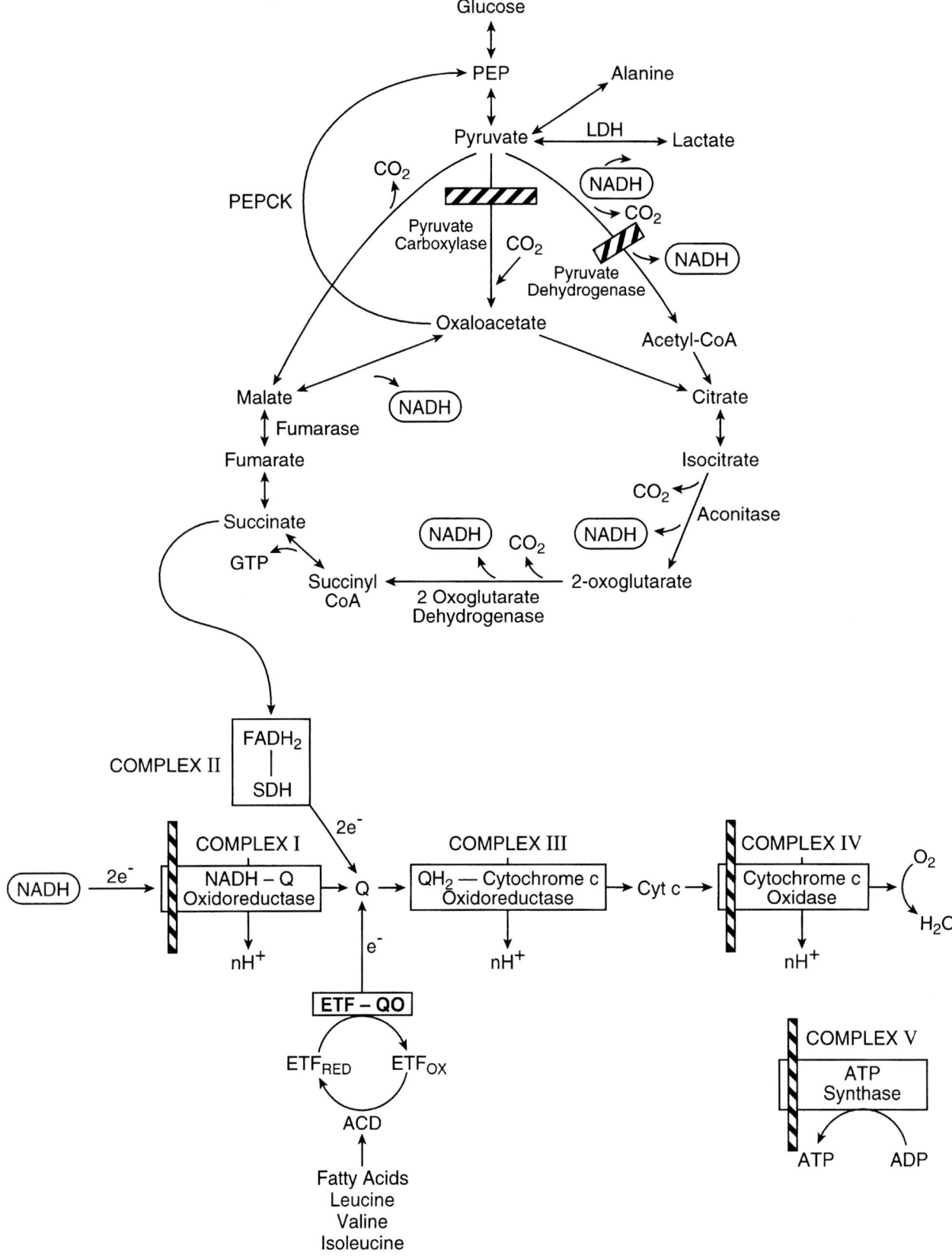

FIGURE 68.14 Overview of oxidative metabolism and the biochemical defects of Leigh disease (*hatched bars*). (ACD = mitochondrial acyl–coenzyme A (CoA) dehydrogenase; ADP = adenosine diphosphate; ATP = adenosine triphosphate; Cyt c = cytochrome c; ETF = electron transfer factor; ETF-QO = ETF-coenzyme Q oxidoreductase; $FADH_2$ = reduced flavine adenine dinucleotide; GTP = guanosine triphosphate; LDH = lactic dehydrogenase; NADH = reduced nicotinamide adenine dinucleotide; ox = oxidase; PEP = phosphoenolpyruvate; PEPCK = phosphoenolpyruvate carboxykinase; Q = coenzyme Q; RED = reductase; SDH = succinic dehydrogenase.)

even when blood levels are normal and should be measured in all patients. Lactic acidosis caused by organic acid disorders or amino acid disorders must be excluded by measuring quantitative urine organic acids and blood amino acids. Blood biotinidase and ammonia also should be measured. In patients with intermittent lactic acidosis, carbohydrate loading with glucose and fructose may confirm abnormal lactate production. These tests may be helpful therapeutically (see Treatment, later in this chapter).

Family history must be recorded, searching for familial, and particularly maternally inherited, mitochondrial phenotypes. Complete definition of the clinical phenotype requires MRI to determine the extent of CNS involvement and electrocardiography and echocardiography to search for cardiomyopathy (present in up to 15% of patients with lactic acidosis). Renal tubular acidosis is common.

The presence of true lactic acidemia requires a 24-hour inpatient fasting study with glucagon stimulation to exclude glycogen storage disease, defects of gluconeogenesis, and defects of fatty acid oxidation. Urine organic acids and blood ketones are measured during fasting. Patients who can fast without hypoglycemia probably have a mitochondrial disorder and need a skin biopsy for fibroblast enzymatic studies and muscle biopsy for histochemical and ultrastructure studies of mitochondria. In some mitochondrial disorders such as COX deficiency, fasting hypoglycemia is common (Haas and Barshop 1998). Special studies of leukocyte and platelet or muscle mitochondrial electron transport activities may be necessary. The blood lactate to pyruvate ratio and the clinical phenotype can help determine the selection of enzymatic assays. Mitochondrial DNA analysis in blood and muscle is usually needed.

Treatment.   Acute, life-threatening lactic acidosis requires alkali therapy, usually with intravenous sodium bicarbonate. Peritoneal dialysis with bicarbonate is lifesaving in some cases. A few patients, particularly those with renal tubular acidosis, require long-term oral bicarbonate supplementation. An experimental agent, dichloroacetic acid, is available in a few centers for the treatment of acute and chronic lactic acidosis. Vitamin and cofactor therapies, such as thiamine, riboflavin, biotin, ascorbic acid, and coenzyme Q_{10} are recommended for severe lactic acidosis: L-carnitine may be beneficial. These agents are effective in some of the specific enzymatic deficiencies that cause lactic acidosis. Children with carbohydrate sensitivity may benefit from glucose or fructose restriction or from a high-fat or ketogenic diet (Haas and Barshop 1998).

Pyruvate Dehydrogenase Deficiency

Pathophysiology.   PDH deficiency is a cooperative mitochondrial enzyme complex composed of five subunits. The three main components of the complex are termed E1, E2, and E3. This configuration is shared by the three ketoacid dehydrogenases: PDH, 2-oxoglutarate dehydrogenase, and BCKA dehydrogenase. Thiamine is a cofactor for E1 and lipoic acid for E3. Two regulatory enzymes, a phosphatase and a kinase, activate and inactivate the E1 component of PDH. E1 consists of two α-subunits encoded on the X chromosome and two beta subunits. The drug dichloroacetic acid activates PDH by inhibiting the kinase. PDH is the major flux-regulating step for entry of carbohydrate carbon skeletons into the citric acid cycle and provides the fine control needed for oxidative metabolism. The available amount of cerebral PDH activity is equivalent to the maximal measured carbohydrate metabolic flux rate; therefore, a partial deficiency has serious effects. Human deficiencies of all three PDH components and both E1 subunits have been reported.

Clinical Features.   E1 deficiency is the best studied and most common form of PDH deficiency. More than 90% of PDH-deficient patients (both male and female) have an E1 alpha gene defect. Disease severity correlates with enzyme activity. The clinical features range from severe neonatal lactic acidosis and death to episodic ataxia with lactic and pyruvic acidosis and spinocerebellar degeneration. Approximately 25% of patients with Leigh disease have PDH deficiency. Children with PDH deficiency who survive the neonatal period often are mentally retarded. Agenesis of the corpus callosum and cystic lesions of the basal ganglia, cerebellum, and brainstem are seen often on MRI or during postmortem examination. Chronic growth delay and hypotonia that often evolves into an athetoid cerebral palsy syndrome may be seen. (see Chapter 66). Demyelinating polyneuropathy (which may be misdiagnosed as Guillain-Barré syndrome [Chabrol et al. 1994]) and seizures are common. Episodic deterioration often occurs at the time of intercurrent infection. Mild elevations of blood and CSF concentrations of lactate, pyruvate, and alanine may be constant or episodic.

Deficiency of the phosphatase-activating enzyme of E1 is described in children with the Leigh phenotype. E3 defects are associated with multiple oxoacid dehydrogenase deficiencies (PDH, 2-oxoglutarate dehydrogenase, and 2-oxo-branched-chain dehydrogenase); the result is severe psychomotor retardation, hypotonia, and moderate, persistent lactic acidosis. A null mouse model for E3 deficiency was lethal to embryos in homozygotes, perhaps explaining the rare occurrence of E3 deficiency in humans (Johnson et al. 1997)

Diagnosis.   PDH deficiency should be suspected in children with lactic acidosis, hypotonia, progressive or episodic ataxia, the Leigh disease phenotype, and recurrent polyneuropathy. Pyruvic acid concentrations are elevated above the normal range (0.04–0.10 mmol/liter), and the lactate to pyruvate ratio is low. Blood lactate and pyruvate concentrations increase at least two- to threefold after a 1.75 g/kg oral glucose load. During fasting, blood ketone and glucose concentrations are normal, and lactate and pyruvate concentrations tend to decrease. Alanine loading increases lactate and pyruvate concentrations. Definitive diagnosis requires enzy-

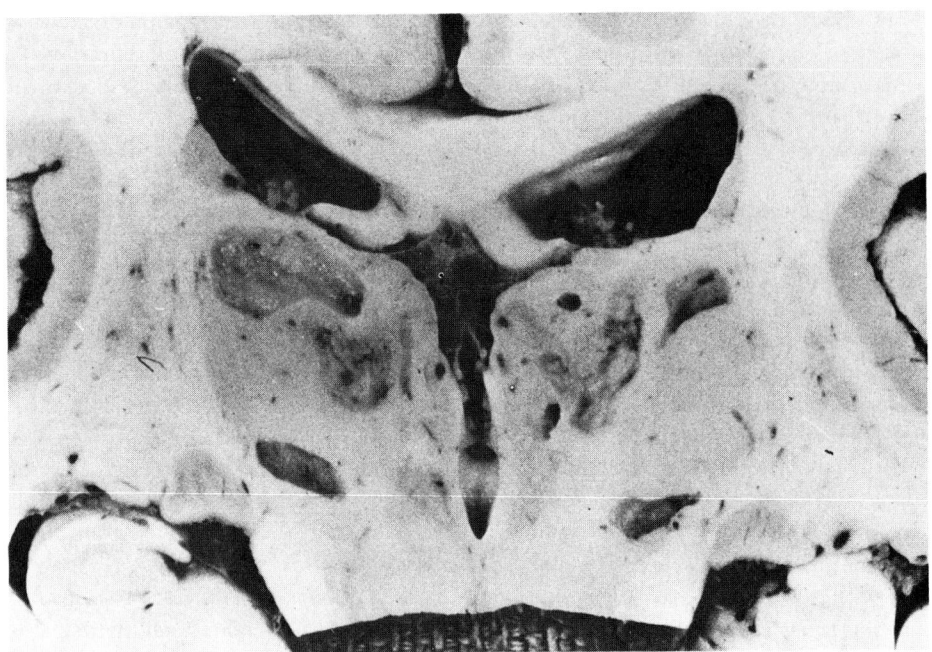

FIGURE 68.15   Cavitary lesions of thalamus and basal ganglia in a patient with Leigh disease.

matic study of muscle, leukocytes, or fibroblasts. Molecular studies of DNA may allow precise characterization of the defect and allow antenatal screening.

Treatment.   Patients usually are treated with thiamine (100–600 mg/day) and a high-fat (>55%), low-carbohydrate diet. Although often recommended, the roles of carnitine, coenzyme Q_{10}, and antioxidants as mitochondrial protectants are not established. Aspartic acid supplementation has been used, and E3-deficient patients should receive lipoic acid. The experimental drug, dichloroacetate, is under study. Unfortunately, current treatments do not prevent disease progression in most patients.

Severe acidosis (pH <7.10) is managed with alkali therapy. Peritoneal dialysis with bicarbonate in the dialysate may be needed for persistent, life-threatening acidosis.

Leigh Disease

Pathophysiology.   Leigh first described this condition in 1951 as a subacute necrotizing encephalomyelopathy. The Leigh disease phenotype usually is caused by failure of brain oxidative metabolism during infancy or early childhood. The neuropathological features are similar to thiamine deficiency (Figure 68.15). Thiamine is a cofactor for E1 of PDH. The basal ganglia usually are affected early; extrapyramidal dysfunction is associated with characteristic bilateral putaminal and globus pallidus necrosis on MRI. Lesions also are found in the caudates, thalamus, midbrain (particularly periaqueductal gray matter), brainstem, cerebellum, and spinal cord; however, in contrast to Wernicke's

encephalopathy, the mammillary bodies are spared. Histologically, the lesions show capillary proliferation, neuronal loss, gliosis, and demyelination with axonal sparing. Cortical atrophy may occur later in the course. White matter T2 signal hyperintensity suggesting leukodystrophy is a particular feature of patients with the neuropathy, ataxia, and retinitis pigmentosa (NARP) syndrome.

Approximately 25% of Leigh disease patients suffer from PDH deficiency, 25% from COX deficiency, 25% from complex I deficiency, and 10–15% from ATP synthase (complex V) deficiency (see Neuropathy, Ataxia, and Retinitis Pigmentosa Syndrome, later in this chapter). Less frequently associated defects include mtDNA deletions, point mutations other than NARP, and biotinidase deficiency.

Clinical Features.   The clinical presentation is heterogeneous. The usual onset in infancy is characterized by failure to thrive and developmental delay. Onset may be delayed until childhood and even adult life. Rapidly progressive deterioration may occur, but the usual course is one of episodic neurological deterioration at the time of intercurrent infection. Apnea is common and a frequent cause of death. Ataxia, neuropathy, ophthalmoplegia, and pyramidal signs are more frequent in children with COX deficiency (Santorelli et al. 1993); seizures and polyneuropathy occur more often in children with NARP syndrome and PDH deficiency. Retinitis pigmentosa is seen only in the NARP syndrome. Inheritance in most cases is autosomal recessive, but the NARP mutation, some complex I deficiencies, and a few cases of COX deficiency are transmitted by maternal inheritance. PDH E1 α deficiency is X-linked.

Diagnosis.   The diagnosis of Leigh disease is based on the clinical and computed tomographical or MRI features. Lactate and pyruvate concentrations are usually mildly elevated in the blood and CSF, but may be further increased by an oral glucose load. Enzyme analysis is useful for diagnosis, genetic counseling, and specific treatment design. Blood or muscle polymerase chain reaction mtDNA analysis is necessary to confirm the T8993G and T8993C point mutations responsible for NARP. Brain neuropathological findings are diagnostic.

Treatment.   Treatment is similar to that suggested for PDH deficiency, except that using carnitine and coenzyme Q_{10} and B-complex vitamins is recommended before identifying the specific biochemical defect because more than 50% of cases have an electron transport defect. Dietary treatment must be individually tailored to the patient and may include glucose, fructose, or glucose and fructose restriction (Haas and Barshop 1998). The experimental drug dichloroacetate is under study in cases with high lactate levels. Unfortunately, treatment is not curative and may have little effect on the course of the disease.

Pyruvate Carboxylase and Biotinidase Deficiency

Pathophysiology.   PC is the gluconeogenetic enzyme responsible for supplying 4-carbon skeletons to the citric acid cycle by catalyzing the condensation of CO_2 with pyruvate to form oxaloacetate (see Figure 68.14). PC consists of four identical subunits. Each subunit covalently binds one molecule of biotin, an essential cofactor. Deficiency of biotin or of biotinidase, the enzyme responsible for recycling biotin, reduces PC activity. PC deficiency has a particular effect on the developing brain; low levels of oxaloacetate seriously affect brain energy metabolism and transmitter synthesis. The CSF concentrations of lactic acid and pyruvic acid may be elevated.

Clinical Features.   Two distinct phenotypes are caused by primary PC deficiency; low PC activity undoubtedly contributes to the neurological manifestations of multiple carboxylase deficiency and biotinidase deficiency. Absence of the PC protein causes severe neonatal lactic acidosis, hypoglycemia, and elevated blood alanine, citrulline, lysine, and ammonia concentrations. 2-Oxoglutaric acid is increased in the urine. Lipid accumulation causes hepatomegaly. Death occurs by 3 months of age.

The juvenile form of PC deficiency is caused by a functionally abnormal carboxylase protein that produces low enzymatic activity. It presents with episodic lactic acidosis and fasting hypoglycemia, usually associated with intercurrent infection. Affected children are severely retarded, fail to thrive, and often develop seizures and spasticity. Early reports that PC was deficient in the tissues of children with Leigh disease at postmortem examination may have been artifactual because of enzyme instability.

PC deficiency occurs in biotin deficiency, biotinidase deficiency, and holocarboxylase synthetase deficiency. Biotin is necessary for the biotin-dependent carboxylases: PC, propionyl-CoA carboxylase, beta-methylcrotonyl-CoA carboxylase, and acetyl-CoA carboxylase. All biotin-dependent carboxylases except acetyl-CoA carboxylase are mitochondrial enzymes. Holocarboxylase synthetase binds biotin to the biotin-dependent enzymes; biotinidase is necessary to recycle biotin. Deficiency of biotin or its related enzymes can cause erythematous skin rash, developmental delay, seizures, hypotonia, ataxia, and metabolic acidosis. The presentation is in infancy or early childhood but later atypical presentation of biotinidase deficiency with optic atrophy and progressive paraparesis has been reported (Lott et al. 1993; Ramaekers et al. 1993).

Diagnosis.   PC deficiency should be considered in children with lactic acidosis and hypoglycemia and in those with compatible clinical features. The blood concentrations of lactate and pyruvate are increased markedly by an oral glucose load; alanine loading may produce a flat glucose response. Final diagnosis requires PC measurement in leukocytes or fibroblasts. DNA studies may be helpful for diagnosis and genetic screening.

Biotinidase deficiency is a treatable disease that must be considered in any child with intractable seizures and in those with ataxia or unexplained encephalopathy. Some degree of lactic acidosis is present usually. It is easily diagnosed by direct measurement of enzyme activity on a blood sample, and biotinidase measurement is included in the neonatal screening panel in some locales.

Treatment.   Biotin supplementation, 10–20 mg per day, is recommended.

Citric Acid Cycle and Related Defects

Phosphoenolpyruvate carboxykinase is an important gluconeogenetic enzyme located in the cytosol and in mitochondria. Phosphoenolpyruvate carboxykinase deficiency often is associated with lower overall mitochondrial activity in fibroblasts. Most affected children have hepatomegaly, failure to thrive, and lactic acidosis. Uncontrollable hypoglycemia, severe liver disease, peripheral edema, unexplained fevers, and hypotonia with myopathy are additional features in severely affected patients.

2-Oxoglutarate dehydrogenase, like PDH, is composed of three major subunits: E1, E2, and E3. This important citric acid cycle enzyme catalyzes the conversion of oxoglutarate to succinyl-CoA. Oxoglutarate dehydrogenase is believed to be a flux-controlling step; the brain abnormalities associated with thiamine deficiency (a cofactor for E1) and alcoholic thiamine deficiency (Wernicke's encephalopathy) may be caused largely by oxoglutarate dehydrogenase deficiency. E3 (lipoamide dehydrogenase) deficiency affects oxoglutarate dehydrogenase as well as PDH and 2-oxo-branched-chain dehydrogenase. Infants with E3 deficiency have microcephaly, optic atrophy, hypotonia, hyperreflexia, seizures, and suffer an early death from dyspnea. The urine concentrations of lactate, pyruvate, alpha-ketoglutarate, α-hydroxybutyrate, α-isovalerate, and α-keto-isocaproate are elevated. The gene for E3 is located on chromosome 7. Lipoic acid has been used as a treatment.

An isolated defect of oxoglutarate dehydrogenase occurred in two siblings with selective motor developmental delay and a degenerative neurological course characterized first by ataxia and then progressive spasticity. The urinary concentration of oxoglutaric acid was elevated in both children, and mild lactic acidosis was present in one. This condition is difficult to diagnose because elevated urine concentrations of oxoglutaric acid is a nonspecific feature in several mitochondrial diseases and also is seen with urinary tract infections.

Fumarase catalyzes the conversion of fumarate to malate in the citric acid cycle. Infants with fumarase deficiency fail to thrive; are developmentally delayed, hypotonic, and hyporeflexic; have cerebral and optic atrophy; and do not survive. A later onset form with choreoathetosis, dystonia, and mental retardation may be a more common presentation (Bourgeron et al. 1994). The biochemical features are mild lactic acidosis with minimal elevation of blood pyruvate concentrations and fumaric aciduria and elevated concentrations of citric acid cycle intermediates. The gene defect is located on chromosome 1, and both cytosolic and mitochondrial isoforms of the enzyme are deficient. Treatment is not available.

Succinic dehydrogenase forms part of complex II of the electron transport chain. This flavoprotein-containing enzyme is responsible for the entry of reducing equivalents into the electron transport chain and catalyzes the conversion of succinate to fumarate. Succinic dehydrogenase (complex II) deficiency has been described in children with a leukodystrophy, Leigh disease, and accompanied other defects of the respiratory chain in a family with myopathy and encephalopathy.

Disorders of Fatty Acid Oxidation

This section deals with the transport and beta-oxidation of long-, medium-, and short-chain fatty acids. The metabolism of branched-chain fatty acids is linked closely to the propionic and methylmalonic acidemias and is discussed in the section on organic aciduria. The metabolism of very-long-chain fatty acids (VLCFA) is discussed in the section on peroxisomal disorders.

Acylcarnitine Transferase Deficiency

The primary oxidative pathway for fatty acids is beta-oxidation within the mitochondrion. After entering the cell,

the long-chain fatty acids are activated to acyl-CoA by specific acyl-CoA synthetases. Acyl-CoA does not cross the inner mitochondrial membrane easily and must be converted to an acylcarnitine ester by carnitine palmitoyltransferase I. The acylcarnitine ester is transported across the inner mitochondrial membrane by carnitine and acylcarnitine translocase where it is converted back to acyl-CoA by an inner mitochondrial membrane carnitine palmitoyltransferase II (see Figure 68.5).

Several different disorders result from deficiencies of acylcarnitine transferase enzymes. Hepatic carnitine palmityl transferase I deficiency causes hypoglycemia and episodic encephalopathy; the syndrome is clinically and biochemically similar to carnitine deficiency. Fasting impairs ketogenesis, but does not affect blood carnitine concentrations, and symptoms do not respond to carnitine therapy. Protective treatment against episodic encephalopathy and hypoglycemia includes frequent feedings to avoid fasting, which activates fatty acid mobilization, and dietary supplementation with medium-chain triglycerides, which use a different acyl-carnitine transferase. Muscle carnitine palmityl transferase I deficiency, characterized by rhabdomyolysis and muscle pain during strenuous exercise, is discussed in Chapter 83.

Acyl–coenzyme A Dehydrogenase Deficiency

Fatty acids are oxidized by beta-oxidation to acetyl-CoA within the mitochondrion by specific very-long-, long-, medium-, and short-chain acyl-CoA dehydrogenases. Fatty acid oxidation is the major energy source for cardiac and skeletal muscle. The products of beta-oxidation are ketone bodies and acetyl-CoA, which enter the Krebs cycle to produce ATP, plus reduced ETF and NADF. The major clinical features are liver, heart, and skeletal muscle disease, alone or in combination.

The most common defect of beta-oxidation is medium-chain acyl-CoA dehydrogenase (MCAD) deficiency. The clinical features are episodic coma, hypoketotic hypoglycemia, hyperammonemia, and fatty liver with little or no acidosis (Stanley 1995). A prior history of a recent viral illness or a prolonged fast is common. Children with MCAD deficiency may be misdiagnosed as having Reye's syndrome. They may have low blood concentrations of free and total carnitine and impaired ketogenesis on fasting.

The urinary excretion of medium-chain dicarboxylic acids (adipic, suberic, and sebacic) is increased during periods of metabolic stress, indicating a compensatory increase in omega oxidation of fatty acids. The plasma acylcarnitine profile for MCAD deficiency is diagnostic and a useful screen for the disease. Hexanoyl-, octanoyl-, octenoyl-, and decenoylcarnitine are present in the urine even when the patient is well.

Very-long-chain acyl-CoA dehydrogenase deficiency often presents as hypoketotic hypoglycemic encephalopathy in the neonate. It can present later as hypertrophic cardiomyopathy, pericardial effusion, and death. Patients can

Table 68.14:   A classification of mitochondrial DNA (mtDNA) disorders

mtDNA defect	Inheritance	Examples	Proposed mechanism
Large-scale deletions and reduplications	Sporadic, acquired	Kearns-Sayre syndrome, Pearson's syndrome, progressive external ophthalmoplegia	Sporadic germ line mutation
Point mutations	Maternal	Mitochondrial encephalomyopathy with lactic acidosis and strokelike episodes, myoclonus epilepsy with ragged-red fibers, neuropathy, ataxia, and retinitis pigmentosa, maternal inherited myopathy with cardiomyopathy	Inherited point mutation Leber's hereditary optic neuropathy
Multiple deletions	Dominant	Dominantly inherited mitochondrial myopathy with multiple mtDNA deletions	Nuclear and mitochondrial signaling defect
Copy number decrease	Recessive	mtDNA depletion syndrome with variable tissue expression, drug induced	Nuclear and mitochondrial signaling defect

have hepatic disease, metabolic acidosis, dicarboxylic aciduria, high plasma creatine kinase, and hyperammonemia. The acylcarnitine profile shows accumulations of 12 and 14 carbon intermediates.

Long chain L-3-hydroxyacyl-CoA dehydrogenase deficiency is one of the enzymes belonging to the membrane-bound trifunctional protein that participates in fatty acid oxidation. Clinical features vary among patients and may include episodic metabolic crisis with encephalopathy and myopathy, hypertrophic or dilatated cardiomyopathy, liver disease, sudden death, sensorimotor neuropathy, and pigmentary retinopathy (Tyni et al. 1996). Episodic deterioration can occur with fasting or catabolic stress with hypoketotic hypoglycemia, dicarboxylic and hydroxydicarboxylic aciduria, and secondary carnitine deficiency. The 16- and 18-carbon, 3-hydroxy monocarboxylic plasma acylcarnitines are elevated. Mothers of affected infants can have serious complications during pregnancy, including fatty liver of pregnancy or HELLP syndrome (*h*ypertension, *e*levated *l*iver enzymes, and *l*ow *p*latelets).

Short chain acyl-CoA dehydrogenase deficiency has a variable presentation that includes acute encephalopathy, developmental delay, growth failure, myopathy, and hepatocellular disease. Laboratory abnormalities that may be present are acidosis, hypoglycemia, hyperammonemia, organic aciduria (ethylmalonate, adipate, butyrate, and lactate), and secondary carnitine deficiency.

Although patients with acyl-CoA dehydrogenase deficiencies have similar clinical presentations, ethylmalonic aciduria presents a striking phenotype. Patients are hypotonic, globally retarded, and have a petechial and purpuric skin rash, apparently resulting from capillary fragility. Lactic acidemia can be marked. The urine contains ethylmalonic acid in large quantities, without other striking changes. The biochemical defect is unknown although COX deficiency has been reported (Garcia-Silva et al. 1997).

Acyl-CoA dehydrogenase deficiency should be suspected in children with hypoglycemia, dicarboxylic aciduria, and carnitine deficiency. The diagnosis is confirmed by enzyme assays of liver biopsy tissue, cultured fibroblasts, or monocytes. DNA analysis is available for MCAD and LCHAD.

Neurological sequelae are lessened by a high-carbohydrate and low-fat diet, avoiding fasting, and cautious carnitine supplementation. Cardiac storage of long chain acyl-CoA carnitine esters has been implicated as a cause of arrhythmias. Medium-chain triglycerides are beneficial as fat supplements for patients with long chain acyl-CoA dehydrogenase and long chain L-3-hydroxyacyl-CoA dehydrogenase deficiency.

Mitochondrial Encephalomyopathies and Other Mitochondrial Cytopathies

The term *mitochondrial encephalomyopathy* is reserved for disorders of primary oxidative mitochondrial metabolism. They usually cause multisystem diseases. The major organs affected are brain and skeletal muscle, but other tissues that require intact oxidative metabolism are affected frequently (Table 68.14).

Pathophysiology

Pyruvate generated from glycolysis or other pathways shuttles across the outer mitochondrial membrane and is converted to acetyl-CoA by PDH. NADH is generated in the process. Acetyl-CoA enters the tricarboxylic cycle, where three NADH molecules and $FADH_2$ are produced (see Figure 68.14). Fatty acids are metabolized primarily by beta-oxidation within the mitochondrial matrix. Each step produces one molecule of acetyl-CoA, which enters the tricarboxylic cycle; one molecule of $NADH^+H$; and one molecule of $FADH_2$, which is carried on the electron transfer flavoprotein. The reduced nucleotide $NADH^+H$ delivers hydrogen to NADH dehydrogenase (complex I) and $FADH_2$ delivers electrons to electron transfer flavoprotein dehydrogenase and complex II of the electron transport chain located on the inner mitochondrial membrane. Electrons transported from these enzymes reduce coenzyme Q (ubiquinone), which in turn passes the electrons to complex III. Complex III delivers the electrons to cytochrome c, which is oxidized by cytochrome c oxidase (COX, complex

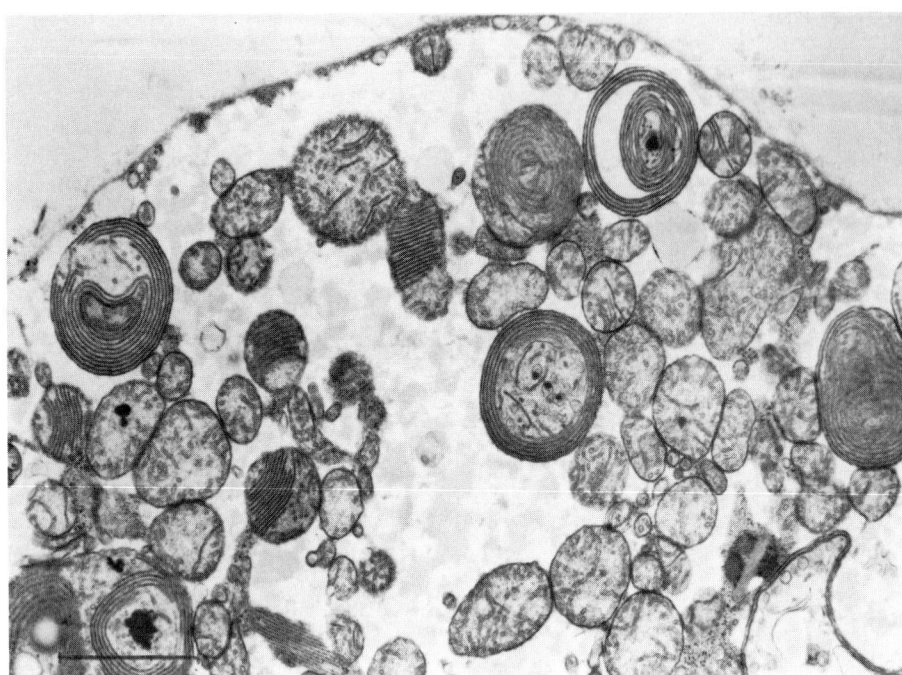

FIGURE 68.16 Morphological abnormalities of mitochondria in a patient with mitochondrial myopathy. The mitochondria are enlarged and contain concentric and rectangular arrays of cristae. (Calibration bar = 1.0 mm.)

IV). Electrons then are passed through cytochromes a and a_3 of complex IV, finally combining with oxygen and hydrogen ions to produce water. During the process of electron transport, protons are pumped out across the mitochondrial matrix membrane creating the proton-motive force across the membrane. This proton gradient is used by complex V (ATP synthase) to generate ATP (see Figure 68.14).

Defects of each of the five complexes, as well as coenzyme Q, are associated with human diseases. The individual complexes each are composed of many polypeptide subunits (14 in complex V, 13 in complex IV, 11 in complex III, 4 in complex II, and at least 42 in complex I). Greater than 97% of mitochondrial proteins, including most electron transport chain subunits, are nuclear encoded. Mitochondria contain their own DNA (mtDNA), however. The double-stranded, circular mtDNA, with 16,569 base pairs, encodes 13 critical polypeptide subunits of the electron transport complexes, including seven subunits in complex I, cytochrome b in complex III, three subunits in complex IV, two subunits in complex V, ribosomal RNA, and 22 tRNAs. Deletions or duplications and point mutations of mtDNA in protein, RNA, and tRNA genes are a relatively common cause of human disease and may contribute to the aging process. Characteristics of mtDNA that contribute to the pathophysiology and heterogeneity of mitochondrial diseases are a high mutation rate, the potential for heteroplasmy (a mixture of wild-type and mutant DNA within the same mitochondrion, cells, and tissues), a threshold effect of abnormal mtDNA necessary to produce disease, and predominantly maternal inheritance. The remarkable phenotypical heterogeneity of mitochondrial disorders is expanded further by the differential susceptibility of organs to oxidative phosphorylation

defects: Decreasing order of sensitivity is seen in the brain, kidney, heart, and liver, according to Wallace in 1992.

Muscle involvement is a common but not invariable characteristic of mitochondrial diseases. Defective oxidative phosphorylation in muscle often results in mitochondrial proliferation in type I and IIA fibers. Mitochondria can have unusual shapes, sizes, structures (particularly the cristae), and grouping and many contain abnormal inclusions (Figure 68.16). Fibers with the most severe biochemical defects may degenerate. Adjacent fibers with less severe or no defect may appear normal. In the most severe form of muscle involvement, the combination of a patchy moth-eaten appearance in individual muscle fibers along with mitochondrial proliferation gives rise to the ragged-red fiber seen on Gomori's trichrome staining. Ragged-red fibers are seen frequently in mtDNA disorders. It appears that overproduction of mitochondria in muscle is rare in nuclear DNA abnormalities; in fact, an underproduction disorder caused by a nuclear defect, the mtDNA depletion syndrome, has been described. Ultrastructural abnormalities of mitochondria may be seen in affected tissues in mitochondrial cytopathies.

Mitochondrial encephalomyopathies are systemic disorders with a wide clinical phenotype. The term *mitochondrial cytopathy* has been used to emphasize multisystem involvement. There are three well-characterized phenotypes and a growing group of less commonly identified disorders (Table 68.15).

Kearns-Sayre Syndrome

The Kearns-Sayre syndrome (KSS) is a progressive multisystem disorder whose diagnostic features are childhood

Table 68.15:   Clinical and laboratory features of mitochondrial encephalomyopathy syndromes

Features	KSS	MERRF	MELAS
Ophthalmoplegia	+	–	–
Retinal degeneration	+	–	–
Heart block	+	–	–
Cerebrospinal fluid protein >100 mg/dl	+	–	–
Myoclonus	–	+	–
Ataxia	+	+	–
Weakness	+	+	+
Seizures	–	+	+
Dementia	+	+	+
Short stature	+	+	+
Episodic vomiting	–	–	+
Cortical blindness	–	–	+
Hemiparesis, hemianopia	–	–	+
Sensorineural hearing loss	+	+	+
Lactic acidosis	+	+	+
Positive family history	–	+	+
Ragged-red fibers	+	+	+
Spongy degeneration of the brain	+	+	+

KSS = Kearns-Sayre syndrome; MELAS = mitochondrial encephalopathy, myopathy, lactic acidosis, and strokelike episodes; MERRF = myoclonus epilepsy with ragged-red fibers; + = usually present; – = usually absent.
Source: S DiMauro, E Bonilla, M Zevani, et al. Mitochondrial myopathies. Ann Neurol 1985;17:525. Reproduced with permission from Little, Brown and Company.

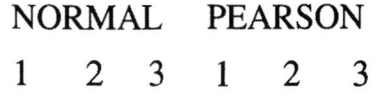

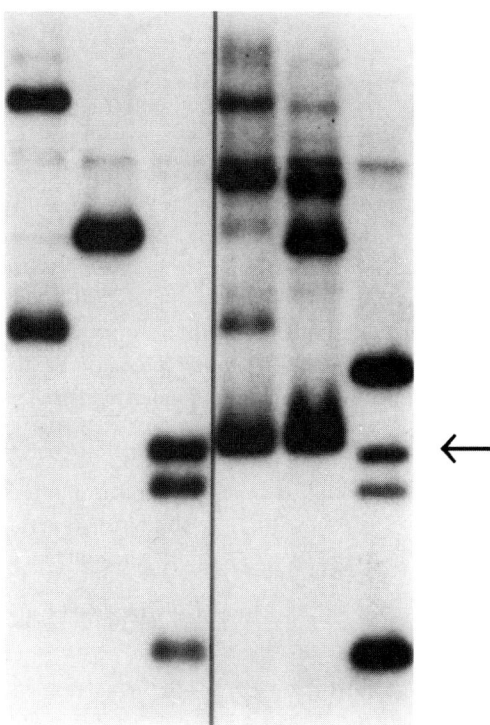

FIGURE 68.17   Southern blot of mitochondrial DNA extracted from the blood of a patient with Pearson's marrow syndrome compared with a control sample. Lane 1 is uncut, lane 2 is DNA linearized by digestion with Bam HI, lane 3 is cut with Bam HI and Eco RV. The Pearson's patient sample shows an extra band, 6.6 Kb in size, visible in lanes 1 and 2 (*arrow*), indicating the presence of a large deletion.

onset, progressive external ophthalmoplegia, cardiac conduction block, atypical pigmentary retinal degeneration, dementia, and a CSF protein concentration greater than 100 mg/dl. Ragged-red fibers are seen on muscle biopsy. Other common features are deafness, ataxia, episodic coma, and endocrine abnormalities (diabetes mellitus, hypoparathyroidism, and growth hormone deficiency). MRI shows predominantly white matter damage that correlates with spongiform degeneration on postmortem examination. Most typical cases of KSS have large mtDNA deletions, and a few have reduplications. Patients with only progressive external ophthalmoplegia have a high incidence of mtDNA deletions, although this phenotype may also occur with the A3243G tRNA^{leu} point mutation responsible for the syndrome of mitochondrial encephalomyopathy with ragged-red fibers and strokelike episodes (MELAS).

Pearson's syndrome is a rare sporadic disorder characterized by bone marrow failure with sideroblastic anemia, pancreatic dysfunction, and death in infancy. Some patients present with renal disease characterized by Toni-Debré-Fanconi tubulopathy (Niaudet et al. 1994). In other cases of large mtDNA deletion, interstitial nephritis has occurred. The few children who survive infancy later may develop features of KSS type. In 1991, McShane and colleagues reported that Pearson's syndrome is caused by a large mtDNA deletion similar to KSS. Diagnosis is by Southern blotting analysis of mtDNA extracted from blood or muscle. An example of mtDNA deletions that characterize this disorder is seen in Figure 68.17.

Mitochondrial Encephalomyopathy with Lactic Acidosis and Strokelike Episodes

MELAS appears to be the single most common mitochondrial disorder. Most cases result from a point mutation in the tRNA$^{leu(UUR)}$ gene at position 3243 when adenine is replaced by guanine. Another mutation accounting for less than 10% of cases is the A3271G mutation also located on the tRNA^{leu} gene. Other tRNA mutations have been associated with the MELAS phenotype (Taylor et al. 1996) and a point mutation in the ND5 complex I gene has been identified (Santorelli et al. 1997). MELAS phenotypes range from asymptomatic to severe childhood multisystem disease with lactic acidosis. The first presentation may be in adulthood as a stroke, retinopathy, or commonly diabetes with or without deafness. The MELAS A3243G mutation is thought to account for 1–2% of cases of diabetes mellitus (Van den Ouweland et al. 1994).

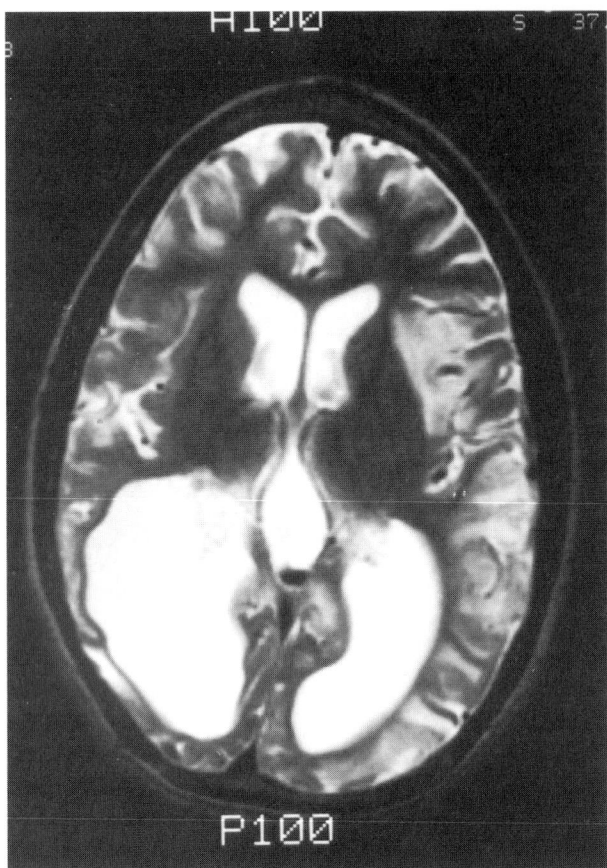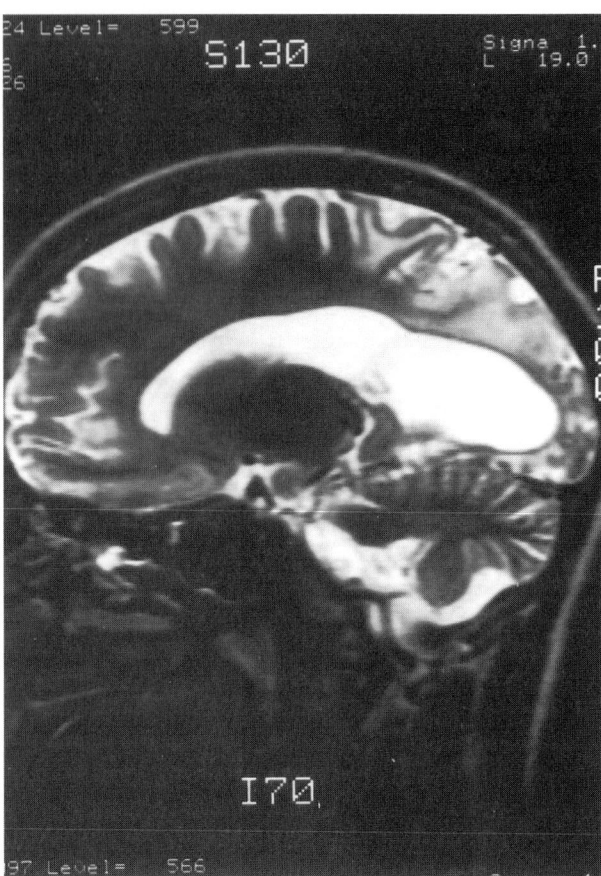

FIGURE 68.18 Magnetic resonance imaging (MRI, T2-weighted axial and sagittal images) of a 14-year-old boy with mitochondrial encephalomyopathy with lactic acidosis and strokelike episodes caused by the A3243G mutation. The child suffered three separate strokelike episodes. The typical occipital distribution of tissue loss is apparent and there is also abnormal high T2 signal in the left parieto-occipital gray matter.

Some children with MELAS have short stature, but their early development is otherwise normal. In this common presentation, episodic seizures, vomiting, and recurrent strokelike episodes of hemiparesis and hemianopia, often associated with severe migrainous headache, begin in childhood. Strokes typically occur in a nonvascular distribution. Occipital infarcts, which eventually become bilateral, are particularly common (Figure 68.18). Severe neurological decline, often with dementia and blindness, does not usually occur until adolescence or adulthood. Most patients have lactic acidosis, and muscle biopsy shows ragged-red fibers. Partial defects of complex IV in muscle have been identified in some cases, but complex I deficiency is usual and can be profound. This appears to be caused by inhibition of translation of the ND1 complex I polypeptide gene, which is adjacent to the MELAS tRNA. Maternal inheritance is found usually if a careful radiolabeled polymerase chain reaction study of the RNA[leu] mutation is made (Smith et al. 1997).

Treatment of MELAS syndrome with B-complex vitamins, niacin, and coenzyme Q_{10} usually is advocated. Increasing evidence suggests that dichloroacetate can be helpful (Kuroda et al. 1997), but drug-induced peripheral neuropathy may limit its usefulness.

Myoclonus Epilepsy with Ragged-Red Fibers

The major clinical features of myoclonus epilepsy with ragged-red fibers (MERF) are muscle weakness and seizures. MERF shares clinical features with MELAS, but strokelike episodes are rare. The range of clinical features in a single family extends from severe CNS dysfunction (deafness, ataxia, spasticity, myoclonus, and dementia) to asymptomatic myopathy with ragged-red fibers (see Table 68.15).

As with MELAS, muscle electron transport activities may be low, with abnormalities of complexes I, II, III, and IV. Most cases are caused by a point mutation in a tRNA encoded by mtDNA. The variable expression is thought to correlate with the load of mutant mtDNA. The tRNA[lys] mutation reported in MERF is a nucleotide substitution at position A8344G. Less commonly a tRNA[lys] mutation at position T8356C is implicated.

Neuropathy, Ataxia, and Retinitis Pigmentosa Syndrome

The point mutation of T to G at position 8893 of mtDNA affects the complex V (ATP synthase) subunit 6 gene. This mutation was first reported in a family with maternally inherited NARP syndrome. It is also responsible for as many as 10–15% of Leigh disease cases (Santorelli et al. 1993). As with other mtDNA disorders, the phenotype is variable. Children with cerebral palsy and recurrent neuropathy, attention deficit-hyperactivity disorder, and learning disabilities have been identified in separate children within the same family.

Maternally Inherited Myopathy with Cardiomyopathy

The clinical features of maternally inherited myopathy with cardiomyopathy are lactic acidosis, ragged-red fiber myopathy, and hypertrophic cardiomyopathy. The CNS is spared. The tRNA$^{leu(UUR)}$ responsible for MELAS is the cause of maternally inherited myopathy with cardiomyopathy, but the mutation is at site np 3260, which differs from the usual MELAS mutation.

Leber's Hereditary Optic Neuropathy

Leber's hereditary optic neuropathy is maternally inherited in some cases and arises de novo in others. The predominant clinical feature is acute or subacute blindness in a young adult. Other features may include psychiatric disorders, ataxia, spasticity, peripheral neuropathy, and cardiac conduction defects. Several mtDNA point mutations in complex I subunit genes are responsible for complex I deficiency and the Leber's hereditary optic neuropathy phenotype (Shoffner et al. 1995). A mutation in the mtDNA cytochrome b gene for complex III also is found in Leber's hereditary optic neuropathy pedigrees. Infantile bilateral striatal necrosis, reported in some families with Leber's hereditary optic neuropathy, may be caused by an unrecognized mtDNA mutation.

Nuclear Mitochondrial DNA Signaling Defects

Nuclear genes affect many aspects of mitochondrial function, including the proteins for mitochondrial biogenesis, replication, transcription, and translation factors. Many mitochondrial diseases probably are caused by defective nuclear-mitochondrial interactions. Two of the first described disorders are a dominantly inherited condition with multiple deletions of mtDNA and a recessively inherited condition associated with a quantitative decrease in mtDNA.

The original phenotype of the dominantly inherited disease is a CNS degenerative disorder with onset in the third decade. The clinical features are lactic acidosis, progressive external ophthalmoplegia, and cataracts. The phenotype has been expanded to include early childhood-onset weakness, with neuropathy and optic atrophy, and intermittent coma, with ketoacidosis and ataxia.

The clinical features of the recessively inherited mtDNA depletion syndrome are also heterogeneous. A congenital-onset form includes myopathy, ragged-red fibers, renal disease, hepatomegaly, lactic acidosis, and death in the first year. The late infantile form is primarily a mitochondrial myopathy. Infantile and juvenile onset also has been associated with severe liver disease and encephalopathy and in some cases with intractable seizures.

Mitochondrial DNA replication requires a replisome complex consisting of a group of enzymes including mtDNA polymerase. There are many possibilities for genetic defects in this system.

Electron Transport Defects

Although decreased activity of various electron transport complexes accompanies many mtDNA defects, other patients with electron transport abnormalities do not have an identifiable mtDNA defect. There may be an unidentified nuclear DNA defect in these patients. Complex I deficiency is one of the most commonly identified defects. This is not surprising in view of the large number of polypeptide subunits (>42) in this protein. COX deficiency is also common, and the great majority of cases are recessively inherited nuclear defects. Interestingly, despite extensive studies of all of the nuclear-encoded COX subunit genes, no defects have been identified. This suggests that most cases of COX deficiency are the result of protein importation or assembly failure.

Oxidative phosphorylation defects cannot always be identified, even when mitochondrial disease is established definitely. The clinical features of patients with various electron transport defects are listed in Table 68.16.

Leigh disease and Alper's syndrome (progressive infantile poliodystrophy) are associated with generalized defects of complex I and complex IV. Alper's syndrome is a progressive gray matter degeneration of infancy characterized by seizures (frequently epilepsia partialis continua), developmental regression, and progressive motor abnormalities. Rare cases have hepatic cirrhosis.

In Menkes' syndrome there is a secondary impairment of complex IV activity because of copper depletion.

Aging and Late-Onset Degenerative Diseases

The mitochondrial electron transport chain produces the majority of cellular free radicals. It is estimated that 2–4% of the oxygen used by mitochondria is for the generation of free radical species. Progressive damage to mtDNA is part of aging. This is thought to occur because of relative inadequacy of mtDNA repair systems in the face of large amounts of accumulated free-radical oxidative damage. Lowered electron transport complex activity and large mitochondrial deletions are increased in tissues from aged individuals. The percentage of the "common" mtDNA deletion at position 4977 increases in aged human hearts progressively from age 30 years, but much larger numbers of deletions are seen in ischemic hearts. After the discovery of complex I inhibition as the mechanism underlying 1-methyl-4-phenyl-1,2,3,6-

Table 68.16: Disorders with defective electron transport chain activity

Complex I (NADH–coenzyme Q (CoQ) oxidoreductase)
  Mitochondrial myopathy with exercise intolerance and myalgia
  Fatal infantile mitchondrial cytopathy with lactic acidosis
  Late-onset encephalomyopathy, with deafness, ataxia, retinitis
    pigmentosa, neuropathy, and dementia
  Mitochondrial encephalomyopathy with lactic acidosis and
    strokelike episodes
  Leber's hereditary optic neuropathy
  Progressive infantile poliodystrophy (Alper's syndrome)
  Parkinson's disease
  1-Methyl-4-phenyl-1,2,3,6-tetrahydropyridine toxicity
Complex II (succinate-CoQ oxidoreductase)
  Myopathy with combined aconitase deficiency
  Infantile encephalomyopathy
  Juvenile myoclonus with ragged-red fiber–like encephalomyopathy
  Familial encephalomyopathy
  Leigh disease with leukodystrophy
  CoQ (ubiquinone) deficiency
  Myopathy with lactic acidemia, learning disability, and ataxia
  Kearns-Sayre syndrome
Complex III (CoQ-cytochrome c oxidoreductase)
  Mitochondrial myopathy
  Cardiomyopathy
  Multisystem disorder with encephalomyopathy, myoclonus
    with ragged-red fibers
Complex IV (cytochrome c oxidase)
  Fatal and benign infantile myopathy, infantile lactic acidosis,
    myopathy, and cardiomyopathy
  Leigh disease
  Alper's syndrome
  Myoneurogastrointestinal disorder and encephalopathy
  Kearns-Sayre syndrome
  Myoclonus with ragged-red fibers
  Mitochondrial encephalomyopathy with lactic acidosis and
    strokelike episodes
Complex V (ATP synthase)
  Mitochondrial myopathy
  Neuropathy, ataxia, retinitis pigmentosa
  Leigh disease
  Kearns-Sayre syndrome

ATP = adenosine triphosphate; NADH = nicotinamide adenine dinucleotide.

tetrahydropyridine–induced parkinsonism, low complex I activity was found in brain, muscle, and platelets of patients with idiopathic Parkinson's disease. Low complex IV activity has been reported in Alzheimer's disease. Several mtDNA deletions and point mutations have been reported in Parkinson's and Alzheimer's tissues, and mtDNA changes with associated failure of oxidative phosphorylation may be etiologically important in these and other age-related neurodegenerative diseases.

Diagnosis. Because the clinical features of mitochondrial encephalomyopathies and cytopathies are so variable, a high index of suspicion and a comprehensive clinical and biochemical evaluation are needed. Blood lactate, measured after fasting and after a glucose load, is an appropriate screening test. CSF analysis for protein and lactic acid can be helpful.

The clinical evaluation should include electrocardiography, echocardiography, brain MRI, and electroencephalography (EEG) to assess the extent of multisystem involvement. In phenotypes such as MELAS, myoclonus epilepsy with ragged-red fibers, and KSS, a mtDNA analysis can be used for diagnosis by identification of specific point mutations or deletions. Muscle biopsy for histological, electron microscopic, biochemical, and DNA studies should be performed in a center specializing in mitochondrial disorders.

Treatment. Potential treatment strategies are based on supplying electron transport chain cofactors and substrates, L-carnitine, and protein and antioxidants in an attempt to protect against mtDNA free-radical damage. Sodium succinate, lipoic acid, ascorbic acid, niacin, riboflavin, and coenzyme Q_{10} have all been tried. Coenzyme Q_{10} (ubiquinone), 4 mg/kg per day, has the largest literature-supported efficacy in mitochondrial disease. When lactic acidosis is a prominent feature, the experimental agent dichloroacetate may be helpful.

Peroxisomal Disorders

Peroxisomal disorders are neurogenetic diseases in which the peroxisome does not function or fails to form. The peroxisome is a subcellular organelle bounded by a single membrane with an average diameter of 500 nm. It is present in all cells except the mature erythrocyte. Peroxisomes are especially prominent in cells involved with specialized lipid metabolism, such as glial cells. The abundance of peroxisomes in the developing nervous system indicates a role in early myelination and neuronal migration. Patients with absent peroxisomes have severe disturbances of these processes.

The peroxisome originally was thought to be a fossil organelle, with only a limited role in mammals; however, more than 40 enzymatic and metabolic functions are now known to be carried out in the peroxisome. Peroxisomes contain oxidases that produce hydrogen peroxide as well as catalases that degrade it, which led to the organelle being named *peroxisome*. In addition to the hydrogen peroxide–related reactions, oxidation of certain fatty acids, degradation of prostaglandins, formation of bile acids, biosynthesis of cholesterol and ether lipids, and other reactions occur in the peroxisome (Table 68.17). Although some reactions, such as cholesterol biosynthesis, also take place in other organelles, where the role of peroxisomes may be subsidiary, some reactions take place in the peroxisome exclusively. Total absence of peroxisomal function causes severe abnormalities in virtually every organ, particularly the nervous system.

Unlike mitochondria, peroxisomes do not contain DNA but do proliferate by fission. Matrix and membrane proteins that are destined for the peroxisome are synthesized in free polyribosomes, enter the cytosol in the mature form, and are then targeted to preexisting peroxisomes. There are at least 50 matrix proteins that are mostly enzymes. The 10 known membrane proteins are specific for this organelle.

Table 68.17:   Metabolic reactions of peroxisomes

Reaction	Metabolic consequence
Oxidation of VLCFA	VLCFA excess in tissue and plasma
Oxidation of pipecolic acid	Pipecolic acid excess in plasma and urine
Oxidation of pristanic acid	Phytanic and pristanic acid excess in plasma
Beta-oxidation of cholesterol side chain and bile acid synthesis	Di- and trihydroxycholestanoic acid accumulation
First two steps of ether-lipid synthesis	Plasmalogen levels reduced or absent in all tissues

VLCFA = very-long-chain fatty acids.

Information directing many of the proteins into peroxisomes is inherent in the mature polypeptide and consists of peroxisomal targeting signals 1 and 2. Peroxisomal targeting signal 1 has an amino acid sequence of serine, lysine, and leucine at the COOH-terminal of the peptide for many of the peroxisomal matrix proteins with evolutionary conservation. Other proteins such as peroxisomal-3-ketoacyl-CoA-thiolase have a different peptide sequence peroxisomal targeting signal 2 located at the amino terminal of the protein according to Swinkels and colleagues in 1991. Without this sequence the proteins do not reach the peroxisome. Defects in this targeting mechanism exist in Zellweger's syndrome spectrum and rhizomelic chondrodysplasia punctata (RCDP). The import process depends equally on suitable membrane receptors and a shared ATP-dependent translocase; some disorders of peroxisome biogenesis appear to involve these membrane receptors. Table 68.18 summarizes the known gene defects of peroxisomal diseases.

As shown in Table 68.19 the peroxisomal disorders have been subdivided into three major categories. The difference between groups 1 and 2 is fundamental: In group 1 the entire organelle fails to form and all peroxisomal functions are deficient. In group 2 disorders the defect involves single enzyme deficiencies of the peroxisome. Peroxisome structure and other functions are normal. The group 3 disorders, of which RCDP is the prime example, probably represent a more restricted example of failure of biogenesis. Peroxisomes are present but abnormal in structure and more than one enzyme is deficient. Peroxisomal disorders have a combined frequency in excess of 1 in 25,000 and a phenotype that is more varied than previously recognized. Peroxisomal disorders can be diagnosed by noninvasive tests, such as assays of plasma, red blood cells, urine, or cultured skin fibroblasts (Table 68.20). Prenatal diagnosis is possible and therapies are emerging for some of the peroxisomal disorders (Moser 1993).

Disorders of Peroxisomal Biogenesis (Zellweger's Syndrome)

Pathophysiology.   The fundamental defect in Zellweger's syndrome and related diseases is the failure of matrix proteins to be imported into the peroxisome, resulting in mul-

Table 68.18:   Peroxisomal disorders and corresponding gene defects

Disorder	Gene defect
Zellweger's-neonatal adreno-leukodystrophy-infantile Refsum's syndrome	Peroxisome membrane protein (PEX1)
	35-kD peroxisome membrane protein (PEX2)
	Receptor for peroxisome targeting sequence 1 (PEX5)
	AAA family ATPase (PEX6)
Rhizomelic chondrodysplasia punctata	48-kD peroxisome membrane protein (PEX12)
	Receptor for peroxisome targeting sequence 2 (PEX7)
X-linked adrenoleuko-dystrophy	ATP-binding transport protein (ALDP)
Refsum's disease	Alanine-glyoxylate amino transferase
	Phytanoyl-CoA hydroxylase
Peroxisomal acyl-CoA oxidase deficiency	Acyl-CoA oxidase
Peroxisomal bifunctional enzyme deficiency	Peroxisomal bifunctional enzyme
Peroxisomal 3-oxoacyl-CoA thiolase deficiency	Peroxisomal thiolase
DHAP acyltransferase deficiency	DHAP acyltransferase
Akyl-DHAP synthase deficiency	Akyl-DHAP synthase
Acatalasemia	Catalase

ATP = adenosine triphosphate; CoA = coenzyme A; DHAP = dihydroxyacetone phosphate.

Table 68.19:   Peroxisomal disorders

Group 1: disorders of peroxisome biogenesis; peroxisomes absent
    Zellweger's syndrome
    Neonatal adrenoleukodystrophy
    Infantile Refsum's syndrome
    Hyperpipecolic acidemia
Group 2: defects of single peroxisomal enzyme; peroxisomes intact
    X-linked adrenoleukodystrophy
    Acyl-CoA oxidase deficiency
    Bifunctional enzyme deficiency
    Thiolase deficiency
    DHAP acyltransferase deficiency
    Akyl-DHAP synthase deficiency
    Hyperoxaluria type I
    Glutaryl-CoA oxidase deficiency (glutaric aciduria type III)
    Classic Refsum's disease
    Acatalasemia
Group 3: multiple biochemical defects; peroxisomes intact
    Rhizomelic chondrodysplasia punctata

CoA = coenzyme A; DHAP = dihydroxyacetone phosphate.

tiorgan diseases with all of the metabolic consequences outlined in Table 68.17. It has been shown that peroxisomal membranes are formed but consist of empty or partially empty membranous structures, referred to as *peroxisome ghosts.* The first point mutation was demon-

Table 68.20: Biochemical diagnostic assays for peroxisomal disorders

Group 1: disorders of peroxisome biogenesis
    Zellweger's syndrome, neonatal adrenoleukodystrophy,
        infantile Refsum's syndrome, hyperpipecolic acidemia
Group 2: single enzyme defects
    X-linked adrenoleukodystrophy hemizygote
    X-linked adrenoleukodystrophy heterozygote
    Isolated defects of VLCFA degradation
    Classic Refsum's disease
    Hyperoxaluria type 1
Group 3: rhizomelic chondrodysplasia punctata
    Plasma: VLCFA, pipecolic acid, phytanic acid, bile
        intermediates
    Red blood cells: plasmalogens
    Fibroblasts: plasmalogen synthesis, catalase subcellular
        localization
    Plasma: VLCFA
    Red blood cells: VLCFA
    Fibroblasts: VLCFA
    DNA analysis: *ALDP*
    Plasma: phytanic acid
    Fibroblasts: VLCFA, VLCFA oxidation, immunoblot of
        peroxisomal fatty acid oxidation enzymes
    Urine: organic acids
    Liver: alanine-glyoxalate aminotransferase in percutaneous
        liver biopsy
    Fibroblasts: plasmalogen synthesis, phytanic acid oxidation

VLCFA = very-long-chain fatty acid.

strated in one female patient with Zellweger's syndrome in the cDNA of the gene encoding a 35-kD peroxisomal membrane protein. It was called *peroxisomal assembly factor 1* or PAF-1. In current nomenclature, PAF-1 is referred to as PEX2. A total of 14 PEX genes essential for peroxisome biogenesis have been identified (Lazarow 1995). The proteins encoded by PEX genes are referred to as *peroxins*. Mutations in PEX genes have been identified in the various complementation groups, resulting in disorders of

peroxisome biogenesis without a strong correlation between genotype and phenotype (Huhse et al. 1998) (Table 68.21). Neonatal adrenoleukodystrophy (NALD) and infantile Refsum's syndrome are disorders named before their basic nature was understood. It is now known that they are milder variants of Zellweger's syndrome. Complementation analyses indicate that a single genotype can be associated with all three phenotypes.

Tissues show absent or markedly reduced numbers of peroxisomes. Abnormalities in neuronal migration are the major neuropathological features. Areas of pachygyria and polymicrogyria in the opercular region, Purkinje's cell heterotopias in the cerebellum, and laminar discontinuities of the olivary nuclei are characteristic and unique for this disorder. Hepatomegaly and hepatic disease are constant features and often cause prolonged neonatal jaundice. Renal cortical cysts are prevalent at autopsy but have limited clinical significance. Adrenal insufficiency is rare.

Clinical Features.   Classic Zellweger's cerebrohepatorenal syndrome is a severe multisystem disorder associated with multiple congenital anomalies (Table 68.22 and Figure 68.19). The incidence of Zellweger's syndrome and related disorders in the United States is estimated to be 1 in 25,000–50,000. It has an autosomal recessive mode of inheritance. Affected children have hepatomegaly and severely impaired liver function, are profoundly hypotonic, have a virtual failure of psychomotor development, and rarely survive beyond the first year of life. Severe neonatal seizures and the profound psychomotor retardation are caused by the characteristic defect in neuronal migration.

NALD and infantile Refsum's syndrome are milder variants of Zellweger's syndrome. Dysmorphic features may be mild or absent, and psychomotor retardation is at the severe rather than the profound level. Children who are not retarded have been identified. Most patients have impaired hearing, pigmentary degeneration of the retina, enlarged liver, and moderately impaired liver function. Adrenal function often is impaired. Seizures are common, and neu-

Table 68.21:   Complementation groups and phenotypes of peroxisome biogenesis defects in patients at the Kennedy-Krieger Institute

Group	Gene	Zellweger's syndrome	Neonatal adrenoleukodystrophy	Infantile Refsum's disease	Rhizomelic chondrodysplasia punctata	Other	Total
1	PEX1	54	37	6	97	—	—
2	PEX5	1	2	3	—	—	—
3	PEX12	6	2	8	—	—	—
4	PEX6	12	11	3	26	—	—
6	PEX6	1	1	—	—	—	—
7(&5)	?	4	3	7	—	—	—
8	?	3	5	6	14	—	—
9	?	1	1	—	—	—	—
10	PEX2	2	2	—	—	—	—
11	PEX7	55	5	60	—	—	—
Total		83	61	15	55	5	219

Table 68.22:   Prevalence of clinical abnormalities in Zellweger's syndrome

Abnormal feature	Percentage of cases with feature*
Dysmorphism	
Low or broad nasal bridge	100
Shallow orbital ridges	100
Redundant neck skin folds	100
Micrognathia	100
High forehead	97
External ear deformity	97
Enlarged fontanelles	96
High arched palate	95
Epicanthal folds	92
Flat occiput	81
Neurological signs	
Abnormal Moro's response	100
Psychomotor retardation	99
Severe hypotonia	98
Hyporeflexia or areflexia	96
Poor suck	92
Nystagmus	81
Impaired hearing	40
Eye findings	
Cataract or cloudy cornea	87
Brushfield's spots	83
Optic disc pallor	74
Glaucoma	58
Abnormal retinal pigmentation	40
Systemic involvement	
Renal cortical cysts	97
Hepatomegaly	78
Cholestasis	59
Skeletal abnormalities	50
Cirrhosis	37
Adrenal insufficiency	5

*Percentages represent the number of patients with the abnormal feature in which information about the feature was available.
Source: Adapted from HSA Heymans. Cerebro-hepato-renal (Zellweger) syndrome. Clinical and biochemical consequences of peroxisomal dysfunction. Thesis, University of Amsterdam, 1984.

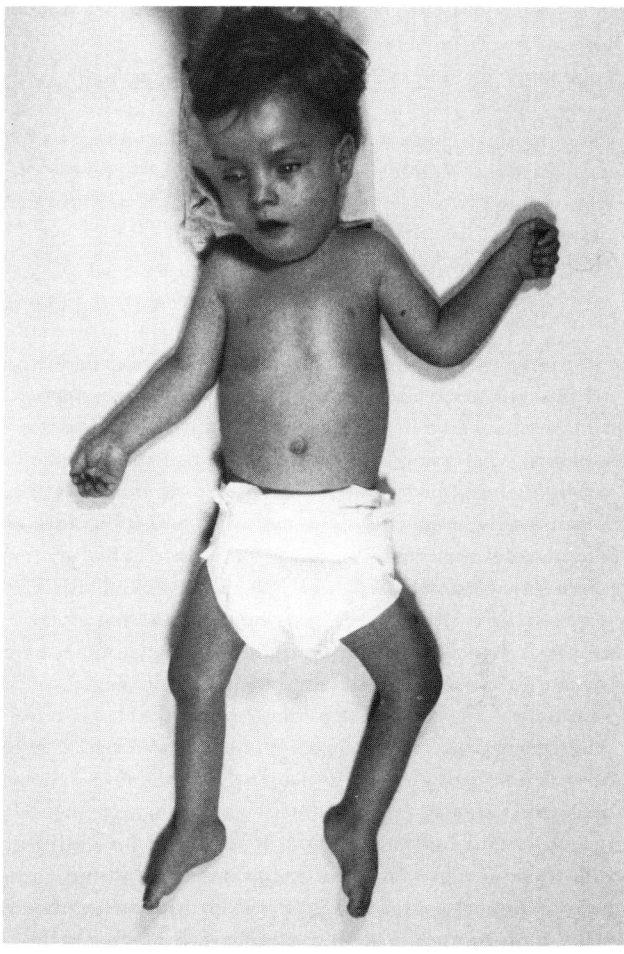

FIGURE 68.19   Morphological features of Zellweger's syndrome.

roimaging studies may show a progressive leukodystrophy. Death usually occurs by age 3–6 years; however, some patients are in stable condition in the second and third decade of life. Laboratory diagnosis depends on similar assays used for Zellweger's syndrome, with results somewhat less abnormal than in classic Zellweger's syndrome.

Diagnosis.   Zellweger's syndrome should be suspected in infants and children presenting with severe psychomotor retardation, hypotonia, characteristic dysmorphic features, and liver disease. Table 68.20 lists the biochemical assays used for the diagnosis of Zellweger's syndrome. Abnormally increased concentrations of VLCFA in plasma is the most frequently used test for diagnosis. Levels of plasmalogens are reduced in red blood cell membranes, and the rate of synthesis of plasmalogens is impaired in cultured skin

fibroblasts. Pipecolic acid levels are increased in plasma and urine, and excessive amounts of bile acid intermediates also are excreted in urine.

Prenatal diagnosis is achieved by demonstrating increased levels of VLCFA and impaired synthesis of plasmalogens in cultured amniocytes or chorionic villus cells.

Treatment.   Therapy for the classic Zellweger's syndrome patients is symptomatic. Anticonvulsants for seizures and vitamin K for the bleeding disorder secondary to cirrhosis may be required. Patients with NALD may benefit from the administration of docosahexaenoic acid (Martinez et al. 1994).

Disorders of Isolated Peroxisomal Enzyme Defects

Diseases of isolated peroxisomal enzymes are outlined in Table 68.19. Of these, X-linked adrenoleukodystrophy (X-ALD) is the most common and therefore is discussed in depth. Other single enzyme disorders that cause severe neurological disability are discussed briefly. Dihydroxyacetonephosphate acyl transferase deficiency is discussed in conjunction with RCDP, which it resembles. Hyperoxaluria

Table 68.23: Phenotypes among X-linked adrenoleukodystrophy hemizygotes

Type	Frequency (%)
Childhood cerebral	48
Adolescent cerebral	5
Adult cerebral	3
Adrenomyeloneuropathy	25
Addison only	10
Asymptomatic and presymptomatic	8

type 1 and acatalasemia do not cause symptoms in most of the affected persons and do not involve the nervous system.

X-Linked Adrenoleukodystrophy

Pathophysiology. The incidence of X-ALD is estimated to be between 1 in 20,000 and 1 in 50,000. It affects all races with approximately equal incidence. The genetic defect causing X-ALD is located in the Xq28 region. The disease results from mutations in the *ALDP* gene, which encodes a peroxisomal membrane protein. The function of this protein, which is a member of the ATP-binding cassette transporter superfamily, is as yet unknown. The heterogeneous genetic mutations cause an inability to form acyl-CoA derivatives of VLCFA. The resulting impaired beta-oxidation of VLCFA causes an accumulation of saturated VLCFA, particularly hexacosanoic acid (C26:0), in body fluids and tissues (Mosser et al. 1993). It is postulated that the basic defect in X-ALD involves the formation of a peroxisomal membrane protein responsible for the transport of lignoceroyl-CoA ligase into the peroxisome. Peroxisomal structure and all other peroxisomal functions are otherwise intact.

X-ALD causes progressive demyelination in brain and atrophy of the adrenal gland, where the adrenocortical cells accumulate C26:0 lipids, mainly in the form of cholesterol esters. In addition, there is testicular atrophy from lipid accumulation in Leydig's cells. The major neuropathological feature is severe demyelination that spares the arcuate fibers and perivascular lymphocytic cuffing.

Clinical Features. Childhood cerebral X-ALD is the most frequent phenotype (Moser et al. 1995) (Table 68.23). Boys develop normally until 4 years of age or later. The initial symptoms resemble those of hyperactivity or attention deficit disorder. The neurological phase may be heralded by seizures, dementia, difficulty in auditory discrimination, loss of vision, or ataxia. Once neurological symptoms occur, the illness advances rapidly and often leads to a vegetative state within 2 years and death at varying intervals thereafter. On neuroimaging studies severe and progressive demyelination is seen, especially in the posterior regions. Evidence exists that the rapid progression is because of a brain inflammatory response. Tumor necrosis factor and other cytokines may play a role in this response.

Adolescent cerebral X-ALD and adult cerebral X-ALD are rare variants of X-ALD. The adolescent form resembles the childhood disease but with later onset. The adult form often presents with dementia or psychiatric disturbances. Neuroimaging studies may reveal focal demyelination. Adrenal insufficiency may be absent, predate the neurological signs, or develop later.

Adrenomyeloneuropathy (AMN) is the second most common form of X-ALD. The mean age of onset is 27 years, with slow progression over decades. Some patients have lived to their 70s. AMN affects the spinal cord, primarily leading to progressive spastic paraparesis and sphincter disturbances. In the past, most of these patients were misdiagnosed as having multiple sclerosis. There is a mild neuropathy with loss of large and small myelinated fibers. Somatosensory evoked potentials are virtually absent. Approximately 88% of patients have Addison's disease, which predates the neurological manifestations in 42%. Cognitive impairment is generally mild, but many have emotional instability and depression. Although most patients eventually become impotent, many have fathered children.

The nervous system appears to be spared in more than 20% of X-linked AMN patients. Some of these patients have adrenal disease, but some are asymptomatic despite having biochemical evidence for the disease. It is important to recognize this disease as a cause of Addison's disease; all male Addison's disease patients should be screened for X-ALD. The various phenotypes frequently occur in the same family and even among brothers. The action of an autosomal modifier gene is the most likely explanation for this. Approximately 20% of female heterozygotes develop a neurological syndrome that resembles AMN.

Diagnosis. X-ALD must be considered in any child or adult with neuroimaging features of a leukodystrophy (Figure 68.20). The clinical features are mainly motor impairments and behavioral or cognitive impairments with or without adrenal insufficiency. The most frequently used and reliable diagnostic test is the demonstration of abnormally high levels of VLCFA in plasma. Approximately 10–15% of carriers may not demonstrate elevated levels of VLCFA and may require DNA analyses, provided there is an informative relative. Prenatal diagnosis is available both by chorionic villus sampling and testing for VLCFA in amniocytes.

Treatment. It is essential that adrenal function be tested at regular intervals in all patients with ALD and that corticosteroid replacement therapy be instituted if deficient. The tests for adrenal function should include the adrenocorticotropic hormone stimulation test. Corticosteroid replacement therapy is effective for the adrenal insufficiency but does not alter the neurological progression. Dietary therapy uses oils containing the monounsaturated oleic and erucic acids, a mixture that is also referred to as *Lorenzo's oil*. This diet has the promising property of normalizing the levels of VLCFA in plasma; however, to date, clinical results in symptomatic patients have been disappointing, because there is no alteration in the rate of progression of the childhood cerebral form of X-ALD or AMN (Aubourg et al. 1993).

Bone marrow transplantation may be remarkably effective but only when neurological involvement is still mild and when a human leukocyte antigen–matched donor is available (Loes et al. 1994). When the disease is moderately or severely advanced, bone marrow transplants have not been effective and may even accelerate the rate of neurological deterioration. The most successful result was in a patient with early neurological involvement with an unaffected nonidentical twin serving as the donor. In this patient, the slight neurological involvement was reversed, and the patient continued to do well 4 years later. Although there is encouragement that it is possible to influence early manifestations of ALD, attempts to modify the common and severe childhood cerebral form of the disease have been unsuccessful. However, downregulation of the inflammatory response and gene therapy are under investigation for potential treatment of X-ALD.

Defects of Fatty Acid Beta-Oxidation

Pathophysiology.   Like mitochondria, peroxisomes catabolize fatty acids by beta-oxidation. Chain-link specific acyl-CoA synthetases, acyl-CoA oxidases, trifunctional enzyme, and thiolyses are similar to mitochondrial beta-oxidation (Figure 68.21). However, the enzymes are specific for the peroxisome. Important differences are the substrate use and end products. Peroxisomes catabolize VLCFA and long-chain fatty acids, partially catabolize medium-chain fatty acids but not small-chain fatty acids at all. The energy produced from mitochondrial fatty acid oxidation is conserved in the production of ATP. The energy produced by peroxisomal beta-oxidation is not conserved but is released as heat. Three disorders have been described in which a deficiency of one of the three enzymes exists in the peroxisomal fatty acid beta-oxidation pathway. Acyl-CoA oxidase deficiency, trifunctional enzyme deficiency, and 3-oxoacyl-CoA thiolase deficiency cause human peroxisomal disease and accumulation of VLCFA and other metabolites in body tissues and fluids.

Clinical Features.   Acyl-CoA oxidase deficiency (also referred to as *pseudoneonatal adrenoleukodystrophy*), trifunctional enzyme deficiency, and 3-oxoacyl-CoA thiolase deficiency (also referred to as *pseudo-Zellweger's syndrome*) phenotypically resemble NALD and Zellweger's syndrome to such an extent that they cannot be distinguished clinically. Laboratory studies permit unequivocal distinction. Biochemical abnormalities are confined to excessive concentrations of VLCFA and bile acid intermediates. Unlike Zellweger's syndrome or NALD, plasmalogen, phytanic acid, and pipecolic acid levels are normal. An important distinction of this group with isolated enzyme defects is that peroxisome structure is preserved. In fact, the peroxisomes often are larger than normal. Approximately 10% of patients with the Zellweger-NALD phenotype have isolated defects of peroxisomal beta-oxidation pathway, the bifunctional enzyme deficiency being the most common.

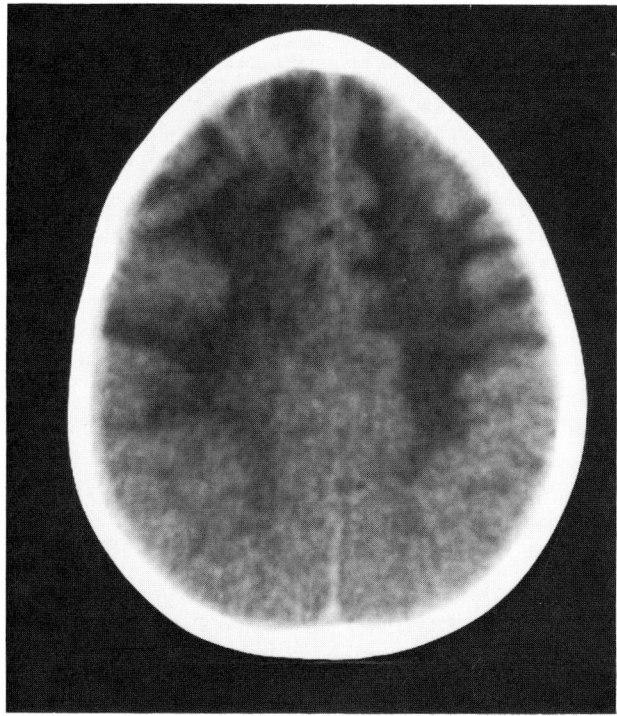

FIGURE 68.20   Diffuse demyelination on computed tomographic scan in a patient with X-linked adrenoleukodystrophy.

Diagnosis and Treatment.   The diagnosis of isolated deficiencies of peroxisomal fatty acid beta-oxidation should be considered in infants presenting with the Zellweger or NALD phenotype. Tissue biopsy shows preserved peroxisomes, which distinguish these disorders from those caused by failure of peroxisomal biogenesis. VLCFA are elevated in the blood. Individual enzymes can be measured in fibroblasts, and prenatal diagnosis is possible. The treatment is similar to that described previously for Zellweger's syndrome and is largely supportive.

Refsum's Disease

Pathophysiology.   Refsum's disease is a rare autosomal recessive disorder of peroxisomes with distinctive clinical and biochemical features related to phytanic acid metabolism. Phytanic acid is a 20-carbon branched-chain fatty acid that is solely derived from dietary phytanic acid phytols. A deficiency in peroxisomal phytanic acid α-oxidase, necessary for degradation of phytanic acid to pristanic acid, causes this disease. The enzyme is targeted to peroxisome by peroxisomal targeting signal 2. The gene is localized to chromosome 10.

Clinical Features.   Refsum's disease is an autosomal recessive disorder with the classic triad of ataxia, retinitis pigmentosa, and polyneuropathy. Increased CSF protein concentration without pleocytosis is a constant feature, and all patients have greatly increased serum concentrations of phytanic acid. Other neurological signs that can be present are sensorineural hearing loss, anosmia, pupillary abnormalities, and nystagmus. Ichthyosis, nonspecific electrocar-

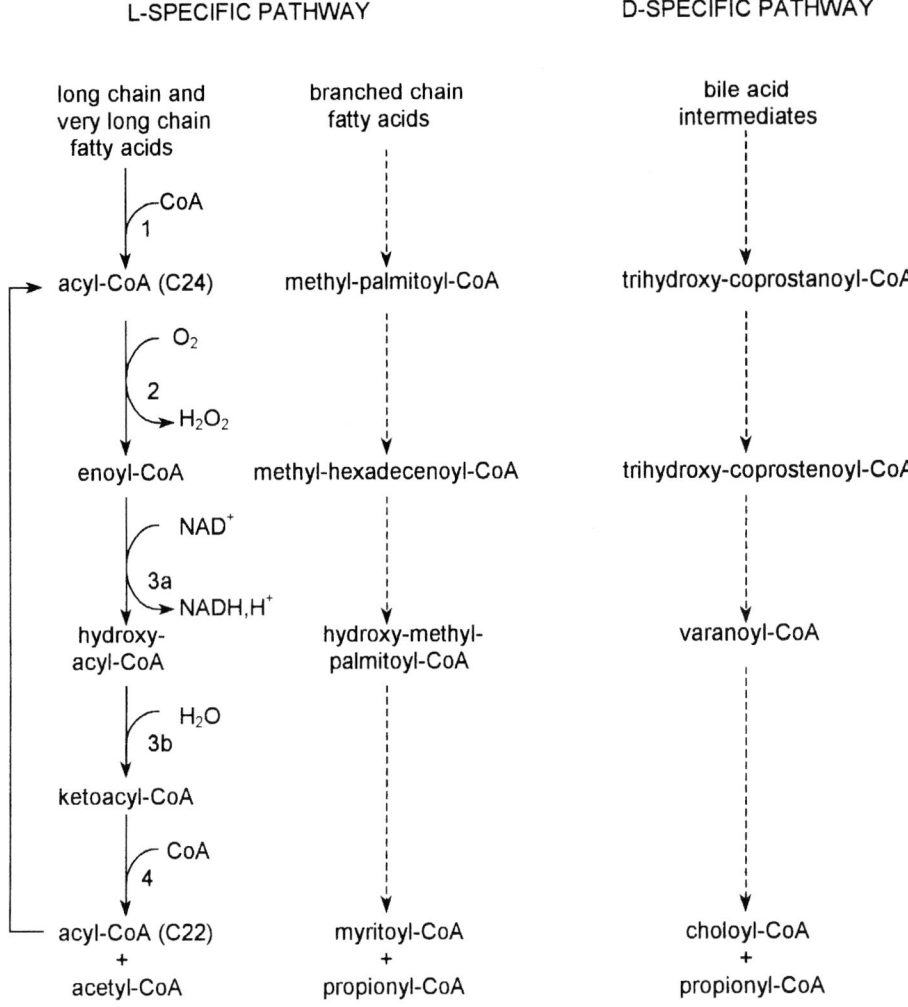

L-SPECIFIC PATHWAY

D-SPECIFIC PATHWAY

FIGURE 68.21 Peroxisomal beta-oxidation pathways. Energy production is in the form of heat and H_2O_2 rather than adenosine triphosphate. Detail is shown for long-chain and very-long-chain fatty acids. Similar steps occur for branched-chain and bile acid catabolism. (1) Acyl–coenzyme A (CoA) synthetase. (2) Acyl-CoA oxidase. (3a) Bifunctional enzyme hydratase. (3b) Bifunctional enzyme dehydrogenase. (4) Thiolase.

diographic changes, and epiphyseal dysplasia are inconstant systemic features. The onset is variable, but most patients become symptomatic in the second decade but occasionally later. The clinical course is also variable, with steady progression interrupted by periods of apparent remission and episodes of acute deterioration. Rapid worsening of symptoms occurs with metabolic stress such as fasting. This is related to temporary tissue release of phytanic acid. Incomplete recovery follows. In general, the clinical severity of the diseases correlates with the degree of phytanic acid elevation in the serum.

Diagnosis. The typical clinical features and the marked increase of serum phytanic acid concentrations are diagnostic in established patients. Early in the course of the disease, not all of the features may be present, and isolated symptoms, such as night blindness, areflexia, or poor coordination, may be the only findings. Serum phytanic acid concentrations are elevated in all cases, however. Enzyme activity can be measured in cultured fibroblasts.

Treatment. Efforts to reduce dietary phytanic acid is effective in arresting progression of the disease, and many complications improve significantly. When combined with

plasmapheresis at the time of diagnosis, improvement is rapid and corresponds with the reduction in serum phytanic acid concentration. Treatment should be initiated as soon as the disease is suspected and continued for life.

Peroxisomal Glutaryl-CoA Oxidase Deficiency. The first patient with this enzyme deficiency was identified at 11 months for failure to thrive and vomiting (in particular, postprandial vomiting) by Bennett and colleagues in 1991. The glutaric aciduria was responsive to riboflavin, 200 mg given twice daily. The activity of peroxisomal glutaryl-CoA oxidase was reduced to less than 10% of control values. This case represents a peroxisomal cause of glutaric aciduria distinct from the well-known mitochondrial disorders, which result in glutaric aciduria types I and II.

Rhizomelic Chondrodysplasia Punctata

Pathophysiology. RCDP has been placed in a separate category because it displays at least three separate peroxisomal biochemical abnormalities, whereas the peroxisome structure appears intact. RCDP has an autosomal recessive mode of inheritance. The main biochemical abnormalities are a severe deficiency and impaired synthesis of plasmalogens, elevated levels and impaired degradation of phytanic acid, and a failure to process the enzyme 3-oxoacyl-CoA thiolase, which fails to be imported into the peroxisomes of patients with RCDP. Demonstration of these abnormalities also can be used for prenatal diagnosis.

The RCDP phenotype also can be associated with a single enzyme defect, namely a deficiency of dihydroxyacetonephosphate acyltransferase, according to Wanders and colleagues in 1992, which results in a severe deficiency of plasmalogens but without a disturbance of phytanic acid or 3-oxoacyl-CoA thiolase. This finding indicates that the plasmalogen defect is the main culprit in the pathogenesis of the RCDP phenotype.

Clinical Features.   Patients with RCDP have severe mental retardation, short stature with disproportionate shortening of the proximal parts of the extremities, microcephaly, peculiar facial appearance, cataracts, and ichthyosis. Radiological findings include shortened limbs, stippled epiphyses and coronal clefts of the vertebral bodies. Other forms of chondrodysplasia punctata do not show abnormalities of peroxisome structure or function.

Diagnosis and Treatment.   RCDP should be suspected in the mentally retarded child with short stature and disproportionately shortened proximal extremities. Radiographical studies show stippled foci of calcification in hyaline cartilage, metaphyseal cupping, and disturbed ossification. Vertebral bodies have a coronal cleft, which is an embryologic remnant. Elevated blood phytanic acid levels and decreased concentrations of blood plasmalogens are virtually diagnostic in this clinical setting. There is no effective therapy.

Lysosomal Storage Disorders

Lysosomes are membrane-bound organelles within the cytosol of the cell that are involved in intracellular digestion. They contain hydrolytic enzymes that function at an acidic pH. Lysosomal disorders may be caused by impaired enzyme synthesis, abnormal enzyme targeting, or a defective accessory factor needed for enzymatic processing. Dysfunctional or absent enzymes result in deficient degradation and storage of cellular products within lysosomes that then increase in size and number. The abnormal storage causes cell injury and death, presumably from mechanical distortion or membrane rupture with toxic injury by the stored material (see psychosine in Krabbe's Disease, later in this chapter). The ruptured lysosomes release hydrolytic enzymes and toxic metabolic by-products into the cytoplasm. The clinical features of lysosomal storage diseases depend on the organ(s) involved and may include neurological impairment, progressive vision loss, visceromegaly, and dysmorphic features.

Abnormal storage material can be recognized in biopsy specimens of skin, conjunctiva, muscle, lymphocytes, and bone marrow. Some diseases can be identified by measuring the concentration of excreted products in the urine. Definitive diagnosis requires enzyme measurement of leukocytes or cultured fibroblasts. Mutation analysis is available for some disorders; prenatal diagnosis and heterozygote detection is available for most.

Glycogen Storage Disorders

Glycogen, a glucose polymer, is found in most cells of the body. The highest concentrations are in liver and then skeletal muscle. Glycogen degradation to glucose requires a series of enzymes that, when absent or dysfunctional, cause abnormal glycogen storage. Glucose is provided by hepatic glycogenolysis during periods of fasting or stress; impaired glycogenolysis is associated with hypoglycemia and lactic acidosis. Deficiency of enzymes responsible for muscle glycogenolysis results in cramps during exercise and myopathy (see Chapter 83).

Pompe's Disease

Pathophysiology.   Pompe's disease is transmitted by autosomal recessive inheritance. The abnormal gene is located on chromosome 17. It is caused by a deficiency of acid α-glycosidase (acid maltase), a lysosomal enzyme found in the CNS and skeletal muscle. The enzyme hydrolyzes maltose and catalyzes the transglucosylation from maltose to glycogen. It does not contribute to the maintenance of normal blood glucose concentrations.

The deficiency state results in a massive accumulation of glycogen within lysosomes, leading to cell damage and necrosis. Infants with Pompe's disease store glycogen in several tissues, especially muscle, heart, and lower motor neurons. Affected tissues have cytoplasmic vacuoles containing material that stains with the periodic–acid Schiff reagent. The vacuoles are membrane-bound and can be identified as distended lysosomes.

Clinical Features.   Four clinical phenotypes are distinguished on the basis of age at onset: infantile, late infantile, juvenile, and adult. The infantile form is characterized by progressive weakness, profound hypotonia, and heart failure. Additional but inconstant features are muscle firmness, hepatosplenomegaly, and macroglossia. Radiography shows massive globular cardiomegaly, and the electrocardiography shows biventricular hypertrophy with a shortened PR interval and very high amplitude QRS complexes. The initial symptoms may be referable to the heart (fatigue with feeding and dyspnea), the skeletal muscles (profound hypotonia and weakness), or both. Developmental delay is out of proportion to muscle weakness. Death usually occurs within several months after symp-

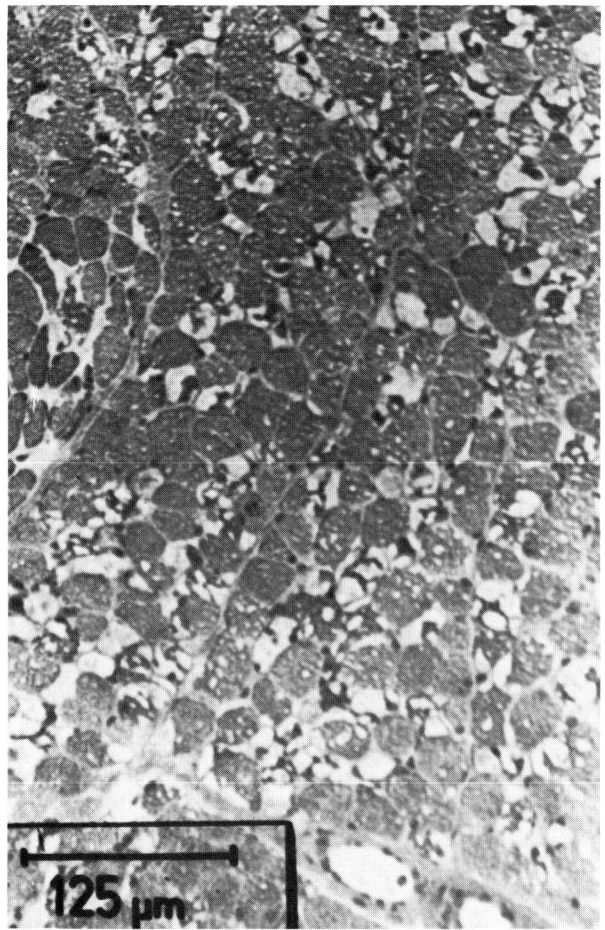

FIGURE 68.22 Muscle biopsy of a patient with glycogen storage disease II (Pompe's disease). (Reprinted with permission from OB Evans. Manual of Child Neurology. New York: Churchill Livingstone, 1987;213.)

toms appear from congestive heart failure. Clinical variability of the adult onset disease occurs within kinships (Felice et al. 1995).

Motor delay and progressive myopathy are the main features of the late infantile, juvenile, and adult forms of acid maltase deficiency. The speed of progression is variable, but the severity of cardiorespiratory involvement correlates with the amount of residual enzyme activity. Visceromegaly is more common in younger cases.

Diagnosis. The infantile form should be considered in hypotonic infants with cardiomegaly or heart failure; the later onset forms should be considered in individuals with progressive myopathies. Electromyography is usually compatible with myopathy but also may have neuropathic features (see Chapter 37B). Myotonic discharges without clinical myotonia suggest the diagnosis. The later onset forms usually are diagnosed by muscle biopsy in

the course of evaluating a progressive myopathy. Biopsy specimens in all forms show the characteristic picture of lysosomal glycogen storage (Figure 68.22): large vacuoles containing material that stains positive on periodic–acid Schiff.

Definitive diagnosis requires measuring the enzyme concentration in muscle, leukocytes, or cultured fibroblasts.

Treatment. Treatment is not available.

Cholesterol Storage Diseases

Cerebrotendinous Xanthomatosis

Pathophysiology. Cerebrotendinous xanthomatosis is transmitted by autosomal recessive inheritance. It is caused by mutations in the sterol 27-hydroxylase gene on the distal portion of chromosome 2q. The affected enzyme is a member of the cytochrome P450 system, which catalyzes the initial steps in the oxidation of sterol intermediate side chains that form bile acids. Enzyme deficiency causes an absence of chenodeoxycholic acid in the bile and a marked increase of cholestanol in plasma and many tissues, particularly in the tendons, neurons, and lungs.

Clinical Features. The onset of symptoms is in late childhood, and the clinical course varies. The major neurological features are spinocerebellar ataxia, spasticity, peripheral neuropathy, dementia, and retardation; the systemic features are tendon xanthomata, juvenile cataracts, osteoporosis secondary to abnormal vitamin D metabolism, and premature atherosclerosis.

Diagnosis. Increased concentrations of cholestanol in the serum and low-to-normal plasma cholesterol concentrations suggest the diagnosis. MRI shows progressive cerebral atrophy and demyelination.

Treatment. Early diagnosis is imperative because effective long-term therapy is available. Daily administration of 750 mg of chenodeoxycholic acid lowers blood cholestanol and improves nerve conduction velocities (Kuriyama et al. 1994). Tendon xanthoma also resolve.

Wolman's Disease and Cholesterol Ester Storage Disease

Pathophysiology. Acid lipase (cholesterol ester hydrolase) hydrolyzes cellular cholesterol esters and triglycerides after uptake of low-density lipoproteins. Acid lipase deficiency results in the intralysosomal storage and abnormal regulation of cellular cholesterol. Wolman's disease and cholesterol ester storage disease (CESD) are autosomal recessive allelic disorders secondary to acid lipase dysfunction (Aslandis et al. 1996).

Extensive storage of cholesterol esters occurs in all organs, especially the liver and spleen. The genetic defect of both disorders is on the long arm of chromosome 10 (Anderson et al. 1993).

Clinical Features.   The onset of Wolman's disease is in early infancy. The features are vomiting, steatorrhea, hepatosplenomegaly, lymphadenopathy, pulmonary insufficiency, and failure to thrive. Adrenal failure sometimes is present and is associated with radiographic evidence of adrenal calcification. Mental regression, spasticity, and clonus, at first mild, progress rapidly; death occurs before age 1 year.

CESD is milder than Wolman's disease because residual enzyme activity is greater. The onset of symptoms is delayed until early adult life. The main features are hepatosplenomegaly, hepatic fibrosis, and premature atherosclerosis. Adrenal calcification is rare.

Diagnosis.   Definitive diagnosis of both Wolman's disease and CESD requires showing the enzyme deficiency in lymphocytes or fibroblasts.

Treatment.   No treatment is considered curative. Bone marrow transplantation is undergoing clinical trials for Wolman's disease, and lovastatin has been shown to be effective in limited cases of CESD.

Niemann-Pick Disease Type C

Pathophysiology.   Niemann-Pick disease type C is transmitted by autosomal recessive inheritance. The abnormal gene has been linked to chromosome 18q11.

Niemann-Pick disease type C is distinguished by a unique defect in the cellular trafficking of cholesterol that allows the lysosomal accumulation of unesterified cholesterol (Carstea et al. 1997).

Niemann-Pick disease type C is biochemically and genetically distinct from the primary sphingomyelinosis (Niemann-Pick disease, types A and B) with which it was previously associated.

Clinical Features.   The clinical spectrum of Niemann-Pick disease type C varies. The usual phenotype is slow developmental progression and then regression.

Niemann-Pick disease type C can present also as just a learning disability. Other invariable features are hepatosplenomegaly, vertical supranuclear gaze palsy, dystonia, dysarthria, dysphagia, and ataxia. Seizures and cataplexy often occur during the course of neurological deterioration.

Fulminant neonatal cholestatic liver disease is a phenotypic variant. Infants who survive the liver disease show gradual improvement of liver function but develop a relentlessly progressive neurological syndrome. Dementia and psychosis are the predominant features when the onset of neurological disease is in adolescence or later.

Diagnosis.   Postmortem examination shows foamy macrophages in the viscera and cytoplasmic ballooning of neurons. Neurofibrillary tangles, most prominent in the hippocampus, are seen (Suzuki et al. 1995). Definitive diagnosis is confirmed by showing a marked decrease in cellular cholesterol esterification; this is shown cytochemically by positive fluorescence after filipin staining in cultured fibroblasts. Enzymatic activity of sphingomyelinase may be normal or partially depressed. Definitive heterozygote determination is not yet available.

Treatment.   Treatment is mainly supportive.

Smith-Lemli-Opitz Syndrome

The Smith-Lemli-Opitz syndrome is an autosomal recessive disorder with an incidence of 1 in 20,000–40,000. The disorder is caused by a defect in 7-dehydrocholesterol-delta-reductase, the enzyme that catalyzes the last reaction of cholesterol synthesis. As a result, a deficiency of cholesterol and an elevation of its precursor, 7-dehydrocholesterol, occurs. The molecular genetic basis for this disorder has not yet been elucidated.

Clinical Features.   Patients with Smith-Lemli-Opitz syndrome suffer from multiple congenital anomalies (Cunniff et al. 1997). Since the discovery of the biochemical defect, the clinical spectrum has broadened. The most common malformation is syndactyly of the second and third toes. Children have a dysmorphic appearance with micrognathia, upturned nares, ptosis, flattened nasal bridge, and prominent epicanthal folds. Other congenital malformations include cleft palate, cataracts, cardiac malformations, renal dysplasia, polydactyly, genital anomalies, gastrointestinal disorders such as Hirschsprung's disease and pyloric stenosis, and growth failure. Microcephaly, holoprosencephaly, and severe mental retardation are the major neurological features of Smith-Lemli-Opitz syndrome.

Diagnosis.   The clinical diagnosis is suspected by the characteristic dysmorphic features and low serum cholesterol and elevated 7-dehydrocholesterol. Measurement of deficient 7-dehydrocholesterol-delta-reductase activity in fibroblasts confirms the diagnosis and can be used for carrier detection and prenatal diagnosis.

Treatment.   The replacement of cholesterol, 60–120 mg/kg per day, with or without additional bile acids has resulted in improvement of growth and neurodevelopment (Irons 1997). The most improvement is seen in patients with initial cholesterol levels less than 40 mg/dl.

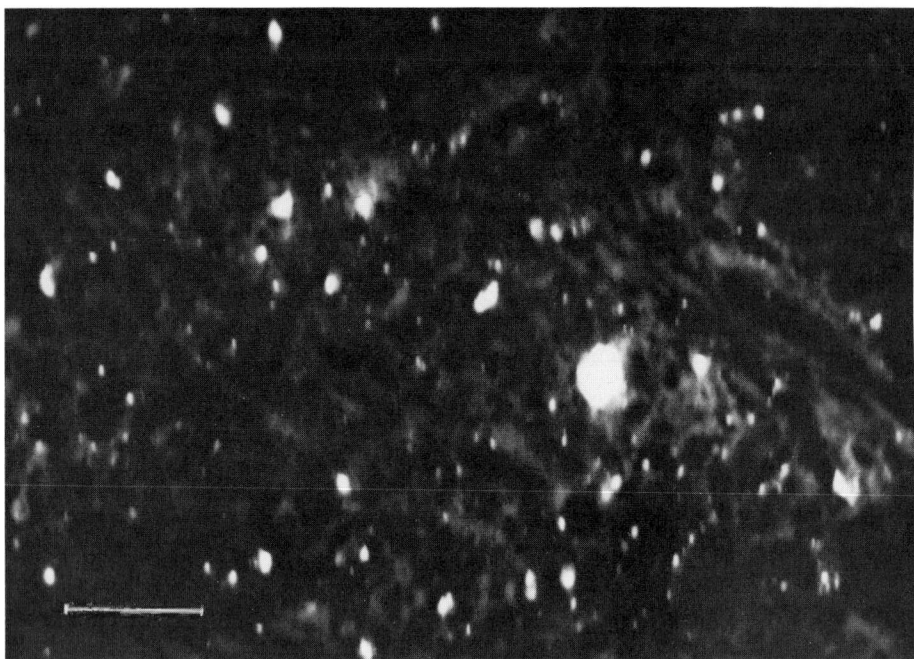

FIGURE 68.23 Autofluorescence of storage material in skeletal muscle from a patient with neuronal ceroid lipofuscinosis (calibration bar = 25 mm).

Farber's Lipogranulomatosis

Pathophysiology

Farber's lipogranulomatosis is caused by a deficiency of the lysosomal enzyme ceramidase. This rare disease is transmitted by autosomal recessive inheritance. Ceramidase hydrolyzes ceramide to sphingosine and fatty acids. When deficient, ceramide accumulates in lysosomes and causes disseminated lipogranulomatosis.

Clinical Features

The initial features have their onset during the first year and include joint pain, stiffness, and subcutaneous nodules of periarticular skin. Nodules also may be located in the larynx (leading to hoarseness), scalp, thoracoabdominal wall, or near pressure points. Additional features are interstitial lung disease, psychomotor regression, lymphadenopathy, hepatosplenomegaly, macroglossia, macular cherry-red spot, conjunctival nodules, and cardiac disease.

Neurological symptoms are caused by lipid storage in the central and peripheral nervous systems and include seizures (especially myoclonus), dementia, hypotonia, muscular wasting, and decreased or absent tendon reflexes. Death occurs during the first decade.

Diagnosis

Lysosomal inclusions are characteristic of Farber's lipogranulomatosis: comma-shaped curvilinear tubular structures (banana bodies) in the lysosomes of the reticuloendothelial system and zebra bodies in the neurons. The former are thought to represent stored ceramide, and the latter stored gangliosides. These characteristic inclusions and assessment of enzyme activity confirm the diagnosis.

Treatment

Treatment is not available.

Neuronal Ceroid Lipofuscinosis

Pathophysiology

The neuronal ceroid lipofuscinosis (NCL) are inherited disorders with lysosomal storage of the autofluorescent lipopigments, ceroid and lipofuscin, and other compounds in neurons and cells of other tissues. The incidence is 1 in 100,000 live births. Most cases are transmitted as an autosomal recessive trait. A characteristic feature is autofluorescence in ultraviolet light (Figure 68.23). The major component of the storage material in all forms of the disease, except the infantile type, is subunit c of the mitochondrial ATP synthase complex. Abnormalities in the sequence or expression of the two known genes for this protein do not account for the subunit c accumulation. Conversely, sphingolipid activator proteins (saposins A and D) are stored in the infantile type, which is genetically and biochemically distinct from later onset forms. The abnormal storage of dolichols (long chain polyisoprenyl alcohols) and dolichyl pyrophosphoryl oligosaccharides was once believed to be the primary abnormality, but is now known to be a nonspecific, secondary disturbance.

Table 68.24:   Classification and clinical summary of the neuronal ceroid lipofuscinoses

Disease	Age of onset (yrs)	Duration (yrs)	Blindness	Myoclonus, seizures	Dementia	EM	Chromosome
Infantile	0–2	5–10	Early	Frequent	Early	GRN	1p32
Late infantile	2–4	5–10	Late	Frequent, typical electroencephalogram	Early	CLB, FPB	—
Juvenile	4–10	5–15	Early	Infrequent	Late	FPB	16p12
Adult	10–20	10–20	Rare	Frequent	Late	GRN	—

CLB = curvilinear bodies; EM = electron microscopic ultrastructural findings; FPB = fingerprint bodies; GRN = granular bodies.

Two major types of cytoplasmic storage bodies are seen by electron microscopy: granular and lamellated. Granular inclusions are osmiophilic and amorphous in appearance; they occur in the infantile form but only rarely in adults. Lamellated inclusions are curvilinear, fingerprint, crystalloid, or tubular in appearance. They occur only in the later onset diseases. Atypical membranous cytoplasmic bodies can be found in variant cases. Other pathological features are cerebral atrophy and neuronal degeneration. Apoptosis has been established as the mechanism of neuronal and photoreceptor cell death in the late infantile and juvenile forms (Lane et al. 1996).

Clinical Features

Dementia, vision loss, ataxia, polymyoclonus, and seizures are the major features of all NCLs. Four primary forms are recognized; however, considerable clinical overlap occurs, and many variant subtypes cannot be classified (Table 68.24). Approximately 20% of the cases have an atypical clinical course. Collectively, the NCLs have often been referred to as *Batten's disease*.

Infantile Neuronal Ceroid Lipofuscinosis.   Infantile NCL (Haltia-Santavouri type) has the earliest onset and is the most severe. It is mainly reported from Finland, where the carrier frequency is 1 in 70. Seizures, especially infantile spasms and myoclonus, begin during the first year and are followed by developmental regression, ataxia, hypotonia, and blindness caused by retinal degeneration and optic atrophy. Death usually occurs within the first decade. The electroretinographical amplitude is absent or markedly diminished early in the disease. The visual evoked response amplitude diminishes and disappears with age.

Granular osmiophilic deposits are seen in circulating lymphocytes and in biopsy specimens of skin, muscle, and conjunctiva. Postmortem examination shows massive loss of cortical neurons with prominent brain atrophy and a peculiar macrophagocytosis. Linkage studies have located the gene to chromosome 1p32. The disorder results from the lysosomal deficiency of palitoyl-protein thioesterase (Hellsten et al. 1997).

Late Infantile Neuronal Ceroid Lipofuscinosis.   The initial features of late infantile NCL (Bielschowsky-Jansky type) is a mixed seizure disorder of generalized tonic-clonic and minor motor seizures beginning at 1–4 years of age. Later, myoclonic jerks become the prominent seizure pattern. Truncal ataxia and hypotonia are early symptoms. Dysarthria and rapidly increasing spasticity soon follow the initial hypotonia. Mental regression is severe. Vision loss from macular degeneration and optic atrophy develop within 2 years of symptom onset. The course is rapid with ultimate spastic quadriparesis, dysphagia, and difficulty handling secretions. Death occurs by age 10 years.

The electroretinographical amplitude is markedly diminished or absent, and the visual evoked response is grossly increased early but diminishes with time. The somatosensory-evoked response also is increased. Photic stimulation at 3 Hz evokes a high-amplitude, polyphasic discharge on EEG. MRI shows an enlarged fourth ventricle and cerebellar atrophy with initial sparing of the occipital lobes early in the course and later shows hydrocephalus *ex vacuo* and evidence of white matter tissue loss and gliosis (Boustany 1993). The affected gene maps to 11p15. A Finnish variant has been mapped to 13q31. The defective protein is a pepstatin-insensitive lysosomal peptidase (Sleat et al. 1997).

Juvenile Neuronal Ceroid Lipofuscinosis.   Juvenile NCL (Spielmeyer-Vogt type) accounts for 50% of NCL cases. Onset of vision loss, often associated with retinitis pigmentosa, is between 4 and 10 years. Dementia is subtle at onset and characterized by slowly progressive personality changes and deteriorating school performance. Generalized tonic-clonic and myoclonic seizures begin in mid-childhood, but are not as frequent as in the infantile and late-infantile forms. Positional myoclonus, rigidity, and dystonia are seen with progressive disease. The results of electrodiagnostic studies are similar to those seen in the other lipofuscinoses, but there is no photoconvulsive response. The inclusions are primarily fingerprint bodies. The abnormal gene locus has been mapped to chromosome 16p12.

Adult-Onset Neuronal Ceroid Lipofuscinosis.   Adult-onset NCL (Kufs' type) is probably heterogeneous and accounts for only 2% of NCL cases. Onset of symptoms is during the second or third decades. Neurological deterioration is slow, vision is preserved, and spasticity is prominent. There are two subtypes: Type A is characterized by seizures and myoclonus, and type B is dominated by dementia, progressive ataxia, spasticity, rigidity, and choreoathetosis, alone or in combination. Dementia is inevitable and can be accompanied by behavioral problems or psychosis. The prominent inclusions are granular, but curvilinear inclusions and fingerprint bodies may be seen as well. Extraneuronal tissue is not always involved. Genetic variation is suggested by families with autosomal dominant inheritance.

Diagnosis

The diagnosis of NCL should be suspected in patients with the triad of seizures, dementia, and progressive vision loss. Fundoscopic examination shows the typical retinal changes. A specific laboratory test is not available, but the combination of typical clinical features and neurophysiological abnormalities is virtually diagnostic. Histological and ultrastructural examination for inclusion bodies provides further confirmation. Lipopigments are most easily found in eccrine sweat glands. Fifteen percent of initial skin biopsies, however, are not diagnostic, and biopsy should be repeated if clinical suspicions persist. Electron microscopy of circulating lymphocytes may help to further classify the inclusions morphologically and assist in clinical subtyping (Goebel 1995). Prenatal diagnosis of the infantile, late infantile, and juvenile types may be accomplished by combined genetic and electron microscopic approach.

Treatment

Treatment is limited to supportive care, seizure management, and genetic counseling.

Mucopolysaccharidoses

The mucopolysaccharidoses (MPS) are hereditary disorders in which specific lysosomal enzyme deficiencies cause the pathological accumulation and increased urinary excretion of incompletely degraded mucopolysaccharides. Mucopolysaccharides are a normal component of cornea, cartilage, bone, connective tissue, and the reticuloendothelial system and are therefore target organs for excessive storage. The incidence of these disorders may be 1 in 10,000 (Wraith 1995).

Pathophysiology

Mucopolysaccharides (glycosaminoglycans) are sulfated polymers composed of a central protein moiety attached to repeating disaccharide branches. They normally are degraded to inorganic sulfated monosaccharides in lysosomes. Dermatan sulfate consists of alternating units of L-iduronic acid and N-acetylgalactosamine. It is normally found in the matrix of many different connective tissues. Heparan sulfate is formed by the joining of a uronic acid (D-glucuronic acid or L-iduronic acid) alternating with N-acetylglucosamine and is associated with the cell plasma membrane in almost all cells. Keratan sulfate is composed of D-galactose residues alternating with N-acetylglucosamine and is found largely in cartilage, nucleus pulposus, and cornea. Chondroitin sulfate consists of alternating units of D-glucuronic acid and N-acetylgalactosamine and also is found largely in cartilage and cornea. Six MPS are recognized, each differing in clinical severity, but all exhibiting some period of normal development followed by a gradual decline of physical and mental function. Table 68.25 summarizes the clinical and biochemical features of the MPS.

Clinical Features

Mucopolysaccharidosis Type I-H (Hurler's Syndrome). Hurler's syndrome is the prototype and most severe form of the MPS. It is transmitted by autosomal recessive inheritance; the genomic clone has been isolated from chromosome 4p16.3. The incidence is 1–2 in 100,000 live births. The disease is caused by deficiency of the enzyme α-L-iduronidase, which cleaves L-iduronic acid from both dermatan and heparan sulfate. Dermatan sulfate and heparan sulfate are excreted in the urine with a ratio of 2 to 1.

Affected newborns appear normal. Macrocephaly, developmental delay, rhinorrhea, and recurrent upper respiratory infections develop late in the first year. The characteristic coarsened facies (frontal bossing, prominent eyes with hypertelorism, open mouth with macroglossia, enlarged lips, and flattened nasal bridge) develop during the second year (MPS phenotype) (Figure 68.24). The hair is thick and coarse, the teeth are small and widely spaced, and the gums are hypertrophic.

Linear growth is stunted, and several skeletal deformities develop that are known collectively as *dysostosis multiplex*: The skull is enlarged and scaphocephalic with a shallow and elongated sella turcica; the vertebral bodies are hypoplastic and hook-shaped in the thoracolumbar region, with anterior beaking (Figure 68.25) often resulting in a gibbus deformity by age 18 months; the ribs are widened and oar-shaped; long bones are shortened and poorly modeled; the joints become stiffened, some to the point of contractures; the hands are broad and short; and fingers are stubby with clawlike deformities.

The liver and spleen are invariably enlarged, and the abdomen is quite protuberant, often with a prominent umbilical hernia. Communicating hydrocephalus can occur as a result of meningeal thickening. Ophthalmological complications include corneal clouding and occasional glaucoma. Deafness also is present. Airway obstruction and secondary sleep apnea are additional complications. Progressive mental deterioration is always present.

Deposition of the mucopolysaccharide by-products in arterial smooth muscle results in cardiovascular compromise. Complete occlusion of the coronary arteries can cause angina pectoris in early childhood. Cardiac valvular involvement also has been described. Death occurs by age 10 years without intervention from respiratory or cardiac disease.

Table 68.25: The mucopolysaccharidoses

Syndrome	Eponym	Enzyme defect	Chromosome	Onset (yrs)	CNS	Bone	Viscera	Cornea	Urine MPS
I-H	Hurler's syndrome	L-Iduronidase	4p16.3	<1	+++	++	++	+	DS, HS
I-S	Scheie's syndrome	L-Iduronidase	4	2–5	−	+	+/−	+	DS, HS
I-H/S		L-Iduronidase	4	1–3	++	+	+	+	DS, HS
II	Hunter's syndrome	Iduronate-2-sulfatase	Xq27/28	2–5	++	+	+	+	DS, HS
III	Sanfilippo's syndrome		Unknown	2–4					
	Type A	Heparan-N-sulfatase	Unknown		+++	+	+	−	HS
	Type B	N-Acetyl-alpha-D-glucosaminidase	Unknown		++	+	+	−	HS
	Type C	Acetyl-CoA: α-glucosaminide	Unknown		++	+	+	−	HS
	Type D	N-Acetyl-alpha-D-glucosaminide-6-sulfatase	12q14		++	+	+	−	HS
IV	Morquio's syndrome			1–3					
	Type A	N-Acetylgalactosamine-6-sulfatase	16q24.3		−	++	−	+	KS
	Type B	β-Galactosidase	3		−	+	+/−	+	KS, HS
VI	Maroteaux-Lamy syndrome	N-Acetyl-galactosamine-4-sulfatase	5q13.3	2–3	−	+	+	+	DS
VII	Sly's disease	β-Glucuronidase	7q21.1–7q22		+	+	+	+	DS, HS

AR = autosomal recessive; CoA = coenzyme A; CNS = central nervous system; DS = dermatan sulfate; HS = heparan sulfate; KS = keratan sulfate; MPS = mucopolysaccharide; XR = X-linked recessive; + = mild abnormality; ++ = moderate abnormality; +/− = variable; − = absent.

Mucopolysaccharidosis Type I-S (Scheie's Syndrome). Mucopolysaccharidosis type I-S (Scheie's syndrome) was classified as MPS V before it was found to be caused by alpha-L-iduronidase deficiency, as in Hurler's syndrome. The biochemical findings are identical to Hurler's syndrome, but the clinical features are less severe. Hurler's and Scheie's syndromes are allelic disorders caused by different mutations within the same gene coding for alpha-L-iduronidase on chromosome 4. The main features are mildly coarsened facies, stiffened joints, and corneal clouding. Intelligence and height are near normal. The skeletal anomalies are most pronounced in the hands, and carpal tunnel syndrome is common. Life expectancy is longer in Scheie's syndrome than in Hurler's syndrome and depends on the degree of cardiovascular involvement.

As with MPS I-H, large amounts of heparan sulfate and dermatan sulfate are excreted in urine.

Mucopolysaccharidosis Type I-H/S (Hurler-Scheie Syndrome). Mucopolysaccharidosis type I-H/S (MPS I-H/S) is an intermediate form between Hurler's and Scheie's syndromes and represents a third phenotype caused by a mutation of the alpha-L-iduronidase gene. The clinical features are moderate mental retardation, corneal clouding, shortened stature, and severe dysostosis multiplex.

Hydrocephalus and arachnoid cysts are seen frequently. Some patients may exhibit unusual facies with micrognathia (Neufeld and Muenzer 1995). Death is in the late teens to early twenties.

Mucopolysaccharidosis Type II (Hunter's Syndrome). Mucopolysaccharidosis type II (Hunter's syndrome) is caused by deficiency of iduronate-2-sulfatase. Unlike other MPS, it is transmitted as an X-linked recessive trait. The iduronate-2-sulfatase gene has been mapped to Xq27/28. Clinical heterogeneity does not correlate with the amount of residual enzyme activity but probably is based on variation at the molecular level. The complete iduronate-2-sulfatase deletion confers a severe phenotype (Froissart et al. 1993).

The clinical course of Hunter's syndrome varies. The onset of symptoms is between 2 and 5 years of age. Corneal clouding, gibbus deformity, and abnormal vertebrae do not usually develop. The most common features are coarsened facies, dwarfism, joint stiffness, shortened neck, deafness, mental retardation, and hepatosplenomegaly. Diarrhea is a common complaint, and a distinctive cutaneous nodular thickening may occur over the scapulae, pectoralis muscles, and limbs. Despite the absence of corneal clouding, blindness can be caused by chronic papilledema and retinal

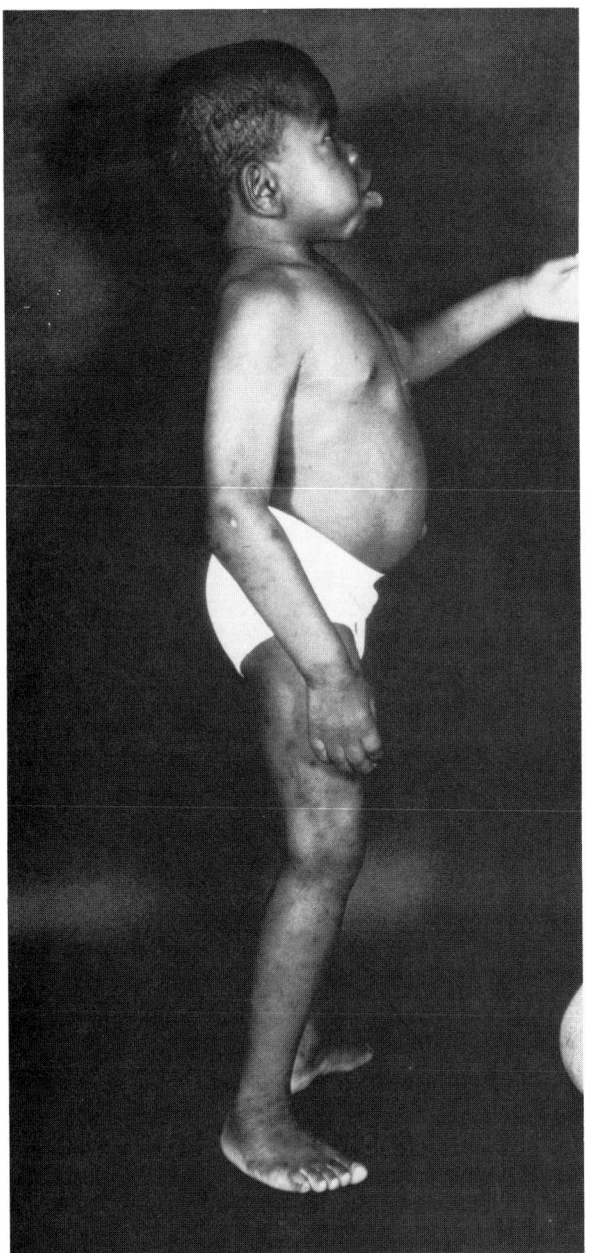

FIGURE 68.24   Typical features of the mucopolysaccharidosis phenotype.

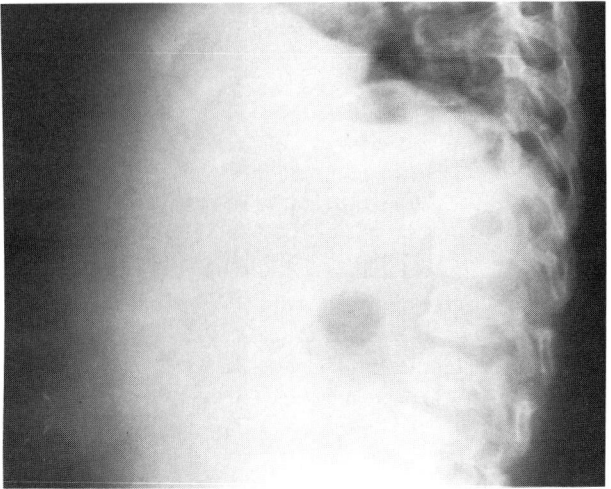

FIGURE 68.25   Radiographic features of dysostosis multiplex of the spinal vertebrae in a patient with Hurler's syndrome.

Mucopolysaccharidosis Type III (Sanfilippo's Syndrome). The four recognized types of mucopolysaccharidosis type III (Sanfilippo's syndrome) are clinically similar but biochemically distinct (see Table 68.25). All are transmitted by autosomal recessive inheritance. The function of the deficient enzymes is to degrade the glucosaminide residue at the nonreducing terminus of heparan sulfate. Excessive amounts of heparan sulfate are excreted in the urine.

Clinical expression is heterogeneous, even within the same family. The typical course is normal development until age 2–8 years, then slowed development, and finally regression. Affected children become hyperactive and aggressive. The dementia is relentlessly progressive and associated with spastic quadriplegia and a movement disorder.

The non-neurological features are mild: coarsening of facial features, shortened neck, and stiffness of the joints. Dysostosis multiplex is not pronounced, but increased thickness of the posterior calvarium is characteristic. Linear growth is normal, corneal clouding and cardiovascular impairment do not occur, and hepatosplenomegaly is mild. Diarrhea is a frequent complaint. Death usually occurs before age 20.

The four types can be distinguished only by enzymatic quantitation. Spot urine screening results may be negative; a 24-hour urine specimen is needed for diagnosis. The diagnosis of milder phenotype often is delayed because the symptoms are subtle and the urine screen result is negative. MPS type III should be considered in children with progressive hyperactivity and mild coarsening of facial features.

Mucopolysaccharidosis Type IV (Morquio's Syndrome). Mucopolysaccharidosis type IV (Morquio's syndrome) is transmitted by autosomal recessive inheritance. It is one of the least common of the MPSs. Two biochemical variants, type A and type B, are both caused by deficiency of enzymes involved in the degradation of keratan sulfate. Increased concentrations of keratan sulfate are excreted in

degeneration caused by direct involvement of the optic nerve sheath. Cardiac and respiratory compromise develops from chest wall deformity, obstructive airway disease, pulmonary hypertension, coronary artery narrowing with ischemia or infarction, myocardial hypertrophy, and valvular dysfunction.

The more severely affected children have progressive dementia, hyperkinesis, and behavioral problems and usually die before puberty. Those with the milder variants have less profound mental retardation and die in the second or third decade.

Excessive concentrations of heparan sulfate and dermatan sulfate are excreted in the urine, with a relative proportion of 1 to 1.

the urine as a result of this syndrome. Type A is caused by a lack of N-acetylgalactosamine-6-sulfatase, which is encoded on chromosome 16q24. Type B is caused by β-galactosidase deficiency, which is encoded on chromosome 3. Other allelic disorders of β-galactosidase deficiency are discussed later in this chapter.

The onset occurs between 1 and 3 years of age. The constant features are short stature caused by short-trunk dwarfism, although the limbs also can be involved. Cervical cord compression is the most severe complication, which results from hypoplasia of the odontoid with secondary atlantoaxial instability. Radiographic studies show spondyloepiphyseal dysplasia with hypoplastic vertebrae, kyphosis, broad ribs, pectus carinatum, sternal gibbus, genu valgum, and shortened long bones. The joints are remarkably loose. The face is only mildly coarsened, and the teeth are widely spaced with thin enamel. Intelligence is normal unless hydrocephalus develops and is not treated. The cranial deformities, however, may cause progressive deafness. Slit-lamp examination often is required to show corneal opacities. Hepatomegaly sometimes is associated.

Cervical instability is the major cause of early death; cardiovascular involvement and respiratory compromise occur later in life. Morquio's syndrome type B is generally milder than type A despite some overlap.

Mucopolysaccharidosis Type VI (Maroteaux-Lamy Syndrome). Mild, intermediate, and severe forms of mucopolysaccharidosis type VI (Maroteaux-Lamy syndrome or MPS type VI) are distinguished. Arylsulfatase B (N-acetylgalactosamine-4-sulfatase) is deficient; excess dermatan sulfate is excreted in the urine. The abnormal gene is located on chromosome 5q13.3.

The initial feature usually is stunted linear growth in early childhood. The typical skeletal anomalies of MPS are severe, as is the limitation of joint movement. A shortened trunk is characteristic. Deficient ossification of the femoral capital epiphysis and coxa valga is common. Patients have the typical Hurler phenotype, corneal clouding, and hepatosplenomegaly. Deafness is frequent but normal intelligence is maintained. Neurological complications include hydrocephalus secondary to pachymeningitis and nerve entrapment syndromes. A myelopathy may result from dural thickening, vertebral body abnormalities, or both. Death typically results from heart failure.

Mucopolysaccharidosis Type VII (Sly's Disease). Mucopolysaccharidosis type VII (Sly's disease) is caused by a deficiency of beta-glucuronidase. Excess dermatan sulfate and heparan sulfate are excreted in the urine. The trait is transmitted by autosomal recessive inheritance. The abnormal gene is located on chromosome 7q21.1-q22.

The gene expression varies from minimal symptoms to the complete Hurler phenotype. Prenatal onset of symptoms causes hydrops fetalis. Characteristic features include variable degrees of corneal clouding, hepatosplenomegaly, umbilical hernia, and skeletal anomalies. The amount of intellectual

Table 68.26: Differential diagnosis of the mucopolysaccharidosis (MPS) phenotype (type in parentheses)

Mucopolysaccharidoses
Hurler's syndrome (MPS I-H)
Scheie's syndrome (MPS I-S)
Hurler-Scheie syndromes (MPS I-H/S)
Hunter's syndrome (MPS II)
Sanfilippo's syndrome (MPS III)
Morquio's syndrome (MPS IV)
Maroteaux-Lamy syndrome (MPS VI)
Shy's disease (MPS VII)
Mucolipidoses
Type II (I-cell disease)
Type III
Type IV
β-Galactosidosis
Infantile GM_1 gangliosidosis
Galactosialidosis
Sialidosis
Fucosidosis
Mannosidosis
Aspartylglucosaminuria
Kniest's syndrome
Multiple sulfatase deficiency
Cretinism

compromise also varies. All patients exhibit inclusions in circulating leukocytes (Neufeld and Muenzer 1995).

Diagnosis

The diagnosis of MPS is suggested by the typical morphological and radiographical features. The differential diagnosis is considerable because several diseases have similar clinical features (Table 68.26). Rapid screening tests for urinary mucopolysaccharides are available but not very reliable, and quantitative measurements should be performed as well. Thin-layer chromatography distinguishes the compounds, and the pattern of urinary excretion helps determine the diagnosis. High-resolution electrophoresis is also available.

Definitive diagnosis requires an enzymatic assay of leukocytes or cultured fibroblasts. Prenatal diagnosis from chorionic villus sampling or cultured amniocytes and heterozygote identification is available.

Treatment

Bone marrow transplantation has been attempted in several patients with MPS with varying success. In one large study of Hurler's syndrome, successful transplantation was associated with an increase in the serum level of L-iduronidase, almost normal urinary excretion of glycosaminoglycan, and marked improvement of communicating hydrocephalus (Whitley et al. 1993). The most promising results are when transplantation is performed early in children with normal intelligence. The procedure, however, is associated with significant morbidity and mortality. Trials of enzyme replacement therapy are being conducted.

Multiple Sulfatase Deficiency

Multiple sulfatase deficiency is a variable deficiency of at least seven different sulfatases that results in the accumulation of sulfatides, mucopolysaccharides, and cholesterol sulfates. It is transmitted as an autosomal recessive trait. The primary defect is unknown, but probably involves the posttranslational modification necessary for the enzymatic activity of sulfatases. The clinical features suggest late-infantile metachromatic leukodystrophy combined with findings of a mucopolysaccharide storage disorder and ichthyosis. Arylsulfatase A and B are both deficient.

Mucolipidoses

Pathophysiology

The mucolipidoses (ML) are uncommon; both mucopolysaccharides and lipids accumulate in lysosomes. The clinical features are similar to both the MPS and the sphingolipidoses. All four types of ML are inherited as autosomal recessive traits (Gilbert-Barness and Barness 1993).

Clinical Features

Mucolipidose Type I (Sialidosis).   ML type I (sialidosis) is caused by deficiency of the glycoprotein-specific N-acetyl-neuraminidase and described in the section on disorders of glycoprotein metabolism.

Mucolipidose Type II (I-Cell Disease).   ML type II (I-cell disease) is caused by deficiency or dysfunction of the enzyme N-acetylglucosamine phosphotransferase, which is normally responsible for the addition of the mannose-6-phosphate lysosomal recognition marker to several acid hydrolases. It is named for the typical inclusions seen on microscopic examination of tissues. The absence of acid hydrolases causes lysosomal storage of many mucolipid materials. At least three different genes are involved in the normal functioning of N-acetylglucosamine phosphotransferase. The gene responsible for I-cell disease is located on chromosome 4q.

Affected infants show a severe MPS phenotype, developmental delay, and poor growth in the first months of life. Skeletal abnormalities are prominent, and many affected infants have congenital hip dislocations. Corneal haziness, if present, is subtle and seen only with slit-lamp examination. Gingival hypertrophy is quite striking. Abnormal storage results in firm subcutaneous nodules and prominent hepatomegaly with less prominent splenomegaly. Death usually occurs between the ages of 5 and 8 years.

Mucolipidose Type III (Pseudo-Hurler's Syndrome).   ML type III (Pseudo-Hurler's syndrome or ML type III), like ML type II, is caused by deficiency or dysfunction of the enzyme N-acetylglucosamine phosphotransferase. The clinical expression is less severe than with MPS type II. Onset is later in childhood and progression is slower. Intelligence is normal or only borderline retarded.

Mucolipidose Type IV.   The biochemical and gene defects of ML type IV are unknown. However, all patients are achlorhydric and have elevated serum gastrin concentrations (Schiffmann et al. 1998), which can be used as a biological marker of the disease. Profound mental retardation and visual disturbances begin during the first year of life. The neurological course is usually static or less often slowly progressive despite the early onset. The retinal degeneration does progress, but the corneal opacifications are often static and sometimes may improve. Inconstant ophthalmological features are strabismus, photophobia, and myopia. Children do not stand or walk without support and are often very hypotonic. Expressive language often never develops despite normal hearing. Some children learn sign language. Organomegaly never occurs. The EEG is usually abnormal, but seizures are not typical. There are many milder variants and the disorder is probably underdiagnosed. The MRI shows characteristic features of hypoplastic corpus callosum with absent rostrum and an absent or dysplastic splenium. There are also white matter abnormalities and increased ferritin deposition in the thalamus and basal ganglia (Frei et al. 1998). Most reported cases have been predominantly of Ashkenazi Jewish heritage, although a few have not.

Diagnosis and Treatment

ML should be considered in children with the Hurler phenotype without excessive urinary excretion of mucopolysaccharides. The diagnosis is confirmed by enzymatic analysis of fibroblasts. There is no specific therapy at this time; however, therapies that are being developed for the MPS and sphingolipidoses should be applicable to the ML.

Disorders of Glycoprotein Catabolism

Glycoproteins are ubiquitous, complex molecules with oligosaccharides attached to a protein structure. The major sugars of the oligosaccharide side chain are galactose, fucose, mannose, sialic acid, N-acetylgalactosamine, and aspartylglucosamine. Disorders of glycoprotein degradation are uncommon and are transmitted as autosomal recessive traits.

Pathophysiology

The protein core of glycoproteins is degraded by several proteases and the oligosaccharide by specific lysosomal hydrolases that split the sugar linkages. Deficiency of the sugar hydrolase causes the accumulation of a partially degraded glycoprotein with excessive sugar linkages that cannot be broken. Because these oligosaccharides are components of other complex structures, such as glycolipids

Table 68.27:   Clinical features of the disorders of glycoprotein catabolism

Disease	Enzyme deficiency	Age onset	Neurological features	Mucopolysac-charidoses phenotype	Eye findings	Other
Fucosidosis	α-Fucosidase					
Type I		3–18 mos	MR, seizures, early hypotonia, late hypotonia	++	–	Chromosome 1p34
Type II		1–2 yrs	MR, ataxia, behavorial problems	++	Tortuous conjunctival vessels	Angiokeratoma, anhydrosis, chromosome 19
α-mannosidosis	α-Mannosidase					
Type I		3–12 mos	Severe MR	+++	Cataracts, corneal opacities	Hearing loss, early death
Type II		1–4 yrs	Ataxia, MR	++	Cataracts, corneal opacities	Hearing loss
β-Mannosidosis	β-Mannosidase	1–2 yrs	MR	–	–	Hearing loss
Sialidosis	N-Acetyl-neuraminidase					
Type I		10–20 yrs	Myoclonic epilepsy, ataxia	–	Nystagmus, CRS, corneal or lens opacities	CRS, myoclonus syndrome
Type II						
Congenital		Birth	MR	++	Corneal clouding	Hydrops fetalis
Infantile		0–12 mos	MR	++	CRS	Renal disease
Juvenile		2–20 yrs	Myoclonus, MR	+	CRS	Angiokeratoma
Free sialic acid storage disease (infantile)	Defective membrane transport of sialic acid	0–3 mos	Hypotonia	++	–	Failure to thrive, early death
Salla disease	Unknown	3–6 mos	Early hypotonia, late hypotonia, ataxia, MR	–	–	Finnish ancestry, growth delay
Aspartyl-glucosaminuria	Aspartyl-glucosaminidase	1–5 yrs	MR, behavioral disturbances	+	Lens opacities	Chromosome 4q, photosensitivity, angiokeratoma, acne, Finnish ancestry
Galactosialidosis	Carboxipeptidase protective protein					
Infantile		0–12 mos	MR	+++	Corneal clouding	–
Juvenile		1–6 yrs	Myoclonus	–	CRS	Angiokeratoma, Japanese ancestry
Schindler's disease	N-Acetylgalactos-aminidase	6–24 mos	MR, seizures, weakness	–	Optic atropy, nystagmus, strabismus	Chromosome 22, neuroaxonal dystrophy

CRS = cherry-red spot; MR = mental retardation; + = mild; ++ = moderate; +++ = marked; – = absent.

and proteoglycans, hydrolase deficiencies often cause more than one class of compounds to accumulate. Therefore, the ML, MPS, and disorders of glycoprotein degradation share several clinical features.

Clinical Features

Table 68.27 summarizes the clinical features of glycoprotein disorders. In general, the clinical features are either a Hurler phenotype or a myoclonus-dementia complex; some patients have macular degeneration (cherry-red spot). Angiokeratoma can be present. The clinical features do not distinguish these disorders from many other lysosomal storage diseases.

Diagnosis and Treatment

The urine shows excessive excretion of oligosaccharides or glycoasparagines. The absence of urinary mucopolysaccharide excretion in children with the Hurler phenotype directs

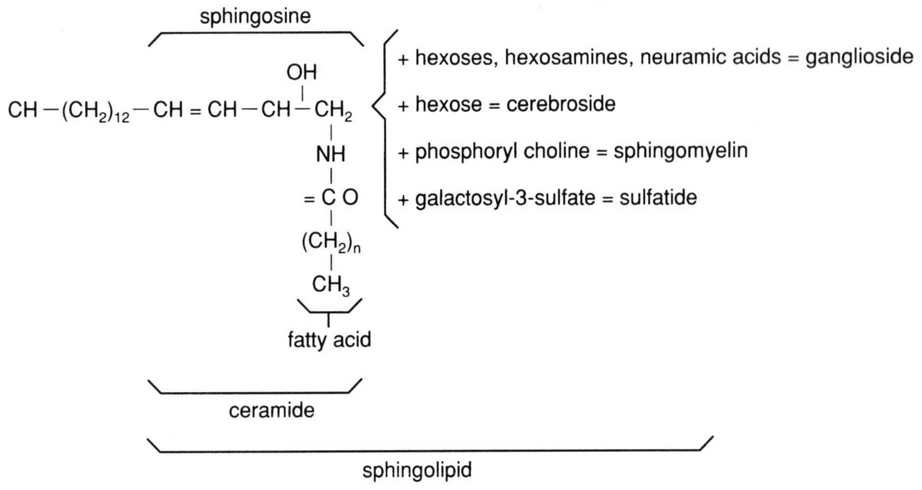

FIGURE 68.26 Structure of sphingolipids.

attention to glycoprotein disorders. Biopsy of the skin and other tissues shows membrane-bound vacuoles containing amorphous material. Tissue concentrations of glycoproteins, and often glycolipids, are increased.

Treatment is not available for the underlying metabolic defect, and the seizures are usually refractory.

Carbohydrate-Deficient Glycoprotein Syndrome

Pathophysiology

The carbohydrate-deficient glycoprotein syndrome is an autosomal recessive multisystem disorder associated with glycoproteins that are partially deficient in their carbohydrate components (Krasenewich and Gahl 1997). Most patients are of Northern European descent. The etiology is unknown.

Clinical Features

The CNS is the primary target organ. The severity of the syndrome varies with its age of onset. Infants are difficult to feed and fail to thrive. Other features are axial hypotonia, lipodystrophy, alternating exotropia, and inverted nipples. Less common features are pericardial effusion; hepatic dysfunction (often with hepatomegaly); nephropathy (with proteinuria); and large, restricted limb joints.

The initial features when onset is during childhood are ataxia and mental retardation; maximum IQ is 40–60. Other features that develop are polyneuropathy with weakness and contractures, kyphoscoliosis, olivopontocerebellar degeneration, and transient strokelike episodes. Fifty percent of patients have seizures, usually exacerbated by stress, such as fever. Some children ambulate with a walker. Retinitis pigmentosa is present by mid-childhood. Systemic involvement is more common in children than in infants. Hepatic and renal disease and the strokelike episodes do not occur after age 14. By adolescence, the ataxia stabilizes,

and the peripheral neuropathy slowly leads to progressive limb weakness and atrophy. The typical appearance is a shortened trunk with long thin limbs.

By adulthood there is no further regression. Primary hypogonadism occurs in female subjects but not always in male subjects. Life expectancy varies.

Diagnosis

Serum transferrin shows a pronounced carbohydrate defect and serves as a highly specific marker of the disorder. Liver biopsies show hepatic fibrosis with mild cirrhosis and intracellular lipid vacuoles. Ultrastructure examination shows lysosomal vacuoles with concentric electron-dense membranes. Nerve conduction velocities are moderately slowed. Sural nerve biopsy shows an attenuation of myelin sheaths and inclusion bodies in Schwann's cells, suggesting abnormal myelin metabolism. Some primary axonal degeneration is present as well. MRI shows cerebellar and pontine atrophy in all patients, and generalized cerebral atrophy in one-third. The protein concentration of the CSF is mildly elevated.

Biochemical diagnosis is by isoelectric focusing of serum transferrin or quantitative analysis of carbohydrate-deficient transferrin. Indirect prenatal diagnosis is possible.

Treatment

There is no treatment for the underlying defect.

Sphingolipidoses

Sphingolipids are complex compounds whose major building block is sphingosine, which is attached to a long-chain fatty acid by an amide linkage, forming a ceramide (Figure 68.26). Further additions to the ceramide produce various sphingolipids, such as hexose to form a cerebroside and phosphorylcholine to form sphingomyelin.

FIGURE 68.27 Metabolism of sphingolipids. (1) Ganglioside sialidase. (2) β-Galactosidase (Gal). (3) Hexosaminidase A. (4) β-Glucosidase (Glu). (5) Ceramidase. (6) α-Galactosidase. (7) Sulfatase. (8) Galactosylceramide β-galactosidase. (9) Sphingomyelinase. (NAcGal = N-acetyl-galactosamine; NANA = N-acetyl-neuraminic acid.)

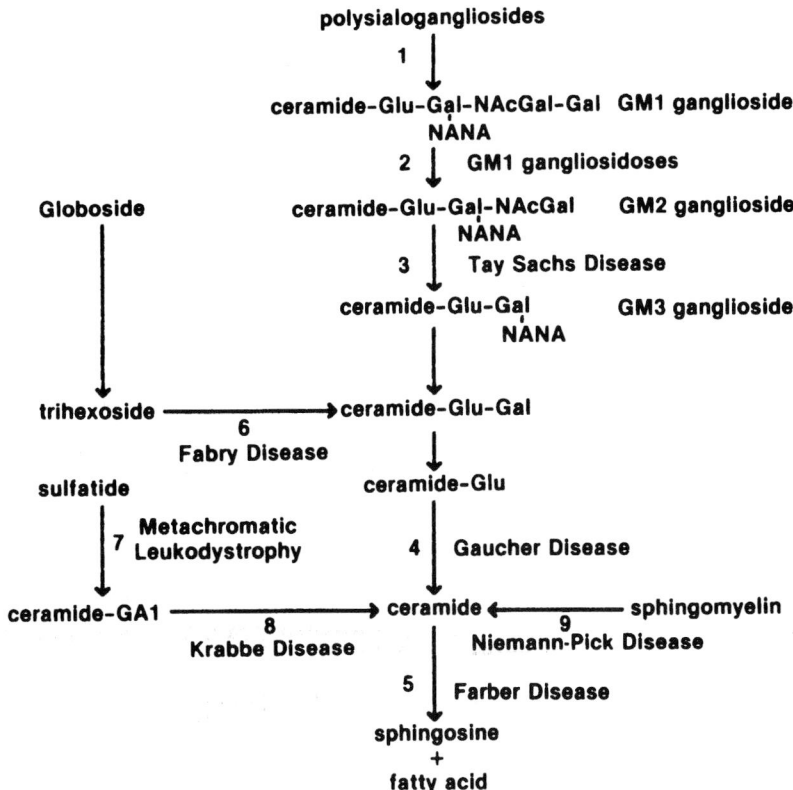

Sphingolipid catabolism requires an ordered stepwise removal of sugar moieties from the oligosaccharide group (Figure 68.27). Lysosomal enzyme deficiencies that prevent the removal of a sugar moiety stop the molecule's further catabolism even if all other required enzymes are present. The subsequent accumulation of intermediary metabolites causes a progressive decline of psychomotor skills associated with varying degrees of visceral involvement. The diseases are classified by the type of lipid stored.

Gangliosidoses

Gangliosides are composed of ceramide and a sialic acid (an oligosaccharide containing N-acetylneuraminic acid) (see Figure 68.27). They are an important constituent of CNS lipids, especially in gray matter and nerve terminals. Blocks at various intermediate steps of ganglioside metabolism cause the accumulation of the specific gangliosides GM_1, GM_2, and GM_3. The storage of these gangliosides in the nervous system and other tissues is responsible for the disease state; their identification on biopsy specimens is important for diagnosis (Figure 68.28).

Beta-Galactosidoses (GM_1 Gangliosidoses)

Pathophysiology. The β-galactosidoses are caused by deficiency of lysosomal acid β-galactosidase, the enzyme that cleaves the terminal galactose moiety from GM_1 ganglioside and other galactose-containing compounds (see

Figure 68.27). The trait is inherited autosomal recessively; the abnormal gene is on chromosome 3p. Depending on the mutation, the defective enzyme may retain activity toward either GM_1 or mucopolysaccharides and other galactose-containing compounds. The amount and type of residual activity determine whether the clinical syndrome is a generalized gangliosidosis, as in GM_1 gangliosidosis, or visceral storage of mucopolysaccharides and relatively little brain disease, as in Morquio's syndrome type B.

Neurons swollen with storage material are present throughout the CNS. Cerebral atrophy is restricted to the cerebral cortex and cerebellar folia. The pathology is similar to that of Tay-Sachs disease but differs in that storage bodies also are found in the visceral organs.

β-Galactosidase is incorporated into a multimolecular complex consisting of neuraminidase (deficiency of which results in the sialidoses) and a protective protein/carboxypeptidase. Saposin B (sphingolipid activator protein B) also may be involved in this complex. Absence of the protective protein causes a clinical disorder similar to GM_1 gangliosidosis.

Clinical Features. Three clinical types form a continuum that differs in the degree of CNS involvement, the rapidity of progression, and the extent of visceral organ involvement. The severity of the disease correlates with the degree of enzyme deficiency.

Infantile GM_1 gangliosidosis also is called *pseudo-Hurler's syndrome* because of its clinical similarity to Hurler's syn-

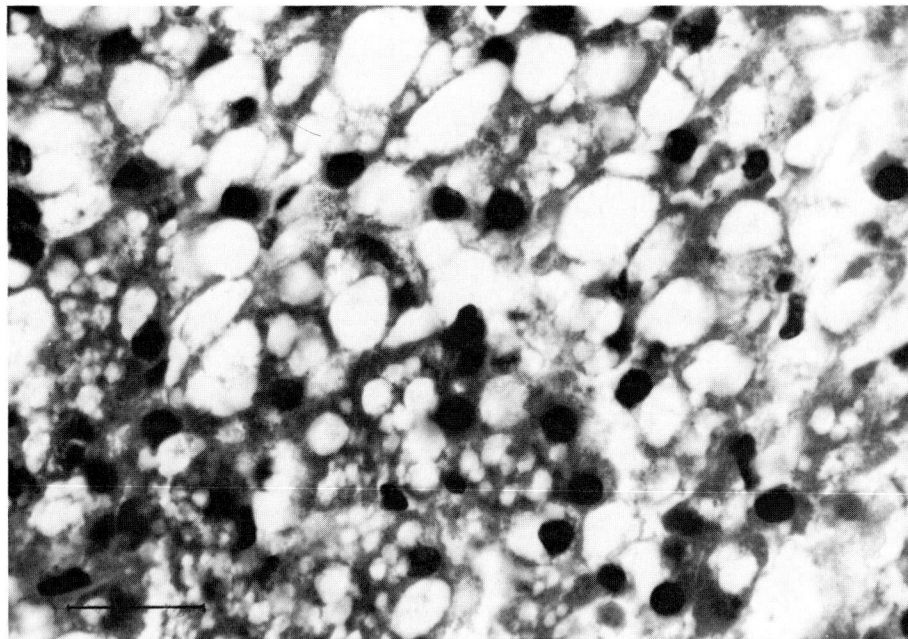

FIGURE 68.28 Ganglioside storage in a liver biopsy specimen (calibration bar = 2.5 mm).

drome. The onset of infantile GM_1, however, is at birth or shortly after. The infants have coarsened facies, enlarged tongues, abdominal distention with hepatosplenomegaly, umbilical hernias, severe dysostosis multiplex, and, occasionally, macrocephaly. Fifty percent of affected infants have a macular cherry-red spot (Figure 68.29). Mental retardation, seizures, diffuse spasticity, blindness, and deafness become progressively worse; death occurs by 2–3 years.

The onset of juvenile GM_1 gangliosidosis is between 6 and 18 months. There is no visceral storage or severe bone

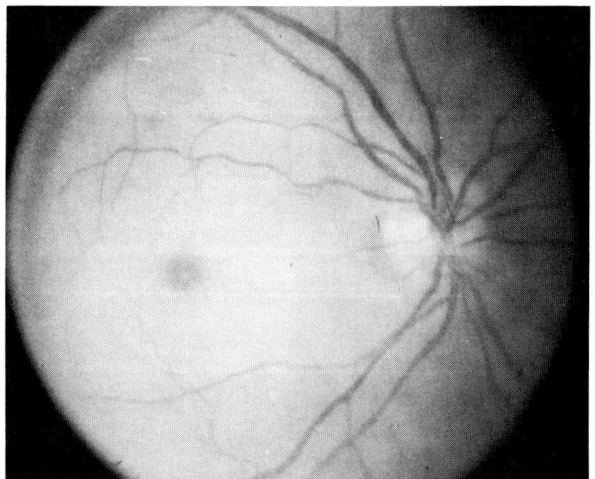

FIGURE 68.29 Macular cherry-red spot. (Reprinted with permission from OB Evans. Manual of Child Neurology. New York: Churchill Livingstone, 1987;26.)

involvement, and vision is preserved. Initial symptoms are weakness and incoordination that progresses to diffuse spasticity, mental retardation, and seizures. Death occurs between the ages of 3 and 7 years.

Adult GM_1 gangliosidosis begins in mid-childhood to adolescence with progressive spasticity, cerebellar ataxia, and dysarthria. Dystonia and mild dementia are inconstant. Organomegaly is absent, radiological changes are minimal, and survival is prolonged.

Diagnosis. The diagnosis of GM_1 gangliosidosis should be suspected in all children with degenerative neurological disorders, especially those with the Hurler phenotype. Biopsy of involved viscera shows vacuolated cells and foamy histiocytes. Definitive diagnosis is accomplished by enzymatic analysis. Prenatal and carrier state detection are possible.

Treatment. There is no specific treatment.

Galactosialidosis

Pathophysiology. Galactosialidosis is caused by deficiency of the β-galactosidase protective protein. Both β-galactosidase and neuraminidase are deficient. The abnormal gene is on chromosome 20.

Clinical Features. Phenotypic variation is considerable, and the types are grouped by age of onset. The infantile form resembles infantile GM_1 gangliosidosis. The juvenile form is most common among ethnic Japanese children and characterized by skeletal dysplasia, dysmorphism, corneal clouding, cherry-red spots, and angiokeratomatous rash in the buttocks and inguinal regions. Pyramidal, extrapyramidal, and cerebellar signs with or without visual disturbance and myoclonus occur.

GM$_2$ Gangliosidoses

Pathophysiology.   GM$_2$ ganglioside accumulates when the activity of hexosaminidase A, a heteropolymer of alpha and beta polypeptides, is deficient. Failure to remove the terminal N-acetylgalactosamine from the parent compound prevents further degradation of these molecules by lysosomal exoglycosidases (see Figure 68.27). The abnormal gene, transmitted by autosomal recessive inheritance, may be a mutation in the gene for the α-subunit on chromosome 15, the β-subunit on chromosome 5, or the glycoprotein activator for hexosaminidase (AB variant) on chromosome 5. Tay-Sachs disease, or infantile GM$_2$ gangliosidosis, is caused by a severe deficiency of hexosaminidase A caused by a mutation of the alpha locus. The juvenile and adult types of GM$_2$ gangliosidosis are caused by a hexosaminidase A deficiency but with some residual function. Sandhoff's disease is caused by an abnormality of the β-subunit, leaving no residual function of hexosaminidase A or hexosaminidase B, which is a tetramer of β-subunits. Patients with combined hexosaminidase A and B deficiency have visceral storage of globoside, especially in the kidneys and spleen, and of other N-acetylglucosaminyl conjugates in addition to the GM$_2$ storage. All types have widespread neuronal storage within the CNS.

Accumulation of the metabolic by-products within the ganglion cell layers of the retina produces a white ring, or halo, around the reddish macula, which is commonly called a *cherry-red spot* (see Figure 68.29). This finding fades with age as the cells are lost, leaving only optic atrophy. Other causes for a cherry-red spot are listed in Table 68.28.

Clinical Features.   The typical features of GM$_2$ gangliosidoses are progressive dementia and vision loss (amaurotic idiocy). The clinical spectrum of hexosaminidase deficiency disease has expanded considerably.

Tay-Sachs disease is the prototype for the ganglioside storage diseases. The onset is between 3 and 6 months, characterized by marked irritability and an excessive startle response (hyperacusis). Weakness and hypotonia are evident by 6 months and followed by developmental regression, progressive blindness, deafness, seizures, and spasticity. Macrocephaly develops but not visceromegaly. More than 95% of children with Tay-Sachs disease have a cherry-red spot. Death is usually before 3 years of age. People with Ashkenazi Jewish ancestry have an estimated heterozygote frequency of 1 in 30.

Sandhoff's disease is phenotypically similar to Tay-Sachs disease in age of onset, neurological features, and macular degeneration. The difference is visceral involvement. Intracytoplasmic storage occurs in liver, kidneys, lymph nodes, spleen, and lung. Sandhoff's disease should be suspected in children with a Tay-Sachs phenotype and visceromegaly, especially in children without Jewish lineage. Hexosaminidase activity is completely absent.

Juvenile GM$_2$ gangliosidosis is uncommon and results from mutations in the α-subunit that allow some residual level of hexosaminidase A. The onset, characterized by gait

Table 68.28:   Storage diseases associated with a macular cherry-red spot

Disease	Frequency of cherry-red spot (%)
β-Galactosidoses (GM$_1$ gangliosidosis)	50
Galactosidoses (GM$_2$ gangliosidosis)	95
Niemann-Pick disease	50
Infantile	25
Late infantile	50
Adult (type E)	Rare
Metachromatic leukodystrophy	Rare
Sialidoses	
Cherry-red spot myoclonus syndrome	100
Other sialidoses	Rare
Farber's lipogranulomatosis	Rare
Infantile Gaucher's disease	Rare

Source: Adapted from J Kivlin, G Serborn, G Myers. The cherry-red spot in Tay-Sachs and other storage diseases. Ann Neurol 1985;17:356–360.

difficulty, ataxia, and intellectual decline, is between 2 and 6 years. The disease progresses to spasticity, decerebrate rigidity, marked mental retardation, and seizures. Vision loss is a late complication, and the viscera are not involved. Death occurs in late childhood or adolescence. MRI shows mild to moderate cerebral and cerebellar atrophy.

In adult-onset GM$_2$ gangliosidosis, the α-subunit precursor is synthesized but not the mature enzyme product. The clinical syndrome is a slowly progressive multisystem degeneration and motor neuron disease similar to a spinocerebellar degeneration. Some cases resemble a juvenile spinal muscular atrophy, and others have had psychotic features with normal cognitive function. The viscera are not involved. The MRI is similar to juvenile GM$_2$ gangliosidosis.

Diagnosis.   The clinical diagnosis of GM$_2$ gangliosidosis is not difficult in children with the complete phenotype of progressive neurological disease and a macular cherry-red spot. The electroretinographical result may be abnormal, and the latency of the visual evoked response usually becomes prolonged or is absent. The diagnosis is more problematic in the late-onset variants, however, and should be considered in the differential diagnosis of spinocerebellar degenerations and spinal muscular atrophies.

Definitive diagnosis requires the measuring hexosaminidase activity in leukocytes and cultured fibroblasts. Heterozygote identification is accurate using an automated screening test. Oral contraceptives and pregnancy may result in a false-positive result. Prenatal diagnosis is possible.

Treatment.   There is no treatment for the underlying disease.

Niemann-Pick Disease Types A and B

Pathophysiology.   Niemann-Pick disease types A and B are caused by deficiency of sphingomyelinase, the enzyme that

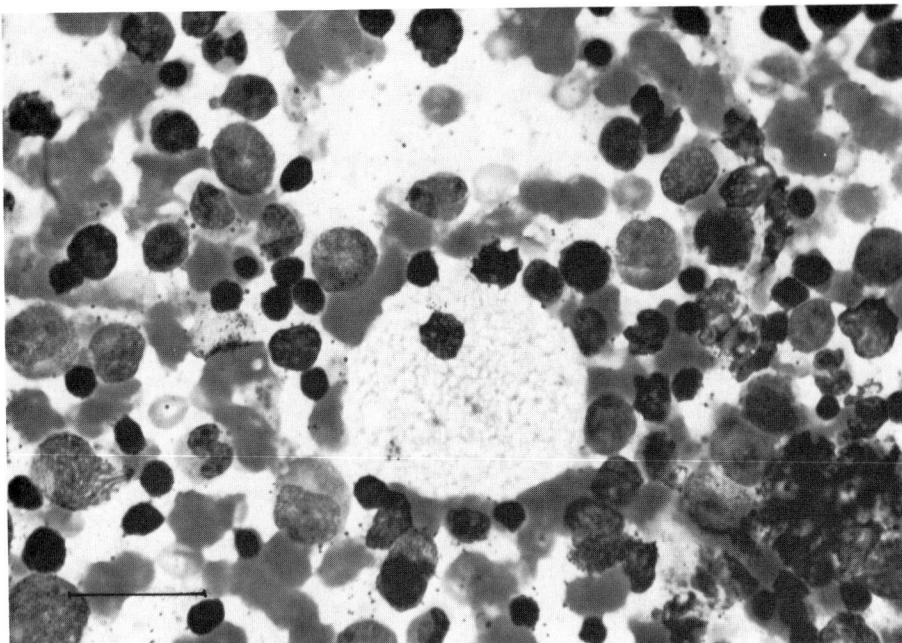

FIGURE 68.30 Foamy histiocyte in a bone marrow aspirate from a patient with Niemann-Pick disease (calibration bar = 25 mm).

catabolizes sphingomyelin to phosphocholine and ceramide. The abnormal gene has been cloned and is found on chromosome 11p15. Sphingomyelin, cholesterol, glycolipids, or bis(monoacylglycero)phosphate accumulates within the cells of the reticuloendothelial system. In Niemann-Pick disease type A, lysosomal storage occurs in the nervous system. The brain stores excessive amounts of GM_2 and GM_3 gangliosides in addition to sphingomyelin. Most tissues, such as bone marrow, show foamy, lipid-laden cells.

Clinical Features.   Niemann-Pick disease type A (infantile form) is more common than type B. The highest incidence is in children of Ashkenazi Jewish ancestry. Sphingomyelinase activity is almost absent. Affected infants fail to thrive and have hepatosplenomegaly, hypotonia, and pulmonary interstitial disease that appears as a diffuse granular pattern on radiography. Approximately 50% have a cherry-red spot. Eye movements are normal. Sitting is achieved rarely, and psychomotor regression is relentless. Seizures and diarrhea are common. Death occurs by age 5 years from infection or fulminant liver failure that progresses over a few weeks.

Children with type B disease are neurologically normal despite the same deficiency of sphingomyelinase found in type A. The clinical features are hepatosplenomegaly and pulmonary infiltration. Life expectancy is usually normal but can be shortened by frequent respiratory infections.

Diagnosis.   Niemann-Pick disease types A and B should be suspected in children with visceromegaly and neurological regression. Foamy cells may be seen on liver or bone marrow specimens (Figure 68.30). The definitive diagnosis is made by measuring the enzymes in leukocytes or cultured fibroblasts. Patients with both types A and B have less than 5% of the normal amount of enzyme activity. Heterozygote detection is possible, as is prenatal diagnosis.

Treatment.   Therapy is supportive.

Gaucher's Disease (Glucosylceramide Lipidosis)

Pathophysiology.   Gaucher's disease is the most prevalent lysosomal storage disease. It is transmitted by autosomal recessive inheritance. Deficiency of the enzyme glucocerebrosidase (glucosylceramide β-glucosidase) causes the lysosomal storage of glucocerebrosides (glucosylceramide), a glucose molecule attached to a ceramide. Rare cases are caused by deficiency of saposin C, a heat-stable enzymatic cofactor. The abnormal gene is on chromosome 1q21. Residual enzymatic activity is generally lower in patients with neurological disease.

Lipid-laden macrophages, Gaucher's cells, are stored throughout the reticuloendothelial system. Gaucher's cells have an eccentric nucleus surrounded by small inclusion bodies that give the cytoplasm a crumpled tissue-paper appearance (Figure 68.31).

Clinical Features.   Several phenotypes are described. Type I disease is the most common but has no neurological involvement. Approximately 60% of patients are of Ashkenazi Jewish heritage. Visceromegaly, most commonly involving the spleen, develops at any time in childhood. Hypersplenism can be symptomatic. Children who require splenectomy then have increased bone marrow storage that may cause pathological fractures or chronic pain. Radiog-

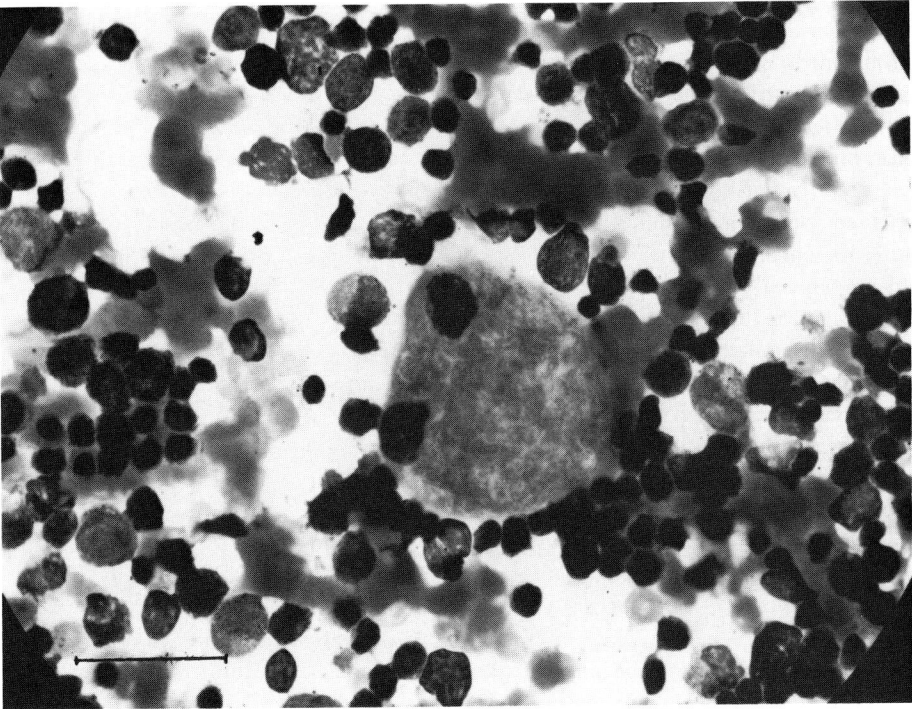

FIGURE 68.31 Gaucher's cell in a bone marrow aspirate from a patient with Gaucher's disease (calibration bar = 25 mm).

raphy of the distal femur shows the Erlenmeyer flask deformity that typifies the disease. Life expectancy is normal.

Types II and III Gaucher's disease are associated with variable neurological features. A horizontal supranuclear gaze palsy is a constant feature. Type II Gaucher's disease also is called the *acute neuronopathic type* because of its early onset and rapidly progressive course. Hepatosplenomegaly brings the child to medical attention within the first few months. Brainstem involvement is pronounced, accompanied by strabismus, horizontal supranuclear gaze palsy, trismus, opisthotonic posturing with noxious stimulation, and swallowing difficulties. Developmental regression, diffuse spasticity, and increasingly frequent episodes of laryngospasm follow. Death is inevitable by age 2 years. Postmortem examination shows CNS neuronophagia and nerve cell loss as well as the perivascular lipid-laden cells.

The onset of type III Gaucher's disease, the subacute neuronopathic form, is from early to mid-childhood. Some children with type II disease have relatively mild systemic involvement and slowly progressive neurological deterioration. Refractory myoclonic seizures and generalized tonic-clonic seizures are a prominent feature. The EEG shows spike and wave discharges. Dementia is also prominent, but ataxia and spasticity are variable. Other children with type III Gaucher's disease have a more severe systemic disease with hepatic cirrhosis and portal hypertension leading to esophageal varices, digital clubbing from pulmonary interstitial involvement, and heart disease. Horizontal supranuclear gaze palsy may be the only neurological abnormality. Some patients have intellectual impairment. Postmortem examination shows neuronophagia, nerve cell loss, and

perivascular infiltration of Gaucher's cells. The perivascular spaces of the CNS contain storage material. Perivascular gliosis and meningeal fibrosis may cause communicating hydrocephalus.

The Norrbottnian type of Gaucher's disease is a genetic isolate from Sweden. The clinical features are similar to both types II and III diseases. Severe skeletal and CNS disease are caused by lipid storage in these tissues.

Diagnosis. Gaucher's disease should be considered in any child with hepatosplenomegaly and neurological disease, especially in the presence of a horizontal supranuclear gaze palsy. Definitive diagnosis is made by enzymatic analysis of leukocytes or cultured fibroblasts. Gaucher's cells can be seen on bone marrow aspirate but are not necessary for diagnosis. Carrier detection and prenatal diagnosis are available.

Treatment. Intravenous enzyme replacement therapy is available using recombinantly produced glucocerebrosidase. The therapy is universally effective in treating the systemic disease of types I and III. Its efficacy in stopping neurological progression is still in question, and it is not recommended for type II disease. Enzyme replacement therapy appears to reduce the burden of Gaucher's cells in the brain and CSF compartments.

Krabbe's Disease (Globoid Cell Leukodystrophy)

Pathophysiology. Krabbe's disease (globoid cell leukodystrophy or galactosylceramide lipidosis) is caused by deficiency of galactocerebroside β-galactosidase. It is transmitted by autosomal recessive inheritance. The gene has been cloned and is found on chromosome 14.

Impaired cleavage of galactose from galactocerebroside causes storage of galactosylceramide within multinucleated macrophages of the CNS white matter, forming globoid cells. Psychosine, a metabolite of galactocerebroside, results in toxic destruction of the oligodendroglia. Demyelination is diffuse, and the disease traditionally is classified as a leukodystrophy.

Clinical Features.   Three types of globoid cell leukodystrophy are recognized based on age at onset. The most common and severe is the infantile form, which begins within the first 6 months of life. Demyelination occurs in the central and peripheral nervous systems. Symptoms vary depending on the relative severity of central or peripheral involvement. Central features are marked irritability, spasticity, opisthotonic posturing on noxious stimulation, ataxia, and seizures. Peripheral features are hypotonia, weakness, and decreased or absent tendon reflexes. Optic atrophy, cortical blindness, and hearing loss are additional features. The viscera are not enlarged. Recurrent low-grade fever without obvious infection may be part of the syndrome. Affected infants have progressive psychomotor decline ending in severe spastic quadriplegia and death within a few years.

Peripheral nerve demyelination is documented by studies of nerve conduction slowing. Examination of the CSF shows an increased protein concentration. Progressive demyelination, most prominently in the periventricular and centrum semiovale regions with sparing of the subcortical U fibers, is documented by serial MRI.

The onset of the late infantile and juvenile form is between the ages of 2 and 10 years, and the onset of the adult form is after age 10. Ataxia is more prominent in younger children; weakness and spasticity are more common in older children. Neurological features may be asymmetric, and the rate of progression is slower than in the infantile form. Bulbar palsy causes speech and swallowing disturbances. Visual complaints vary; optic atrophy or slowing of the visual evoked response latency may be the only finding. Dementia is more common in children with younger age at onset. Nerve conduction velocity and CSF protein concentration are normal or only mildly increased. The MRI shows central white matter abnormalities with a tendency to preferential involvement of the parieto-occipital periventricular white matter. The MRI may be normal if performed early in the course of the disease.

Diagnosis.   Definitive diagnosis requires enzyme analysis on leukocytes or cultured fibroblasts. It is not possible to distinguish the various subtypes by the amount of residual enzyme activity. Prenatal and heterozygote detection are available.

Treatment.   Bone marrow transplantation has been shown to reverse the neurological manifestations of globoid cell leukodystrophy (Krivit et al. 1998).

Fabry's Disease

Pathophysiology.   Fabry's disease is caused by deficiency of α-galactosidase A; ceramide trihexoside accumulates in lysosomes. It is inherited as an X-linked recessive trait, the abnormal gene being on chromosome Xq22. Ceramide trihexoside storage is mainly in endothelial cells, which causes secondary vascular complications. Ganglion cells, kidneys, eyes, and the heart are affected.

Clinical Features.   Clustered, nonblanching angiectases of the skin (angiokeratoma corporis diffusum universale), primarily on the scrotum, buttocks, thighs, and back, appear during childhood and adolescence. Mucosal surfaces can be involved; in rare cases, the skin is not affected. Similar angiokeratoma are found in glycoprotein disorders and sialidosis. Ocular lesions include whorl-like corneal opacifications, cataracts, and tortuosity of the conjunctival and retinal vessels.

A polyneuropathy involving mainly small myelinated and unmyelinated fibers develops in the second decade. Involvement of the vasa nervorum or the cytoplasm of the nerve cells may cause the neuralgia. Burning pain, dysesthesias, and dysautonomia can be associated with low-grade fever. Anhidrosis and heat intolerance are additional problems. The cerebrovascular complications of the disease are caused by an obstructive vasculopathy, predominantly of the vertebrovascular circulation. There is progressive accumulation of ceramide trihexoside within the media and intima of cerebral blood vessels. In one study, no patients had MRI evidence of cerebrovascular disease before age 26 whereas every patient older than 54 years had MRI abnormalities. Only 37.5% of those with MRI evidence of cerebrovascular disease had neurological symptoms (Crutchfield et al. 1998). Involvement of multiple small penetrating vessels causes early dementia.

Systemic complications of the vasculopathy include progressive renal disease, leading to hypertension and eventual renal failure, myocardial ischemia and infarction, lymphedema, respiratory compromise, arthritis, and episodic gastrointestinal disturbances. Degenerative changes of the distal interphalangeal joints of the fingers sometimes can be seen radiographically. Death usually occurs by the fifth decade. Female carriers may be completely asymptomatic or have limited symptoms but some have significant manifestations of the disease.

Diagnosis.   Fabry's disease is part of the differential diagnosis in boys with painful neuropathies. The presence of angiectases and a slit-lamp examination revealing the corneal opacities are virtually diagnostic. Skin biopsy shows lipid inclusions in vascular epithelial cells. Definitive diagnosis requires measuring enzyme activity. Prenatal diagnosis and carrier detection are available. Approximately 80% of female carriers have a significant decrease in the enzymatic activity; 90% have a typical corneal whorl on slit-lamp examination.

Treatment.   Carbamazepine or gabapentin may help relieve the painful neuropathy. Renal transplantation for renal failure does not provide sufficient enzyme replacement to cure the disease. Enzyme replacement therapy is under investigation.

Schindler's Disease

Pathophysiology.   Schindler's disease is caused by deficiency of the enzyme α-N-acetylgalactosaminidase. It is transmitted as an autosomal recessive trait. The abnormal gene, which is on chromosome 22q, is homologous with the α-galactosidase gene, suggesting a common ancestry.

Clinical Features.   The disease is a type of infantile neuroaxonal dystrophy. Children present with developmental delay and loss of milestones. Progressive neurological deterioration is rapid and includes optic atrophy, strabismus, nystagmus, hypotonia, hyperreflexia, and intractable seizures. Spastic quadriparesis, blindness, and deafness develop later. The viscera and bones are not involved.

Typical lysosomal spheroids are seen in dystrophic axons. α-N-Acetylgalactosamine, which contains oligosaccharides, accumulates in tissues and is excreted in the urine.

Diagnosis.   Urine excretion of oligosaccharides can be used for screening, but definitive diagnosis requires enzyme analysis. Heterozygote identification and prenatal diagnosis are possible.

Treatment.   Therapy is supportive.

Metachromatic Leukodystrophy

Pathophysiology.   Metachromatic leukodystrophy (MLD) is caused by a deficiency of either aryl-sulfatase A or its sphingolipid activator protein B (saposin B); together they form cerebroside sulfatase. Sulfated sphingolipids and other sulfated lipids accumulate in neurons of the central and peripheral nervous systems. MLD is transmitted as an autosomal recessive trait. The mutated gene has been cloned and is on chromosome 22.

MLD was named because of the stored sulfatides that change from blue to brown or red (metachromasia) when they are stained with toluidine blue and cresyl violet. The major pathological features are marked demyelination of the CNS with sparing of the subcortical U fibers and a demyelinating polyneuropathy. MLD traditionally is classified as a leukodystrophy. Oligodendroglial cells are markedly reduced in number, and neurons and Schwann cells show the typical metachromatic inclusions.

Clinical Features.   Despite considerable heterogeneity, MLD traditionally is divided into three groups depending on age at onset. Phenotypic variation is probably caused by allelic mutations, with variable levels of residual enzyme activity. The incidence of all forms in the United States is 1 in 40,000–100,000, with the infantile form representing two-thirds of the total. Pseudodeficiency alleles in the gene cause low levels of enzyme activity that are detectable with artificial substrates, but cause no symptoms. DNA analysis of the gene is possible (Francis et al. 1993).

The onset of late infantile MLD is before age 2 years. Initial features of spasticity, ataxia, or both impair motor development. Approximately one-half of patients have depressed ankle tendon reflexes; 20% have extrapyramidal signs. Weakness, dementia, and blindness with optic atrophy are progressive. A cherry-red spot is unusual. Seizures are a late complication in 25%; death occurs within several years after onset.

Juvenile MLD begins later and has a slower course than the late infantile disease. The clinical syndrome of saposin B deficiency is typically the juvenile form. Development stagnates and then declines between the ages of 3 and 10 years. Initial symptoms are poor school performance, behavioral change, and a gait disturbance. The older the child, the more likely behavioral and cognitive disturbances occur first. Ataxia, spasticity, and extrapyramidal signs follow the mental changes and become progressively worse. Peripheral nerve involvement may occur, but not to the extent as in the late infantile disease. After 5–10 years, the child is demented, quadriplegic, incontinent of urine, and dysarthric. Seizures occur in 80% of patients. Life expectancy from time of onset is 3–15 years.

Adult-onset MLD usually is characterized by psychosis, personality change, or dementia. Neurological features are similar to the younger onset types but evolve slowly. The course is prolonged, and survival into the fifth or sixth decade is possible.

Diagnosis.   The diagnosis of MLD should be considered in any child with symptoms of progressive central and peripheral demyelinating disease, in older children with polyneuropathy, and in adults with progressive mental changes, especially with a family history of neurological deterioration. Multiple sulfatase deficiency has features of late infantile MLD plus features of mucopolysaccharidosis (see Mucopolysaccharidoses, previously in this chapter).

MRI shows diffuse subcortical demyelination. A posterior predominance of white matter abnormalities is found in late infantile MLD (Kim et al. 1997). Visual, auditory, brainstem, and somatosensory-evoked responses are abnormally prolonged or absent. Nerve conduction velocities are slowed to less than 30 m per second, even in patients with brisk reflexes. CSF protein concentration is elevated, sometimes greater than 2,000 mg/dl in 90% of patients. Urine samples and nerve biopsy to show metachromatic granules are no longer a standard for diagnosis. Definitive diagnosis requires measuring enzyme activity in leukocytes or fibroblasts. Carrier detection and prenatal diagnosis are possible.

Treatment.   Bone marrow transplantation slows progression in some cases.

REFERENCES

Anderson HC, Shapira E. Biochemical and clinical response to hydroxycobalamin versus cyanocobalamin treatment in patients with methylmalonic acidemia and homocystinuria (cblC). J Pediatr 1998;132:121–124.

Anderson RA, Rao N, Byrum R, et al. In situ localization of the genetic locus encoding the lysosomal acid lipase/cholesteryl esterase (LIPA) deficient in Wolman disease to chromosome 10q23.3-q23.3. Genomics 1993;15:245–247.

Aslandis C, Reis S, Fehringer P, et al. Genetic and biochemical evidence that CESD and Wolman disease are distinguished by residual lysosomal acid lipase activity. Genomics 1996;33:85–93.

Aubourg P, Adamsbaum C, Lavallard-Rousseau MC, et al. A two-year trial of oleic and erucic acids ("Lorenzo's oil") as treatment for adrenomyeloneuropathy. N Engl J Med 1993;329:745–752.

Batshaw ML. Inborn errors of urea synthesis. Ann Neurol 1994;35:133–141.

Bourgeron T, Chretien D, Poggi-Bach J, et al. Mutation of the fumarase gene in two siblings with progressive encephalopathy and fumarase deficiency. J Clin Invest 1994;93:2514–2518.

Boustany RM. Neurology of the neuronal ceroid-lipofuscinoses: late infantile and juvenile types. Am J Med Genet 1993;42:533–535.

Brewer GJ. Practical recommendations and new therapies for Wilson's disease. Drugs 1995;50:240–249.

Brusilow SW, Clissold DB, Bassett SS. Long-term treatment of girls with ornithine transcarbamylase deficiency. N Engl J Med 1996;335:855–859.

Brusilow SW, Maestri NE. Urea cycle disorders: diagnosis, pathophysiology, and therapy. Adv Pediatr 1996;43:127–170.

Burlina AB, Dionisi-Vici C, Bennett MJ, et al. A new syndrome with ethylmalonic aciduria and normal fatty acid oxidation in fibroblasts (see comments). J Pediatr 1994;124:79–86.

Burns SP, Iles RA, Saudubray JM, et al. Propionylcarnitine excretion is not affected by metronidazole administration to patients with disorders of propionate metabolism. Eur J Pediatr 1996;155:31–35.

Carstea ED, Morris JA, Coleman KG, et al. Niemann-Pick C1 disease gene: homology to mediators of cholesterol homeostasis. Science 1997;277:228–231.

Chabrol B, Mancini J, Benelli C, et al. A Leigh syndrome: pyruvate dehydrogenase defect. A case with peripheral neuropathy. J Child Neurol 1994;9:52–55.

Chuang DT, Shih VE. Disorders of Branched Chain Amino Acid and Keto Acid Metabolism. In CR Scriver, AL Beaudet, WS Sly, et al. (eds), The Metabolic and Molecular Basis of Inherited Disease (7th ed). New York: McGraw-Hill, 1995;1187–1232.

Crutchfield KE, Patronas NJ, Dambrosia JM, et al. Quantitative analysis of cerebral vasculopathy in Fabry disease patients. Neurology 1998;50:1746–1749.

Cunniff C, Kratz LE, Moser A, et al. Clinical and biochemical spectrum of patients with RSH/Smith-Lemli-Opitz syndrome and abnormal cholesterol metabolism. Am J Med Genet 1997;68:263–269.

DiDonato M, Sarkar B. Copper transport and its alterations in Menkes and Wilson diseases. Biochimica et Biophysica Acta 1997;1360:3–16.

Felice KJ, Alessi AG, Grunnet ML. Clinical variability in adult-onset acid maltase deficiency: report of affected sibs and a review of the literature. Medicine 1995;74:131–135.

Fenton WA, Rosenberg LE. Disorders of Propionate and Methylmalonate Metabolism. In CR Scriver, AL Beaudet, WS Sly, et al. (eds), The Metabolic and Molecular Basis of Inherited Disease (7th ed). New York: McGraw-Hill, 1995;1423–1450.

Fletcher JM, Bye AM, Nayanar V, et al. Non-ketotic hyperglycinemia presenting as pachygyria. J Inherit Metab Dis 1995;18:665–668.

Francis GS, Bonni A, Shen N, et al. Metachromatic leukodystrophy: multiple nonfunctional and pseudodeficiency alleles in a pedigree: problems with diagnosis and counseling. Ann Neurol 1993;34:212–218.

Frei KP, Patronas NJ, Crutchfield KE, et al. Mucolipidosis type IV: characteristic MRI findings. Neurology 1998;51:565–569.

Fries MH, Rinaldo P, Schmidt-Sommerfield E, et al. Isovaleric acidemia: response to leucine load after three weeks of supplementation with glycine, L-carnitine, and combined glycine-carnitine therapy. J Pediatr 1996;129:449–452.

Froissart R, Blond JL, Maire I, et al. Hunter syndrome: gene deletions and rearrangements. Hum Mutat 1993;2:138–140.

Garcia L, Ozand P, Rashed M. Diagnosis of organic aciduria. Rev Neurol 1995;23(Suppl. 3):325–329.

Garcia-Silva MT, Ribes A, Campos Y, et al. Syndrome of encephalopathy, petechiae, and ethylmalonic aciduria. Pediatr Neurol 1997;17:165–170.

Gilbert-Barness EF, Barness LA. The Mucolipidoses. In BH Landing, MD Haust, J Bernstein, et al. (eds), Genetic Metabolic Disease. Perspect Pediatr Pathol. Basel: Karger, 1993;148–184.

Goebel HH. The neuronal ceroid lipofuscinoses. J Child Neurol 1995;10:424–437.

Haas RH, Nasirian F, Nakano K, et al. Low platelet mitochondrial complex I and II/III in early untreated Parkinson's disease. Ann Neurol 1995;37:714–722.

Haas RH, Barshop BA. Diet change in the management of metabolic encephalomyopathies. Biofactors 1998;7:259–262.

Hamosh A, Maher JF, Bellus GA, et al. Long term use of high-dose benzoate and dextromethorphan for the treatment of nonketotic hyperglycinemia. J Pediatr 1998;132:709–713.

Hayashi Y, Hanioka K, Kanomata N, et al. Clinicopathologic and molecular-pathologic approaches to Lowe's syndrome. Pediatr Pathol Lab Med 1995;15:389–402.

Hellsten E, Vesa J, Jalanko A, et al. From locus to cellular disturbances: positional cloning of the infantile ceroid lipofuscinosis gene. Neuropediatrics 1997;28:9–11.

Huhse B, Rehling P, Albertini M, et al. PEX 17p of Saccharomyces cerevisiae is a novel peroxin and component of the peroxisomal protein translocation machinery. J Cell Biol 1998;140:49–66.

Irons M, Elias ER, Abuelo D, et al. Treatment of Smith-Lemli-Opitz syndrome: results of a multicenter trial. Am J Med Genet 1997;68:311–314.

Jain A, Buist NRM, Kennaway NG, et al. Effect of ascorbate or N-acetylcysteine treatment in a patient with hereditary glutathione synthetase deficiency. J Pediatr 1994;124:229–233.

Johnson MT, Yang HS, Magnuson T, et al. Targeted disruption of the murine dihydrolipoamide dehydrogenase gene Dld results in perigastrulation lethality. Proc Natl Acad Sci U S A 1997;94:14512–14517.

Kalish JE, Keller GA, Morrell JC, et al. Characterization of a novel component of the peroxisomal protein import apparatus using fluorescent peroxisomal proteins. EMBO J 1996;15:3275–3285.

Kane JP, Havel RJ. Disorders of the Biogenesis and Secretion of Lipoproteins Containing the B Apolipoproteins. I. In CR Scriver,

AL Beaudet, WS Sly, et al. (eds), The Metabolic and Molecular Basis of Inherited Disease (7th ed). New York: McGraw-Hill, 1995;1853–1886.

Kappas A, Sassa S, Gallbraith RA, et al. The Porphyrias. In CR Scriver, AL Beaudet, WS Sly, et al. (eds), The Metabolic and Molecular Basis of Inherited Disease (7th ed). New York: McGraw-Hill, 1995;2103–2160.

Kim TS, Kim IO, Kim WS, et al. MR of childhood metachromatic leukodystrophy. Am J Neuroradiol 1997;18:733–738.

Krasenewich D, Gahl WA. Carbohydrate-deficient glycoprotein syndrome. Adv Pediatr 1997;47:1098–1140.

Krivit W, Shapiro EG, Perters C, et al. Hematopoietic stem-cell transplantation in globoid-cell leukodystrophy. N Engl J Med 1998;338:1119–1126.

Kuriyama M, Tokimura Y, Fujiyama J, et al. Treatment of cerebrotendinous xanthomatosis: effects of chenodeoxycholic acid, pravastatin, and combined use. J Neurol Sci 1994;125: 22–28.

Kuroda Y, Ito M, Naito E, et al. Concomitant administration of sodium dichloroacetate and vitamin B_1 for lactic acidemia in children with MELAS syndrome. J Pediatr 1997;131:450–452.

Lane SC, Jolly RD, Schmechet DE, et al. Apoptosis as the mechanism of neurodegeneration in Batten's disease. J Neurochem 1996;67:677-683.

Lazarow PB. Peroxisome structure, function and biogenesis—human patients and yeast mutants show strikingly similar defects in peroxisomal biogenesis. J Neuropathol Exp Neurol 1995;54:720–725.

Loes DJ, Stillman AE, Hite S, et al. Childhood cerebral form of adrenoleukodystrophy: short term effect of bone marrow transplantation on brain MR observations. Am J Neuroradiol 1994;15:1767–1771.

Lott IT, Lottenberg S, Nyhan WL, et al. Cerebral metabolic change after treatment in biotinidase deficiency. J Inherit Metab Dis 1993;16:399–407.

Martinez M, Mougan I, Roig M, et al. Blood polyunsaturated fatty acids in patients with peroxisomal disorders. A muticenter study. Lipids 1994;29:273–280.

Martinez M, Pineda M, Vidal R, et al. Docosahexaenoic acid: a new therapeutic approach to peroxisomal patients. Experience with two cases. Neurology 1993;43:1389–1397.

Matalon R, Kaul R, Michals K. Canavan disease: biochemical and molecular studies. J Inherit Metab Dis 1993;16:744–752.

Mitchell GA, Lambert M, Tanguay RM. Hypertyrosinemia. In CR Scriver, AL Beaudet, WS Sly, et al. (eds), The Metabolic and Molecular Basis of Inherited Disease (7th ed). New York: McGraw-Hill, 1995;1077–1106.

Moser HW. Peroxisomal Diseases. In H Harris, K Hirschhorn (eds), Advances in Human Genetics. New York: Plenum, 1993; 21:1–106.

Moser HW, Smith KD, Moser AB. X-linked Adrenoleukodystrophy. In CR Scriver, AL Beaudet, WS Sly, et al. (eds), The Metabolic and Molecular Basis of Inherited Disease (7th ed). New York: McGraw-Hill, 1995;2325–2350.

Mosser J, Douar AM, Sarde CO, et al. Putative X-linked adrenoleukodystrophy gene shares unexpected homology with ABC transporters. Nature 1993;361:726–730.

Neufeld EF, Muenzer J. The Mucopolysaccharidoses. In CR Scriver, AL Beaudet, WS Sly, et al. (eds), The Metabolic and Molecular Basis of Inherited Disease (7th ed). New York: McGraw-Hill, 1995;2465–2494.

Niaudet P, Heidet L, Munnich A, et al. Deletion of the mitochondrial DNA in a case of de Toni-Debre-Fanconi syndrome and Pearson syndrome. Pediatr Nephrol 1994;8:164–168.

Northrup H, Sigman ES, Hebert AA. Exfoliative erythroderma resulting from inadequate intake of branched-chain amino acids in infants with maple syrup urine disease. Arch Dermatol 1993;129:385–389.

Online Mendelian Inheritance in Man, OMIM. Center for Medical Genetics, Johns Hopkins University (Baltimore, MD) and National Library of Medicine (Bethesda, MD) 1998. World Wide Web URL: http://www.ncbi.nlm.nih.gov/omim/.

Patterson MC, DiBiscegli AM, Higgins JJ, et al. The effect of cholesterol-lowering agents on hepatic and plasma cholesterol in Niemann-Pick disease type C. Neurology 1993a;43:61–64.

Patterson MC, Horowitz M, Abel RB, et al. Isolated supranuclear gaze palsy as a marker of severe systemic involvement in Gaucher's disease. Neurology 1993b;43:993–997.

Ramaekers VT, Brab M, Rau G, et al. Recovery from neurological deficits following biotin treatment in a biotinidase Km variant. Neuropediatrics 1993;24:98–102.

Rogers PD. Cimetidine in the treatment of acute intermittent porphyria. Ann Pharmacother 1997;31:365–367.

Santorelli FM, Shanske S, Macaya A, et al. The mutation at nt 8993 of mitochondrial DNA is a common cause of Leigh's syndrome. Ann Neurol 1993;34:827–834.

Santorelli FM, Tanji K, Kulikova R, et al. Identification of a novel mutation in the mtDNA ND5 gene associated with MELAS. Biochem Biophys Res Commun 1997;238:326–328.

Schiffmann R, Dwyer NP, Lubensky IA, et al. Constitutive achlorhydria in mucolipidosis type IV. Proc Natl Acad Sci U S A 1998;95:1207–1212.

Scriver CR, Beaudet AL, Sly WS, et al. (eds). The Metabolic and Molecular Basis of Inherited Disease (7th ed). New York: McGraw-Hill, 1995.

Scriver CR, Kaufman S, Eisensmith RC, et al. The hyperphenylalaninemias. In CR Scriver, AL Beaudet, WS Sly, et al. (eds), The Metabolic and Molecular Basis of Inherited Disease (7th ed). New York: McGraw-Hill, 1995;1015–1106.

Shoffner JM, Brown MD, Stugard C, et al. Leber's hereditary optic neuropathy plus dystonia is caused by a mitochondrial DNA point mutation. Ann Neurol 1995;38:163–169.

Shoffner JM, Brown MD, Torroni A, et al. Mitochondrial DNA variants observed in Alzheimer disease and Parkinson disease patients. Genomics 1993;17:171–184.

Sleat DE, Donnelly RJ, Lackland H, et al. Association of mutations in a lysosomal protein with classical late-infantile neuronal ceroid lipofuscinosis. Science 1997;277:1802–1805.

Smith ML, Hua XY, Marsden DL, et al. Diabetes and mitochondrial encephalopathy with lactic acidosis and stroke-like episodes (MELAS): radiolabeled polymerase chain reaction is necessary for accurate detection of low percentages of mutation. J Clin Endocrinol Metab 1997;82:2826–2831.

Stanley CA. Carnitine disorders. Adv Pediatr 1995;42:209–242.

Suzuki K, Parker CC, Pentchev PG, et al. Neurofibrillary tangles in Niemann-Pick disease type C. Acta Neuropathol 1995;89: 227–238.

Svensson E, von Dobeln U, Eisensmith RC, et al. Relation between genotype and phenotype in Swedish phenylketonuria and hyperphenylalaninemia patients. Eur J Pediatr 1993;152:132–139.

Sweetman L, Williams JC. Branched Chain Organic Acidurias. In CR Scriver, AL Beaudet, WS Sly, et al. (eds), The Metabolic and Molecular Basis of Inherited Disease (7th ed). New York: McGraw-Hill, 1995;1387–1422.

Tada K, Kure S. Nonketotic hyperglycinemia: molecular lesion and pathophysiology. Int Pediatr 1993;8:52–59.

Tatum WO, Zachariah SB. Gabapentin treatment in acute intermittent porphyria. Neurology 1996;46:1497–1498.

Taylor RW, Chinnery PF, Haldane F, et al. MELAS associated with a mutation in the valine transfer RNA gene of mitochondrial DNA. Ann Neurol 1996;40:459–462.

Tyni T, Majander A, Kalimo H, et al. Pathology of skeletal muscle and impaired respiratory chain function in long chain 3 hydroxy-acyl-CoA dehydrogenase deficiency with the Gl528C mutation. Neuromuscul Disord 1996;6:327–337.

Van den Ouweland JMW, Lemkes HHPJ, Trembath RC, et al. Maternally inherited diabetes and deafness is a distinct subtype of diabetes and associates with a single point mutation in the mitochondrial tRNA Leu(UUR). Gene Diabet 1994;43:746–751.

Van Gennip AH, Abeling NGGM, Vreken P, et al. Inborn errors of pyrimidine degradation. Clinical, biochemical and molecular aspects. J Inherit Metab Dis 1997;20:203–213.

Waggoner DD, Buist NR. Long-term complications in treated galactosemia. Int Pediatr 1993;81:97–100.

Welch GN, Loscalzo J. Homocysteine and atherothrombosis. N Engl J Med 1998;338:1042–1050.

Whitley CB, Belani KG, Chang PN, et al. Long-term outcome of Hurler syndrome following bone marrow transplantation. Am J Med Genet 1993;46:209–218.

Wraith JE. The mucopolysaccharidoses: a clinical review and guide to management. Arch Dis Child 1995;72:263–267.

Chapter 69
Neurocutaneous Syndromes

Van S. Miller and E. Steve Roach

Congenital or hereditary conditions that feature lesions of both the skin and nervous system have been traditionally considered as neurocutaneous disorders (also phakomatosis). Although these conditions are very different and each has a distinct pathophysiology, the concept of neurocutaneous disorders does serve to unify neurological disorders whose identification depends predominantly on simple visual diagnosis. These disorders may be inherited or sporadic. Advances in clinical genetics have established the molecular basis for some, although recognition and treatment still requires an appreciation of the cutaneous and systemic symptoms. This chapter reviews the clinical features of the more common neurocutaneous syndromes (Table 69.1).

Table 69.1:   Neurocutaneous disorders

Tuberous sclerosis
Neurofibromatosis
Ehlers-Danlos syndrome
Pseudoxanthoma elasticum
Osler-Weber-Rendu syndrome
Progeria
Fabry's disease
Lesch-Nyhan syndrome
Sturge-Weber syndrome
Progressive facial hemiatrophy
Ataxia-telangiectasia
Kinky hair syndrome
Cerebrotendinous xanthomatosis
Epidermal nevus syndrome
Hypomelanosis of Ito
Neurocutaneous melanosis
Von Hippel–Lindau syndrome
Wyburn-Mason syndrome
Xeroderma pigmentosum

Table 69.2:   Revised diagnostic criteria for tuberous sclerosis complex

Major features
   1. Facial angiofibromas or forehead plaque
   2. Nontraumatic ungual or periungual fibroma
   3. Hypomelanotic macules (more than three)
   4. Shagreen patch (connective tissue nevus)
   5. Multiple retinal nodular hamartomas
   6. Cortical tuber[a]
   7. Subependymal nodule
   8. Subependymal giant cell astrocytoma
   9. Cardiac rhabdomyoma, single or multiple
  10. Lymphangiomyomatosis[b]
  11. Renal angiomyolipoma[b]
Minor features
   1. Multiple randomly distributed pits in dental enamel
   2. Hamartomatous rectal polyps[c]
   3. Bone cysts[d]
   4. Cerebral white matter radial migration lines[a,d,e]
   5. Gingival fibromas
   6. Nonrenal hamartoma[c]
   7. Retinal achromic patch
   8. Confetti skin lesions
   9. Multiple renal cysts[c]
Definite tuberous sclerosis complex: either two major features or one major feature plus two minor features
Probable tuberous sclerosis complex: one major plus one minor feature
Possible tuberous sclerosis complex: either one major feature or two or more minor features

[a]When cerebral cortical dysplasia and cerebral white matter migration tracts occur together, they should be counted as one rather than two features of tuberous sclerosis.
[b]When both lymphangiomyomatosis and renal angiomyolipomas are present, other features of tuberous sclerosis should be present before a definite diagnosis is assigned.
[c]Histological confirmation is suggested.
[d]Radiographical confirmation is sufficient.
[e]One panel member felt strongly that three or more radial migration lines should constitute a major sign.
Source: Reprinted with permission from ES Roach, MR Gomez, H Northrup. Tuberous sclerosis consensus conference: revised clinical diagnostic criteria. J Child Neurol 1998;13:624–628.

TUBEROUS SCLEROSIS

Tuberous sclerosis complex (TSC) is a disorder of cellular differentiation and proliferation that can affect the brain, skin, kidneys, heart, and other organs. Many of the clinical manifestations of TSC result from hamartomas; true neoplasms also occur, particularly in the kidney and brain. Abnormal neuronal migration plays a major additional role in neurological dysfunction.

Population-based studies suggest a prevalence of 1 per 6,000–9,000 individuals. However, because of its striking variability of clinical expression and severity, the diagnosis of TSC can be difficult in individuals with subtle findings, and the true prevalence may be considerably higher. Cutaneous findings are usually the first clue that a patient has TSC, but other typical features may lead to the diagnosis; current revised criteria for TSC are presented in Table 69.2 (Roach et al. 1998).

Genetics

Tuberous sclerosis is inherited as an autosomal dominant trait with variable penetrance (Weiner et al. 1998). The estimated spontaneous mutation rate for TSC varies from 66% to 86%, depending in part on the completeness of investigation of the extended family.

Two genes are responsible for TSC. One gene (*TSC1*) is located at chromosome 9q34, and the other (*TSC2*) is adjacent to the gene for adult polycystic kidney disease at chromosome 16p13.3. Unlike neurofibromatosis (NF) types 1 and 2, there are no obvious phenotypic differences between *TSC1* and *TSC2*. Tuberin, the gene product of *TSC1*, has a homologous area with the GTPase activating protein of rap1GAP. Now that both genes have been identified, however, *TSC1* seems to be

more likely than *TSC2* to account for familial cases and is generally less severe (Jones et al. 1997). Multiple mutation types found in different regions of the gene are described.

Cutaneous Features

The cutaneous lesions of TSC include hypomelanotic macules, the shagreen patch, ungual fibromas, and facial angiofibromas. Hypomelanotic macules (ash leaf spots) are found in up to 90% of patients (Figure 69.1). The lesions usually are present at birth but are often difficult to see in the newborn without an ultraviolet light. Other pigmentary abnormalities include confetti lesions (an area with stippled hypopigmentation, typically on the extremities) and poliosis

FIGURE 69.1 A hypomelanotic macule (ash leaf spot) (*arrow*) from the leg of a patient with tuberous sclerosis. (Reprinted with permission from ES Roach. Diagnosis and management of neurocutaneous syndromes. Semin Neurol 1988;8:83–96.)

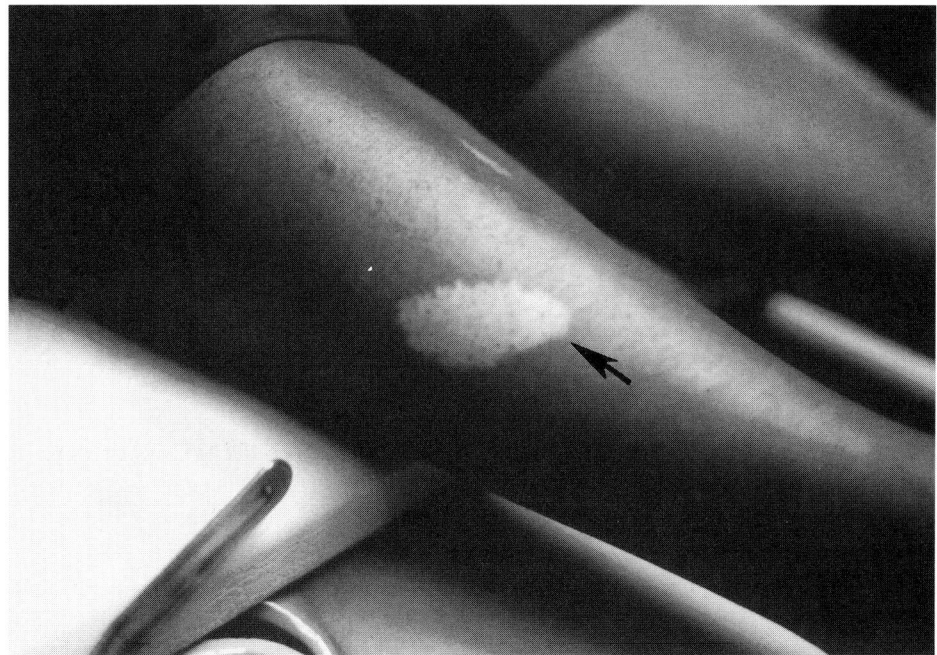

(a white patch or forelock) of the scalp hair or eyelids (Figure 69.2). Hypomelanotic macules are not specific for TSC; one or two of these lesions are common in normal individuals (Vanderhooft et al. 1996).

Facial angiofibromas (adenoma sebaceum) are made up of vascular and connective tissue elements. Although these lesions are considered specific for TSC, they are found in only approximately three-fourths of patients and often appear several years after the diagnosis has been established by other means. The lesions typically become apparent during the preschool years as a few small red papules on the malar region; they gradually become larger and more numerous, sometimes extending down the nasolabial folds or onto the chin (see Figure 69.2).

The shagreen patch is most often found on the back or flank area; it is an irregularly shaped, slightly raised, or textured skin lesion (see Figure 69.2). The lesion is found in only 20–30% of patients with TSC and may not be apparent in young children. Ungual fibromas are nodular or fleshy lesions that arise adjacent to or underneath the nails (see Figure 69.2). This lesion is usually considered specific for TSC, although a single lesion occasionally occurs after trauma in patients with TSC. Ungual fibromas are seen in only 15–20% of unselected patients with TSC and are more likely to be found in adolescents or adults.

Neurological Features

The predominant neurological manifestations of TSC are mental retardation, seizures, and behavioral abnormalities, although milder forms of the disease with little or no neurological impairment are common. Neurological lesions probably result from impaired cellular interaction resulting in disrupted neuronal migration along radial glial fibers and abnormal proliferation of glial elements. Neuropathological lesions of TSC include subependymal nodules, cortical hamartomas, areas of focal cortical hypoplasia, and heterotopic gray matter.

Various types of seizures occur in 80–90% of patients. Most mentally retarded patients have epilepsy. On the other hand, many patients with TSC have seizures but are not retarded. The most abnormal regions seen on magnetic resonance imaging (MRI) tend to coincide with focal abnormalities of the electroencephalogram (EEG). The number of subependymal lesions does not correlate with the clinical severity of TSC. However, patients who have numerous lesions of the cerebral cortex shown by MRI tend to have more cognitive impairment and more difficulty with seizure control. Children with infantile spasms have more cortical lesions demonstrated by MRI and are more likely to exhibit long-term cognitive impairment (Jozwiak et al. 1998).

The likelihood of mental retardation in patients with TSC is probably overestimated. One population survey found only 10 mentally retarded patients among 26 patients with TSC. The severity of intellectual dysfunction ranges from borderline to profound mental retardation. However, in addition to frank mental retardation, many children have serious behavioral disorders. Autism, hyperkinesis, aggressiveness, and frank psychosis are sometimes noted, either as isolated problems or in combination with epilepsy or intellectual deficit (Curatolo 1996).

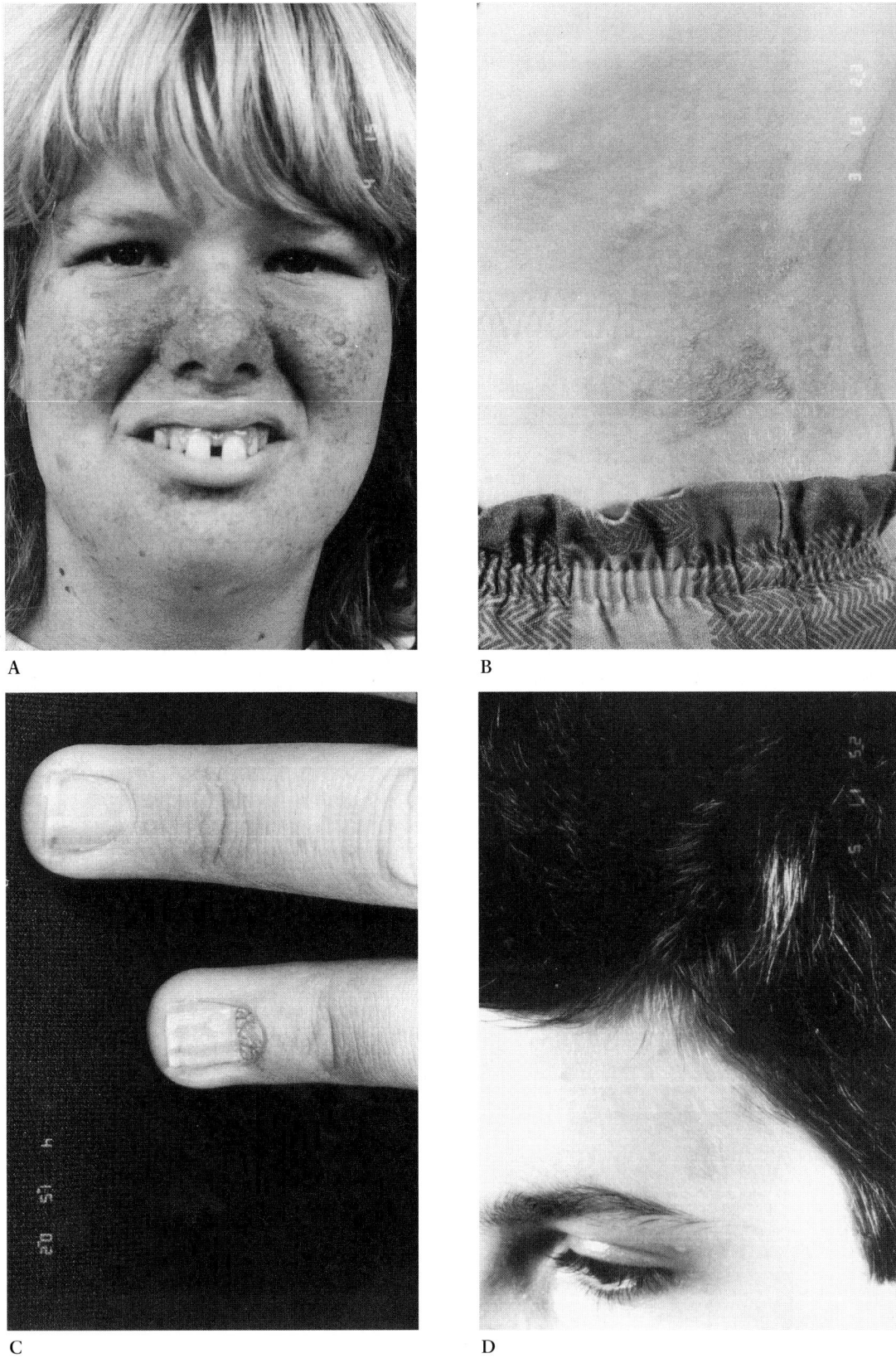

FIGURE 69.2   Classic cutaneous manifestations of tuberous sclerosis include (**A**) facial angiofibromas; (**B**) shagreen patch; (**C**) ungual fibromata; and (**D**) poliosis. (Reprinted with permission from ES Roach, MR Delgado. Tuberous sclerosis. Dermatol Clin 1995;13:151–161.)

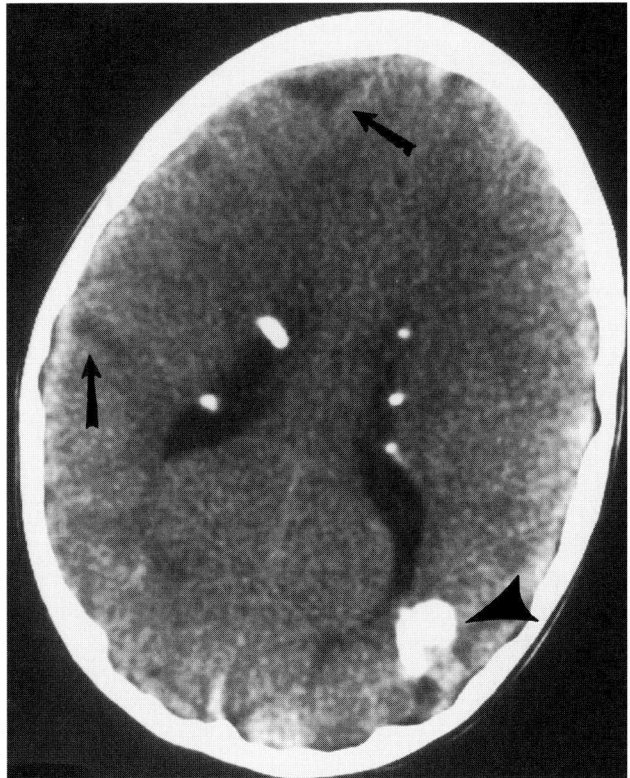

FIGURE 69.3   Computed cranial tomography scan from a child with tuberous sclerosis complex demonstrates typical calcified subependymal nodules; a large calcified parenchymal lesion (*arrowhead*) and low-density cortical lesions (*arrows*) are seen as well. (Reprinted with permission from ES Roach, J Kerr, D Mendelsohn, et al. Diagnosis of symptomatic and asymptomatic gene carriers of tuberous sclerosis by CT and MRI. Ann N Y Acad Sci 1991;615:112–122.)

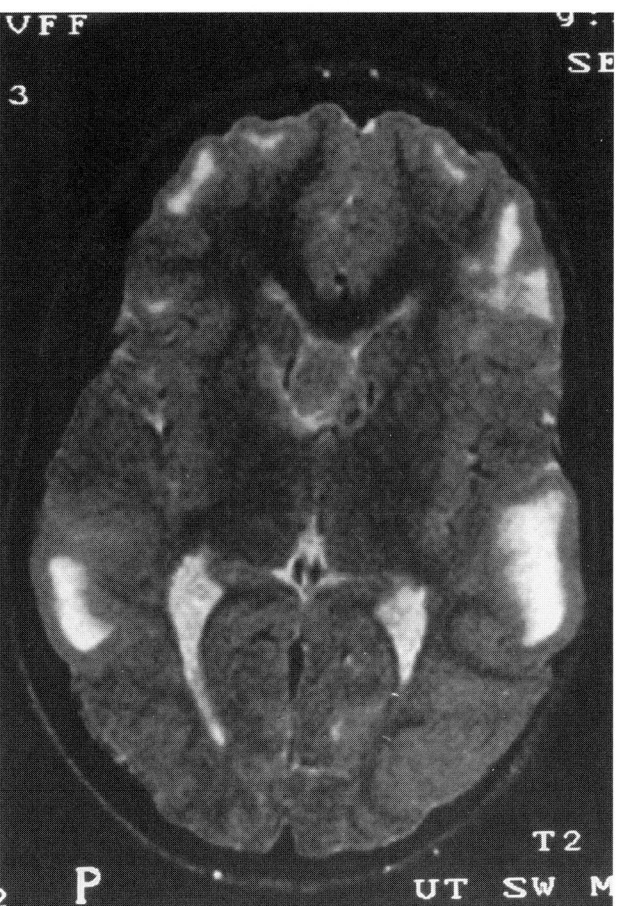

FIGURE 69.4   Noncontrast T2-weighted magnetic resonance imaging scan from a child with tuberous sclerosis demonstrates extensive high-signal cortical lesions typical of tuberous sclerosis.

The calcified subependymal nodules that characterize TSC are best demonstrated with computed tomography (CT) (Figure 69.3). Superficial cerebral lesions can sometimes be seen with CT, but are far more obvious with T2-weighted MRI (Figure 69.4). Cerebellar anomalies can be shown in over one-fourth of patients with TSC. Nodular subependymal lesions that have not yet calcified produce a high-signal lesion with T2-weighted scans. Evidence of abnormal neuronal migration can be seen in some patients as high-signal linear lesions running perpendicular to the cortex on T2-weighted scans.

Subependymal giant cell astrocytomas (SEGAs) develop in 6–14% of patients with TSC. Unlike the more common cortical tubers, giant cell astrocytomas can enlarge (Figure 69.5) and cause symptoms of increased intracranial pressure (Torres et al. 1998). Clinical features include new focal neurological deficits, increased intracranial pressure, unexplained behavior change, or deterioration of seizure control. Acute or subacute onset of neurological dysfunction may result from sudden obstruction of the ventricular sys-

tem by an intraventricular SEGA. Rarely, acute deterioration occurs because of hemorrhage into the tumor itself.

The presence of contrast enhancement on either CT or MRI may help to distinguish a SEGA from the other cerebral lesions seen with TSC. Giant cell tumors are usually benign but locally invasive, and surgery performed early can be curative. Identification of an enlarging SEGA before the onset of symptoms of increased intracranial pressure or new neurological deficits may improve surgical outcome.

Retinal Features

The frequency of retinal hamartomas in TSC has varied from almost negligible to 87% of patients, probably reflecting the expertise and technique of the examiner. Retinal lesions may be difficult to identify without pupillary dilatation and indirect ophthalmoscopy, particularly in uncooperative children. Retinal lesions vary from the classic mulberry lesions adjacent to the optic disc (Figure 69.6) to the plaquelike hamar-

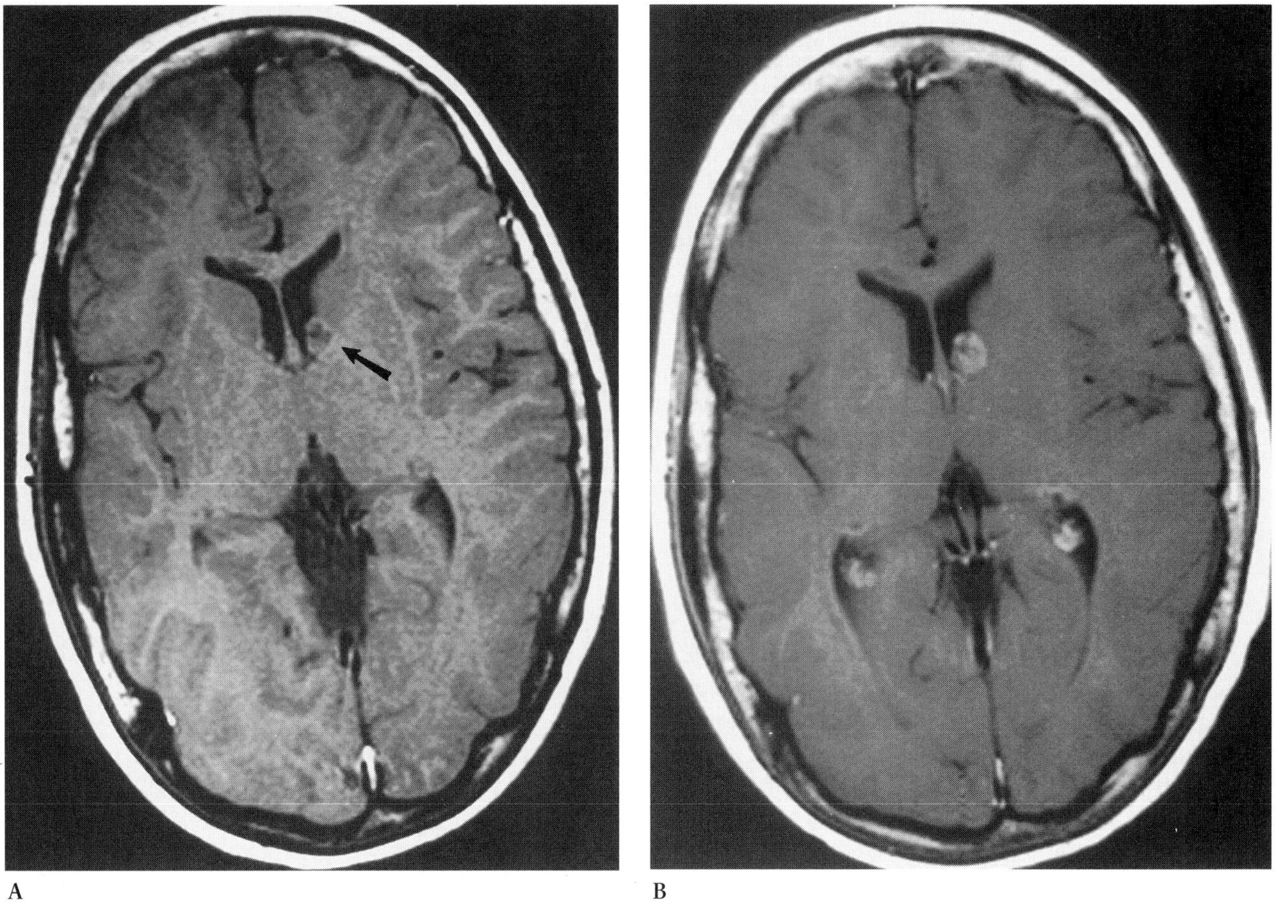

A

B

FIGURE 69.5   (**A**) Noncontrast T1-weighted magnetic resonance imaging scan from a child with tuberous sclerosis shows an irregular mass (*arrow*) with a central signal void caused by calcification protruding into the left frontal horn. (**B**) Another scan with gadolinium a few months later shows contrast enhancement and minimal tumor growth.

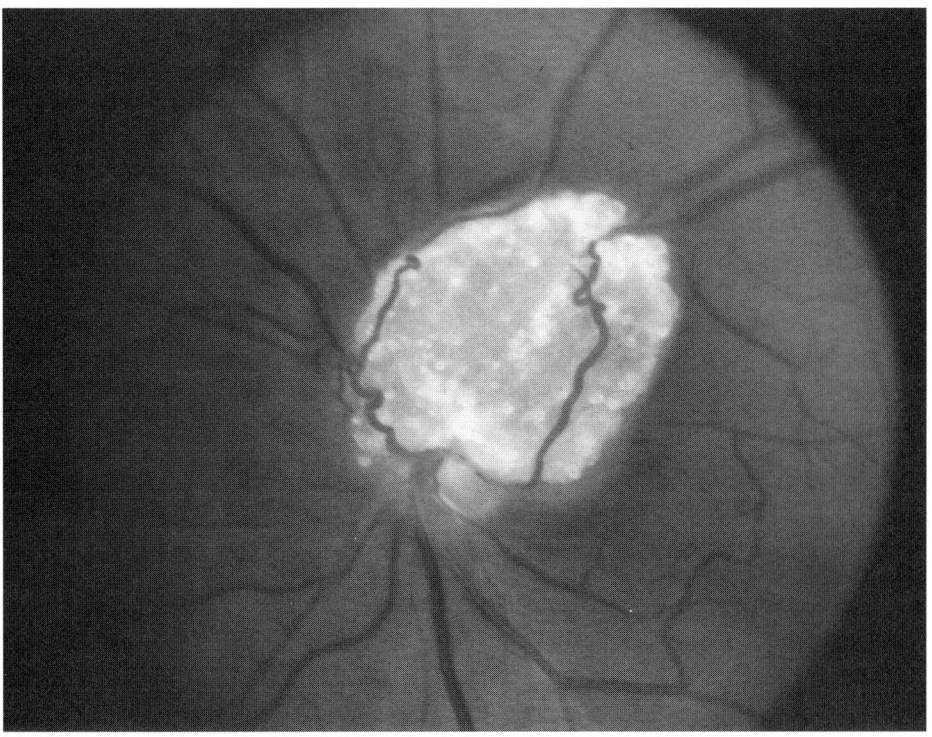

FIGURE 69.6   A retinal astrocytoma (mulberry lesion) adjacent to the optic nerve is typical of those found with tuberous sclerosis. (Reprinted with permission from ES Roach. Neurocutaneous syndromes. Pediatr Clin North Am 1992;39:591–620.)

toma or depigmented retinal lesions. Most retinal lesions are clinically insignificant, but occasional patients have visual impairment caused by a large macular lesion, and rare patients have visual loss caused by retinal detachment, vitreous hemorrhage, or hamartoma enlargement. Occasional patients have a pigmentary defect of the iris.

Systemic Features

Cardiac

Approximately two-thirds of patients with TSC have a cardiac rhabdomyoma, but few of these lesions are clinically important. Cardiac rhabdomyomas are hamartomas; they tend to be multiple, and evidence exists that their frequency diminishes with age. These lesions are sometimes evident on prenatal ultrasound testing (Figure 69.7), and most of the patients with cardiac dysfunction present soon after birth with heart failure. A few children later develop cardiac arrhythmias or cerebral thromboembolism from the rhabdomyomas. Congestive heart failure is caused by either obstruction of blood flow by intraluminal tumor or lack of sufficient normal myocardium to maintain perfusion. Some patients stabilize after medical treatment with digoxin and diuretics and eventually improve; others require surgery.

Renal

Renal angiomyolipomas occur in up to three-fourths of patients with TSC; most of these lesions are histologically

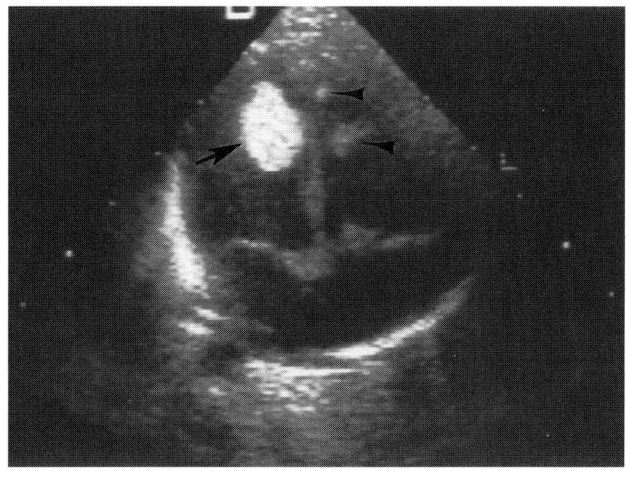

FIGURE 69.7 Prenatal ultrasound study reveals a large cardiac rhabdomyoma (*arrow*) and two smaller rhabdomyomas (*arrowheads*) in a child who subsequently proved to have tuberous sclerosis. (Reprinted from DM Weiner, DE Ewalt, ES Roach, TW Hensle. Tuberous sclerosis complex: a comprehensive review. J Am Coll Surg 1998;187:548–561, with permission from the American College of Surgeons.)

benign tumors with varying amounts of vascular tissue, fat, and smooth muscle (Figure 69.8). Bilateral tumors or multiple tumors in a kidney are common. The prevalence of renal tumors increases with age, and tumors larger than 4 cm are much more likely to become symptomatic than smaller tumors (Ewalt et al. 1998). Renal cell carcinoma or other malignancies are less common.

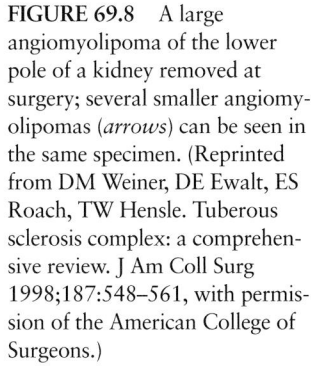

FIGURE 69.8 A large angiomyolipoma of the lower pole of a kidney removed at surgery; several smaller angiomyolipomas (*arrows*) can be seen in the same specimen. (Reprinted from DM Weiner, DE Ewalt, ES Roach, TW Hensle. Tuberous sclerosis complex: a comprehensive review. J Am Coll Surg 1998;187:548–561, with permission of the American College of Surgeons.)

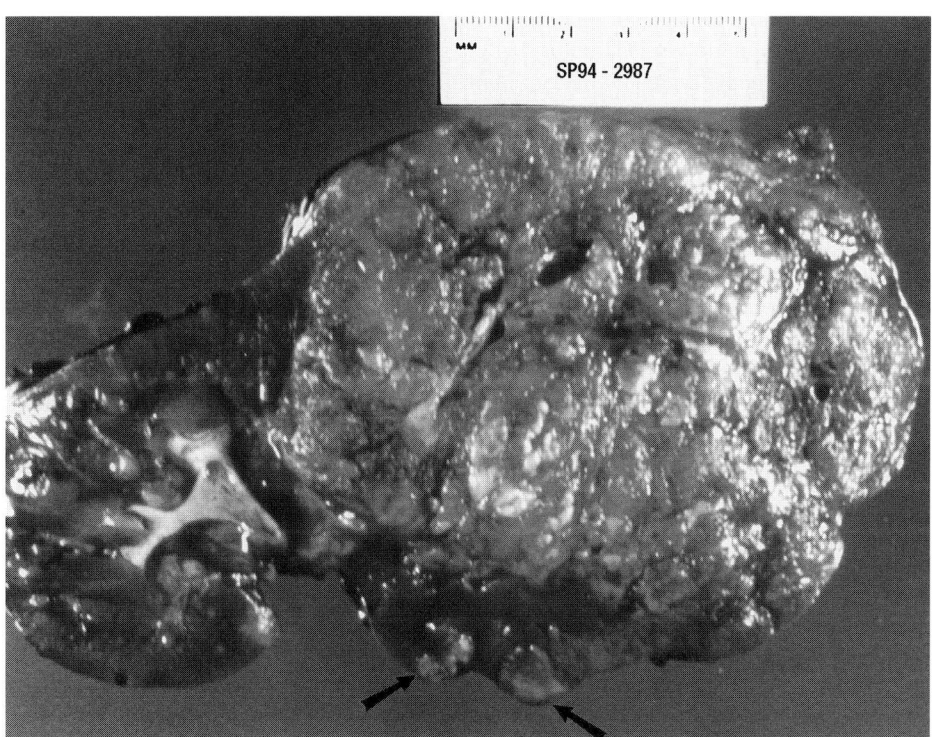

Single or multiple renal cysts are also a feature of TSC; these tend to appear earlier than the renal tumors. Larger cysts are easily identified with ultrasound or with cranial CT, and the combination of renal cysts and angiomyolipomas is characteristic of TSC. Individual renal cysts may disappear.

Pulmonary

An estimated 1% of patients with TSC develop lung disease. Pulmonary disease is five times more common in female than in male subjects. Spontaneous pneumothorax, dyspnea, cough, and hemoptysis are typical symptoms of pulmonary TSC, although these do not often develop before the third or fourth decade (Scully et al. 1994). Almost two-thirds of these patients die within 5 years of the onset of symptoms. Tamoxifen and progesterone may be helpful in some patients, but no treatment is universally effective.

NEUROFIBROMATOSIS

NF is actually two separate diseases, each caused by a different gene: NF type 1 (NF1), or von Recklinghausen's disease; and NF type 2 (NF2), which is characterized by bilateral vestibular schwannomas and is often associated with other brain or spinal cord tumors. The clinical manifestations of both conditions are highly variable (Friedman and Birch 1997). NF1 is the most common of the neurocutaneous syndromes, occurring in approximately 1 in 3,000 people. Approximately one-half of the cases of NF1 result from a spontaneous mutation. In contrast, NF2 occurs in only 1 in 50,000 people.

Molecular Biology

NF1 is caused by a mutation of the 60 exon NF1 gene on chromosome 17q. The NF1 gene product, *neurofibromin*, is partially homologous to GTPase-activating protein. Approximately 100 mutations of NF1 have been identified in various regions of the gene.

Several patients have developed a somatic NF1 mutation affecting only a limited region of the body. With this segmental NF, one extremity may have café au lait lesions, subcutaneous neurofibromas, and other signs of NF, but the rest of the body is unaffected (Hager et al. 1997). Similarly, patients with gonadal mosaicism have been described. These individuals have no outward manifestations of NF1, but have multiple affected offspring.

NF2 is caused by a mutation of the *NF2* gene on chromosome 22. The NF2 protein product is known as *schwannomin*. The *NF2* gene suppresses tumor function, and its dysfunction accounts for the common occurrence of central nervous system (CNS) tumors in patients with NF2 (Gutmann et al. 1998). Multiple different mutations of the *NF2* gene have been described. The clinical severity may be related to the nature of the NF2 mutation; missense mutations that allow some protein function tend to produce milder clinical forms, whereas frame shift and nonsense mutations that produce stop codons that prevent the production of any protein often cause severe disease.

Cutaneous Features of Neurofibromatosis Type 1

Cutaneous lesions of NF1 include café au lait spots, subcutaneous neurofibromas, plexiform neurofibromas (Figure 69.9), and axillary freckling. Café au lait spots are flat, light to medium brown areas that vary in shape and size. They are typically present at birth, but increase in size and number during the first few years. Additional frecklelike lesions, 1–3 mm in diameter, often occur in the axillae or intertriginous regions.

Neurofibromas are benign tumors arising from peripheral nerves (Figure 69.9). These tumors are composed predominantly of Schwann cells and fibroblasts, but contain endothelial, pericytes, and mast cell components. Neurofibromas can develop at any time; the size and number often increase after puberty.

Plexiform neurofibromas often occur on the face and can cause substantial deformity (see Figure 69.9). In one series, plexiform neurofibromas progressed in 46% of the patients. Patients with plexiform tumors of the head, face, or neck and those who presented before 10 years of age were more likely to do poorly (Needle et al. 1997). Plexiform neurofibromas have a 5% lifetime risk of malignant degeneration.

Systemic Features of Neurofibromatosis Type 1

Lisch nodules are pigmented iris hamartomas (Figure 69.10) that are pathognomonic for NF1. Lisch nodules do not cause symptoms; their significance lies in their implications for the diagnosis of NF1. Lisch nodules are often not apparent during early childhood, and so their absence does not exclude the diagnosis of NF1. Rare children with NF1 have retinal hamartomas, but these usually remain asymptomatic.

Dysplasia of the renal or carotid arteries occurs in a small percentage of patients with NF1. Renal artery stenosis causes systemic hypertension. Another potential cause of hypertension is pheochromocytoma. Several forms of cerebral artery dysplasia occur, most commonly moyamoya syndrome, which promotes cerebral infarction in children and brain hemorrhage in adults.

Neurological Features in Neurofibromatosis Type 1

NF1 affects the nervous system in several ways, but the clinical features vary even among affected members of the

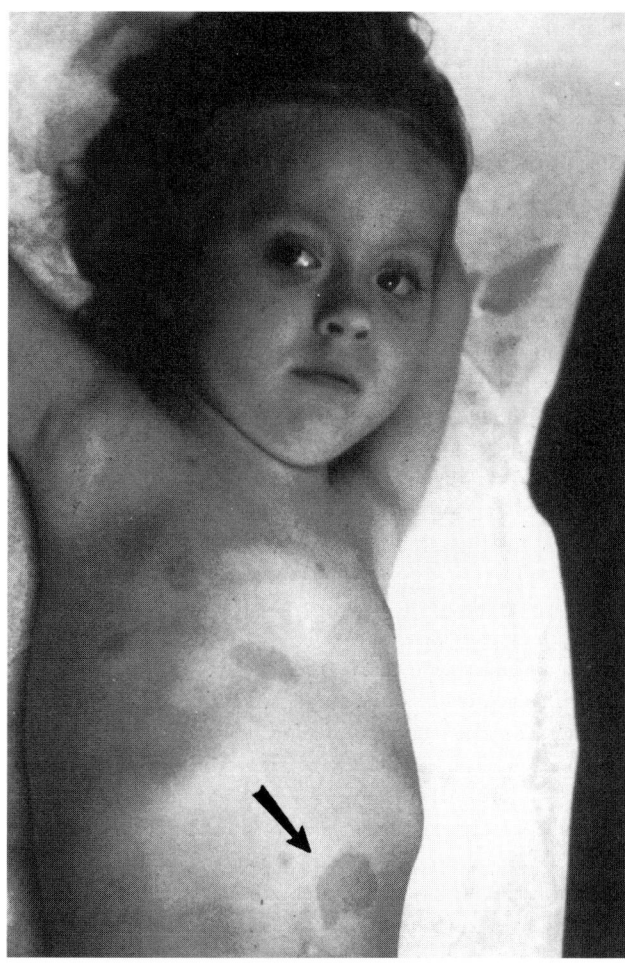

A

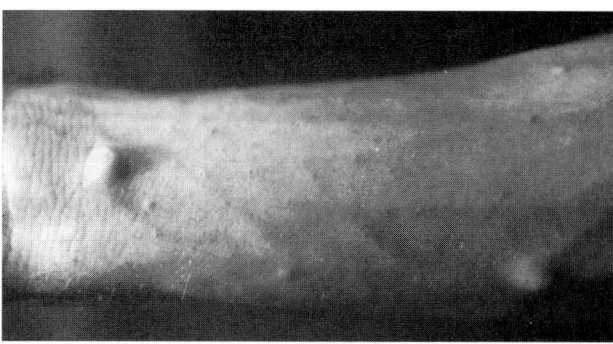

B

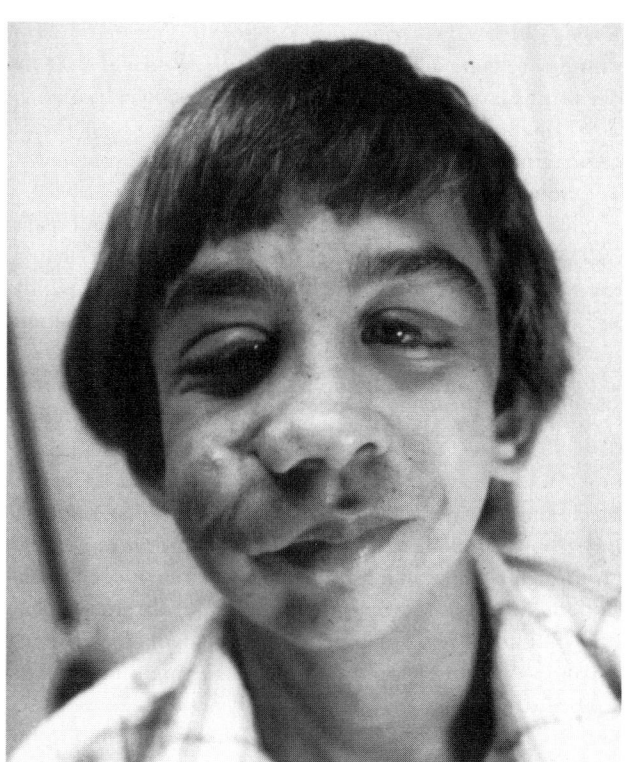

C

FIGURE 69.9 (A) Typical café au lait spots (*arrow*) in a child with neurofibromatosis type 1. (B) Subcutaneous neurofibromata in a patient with neurofibromatosis type 1. (C) Plexiform neurofibroma in a boy with neurofibromatosis type 1. (Reprinted with permission from ES Roach. Diagnosis and management of neurocutaneous syndromes. Semin Neurol 1988;8:83–96.)

same family. Tumors occur in the brain, spinal cord, and peripheral nerves, though not as frequently as with NF2.

Optic nerve glioma (Figure 69.11) is the most common CNS tumor caused by NF1. Approximately 15% of patients with NF1 have unilateral or bilateral optic glioma. The rate of growth of these optic nerve gliomas varies, but they tend to behave less aggressively in patients with NF1 than those without NF1. Optic atrophy and progressive vision loss are more common than pain or proptosis. Precocious puberty is a common presenting sign of optic nerve tumors in patients with NF1, although occasional children with NF1 present with precocious puberty even in the absence of optic tumors (Zacharin 1997).

Ependymomas, meningiomas, and astrocytomas of the CNS occur in patients with NF1 less often than in patients with NF2. Neurofibromas and schwannomas are common, but not always symptomatic; they develop on either cranial nerves or spinal nerve roots. The symptoms from these tumors reflect their size, location, and rate of growth.

Approximately 60–78% of patients with NF1 have increased signal lesions within the basal ganglia, thalamus, brainstem, and cerebellum on T2-weighted MRIs (Figure 69.12) (Menor et al. 1998). These areas are not routinely visible with CT. The origin and significance of these radiographic lesions is unclear. Whether these MRI lesions correlate with the likelihood of cognitive impairment is still debated. Patients with NF1 tend to have full-scale IQ scores within the low normal range, and it is estimated that 40% of patients with NF1 have some type of learning disability or behavioral problem.

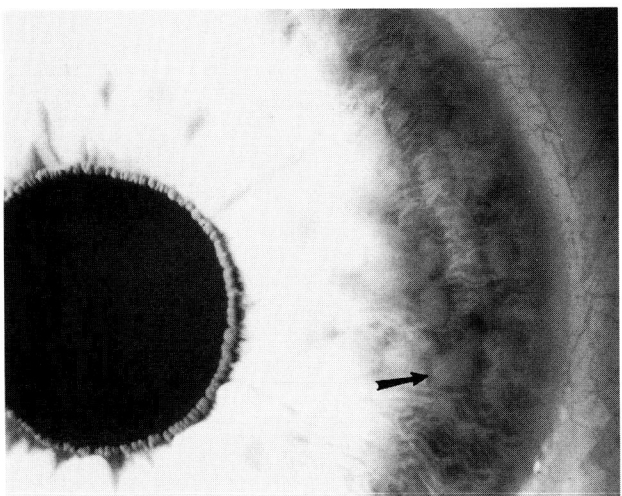

FIGURE 69.10   Lisch nodules (*arrow*) of the iris in a patient with neurofibromatosis type 1. (Reprinted with permission from ES Roach. Neurocutaneous syndromes. Pediatr Clin North Am 1992;39:591–620.)

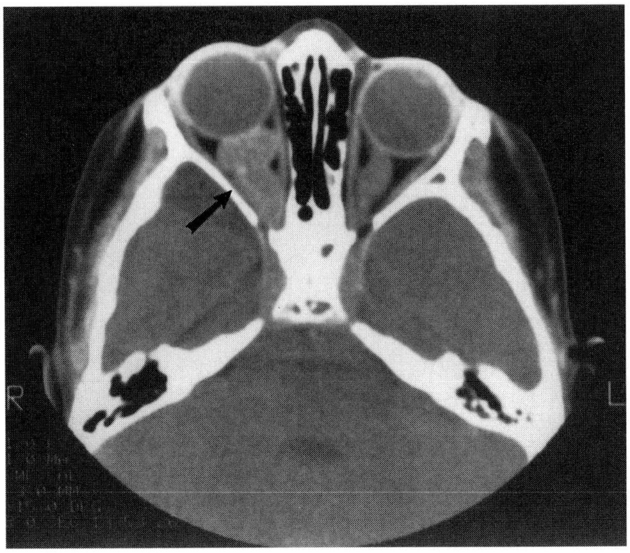

FIGURE 69.11   Computed cranial tomography scan (from a child with neurofibromatosis type 1) shows bilateral optic nerve gliomas, larger in the right optic nerve (*arrow*) than the left. (Reprinted with permission from ES Roach. Neurocutaneous syndromes. Pediatr Clin North Am 1992;39:591–620.)

Clinical Features of Neurofibromatosis Type 2

Patients with NF2 have few cutaneous lesions. Instead, these patients often have multiple types of tumors of the CNS (thus, it is sometimes designated as *central NF*). Café au lait spots are uncommon. Lisch nodules are not typically seen in NF2, and subcutaneous neurofibromas are much less common. NF1 and NF2 do not occur in different members of the same family because they are caused by mutations of different genes.

Most patients who meet established diagnostic criteria for NF2 (Table 69.3) eventually develop bilateral vestibular schwannomas (Figure 69.13). Symptoms of NF2 typically develop in adolescence or early adulthood, although children can be affected also. Common complaints with large acoustic tumors include hearing loss, tinnitus, vertigo, facial weakness, and headache. Unilateral hearing loss is relatively common in the early stages.

Various other tumors of the CNS occur, although much less often than acoustic schwannomas. The clinical features of these tumors depend primarily on the lesion's location within the brain and spinal cord. Schwannomas of other cranial nerves occur in some patients, and meningiomas, ependymomas, and astrocytomas also occur with increased frequency. Patients with NF2 may develop multiple simultaneous tumor types.

Diagnostic Criteria for Neurofibromatosis

If several characteristics are present, the diagnosis of either NF1 or NF2 is obvious, especially when another family member is affected. But when the clinical features are not

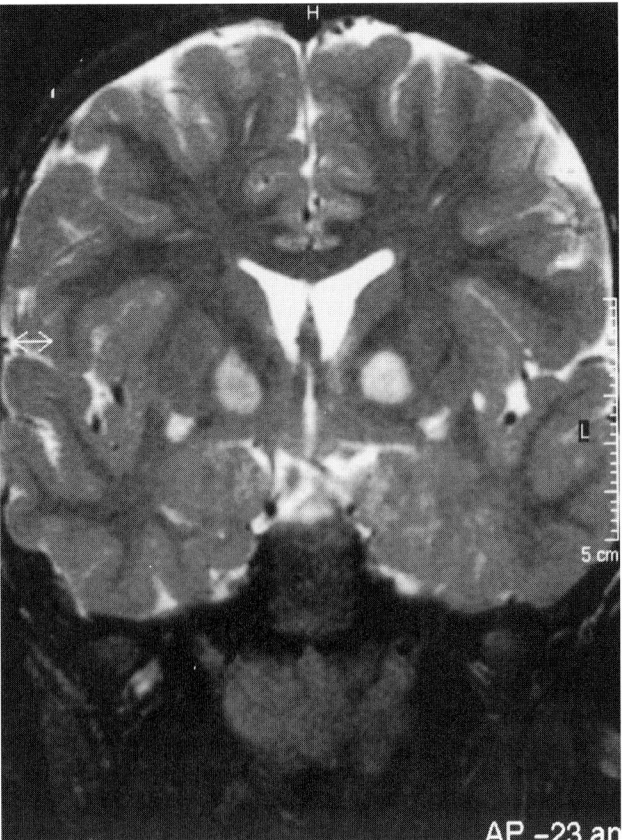

FIGURE 69.12   Coronal T1-weighted magnetic resonance imaging scan shows bilateral high-signal lesions in the basal ganglia, abnormalities typical of neurofibromatosis type 1.

Table 69.3: Diagnostic criteria for neurofibromatosis

Neurofibromatosis type 1 (any two or more)
    Six or more café au lait lesions over 5 mm in diameter before
        puberty and over 15 mm in diameter afterward
    Freckling in the axillary or inguinal areas
    Optic glioma
    Two or more neurofibromas or one plexiform neurofibroma
    A first-degree relative with neurofibromatosis type 1
    Two or more Lisch nodules
    A characteristic bony lesion (sphenoid dysplasia, thinning of
        the cortex of long bones, with or without pseudarthrosis)
Neurofibromatosis type 2
    Bilateral VIII nerve tumor (shown by magnetic resonance imag-
        ing, computed tomography, or histological confirmation)
    A first-degree relative with neurofibromatosis type 2 and a
        unilateral eighth nerve tumor
    A first-degree relative with neurofibromatosis type 2 and any
        two of the following lesions: neurofibroma, meningioma,
        schwannoma, glioma, or juvenile posterior subcapsular
        lenticular opacity

Source: Data from Neurofibromatosis. Conference statement. National Institutes of Health Consensus Development Conference. Arch Neurol 1988;45:575–578.

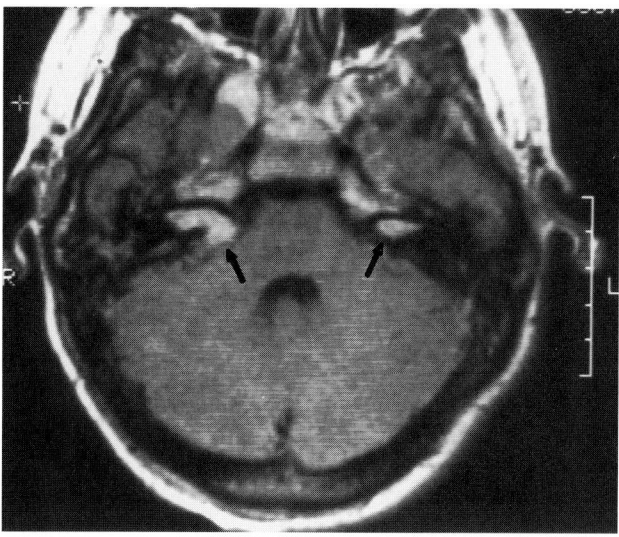

FIGURE 69.13 Cranial magnetic resonance imaging scan from a child with neurofibromatosis type 2 shows bilateral vestibular tumors (*arrows*). (Reprinted with permission from ES Roach. Neurocutaneous syndromes. Pediatr Clin North Am 1992;39:591–620.)

typical and the family history is negative, the diagnosis can be difficult. Very young children may have fewer apparent lesions, and definitive diagnosis can be difficult in these children. Diagnostic criteria (see Table 69.3) help to resolve some of these questionable cases, but the criteria are now being replaced by specific gene testing. Screening for the *NF1* gene is technically difficult because the gene is large and several different mutations have been identified. Commercially available studies have a 30% false-negative rate.

EHLERS-DANLOS SYNDROME

Several subtypes of Ehlers-Danlos syndrome can be defined by the clinical manifestations, inheritance pattern, and, in some instances, specific molecular defects. Together these syndromes are characterized by fragile or hyperelastic skin (Figure 69.14), hyperextensible joints, vascular lesions, easy bruising, and excessive scarring after injuries. Occasional patients develop peripheral neuropathy caused by lax ligaments, but vascular lesions such as aneurysm (Figure 69.15) and arterial dissection are the most serious threat to the nervous system.

Over 80% of the patients have types I, II, or III, and the other subtypes are individually uncommon. It is type IV that most often leads to neurovascular complications. All familial type IV Ehlers-Danlos cases with a documented abnormality of type III collagen are transmitted by autosomal dominant inheritance. Various defects of the *COL3A1* gene (which codes for the α-1 chain of type III collagen) on chromosome 2 have been identified (Schwartze et al. 1997).

Intracranial Aneurysm

The initial report of Ehlers-Danlos syndrome was an adult woman who had aneurysms of both the internal carotid and vertebral arteries. Subsequent patients with extracranial and intracranial aneurysms have been reported, including several individuals with multiple intracranial aneurysms. Most individuals become symptomatic in early adulthood, but onset in childhood and adolescence is reported (see Figure 69.15).

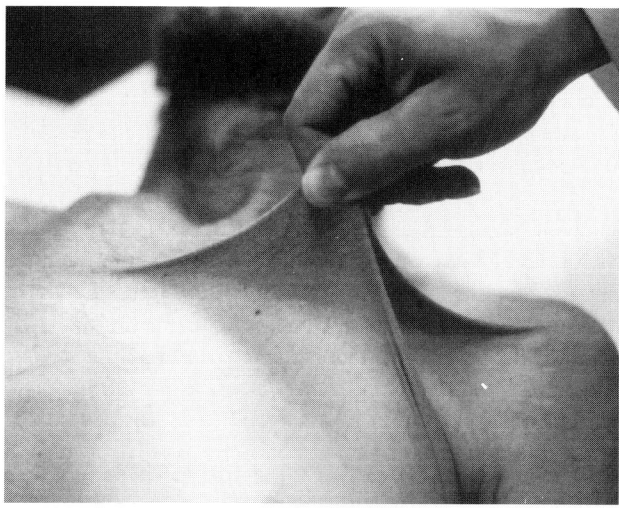

FIGURE 69.14 Cutaneous hyperelasticity of the anterior chest in a patient with Ehlers-Danlos syndrome without cerebrovascular disease. (Reprinted with permission from ES Roach. Congenital Cutaneovascular Syndromes. In PV Vinken, GW Bruyn, HL Klawans [eds], Handbook of Clinical Neurology [Vol. 11]. Vascular Diseases. Amsterdam: Elsevier, 1989;443–462.)

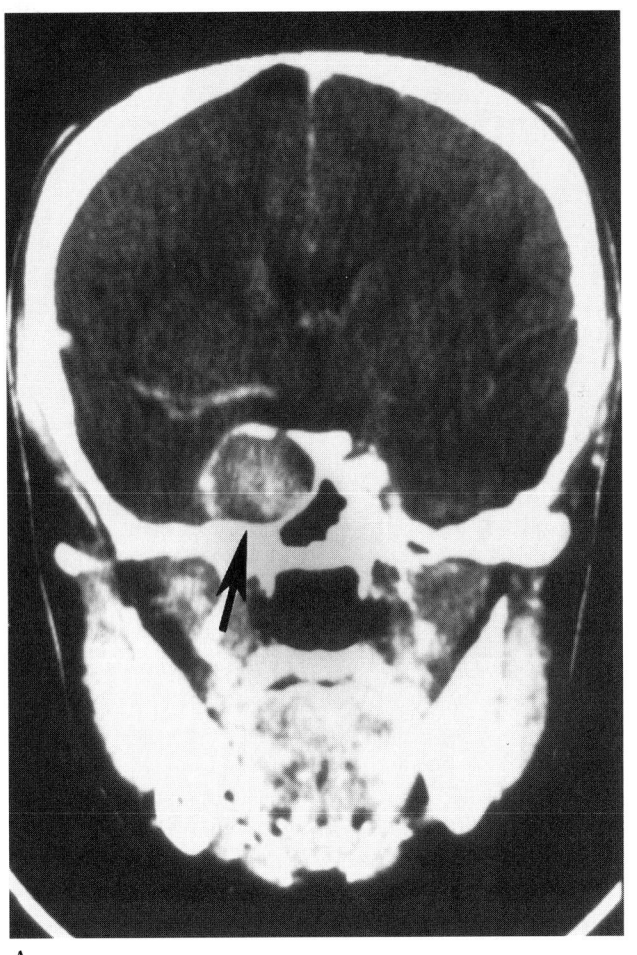
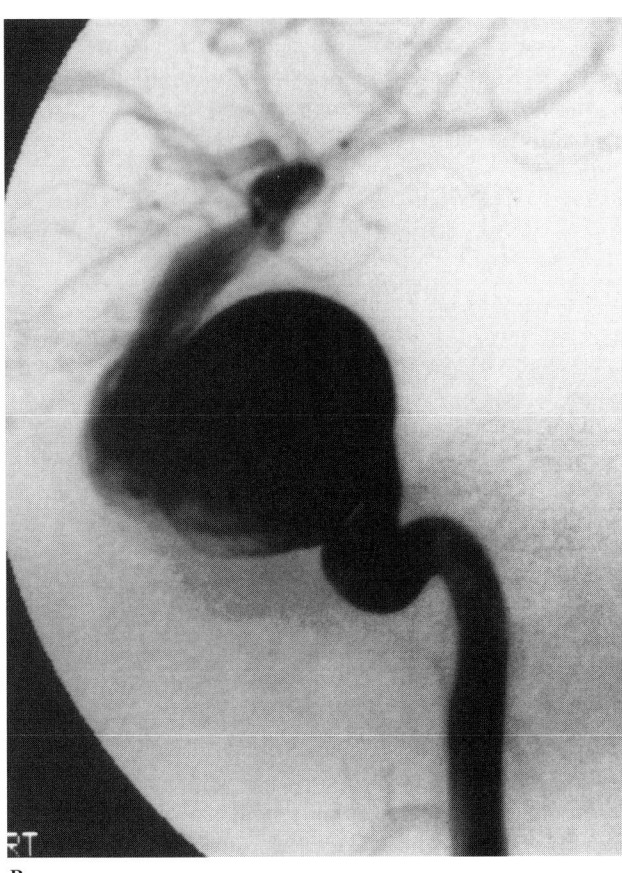

A

B

FIGURE 69.15   (A) Computed tomographic scan with contrast from an 18-year-old patient with a family history of Ehlers-Danlos syndrome type IV and headache reveals a giant aneurysm (*arrow*) of the right intracavernous carotid artery. (B) Right internal carotid angiogram confirms the giant aneurysm of the intracavernous carotid artery. (Reprinted with permission from ES Roach, CF Zimmerman. Ehlers-Danlos Syndrome. In J Bogousslavsky, LR Caplan [eds], Stroke Syndromes. London: Cambridge University Press, 1995;491–496.)

The most common intracranial vessel to develop an aneurysm is the internal carotid artery, typically in the cavernous sinus or just after it emerges from the sinus. Rupture of the aneurysm can occur spontaneously or during vigorous activity. Because the aneurysm is often within the cavernous sinus (see Figure 69.15), rupture often creates a carotid-cavernous fistula. Less often the aneurysm occurs in other intracranial arteries, and these are more likely to present with subarachnoid hemorrhage. In one family, members of three different generations suffered subarachnoid hemorrhage.

Carotid-Cavernous Fistula

Some patients with Ehlers-Danlos syndrome develop a fistula after minor head trauma, but in most it occurs spontaneously. The clinical features of carotid-cavernous fistulae include proptosis, chemosis, diplopia, and pulsatile tinnitus.

Intracranial aneurysms and carotid-cavernous fistulae often occur together. Rupture of an internal carotid artery aneurysm within the cavernous sinus probably causes many of the fistulae, although spontaneous fistula formation without an aneurysm does occur. Postmortem examination of such cases reveals fragmentation of the internal elastic membrane and fibrosis of portions of the carotid wall. Several other arteries may show microscopic ruptures between the media and adventitia. The vascular fragility of type IV Ehlers-Danlos syndrome makes both standard angiography and intravascular occlusion of the fistula difficult. Nevertheless, interventional endovascular occlusion is sometimes successful (Kashiwagi et al. 1993).

Arterial Dissection

Arterial dissection has been documented in most intracranial and extracranial arteries, and the clinical presentation depends primarily on which artery is affected. One patient with a vertebral dissection developed a painful, pulsatile mass of the neck. Dissection of an intrathoracic artery can secondarily occlude cervical vessels, and distal embolism from a dissection can cause cerebral infarction. One adolescent girl with headache and transient hemiparesis had an infarction involving the right internal capsule caused by a dissection of the internal carotid artery.

Surgery is difficult because the arteries are friable and difficult to suture, and handling the tissue leads to tears of the artery or separation of the arterial layers.

PSEUDOXANTHOMA ELASTICUM

Pseudoxanthoma elasticum is a hereditary connective tissue disorder with skin, ophthalmic, and vascular manifestations. The clinical presentation and rate of progression vary considerably, even among affected members of the same family.

Autosomal dominant and autosomal recessive forms of pseudoxanthoma elasticum exist. Both autosomal dominant and autosomal recessive pseudoxanthoma elasticum have been linked to chromosome 16p13.1, suggesting that allelic heterogeneity of a single gene could account for all of the cases (Struk et al. 1997).

Clinical Features

Cutaneous signs consist of yellowish plaques or papules affecting the neck, axilla, abdomen, or the inguinal, decubital, or popliteal areas. Similar looking lesions have been observed in the mucous membranes or intestinal mucosa. Older patients share a facial resemblance because of the lax redundant cutaneous changes of the face and neck. Pregnancy, puberty, and stressful emotional situations may increase the rate of progression of the cutaneous lesions. Although the skin lesions of pseudoxanthoma elasticum become apparent before age 10 in approximately one-half of the patients, occlusive or hemorrhagic vascular complications occur primarily in adults (van Soest et al. 1997).

Angioid streaks of the ocular fundus, the result of ruptures of Bruch's membrane, are found in 85% of patients with pseudoxanthoma elasticum. These ocular lesions are gray or red irregular lines that radiate away from the optic disc. Gradual vision loss may develop from macular degeneration, or vision loss can develop acutely from retinal hemorrhage.

Most of the systemic complications of pseudoxanthoma elasticum result from arterial degeneration and occlusion, but the exact clinical presentation depends largely on which organ system is affected. Progressive occlusion of the large arteries of the limbs may lead to intermittent claudication. Large arteries are sometimes palpably rigid, and radiographs of the extremities sometimes show arterial calcification. Coronary artery disease may occur in young patients with pseudoxanthoma

elasticum (Kevorkian et al. 1997). Gastrointestinal hemorrhage occurs primarily in adults, but also occurs in children. Pregnancy may increase the frequency of gastrointestinal hemorrhage. Epistaxis, hematuria, and hemoptysis occur but less often than gastrointestinal hemorrhage.

Neurological Features

Neurological signs are secondary to vascular compromise. As in other parts of the body, brain dysfunction can result directly from arterial occlusion or rupture or indirectly from systemic hypertension or cardiovascular disease. The onset of cerebrovascular lesions is usually delayed until adulthood, when patients typically present with single or multiple cerebrovascular occlusions resulting from progressive narrowing and then occlusion of an artery. The angiographic pattern resembles that of severe atherosclerosis, but if the occlusion occurs gradually, sufficient collateral flow may develop to prevent stroke. Aneurysms of the intracranial carotid artery are more common than aneurysms of other intracranial arteries.

Early reports of frequent behavioral and psychiatric disturbances were not confirmed by objective psychological testing. Similarly, the percentage of patients with pseudoxanthoma elasticum who have epilepsy does not differ markedly from the general population.

Treatment

Careful control of the systemic blood pressure and avoidance of factors that could exacerbate the vascular lesions might help to minimize arterial complications. Surgery may be required for gastrointestinal bleeding, and surgical bypass grafts may be helpful in restoring blood flow to affected limbs. Surgical correction of intracranial aneurysms may be required. Genetic counseling for the patient and family is recommended.

OSLER-WEBER-RENDU SYNDROME

Hereditary hemorrhagic telangiectasia (HHT), also known as *Osler-Weber-Rendu syndrome*, is an autosomal dominant disorder characterized by telangiectasias of the skin, mucous membranes, and various internal organs. Up to 30% of cases arise from spontaneous mutations. Identical twins with both HHT and intracranial arteriovenous malformation (AVM) have been described, but in general the clinical manifestations and the age of presentation are highly variable.

Cutaneous telangiectasias most often occur on the face, lips, and hands and are less common on the trunk. Telangiectasias of the nasal mucosa cause epistaxis in many patients well before other complications of the disease occur. Approximately one-third of patients have conjunctival telangiectasias and 10% have retinal vascular malformations, although vision loss from these lesions is not common. Telangiectasias are not prominent during the first decade, but thereafter they tend to enlarge and multiply.

Widespread vascular lesions of the lungs, gastrointestinal tract, or genitourinary system can, depending on which site is predominantly affected, produce hemoptysis, hematemesis, melena, or hematuria.

Neurological Features

Neurological complications are common. Frequent complaints include headache, dizziness, and seizures. Less common complications include paradoxical embolism with stroke, intraparenchymal or subarachnoid hemorrhage, and meningitis or cerebral abscess.

Paradoxical embolism through a pulmonary arteriovenous fistula leads to cerebral infarction, although rarely a clot may form within the fistula itself before migrating into the arterial circulation. Intermittent symptoms result from repeated small emboli with subsequent improvement. Transient ischemic attacks during hemoptysis may be caused by air embolism from a bleeding pulmonary arteriovenous fistula. Air within the retinal vessels was noted in one such patient. Approximately 1% of patients develop cerebral abscess or meningitis, probably because septic microemboli bypass the normal filtration of the pulmonary circulation via a pulmonary arteriovenous fistula.

Vascular anomalies may be found anywhere in the brain, spinal cord, or meninges, and more than one type of lesion may be present in the same patient. Intracerebral vascular anomalies occur more often than once suspected. One summary of 90 patients with HHT from the literature listed 17 (19%) with AVMs and 36 (40%) with telangiectasias or angiomas. Although many of these patients remained asymptomatic, others developed either subarachnoid or intracerebral hemorrhage (Kikuchi et al. 1994). HHT should be considered in patients with multiple cerebrovascular malformations.

Intracranial aneurysms are much less common in patients with HHT than AVMs. The number of individuals with both HHT and intracranial aneurysm is so small, in fact, that the association could be purely coincidental. The same is true of spontaneous carotid cavernous fistula. One adult had a fatal subarachnoid hemorrhage from a mycotic aneurysm.

Treatment

As with most of the neurocutaneous syndromes, treatment of HHT is limited to the management of complications. Because many of the neurological complications of the disease arise because of a pulmonary arteriovenous fistula, resection or occlusion of the fistula has been recommended.

Periodic transfusion and chronic iron administration may be necessary. One child with HHT and platelet sequestration syndrome was treated successfully with aspirin.

PROGERIA

Hutchinson-Gilford syndrome or progeria (derived from *pro*, before, and *geras*, old age) is a rare condition characterized by premature aging (Figure 69.16) and the early occurrence of age-related complications. The estimated prevalence is 1 in 8 million.

Patients with progeria do not reproduce and most do not have affected family members. Some of the children with affected siblings have had atypical features leading to debate about the genetic nature of progeria. Both autosomal dominant and recessive traits have been proposed, but the clinical pattern is perhaps best explained by a dominant trait, usually arising via spontaneous mutation, with occasional instances of germline mosaicism in the families with affected siblings.

The pathogenesis of progeria has not been well characterized. In one study, cultured fibroblasts derived from a person with progeria reached senescence earlier than control cells, and patient fibroblasts had reduced levels of mRNA coding for the macromolecules of the extracellular matrix. It is tempting to speculate that progeria could result from an abnormality of telomerase, shown to determine the number of cell replications before cellular senescence.

Clinical Features

Clinical changes of progeria usually become apparent during the first 2 years of life. Some features may be subtle initially but become progressively more severe over time. Alopecia, for example, may not be present at first, but is almost universal by adolescence. The most common early features are short stature, decreased subcutaneous fat stores, joint restriction, and alopecia (see Figure 69.16). Skeletal changes include thinning of the bones, coxa valga, and small clavicles; some children have repeated poorly healing fractures. The characteristic physical appearance of progeria results from a combination of postural changes, decreased subcutaneous fat, alopecia, and facial hypoplasia and micrognathia.

Children with progeria eventually develop premature atherosclerosis, leading to coronary artery disease or stroke (see Figure 69.16) (Matsuo et al. 1994). Heart disease is the chief cause of death. Survival into middle age has been described, but death during the second decade is typical.

Other syndromes that cause signs of premature aging or carotid occlusion constitute the differential diagnosis of progeria. Werner's syndrome is an autosomal recessive disorder characterized by cataracts, scleroderma with subcutaneous calcium deposition, a beaklike nose, and the

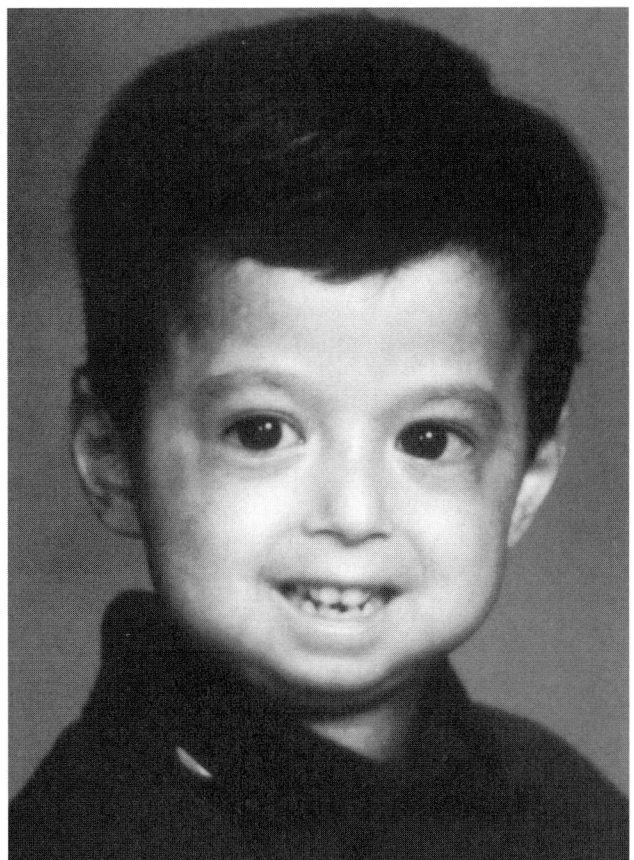

A

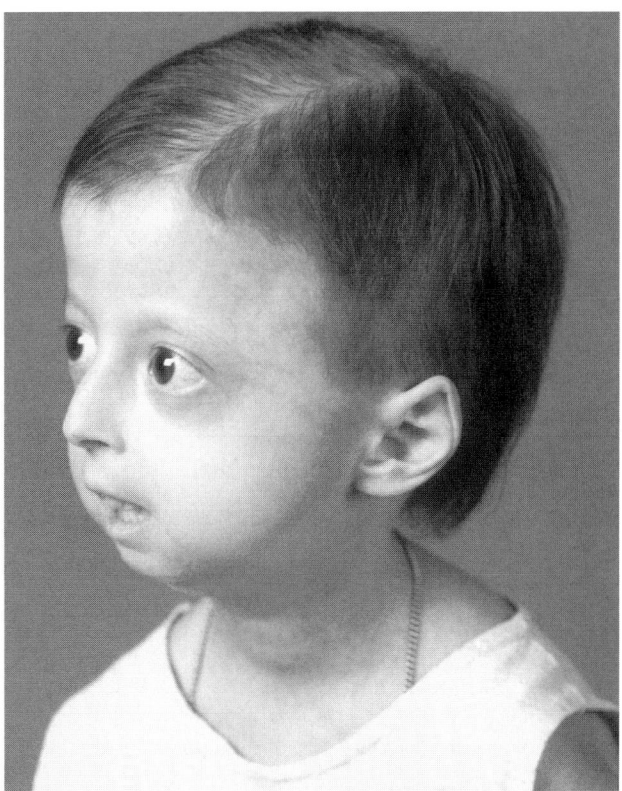

B

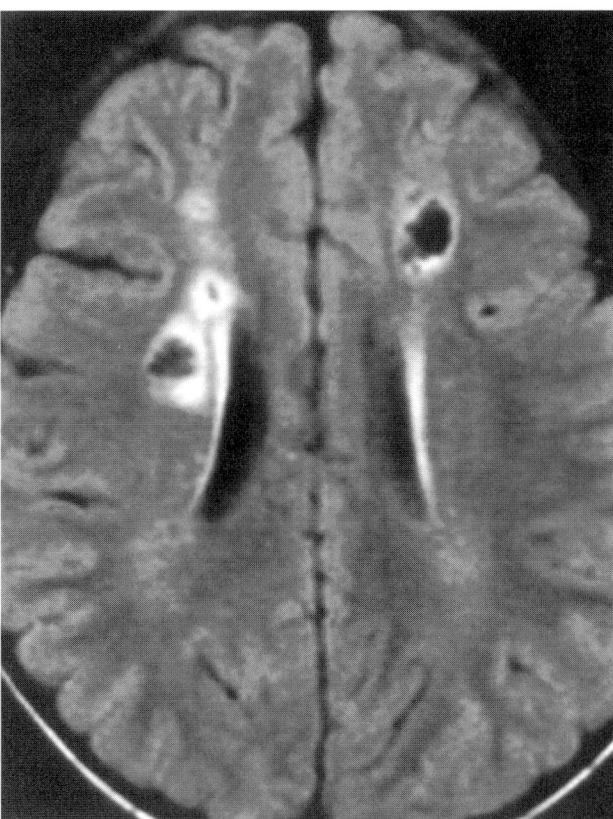

C

FIGURE 69.16 Premature aging syndrome in a young boy. (A) School picture before onset of neurological symptoms. (B) Later picture showing hair thinning, loss of subcutaneous fat, and stooped posture. (C) Magnetic resonance imaging scan showing bilateral cerebral infarctions of varying ages.

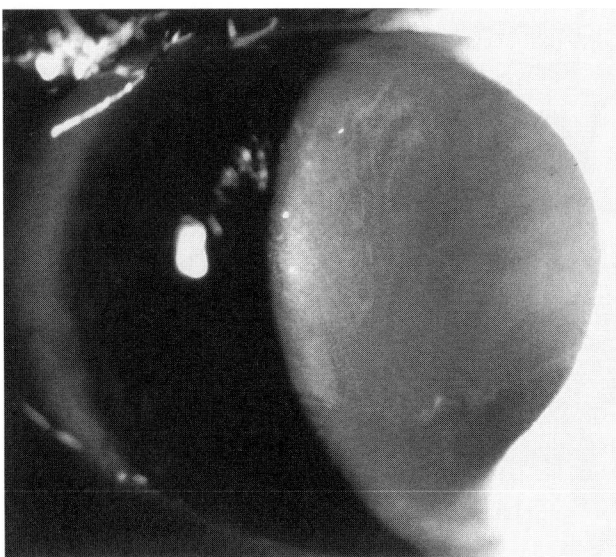

FIGURE 69.17 Characteristic swirling corneal opacity in a patient with Fabry's disease. (Courtesy of Dr. Carol F. Zimmerman.)

premature appearance of disorders usually associated with aging, such as graying of the hair, senile macular degeneration, osteoporosis, diabetes, malignancies, and atherosclerosis. Werner's syndrome has been described as adult progeria. Affected individuals often live well into adulthood, and, even so, death from cardiac disease and stroke seem to be less common than in patients with progeria. Mandibuloacral dysplasia is another autosomal recessive disorder that features alopecia and short stature, along with clavicular and mandibular hypoplasia, stiff joints, and persistently open cranial sutures. Whether this is an entirely distinct condition is still in question.

FABRY'S DISEASE

Fabry's disease (angiokeratoma corporis diffusum) is caused by deficiency of α-galactosidase A. Fabry's is an X-linked lysosomal storage disease with minimal penetrance in female subjects and complete penetrance in male subjects. The diagnosis is confirmed by enzyme analysis in cultured leukocytes or fibroblasts.

Clinical Features

Patients with Fabry's disease develop dark red or purple papules that tend to occur in clusters around the umbilicus or on the buttocks, scrotum, hips, or thighs. The size and number of the cutaneous lesions gradually increase with age, though the lesions themselves are asymptomatic.

Ocular abnormalities caused by Fabry's disease do not usually result in vision loss but may lead one to suspect the disease. Corneal deposits with a whorl-like pattern (Figure 69.17) are characteristic. In addition, the anterior capsule deposits and abnormalities of the conjunctival vessels are sometimes apparent.

The symptoms of Fabry's disease usually begin during the first decade with temperature-sensitive painful dysesthesias of the distal limbs. The pain often develops before the appearance of the characteristic cutaneous lesions or when the cutaneous findings are subtle.

Both cerebral thrombosis and hemorrhage occur with Fabry's disease, although thrombosis is more common. Brain hemorrhage can occur even without systemic hypertension from renal failure. Most of the patients with cerebrovascular complications are in their third or fourth decade, but occasional teenagers are affected. Cerebral hemispheric lesions with hemiplegia and aphasia are the most common deficits but various brainstem lesions have been described. Rarely, a stroke is the first manifestation of Fabry's disease (Grewal 1994).

The painful dysesthesias result from the sensory neuropathy caused by Fabry's disease. Nerve biopsies reveal preferential loss of small myelinated and unmyelinated nerve fibers and also loss of the smaller cell bodies of the spinal ganglia. Glycolipid inclusion granules are deposited within the cytoplasm of the perineural and vascular endothelial cells.

As the disease progresses, the accumulation of glycolipid in the arterial endothelium and vascular smooth muscle cells results in progressive narrowing and occlusion of the vascular lumen. Vascular changes can be found throughout the body, including the kidney, and renal failure (beginning in early adulthood) is the most common cause of death in Fabry's disease.

Treatment

No completely effective treatment is available for Fabry's disease. Infusion of the deficient enzyme reduces the ceramide trihexoside level but is not clinically useful. Likewise, plasmapheresis reduces the level of circulating ceramide trihexoside, but it has not been determined whether the procedure will reduce the long-term complications of the disease. Renal transplantation alleviates renal failure; in some patients, renal transplantation also provides enough enzyme activity to improve symptoms and possibly delay the systemic complications. Carbamazepine or phenytoin may offer symptomatic relief from the painful paresthesias, but they do not reduce the vascular complications. Bone marrow transplantation is a potentially useful treatment.

LESCH-NYHAN DISEASE

Lesch-Nyhan disease is an X-linked disorder of purine metabolism resulting from deficiency of hypoxanthine guanine-phosphoribosyl transferase. The clinical features include hypotonia, delayed developmental milestones, choreoathetosis, and nonprogressive mental deficiency. Self-mutilation (Figure 69.18) eventually develops in virtually all patients, although usually after hypotonia, chorea, or developmental delay.

Although self-abusive behavior is a nonspecific feature of various neurological and psychiatric conditions, children with mental retardation or behavioral disorders typically exhibit head banging, face slapping, or other nondirected behavior. Abuse targeted to the digits, tongue, and lips suggests Lesch-Nyhan disease or congenital sensory neuropathy. Children with acquired sensory neuropathy occasionally develop self-mutilation as well.

Pathogenesis

Brain histopathology and electron microscopy are usually normal or show only nonspecific abnormalities. One adult had abnormal sural nerve findings at autopsy, but sensory nerve biopsies in younger patients are usually normal or exhibit only minor nonspecific changes (Roach et al. 1996).

Various lines of evidence suggest that self-mutilation by Lesch-Nyhan patients may be caused by an imbalance of dopaminergic activity in the striatum (Ernst et al. 1996), but therapeutic measures based on this dopaminergic model have been disappointing in clinical trials on human subjects.

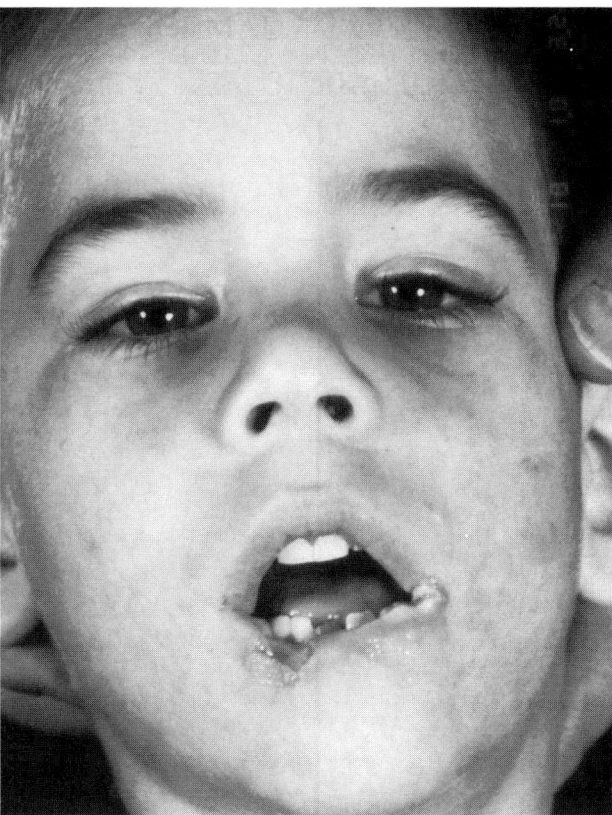

FIGURE 69.18 A child with Lesch-Nyhan disease with self-mutilation of his lower lip. (Courtesy of Dr. Mauricio R. Delgado.)

Treatment

Numerous medications (including L-5-hydroxytryptophan, haloperidol, pimozide, diazepam, L-dopa, and many others) and behavior management techniques have been tried without success. Allopurinol prevents the formation of uric acid renal stones but does not affect either the self-mutilation or the neurological impairment. An uncontrolled trial with four patients suggested that carbamazepine might reduce self-abusive behavior caused by Lesch-Nyhan disease (Roach et al. 1996). Most patients require dental extraction and constant restraint of the arms to prevent trauma.

STURGE-WEBER SYNDROME

Sturge-Weber syndrome (SWS) is characterized by a facial cutaneous angioma (port-wine nevus) and an associated leptomeningeal and brain angioma, typically ipsilateral to the facial lesion. In addition to the facial nevus, other findings include mental retardation, contralateral hemiparesis and hemiatrophy, and homonymous hemianopia (Bodensteiner and Roach 1998). However, the clinical features are highly variable, and patients with the cutaneous lesion and seizures but with normal intelligence and no focal neurological deficit are common. The syndrome occurs sporadically and in all races.

Cutaneous Features

The nevus classically involves the forehead and upper eyelid, but it often affects both sides of the face and may extend onto the trunk and extremities (Figure 69.19). Patients whose nevus involves only the trunk, or the maxillary or mandibular area but not the upper face, have little risk of an intracranial angioma. The facial angioma is usually obvious at birth, but occasional patients have the characteristic neurological and radiographic features of SWS, yet have no skin lesion. More frequently, the typical cutaneous and ophthalmic findings are present without clinical or radiographic evidence of an intracranial lesion. Only 10–20% of children with a port-wine nevus of the forehead have a leptomeningeal angioma. Although the leptomeningeal angioma is typically ipsilateral to a unilateral facial nevus, bilateral brain lesions occur in at least 15% of patients, including some with a unilateral cutaneous nevus.

Ocular Features

Glaucoma is the main ophthalmologic problem of patients with SWS (Sujansky and Conradi 1995a). In one study, 36 of 51 patients (71%) had glaucoma; in 26, glaucoma devel-

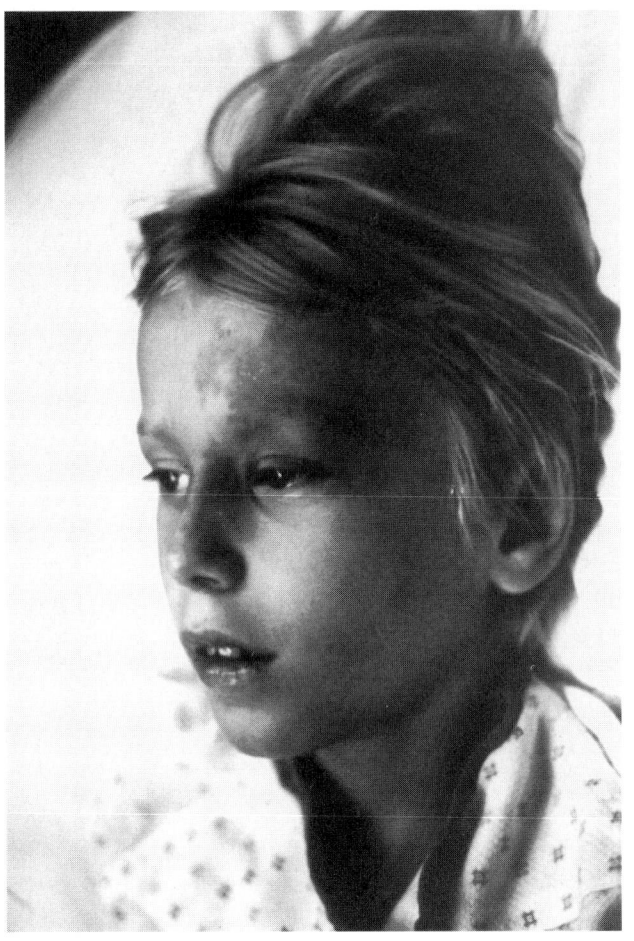
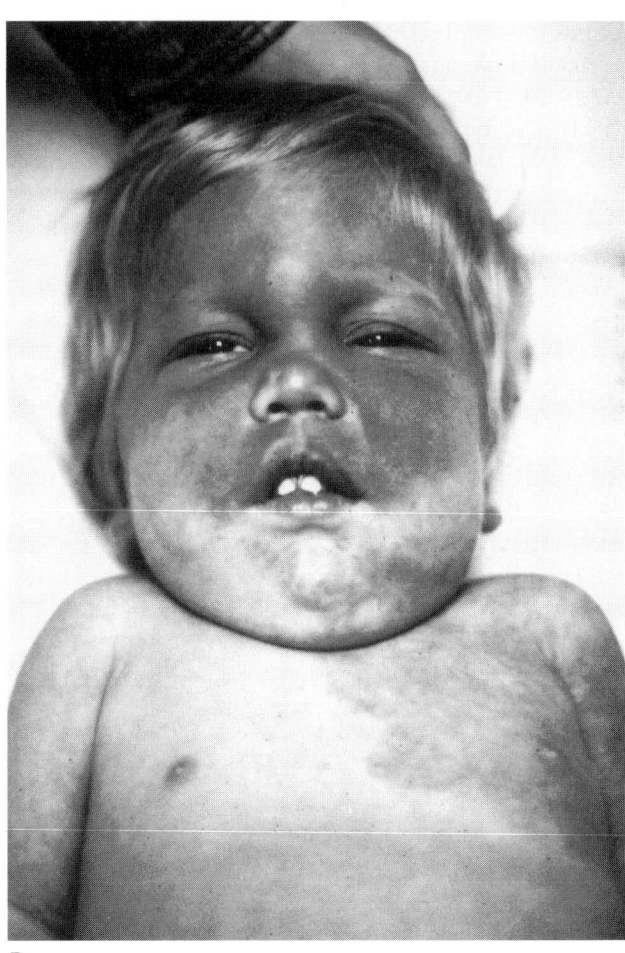

A   B

FIGURE 69.19   **(A)** A patient with the classic distribution of the port-wine nevus of Sturge-Weber syndrome on the upper face and eyelid. (Reprinted with permission from ES Roach. Congenital Cutaneovascular Syndromes. In PV Vinken, GW Bruyn, HL Klawans [eds], Handbook of Clinical Neurology [Vol. 11]. Vascular Diseases. Amsterdam: Elsevier, 1989;443–462.) **(B)** Another patient whose port-wine nevus involves both sides of the face and extends onto the left trunk and arm. (Reprinted with permission from ES Roach, AR Riela. Pediatric Cerebrovascular Disorders [2nd ed]. New York: Futura, 1995.)

oped by age 2 years. The risk of developing glaucoma is highest in the first decade, but young adults occasionally develop glaucoma. Buphthalmos and amblyopia are present in some newborns, evidently caused by an anomalous anterior chamber angle. In other patients, the glaucoma becomes symptomatic later and, if not treated, causes progressive blindness. Periodic measurement of the intraocular pressure is mandatory, particularly when the nevus is near the eye.

Neurological Features

Epileptic seizures, mental retardation, and focal neurological deficits are the principal neurological abnormalities of SWS. Seizures usually start acutely in conjunction with hemiparesis. The age when symptoms begin and the overall clinical severity are variable, but onset of seizures before 2 years of age tends to increase the likelihood of future men-

tal retardation and refractory epilepsy. Patients with refractory seizures are more likely to be mentally retarded, whereas patients who have never had seizures are typically normal. Few patients who remain normal past age 3 later develop severe intellectual impairment.

Seizures eventually develop in 72–80% of patients with SWS with unilateral lesions and in 93% of patients with bihemispheric involvement. Seizures can begin anytime from birth to adulthood, but 75% of seizures begin during the first year, 86% by age 2, and 95% before age 5. Thus, the risk of a child developing seizures is highest in the first 2 years and thereafter diminishes.

Focal motor seizures or generalized tonic-clonic seizures are most typical of SWS initially, but infantile spasms, myoclonic seizures, and atonic seizures occur. The first few seizures are often focal even in patients who later develop generalized tonic-clonic seizures or infantile spasms. Older children and adults are more likely to have complex partial seizures or focal motor seizures. Some patients continue to have daily seizures after the initial deterioration in spite of various daily anticonvulsant medications, whereas others have long seizure-free intervals, sometimes even without medication, punctuated by clusters of seizures.

The neurological impairment caused by SWS depends in part on the site of the intracranial vascular lesion. Because the occipital region is frequently involved, visual field deficits are common. Hemiparesis often develops acutely, in conjunction with the initial flurry of seizures. Although often attributed to post-ictal weakness, hemiparesis may be permanent or persist much longer than the few hours typical of a postictal deficit. Some children suddenly develop weakness without seizures, either as repeated episodes of weakness similar to transient ischemic attacks or as a single strokelike episode with persistent deficit. In patients with both hemiparesis and seizures, it is difficult to establish which came first. Not all patients have permanent focal neurological signs.

Early developmental milestones are usually normal, but mild to profound mental deficiency eventually develops in approximately one-half of patients with SWS (Sujansky and Conradi 1995b). Only 8% of the patients with bilateral brain involvement are intellectually normal. Behavioral abnormalities are often a problem even in patients who are not mentally retarded. The clinical condition eventually stabilizes, leaving a patient who has residual hemiparesis, hemianopia, retardation, and epilepsy but without further deterioration. Contrary to what might be expected, intracranial hemorrhage is rare.

Diagnostic Studies

Most of the children with facial port-wine nevi do not have an intracranial angioma, and neuroimaging studies and other tests help to distinguish the children with SWS from those with an isolated cutaneous lesion. Although gyral calcification is a typical feature of SWS, the trolley track appearance first described on standard radiographs is uncommon and is almost never present in neonates. Intracranial calcification can be demonstrated much earlier with CT (Figure 69.20) than with standard skull films. Extensive cerebral atrophy is apparent even with CT, but subtle atrophy is more readily demonstrated by MRI.

MRI with gadolinium contrast (Figure 69.21) effectively demonstrates the abnormal intracranial vessels in patients with SWS and is currently the best test to determine intracranial involvement. MR angiography has been used to directly image the larger abnormal vessels. Functional imaging with positron emission tomography (see Chapter 38E) demonstrates reduced metabolism of the brain adjacent to the leptomeningeal lesion. However, patients with recent-onset seizures may have increased cerebral metabolism near the lesion. Single-photon emission tomography shows reduced perfusion of the affected brain. Both positron emis-

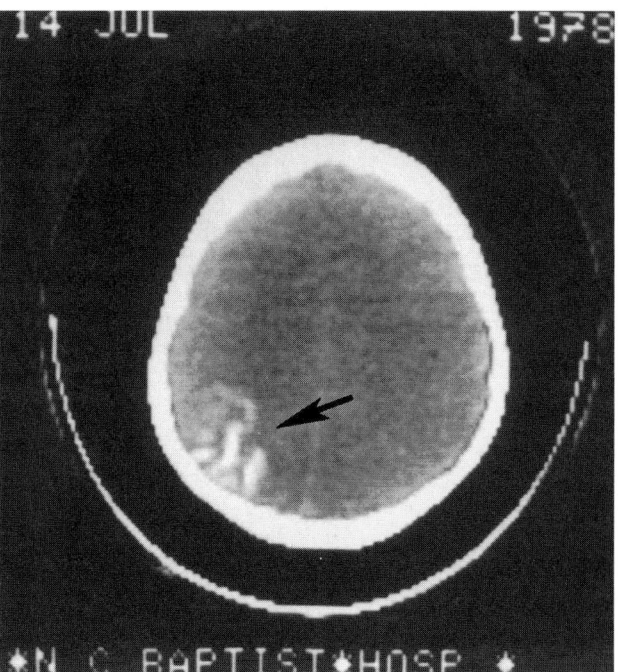

FIGURE 69.20 Computed tomographic scan from a typical patient with Sturge-Weber syndrome; the gyriform calcification pattern (*arrow*) is easily seen in the left occipital area. (Reprinted with permission from JC Garcia, ES Roach, WT McClean. Recurrent thrombotic deterioration in the Sturge-Weber syndrome. Childs Brain 1981;8:427–433.)

sion tomography and single-photon emission tomography often reveal vascular changes extending well beyond the area of abnormality depicted by CT (Maria et al. 1998). Although functional imaging may not be necessary for all patients, these tests may help to initially establish a diagnosis and may help localize the lesion before surgery.

Cerebral arteriography (see Chapter 38C) is no longer a routine procedure in the evaluation of SWS, but it is sometimes useful in atypical patients or prior to surgery for epilepsy. The veins are more abnormal than the arteries. The subependymal and medullary veins are enlarged and tortuous, and the superficial cortical veins are sparse. Failure of the sagittal sinus to opacify after ipsilateral carotid injection may be secondary to obliteration of the superficial cortical veins by thrombosis, and the abnormal deep venous channels probably have a similar origin as they form collateral conduits for nonfunctioning cortical veins.

Treatment

Generally, the more extensive the intracranial lesion, the more difficult it is to fully control seizures with medication. Nevertheless, complete seizure control is possible in some children. In one study, one-half of the patients achieved complete seizure control and an additional 39% had partial control.

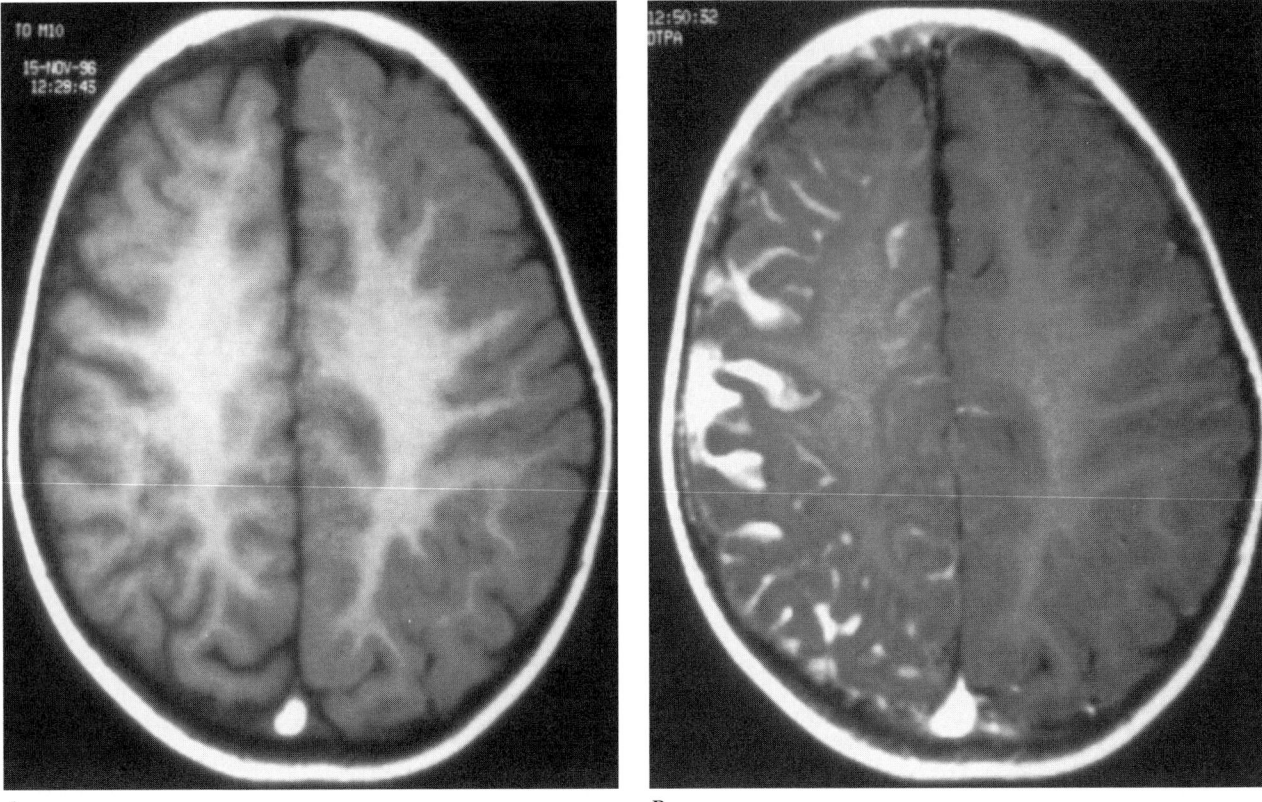

A   B

FIGURE 69.21 (A) Magnetic resonance imaging study from a child with Sturge-Weber syndrome; this T1-weighted axial view without contrast infusion is normal. (B) On the coronal view with gadolinium, the scan reveals a left frontal leptomeningeal and intraparenchymal angioma.

Hemispherectomy sometimes improves seizure control and may promote more normal intellectual development (Carson et al. 1996). Early hemispherectomy has been recommended for patients whose seizures begin in infancy. Resection of the area predominantly affected can be effective, and corpus callosum section may be useful for occasional patients with extensive disease. Despite the general agreement that surgical resection is effective, there remains some debate about patient selection and the timing of surgery. Almost one patient in five has bilateral cerebral lesions, limiting the surgical options unless one hemisphere is clearly causing most of the seizures. Most physicians do not feel comfortable recommending surgery in a patient who has not yet developed seizures or one whose seizures are fully controlled with medication, and there is also understandable reluctance to resect a still functional portion of the brain and thereby cause a deficit. Thus, surgery is usually reserved for patients with severe seizures who do not respond to medication and who already have clinical dysfunction of the area to be removed (e.g., hemiparesis or hemianopia).

Surgical guidelines have been developed for patients with SWS. Hemispherectomy should be reserved for patients with clinically significant seizures who fail to respond to an adequate trial of anticonvulsants. Surgery should not be done automatically just because the diagnosis of SWS is made. Surgery should only be done in a center with an ongoing program in pediatric epilepsy surgery and age-appropriate facilities for preoperative and postoperative care. Patients with less extensive lesions should have a limited resection, rather than a complete hemispherectomy, that preserves as much normal brain as possible, even at the risk of having to do another operation later. Corpus callosotomy should be reserved for patients with refractory tonic or atonic seizures. In effect, a similar approach should be used in children with SWS as with other epileptic patients.

PROGRESSIVE FACIAL HEMIATROPHY

Progressive facial hemiatrophy (Parry-Romberg syndrome) occurs sporadically. The relationship of this disorder to *en coup de sabre*, morphea, and linear scleroderma is still debated (Peterson et al. 1996). Traditionally, progressive facial hemiatrophy is said to have more involvement of the upper cranium, whereas *en coup de sabre* tends to affect the lower face as well. Scleroderma and morphea affect other parts of the body. However, the pathogenesis of the conditions is poorly understood, and they may prove to have a similar origin. An arbitrary distinction based on the anatomical distribution does have at least one practical use: As a rule, only patients whose upper face and head are affected are likely to develop cerebral complications.

Clinical Features

Progressive facial hemiatrophy is characterized by unilateral atrophy of the skin, subcutaneous tissue, and adjacent bone. The atrophic area is characteristically oblong or linear and sometimes begins as a raised erythematous lesion. The lesion sometimes begins after trauma to the area. The atrophy eventually stabilizes, leaving the patient disfigured.

Epilepsy is probably the most common neurological problem in patients with progressive facial hemiatrophy, and several patients have developed a usually mild hemiparesis. Various other neurological signs and symptoms occur less frequently, including cognitive impairment, cranial neuropathy, or even brainstem signs. One patient developed an intracranial arterial aneurysm (Schievink et al. 1996). Both cerebral calcifications and white matter lesions are probably common (Fry et al. 1992) (Figure 69.22).

The cause of progressive facial hemiatrophy and related disorders is poorly understood. Various mechanisms (e.g., cortical dysgenesis, dysfunction of the sympathetic nervous system, chronic localized meningoencephalitis) have been proposed, but none of these mechanisms adequately explains all of the clinical findings of the syndrome. Others have suggested that progressive facial hemiatrophy results from an autoimmune process. Nevertheless, the pathogenesis remains obscure (Fry et al. 1992).

ATAXIA-TELANGIECTASIA

Ataxia-telangiectasia (AT) is a neurodegenerative disorder whose onset is marked by slowly progressive ataxia that usually begins in early childhood, telangiectases (dilated small blood vessels), immunodeficiency, and cellular sensitivity to ionizing radiation. The classic skin findings of AT are distinctive telangiectases most prominently involving the sclerae, earlobes, and bridge of the nose. Less common sites of telangiectases include the eyelids, neck, and antecubital and popliteal fossae. The occurrence of these telangiectases in a child with progressive ataxia is probably pathognomonic for AT. The most striking non-neurological feature of AT is an increased frequency of sinopulmonary infections and a dramatically increased risk for malignancy of the lymphoreticular system, especially leukemia and lymphoma. Estimates of the prevalence of AT, an autosomal

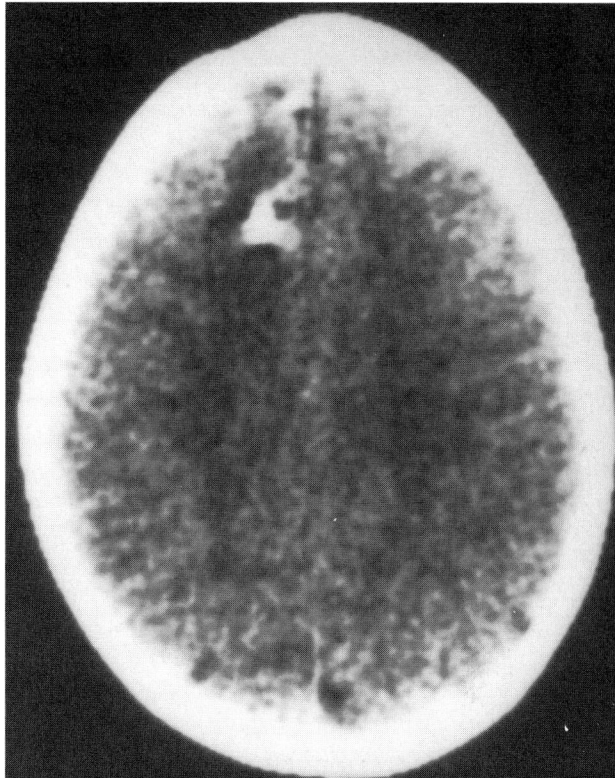

FIGURE 69.22   Computed tomographic scan revealing right frontal encephalopatitis and calcification in a patient with progressive facial hemiatrophy.

recessive disorder affecting male and female subjects equally, range from 1 in 40,000 to 1 in 100,000. The gene frequency is as high as 1% in the general population.

Cutaneous Features

Telangiectases typically do not develop until early childhood, years after the onset of ataxia, usually between the ages of 3 and 6 years. Two other dermatological features of AT that may be overlooked are hypertrichosis and infrequent gray hairs (Gatti 1995). Hypertrichosis is noticeable particularly over the forearms. These features are often overlooked but in the context of a child with slowly progressive ataxia they provide clues to the correct diagnosis. Progeric changes such as poikiloderma, loss of subcutaneous fat, and sclerosis also have been associated with AT. Other skin lesions rarely are associated with AT, including seborrheic dermatitis, café au lait macules, vitiligo, acanthosis nigricans, and eczema, though whether these lesions are causally linked to AT is uncertain. Basal cell carcinomas in young adults have been reported and may be caused by abnormal radiosensitivity. Cutaneous granulomas, commonly associated with immunodeficiency states such as severe combined immunodeficiency and X-linked hypogammaglobulinemia, may appear as the initial cutaneous manifestation of AT.

Neurological Features

Ataxia is usually the first manifestation of AT and it appears approximately when the child learns to walk, around 12 months. Truncal ataxia predominates, especially early in the course of the disorder, so that sitting balance and gait are primarily affected. Muscle strength is normal and early gross motor milestones tend to be reached on time. The ataxia is slowly progressive, and children typically require a wheelchair by the age of 12 years. As the child matures, limb ataxia, intention tremor, and segmental myoclonus become apparent. Choreoathetosis may be difficult to distinguish from dysmetria and intention tremor, but it may dominate the clinical picture in older children. At times the choreoathetosis may resemble segmental myoclonus of the extremities or trunk. Progressive dystonia of the fingers may appear as the child matures into the second and third decades of life. Axial muscles are affected also, and the patient gradually develops a stooped posture.

Abnormal eye movements are nearly universal in children with AT. Voluntary ocular motility is impaired; nystagmus and apraxias of voluntary gaze such as disorders of smooth pursuit and limitation of upgaze are the most common abnormalities. Oculomotor apraxia may precede appearance of the telangiectases but is often misidentified as an "attention-getting" behavior. Strabismus is seen in many young children with AT, but it is often transient and corrective surgery is not required.

In adult patients with AT the neurological symptoms include progressive distal muscular atrophy with fasciculations, although proximal strength is relatively preserved. Involvement of the spinal cord dorsal columns in AT is indicated by the gradual loss of vibration and position sense, and neuropathological and electrophysiological studies reveal a peripheral polyneuropathy.

Serial brain imaging in older children and adults shows nonprogressive cerebellar and panvermian atrophy (Sardanelli et al. 1995). Autopsy studies have confirmed the radiographical impression of cerebellar degeneration, with reduced numbers of Purkinje cells, granular and basket cells of the cortex, and neurons in the vermal nuclei. In older patients more extensive degenerative changes are seen, including the substantia nigra, brainstem nuclei, and spinal cord. The cerebral cortex is relatively spared, which one would expect given that significant neuropsychological deficits are unusual in AT.

Immunodeficiency and Cancer Risk

Approximately 10–15% of patients with AT develop a lymphoid malignancy by early adulthood (Taylor et al. 1996). T-cell acute lymphatic leukemia and T-cell lymphomas are more common than B-cell tumors, although both are more frequent than in the general population. This increased risk of T-cell tumors may be caused by the increase in chromosomal rearrangement observed in T lymphocytes from patients with AT. Presumably, the AT mutation allows a large increase in the number of translocations formed during recombination that leads to an increased risk of leukemia. T-cell tumors may occur at any age, whereas B-cell lymphomas tend to arise in older children.

Many other tumor types have been reported in association with AT, including dysgerminoma, gastric carcinoma, liver carcinoma, retinoblastoma, and pancreatic carcinoma. In fact, nonlymphoid tumors, primarily carcinomas, represent approximately 20% of all malignancies in patients with AT. Solid gynecological tumors (ovarian and uterine) are common in patients with AT, and female relatives of patients with AT appear to have an increased risk of breast cancer. Cerebellar astrocytoma, medulloblastoma, and glioma also have been linked to AT in case reports.

Frequent sinopulmonary infections are another characteristic of AT. Recurrent or chronic sinusitis, bronchitis, pneumonia, and chronic progressive bronchiectasis were frequent causes of death in patients with AT in previous years but now usually respond to antibiotic treatment. However, bronchiolitis obliterans was noted in four immunodeficient AT patients who died of respiratory failure associated with pulmonary infection by cytomegalovirus, mycoplasma, and *Pseudomonas aeruginosa*. The thymus gland in patients with AT is often small or absent on chest roentgenography and at autopsy may be only rudimentary.

Nijmegen breakage syndrome (NBS), a rare autosomal recessive disorder, is one of a family of disorders including Bloom's syndrome, Fanconi's anemia, and AT that are characterized by specific cellular defects in response to DNA-damaging agents. Clinically, NBS is characterized by microcephaly, a birdlike facial appearance, growth retardation, immunodeficiency, frequent sinopulmonary infections, chromosomal instability, radiation sensitivity, and an increased susceptibility to malignancies, particularly lymphomas. However, patients with NBS lack many of the clinical hallmarks of AT such as progressive cerebellar ataxia, oculocutaneous telangiectasia, and elevated serum α-fetoprotein levels. Abundant evidence now exists from genetic and cell biology studies that NBS is a separate disorder from AT that arises from mutations in a yet unidentified gene.

Laboratory Diagnosis

Useful laboratory tests in the diagnosis of AT include serum α-fetoprotein, immunoglobulins, and cellular radiosensitivity tests. Nearly all patients with AT have an elevated α-fetoprotein, and approximately 80% have decreased serum IgA, IgE, or IgG. Especially characteristic is a selective deficiency of the IgG2 subclass. Some patients with clinical features of AT (progressive childhood-onset ataxia with typical telangiectases) have normal serum α-fetoprotein and immunoglobulin levels. Characteristic cellular features of AT are reduced cell life span in culture, cytoskeletal abnormalities, chromosomal instability, hypersensitivity to ionizing radiation and radiomimetic agents, defective radiation-induced checkpoints at the G_1, S, and G_2 phases of the cell cycle, and defects in several signal transduction pathways (Rotman and Shiloh 1997).

The gene associated with AT (*ATM*) is a large gene located at chromosome 11q22-23 and more than 100 *ATM* mutations occurring in patients with AT have been discovered. These mutations are broadly distributed throughout the *ATM* gene. Although the function of the *ATM* gene product is not completely understood, it belongs to a family of large proteins involved in cell-cycle progression and checkpoint response to DNA damage. It is postulated that *ATM* is activated specifically by oxidative damage or stress, initiating signal transduction pathways responsible for protecting cells from such insults. Thus, the production of reactive oxygen species by ionizing radiation may play an important role in mutagenesis in cells with absent or abnormal *ATM*.

The high risk of malignancy in AT underscores the importance of early diagnosis in affected individuals and subsequent routine surveillance for leukemia and lymphoma. Treatment of the neurological deficits is symptomatic at present. Whether neuroprotective medications such as calcium-channel blockers, antioxidants, and medications that modulate neuronal growth factors can slow neurodegeneration in AT is unknown.

Table 69.4: Neurological and systemic features of infantile-onset kinky hair syndrome

Premature birth, low birth weight
Neonatal jaundice
Hypothermia
Decreased facial expression
Prominent forehead
Full cheeks
Narrow palate
Hypopigmented skin
Cutis laxa
Pili torti
Inguinal hernia
Hepatomegaly
Deafness
Bladder diverticula
Joint laxity
Skeletal anomalies
    Pectus excavatum
    Wormian skull bones
    Metaphyseal spurring of long bones
Ataxia
Seizures
Intracranial hemorrhage
Neuroimaging findings
    Cerebellar and cerebral atrophy
    White matter abnormalities
    Subdural fluid collections
    Dilatated and tortuous intracranial and extracranial blood vessels
    Cerebral edema

KINKY HAIR SYNDROME

Kinky hair syndrome, also known as *Menkes' disease* or *trichopoliodystrophy*, is an X-linked disorder of connective tissue and neuronal metabolism caused by inborn disorders of copper metabolism. The frequency of kinky hair syndrome is estimated to be 1 in 40,000 to 1 in 298,000 live births. In the classic form of kinky hair syndrome the neurological symptoms begin in the first year of life and the course is rapidly progressive, but late-onset cases and apparently asymptomatic individuals have been described. Typical findings are listed in Table 69.4.

Cutaneous Features

Connective tissue abnormalities are a major feature of kinky hair syndrome, leading to symptoms such as loose skin, hyperextensible joints, bladder diverticula, and skeletal anomalies. The hair is light colored and brittle and on microscopic examination (Figure 69.23) appears as pili torti (twisted hair) and trichorrhexis nodosa (complete or incomplete fractures of the hair shafts at regular intervals). Trichorrhexis nodosa is not pathognomonic of kinky hair syndrome; it is also seen in biotinidase deficiency and argininosuccinic aciduria. Skin may be normal or diffusely hypopigmented.

Other Clinical Features

Variants of kinky hair syndrome have been described, with symptoms covering a clinical continuum from nearly normal to the severe classic infantile-onset form. One allelic variant of kinky hair syndrome is the occipital horn syndrome (also known as *type IX Ehlers-Danlos* or *X-linked cutis laxa*) in which the connective tissue symptoms predominate. This disorder is named for the characteristic exostoses resulting from calcification of the trapezius and sternocleidomastoid muscles at their attachment to the occipital skull. Metaphyseal fractures may occur, and bladder diverticula and skeletal changes (osteoporosis, coxa valga, short clavicles with hammer-shaped distal ends, and deformations of the long bones) are additional symptoms. Cognitive and motor development in this variant may be normal, slightly delayed, or severely affected. Mutations of the *ATP7A* gene in the patients with the occipital horn syndrome have been base pair substitutions affecting normal mRNA splicing (Tumer and Horn 1997).

Neurological Features

In early-onset cases, infants are normal at birth except for temperature instability. Within a few weeks or months affected infants become hypotonic, and poor feeding may

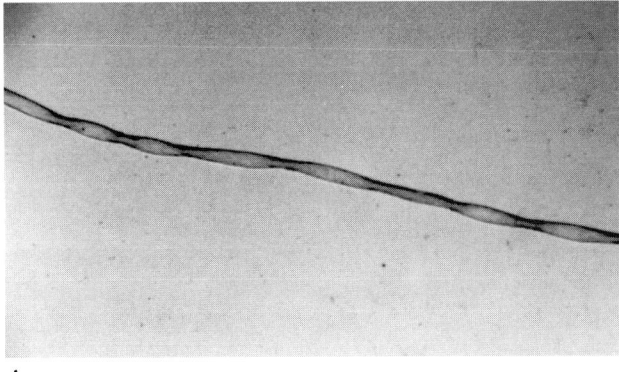

A

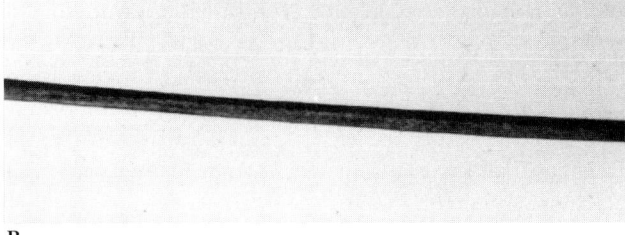

B

FIGURE 69.23   (A) Hair shaft from a patient with kinky hair disease. (B) Normal hair.

lead to failure to thrive. Infants appear unusually suscepti- ble to sepsis and are often intolerant of heat. Chronic diar- rhea is common but not invariable. Hypotonia gradually develops into spastic quadriparesis with clenched fists, opisthotonus, and scissoring. Seizures are a prominent fea- ture of this disorder and may be partial or generalized; myoclonic seizures are especially common. Some of the neu- roimaging findings are diffuse brain atrophy, subdural effu- sions or hemorrhages, infarction, edema, and abnormal white matter signal. One infant who developed neurological symptoms shortly after birth had cranial MRI at 5 weeks of age that showed early cerebellar atrophy and hypomyelina- tion (Geller et al. 1997).

Less common is a later-onset variant with milder symp- toms. This indicates that symptoms of this disorder form a continuum from neonatal onset with rapid deterioration to adult onset with slow progression of symptoms and long- term survival. A few affected female subjects have been described; diagnosis was confirmed on the basis of low cop- per content in liver and high copper content in an intestinal biopsy sample. Clinical features in these girls were similar to but milder than those seen in typical neonatal-onset cases, and genetic analysis indicated that the normal X chromosome in these girls was inactivated.

Intracranial and extracranial blood vessels may be tortu- ous, kinked, and dilated (Kim and Suh 1997), which may be caused by defective or deficient elastin fibers in the walls of these blood vessels. Neuropathological studies show diffuse neuronal loss and gliosis that is particularly prominent in the cerebrum and cerebellum. Microscopic findings include abnormal dendritic arborization in the cerebellar cortex; Purkinje cells may have a Medusa-head appearance, and cells in the molecular layer may resemble weeping willows.

Neuroimaging

Cranial MRI and CT studies show diffuse cerebral atrophy with secondary subdural fluid collections, which may be large enough to cause mild compression of the ventricular system. The occurrence of large subdural fluid collections

and metaphyseal fractures in an infant can lead to the erro- neous diagnosis of child abuse. In older children, MRI stud- ies typically reveal diffuse white matter signal abnormalities suggestive of demyelination and gliosis, whereas in infants the white matter may be only focally affected. Tortuous intracranial blood vessels can be seen on routine MRI but are better demonstrated with MR angiography. Conven- tional angiography shows markedly elongated, tortuous, and dilated cerebral blood vessels. Wormian bones may be seen on skull radiographs.

Genetic Studies

A gene involved in transmembrane copper transport (*ATP7A*, also referred to as *MNK*) has been implicated in both kinky hair disease and occipital horn syndrome. *ATP7A* maps to Xq13.3 and is highly homologous to the gene impli- cated in Wilson's disease. Infantile-onset kinky hair syndrome results from extensive mutations of *ATP7A* (e.g., large dele- tions and frame shift mutations), whereas occipital horn syn- drome is associated with promoter and splicing efficiency mutations, possibly leading to reduced levels of an otherwise normal protein product. Copper deficiency impairs function of several enzymes that require copper as a cofactor. Neu- ronal degeneration is likely caused by abnormal function of some of these cuproenzymes: tyrosinase, cytochrome C oxi- dase, dopamine β-hydroxylase, and Cu/Zn superoxide dis- mutase. Connective tissue abnormalities seen in kinky hair syndrome are probably related to deficiency of lysyl oxidase, which helps to cross-link collagen and elastin. Evidence sup- ports the supposition that lysyl oxidase is particularly impor- tant in the occipital horn syndrome. Autonomic symptoms such as diarrhea and temperature instability may be caused by deficiency of dopamine β-hydroxylase.

The structure of the *ATP7A* gene is similar to that of the Wilson's disease locus. The *ATP7A* gene encodes for a P- type ATPase (*ATP7A*), one of a family of integral mem- brane proteins that uses an aspartyl phosphate intermediate to transport cations across cell membranes. *ATP7A* mRNA is present in a variety of cell types and organs except liver, which explains the clinical observations that liver does not accumulate excess copper and therefore is largely unaffected in kinky hair syndrome.

Treatment

Treatment approaches have focused on trying to restore copper to normal levels in brain and other tissues. Copper-histidine administered subcutaneously is the most promising treatment, and substantial clinical improvement in a small number of patients has been reported. Undoubtedly, response to copper-histidine treatment partly depends on the specific mutation of *ATP7A* involved, but such correlations are only now beginning to be made.

Aggressive copper replacement beginning in early infancy may be necessary to significantly improve neurological outcome, but the outcome may be spectacular. A promising outcome in a patient with kinky hair disease was reported in an infant with two affected relatives (Kaler et al. 1996). This infant was diagnosed by analysis of umbilical cord blood and was found to have a splice acceptor site mutation, which yields a partially functional enzyme. Parenteral copper replacement was begun at 8 days of life. During infancy he showed normal head growth, brain myelination, and age-appropriate neurodevelopment, including independent walking at 14 months of age. In contrast, his half-brother and first cousin had the same mutation but were not treated from an early age; these children showed slow head growth, cerebral atrophy, delayed myelination, and abnormal neurodevelopment. Preservation of some residual activity of ATPase may be required for significant clinical efficacy from copper replacement treatment. Early copper histidine therapy did not normalize neurological outcome in two children with the *Q724H* splicing mutation, which yields a nonfunctioning ATPase. Interestingly, the connective tissue abnormalities in kinky hair syndrome do not appear to be helped by copper replacement treatment.

CEREBROTENDINOUS XANTHOMATOSIS

Cerebrotendinous xanthomatosis (CTX) is an autosomal recessive disorder characterized by tendon xanthomas, cataracts, and progressive neurological deterioration. In this disorder deposits of cholesterol and cholestanol are found in virtually every tissue, particularly the Achilles tendons, brain, and lungs (Berginer et al. 1994).

Neurological Features

The clinical features of CTX are summarized in Table 69.5. Personality changes and decline in school performance may be the earliest neurological manifestations of this syndrome.

Table 69.5:   Clinical features of cerebrotendinous xanthomatosis

Neurological
  Progressive dementia
  Ataxia
  Nystagmus
  Dysarthria
  Hyperreflexia
  Bulbar symptoms
  Palatal and pharyngeal myoclonus
  Peripheral neuropathy
  Electroencephalographical abnormalities
  Parkinsonism
  Cerebral and cerebellar atrophy
  Cataracts
Behavioral abnormalities
  Personality changes
  Irritability
  Agitation
  Aggressiveness
  Paranoid ideation
  Auditory hallucinations
  Catatonia
Musculoskeletal
  Xanthomas
  Osteoporosis and bone fractures
  Large paranasal sinuses

Progressive loss of cognitive function typically begins in childhood, but some patients remain intellectually normal for many years. Ataxia with gait disturbance, dysmetria, nystagmus, and dysarthria are common. Psychosis with auditory hallucinations, paranoid ideation, and catatonia occur rarely, but examination for cataracts and tendon xanthomas should be included in the evaluation of patients with new-onset psychosis. Parkinsonism may be the only neurological abnormality. Cranial MRIs typically show cerebral and cerebellar atrophy and diffuse abnormal signal of the cerebral white matter, presumably reflecting sterol infiltration with demyelination. Focal lesions of the cerebral white matter and globus pallidus are sometimes demonstrable on MRI.

Peripheral neuropathy is a prominent feature of CTX as evidenced by pes cavus deformities, loss of deep tendon reflexes, and loss of vibration perception. Sural nerve biopsy may show reduced densities of both myelinated and unmyelinated axons, and teased fibers show axonal regeneration and remyelination. Large diameter myelinated nerve fibers are particularly affected. Foamy macrophages and lipid droplets are found in Schwann cells. Electrophysiological studies show prolonged central conduction times in short latency somatosensory evoked potentials with tibial nerve stimulation but normal conduction velocities with median nerve stimulation. Brainstem auditory evoked potentials and visual evoked potentials are abnormal in approximately one-half of patients studied. These electrophysiological parameters correlate with the ratio of serum cholestanol to cholesterol concentration and may improve with treatment with chenodeoxycholic acid.

Xanthomas

Achilles tendon is the most common site of tendon xanthomas, but quadriceps, triceps, and finger extensor tendons can be involved also. Tendon xanthomas usually appear after the age of 10 years but occasionally occur in the first decade of life. Although they have the same appearance as xanthomas found in patients with familial hypercholesterolemia or hyperlipoproteinemia, biochemical analysis reveals that they contain high amounts of cholestanol and little cholesterol. Biopsy of the tendon xanthomas is rarely necessary for diagnosis. The presence of early-onset cataracts, progressive dementia, and tendon xanthomas is pathognomic of CTX syndrome, though all patients may not have the complete triad of symptoms early in the course of the disorder. Patients without subcutaneous xanthomas may be diagnosed mistakenly with Marinesco-Sjögren syndrome, an autosomal recessive disorder characterized by cerebellar ataxia, congenital cataract, and mental retardation (Siebner et al. 1996).

Other Clinical Features

Early-onset cataracts are characteristic of CTX. Osteoporosis may lead to an increased risk of skeletal and vertebral fractures. Large paranasal sinuses have been reported in association with CTX. Renal disorders reported in patients with CTX include nephrolithiasis, nephrocalcinosis, and renal tubular acidosis.

Biochemical Features

Cholestanol, a metabolic derivative of cholesterol, is elevated in serum and tissue in individuals with CTX. Levels of cholestanol are particularly high in bile, xanthomas, and brain. Bile acid production is decreased markedly, which leads to reduced chenodeoxycholic acid concentration in bile. Excretion of bile acid precursors is increased in bile and urine. Serum cholesterol levels are typically not elevated in CTX syndrome.

CTX results from mutations in the gene (CYP27) encoding sterol 27-hydroxylase, an enzyme that catalyzes the oxidation of sterol intermediates during bile acid synthesis. Loss of this enzyme results in accumulation of cholestanol in the nervous system and other tissues.

Treatment

Treatment of CTX focuses on lowering cholestanol levels, primarily with chenodeoxycholic acid and other lipid-lowering agents. Plasmapheresis to lower low-density lipoproteins also has been attempted with equivocal success. Long-term treatment with chenodeoxycholic acid can lead to striking improvement in neurological function, resolution of peripheral and intracranial xanthomas, and improvement of EEG and peripheral nerve conduction abnormalities and visual and somatosensory evoked potentials. However, most studies have not found significant clinical or neuroradiographical improvement with chenodeoxycholic acid (Kuriyama et al. 1994). It may be that early treatment is required, which ideally would begin before onset of clinical symptoms in individuals with a family history of CTX, but this has yet to be established. The possibility that early treatment may improve the neurological symptoms of CTX underscores the importance of careful screening and genetic counseling of asymptomatic relatives of patients with this disorder.

EPIDERMAL NEVUS SYNDROME

The term *epidermal nevus syndrome* (ENS) refers to various disorders that have in common an epidermal nevus and neurological manifestations such as seizures or hemimeganencephaly. The syndrome may be named after the predominant cell type of the nevus, e.g., nevus verrucosus (keratinocytes), nevus comedonicus (hair follicles), and nevus sebaceous (sebaceous glands). When neurological findings dominate the clinical picture in a patient with a sebaceous nevus, terms such as *Schimmelpenning's syndrome*, *organoid nevus syndrome*, and *Jadassohn's nevus phakomatosis* have been used. Obviously, the present nomenclature of disorders with epidermal nevi is unsatisfactory. It is debatable whether all patients with epidermal nevi should be subsumed under the term ENS. Clearly, the nosology of these disorders will remain arbitrary until the genetic bases of epidermal nevi are known. In 1992, Meschia and colleagues reported that familial epidermal nevi are rare, and nearly all reported cases are sporadic. No evidence yet supports the hypothesis that ENS is caused by an autosomal lethal mutation that survives by mosaicism, as karyotypes reported in patients with ENS have been normal.

Cutaneous Features

Epidermal nevi are linear or patchy slightly raised lesions that typically are present at birth, although they may first appear in early childhood. The most common location of these nevi is on the head or neck. Only 16% of congenital nevi subsequently enlarge, compared with 65% of nevi arising after birth. Nevi on the head and neck enlarge only 4% of the time, whereas over one-half of the lesions elsewhere extend beyond their original boundaries.

Most nevi contain more than one tissue type, which may complicate dermatological classification, but the nevus typically is named according to the predominant tissue. Verrucous nevi are the most common type. Sebaceous nevi may be small or quite large and on histological examination have hyperplasia of sebaceous glands. Many other skin lesions have been noted in patients with ENS, including café au lait spots, localized acanthosis nigricans, hemangiomas, congenital hypopigmented macules, and atopic dermatitis, but these are common skin lesions in the general population and the association of these lesions with ENS is likely coincidental.

Neurological Features

Between 50% and 80% of patients with ENS have neurological deficits. The location of the nevus appears to correlate with the likelihood of neurological symptoms. A review of the neurological complications of ENS found that 31 of 33 patients had an epidermal nevus on the face or scalp. Cognitive deficits are common, and many patients are mentally retarded. Seizures occur in more than one-half of the patients. Focal epileptiform discharges and focal slowing are the most common EEG abnormalities, and the EEG abnormality is usually ipsilateral to the nevus. Infantile spasms with a hypsarrhythmic EEG may occur. Other neurological symptoms associated with ENS include cranial nerve palsies, hemiparesis (especially in patients with hemimeganencephaly), microcephaly, and behavior problems. Cranial nerves VI, VII, and VIII are most likely to be affected but the reason is unknown. Hemimeganencephaly, agenesis of the corpus callosum, and Dandy-Walker malformation have been reported in a child with a facial sebaceous nevus (Dodge and Dobyns 1995). Spina bifida and encephaloceles are seen rarely in ENS.

Cerebrovascular anomalies are seen in approximately 10% of patients with ENS. Intracranial blood vessels may be dysplastic, dilated, or occluded. For example, a leptomeningeal hemangioma extending into the right temporal lobe was noted in a patient with a facial epidermal nevus. AVMs and aneurysms have been reported in a few patients. Ischemia or hemorrhage from intracranial blood vessel anomalies may result in porencephaly, infarctions, and dystrophic calcification.

Other Features

Tumors have been reported with moderate frequency in association with ENS, and several have involved the brain. Low-grade astrocytomas of the hypothalamus, optic glioma, choroid plexus papilloma, and cerebral glioma have been reported in a single patient each (Sato et al. 1994). Skeletal abnormalities are quite frequent, but many of them are probably secondary to neurological dysfunction that alters skeletal development. For example, a congenital hemiparesis may lead to kyphoscoliosis and poor lingual movement in utero may result in a narrow, high-arched palate. Nonetheless, certain skeletal anomalies may be a primary part of ENS. Limb anomalies include clinodactyly, limb reduction defects, syndactyly, polydactyly, bifid thumbs, and talipes equinovarus. Abnormal vertebrae have been reported in a few patients.

Ocular abnormalities occur in approximately one-half of the patients with ENS. Colobomas are the most frequent eye anomaly. Disorders of globe growth include either microphthalmia or macrophthalmia. Retinal lesions such as scarring, degeneration, and detachment may occur. Strabismus and lipodermoid lesions of the conjunctivae are more frequent but less serious findings.

Cardiovascular and genitourinary malformations are found in approximately 10% of patients with ENS. Hypoplastic left-sided heart, ventricular septal defect, coarctation of the aorta, pulmonic stenosis, patent ductus arteriosus, and dilated pulmonary artery have been reported, most in a single patient each. Horseshoe kidney, cystic kidneys, duplicated collecting system, and ureteropelvic junction obstruction have been described. Hypophosphatemic vitamin D–resistant rickets and precocious puberty have been reported in a newborn with an epidermal nevus (Ivker et al. 1997). Interestingly, the hypophosphatemia resolved when the nevus was surgically removed, implicating a hormonal agent produced by the nevus.

Neuroimaging

Megalencephaly ipsilateral to the epidermal nevus is the most frequent finding on neuroimaging; the left and right hemispheres often are involved equally. In some patients megalencephaly results from asymmetric growth of the skull, with the brain being of normal size. MRI of the skull may show a widened diploic space. Often enlargement of the calvarium and the ipsilateral cerebral hemisphere are present together. In addition, several types of cerebral dysplasia are associated with ENS, and as with megalencephaly these occur primarily ipsilateral to the epidermal nevus. Focal pachygyria is the most common type of cortical dysplasia in ENS. The surface of the affected hemisphere may be smooth, the cortical mantle thickened, and the adjacent white matter abnormal.

HYPOMELANOSIS OF ITO

Hypomelanosis of Ito (HI) is a heterogeneous and complex neurocutaneous disorder affecting the skin, brain, eye, and skeleton, as well as other organs. HI was first described by Ito as *incontinentia pigmenti achromians*, but it is now commonly known as *HI* to avoid confusion with incontinentia pigmenti. No reliable estimates of the population frequency of HI are available, but according to Ruiz-Maldonado and colleagues in 1992 at the National Institute of Pediatrics in Mexico City, 1 of every 7,805 general pediatric outpatients was diagnosed with HI. HI affects male and female subjects equally and is usually a sporadic disorder with minimal recurrence risk.

Cutaneous Features

The skin findings are distinctive and in fact are the only constant feature of HI; hypopigmented whorls, streaks, and patches are present at birth and tend to follow Blaschko's lines. Blaschko's lines form a V-shaped pattern over the back, an S-shaped pattern over the anterior trunk, and linear streaks over the extremities (Plate 69.I). In HI the hypopigmented skin lesions are usually multiple and involve several body segments, and they may be unilateral or bilateral. They may be observable at birth but commonly develop in infancy, depending on the degree of skin pigmentation. Wood's lamp examination may enable detection of hypopigmented lesions in light-skinned individuals. The degree or distribution of skin depigmentation does not appear to correlate with either the severity of neurological symptoms or associated organ pathology. The hypopigmented lesions follow the lines of Blaschko in only approximately two-thirds of patients; in others the lesions are patchy without any specific distribution pattern. Other skin findings in patients with HI include café au lait spots, cutis marmorata, aplasia cutis, nevus of Ota, trichorrhexis, focal hypertrichosis, and nail dystrophy. Electron microscopy of the hypopigmented lesions consistently shows a marked reduction of melanocytes in the hypopigmented areas (Cavallari et al. 1996). In the proximity of preserved melanocytes, a nearly normal content of melanosomes is detected in basal keratinocytes. Increased numbers of Langerhans' cells are seen in depigmented areas.

Many different cytogenetic anomalies have been reported in HI. The most common karyotype pattern is autosomal mosaicism, but the X chromosome is often involved. Most patients are mosaic for aneuploidy or unbalanced translocations, with two or more chromosomally distinct cell lines either within the same tissue or between tissues. Genetic alterations in HI are varied and include ring chromosome 22, mosaic trisomy 18, 18/X translocation, among others. Mosaicism for sex chromosome aneuploidy also occurs. Normal lymphocyte karyotypes have been reported in many individuals with HI, but it is important to recognize that mosaicism may be tissue specific, so that, for example, karyotype abnormalities may be demonstrable in fibroblasts but not in lymphocytes.

The lack of correlation between cytogenetic anomalies and the noncutaneous manifestations of pigmentation disorders, as well as the wide diversity of neurological and systemic findings make it doubtful that HI is caused by a specific genetic anomaly. Rather, HI and similar pigmentation disorders may be caused by a general effect of mosaicism on determination of skin pigment distribution. Uniparental disomy has been described in several patients

with HI (Crowe et al. 1997), indicating that molecular cytogenetic analysis should be considered in all patients with HI.

Neurological Features

The frequency of neurological abnormalities in patients with skin lesions typical for HI is not established and estimates range from 50–80% (Nehal et al. 1996). Ascertainment bias also may contribute to the variability of incidence estimates, as patients with normal neurological development may have abnormal cranial MRI. Most case series have not included MRI in patient evaluations.

Seizures and mental retardation are the most common neurological abnormalities. In a series that included systematic neuropsychological testing, IQ scores are below 70 in more than one-half of patients with HI, although approximately 20% have IQ scores above 90. Approximately one-half of patients with HI have seizures, usually with onset in the first year of life. Focal seizures are most common, although occasional patients with infantile spasms (Ogino et al. 1994) and Lennox-Gastaut have been described. No specific EEG or evoked response patterns have been identified.

It is unclear how (or whether) HI is related to the conditions of linear and whorled nevoid hyperpigmentation and nevus depigmentosus. Approximately 10% of patients referred for analysis of swirling or patchy skin pigmentation have areas of hypopigmentation and hyperpigmentation. Neurological and systemic abnormalities are distinctly less common in linear and whorled nevoid hyperpigmentation and nevus depigmentosus than in HI, so these conditions are not usually classified as neurocutaneous disorders.

Macrocephaly is more common than microcephaly. Neuroimaging studies, primarily using CT, have revealed disparate findings. Generalized cerebral or cerebellar hypoplasia is the most common abnormality. Severe cortical neuronal migration anomalies are reported (Malherbe et al. 1993), and hemimeganencephaly and lissencephaly are seen also. Hemimeganencephaly may be ipsilateral or contralateral to the cutaneous hypopigmentation. As expected, MRI studies have shown more subtle abnormalities of cerebral architecture that appear to be stable over time. Extensive periventricular white matter lesions are another common finding. Small periventricular cysts and gray matter heterotopias are seen also. Polymicrogyria with brachycephaly has been noted in one autopsied case. Approximately one-third of patients with HI have normal cranial MRI studies.

Systemic Features

Noncutaneous defects involving nearly every organ system are found in 50–75% of patients with HI. Ocular findings include microphthalmia, heterochromia iridis, dacryostenosis, pannus, corneal opacities, cataract, optic atrophy, retinal detachment, and pigmentation anomalies of the retina. The most common musculoskeletal anomaly is hemihypertrophy, but short stature, pectus carinatum and excavatum, cleft palate, butterfly vertebrae, scoliosis, and clinodactyly and polysyndactyly are described also. Dental anomalies are frequent, including conical or hypoplastic teeth, hypoplastic dental enamel, and cleft lip and palate. Cardiac defects include tetralogy of Fallot, pulmonary stenosis, and septal defects. Disorders of endocrine and renal development occur infrequently, and one patient with HI and neuroblastoma has been reported.

NEUROCUTANEOUS MELANOSIS

Neurocutaneous melanosis (NCM) is a congenital disorder of melanotic cell development that involves the CNS, especially the leptomeninges. Congenital melanocytic nevi may occur without CNS involvement, and conversely, melanin is found normally in the CNS in the absence of congenital nevi. NCM is apparently not hereditary and affects male and female subjects with equal frequency. The incidence of NCM is unknown, but it is very uncommon.

Cutaneous Features

The characteristic lesions are dark to light brown hairy nevi present at birth (Plate 69.II). Multiple small nevi (satellite nevi) are usually present around one giant nevus that most commonly appears on the lower trunk and perineal area (swimming trunk nevus). A giant nevus is absent in 34% of patients with NCM. Approximately one-third of patients have a large nevus over the upper back (cape nevus). The giant nevi may fade over time, but satellite nevi continue to appear during the first few years of life.

Diagnostic criteria for NCM have been suggested: (1) Large or multiple (three or more) congenital nevi in which large is defined as equal to or greater than 20 cm in an adult, 9 cm on the scalp of an infant, or 6 cm on the body of an infant; (2) no evidence of cutaneous melanoma, except in patients in whom the examined portions of the meningeal lesions are benign; and (3) no evidence of meningeal melanoma, except in patients in whom the examined areas of the cutaneous lesions are benign. Some authors argue that a definitive diagnosis of NCM requires histological confirmation of the CNS lesions, but in the context of the typical melanocytic cutaneous nevi and characteristic neuroimaging findings it is doubtful that leptomeningeal or brain biopsy is necessary.

Biopsy of a congenital nevus reveals extension of the nevus cells into the deep dermis or even the subcutis between collagen bundles and around nerves, hair follicles, and blood vessels. Nevus cells tend to form cords or nests. In addition, sheets of nevomelanocytes in the dermis may display a few mitoses and large atypical cells positive for S-100 and HMB-45 antibodies and formalin-induced green specific fluorescence. The occurrence of atypical mitoses in the dermis may constitute an early stage of malignant melanoma (Sasaki et al. 1996). The greatest risks in NCM are the high incidence of transformation of melanotic cells into malignant melanoma and spinal and intracranial pathology.

Neurological Features

Neurological symptoms may result from leptomeningeal melanosis, intracranial melanoma, intracerebral or subarachnoid hemorrhage, and vertebral column, spinal, or cerebral malformations. Neurological symptoms present at a median age of 2 years but infants as young as 1 month may be affected (DeDavid et al. 1996). Leptomeningeal melanosis tends to occur at the base of the brain along the interpeduncular fossa, ventral brainstem, upper cervical cord, and ventral surface of the lumbosacral cord and is probably the most common cause of neurological symptoms, especially in children. In one series marked leptomeningeal melanosis was present in 97% of patients with NCM. Leptomeningeal melanosis is associated with the interruption of cerebrospinal fluid flow, which leads to hydrocephalus and increased intracranial pressure that presents with irritability, vomiting, seizures, and papilledema. In infants, the head circumference may increase rapidly and the anterior fontanel may become tense. Cranial nerve deficits such as limitation of upgaze and abducens nerve weakness are common in such patients.

The likelihood of symptomatic neurological involvement correlates with location of large nevi. Large congenital melanocytic nevi occur on the back in nearly 80% of patients. In one large series all 33 patients with neurological symptoms had a nevus over the back, whereas none of 26 patients with nevi restricted to the extremities had neurological findings. Patients with leptomeningeal melanosis confirmed by biopsy and CNS involvement but without skin lesions have been reported.

The pathogenesis of NCM is poorly understood although it clearly is a disorder of melanocyte embryogenesis. The prominent involvement of the leptomeninges and skin over the spine supports the suggestion that the primary defect is abnormal migration of nevus cell precursors, although the embryological origin of nevus cells has not been determined. Alternatively, melanin-producing cells may be produced in excessive numbers. It has been speculated also that nevi located over the spine result from an error early in nevus cell migration or differentiation, whereas nevi are restricted to the extremities if the error occurs later in development.

Laboratory Diagnosis

Analysis of cerebrospinal fluid from patients with neurological symptoms may show a mild pleocytosis and elevated

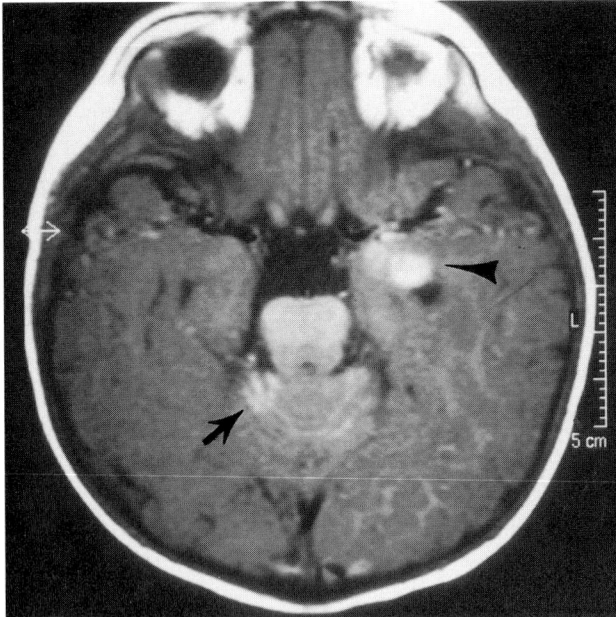

FIGURE 69.24 T1-weighted cranial magnetic resonance imaging scan showing leptomeningeal melanosis over the cerebellum (*arrow*) and focal melanosis or melanoma in the temporal lobe (*arrowhead*).

Table 69.6: Risk categories of von Hippel–Lindau groups

Pheochromocytoma	Hemangioblastoma risk	Renal cell carcinoma risk
No	High	High
Yes	High	Low
Yes	High	High
Yes	Low	Low

Unfortunately, melanoma may not exhibit any of these findings until late in its course, when metastasis is likely to have already occurred.

VON HIPPEL–LINDAU SYNDROME

Von Hippel–Lindau syndrome (VHL) is an autosomal dominantly inherited disorder characterized by hemangioblastomas arising in the retina and CNS and visceral cysts and tumors. Hemangioblastomas may occur sporadically, but in VHL are usually multiple and more likely to occur in young persons. Current prevalence estimates of this disorder are approximately 1 in 40,000–100,000 population (Maher and Kaelin 1997).

Clinical Features

The initial symptoms of VHL usually arise from effects of the vascular anomalies in the CNS, but occasional patients may present with pheochromocytoma or renal, pancreatic, hepatic, or epididymal tumors. One classification system categorizes patients according to whether pheochromocytoma is present (Table 69.6). The most common pattern of VHL findings includes retinal and CNS hemangioblastomas and pancreatic cysts. Childhood onset of symptoms is unusual, but retinal hemangioblastomas may occur in children as young as 1 year. Cerebellar hemangioblastomas may begin in the second decade of life.

Hemangioblastomas are benign, slow-growing vascular tumors that cause symptoms from hemorrhage or local mass effect. Histologically, hemangioblastomas are composed of endothelium-lined vascular channels surrounded by stromal cells and pericytes. Mast cells are present and may produce erythropoietin.

Retinal hemangioblastomas may be asymptomatic, especially if they occur in the periphery of the retina. Vision loss occurs when the lesions are large and centrally located, even in the absence of hemorrhage. Arteriovenous shunting leads to fluid extravasation. Hemorrhage may lead to retinal injury and detachment, glaucoma, uveitis, macular edema, and sympathetic ophthalmitis. In the CNS the most common site of hemangioblastomas is the cerebellum, in approximately one-half of patients, followed by spinal and medullary sites. Cerebral hemangioblastomas are present in less than 5% of

pressure and protein. Cerebrospinal fluid cytopathology shows numerous round cells with abundant cytoplasm and ovoid nuclei and light brown cytoplasmic granules (presumably melanin) may be seen. The most characteristic histological feature is the presence of numerous irregular fingers projecting from the cell body, which may aid in diagnosis of NCM.

Neuroimaging studies are important in the evaluation of a patient with giant melanotic nevi. Approximately one-half of neurologically asymptomatic children with NCM have abnormal cranial neuroimaging study results. Cranial MRI demonstrates lesions with T1 shortening in the cerebellum, anterior temporal lobe (especially the amygdala), and along the basilar meninges (Figure 69.24). Some of these lesions also show T2 shortening as well. The pons, medulla, thalami, and base of the frontal lobe are also typically affected. Gadolinium-enhanced MRIs may rarely show enhancement of the pia-arachnoid (Byrd et al. 1997). Leptomeningeal thickening and enhancement were seen in all five children with neurological symptoms of increased intracranial pressure in one study. Conversely, leptomeningeal thickening was not seen in any asymptomatic children. Spinal MRI study results are usually normal.

Care must be taken to distinguish radiological evidence of CNS melanoma from benign melanin deposits. This may be difficult; serial imaging studies are the best way to follow clinically suspect MRI lesions. Certain neuroimaging findings help distinguish benign intracranial melanosis from melanoma: The presence of necrosis, perilesional edema, contrast-enhancement, or hemorrhage are features of melanoma.

patients with VHL. The cerebellar hemispheres are affected far more frequently than the cerebellar vermis.

Early symptoms of cerebellar and brainstem hemangioblastomas include headache, the most common symptom, followed by ataxia, nausea and vomiting, and nystagmus. Symptoms are often intermittent or slowly progressive, but up to 20% of patients have an acute onset of symptoms following mild head trauma. Spinal hemangioblastomas typically present with focal back or neck pain and sensory loss or weakness in a spinal cord distribution. Because of their typical intramedullary location, spinal hemangioblastomas frequently lead to syringomyelia (Choyke et al. 1995). The conus medullaris and the cervicomedullary junction are the most common sites. Extensive involvement of the spinal cord can occur. Brainstem hemangioblastomas tend to arise in the area postrema in the medulla, where they may be associated with syringobulbia. Occasionally hemangioblastomas occur in sites near the third ventricle, such as the pituitary gland or its stalk, the hypothalamus, optic nerve, wall of the third ventricle, and in the cerebral hemispheres. The incidence of cerebellar hemangioblastomas increases with age so that 84% of patients with VHL have at least one such tumor by age 60 years.

Cerebellar hemangioblastomas are best imaged with contrast-enhanced MRI. Routine screening of the brain and spinal cord should include precontrast and postcontrast T1-weighted images with thin sections through the posterior fossa and spinal cord and surface coil imaging of the entire spinal cord. Arteriography is not necessary for diagnosis but is valuable in demonstrating the feeding vessels if surgical resection is planned.

Systemic Features

Renal cysts are present in over one-half of individuals with VHL, although as with CNS and retinal hemangioblastomas the patients may be asymptomatic. If the renal cysts are extensive they may lead to renal failure, but this is unusual. Of greater concern is that renal cell carcinoma develops in over 70% of patients with VHL and is the leading cause of death. These tumors are usually multiple, and they tend to occur at a younger age than sporadic renal cell carcinoma. Simple renal cysts arise from distal tubular epithelium, whereas renal cell carcinoma tumors arise from proximal tubular epithelium.

Pheochromocytomas are seen in from 7–19% of patients with VHL and may be the only clinical manifestation of the disorder, even in carefully screened individuals (Ritter et al. 1996). In one study, 20% of patients with apparently sporadic pheochromocytoma actually had VHL. In patients with VHL pheochromocytomas may be bilateral and occur outside the adrenal glands. Rarely, they may become malignant. Symptoms of pheochromocytoma include episodic or sustained hypertension, severe headache, and flushing with profuse sweating. In advanced stages pheochromocytomas can lead to hypertensive crises, stroke, myocardial infarction, and heart failure. Pheochromocytomas are also a distinctive feature of multiple endocrine neoplasia type 2 and NF, and VHL and NF1 have been reported in the same patient. Diagnosis is made by showing excessive catecholamines in serum and urine. Norepinephrine and epinephrine are elevated in both serum and urine, and vanillylmandelic acid is elevated in urine.

Cysts and tumors of the pancreas and epididymis are also features of VHL. In the pancreas, nonsecretory islet cell tumors, simple cysts, serous microcystic adenomas, and adenocarcinomas are found. Fortunately, pancreatic cysts are the most common of these lesions and they are asymptomatic unless they obstruct the bile duct or become so numerous that pancreatic insufficiency occurs. Islet cell tumors are frequent in patients with pheochromocytomas, an observation that may be linked to the fact that these tumors are derived from neural crest cells, as are pheochromocytomas.

Molecular Genetics

The VHL gene is a tumor-suppressor gene located on chromosome 3 (Latif et al. 1993). Hundreds of mutations have thus far been discovered, and although the genotype-phenotype relationship is complex, some clinical correlations are beginning to be possible. Missense mutations in this gene are associated with pheochromocytoma, whereas nonsense, frame shift, splice site, and deletions predominate in families without pheochromocytomas (see Table 69.6). Microdeletions and microinsertions, nonsense mutations, or deletions were found in 56% of families with VHL type 1; missense mutations accounted for 96% of those responsible for VHL type 2 (Chen et al. 1995). Specific mutations in codon 238 accounted for 43% of the mutations responsible for VHL type 2, and one group of patients (type 2C) appears to be at low risk for any of the manifestations of VHL except pheochromocytoma. The function of the VHL protein (pVHL) appears to be related to tumor regulation. Inactivation or loss of the normal allele leads to tumor development. The propensity for hemangioblastomas in this disorder is likely related to the observation that VHL tumor-suppressor gene regulates the expression of vascular endothelial growth factor. Vascular endothelial growth factor levels in ocular fluid of patients is significantly higher than in unaffected subjects.

The tumorigenic properties of VHL mutations have been linked to a characteristic feature of cancer cells, which is their failure to exit the cell cycle under conditions of cell-cell contact or withdrawal of serum. VHL-negative renal cell carcinoma cells fail to exit the cell cycle on serum withdrawal; reintroduction of the wild-type VHL gene restores this ability. This suggests that the loss of wild-type VHL gene results in a specific cellular defect in serum-dependent growth control, which may initiate tumor formation.

Table 69.7: Cambridge screening protocol for
von Hippel–Lindau disease

Affected patient
    Annual physical examination and urine testing
    Annual direct and indirect ophthalmoscopy with fluorescein
        angioscopy or angiography
    Cranial magnetic resonance imaging or computed tomog-
        raphy every 3 years to age 50 and every 5 years thereafter
    Annual renal ultrasound, with abdominal computed tomog-
        raphy scan every 3 years (more frequently if multiple renal
        cysts are discovered)
    Annual 24-hour urine collection for vanillylmandelic acid
At-risk relative
    Annual physical examination and urine testing
    Annual direct and indirect ophthalmoscopy from age 5 years
    Annual fluorescein angioscopy or angiography from age 10
        years until age 60
    Cranial magnetic resonance imaging or computed tomog-
        raphy every 3 years from age 15–40 and every 5 years
        until age 60
    Annual renal ultrasound, with abdominal computed tomog-
        raphy scan every 3 years from age 20–65 years
    Annual 24-hour urine collection for vanillylmandelic acid

---

Treatment

Careful screening is the most important aspect of management of patients with VHL, and several protocols for at-risk
asymptomatic patients, such as a first-degree relative of a
patient with VHL, have been published (Lesho 1994) (Table
69.7). If a family history of VHL or pheochromocytoma is
present, then all first-degree relatives should be screened.
Other indications for clinical screening include pancreatic
cysts, multiple or bilateral renal cell tumors, multiple (and
perhaps single) retinal hemangiomas, and cerebellar hemangioblastomas. The clinical availability of molecular analysis
for the VHL gene now reduces the number of asymptomatic
relatives requiring surveillance; only relatives who have
inherited the VHL mutation need annual screening.

WYBURN-MASON SYNDROME

Wyburn-Mason syndrome is a rare neurocutaneous syndrome characterized by retinal, facial, and intracranial
AVMs. In contrast to VHL, in which intracranial vascular
malformations are also a prominent feature, Wyburn-
Mason syndrome does not seem to be inherited.

Clinical Features

The vascular malformations of the retina and intracranial
blood vessels may occur independently, but there is a general relationship between severity of the retinal lesion and
the likelihood of an intracranial AVM. Three groups of
patients with retinal AVMs have been recognized according
to the pattern of the vascular malformation. In group one,
the vascular malformation is usually focal and an arteriolar
capillary bed is interposed between the retinal arteries and
veins. Vision may be unaffected and intracranial vascular
malformations are uncommon. In group two, direct arteriovenous communication leads to higher blood flow and
intravascular pressure, which produces retinal hemorrhages
and exudates that may impair vision. Group three is characterized by large convoluted retinal AVMs with high blood
flow and significant retinal degeneration. Vision may be
compromised seriously from the retinal involvement, and
the incidence of intracranial vascular anomalies is highest in
this group.

Approximately 25% of patients with retinal lesions also
have intracranial vascular malformations. Retinal lesions
range in magnitude from small asymptomatic lesions to
massive vascular anomalies that involve most of the retina.
Skin lesions in this disorder occur in a minority of cases and
usually take the form of facial angiomas in the trigeminal
nerve distribution. Facial angiomas are usually unilateral
but may be bilateral. AVMs also occur in the mandible and
maxilla, and hemorrhage from these vessels may be the first
clue to the syndrome; it is unknown how often AVMs of
the subcutaneous facial tissues are associated with intracranial vascular anomalies. Retinal and intracranial vascular
malformations tend to occur ipsilaterally.

Neurological and visual symptoms may begin at birth but
usually do not develop until adulthood. Proptosis and catastrophic or slowly progressive visual loss may be the presenting symptoms of retinal AVMs. These symptoms may
be caused by retinal edema, exudate, or hemorrhage. Visual
field defects may be caused by ischemia or direct compression of visual pathway tracts by a vascular malformation.
Other ocular manifestations of Wyburn-Mason syndrome
include glaucoma, optic atrophy, and enlargement of the
optic foramen. Alternatively, neurological symptoms such as
seizures, headache, and subarachnoid hemorrhage may be
the initial manifestations of this disorder. Dandy-Walker
malformation associated with obstructive hydrocephalus has
occurred in one newborn with retinal and facial vascular
anomalies, but this association may have been incidental.

Retinal vascular malformations are demonstrated well by
fluorescein angiography. Vascular malformations of the face
and brain can be demonstrated with conventional arteriography or with MR angiography. The internal carotid vessels are more often involved than the external carotid
vessels or the posterior cerebral circulation.

Treatment

Treatment of the AVMs in Wyburn-Mason syndrome is the
same as for sporadically occurring vascular malformations.
Photocoagulation of a retinal AVM is possible but results
have not been encouraging. Treatment options for intracranial vessels include surgical resection, endovascular

embolization, and radiosurgery; some patients may require a combination of these therapies. Surgical resection offers definitive and immediate removal of an AVM, although surgery carries significant risks. The risk for a given patient depends on several factors, such as age, general health, and the location of the AVM. Lesions located deep within the brain such as in the thalamus or brainstem or in eloquent cortex carry a higher risk of significant postoperative disability, and larger AVMs and those whose venous drainage is carried deep into the brain's venous system are difficult to remove surgically.

Endovascular treatments use interventional radiological techniques to embolize an AVM with clot-enhancing material such as glue or coils. Endovascular techniques are often used to prepare an AVM for subsequent surgical resection. Embolization of one or more of the feeding vessels of the AVM can make its resection easier and safer. Embolization also may make an AVM more amenable to radiosurgery. Radiosurgery involves focusing gamma radiation to a targeted lesion, rather than subjecting a large area to the damaging effects of radiation. When gamma radiation is applied to an AVM the lesion gradually scars and eventually may be obliterated. This obliteration occurs slowly, taking up to 2 years, and during this time hemorrhage may occur. Also, radiosurgery is less effective in AVMs larger than approximately 2 cm in diameter than in smaller AVMs.

XERODERMA PIGMENTOSUM

Xeroderma pigmentosum (XP) is a group of uncommon neurocutaneous disorders characterized by susceptibility to sun-induced skin disorders and variable but typically progressive neurological deterioration. XP is inherited in an autosomal recessive manner and occurs in from 1 in 30,000 to 1 in 250,000 population. Several gene mutations have been associated with XP and related syndromes such as Cockayne's syndrome, trichothiodystrophy, and DeSanctis-Cacchione syndrome.

Complementation Groups

Complementation analysis has been important in understanding the genetic basis of XP. If two particular cell types with different metabolic abnormalities are fused, the cell produced may function normally. These two cell types are said to be in different complementation groups and presumably have a different genetic basis. In XP eight complementation groups have been identified (XP-A through XP-G and a variant group). Although some general genotype-phenotype correlations among these complementation groups can be made, considerable clinical overlap exists between these groups (Copeland et al. 1997). Complementation groups XP-A, XP-C, and XP-D are the most common in the published literature; XP-A predominates in Japan but is uncommon in the United States. The gene linked to this group is termed *XPAC* and has been mapped to chromosome 9q34. The *XPAC* protein's function has not been fully elucidated, but it is involved in nucleotide excision repair. Only a few patients with XP-B have been described, but the responsible gene (*XPBC*) has been cloned. The *XPBC* gene is located on chromosome 2q21 and encodes a protein that is a component of the basal transcription factor TFIIH/BTF2. This protein helps regulate both DNA transcription initiation and nucleotide excision repair.

Complementation group C is caused by mutations in the *XPCC* gene, located on chromosome 3p25.1. Patients with XP-C generally do not have prominent neurological dysfunction. The *XPCC* gene codes for a protein involved in global genome repair although its exact role is not yet understood. Complementation group D is the third most common complementation group, and it is characterized by mild to severe neurological dysfunction. The gene associated with XP-D is at chromosome 9q13. The gene product in XP-D is a component of TFFIIH/BTF2, as is XP-B, and accordingly, XP-B and XP-D have similar clinical features. Complementation group E (XP-E) is uncommon and associated with mild neurological and cutaneous symptoms. The XP-E gene has not been precisely localized and the function of its associated protein XPEC has not been determined. Neurological symptoms have not been described in patients from complementation groups F, G, or the variant group.

Related Syndromes

DeSanctis-Cacchione syndrome is a variant of XP in which patients have severe and progressive cognitive deficiency, dwarfism, and gonadal hypoplasia. Trichothiodystrophy and similar syndromes have been linked to XP complementation groups B and D. Patients with trichothiodystrophy have brittle hair and nails because of sulfur-deficient matrix proteins, ichthyosis, and mental retardation. Patients with photosensitivity (P), ichthyosis (I), brittle hair (B), impaired intelligence (I), possibly decreased fertility (D), and short stature (S) fit into the PIBI(D)S syndrome. DNA repair studies of patients with trichothiodystrophy demonstrate reduced ultraviolet-induced DNA repair synthesis, and one patient has been assigned to XP-D. A variant of trichothiodystrophy is Tay's syndrome, in which dysplastic nails and lack of subcutaneous fatty tissue are characteristic. Low birth weight, short stature, and mental retardation are also features of this disorder.

Similarly, the finding of patients combining features of XP and Cockayne's syndrome within complementation groups XP-B, XP-D, and XP-G indicate that there is considerable clinical heterogeneity and phenotypic overlap within the subsets of these complementation groups. The close relationship between Cockayne's syndrome and XP is emphasized by the report of a patient with the clinical fea-

Table 69.8: Cutaneous and ocular features of xeroderma pigmentosum

Cutaneous features
  Sunlight sensitivity
  Freckling
  Atrophy
  Xerosis and scaling
  Telangiectasia
  Actinic keratosis
  Angioma
  Keratoacanthoma
  Fibroma
  Malignant tumors
  Basal cell carcinoma
  Squamous cell carcinoma
  Melanoma
  Fibrosarcoma
Ocular features
  Eyelids
    Atrophy leading to loss of lashes, ectropion, entropion
    Neoplasm
  Conjunctiva
    Conjunctivitis
    Inflammatory lesions such as pinguecula
    Pigmentation, telangiectases, dryness
    Symblepharon, inflammatory nodules
    Neoplasm
  Cornea
    Exposure keratitis leading to corneal clouding, dryness,
      ulceration, scarring, and vascularization
    Neoplasm
  Iris
    Iritis, synechiae, atrophy

tures of XP but who was assigned to a Cockayne complementation group (CS-B) (Itoh et al. 1996).

Cutaneous and Ocular Features

Cutaneous and ocular features of XP result primarily from ultraviolet light exposure (Table 69.8). The onset of cutaneous symptoms in XP is usually quite early; the median age of onset of cutaneous symptoms is 1–2 years, typically freckling or erythema and bullae formation after sun exposure. Nearly one-half of reported patients had developed malignant skin lesions, with the median age of first skin neoplasm being only 8 years. The incidence of basal cell carcinoma or squamous cell carcinoma of the skin is estimated to be 4,800 times greater than that observed for the general United States population. Light-skinned infants develop erythema and bullae after even brief sun exposure. Sun exposure also induces prominent macule formation (freckling), which over time enlarge and coalesce. Telangiectasias and epidermal and dermal atrophy develop in later years, and the skin becomes dry. Actinic keratosis, angiomas, keratoacanthomas, and fibromas are described

also. Ocular tissues are particularly susceptible to ultraviolet damage. Keratitis and conjunctivitis with photophobia are common in patients with XP. Atrophy of the eyelids leads to loss of lashes and ectropion or entropion. Neoplasms of the eyelid, conjunctiva, and cornea include squamous cell carcinoma, epithelioma and basal cell carcinoma, and melanoma.

Neurological Features

Most of what is known about the neurological findings in XP comes from studies of Japanese patients with XP-A. Research indicates that the severity of neurological symptoms correlates with particular mutations within the *XPAC* gene, and presumably this is true in other types of XP (Maeda et al. 1995). The principal neurological symptoms in XP-A are progressive dementia, sensorineural hearing loss, tremor, choreoathetosis, and ataxia. Progressive dementia begins in patients with XP-A during the preschool years, and IQ scores after 10 years of age are invariably less than 50. Sensorineural hearing loss has a later onset but most patients older than 10 years have hearing impairment. Cerebellar signs develop at approximately the same time as the hearing loss. Microcephaly is present in approximately one-half of patients.

EEG studies most often show generalized slowing but focal slow-wave and focal spike discharges are occasionally seen; these findings are seen in many other neurological disorders and are not pathognomonic of XP. Peripheral neuropathy is a prominent feature that may begin in the first decade of life. Deep tendon reflexes are absent in nearly all patients older than 6 years. Motor nerve conduction velocities are normal during the first 3 years of life but by age 6 years become slow. Similarly, all patients over 6 years of age had either absent or prolonged sensory nerve conduction velocities.

Electromyography shows a neuropathic pattern with large, prolonged, polyphasic motor unit potentials and incomplete recruitment of motor units. Nerve biopsy may show an age-dependent decrease of myelinated fibers, which was associated with rare acute axonal degeneration, sparse axonal regeneration, rare axonal atrophy, and few onion bulb formations. These findings are consistent with a neuropathic process.

Neural tissue is shielded from sunlight-induced DNA damage, so the cause of neurodegeneration in patients with XP remains unexplained. The high frequency of neurological symptoms in XP-B and XP-D but not in XP-C, XP-D, XP-G, and the variant group supports the notion that one cause of the neurological dysfunction in XP is dysfunction of DNA transcription rather than nucleotide excision repair. Deficits in excision repair may be more closely linked to skin cancer susceptibility characteristic of some of the other complementation groups. In addition, recent work suggests that in XP neurological injury is at least partly caused by defective repair of lesions that are produced in nerve cells by reactive oxygen species generated as by-products of an active oxidative metabolism. Specifically, two major oxidative DNA lesions, 8-oxoguanine and thymine glycol, are excised from DNA in vitro by the same enzyme system responsible for removing pyrimidine dimers and other bulky DNA adducts.

Treatment

As the previous discussion indicates, cancer surveillance and avoidance of precipitating factors is the most important aspect of health screening of individuals with XP, but optimism exists for genetic therapy to reduce cancer risk and perhaps improve neurological outcome. In vitro studies offer hope that recombinant retroviruses can transfer and stably express the human DNA repair genes in XP cells in order to correct defective DNA repair seen in XP (Zeng et al. 1997), but such technology is in its infancy. The recombinant retroviral vector LXSN has been used to transfer human XP-A, XP-B, and XP-C cDNAs into primary and immortalized fibroblasts obtained from patients with XP-A, XP-B, and XP-C. After transduction, the complete correction of DNA repair deficiency and functional expression of the transgenes were monitored by ultraviolet survival, unscheduled DNA synthesis and recovery of RNA synthesis, and Western blots. In a similar study, XP-F cDNA was cloned into a mammalian expression vector plasmid and introduced into group F XP (XP-F) cells. The XP-FR2 cells expressed a high level of XP-F protein, as well as ERCC1 protein. They showed ultraviolet resistance comparable with normal human cells and had normal levels of ultraviolet-induced unscheduled DNA synthesis and normal capability to remove DNA adducts. This demonstrates that the nucleotide excision repair defect in XP-F cells is fully corrected by overexpression of XP-F cDNA alone.

REFERENCES

Berginer VM, Berginer J, Korczyn AD, Tadmor R. Magnetic resonance imaging in cerebrotendinous xanthomatosis: a prospective clinical and neuroradiological study. J Neurol Sci 1994;122:102–108.

Bodensteiner J, Roach ES. Sturge-Weber Syndrome. Mt. Freedom, NJ: Sturge-Weber Foundation, 1999.

Byrd SE, Darling CF, Tomita T, et al. MR imaging of symptomatic neurocutaneous melanosis in children. Pediatr Radiol 1997;27:39–44.

Carson BS, Javdan SP, Freeman JM, et al. Hemispherectomy: a hemidecortication approach and review of 52 cases. J Neurosurg 1996;84:903–911.

Cavallari V, Ussia AF, Siragusa M, Schepis C. Hypomelanosis of Ito: electron microscopical observations on two new cases. J Dermatol Sci 1996;13:87–92.

Chen F, Kishida T, Yao M, et al. Germline mutations in the von Hippel-Lindau disease tumor suppressor gene: correlations with phenotype. Hum Mutat 1995;5:66–75.

Choyke PL, Glenn GM, Walther MM, et al. von Hippel-Lindau disease: genetic, clinical, and imaging features. Radiology 1995;194:629–642.

Copeland NE, Hanke CW, Michalak JA. The molecular basis of xeroderma pigmentosum. Dermatol Surg 1997;23:447–455.

Crowe CA, Schwartz S, Black CJ, Jaswaney V. Mosaic trisomy 22: a case presentation and literature review of trisomy 22 phenotypes. Am J Med Genet 1997;71:406–413.

Curatolo P. Neurological manifestations of tuberous sclerosis complex. Child Nerv Syst 1996;12:515–521.

DeDavid M, Orlow SJ, Provost N, et al. Neurocutaneous melanosis: clinical features of large congenital melanocytic nevi in patients with manifest central nervous system melanosis. J Am Acad Dermatol 1996;35:529–538.

Dodge NN, Dobyns WB. Agenesis of the corpus callosum and Dandy-Walker malformation associated with hemimeganencephaly in the sebaceous nevus syndrome. Am J Med Genet 1995;56:147–150.

Ernst M, Zametkin AJ, Matochik JA, et al. Presynaptic dopaminergic deficits in Lesch-Nyhan disease. N Engl J Med 1996;334:1568–1572.

Ewalt DE, Sheffield E, Delgado MR, Roach ES. Longitudinal study of renal lesions in children with tuberous sclerosis complex. J Urol 1998; 160:141–145.

Friedman JM, Birch PH. Type 1 neurofibromatosis: a descriptive analysis of the disorder in 1,728 patients. Am J Med Genet 1997;70:138–143.

Fry JA, Alvarellos A, Fink C, et al. Intracranial findings in progressive facial hemiatrophy. J Rheumatol 1992;19:952–956.

Gatti RA. Ataxia-telangiectasia. Dermatol Clin 1995;13:1–6.

Geller TJ, Pan Y, Martin DS. Early neuroradiologic evidence of degeneration in Menkes' disease. Pediatr Neurol 1997;17:255–258.

Grewal RP. Stroke in Fabry's disease. J Neurol 1994;241:153–156.

Gutmann DH, Geist RT, Xu HM, et al. Defects in neurofibromatosis 2 protein function can arise at multiple levels. Hum Mol Genet 1998;7:335–345.

Hager CM, Cohen PR, Tschen JA. Segmental neurofibromatosis: case reports and review. J Am Acad Dermatol 1997;37:864–869.

Itoh T, Cleaver JE, Yamaizumi M. Cockayne syndrome complementation group B associated with xeroderma pigmentosum phenotype. Hum Genet 1996;97:176–179.

Ivker R, Resnick SD, Skidmore RA. Hypophosphatemic vitamin D-resistant rickets, precocious puberty, and the epidermal nevus syndrome. Arch Dermatol 1997;133:1557–1561.

Jones AC, Daniells CE, Snell RG, et al. Molecular genetic and phenotypic analysis reveals differences between TSC1 and TSC2 associated tuberous sclerosis. Hum Mol Genet 1997;6:2155–2161.

Jozwiak S, Goodman M, Lamm SH. Poor mental development in TSC patients: clinical risk factors. Arch Neurol 1998;55:379–384.

Kaler SG, Das S, Levinson B, et al. Successful early copper therapy in Menkes disease associated with a mutant transcript containing a small In-frame deletion. Biochem Molec Med 1996;57:37–46.

Kashiwagi S, Tsuchida E, Goto K, et al. Balloon occlusion of a spontaneous carotid-cavernous fistula in Ehlers-Danlos syndrome type IV. Surg Neurol 1993;39:187–190.

Kevorkian JP, Masquet C, Kural-Menasche S, et al. New report of severe coronary artery disease in an eighteen-year-old girl with pseudoxanthoma elasticum. Angiology 1997;48:735–741.

Kikuchi K, Kowada M, Sasajima H. Vascular malformations of the brain in hereditary hemorrhagic telangiectasia (Rendu-Osler-Weber disease). Surg Neurol 1994;41:374–380.

Kim OH, Suh JH. Intracranial and extracranial MR angiography in Menkes disease. Pediatr Radiol 1997;27:782–784.

Kuriyama M, Tokimura Y, Fujiyama J, et al. Treatment of cerebrotendinous xanthomatosis: effects of chenodeoxycholic acid, pravastatin, and combined use. J Neurol Sci 1994;125:22–28.

Latif F, Tory K, Gnarra J, et al. Identification of the von Hippel-Lindau disease tumor suppressor gene. Science 1993;260:1317–1320.

Lesho EP. Recognition and management of von Hippel-Lindau disease. Am Fam Physician 1994;50:1269–1272.

Maeda T, Sato K, Minami H, et al. Chronological difference in walking impairment among Japanese group A xeroderma pigmentosum (XP-A) patients with various combinations of mutation sites. Clin Genet 1995;48:225–231.

Maher ER, Kaelin WGJ. von Hippel-Lindau disease. Medicine 1997;76:381–391.

Malherbe V, Pariente D, Tardieu M, et al. Central nervous system lesions in hypomelanosis of Ito: an MRI and pathological study. J Neurol 1993;240:302–304.

Maria BL, Neufeld JA, Rosainz LC, et al. High prevalence of bihemispheric structural and functional defects in Sturge-Weber syndrome. J Child Neurol 1998;13:595–605.

Matsuo S, Takeuchi Y, Hayashi S, et al. Patient with unusual Hutchinson-Gilford syndrome (progeria). Pediatr Neurol 1994;10:237–240.

Menor F, Marti-Bonmati L, Arana E, et al. Neurofibromatosis type 1 in children: MR imaging and follow-up studies of central nervous system findings. Eur J Radiol 1998;26:121–131.

Meschia JF, Junkins E, Hofman KJ. Familial systematized epidermal nevus syndrome. Am J Med Genet 1992;44:664–667.

Needle MN, Cnaan A, Dattilo J, et al. Prognostic signs in the surgical management of plexiform neurofibroma: the Children's Hospital of Philadelphia experience, 1974–1994. J Pediatr 1997;131:678–682.

Nehal KS, PeBenito R, Orlow SJ. Analysis of 54 cases of hypopigmentation and hyperpigmentation along the lines of Blaschko. Arch Dermatol 1996;132:1167–1170.

Ogino T, Hata H, Minakuchi E, et al. Neurophysiologic dysfunction in hypomelanosis of Ito: EEG and evoked potential studies. Brain Dev 1994;16:407–412.

Peterson LS, Nelson AM, Su WPD. Classification of morphea (localized scleroderma). Mayo Clin Proc 1996;70:1068–1076.

Ritter MM, Frilling A, Crossey PA, et al. Isolated familial pheochromocytoma as a variant of von Hippel-Lindau disease. J Clin Endocrin Metab 1996;81:1035–1037.

Roach ES, Delgado MR, Anderson L, et al. Carbamazepine trial for Lesch-Nyhan self-mutilation. J Child Neurol 1996;11:476–478.

Roach ES, Gomez MR, Northrup H. Tuberous sclerosis consensus conference: revised clinical diagnostic criteria. J Child Neurol 1998;13:624–628.

Rotman G, Shiloh Y. The ATM gene and protein: possible roles in genome surveillance, checkpoint controls and cellular defence against oxidative stress. Cancer Surv 1997;29:285–304.

Sardanelli F, Parodi RC, Ottonello C, et al. Cranial MRI in ataxia-telangiectasia. Neuroradiology 1995;37:77–82.

Sasaki Y, Kobayashi S, Shimizu H, Nishikawa T. Multiple nodular lesions seen in a patient with neurocutaneous melanosis. J Dermatol 1996;23:828–831.

Sato K, Kubota T, Kitai R. Linear sebaceous nevus syndrome (sebaceous nevus of Jadassohn) associated with abnormal neuronal migration and optic glioma: case report. Neurosurgery 1994;35:318–320.

Schievink WI, Mellenger JF, Atkinson JLD. Progressive intracranial aneurysmal disease with progressive hemifacial atrophy (Parry-Romberg disease): case report. Neurosurgery 1996;38:1237–1241.

Schwartze U, Goldstein JA, Byers PH. Splicing defects in the COL3A1 gene: marked preference for 5' (donor) splice-site mutations in patients with exon-skipping mutations and Ehlers-Danlos syndrome type IV. Am J Hum Genet 1997;61:1276–1286.

Scully RE, Mark EJ, McNeely WF, McNeely BU. Case records of the Massachusetts General Hospital—Case 18-1994. N Engl J Med 1994;330:1300–1306.

Siebner HR, Berndt S, Conrad B. Cerebrotendinous xanthomatosis without tendon xanthomas mimicking Marinesco-Sjögren syndrome: a case report. J Neurol Neurosurg Psychiatry 1996;60:582–585.

Struk B, Neldner KH, Rao VS, et al. Mapping of both autosomal recessive and dominant variants of pseudoxanthoma elasticum to chromosome 16p.13.1. Hum Mol Genet 1997;6:1823–1828.

Sujansky E, Conradi S. Outcome of Sturge-Weber syndrome in 52 adults. Am J Med Genet 1995b;57:35–45.

Sujansky E, Conradi S. Sturge-Weber syndrome: age of onset of seizures and glaucoma and the prognosis for affected children. J Child Neurol 1995a;10:49–58.

Taylor AM, Metcalfe JA, Thick J, Mak YF. Leukemia and lymphoma in ataxia telangiectasia. Blood 1996;87:423–438.

Torres OA, Roach ES, Delgado MR, et al. Early diagnosis of subependymal giant cell astrocytoma in patients with tuberous sclerosis. J Child Neurol 1998;13:173–177.

Tumer Z, Horn N. Menkes disease: recent advances and new aspects. J Med Genet 1997;34:265–274.

van Soest S, Swart J, Tijmes N, et al. A locus for autosomal recessive pseudoxanthoma elasticum, with penetrance of vascular symptoms in carriers, maps to chromosome 16p.13.1. Genome Res 1997;7:830–834.

Vanderhooft SL, Francis JS, Pagon RA, Smith LT. Prevalence of hypopigmented macules in a healthy population. J Pediatr 1996;129:355–361.

Weiner DM, Ewalt DE, Roach ES, Hensle TW. The tuberous sclerosis complex: a comprehensive review. J Am College Surg 1998;187:548–561.

Zacharin M. Precocious puberty in two children with neurofibromatosis type 1 in the absence of optic chiasmal glioma. J Pediatr 1997;130:155–157.

Zeng L, Quilliet X, Chevallier-Lagente O, et al. Retrovirus-mediated gene transfer corrects DNA repair defect of xeroderma pigmentosum cells of complementation groups A, B and C. Gene Ther 1997;4:1077–1084.

Chapter 70
The Dementias

Martin N. Rossor

All definitions of dementia include three essential features:

1. The cognitive impairment should be acquired.
2. The impairment should involve multiple domains of cognitive function rather than a discrete neuropsychological deficit.
3. The patient should not have impairment of arousal, in contrast to delirium, in which this is a prominent feature.

This definition is from the *Diagnostic and Statistical Manual of Mental Disorders*, 4th edition (*DSM-IV*). Table 70.1 provides criteria for these features. These criteria include more detail of the memory impairment than the third edition (*DSM-III*) and importantly define the terms *short-term* and *long-term memory*. Two assessments may be needed to demonstrate evidence of progressive memory loss, but this can be assumed from an informant's history. The *International Classification of Diseases 10* (*ICD 10*) classification, and that of its neurological adaptation (*ICD 10NA*), are similar and also provide criteria for severity. The distinction between dementia and a confusional state or delirium can be difficult to make. Patients with dementia may have impairment of selective attention; if arousal mechanisms are involved, however, then widespread cognitive deficits may arise. This may be easy to identify with acute onset, but distinguishing between a chronic confusional state and a dementia may be impossible.

In the past, there was a tendency to view dementia only as a global impairment of cognitive function, but it is possible to recognize characteristic features among the many different dementias. This applies both to the primary degenerative dementias, in which the cognitive impairment is either the sole or the major feature, and to the dementias arising within the context of more widespread neurological disturbance, the dementia-plus syndromes. Thus, in addition to the criteria for dementia (*DSM-IV*, *ICD 10*), operational criteria also have been developed for Alzheimer's disease (National Institute of Neurological and Communicative Disorders and Stroke; Alzheimer's Disease and Related Disorders Association), vascular dementia (National Institute of Neurological Disorders and Stroke; Association Internationale pour la Recherche et L'Enseignement en Neurosciences) (Román et al. 1993), dementia with Lewy bodies (McKeith et al. 1996), and the frontotemporal dementias (Lund-Manchester criteria) (Brun et al. 1994).

A major clinical distinction has been proposed between cortical and subcortical dementias. The term *subcortical dementia* was originally applied to the cognitive impairment seen in progressive supranuclear palsy and Huntington's disease. The distinction is that patients with subcortical dementia show marked slowness (bradyphrenia), with disturbance of motivation and attention. In contrast, patients with cortical dementia show, in addition to the amnesia, variable combinations of aphasia, apraxia, and agnosia, which can most readily be related to damage to the association cortices (Pate and Margolin 1994). Slowness is a key feature of subcortical dementia, and the memory deficit may show differences from that of cortical dementia in that recall of new information is partially aided by cues. This suggests that there is a greater deficit in recollection than in encoding, again in contrast to cortical dementia. In addition to the cognitive impairment, apathy, irritability, and depression are features of subcortical dementia (Table 70.2). Subcortical damage may be seen in the prototypical cortical dementia of Alzheimer's disease, but it is much more prominent in those disorders associated with subcortical dementia, in which intrinsic damage to the cerebral cortex is not prominent. Subcortical dementia may be seen in a wide variety of pathological processes, including degenerative, vascular, infective, and inflammatory disease, that affect the basal ganglia and the basal forebrain.

The concept of *subcortical dementia* has been criticized, particularly the semantic difficulty posed by the term, which implies a strict distinction between cortical and subcortical pathology. It has been argued that a clear distinction cannot be demonstrated clinically, although failures to establish clear differences from patients with cortical dementia may relate to insensitive testing and inadequate matching of groups with subcortical dementia. Moreover, not all dementias can be classified according to whether they are cortical or subcortical, but it does remain a useful clinical distinction and most of the reversible dementias are associated with a subcortical pattern.

Although different dementias may demand specific strategies of investigation and assessment, the overall approach to investigation is similar. A common strategy is a detailed neuropsychological assessment of the patient that explores the major domains of cognitive function (see Chapter 39). In clinical practice, such an assessment is made by a clinical psychologist and tailored to the patient, as opposed to using a standard battery. However, to achieve comparability in research studies, defined assessment protocols have been developed for specific diseases (e.g., the Consortium to Establish a Registry for Alzheimer's Disease) or as diagnostic aids, primarily to assist with the broader differential diagnosis of depression or degenerative or vascular dementia. Composite cognitive assessments can give an overall indication of dementia severity, which is of value in following patients

Table 70.1: DSM-IV criteria for dementia

The development of multiple cognitive deficits that include
    memory impairment and at least one of the following:
    Aphasia
    Apraxia
    Agnosia
    Disturbance in executive functioning
The cognitive deficits must
    Be sufficiently severe to cause impairment in occupational or
        social functioning
    Represent a decline from a previous higher level of functioning
Diagnosis should not be made if the cognitive deficits occur
    exclusively during the course of a delirium. However, a
    dementia and a delirium may both be diagnosed if the demen-
    tia is present at times when the delirium is not present.
Dementia may be etiologically related to a general medical condi-
    tion, to the persisting effects of substance abuse (including
    toxin exposure), or to a combination of these factors.

Source: Adapted from Diagnostic and Statistical Manual of Mental Disorders (DSM-IV) (4th ed). Washington, DC: American
Psychiatric Association, 1994.

(e.g., the Alzheimer's Disease Assessment Scale). Brief assessments, such as the Blessed Dementia Scale, the Mini-Mental
State Examination, and the Mattis Rating Scale, have the
advantage of brevity but can only provide crude overall measures. In addition, functional scales may measure the effect
of dementia on everyday function, either on basic skills
assessed in activities of daily living or on more complex tasks,
such as shopping and cooking, explored with instrumental
activities of daily living measures (e.g., the Interview for
Deterioration in Daily Living Activities in Dementia).

In addition to the assessment of higher cortical function,
a general neurological and physical examination is essential.
Evidence of additional neurological dysfunction with pyramidal, extrapyramidal, or cerebellar signs would place the
patient in one of the dementia-plus categories. Systemic disturbance also may provide valuable information, not only in
identifying potential causes (e.g., neoplasm), but also the
cause of deterioration in a patient with established dementia. Investigations are still aimed primarily at treatable or
reversible causes of dementia (Small et al. 1997). Routine
biochemistry, hematology, syphilis and *Borrelia* serology, thyroid function, and vitamin B_{12} estimations identify many of
the common and reversible dementias. Mutation screening
can provide a specific diagnosis in a number of hereditary

dementias (e.g., huntingtin, presenilin, amyloid precursor
protein [APP], prion and tau genes). Neuroimaging with
computed tomography or magnetic resonance imaging scanning is essential, not only to identify space-occupying lesions
and hydrocephalus, but increasingly to assess regional distribution of atrophy in the degenerative dementias that may be
of diagnostic value. Functional imaging with single-photon
emission computed tomography or, less commonly, positron
emission tomography can also provide information on the
regional distribution of metabolic deficits. Electroencephalography is of value in identifying subclinical seizure activity
resulting in memory impairment, slowing in Alzheimer's disease in contrast to many of the frontal dementias, or the
characteristic periodic complexes in Creutzfeldt-Jakob disease. Examination of the cerebrospinal fluid is necessary in
atypical cases to identify inflammatory causes. More specific
tests may be required, depending on the clinical picture. Ultimately, in a few selected cases, cerebral biopsy may be necessary to exclude treatable causes such as granulomatous
angiitis. Careful investigation to achieve a precise diagnosis is
important, not only to identify causes that are potentially
treatable, but also to provide prognosis, explanation, and
planning for long-term management.

REFERENCES

Brun A, Englund E, Gustafson L, et al. Clinical and neuropatho-
    logical criteria for frontotemporal dementia. The Lund and
    Manchester Groups. J Neurol Neurosurg Psychiatry 1994;57:
    416–418.
Diagnostic and Statistical Manual of Mental Disorders (4th ed).
    Washington, DC: American Psychiatric Association, 1994.
McKeith LG, Galasko D, Kosaka K, et al. Consensus guidelines
    for the clinical and pathologic diagnosis of dementia with Lewy
    bodies (DLB): report of the consortium on DLB international
    workshop. Neurology 1996;47:1113–1124.
Pate DS, Margolin DI. Cognitive slowing in Parkinson's and
    Alzheimer's patients: distinguishing bradyphrenia from demen-
    tia. Neurology 1994;44:669–674.
Román GC, Tatemichi TK, Erkinjuntti T, et al. Vascular dementia:
    diagnostic criteria for research studies. Report of the NINDS-
    AIREN International Workshop. Neurology 1993;43:250–260.
Small GW, Rabins PV, Barry PP, et al. Diagnosis and treatment of
    Alzheimer disease and related disorders. Consensus statement
    of the American Association for Geriatric Psychiatry, the
    Alzheimer's Association, and the American Geriatrics Society.
    JAMA 1997;278:1363–1371.

Table 70.2: Distinctions between cortical and subcortical dementia

	Subcortical dementia	*Cortical dementia*
Severity	Mild to moderate	More severe earlier in course
Speed of cognition	Slow	Normal
Neuropsychological deficits	Frontal memory impairment (recall aided by cues)	Dysphasia, dyspraxia, agnosia
Neuropsychiatry	Apathy, depression	Depression less common
Motor abnormalities	Dysarthria, extrapyramidal	Uncommon, gegenhalten
Pathology	Prominent changes in striatum and thalamus	Prominent changes in cortical association areas

Source: Adapted from JL Cummings. Subcortical dementia: neuropsychology, neuropsychiatry and pathophysiology. Br J Psychiatry
1986;149:682–697.

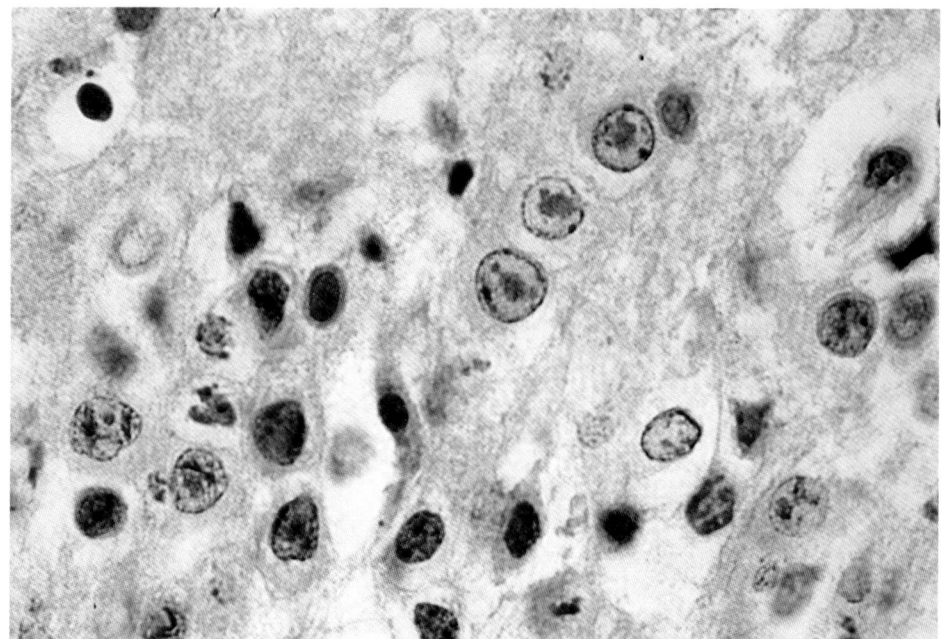

PLATE 59B.I Hippocampal granule cell neurons in herpes simplex 1 encephalitis. Many of the nuclei contain acidophilic Cowdry type A intranuclear inclusions, which are surrounded by haloes and which marginate the nuclear chromatin. (Hematoxylin-eosin stain; ×350; courtesy of R. Kim.)

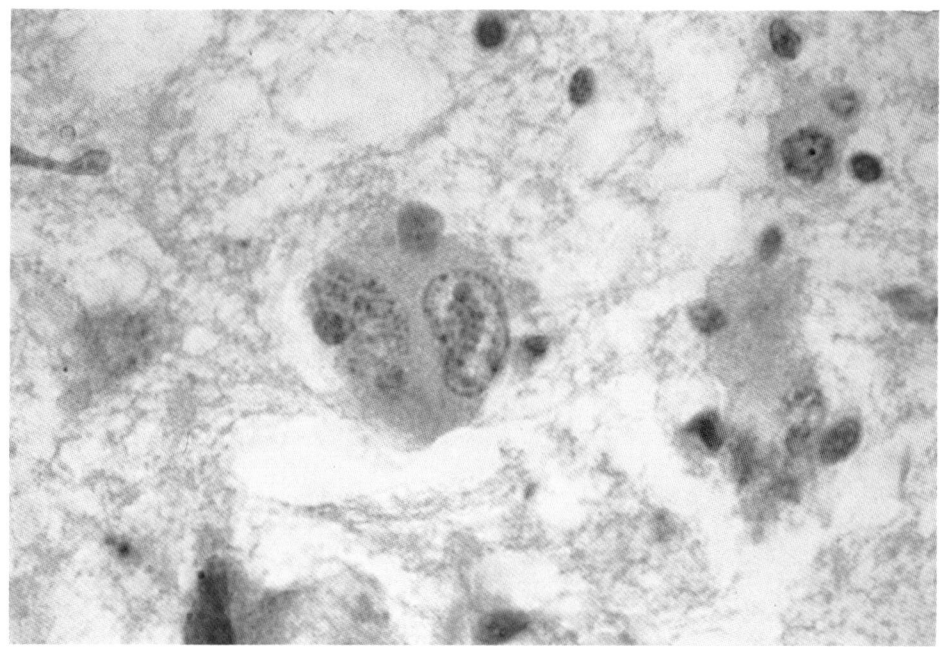

PLATE 59B.II Ballooned cell with eccentric nucleus in human cytomegalovirus encephalitis. An acidophilic Cowdry type A intranuclear inclusion body, with its surrounding halo, marginates the nuclear chromatin. The cytoplasm also contains granular inclusion material. (Hematoxylin-eosin stain; ×350; courtesy of R. Kim.)

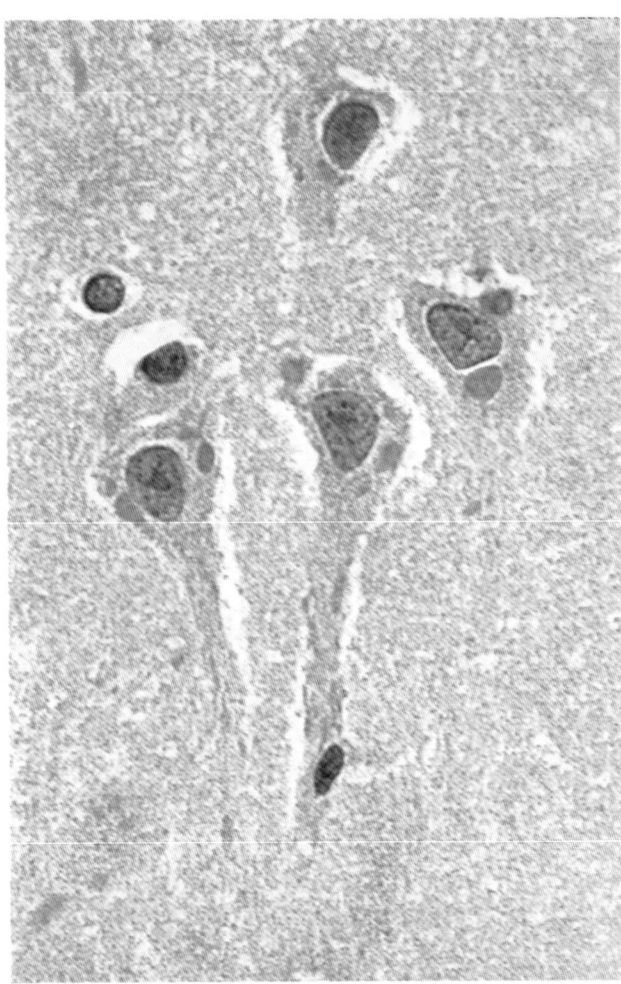

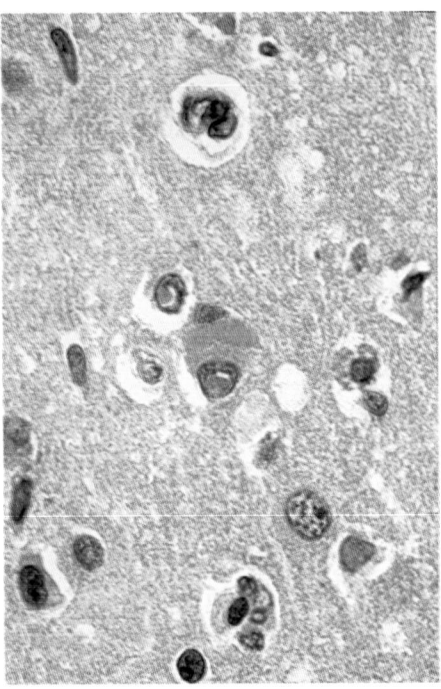

PLATE 59B.IV Cerebral cortex in subacute sclerosing panencephalitis. A pyramidal neuron contains both a Cowdry type A intranuclear inclusion and a cigar-shaped cytoplasmic inclusion. Cowdry A inclusions are present also in the nuclei of several nearby glia cells. (Hematoxylin-eosin stain; ×350; courtesy of R. Kim.)

PLATE 59B.III Hippocampal neurons in human rabies encephalitis. The cytoplasm of these neurons bears one or more rounded or oval Negri inclusion bodies. (Hematoxylin-eosin stain; ×350; courtesy of R. Kim.)

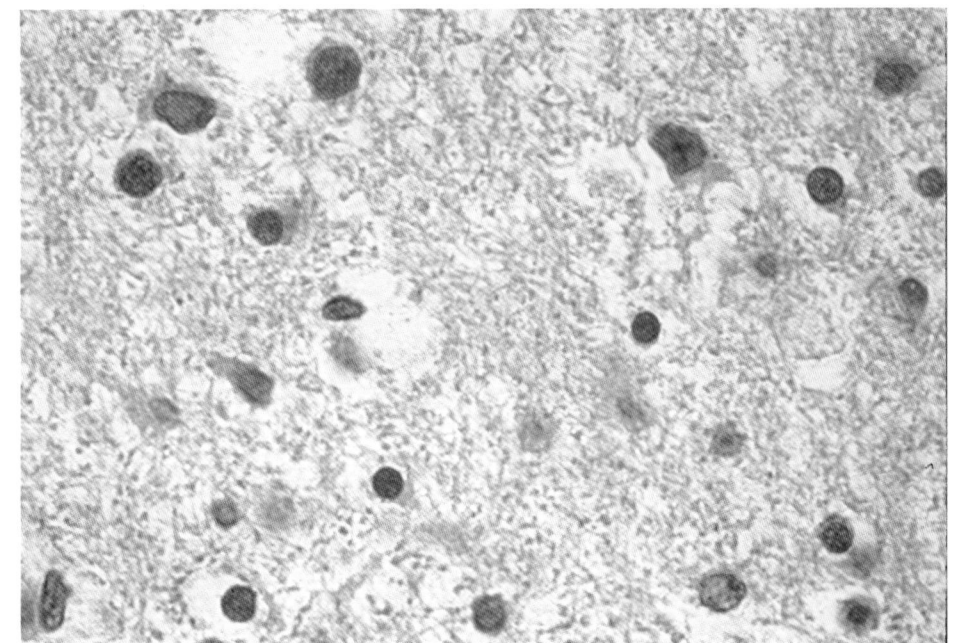

PLATE 59B.V Cerebral white matter in progressive multifocal leukoencephalopathy. Oligo-dendroglial cell nuclei are greatly enlarged and their nuclear chromatin replaced by glassy acidophilic material. (Hematoxylin-eosin stain; ×350; courtesy of R. Kim.)

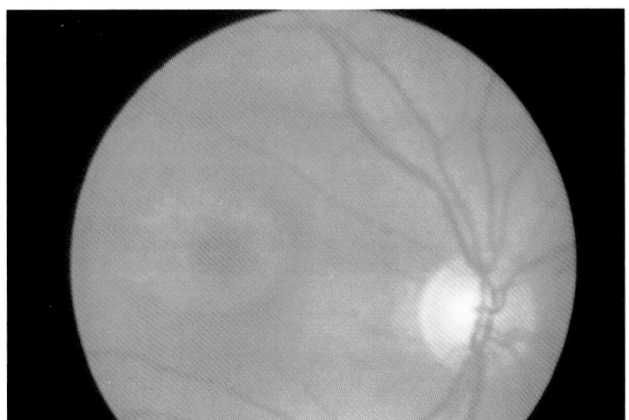

PLATE 59D.I Chloroquine retinopathy. Bull's-eye appearance of chloroquine retinopathy with increased pigmentation in the macula, a ring of depigmentation surrounded by mildly increased pigmentation. (Courtesy of Caygill Ophthalmic Library, Department of Ophthalmology, University of California, San Francisco.)

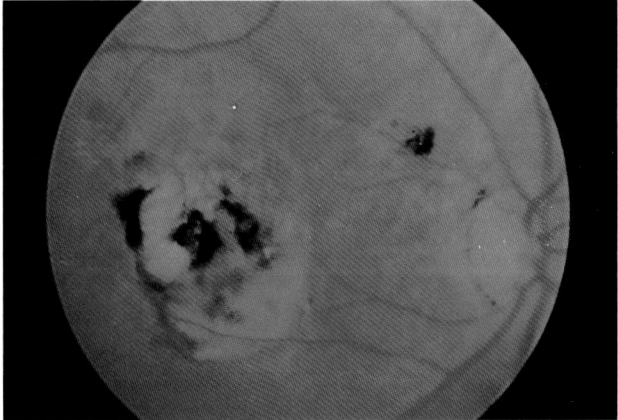

PLATE 59D.II Toxoplasmosis chorioretinitis. Chorioretinal scar surrounded by pigmentation in healed toxoplasmosis. The central white area is the sclera, seen after necrosis of the retina and choroid. (Courtesy of Caygill Ophthalmic Library, Department of Ophthalmology, University of California, San Francisco.)

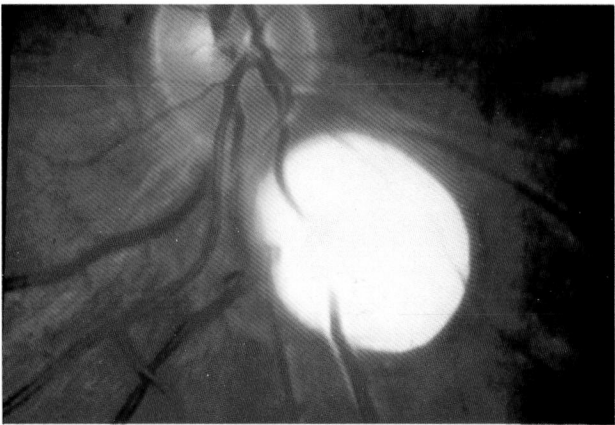

PLATE 59D.III Ocular toxocariasis. *Toxocara canis* chorioretinitis with granuloma elevated above the retina. (Courtesy of Caygill Ophthalmic Library, Department of Ophthalmology, University of California, San Francisco.)

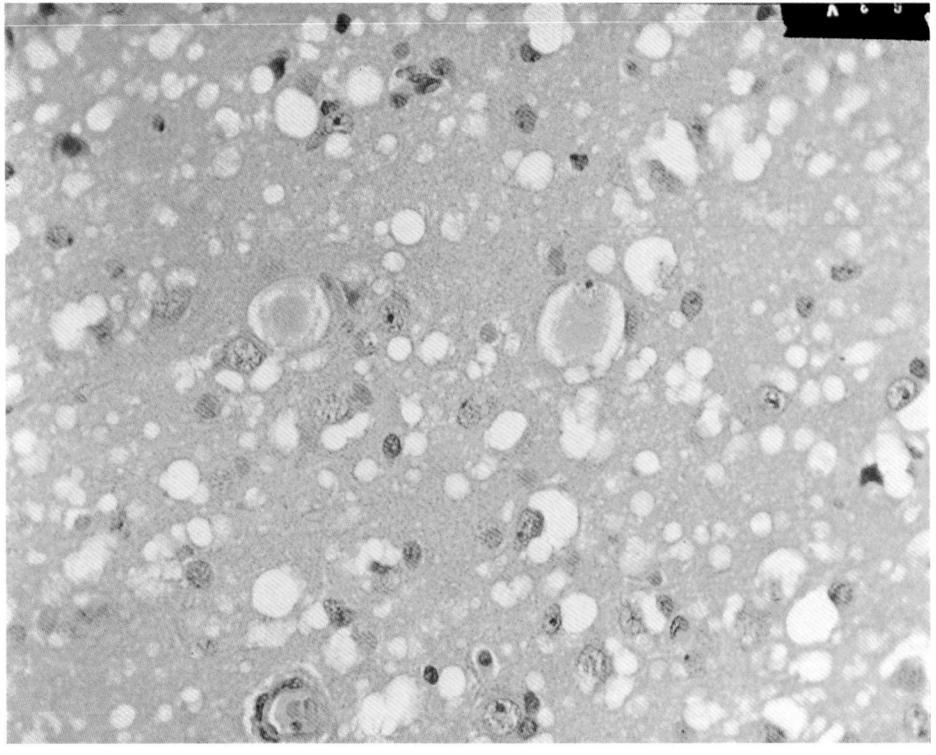

A

PLATE 59F.I Various appearances of spongiform change in patients with Creutzfeldt-Jakob disease. (A) The most characteristic distribution of translucent oval vacuoles is seen. (B) A coalescent focus of vacuoles. (C) A virtual replacement of normal brain tissue by vacuoles.

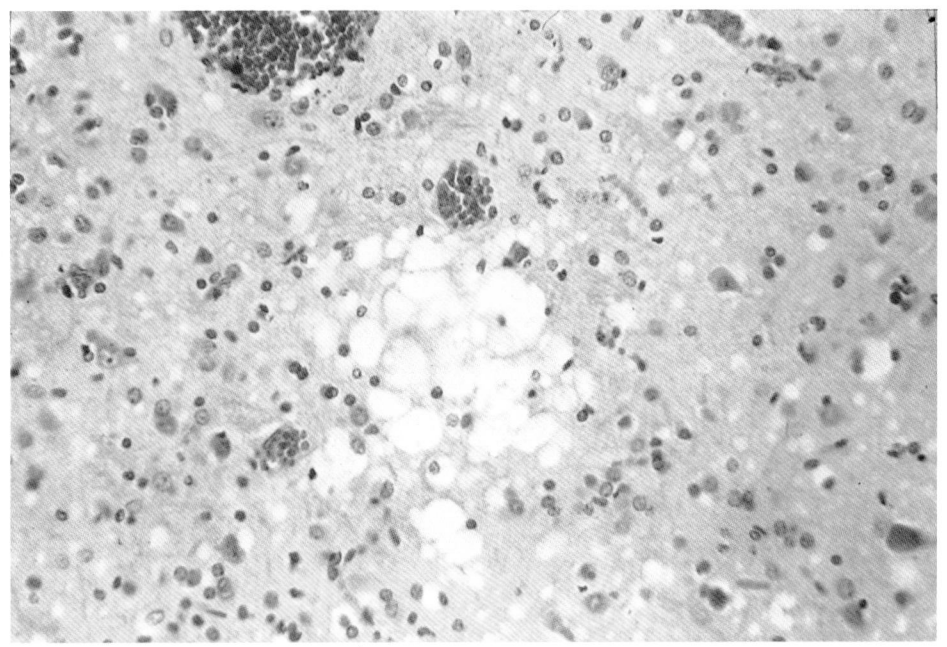

B

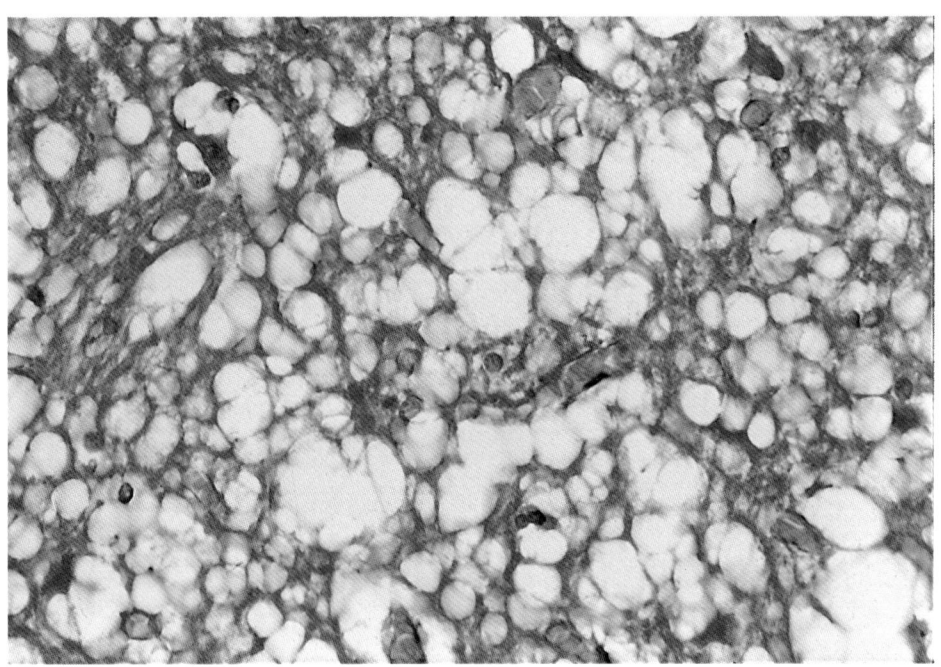

C

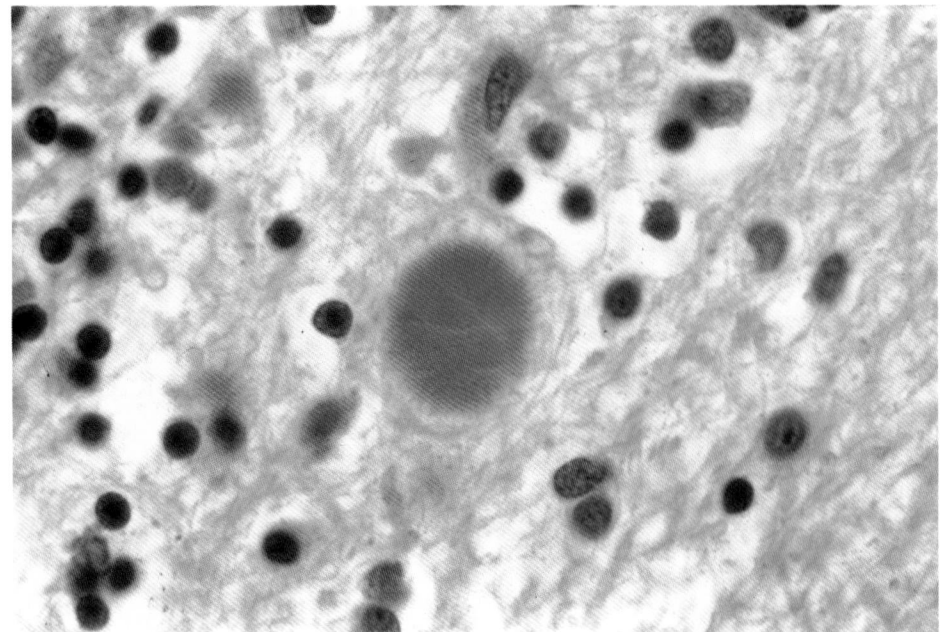

A

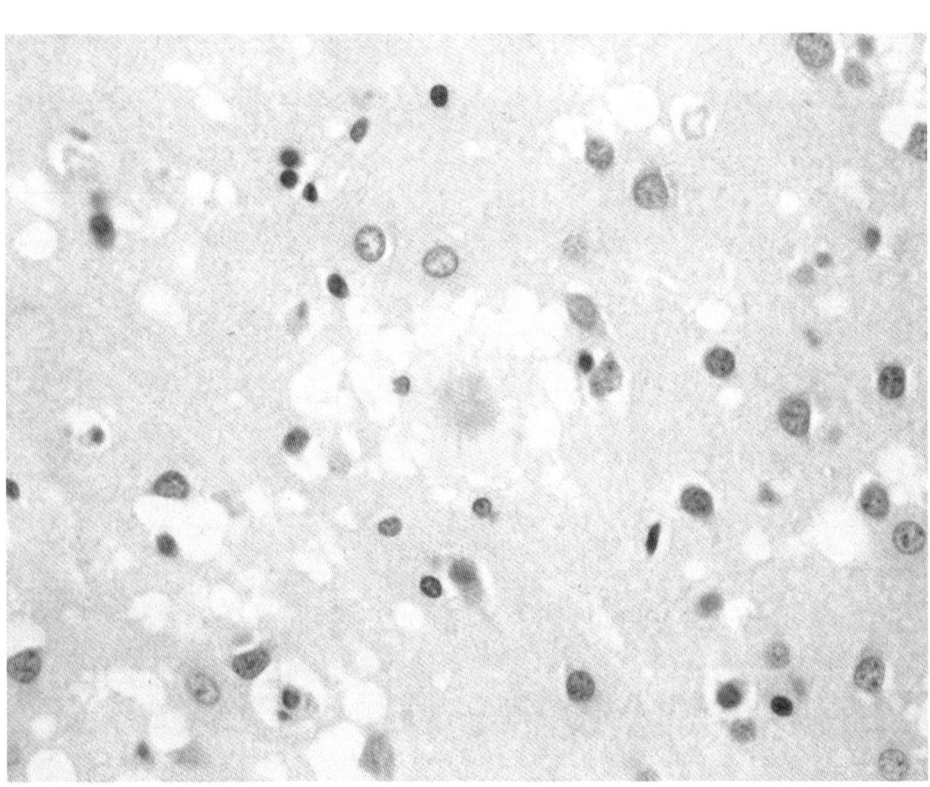

B

PLATE 59F.II Various types of amyloid plaques seen in transmissible spongiform encephalopathies (TSE). (A) A kuru-type unicentric plaque may occur in any form of TSE. (B) A daisy plaque (a unicentric plaque surrounded by a halo of vacuoles) that is characteristic of new variant Creutzfeldt-Jakob disease. (C) A multicentric plaque is characteristic of Gerstmann-Sträussler-Scheinker syndrome.

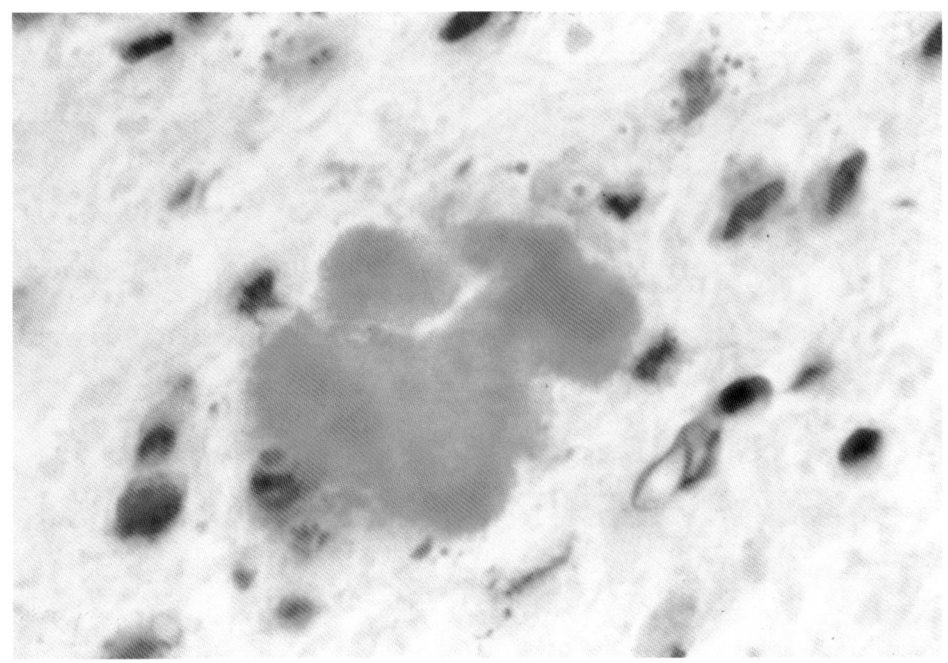

C

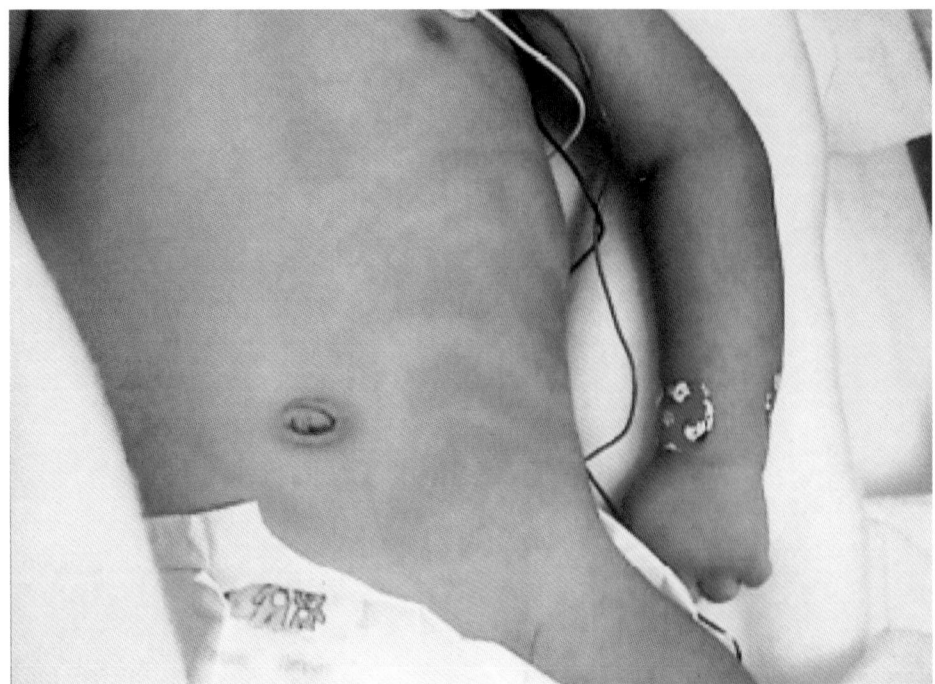

PLATE 69.I Characteristic swirling pigmentation of the trunk of a 4-month-old infant with hypomelanosis of Ito. This patient also had seizures and cataracts.

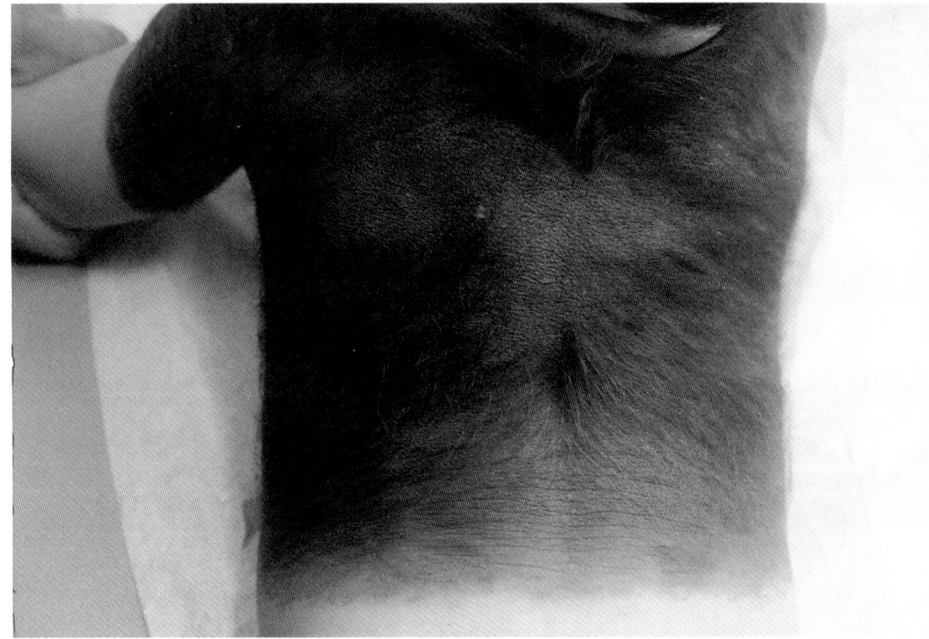

PLATE 69.II Large, dark, hairy nevus covering most of the back of an infant with neurocutaneous melanosis.

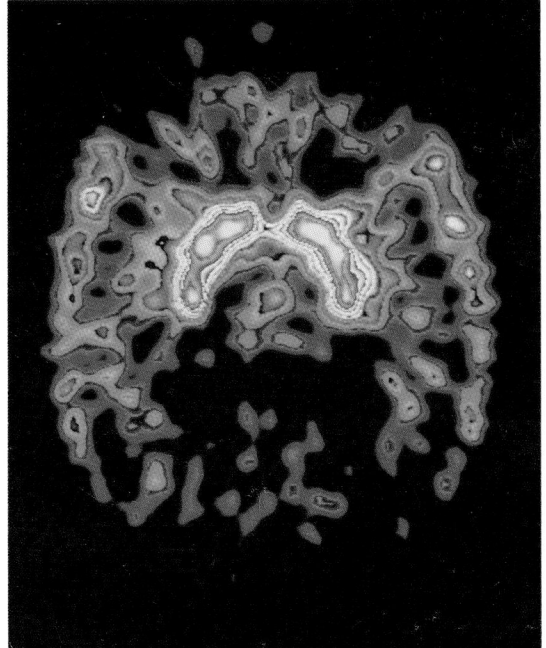

A

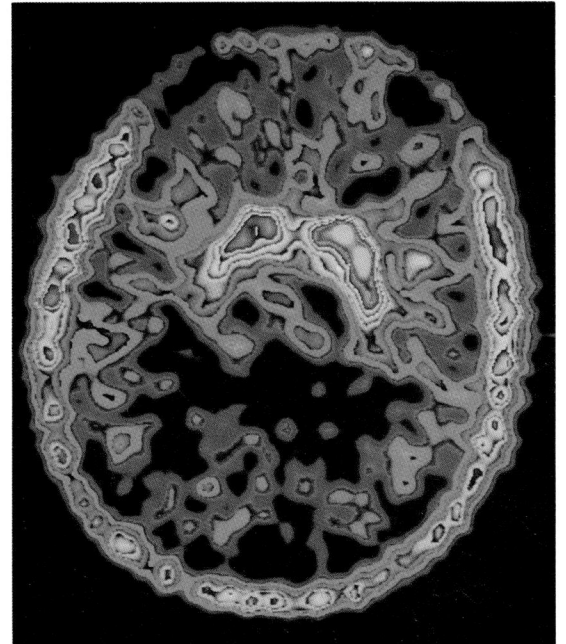

B

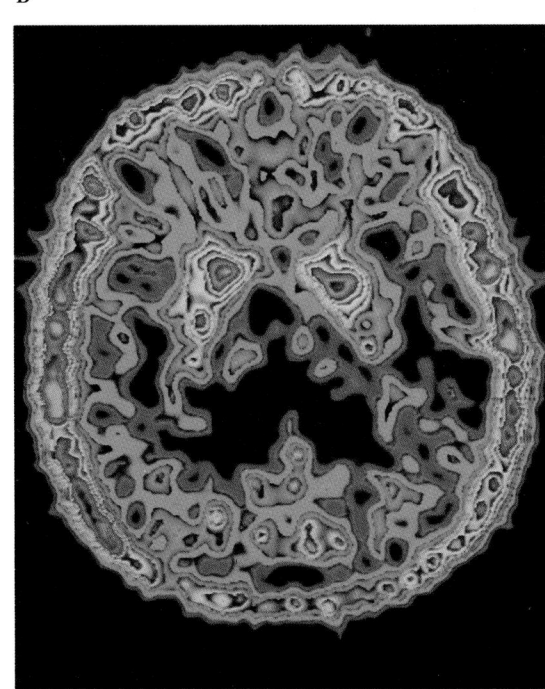

C

PLATE 75.I Positron emission tomography using 6-[^{18}fluorine] fluorolevodopa in Parkinson's disease. **(A)** Normal. The comma-shaped striata show intense accumulation of radioactivity relative to other structures (colors in order of decreasing activity: pink, red, orange, yellow, green, and blue). **(B)** Early Parkinson's disease. Left hemiparkinsonism with loss of radioactivity in the right striatum (shown on the left in the photograph), particularly the putamen. **(C)** Advanced Parkinson's disease. Bilateral parkinsonism with decreased isotope accumulation in both striata. Note that the color representations are relative, not absolute, values, and that there is now proportionately more activity in the temporalis muscles than in the caudate nucleus or putamen. (Courtesy of the late Dr. Steve Garnett.)

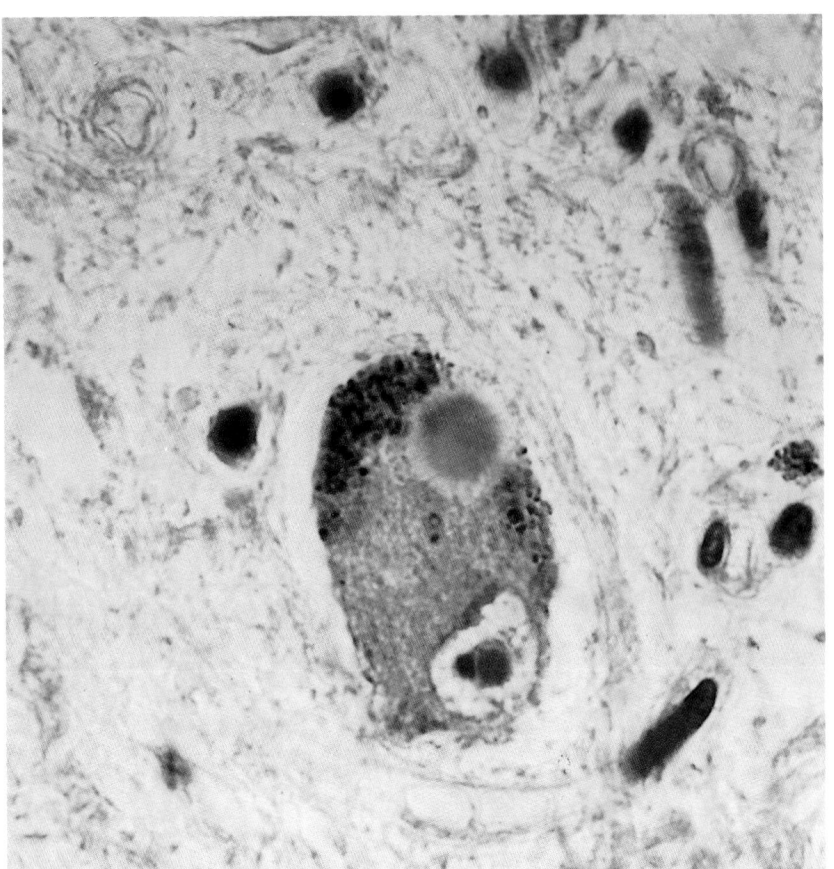

PLATE 75.II Lewy body. A typical eosinophilic inclusion with a clear halo is present in the cytoplasm of this pigmented substantia nigra neuron from a patient with Parkinson's disease. The Marinesco inclusion body in the nucleus is an incidental finding. (Courtesy of Dr. Lothar Resch.)

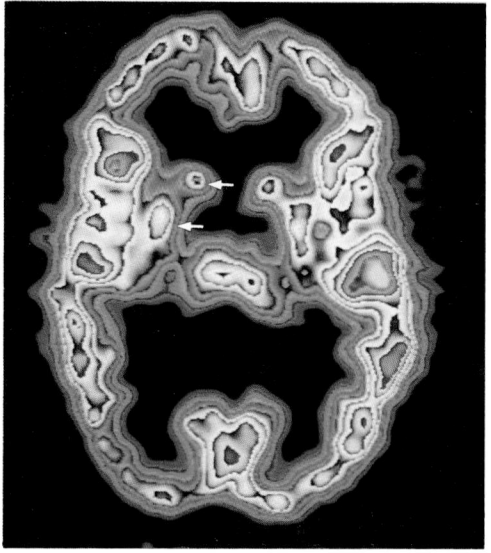

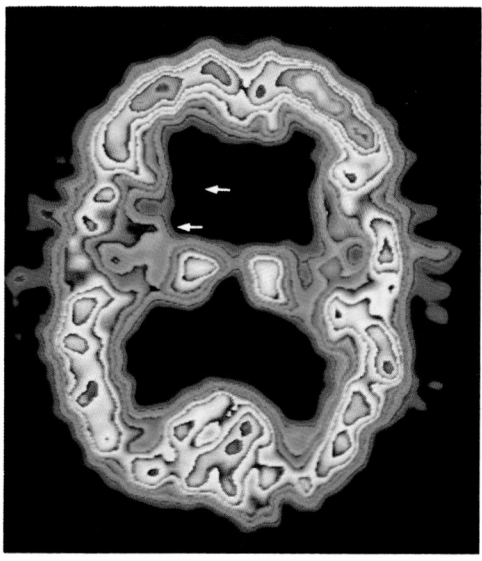

A   B

PLATE 75.III Positron emission tomography using [18fluorine]-fluorodeoxyglucose in Huntington's disease. (**A**) Normal isotope accumulation in the striata (*arrows* indicate right caudate nucleus [upper] and putamen [lower]). (**B**) Absence of radioactivity in the striata in a patient with Huntington's disease without significant caudate atrophy on computed tomographic scan (*arrows* directed at sites corresponding to those indicated in [**A**]). (Courtesy of the late Dr. Steve Garnett.)

Chapter 70
The Dementias

A. PRIMARY DEGENERATIVE DEMENTIA
Martin N. Rossor

The term *primary degenerative dementia* applies to those neuronal degenerations for which a cause is not established. As knowledge increases, more cases will be attributed to a specific cause, and as clinical diagnosis becomes more precise, cases may be assigned with greater confidence to diseases within this group, such as Alzheimer's disease (AD), dementia with Lewy bodies (DLB), and the frontotemporal dementias including Pick's disease. Most cases of primary degenerative dementia are caused by AD, although the exact proportion depends on the age of the patient. In autopsy and in clinical series of elderly patients, 15–20% are believed to be caused by DLB (Perry et al. 1996). DLB may be less common in younger patients, and frontotemporal dementia (see Chapter 70D) is the second most common after AD, constituting approximately 25% (Snowden et al. 1996).

ALZHEIMER'S DISEASE

History

In 1907, Alois Alzheimer described the case of a 51-year-old woman who developed paranoid delusions with memory impairment and subsequent disintegration of language (Maurer et al. 1997). Postmortem examination of the brain using the newly available silver stains revealed an abnormal pattern of staining. This staining revealed the senile plaques, consisting of dystrophic neurites, which, as was demonstrated subsequently, are clustered around a central amyloid core. Dense perikaryal staining was termed the *neurofibrillary tangle*. The cerebral cortex was also atrophic, which was assumed to be caused by cell loss. Initially, there was doubt about the distinction from the effects of old age, although subsequently Kraepelin considered this to be a distinct entity and introduced the eponym *Alzheimer's disease*. The disease was considered to be a rarity, occurring only within the presenile age group, and until 1960 only approximately 100 cases of AD were reported in the literature.

In the 1960s, pioneer prospective studies in Newcastle by Blessed, Tomlinson, and Roth showed an overall association between the number of senile plaques in the cerebral cortex and the severity of cognitive impairment; moreover, no qualitative difference was found between presenile and senile cases. From being a rarity, AD has become one of the most common diseases of the aging population and is now the fourth most common cause of death. Consequent to this have been advances in the description of the neuropathology and neurotransmitter abnormalities, the elucidation of the molecular pathology of senile plaques and neurofibrillary tangles (Selkoe 1998), and the appreciation of an important genetic role in the disease. The first example of familial AD (FAD) was not reported until 1932, but since then extensive pedigrees have been described and a family history of dementia is found in approximately 25% of cases. The genetic mutations associated with these autosomal dominant FAD cases are being elucidated and to date include the *presenilin 1* and *2* and amyloid precursor protein (*APP*) genes (Hardy 1997). The importance of genetic risk factors and in particular the inheritance of the E4 allele of apolipoprotein E (apo E) are also now recognized. However, despite advances in the pathophysiology of AD, the initial question of its relationship to aging remains unanswered. It has, however, been pragmatic to consider old age and AD as separate conditions for the management of individual patients.

Clinical Features

The disease is predominantly one of middle and late life. It is rare below age 45, and although patients as young as 30 years are seen, this is usually within the context of *presenilin 1* mutation FAD. The disease may be difficult to diagnose in the elderly, in whom memory inefficiency is common; in order to make the diagnosis, follow-up may be necessary to establish deterioration. Although a typical case may be described, with prominent early memory disturbance and subsequent language and visuospatial impairment, variation is wide, and in unselected series diagnostic accuracy is relatively low when tested against autopsy diagnosis. If atypical cases are excluded and criteria such as those of the National Institute of Neurological and Communicative Diseases and Stroke are used, high accuracies of 80–90% can be anticipated.

At the initial assessment, the history may be unreliable, particularly in the presence of anosagnosia (a patient's lack of recognition of the illness), and it is essential to obtain an independent description from a relative. Even the relative's history may be inaccurate, however, often in an attempt to protect the patient. A useful guide can be obtained from work performance and the ability to deal with everyday family affairs.

In many early reports, broad clinical descriptions were used. Increasingly, the neuropsychological deficits have been dissected to explore the disintegration of modular function. However, although discussed individually, these do not of course occur in isolation once the disease is established. At presentation, the deficit may be discrete and usually involves memory, but as cognitive function deteriorates, islands of relative preservation such as motor skills are seen before final deterioration into a bedridden, mute, incontinent, and unresponsive state, which mimics the persistent vegetative state, and then to death.

Memory

Memory impairment has been a major feature in all studies in which the diagnosis has been confirmed at autopsy or biopsy. Because memory impairment is an essential compo-

nent of the dementia criteria, there is a danger of circular argument unless cases are independently confirmed neuropathologically. Indeed, AD can rarely present with neuropsychological deficits other than in memory, for example, aphasia, but memory tasks in general are the earliest deficits to be reported.

It is not clear which tests were used to investigate memory in many earlier studies, and more recently interest has been directed at the different components such as short-term or primary memory versus long-term or secondary memory; episodic versus semantic memory; and procedural memory. Short-term, or primary, memory has limited storage capacity and can be assessed by digit span, word span, and block span tasks. Patients with early AD show only a mild deficit, compared with long-term memory. Long-term memory (i.e., remembering material over intervals longer than 30 seconds) is more severely and earlier affected and underpins the clinically salient impairment of everyday episodic memory. The observed long-term memory impairment involves impairment of both encoding and retrieval.

Remote memory, memory for events in a person's distant past, is often claimed to be preserved in dementia, but this is difficult to substantiate at bedside. When remote memory is scrutinized in detail, it is found to be impaired.

In 1972, Tulving proposed a distinction between episodic and semantic memory. Most of the tests described here relate to episodic memory, although semantic memory is also impaired. Indeed, some of the language impairments seen in AD can be related to disintegration of semantic memory (Hodges and Patterson 1995). A further classification of memory systems emphasizes the difference between declarative and procedural knowledge. With procedural knowledge, there may be implicit learning of which the patient is unaware (e.g., patients with Korsakoff's psychosis may learn a motor task without being aware of having done so). In AD, there is evidence of relative preservation of procedural memory, and patients can be shown to exhibit procedural or implicit learning in the absence of any apparent parallel declarative learning. It is of interest, in light of the observed cholinergic deficit, that these two systems may be dissociated neurochemically; the administration of the anticholinergic scopolamine reduces declarative but not procedural memory.

Aphasia, Apraxia, and Visuospatial Impairment

Language disturbance is generally an early feature of AD. It has been claimed that this is more prominent in early-onset cases, in contrast to a salient memory disturbance with visuospatial problems in later onset cases. In some patients, aphasia may be a prominent early feature, with more widespread cognitive disturbance occurring only later. Impairment of verbal fluency and confrontation naming are often observed early. On the latter task, semantic constraints, such as examples of categories (i.e., animals, are more difficult than orthographically constrained tasks, e.g., words starting with a particular letter). This may be attributed to the breakdown in semantic memory, auditory comprehension, and, in particular, to difficulty comprehending complex linguistic structures. In general, apraxia occurs late in the course of the disease, after memory and language disturbances are established and appears to progress relatively slowly, although in some cases apraxia may be a prominent feature.

Impairment of visuoperceptual and visuospatial skills are frequently found and reported to be more common in older patients. Apperceptive agnosias are more commonly observed than associative agnosias, but early visual processing deficits may contribute to perceptual difficulties. Assessment of visuospatial skills can be difficult in the presence of apraxia but are seen commonly as the disease progresses. Perceptual deficits can be a prominent early feature, and some patients present with visual disorientation. Frontal lobe deficits tend to occur later, in contrast to the frontotemporal dementias. Anosognosia, or unawareness of the cognitive deficit, can be an early feature and present a difficult management problem.

Neuropsychiatric Symptoms

In general, the neuropsychiatric symptoms of AD fall into four groups: mood disturbances, delusions and hallucinations, personality change, and disorders of behavior.

Depression is common in all forms of dementia, although its prevalence varies with the type of dementia. From a study of 1,700 elderly patients with memory complaints, the rate of depression was 25–30% in those with possible or probable AD, compared with 40% in mixed dementia (Coreybloom et al. 1993). By contrast, the frequency of manic symptoms in AD is rare, with a rate of approximately 3%. Two-thirds of patients with AD have at least one symptom of depression. Depression can be difficult to diagnose as language declines and may be manifested as agitation or importuning behaviors. In a study of patients referred to a dementia clinic who were thought to be suffering from depressive pseudodementia, a proportion later developed an organic dementia. There is now good evidence that the depression associated with AD is a direct result of neurological damage rather than a psychological reaction to the disease. On neuropathological examination, depressed patients with AD have a greater loss of neurons from the locus ceruleus, resulting in catecholamine depletion and a possible explanation for the clinical features of depression. There is no association of depression with presence or absence of anosognosia.

Delusions and hallucinations are common in AD. Reported prevalences for delusions are up to 30% (Allen and Burns 1995). Simple delusions of theft and suspicion are most common and are more prevalent in men. The reported prevalence of hallucinations is up to 20% but this is higher in DLB. Hallucinations may be in the visual, auditory, or, less commonly, olfactory domain. Misidentification syndromes are found in up to 15% of patients. The type of psychotic symptoms to some extent predicts the course of the disease: Subjects with misidentification syndromes are younger and have an earlier age at onset and a lower death rate; those with hallucinations have a more rapid cognitive decline; whereas the presence of delusions has no relationship with cognitive function or rate of progression.

Personality changes occur in at least three-fourths of even mildly demented AD patients. The changes are apathy, disengagement, and disinhibition and are often associated with depression.

Behavioral disturbance is found in 30–85% of patients. The types found include verbal and physical aggression, wandering, agitation, inappropriate sexual behavior, uncooperativeness, urinary incontinence, binge eating, catastrophic reactions, and attempts at self-inflicted harm. Unlike delusions and hallucinations, behavioral disturbances have a positive correlation with severity of dementia. Aggressive behavior in particular can pose major management problems and cause great strain on caregivers.

Physical Examination

Generally, with primary degenerative dementias the prominent abnormalities are found on examination of higher cortical function, and the general neurological examination is relatively normal. Extrapyramidal abnormalities have been reported in as many as 60% of patients in some series. Increased muscle tone is the main feature, and it may be difficult to distinguish extrapyramidal rigidity in these patients from paratonia, or *gegenhalten* (*to hold against* or *resist*, a term used to describe the variable resistance to passive movement that increases with the extent of displacement). Other patients with akinesia are usually found to have additional Lewy bodies, but tremor is rare. Primitive developmental reflexes, such as grasping, rooting, and sucking, may be seen later, but pouting and palmomental reflexes appear to be common in the aged population generally and do not clearly distinguish those with dementia. In general, there appears to be a poor correlation between the emergence of primitive reflexes and the severity of the cognitive impairment in patients with AD.

Generalized seizures have a 10–20% prevalence rate among patients with AD and may be more common in early-onset AD. Myoclonus is seen in a mild form in as many as 10% of those with AD, but in some patients it may be a prominent feature, creating confusion clinically with Creutzfeldt-Jakob disease. The reports of occasional pyramidal signs with increased tendon reflexes and extensor plantar responses may be difficult to interpret in an elderly population in which cervical spondylotic myelopathy and vascular disease may coexist. Exceptions are rare cases of *presenilin 1* FAD. Late in the disease the patient is mute, incontinent, and bedridden, with flexion deformities of the limbs and impaired swallowing. Weight loss is also common at this stage.

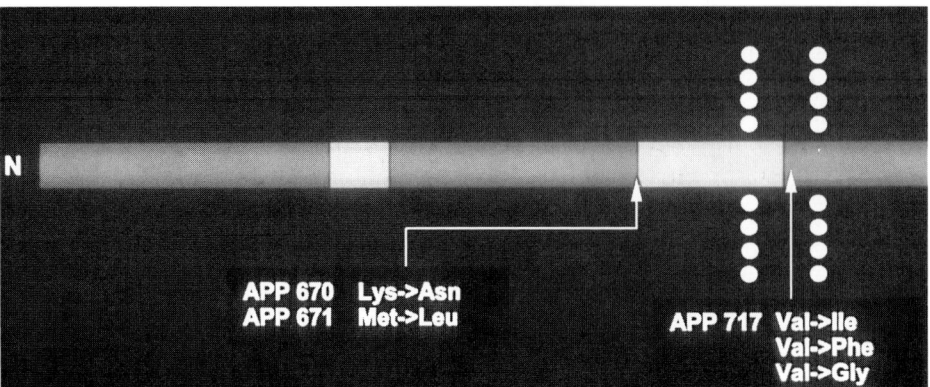

FIGURE 70A.1   Ideogram of the amyloid precursor protein (APP) molecules showing sites of mutations.

Heterogeneity of Alzheimer's Disease

AD exhibits clinical, pathological, and biochemical heterogeneity. One potential subdivision, which dates back to the original observations of Alzheimer, is between early- and late-onset cases, which are generally divided at age 65. It is still argued whether early- and late-onset cases are fundamentally different or merely show an association with age rather than a precise age cutoff. It has been claimed that prominent language disturbances occur more in the young-onset cases, in contrast to visuospatial deficits in late-onset cases. A subtype has been suggested on the basis of extrapyramidal features, which appear to be associated with more severe dementia and a poorer prognosis. Some of these cases have additional cortical Lewy bodies at autopsy and have been referred to as the *Lewy body variant of AD*; these cases are now usually considered under the rubric of DLB. Some patients also have a strikingly focal onset; reference has already been made to onset with aphasia or visual disorientation, but patients also have been described with hemiparesis and cortical sensory disturbance. Although different patterns may be identified, these need not imply separate causation. Recent advances in molecular genetics, however, have identified categorical differences within FAD.

Familial Alzheimer's Disease

It is difficult to determine the prevalence of FAD, and considerable variation in prevalence figures are quoted. Large autosomal dominant pedigrees of early onset are relatively rare, accounting for less than 5%. However, late-onset pedigrees may be censored, by early death from other causes, and could be much more common. As a group, no consistent differences between FAD and sporadic AD disease have been identified, although within the FAD group phenotypic heterogeneity, primarily in age at onset, can be observed. This in part reflects the molecular genetic heterogeneity, in that at least five different loci have now been identified. In rare families, the disease is associated with mutations in the amyloid precursor protein (APP) gene (Fig-

ure 70A.1); the age at onset is approximately 50 years. The majority of early-onset pedigrees are caused by mutations in the *presenilin 1* gene on chromosome 14, of which more than 40 have been described (Cruts and VanBroeckhoven 1998); onset age is variable but can be as young as 30. Mutations in a homologous *presenilin 2* gene are mainly associated with the Volga German pedigrees. Some, but not all, late-onset pedigrees are associated with inheritance of the E4 allele of apo E (Corder et al. 1993), which also contributes to apparent sporadic disease. Increased amyloid load and earlier age at onset are related to the apo E4 gene dosage. The apo E4 genotype is, however, only a risk factor, being neither sufficient nor necessary for disease development. The odds ratio of developing cognitive impairment in population studies is up to 3.7 for the E4 allele. Other risk factors include allelic variance of the 1-antichymotrypsin and very-low-density lipoprotein receptor genes.

Laboratory Studies

Acute-phase protein, hematological, biochemical, and immunological measurements are normal. Cerebrospinal fluid (CSF) opening pressure, cell count, and protein and sugar concentrations are within normal limits. Measurements of the concentrations of CSF neurotransmitters, neuropeptides, amino acids, and trace elements have not proved to be of diagnostic value. Ubiquitin and tau levels in CSF have been reported to be raised in AD, but the levels are similar to those found in other neurodegenerative disorders. The CSF concentrations of Aβ42 (see Pathology, later in this chapter) are reduced and assay of this analyte in combination with tau has been suggested as a diagnostic marker (Motter et al. 1995). The electroencephalogram (EEG) shows abnormalities on single awake testing in approximately 80% of patients with AD of less than 4 years' duration. These changes increase with disease severity and consist of a slowing of the posterior dominant rhythm (loss of alpha activity) and an increase in diffuse slow waves (theta and delta activity) that contrasts with the relatively normal EEG found in frontotemporal dementia. In rare families, identification of specific *APP* and *presenilin* mutations may be diagnostic. In the differential diagnosis of dementia, apo E genotyping may contribute to diagnostic accuracy if an apo E4 allele is present. As with all genetic testing, appropriate pretest advice and counseling should be available to family members because positive results have risk implications.

Neuroimaging

The main role of neuroimaging in the patient with presumed AD is still to exclude a structural and potentially reversible cause. Structural imaging, either computed tomography (CT) or magnetic resonance imaging (MRI), is widely used to exclude cerebral tumors, hydrocephalus, cerebrovascular disease, or subdural hemorrhage. Generalized cerebral atrophy, more than would be expected in normal aging, is common with moderate or greater disease severity, but in the early stages scans may be reported as normal. Such visual assessment is dependent on the rater, and volumetric measures have better sensitivity than either linear or visual assessments. With single scans, measures of ventricular size and cerebral atrophy are approximately 80% reliable in distinguishing Alzheimer patients from controls. CT measurements have shown almost a 50% reduction of medial temporal lobe width in severe AD and significantly different rate of atrophy in mild disease according to Jobst et al. in 1992. Localized lobar atrophy is a pointer away from AD and toward a diagnosis of Pick's disease or other causes of focal cortical atrophy. MRI, with its improved resolution, allows better quantification of cerebral structures and better discrimination of normal from mildly affected AD subjects than CT. In clinically diagnosed AD of moderate severity, MRI-based volumetric measurements show a reduction of up to 40% in the size of several cerebral structures, including the hippocampus, hippocampal formation, amygdala, thalamus, and anterior temporal lobe (Figure 70A.2). Measurement of the hippocampal formation is more sensitive than temporal lobe measurements in separating controls from AD subjects. It is unclear when the earliest changes are detectable; small studies claim to be able to identify mild (mean Mini-Mental State Examination of 23) or early (>2 years' symptom duration) AD. Determination of rates of tissue loss by serial scanning may be the most valuable because it avoids the variability of single scans (Fox et al. 1996). White matter lesions are found commonly in AD; they are best seen as signal hyperintensities on T2-weighted MRI, but also are shown on CT, particularly surrounding the ventricles. Such white matter changes are associated with age and with vascular risk factors, as well as with AD, and are not diagnostic (Erkinjuntti et al. 1994).

Functional neuroimaging using positron emission tomography (PET) or single-photon emission computed tomography (SPECT) to quantify metabolism or to assess cerebral blood flow has been limited largely to research studies. It is useful in distinguishing AD from other dementias, but does not replace structural imaging. PET scans in AD show a characteristic, but not specific, bilateral temporoparietal hypometabolism and hypoperfusion, and a sensitivity of 90% and a specificity of 80% are reported when a composite metabolic ratio of affected to unaffected areas is used (Herholz et al. 1993). SPECT studies have reproduced the bilateral temporoparietal deficits seen with PET but lack the precise quantitation of PET (Read et al. 1995). Combination of a temporoparietal deficit on SPECT and hippocampal atrophy on MRI is claimed to be more accurate for diagnosis. Attempts at imaging some of the biochemical changes, and in particular the cholinergic deficit, have identified reductions in cholinergic terminals and cholinesterase activity (Iyo et al. 1997). The value of MRI and MR spectroscopy in clinical management remains to be established.

Accuracy of Clinical Diagnosis

Laboratory investigations are directed primarily toward the exclusion of other causes of dementia, but increasingly the goal is to find techniques that are diagnostic. At present, clinical diagnosis with simple laboratory measures provide a relatively high specificity of diagnosis, provided atypical cases are excluded. Guidelines using the criteria of probable and possible AD have been developed (National Institute of Neurological and Communicative Diseases and Stroke and Alzheimer's Disease and Related Disorder Association [ARRDA] criteria) and provide a high degree of accuracy when patients are followed to biopsy. This reflects in part the high prior probability of a patient with dementia suffering from AD. Using a modified ischemia score and clinical features or simple clinical assessment by a clinical neurologist, high sensitivity and specificity can be achieved, but in general, early-onset, atypical, and mild early disease diagnosis remains a challenge. Molecular genetic markers have the potential for specific and presymptomatic diagnosis in the rare presenilin and APP pedigrees. Apo E genotyping has been claimed to be of value in that the identification of an apo E4 genotype in a patient with cognitive impairment makes AD very likely. As yet, uncertainty about its ability to alter management and about the implications for at-risk family members has limited widespread application.

Pathology

The major pathological features of AD are brain atrophy with neuron loss, neurofibrillary tangles, senile plaques, and cerebrovascular amyloid (Figure 70A.3). Atrophy is prominent in younger patients but may be difficult to demonstrate with advancing age, when it may be confined to the

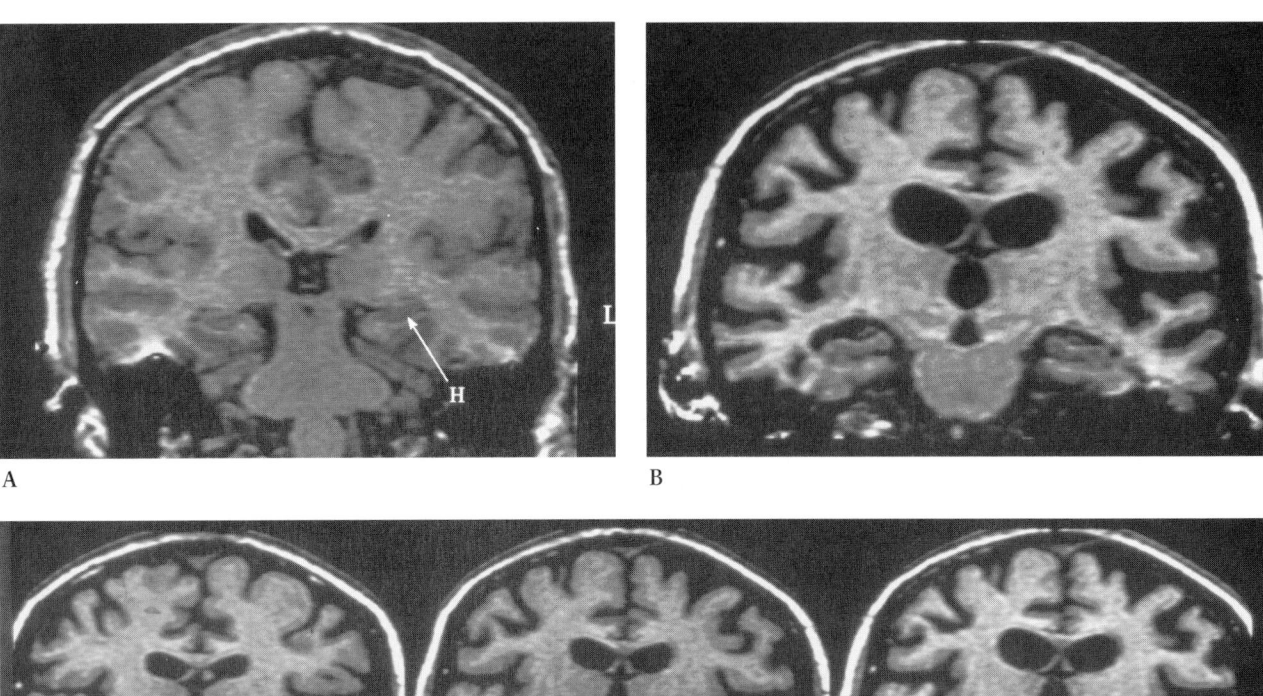

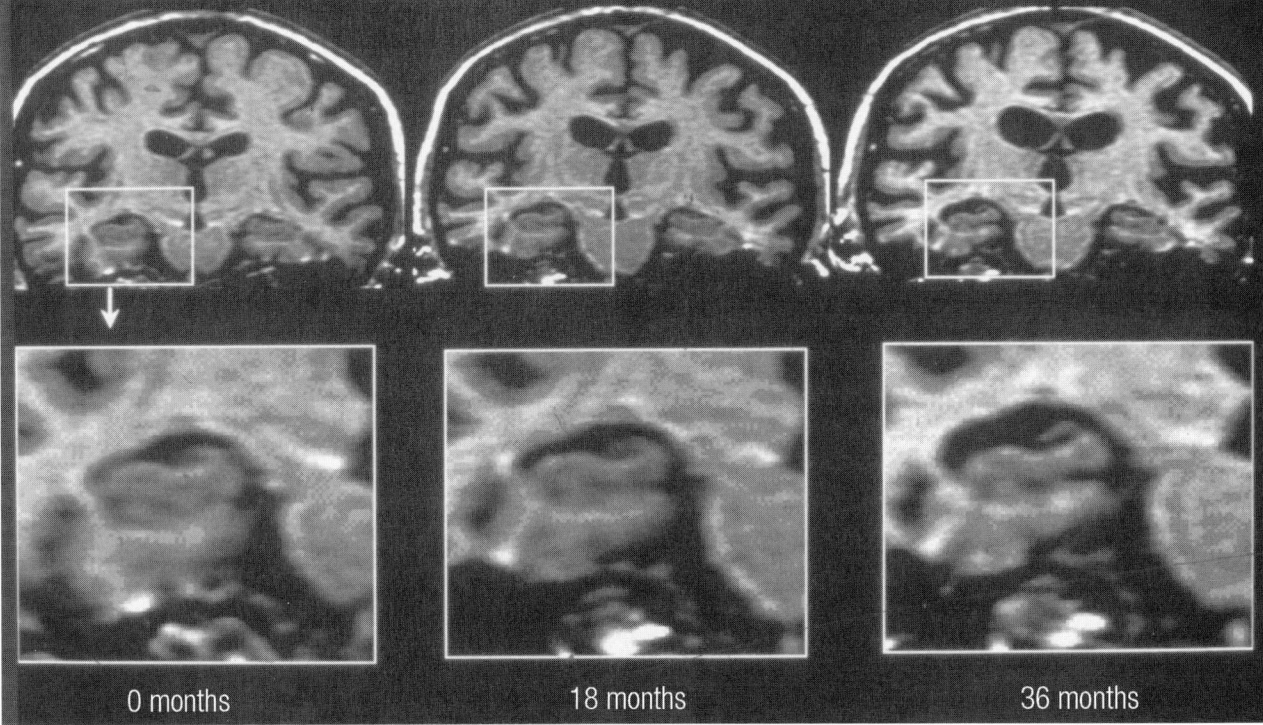

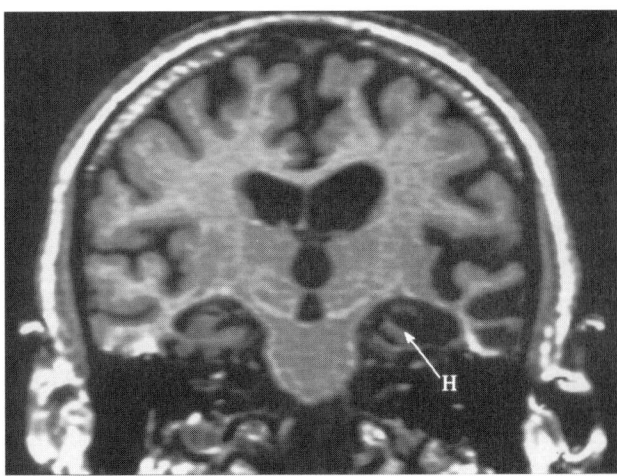

FIGURE 70A.2 (A) A control subject with normal-sized hippocampi (H). (B) A patient with Alzheimer's disease showing symmetrical and generalized cortical atrophy with marked widening of cerebral sulci, ventricular enlargement, and prominent hippocampal atrophy. (C) Serial imaging of the same patient with Alzheimer's disease showing how the scan may initially appear normal but hippocampal and generalized atrophy rapidly progressed. (D) A patient with Pick's disease showing selective and severe left temporal lobe atrophy; the gyri have a knife-edge appearance and the anterior inferior medial temporal lobe structures are almost completely atrophied. (Courtesy of Dr. N. Fox.)

FIGURE 70A.3 A section of temporal neocortex from the brain of a 62-year-old man with Alzheimer's disease. Glee's silver stain reveals argyrophilic intraneuronal neurofibrillary tangles and the dystrophic neurites of senile plaques. (Courtesy of Dr. C. Mountjoy.)

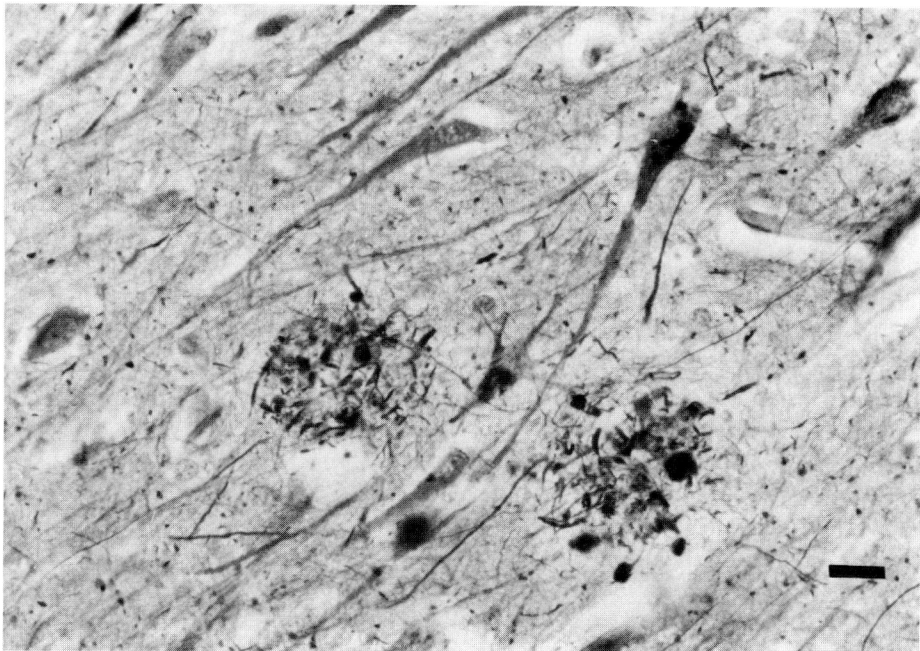

temporal lobes. Cell loss occurs particularly from the deeper layers of the cortex and preferentially involves large neurons. Neurofibrillary tangles are found especially in the allocortex and the temporoparietal neocortex. There is a predilection for the pyramidal cells of layers 3 and 5 in the neocortex and for the CA1 layer of the hippocampus, subiculum, and layers 2 and 5 of the entorhinal cortex, but as the disease progresses, tangles become more widespread. Ultrastructurally, the neurofibrillary tangles consist of paired helical filaments, with an individual filament diameter of 10 nm, wound together in a double helix with a total diameter of 200 nm and a periodicity of 160 nm. Neurofibrillary tangles are not exclusive to AD and can be found in other conditions, such as dementia pugilistica, prion disease, and Kufs' disease. Paired helical filaments are found also within neurites of senile plaques. Neuropil threads, or curly fibers, are another feature and represent paired helical filament–containing neurites. They usually parallel the severity of neurofibrillary tangle formation.

Senile plaques are found predominantly in the cerebral cortex and, as with neurofibrillary tangles, especially in the association areas. They vary in diameter between 25 and 200 μm and consist of three components: abnormal nerve processes, often referred to as dystrophic neurites; glial processes; and a central core of β-amyloid. Diffuse or immature plaques are not associated with dystrophic neurites or with fibrillary amyloid, although immunostaining reveals the presence of the Aβ protein predominantly of the larger Aβ42 species (Iwatsubo et al. 1995). It is believed that diffuse plaques precede classical neuritic plaques. The classical plaque contains a central amyloid core and rim of dystrophic neurites. Some authors refer to burnt-out plaques in which there is a prominent amyloid core

and only a very thin rim of dystrophic neurites. β-amyloid is found also in cerebral and leptomeningeal vessels with increasing age but is more prevalent in AD.

Other histological features include granulovacuolar degeneration of neurons, which consists of clear, round cytoplasmic zones 4–5 mm in diameter. These are found particularly within the hippocampus and may coexist with neurofibrillary tangles. Hirano bodies, eosinophilic inclusions, are found particularly within the pyramidal layer of the hippocampus. In addition to these features, a mild spongiosis may occur in severe cases of AD but is distinct from the status spongiosis found in Creutzfeldt-Jakob disease. The overall distribution of the histological abnormalities follows the association cortices, with sparing of the primary sensory and motor cortex, although the distribution of Aβ immunostaining is more extensive. Cell loss and neurofibrillary tangle formation also occur within the nucleus basalis of Meynert, which is the origin of the cholinergic projection to cerebral cortex, and, to a lesser extent, within the locus ceruleus and the nucleus raphe. There is an overall correlation between the number of plaques and of neurofibrillary tangles and the severity of the disease, although cases with predominantly tangles are seen as well as cases with senile plaques and absence of dementia. Loss of synapses may provide a better marker of dysfunction and cognitive impairment. The major diagnostic problem is that similar histological features can be found to a limited extent, particularly within the hippocampus, in normal aging. This has led to neuropathological criteria for diagnosis based either on plaque and tangle numbers in relation to age, or on neuritic plaque numbers alone (Consortium to Establish a Registry for Alzheimer's Disease criteria).

Biochemistry

Biochemical studies have aimed to identify the components of the histological change and to elucidate the consequent transmitter deficits. A major component of the neurofibrillary tangle is the microtubule-associated protein tau. The tau is abnormally hyperphosphorylated and has reduced binding to microtubules and thus disrupts the cytoskeleton. Tau exists as six isoforms because of a variable N terminus and three or four microtubule-binding domains. All six isoforms contribute in AD but variations on Western blotting of tau isolated from AD and Pick's disease, corticobasal degeneration, and hereditary tauopathy suggest differential deposition of isoforms (Spillantini et al. 1998). Ubiquitin is found also in association with tangles, which may represent an attempt by the cell to degrade the abnormal protein.

Amyloid protein isolated from plaque cores is predominantly a 40 amino acid peptide derived from a larger APP, the gene for which is on the long arm of chromosome 21 (Selkoe 1994). APP is a transmembrane protein and widely expressed in neural and non-neural tissue, although its physiological role is unclear. The β-amyloid domain straddles the membrane. There are various metabolic pathways for the processing of APP, including production of a soluble form (Aβ) of the β-amyloid protein sequence (Figure 70A.4). α-Secretase cleaves within the β-amyloid domain precluding Aβ production. β- and γ-secretases cleave at the N and C termini, respectively. There is variability in the cleavage at the C terminus with a small proportion of Aβ1-42, in addition to the predominant Aβ1-40. The Aβ1-42 has a greater propensity to fibril formation and is also the predominant form in early plaques. Vascular amyloid is predominantly Aβ1-40. This suggests that post-translational modification to allow amyloid fibril formation may be important. Many other molecules have been reported in association with the plaque core including inflammatory markers. Notable also is apo E, in view of the genetic risk for AD associated with the E4 allele.

The success of neurotransmitter replacement therapy in Parkinson's disease has directed interest toward the neurotransmitter systems that are damaged in AD. Choline acetyltransferase activity is reduced in the cerebral cortex, particularly in the temporal neocortex and hippocampus, reflecting damage to the cholinergic projection from the basal forebrain. It is clear, however, that this is not a specific defect and that a number of other subcortical ascending systems are involved, in particular the noradrenergic and serotonergic ones. Of equal importance are the changes within the cerebral cortical neurons, particularly the glutamatergic pyramidal neurons, which bear the brunt of cell loss and neurofibrillary tangle formation. The muscarinic cholinergic receptors are relatively preserved, which is important in terms of potential cholinergic replacement treatments, but in general other neurotransmitter receptor systems are damaged. The available evidence indicates that there is no specific neurotransmitter deficit in AD, but nevertheless not all systems appear to be equally vulnerable. Moreover, the consistent cholinergic deficit has led to the first rational treatment for AD (see Treatment and Management, later in this chapter). In general, young patients with AD appear to have more widespread neurotransmitter deficits compared with older patients.

Pathogenesis

The discovery of FAD in association with mutations of the APP gene has contributed substantially to our understanding of the pathophysiology of familial and, by implication, sporadic AD. The amyloid cascade hypothesis proposes that the histopathological abnormalities of senile plaques, neurofibrillary tangles, and neuronal loss are all secondary to amyloid deposition. In vitro studies of cells transfected with constructs containing the known APP mutations (see Figure 70A.1) have identified possible mechanisms whereby abnormal APP metabolism results in increased β-amyloid deposition. Thus, the Swedish mutation ($APP\ 670/671_{lys-met \rightarrow asn-leu}$) results in increased production of the soluble Aβ protein and by implication increased formation of β-amyloid fibrils. By contrast, cells transfected with $APP\ 717_{val \rightarrow ile}$ constructs produce a normal amount of soluble Aβ protein, but with a subtle shift toward molecules that are extended at the C terminus and that may theoretically predispose to fibril formation. Further support for the central role of amyloid processing is provided by studies in presenilin mutation families. At least one-half of young-onset FAD can be attributed to mutations in the presenilin 1 gene on chromosome 14; a few families carry mutations on the homologous presenilin 2 gene on chromosome 1 (Cruts and VanBroeckhoven 1998). The presenilins are transmembrane proteins that are located primarily in the neuronal Golgi apparatus and endoplasmic reticulum, where they interact with APP. In vitro and in vivo studies demonstrate an increase in Aβ1-42 with presenilin mutations.

The post-translational modification from physiological soluble Aβ protein to fibrillary β-amyloid is important for the neurotoxicity, but the basis of the latter is still unclear. Some evidence exists that β-amyloid may alter calcium homeostasis or enhance free radical generation. However, the extent to which sporadic disease may be related directly to abnormal amyloid metabolism is as yet unknown.

The other major genetic risk factor, namely inheritance of the apo E4 genotype, may be associated with amyloid mismetabolism insofar as apo E4 is associated with increased amyloid deposition neuropathologically and purified apo E4 may enhance amyloid aggregation.

Although amyloid is considered to have a major role, this is only established in FAD. Moreover, the link between amyloid deposition, tangle formation, and neuronal death remains obscure.

FIGURE 70A.4 Ideogram showing APP processing by α, β, and γ secretases. (A) The predominant Aβ species is Aβ1-40, which had a low propensity for the formation of β-amyloid fibrils. (B) APP 717 and presenilin mutations increase the proportion of Aβ1-42, which has a greater propensity to β-amyloid fibril formation.

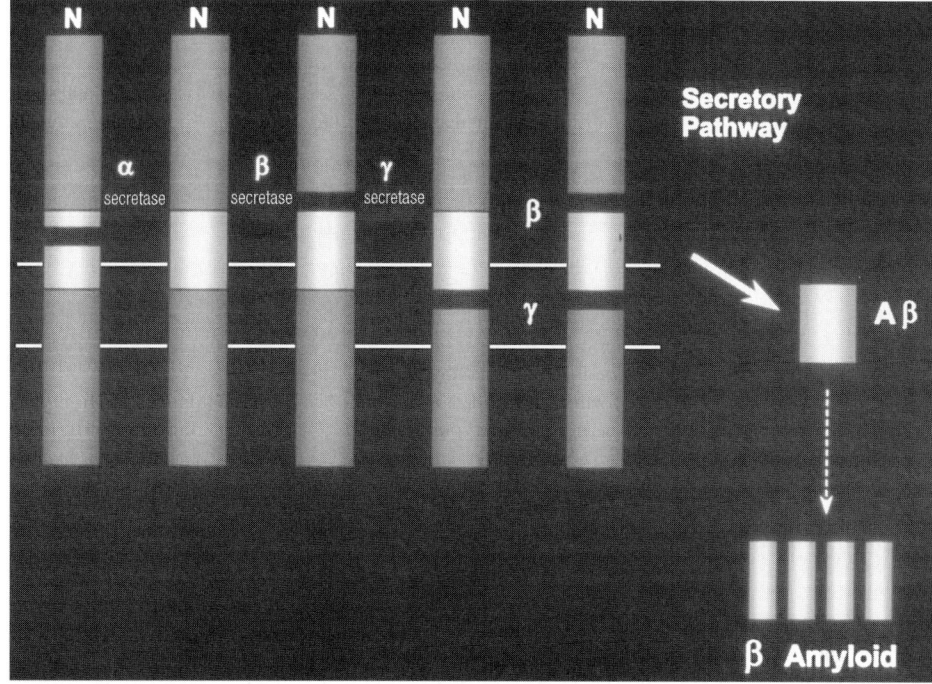

Epidemiology and Etiology

The single most important risk factor for the development of AD is age. Dementia is common in old age, with rates approaching 50% in the very elderly (Skoog et al. 1993).

Autopsy studies of patients with dementia implicate AD in approximately 50%, and a further 20% have AD together with other diseases, particularly vascular disease. There are difficulties with extrapolating from autopsy figures, but community studies using clinical criteria indicate a doubling of AD prevalence for every 5 years over the age of 65 with a prevalence of approximately 4% at 75 years. This does suggest that AD is one of the most common neurological disorders of old age. In 1950, there were some 214 million people in the world over 60 years old; by the year 2025, it is predicted there will be 1 billion. AD presents a major public health problem.

A family history is a major risk factor. Pathogenic *APP* and *presenilin* mutations confer 50% risk in young-onset pedigrees. Apo E genotype also determines risk in late-onset familial and apparent sporadic disease; inheritance of an apo E4 allele represents an odds-ratio risk of approximately 4. A history of head trauma is associated with increased risk, which has been attributed to increased *APP* expression in response to neuronal injury (Roberts et al. 1994). Reported protective factors are education, wine consumption, and inheritance of the apo E2 allele. The effect of smoking is complex. Early reports of a protective effect were probably caused by censoring by early vascular deaths and recent data suggest an increased risk (Ott et al. 1998).

Course and Prognosis

Although there is considerable variability, and, occasionally, there may be apparent plateaus, there is generally an inexorable decline of function in AD. The increased mortality from AD makes it the fourth leading cause of death in patients over the age of 65. Survival has increased with improved general care, the mean survival being 8.1 years from onset of the disease, compared with 6.7 years for multi-infarct dementia. Reported average rates of decline are four to five points on the Mini-Mental State score and six points on the Alzheimer's Disease Assessment Scale annually. However, it cannot be assumed that the rate of decline is linear. The cause of death is usually bronchopneumonia.

Treatment and Management

The disorientation experienced by AD patients may be reduced by providing a quiet, familiar environment, with clear labels on doors and other objects throughout the house. At night, efficient lighting to the bathroom or other amenities is important to reduce disorientation. Patients are also liable to develop confusional episodes because of intercurrent medical problems. Even minor urinary tract infections may cause a marked confusion. Any patient presenting with a sudden deterioration of cognition should undergo careful clinical examination and investigation for signs of medical or surgical disease. Depression in dementia is common, and improvement in mood can be associated with improvement of other associated symptoms such as irritability, anxiety, restlessness, and confusion. The anticholinergic side effects of tricyclic antidepressants such as imipramine can adversely affect cognition, and selective serotonin-reuptake inhibitors are preferable.

Aggressive behavior may pose considerable management problems and should always involve a thorough clinical assessment to determine the etiology of the symptoms. Psychological intervention includes specific training for professional and family caregivers in dealing with aggression, the need for alertness to the signs of an impending crisis, and the use of positive and clear language to reassure and distract the patient (Patel and Hope 1993). Despite these interventions, drug treatment may be required; neuroleptics and short-acting benzodiazepines are the most widely used drugs in the treatment of acute behavioral disturbance. The high frequency of side effects from neuroleptics should restrict their continued use to alleviating psychotic symptoms, and the newer atypical neuroleptics such as risperidone and olanzapine have less propensity for extrapyramidal side effects. Despite the widespread use of neuroleptics, there is a paucity of evidence of efficacy and some data suggest a deterioration clinically in patients with AD (McShane et al. 1997). For chronic aggression and behavioral disturbance, other drugs, including propranolol, serotonergic agents, and carbamazepine have been reported to be beneficial.

Sexual problems often cause great strain in caregivers and have received little attention in the literature. As with aggressive behavior, management depends on thorough assessment and is based on psychological and physical principles. Caregivers require sensitive support and often simple advice such as sleeping in a different bed or different room from the patient may resolve the problem.

Considerable efforts have been directed toward rectifying the cholinergic deficit in AD. So far only acetylcholinesterase inhibitors have been shown to have an effect in AD. Three drugs have been licensed in the United States and Europe. Tacrine (Cognex), the first to be licensed, has the disadvantage of hepatotoxicity. Donepezil (Aricept) and rivastigmine (Exelon) have better side-effect profiles. Efficacy is similar in all drugs of this class and can be demonstrated on the ADAS(Cog) and global measures. Improvements of four points on the ADAS(Cog), equivalent to the change seen in 6–8 months, and no deterioration or improvement in global measures is seen in approximately 20–25% of patients over and above the placebo response (therapeutic gain) (Rogers et al. 1998). The symptomatic effects reverse on cessation. A trial of selegiline and vitamin E alone and in combination demonstrated an apparent delay in progression of dementia severity (Sano et al. 1997), and many patients take vitamin E supplementation.

DOWN SYNDROME

Neuropathologically, Alzheimer's-type changes have been reported in as many as 90% of Down syndrome patients who die after the age of 30, and it has been suggested that the neuropathological changes may be a consistent finding in all elderly cases. Ultrastructurally, neurofibrillary tangles are identical to those found in AD, and biochemically there are similar neurotransmitter changes and prominent cholinergic deficits.

Comparison of brains of people with Down syndrome dying at different ages has established progression from early appearance of diffuse amyloid plaques to neuritic plaques and tangles. In the presence of learning difficulties, cognitive decline may be difficult to measure, but dementia prevalence rates are as high as 75% in those older than 60. The parsimonious explanation for the early development of plaques at around age 30 is that trisomy 21 results in overexpression of the *APP* gene and thus increased β-amyloid deposition.

DEMENTIA WITH LEWY BODIES

Although there had been earlier descriptions in the German literature, the first detailed report by Okazaki in 1961 described cortical Lewy bodies in two patients with dementia (Perry et al. 1996). This disorder was thought to be a rarity but is now increasingly recognized as a cause of dementia. However, cortical Lewy bodies are often found in association with AD histopathology, especially senile plaques.

A variety of terms have been applied to this disorder, including cortical Lewy body disease, diffuse Lewy body disease, Lewy body dementia, senile dementia of the Lewy body type, and in those cases with AD histopathology, the Lewy body variant of AD. *Dementia with Lewy bodies* is currently the preferred term.

Clinical Features

The clinical picture of established cases of DLB is that of a parkinsonian dementia syndrome (McKeith et al. 1996). Cognitive deficits may emerge in the course of Parkinson's disease (see Chapter 70B), but the presenting feature is usually the cognitive impairment with later emergence of parkinsonism. The latter is rarely asymmetrical and resting tremor less prominent than with brainstem Lewy body Parkinson's disease. The cognitive impairment is similar to AD, although visuospatial function and visual memory are impaired more severely. The key clinical features, in addition to the emergence of an extrapyramidal syndrome, are fluctuations and visual hallucinations. Fluctuations in performance are usual and can occur suddenly. They often lead to an erroneous diagnosis of vascular dementia. Caregiver reports of periods of lucidity occur even into advanced disease. Visual hallucinations occur in up to 80% of patients (Klatka et al. 1996). These features have been incorporated into criteria for diagnosis (McKeith et al. 1996) but await formal validation against neuropathology. Another diagnostic clue is marked neuroleptic sensitivity: Some patients

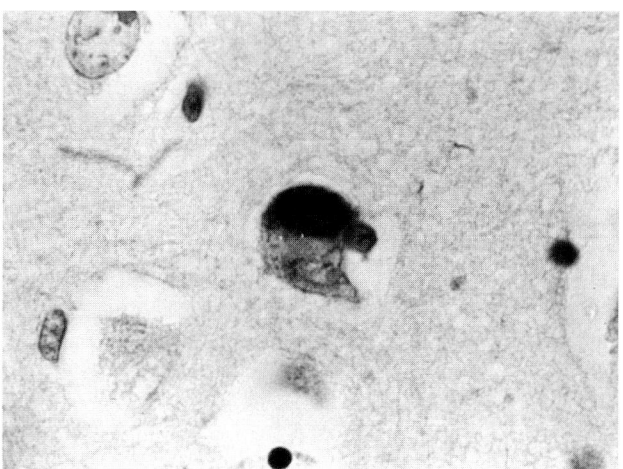

FIGURE 70A.5   Photomicrograph showing a Lewy body in the insular cortes. α-Synuclein immunohistochemistry. (Antibody courtesy of Professor B. H. Anderton.) (Magnification ×900.) (Courtesy of Dr. T. Revesz.)

have prominent sleep disturbances and others have falls and syncopal episodes. Myoclonus is not unusual and rarely individuals may have prominent myoclonus and rapid deterioration suggestive of Creutzfeldt-Jakob disease.

Investigations

Routine blood test results are normal as is the CSF. EEG usually shows nonspecific abnormalities such as diffuse slowing. This is similar to AD but may help to distinguish patients with DLB with a frontal presentation from cases of Pick's disease and other frontotemporal degenerations. Structural neuroimaging often shows atrophy and commonly additional white matter changes often attributed to ischemia. Few studies of functional imaging have been done, although Albin et al. (1996) demonstrated a temporoparietal pattern, as is found with AD, but in addition more posterior changes including the occipital cortex; this may be relevant to the hallucinations.

Pathology

The pathological hallmark is the Lewy body, which is identical to that found in the brainstem in Parkinson's disease, namely eosinophilic inclusion on hematoxylin and eosin stain with a core halo. These can be better demonstrated with anti-ubiquitin immunostaining. A major component of Lewy body has been demonstrated to be α-synuclein (Spillantini et al. 1997) (Figure 70A.5). In association with Lewy bodies, the neurons show neuritic change, demonstrated both with ubiquitin and synuclein immunostaining, sometimes referred to as *Lewy neurites.*

The Lewy bodies are found throughout the cerebral cortex as well as the brainstem and other subcortical nuclei. They are found in greatest number in the parahippocampal entorhinal and insular cortices. The neuritic changes follow the distribution of Lewy bodies and within the hippocampus are seen primarily in the CA2-3 regions, which is different from the neuritic changes in AD. Many cases have associated senile plaques but these tend to be diffuse and lack the tau immunoreactive neuritic component, suggesting that the pathogenesis is different from AD. Up to 50% of cases also have tangle formation. Undoubtedly, some of these indicate coincidental AD but in group studies, tangles tend to spare the hippocampus in DLB, again in contrast to AD.

Epidemiology and Etiology

Estimates of prevalence are difficult because of lack of histological confirmation. However, in autopsy series, DLB accounts for between 15% and 25% of cases, and application of the DLB criteria suggests a similar proportion in clinical studies. This makes it the second most common cause of dementia; most of these series are in elderly patients and the disease appears less common in young-onset dementia. The etiology is unknown. No clearly established risk factors exist. The overlap between brainstem Lewy body Parkinson's disease and AD have suggested shared pathogenesis but this remains controversial. However, the observation of cortical Lewy bodies in families with FAD caused by $APP\ 717_{val\rightarrow ile}$ mutation disease suggests that amyloid mismetabolism can ultimately lead to Lewy body formation. Families with typical Parkinson's disease and a variable cognitive deficit have been shown to be associated with mutations in the α-synuclein gene (Polymeropoulos et al. 1997). Although there are reports of familial DLB, these have not yet been associated with α-synuclein mutations. A weak association with allelic variation in cytochrome P450 gene *CYP2D6* has been reported in patients with Lewy bodies and associated Alzheimer histopathology (Saitoh et al. 1995).

Management and Treatment

Management is difficult. Anti-parkinsonian medication may help the akinesia but usually at the expense of worsening hallucinations and confusion. Conversely, dopamine-blocking neuroleptics can markedly worsen the extrapyramidal syndrome and worsen cognitive function. A few patients experience life-threatening deterioration. Patients are sometimes best managed with no medication. If the motor symptoms are prominent, these are best managed with small doses of L-dopa, and anticholinergic drugs should be avoided. Similarly, neuroleptics should be avoided, although some evidence exists that the newer atypical neuroleptics such as olanzapine may be safer, at least in the management of psychosis in classical

Parkinson's disease (Wolters et al. 1996). Anecdotal evidence is emerging that acetylcholinesterase inhibitors may be beneficial, but confirmation awaits the outcome of randomized trials.

FRONTOTEMPORAL DEGENERATIONS

The main disorders that present as frontotemporal dementias caused by the regional selectivity of the disease process are presented here. For a general description of the clinical features of frontotemporal dementias see Chapter 70D.

Pick's Disease

Pick's disease is far less common than AD. It is characterized by circumscribed frontotemporal lobar atrophy with argyrophilic inclusion bodies within the neuronal cytoplasm and by swollen chromatolytic neurons. The disease was originally described in 1892 by Arnold Pick, in Prague, who drew attention to the prominent aphasia in his patients. He noted the circumscribed atrophy and used this case to argue against Wernicke's proposal that all degenerations in the elderly were diffuse. The histological features awaited Alzheimer's description in 1911. However, the relationship between the histological features of argentophilic cellular inclusions (Pick bodies), chromatolytic ballooned neurons (Pick cells), and lobar atrophy is inconsistent, and lobar atrophy can be associated with a variety of histopathologies. Historically, authors have used the term *Pick's disease* for cases with lobar atrophy alone, as well as for the more restricted sense of lobar atrophy plus Pick cells and Pick bodies. The latter definition is used here.

Clinical Features

Reports of the clinical features of Pick's disease are often based on clinical diagnoses; there are few reports of clinical features specifically relating to the presence of Pick bodies and Pick cells. The common presentations are of frontal or temporal lobe syndromes, depending on the location of maximal lobar atrophy. The described features thus reflect the regional atrophy, and the presentation of a progressive frontal or temporal lobe syndrome does not automatically relate to the presence of Pick cells and Pick bodies and a precise diagnosis of Pick's disease. Patients with frontal atrophy have prominent and early personality change, often with apathy and abulia or lack of initiative. Obsessive or compulsive behavior may be seen. Speech output diminishes, but in the early stages patients may perform well on simple psychometric measures. As the disease progresses, speech deteriorates further, and patients may develop an orofacial apraxia with speech production deficits and, later, palilalia and echolalia. By contrast, cases with predominant temporal lobe atrophy present with a prominent aphasia. This is usually fluent with a semantic memory impairment (see Chapter 41), and with progression patients may develop a visual agnosia. Thus, cases of semantic dementia may be associated with Pick's disease. In some patients, oral exploratory behavior with gross overeating is prominent and has been related to degeneration extending to the amygdala, by analogy with the Klüver-Bucy syndrome seen in monkeys that have undergone bilateral amygdaloidectomy. Rarely, the disease process may extend to involve subcortical structures, particularly the caudate nucleus. Such patients tend to be younger and exhibit extrapyramidal features and occasionally pyramidal signs. Otherwise, physical examination usually is unremarkable or reveals frontal signs such as grasp reflexes and utilization behavior. Autosomal dominant pedigrees have been reported but only rarely. Most reported pedigrees do not have Pick bodies on histological examination.

Laboratory Studies

Routine blood test results and CSF examination are normal. The EEG is relatively normal by contrast to AD. The CT or MRI scan (see Figure 70A.2B) shows prominent frontotemporal atrophy, often asymmetrical. Functional imaging confirms frontotemporal patterns of hypometabolism.

Biochemistry

In the relatively few cases that have been analyzed postmortem, there was relative preservation of choline acetyltransferase activity, in contrast to the severe loss in AD, but prominent loss of the muscarinic acetylcholine receptor. Abnormalities of serotonin receptors also have been reported. More recent studies have focused on the molecular pathology of the tau-positive Pick bodies. Western blotting of tau extracted from brains of patients with Pick's disease reveals a characteristic doublet indicative of predominant deposition of isoforms containing the triplet repeat microtubule-binding domain (Delacourte et al. 1998). The pattern of isoform deposition is distinct from AD, corticobasal degeneration, progressive supranuclear palsy, and chromosome 17 hereditary tauopathy and confirms the view that Pick's disease is a separate nosological entity. The underlying pathophysiology remains unknown.

Pathology

Affected gyri within the areas of circumscribed atrophy in the frontal and temporal lobes may be extremely thin, but the superior temporal gyrus is usually spared (Figure 70A.6). The atrophy can extend to the hippocampus, amygdala, and, more rarely, caudate and thalamus. The white matter also is reduced in volume. Microscopically, there is a loss of neurons, particularly in cortical layers I–III, with the characteristic argentophilic Pick bodies. Widespread astro-

cytic gliosis in both the cortex and the subcortical white matter also occurs. On electron microscopy, the Pick bodies consist of randomly arranged straight filaments of 10–20 nm in width. Immunocytochemistry reveals staining of Pick bodies with both anti-ubiquitin and anti-tau antibodies.

Epidemiology and Etiology

Pick's disease is rare. There are no reliable prevalence figures based on histological diagnosis, and estimates vary considerably. The underlying cause is unknown. Pedigrees with autosomal dominant Pick's disease have rarely been reported, but the causative gene has not been identified. Chromosome 17 hereditary tauopathy caused by mutations in the *tau* gene do not have the histological features of typical Pick's disease (Hutton et al. 1998).

Progress and Management

The disease usually progresses inexorably, but length of history varies widely (3–15 years). Some patients with aphasia remain independent for many years. At present no specific treatment exists, but selective serotonin reuptake inhibitors may help in behavioral management.

FRONTAL LOBE DEGENERATION

In 1992, Gustafson and Brun described a clinical syndrome distinct from AD that they referred to as frontal lobe degeneration of non-Alzheimer type (see Chapter 71D). The onset is typically in the 50s, with insidious change of personality and disinhibition followed by gradual loss of speech output. Approximately 50% of cases are familial. Although the clinical picture would suggest Pick's disease, the majority did not have Pick cells or Pick bodies but rather frontal cortical neuronal loss, mild spongiosis, some loss of myelin, and astrocytic gliosis in the white matter. Similar cases have been referred to as dementia lacking distinctive histological features. Approximately 10% of Brun and Gustafson's dementia autopsy series were categorized as frontal lobe degeneration. Approximately 20% of patients in a specialist neurology referral clinic in the United Kingdom had a progressive frontal lobe dementia. Although some of these had Pick bodies and cells, the majority had a nonspecific cell loss from the frontal cortex similar to that described by Gustafson et al. A number of cases of primary progressive aphasia have a similar pathology.

MOTOR NEURON DISEASE AND FRONTOTEMPORAL DEGENERATION

Rarely, frontotemporal degeneration can be seen in association with anterior horn cell degeneration. Although frontal

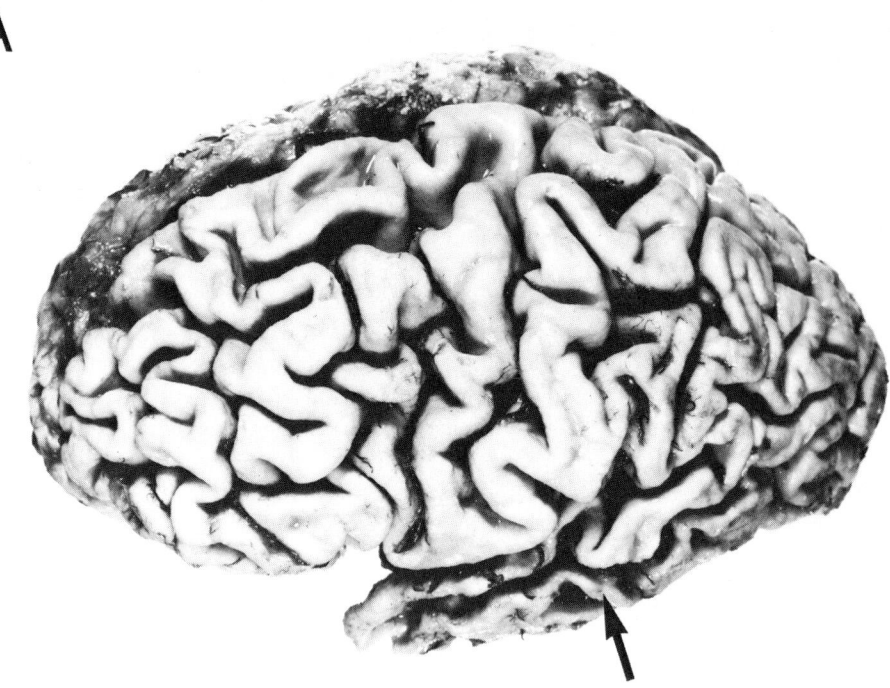

A

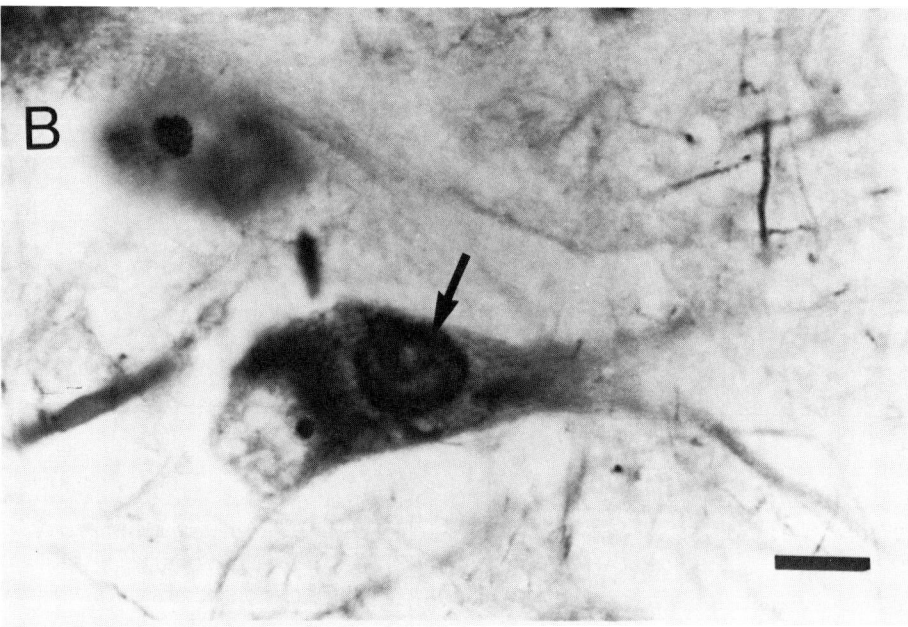

B

FIGURE 70A.6 (A) The brain of a 62-year-old woman with Pick's disease after removal of the leptomeninges. There is widening of the sulci and gyral atrophy in the frontal and temporal lobes. This is particularly severe in the temporal lobe, giving the gyri a knife-edged appearance (*arrow*). (B) The arrow indicates a darkly stained argyrophilic Pick's body in a neuronal perikaryon from the subiculum of the same patient. (Von Braunmuhl silver impregnation of a frozen section. Calibration bar = 25 m.) (Courtesy of L. Duchen.)

lobe deficits can be found on careful testing in patients with motor neuron disease, this is not the salient feature. By contrast, patients may present with a frontal lobe syndrome or a nonfluent aphasia who subsequently developed features of anterior horn cell dysfunction. Long tract signs emerge only late and typically fasciculation is seen in the proximal upper limbs. Such patients have ubiquitin-positive, tau-negative, motor neuron disease inclusion bodies not only in the anterior horn cells but also in the frontal cortex. Jackson et al. (1996) have reported a series of patients with a frontal dementia in whom there were ubiquitin-positive tau-negative motor neuron disease inclusion bodies in the frontotemporal cortex but without evidence of anterior horn cell degeneration.

THALAMIC DEMENTIA

Degenerative disease of the thalamus appears to be rare, but in such cases dementia may be the overwhelming feature, with few other abnormalities. In 1939, Stern reported severe dementia with bilateral symmetrical degeneration of the thalamus in a patient with pupillary abnormalities who subsequently developed hypersomnia; occasional cases have been reported subsequently. More recently, patients with dementia and subcortical gliosis involving the thalamic nuclei have been reported, although the overlap with Neumann's subcortical gliosis is unclear. Some of these cases may be caused by prion disease. Fatal familial insomnia with thalamic degeneration is now attributable to a mutation in the prion protein gene.

MISCELLANEOUS DEGENERATIVE DEMENTIAS

Families with an autosomal dominant frontal dementia and variable combinations of extrapyramidal and lower motor neuron features were found to have deposition of tau distinct from the isoform pattern of tau deposition in Pick's disease. The genetic locus was shown to be on chromosome 17 and subsequently referred to as chromosome 17 hereditary tauopathy or dementia disinhibition parkinsonism amyotrophy complex. Some of these families have been found to carry mutations in the tau gene that disturb the normal frequency of the different tau isoforms (Hutton et al. 1998; Poorkaj et al. 1998; Spillantini et al. 1998).

Some patients show prominent subcortical gliosis out of proportion to cortical changes. These were initially thought to be a variant of Pick's disease but are now considered to form a separate entity, progressive subcortical gliosis. Patients develop a frontal dementia, often with additional extrapyramidal features; some cases are familial. Argyrophilic grain dementia has been described in an autopsy series. Spindle-shaped grains are demonstrated with silver stains especially in hippocampus, entorhinal, and frontotemporal cortex. The clinical features are not well delineated at present. Kosaka (1994) described a number of patients with dementia with basal ganglia calcification and cortical neurofibrillary tangles.

REFERENCES

Albin RL, Minoshima S, D'Amato CJ, et al. Fluoro-deoxyglucose positron emission tomography in diffuse Lewy body disease. Neurology 1996;47:462–466.

Allen NHP, Burns AB. The non-cognitive features of dementia. Rev Clin Gerontol 1995;5:57–75.

Anonymous. Statement on use of apolipoprotein E testing for Alzheimer disease. American College of Medical Genetics/American Society of Human Genetics Working Group on ApoE and Alzheimer disease. JAMA 1995;274:1627–1629.

Corder EH, Saunders AM, Strittmatter WJ, et al. Gene dose of apolipoprotein E type 4 allele and the risk of Alzheimer's disease in late onset families [see comments]. Science 1993;261:921–923.

Coreybloom J, Galasko D, Hofstetter CR, et al. Clinical features distinguishing large cohorts with possible Alzheimer's disease, probable Alzheimer's disease, and mixed dementia. J Am Geriatr Soc 1993;41:31–37.

Cruts M, VanBroeckhoven C. Presenilin mutations in Alzheimer's disease. Hum Mutat 1998;11:183–190.

Delacourte A, Sergeant N, Wattez A, et al. Vulnerable neuronal subsets in Alzheimer's and Pick's disease are distinguished by their tau isoform distribution and phosphorylation. Ann Neurol 1998;43:193–204.

Erkinjuntti T, Gao F, Lee DH, et al. Lack of difference in brain hyperintensities between patients with early Alzheimer's disease and control subjects. Arch Neurol 1994;1:260–268.

Fox NC, Freeborough PA, Rossor MN. Visualisation and quantification of atrophy in Alzheimer's disease. Lancet 1996;348:94–97.

Hardy J. Amyloid, the presenilins and Alzheimer's disease. Trend Neurosci 1997;20:154–159.

Herholz K, Perani D, Salmon E, et al. Comparability of FDG PET studies in probable Alzheimer's disease. J Nucl Med 1993;34:1460–1466.

Hodges JR, Patterson K. Is semantic memory consistently impaired early in the course of Alzheimer's disease? Neuroanatomical and diagnostic implications. Neuropsychologia 1995;33:441–459.

Hutton M, Lendon C, Rizzu P, et al. Association of missense and 5'-splice-site mutations in tau with the inherited dementia FTDP-17. Nature 1998;393:702–705.

Iwatsubo T, Mann DM, Odaka A, et al. Amyloid b protein (Ab) deposition: Ab42(43) precedes Ab40 in Down syndrome. Ann Neurol 1995;37:294–299.

Iyo M, Namba H, Fukushi K, et al. Measurement of acetylcholinesterase by positron emission tomography in the brains of healthy controls and patients with Alzheimer's disease. Lancet 1997;349:1805–1809.

Jackson M, Lennox G, Lowe J. Motor neurone disease-inclusion dementia. Neurodegeneration 1996;5:339–350.

Klatka LA, Louis ED, Schiffer RB. Psychiatric features in diffuse Lewy body disease: a clinicopathologic study using Alzheimer's disease and Parkinson's disease comparison groups. Neurology 1996;47:1148–1152.

Kosaka K. Diffuse neurofibrillary tangles with calcification—a new presenile-dementia. J Neurol Neurosurg Psychiatry 1994;57:594–596.

Maurer K, Volk S, Gerbaldo H. Auguste D and Alzheimer's disease. Lancet 1997;349:1546–1549.

McKeith IG, Galasko D, Kosaka K, et al. Clinical and pathological diagnosis of dementia with Lewy bodies (DLB): report of the CDLB international workshop. Neurology 1996;47:1113–1124.

McShane R, Keene J, Gedling K, et al. Do neuroleptic drugs hasten cognitive decline in dementia? Prospective study with necropsy follow up [see comments]. BMJ 1997;314:266–270.

Motter R, Vigo PC, Kholodenko D, et al. Reduction of beta-amyloid peptide 42 in the cerebrospinal fluid of patients with Alzheimer's disease. Ann Neurol 1995;38:643–648.

Ott A, Slooter AJ, Hofman A, et al. Smoking and risk of dementia and Alzheimer's disease in a population-based cohort study: the Rotterdam Study. Lancet 1998;351:1840–1843.

Patel V, Hope T. Aggressive behaviour in elderly people with dementia: a review. Int J Geriatr Psychiatry 1993;8:457–472.

Perry RH, McKeith IG, Perry EK. Dementia with Lewy Bodies. Cambridge: Cambridge University Press, 1996.

Polymeropoulos MH, Lavedan C, Leroy E, et al. Mutation in the alpha-synuclein gene identified in families with Parkinson's disease [see comments]. Science 1997;276:2045–2047.

Poorkaj P, Bird TD, Wijsman E, et al. Tau is a candidate gene for chromosome 17 frontotemporal dementia. Ann Neurol 1998;43: 815–825.

Read SL, Miller BL, Mena I, et al. SPECT in dementia: clinical and pathological correlation. J Am Geriatr Soc 1995;43: 1243–1247.

Roberts GW, Gentleman SM, Lynch A, et al. Beta amyloid protein deposition in the brain after severe head injury: implications for the pathogenesis of Alzheimer's disease. J Neurol Neurosurg Psychiatry 1994;57:419–425.

Rogers SL, Farlow MR, Doody RS, et al. A 24-week, double-blind, placebo-controlled trial of donepezil in patients with Alzheimer's disease. Donepezil Study Group. Neurology 1998; 50:136–145.

Saitoh T, Xia Y, Chen X, et al. The CYP2D6B mutant allele is overrepresented in the Lewy body variant of Alzheimer's disease. Ann Neurol 1995;37:110–112.

Sano M, Ernesto C, Thomas RG, et al. A controlled trial of selegiline, alpha-tocopherol, or both as treatment for Alzheimer's disease. The Alzheimer's Disease Cooperative Study [see comments]. N Engl J Med 1997;336:1216–1222.

Selkoe DJ. Molecular Pathology of Alzheimer's Disease: The Role of Amyloid. In JH Growdon, MN Rossor (eds), The Dementias. Boston: Butterworth–Heinemann, 1998;257–284.

Selkoe DJ. Normal and abnormal biology of the beta-amyloid precursor protein [review]. Annu Rev Neurosci 1994;17:489–517.

Skoog I, Nilsson L, Palmertz B, et al. A population-based study of dementia in 85-year-olds. N Engl J Med 1993;328:153–158.

Snowden JS, Neary D, Mann DMA. Fronto-temporal Lobar Degeneration. Edinburgh: Churchill Livingstone, 1996.

Spillantini MG, Bird TD, Ghetti B. Frontotemporal dementia and parkinsonism linked to chromosome 17: a new group of tauopathies. Brain Pathol 1998;8:387–402.

Spillantini MG, Schmidt ML, Lee VM, et al. Alpha-synuclein in Lewy bodies [letter]. Nature 1997;388:839–840.

Wolters EC, Jansen EN, Tuynman QH, Bergmans PL. Olanzapine in the treatment of dopaminomimetic psychosis in patients with Parkinson's disease. Neurology 1996;47:1085–1087.

Chapter 70
The Dementias

B. DEMENTIA AS PART OF OTHER DEGENERATIVE DISEASES
Martin N. Rossor

Dementia occurs in several neurological disorders in which it is not the major feature. These disorders are referred to briefly here and covered in greater detail in other sections of this book.

PARKINSON'S DISEASE

In first describing Parkinson's disease, James Parkinson referred to the senses and intellect being uninjured (see Chapter 75). In contrast to Alzheimer's disease, this is undoubtedly so, but some degree of cognitive impairment is frequent. The features of motor slowness and bradyphrenia (cognitive slowing) are characteristic of subcortical dementia, but what is less clear is how frequently dementia, as defined by the criteria of the *Diagnostic and Statistical Manual of Mental Disorders*, 4th edition, occurs. The probable frequency of dementia in Parkinson's patients is approximately 15–20%, but problems exist both with the definition of dementia and with the differential diagnosis of idiopathic Parkinson's disease from other akinetic-rigid syndromes in which a dementia may coexist. Age, depression, and more severe akinesia are all risk factors for associated dementia; it is relatively uncommon in the tremor predominant form (Roos et al. 1996).

The pathological substrate of the dementia in Parkinson's disease is complex. Alzheimer's-type pathology may be seen, but this may only be because of the coincidence of Alzheimer's and Parkinson's diseases, and there is no consistent increase in apolipoprotein E4 allele frequency in Parkinson's disease with dementia (Koller et al. 1995). In some, there are cortical Lewy bodies, usually with diffuse senile plaques, and these form part of the Lewy body dementia spectrum. Prominent dementia, however, may occur in the absence of such cortical changes. Cognitive impairment in the younger patient with brainstem Lewy body disease is more subtle and is a predominantly frontal-subcortical syndrome with bradyphrenia (Pate and Margolin 1994). Patients with Parkinson's disease caused by 1-methyl-4 phenyl-1,2,3,6-tetra hydropyridine (MPTP) which represent a pure dopaminergic deficit, also show subtle intellectual changes.

L-Dopa improves performance on some frontal lobe tasks in experimental situations, but with progression of disease L-dopa can be associated with psychosis, hallucinations, and a confusional state, all of which are exacerbated by anticholinergic drugs especially in the elderly.

PROGRESSIVE SUPRANUCLEAR PALSY

Progressive supranuclear palsy is the prototypical subcortical dementia. The memory impairment may be more apparent than real; given enough time to initiate and complete the task, the patient may perform relatively well. Frontal lobe deficits are prominent. Associated frontal lobe features such as grasp reflexes, utilization behavior (i.e., automatic use of objects), and motor impersistence may be seen also. In general, the cognitive features are more prominent than in Parkinson's disease. In some patients, dementia can be a prominent early feature, creating diagnostic confusion before the characteristic motor abnormalities emerge.

The correlates of cognitive impairment in progressive supranuclear palsy are not established. There is no obvious cortical atrophy, and ascending dopaminergic systems are spared, although the cholinergic projection is involved to a minor extent. Many of the frontal lobe features may relate to deafferentation from the basal ganglia. Positron emission tomography shows marked frontal hypometabolism.

HUNTINGTON'S DISEASE

Cognitive impairment is a characteristic feature of Huntington's disease, although the severity is variable in relation to the movement disorder (see Chapter 75). It is usually accompanied by behavioral disturbances, most commonly apathy and depression, but also, rarely, a schizophreniform psychosis. These can precede the motor features of the disease by many years. The cognitive impairment of Huntington's disease has the characteristics of a subcortical dementia with impairments of frontal executive function. In contrast to Alzheimer's disease, patients with Huntington's disease may develop dysarthria and reduced verbal fluency, but the linguistic structure of their language is relatively preserved. In general, the memory deficit is less severe than in Alzheimer's disease and performance on recognition tasks is better, reflecting impairment of concentration. Cognitive impairment can be demonstrated in presymptomatic mutations when compared with controls (Lawrence et al. 1998). The subcortical pathology no doubt contributes to the cognitive profile, but cortical cell loss also occurs, particularly from layers III–V. This occurs later with frontal lobe atrophy only apparent on volumetric magnetic resonance imaging with moderate disease severity (Aylward et al. 1998).

PRION DEMENTIA

The varied phenotype of prion disease is now recognized; for example, not all cases show spongiform changes but can be characterized by the presence of the scrapie isoform of prion protein (see Chapter 59F). Cortical dementia as part of a rapidly progressive and fatal multisystem degeneration is the characteristic presentation of Creutzfeldt-Jakob disease; some cases may present focally, for example, as aphasia. Some cases of prion disease, particularly familial, may present as a slowly progressive presenile dementia and, as such, enter into the differential diagnosis of many patients presenting with dementia. Cases of new variant Creutzfeldt-Jakob disease occur in younger patients and may have florid behavioral disturbance with anxiety and depression as early features (Zeidler et al. 1997).

AMYOTROPHIC LATERAL SCLEROSIS

Cognitive impairment is not normally a salient feature of amyotrophic lateral sclerosis, although subtle abnormalities in tasks sensitive to frontal lobe function such as verbal fluency are found in association with reduced activation in frontolimbic systems demonstrated by positron emission tomography (see Chapter 78). In 2–3% of cases a promi-

nent frontal dementia develops and can precede the motor neuron degeneration. Speech output is frequently reduced over and above the effect of any bulbar palsy. Rarely, there may be associated extrapyramidal features. A family history is more common (approximately one-third) in these cases than in uncomplicated amyotrophic lateral sclerosis.

CORTICOBASAL DEGENERATION

Corticobasal degeneration characteristically presents with an asymmetric motor syndrome of apraxia, dystonia, and action myoclonus. By contrast to the subcortical cognitive impairment of other motor disorders, corticobasal degeneration has prominent cortical features such as cortical sensory loss and the alien hand sign. Dementia often develops, typically with a parietal cluster of acalculia and visuospatial deficits in addition to the apraxia. Some cases with this pathology have focal cognitive syndromes such as primary progressive aphasia.

OTHER DEGENERATIVE DISEASES

Cognitive impairment may occur in many other degenerative disorders, some of which usually present in childhood or adolescence, such as Lafora body disease and Hallevorden-Spatz disease. Others, such as cerebellar degenerations, present later in life (see Chapter 76) and, in general, dementia develops late in the disease, after the appearance of other neurological features.

REFERENCES

Aylward EH, Anderson NB, Bylsma FW, et al. Frontal lobe volume in patients with Huntington's disease. Neurology 1998; 50:252–258.

Koller WC, Glatt SL, Hubble JP, et al. Apolipoprotein E genotypes in Parkinson's disease with and without dementia. Ann Neurol 1995;37:242–245.

Lawrence AD, Hodges JR, Rosser AE, et al. Evidence for specific cognitive deficits in preclinical Huntington's disease. Brain 1998;121:1329–1341.

Pate DS, Margolin DI. Cognitive slowing in Parkinson's and Alzheimer's patients: distinguishing bradyphrenia from dementia. Neurology 1994;44:669–674.

Roos RA, Jongen JC, van der Velde EA. Clinical course of patients with idiopathic Parkinson's disease. Mov Disord 1996;11:236–242.

Zeidler M, Johnstone EC, Bamber RW, et al. New variant Creutzfeldt-Jakob disease: psychiatric features. Lancet 1997;350:908–910.

Chapter 70
The Dementias

C. VASCULAR DEMENTIA
Albert Hijdra

Vascular disease is the second most common cause of dementia after Alzheimer's disease. In clinical and pathological surveys of demented patients, vascular disease is considered to be the cause of the dementia in 10–20% and to be an important contributing cause in approximately the same percentage. This means that in one of every four demented patients, vascular disease is either a primary cause or a contributing factor.

When dementia is presumed to be caused by vascular disease, the diagnostic term *vascular dementia* is now generally used. Patients diagnosed as having vascular dementia, however, do not constitute a homogeneous group. The most important subgroups are dementia caused by a single brain lesion, multi-infarct dementia (MID), and subcortical arteriosclerotic encephalopathy (SAE).

CLINICAL FEATURES

Mental Changes and Dementia with Single Brain Lesions

Strategically localized single brain lesions may profoundly affect mental function and behavior. When presenting with hemiparesis, hemianopia, or hemisensory symptoms, such lesions are not a diagnostic problem. In some patients, however, mental signs and symptoms are the only manifestation of the stroke. Occult or nonobvious strokes with behavioral signs and symptoms and only minor and mostly transient motor signs constitute approximately 5% of fully conscious nonaphasic stroke patients. In such patients, a vascular or degenerative dementia may be suspected. The clinical manifestations of these small cortical or subcortical infarcts or hemorrhages are mainly determined by the location of the lesion.

Middle Cerebral Artery Territory Lesions

Patients with aphasia caused by a single lesion in the left middle cerebral artery distribution are often thought to be demented by laypersons. They may have a decline in intelligence (as measured with nonlinguistic tests), but these patients rarely exhibit true dementia. In general, the language disorder is easily recognized as an isolated aphasia, even when other localizing signs are absent. With lesions of the angular gyrus, the signs and symptoms may suggest Alzheimer's disease. Complaints of difficulty in remembering are accompanied by fluent, paraphasic, and empty speech; agraphia; alexia; acalculia; left-right disorientation; finger agnosia; and constructional disturbances. Intact memory (except in verbal tests) and topographic orientation and the aphasic disturbance in patients with angular gyrus lesions are important features distinguishing them from those with dementia.

An acute confusional state is well documented in stroke patients, most often with lesions in the right middle cerebral artery distribution. It occurs with infarction of the middle frontal gyrus, middle temporal gyrus, or inferior parietal lobule—heteromodal cortical structures that all serve as convergence areas for association cortices. A global deficit in selective attention probably is the underlying mechanism for the confusion. These patients are inattentive to relevant stimuli and are easily distracted, although arousal is intact. They do not seem to grasp their current situations and show lack of concern for their illness. Inability to maintain a coherent stream of thought, disorientation, inappropriate behavior, and anomia are further characteristics. Deficits in memory and abstract thinking also occur, probably secondary to the attention disorder. The patients are often restless and sometimes agitated and aggressive. Such confusional states are generally short-lived (days to weeks), but they also may be irreversible.

Anterior Cerebral Artery Territory Lesions

Frontal lobe lesions, especially those in the distribution of the frontopolar or callosomarginal arteries causing destruction of the orbital and medial cortex, may lead to indifference and apathy, emotional blunting, and loss of self-criticism. Despite severe mental inertia, behavior may be appropriate when a patient is instructed to carry out a certain task or when it is triggered by environmental stimuli. Neuropsychological examination may demonstrate intact cognition, or it may only reveal defects with less conventional tests of divergent thinking, temporal organization, and planning behavior. The loss of intellectual control of behavior, and the dependence on social and physical environment, may manifest as a tendency to imitate the behavior of others and to automatically use objects presented, without being asked to do so (imitation and utilization behavior).

Posterior Cerebral Artery Territory Lesions

Lesions in the posterior cerebral artery distribution may affect behavior through occipital, mediotemporal, deep mesencephalic, and thalamic damage. Apart from visual field defects, occipital lobe lesions may cause disturbances in color vision and color naming, and alexia without agraphia. Visual distortions and pseudohallucinations may be perceived either in the hemianopic field defect or in the entire visual field. Visual images may totally or partly persist for some time after the stimulus has been removed, and such cortical afterimages may be incorporated in the present environment (palinopsia) (see Chapter 16). Bilateral lesions may cause visual agnosia or cortical blindness without awareness of the defect (Anton's syndrome). Inability to recognize faces (prosopagnosia) may occur in the context of a more extensive visual agnosia but is sometimes seen as a relatively isolated defect (see Chapter 11B).

A patient with a vertebrobasilar occlusion causing bilateral medial temporal lobe infarction in the distribution of the posterior cerebral arteries can appear to have an acute dementia because of the severe amnesia that occurs with bilateral lesions of the hippocampus (Ott and Saver 1993).

The amnesia probably never occurs in isolation (in contrast to lesions caused by global ischemia, for example, after cardiac arrest) and is accompanied by other posterior cerebral artery manifestations. Patients with medial temporo-occipital infarcts also may present with agitated confusion.

Subcortical Infarcts

Thalamic infarcts, even when unilateral, can lead to disturbances in attention, memory, language, and abstract thinking. The lesions are caused by occlusion of any of the small arteries arising from the proximal posterior cerebral or the posterior communicating arteries; the lesions include intralaminar, parafascicular, median, and central nuclei as well as the mamillothalamic tract, and sometimes extend into the mesencephalon and the hypothalamus. When the lesions are bilateral, the clinical picture is often dominated by disturbances of consciousness, ocular motor palsies, and bilateral motor signs, at least in the acute stage. With unilateral lesions, behavioral signs are more important and include severe inattention, decreased motor initiative, and anterograde amnesia. With left-sided lesions, aphasia characterized by fluent paraphasic speech, anomia, and intact repetition, marked fluctuation of performance may be present also. With right-sided lesions, hemineglect may simulate a parietal defect.

A syndrome reminiscent of frontal lobe disease, with obsessive-compulsive behavior and severe apathy and lack of initiative, but with no cognitive deficits, may occur in bilateral basal ganglia lesions, mainly within the globus pallidus. Lesions of the head of the caudate nucleus may be responsible for mental signs and symptoms, including apathy with decreased spontaneous verbal and motor activity, disinhibition with inappropriate and aggressive behavior, and affective symptoms with psychotic features.

Infarcts restricted to the genu of the internal capsule may present with fluctuating alertness, inattention, memory loss, apathy, and psychomotor retardation, with no or minimal motor disturbances.

Dementia after Stroke

In one study in which dementia was diagnosed according to the criteria of the *Diagnostic and Statistical Manual of Mental Disorders*, 3rd edition, 26% of stroke patients met the criteria 3 months after their strokes. In most of these patients, mental and behavioral changes were not the only manifestation of the stroke; 70% had a hemiparesis, walking was disturbed in 80%, and one-third had urinary incontinence. Most of these patients, therefore, look like stroke patients. In their activities of daily living, the demented patients were more disturbed than the nondemented stroke patients. One-third of these patients already had memory disturbances before the stroke; in these patients primary degenerative disease and vascular disease were probably combined. The other two-thirds had been cognitively intact before the stroke.

Multi-Infarct Dementia

The most common type of vascular dementia is caused by the accumulation of defects through multiple, bilaterally localized supratentorial infarcts. Demented stroke patients with severe physical disability, e.g., a dense hemiplegia with neglect, are generally not included in tabulations of MID, because the dementia was not the presenting problem. The following description, therefore, does not apply to these more common stroke patients.

Patients with MID are usually over 50 and are more often men than women. Over a number of years, episodes of focal neurological dysfunction occur with hemiparesis, hemisensory symptoms, hemianopia, aphasia, confusion, ataxia, diplopia, dysarthria, and dizziness, with either complete or partial recovery and only minor residual symptoms. Cognitive symptoms may be present early or late in the disease, according to the location of the infarcts. Urinary disturbances, with increased frequency and urgency or incontinence, and gait disturbances often occur early in the disease, even before cognitive decline.

Because MID is most frequent in the setting of generalized vascular (most often atherosclerotic) or cardiac valvular disease, patients often have a history of hypertension, diabetes, angina and myocardial infarction, congestive heart failure, intermittent claudication, and vascular surgery. Some vascular conditions are genetically determined, and a family history of strokes and dementia may exist (Dichgans et al. 1998; Jen et al. 1997).

The type of cognitive decline depends on the predominant locations of the lesions. With multiple deep subcortical infarcts (lacunar state; Figure 70C.1, top and middle), psychomotor functions are slowed, with inertia, decreased attention and concentration, and memory deficits. Patients with cortical infarcts have aphasia, apraxia, amnesia, and visuospatial disturbances (Figure 70C.1, bottom). The subcortical type of dementia is often accompanied by motor signs, with slowness and instability of gait, stooped posture, lack of facial features, and soft voice, sometimes with pseudobulbar features such as forced laughing, crying, or choking. Most of these features are absent in patients with a cortical type of dementia. Combinations of cortical and subcortical features may occur.

Hypertension, carotid bruits and cardiac murmurs, and retinal vascular lesions are frequently present. Neurological examination often reveals minor signs: visual field abnormalities, pseudobulbar reflexes, subtle hemiparesis or clumsiness, increased tone, asymmetrical reflexes, and extensor plantar responses.

In most patients with MID, the clinical course is progressive, and cognitive decline is as severe as in Alzheimer's disease. In one study 50% of patients survived 6–7 years after the initial signs of disease, 2 years less than in patients with Alzheimer's disease in the same study, presumably because of death from other complications of vascular disease. Clinically important fluctuations in cognitive performance often occur.

Subcortical Arteriosclerotic Encephalopathy

SAE, first described by Otto Binswanger as a periventricular demyelination of the cerebral white matter of demented patients with a history of hypertension (and also known as *Binswanger's disease*), was always considered rare. Because computed tomography (CT) or magnetic resonance imaging (MRI) easily detect the white matter changes during life, the diagnosis is now made more often (see Figure 70C.1, top and middle). However, nonspecific white matter changes (see Leukoaraiosis, later in this chapter) are a frequent finding in nondemented elderly persons, and a diagnosis of SAE should only be considered in patients with leukoaraiosis who are demented, with no other obvious cause for the dementia.

Demented patients with SAE have a clinical history that is not very different from those with MID. A gradual onset, however, is a feature in most patients, with mental deterioration as the first sign in as many as two-thirds. Memory deficits, apathy, and increasing slowness of thinking and conduct are frequent complaints. Many patients also have acute episodes of neurological dysfunction, either at the onset or during the course of the disease, with paresis, clumsiness, or slurred speech. Apart from these episodes, frequent falls are often reported. A slowly progressing mental deterioration without acute exacerbations is also possible.

Although the mental symptoms may seriously interfere with activities of daily living, dementia may be mild on the scores of simple bedside tests. However, with neuropsychological studies, apathy, defective attention and concentration, memory dysfunction with severely impaired retrieval of information and relatively intact cognition, word-finding difficulties in conversational speech, reduced word fluency, and visuospatial and visuoconstructional deficits are found. The patient speaks with a soft voice and is often dysarthric. Lack of facial expression, shuffling gait, and a generally unkempt appearance are further characteristics.

Motor signs are almost always present in the later stages of the disease, with clumsiness, slowness of conduct, and gait disturbances. Asymmetrical reflexes, extensor plantar responses, and released pseudobulbar reflexes are often present, as is urinary incontinence. The average duration of the disease from the first symptoms to death is 5 years, with a range of 2 months to 22 years. A fluctuating course with periods of improvement and plateaus is more common than a slowly progressive course. Because the clinical picture of SAE is similar to that of MID, cases with SAE are probably included as MID in population surveys. The incidence and prevalence of SAE is unknown.

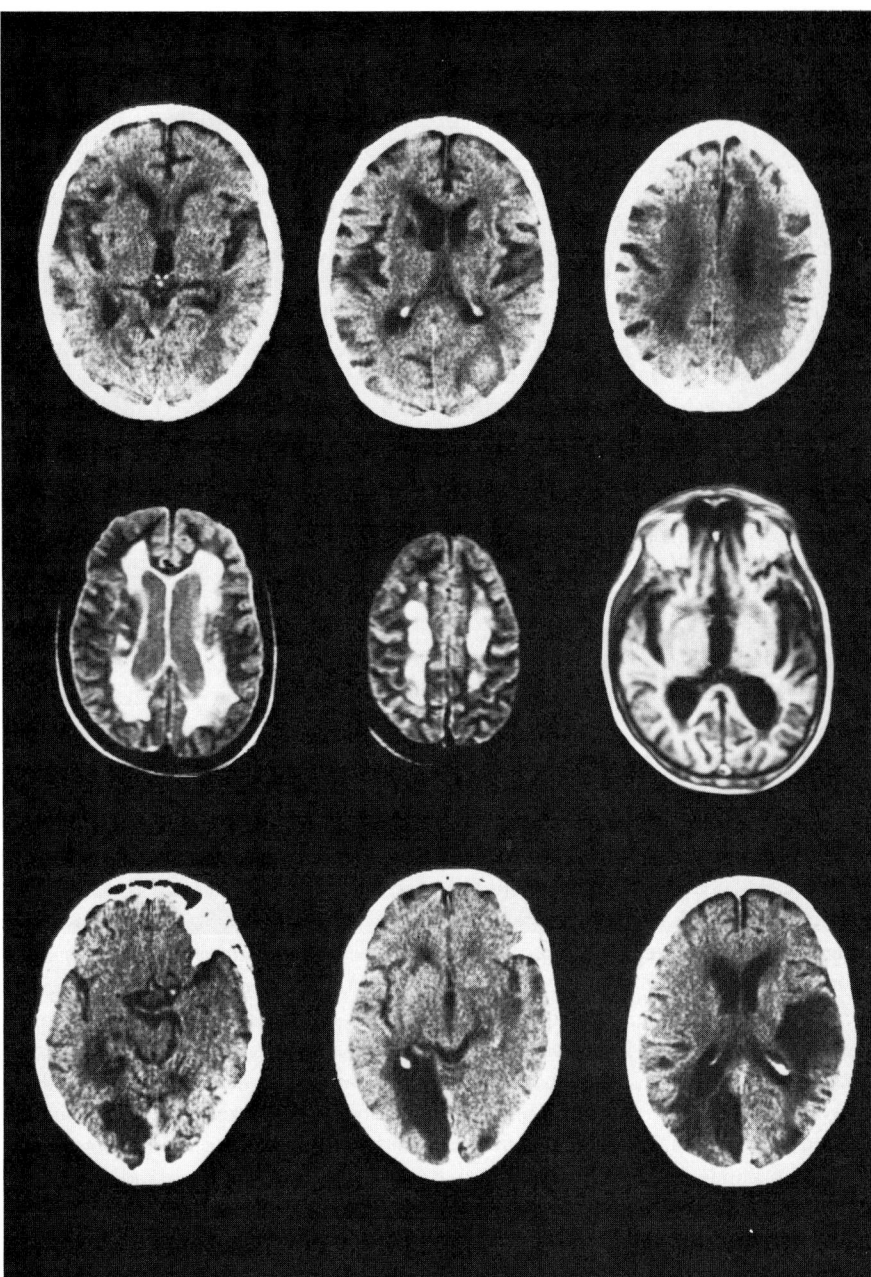

FIGURE 70C.1   (Top) Computed tomographic scans of a 77-year-old man with a moderately severe subcortical type of dementia. Several lacunar infarctions are visible in the basal ganglia and internal capsule (left and middle scans). A right occipital hemorrhagic infarct is visible in the middle and right scans. The right scan also shows low attenuation of the periventricular white matter. (Middle) Magnetic resonance imaging of a 57-year-old man with a severe subcortical type of dementia. The left and middle images (T2-weighted) show a high-intensity signal of the periventricular white matter. On the right image (T1-weighted), several small low-signal lesions are visible bilaterally in the thalamus. (Bottom) Computed tomographic scans of a 71-year-old woman with a moderately severe cortical type of dementia. Bilateral cortical infarctions are present in the middle and posterior cerebral artery distributions. In the middle scan, a lacunar infarct is visible near the left frontal horn, and the left external capsule region is hypodense.

PATHOGENESIS

Focal Lesions

In most types of vascular diseases, focal lesions (most frequently infarcts, sometimes hemorrhages) are the final mechanism that leads to brain damage and dementia (Table 70C.1). The nature and severity of the functional deficits caused by focal brain lesions are determined by the combination of location, volume, and multiplicity of lesions. Investigations in demented and nondemented patients with

brain infarcts have repeatedly demonstrated that total volume of brain tissue loss is an important determinant of dementia. In both groups, however, the variation in tissue loss is wide, and some demented patients only have small lesion volumes. This can be explained by the strategic location of some lesions or, in patients who already have diffuse tissue loss from other conditions, by a summation effect. In patients with infarcts, ventricular size contributes to the risk of dementia independent from other factors. Another factor is increasing age. Older patients often have neuronal loss, either from normal aging (see Chapter 86) or primary degenerative disease, which may not have led to manifest cognitive deterioration, and the focal brain lesion may cause an apparently exaggerated mental deterioration. Indicators of atherosclerosis in the general population are not only associated with an increased risk of vascular dementia, but also with an increased risk of Alzheimer's disease (Hofman et al. 1997), which might be additional evidence for the summation hypothesis.

Most patients with a clinical diagnosis of vascular dementia have multiple infarcts distributed in both cerebral hemispheres. The infarcts are more often lacunar than cortical, with the most frequent location in the basal ganglia and thalamus. Compared with nondemented stroke patients, demented patients more often have dominant hemisphere infarcts, more white matter changes, and larger ventricles. In patients with cortical infarcts, dementia occurs more often with anterior and posterior cerebral artery infarcts than with middle cerebral artery infarcts, possibly because of the involvement of limbic structures.

Patients with multiple infarcts have a multifocal decrease of cerebral blood flow (CBF). CBF reduction occurs most frequently in the thalamus, basal ganglia, and frontal and temporal cortices, in accordance with the location of infarcts. Blood flow in the cervical carotid arteries is consequently reduced, unrelated to the presence of stenosis. Vascular CO_2 reactivity and autoregulation are generally intact or only marginally disturbed. With positron emission tomography, there is a multifocal decrease in glucose use with normal oxygen extraction ratios, indicating that the decrease of flow is secondary to diminished metabolic demands. Areas with depressed metabolism are usually larger than the structural lesions seen on CT scan and are caused by microscopic ischemic lesions and disconnection of remote structures attributable to degeneration of fiber tracts.

Leukoaraiosis

Nonspecific periventricular white matter abnormalities are recognized increasingly as a risk factor for dementia, although the relation between the two is not simple. Cerebral white matter changes are present in multiple sclerosis, leukodystrophies, mitochondrial encephalopathies, certain infections, and after cerebral anoxia from cardiac arrest or carbon monoxide poisoning, but in elderly subjects they can only rarely be attributed to these conditions. For such nonspecific white matter changes on CT scan or MRI, the term *leukoaraiosis* is applied.

On CT scan, leukoaraiosis consists of ill-defined regions with low attenuation values around the frontal and occipital horns of the lateral ventricles, often extending into the frontal subinsular white matter and into the white matter of the centrum semiovale. It may extend to the cortex, with sparing of the corticocortical U-fibers. The internal capsule is never involved. In some patients with atherosclerosis, leukoaraiosis is associated with similar white matter changes

Table 70C.1: Types of cerebrovascular brain damage that may cause or contribute to dementia*

Lacunar infarct
Cortical infarct
Intracerebral hemorrhage
Leukoaraiosis
Intraventricular or subarachnoid hemorrhage
Neuronal loss in hippocampus, neocortex, and basal ganglia after global cerebral anoxia or ischemia

*Combinations often occur.

in the pons (Kwa et al. 1997). The lateral ventricles are often moderately enlarged. In most patients, lacunar and cortical infarcts are present also. On T2-weighted MRI, the white matter changes have an increased signal (see Figure 70C.1, middle). Those around the frontal and occipital horns are homogeneous, whereas those in the periventricular white matter frequently consist of a conglomerate of multiple smaller lesions. CBF studies show a decrease of CBF in the location of the white matter changes.

On pathological examination, the boundaries between lesions and normal white matter are ill defined. Demyelination is present, with or without loss of axons, and with varying amounts of gliosis. Widened perivascular spaces are often found (état criblé). The arterioles in affected and unaffected regions are often tortuous and show medial hypertrophy, hyalinosis, and fibrinoid necrosis indicative of hypertension. In some patients, there is a prominent amyloid angiopathy. Lacunar and cortical infarcts are present in most patients, and some show, in addition to the vascular pathology, typical Alzheimer's-type changes.

The most important risk factors for the development of leukoaraiosis are increasing age, hypertension, and cerebral vascular disease. Age is the most important; under age 50 the frequency on CT is only a few percent, and over 50 it increases two to three times with every decade. Hypertension is the next most important factor, occurring two times more often in demented and nondemented patients with leukoaraiosis compared with patients with normal CT scans. The third factor is cerebrovascular disease; most patients with leukoaraiosis have a history of stroke or transient ischemic attacks and have infarcts on their scans.

The frequency of leukoaraiosis varies considerably depending on age, disease, and many unknown factors; it is present in normal subjects in from 1–10% when studied with CT scan, and up to 27% when studied with MRI (Breteler et al. 1994). In demented and stroke patients, these figures are variable, but they are consistently higher. Apart from the imaging modality used, patient selection, age composition of the study population, and criteria for leukoaraiosis account for this substantial variability.

Hypoxia and ischemia are implicated by most authors as the cause of the changes, but exactly how this occurs is uncertain. Occlusion of the long penetrating arterioles may be an explanation. However, the lumina of the long arterioles, which penetrate the cortical surface and serve the main blood supply to the periventricular white matter, are most often found to be patent. Furthermore, the white matter lesions often contain normal tissue elements and cannot be considered as infarcts. Because the periventricular region is the end zone for the long cortical arterioles, this region may suffer from distal field ischemia caused by repeated hypotensive episodes, especially in patients with hypertension in whom the autoregulation curve has shifted to higher values. Another possible mechanism is rarefaction of the white matter by increasing tortuosity of the pulsatile arterioles with widening of the perivascular spaces. Embolism is considered an unlikely mechanism. Leukoaraiosis is a prominent feature in some hereditary cerebrovascular conditions such as cerebral autosomal dominant arteriopathy with subcortical infarcts and leukoencephalopathy (Dichgans et al. 1998), hereditary cerebral hemorrhage with amyloidosis (Bornebroek et al. 1996), and hereditary endotheliopathy with retinopathy, nephropathy, and stroke (Jen et al. 1997).

The mental status of patients with leukoaraiosis may vary from normal to that of a severe dementia that cannot always be attributed to concomitant cerebral pathology. In several population-based studies with nondemented volunteers, leukoaraiosis was associated with significantly lower scores on neuropsychological test batteries (Breteler et al. 1994). Furthermore, in a number of studies of determinants of dementia in patients with cerebrovascular disease, leukoaraiosis emerged as an independent risk factor for dementia. In stroke patients, leukoaraiosis is associated with a decline in speed and flexibility of mental processing. Although a correlation between the presence of leukoaraiosis and defective mental functioning has not been confirmed in all studies, the evidence indicates that leukoaraiosis in itself can impair mental function.

CT and MRI have greatly improved the possibility for prospective clinicoanatomical studies of leukoaraiosis, but pathological studies still remain of great importance, because CT and MRI cannot differentiate between demyelination, necrosis, gliosis, or état criblé; leukoaraiosis also may be associated with Alzheimer's disease and cerebral amyloid angiopathy. This pathological variability may account for the clinically heterogeneous correlates of the CT and MRI findings.

Other Types of Pathology Causing Vascular Dementia

After massive intraventricular or subarachnoid hemorrhage, diffuse brain damage may occur from severe temporary decrease in cerebral perfusion or from a concussion effect of the hemorrhage on the brain. Patients with aneurysmal subarachnoid hemorrhage may develop cerebral ischemia that is often multifocal. Further deterioration after a stable period may indicate normal pressure hydrocephalus.

The brain damage after global cerebral ischemia (see Chapter 61), such as occurs in cardiac arrest, near-drown-ing, severe shock, or carbon monoxide poisoning, is generally diffuse with hippocampal cell loss and cortical laminar necrosis. There also may be prominent focal features caused by border zone infarcts in the parietotemporal cortex or basal ganglia.

It is uncertain whether small ischemic lesions restricted to the cortex play an important role in the vascular dementia associated with hypertension and atherosclerosis. In theory, such lesions may lead to dementia when they are scattered throughout the cortex. Such granular cortical atrophy without concomitant large cortical and subcortical infarcts does occur in some relatively rare types of vascular disease, such as vasculitis.

Clinicopathological Correlations

Because the location of pathological changes in most patients with vascular dementia is different from that in patients with primary degenerative diseases such as Alzheimer's disease (with pathological changes in subcortical structures, rather than in the cerebral association cortex), the dementia syndrome resulting from vascular disease should be different from that caused by primary degeneration of the cerebral association cortex. Indeed, in many neuropsychological studies in patients with vascular dementia, defects in executive rather than instrumental functions were demonstrated, with reduced initiative, cognitive speed, and cognitive flexibility in the absence of aphasia, apraxia, and agnosia (see Chapter 11). Furthermore, in contrast to patients with Alzheimer's disease, patients with vascular dementia often have motor symptoms such as dysarthria, swallowing disturbances, forced crying and laughing, gait disorders, urinary urgency and incontinence, pyramidal signs, hypokinesia, and rigidity.

INVESTIGATIONS

Imaging with either CT or MRI is important to confirm the cerebrovascular pathology (see Figure 70C.1). The distribution and nature of the lesions also may give important clues for the pathogenetic mechanisms involved. Multiple cortical infarcts suggest repeated embolism; a lacunar state may be associated with poorly controlled hypertension; and a frontal watershed lesion points to ipsilateral carotid disease. Differential diagnosis can then be further refined by the appropriate ancillary investigations.

One or multiple infarcts may be found on CT in up to one-third of patients presenting with dementia. In patients clinically diagnosed as having MID, this figure may rise to 90%. MRI is even more sensitive, especially in the detection of small deep infarcts. Infarcts may be associated with ventricular widening, which occurs significantly more often in demented than in nondemented patients. Whether focal widening of sulci represents restricted cortical lesions, incomplete infarcts, or subcortical atrophy cannot be decided with CT and MRI. Leukoaraiosis often occurs in combination with other cerebrovascular lesions, most often with lacunar infarcts or hemorrhages, but also with cortical infarcts.

In an elderly population, infarcts, brain atrophy, and leukoaraiosis may all be incidental findings. Volume, multiplicity, and location of infarcts are required for clinicopathological correlation. Brain atrophy, also found in patients with Alzheimer's disease, is more strongly related to the severity of dementia than to its cause.

Positron emission tomography and single-photon emission computed tomography may reveal multifocal decreases in CBF and metabolism in patients with vascular dementia, whereas in patients with Alzheimer's disease these changes are found in the temporoparietal regions. CT or MRI may help differentiate the two patient groups. Electroencephalography shows generalized slowing in most patients with vascular dementia, with asymmetrical or focal slowing in many.

Ultrasound evaluation of the extracranial arteries and cerebral angiography usually reveal nonspecific atherosclerotic lesions in the extracranial and intracranial vessels. Unless specific remediable vascular lesions, such as vasculitis or vascular malformations, are a possibility, ultrasound evaluation and angiography are generally not indicated in patients with vascular dementia. When cerebral embolism is suggested by the history or CT or MRI findings, cardiac evaluation with electrocardiography, chest roentgenography, echocardiography, and Holter monitoring may be indicated. Laboratory evaluation for specific vascular or thrombotic disorders (blood lipids, erythrocyte sedimentation rate, serological markers of syphilis or connective tissue disease, prothrombin time, partial thromboplastin time, lupus anticoagulant, anticardiolipin antibodies, protein C, protein S, and antithrombin III) may be indicated in selected patients. Cerebrospinal fluid examination is of no value unless intracranial neoplasms, infections, vasculitis, or neurosyphilis are suspected.

DIAGNOSTIC CRITERIA AND DIFFERENTIAL DIAGNOSIS

The clinical diagnosis of vascular dementia in a demented person is often based on the presence of factors believed to be characteristic for a vascular etiology, summarized in an ischemic score (Table 70C.2). The presence of cerebrovascular disease, however, does not necessarily imply that stroke caused the dementia or even contributed to it, especially because concomitant Alzheimer's disease frequently occurs. When the diagnosis of vascular dementia is based only on the ischemic score, it will certainly be overdiagnosed. The duration of the dementia and the signs of cerebrovascular disease, and the results of brain imaging should be considered. In the *Diagnostic and Statistical Manual of Mental Disorders*, 4th edition, criteria for vascular dementia, both preconditions are poorly defined, but other for-

Table 70C.2: The ischemic score

Feature	Score[a]
Abrupt onset[b]	2
Stepwise deterioration	1
Fluctuating course[b]	2
Nocturnal confusion	1
Relative preservation of personality	1
Depression	1
Somatic complaints	1
Emotional incontinence	1
History of hypertension	1
History of strokes[b]	2
Evidence of associated atherosclerosis	1
Focal neurological symptoms[b]	2
Focal neurological signs[b]	2

[a]A score of ≤4 is considered suggestive of primary degenerative dementia, and a score of ≥7 of multi-infarct dementia. Ischemic scores are similar in patients with predominantly cortical or subcortical infarcts on computed tomography.
[b]Found to be one of the most important features for discriminating primary degenerative dementia and vascular dementia.
Source: Reprinted with permission from VC Hachinski, LD Illiff, H Zilhka, et al. Cerebral blood flow in dementia. Arch Neurol 1975;32:632–637.

mulated sets of criteria contain more explicit guidelines (Román et al. 1993). According to the American-European criteria (Table 70C.3), dementia should be present within 3 months after the clinical signs of a stroke. When such a time relationship is not present, the dementia should have had a sudden onset or a fluctuating course. Brain imaging is thought to be essential for the diagnosis, and when cerebrovascular lesions cannot be demonstrated with CT or MRI, the diagnosis of vascular dementia is not tenable.

The diagnosis of dementia in patients with cerebrovascular disease may be complicated by the presence of focal neuropsychological signs. The definition of dementia used in the American-European criteria (Román et al. 1993) is therefore more restrictive than usual. Apart from memory disturbances, cognitive changes should be present in at least two domains instead of one, to allow for the possible effect of the focal lesion alone. Careful neurobehavioral or neuropsychological evaluation of the patients is therefore necessary.

The following criteria have been suggested for the diagnosis of SAE: (1) dementia; (2) leukoaraiosis on CT or MRI; and (3) two of the following three characteristics—presence of a vascular risk factor or evidence of systemic vascular disease, evidence of focal cerebrovascular disease, or evidence of subcortical cerebral dysfunction (gait disorder, urinary incontinence).

Despite differences in the profile of cognitive decline between patients with vascular dementia and those with Alzheimer's disease (see Clinicopathological Correlations, previously in this chapter), it is still uncertain whether patients may be reliably discriminated on the basis of these differences alone. Because motor symptoms are absent in Alzheimer's disease until the late stages and are common in

Table 70C.3: Main features of the criteria for vascular dementia of the National Institute of Neurological Disorders and Stroke and the Association Internationale pour la Recherche et L'Enseignement en Neurosciences

1[a]	2[b]	3[c]	4[d]	5[e]	Degree of confidence for diagnosis of vascular dementia
+	+	+	NP	NP	Possible
+	+	−	+	NP	Possible
+	+	+	+	NP	Probable
+	+	+	+/NP	+	Certain
+	+	+	−	NP	No vascular dementia

(+) = factor present; (−) = factor absent; NP = not performed.
[a]Clinical characteristics of dementia
[b]Clinical characteristics of cerebral vascular disease
[c]Temporal relation between 1 and 2 or sudden onset, fluctuating course of the dementia, or both
[d]Confirmation of cerebrovascular pathology with brain imaging (computed tomography or magnetic resonance imaging)
[e]Histopathological confirmation of ischemic/hemorrhagic brain damage and exclusion of other pathological changes associated with dementia
Source: Reprinted with permission from GC Román, TK Tatemichi, T Erkinjuntti, et al. Vascular dementia: diagnostic criteria for research studies. Report of the NINDS-AIREN International Work Group. Neurology 1993;43:250–260.

patients with vascular dementia, these may be a more reliable discriminating criterion. When motor symptoms are prominent in patients with dementia, alternative diagnoses include Parkinson's disease, multiple system atrophy, progressive supranuclear palsy, and normal pressure hydrocephalus. When infarcts or leukoaraiosis are present on CT or MRI of these patients, they may only be incidental findings or may explain the dementia. These considerations are also of importance in patients with possible diffuse Lewy body disease, in whom a fluctuating course may suggest vascular dementia, and in patients with possible SAE, who may present with a clinical course reminiscent of Alzheimer's disease.

Because of the heterogeneous pathophysiology and pathology of vascular dementia, diagnostic criteria for vascular dementia might never be simple. This may be different for the primary degenerative diseases leading to dementia, in which rather specific pathology is present. Because primary degenerative and vascular diseases in the elderly are often combined, the diagnosis of vascular dementia will probably become more valid when specific diagnostic tests for the different degenerative diseases become available.

PREVENTION AND TREATMENT

Most vascular dementias arise as complications of atherosclerosis, and the same principles of treatment that are applied in the secondary prevention of atherothrombotic strokes may be of use to ameliorate the clinical course of dementia in MID patients (i.e., treatment of hypertension,

anticoagulants in cardiac embolic disease, and aspirin). The effects of aspirin and ticlopidine in patients with large vessel disease and embolic cortical infarcts have not been studied in patients with small vessel disease and lacunar infarction.

Treatment of isolated systolic hypertension in elderly people reduces the incidence of dementia by 50% (Forette et al. 1998). Only a few small studies have specifically addressed the efficacy of antihypertensive treatment in patients with vascular dementia, and short-term arrest of progression of cognitive decline, or even amelioration, may be achieved. However, an acute deterioration has often been the reason for the start of treatment and partial recovery usually occurs spontaneously after each infarct.

Treatment of hypertension may be as important in preventing the progression of periventricular leukoencephalopathy as in preventing repeated infarction, but this has not been demonstrated specifically. The suggested worsening of the clinical condition with antihypertensive therapy has, again, not been demonstrated.

The clinical features of SAE in combination with the enlarged lateral ventricles on CT scan may suggest the presence of a normal pressure hydrocephalus (see Chapter 86). A few patients with vascular dementia had short-term improvement after ventricular shunting, then deteriorated after 6 months to 1 year. With MRI, better identification of parenchymal lesions is now possible, and when these are present, shunting is not recommended (Vanneste et al. 1993).

Because of apathy and slowness of behavior, sometimes combined with forced crying, patients with vascular dementia may give the impression of being depressed. However, more specific symptoms of depression such as feelings of sadness, suicidal ideation, fluctuations in mood, and sleep disturbances are mostly absent, and treatment with antidepressants is not indicated. Forced crying and laughing may respond to specific serotonin reuptake inhibitors such as sertraline (50–150 mg/day) or to amitriptyline (25–75 mg/day).

In patients with swallowing disturbances, choking may be prevented by replacing drinks with thick fluids such as milkshakes and yogurt. When oral hydration and feeding become insufficient, the patient should receive additional tube feeding. The most convenient way (for the patient and caregivers) to achieve this is through a percutaneous endoscopic gastrostomy. Urinary incontinence can be partly prevented by a regimen of regular micturition. Motor disabilities may require formal rehabilitation.

REFERENCES

Bornebroek M, Haan J, Van Buchem M, et al. White matter lesions and cognitive deterioration in presymptomatic carriers of the amyloid precursor protein gene codon 693 mutation. Arch Neurol 1996;53:43–48.
Breteler MMB, Van Swieten JC, Bots ML, et al. Cerebral white matter lesions, vascular risk factors, and cognitive function in a population-based study: The Rotterdam Study. Neurology 1994;44:1246–1252.

Dichgans M, Mayer M, Uttner I, et al. The phenotypic spectrum of CADASIL: clinical findings in 102 cases. Neurology 1998;44: 731–739.

Forette F, Seux ML, Staessen JA, et al. Prevention of dementia in radomized double-blind placebo-controlled Systolic Hypertension in Europe (Syst-Eur) trial. Lancet 1998;352:1347–1351.

Hofman A, Ott A, Breteler MB, et al. Atherosclerosis, apolipoprotein E, and prevalence of dementia and Alzheimer's disease in the Rotterdam Study. Lancet 1997;349:151–154.

Jen J, Cohen AH, Yue Q, et al. Hereditary endotheliopathy with retinopathy, nephropathy, and stroke (HERNS). Neurology 1997;49:1322–1330.

Kwa VI, Stam J, Blok LM, Verbeeten Jr B. T2-weighted hyperintense MRI lesions in the pons in patients with atherosclerosis. Stroke 1997;28:1357–1360.

Ott BR, Saver JL. Unilateral amnesic stroke. Stroke 1993;24: 1033–1042.

Román GC, Tatemichi TK, Erkinjuntti T, et al. Vascular dementia: diagnostic criteria for research studies. Report of the NINDS-AIREN International Work Group. Neurology 1993;43: 250–260.

Vanneste J, Augustijn P, Tan WF, et al. Shunting normal pressure hydrocephalus: the predictive value of combined clinical and CT data. J Neurol Neurosurg Psychiatry 1993;56:251–256.

Chapter 70
The Dementias

D. PROGRESSIVE FOCAL CORTICAL SYNDROMES
David Neary and Julie S. Snowden

The term *progressive focal cortical syndrome* refers to a relatively circumscribed neuropsychological disorder arising from degenerative brain disease that, although progressive, remains selective in the functions affected until relatively late in the evolution of disease. The particular neuropsychological syndrome is determined by the topographical distribution of pathological change within the brain and is characterized either by a predominance of atrophy in one or more lobes or by an asymmetrical distribution of atrophy between the two hemispheres. In one sense, all cortical atrophies leading to dementia syndromes are focal in that they have a preferential site of disease onset. For example, Alzheimer's disease has an affinity for the limbic system and parietotemporal association cortex and may present with selective disorders of memory, language, or perceptuospatial function. Occasionally, such focal symptomatology persists over several years, giving rise to descriptive designations such as progressive amnesia, posterior cortical atrophy, progressive aphasia, and progressive agnosia. In Alzheimer's disease, selective deficits are typically short-lived, and a constellation of characteristic neuropsychological deficits, which includes amnesia, visuospatial disorientation, apraxia, and aphasia, accrues within a relatively short time. In contrast, in non-Alzheimer's disease forms of cerebral atrophy the cerebral pathology commonly remains restricted for many years. The atrophy may be highly localized or asymmetrical on neuroimaging studies such as computed tomography, magnetic resonance imaging, positron emission tomography, and single-photon emission computed tomography (SPECT). The areas of focal atrophy or maximal hypometabolism usually reflect the particular neuropsychological deficit.

Focal non-Alzheimer's cortical syndromes take many forms. Examples of a predominance of atrophy on one or more lobes are frontotemporal dementia (FTD), which involves the frontal and anterior temporal lobes, and semantic dementia, which involves the temporal lobes. An asymmetrical distribution of atrophy between the two hemispheres is exemplified by progressive nonfluent aphasia that involves the left dominant perisylvian cortex and progressive prosopagnosia, affecting the right temporal lobe. Other focal syndromes are progressive (limb) apraxia, involving the pre-motor and superior parietal lobes and buccofacial dyspraxia, in which frontal hypometabolism is demonstrated. Given the highly asymmetrical distribution of pathology in the frontoparietal cortex as well as the basal ganglia, cortical-basal ganglionic degeneration, in which there is profound limb apraxia and other cortical signs, can reasonably be incorporated within the rubric of focal cortical syndromes. These distinct clinical syndromes appear to share a common non-Alzheimer's pathology.

FRONTOTEMPORAL DEMENTIA

Clinical Features

FTD is a disorder of behavior, characterized by profound alteration in personality and social conduct about which the patient has no insight and shows no concern (Snowden et al. 1996). Patients neglect domestic and occupational responsibilities and behavior is purposeless and lacking in goals. Planning, judgment, and mental flexibility are impaired. Affect is shallow, and sympathy and empathy with others is lost. Behavioral characteristics are not identical in all patients. Some patients are disinhibited, overactive, and restless, with a fatuous affect. They may clown, pun, or sing, usually according to a restricted and stereotyped repertoire. Other patients are apathetic and inert, lacking in drive and initiative and minimally responsive to external stimuli. These behavioral types represent opposite poles of a spectrum of behavioral disorder, determined by the part of the frontal lobes predominantly affected by the disease: orbitofrontal involvement in overactive, disinhibited patients, and widespread frontal involvement including dorsolateral cortex in apathetic patients. Patients who present with extreme overactivity and disinhibition may become increasingly apathetic and inert with disease progression.

Behavioral change in FTD may include altered food preferences, particularly an increased liking for sweet foods. Hyperoral behavior in which the patient mouths inedible objects may occur also, although usually only in the late stages. Environmental dependency, in which patients are drawn and react to objects in the visual environment, may be evident. Utilization behavior, an extreme form of environmental dependency in which the patient carries out the action pertinent to an object despite its irrelevance to the social context (e.g., repeated drinking from an empty cup) occurs in a minority of patients. Stereotypic features, such as repeated wandering following an identical route, are common. In a minority of patients, however, the stereotypic, ritualistic nature of the patient's behavior is the dominant presenting feature. These patients typically adhere to a rigid daily routine and may develop elaborate procedures for dressing or toileting and behavioral rituals such as not walking on cracks in the pavement.

Language in FTD is characterized by a marked economy of speech output, particularly in apathetic patients, bearing resemblance to a dynamic aphasia. Occasionally, disinhibited patients may show pressure of speech, but content is repetitive and stereotyped. Additional speech abnormalities are concreteness of thought, echolalia, and perseveration. Structural aspects of language, such as phonology, morphology, and semantics are generally well preserved, although word errors in naming may occur with disease progression. Mutism invariably occurs in middle to late stage disease. Perceptual, spatial, and praxic skills remain strikingly well preserved throughout the illness. Patients have no difficulty localizing and recognizing objects and in negotiating their environment. Constructional tasks such as drawing and block design may be performed poorly for strategic and organizational, rather than primarily spatial, reasons. Memory is patchy and variable and patients exhibit a frontal type of amnesia. They typically remain oriented in time and place. However, they perform poorly on formal memory tests, as a result of their failure to implement effortful encoding and retrieval strategies. Recall performance can generally be enhanced by provision of

directed rather than open-ended questions and multiple-choice response alternatives. Formal neuropsychological assessment reveals the most profound deficits on frontal lobe executive tests, these being more striking in apathetic patients than in orbitofrontal, disinhibited patients. Abnormal characteristics are attention failures; concreteness of thought; strategic, organizational, and sequencing difficulties; verbal and motor perseveration and failures in mental set shifting; and strategic, organizational, and sequencing difficulties. Some impairment may be demonstrated, however, on nonfrontal lobe executive tasks, reflecting patients' cursory mode of responding, lack of concern for accuracy, and failure of self-monitoring. It is because of such widespread test failures that the focal nature of the disorder may sometimes fail to be recognized.

Initially, neurological signs are few, limited to the presence of primitive reflexes, but with progression, striatal signs of akinesia and rigidity emerge. In those patients in whom stereotypical, ritualistic behavior dominates the clinical presentation, akinesia and rigidity occur relatively early in the course of the illness. Electroencephalography remains substantially normal in all patients. Functional brain imaging, using xenon 133 inhalation, positron emission tomography, and SPECT, reveals abnormalities in the anterior cerebral hemispheres.

Onset of disease is most commonly between 45 and 65 years, although the range is wide. FTD occasionally has its onset in the elderly. The youngest recorded onset is 21 years of age. Both genders are affected equally. The mean duration of illness is approximately 8 years, although the range is from 2–15 years. A family history of a similar disorder in a first-degree relative occurs in approximately one-half of cases. Strong evidence exists in some families of an autosomal dominant mode of inheritance. No known geographical influences on prevalence exist. The presence or absence of a family history does not determine the behavioral pattern; familial cases occur in the disinhibited, inert, and stereotypical forms of the disorder.

Anatomical Correlates and Histology

The brains of patients with FTD are characterized by frontotemporal cortical atrophy (Mann et al. 1993). In overactive, disinhibited patients the orbitomedial frontal lobe is preferentially affected, with relative sparing of the dorsolateral frontal convexity. Inert, apathetic patients, in contrast, have severe atrophy extending into the dorsolateral frontal cortex. In a minority of patients, the brunt of the pathology is borne by the striatum, with usually severe limbic involvement but variable cortical and nigral involvement. This subgroup with predominant striatal pathology conforms clinically to those patients in whom stereotypical, ritualistic behavior dominates the clinical picture, and in whom striatal neurological signs develop early in the disease course.

Two characteristic histopathological processes underlie cases with frontotemporal atrophy. The most common histological change is loss of large cortical nerve cells (chiefly from layers III and V), and a spongiform degeneration or microvacuolation of the superficial neuropil (layer II); gliosis is minimal and restricted to subpial regions. No distinctive changes (swellings or inclusions) within remaining nerve cells are seen. The limbic system and striatum are affected, but to a much lesser extent.

The second and less common histological process is characterized by a loss of large cortical nerve cells with widespread and abundant gliosis but minimal or no spongiform change or microvacuolation. Swollen neurons or inclusions that are both tau- and ubiquitin-positive are present in some cases, and the limbic system and striatum are more seriously damaged. The two differing histologies nevertheless share a similar distribution within the frontal and temporal cortex and cannot be distinguished on the basis of the behavioral disorder or the familial incidence. Cases with predominant striatal pathology appear to share features of both histological types.

FRONTOTEMPORAL DEMENTIA AND MOTOR NEURON DISEASE

Clinical Syndrome

An association between dementia and motor neuron disease (MND) or amyotrophic lateral sclerosis has long been recognized, although it is relatively recently that a link has been drawn between the form of dementia and FTD. Typically, personality and behavioral changes consistent with FTD emerge first and are often of the overactive, disinhibited type, although increased apathy occurs with disease progression. After some months, patients develop the amyotrophic form of MND with widespread fasciculations, muscular weakness, wasting, and bulbar palsy. The bulbar palsy is responsible for death, which takes place within 3 years of onset. Extrapyramidal signs of akinesia and rigidity emerge in patients with disease of longer duration. Neurophysiological investigations demonstrate widespread muscular denervation, the electroencephalogram remains normal, and SPECT imaging reveals reduced tracer in the anterior hemispheres as with FTD.

Anatomical and Histological Changes

Cerebral atrophy is less marked in FTD with MND than without MND, presumably reflecting the short duration of illness. The atrophy is mostly frontal, involving the orbitomedial regions with some temporal lobe involvement. The histology in the majority of cases is characterized by loss of large cortical nerve cells, microvacuolation, and mild gliosis. Limbic involvement is slight, though nigral damage is

severe, with heavy loss of pigmented nerve cells and intense reactive fibrous astrocytosis. Ubiquitinated but not tau-immunoreactive inclusions are present within the frontal cortex and hippocampus (dentate gyrus). In the brainstem, the hypoglossal nucleus shows atrophy with loss of neurons. Large Betz's cells of the precentral gyrus are preserved in number, and no obvious axonal loss occurs within the corticospinal tracts. A gross loss of anterior horn neurons occurs at all levels, and many of the surviving anterior horn cells contain large pale ubiquitinated inclusions within the cytoplasm. No Lewy- or Pick-type inclusions are observed in any cortical or subcortical neurons. Spongiform or microvacuolar changes are highly characteristic of this syndrome, although more rarely the histological findings are of gliosis and neuronal cell loss and ballooned neurons may be present.

PROGRESSIVE NONFLUENT APHASIA

Clinical Syndrome

Several forms of language disorder have been described under the broad rubric of slowly progressive aphasia. However, the designation was originally introduced to refer to a syndrome of nonfluent, anomic aphasia. The dominant presenting feature is in the domain of speech production; output is nonfluent, effortful, and hesitant, often with a stuttering quality, and there are phonemic (sound based) and some verbal (semantic) errors. Word finding and repetition is impaired severely. Reading is also effortful and nonfluent, with phonological errors. Writing is telegrammatic and spelling is poor. Comprehension, particularly of individual lexical terms, is relatively preserved initially, and patients retain insight into their language disorder. This, together with the fact that nonlanguage cognitive skills, including memory function, are strikingly preserved, accounts for the observation that patients may continue in productive employment for many years after onset of symptoms. With progression of disease speech output becomes increasingly attenuated, leading ultimately to mutism. Patients also may manifest a gestural dyspraxia, so that effective communication is impossible. Comprehension skills gradually deteriorate over the course of the illness, although the extent of this is difficult to determine in view of the patient's profound communication disorder. However, evidence exists that patients retain some understanding of language at a time when their own powers of oral and gestural expression are negligible. Social skills are typically extremely well preserved in the early stages, although behavioral changes akin to those of FTD may occur late in the disease.

Neurological signs are absent usually, although there are pathologically confirmed cases in which a progressive, asymmetrical akinesia, rigidity, and tremor affecting the right arm and leg emerged over the course of disease. Electroencephalography is usually normal, and left perisylvian hypometabolism is seen on functional imaging using positron emission tomography and SPECT. Demographical characteristics are similar to those of FTD.

A link between the syndromes of progressive aphasia and FTD is demonstrated clinically by the finding of the two syndromes occurring within the same family. Moreover, there may be overlap between the clinical syndromes with disease progression. The link is further reinforced by the finding that progressive aphasia also may occur in association with MND (Caselli et al. 1993).

Anatomical and Histological Findings

The brain in progressive nonfluent aphasia (Snowden et al. 1996) shows markedly asymmetrical atrophy, being slight and generalized on the right but gross on the left side, particularly affecting frontotemporal, frontoparietal, and lateral parieto-occipital regions. The left anterior temporal cortex shows knife-edge atrophy of gyri. The pattern of atrophy involves the hippocampus, amygdala, caudate, putamen, globus pallidus, and thalamus on the left side alone. Histologically, frontal, frontoparietal, and anterior temporal cortices on the left side are affected severely and show a virtually complete loss of large pyramidal cells from layers III and V. Typically, there is widespread spongiform change, particularly in layers II and III, caused by neuronal fallout. Reactive astrocytosis is mild, even in severely affected regions, and typically no Pick- or Lewy-type inclusion bodies are present in surviving nerve cells in any region of the cortex or subcortex. Although the majority of cases of progressive aphasia conform to the microvacuolar spongiform type of change, a smaller group are characterized by histological appearances of severe gliosis.

SEMANTIC DEMENTIA

Clinical Syndrome

The term *semantic dementia* was introduced to denote a syndrome distinct from FTD and progressive aphasia but sharing a common pathology. The prominent feature of the disorder is a profound loss of meaning, encompassing both verbal and nonverbal material (Snowden et al. 1996). Typically, patients present with difficulties in naming and word comprehension, and speech becomes increasingly empty and lacking in substance. Nevertheless, speech output is fluent, effortless, grammatically correct, and free from phonemic paraphasias. This superficial facility with language belies the profound underlying anomia and word comprehension deficit, which is apparent on formal testing. Repetition and recitation of overlearned verbal series is essentially preserved. Reading and writing are fluent and

effortless, but regularization errors in reading aloud and written spelling occur for words with irregular spelling-to-sound correspondence, reflecting failure of comprehension of written material. With the progression of disease, the patients' understanding of words systematically deteriorates, and their conversational repertoire becomes increasingly restricted and stereotyped. Echolalia may occur and eventually mutism. At no time is speech output nonfluent or effortful; there is simply a contraction of speech repertoire until no interactive communication is possible.

Many patients with progressive failure of word comprehension and naming reported in the literature have been subsumed within the rubric of progressive aphasia because of the prominence of language symptoms. The semantic disorder is, however, rarely confined to language. Failure of face recognition is ubiquitous, and patients also exhibit difficulties in recognizing the significance of objects. These difficulties in face and object identity occur in the context of well-preserved elementary perceptual skills; patients perform normally on perceptual matching and copying tasks. In some patients a disorder of face or object recognition may be the earliest presenting feature, preceding symptoms of language breakdown, giving rise to focal syndromes of progressive prosopagnosia and associative agnosia. Typically, however, widespread impairments of semantic knowledge, affecting all sensory modalities, emerge with disease progression.

Behavior in the early and middle stages of the illness may be eccentric, and patients may exhibit obsessional traits, preoccupations, and behavioral stereotypes. The gross asocial and disinhibited behavior of FTD is, however, typically absent. Nevertheless, with disease progression an increase in frontal-type behavioral features may occur with overlap in symptomatology with FTD.

Neurological signs are usually absent, the electroencephalogram is normal, and structural and functional brain imaging indicate bilateral temporal lobe atrophy, which may be asymmetrical, with the predominance of left or right temporal atrophy reflecting the relative severity of the semantic deficit for verbal and nonverbal material.

Demographical characteristics are similar to those of FTD and progressive aphasia. Onset is typically between 45 and 65 years and the syndrome may be familial.

Anatomical and Histological Findings

The temporal lobes are severely atrophied, particularly the middle and inferior temporal gyri, with preservation of the superior temporal gyrus, parietal, and occipital cortices. The frontal lobes are moderately atrophied, as are the corpus striatum, globus pallidus, and thalamus. The histological changes consist of large pyramidal cell loss, spongiform change, and mild reactive astrocytosis with no Pick- or Lewy-type inclusions in surviving neurons.

PROGRESSIVE APRAXIA

Clinical Features

Some authors have drawn attention to the presence of buccofacial apraxia as a dominant presenting feature in patients with focal cerebral atrophy. Typically, the apraxia occurs in the context of an expressive language disorder and is associated with predominant frontal lobe atrophy. Rather less common but more striking in view of the selective nature of the disorder is the syndrome of slowly progressive limb apraxia. Patients present initially with an upper limb apraxia that affects both left and right side, albeit on occasions somewhat asymmetrically. The disorder severely compromises the ability to use objects in activities of daily living. Difficulties are particularly marked for bimanual actions, such as using a knife and fork, for which there is intermanual interference. The apraxia is of an ideomotor type, and patients retain the ability to describe the actions that they are unable to produce and display appropriate distress at their difficulties into which they retain full insight. Lower limb movements are initially much less affected than upper limb movements, although these too become increasingly affected with disease progression. Buccofacial movements are compromised relatively late in the disease course. Eventually, however, all voluntary movements are impaired. The profound apraxia stands in striking contrast to the patients' preserved language, visuoperceptual, spatial, and memory skills. In the later stages of illness, however, communication may be precluded because of patients' buccofacial apraxia and inability to convey information by gesture and pantomime, so that evaluation of cognitive skills outside the realm of apraxia becomes difficult to determine.

Neurological examination in the early stages is normal, although striatal signs of akinesia and rigidity emerge with disease progression. Electroencephalography is normal, and SPECT imaging reveals reduced tracer uptake in the superior parietal areas.

Anatomical and Histological Findings

Atrophy is bilateral and symmetrical, affecting predominantly the frontal pre-motor and parietal areas (Snowden et al. 1996). Prefrontal, superior temporal, and occipital cortex are essentially preserved. Cases are described in which Pick-type histology is demonstrated, with severe astrocytic gliosis in parietal and insular cortex and in layer 11 of the motor cortex, neuronal inclusions, and swollen neurons.

NOSOLOGY OF LOBAR DEGENERATION

The focal cortical syndromes described previously appear to reflect the topographic distribution of the non-Alzheimer's pathology. When the frontal lobes are bilaterally, symmetrically, and predominantly affected, the syndrome of FTD emerges, with breakdown in problem solving and regulation of social conduct. When the left cerebral hemisphere is affected predominantly, involving the frontoparietal regions of the perisylvian cortex, the syndrome of progressive nonfluent aphasia occurs, with failure in phonological and syntactic aspects of language. Predominant involvement of the temporal lobes bilaterally leads to the loss of word and object meaning of semantic dementia. Asymmetrical involvement of the right temporal lobe is associated with loss of meaning of faces (prosopagnosia). Progressive limb apraxia is associated with involvement of frontal pre-motor and parietal regions. When, in progressive aphasia and semantic dementia, the pathology spreads into the frontal lobes, the behavioral changes of FTD emerge as a late consequence. MND is associated with FTD and progressive aphasia and presumably also may occur in other forms of lobar degeneration.

Neither the clinical syndrome nor familial incidence dictates the underlying type of histology, which falls into three classes: (1) the microvacuolar or spongiform change; (2) gliosis with or without inclusion bodies and swollen neurons; and (3) MND type. Confusion in the literature has occurred because of uncertainty regarding the different clinical syndromes arising from frontotemporal lobe degeneration and lack of agreement concerning the pathological criteria for Pick's disease: whether the presence of focal atrophy of the frontal and anterior temporal lobes is sufficient for the diagnosis or whether the histological characteristics of swollen neurons and inclusion bodies need to be present. Workers in Sweden and the United Kingdom shared their clinical and pathological material and published consensus criteria (Brun et al. 1994) for the clinical syndrome of FTD and the three major histological changes (see Appendix to this chapter). The microvacuolar or spongiform appearances have been designated frontal lobe degeneration type. Gliosis with or without inclusion bodies and swollen neurons has been designated Pick-type histology. The amyotrophic histology has been referred to as MND type. This range of histology also underlies the syndromes of progressive aphasia and presumably semantic dementia and progressive apraxia. Revised clinical criteria for FTD, progressive aphasia, and semantic dementia have been established subsequently by a consensus of investigators from the United States, Canada, and Europe (Neary et al. 1998).

Currently, it is not certain whether the histologies underlying these focal syndromes are etiologically distinct or represent a range of pathological phenotypes. The microvacuolar type of histology seems to be associated with the splice-site mutations that increase the use of exon 10 when transcribing tau (Hutton et al. 1998), at least in families with disease previously linked to chromosome 17 (Foster et al. 1997). Whether the Pick-type histology is associated also with mutations in tau is currently not known; the histological changes may only represent a post-translational alteration. The issue is likely to be resolved by genetic and molecular biological studies.

In general, the focal cerebral atrophies favor the anterior-superior cortex (frontotemporal and superior parietal lobes). The majority of instances of these anterior-superior atrophies exhibit the non-Alzheimer's disease form of cerebral atrophy described previously. The non-Alzheimer's disease pathology is associated with a high familial incidence, and the different clinical syndromes may be linked by common genetic influences.

In Alzheimer's disease, in contrast, a predilection exists for posterior-inferior cortex (inferior parietal-temporal lobes). It is perhaps not surprising that the posterior cortical atrophy syndrome, in which perceptuospatial abnormalities occur in the absence of memory loss, has been associated with instances of Alzheimer's disease and that some patients with a progressive disorder of language or praxis also may prove ultimately to have Alzheimer's disease.

CONCLUSION

Focal cortical syndromes are commonly differentiated conceptually from dementia on the grounds that the neuropsychological deficit in the former is selective and circumscribed, whereas in the latter it is diffuse and nonspecific. Such premises are inaccurate and misleading. Dementing disorders such as Alzheimer's disease have a predilection for certain brain regions and as such give rise to characteristic and identifiable patterns of cognitive disturbance and not undifferentiated impairment. In some instances that pattern of deficit is sufficiently selective that it is appropriately described as a focal syndrome. The symptom-cluster characteristic of the dementia syndrome typically evolves gradually with disease progression. In non-Alzheimer's forms of focal atrophy, the selective nature of the psychological deficits may persist for many years, yet even in these conditions, typically spread of the degenerative process occurs with disease progression. In progressive aphasia, for example, extension of pathology into the parietal areas may give rise to late symptoms of apraxia. Moreover, at autopsy the degenerative change is typically demonstrated to be bilateral, albeit affecting the left side more than the right. At end-stage disease, even in focal cerebral atrophy, clinical differences become submerged. If *dementia* is conceived of as a generic term embracing the neuropsychological syndromes characteristic of particular brain diseases, then the apparent dichotomy between focal atrophy syndromes and dementia no longer holds.

REFERENCES

Brun A, Mann DMA, Englund B, et al. Clinical and neuropathological criteria for fronto-temporal dementia. J Neurol Neurosurg Psychiatry 1994;4:416–418.

Caselli RJ, Windebank AJ, Petersen RC, et al. Rapidly progressive aphasic dementia and motor neuron disease. Ann Neurol 1993;33:200–207.

Foster NL, Wilhelmsen K, Sima AAF, et al. Frontotemporal dementia and parkinsonism linked to chromosome 17: a consensus conference. Ann Neurol 1997;41:706–715.

Hutton M, Lendon CL, Rizzu P, et al. Association of missense and 5'-splice-site mutations in tau with the inherited dementia FTDP-17. Nature 1998;393:702–705.

Mann DMA, South PW, Snowden JS, et al. Dementia of frontal lobe type; neuropathology and immunohistochemistry. J Neurol Neurosurg Psychiatry 1993;56:605–614.

Neary D, Snowden JS, Gustafson L, et al. Frontotemporal lobar degeneration. A consensus on clinical diagnostic criteria. Neurology 1998;51:1546–1554.

Snowden JS, Neary D, Mann DMA. Frontotemporal lobar degeneration: frontotemporal dementia, progressive aphasia, semantic dementia. London: Churchill-Livingstone, 1996.

APPENDIX: Neuropathological Diagnostic Features of Frontotemporal Dementia

I. Frontal lobe degeneration type

Gross changes: These include slight symmetrical convolutional atrophy in frontal and anterior temporal lobes, neither circumscribed nor of a knife blade–type; atrophy can be severe in a few cases. The ventricular system is widened frontally. Usually, no gross atrophy of the striatum, amygdala, or hippocampus exists, although, in some instances, severe involvement of these regions can occur.

Distribution of microscopic changes: Changes are seen in the frontal convexity cortex, sometimes in the orbitofrontal cortex, often in the anterior one-third of the temporal cortex, and the anterior, but rarely posterior, cingulate gyrus. The superior temporal gyrus is conspicuously spared. The parietal cortex is mildly involved in a few patients, more so in rare advanced cases. In some patients with pronounced stereotypical behaviors, there is less neocortical involvement with mostly striatal, amygdala, and hippocampal changes. These may represent a possible subtype.

Microscopic characteristics, gray matter: Microvacuolation and mild to moderate astrocytic gliosis affecting chiefly laminae I–III are seen, sometimes one or the other change prevailing. There is atrophy or loss of neurons in laminae II and III, whereas those of lamina V are mildly affected, being atrophic rather than lost. Occasionally, there are a few dystrophic neurites. There are no Pick's bodies, ballooned neurons, or Lewy bodies. In the substantia nigra of some patients, there is mild to moderate loss of pigmented neurons.

Microscopic characteristics, white matter: White matter astrocytic gliosis, moderate to mild, is seen in subcortical U-fibers. There is mild astrocytic gliosis in deeper white matter, sometimes with slight attenuation and loss of myelin. The distribution is related to gray matter changes. Sometimes also ischemic white matter attenuation exists.

II. Pick's disease type

Gross changes: These have the same topographical localization as frontal lobe degeneration, but are generally more intense and usually more circumscribed. Asymmetry and striatal atrophy are common. The distribution of microscopic changes is the same as frontal lobe degeneration, in agreement with the gross distribution.

Microscopic characteristics of gray and white matter: The main characteristics are the same as frontal lobe degeneration, but with intense involvement of all cortical layers. Ballooned neurons and Pick's bodies, which are silver-positive, tau- and ubiquitin-immunoreactive, are present. There is more intense white matter involvement. Patients with intense astrocytosis but without ballooned neurons or inclusions, or both, may for the present be included.

III. Motor neuron disease type

Gross changes: These are the same as frontal lobe degeneration, although usually less severe.

Distribution of microscopic changes and microscopic characteristics in gray and white matter: These are the same as for frontal lobe degeneration, affecting cervical and thoracic levels more than lumbar or sacral. There is greater cell loss in medial than lateral cell columns. Motor neurons, layer II neurons in frontal and temporal cortex, and hippocampal dentate gyrus neurons show inclusions that are ubiquitin-positive but not silver- or tau-reactive. Nigral cell loss is severe in many cases. There is also hypoglossal degeneration in some.

Diagnostic exclusion features

There are senile plaques, diffuse amyloid deposits, and amyloid angiopathy with anti–beta-protein antibodies, tangles, and neuropil threads, with anti-tau and ubiquitin antibodies, more than normal for the age of the patient. Prion protein is present with antiprion antibodies.

Source: Reprinted with permission from Consensus statement: the Lund and Manchester Groups. Clinical and neuropathological criteria for frontotemporal dementia. J Neurol Neurosurg Psychiatry 1994;57:416–418.

Chapter 70
The Dementias

E. OTHER CAUSES OF DEMENTIAS
Martin N. Rossor

INFECTIONS

Human Immunodeficiency Virus

Patients with human immunodeficiency virus (HIV) infection are at risk from opportunistic infections and neoplasms, both of which may cause cognitive impairment. In addition, patients may develop an encephalopathy associated with dementia, known as the acquired immunodeficiency syndrome (AIDS)-dementia complex, HIV dementia, or HIV-1–associated motor/cognitive complex. It may be the only manifestation of HIV infection. Early features of forgetfulness and poor concentration present the clinical picture of a subcortical dementia. Later, however, ataxia, occasionally paraparesis, and increasing psychomotor slowing occur. The rate of progression is, however, variable (Bouwman et al. 1998). Investigations reveal an increased cerebrospinal fluid (CSF) protein and a mild pleocytosis, often with oligoclonal bands. White matter changes may be apparent in the computed tomographic (CT) scan and are prominent in magnetic resonance imaging (MRI) scans, together with cortical atrophy and ventricular dilatation. Neuropathologically, the white matter and subcortical gray matter are most affected, with relative sparing of the cerebral cortex, although dendritic injury is widespread. In these areas macrophages and multinucleate giant cells are seen with a reactive astrocytosis. Zidovudine can delay cognitive decline, and evidence exists that dementia may have become less common (Melton et al. 1997), but HIV remains an important cause of dementia, especially in younger people.

Other Chronic Viral Encephalitides

A static cognitive deficit can be seen following recovery from a viral encephalitis, most commonly amnesia after herpes simplex encephalitis treated with acyclovir. In these instances the cause of dementia is usually obvious. However, chronic viral encephalitis can cause diagnostic confusion. Subacute sclerosing panencephalitis and progressive rubella panencephalitis are both persistent viral infections that can cause cognitive impairment and present as dementia. Subacute sclerosing panencephalitis usually occurs in children, but can present as dementia in adults. Chronic rubella panencephalitis, though usually occurring after congenital rubella injection, also may follow acquired infection in the adult. Progressive multifocal leukoencephalopathy results from chronic infection with JC virus and occurs as an opportunistic infection in immunocompromised patients, most commonly those with AIDS. The initial cerebral infection is probably from hematogenous spread via lymphocytes; this may follow reactivation of latent virus. White matter damage with abnormal oligodendrocytes occurs. The cognitive impairment occurs in the setting of immunodeficiency, often together with limb weakness, ataxia, and field defects. The disease usually progresses to death in 6 months.

Spirochetal Disease

Neurosyphilis, now a rare cause of dementia, was once a major cause of admission to mental hospitals. Patients with general paresis or meningoencephalitis develop cognitive impairment, which usually occurs some 15–20 years after the original infection. Diagnosis in the preparalytic stage, when insidious memory failure is the only feature, is difficult and may be confused with Alzheimer's disease. Patients also exhibit apathy in the early stages, but as the disease progresses may develop seizures, dysarthria, tremor, and hypertonia. The dementia becomes more apparent with development of cortical features such as dysphasia and dyspraxia. The blood serology result is positive, and the CSF shows an increase in protein, a pleocytosis, and positive serology. MRI may show foci of increased signal on T2-weighted images together with atrophy (Russouw et al. 1997). Treatment with penicillin results in improvement but needs to be instituted early. There may still be progression of the disease, necessitating close monitoring. Late stages of infection with *Borrelia burgdorferi* (Lyme disease) can be associated with significant cognitive impairment and behavioral disturbance, and fatigue and mild memory deficits are common after the acute illness (Gaudino et al. 1997).

Chronic Bacterial Meningitides

The cognitive deficits associated with acute bacterial meningitis are those of a toxic confusional state with fluctuating or deteriorating consciousness. Chronic meningitis with tuberculosis or cryptococcosis may present with cognitive impairment, usually of a subcortical type, and apathy. In some this is secondary to the development of hydrocephalus. Brucellosis may be associated with prominent behavioral change.

Whipple's Disease

Whipple's disease is a rare multisystem disorder and dementia may feature prominently among the neurological manifestations. It occurs particularly in middle-aged men, normally in association with gastrointestinal malabsorption. Abnormal macrophages and *Tropheryma whippleii* may be apparent on jejunal biopsy. Detection of bacilli in CSF and biopsy tissues is increased using polymerase chain reaction technology. Rarely, neurological manifestations may occur in the absence of other clinical features, and even in patients without neurological involvement, histological changes may be found throughout the central nervous system at autopsy. The dementia is usually seen in association with ocular palsies and ataxia or with a hypothalamic syndrome. The cognitive impairment may be reversible with appropriate antibiotic treatment (Singer 1998).

METABOLIC DISORDERS

Acquired Metabolic Disorders

Many electrolyte and biochemical disturbances cause impaired cognition by effects on arousal and present as a con-

fusional state (see Chapter 62). The following, however, may give rise to impairment that resembles a dementia, although this is usually subcortical rather than cortical in type.

Vitamin Deficiencies

In addition to the spinal cord and peripheral nerve features of subacute combined degeneration arising from vitamin B_{12} deficiency, there are frequently mental changes ranging from apathy, which is the most common, to a gradual intellectual deterioration (see Chapter 63). This disorder responds to treatment if vitamin B_{12} is replaced early. In some patients the mental changes may be prominent in the absence of other neurological deficits or anemia. Folic acid deficiency also may be associated with some cognitive impairment, although the changes are slight and controversial. Thiamine deficiency underlies the Wernicke-Korsakoff syndrome. Wernicke's encephalopathy is associated with a confusional state and is seen most commonly with alcoholism but occasionally also with hyperemesis gravidarum. The emergent Korsakoff's syndrome is characterized by a profound amnesia with relatively intact long-term and procedural memory. Pellagra, caused by deficiency of nicotinic acid, also can be associated with dementia.

Hypothyroidism

Hypothyroidism is associated frequently with apathy and cognitive slowing. The clinical features suggest a subcortical disturbance, and with progression of the hypothyroidism, drowsiness may supervene rather than the development of a cortical dementia. Impaired cognition may remain despite treatment if not instituted early.

Chronic Hypoglycemia

Acute and subacute hypoglycemia give rise to a confusional state, but chronic mild recurrent hypoglycemia may cause a gradual deterioration in intellect suggestive of dementia. It is usually found in association with ataxia and involuntary movements.

Abnormalities of Calcium and Corticosteroid Homeostasis

Both hypocalcemia and hypercalcemia may be associated with cognitive dysfunction (see Chapter 62). Hypercalcemia tends to give rise to prominent lethargy, progressing to stupor rather than dementia. Hypocalcemia may give rise to cognitive impairment, usually in the setting of an extrapyramidal disturbance. Behavioral abnormalities, sometimes with the development of a frank psychosis, may occur with Cushing's syndrome or iatrogenically as a result of high-dose corticosteroid medication. Patients also may develop cognitive impairment, usually due to impaired attention, with a picture of a subcortical disturbance. In Addison's disease, patients may develop changes in personality and become apathetic with poorly defined cognitive impairment.

Renal Impairment

Uremic encephalopathy presents as a confusional state rather than as a dementia, but dialysis dementia may present with intellectual decline with dysphasia, in addition to a characteristic picture of dysarthria, myoclonus, and seizures (see Chapter 62). The electroencephalogram result is abnormal, with paroxysmal sharp waves or polyspike and wave formation. The neuropathological feature is spongiform changes in the superficial layers of the cerebral cortex. The condition is believed to be caused by aluminum toxicity, arising both from the dialysate fluid and from the use of aluminum antacids. This is now rare because the aluminum excess is avoided. However, mild cognitive impairment has been reported with mildly raised aluminum levels, and abnormalities of tau similar to those of Alzheimer's disease have been reported in association with aluminum accumulation in brains of patients on routine renal dialysis (Harrington et al. 1994).

Hepatic Disturbance

Although acute hepatic encephalopathy gives rise to a confusional state, many patients may develop reversible psychomotor deficits without overt encephalopathy. A smaller proportion of patients may develop a permanent progressive neurological deficit after repeated episodes of hepatic coma, which has been termed *hepatocerebral degeneration*. Dementia may occur, but usually the picture consists of dysarthria, ataxia, and involuntary movements. Portosystemic shunting can usually be demonstrated, and neuropathologically necrosis occurs within the cerebral cortex, particularly within the parietal and occipital lobes, with loss of cells and an astrocytic hyperplasia.

Inherited Metabolic Disorders

Several inborn errors of metabolism feature dementia as part of the clinical picture (see Chapter 68). Most of these present during childhood or adolescence, but many have their onset in adulthood. The following are notable for adult onset. They may present as cognitive impairment but are usually associated with other neurological features.

Wilson's disease may present in adulthood and even into late middle age, with tremor, dysarthria, and dystonia. Rarely, impairment of cognition may be an early feature, although behavioral and cognitive changes are common in established disease.

Metachromatic leukodystrophy can present with cognitive impairment as a prominent or early feature, but the development of extensor plantar responses and the loss of tendon reflexes may suggest the diagnosis, which can be confirmed by the demonstration of reduced activity of arylsulfatase A in white cells. A case has been documented of onset at the age of 62 years with dementia. Rarely, adrenoleukodystrophy can present in adult life with dementia as a major feature. Adult-onset neuronal ceroid-lipofuscinosis (Kufs' disease) may present with early behavioral and personality changes, which can progress to a frank dementia, usually with extrapyramidal features. Membranous lipodystrophy is characterized by bone cysts with pathological fractures, seizures, and presenile dementia.

The lysosomal storage disorders, Gaucher's disease, Niemann-Pick disease, GM_2 gangliosidosis, cerebrotendinous xanthomatosis, and the polysaccharidoses, may all present in late adolescence or early adulthood with cognitive impairment, although usually the other neurological features associated with these diseases provide the clues to diagnosis. Adult polyglucosan body disease is notable because of late-onset dementia with peripheral neuropathy. The mitochondrial encephalopathies are recognized increasingly as a cause of dementia in adults. Both mitochondrial encephalomyelopathy with lactic acidosis and strokelike episodes (MELAS) and myoclonus epilepsy with ragged-red fibers (MERFF) are commonly associated with cognitive impairment in adulthood, but this is usually in the context of widespread neurological dysfunction.

NEOPLASMS

Both malignant and benign neoplasms may result in a dementia syndrome, which is largely determined by the site of the lesion (see Chapter 58). Slow-growing tumors, especially those in the midline (i.e., colloid cysts, pinealomas, or even pituitary tumor) are more likely to cause diagnostic confusion (Figure 70E.1). Gliomas that arise in the frontal lobe, corpus callosum, or midline thalamus may cause prominent cognitive impairment. Before CT and MRI became available, callosal gliomas were particularly difficult to diagnose because they are rarely associated with abnormal neurological signs. Diffuse involvement of an entire cerebral hemisphere with gliomatosis cerebri may also cause prominent cognitive impairment, but there are usually features of raised intracranial pressure. Cerebral neoplasms are commonly treated by irradiation, which itself may lead to cognitive impairment. Deficits in memory and cognitive slowing may occur after cerebral irradiation has been completed and without apparent increase in tumor bulk (Keime-Guibert et al. 1998).

Cognitive impairment may also arise as a paraneoplastic effect of systemic neoplasia (see Chapter 59C). This is most commonly seen in association with carcinoma of the bronchus and occasionally of the breast. Memory impairment is prominent, and its development can precede the diagnosis of the tumor by as long as 2 years. Neuropathologically, there is cell loss in the hippocampus and cingulate

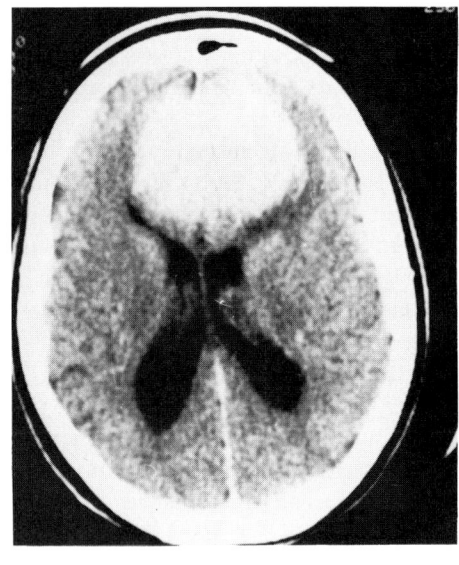 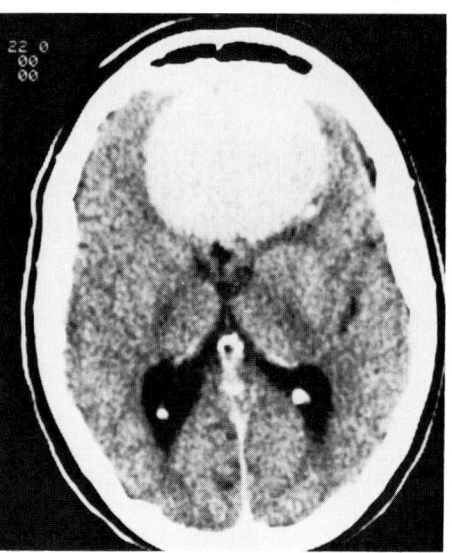

A   B

FIGURE 70E.1 (A) Computed tomographic scan of a 72-year-old man presenting with poor memory and features of a frontal lobe syndrome on examination. The scan shows a large front meningioma. (B) Unenhanced computed tomographic scan of a 68-year-old woman who presented with dementia. The scan shows a nonenhancing calcified oligodendroglioma that infiltrates across the corpus callosum.

gyrus with lymphocytic perivascular cuffing. This is termed *limbic encephalitis*. The CSF often shows an increase in cells and protein and occasionally oligoclonal bands.

DRUGS AND TOXINS

Alcohol-induced Korsakoff's psychosis causes a memory disorder out of proportion to other cognitive deficits. Short-term memory is intact, and confabulation may be associated (Kopelman 1995) (see Chapter 63). Many patients, however, develop more widespread cognitive impairment, referred to as *alcoholic dementia*. In contrast to the clinicopathological correlates of the Wernicke-Korsakoff syndrome, the pathological substrate of this more widespread cognitive impairment is not clear, although cortical shrinkage and large ventricles may be seen on CT or MRI. Hepatocerebral degeneration and nicotinic acid deficiency also may contribute to cognitive impairment.

Many centrally acting drugs may impair cognitive function, usually through effects on arousal. Chronic barbiturate ingestion, in particular, may cause prominent psychomotor slowing. Of the many toxins that may give rise to neurological disturbance, lead can cause a prominent encephalopathy with intellectual deterioration. This is seen predominantly in children but in rare cases can occur in adults. Arsenic intoxication may cause prominent memory impairment, and manganese poisoning is reported to cause early cognitive impairment before the development of extrapyramidal features. Mercury also may cause prominent behavioral changes with confusion and irritability, hence the term *mad as a hatter* from the use of elemental mercury in the manufacture of felt hats. A variety of industrial toxins also may cause cognitive impairment; some of these, such as toluene, are found in glues and may be encountered as recreational drugs, giving rise to irreversible cognitive impairment.

TRAUMA

Widespread cognitive impairment may occur following severe closed-head injury, usually causing coma. Trauma also may cause subdural hematomas that may not be readily recognized in the elderly. Of particular interest is the cognitive impairment that may occur after repeated head trauma, dementia pugilistica, which was described originally in professional boxers. The cognitive impairment characteristically occurs in association with dysarthria and sometimes with akinesia. Ventricular dilatation and a cavum septum pellucidum may be seen on the CT scan, and neurofibrillary tangles are found throughout the cerebral cortex, especially in the medial temporal lobes. β-amyloid immunoreactivity can be demonstrated in severe head injury, which may reflect increased expression of the amyloid precursor protein in response to neuronal injury (Roberts et al. 1994).

MULTIPLE SCLEROSIS

Nearly one-half of patients with multiple sclerosis develop some cognitive impairment during the course of their disease (Rao 1995) (see Chapter 60). Impairment in memory can be demonstrated in patients with only mild physical disability, although this does not necessarily fulfill the criteria of dementia. It is more frequent in patients with chronic progressive disease. In some patients cognitive impairment may be the presenting or major feature. In general, the features are those of a subcortical dementia without dysphasia or dyspraxia. Patients may show atrophy in the CT and MRI scans, but there is no clear correlation with the distribution of multiple sclerosis plaques. Atrophy of the corpus callosum has been shown to correlate with the severity of dementia; this cannot explain the dementia *per se*, but it may reflect the widespread involvement of cortical association tracts. Follow-up of patients with relapsing and remitting disease does suggest that the appearance of cognitive impairment relates to increased abnormalities on MRI (Feinstein et al. 1993).

NORMAL PRESSURE HYDROCEPHALUS

Considerable optimism was generated by the initial description of the triad of gait impairment, urinary incontinence, and impaired mental function caused by a compensated hydrocephalus, which could be reversed by CSF shunting (see Chapter 66). However, the results of shunting in terms of reversal of the cognitive impairment were extremely variable, and some of the negative responses may have been caused by the overenthusiastic inclusion of patients with degenerative diseases. Clinically, the cognitive impairment shows a psychomotor slowing with a prominent subcortical picture and is associated with reduced cerebral metabolism. The causes of normal pressure hydrocephalus include trauma, subarachnoid hemorrhage, and meningitis, and some are idiopathic. Patients with a known cause and a short history, and those in whom imaging shows small cortical sulci and periventricular lucencies (i.e., those in whom an additional degenerative dementia is unlikely), respond best to shunting with respect to the dementia.

PSEUDODEMENTIA

A group of disorders caused by functional disease rather than an organic dementia have been grouped under the heading pseudodementia. Use of the term *pseudodementia* has some disadvantages, however, because the cognitive disturbance, for example, in depression, may share similar biochemical disturbances of ascending projections to cerebral cortex with the organic dementias. Cognitive impairment, particularly with psychomotor slowing, is well recognized in depression. This is the most common cause of diagnostic confusion with the primary degenerative dementias and usually forms the major group of reversible dementias in reported series. The abnormality may be caused by incomplete encoding strategies, making events less memorable. Depressive pseudodementia may be an important differential diagnosis in primary degenerative dementia, but depression also may occur early in the course of degenerative dementia. A significant proportion of the patients presenting to a dementia clinic who are diagnosed as suffering from depression subsequently go on to develop presumed Alzheimer's disease.

Hysterical dementia and psychogenic amnesia present less diagnostic confusion. The apparent cognitive impairment is inconsistent, and often patients find their way around the ward and function adequately, although on formal testing they may show dramatic impairment. Simulated dementia is rare and tends to overlap with hysterical dementia. In a study of students asked to simulate cognitive impairment, it was noted that perseveration was rare, in contrast to organic dementia. In addition, with persistent testing and with development of fatigue, people who are simulating dementia begin to respond more normally. Nonetheless, it may be difficult to distinguish between hysterical and simulated dementia. In general, however, if the inconsistencies are pointed out to patients with hysteria, they appear unconcerned, whereas patients who are simulating dementia may become angry or upset.

REFERENCES

Bouwman FH, Skolasky RL, Hes D, et al. Variable progression of HIV-associated dementia. Neurology 1998;50:1814–1820.

Feinstein A, Ron M, Thompson A. A serial study of psychometric and magnetic-resonance-imaging changes in multiple-sclerosis. Brain 1993;116:569–602.

Gaudino EA, Coyle PK, Krupp LB. Post-Lyme syndrome and chronic fatigue syndrome. Neuropsychiatric similarities and differences. Arch Neurol 1997;54:1372–1376.

Harrington CR, Wischik CM, McArthur FK, et al. Alzheimer's disease–like changes in tau protein processing: association with aluminium accumulation in brains of renal dialysis patients. Lancet 1994;343:993–997.

Keime-Guibert F, Napolitano M, Delattre JY. Neurological complications of radiotherapy and chemotherapy. J Neurol 1998;245:695–708.

Kopelman MD. The Korsakoff syndrome. Br J Psychiatry 1995; 166:154–173.

Melton ST, Kirkwood CK, Ghaemi SN. Pharmacotherapy of HIV dementia. Ann Pharmacother 1997;31:457–473.

Rao SM. Neuropsychology of multiple sclerosis. Curr Opin Neurol 1995;8:216–220.

Roberts GW, Gentleman SM, Lynch A, et al. Beta amyloid protein deposition in the brain after severe head injury: implications for the pathogenesis of Alzheimer's disease. J Neurol Neurosurg Psychiatry 1994;57:419–425.

Russouw HG, Roberts MC, Emsley RA, Truter R. Psychiatric manifestations and magnetic resonance imaging in HIV-negative neurosyphilis. Biol Psychiatry 1997;41:467–473.

Singer R. Diagnosis and treatment of Whipple's disease. Drugs 1998;55:699–704.

Chapter 71
The Epilepsies

William H. Trescher and Ronald P. Lesser

Epilepsy has been recognized since antiquity. The word derives from the Greek word meaning "to seize" or "take hold of," indicating that the person having a seizure is "possessed" or at least out of control. The clinical features of epilepsy have often provoked fear. Early treatments ranged from exorcism to blood letting. In the last century, the cumulative observations of many clinical investigators, along with adjunctive neurophysiological, imaging, and genetic tools, have created the well-accepted concept that epilepsy is not a single entity but rather a collection of different and often distinct disorders that have in common the occurrence of seizures.

Seizures are often described as *convulsive* or *nonconvulsive*, depending on the prominence of motor features. This distinction omits the diversity of nonconvulsive seizures and the more important distinction between seizures of *focal* and of *nonfocal* cortical origin. Furthermore, seizures with an immediate and proximate cause, such as an acute metabolic disturbance, infection, or head trauma, can be considered symptomatic or provoked. In other instances, seizures may be due to past brain injury. Such episodes can be described as *remote symptomatic*. In a large number of seizures, however, no cause can be identified. These seizures can be called either *idiopathic* or *cryptogenic*. Idiopathic seizures are presumed to have a genetic basis (Sander and Shorvon 1996). They occur in partial or generalized epileptic syndromes that have particular clinical and electroencephalographic (EEG) characteristics. The term *cryptogenic*, on the other hand, implies a symptomatic cause that cannot be diagnosed with currently available medical technology.

EPIDEMIOLOGY

Incidence and Prevalence

Epilepsy is a relatively common neurological disorder. Problems with case definition, exclusion criteria, and methods of case ascertainment, as well as regional population differences, however, complicate the comparison of incidence and prevalence rates across studies. In most developed countries, incidence rates range from 40–70 per 100,000, but in developing countries, the rates may be as high as 100–190 per 100,000 (Sander and Shorvon 1996). Similarly, the prevalence of active epilepsy, defined as persons who take anticonvulsant drugs or who have had a seizure in the past 5 years, ranges from 4–10 per 10,000 in developed countries and up to 57 per 10,000 in developing countries. Studies have estimated that 1.5–5.0% of any population will have a seizure at some time. Partial seizures, with or without secondary generalization, are the most common seizure type, followed by generalized tonic-clonic seizures. Other seizure types, such as absence, pure tonic, atonic, or myoclonic, are relatively uncommon.

A number of factors contribute to the higher incidence and prevalence of epilepsy in developing countries (de Bittencourt et al. 1996a). Limited access to health care compounds the problems of birth injury and head trauma. Poor sanitation leads to the high rate of infectious disorders that affect the central nervous system (CNS) and cause seizures. Poverty and illiteracy increase the risk of social diseases, such as alcohol and substance abuse, which indirectly contribute to epilepsy. Furthermore, a combination of local social perceptions, government policies, and antiepileptic drug availability influence the treatment of epilepsy in developing countries.

Most studies show a bimodal age distribution of the incidence of epilepsy. Traditionally, epilepsy has been more common in children than in adults. Rates are high in the first decade, particularly under the age of 1 year, with a decline during the first decade. Rates are low during most of adulthood, and there is a secondary rise after age 60 years. Studies suggest that changes in the age-specific incidence may be occurring with a shift to older age groups. In developing countries, this bimodal distribution is not as evident because the age-specific incidence of epilepsy remains high throughout adulthood.

In studies of hospital- and clinic-based populations, as well as in field studies, the etiology for epilepsy can be identified in only approximately one-fourth to one-third of cases. Perinatal disorders, mental retardation, cerebral palsy, head trauma, infections of the CNS, cerebrovascular disease, brain tumors, Alzheimer's disease, and alcohol or heroin use are all associated with an increased risk for epilepsy. Men are 1.0–2.4 times more likely to have epilepsy than women. Several studies show higher rates of epilepsy in black African populations, but this may be related to differences in socioeconomic status (Sander and Shorvon 1996).

Prognosis

The risk of seizure recurrence after the first seizure ranges from 27% to 80%, with lower rates typically reported from hospital-based estimates and higher rates from population-based studies (Sander 1993). Most recurrences happen within 6 months of the first seizure. The risk for further seizures decreases with longer interval from the initial event. Seizures associated with CNS insults, particularly those that occur in the neonatal period, have a high rate of recurrence.

Once the diagnosis of epilepsy is established with the occurrence of two or more seizures, the prognosis for remission overall is good, but it depends on the wide range of heterogeneous disorders that are subsumed under the definition of epilepsy. In a review, Sander suggested that patients developing epileptic seizures fall into four prognostic groups (Sander 1993). Excellent prognosis is expected in approximately 20–30% of individuals who have one of a number of conditions, such as benign neonatal seizures, benign childhood epilepsy with centrotemporal spikes, or benign myoclonic epilepsy of childhood. Often, remission occurs without antiepileptic drug treatment. Good prognosis characterizes approximately 30–40% of people with epilepsy, whose seizures are easily controlled with antiepileptic drugs. Remission is often permanent when medications are discontinued. Some of the conditions with good prognosis include childhood absence epilepsy, epilepsy with generalized tonic-clonic seizures on awakening, and even a small subset of localization-related epilepsies. In an uncertain prognosis group, comprising approximately 10–20% of people with epilepsy, antiepileptic drugs are suppressive rather than curative. Individuals with juvenile myoclonic epilepsy (JME) and the majority of those with localization-related epilepsy fall into this category. A subset of the latter group may benefit from epilepsy surgery. As many as 20% of individuals with epilepsy have a bad prognosis, meaning that most treatments, including surgery, are only palliative. Individuals in this group often have a history of infantile spasms, Lennox-Gastaut syndrome, or localization-related seizures associated with extensive structural brain damage or congenital disorders, such as tuberous sclerosis.

CLASSIFICATION OF SEIZURES AND EPILEPTIC SYNDROMES

Epilepsy encompasses a heterogeneous group of disorders with multiple causes and manifestations. Classification has

Table 71.1: The International League Against Epilepsy classification of epileptic seizures

I. Partial (focal, local) seizures
  A. Simple partial seizures (consciousness not impaired)
    1. With motor symptoms
    2. With somatosensory or special sensory symptoms
    3. With autonomic symptoms
    4. With psychic symptoms
  B. Complex partial seizures (with impairment of consciousness)
    1. Beginning as simple partial seizures and progressing to impairment of consciousness
    2. With no other features
    3. With features as in simple partial seizures
    4. With automatisms
  C. With impairment of consciousness at onset
    1. With no other features
    2. With features as in simple partial seizures
    3. With automatisms
  D. Partial seizures evolving to secondarily generalized seizures
    1. Simple partial seizures evolving to generalized seizures
    2. Complex partial seizures evolving to generalized seizures
    3. Simple partial seizures evolving to complex partial seizures to generalized seizures
II. Generalized seizures (convulsive or nonconvulsive)
  A. Absence seizures
    1. Absence seizures
    2. Atypical absence seizures
  B. Myoclonic seizures
  C. Clonic seizures
  D. Tonic seizures
  E. Tonic-clonic seizures
  F. Atonic seizures (astatic seizures)
III. Unclassified epileptic seizures (includes all seizures that cannot be classified because of inadequate or incomplete data and some that defy classification in hitherto described categories. This includes some neonatal seizures, such as rhythmic eye movements, chewing, and swimming movements.

Table 71.2: The International League Against Epilepsy classification of epilepsies and epileptic syndromes

I. Localization-related (focal, local, partial) epilepsies and syndromes
  A. Idiopathic (with age-related onset). At present, two syndromes are established:
    1. Benign childhood epilepsy with centrotemporal spike
    2. Childhood epilepsy with occipital paroxysms
  B. Symptomatic. This category comprises syndromes of great individual variability.
II. Generalized epilepsies and syndromes
  A. Idiopathic (with age-related onset, in order of age appearance)
    1. Benign neonatal familial convulsions
    2. Benign neonatal convulsions
    3. Benign myoclonic epilepsy in infancy
    4. Childhood absence epilepsy (pyknolepsy, petit mal)
    5. Juvenile absence epilepsy
    6. Juvenile myoclonic epilepsy (impulsive petit mal)
    7. Epilepsy with grand mal seizures on awakening
  B. Idiopathic, symptomatic, or both (in order of age of appearance)
    1. West's syndrome (infantile spasms)
    2. Lennox-Gastaut syndrome
    3. Epilepsy with myoclonic-astatic seizures
    4. Epilepsy with myoclonic absences
  C. Symptomatic
    1. Nonspecific cause. Early myoclonic encephalopathy
    2. Specific syndromes. Epileptic seizures may complicate many disease states. Under this heading are included those diseases in which seizures are a presenting or predominant feature.
III. Epilepsies and syndromes undetermined as to whether they are focal or generalized
  A. With both generalized and focal seizures
    1. Neonatal seizures
    2. Severe myoclonic epilepsy in infancy
    3. Epilepsy with continuous spikes and waves during slow-wave sleep
    4. Acquired epileptic aphasia (Landau-Kleffner syndrome)
  B. Without unequivocal generalized or focal features
IV. Special syndromes
  A. Situation-related seizures (Gelegenheitsanfalle)
    1. Febrile convulsions
    2. Seizures related to other identifiable situations, such as stress, hormones, drugs, alcohol, or sleep deprivation
  B. Isolated, apparently unprovoked epileptic events
  C. Epilepsies characterized by the specific modes of seizures precipitated
  D. Chronic progressive epilepsia partialis continua of childhood

been attempted on the basis of clinical events, EEG characteristics, etiology, pathophysiology, anatomy, or age (Sander and Shorvon 1996). The International League Against Epilepsy (ILAE) introduced a classification scheme in 1969 and published a revised version in 1981 (Wyllie and Luders 1997). The ILAE classified seizures as partial, generalized, and unclassifiable (Table 71.1). This is now a widely accepted guide for clinical management and research. The latest ILAE classification recognizes epilepsies and epileptic syndromes by incorporating the basic categories of partial and generalized seizures while taking into account seizure type, EEG findings, prognostic, and pathophysiological and etiological information (Table 71.2). Additional categories were included for epileptic syndromes that were not clearly focal or generalized and for special syndromes. The ILAE viewed the classifications as guides for the understanding of epilepsy rather than as definitive documents.

Essential to an understanding of epilepsy is an accurate characterization of seizures. Subtle features of a seizure help

to localize the site of seizure origin and, when taken in the context of other characteristics of the total clinical picture, may point to a specific syndrome.

Partial Seizures

The category of partial seizures was and continues to be one of the most controversial aspects of the ILAE classification (Luders et al. 1993). The ILAE definition of *partial seizures* is "those in which, in general, the first clinical and

EEG changes indicate initial activation of a system of neurons limited to part of one cerebral hemisphere" (Wyllie and Luders 1997). Other terms, such as *focal* and *local*, however, are not synonymous and do not apply to all partial seizures.

Classifying partial seizures as either simple or complex causes sufficient confusion that some epileptologists avoid the terms (Kotagal 1997). The original ILAE classification defined a *complex partial seizure* as one associated with impairment of consciousness and defined a *simple partial seizure* as one without impairment of consciousness, regardless of the complexity of the clinical features. This distinction is often difficult to make in clinical practice. *Consciousness* has been defined operationally as the level of awareness or responsiveness, or both, of the individual to external stimuli. Seizures may preserve awareness but compromise responsiveness. Furthermore, historical recall from the individual or observers is often misleading. Many individuals who seem alert during a seizure may prove to be impaired when tested.

An important concept of the 1981 ILAE classification was the recognition of the sequential evolution of seizure phases. Accurate classification of seizures requires recognition of the initial features and progression of the seizure. The ILAE classification recognizes six basic combinations of partial seizure progression: (1) simple partial seizures, (2) simple partial seizures that develop into complex partial seizures, (3) complex partial seizures, (4) simple or (5) partial seizures that progress into generalized tonic-clonic seizures, and (6) simple partial seizures that progress to complex partial seizures and then secondarily generalize. This classification does not encompass the full spectrum of seizures and seizure progression encountered in clinical practice. The scheme has been criticized for a variety of reasons, including its limited ability to describe seizure progression, lack of specificity in lateralizing and somatotopic information, and complexity of terminology (Luders et al. 1993). Furthermore, in some clinical series, as many as one-third of seizures encountered in clinical practice cannot be classified (Sander and Shorvon 1996). These criticisms highlight an important point made by the ILAE Commission on Classification: The classification is not sacrosanct, and "with increasing knowledge, the categories may change, the skeleton will be 'fleshed out' and the nuances elaborated" (Wyllie and Luders 1997). Nevertheless, changes will of necessity be slow to occur, if for no other reason than that the current classification provides a stable communication framework for clinicians and investigators in the field of epilepsy.

Simple Partial Seizures

The ILAE classification divides simple partial seizures into four major categories: (1) those with motor signs, (2) those with somatosensory or special sensory symptoms, (3) those with autonomic symptoms or signs, and (4) those with psychic symptoms (see Table 71.1). The clinical features of simple partial seizures depend on the brain region activated. The initial discharge is thought to be relatively localized, but ictal activity then spreads to adjacent brain areas, producing a progression of the clinical seizure pattern. Despite very elaborate clinical features, the seizure remains classified as simple partial if consciousness is preserved (Luders et al. 1993). Two other points are important when evaluating the clinical features of partial seizures: The ictal onset may be clinically silent and all features of the seizure may be attributed to subsequent spread of ictal activity, and identical clinical features can arise from ictal activation of different brain regions. The most common simple partial seizure patterns are those with motor symptoms and those with sensory symptoms.

Simple Partial Motor Seizure

Epileptic activity that starts in one area of the motor cortex and spreads to contiguous regions produces progressive jerking of successive body parts in what are often called *jacksonian seizures*, after Hughlings Jackson. The clinical features are associated with seizure foci in different areas of the cortex. The motor strip produces clonic activity of the contralateral arm or leg or the face. The prerolandic area impairs speech and causes tonic-clonic movements of the contralateral face or repetitive swallowing. The opercular region causes clonic movements of the face that may be ipsilateral, accompanied by mastication, salivation, and swallowing. The dorsolateral prefrontal cortex causes forced turning of the eyes and head to the opposite side as well as speech arrest. The paracentral lobule causes tonic movement of the ipsilateral foot and, often, contralateral involvement of the legs. The supplementary motor cortex causes head turning with arm extension on the same side (fencer's posture). Consciousness usually is not impaired, but speech arrest and tonic or dystonic posturing may incorrectly suggest impaired consciousness.

Simple Partial Sensory Seizure

Parietal Lobe Seizures. Simple partial sensory seizures usually originate in the parietal lobe. Tingling or numbness usually is confined to one body region but can progress in a jacksonian fashion. The likelihood that a specific body area is involved probably correlates with the size of its cortical representation. Tongue sensations of crawling, stiffness, or coldness and facial sensory phenomena, such as tingling or numbness, often are bilateral. Other sensory seizures are characterized by a desire to move a body part or a feeling that a part is being moved. Negative seizure phenomena are a sense that a body part is absent or that awareness is lost of a part or even a whole side of the body (asomatognosia), particularly with nondominant hemisphere involvement. A sensation of sinking, choking, or nausea usually indicates that the seizure originates in the inferior and lateral parietal lobe. Severe vertigo or disorientation in space indicates inferior parietal lobe seizures. Rudimentary, vague sensations of pain or coldness usually indicate opercular seizures in the second sensory area; these may be bilateral, contralateral, or ipsilateral to the ictal activity. Seizures in the dominant parietal lobe also can cause receptive or conductive language disturbances.

Occipital Lobe Seizures.   Occipital lobe seizures are associated with visual symptoms. The epileptic images usually are elementary: flashes of light, scotomata, hemianopia, or amaurosis. These symptoms may be isolated to one portion of the visual field or may spread. Seizures from the occipital-temporal-parietal junction produce complex imagery. Objects may be distorted in size (micropsia or macropsia), shape (metamorphopsia), or perceived distance from the individual. Visual hallucinations also occur and usually consist of previously experienced imagery. These are sometimes distorted but often are complex and colorful. Imagery of the person having the seizure (autoscopy) is unusual. Occipital lobe seizures also may produce tonic or clonic contraversion of the eyes (oculoclonic or oculogyric deviation), clonic palpebral jerks, or forced closure of the eyelids. Forced eye turning (versive movement) usually is associated with simple partial seizures of frontal lobe origin but also may occur during seizures of parietal-occipital origin.

Temporal Lobe Seizures.   Sensory seizures of temporal lobe origin often are difficult to recognize as epileptic events: They may include auditory or olfactory hallucinations, emotional or psychic symptoms, sensations of movement or rotation, or autonomic symptoms. The focus is usually in the superior temporal gyrus. Auditory hallucinations may range from the very simple sounds to the perception of complex language (So 1997). Olfactory seizures, usually an unpleasant odor, are caused by discharges in the medial temporal lobe and are called *uncinate fits*; gustatory seizures are caused by discharges deep in the sylvian fissure or the operculum. Epigastric sensations of nausea, "butterflies," emptiness, or tightness are usually, but not exclusively, caused by temporal lobe activity.

Emotional changes and psychic phenomena sometimes are attributed to simple partial seizures of temporal lobe origin, but they are more common with complex partial seizures. Distortions of memory include dreamy states, flashbacks, sensations of familiarity with unfamiliar events (déjà vu), or sensations of unfamiliarity with previously experienced events (jamais vu). When these sensations refer to auditory experiences, they are known as *déjà entendu* or *jamais entendu*.

Occasionally, patients experience during the seizure a form of forced thinking, characterized by a rapid recollec-tion of episodes from past life experiences (panoramic vision). Other possible seizure manifestations are alterations of cognitive state (distortions of time sense and sensations of unreality, detachment, or depersonalization) or affect (feelings of extreme pleasure or displeasure, fear or terror, and intense depression with feelings of unworthiness and rejection). Epileptic anger or rage is rare. When it occurs, it differs from temper tantrums because it is unprovoked and abates rapidly.

Epileptic Aura

The word *aura* is used to describe a sensation that precedes a seizure. Auras are simple partial seizures that last seconds to minutes (So 1997). They should be distinguished, however, from "premonitions" or prodromes, which are not ictal events. A premonition or prodrome is a sense of nervousness or anxiety for hours or even days before a seizure. Subtle changes in behavior, such as increased irritability, also may occur.

Complex Partial Seizures

Complex partial seizures are characterized by impaired consciousness without generalized tonic-clonic activity. The two essential features are partial or complete lack of awareness and amnesia for the event. Impaired awareness must be distinguished from a transitory block of motor or verbal output or of verbal comprehension despite maintained consciousness (Kotagal 1997). Some responses to external stimuli, such as resistance to restraint, can occur during a complex partial seizure. Individuals are usually either unaware that they had a seizure or are unable to recall events that occurred during the seizure. Most complex partial seizures arise from the temporal lobe and were previously designated *temporal lobe epilepsy*. Epilepsy monitoring unit studies have shown that 10–30% of complex partial seizures arise from extratemporal locations, most commonly the frontal lobe but also the parietal and occipital lobes.

Automatisms

Automatisms are more or less coordinated, involuntary motor activity that occurs during a state of impaired consciousness either in the course of or after an epileptic seizure and usually followed by amnesia. Several types have been recognized (Kotagal 1997). De novo automatisms are behaviors that begin spontaneously after the onset of the seizure and seem to be release phenomenon. Reactive automatisms also begin after the onset of the seizure but appear to be reactions to external stimuli. For example, a patient may chew gum placed in the mouth or hold and even drink from a cup placed in the hand. Perseverative

Table 71.3: Differential features of partial complex and absence seizures

Feature	Partial complex	Absence
Age of onset	Any age; rare in childhood	Childhood
Aura	Frequent	None
Caused by hyperventilation	Rare	Often
Electroencephalogram	Temporal slowing or sharp activity	3-Hz spike wave
Postictal confusion	Common	Never
Precipitation by photic stimulation	Very rare	Occasionally
Characteristic of seizure event		
Automatisms	Simple complex	Simple or complex
Duration	Minutes	Seconds
Level of consciousness	Out of contact	Out of contact
Sounds	Often incoherent dysphasic speech	Never speaks, rarely hums
Staring	Common	Common

Source: Reprinted with permission from RJ DeLorenzo. The Epilepsies. In WG Bradley, RB Daroff, GM Fenichel, CD Marsden (eds), Neurology in Clinical Practice. Boston: Butterworth–Heinemann, 1991;1443–1477.

automatisms are continuations of complex acts that were engaged in before the seizure started. Automatisms are often associated with temporal lobe seizures but also occur during complex partial seizures of extratemporal origin and with typical and atypical absence seizures.

Temporal Lobe Seizures

Complex partial seizures may begin with impairment of consciousness or may be preceded by a simple partial seizure or an aura. Auras vary in duration from seconds to several minutes before impairment of consciousness. Most complex partial seizures last longer than 30 seconds, usually up to 1–2 minutes; few last less than 10 seconds, which is a distinguishing characteristic from absence seizures (Table 71.3). Postictal recovery is usually slow, with significant confusion that may last for several minutes or longer. A correlation of clinical features and site of seizure discharge has been suggested but is not universally accepted (Kotagal 1997). Within the temporal lobe, seizures may arise from different regions—that is, from mesial temporal structures (amygdala and hippocampus) or neocortical regions. Some have suggested that clinical symptomatology at the very onset of the seizure occasionally can provide clues about the site of ictal onset in the temporal lobe.

With mesial temporal lobe onset, an initial behavioral arrest or brief motionless stare may occur with an epigastric sensation, emotional symptoms, and olfactory or gustatory hallucinations (Kotagal 1997). Auditory hallucinations or vertigo suggest neocortical onset. Opercular seizures may be accompanied by auditory or visceral auras and visceral motor phenomena, such as salivation, spitting, retching, and vomiting. Rapid seizure propagation through the temporal lobe, however, often makes difficult the clear delineation of site of origin based solely on clinical symptomatology.

Frontal Lobe Seizures

Complex partial seizures that begin abruptly, are brief in duration, show minimal postictal confusion, and occur in clusters are more often of frontal lobe origin (Kotagal 1997). The attacks are often bizarre, with motor automatisms in which the legs make bicycling or pedaling movements. Stereotyped sexual automatisms and vocalizations also occur. The clinical features vary with the region of involved frontal lobe. Cingulate seizures cause complex motor gestural automatisms with changes in mood and affect and autonomic signs. Anterior frontopolar seizures cause forced thinking, adversive movements of the head, contraversive movements, and axial clonic jerks, which may make the patient fall. Orbitofrontal seizures cause motor and gestural automatisms and olfactory hallucinations and illusions. Dorsolateral frontal seizures cause tonic posturing or, less commonly, clonic activity with versive eye movements and speech arrest.

Violent Behavior

Epileptic activity, particularly involving the temporal lobe, may cause emotional symptoms, such as fear, agitation, and, occasionally, undirected aggressive or violent behavior. Most violent behavior during a seizure occurs in response to being restrained. The consensus of several international conferences has been that the following criteria should be fulfilled before concluding that a specific violent crime was the result of a seizure (Kotagal 1997):

1. The diagnosis of epilepsy must be firmly established.
2. The presence of aggression during epileptic automatisms should be verified by epilepsy monitoring.
3. The aggressive or violent act should be a difficult action with complex activity.
4. A clinical neurologist with special expertise in epilepsy should be involved in making the determination of

whether the violence that occurred during the seizure could have contributed to the crime.

Electroencephalographic Characteristics of Partial Seizures

The temporal lobe, most commonly the anterior temporal lobe, is the area of onset in approximately 80% of patients with partial seizures (Kotagal 1997). During the interictal period, abnormalities of rhythm or transient epileptiform discharges suggest a seizure focus (see Chapter 37A). A single routine EEG record may be normal in 30–50% of patients with probable epilepsy, but the yield for abnormalities increases with multiple records. Interictal epileptiform activity correlates fairly well with the site of ictal onset, but temporal sharp wave activity can be bilateral in one-third of cases. Abnormal interictal activity tends to be distributed more diffusely in patients with partial seizures from extratemporal foci. The interictal activity in children with benign epilepsies is often characteristic (see Benign Childhood Epilepsy with Centrotemporal Spikes and Childhood Epilepsy with Occipital Paroxysms, later in this chapter).

Scalp EEG recordings during simple partial and even some complex partial seizures may be normal (Chabolla and Cascino 1997). During an aura, the EEG background rhythms may attenuate before the onset of ictal activity. The EEG patterns that occur during complex partial seizures of temporal lobe origin include (1) rhythmic activity, often 5–7 Hz without spike or sharp wave activity; (2) rhythmic spike or sharp wave activity; and (3) focal attenuation of normal activity. However, the ictal activity on scalp recording may be bilateral or poorly localized in as many as 50% of cases.

EEG activity is often more poorly localized during seizures from extratemporal foci, particularly with frontal lobe onset, than during temporal lobe seizures (Chabolla and Cascino 1997). Brief frontal lobe seizures may not have a clearly defined ictal pattern, especially with standard montages that do not have adequate coverage of the frontal regions.

PARTIAL EPILEPTIC SYNDROMES

The International Classification of the Epilepsies recognizes two "localization-related disorders": benign childhood epilepsy with centrotemporal spikes (benign rolandic epilepsy) and childhood epilepsy with occipital paroxysms (benign occipital epilepsy). The spectrum of benign childhood epilepsies is probably broader than just these two syndromes. In a 1992 review by Dalla Bernardina and colleagues of 260 patients with benign partial epilepsy, the syndromes classified were benign rolandic epilepsy, 62%; benign psychomotor epilepsy, 10%; benign occipital epilepsy, 7%; and others, 20%. The clinical features of these syndromes are similar. Onset occurs in childhood with minor variations in the pre-

cise age of onset, which may not be significant for the different disorders (Holmes 1993). Development, neurological examinations, and neuroradiological studies at the time of diagnosis are normal. Seizures are typically nocturnal but can occur during the day. Headache and vomiting may be associated. Seizures usually stop in adolescence, and the outcome is favorable. A family history of epilepsy is recorded in approximately 40% of cases.

Because the overall prognosis for benign childhood epilepsy is good, treatment is not recommended after the first or even the second seizure, and it may not be needed at all in some patients. Most anticonvulsant drugs are effective as monotherapy.

Benign Childhood Epilepsy with Centrotemporal Spikes

The seizures are usually characterized by somatosensory disturbance of the mouth, preservation of consciousness, excessive pooling of saliva and tonic or tonic-clonic activity of the face, and speech arrest when the dominant hemisphere is affected (Holmes 1993). The somatosensory or motor activity may spread to the arm. Secondary generalization may occur, especially when the seizures are nocturnal.

The EEG consists of a normal background with midtemporal and central, high-amplitude, often diphasic spikes and sharp waves with increased frequency during sleep (Niedermeyer 1993). The spikes and sharp waves are usually unilateral, but they may be bilateral (see Chapter 37A).

Childhood Epilepsy with Occipital Paroxysms

Partial motor or generalized tonic-clonic seizures occur during sleep, and visual seizures occur during wakefulness. The visual symptoms are amaurosis, elementary visual hallucinations, complex visual hallucinations, or illusions, including micropsia, metamorphopsia, or palinopsia (Holmes 1993). The EEG shows high-voltage occipital spikes occurring in 1- to 3-Hz bursts or trains. The spikes disappear with eye opening and reappear 1–20 seconds after eye closure or darkness.

Benign Psychomotor Epilepsy

The seizure in benign psychomotor epilepsy is a sudden onset of fear. The child yells for a parent or clings to someone nearby. Automatic behaviors often accompany the seizure, and consciousness may be impaired.

Epilepsia Partialis Continua

Prolonged focal seizures are called *epilepsia partialis continua*. Typical features are repeated focal motor or jacksonian seizures that occur in clusters (Blume 1997). Focal seizures sometimes become secondarily generalized. Myoclonic activity may persist between attacks. The usual cause of epilepsia partialis continua is focal injury to the cortex from anoxia, inflammation, or a metabolic disturbance.

Rasmussen's Encephalitis

Rasmussen's encephalitis is a disorder of previously healthy children usually younger than 10 years of age (Vining et al. 1993). Histopathological analysis shows a characteristic pattern of inflammation, but a cause has not been established. Seizures are limited to one hemisphere at onset but may become bilateral late in the course. The initial feature is often continuous motor seizures of one limb. Episodes of secondary generalization are common. The seizures soon spread, and progressive hemiplegia is the rule. At first, the seizures respond to standard anticonvulsant therapy but then become refractory. An antibody to the GluR-3 subunit of one of the glutamate receptors has been identified in some patients, implicating an autoimmune process (Rogers et al. 1994). Corticosteroids, intravenous (IV) immunoglobulin, and plasmapheresis are reported as beneficial in some patients, but their efficacy is not established. Most affected children require hemispherectomy for seizure control.

GENERALIZED SEIZURES: GENERALIZED TONIC-CLONIC SEIZURES

The most common type of generalized seizure is generalized tonic-clonic seizure (Sander and Shorvon 1996). This was previously called *grand mal*, and the term is still in common use, despite efforts to discard it.

Clinical Features

The clinical features of generalized tonic-clonic seizures can be divided into five phases (Fisch 1997). Not all five phases occur in every person with generalized tonic-clonic seizures or with every generalized seizure in the same patient. The first phase is premonition. It is characterized by a vague sense that a seizure is imminent, and it may last for hours or days. Mood changes often occur, which are recognized by the individual or others. An increased level of irritability and headaches are thought to arise from "heightened cortical irritability" (Fisch 1997). Premonitions are not auras and do not have localizing value.

The second phase is the immediate pre–tonic-clonic phase. A few myoclonic jerks or brief clonic seizures may occur at this time, either with primary generalized seizures or in the transition from another seizure type. Some patients experience deviations of the head and eyes; however, the localizing value of this activity is uncertain.

The third (tonic) phase usually begins with a sudden tonic contraction of the axial musculature, accompanied by upward eye deviation and pupillary dilatation. Tonic contraction of the limbs follows quickly. Involvement of the respiratory muscles produces a forced expiration of air, often resulting in an "epileptic cry" or moan at the onset of the seizure. Tonic contracture of the muscles of the jaw causes injury to the mouth or tongue. Cyanosis develops due to restricted respiratory function.

The progression from the tonic to the fourth (clonic) phase is gradual. Initially, the clonic activity is low amplitude, with a relatively fast frequency of approximately 8 jerks per second. The clonic jerks progressively increase in amplitude and slow to approximately 4 jerks per second. As the seizure continues, periods of atonic inhibition increase in duration and interrupt the clonic contractions until they stop, with complete relaxation of all muscles. It is at this stage that incontinence of urine and occasionally stool may occur with relaxation of the sphincter muscles.

In the final (postictal) period, the individual is generally unresponsive, but respiration returns. Muscle tone is generally decreased but is sometimes tonic with opisthotonos and trismus. The individual may awaken briefly and then fall asleep or remain awake but lethargic. Generalized headache and muscle soreness are common complaints.

Some generalized seizures are only tonic or clonic. Clonic seizures generally carry no special significance compared with tonic-clonic seizures, but tonic seizures are more common with secondary generalized epilepsy than primary generalized epilepsy (Farrell 1997b). Infants and children with tonic seizure often have other seizure types and mental retardation. Tonic seizures that develop in late childhood or in adults are more likely to be a variant of generalized tonic-clonic seizures.

Arterial blood gas determinations during or immediately after a generalized motor seizure show a mixed respiratory and metabolic acidosis. The arterial pH is seldom lower than 7.0, and acid-base equilibrium returns to normal within 1 hour (Fisch 1997). A transient mild hyperglycemia may occur during a brief seizure, but hypoglycemia may occur during status epilepticus. Endocrine changes also can occur after brief generalized motor seizures. Prolactin levels increase in 90% of generalized tonic-clonic seizures and can reach a peak of up to 20–30 times baseline values approximately 20 minutes after the seizure.

Examination of the CSF after a generalized seizure may show a transitory pleocytosis of 9–80 white blood cells/µl, reaching a peak 1 day after the seizure.

Injuries during Seizures

Laceration of the tongue, cheeks, and lips are common, but additional injury occurs when observers attempt to place objects in the mouth in the mistaken belief that a person having a seizure will "swallow the tongue." Head trauma may result from unprotected falls or seizures near furniture or other hard objects. Vertebral compression fractures occur in approximately 5–15% of people having seizures, usually older individuals (Fisch 1997). Eighty percent of fractures are asymptomatic.

Aspiration pneumonia occurs because mechanisms to protect the airway are compromised during the seizure and individuals fall supine, which increases the chance of aspiration of saliva or stomach contents. Pulmonary edema is rare, as is sudden death. Death from generalized tonic-clonic seizures usually occurs during sleep, and the precise cause is often unexplained.

Electroencephalographic Characteristics of Generalized Tonic-Clonic Seizures

Interictal

The interictal EEG is often abnormal in idiopathic epilepsy. Some anticonvulsant drugs slow the normal background rhythms, whereas others, particularly barbiturates and benzodiazepines, may increase beta activity in the 14- to 20-Hz range (Fisch 1997). Excessive diffuse slowing suggests the possibility of drug toxicity. Approximately one-half of the interictal EEGs in patients with generalized tonic-clonic seizures contain epileptiform activity, especially if the EEG was obtained within 5 days after a seizure (Niedermeyer 1993). The epileptiform activity is usually one or more of four main patterns: (1) typical 3-Hz spike-and-wave complexes, (2) irregular spike-and-wave complexes, (3) 4- to 5-Hz spike-and-wave complexes, and (4) multifocal spike complexes. These interictal epileptiform discharges are usually bilateral, with anterior or frontocentral predominance, but they may have a posterior dominance in children. Subtle interhemispheric asymmetries of the interictal epileptiform discharges do not necessarily suggest focal, symptomatic seizures unless they are accompanied by clearly defined focal epileptiform abnormalities. Interictal EEG also may include intermittent runs of epileptiform activity in the occipital or frontal regions bilaterally or prolonged runs of parietal theta activity. Focal brain lesions may give rise to generalized epileptiform activity (secondary bilateral synchrony). The lesions are usually mesial frontal, but other cortical areas produce the same activity.

Ictal

The EEG hallmark of idiopathic generalized tonic-clonic seizures is bihemispheric involvement at the onset. However, computerized analysis of scalp recordings shows that the activity between the two hemispheres is seldom bisynchronous (Niedermeyer 1993). Therefore, asynchronous ictal activity at seizure onset does not necessarily exclude primary generalized epilepsy but sometimes makes the distinction between focal and generalized seizures difficult on scalp EEG (Fisch 1997).

The tonic phase of a primary generalized tonic-clonic seizure usually begins with an abrupt decrease in the voltage lasting 1–3 seconds, accompanied by diffuse, low-voltage, 20- to 40-Hz activity, referred to as a desynchronization pattern (Niedermeyer 1993). This pattern may be preceded by generalized bursts of spike and polyspike activity that accompanies myoclonic or initial clonic activity. After the desynchronization phase, lasting 1–3 seconds, the record is usually obscured by muscle artifact. When muscle artifact is prevented by pharmacological paralysis, a characteristic EEG progression of the generalized seizure is recorded. As the tonic phase continues, the ictal sharp waves build in amplitude to rhythmic 8–10 Hz. The rhythmic ictal activity then is gradually replaced by high-amplitude repetitive polyspike-and-wave complexes that gradually decrease in frequency. The clonic phase of the seizure develops when the polyspike-and-wave complexes slow to approximately 4 Hz (Niedermeyer 1993). The ictal activity ends with diffuse suppression of EEG activity or low-voltage delta waves. After a variable period of time, there is a gradual resumption of normal rhythms.

The ictal EEG of secondarily generalized seizures has a similar pattern during the tonic and clonic phases, but seizure onset may be preceded by one of three patterns: (1) focal rhythmic or arrhythmic epileptiform spike discharges; (2) brief, localized voltage attenuation or low-voltage fast activity; or (3) a buildup of focal rhythmic activity (Fisch 1997).

ABSENCE SEIZURES

Clinical Features

The simplest clinical feature of a typical absence seizure is the sudden onset of a blank stare, usually lasting 5–10 seconds. Speech may be interrupted or slowed in midsentence. Ongoing activity, such as chewing or walking, may stop abruptly. The individual does not respond to external stimuli and is unaware of having had the seizure. Recovery is as sudden as onset, and previous activity or speech continues as though nothing had happened. Less than 10% of absence seizures occur in this simple form; most have other features, such as clonic movements of the eyelids or mouth, which may be asymmetrical, or varying degrees of clonic, tonic, myoclonic, or atonic activity (Porter 1993). Objects held in the hand may be thrown or dropped. The head may nod slightly, or the shoulders or trunk may droop. Complete collapse is rare, but tonic activity of the trunk and limbs can cause falling. Absence seizures may be accompanied by automatisms that range from simple lip smacking to semipurposeful responses to tactile stimuli and even walking. The automatisms of absence may suggest a complex partial seizure (see Table 71.3).

The onset of atypical absence seizures is usually less abrupt. They last longer than the typical absence seizures, and they are often associated with loss of postural tone

(Porter 1993). Patients with atypical absence seizures usually have other seizure types, such as generalized tonic-clonic, myoclonic, and atonic seizures. Whereas almost all individuals with typical absence seizures are of normal intelligence, most with atypical absence seizures are mentally retarded.

Electroencephalographic Characteristics of Absence Seizures

The background rhythms in patients with typical absence seizures usually are normal. The ictal EEG pattern for typical absence seizures is a characteristic 3-Hz spike-and-wave pattern. Discharges lasting less than 3 seconds may cause no clinical changes. The frequency of the spike-and-wave activity may be slightly faster than 3 Hz at seizure onset, slowing to 2.5–3.0 Hz as the seizure progresses.

The EEG background is often abnormal in patients with atypical absence seizure because of diffuse slowing and focal or multifocal spike discharges. The ictal EEG consists of generalized slow spike-and-wave discharges in the range of 0.5–2.5 Hz.

MYOCLONIC SEIZURES

Myoclonus is a sudden, involuntary, shocklike muscle contraction arising from the CNS that causes a generalized jerk or a focal jerk (see Chapter 75). Focal jerks may be confined to a single muscle or a group of muscles. The jerks may be isolated or occur in clusters (Delgado-Escueta et al. 1997b). Myoclonus can be epileptic or nonepileptic. The primary distinguishing factor is that in epileptic myoclonus the jerk occurs concurrently with an ictal EEG discharge. The EMG bursts in epileptic myoclonus tend to be shorter and muscle activation more synchronous. Epileptic myoclonus has been divided into cortical reflex myoclonus, reticular reflex myoclonus, and primary generalized epileptic myoclonus (Niedermeyer 1993).

Cortical Reflex Myoclonus

The myoclonic jerk is caused by a discharge from a small cortical area in hyperexcitable sensorimotor cortex. A time-locked focal EEG event in the contralateral sensorimotor strip produces impulses that travel down the brainstem and spinal cord to cause the myoclonic jerk.

Reticular Reflex Myoclonus

The jerk is initiated by impulses originating in the caudal brainstem reticular formation. A generalized spike discharge is associated with, but is not time-locked to, the myoclonic jerk. The cortical manifestation may occur after the EMG evidence of activity in the muscle.

Primary Generalized Epileptic Myoclonus

Myoclonic jerks come from diffuse epileptic discharges in the cerebral cortex. They are preceded by diffuse bursts of polyspike or spike-wave discharges on the EEG.

TONIC AND ATONIC SEIZURES

Tonic and atonic seizures are electrophysiologically and usually clinically distinct, but the two may be difficult to distinguish without video and EEG correlation. Both occur most commonly in secondarily generalized epilepsy, particularly as part of the Lennox-Gastaut syndrome.

Tonic Seizures

Clinical Features

Tonic seizures last an average of 10 seconds but may persist for up to 1 minute (Farrell 1997b). The onset of clinical features may be gradual or abrupt. A myoclonic jerk may occur at the beginning, followed by a generalized tonic contraction. Movement may be limited to the axial musculature (tonic axial seizure), extend to the proximal muscles of the arms and legs (tonic axorhizomelic seizure), or involve proximal and distal limb muscles in addition to axial muscles (global tonic seizure). Tonic seizures sometimes cause a fall and are confused with atonic seizures. Involvement of the respiratory musculature produces apnea. Long tonic seizures may have a vibratory quality that gives them the appearance of a clonic seizure. Tonic status epilepticus can occur in patients with Lennox-Gastaut syndrome. It can last for hours to weeks and is often resistant to standard treatments for status epilepticus (see Status Epilepticus, later in this chapter).

Electroencephalogram

Four EEG patterns are associated with tonic seizures: (1) diffuse attenuation of activity (desynchronization) during the episode; (2) bilaterally synchronous, generalized rhythmic 15- to 25-Hz activity, initially at low amplitude, then gradually building to 50–100 µV; (3) generalized high-voltage rhythmic 10-Hz activity; and (4) diffuse theta or delta activity (Farrell 1997b). Progression may occur from one pattern to another.

Atonic Seizures

Clinical Features

Atonic seizures, commonly called *drop attacks*, occur abruptly and without warning and usually last 1–2 seconds. The main clinical feature is a sudden loss of tone, which may be limited to eye blinks or head drops but can involve the entire body. A severe seizure in someone who is standing is likened to suddenly cutting the strings of a marionette. Atonic seizures pose a high risk of injury because of the suddenness and forcefulness of the fall.

A myoclonic jerk may precede or accompany the seizure. Loss of consciousness is very brief and often unnoticed, and there is little postictal confusion. Long seizures cause several seconds of flaccid paralysis. Atonic seizures usually begin in late infancy, childhood, or as late as adolescence. Onset in adulthood is rare (Niedermeyer 1993).

Akinetic seizures are similar to atonic seizures, except that tone is preserved; the patient remains motionless, with impaired consciousness. These seizures are less strongly linked to Lennox-Gastaut syndrome (Niedermeyer 1993).

Electroencephalogram

The EEG during a brief atonic seizure may consist of poly-spike-and-wave discharges or generalized spike-and-wave discharges associated with a myoclonic jerk. The spike-and-wave burst is followed by diffuse slowing that is maximal in the vertex and central regions. During a prolonged atonic seizure, the EEG consists of generalized spikes, sharp waves, slow waves, and activity in the range of 10 Hz (Niedermeyer 1993).

GENERALIZED EPILEPTIC SYNDROMES

The generalized epileptic syndromes are diverse in severity and etiology. One seizure type often predominates in a given syndrome and patient, but several types usually occur. After recognition of the seizure type, the next most important distinction is between conditions that have relatively good and bad outcomes. Benign epilepsies are discussed first.

Benign Generalized Epileptic Syndromes

Febrile Seizures

Febrile seizures occur in 2–4% of children, making them the most common form of seizures in children (Hirtz 1997). Many people with epilepsy may have their first seizure during a fever, but febrile seizures are part of a benign syndrome that is distinct from epilepsy (Berg et al. 1997).

Clinical Features.   First febrile seizures usually occur between 3 months and 5 years of age, but the range is from 1 month to 10 years. Any evidence of intracranial infection or a defined cause precludes the diagnosis of febrile seizures. The majority of first febrile seizures occur during the first day of the fever, often before the parent is aware of temperature elevation. Predictors of increased risk for a first febrile seizure include a family history of febrile seizures, neonatal hospitalization for 28 days or longer,

delayed development, day care attendance, and high fever. Additionally, an association of a first febrile seizure has been made with low serum sodium and independently with the presence of human herpesvirus 6 infection (Hirtz 1997).

Most febrile seizures are simple—that is, single, generalized, and lasting less than 15 minutes. Approximately 20% are complex, which is defined as having any focal features, lasting longer than 15 minutes, having more than one seizure in 24 hours, or showing new postictal neurological signs. Fewer than 8% of febrile seizures last longer than 15 minutes.

Approximately one-third of children with febrile seizures have at least one recurrence, but less than 10% have three or more. The risk for recurrent seizures increases if the first febrile seizure occurs before age 12–18 months, if the duration of fever before the seizure is short, if the temperature elevation is low, or if other family members have had febrile seizures. Complex febrile seizures increase the risk of later epilepsy, but it is not established that they increase the risk of febrile seizure recurrence.

The prognosis is excellent. Children who were neurologically normal before the seizure, even before several febrile seizures, develop normally afterward. There is, however, a relationship between febrile seizures and later risk of epilepsy. Approximately 15% of individuals with epilepsy report a history of febrile seizures, but overall, less than 5% of children with febrile seizures develop epilepsy. Factors that increase the risk of later afebrile seizures are (1) neurological or developmental abnormality before the febrile seizure, (2) family history of afebrile seizure, and (3) a complex febrile seizure. The presence of one of these factors does not increase the risk of epilepsy, but the concurrence of two factors increases that risk to 2%, and three factors increases the risk to 10%.

Genetics.   A familial association of febrile seizures exists, but the exact mode of genetic inheritance is not known. Febrile seizures are two to three times more likely in family members of affected children than in the general population, whereas no clear association exists between febrile seizures and a family history of afebrile seizures.

Management.   The usual standards of management apply for the child who presents with active seizures. The most important consideration is the exclusion of infections of the CNS. An otherwise well child, who recovers quickly from the seizure, does not have meningitis; lumbar puncture and imaging studies are not needed. The source of the infection should be sought and treated. Hospitalization is not required for a febrile seizure.

Prophylactic anticonvulsant therapy is not indicated for febrile seizures (Hirtz 1997). Phenobarbital and valproic acid decrease the risk of recurrence of febrile seizures, but their use is not justified: The side effects are potentially more harmful than the seizures. Oral diazepam (1 mg/kg body weight in three divided doses/day) given intermittently with onset of fever reduces the risk of recurrent febrile seizures. It is an option for children whose febrile seizures are prolonged but is not routinely recommended because of its high rate of side effects.

Benign Neonatal Familial Convulsions

Clinical Features.   Brief clonic seizures develop during the first week of life, sometimes associated with apnea (Duchowny 1994). Whether anticonvulsants are given or withheld, the seizures resolve spontaneously by 6 months of age. Growth and development are subsequently normal; 10–14% of patients develop epilepsy later in life.

Genetics.   Benign neonatal convulsions are transmitted by autosomal dominant inheritance. The gene has been linked to a locus on chromosome 20q with a mutation in a potassium channel, but there is evidence of heterogeneity among different families (Berkovic 1997; Biervert et al. 1998).

Benign Myoclonic Epilepsy of Infancy

Clinical Features.   Benign myoclonic epilepsy of infancy develops in otherwise normal children before age 2 years (Delgado-Escueta et al. 1997a). Brief generalized myoclonic seizures of variable intensity are the only seizure type. Severe axial and appendicular involvement can cause falls, but most are characterized by head drops or eye blinks. Attacks can last up to 10 seconds. Consciousness is not completely lost but may be compromised in longer spells.

Electroencephalogram.   The ictal EEG shows diffuse irregular 3-Hz spike-wave or polyspike-and-wave discharges with the myoclonic jerks. The interictal EEG is usually normal. Generalized tonic-clonic seizures may develop later in life.

Treatment.   Myoclonic seizures are easily controlled with valproic acid. Developmental outcome is good when treatment is started early.

Juvenile Myoclonic Epilepsy

JME accounts for 4–10% of all cases of epilepsy, but the diagnosis is often delayed and the prevalence underestimated because symptoms are not recognized (Duchowny 1994). Other names for JME are impulsive petit mal, jerk epilepsy, or myoclonic epilepsy of adolescence.

Clinical Features.   Age at onset is usually between 12 and 18 years but may be from ages 8 to 30 years. The characteristic feature is sudden, mild-to-moderate myoclonic jerks of the shoulders and arms that usually occur after awakening. Generalized tonic-clonic seizures develop in 90% of cases, and approximately one-third have absence seizures. Myoclonic seizures precede generalized tonic-clonic seizures in approximately one-half of patients.

Initially, myoclonic jerks are mild and explained as nervousness, clumsiness, or tics. They may not be recognized

as seizures until a generalized tonic-clonic seizure brings the patient to medical attention. Seizures are precipitated by sleep deprivation, alcohol intake, and fatigue. Affected individuals are of normal intelligence, and there is no evidence of neurological deterioration.

A seizure disorder with onset between ages 1 and 5 years has been recognized that may represent a bridge between benign myoclonic epilepsy of infancy and JME. It is characterized by myoclonic-astatic, myoclonic, absence, and tonic-clonic or clonic-tonic-clonic seizures. Development and intelligence are normal.

Genetics.   JME is familial; it is presumed to be transmitted as an autosomal dominant trait. The gene locus has been mapped to the short arm of chromosome 6. The same locus may be responsible for other forms of epilepsy. Heterogeneity may be due to different alleles at the same locus or the influence of another locus (Delgado-Escueta et al. 1997a).

Electroencephalogram.   The interictal EEG in JME consists of bilateral, symmetrical spike and polyspike-and-wave discharges of 3–5 Hz, usually maximal in the frontocentral regions. The EEG correlate of the myoclonic jerks is a burst of high-voltage, 10- to 16-Hz polyspikes followed by irregular 1- to 3-Hz slow waves and single spikes or polyspikes. Focal EEG abnormalities occur in a significant number of patients with JME.

Treatment.   Seizures usually are controlled with valproic acid, but lifetime treatment is necessary. Lamotrigine may be considered in patients who do not tolerate valproic acid. Ethosuximide can be used to treat uncontrolled absence seizures (Delgado-Escueta et al. 1997a).

Epilepsy with Generalized Tonic-Clonic Seizures on Awakening

Epilepsy with generalized tonic-clonic seizures on awakening is probably distinct from JME. Onset occurs in the second decade, and 90% of seizures occur on awakening, regardless of the time of day. Seizures also occur with relaxation in the evening. Absence and myoclonic seizures may occur. The syndrome is familial, but the mode of inheritance is unknown. The EEG shows a pattern of idiopathic generalized epilepsies. Treatment is similar to that of JME (Delgado-Escueta et al. 1997b).

Absence Syndromes

Clinical Features.   Several absence syndromes have been recognized in the ILAE classification of syndromes. Childhood absence epilepsy (pyknolepsy) was previously called *petit mal*, a term that is still used. The onset of childhood absence epilepsy is usually between ages 5 and 10 years, but it may begin as early as 3 years of age (Duchowny 1994). Untreated seizures are very frequent, sometimes up to 100 per day. Juvenile absence epilepsy, with onset around puberty, may represent a distinct but related syndrome. The absences are less frequent, but myoclonic and generalized tonic-clonic seizures are more frequent. Approximately one-half of patients with absence epilepsy become free of seizures 10 years after onset, but many continue to relapse or have poor seizure control. Good prognostic factors include normal or above-average intelligence, normal neurological examination, male gender, and lack of hyperventilation-induced spike waves on the EEG.

Children who have stereotyped absences associated with bilateral rhythmic clonic jerking of the arms probably have a separate, rare disorder, epilepsy with myoclonic absences. Age of onset is similar to childhood absence epilepsy, but the prognosis is worse; seizures are often resistant to therapy, and mental deterioration may occur.

Genetics.   The mode of genetic transmission of childhood absence epilepsy was thought to be autosomal dominant but may be multifactorial (Porter 1993). Girls are affected more often than are boys.

Electroencephalogram.   See Electroencephalographic Characteristics of Absence Seizures, earlier in this chapter.

Treatment.   Ethosuximide is generally considered the initial medication of choice for absence seizures, unless other seizure types also occur, in which case valproic acid is used (Porter 1993). Children who do not respond to ethosuximide should be switched to valproic acid. A small number of children with absence epilepsy require both drugs. Children with both absence and myoclonic seizures who do not respond to valproic acid alone may benefit from the addition of clonazepam.

Severe Generalized Epileptic Syndromes

Early Infantile Myoclonic Encephalopathy (Ohtahara Syndrome)

Clinical Features.   The onset of myoclonic seizures before 3 months of age is always associated with serious underlying disorders (Duchowny 1994). Myoclonic seizures in the newborn are caused by inborn errors of metabolism (see Chapter 68). Some cases are familial, indicating an underlying genetic disorder. A cause-and-effect relationship between early myoclonic encephalopathy and routine childhood immunization has never been established, in spite of the temporal relationship. The initial seizures are myoclonic. These are followed by partial seizures, massive myoclonic or tonic spasms, and generalized tonic-clonic seizures. Psychomotor arrest and regression are constant features.

Electroencephalogram.   Infants with myoclonic encephalopathy show a burst-suppression pattern. Newborns have a burst-suppression pattern alternating with bursts of diffuse, high-amplitude, spike-wave complexes.

Treatment.   These seizures are refractory to most anticonvulsant drugs. Valproic acid and clonazepam are often used for myoclonic seizures, and carbamazepine is contraindicated.

West's Syndrome

Clinical Features.   West's syndrome is the clinical triad of infantile spasms, arrest of psychomotor development, and hypsarrhythmia on EEG (Duchowny 1994). Its incidence is estimated to be 1 per 4,000–6,000 live births. The identified causes of infantile spasms are divided into prenatal (cerebral dysgenesis, genetic disorders, intrauterine infection), perinatal (anoxic injury, head trauma, infection), and postnatal (metabolic disorders, trauma, infection). No etiology (cryptogenic) can be identified in as many as 40% of cases, but this percentage should be reduced by improvements in technology, especially with regard to imaging and biochemical and genetic analyses.

The onset of almost all cases occurs before age 1 year, with peak onset between 3 and 7 months of age. The spasms occur in clusters and are characterized by sudden flexor or extensor movements of the trunk. They have a myoclonic quality but are somewhat longer in duration. Flexor spasms consist of sudden flexion of the head and legs with adduction of the arms, a pattern that has been described as a *jackknife convulsion*. The less common extensor spasms consist of extension of the head and trunk and abduction of the arms, which may mimic Moro's reflex. Both extensor and flexor spasms may occur in combination.

At first, the spasms are subtle and may not be recognized as seizures. Primary care physicians may misdiagnosis the spasms as colic or gastroesophageal reflux because clusters often occur in the morning at the time of feeding. Conversely, gastroesophageal reflux can be mistaken for epilepsy.

Developmental arrest and regression begins with or before the spasms. This may be difficult to ascertain when spasms begin before 6 months because only a few skills are normally achieved and the normal range is considerable. Furthermore, many children with West's syndrome have developed slowly from birth, and deterioration is difficult to discern.

The prognosis for children with infantile spasms is extremely poor, but the major determinant of outcome is the underlying cause of the spasms. Only 5% of children develop normally, and these are mainly from the cryptogenic group. The belief that early treatment improves prognosis has never been substantiated.

Electroencephalogram.   The third defining feature is the pattern of hypsarrhythmia on interictal EEG recordings. On the waking record, hypsarrhythmia consists of disorganized high-voltage slow waves, spikes, and sharp waves that occur diffusely with a somewhat posterior predominance. Hypsarrhythmia may not be fully developed at the onset of the spasms, but the persistence of a normal interictal background on the EEG is against the diagnosis and suggests benign myoclonus of infancy.

Treatment. Corticosteroids, in the form of adrenocorticotropic hormone (ACTH), prednisone, or prednisolone, are the treatment of choice for infantile spasms. Benzodiazepines, in the form of clonazepam, provide some benefit but are not as effective as corticosteroids. Valproic acid is also effective, but the risk of hepatotoxicity in this age group must be considered. Vigabatrin has been used to treat infantile spasms effectively (Duchowny 1994).

Lennox-Gastaut Syndrome

The defining features of Lennox-Gastaut syndrome are (1) the presence of several seizure types, (2) a characteristic interictal EEG abnormality, and (3) diffuse cognitive dysfunction. The causes of Lennox-Gastaut syndrome are similar to those of West's syndrome and can be divided into the symptomatic and the cryptogenic. Cerebral malformations are less common as a cause of Lennox-Gastaut than of West's syndrome (Farrell 1997b). Abnormalities of the frontal lobe are more often associated with Lennox-Gastaut syndrome than with any other region of the brain.

Clinical Features. Seizure onset occurs between 1 and 7 years of age. The seizures types are usually generalized (axial tonic, atypical absence, generalized tonic-clonic, and atonic), but partial seizures may occur as well. Cognitive function is normal in 40% of children at the onset of seizures, but it deteriorates in most affected children.

Electroencephalogram. The waking interictal EEG consists of an abnormally slow background with characteristic 1.5- to 2.5-Hz slow spike-and-wave interictal discharges, often with an anterior predominance (Farrell 1997b). Bursts of rhythmic 10-Hz activity characteristically occur during sleep.

Treatment. The seizures of Lennox-Gastaut syndrome are often refractory to anticonvulsant drugs. Valproic acid and benzodiazepines are the mainstay of therapy (Farrell 1997b). Lamotrigine and topiramate may have a role in the treatment of seizures associated with Lennox-Gastaut syndrome (Dichter and Brodie 1996). The addition of felbamate to existing therapy improves seizure control in approximately 30% of patients with Lennox-Gastaut syndrome, but routine use is not indicated due to the risk of aplastic anemia and hepatotoxicity. Corticosteroids and ACTH are beneficial in some cases, and the ketogenic diet may be useful (Swink et al. 1997).

Epilepsy with Myoclonic-Astatic Seizures

Absence and myoclonic-astatic seizure predominate in this seizure disorder, which usually presents between 1 and 6 years of age (Duchowny 1994). Generalized tonic-clonic seizures may occur, but tonic seizures are uncommon and usually occur only in sleep. The multiple seizures are similar to those with Lennox-Gastaut syndrome, but most individuals are neurologically normal at the time of seizure onset. One-half of children exhibit cognitive deterioration, but overall the prognosis is better than for Lennox-Gastaut syndrome. Early treatment with agents directed against generalized seizure disorders may be associated with a better prognosis.

Landau-Kleffner Syndrome

Patients with Landau-Kleffner syndrome typically present between 3 and 9 years of age with an acquired aphasia that is usually, but not always, associated with seizures. A variety of seizure types occur, including generalized tonic-clonic, partial, and myoclonic seizures (Duchowny 1994). The severity of the seizure disorder does not correlate with the language loss. Characteristically, children exhibit word deafness in the face of otherwise normal hearing. The EEG may show spike activity over the temporal-central regions, often bilateral. Other EEG patterns occur, such as multifocal spike and slow waves. The seizures are usually controlled with standard antiepileptic drug treatment, but recovery of language is variable. High-dose steroids have been used with variable success.

Electrical Status Epilepticus during Slow-Wave Sleep

Patients with electrical status epilepticus during slow-wave sleep present between 1 and 12 years of age with neuropsychological regression, with or without seizures (Duchowny 1994). The disorder appears to be distinct from Landau-Kleffner syndrome. The EEG characteristically shows continuous spike and slow waves during non–rapid eye movement sleep. A variety of seizure types occur, but they are commonly nocturnal. Seizures and EEG changes usually disappear in the second decade, but cognitive and language function often remain impaired.

Progressive Myoclonic Epilepsies

The progressive myoclonic epilepsies are a heterogeneous group of genetic disorders (Delgado-Escueta et al. 1997b). Most are caused by inborn errors of metabolism. The main features are myoclonus, epilepsy, cognitive impairment, and progressive neurological disorders. The rate and degree of progression varies between disorders. They are better classified by the underlying biochemical abnormality than as epileptic syndromes. Progressive myoclonic epilepsies occurs in lysosomal storage diseases, mitochondrial disorders, and biotin-responsive encephalopathy (see Chapter 68) and in Hallervorden-Spatz disease, action myoclonus-renal failure syndrome, and hereditary dentatorubral-pallidoluysian atrophy (see Chapters 75 and 76). Unverricht-Lundborg disease and Lafora's disease are traditionally classified as progressive myoclonic encephalopathies and are discussed here.

Unverricht-Lundborg Disease

Unverricht-Lundborg disease was first described in families in Estonia and Sweden and was called Baltic myoclonus (Delgado-Escueta et al. 1997b). It is now recognized that the disorder occurs worldwide. Inheritance is autosomal recessive in Finnish families. Mutations in the human *EPM1* gene are responsible for Unverricht-Lundborg disease (Hosford et al. 1997). *EPM1* encodes for cystatin B, an intracellular protein that competitively inhibits intralysosomal cysteine proteases known as *cathepsins*. How the defect results in progressive deterioration or seizures is not yet clear. Inheritance is autosomal recessive. Myoclonus, which may be spontaneous, action induced, or stimulus sensitive, begins insidiously in childhood between ages 6 and 16 years. Tonic-clonic seizures and cerebellar signs also occur. Dementia is mild and very slowly progressive. The myoclonus gradually becomes incapacitating, affecting gait, swallowing, and speech. Valproic acid and benzodiazepine are used to treat the seizures and myoclonus. Phenytoin may exacerbate the condition.

Lafora's Disease

Lafora's disease is transmitted by autosomal recessive inheritance. The biochemical defect is unknown, but characteristic "amyloid" deposits (Lafora's bodies) are seen in cerebral cortex, liver, skeletal muscle, and skin (Delgado-Escueta et al. 1997b). The onset of generalized tonic-clonic seizures occurs in late childhood and adolescence. Characteristic visual seizures involving simple hallucinations, scotomas, or occipital complex partial seizures are reported in one-half of cases. Progressive development of resting and action myoclonus is accompanied by cognitive decline that is more severe than that seen in Unverricht-Lundborg disease. A fluctuating course may be associated with periods of cortical pseudoblindness. Death occurs 2–10 years after onset of symptoms.

STATUS EPILEPTICUS

Status epilepticus is defined as occurring when a seizure continues for longer than 30 minutes or when seizures recur within 30 minutes without the patient regaining consciousness between seizures (Dodson et al. 1993). In practice, however, most clinicians recognize status epilepticus as a medical emergency that requires prompt, vigorous treatment well before 30 minutes elapse (Lowenstein and Alldredge 1998).

Clinical Features

Any type of seizure can evolve into status epilepticus. The most commonly recognized form of status epilepticus is the generalized tonic-clonic or convulsive type. Most common are repeated tonic-clonic seizures lasting 2–3 minutes without regaining of consciousness between seizures, but continuous seizures also occur. Tonic status epilepticus occurs in children and adolescents with Lennox-Gastaut syndrome, and myoclonic status epilepticus occurs in patients with JME. Continuous nonepileptic myoclonus is seen in some systemic disorders, after cerebral anoxia, or in Creutzfeldt-Jakob disease, and it must be distinguished from epileptic myoclonus. Generalized nonconvulsive (absence) status epilepticus is characterized by stupor, a confused state, clouding of consciousness, and little or no motor activity. Complex partial status epilepticus is clinically similar, with features that range from partial responsiveness and semipurposeful automatisms to total unresponsiveness, speech arrest, and stereotypical automatisms. Simple partial status epilepticus often appears as repeated clonic or myoclonic jerks, often limited to one extremity, with preserved consciousness (see Epilepsia Partialis Continua, earlier in this chapter).

Epidemiology

The annual number of cases of status epilepticus in the United States is estimated to be 102,000–152,000 (Lowenstein and Alldredge 1998). Approximately one-half of the cases of status epilepticus occur in young children, but adults older than 60 years have a high risk (Dodson et al. 1993). Status epilepticus occurs in three broad settings: (1) in patients who sustain an acute process that affects the brain, such as metabolic disturbances, hypoxia, CNS infection, head trauma, or drug intoxication; (2) in epileptic patients having an exacerbation of seizures, often due to abrupt reduction in antiepileptic medication; and (3) as a first unprovoked seizure, often heralding the onset of epilepsy. This third, or idiopathic, group accounts for approximately one-third of cases of status epilepticus.

Morbidity and Mortality

The mortality associated with status epilepticus has declined dramatically during the last century, but rates remain in the range of 3% to 35% (Dodson et al. 1993).

Table 71.4:   A suggested timetable for the treatment of status epilepticus*

Time (mins)	Action
0–5	Diagnose status epilepticus by observing continued seizure activity or one additional seizure.
	Give oxygen by nasal cannula or mask; position patient's head for optimal airway patency; consider any abnormalities as necessary; initiate ECG monitoring.
	Obtain and record vital signs at onset and periodically thereafter; control any abnormalities as necessary; initiate ECG monitoring.
	Establish IV access; draw venous blood samples for glucose level, serum chemistries, hematology studies, toxicology screens, and determinations of antiepileptic drug levels.
	Assess oxygenation with oximetry or periodic arterial blood gas determinations.
6–9	If hypoglycemia is established or a blood glucose determination is unavailable, administer glucose; in adults, give 100 mg of thiamine first, followed by 50 ml of 50% glucose by direct push into the IV line; in children, the dose of glucose is 2 ml/kg of 25% glucose.
10–20	Administer either lorazepam, 0.1 mg/kg IV at 2 mg/min, or diazepam, 0.2 mg/kg IV at 5 mg/min. If diazepam is given, it can be repeated if seizures do not stop after 5 minutes; if diazepam is used to stop the status, phenytoin should be administered next to prevent recurrent status.
21–60	If status persists, administer phenytoin, 15–20 mg/kg IV, no faster than 50 mg/min in adults and 1 mg/kg/min IV in children; monitor ECG and blood pressure during the infusion; phenytoin is incompatible with glucose-containing solutions; the IV line should be purged with normal saline before the phenytoin infusion. Alternatively, fosphenytoin, 20 mg/kg phenytoin equivalents at 150 mg/min in adults or 3 mg/kg/min in children, can be used.
40–60	If status does not stop after 20 mg/kg of phenytoin or fosphenytoin, give additional doses of 5–10 mg/kg of phenytoin or fosphenytoin to a maximal dose of 30 mg/kg.
50–70	If status persists, give phenobarbital, 20 mg/kg IV at 50–100 mg/min; when phenobarbital is given after a benzodiazepine, the risk of apnea or hypopnea is great, and assisted ventilation is usually required. If seizures continue, give an additional 5–10 mg/kg of phenobarbital.
>70	If status persists, give anesthetic doses of drugs such as midazolam (loading dose of 0.2 mg/kg by slow intravenous bolus, then 0.75–10.00 μg/kg/min), propofol (loading dose of 1–2 mg/kg IV, followed by 2–10 mg/kg/hr) or pentobarbital (5–15 mg/kg IV bolus over 1 hr, followed by 0.5–3.0 mg/kg/hr); ventilatory assistance and vasopressors are virtually always necessary. Continuous EEG monitoring is indicated throughout therapy, with the primary end point being suppression of EEG spikes or a burst-suppression pattern with short intervals between bursts.

ECG = electrocardiogram; EEG = electroencephalogram.
*Time starts at seizure onset. Note that a neurological consultation is indicated if the patient does not wake up, convulsions continue after the administration of a benzodiazepine and phenytoin, or confusion exists at any time during evaluation and treatment.
Source: Reprinted with permission from WE Dodson, RJ DeLorenzo, TA Pedley, et al. Treatment of convulsive status epilepticus—recommendations of the Epilepsy Foundation of America's Working Group on Status Epilepticus. JAMA 1993;270:854–859.

Children have lower mortality rates than adults. Prolonged seizure duration and an identified acute brain insult are associated with higher mortality and morbidity. Systemic alterations, including respiratory compromise, acidemia, hypoglycemia, and hypotension, become progressively worse when the seizures last longer than 30 minutes. Furthermore, prolonged electrical activity itself may contribute to neuronal injury. Among survivors, the risk of intellectual impairment from status epilepticus has been difficult to document, mainly because controlled studies with adequate neuropsychological evaluations are difficult to do. Prolonged status epilepticus, however, may have subtle to severe adverse effects on intellectual development in children and on memory and cognitive function in adults, independent of the underlying neurological condition (Dodson et al. 1993). In general, however, idiopathic status epilepticus of short duration is associated with a favorable outcome, especially in children.

Management

Time is a critical factor in the treatment of status epilepticus. Diagnosis and treatment should proceed in a rapid and organized manner. The initial steps are a rapid assessment and stabilization of cardiovascular and respiratory function. A brief history and physical examination are directed toward identifying an immediate and potentially treatable cause. Table 71.4 outlines the recommended method for managing status epilepticus.

The pharmacological management of status epilepticus requires close attention to the potential cardiorespiratory and neurological reaction caused by anticonvulsant drugs (Table 71.5). Benzodiazepines rapidly enter the CNS and are, with phenytoin, the drugs of first choice. Diazepam is highly lipid soluble and redistributes rapidly; its CNS activity is short. Lorazepam has a higher binding affinity to the benzodiazepine receptor. Its CNS activity is longer, and it is therefore

Table 71.5:   Major drugs used to treat status epilepticus: intravenous doses, pharmacokinetics, and major toxicity

	Diazepam	*Lorazepam*	*Phenytoin*	*Phenobarbital*
Adult IV dose in mg/kg (range [total dose])	0.15–0.25 [10 mg]	0.1 [4–8 mg]	15–20	20
Pediatric IV dose in mg/kg (range [total dose])	0.1–1.0 [10 mg]	0.05–0.50 [1–4 mg]	20	20
Pediatric per rectum dose in mg/kg	0.5 [20 mg maximum]	—	—	—
Maximal administration rate in mg/min	5.0	2.0	50	100
Time to stop status in minutes	1–3	6–10	10–30	20–30
Effective duration of action in hours	0.25–0.50	>12–24	24	>48
Potential side effects				
Depression of consciousness	10–30 mins	Several hours	None	Several days
Respiratory depression	Occasional	Occasional	Infrequent	Occasional
Hypertension	Infrequent	Infrequent	Occasional	Infrequent
Cardiac arrhythmia	—	—	In patients with heart disease	—

Source: Reprinted with permission from WE Dodson, RJ DeLorenzo, TA Pedley et al. Treatment of convulsive status epilepticus—recommendations of the Epilepsy Foundation of America's Working Group on Status Epilepticus. JAMA 1993;270:854–859.

preferable to diazepam. Midazolam, a water-soluble benzodiazepine, can be given intramuscularly as well as intravenously for the treatment of refractory status epilepticus. Benzodiazepines can cause significant respiratory depression, especially when given with barbiturates, and respiratory support, including intubation, is sometimes necessary. In carefully selected patients at risk for status epilepticus, diazepam can be administered rectally to effectively limit the recurrence of acute repetitive seizures and potentially decrease the risk of progression to status epilepticus (Dooley 1998).

Phenytoin is usually administered intravenously before or with the benzodiazepines. Rapid IV administration of phenytoin may be associated with cardiac arrhythmia and hypotension; therefore, the rate should not be faster than 50 mg per minute in adults or 1 mg/kg per minute in children, and heart rate or the electrocardiogram should be monitored during administration. Fosphenytoin, a water-soluble prodrug of phenytoin, is administered as phenytoin equivalents at rates up to 150 mg per minute. At this infusion rate, the risk of hypotension and adverse cardiac effects is similar to that of phenytoin administered at slower rates, but infusion site reactions are dramatically less frequent with fosphenytoin (Lowenstein and Alldredge 1998). IV phenobarbital can be administered faster than phenytoin, but it has both a cardiorespiratory- and CNS-depressing effect. Status epilepticus that is refractory to IV benzodiazepines, phenytoin, and phenobarbital requires more aggressive treatment. In an intensive care setting, continuous IV infusions of anesthetic doses of midazolam, propofol, or short-acting barbiturates may be necessary, usually with ventilatory support and continuous EEG monitoring (Lowenstein and Alldredge 1998). The short-acting barbiturates often produce hypotension, which limits their safety. Patients who do not wake up after convulsive status is stopped should have an EEG to determine if they are in nonconvulsive status.

CAUSES OF SEIZURES

Symptomatic epilepsy can be caused by almost all diseases and injuries of the brain. Some medical conditions that cause seizures are reviewed in Chapters 55 and 59. Brain tumors and paraneoplastic disorders that cause seizures are reviewed in Chapter 58 and neonatal seizures in Chapter 84.

POST-TRAUMATIC EPILEPSY

Head trauma is associated with an increased susceptibility to subsequent seizures (see Chapter 56A). The onset of seizures may be early (<1 week) or late (>1 week) after the injury. Factors that increase the risk of early seizures are the severity of the injury, frontoparietal location, and depression of the fractured bone (Willmore 1997). Intracranial hematoma increases the risk of early seizures independent of the duration of post-traumatic amnesia or focal neurological signs. Age is also an important risk factor; young children have the highest risk of early post-traumatic seizures, and the risk progressively decreases through adult life.

The reported rates of late post-traumatic epilepsy vary considerably. Reports from the military series, which include missile injuries, are 28–53%, whereas civilian rates after closed head injuries are 3–14% (Willmore 1997). Risk factors for late-onset post-traumatic epilepsy are the type and severity of injury and the occurrence of early post-traumatic seizures. Post-traumatic epilepsy followed 34% of missile injuries but only 7.5% of nonmissile injuries. Late seizures after closed head injury are more likely to occur in association with intracranial hematoma or depressed skull fracture.

It had been customary to start prophylactic anticonvulsant therapy after a head injury to prevent post-traumatic seizures. However, studies have shown that phenytoin prophylaxis can decrease the risk of early post-traumatic seizures but not late post-traumatic seizures (Willmore 1997). Long-term post-traumatic prophylactic antiepileptic drug treatment is rarely indicated.

INFECTIOUS CAUSES OF SEIZURES

Neurocysticercosis is a leading cause of epilepsy in tropical countries, but it is not limited to countries with hot or tropical climates (de Bittencourt et al. 1996a). In areas of poor sanitation, the causative organism, *Taenia solium*, comes from a variety of contaminated foods, including vegetables and undercooked meat. In developing countries, approximately 30% of epilepsy is related to neurocysticercosis. Seizures are the presenting symptom in up to 90% of individuals with intraparenchymal lesions. Partial seizures with or without secondary generalization are the most common seizure type. In children and adolescents, an acute encephalitic form of neurocysticercosis occurs due to widely disseminated intraparenchymal cysts (de Bittencourt et al. 1996b). These patients have frequent seizures and acutely evolving intracranial hypertension. Prognosis for seizure control is good for both the encephalitic form and the more localized cystic form. Appropriate treatment of the underlying infection, however, is critical in addition to antiepileptic drugs.

Cerebral hydatidosis is similar to cysticercosis (de Bittencourt et al. 1996a). The reservoir for the causative organism, *Echinococcus granulosus*, is sheep rather than pigs. The cerebral cysts often become quite large, in contrast to the usually more localized cysts of cysticercosis. Seizures more commonly occur after drainage of the large cerebral cysts.

In African trypanosomiasis, chronic meningoencephalitis occurs after the lymphosanguine phase (de Bittencourt et al. 1996). Presenting symptoms are motor, sensory, and psychiatric in nature, which then progress to disturbances of consciousness and sleep. Seizures usually occur only in the terminal phase. In American trypanosomiasis, seizures occur only rarely and are usually secondary to the effects of emboli from the involved heart (de Bittencourt et al. 1996a).

Cerebral malaria occurs with *Plasmodium falciparum* (de Bittencourt et al. 1996a). Acute symptomatic generalized seizures occur in 40% of adults and the majority of children. Chronic, remote symptomatic epilepsy may be related to astrocytosis that develops after vascular invasion by the organisms. In children, fever associated with malaria contributes to a high proportion of febrile convulsions in endemic areas. Differentiating cerebral malaria from febrile convulsions with malaria can be difficult. In addition, seizures due to these treatments can be confused with the underlying disorder. Chloroquine and mefloquine can cause seizures. Quinine can cause hypoglycemia, which indirectly leads to seizures.

Congenital toxoplasmosis is associated with seizures in approximately 50% of affected children (de Bittencourt et al. 1996b). The majority have varying manifestations of chorioretinitis, hydrocephalus, cerebral calcifications, cerebral palsy,

and blindness. Toxoplasmosis infection with human immunodeficiency virus infection is associated with acute symptomatic seizures in approximately 25% of patients.

With tuberculosis, seizures may occur with cerebral intraparenchymal involvement after systemic infection. Pyogenic meningitis contributes to late seizure in less than 10% of cases, but other focal neurological abnormalities usually are present (de Bittencourt et al. 1996a).

Seizures occur uncommonly with filariasis, paragonimiasis, and schistosomiasis (de Bittencourt et al. 1996a). *Angiostrongylus cantonensis* and *Gnathostoma spinigerum* can involve the CNS but do not cause seizures. Cerebral amebiasis causes suppurative brain abscesses that may be associated with seizures.

PSYCHOGENIC SEIZURES

Psychogenic seizures are emotionally triggered, episodic, but nonepileptic events or spells that can be extremely difficult to distinguish from epileptic seizures, even for trained observers (Lesser 1996). They can occur in people with and without epilepsy. Psychogenic seizures also are called *hysterical seizures*, but this term is best avoided because *hysterical* implies an etiological basis that does not apply to all individuals with psychogenic seizures.

Diagnosis

Four patterns of behavior are seen during psychogenic seizures: (1) sustained or repetitive muscular contractions that can be unilateral or bilateral, (2) muscle inactivity or loss of tone, (3) unresponsiveness without the presence of other observable behavioral phenomena, and (4) unresponsiveness in association with apparently purposeful or semipurposeful or apparently automatic or semiautomatic behaviors. One patient may show more than one pattern. An aura before the episode is sometimes reported.

The phenomenology of the events must be carefully analyzed to determine whether the episode is epileptic or psychogenic. Although no rule works consistently, the following features are more likely to occur in psychogenic than in epileptic seizures:

1. Gradual onset or progression from the initial symptoms to the complete episode
2. Symptoms such as palpitations, malaise, choking, dizziness, or acral paresthesias
3. Quivering, side-to-side movements of the head, pelvic thrusting, and uncontrolled flailing, thrashing, or asynchronous rhythmic movements of the limbs
4. Quasi-volitional speech or movements in response to observers during periods of apparent unresponsiveness

Similar behaviors, however, can be seen in some complex partial seizures. Self-injury and incontinence of urine or stool are uncommon but do occur with psychogenic seizures. Psychogenic seizures can be very stereotyped, and epileptic seizures can have variable expression; therefore, relative consistency of the pattern of the events cannot always be used to make a distinction.

Two observational tools can be used by clinicians to help make a diagnosis. One is avoidance testing maneuvers, such as releasing the patient's hand over the face, which may produce resistance or terminate a psychogenic seizure, although some patients might allow themselves to be traumatized. An unconscious individual during an epileptic seizure is not likely to respond. The other observational tool is inducing the psychogenic seizures by suggestion. A variety of methods are available, such as hyperventilation, flashing lights, and saline injections. When such techniques are used, however, care must be taken not to "trick" the patient but rather to create a permissive setting that allows an event to occur. Controlled induction of epileptic seizure is unusual, except in special circumstances, such as absence seizures provoked by hyperventilation or in some forms of stimulus-sensitive epilepsy. The ability to "bring on" a seizure is especially useful because it allows evaluation with EEG monitoring.

Electroencephalogram

The EEG is useful to determine the presence of interictal epileptiform activity and to document brain activity during the seizure. The presence of interictal epileptiform activity does not rule out the diagnosis of psychogenic seizures because epileptic seizures and psychogenic seizures may coexist in the same patient.

The ictal EEG, preferably with video monitoring, usually can distinguish psychogenic from epileptic seizures. The absence of ictal epileptiform activity and a preserved posterior alpha rhythm during a seizure manifested by unresponsiveness is diagnostic of a psychogenic seizure. Simple partial seizures can occur without clear ictal EEG activity recorded from the scalp, but generalized seizures do not. Movement artifact is sometimes confused with epileptiform activity or obscures the background. The background activity should be suppressed or slowed after a generalized tonic-clonic seizure but not after a psychogenic seizure.

Seizures that are difficult to diagnose through routine outpatient EEG may be clarified by prolonged video and EEG monitoring. These can be done on an outpatient basis, but sometimes hospitalization is needed to stop anticonvulsant drugs.

Serum Prolactin

Serum prolactin concentrations are increased for 15–30 minutes after some generalized tonic-clonic and some complex partial seizures. The rise is not constant, and lack of change in prolactin concentration does not exclude epileptic seizures. Furthermore, some patients with epilepsy have elevated prolactin concentrations, and an increased concentration does not exclude concurrent psychogenic seizures.

Treatment

When a diagnosis is established within reasonable certainty, it should be presented to the patient. An extended and supportive counseling session is beneficial to explain the differential diagnosis, the psychogenic basis of the patient's condition, and treatment alternatives. If there is no evidence of epilepsy, anticonvulsants should be stopped. Occasionally, a simple explanation of the condition brings an end to the psychogenic seizures, but more often a well-coordinated counseling program is necessary.

OTHER PAROXYSMAL CONDITIONS

Several nonepileptic conditions cause paroxysmal events that may be confused with epilepsy (see Chapters 2, 9, 58F, 75, 55A, and 55B). Nonepileptic episodes in infants and young children include breath-holding spells, jitteriness, head banging, masturbation, spasmodic torticollis, spasmus nutans, opsoclonus, shuddering attacks, benign paroxysmal vertigo, and night terrors. In older children and adults, rage attacks, panic attacks (often with hyperventilation), syncope, paroxysmal choreoathetosis, and myoclonus should be considered.

PREGNANCY

For a fuller discussion of epilepsy during pregnancy, see Chapter 85. Approximately 400,000 women with epilepsy are of childbearing age in the United States. Only one-third of them experience a significant increase in seizure frequency during pregnancy (Yerby 1997). This does not happen at any specific time during pregnancy.

Anticonvulsant Concentrations

One important factor contributing to the increased seizure frequency is a decrease in anticonvulsant blood concentrations during pregnancy. Some cases are the result of not taking medicine out of concern for adverse effects on the fetus. These concerns should be addressed before or early in the pregnancy and balanced with the effects of maternal seizures on the fetus.

Even with full compliance, anticonvulsant levels decline during pregnancy, primarily because of decreased plasma protein binding. The proportion of unbound to bound drug increases in the plasma and, at a constant dose, is metabolized at a faster rate. During pregnancy, total concentrations of carbamazepine, phenytoin, valproic acid, and phenobarbital decrease, but only unbound phenobarbital decreases; unbound valproic acid actually increases. For this reason, it is important that unbound concentrations are measured and that the goals of therapy be based on the unbound concentration rather than total anticonvulsant blood concentrations.

Other factors that may contribute to the changes in the anticonvulsant blood concentrations include increased hepatic and renal clearance rates, increased volume of distribution, and possibly malabsorption. Anticonvulsant blood concentrations may decline at the time of delivery, usually because of missed doses of medication. Then, in the first few weeks after delivery, doses may need to be decreased to avoid toxic levels.

Pregnancy Complications

Several studies have documented that the risk of complications is approximately 1.5–3.0 times greater in women with epilepsy than without epilepsy. The possible complications are toxemia, preeclampsia, bleeding, anemia, placental abruption, and premature labor. Although most women with epilepsy have a normal labor and delivery, rates of prolonged labor and bleeding at delivery are increased. Anticonvulsants, particularly phenytoin, are suspected to weaken uterine muscle contractility and interfere with coagulation factors.

Fetal Complications

Maternal epilepsy has an unfavorable effect on the fetus. Perinatal mortality is increased up to threefold. The healthy fetus is remarkably tolerant to maternal tonic-clonic convulsions, but generalized tonic-clonic seizures and trauma from falls may cause fetal injury and premature labor. Generalized tonic-clonic seizures during labor can cause a transient fetal asphyxia.

Newborns exposed to anticonvulsant drugs during gestation are at risk for hemorrhagic disease. Deficiencies of vitamin K–dependent clotting factors are associated with several anticonvulsant drugs and especially with polytherapy. Some experts believe that women on anticonvulsant drugs should be treated prophylactically with vitamin K_1 (20 mg/day) during the last week of pregnancy. Others disagree and believe that routine intramuscular (IM) vitamin K administration to the newborn is satisfactory.

Congenital malformations are the most frequently reported and intensively studied of the adverse outcomes in infants of mothers with epilepsy (Yerby 1997). The risk of congenital malformations in newborns of mothers with epilepsy is 5–7%, compared with 1–3% in the general population. The contribution of anticonvulsant drugs to increased risk is an important question. The four major anticonvulsant drugs in common use (phenytoin, carbamazepine, valproic acid, and phenobarbital) each have been associated with neural tube defects, congenital heart disease, orofacial clefts, intestinal atresia, and urinary tract malformations. Although conclusive evidence is lacking for any one anticonvulsant producing major malformations, the evidence suggests that polytherapy may be the major factor. Carbamazepine and valproate, however, may carry a higher risk of neural tube defects.

In addition to major malformations, infants born to mothers with epilepsy have several minor malformations and dysmorphisms. A constellation of features consisting of craniofacial anomalies, distal digital hypoplasia, intrauterine growth retardation, and mental deficiency was originally attributed to phenytoin and called the fetal hydantoin syndrome. Similar mild dysmorphic abnormalities have been associated with most anticonvulsant drugs, which suggests that the syndrome is not caused by phenytoin but rather is part of a fetal antiepileptic drug syndrome or may be caused by maternal epilepsy rather than anticonvulsant drugs (Yerby 1997). Fetal exposure to anticonvulsant drugs was considered a risk factor for later mental retardation, but studies that control for maternal factors and socioeconomic status have not supported that association.

The continuing search for mechanisms underlying congenital malformations is directed at a better understanding of the genetics of epilepsy and the metabolism of antiepileptic drugs. Some inherited forms of epilepsy may predispose the fetus to malformations or to alteration of the metabolism of drugs in a way that causes toxic metabolites, particularly epoxide derivatives, to accumulate. Folate supplementation decreases the risk of neural tube defects, and the relative folate deficiency induced by anticonvulsant drugs may contribute to the increased risk of neural tube defects in children of mothers taking anticonvulsant drugs. Folate supplementation (1–4 mg/day) for all women of childbearing age is recommended by the United States Public Health Service, who ensure this by fortifying cereal grains with folate.

Treatment of the Mother

Consensus guidelines for counseling and treating women with epilepsy who are planning pregnancy are outlined in Tables 71.6 and 71.7. Generalized tonic-clonic seizures at the time of labor and delivery are best treated with benzodiazepines because phenytoin impairs uterine contractions. If the seizures cannot be controlled, or if the mother's cooperation is impaired, a cesarean section is recommended to minimize the effects of repeated seizures on the fetus.

Magnesium is often used for eclampsia, and it appears to be more effective for treating the associated seizures than diazepam or phenytoin (Duley et al. 1995). After delivery, anticonvulsant drug concentrations are monitored and usually require downward adjustment. Although all anticonvulsant drugs appear in breast milk, breast-feeding is not contraindicated. The possible sedative effects of barbitu-

Table 71.6: Guidelines for counseling women with epilepsy who plan pregnancy

1. The risk of major malformations, minor anomalies, and dysmorphic features is twofold to threefold higher in infants of mothers with epilepsy who receive treatment with AEDs compared with the risk in infants of mothers without epilepsy.
2. A possibility exists that some of the risk is caused by a genetic predisposition for birth defects inherent in certain families. Both parents' family histories should be reviewed for birth defects.
3. Possibilities for prenatal diagnosis of major malformations should be discussed. If valproate or carbamazepine is the necessary AED, the likelihood of amniocentesis and ultrasound examinations during pregnancy should be discussed. Ultrasound examination for a variety of major malformations can be done during weeks 18–22.
4. Effects of tonic-clonic seizures on the fetus during pregnancy are not well established. However, tonic-clonic convulsions might be deleterious to the fetus, injure the mother, and lead to miscarriage.
5. The diet before conception should contain adequate amounts of folate.
6. If the patient is seizure free for at least 2 yrs (e.g., free from absences, complex partial, or tonic-clonic attacks), withdrawal of AED should be considered.
7. If AED treatment is necessary, a switch to monotherapy should be made if possible.
8. The lowest AED dose and plasma level that protects against tonic-clonic, myoclonic, absence, or complex partial seizures should be made if possible. Closed-circuit television electroencephalographic monitoring should be used if necessary.

AED = antiepileptic drug.
Source: Reprinted with permission from AV Delgado-Escueta, D Janz. Consensus guidelines: preconception counseling, management, and care of the pregnant woman with epilepsy. Neurology 1992;42(Suppl. 5):149–160.

Table 71.7: Guidelines for antiepileptic drug (AED) use during pregnancy

1. Use first-choice drug for seizure type and epilepsy syndrome.
2. Use AED as monotherapy at lowest dose and plasma level that protects against tonic-clonic seizures.
3. Avoid valproate and carbamazepine when there is a family history of neural tube defects.
4. Avoid polytherapy, especially the combination of valproate, carbamazepine, and phenobarbital.
5. Monitor plasma AED levels regularly and, if possible, free or unbound plasma AED levels.
6. Continue folate daily supplement, and ensure normal plasma and red cell folate levels during the period of organogenesis in the first trimester.
7. In cases of valproate treatment, avoid high plasma levels of valproate. Divide doses over 3–4 administrations per day.
8. In cases of valproate or carbamazepine treatment, offer amniocentesis for α-fetoprotein at 16 wks and real-time ultrasonography at 18–19 wks, looking for neural tube defects. Ultrasonography at 22–24 wks can detect oral clefts and heart anomalies.

Source: Reprinted with permission from AV Delgado-Escueta, D Janz. Consensus guidelines: preconception counseling, management, and care of the pregnant woman with epilepsy. Neurology 1992;42(Suppl. 5):149–160.

rates and benzodiazepines must be considered, however, and balanced against the absolute amounts absorbed (see Table 71.7).

PATHOPHYSIOLOGY

The pathophysiology of epilepsy is incompletely understood, but a single mechanism is unlikely, given the diversity of seizure types and causes.

Morphological Studies

Postmortem examination of the brain has been the traditional method of studying epilepsy, but epilepsy surgery has increased the amount of tissue available for study. A major problem with morphological studies is the difficulty in determining if changes are the cause or effect of recurrent seizures. This is best exemplified by mesial temporal sclerosis, which is the most common and consistent change in

specimens from patients with complex partial seizures involving the temporal lobe.

Mesial temporal sclerosis is characterized by neuronal dropout and astrocytosis of the granule cell layer of the dentate gyrus and hilar region as well as loss of CA1 and CA3 pyramidal cells (Babb and Pretorius 1997). Ischemia was thought to produce the injury and cause epilepsy, but the morphological features are slightly different from those seen after acute ischemic injury to the hippocampus. The neuropathology of mesial temporal sclerosis can be produced in animal models by kindling, which suggests that frequent seizures may be the cause rather than the effect (Sutula 1993).

Pathological studies of resected epileptic foci from temporal and extratemporal regions have shown a wide range of abnormalities. They support the hypothesis that focal pathology may be the cause of partial and secondarily generalized seizures and suggest that diffuse cortical microdysgenesis may play a role in the pathophysiology of the primary generalized epilepsies.

Epileptogenesis

The morphological abnormalities associated with epilepsy do not explain how seizures develop or propagate. The hypothesis that single or small groups of "epileptic" neurons produce abnormal electrical activity and drive normal neurons into seizure activity is being challenged by concepts involving the plasticity of normal neurons in adapting to changes in their environment.

Neuronal Plasticity

At the extremes, neuronal plasticity may be responsible for the neuronal hyperexcitability and hypersynchrony that are primary features of epileptiform activity (Schwartzkroin 1993). Neuronal plasticity has been shown in mesial temporal sclerosis and in experimental models of hippocampal injury after kindling. When neurons are lost, abnormal sprouting of fiber terminals with synaptic reorganization occurs. The pattern of reorganization is not random but occurs in a way that may support epileptic activity of the abnormal hippocampus. Although synaptic reorganization has been most extensively studied in the hippocampus, it also may play a role in epileptic activity in the cortex (Babb and Pretorius 1997).

Investigations of the mechanisms of epileptic activity are beginning to address the interplay of the intrinsic electrical properties of the neurons against a background of the activity of entire cell populations, or what Schwartzkroin has called *ensemble interactions* (Schwartzkroin 1993). The electrical behavior of the cells, which is central to the normal as well as the abnormal activity of the neurons, depends on ion conductances, primarily of sodium, calcium, potassium, and chloride. The ion conductances depend on the intra- and extracellular concentrations of these ions as well as the ionic flux across the cell membrane. Ion flux across the cell membrane is controlled by a combination of energy-dependent pumps, voltage-gated channels, and neurotransmitter-controlled channels.

Neurotransmitter Systems

Neuronal interactions depend to a large degree on neurotransmitter systems. γ-Aminobutyric acid (GABA) is the major inhibitory neurotransmitter in the brain (see Chapter 50). GABA subclass A ($GABA_A$) receptors mediate flux of chloride across the membrane, which typically produces a membrane hyperpolarization and inhibition of neuronal activity. $GABA_A$ receptor blockade produces epileptic activity in experimental models, but the role of GABA inhibition in chronic epilepsy is less clear (Schwartzkroin 1993). Benzodiazepines bind to a modulatory site of the $GABA_A$ receptor complex to increase the binding efficacy of the receptor for GABA. The GABA subclass B ($GABA_B$) receptor also produces hyperpolarization but through a different mechanism, specifically modulation of potassium channels via a guanosine triphosphate–binding protein-mediated intracellular messenger system. Many of the cortical GABAergic neurons are interneurons that participate in both feed-forward and feed-backward inhibition. These interneurons may have an important role in controlling epileptic activation of neurons.

Glutamate is the major excitatory neurotransmitter in the CNS. It activates several receptor subtypes. The N-methyl-D-aspartate (NMDA) receptor is an ionophore complex that mediates calcium flux (Johnston 1997). Antagonists of the NMDA receptor have antiepileptic activity, but several in vitro and in vivo studies suggest that the NMDA receptor has a greater role in epileptogenesis than in maintaining already developed seizures. The non-NMDA ionotropic receptors primarily mediate fast synaptic transmission through sodium and potassium flux. The role of these non-NMDA receptors in epilepsy is less clear but is under active investigation. Other neurotransmitter systems play a modulating role in epileptogenesis. In addition to abnormalities of the receptors themselves, dysfunction of neurotransmitter transport, particularly glutamate and GABA, may contribute to seizures (Meldrum 1997).

Ion Channels

The identification of an abnormality in a potassium channel as an underlying defect in benign familial neonatal convulsions highlights the importance of ion channels in epilepsy (Biervert et al. 1998). Many of the anticonvulsants influence the voltage-dependent sodium channel, and abnormalities in this channel may underlie some heritable forms of epilepsy (Meldrum 1997). Similarly, calcium channels may influence epilepsy through their role in modulating neurotransmitter release.

Ion Exchangers

Na^+/H^+ and H^+/HCO_3^- exchangers have been implicated in experimental absence seizure models (Meldrum 1997). The antiepileptic effect of carbonic anhydrase inhibitors may be explained in part by the block of the depolarizing effects of intracellular HCO_3^- with intense GABA receptor activation.

Regional Differences

Regional differences exist for seizure susceptibility and propagation. Even specific neuronal populations within regions, such as pyramidal neurons in the hippocampus or layer V cortical neurons, have a greater propensity to spontaneous bursting, possibly akin to interictal epileptiform activity (Schwartzkroin 1993). Other regions, such as the entorhinal cortex or the area tempestas in the piriform cortex, may actually be trigger zones for seizure activity. In addition to these seizure-prone regions, other regions, such as the granule cell layer of the dentate gyrus or substantia nigra pars reticulata, serve as gating regions that may control seizure spread.

GENETICS

In the last two decades, increasing attention has been directed to genetics in attempting to determine the underlying pathophysiology of several epilepsies. The hereditary basis of many epilepsy syndromes has long been suspected, but progress in identification of the molecular genetic defects has been slow. Most of the common epilepsy syndromes show complex rather than simple (mendelian) inheritance patterns, which makes linkage analysis difficult (Berkovic 1997). Linkage has been established for some rare syndromes that do follow mendelian inheritance, including benign familial neonatal convulsions (chromosomes 20q and 8q), benign familial infantile convulsions (chromosome 19q), autosomal dominant nocturnal frontal lobe epilepsy (20q), and partial epilepsy with auditory features (chromosome 10q). The precise genetic defect has been determined for benign familial neonatal convulsions (potassium-channel gene located on chromosome 20q) and for autosomal dominant nocturnal frontal lobe epilepsy (α_4 subunit of the neuronal nicotinic acetylcholine receptor located on chromosome 20q) (Berkovic 1997; Biervert et al. 1998). Similarly, a defect in cystatin B occurs in Unverricht-Lundborg disease, but how this contributes to the myoclonic epilepsy is not clear (Berkovic 1997). Other genes will certainly be determined. Understanding the gene function or abnormal gene product will provide a foundation for understanding the pathophysiology of epilepsy.

EVALUATION OF SEIZURES

History and Physical Examination

The initial evaluation of a patient with suspected seizures begins with a thorough history and physical examination. In many cases, the history must be supplemented with information from witnesses who have not accompanied the patient. The patient usually has no recall for the seizure but brings an account by witnesses who have no medical training and may have been so unnerved by the seizure that they cannot accurately provide precise details. An inadequate or faulty description of the event is the leading cause of misdiagnosis; nonepileptic spells are often thought to be epileptic, and epileptic seizures are thought to be nonepileptic spells. A home videotape of the spell often can resolve the issue.

The review of the past history in children and adults should include birth history, developmental milestones, early seizures, history of febrile seizures, and events such as head trauma or CNS infection. Family history of seizures should be thoroughly investigated, often requiring contact with grandparents and children. Finally, a medial history and review of systems should be directed at conditions that have a high likelihood of causing seizures.

On physical examination, special attention should be directed toward careful examination of the skin for neurocutaneous disorders (see Chapter 69), dysmorphic features for chromosome disorders, and subtle impairments or asymmetries of fine motor skills and coordination, indicating CNS abnormalities that cause the seizures.

Electroencephalogram

The EEG remains central to the diagnosis of epilepsy. Routine EEGs generally last 20–40 minutes and represent only a snapshot of brain activity. They can be normal, even in patients with established seizure disorders (Chabolla and Cascino 1997). When the EEG is abnormal, it is useful to localize the epileptogenic region in patients with partial seizures and to classify seizures, particularly in the case of absence versus complex partial seizures. Routine EEG should be recorded during wakefulness and sleep to maximize the chance of seeing epileptiform activity.

Prolonged Recordings

It was previously good practice to repeat the study when the initial routine EEG was not diagnostic. The use of ambulatory recordings is now a better strategy. They allow prolonged recordings and increase the chance of capturing abnormal interictal activity or actual seizures. The main limitation of these systems is the often limited number of channels available (generally 8–16), the lack of visual correlation with clinical behavior, and the frequent presence of artifacts.

When the diagnosis remains in doubt, inpatient evaluation with continuous video and EEG monitoring should be considered. Most units use time-synchronized video and EEG recording, usually in combination with computer-enhanced analysis of the recording. Patients are evaluated for days to weeks to capture a sufficient number of events to correlate clinical events and EEG activity. A computerized system decreases reliance on the vast amounts of paper generated by traditional EEG machines and also enhances data analysis. Many monitoring units have 32, 64, or more EEG recording channels; this permits adding leads to the standard International Ten–Twenty System that are often of benefit in localizing the seizure focus.

Intracranial Monitoring

More precise localization of the epileptogenic region is often required in patients with intractable seizures who are being considered for surgery (Wyler 1994). The most commonly used invasive methods for intracranial monitoring are (1) depth electrodes, (2) epidural or subdural grid electrodes, and (3) subdural strip electrodes. Depth electrodes are fine wires that are specially insulated, except at recording points. The recording points are spaced such that, when the electrodes are inserted into the brain, activity can be measured from both the deep nuclei and the cortical surface. Depth electrodes are especially suited for recording activity from medial temporal structures, such as the amygdala and hippocampus, and from the basal frontal region.

Epidural or subdural grids and subdural strips are designed for recording over the surface of the brain. The electrodes are embedded in plastic sheets or strips with spacing of approximately 0.5–1.0 cm between electrodes. When the arrays are surgically placed over the surface of the brain, the electrodes can be used for recording electrical activity. When placed subdurally, the electrodes also can be used for cortical stimulation and functional mapping, which allow extraoperative localization of regions (such as motor, sensory, or language areas) that the surgical team wishes to avoid removing during surgery.

The use of implanted electrodes has a complication rate of approximately 4%. Problems include hematoma, infection, severe headaches, irritative meningitis, and difficulty removing electrodes.

Magnetoencephalography

Magnetoencephalography (MEG) measures the extracranial magnetic fields produced by electrical current, mostly intracellular, within the brain (Ebersole 1997). The currents are extremely small, requiring special sensors that detect and convert the magnetic field into current and output voltage. The technique noninvasively measures tangential source activity and can be used for dipole source localization, as can EEG. In many ways, MEG and EEG are complementary, and source modeling in epilepsy evaluations can combine the two techniques. At present, MEG remains very expensive and has limited availability.

Neuroimaging

Neuroimaging has become increasingly important in the diagnosis and management of epilepsy, especially in patients with intractable seizures who are being considered for surgery (see Chapter 38). Computed tomography (CT), the first of the new imaging modalities, has been important in the identification of tumors or other major structural changes that can cause seizures, but CT scans are normal in most patients with epilepsy. Developments in magnetic resonance imaging (MRI), single-photon emission CT (SPECT), and positron emission tomography (PET) have opened up new opportunities for noninvasive brain imaging (Jackson 1994; Spencer 1994).

Magnetic Resonance Imaging

MRI has become the most important imaging technique in the evaluation of the patient with seizures, particularly the partial epilepsies. High-resolution structural scanning can assist in the detection of pathological abnormalities in up to 90% of patients with intractable epilepsy (Jackson 1994). MRI is particularly useful in the diagnosis of mesial temporal sclerosis and hippocampal atrophy ipsilateral to the epileptogenic region. Detection of abnormalities in the hippocampus has begun to approach the resolution seen with microscopic analysis. Concordance of MRI abnormalities and EEG findings also approaches 90% with temporal lobe epilepsy, but it is less with extratemporal abnormalities (Spencer 1994). This may change as more attention is directed toward neocortical dysplasia and other abnormalities.

Magnetic Resonance Spectroscopy

Magnetic resonance spectroscopy (MRS) technology remains in the investigational phases with respect to epilepsy. Proton (^{1}H) signals distinguished from water on the basis of frequency and chemical shift permits detection of various brain substances, such as N-acetyl aspartate (NAA), creatine plus phosphocreatine choline–containing compounds, as well as other compounds, such as lactate, glutamate, and GABA (Jackson 1994). Multiple lines of evidence suggest that in the brain, NAA is located almost entirely within neurons. Reductions in NAA signal intensity in the temporal lobes ipsilateral to the seizure focus in patients with epilepsy compared with controls are consistent with neuronal loss in the affected regions. Sodium flux measured with sodium-23 spectroscopy and changes in high-energy metabolites monitored with phosphorus-31 spectroscopy will further extend the role of MRS.

Functional Magnetic Resonance Imaging

Functional MRI (also in the investigational stages) indirectly measures neuronal function based on changes in blood flow and the oxygen content of venous blood. Cortical activation can be detected during a variety of cognitive tasks as well as during seizures (Jackson 1994). This technique will play an increasingly important role in the management of epilepsy.

Positron Emission Tomography

PET and SPECT permit physiological evaluation of patients with epilepsy. PET uses positron-emitting isotopes, including carbon-11, nitrogen-13, oxygen-15, and fluorine-18. Most studies in humans with epilepsy have examined cerebral metabolism with fluorodeoxyglucose. Hypometabolic areas in the interictal period correlate well with areas of seizure onset in the temporal lobe documented with EEG (Spencer 1994). Some cases show multiple areas of hypometabolism. PET studies using neurotransmitter receptor markers may allow even more precise localization of the seizure focus. PET is an expensive study and requires a cyclotron to make isotopes and a large support staff. Only a few research centers have the instrument.

Single-Photon Emission Computed Tomography

SPECT also allows for functional imaging of the brain but uses ordinary gamma-emitting isotopes and scanners that are relatively inexpensive compared to those used for PET studies (Spencer 1994). The resolution of SPECT generally is inferior to PET, but scans using hexamethylpropyleneamineoxime (HMPAO) label with technetium-99 are satisfactory for epilepsy studies. Interictal SPECT, like PET, shows hypometabolism in the areas of seizure focus but with a relatively low sensitivity when correlated with EEG localization. Flumazenil SPECT, targeting benzodiazepine receptors, may be superior to technetium-99-HMPAO SPECT. SPECT studies obtained after injection during a seizure (ictal SPECT) show increased metabolism in the area of the seizure focus. Ictal SPECT is superior to interictal SPECT in localization of a seizure focus. The availability of newer radiopharmaceuticals with greater stability has made ictal studies easier.

TREATMENT

The decision to initiate prophylactic anticonvulsant drug therapy requires careful assessment of the probability and risks of continued seizures against the risks and benefits of the medication. Other than the benign epilepsies of childhood, epilepsy usually is a chronic condition that does not remit spontaneously, and treatment is required.

The overall risk of seizure recurrence after a first unexplained seizure ranges from 27% to 80% (Sander 1993). After a second seizure, the risk of further seizures increases to 80–90%. Treatment after a first seizure risks exposing an individual to unneeded medication and must be balanced against the danger of further seizures in that individual. Of course, the risk of recurrence is not uniform in all epileptic syndromes and conditions. The important risk factors for seizure recurrence are pre-existing neurological conditions, partial seizures, and epileptiform discharges on the interictal EEG.

Principles of Drug Therapy

The likelihood of achieving seizure control without drug toxicity is greatly increased by following these basic principles (Pippenger and Lesser 1994):

1. Use a single drug whenever possible.
2. Increase the dose of that drug to either seizure control or toxicity (decreasing the dose if toxicity occurs).
3. If a drug does not control seizures without toxicity, switch to another appropriate drug used alone, and again increase the dose until seizure control occurs or toxicity intervenes.
4. Remember that the "therapeutic range" is a guideline and not an absolute. Some patients achieve seizure control with blood concentrations below the range, and others tolerate concentrations above the range without toxicity.
5. Consider using two drugs only when monotherapy is unsuccessful. Keep in mind that some patients may have more seizures when taking two drugs rather than one drug because of drug interactions.

6. Be aware that the ability to metabolize anticonvulsant drugs is different in the young, the elderly, pregnant women, and people with certain chronic diseases, especially hepatic and renal disease, than in healthy, nonpregnant adults.

Antiepileptic Drugs

Benzodiazepines

Benzodiazepines are heterocyclic compounds originally used clinically as anxiolytic agents. In 1965, diazepam was shown to effectively treat status epilepticus (Henriksen 1998). Most of the benzodiazepines in clinical use are benzo-1,4-diazepines, except for clobazam, which is a benzo-1,5-diazepine. The primary mechanism of anticonvulsant action of these drugs appears to be through binding to a modulatory site on the $GABA_A$ receptor. Benzodiazepines enhance GABA-dependent chloride conductance, hyperpolarizing the neuron, which produces inhibition.

Metabolism. Alterations in the structure of the benzodiazepine ring through the changing of side group substitutions modifies the pharmacokinetic properties. One important factor is the lipid solubility of the various compounds—a critical factor in the medications administered by IV route. Diazepam and midazolam are very lipophilic, which allows them to cross rapidly into the brain, but they have a relatively short duration of action due to rapid redistribution. Lorazepam is less lipophilic, but its volume of distribution is less; thus, it has a longer duration of action. The rapid redistribution of these compounds, however, results in a long elimination half-life. With repeated doses, side effects become cumulative. The other benzodiazepines are not all universally available in IV preparations. All the compounds are metabolized in the liver.

Administration. The main indication for the benzodiazepines in epilepsy is in the treatment of status epilepticus (see Status Epilepticus, earlier in this chapter). Diazepam and lorazepam are commonly administered by the IV route. Midazolam is water soluble at physiological pH, but it becomes lipid soluble after injection (Shorvon 1998). It is the only benzodiazepine that produces consistent tissue levels after IM administration, and it can be effective in situations in which IV or rectal administration is not possible. Diazepam, lorazepam, and midazolam can all be administered by continuous IV infusion in an intensive care setting for refractory status epilepticus. The major adverse effects of IV or IM administration of these drugs are respiratory depression and sedation.

Rectal administration of benzodiazepines, particularly diazepam, is available for individuals with demonstrated tendency to develop status epilepticus or frequent, repeti-

Table 71.8:   Antiepileptic drugs approved for use in North America, Europe, or Japan

Drug	Absorption	Protein binding (%)	Elimination half-life (hrs)	Route of elimination	Adult starting dose (mg)	Adult maintenance dose (range in mg)	No. of doses/day	Target plasma drug concentration (range µg/ml)
Carbamazepine	Slow	70–80	8–24	Hepatic	200	400–2,000	1–4[a]	6–12
Ethosuximide	Rapid	0	20–60	Hepatic	500	500–2,000	1 or 2	40–100
Felbamate	Rapid	22–25	20–23	90% Renal	400–800	2,800–4,800	2–4	Not defined
Gabapentin	Dose related	0	5–7	Renal	300	1,200–2,400	3–4	Not defined
Lamotrigine	Rapid	54	25[c]	Hepatic	25–50[b]	Up to 700[b]	2	Not defined
Oxcarbazepine	Rapid	40	8–24	Hepatic	600	1,200–2,400	2–3	Not defined
Phenobarbital	Slow	48–54	72–144	Hepatic	60	60–250	1 or 2	10–40
Phenytoin	Slow	90–93	9–40	Hepatic	200	100–700	1 or 2	10–20
Primidone	Rapid	20–30	4–12	Hepatic	250	250–1,500	1 or 2	5–12[d]
Tiagabine	Rapid	96	6–8	Hepatic	4–8	32–56	3–4	Not defined
Topiramate	Rapid	10–20	20–24	70% Renal	50	400–1,000	2	Not defined
Valproic acid	Rapid	88–92	7–17	Hepatic	500	500–3,000	2 or 3	50–100[e]
Vigabatrin	Rapid	Minimal	4–8[f]	Renal	1,000	Up to 3 g	2	Not defined
Zonisamide	Rapid	38–40	50–68	Hepatic	100–200	400–600	2	Not defined

[a]Only one to two doses required with modified-release preparations.
[b]With valproic acid, 25 mg every other day; increase by 25 mg/day every other day and increase by 25 mg/day every 1–2 wks. Maintenance dose is 100–150 mg/day.
[c]With enzyme inducers, 12–14 hrs; with valproic acid, 60 hrs.
[d]Phenobarbital level 20–40 µg/ml.
[e]Commonly published values, but many patients tolerate higher levels without discernible side effects.
[f]Effective action longer due to irreversible inhibition of γ-aminobutyric acid-transaminase.
Source: Reprinted with permission from MJ Brodie, MA Dichter. Antiepileptic drugs. N Engl J Med 1996;334:168–175; and MA Dichter, MJ Brodie. New antiepileptic drugs. N Engl J Med 1996;334:1583–1590.

tive seizures (Henriksen 1998). With appropriate training, family or caregivers of individuals with epilepsy can give rectal diazepam at home and thus decrease the need for emergency department treatment of seizures. Patients using this mode of therapy should be followed closely by a physician well versed in the use, and potential for misuse, of rectal administration of benzodiazepines.

The benzodiazepines also can be used for long-term therapy. Clonazepam and nitrazepam are effective as prophylactic therapy for several seizure types but are used commonly for the treatment of Lennox-Gastaut syndrome, myoclonic epilepsy, and infantile spasms. They are used in combination with other drugs. Clorazepate usually is ineffective by itself and is used for adjunctive therapy. Clobazam originally was expected to be more effective, less sedating, and with decreased tendency toward the development of tolerance, but its spectrum of activity and side effects may be similar to the other benzodiazepines (Henriksen 1998).

Adverse effects are drowsiness, ataxia, diplopia, blurred vision, personality changes, irritability, memory disturbances, hypotonia, and hypersecretion in children. Additionally, tolerance may develop to the anticonvulsant effects as well as to the side effects. Cross-tolerance can occur between different benzodiazepines. Finally, dependence occurs, and abrupt discontinuation of benzodiazepines can cause withdrawal symptoms and seizures. In general, no

clear correlation exists between plasma levels of these compounds and their therapeutic effect (Henriksen 1998). Following levels on a regular basis is not warranted.

Carbamazepine

Carbamazepine is structurally related to tricyclic antidepressants. In the United States, it was originally approved for treatment of trigeminal neuralgia, but its antiepileptic activity has been well established for treatment of partial and generalized tonic-clonic seizures. It is not effective against and may even exacerbate absence and myoclonic seizures. Carbamazepine acts by preventing repetitive firing of action potentials in depolarized neurons through blockade of voltage-dependent sodium channels (Brodie and Dichter 1996).

Metabolism.   Absorption of carbamazepine from the gastrointestinal tract is moderately slow (Table 71.8). Hepatic metabolism produces an epoxide metabolite, which itself has anticonvulsant activity. Carbamazepine induces its own hepatic metabolism, so that the starting half-life of 24 hours falls by more than one-half during the first 20–30 days of treatment. Increments in the dose after the first month are often necessary to maintain a therapeutic effect. Carbamazepine has significant, complex, and often unpredictable interactions with other antiepileptic medications and a wide range of other drugs, including corticosteroids, theophylline, haloperidol, warfarin, and estrogen-containing oral contraceptives. Most women on oral contraceptive and carbamazepine require a higher estrogen dose. Even with this change, carbamazepine and other enzyme-inducing antiepileptic drugs may render the oral contraceptives ineffective. Furthermore, a number of drugs inhibit carbamazepine metabolism, and coadministration can precipitate dose-related carbamazepine toxicity. This occurs particularly with cimetidine, propoxyphene, diltiazem, clarithromycin, erythromycin, isoniazid, and verapamil. Carbamazepine also may interact with lithium to produce confusion, drowsiness, ataxia, tremor, and hyperreflexia without a change in the level of either drug (Brodie and Dichter 1996).

Administration. In adults, a starting dose of 200 mg is often necessary to minimize CNS side effects. The dose is increased gradually over days to weeks. In the maintenance phase, high peak plasma concentrations can produce intermittent CNS side effects within a couple hours of drug administration. At least three-times-daily dosing of a regular preparation or twice-daily administration of an extended release preparation may be necessary. Dose-related CNS side effects include diplopia, dizziness, headache, nausea, and somnolence. This neurotoxicity often occurs at the initiation of therapy unless a lower dose is started and gradually increased over days to weeks. Other side effects are an allergic morbilliform rash, which can progress to a Stevens-Johnson syndrome; a reversible mild leukopenia; and an antidiuretic hormone–like action, which causes fluid retention and hyponatremia. Toxic hepatitis, orofacial dyskinesia, cardiac arrhythmia, and severe idiosyncratic blood dyscrasias are rare. The severe hematological reactions cannot be predicted by routine blood monitoring.

Ethosuximide

Ethosuximide is used in the treatment of uncomplicated absence seizures. It is not effective in the treatment of generalized tonic-clonic seizures that may accompany absence seizures, and valproic acid is preferred in such cases. It acts by reducing low-threshold, transient, voltage-dependent calcium conductance in thalamic neurons (Brodie and Dichter 1996).

Metabolism. Ethosuximide has rapid bioavailability, is not significantly bound to plasma proteins, and is metabolized in the liver with approximately 25% excreted unchanged. Hepatic enzyme inducers, such as carbamazepine and phenytoin, and enzyme inhibitors, such as valproic acid, affect the levels.

Administration. In children older than 6 years, a usual starting dose of ethosuximide is 500 mg in at least two divided doses, with gradual increases up to 2 g per day,

depending on the clinical response and EEG response. Adverse effects are gastrointestinal (nausea, vomiting, abdominal pain) or CNS related (lethargy, dizziness, ataxia, psychosis) (Brodie and Dichter 1996).

Felbamate

Felbamate was approved for clinical use the United States in 1993 for adults with partial seizures and as add-on therapy in children with Lennox-Gastaut syndrome. In 1994, however, cases of aplastic anemia and hepatotoxicity were reported; therefore, its use has been greatly restricted. The mechanism of action is not completely understood, but felbamate reduces sodium currents, enhances the inhibitory action of GABA, and blocks NMDA receptors (Dichter and Brodie 1996).

Metabolism. Felbamate is well absorbed from the gastrointestinal tract and has linear absorption and elimination (Dichter and Brodie 1996). Most of the drug is excreted in the urine unmetabolized. Felbamate does not appear to induce its own metabolism. Its half-life is approximately 20 hours after both single dosing and chronic administration. Protein binding is 22–25%, so that protein-binding interactions are unlikely. Felbamate has significant interactions with other anticonvulsant drugs. Valproic acid increases the concentration of felbamate; carbamazepine and phenytoin decrease its concentration. Felbamate increases the blood concentration of phenytoin and valproic acid by reducing their clearance. The interaction with carbamazepine is more complex: Carbamazepine blood concentrations are reduced, but the epoxide metabolite concentration is increased.

Administration. Due to the risks of aplastic anemia and hepatotoxicity, the United States Food and Drug Administration recommends that felbamate be given only to patients who have seizures that are refractory to treatment with all other medications and in whom the risk-benefit considerations warrant its use (Dichter and Brodie 1996). Additional common side effects are headache, nausea, weight loss, dyspepsia, vomiting, dizziness, and insomnia.

Gabapentin

Gabapentin is effective for the treatment of partial and secondarily generalized tonic-clonic seizures. Designed as a structural analogue of GABA, it does not appear to act directly at GABA-binding sites in the CNS but seems to have a distinct binding site (Dichter and Brodie 1996). The mechanism of action is unknown, although it appears to inhibit voltage-dependent sodium currents, and it may enhance the release or activity of GABA.

Metabolism. Absorption through the gastrointestinal tract depends on an active L-amino acid transport system.

Bioavailability is dose dependent and deviates from proportionality at dosages exceeding 1.8 g per day (Mclean 1994). The drug is not significantly protein bound nor is it metabolized in the liver, and it is eliminated through the kidneys as unchanged drug. The half-life, which does not change with chronic treatment, is approximately 5–7 hours.

Administration.   Gabapentin does not affect the metabolism of other antiepileptic agents and is ideally suited as an add-on agent in the treatment of partial and secondarily generalized seizures. Adverse effects are fatigue, nausea, somnolence, dizziness, slurred speech, and unsteady gait. These adverse effects are usually mild, and hematological abnormalities are not reported.

Lamotrigine

Lamotrigine is similar in structure to drugs that inhibit dihydrofolate reductase. It has relatively weak antifolate activity. It is effective against partial and generalized tonic-clonic seizures, but it is also effective for other seizure types associated with the Lennox-Gastaut syndrome. Structurally different from carbamazepine or phenytoin, it also inhibits voltage-dependent sodium currents (Dichter and Brodie 1996).

Metabolism.   Gastrointestinal absorption is complete. The drug is approximately 55% protein bound. It undergoes hepatic metabolism and is excreted in the urine as the 2-*N*-glucuronide metabolite. The half-life during monotherapy is approximately 30 hours. When used in combination with carbamazepine or phenytoin, half-life decreases to approximately 15 hours. In contrast, valproic acid inhibits metabolism of lamotrigine and increases the half-life to approximately 60 hours (Ramsay 1993). Lamotrigine does not affect the metabolism or plasma levels of carbamazepine, phenytoin, phenobarbital, primidone, or valproate.

Administration.   The starting dose of lamotrigine needs to be low, gradually building up over 6–8 weeks to minimize the risk of developing a rash that can progress to Stevens-Johnson syndrome. The risk seems to be higher in children. Other adverse effects are drowsiness, dizziness, unsteady gait, headache, tremor, and nausea. Some patients report a sense of well-being on the medication that is separate from the anticonvulsant effect.

Oxcarbazepine

Oxcarbazepine is a keto-homologue of carbamazepine. Effectively, it is a prodrug of carbamazepine, and it has a similar spectrum of antiepileptic activity (Dichter and Brodie 1996). The altered structure changes the metabolism of the drug.

Metabolism.   Oxcarbazepine is reduced almost completely in the liver to a monohydroxylated derivative, in contrast to carbamazepine, which is oxidized to an epoxide derivative. Elimination of oxcarbazepine occurs through renal excretion and glucuronidation of the monohydroxylated derivative. Oxcarbazepine does not induce its own metabolism. Preliminary observations indicate little interaction with other drugs or anticonvulsants.

Administration.   Dosing is similar to carbamazepine. The adverse effects of oxcarbazepine are similar to those of carbamazepine but are less frequent and less severe. The exception is the antidiuretic effect, which seems to occur at least as frequently as with carbamazepine (Dichter and Brodie 1996).

Phenobarbital

Phenobarbital is the oldest of the commonly used antiepileptic drugs with established efficacy against partial and generalized tonic-clonic seizures. Its mechanism of action is to prolong inhibitory postsynaptic potentials by increasing the mean chloride-channel opening time and duration of GABA-induced bursts of neuronal activity (Brodie and Dichter 1996).

Metabolism.   The half-life is 72–96 hours in adults and longer in children (Brodie and Dichter 1996). It is moderately protein bound, but it induces hepatic enzymes, causing significant interactions with the metabolism of other drugs.

Administration.   One major advantage of phenobarbital, along with phenytoin, is that it can be administered intravenously for treatment of status epilepticus. In chronic therapy, however, side effects limit its role as a first-line agent. The common adverse reactions are sedation or a sense of fatigue and tiredness in adults and hyperactivity and irritability in children. Phenobarbital sometimes precipitates depression.

Phenytoin

Phenytoin was discovered more than 50 years ago to have anticonvulsant properties with established efficacy for the control of partial and generalized tonic-clonic seizures. It appears to act by inducing voltage-dependent blockade of sodium channels (Brodie and Dichter 1996).

Metabolism.   Gastrointestinal absorption is relatively slow and can be erratic in young children. As with carbamazepine and barbiturates, metabolism is through the hepatic P450 mixed oxidase system. The catabolic enzymes for phenytoin are saturable, which gives rise to zero-order kinetics; at the point of saturation, a small increase in the dose produces large changes in the serum concentration. Phenytoin is highly protein bound, so that systemic diseases and interaction with other drugs can change the concentration of its unbound fraction.

Administration. Phenytoin has a relatively long half-life (9–40 hours) allowing for once-daily dosing in adults and twice-daily dosing in children. Adverse effects are dose-related neurotoxicity (nystagmus, dizziness, unsteady gait, and lethargy), hypersensitivity skin reactions, gingival hyperplasia, hirsutism, and coarsening of facial features. Phenytoin causes hypocalcemia in nonambulatory patients by impairing vitamin D absorption and causes megaloblastic anemia by interfering with folate metabolism. Folate supplementation is recommended, especially in women of childbearing age. Phenytoin and other antiepileptic drugs metabolized in the liver can alter metabolism of oral contraceptive agents and reduce their efficacy.

Fosphenytoin, a water-soluble prodrug of phenytoin, is available for IV and IM administration (see Status Epilepticus, earlier in this chapter). It is less irritating than phenytoin and in many cases may be the preferable form for parenteral administration (Dichter and Brodie 1996).

Primidone

Primidone is structurally related to the barbiturates, and it is metabolized to phenobarbital and phenylethyl malonamide (PEMA). The drug itself and its metabolites have antiepileptic activity (Brodie and Dichter 1996). This allows for anticonvulsant activity at lower levels of phenobarbital, but concurrent use of other drugs may increase the rate of conversion to phenobarbital.

Tiagabine

Tiagabine appears to act by blocking the uptake of GABA, thereby prolonging its synaptic activity. In addition to the expected enhancement of inhibition, the presynaptic effects of GABA may have effects on other neurotransmitter systems, thus complicating its mechanism of action. Tiagabine appears to be effective for partial and secondarily generalized tonic-clonic seizures (Dichter and Brodie 1996).

Metabolism. Metabolism occurs in the liver through a combination of cytochrome P450 oxidation and glucuronidation in the liver. There is evidence that its metabolism is induced. Interactions appear to occur with other hepatic enzyme–inducing drugs.

Administration. In adolescents older than 12 years and adults, the recommended starting dose is 4 mg per day, with gradual 4- to 8-mg increases at weekly intervals, to 32 mg per day in adolescents or 56 mg per day for adults in divided doses. Reported side effects include tiredness, dizziness, confusion, and gastrointestinal upset.

Topiramate

Topiramate is a weak carbonic anhydrase inhibitor, which in clinical trials was effective against partial and secondarily generalized seizures. Additionally, it may have a role in Lennox-Gastaut syndrome. The mechanisms of action include blockade of sodium channels, attenuation of kainate-induced responses at glutamate receptors, and enhancement of GABA inhibition (Dichter and Brodie 1996).

Metabolism. The pharmacokinetics of topiramate are linear, and the drug is excreted essentially unchanged in the urine. As with other drugs with renal elimination, the dose must be adjusted with impaired renal function. Phenytoin and carbamazepine may enhance the clearance. Topiramate may weakly induce hepatic enzymes.

Administration. In adults, the recommended starting dose of topiramate is 50 mg, which can be increased gradually, weekly or biweekly, in 25- to 50-mg increments to 400 mg in two divided doses. Cognitive side effects can be limiting and exacerbated by too high a starting dose or too rapid an increase in the dose. Other side effects include tremor, dizziness, ataxia, headache, fatigue, gastrointestinal upset, and renal calculi.

Valproic Acid

Valproic acid is a versatile drug with demonstrated efficacy against primary generalized tonic-clonic, absence, and myoclonic seizures. It is also effective for partial seizures (Brodie and Dichter 1996). It acts by limiting sustained, repetitive neuronal firing through voltage-dependent blockade of sodium channels, although it likely has other mechanisms of action, such as enhancing GABA inhibition.

Metabolism. Valproic acid is rapidly absorbed in the gastrointestinal tract and has a half-life of between 7 and 17 hours (Brodie and Dichter 1996). Valproic acid is metabolized in the liver but does not produce enzyme induction. It can inhibit several hepatic metabolic functions, including oxidation, conjugation, and epoxidation. Furthermore, it is highly protein bound. These characteristics contribute to complex interactions with other anticonvulsant drugs. In general, valproic acid blood concentrations are lower with monotherapy than with polytherapy.

Administration. Valproic acid can be administered twice daily; more frequent administration of lower doses limits gastrointestinal side effects, especially in children (Brodie and Dichter 1996). Unlike some other antiepileptic drugs, plasma concentrations of valproic acid are not clearly related to its effect or toxicity. In clinical practice, many patients tolerate concentrations as high as 150–200 µg/ml.

Relatively common side effects are tremor, weight gain, thinning of the hair, and ankle swelling. Valproic acid formulations produce gastrointestinal discomfort more commonly than sodium valproate or divalproex sodium preparations. Sedation can be a problem, most commonly with initiation of therapy or at high doses. More severe reactions include pancreatitis, bone marrow suppression, and hepatotoxicity. The hepatotoxicity is rare in adults but can be seen on the order of 1 in 700 cases in infants less than 2–3 years of age. Its clinical features are similar to Reye's syndrome. The main risk factors for the hepatotoxicity are coadministration of other drugs metabolized in the liver and underlying inborn errors of metabolism. Mild-to-moderate chronic elevations of liver enzymes are common and do not indicate severe hepatotoxicity. Valproic acid interferes with the urea cycle and causes a mild-to-moderate increase in serum ammonia concentration, which is often asymptomatic. It also suppresses bone marrow and impairs platelet function. Valproate is a versatile drug with demonstrated efficacy against primary generalized tonic-clonic, absence, and myoclonic seizures. It is used as a second-line agent against partial seizures.

Vigabatrin

Vigabatrin enhances GABAergic action through irreversible inhibition of the catalytic enzyme, GABA-transaminase. It is effective in the treatment of partial and secondarily generalized seizures as well as infantile spasms (Dichter and Brodie 1996). The drug has been used in Europe and Canada, but introduction into the United States has been delayed due to the observation that vigabatrin produces a dose-related, reversible microvascularization of the myelin in the white matter of the brains of several animal species. These changes have not been observed in the human brain.

Metabolism.   Vigabatrin is water soluble, and gastrointestinal absorption is not affected by food. The elimination of the drug is primarily through the kidneys. As the mechanism of action is through irreversible inhibition of GABA-transaminase, the anticonvulsant effect may be prolonged and not completely dependent on the metabolism of the drug. Regeneration of GABA-transaminase activity may take 3 days or longer after discontinuation of vigabatrin.

Administration.   The efficacy of vigabatrin in controlling partial seizures has been shown in several studies. Side effects are drowsiness, dizziness, and weight gain. It may produce agitation, confusion, and psychosis; it is not recommended for use in patients with a history of mental illness (Dichter and Brodie 1996). More recently, retinal cone dysfunction has been noted with vigabatrin (Krauss et al. 1998).

Zonisamide

Zonisamide has a spectrum of activity similar to that of carbamazepine and phenytoin. The mechanism of activity is not known, but it can block sodium and calcium channels. It is available in Japan and in clinical trials in the United States.

Metabolism.   Zonisamide is well absorbed through the gastrointestinal tract. It has a relatively long elimination half-life of 50–68 hours, which is shortened to 27–38 hours in patients taking enzyme-inducing antiepileptic drugs (Dichter and Brodie 1996).

Administration.   Side effects include somnolence, headache, dizziness, and ataxia. Additionally, renal calculi can develop in a relatively high proportion of individuals taking the drug.

Choosing a Drug

Anticonvulsant drugs are primarily chosen on the basis of their efficacy against a specific seizure type. Other considerations are expense, dosing schedule, and available preparations. Generic preparations of anticonvulsant drugs generally are less expensive than brand-name drugs. However, bioavailability of different preparations of the same drug can differ greatly and cause changes in seizure control. In addition to the immeasurable effect of increased seizures on the patient, the cost of added physician visits and blood monitoring offsets the potential cost savings of the generic preparation.

Partial and Secondarily Generalized Seizures

Carbamazepine, phenytoin, and valproic acid are the first-line agents among most specialists for partial and secondarily generalized seizures (Brodie and Dichter 1996). Gabapentin, lamotrigine, oxcarbazepine, tiagabine, topiramate, and vigabatrin are new anticonvulsants that are recommended for treatment of partial seizures. Experience with these drugs is limited, and their place in relation to the more established anticonvulsant drugs is not yet defined. With increased experience, however, the newer drugs are finding an increased role in the treatment of epilepsy. Some of them may have fewer side effects or at least a different profile in some patients. Phenobarbital and primidone are effective antiepileptic drugs, but adverse side effects limit their effectiveness as first- or even second-line agents.

Primary Generalized Seizures

The primary generalized epilepsies, including myoclonic, tonic-clonic, and absence seizures, typically have their onset in childhood or adolescence. Valproic acid is accepted on empirical studies to be effective in controlling all types of generalized seizures (Brodie and Dichter 1996). Randomized controlled studies comparing valproic acid to other drugs have not been performed; however, lamotrigine and topiramate appear to have a broad spectrum of antiepileptic activity (Dichter and Brodie 1996). Felbamate similarly has a broad spectrum of antiepileptic activity, but its use has been extremely limited due to the severity of side effects. Ethosuximide and valproic acid are equally effective for treating absence seizures, but ethosuximide is not effective for treatment of primary generalized tonic-clonic seizures.

Table 71.9: Guidelines for therapeutic monitoring on antiepileptic drugs (AEDs)

A. Routine determination in all patients receiving AEDs has been suggested on theoretical grounds
 1. After initiation of AED therapy, usually some weeks later, to confirm the first value
 2. Once or twice yearly to verify compliance
 3. After each change in AED regimen (change in dosage or change of AED or other medication)
 4. In the situations listed below
B. Tailored determinations, with specific purposes
 1. When a patient complains of toxic signs, possibly dosage related, or is insidiously deteriorating, and it is not clear whether the condition is disease- or AED-related
 2. To check for compliance, when seizures are not controlled despite an adequate prescription
 3. When a patient receiving an AED exhibiting zero-order kinetics is not controlled, for calculation of the dosage increment
 4. When a particular rate of metabolism is suspected: persisting seizures despite large doses of an appropriate AED, relapse concomitant with hepatic or renal disease, with prescription of non-AEDs, and during pregnancy
 5. In polytherapy, to monitor drug-to-drug interactions (optional only when a problem of inefficiency or toxicity occurs) and also when an AED is discontinued
 6. When an abnormal ratio between total and free plasma level is suspected (e.g., in special physiological or pathological states, such as pregnancy or renal failure)
 7. When a metabolite is suspected of playing a significant role in the clinical condition

Source: Reprinted with permission from Commission on Antiepileptic Drugs of the International League Against Epilepsy. Guidelines for Therapeutic Monitoring on Antiepileptic Drugs. Epilepsia 1993;34:585–587.

Table 71.10: Blood monitoring in patients with epilepsy

Routine
 Complete blood cell count, differential white cell count, platelets
 Serum chemistry—glucose, blood urea nitrogen, electrolytes, calcium, phosphorus, magnesium, creatinine, urate, iron, cholesterol, bilirubin, alkaline phosphatase, aspartate aminotransferase, alanine aminotransferase, total protein, albumin, globulin
 Prothrombin time, partial thromboplastin time
High-risk patients
 Lactate, pyruvate, arterial blood gases
 Urine metabolic screen organic acids
 Ammonia
 Carnitine
 Specific tests for suspected underlying disease

Source: Reprinted with permission from JM Pellock, LJ Willmore. A rational guide to routine blood monitoring in patients receiving antiepileptic drugs. Neurology 1991;41:961–964.

Monitoring Anticonvulsant Blood Concentrations

The most basic principle of anticonvulsant therapy is to use enough medicine to control seizures without producing toxicity. The accurate measurement of drug concentrations in biological fluids has established therapeutic ranges, in which most patients achieve seizure control without toxicity. The ILAE guidelines for anticonvulsant drug monitoring are summarized in Table 71.9. The guidelines specifically advise against "indiscriminate" determinations of anticonvulsant drug blood concentrations and emphasize the need for logic and clinical judgment in their use (Commission on Antiepileptic Drugs of the ILAE 1993).

Monitoring for potential adverse effects is equally important (Table 71.10). Several anticonvulsant drugs cause dangerous hematological, hepatic, and even electrolyte disturbances. Routine schedules of laboratory monitoring have been recommended for virtually all the antiepileptic medications in common use. However, routine testing does not detect or prevent severe reactions, most of which are idiosyncratic. Several authorities do not recommend routine laboratory monitoring but instead suggest screening laboratory studies before starting treatment to evaluate specific medical conditions that may influence the metabolism of anticonvulsant drugs. Subsequent monitoring is guided by clinical evaluation rather than routine schedules. Exceptions are patients who cannot communicate or who live in institutions.

Discontinuation of Therapy

Long-term anticonvulsant therapy has potential morbidity: therefore, the possibility of discontinuing therapy should be balanced against the risk and danger of seizure recurrence. In general, seizures are less dangerous to children than adults because children are usually supervised and not driving. Overall, approximately two-thirds of patients remain seizure-free after anticonvulsant drugs are withdrawn (Gross-Tsur and Shinnar 1997). Several known risk factors for recurrence have been established. First and most important is the abnormal neurological or developmental evaluation. Seizures are much more likely to recur in patients with remote symptomatic epilepsy than in those with idiopathic epilepsy. Patient age is also important. The recurrence rate in children is between 8% and 40%, compared with 28–66% in adults. Among children, seizure onset before age 2 years increases the risk of recurrence when anticonvulsant therapy is stopped. Partial seizures have a very low risk of seizure recurrence when caused by benign epilepsies of childhood and a high risk when caused by a focal brain abnormality. Of the generalized seizure disorders, absence epilepsy has a favorable prognosis and JME a poor prognosis for long-term seizure control after anticonvulsants are discontinued. Most studies in children and adults have shown that EEG abnormalities, not just epileptiform activity, detected just before stopping therapy, increases the risk of recurrence. Other factors for recurrence are a long duration of epilepsy and the total number of seizures.

The importance of total duration of therapy is not established. Seizure control for 2 years and for 4 years has a similar risk of recurrence. Pediatric neurologists generally favor 2 years of seizure control before attempting withdrawal of anticonvulsant drugs, but shorter durations of treatment may be possible in some circumstances. The period in adults is more variable.

The method of drug withdrawal may affect the risk of recurrence. Abrupt discontinuation of anticonvulsant drugs is believed to be associated with increased seizures and status epilepticus. Most agree that a tapered withdrawal is advisable, but the rate at which to taper is not established (Gross-Tsur and Shinnar 1997). Indeed, the important factor for recurrence may be the absolute blood concentration rather than the rate at which the blood concentration was attained.

Other Therapies for Epilepsy

In a significant number of patients, seizures remain refractory to antiepileptic drugs. A number of agents can be used for the treatment of seizures in special circumstances.

Corticosteroids

Corticosteroids have a specialized role in the treatment of seizure disorders. Both ACTH and prednisone have been used as first-line treatment of infantile spasms (Duchowny 1994). Whether newer antiepileptic drugs will relegate these to second-line agents remains to be determined. Additionally, corticosteroids are used in refractory cases of Lennox-Gastaut syndrome and acquired epileptic aphasia. The major limitation is their severe adverse side effects.

Carbonic Anhydrase Inhibitors

Acetazolamide is used as an adjunctive therapy for treatment of Lennox-Gastaut syndrome and absence seizures (Farrell 1997b). Its mechanism of action may be to block the depolarizing effects of HCO_3^- due to intense GABA-receptor activation (Meldrum 1997).

Ketogenic Diet

The beneficial effect of fasting on seizures has been recognized since antiquity (Swink et al. 1997). In the early 1900s, prolonged fasting was used for the treatment of severe seizures. At that time, investigators recognized the ability of a high-fat, low-protein, and low-carbohydrate diet to maintain a stable state of ketosis and mild acidosis mimicking starvation. Early reports documented the effectiveness of the diet; however, the availability of antiepileptic drugs led to decreased use of the diet. In the 1990s, a resurgence of interest occurred. The basic protocol calls for a diet with a fat-to–carbohydrate-plus-protein ratio of 4 to 1 on a caloric basis. A modification of the diet uses medium-chain triglyceride (MCT) oil and allows for a greater amount of carbohydrate. The MCT oil diet is not clearly more beneficial, nor is it better tolerated. Controlled studies of the diet are limited, but in clinical practice, it is clearly beneficial in a subset of patients who have not responded to antiepileptic drugs. It is used predominantly in children. One-third to one-half of patients discontinue the diet within 3–6 months without benefit. Side effects include lethargy, abdominal discomfort, acidosis, nephrolithiasis, and the potential for exacerbation of metabolic disorders.

Surgery

Approximately 20–30% of patients with epilepsy do not respond to anticonvulsant drugs (Sander and Shorvon 1996). When medication is unsuccessful in controlling seizures, properly selected patients have an excellent chance of achieving improved or complete seizure control with surgery (Table 71.11) (Engel 1993; Vickrey et al. 1993). The completeness of seizure control correlated directly with the eventual quality of psychosocial outcome, but some patients have difficulty adjusting to life without seizures and require counseling (Lesser 1994).

Selection Criteria

The following steps are critical in evaluating the potential benefits of epilepsy surgery (Sperling 1994):

1. A precise diagnosis of seizure type and exclusion of patients with nonepileptic events.
2. Documented failure of seizure control on adequate blood concentrations of appropriate anticonvulsant drugs.
3. The seizure focus is defined in a part of the brain that can be resected with a low probability of causing a functional impairment that is worse than the intractable seizures.
4. Adequate time to establish that seizures are refractory to medical treatment. In adults, this is usually 6 months to 2 years, but in special circumstances, such as epilepsia partialis continua, less time is needed. In children, shorter waiting periods are indicated when seizures are causing developmental delay.

The decision that medical therapy has failed is not absolute but is a joint conclusion of the physician, patient, and family. Complete control of seizures is desirable but not necessary in all cases. Seizures that are infrequent or do not significantly interfere with activities of daily living, such as brief simple partial seizures or nocturnal seizures, may not justify surgery.

Several psychosocial factors affect a patient's suitability for surgery. The surgical evaluation requires considerable cooperation, and surgery should not be considered in patients who cannot cooperate fully. A history of noncom-

Table 71.11:   Seizure control after epilepsy surgery*

Operation	No. of patients	% seizure-free	% improved	% not improved
Anterior temporal lobectomy	3,579	67.9	24.0	8.1
Amygdalohippocampectomy	413	68.8	22.3	9.0
Extratemporal resection	805	45.1	35.2	19.8
Lesionectomy	293	66.6	21.5	11.9
Hemispherectomy	190	67.4	21.1	11.6
Large multilobar resections	166	45.2	35.5	19.3
Corpus callosotomy	563	7.6	60.9	31.4

*The table indicates the percentage of patients rendered seizure-free, with meaningful improvement in seizure control, or with no meaningful improvement in seizure control. The patients represent pooled data from 67 centers, accumulated as a part of the Second Palm Desert Conference on the Surgical Treatment of the Epilepsies.
Source: Reprinted with permission from JJ Engel. Update on surgical treatment of the epilepsies. Summary of the Second International Palm Desert Conference on the Surgical Treatment of the Epilepsies, 1992. Neurology 1993;43:1612–1617.

pliance with medication not only suggests that medical therapy may control the seizures but also indicates an uncooperative patient who may not comply with the presurgical evaluation. Severe behavioral or emotional disturbances may interfere with the evaluation and treatment process. Some patients and families have unrealistic expectations of surgery. Social and psychological disturbances may be related to the seizure disorder but are not necessarily cured by the surgery. Mental retardation is not an absolute contraindication to surgery, but a basic level of comprehension of the evaluation process is often necessary for surgery to be successful. Finally, patients often require significant support during the evaluation process and in the postoperative period. Severe dysfunction in the family or in the patient's support structure must be considered carefully when deciding whether to perform surgery.

Surgical Procedures

Focal Cortical Resection.   Focal cortical resections, usually involving the temporal lobe, are the most common surgical procedures for the treatment of epilepsy (Engel 1993; Vickrey et al. 1993). The term *temporal lobectomy* has become somewhat anachronistic because modern localization techniques have permitted very precise delineation of the focus of epileptic activity. The tissue removed is usually limited to only a portion of the temporal lobe, depending on the seizure focus and the underlying pathology.

In general, an anterior temporal lobectomy is performed for mesial temporal lobe seizures, but variations include an anterior medial resection or, in some cases, an amygdalohippocampectomy. When a specific structural lesion is identified, such as a tumor or malformation, the goals of surgery are removal of the abnormality and resection of epileptogenic tissue with careful attention to sparing functional tissue.

Extratemporal cortical resections are less common because extratemporal epileptic foci are less common and more difficult to localize, and resection is more likely to cause a functional deficit (Olivier 1997). Some patients with extratemporal foci do quite well.

Hemispherectomy.   Hemispherectomy is used in conditions in which the seizure focus is not localized but is limited to one hemisphere. Examples are Sturge-Weber syndrome, diffuse cortical dysplasias, hemimeganencephaly, unilateral congenital injuries, and Rasmussen's encephalitis. Hemispherectomy provides complete or partial seizure control in 60–75% of patients and may improve cognitive function by decreasing seizure frequency (Vining et al. 1997). Because the involved cortex is already dysfunctional, hemispherectomy usually does not significantly increase motor, sensory, or cognitive impairment.

Corpus Callosotomy.   Corpus callosotomy is used to interrupt pathways of spread of seizure activity rather than to eliminate the focus. Indications for callosotomy are not clearly defined (Wyler 1997). Generalized seizures, especially atonic seizures, show the greatest benefit from callosal section. Partial sectioning is often as effective, and it is not clear that complete callosotomy or even total commissurotomy is necessary for seizure control.

REFERENCES

Babb TL, Pretorius JK. Pathological Substrates of Epilepsy. In E Wyllie (ed), The Treatment of Epilepsy: Principles and Practice (2nd ed). Baltimore: Williams & Wilkins, 1997;106–121.

Berg AT, Shinnar S, Darefsky AS, et al. Predictors of recurrent febrile seizures: a prospective cohort study. Arch Pediatr Adolesc Med 1997;151:371–378.

Berkovic SF. Epilepsy genes and the genetics of epilepsy syndromes: the promise of new therapies based on genetic knowledge. Epilepsia 1997;38:S32–S36.

Biervert C, Schroeder BC, Kubisch C, et al. A potassium channel mutation in neonatal human epilepsy. Science 1998;279:403–406.

Blume WT. Focal Motor Seizures and Epilepsia Partialis Continua. In E Wyllie (ed), The Treatment of Epilepsy: Principles and Practice (2nd ed). Baltimore: Williams & Wilkins, 1997; 393–400.

Brodie MJ, Dichter MA. Antiepileptic drugs. N Engl J Med 1996; 334:168–175.

Chabolla DR, Cascino GD. Interpretation of Extracranial EEG. In E Wyllie (ed), The Treatment of Epilepsy: Principles and Practice (2nd ed). Baltimore: Williams & Wilkins, 1997;264–279.

Commission on Antiepileptic Drugs of the International League Against Epilepsy. Guidelines for therapeutic monitoring on antiepileptic drugs. Commission on Antiepileptic Drugs, ILAE. Epilepsia 1993;34:585–587.

de Bittencourt PRM, Adamolekum B, Bharucha N, et al. Epilepsy in the tropics. 1. Epidemiology, socioeconomic risk factors, and etiology. Epilepsia 1996a;37:1121–1127.

de Bittencourt PRM, Adamolekum B, Bharucha N, et al. Epilepsy in the tropics. 2. Clinical presentations, pathophysiology, immunologic diagnosis, economics, and therapy. Epilepsia 1996b;37:1128–1137.

Delgado-Escueta AV, Serratosa JM, Medina MT. Juvenile Myoclonic Epilepsy. In E Wyllie (ed), The Treatment of Epilepsy: Principles and Practice (2nd ed). Baltimore: Williams & Wilkins, 1997a;484–501.

Delgado-Escueta AV, Serratosa JM, Medina MT. Myoclonic Seizures and Progressive Myoclonus Epilepsy Syndromes. In E Wyllie (ed), The Treatment of Epilepsy: Principles and Practice (2nd ed). Baltimore: Williams & Wilkins, 1997b;467–483.

Dichter MA, Brodie MJ. New antiepileptic drugs. N Engl J Med 1996;334:1583–1590.

Dodson WE, Delorenzo RJ, Pedley TA, et al. Treatment of convulsive status epilepticus—recommendations of the Epilepsy Foundation of America's Working Group on Status Epilepticus. JAMA 1993;270:854–859.

Dooley JM. Rectal use of benzodiazepines. Epilepsia 1998;39: S24–S27.

Duchowny M. A pragmatic approach to epilepsy syndromes. Int Pediatr 1994;9:62–77.

Duley L, Carroli G, Belizan J, et al. Which anticonvulsant for women with eclampsia? Evidence from the collaborative eclampsia trial. Lancet 1995;345:1455–1463.

Ebersole JS. Magnetoencephalography/magnetic source imaging in the assessment of patients with epilepsy. Epilepsia 1997;38:S1–S5.

Engel JJ. Update on surgical treatment of the epilepsies. Summary of the Second International Palm Desert Conference on the Surgical Treatment of the Epilepsies, 1992. Neurology 1993;43:1612–1617.

Farrell K. Generalized Tonic and Atonic Seizures. In E Wyllie (ed), The Treatment of Epilepsy: Principles and Practice (2nd ed). Baltimore: Williams & Wilkins, 1997a;522–529.

Farrell K. Secondary Generalized Epilepsy and Lennox-Gastaut Syndrome. In E Wyllie (ed), The Treatment of Epilepsy: Principles and Practice (2nd ed). Baltimore: Williams & Wilkins, 1997b;530–539.

Fisch BJ. Generalized Tonic-Clonic Seizures. In E Wyllie (ed), The Treatment of Epilepsy: Principles and Practice (2nd ed). Baltimore: Williams & Wilkins, 1997;502–521.

Gross-Tsur V, Shinnar S. Discontinuing Antiepileptic Drug Treatment. In E Wyllie (ed), The Treatment of Epilepsy: Principles and Practice (2nd ed). Baltimore: Williams & Wilkins, 1997;799–807.

Henriksen O. An overview of benzodiazepines in seizure management. Epilepsia 1998;39:S2–S6.

Hirtz DG. Febrile seizures. Pediatr Rev 1997;18:5–8.

Holmes GL. Benign focal epilepsies of childhood. Epilepsia 1993;34(Suppl. 3):S49–S61.

Hosford DA, Caddick SJ, Lin FH. Generalized epilepsies: emerging insights into cellular and genetic mechanisms (Review). Curr Opin Neurol 1997;10:115–120.

Jackson GD. New techniques in magnetic resonance and epilepsy. Epilepsia 1994;35:S2–S13.

Johnston MV. Neurotransmitters and Epilepsy. In E Wyllie (ed), The Treatment of Epilepsy: Principles and Practice (2nd ed). Baltimore: Williams & Wilkins, 1997;122–138.

Kotagal P. Complex Partial Seizures with Automatisms. In E Wyllie (ed), The Treatment of Epilepsy: Principles and Practice (2nd ed). Baltimore: Williams & Wilkins, 1997;385–400.

Krauss GL, Johnson MA, Miller NR. Vigabatrin-associated retinal cone system dysfunction: electroretinogram and ophthalmologic findings. Neurology 1998;50:614–618.

Lesser RP. The role of epilepsy centers in delivering care to patients with intractable epilepsy. Neurology 1994;44:1347–1352.

Lesser RP. Psychogenic seizures. Neurology 1996;46:1499–1507.

Lowenstein DH, Alldredge BK. Current concepts: status epilepticus. N Engl J Med 1998;338:970–976.

Luders HO, Burgess R, Noachtar S. Expanding the international classification of seizures to provide localization information. Neurology 1993;43:1650–1655.

Mclean MJ. Clinical pharmacokinetics of gabapentin. Neurology 1994;44:17–22.

Meldrum BS. Identification and preclinical testing of novel antiepileptic compounds. Epilepsia 1997;38:S7–S15.

Niedermeyer E. Epileptic Seizure Disorders. In E Niedermeyer, FH Lopes da Silva (eds), Electroencephography: Basic Principles, Clinical Applications, and Related Fields (3rd ed). Baltimore: Williams & Wilkins, 1993;461–564.

Olivier A. Surgery of Extratemporal Epilepsy. In E Wyllie (ed), The Treatment of Epilepsy: Principles and Practice (2nd ed). Baltimore: Williams & Wilkins, 1997;1060–1073.

Pippenger CE, Lesser RP. Principles of Antiepileptic Drug Monitoring. Current Trends in Epilepsy: A Self-Study Course for Physicians. New York: Epilepsy Foundation of America, 1994.

Porter RJ. The absence epilepsies. Epilepsia 1993;34(Suppl. 3): S42–S48.

Ramsay RE. Advances in the pharmacotherapy of epilepsy. Epilepsia 1993;34:S9–S16.

Rogers SW, Andrews PI, Gahring LC, et al. Autoantibodies to glutamate receptor GluR3 in Rasmussen's encephalitis. Science 1994;265:648–651.

Sander JWAS. Some aspects of prognosis in the epilepsies—a review. Epilepsia 1993;34:1007–1016.

Sander JWAS, Shorvon SD. Epidemiology of the epilepsies. J Neurol Neurosurg Psychiatry 1996;61:433–443.

Schwartzkroin PA. Basic Mechanisms of Epileptogenesis. In Wyllie E (ed), The Treatment of Epilepsy: Principles and Practice. Philadelphia: Lea & Febiger, 1993;83–98.

Shorvon SD. The use of clobazam, midazolam, and nitrazepam in epilepsy. Epilepsia 1998;39:S15–S23.

So NK. Epileptic Auras. In E Wyllie (ed), The Treatment of Epilepsy: Principles and Practice (2nd ed). Baltimore: Williams & Wilkins, 1997;376–384.

Spencer SS. The relative contributions of MRI, SPECT, and PET imaging in epilepsy. Epilepsia 1994;35:S72–S89.

Sperling MR. Who Should Consider Epilepsy Surgery? Medical Failure in the Treatment of Epilepsy. In AR Wyler, BR Herman (eds), The Surgical Management of Epilepsy. Boston: Butterworth–Heinemann, 1994;26–31.

Sutula TP. The Pathology of the Epilepsies: Insights into the Causes and Consequences of Epileptic Syndromes. In WE Dodson, JM Pellock (eds), Pediatric Epilepsy: Diagnosis and Therapy. New York: Demos, 1993;37–44.

Swink TD, Vining EPG, Freeman JM. The ketogenic diet: 1997. Adv Pediatr 1997;44:297–329.

Vickrey BG, Hays RD, Hermann BP, et al. Outcomes with Respect to Quality of Life. In JJ Engel (ed), Surgical Treatment of the Epilepsies (2nd ed). New York: Raven, 1993;623–635.

Vining EPG, Freeman JM, Brandt J, et al. Progressive unilateral encephalopathy of childhood (Rasmussen's syndrome): a reappraisal. Epilepsia 1993;34:639–650.

Vining EPG, Freeman JM, Pillas DJ, et al. Why would you remove half a brain? The outcome of 58 children after hemispherectomy—the Johns Hopkins experience: 1968 to 1996. Pediatrics 1997;100:163–171.

Willmore LJ. Posttraumatic Epilepsy. In E Wyllie (ed), The Treatment of Epilepsy: Principles and Practice (2nd ed). Baltimore: Williams & Wilkins, 1997;629–635.

Wyler AR. Chronic Intracranial Monitoring Techniques. In AR Wyler, BP Hermann (eds), The Surgical Management of Epilepsy. Boston: Butterworth–Heinemann, 1994;62–69.

Wyler AR. Corpus Callosotomy. In E Wyllie (ed), The Treatment of Epilepsy: Principles and Practice (2nd ed). Baltimore: Williams & Wilkins, 1997;1097–1102.

Wyllie E, Luders HO. Classification of Seizures. In E Wyllie (ed), The Treatment of Epilepsy: Principles and Practice (2nd ed). Baltimore: Williams & Wilkins, 1997;355–363.

Yerby MS. Treatment of Epilepsy during Pregnancy. In E Wyllie (ed), The Treatment of Epilepsy: Principles and Practice (2nd ed). Baltimore: Williams & Wilkins, 1997;785–798.

Chapter 72
Sleep Disorders

Sudhansu Chokroverty

Scientific progress in the areas of sleep and its disorders has been slow. The invention of the electroencephalogram (EEG) in 1929; fundamental physiological studies to understand consciousness, sleep, and wakefulness in the 1930s and 1940s; and the discovery of rapid eye movement (REM) sleep in 1953 ushered in the golden age of sleep medicine. In the second half of this century, great advances have been made in the scientific understanding of sleep and its disorders, and sleep medicine has been established as an important clinical discipline. Awareness of the importance of sleep and its disorders is increasing among the medical profession and the public.

This chapter begins with a review of physiological changes in sleep, circadian rhythms, the function of sleep, and the neurobiology of sleepiness. It also discusses the classification of sleep disorders, the approach to a patient with sleep complaints, and a brief description of some important sleep disorders and their management. For a brief review of the basic science of sleep, which is required to understand clinical sleep disorders, see Chapter 6. For

Table 72.1: Physiological changes during wakefulness, NREM sleep, and REM sleep

Physiology	Wakefulness	NREM sleep	REM sleep
Parasympathetic activity	++	+++	++++
Sympathetic activity	++	+	Decreases or variable (++)
Heart rate	Normal sinus rhythm	Bradycardia	Brady-tachyarrhythmia
Blood pressure	Normal	Decreases	Variable
Cardiac output	Normal	Decreases	Decreases further
Peripheral vascular resistance	Normal	Normal or decreases slightly	Decreases further
Respiratory rate	Normal	Decreases	Variable; apneas may occur
Alveolar ventilation	Normal	Decreases	Decreases further
Upper airway muscle tone	++	+	Decreases or −
Upper airway resistance	++	+++	++++
Hypoxic and hypercapnic ventilatory responses	Normal	Decreases	Decreases further
Cerebral blood flow	++	++ or +++	++++
Thermoregulation	++	+	−
Gastric acid secretion	Normal	Variable	Variable
Gastric motility	Normal	Decreases	Decreases
Swallowing	Normal	Decreases	Decreases
Salivary flow	Normal	Decreases	Decreases
Migrating motor complex (a special type of intestinal motor activity)	Normal	Slow velocity	Slow velocity
Penile or clitoral tumescence	Normal	Normal	Markedly increased

NREM = non–rapid eye movement; REM = rapid eye movement; + = mild; ++ = moderate; +++ = marked; ++++ = very marked; − = absent.

in-depth information, consult a text on sleep medicine (see Further Reading and Chokroverty 1999a).

GENERAL COMMENTS ON SLEEP

The three states in the human wake-sleep cycle are wakefulness, non-REM (NREM) sleep, and REM sleep (Chokroverty 1999b). The neuroanatomical substrates as well as the physiological mechanisms of these three states are distinct, each having its own controls and functions (Table 72.1). Shortly after the invention of the EEG, sleep was subdivided into stages based on EEG criteria (see Chapter 6). Modern understanding about sleep states began after the discovery of REM sleep. In 1968, Rechtschaffen and Kales devised a system for defining and scoring sleep stages that set the standard for scientific investigations throughout the world, despite some limitations. Their system scores adult sleep; for infants, there is a different scoring system, devised by Anders and colleagues in 1971. To understand the pathophysiology of clinical sleep disorders, it is essential to know the neurobiology of sleep and wakefulness and the physiological changes that occur during NREM and REM sleep. A classic example is upper airway obstructive sleep apnea (OSA) syndrome (OSAS), in which profound physiological changes in the upper airway and respiratory control systems in the central nervous system (CNS) cause upper airway obstructive apneas and increased arousals during sleep, sleep fragmentation, and excessive somnolence during wakefulness.

PHYSIOLOGICAL CHANGES IN SLEEP

Various physiological changes occur during NREM and REM sleep that are different from those noted during wakefulness (Chokroverty 1999e). These changes are observed in somatic and autonomic nervous systems and include respiratory, cardiovascular, and gastrointestinal systems; endocrine, renal, and sexual function; and thermoregulation (see Table 72.1).

Somatic Central Nervous System

Firing rates of many neurons in the CNS decrease during NREM sleep but increase during REM sleep.

Autonomic Nervous System

During sleep, the autonomic nervous system undergoes several changes that may have implications for the pathophysiology of autonomic failure and sleep disorders in humans. Most of the autonomic changes involve respiration, circulation, thermoregulation, and pupils (e.g., pupilloconstriction during sleep). During NREM sleep, there is an overall tonic increase in parasympathetic activity, which increases further during tonic REM sleep. In addition, during phasic REM sleep, sympathetic activity decreases. Sympathetic activity during REM sleep, however, increases intermittently, which results in swings of blood pressure and heart rhythm, causing brady-tachyarrhythmias.

Respiratory

Two systems—metabolic (or automatic) and voluntary (or behavioral)—control respiration during sleep and wakefulness. Both metabolic and voluntary systems operate during wakefulness, whereas only the metabolic system operates during NREM sleep. The wakefulness stimuli that act through the ascending reticular activating system (ARAS) also act as tonic stimuli to ventilation. Activity decreases in the respiratory neurons in the parabrachial and Kolliker-Fuse nuclei in the pons, the nucleus tractus solitarius, nucleus ambiguus, and nucleus retroambigualis in the medulla. Respiratory muscle activity decreases slightly during NREM sleep but markedly during REM sleep. A marked decrement, or even temporary suppression of intercostal muscle tone, occurs during REM sleep, whereas tonic activity of the diaphragm diminishes and phasic activity continues. Muscle tone in the upper airway decreases in NREM and disappears in REM sleep, resulting in an increase in upper airway resistance. The decreased sensitivity of the respiratory neurons to carbon dioxide, inhibition of the reticular activating system, and alteration of metabolic control of respiratory neurons during sleep result in a decrement of tidal volume, minute ventilation, and alveolar ventilation. In normal individuals, diminished alveolar ventilation causes arterial carbon dioxide tension (Pco_2) to rise by 2–8 mm Hg, the arterial oxygen tension (Po_2) to decrease by 3–10 mm Hg, and oxygen saturation (So_2) to decrease by less than 2% during sleep. These blood gas changes are noted despite a fall in oxygen consumption and carbon dioxide production during sleep. Both hypercapnic and hypoxic ventilatory responses decrease during REM and NREM sleep, with a more marked decrease during REM sleep. These decrements result from a combination of factors: fewer functional medullary respiratory neurons during sleep, decreased sensitivity of the central chemoreceptors subserving medullary respiratory neurons, and increased resistance in the upper airway. Arousal responses also decrease, particularly during REM sleep. The voluntary respiratory control system may be active during some portion of REM sleep.

Respiration is therefore vulnerable during sleep in normal individuals. Mild respiratory irregularity with few apneic episodes (apnea index <5) may occur at sleep onset and during REM sleep. In disease states, however, apneas may become more frequent, prolonged, and pathologically significant.

Cardiovascular

Heart rate, blood pressure, cardiac output, and peripheral vascular resistance decrease during NREM sleep and decrease still further during REM sleep. During phasic REM, blood pressure and heart rate are unstable because of phasic vagal inhibition and sympathetic activation caused by alterations in brainstem neural activity. Heart rate and blood pressure fluctuate during REM sleep.

Cerebral blood flow and cerebral metabolic rate for glucose and oxygen decrease by 5–23% during NREM stages I to IV (see Chapter 6), whereas these values increase by 10–41% above waking levels during REM sleep. These data indirectly suggest that NREM sleep is the state of resting brain, with reduced neuronal activity, decreased synaptic transmission, and depressed cerebral metabolism. The data also are consistent with the assumption that REM sleep represents an active brain state with increased neuronal activity and increased brain metabolism. The largest increases during REM sleep are noted in the hypothalamus and the brainstem structures, and the smallest increases are in the cerebral cortex and white matter.

Because of all the hemodynamic and sympathetic alterations, REM sleep, which is prominent during the third part of the night's sleep, could initiate increased platelet aggregation, plaque rupture, and coronary artery spasm. These increases may act as triggering mechanisms for thrombotic events, causing myocardial infarction, ventricular arrhythmias, or even sudden cardiac death.

Gastrointestinal

Gastric acid secretion shows a variable response during sleep in normal individuals, but patients with duodenal ulcer show a striking increase in acid secretion and no inhibition of secretion during the first 2 hours of sleep. Swallowing is suppressed during sleep, and there is prolonged acid clearance; these factors are important in the pathogenesis of esophagitis caused by nocturnal gastroesophageal reflux. Esophageal motility is also reduced during sleep. The studies of intestinal motility during sleep are contradictory. A special pattern of motor activity, called migrating motor complex, shows a circadian rhythm in its propagation with the slowest velocity during sleep.

Endocrine Function

Profound changes in neuroendocrine secretions are found during sleep (Figure 72.1). Growth hormone secretion exhibits a pulsatile increase during NREM sleep in the first one-third of the night. Prolactin secretion also rises 30–90 minutes after the onset of sleep. Sleep inhibits cortisol secretion. Secretion of thyroid-stimulating hormone reaches a peak in the evening and then decreases throughout the night.

Testosterone levels in adult men continue to be highest during sleep, but no clear relation has been demonstrated between levels of gonadotropic hormones and sleep-wake cycle in children or adults. During puberty, gonadotropin levels increase in sleep. Melatonin, which is synthesized and released by the pineal gland and derived from serotonin, begins to show a rise in the evening, attaining maximal values between 3:00 AM and 5:00 AM, and decreases to low levels during the day.

Other endocrine changes include a maximum rise of aldosterone just before awakening in the early hours of the morning and a marked decrease of plasma renin activity during REM sleep.

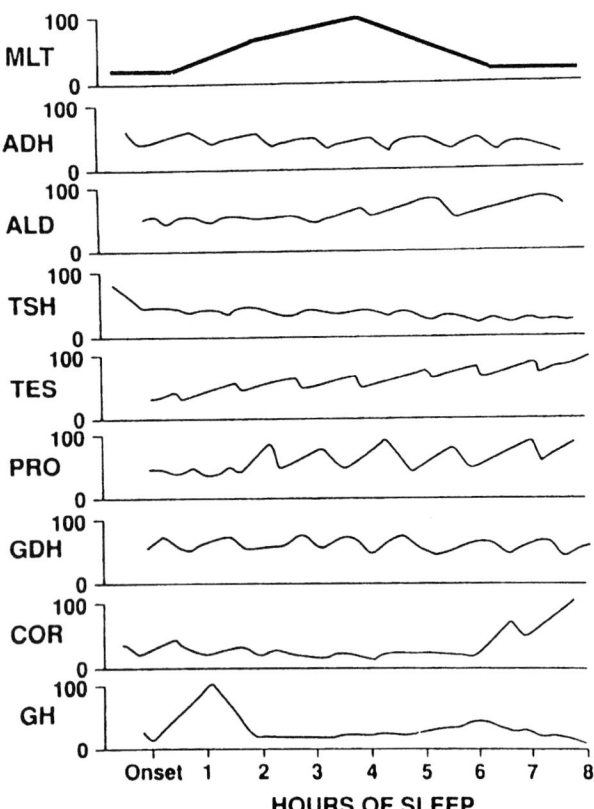

FIGURE 72.1 Schematic diagram to show plasma levels of hormones during 8 hours of sleep in an adult. (ADH = antidiuretic hormone; ALD = aldosterone; COR = cortisol; GDH = gonadotropic hormone; GH = growth hormone; MLT = melatonin; PRO = prolactin; TES = testosterone; TSH = thyroid-stimulating hormone. Zero indicates lowest secretory episode, and 100 indicates peak secretion.) (Reproduced with permission from S Chokroverty. Physiological Changes in Sleep. In S Chokroverty [ed], Sleep Disorders Medicine: Basic Science, Technical Considerations, and Clinical Aspects. Boston: Butterworth–Heinemann, 1999.)

Sexual Function

The most striking finding is increased penile tumescence in men during REM sleep. In women, there is increased clitoral tumescence during REM sleep.

Thermoregulation

Body temperature has been linked intimately to the sleep-wake cycle, but it follows a circadian rhythm that is independent of the sleep-wake rhythm. At the onset of sleep, body temperature begins to fall. Body temperature reaches its lowest point during the third sleep cycle. Thermoregulation is maintained during NREM sleep but is nonexistent in REM sleep, and experimental animals become poikilothermic. Thus, physiological responses (e.g., shivering, panting, sweating, and piloerection) to thermal stimuli are depressed or absent during REM sleep.

CIRCADIAN RHYTHMS

Circadian means a period of approximately 24 hours. The human circadian rhythm is a cycle of approximately 25 hours (range, 24.7–25.2 hours). The eighteenth-century French astronomer de Mairan noted that a heliotrope plant displayed a diurnal rhythm manifested by opening of the leaves at sunrise, even when the plants were placed in total darkness. This suggested an internal clock controlling the 24-hour rhythm. Modern scientists have confirmed the existence of circadian rhythm in human beings and other animals.

The site of the biological clock is in the suprachiasmatic nucleus (SCN) of the hypothalamus above the optic chiasm (Kilduff and Kushida 1999). Experimental stimulation, ablation, and lesions of these nuclei alter circadian rhythms. A neuroanatomical connection from the retina to SCN—the retinohypothalamic pathway—sends environmental cues of light to the SCN. The SCN serves as a pacemaker, and the neurons in the SCN are responsible for generating circadian rhythms. Several neurotransmitters have been located within terminals of SCN afferents and interneurons. Time isolation experiments have clearly shown the presence of daily rhythms in many physiological processes, such as sleep, basic rest-activity, body temperature rhythm, and neuroendocrine secretion. The most important of these is body temperature rhythm, which follows closely the circadian rhythm of sleep and wakefulness. During free-running experiments (external cues removed), the internal clock is desynchronized from the outside environment, and body temperature rhythm dissociates from the sleep rhythm as a result of that desynchronization. Dysfunction of circadian rhythm results in some important human sleep disorders, such as jet lag resulting from changing time zones, which sets off the internal circadian clock. Jet lag is more severe in those traveling eastward and in the elderly.

Melatonin, the hormone synthesized by the pineal gland, is secreted maximally during the night and may be an important modulator of human circadian rhythm entrainment by the light-dark cycle (Brzezinski 1997). Melatonin is synthesized from L-tryptophan. Tryptophan is converted to 5-hydroxytryptophan by the enzyme tryptophan hydroxylase, which is then decarboxylated to serotonin. Serotonin is then catalyzed by acetyltransferase and hydroxyindol-O-methyltransferase, and converted to melatonin. Evidence indicates that the environmental light-dark cycle and the SCN act in concert to produce the daily rhythm of melatonin production. The neural pathways involved in this process include the retino-hypothalamic tract from the retinal ganglion cells to the SCN, efferent fibers from the SCN to the superior cervical ganglia through multiple synaptic connections, and the postganglionic efferent fibers from the superior cervical ganglia to the pineal gland. This neural pathway is activated during the night, triggering melatonin production, which is suppressed by exposure to bright light. A circadian rhythm generated by the rhythmic SCN output is responsible for the melatonin circadian rhythm.

Administration of melatonin has some beneficial effects on the symptoms of jet lag as well as improving nighttime alertness and daytime sleep of shift workers. In some primary circadian rhythm sleep disorders, such as delayed sleep-phase syndrome (DSPS) and non–24-hour sleep-wake syndrome, administration of melatonin was found to be beneficial in some reports. However, placebo-controlled, double-blind studies using a large number of subjects are necessary before accepting melatonin as a treatment for various sleep disorders.

FUNCTION OF SLEEP

Several theories (Table 72.2) have been proposed to explain the biological function of sleep (Crick and Mitchison 1995; Kavanau 1997; Krueger et al. 1995; Mahowald et al. 1997).

The restorative theory suggests that sleep is needed to restore cerebral function after periods of waking. The findings of increased secretion of anabolic hormone (e.g., growth hormone, prolactin, testosterone, and luteinizing hormone) and decreased levels of catabolic hormone (e.g., cortisol) during sleep, as well as the subjective feeling of being refreshed after sleep, may support the theory of body and brain tissue restoration by sleep. The role of NREM sleep in restoring the body is further supported by the presence of increased slow-wave sleep (SWS) after sleep deprivation. The critical role of REM sleep for CNS development in young organisms and increased protein synthesis in the brain during REM sleep may support the theory of restoration of brain function by REM sleep. Although data remain scant and controversial, studies of brain basal metabolism that suggest an enhanced synthesis of macromolecules during sleep, such as nucleic acids and proteins in the brain, provide an argument in favor of the restorative theory of sleep.

The energy conservation theory is somewhat inadequate. The fact that animals with high metabolic rate sleep longer than those with slower metabolism has been cited in support of this theory. It should, however, be noted that during 8 hours of sleep, only 120 calories are conserved.

The adaptive theory suggests that sleep is an instinct that allows creatures to survive under a variety of environmental conditions.

The memory reinforcement and consolidation theory suggests that memory reinforcement and consolidation take place during REM sleep. It has been strengthened by the observation that, after REM and SWS sleep-deprivation experiments in six young adults, perceptual learning during REM deprivation was significantly less than it was with SWS deprivation. These data suggest that REM deprivation affected the consolidation of the recent perceptual experience.

The synaptic neuronal network integrity theory is an emerging theory proposing that the primary function of sleep is the maintenance of synaptic and neuronal network integrity. Intermittent stimulation of neural network synapses is necessary to preserve CNS function. The concept of dynamic sta-

Table 72.2: Biological functions of sleep

Body and brain tissue restoration
Energy conservation
Adaptation
Memory reinforcement and consolidation
Synaptic neuronal network integrity
Thermoregulation

bilization (repetitive activation of brain synapses and neural circuitry) suggests that REM sleep maintains motor circuits, whereas NREM sleep maintains nonmotor activities.

The thermoregulatory function theory is based on the observation that thermoregulatory homeostasis is maintained during sleep, whereas severe thermoregulatory abnormalities follow total sleep deprivation. The influence of the preoptic and anterior hypothalamic thermosensitive neurons on sleep and arousal can be cited as evidence for the thermoregulatory function of sleep.

NEUROBIOLOGY OF SLEEP AND WAKEFULNESS

The neuroanatomical substrates for REM sleep and NREM sleep are located in separate parts of the CNS (McCarley 1999; Steriade 1999). NREM and REM sleep generation depends on both active and passive mechanisms. Earlier in this century, sleep physiologists emphasized the passive theory of sleep, but beginning in the late 1950s, the emphasis shifted toward active sleep mechanisms. Proponents of active and passive theories base their conclusions on stimulation, ablation, or lesion experiments. Later in this century, intracellular and extracellular recordings, combined with injections of chemicals into discrete areas of the brain, were used to support the various mechanisms of sleep, which most likely result from both passive and active processes.

In cerveau isolé preparations (midcollicular transection) in cats, all specific sensory stimuli are withdrawn and animals are somnolent. In encephale isolé preparations (transection at C1 vertebral level to disconnect the entire brain from the spinal cord), such specific sensory stimuli maintained the activation of the brain, and the animals were awake. Later studies postulated that withdrawal of the nonspecific sensory stimuli of the ARAS was responsible for somnolence in cerveau isolé preparation. Wakefulness results from activation of the ARAS and diffuse thalamocortical projections. Subsequently, two preparations in the brainstem in cats challenged this passive theory (that postulates withdrawal of sensory stimuli). Midpontine pretrigeminal sections produced EEG and behavioral signs of wakefulness. Thus, it was concluded that neurons in the brain located between the midcollicular and midpontine regions are responsible for wakefulness.

The active hypnogenic neurons for NREM sleep are located primarily in the preoptic area of the hypothalamus and the basal forebrain area as well as in the neurons in the region of the nucleus tractus solitarius in the medulla. The evidence is based on stimulation, lesion, and ablation studies and recently on extracellular and intracellular recordings. The active inhibitory role of lower brainstem hypnogenic neurons on the upper brainstem ARAS was clearly demonstrated by Batini's experiment of midpontine pretrigeminal section. Similarly, electrical stimulation of the preoptic area, which produces EEG synchronization and behavioral state of sleep, supports the idea of the existence of active hypnogenic neurons in the preoptic area. Experiments showing insomnia after lesion of the preoptic region also supported the hypothesis of active hypnogenic neurons in the forebrain preoptic area. Ibotenic lesions in the preoptic region have been found to produce insomnia, and these results support the active hypnogenic role of preoptic area. In the same experiments, however, injections of a γ-aminobutyric acid agonist (Muscimol) in the posterior hypothalamus transiently recovered sleep, which suggests that the sleep-promoting role of the anterior hypothalamus depends on inhibition of posterior hypothalamic histaminergic-awakening neurons.

The concept of active hypnogenic neurons in the preoptic area was again challenged by intracellular studies of forebrain neurons. These neurons were found to be state indifferent or waking active. Other studies have clearly shown increased firing rates of basal forebrain neurons during EEG desynchronization associated with behavioral sleep. It was concluded that the idea of an active hypnogenic center or group of neurons still awaits confirmation at the cellular level. However, the search for active hypnogenic neurons should be conducted in the region of the basal forebrain rather than any other brain region because cholinergic pathways were shown to descend from the basal forebrain to the pedunculopontine tegmental (PPT) nucleus in the mesopontine junction. Sleep therefore most likely results from passive and active mechanisms.

Data clearly demonstrate that REM sleep–generating neurons are located in the pontomesencephalic region (McCarley 1999). In fact, neurons in the PPT and the laterodorsal tegmental (LDT) nucleus in the pontomesencephalic region are cholinergic and are the "REM-on" cells, which are responsible for REM sleep. The "REM-off" cells are located in the locus ceruleus and raphe nucleus; they are aminergic neurons that are quite inactive during REM sleep. Thus, a reciprocal interaction between REM-on and REM-off neurons in the brainstem is responsible for REM generation and maintenance. The cholinergic neurons of PPT and LDT project to the thalamus and basal forebrain regions as well as to the medial pontine reticular formation. These neurons are likely responsible for activation and generation of REM sleep. The forebrain cholinergic neurons from the basal nucleus of Meynert project to the cerebral hemisphere, particularly to the sensorimotor cortex. Lesions in these regions disrupt the EEG waves and elicit diffuse slow waves. The finding of cholinergic neurons at the mesopontine junction confirms the conclusions drawn after midpontine pretrigeminal transections. Transection

experiments through different regions of the midbrain, pons, and medulla clearly show the existence of REM sleep–generating neurons in the pontine cat brain. Muscle hypotonia during REM sleep is thought to depend on the inhibitory postsynaptic potentials generated by dorsal pontine descending axons.

The role of neurotransmitters and neuropeptides is not clearly delineated; they are thought to modulate various sleep stages and cycles. It has been shown that adenosine may fulfill the major criteria for neural sleep factor, which mediates the somnogenic effects of prolonged wakefulness (Porkka-Heiskanen et al. 1997).

Two major systems are thought to be responsible for arousal and cognition: (1) ARAS in the upper brainstem and its projection to the posterior hypothalamic region and (2) the system responsible for cognition in the cerebral cortex and its subcortical connections. Marked impairment of the arousal and cognition systems may result in coma or severe sleepiness. The reversibility of this state of awareness differentiates sleep from coma. There are also physiological and metabolic differences between sleep and coma. Coma is a passive process (loss of function), whereas sleep is an active state resulting from physiological interactions of various systems in the brainstem and cerebral cortex. Metabolic depression of the cerebral cortex and brainstem characterizes coma and stupor, whereas in sleep, oxygen use and metabolism remain intact.

By disrupting the arousal system or stimulating the sleep-promoting regions, focal neurological lesions may also cause excessive sleepiness. For example, lesions of the brainstem, thalamus, hypothalamus, and periaqueductal region may produce excessive sleepiness, stupor, and coma. These regions may also affect REM-generating neurons in the pons and cause various REM sleep alterations. Thus, these lesions may cause symptomatic narcolepsy.

CIRCADIAN AND HOMEOSTATIC FACTORS IN SLEEP

Sleep and wakefulness are controlled by both homeostatic and circadian factors. The duration of prior wakefulness determines the propensity to sleepiness (homeostatic factor), whereas circadian factors determine the timing, duration, and characteristics of sleep. There are two types of sleepiness: physiological and subjective (Dinges 1995). Physiological sleepiness is the body's propensity to sleepiness. There are two highly vulnerable periods of sleepiness: 2:00–6:00 AM, particularly 3:00–5:00 AM, and 2:00–6:00 PM, especially 3:00–5:00 PM. The propensity to physiological sleepiness (e.g., mid-afternoon and early morning hours) depends on circadian factors. The highest number of sleep-related accidents have been observed during these periods. Subjective sleepiness is the individual's perception of sleepiness; it depends on several external factors, such as a stimulating environment and ingestion of coffee and other caffeinated beverages. Physiological sleepiness depends on two processes: sleep factor and circadian phase. Sleep factor refers to a prior period of wakefulness and sleep debt. After a prolonged period of wakefulness, there is an increasing tendency to sleep. The recovery from sleep debt is aided by an additional amount of sleep, but this recovery is not linear. Thus, an exact number of hours of sleep are not required to repay sleep debt; rather, the body needs an adequate amount of SWS for restoration. The circadian factor determines the body's propensity to maximal sleepiness, between 3:00 AM and 5:00 AM. The second period of maximal sleepiness (3:00–5:00 PM) is not as strong as the first. Sleep and wakefulness and the circadian pacemaker have a reciprocal relationship: The biological clock can affect sleep and wakefulness, and sleep and wakefulness can affect the clock. The neurological basis of this interaction is unknown, however.

The role of various sleep factors in maintaining homeostasis has not been clearly established (Krueger and Obal 1994). Several cytokines have been shown to promote sleep in animals, including interleukin-1, interferon-α, and tumor necrosis factor. Other sleep-promoting substances, called sleep factors, increase in concentration during prolonged wakefulness or during infection. Other endogenous compounds that enhance sleep include delta-sleep–inducing peptides, muramyl peptides, cholecystokinin, arginine vasotocin, vasoactive intestinal peptide, growth hormone–releasing factor, and somatostatin. It has been shown that adenosine may fulfill the major criteria for a neural sleep factor that mediates the somnogenic effects of prolonged wakefulness.

CLASSIFICATION OF SLEEP DISORDERS

The original diagnostic classification of sleep and arousal disorders by the Association of Sleep Disorder Centers categorized sleep-wake disorders into four classes: (1) disorders of initiating and maintaining sleep, (2) disorders of excessive somnolence, (3) disorders of sleep-wake schedule, and (4) dysfunctions associated with sleep, sleep stages, or partial arousals (parasomnias). This classification has been supplanted by the 1990 *International Classification of Sleep Disorders* (ICSD), which was revised slightly in 1997. The ICSD system is the one used by sleep specialists; it lists 84 sleep disorders in four broad categories: dyssomnias, parasomnias, sleep disorders associated with medical or psychiatric disorders, and proposed sleep disorders (Table 72.3).

Dyssomnias are subdivided into intrinsic, extrinsic, and circadian rhythm sleep disorders. Intrinsic disorders result from causes in the body, whereas extrinsic disorders are primarily caused by environmental factors. Circadian rhythm disorders result from disruption of sleep-wake schedule changes.

Parasomnias are characterized by abnormal movements and behavior intruding into sleep without necessarily disturbing sleep architecture. These consist of arousal and sleep-wake transition disorders, REM-related parasomnias, and others.

Medical or psychiatric sleep disorders include those attributable to another condition; they are secondary to mental (psychiatric), neurological, and other medical disorders.

Proposed sleep disorders include disorders for which inadequate or insufficient information is available to substantiate with certainty the existence of that particular disorder.

The ICSD includes descriptive details, specific diagnostic criteria, severity, and duration. There is also coding information for clinical and research purposes.

In addition to the ICSD classification are two other systems: the *International Classification of Diseases* (ICD), ninth revision, clinical modification, and the *ICD*, tenth revision (ICD-10). The *ICD-10NA* is an expansion of *ICD-10* with alphanumeric codes for every neurological disease, including specific sleep disorders. There has been no study to assess the validity and reliability of any classification of sleep disorders.

APPROACH TO A PATIENT WITH SLEEP COMPLAINTS

The approach to a patient with a sleep complaint must begin with a clear understanding about sleep disorders as listed in the *ICSD*. Some common sleep complaints are trouble falling asleep and staying asleep (insomnia); falling asleep during the day (daytime hypersomnolence); and inability to sleep at the right time (circadian rhythm sleep disorders). Other common complaints are thrashing and moving about in bed with repeated leg jerking (parasomnias and other abnormal movements, including nocturnal seizures) and restless legs syndrome (RLS).

Cardinal manifestations in a patient complaining of insomnia include all or some of the following: difficulty falling asleep; frequent awakenings, including early-morning awakening; insufficient or total lack of sleep; daytime fatigue, tiredness, or sleepiness; lack of concentration, irritability, anxiety, and sometimes depression and forgetfulness; and preoccupation with psychosomatic symptoms, such as aches and pains.

Cardinal manifestations of hypersomnia include excessive daytime somnolence (EDS); falling asleep in an inappropriate place and under inappropriate circumstances; no relief of symptoms after an additional sleep at night; daytime fatigue; inability to concentrate; and impairment of motor skills and cognition. Additional symptoms depend on the nature of the underlying sleep disorder (e.g., snoring and witnessed apneas during sleep by a bed partner in patients with OSAS; attacks of cataplexy, hypnagogic hallucinations, sleep paralysis, automatic behavior, and disturbed night sleep in patients with narcolepsy).

Sleeplessness and EDS are symptoms; therefore, every attempt should be made to find a cause for these complaints. Insomnia may be secondary to a variety of causes. The etiological differential diagnosis for EDS may include OSAS; central sleep apnea (CSA); narcolepsy; idiopathic hyper-

Table 72.3: International Classification of Sleep Disorders

Dyssomnias	Parasomnias	Sleep disorders associated with medical
Intrinsic sleep disorders	Arousal disorders	or psychiatric disorders
Psychophysiological insomnia	Confusional arousals	Mental disorders
Sleep-state misperception	Sleepwalking	Psychoses
Idiopathic insomnia	Sleep terrors	Mood disorders
Narcolepsy	Sleep-wake transition disorders	Anxiety disorders
Recurrent hypersomnia	Rhythmic movement disorders	Panic disorders
Idiopathic hypersomnia	Sleep starts	Alcoholism
Obstructive sleep apnea syndrome	Sleep talking	Neurological disorders
Central sleep apnea syndrome	Nocturnal leg cramps	Cerebral degenerative disorders
Central alveolar hypoventilation	Parasomnias usually associated with	Dementia
syndrome	REM sleep	Parkinsonism
Periodic limb movement disorder	Nightmares	Fatal familial insomnia
Restless legs syndrome	Sleep paralysis	Sleep-related epilepsy
Intrinsic sleep disorders NOS	Impaired sleep-related penile erections	Electrical status epilepticus of sleep
Extrinsic sleep disorders	Sleep-related painful erections	Sleep-related headaches
Inadequate sleep hygiene	REM sleep–related sinus arrest	Other medical disorders
Environmental sleep disorder	REM sleep behavior disorder	Sleeping sickness
Altitude insomnia	Other parasomnias	Nocturnal cardiac ischemia
Adjustment sleep disorder	Sleep bruxism	Chronic obstructive pulmonary disease
Insufficient-sleep syndrome	Sleep enuresis	Sleep-related asthma
Limit-setting sleep disorder	Sleep-related abnormal swallowing	Sleep-related gastroesophageal reflux
Sleep-onset association disorder	syndrome	Peptic ulcer disease
Food allergy insomnia	Nocturnal paroxysmal dystonia	Fibromyalgia
Nocturnal eating (drinking) syndrome	Sudden unexplained nocturnal death	Proposed sleep disorders
Hypnotic-dependent sleep disorder	syndrome	Short sleeper
Stimulant-dependent sleep disorder	Primary snoring	Long sleeper
Alcohol-dependent sleep disorder	Infant sleep apnea	Subwakefulness syndrome
Toxin-induced sleep disorder	Congenital central hypoventilation	Fragmentary myoclonus
Extrinsic sleep disorders NOS	syndrome	Sleep hyperhidrosis
Circadian rhythm sleep disorders	Sudden infant death syndrome	Menstrual-associated sleep disorder
Time-zone (jet lag) syndrome	Benign neonatal sleep myoclonus	Pregnancy-associated sleep disorder
Shift-work sleep disorder	Other parasomnias NOS	Terrifying hypnagogic hallucinations
Irregular sleep-wake pattern disorder		Sleep-related neurogenic tachypnea
Delayed sleep-phase syndrome		Sleep-related laryngospasm
Advanced sleep-phase syndrome		Sleep choking syndrome
Non–24-hour sleep-wake disorder		
Circadian rhythm sleep disorders NOS		

NOS = not otherwise specified; REM = rapid eye movement.

somnia; several psychiatric, neurological, and other medical illnesses; drug or alcohol abuse; and periodic hypersomnolence (e.g., Kleine-Levin syndrome, idiopathic recurrent stupor, and catamenial hypersomnolence). Sometimes a patient with RLS may complain of EDS. Abnormal movements and behavior during sleep include REM and NREM parasomnias and other abnormal movements (e.g., periodic limb movements in sleep, or PLMS), some daytime movement disorders that persist during sleep, and nocturnal seizures.

The physician must evaluate the patient first based on the history and physical examination before undertaking laboratory tests, which must be subservient to the clinical diagnosis. The first step in the assessment of a sleep-wakefulness disturbance is careful evaluation of the sleep complaints. The history must include a detailed sleep history, including a sleep questionnaire as well as a sleep log or diary. It must also include psychiatric, neurological, medical, drug-alcohol, and family histories. Several scales (Stanford Sleepiness Scale, Epworth Sleepiness Scale) provide subjective mea-

surement of sleepiness (see Chapter 6). History must be followed by physical examination to uncover various causes of insomnia, hypersomnia, and parasomnias. Further details of history and physical examination are discussed in Chapter 6.

CLINICAL PHENOMENOLOGY

In this section, the clinical characteristics of selected sleep disorders are described.

Insomnia

Insomnia is a symptom rather than a disease and is characterized by an inadequate amount of sleep or impaired quality of sleep. People with insomnia complain of difficulty initiating or maintaining sleep, which causes sleep that does not restore or refresh and impairment of daytime functioning. The National Institute of Mental Health (NIMH) consensus conference in 1984 divided insomnia (Chokroverty 1998) into transient (1 week), short-term (1–3 weeks), and chronic (>3 weeks). The *ICSD* includes 14 categories that may have insomnia as a prominent complaint (included under the category of dyssomnias) and can occur in intrinsic, extrinsic, and circadian rhythm sleep disorders.

Insomnia is the most common sleep disorder in the population. In one survey, 35% of adults between the ages of 18 and 79 years complained of insomnia in the past year (Chokroverty 1998). In the NIMH Epidemiological Catchment Area Study (1981–1985), 10% of the subjects responding to a sleep questionnaire had had problems sleeping for 2 weeks or more in the preceding 6 months; the problems were not related to neurological or psychological conditions. Other surveys have confirmed that insomnia affects about one-third of the adult population in the United States at one time or another, and in 10%, it is a persistent problem. The prevalence of insomnia increases with age, and symptoms were more prevalent in women than in men. There is also a higher prevalence of insomnia among persons of lower socioeconomic status; in divorced, widowed, or separated individuals; and in those experiencing recent stress, depression, and drug or alcohol abuse.

Clinical Manifestations of Insomnia

The symptoms of insomnia frequently interfere with interpersonal relationships or job performance. Decrements in daytime task performance and prolonged reaction times have been reported in patients complaining of insomnia (Chokroverty 1998). Formal cognitive and motor skill tests generally do not detect objective evidence of impairment. The NIMH Epidemiological Catchment Area Study, however, indicated an increased risk of major depression in those with chronic insomnia. A 1991 Gallup survey found that patients who report sleep deprivation due to chronic insomnia have 2.5 times as many automobile accidents as those who report fatigue from other causes. Some of these excessive risks may relate to the increasing proportion of drug or alcohol abuse with insomnia. Long-term detrimental health effects due to insomnia have not been documented, but one prospective study reported an increased chance of deaths from cancer, stroke, or heart disease among persons who reported sleeping for less than 4 hours or more than 10 hours per night (Chokroverty 1999b). These results have not been corroborated and may have been confounded by several factors.

Objective tests for sleepiness (e.g., multiple sleep latency test [MSLT]) document that insomniacs are no more sleepy than age-matched normal controls; in fact, insomniacs are less sleepy than normal controls, which suggests a hyperarousal state. These findings may also be due to an impaired perception of sleep. In one study, more than 70% of patients with chronic insomnia and more than 30% of normals reported being awake if awakened from stage II NREM sleep (Mahowald et al. 1997), and insomniacs tend to overestimate sleep latency (the deviation of time between lights-out and the onset of sleep) after nocturnal awakenings.

Causes of Insomnia

Insomnia is a heterogeneous condition that may result from a wide variety of factors. Multiple causes may contribute to insomnia in an individual, and different causes may be responsible for different types of insomnia (transient, short-term, and chronic).

Transient and Short-Term Insomnia. Factors that can result in transient or short-term insomnia are similar, but the disturbances that produce short-term insomnia are of greater magnitude. Causes of transient and short-term insomnia are listed in Table 72.4.

Jet lag is experienced after travel through several time zones, which disrupts the synchronization between the body's inner clock and external cues (Bearpark 1994). Some of these sleep problems result from "jet" factor and others from "lag" factors. "Jet" factors that may be detrimental to sleep include long periods of travel with limited mobility, dryness of the eyes, headache, fatigue, gastrointestinal disturbances, and nasal congestion. "Lag" factors result in dyssynchrony between the body's internal clock and the sleep schedule of the new environment. Symptoms are usually most pronounced when traveling west to east and are more severe in elderly individuals. Readjustment and resynchronization occur at a rate of about 1 hour per day when traveling eastward and 1.5 hours per day when traveling westward (Bearpark 1994).

Shift work may affect up to 5 million workers in the United States; it can cause sleep disruption, chronic fatigue, gastrointestinal symptoms (including peptic ulcer), an increased chance of traffic accidents, and increased errors on the job. Drug-related insomnia includes rebound insomnia on discontinuation of short- and intermediate-acting hypnotics. Other drugs that may be responsible for insomnia are listed in Table 72.4.

Chronic Insomnia. Chronic insomnia can be caused by the chronic use of drugs or alcohol; various medical, neurological, or psychiatric disorders; or a variety of primary sleep disorders (Table 72.5).

Table 72.4: Causes of transient and short-term insomnia

A change of sleeping environment (the most common cause of transient insomnia, the so-called first night effect)
Jet lag
Unpleasant room temperature
Stressful life events (e.g., loss of a loved one, divorce, loss of employment, preparing to take an examination)
Acute medical or surgical illnesses (including intensive care units)
Stimulant medications (e.g., theophylline, beta blockers, corticosteroids, thyroxine, bronchodilators, or withdrawal of central nervous system depressant medications)

Table 72.5:   Causes of chronic insomnia

General medical disorders
Neurological disorders, including fatal familial insomnia
    and post-traumatic insomnia
Psychiatric disorders
Drug- or alcohol-related insomnia
Primary sleep disorders
Primary or idiopathic (used to be called childhood-onset insomnia)
    Psychophysiological insomnia
    Circadian rhythm disorders associated with insomnia
    Sleep-state misperception
    Restless legs syndrome
    Periodic limb movements in sleep
    Inadequate sleep hygiene
    Altitude insomnia
    Insufficient sleep syndrome
    Central sleep apnea–insomnia syndrome

Table 72.6:   Medical causes of insomnia

Congestive heart failure
Ischemic heart disease
Nocturnal angina
Chronic obstructive pulmonary disease
Bronchial asthma including nocturnal asthma
Peptic ulcer disease
Reflux esophagitis
Rheumatic disorders, including fibromyalgia syndrome
Lyme disease
Acquired immunodeficiency syndrome
Chronic fatigue syndrome

Table 72.7:   Neurological disorders causing insomnia

Cerebral hemispheric and brainstem strokes
Neurodegenerative diseases, including Alzheimer's disease and
    Parkinson's disease
Brain tumors
Traumatic brain injury causing post-traumatic insomnia
Neuromuscular disorders, including painful peripheral
    neuropathies
Headache syndromes (migraine, cluster, hypnic headache, and
    exploding head syndromes)
Fatal familial insomnia, a rare prion disease

Persistent insomnia can result directly from a medical illness (Table 72.6) or indirectly from the medications required for treatment of that illness. For example, sleep disruption may be caused by paroxysmal nocturnal dyspnea in untreated congestive heart failure (CHF), whereas treatment with diuretics may disturb sleep by causing nocturia. Similar situations occur with nocturnal angina, chronic obstructive pulmonary disease (COPD), and bronchial asthma. Asthma may be exacerbated at night, with coughing and wheezing, which is related to several circadian factors (Chokroverty 1999e).

Neurological disorders causing insomnia are listed in Table 72.7. The pathogenesis of insomnia in neurological disorders may be related to direct or indirect mechanisms. For example, lesions of the hypnogenic neurons in the hypothalamic-preoptic nuclei and the lower brainstem area in the region of the nucleus tractus solitarius can alter the balance between waking and sleeping brain, causing sleeplessness. Other neurological conditions can produce pain, confusional episodes, changes in the sensorimotor system, or movement disorders that interfere with sleep. Insomnia in some neuromuscular diseases may be due to sleep-related hypoventilation with consequent sleep fragmentation. Insomnia may also be due to medications used to treat neurological illnesses (e.g., anticonvulsants, dopaminergic agents, and anticholinergics).

Insomnia commonly coexists with or precedes the development of a number of psychiatric illnesses. A large epidemiological study found that individuals with insomnia at baseline were about 34 times more likely than normals to develop a new psychiatric disorder within a year compared with individuals without insomnia (Chokroverty 1998). Insomniacs are also about 40 times more likely than normals to develop a new episode of major depression within 6 months. Individuals with insomnia that resolved within a year had a similar incidence of subsequent psychiatric disorders compared with normal individuals. Specific examples of psychiatric disorders that may be associated with insomnia include depression, anxiety disorders, and schizophrenia.

There is a high prevalence of depression among elderly individuals complaining of insomnia. Early morning awakening is considered to be the biological hallmark of depression. Adolescents and young adults with depression, in contrast, may report difficulty in initiating sleep. Characteristic findings in sleep disorders associated with depression are a short REM latency and maldistribution of REM cycle duration, with the longest nocturnal REM cycle occurring in the first one-third of the night.

Anxiety disorders are the most common psychiatric disorders and include panic, phobic, obsessive-compulsive, post-traumatic stress, and generalized anxiety disorders. Sleep may be disrupted by panic attacks, nightmares, or flashbacks, depending on the underlying anxiety disorder. Major depression coexists in many patients.

In schizophrenia, the severity of sleep disturbances is related to the intensity of psychotic symptoms. There is often extremely prolonged sleep-onset latency during the acute illness, with a reduction of total sleep time.

Primary Sleep Disorders Associated with Chronic Insomnia.
Some patients with chronic insomnia have either idiopathic or psychophysiological insomnia or insomnia as a symptom of another primary sleep disorder.

Idiopathic Insomnia.   Idiopathic or primary insomnia, previously called childhood-onset insomnia, is defined as a life-long difficulty in initiating and maintaining sleep, resulting in poor daytime functioning. The cause of this syndrome is unknown, but a neurochemical imbalance, either in the arousal (hyperactivity) or sleep-promoting neurons (hypoactivity), has been suggested but not proved.

Onset occurs in early childhood, and sometimes the syndrome runs in families. This condition should only be diagnosed after exclusion of concomitant medical, neurological, and psychiatric or other psychological problems.

Psychophysiological Insomnia. Psychophysiological insomnia is defined as a chronic insomnia resulting from learned, sleep-preventing associations and increased tension or agitation. It is estimated that about 15% of all insomniacs attending sleep disorder centers have psychophysiological insomnia. Affected individuals are overly concerned and overly focused on the problem of sleep but do not have generalized anxiety, phobic, or other psychiatric disorders. Onset of these syndromes often occurs in young adults, and symptoms persist for decades. First-degree relatives may have similar sleep problems, suggesting a possible genetic component.

The characteristic feature of psychophysiological insomnia is development of conditioned responses that are incompatible with sleep. The disorder begins in some patients during an initial period of stressful events, but the insomnia persists even after the inciting stressors have resolved. The combination of excessive worry, fear, and frustration about being unable to initiate and maintain sleep and the identification of the bedroom as a signal for arousal contribute to negative conditioning and sleeplessness. Affected patients tend to sleep poorly during polysomnographic (PSG) study, although occasional patients sleep better because they are removed from their usual sleep environment. This condition is distinguishable from generalized anxiety disorder because patients with psychophysiological insomnia have anxiety confined to issues relating to sleep. The condition tends to have a later onset than idiopathic insomnia, which typically begins in childhood.

Sleep-State Misperception. In this disorder, subjects complain of sleeplessness but without objective evidence (e.g., PSG recording of a sleep disorder). Despite complaints of no sleep or poor sleep over many years, actigraphy (a technique that measures patient activity and permits an objective assessment of sleep time) or PSG recordings document a normal sleep pattern (Saadeh et al. 1995).

Inadequate Sleep Hygiene. Good "sleep hygiene" measures promote sleep. These include avoidance of caffeinated beverages, alcohol, and tobacco in the evening; avoidance of intense mental activities and vigorous exercise close to bedtime; avoidance of daytime naps and excessive time spent in bed; and adherence to a regular sleep-wake schedule.

Insufficient Sleep Syndrome. Insufficient sleep is probably the most common cause of sleepiness in the general population. The whole society appears to be sleep deprived (Bonnet and Arand 1995), which results from various factors, such as lifestyle, competitive drive to perform that sacrifices sleep, and environmental light and sound. Chronic sleep deprivation may lead to daytime sleepiness, irritability, lack of concentration, decreased daytime performance, muscle aches and pains, or depression.

Altitude Insomnia. Altitude insomnia refers to sleeplessness that develops in some individuals on ascent to altitudes higher than 4,000 m in conjunction with other features of acute mountain sickness, such as fatigue, headache, and loss of appetite (Coote 1994). The severity of sleep disturbance is directly proportional to the height of ascent. Those who live at higher altitudes become acclimatized and tend to sleep normally, but in some, chronic mountain sickness may develop, causing sleep disturbance.

Affected patients have periodic breathing (Cheyne-Stokes) due to the stimulation of peripheral chemoreceptors by hypobaric hypoxemia. This causes hyperventilation, hypocapnia, and a respiratory alkalosis that suppresses ventilation. The abnormal breathing pattern causes repeated awakenings and sleep fragmentation, which may be exacerbated by stress, uncomfortable sleeping environment, and cold temperature. The best treatment for altitude insomnia is acetazolamide, which promotes a mild metabolic acidosis that compensates for the hypoxemia-driven respiratory alkalosis.

RLS, periodic limb movement disorder (PLMD), and circadian rhythm disorders are some of the important causes of persistent insomnia. In some patients, CSA may cause insomnia.

Narcolepsy

In 1880, the French physician Gélineau coined the term *narcolepsy* and gave a classic description of irresistible sleep attacks. He also described "astasia," which had all the clinical features of what was later termed *cataplexy*. Before Gélineau's description, however, there were isolated cases of hypersomnolence, many of which resembled narcolepsy (although some may have been EDS associated with sleep apnea). In this century, reports of large series of patients brought the entity of narcolepsy to the attention of the medical profession (Bassetti and Aldrich 1996). In 1957, Yoss and Daly listed the narcoleptic tetrad of sleep attacks, cataplexy, sleep paralysis, and hypnagogic hallucinations (Bassetti and Aldrich 1996). The modern era of narcolepsy research began in 1960 with Vogel's discovery of sleep-onset REMs (SOREMs) in narcolepsy syndrome. The observation by Honda and coworkers of the presence of HLA-DR2 and DQw1 (now called DQw15) antigens in 100% of Japanese narcoleptic patients brought narcolepsy research to the field of molecular neurobiology (Mignot 1998).

Epidemiology, Genetics, and Family Studies in Narcolepsy

There is wide variation in the prevalence of narcolepsy throughout the world, and good epidemiological studies are lacking. In the United States, the prevalence is 3–6 per 10,000; in Japan, it is 1 per 600; and in Israel, it is only 1 per 500,000.

Both genetic and environmental factors contribute to the development of narcolepsy. About 1–2% of the first-degree relatives of narcoleptics manifest the illness, compared with 0.02–0.18% in the general population (a difference of 10–40 times) (Mignot 1998). Several reports of familial narcolepsy have appeared in the literature since the first report in 1877. A positive family history of hypersomnolence and, less commonly, of cataplexy was reported in up to 50% of relatives of narcoleptics in the early studies. Early reports were based on symptoms only and not on PSG studies; therefore, cases of sleep apnea causing EDS may have been misdiagnosed as narcolepsy. Reports show that 4.7% of first-degree relatives of people with narcolepsy-cataplexy complain of EDS (Billiard et al. 1994). In view of the fact that the prevalence of EDS in the general population may be about 13%, it can be concluded that most "sleepy" relatives of narcolepsy do not have narcolepsy.

The mode of inheritance is thought to be autosomal dominant in humans, recessive in Doberman pinschers (canarc-1) and Labrador retrievers, and multifactorial in poodles.

Twin studies in narcolepsy do not suggest a strong genetic influence. Approximately 25–31% of monozygotic twins are concordant, but the majority are discordant for narcolepsy, which suggests the influence of environmental factors in the etiology of narcolepsy. Because most monozygotic twin pairs are discordant for narcolepsy-cataplexy and three discordant dizygotic twins were identified in a sample of 11,354 twins in the Finnish study, there may be an interaction of environmental and genetic factors in the development of narcolepsy (Mignot 1998).

Honda and co-workers first directed attention to an association between HLAs of the major histocompatibility complex for narcolepsy-cataplexy. The haplotypes DR15 subtype of DR2 and DQ6 subtype of DQ1 are closely associated with narcolepsy in 95–100% of white and Japanese patients (Bassetti and Aldrich 1996). In blacks with narcolepsy, DR2 antigen is found in only 65%, but DQ1 antigen is present in more than 90% of patients. It has been established that the HLA DQB1*0602 is the narcolepsy subtype gene along with the allele DQA1*0102 located nearby on chromosome 6 in all ethnic groups (Mignot 1998). However, cases of narcolepsy not carrying HLA-DR2 or DQ1 antigens have been reported (Mignot 1998). Also, 12–35% of the general population carry the same HLA alleles, but narcolepsy is present in only 0.02–0.18% of the population. Therefore, the alleles DQB1*0602 and DQA1*0102 are neither necessary nor sufficient for development of narcolepsy.

Clinical Manifestations

The syndrome of narcolepsy is a lifelong neurological condition that generally begins in an adolescent or young adult with EDS and "sleep attacks." Peak incidence occurs during the teens and early 20s (mostly at ages 15–20 years); another peak is seen after the second decade. Rare patients have been described before age 5 years and after age 50. In modern demographic studies, there is no difference in prevalence between men and women. Many precipitating factors have been described, but most of them are probably incidental. After a variable interval of months to years, at least 70% of patients develop the second characteristic feature, cataplexy, which is followed by other symptoms in a certain percentage of patients. Narcolepsy begins before the age of 10 in about 5–15% of patients and after the age of 50 in about 5% of patients. In about 10% of patients, cataplexy precedes EDS by a few months and rarely by as much as 28 years. Any of the other major symptoms may rarely be the first symptom before narcoleptic sleep attacks and cataplexy (Bassetti and Aldrich 1996). Clinical manifestations of narcolepsy syndrome may be described under three headings: major, minor, and miscellaneous.

Major manifestations are narcoleptic sleep attacks and EDS; cataplexy; sleep paralysis; hypnagogic hallucinations; disturbed night sleep; and automatic behavior.

Narcoleptic Sleep Attacks

The patient complains of EDS and characteristic sleep attacks, which are manifested by an irresistible desire to fall asleep. The attacks may come under inappropriate circumstances and inappropriate places, during driving, talking, eating, playing, walking, running, working, in class, sexual intercourse, watching television, sitting, and in conditions of boredom and monotony. Attacks are generally brief, lasting for a few minutes to 15–30 minutes, and on awakening, the patient usually feels fresh, although occasionally, the patient feels tired and drowsy. Frequency of attacks varies widely from one or more attacks daily, weekly, or monthly. Sometimes they occur once every few weeks to months and, occasionally, once every year to every few years. The attacks persist throughout life, although there may be fluctuations and, rarely, temporary remissions. Because of these sleep attacks, EDS, and frequent "microsleeps," performance at school and work declines, resulting in a variety of psychosocial and socioeconomic difficulties.

Cataplexy

Lowenfeld coined the term cataplexy (Bassetti and Aldrich 1996). Cataplexy is characterized by sudden loss of tone in the voluntary muscles, except for respiratory and ocular muscles. The cataplectic attacks are often (>95% of the time) triggered by emotional factors, such as laughter, rage, and anger. The attacks may be complete or partial and, rarely, unilateral (0.5–1.0% of patients). The patient completely loses tone in the limb muscles and falls to the ground. Knees may buckle, there may be head nodding, sagging of the jaw, dysarthria, or loss of voice, and in rare unilateral cases, there may be a loss of power in one arm or leg. These attacks generally last for a few seconds to a minute and sometimes a few minutes. Consciousness is retained completely during the attacks, and there is never any jerking of the limbs or head. Physical examination during these brief spells reveals flaccidity of the muscles and absent or markedly diminished muscle stretch reflexes. H-reflex, which is the electrical counterpart of the muscle stretch reflex, and F responses are decreased or absent.

Cataplexy is the second most important manifestation of narcolepsy syndrome and is present in 60–100% of patients with narcolepsy. In most patients, cataplexy appears months to years after onset of the sleep attacks, but occasionally, cataplexy may be the initial presentation, which causes diagnostic confusion. At the onset, the patient may have attacks daily or weekly; gradually, they decrease in frequency and may even disappear in old age. Rarely, particularly after withdrawal of tricyclic medications, patients may develop status cataplecticus. The EEG shows wakefulness during the brief cataplectic spells, but if these are prolonged to 1–2 minutes, the EEG shows REM sleep and all its manifestations.

Sleep Paralysis

Sleep paralysis is the third major manifestation of narcolepsy. It occurs months to years after onset of narcoleptic sleep attacks and is seen in about 25–50% of patients. There is sudden apparent unilateral or bilateral paralysis or paralysis of one limb, either during sleep onset at night (hypnagogic) or while awakening (hypnopompic) in the morning. The patient is conscious during these paralytic attacks but is unable to move or speak and is often frightened and fearful. As the patient experiences more and more of these episodes, he or she overcomes the fear and anxiety.

Hypnagogic Hallucination

Hypnagogic hallucination is the fourth major manifestation of narcolepsy syndrome and may occur either at the onset of sleep or while awakening early in the morning. The hallucination manifests as vivid, often fearful, visual imagery but sometimes has auditory, vestibular, or somesthetic hallucinatory phenomena. These hallucinations may occur years after the onset of sleep attacks in 20–40% of narcolepsy patients. Narcoleptic sleep attacks, cataplexy, and sleep paralysis or hypnagogic hallucination are seen in about 30% of cases; all four major features (narcoleptic tetrad) may occur together in about 10% of cases.

Disturbance of Night Sleep

Disturbance of night sleep, together with the four major manifestations, may be termed the *narcoleptic pentad*. PSG findings showing disturbed night sleep are seen in 72–80% of patients (see Laboratory Assessment of Sleep Disorders, later in this chapter).

Automatic Behavior

Automatic behavior is included under major manifestation and is found in a large percentage of patients (20–40%). During these episodes, the patient performs the same function repetitively, speaks or writes in a meaningless manner, drives on the wrong side of the road, or drives to a strange place and then forgets the episodes. The behavior resembles fuguelike state and may result from partial sleep episodes, frequent lapses, or "microsleeps."

Minor Manifestations

In addition to major manifestations, many patients have other minor clinical features. These may include psychosocial disturbances, anxiety, depression, morning headache, impotence in men, frigidity and lack of orgasm in women, and recent memory impairment.

Miscellaneous Manifestations

Patients with narcolepsy syndrome may also have sleep apnea and PLMS, which often aggravate sleep attacks in narcoleptics. The incidence of associated sleep apnea in narcolepsy varies, but about 30% of narcoleptic patients may have sleep apnea, which is most commonly central but may be obstructive or mixed. It is important to recognize OSA in narcoleptic patients because they may need additional treatment with continuous positive airway pressure (CPAP) for relief of apneas and EDS. The third important miscellaneous manifestation is REM sleep behavior disorder (RBD), which Schenck and Mahowald reported in 17 patients diagnosed by established criteria for narcolepsy and RBD. These patients ranged in age from 8 to 74 years, and 71% were men. Narcolepsy and RBD most commonly emerged in tandem. In three patients, treatment of narcolepsy-cataplexy with stimulants and tricyclic medications either induced or exacerbated RBD.

Differential Diagnosis

Narcoleptic sleep attacks should be differentiated from other causes of EDS. These include sleep deprivation and insufficient sleep syndrome; OSAS; alcohol- and drug-related hypersomnolence; other medical, neurological, and psychiatric disorders causing hypersomnolence; idiopathic hypersomnia; and circadian rhythm sleep disorders.

OSAS (see Sleep Apnea Sndrome, later in this chapter) is the most common cause of EDS referred to sleep laboratory for evaluation and is characterized by repeated episodes of obstructive and mixed apneas during NREM and REM sleep in overnight PSG recordings. These patients have prolonged daytime sleep episodes, followed by fatigue and drowsiness on awakening, which contrasts with a fresh feeling in narcoleptics on awakening from brief sleep attacks. All patients with hypersomnolence can be excluded after careful history and physical examination and overnight PSG recording.

Idiopathic hypersomnia (see Idiopathic Hypersomnia, later in this chapter) closely resembles narcolepsy syndrome. In contrast to narcolepsy, the sleep episodes in idiopathic hypersomnia are prolonged and the sleep is not refreshing. PSG and MSLTs do not show SOREMs but do show pathological sleepiness. There is no disturbance of REM-NREM organization in PSG. Some patients with idiopathic hypersomnia may have a positive family history.

Cataplexy may be mistaken for partial complex seizure, absence spells, atonic seizures, drop attacks, and syncope. During partial complex seizure, there is altered state of consciousness, but in cataplexy, patients retain consciousness. Patients with partial complex seizures may have secondary generalized tonic-clonic movements and postictal confusion, and the EEG may show characteristic epileptiform discharges in the anterior and midtemporal regions. Absence spells are characterized by staring and vacant expression lasting for a few seconds to 30 seconds and altered state of alertness accompanied by characteristic 3-Hz spike-and-wave discharges on EEG. Atonic seizures are accompanied by transient loss of consciousness, and the EEG may show slow spike-and-wave or polyspike-and-wave discharges. Drop attacks may occur in vertebrobasilar insufficiency (transient ischemic attacks), and the patient may have other evidence of brainstem ischemia, such as vertigo, ataxia, or diplopia. Syncope results from transient loss of consciousness and may have resulted from cardiogenic or other causes, including neurogenic orthostatic hypotension.

Sleep paralysis in narcolepsy should be differentiated from isolated and physiological sleep paralysis and familial sleep paralysis. In all these conditions, other manifestations of narcolepsy are absent.

Automatic behavior and fugue states should be differentiated from the automatism seen in partial complex seizure and psychogenic fugue. History, physical examination, and EEG are helpful in the differentiation.

Differential diagnosis should also include neurological conditions that were thought to be associated with secondary or symptomatic narcolepsy. Secondary narcolepsy has been controversial, and many cases of hypersomnolence resulting from CNS lesions have been described in the past as narcolepsy. Most of these are atypical sleep attacks and did not have the classic features of narcolepsy. Occasional cases of true narcoleptic sleep attacks and cataplexy have been described, however, in association with diencephalic and midbrain tumors. Multiple sclerosis (MS) and narcolepsy may occasionally be seen in the same individual and are associated with a positive HLA-DR2 antigen.

Pathophysiological Mechanisms

Physiological, neurochemical, genetic, and environmental factors all play distinct roles in the pathogenesis of narcolepsy syndrome.

Physiological Mechanisms.   Physiological abnormalities in narcolepsy suggest a disturbance of REM-NREM sleep-wake state boundaries. The hallmark of physiological testing in narcolepsy is the presence of SOREMs (i.e., the onset of REM sleep at sleep onset or within 15 minutes of sleep onset). In most cases, this sign is found in two of four to five nap recordings in MSLT and in approximately 50% of PSG recordings. Other features point to dissociation of REM sleep and intrusion into wakefulness. During cataplexy, there is muscle atonia of REM sleep without other REM features during wakeful EEG. If the episode is prolonged, however, the patient develops full REM sleep. Similarly, in sleep paralysis, muscle atonia is similar to the REM sleep atonia. REM sleep intrusion with dream imagery without other features of REM sleep is noted in hypnagogic hallucinations. In many of these episodes, the sleep state is intermediate between REM and NREM. Many patients also have "microsleeps" during the daytime (i.e., brief episodes of NREM sleep). The time-isolation laboratory experiments conducted by Pollak and co-workers showed strong evidence for circadian disorganization in narcoleptics. Although the total 24-hour sleep, as well as the percentage of REM sleep, is normal in narcoleptics, the intrusion of REM sleep atonia into wakefulness suggests the dissociation of REM sleep regulation. Occasional occurrence of RBD in some narcoleptic patients may be cited as evidence favoring an impairment of state boundary theory in narcolepsy.

Neurochemical Mechanisms.   REM sleep regulatory mechanisms, including cholinergic "REM-on" cells, which are active during REM sleep, are located in the brainstem. Injection of cholinergic drugs (e.g., physostigmine) in narcoleptic dogs (Doberman pinschers are good models of narcoleptic dogs with an autosomal recessive inheritance) increases the cataplectic episodes, whereas atropine and scopolamine (muscarinic-blocking agents) decrease cataplectic episodes (Guilleminault et al. 1998). M_2 subtypes of muscarinic cholinergic receptors are found to be upregulated in the pontine reticular formation of narcoleptic dogs (Guilleminault et al. 1998). Postmortem studies have also shown increased muscarinic M_1 receptor binding in the basal ganglia and the amygdala. These findings, in conjunction with the pharmacological experiments, suggest hypersensitivity of the muscarinic cholinergic system in the cataplectic dog brain. There is also evidence to suggest a defect in monoaminergic regulation of cholinergic REM sleep mechanism contributing to narcoleptic symptoms. "REM-off" cells (serotonergic cells in the raphe and noradrenergic cells in the locus ceruleus) are completely inactive during REM sleep and appear to play a permissive role by modulating cholinergic activity. Therefore, an imbalance of the chemical regulation between the cholinergic and monoaminergic neurons may play a role in narcoleptic symptomatology. The stimulants (amphetamine and others) used for effective treatment of sleepiness in narcolepsy increase the synaptic availability of norepinephrine. Tricyclic antidepressants used in the treatment of cataplexy decrease the reuptake of norepinephrine; fluoxetine decreases the reuptake of serotonin, thus increasing the availability of both of these monoamines. The α_1 antagonist prazosin and α_2 agonists exacerbate cataplexy, whereas α_2 antagonists (e.g., yohimbine) reduce the symptoms of cataplexy. These findings are consistent with an inhibitory role of norepinephrine and serotonin in the control of cataplexy. Therefore, all these findings indicate a disturbance of aminergic mechanism in REM sleep.

In humans, cerebrospinal fluid dopamine and the dopamine metabolite, homovanillic acid, are often decreased. In human autopsy brain samples, there is an increase of striatal dopamine D_2 receptors, although these findings have been contradicted by positron emission tomography (PET) reports. These findings suggest an impairment of dopamine release or an increased turnover. There is also some evidence suggesting an alteration of α-adrenergic receptors in certain brain regions. The primary neurochemical defect, however, is still unknown. Studies using proton spectroscopy in subjects with idiopathic narcolepsy found no evidence of loss of neurons or of gross biochemical abnormality in the ventral pons. However, global biochemical measurements of metabolic pools from the brainstem spectra are not likely to reflect small but functionally important changes in cholinergic or other neurotransmitter mechanisms in brainstem nuclei (Ellis et al. 1998).

Genetic and Environmental Factors. Genetic and environmental factors in narcolepsy are described briefly under Epidemiology, Genetics, and Family Studies in Narcolepsy, earlier in this chapter. The exact environmental factors in narcolepsy are unknown. The question of autoimmunity in narcolepsy is the subject of speculation, but no definite evidence has been uncovered.

Idiopathic Hypersomnia

ICSD (1997) defines idiopathic hypersomnia as a disorder of excessive sleepiness of presumed (but not proved) CNS cause that is associated with normal or prolonged (1–2 hours) NREM sleep episodes. The syndrome has been described under a variety of labels, including NREM narcolepsy, idiopathic CNS hypersomnia, and functional, mixed, or harmonious hypersomnia. Idiopathic hypersomnia occurs insidiously, generally between the ages of 15 and 30 years. It closely resembles narcolepsy and sleep apnea. Although sometimes it is very difficult to distinguish from narcolepsy syndrome, the sleep pattern is different from that in narcolepsy or sleep apnea (Bassetti and Aldrich 1997). Such a patient generally sleeps for hours, and the sleep is not refreshing. The patient does not give a history of cataplexy, snoring, or repeated awakenings throughout the night. Sleep drunkenness (i.e., confusional arousal) is often seen in these patients, and they may have automatic behavior with amnesia for the events. Physical examination uncovers no abnormal neurological or other findings. This

is a very disabling and lifelong condition. MSLT shows evidence of pathological sleepiness without SOREMs.

The differential diagnosis of idiopathic hypersomnia should include other causes of EDS, such as classic narcolepsy-cataplexy, upper airway OSAS, CSA syndrome, upper airway resistance syndrome (UARS), insufficient sleep, drug-induced hypersomnia, and other medical or psychiatric disorders, particularly mood disorders. Post-traumatic hypersomnia, chronic fatigue syndrome, DSPS, and long sleeper syndrome should also be included in the differential diagnosis. Based on a retrospective review of clinical and PSG features as well as questionnaire results derived from a database of 3,618 patients evaluated between 1985 and 1993 at a sleep disorder center, Aldrich (1996) suggested that idiopathic hypersomnia is a heterogeneous syndrome. He contradicted some of the previously reported findings, and in his analysis, these patients did not exhibit prolonged night sleep or sleep drunkenness. Aldrich also questioned the validity of using prolonged or "deep" sleep as a diagnostic criterion for idiopathic hypersomnia. He suggested that clinical heterogeneity may reflect differences in etiologies, such as reports of preceding Epstein-Barr viral infection, infectious mononucleosis, Guillain-Barré syndrome, or human immunodeficiency virus (HIV) infection. The author argued for re-evaluation of the diagnostic criteria for idiopathic disorders of sleepiness not associated with cataplexy. Some of these patients may have a positive family history, but the mode of inheritance is unknown. Unlike narcolepsy, there is no clear association between idiopathic hypersomnia and HLAs.

Sleep Apnea Syndrome

Sleep apnea syndrome encompasses both obstructive and central apneas as well as hypopnea. OSAS is very common but remains underdiagnosed, whereas CSA syndrome is uncommon in the general population. OSAS is the most common sleep disorder studied in the sleep laboratory by overnight PSG recording done to assess EDS. In the general population, however, sleep deprivation or insufficient sleep syndrome is the most common cause of EDS today. The reason for underdiagnosis of OSAS is an inadequate public awareness and insufficient knowledge about the serious consequences of this disorder among physicians and the public. OSAS causes significant morbidity and mortality, and it is important to diagnose the condition because there is effective treatment for most of the individuals who have it. To understand the condition, definition of several terms related to sleep-disordered breathing (SDB) is necessary.

Sleep-Disordered Breathing: Terminology

Apnea (obstructive, central, or mixed), hypopnea, hypoventilation, paradoxical breathing, periodic breathing, increased upper airway resistance, dysrhythmic breathing, apneustic

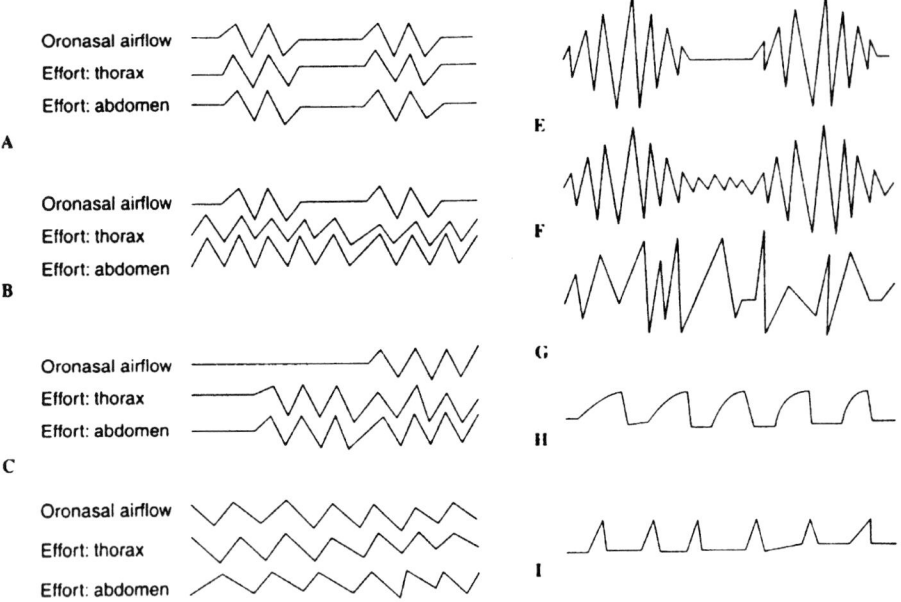

FIGURE 72.2 Patterns of sleep-disordered breathing. (**A**) central apnea; (**B**) upper airway obstructive apnea; (**C**) mixed apnea [initial central followed by obstructive apnea]; (**D**) paradoxical breathing; (**E**) Cheyne-Stokes breathing; (**F**) Cheyne-Stokes variant pattern; (**G**) dysrhythmic breathing; (**H**) apneustic breathing; (**I**) inspiratory gasp.) (Reproduced with permission from S Chokroverty. Sleep, Breathing, and Neurological Problems. In S Chokroverty [ed], Sleep Disorders Medicine: Basic Science, Technical Considerations, and Clinical Aspects. Boston: Butterworth– Heinemann, 1999.)

breathing, inspiratory gasps, and nocturnal stridor may all be grouped under SDB. Figure 72.2 shows some patterns of SDB. The term *sleep apnea* refers to temporary cessation or absence of breathing during sleep. Analysis of the breathing pattern has revealed the presence of three types of sleep apnea: upper airway obstructive, central, and mixed. Normal individuals may experience a few episodes of sleep apnea, particularly central apnea at the onset of NREM sleep and during REM sleep. To be of pathological significance, the sleep apnea should last at least 10 seconds, the apnea index (number of episodes of apnea per hour of sleep) should be at least 5, and the patient should have at least 30 episodes during 7 hours of all-night sleep.

Cessation of airflow with no respiratory effort constitutes central apnea; diaphragmatic and intercostal muscle activities are absent, as is air exchange through the nose or mouth. Upper airway OSA is characterized by cessation of airflow through the nose or mouth with persistence of the diaphragmatic and intercostal muscle activities. Mixed apnea is manifested as an initial cessation of airflow with no respiratory effort (central apnea) followed by a period of upper airway OSA.

Sleep-related hypopnea is characterized by decreased airflow at the mouth and nose and decreased chest movement, which causes a reduction in tidal volume and a reduction of the amplitude of oronasal thermistor or pneumographic signal to half the volume measured during the preceding or following respiratory cycle. Some investigators consider a reduction of one-third of the tidal volume associated with 4% reduction of oxygen saturation to be consistent with a diagnosis of hypopnea. There is, however, no precise standardized definition of hypopnea.

Respiratory disturbance index (RDI) or apnea-hypopnea index (AHI) is defined as the number of apneas and hypopneas per hour of sleep. A normal index is less than 5, but most investigators consider AHI or RDI of 10 or more significant.

Apneas and hypopneas are accompanied by oxygen desaturation and are terminated by an arousal, which is defined as transient (lasting 3–14 seconds) return of alpha activities in the EEG. Repeated arousals causing sleep fragmentation may be the main contributing cause to EDS. Arousals along with repeated hypoxemias are also the most important factors for long-term cardiovascular consequences of OSAS.

During paradoxical breathing, the thorax and abdomen move in opposite directions, thereby indicating increased upper airway resistance. This type of breathing may be noted in patients with OSAS as well as in some patients with UARS.

Periodic breathing includes Cheyne-Stokes breathing and Cheyne-Stokes variant pattern of breathing. Cheyne-Stokes breathing is a special type of central apnea manifested as cyclic changes in breathing, with crescendo-decrescendo sequence separated by central apneas. The Cheyne-Stokes variant pattern of breathing is distinguished by the substitution of hypopneas for apneas. Cheyne-Stokes breathing and the variant pattern are most commonly noted in CHF and neurological disorders.

Dysrhythmic breathing is characterized by nonrhythmic respiration of irregular rate, rhythm, and amplitude that becomes worse during sleep. This type of breathing may result from an abnormality in the automatic respiratory pattern generator in the brainstem.

Apneustic breathing is characterized by prolonged inspiration with an increase in the ratio of inspiratory to expiratory time. This type of breathing may result from a neurological lesion in the caudal pons disconnecting the

FIGURE 72.3   Polysomnographic recording of a patient with upper airway resistance syndrome. Note that peak increase in effort (*solid arrow*) is associated with a small drop in peak flow and tidal volume causing a transient EEG arousal. (ECG = electrocardiogram; EMG_{facial} = facial muscle electromyogram; EOG = electro-oculogram (right and left); Flow = pneumotachometer to quantify airflow; Pes = esophageal manometry to record esophageal pressure; $RESP_{sum}$ = respiratory effort; SaO_2 = oxygen saturation. (Reproduced with permission from A Robinson, C Guilleminault. In S Chokroverty [ed], Sleep Disorders Medicine: Basic Science, Technical Considerations, and Clinical Aspects. Boston: Butterworth–Heinemann, 1999.)

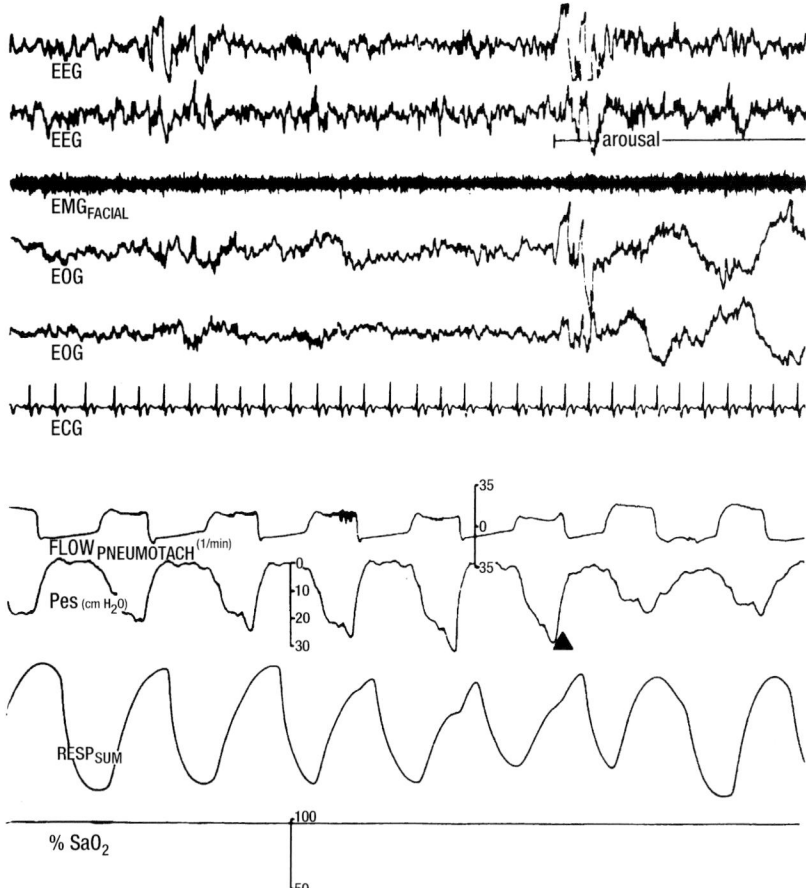

apneustic center in the lower pons from the pneumotaxic center in the upper pons.

Inspiratory gasp is characterized by short inspiratory time and a relatively prolonged expiration and has been noted after a lesion in the medulla.

Hypoventilation refers to reduction of alveolar ventilation accompanied by hypoxemia and hypercapnia; it may be noted in patients with neuromuscular disorders and kyphoscoliosis. Nonapneic breathing refers to hypoxemia without accompanying apneas or hypopneas and may be found in individuals with underlying lung or chest wall abnormalities that impair gas exchange during wakefulness.

Upper Airway Resistance Syndrome

There is a general gradation from increasing upper airway resistance, which is found in normal individuals during sleep, to the limitation of airflow in subjects with loud snoring to a stage of UARS followed by the next stage of complete airway occlusion, seen in patients with OSAS. Patients with UARS show subtle airflow limitations due to increased upper airway resistance followed by repeated arousals during sleep at night. This subtle airflow limitation cannot be identified by the usual recording of respiration using oronasal thermistor or inductance plethysmography to register chest and abdominal wall motions. Intraesophageal balloon manometry, however, reveals increasing efforts, with increasing intraesophageal pressure leading to arousal but without any apneas or hypopneas (Figure 72.3). These patients may or may not have snoring; they do have EDS and all its consequences, as seen in OSAS.

Epidemiology of Obstructive Sleep Apnea Syndrome

No study has been specifically designed to determine the incidence of OSAS in a previously healthy population. Based on a definition of at least five apneas or hypopneas per hour of sleep accompanied by EDS (Young et al. 1993), however, the prevalence of OSAS is 4% in men and 2% in women. There is a strong association between OSAS and male gender, increasing age, and obesity. The condition is common in men older than 40 years, and among women the incidence of OSAS is greater after menopause. About 85% of patients with OSAS are men, and obesity is present in about 70% of OSAS patients. There is an increased relationship found between neck circumference, abdominal measurement, and OSAS. Men with neck circumference measuring more than 17 inches and women measuring more than 16 inches are at risk for OSAS.

Race may be a factor, given that high prevalence of SDB is noted in Pacific Islanders, Mexican-Americans, and African-Americans. There are also family aggregates of OSAS. Other factors with a high association are alcohol, smoking, and drug use.

Consequences of Obstructive Sleep Apnea Syndrome

Short-term consequences of OSAS include impairment of the quality of life and increasing traffic accidents; long-term consequences include cardiovascular and neurological dysfunction. OSAS is associated with increased morbidity and mortality (Pack 1994; Strollo and Rogers 1996).

Prevalence of hypertension in untreated OSAS exceeds 40%, whereas 30% of patients with idiopathic hypertension have OSA. Although no direct causal relationship has been noted, several investigators (Pack 1994) report a clear improvement of hypertension after treatment of OSA. A significant relationship between hypertension and RDI exists even after eliminating obesity and other confounding factors. Factors responsible for hypertension in OSAS include repeated hypoxemia during sleep at night and increased sympathetic activity. Cardiac arrhythmias, pulmonary hypertension, and cor pulmonale, which are noted in severe cases of OSAS, may be related to severe hypoxemia during sleep. There is also a strong relationship between snoring, myocardial infarction, and stroke. The association of supratentorial infarction, infratentorial infarction, and transient ischemic attacks with snoring and sleep apnea has been clearly documented. Neuropsychological measurements document cognitive dysfunction in patients with OSAS who improve after treatment. Vigorous epidemiological studies, however, are needed to clearly document an association between stroke, myocardial infarction, and hypertension.

Pathogenesis of Obstructive Sleep Apnea Syndrome

The pathogenesis of OSAS includes local anatomical factors as well as neurological factors (Douglas and Polo 1994; Robinson and Guilleminault 1999). Collapse of the pharyngeal airway is the fundamental factor in OSA. During sleep, muscle tone decreases, including that of the upper airway dilator muscles, which maintains upper airway patency. As a result of this decreased tone, these muscles relax, causing increased upper airway resistance and narrowing of the upper airway space. This effect becomes more marked during REM sleep because of marked muscle hypotonia or atonia of muscles at this stage. This generates turbulent flow and vibration, causing snoring; in some individuals, there may be significant narrowing or occlusion, causing apnea. Episodes of upper airway narrowing causing apneas, hypopneas, or increased upper airway resistance that are terminated by arousals and sleep fragmentation, with repetition of the cycles numerous times throughout the night, are responsible for the daytime symptoms in OSAS. The site of narrowing in most individuals is at the level of the soft palate. There-fore, decreased tone in the palatal, genioglossal, and other upper airway muscles, causing increased upper airway resistance and decreased airway space, plays an important role in upper airway obstruction in OSAS. Obesity associated with increased fat deposition in the region of the pharynx and soft palate, abnormal facial features (e.g., retrognathia, micrognathia), and other conditions (e.g., myxedema, acromegaly) that cause fatty tissue deposit in the pharyngeal region predispose to upper airway narrowing and OSA. Imaging studies of the upper airway region have shown that in OSA patients, upper airway space is narrower than in those who do not have apnea or hypopnea. In addition to the smaller airway space in OSAS, the activity of the genioglossus muscle is found to be higher than normal during wakefulness in these patients; this may be considered a compensatory mechanism to keep the upper airway patent. Other anatomical abnormalities include adenotonsillar enlargement in children and craniofacial dysostosis. Defective upper airway reflexes may also play a role in upper airway occlusion. In some family members, abnormal facial structures, narrow upper airway, and long uvula have been found.

Neural factors responsible for OSAS include abnormalities of respiratory control in the medullary respiratory neurons. The output of sleep-related medullary respiratory neurons is thought to decrease in normal individuals during sleep. This reduction of the medullary respiratory neuronal activity in sleep causes a loss of tonic and phasic motor output to the upper airway dilator muscles, resulting in an increase in airway resistance. Hypoxic and hypercapnic ventilatory responses, however, are found to be normal in OSAS, but in obesity-hypoventilation syndrome (pickwickian syndrome), which may be considered a very advanced stage of OSAS in obese patients, these responses are depressed, causing hypercapnia and hypoxemia even during wakefulness. Thus, a complex interaction of peripheral upper airway and central neural factors combine to produce the full-blown syndrome of OSAS.

Symptoms

Symptoms of OSAS can be divided into two groups (Table 72.8): those occurring during sleep (nocturnal events) and those occurring during the daytime (diurnal events). Nocturnal sleep symptoms of OSAS include loud snoring (often with a long history), choking, cessation of breathing (witnessed apneas by the bed partner), sitting up fighting for breath, abnormal motor activities with thrashing about in bed, severe sleep disruption, gastroesophageal reflux, nocturia and nocturnal enuresis (seen mostly in children), and occasionally hyperhidrosis.

The major daytime symptom of OSAS is EDS. Patients fall asleep during the day at inappropriate times and in inappropriate places and may be involved in driving accidents. They cannot function adequately during the day, and some patients may complain of morning headaches and forgetfulness; men may report impotence. The prolonged duration and the unrefreshing nature of the EDS attacks differentiate them from narcoleptic sleep attacks.

Snoring is present in most patients, and there is often a gradation from mild snoring for many years to very loud snoring for a period and then to the development of daytime symptoms. A history of witnessed apneas by a bed partner is a strong indicator of the presence of sleep apnea. Occasionally, patients may complain of difficulty falling asleep and numerous awakenings during the night. Excessive sweating in some patients may be related to the increased muscle activity related to abnormal motor activities during sleep at night. Increased release of atrial natriuretic peptide during sleep may be responsible for natriuresis, diuresis, and nocturnal enuresis. Some patients may complain of hearing impairment related to a history of loud snoring for many years. Other complaints include memory impairment, automatic behavior with retrograde amnesia, dryness of mouth on awakening in the morning, decreased libido, personality changes, and hyperactivity in children. Factors that may aggravate symptoms of OSA include alcohol intake, CNS depressants, sleep deprivation, respiratory allergies, and smoking.

Signs

Physical examination should include assessment of respiratory, oropharyngeal, neurological, hematological, and cardiovascular functions. Examination of the oropharyngeal region may detect redundant oropharyngeal tissues, such as large edematous uvula, redundant mucosal folds of the pharyngeal walls, low-hanging long soft palate, or large tonsils and adenoids, especially in children. Other findings may include macroglossia, micrognathia, and retrognathia. Body weight and height measurements are important. Neck circumference correlates with SDB. Physical examination reveals obesity in about 70% of cases. Physical examination may also uncover the risk factors associated with repeated hypoxemia and apnea during sleep, such as hypertension, cardiac arrhythmias, and evidence of CHF.

Evaluation and Assessment

Evaluation and assessment is the same as that for other sleep disorders. Particular attention should be paid to detailed sleep history as well as the daytime history, and careful physical examination should be directed at specific associated and risk factors. The laboratory assessment and management are described later in this chapter, under Laboratory Assessment of Sleep Disorders.

Restless Legs Syndrome

Clinical Manifestations

Thomas Willis gave a graphic clinical description of RLS more than 300 years ago. More than 50 years ago, Ekbom

Table 72.8: Symptoms and signs in obstructive sleep apnea syndrome

Nocturnal symptoms during sleep
  Loud snoring (often with a long history)
  Choking during sleep
  Cessation of breathing (witnessed apneas by the bed partner)
  Sitting up or fighting for breath
  Abnormal motor activities (e.g., thrashing about in bed)
  Severe sleep disruption
  Gastroesophageal reflux causing heartburn
  Nocturia and nocturnal enuresis (mostly in children)
  Insomnia in some cases
  Excessive nocturnal sweating in some cases
Daytime symptoms
  Excessive daytime somnolence
  Forgetfulness
  Personality changes
  Decreased libido and impotence in men
  Dryness of mouth on awakening
  Morning headache (in some patients)
  Automatic behavior with retrograde amnesia
  Hyperactivity in children
  Hearing impairment (in some patients)
Physical findings
  Obesity in the majority of cases
  Increased body mass index (body weight in kg/height in m^2) >25
  Increased neck circumference (>17 in. in men and >16 in. in women)
  In some patients:
    Large edematous uvula
    Low-hanging soft palate
    Large tonsils and adenoids (especially in children)
    Retrognathia
    Micrognathia
    Hypertension
    Cardiac arrhythmias
    Evidence of congestive heart failure

brought the entity to the attention of the medical community (Trenkwalder et al. 1996). RLS remains largely underdiagnosed or undiagnosed. The exact prevalence of RLS is not known because an adequate epidemiological study has not been undertaken. Ekbom gave a prevalence rate of 5% and others gave 1%, but a realistic figure is probably somewhere between the two (approximately 2%), although some surveys indicate that it may be as high as 10%. RLS is a lifelong condition that may begin at any age but is most severe in middle-aged and elderly persons, in whom it has a chronic progressive course. The fundamental problem in RLS is a complex sensorimotor disorder involving predominantly the legs. The essential clinical diagnostic features are listed in Table 72.9. RLS is idiopathic in most cases, but it also may occur secondary to conditions such as iron deficiency, uremia, or polyneuropathy.

The hallmark of idiopathic or primary RLS are intense, disagreeable, creeping sensations (paresthesia or dysesthesia) in the lower extremities that are relieved by moving the legs (Walters et al. 1995). The symptoms are worse when

Table 72.9:   Clinical diagnostic criteria for idiopathic restless legs syndrome

Intense disagreeable feelings (paresthesias or dysesthesias), predominantly in the legs, causing an intense urge to move the limbs that provides relief from these sensations
Motor restlessness
Presence of symptoms or worsening of symptoms at rest or repose, with relief by motor activity
Worsening of the symptoms in the evening and nightfall, suggesting a possible circadian variability
Involuntary movements (both myoclonic and dystonic), which may be periodic or aperiodic limb movements in relaxed wakefulness
Periodic limb movements in sleep and sleep disturbance, especially difficulty in initiating sleep
Autosomal dominant inheritance
Normal neurological examination (in secondary restless legs syndrome, this may be abnormal, depending on the potential causes or associations)
Onset at any age; most severe in middle-aged and elderly individuals
The course is typically chronic and progressive, with occasional remission and frequent aggravation during pregnancy

Table 72.10:   Features of periodic limb movements in sleep

Repetitive, often stereotyped movements during NREM sleep
Usually noted in the legs consisting of extension of the great toe, dorsiflexion of the ankle, and flexion of the knee and hip; sometimes seen in the arms
Periodic or quasi-periodic at an average interval of 20–40 secs (range 5–120 seconds) with a duration of 0.5–5.0 secs and as part of at least four consecutive movements
Occurs at any age but prevalence increases with age
May occur as an isolated condition or may be associated with a large number of other medical, neurological, or sleep disorders and medications
Seen in at least 80% of patients with restless legs syndrome

NREM = non–rapid eye movement.

lying down in bed in the evening and occur most commonly at sleep onset. Additional diagnostic criteria are shown in Table 72.9.

The sensory manifestations include intense, disagreeable feelings that are generally different from the usual paresthesias or dysesthesias encountered in common polyneuropathies or radiculopathies. These creeping sensations occur mostly between the knees and the ankles, causing an intense urge to move the limbs, which relieves the feelings. Occasionally, patients complain of pain. Affected patients generally have severe difficulty in initiating sleep due to paresthesias and restlessness of the legs. Severely affected individuals may also have paresthesias during the day when resting or sitting quietly.

Motor manifestations of RLS can be divided into three groups: voluntary motor restlessness, involuntary movements in wakefulness, and PLMS. The voluntary motor restlessness is seen mostly in the legs but occasionally also in the arms. The movements are usually symmetrical but sometimes may be seen asymmetrically and asynchronously. Motor restlessness generally comprises tossing and turning in bed, floor pacing, leg stretching, leg flexion, foot rubbing, and occasionally marching in place and body rocking. The involuntary movements during relaxed wakefulness include myoclonic jerks and dystonic movements. These movements may be periodic, and these are called periodic limb movements in wakefulness. The myoclonic jerks can also be aperiodic or may occur in clusters. The dystonic movements are more sustained and prolonged in duration than the myoclonic jerks. The salient features of PLMS (Table 72.10) are seen in at least 80% of patients with RLS.

PLMS are mostly dystonic and rarely myoclonic, based on the electromyographic (EMG) criteria of duration of the muscle bursts.

Neurological examination in the idiopathic form of RLS is generally normal because movements are usually noted in the evening, when the patients are resting in bed. In severe cases, however, the movements may be noted during the day while subjects are sitting or lying down, and both voluntary and involuntary movements may be seen during neurological examination. In secondary forms of RLS, clinical signs of associated abnormality may be present. The course is generally chronic and progressive, but remissions sometimes occur. The condition may be exacerbated during pregnancy or by caffeine or iron deficiency. Family history may be present in 30–50% of the patients, which suggests a dominant mode of inheritance.

Differential diagnosis of RLS may be considered under two categories: secondary RLS and the entities that may mimic RLS. In secondary or symptomatic RLS, several conditions may be associated with RLS or may cause symptomatic RLS (Table 72.11). The entities that mimic RLS are listed in Table 72.12. An important and often difficult condition to differentiate from RLS is akathisia. Essential features of akathisia that are important to differentiate from RLS are listed in Table 72.13.

Pathophysiology

The physiological mechanism or the anatomical locus responsible for RLS-PLMS is unknown. Pathophysiological clues may be derived from electrophysiological and imaging studies as well as from state-dependent and circadian factors (Hening et al. 1999). Dopaminergic and peptidergic theories are based on pharmacological response. Based on the implications derived from secondary RLS, a vascular hypothesis, a peripheral neuropathy hypothesis, and deficient and toxic states have been suggested as etiologies, but none has been satisfactory. The most likely hypothesis is a functional alteration in the brainstem region, but the exact location is undetermined.

Table 72.11: Causes of symptomatic or secondary restless legs syndrome

Neurological disorders
  Polyneuropathies
  Lumbosacral radiculopathies
  Amyotrophic lateral sclerosis
  Myelopathies
  Multiple sclerosis
  Parkinson's disease
  Poliomyelitis
  Isaac's syndrome
  Hyperexplexia (startle disease)
Medical disorders
  Anemia: iron and folate deficiency
  Diabetes mellitus
  Amyloidosis
  Uremia
  Gastrectomy
  Cancer
  Chronic obstructive pulmonary disease
  Peripheral vascular (arterial or venous) disorder
  Rheumatoid arthritis
  Hypothyroidism
Drugs and chemicals
  Caffeine
  Neuroleptics
  Withdrawal from sedatives or narcotics
  Lithium
  Calcium-channel antagonists (e.g., nifedipine)

Table 72.12: Entities that may mimic restless legs syndrome

Neuroleptic-induced akathisia
Syndrome of painful legs and moving toes
Muscular pain-fasciculation syndrome
Myokymia
Causalgia-dystonia syndrome
Painful nocturnal leg cramps
Myoclonus (essential myoclonus)
Hypnic jerks ("sleep starts")
Anxiety-depression
Growing pains

Table 72.13: Pertinent features of akathisia that differentiate from restless legs syndrome

Inner restlessness, fidgetiness with jittery feelings, or generalized restlessness
A common side effect of neuroleptics
Can be acute, chronic, or tardive
Characteristic motor restlessness consists of swaying or rocking movements of the body; marching in place; crossing and uncrossing of the legs; shifting body positions in chair; inability to sit still; rhythmic or nonrhythmic, synchronous or asynchronous, symmetrical or asymmetrical limb movements; movements resemble chorea rather than the voluntary movements of restless legs syndrome
Motor restlessness present mostly during the day but may be worse when sitting or standing in one place for a long time
Polysomnography study shows no distinctive features, rarely may show evidence of mild sleep disturbance and periodic limb movements in sleep
No relevant family history
Neurological examination reveals evidence of akathisia and sometimes drug-induced extrapyramidal manifestations
Involuntary movements (e.g., myoclonic jerks) are uncommon and not a prominent feature
Best treated with anticholinergics or β-adrenergic antagonists

Several studies have found inconsistent support for the presence of some hyperexcitable brainstem reflexes. Based on the absence of cortical prepotentials in jerk-locked back averaging study, it is unlikely that the cortex is the generator of PLMS. Studies have shown that RLS was maximum during the falling phase of a body temperature curve, which suggests that there is a circadian factor that modulates RLS severity, independent of activity state. A functional magnetic resonance imaging (MRI) study showed increased activity in the contralateral thalamus and in the red nucleus, bilateral cerebellum, and brainstem reticular formation in patients with PLMS and sensory symptoms. One study found decreased dopamine D_2-receptor binding by iodobenzamide–single-photon emission computed tomography (SPECT), which was reversed with therapy. In contrast, another study found no abnormalities of cerebral metabolism or dopaminergic presynaptic function in a PET study during an asymptomatic period (Trenkwalder et al. 1996).

Periodic Limb Movement Disorder

PLMD is characterized by periodically recurring limb movements during NREM sleep; most commonly, patients dorsiflex the ankles and flex the knees and hips every 20–40 seconds. Occasionally, PLMS is noted in the upper limbs.

In at least 80% of cases of RLS, PLMS is seen, whereas RLS is found in about 30% of cases of PLMS. Additional criteria for PLMS are listed in Table 72.10. Limb movements may be accompanied by partial arousal, causing sleep fragmentation. A PLMS index (number of PLMS/hour of sleep) of 5 is considered within normal range. PLMS accompanied by arousals are thought to be more significant for sleep disruption than those without arousals.

PLMS may occur as a primary disorder, when it is called PLMD, or may be associated with end-stage renal disease or medications such as tricyclic antidepressants or monoamine oxidase inhibitors. In addition, asymptomatic PLMS can occur in normal individuals, particularly elderly subjects, in whom a prevalence of approximately 30% has been reported. PSG study is necessary for diagnosis of this condition. The results should be interpreted in light of the fact that night-to-night variability of the condition has been noted.

Circadian Rhythm Sleep Disorders

Circadian rhythm sleep disorders result from a mismatch between the body's internal clock and the geophysical environment (Mahowald et al. 1997) either because malfunction in the biological clock (primary circadian rhythm disorders) or because the clock is out of phase due to a shift in environment (secondary circadian dysrhythmias). Jet lag and shift work are two common sources of secondary circadian dysrhythmias resulting from exogenous factors.

Delayed Sleep-Phase Syndrome

The ICSD defines DSPS as a condition in which the major sleep episode is delayed in relation to the desired clock time. This causes symptoms of sleep-onset insomnia or difficulty awakening at the desired time. Typically, the patient goes to sleep late (e.g., 2:00–6:00 AM) and awakens in the late morning or afternoon (e.g., 10:00 AM–2:00 PM). Patients with this disorder have great difficulty in functioning adequately in the daytime if they have to wake up early in the morning to go to school or work. They have severe sleep-initiation difficulty and cannot function normally in society because of the disturbed sleep schedule. They often try a variety of hypnotic medications or alcohol in an attempt to initiate sleep sooner. Sleep architecture is generally normal if these individuals are allowed to follow their own uninterrupted sleep-wake schedule.

DSPS may represent 5–10% of cases with complaints of insomnia in some sleep disorders centers. Onset occurs during childhood or adolescence. Sometimes, there is a history of DSPS in other family members. Some patients may have depression. Primary DSPS results from an unusually long intrinsic circadian period due to abnormalities in the biological clock in the SCN. Actigraphic recordings over several days document the characteristic sleep schedule.

Advanced Sleep-Phase Syndrome

Advanced sleep-phase syndrome (ASPS) is the converse of DSPS: The patient goes to sleep in the early evening and wakes up earlier than desired in the morning (e.g., 2:00–4:00 AM). If these patients do not go to sleep at an early hour, they experience sleep disruption and daytime sleepiness.

ASPS is most commonly seen in elderly individuals. The basic mechanism is thought to be an inherent shortening of the endogenous circadian timing. The diagnosis is based on sleep logs and characteristic actigraphic recordings over several days. ASPS is easy to distinguish from the early morning awakening of depression because sleep architecture is normal and does not exhibit the shortened REM latency and other REM sleep abnormalities seen in depressed patients.

Hypernychthemeral Syndrome

Hypernychthemeral syndrome, also called non–24-hour sleep-wake disorder, is characterized by an inability to maintain a regular bedtime. Sleep onset wanders around the clock. Affected patients have a gradually increasing delay in sleep onset by about 1 hour per sleep-wake cycle, causing eventual progression of sleep onset through the daytime hours and into the evening. These individuals fail to be entrained or synchronized by usual time cues, such as sunlight or social activities.

Hypernychthemeral syndrome is an extremely uncommon disorder and is most often associated with blindness. Approximately one-third of blind individuals are affected because of impairment of the retino-hypothalamic pathway, which normally cues circadian patterns. The syndrome also may be associated with hypothalamic tumors. Sometimes depression and anxiety disorders are associated with this syndrome.

NEUROLOGICAL DISORDERS AND SLEEP DISTURBANCE

Sleep disorders are very common in neurological illnesses, which may adversely affect patients' sleep. Thus, there is an interrelationship between sleep and neurological disorders. Sleep dysfunction may result from central or peripheral somatic and autonomic neurological disorders. Neurological diseases may cause insomnia or EDS as well as parasomnias. Neurological causes of excessive sleepiness are described in Chapter 6, and neurological disorders that cause insomnia are described under Insomnia, earlier in this chapter.

Sleep and Epilepsy

There is a distinct and reciprocal relationship between sleep and epilepsy (Chokroverty and Quinto 1999). Sleep affects epilepsy, and epilepsy affects sleep. In the beginning of this century, before the availability of EEG, several authors emphasized that many seizures are predominantly nocturnal and occur at certain times at night. The modern era of combining the clinical and EEG findings on sleep and seizures began with the observation of Gibbs and Gibbs in 1947 that EEG epileptiform discharges were seen more frequently during sleep than during wakefulness (Chokroverty and Quinto 1999). A basic understanding of the mechanism of epileptogenesis and sleep makes it clear why seizures are frequently triggered by sleep. The fundamental mechanism for epileptogenesis includes neuronal synchronization, neuronal hyperexcitability, and a lack of inhibitory mechanism. During NREM sleep, there is an excessive diffuse cortical synchronization mediated by the thalamocortical input, whereas during REM sleep, there is inhibition of the thalamocortical synchronizing influence in addition to a tonic reduction in the interhemispheric impulse traffic through the corpus callosum. Factors that enhance synchronization are conducive to active ictal precipitation in susceptible individuals. NREM sleep thus acts as a convulsant by causing excessive synchronization and activation of seizures in an already hyperexcitable cortex. In contrast, during REM sleep, there is attenuation of epileptiform discharges and limitation of propagation of generalized epileptiform discharges to a focal area.

Sleep deprivation is another important seizure-triggering factor, and the value of sleep-deprived EEG in the diagnosis of seizures is well known. Sleep deprivation increases epileptiform discharges, mostly during the transition period between waking and light sleep. Sleep deprivation causes sleepiness, which is one factor for activating seizures, but it probably also increases cortical excitability, which triggers seizures.

Biorhythmic classification of seizures has shown inconsistencies and contradictions. Seizures have been shown to occur predominantly during sleep (nocturnal seizures), predominantly in the daytime (diurnal seizures), or both during sleep at night and daytime (diffuse epilepsy). Taking into consideration different series, the frequency of sleep epilepsy has been quoted as 22%, but most of these statistics were obtained before the advent of EEG. The most likely figure for nocturnal seizures is about 10%. Because of inconsistencies in biorhythmic classification, modern epileptologists use the International Classification of Epilepsy, which divides seizures into primarily generalized and partial seizures with or without secondary generalization.

Effect of Sleep on Epilepsy

True nocturnal seizures may include tonic seizures, benign focal epilepsy of childhood with rolandic spikes, juvenile myoclonic epilepsy, electrical status epilepticus during sleep or continuous spikes and waves during sleep, and some varieties of frontal lobe seizures, particularly nocturnal paroxysmal dystonia (NPD). Many patients with generalized tonic-clonic and partial complex seizures also have predominantly nocturnal seizures. Nocturnal seizures may be mistaken for motor and behavioral parasomnias or other movement disorders that persist during sleep or reactivate during stage transition or awakenings in the middle of the night.

Tonic Seizure

Tonic seizures are characteristic of Lennox-Gastaut syndrome, which may also include other seizure types, such as myoclonic, generalized tonic-clonic, atonic, and atypical absence. Tonic seizures are typically activated by sleep, are much more frequent during NREM sleep than during wakefulness, and are never seen during REM sleep. The typical EEG finding consists of slow spikes and waves intermixed with trains of fast spikes as interictal abnormalities during sleep.

Benign Rolandic Seizure

Benign rolandic seizure is a childhood seizure disorder seen mostly during drowsiness and NREM sleep and is characterized by focal clonic facial twitching, often preceded by perioral numbness. Many patients may have secondary generalized tonic-clonic seizures. The characteristic EEG finding consists of central-temporal or rolandic spikes or sharp waves. Seizures generally stop by the age of 15–20 years without any neurological sequela.

Juvenile Myoclonic Epilepsy

Onset of myoclonic epilepsy of Janz usually occurs between 13 and 19 years and is manifested by massive bilaterally synchronous myoclonic jerks. The seizures increase shortly after awakening in the morning and occasionally on awakening in the middle of the night. A typical EEG shows synchronous and symmetrical polyspikes and spike-and-wave discharges. The interictal discharges predominate at sleep onset and then on awakening but are virtually nonexistent during the rest of the sleep cycle.

Nocturnal Paroxysmal Dystonia, Paroxysmal Arousals and Awakenings, and Episodic Nocturnal Wanderings

NPD, paroxysmal arousals and awakenings, and episodic nocturnal wanderings all share common features of abnormal paroxysmal motor activities during sleep and respond favorably to anticonvulsants. These entities most likely represent partial seizures arising from discharging foci in the deeper regions of the brain, particularly frontal cortex, without any concomitant scalp EEG evidence of epileptiform activities (Hening et al. 1999). The relationship to seizures, particularly partial complex seizures of temporal or extratemporal origin, however, remains controversial. Nonepileptic seizures or pseudoseizures are not common during sleep at night but sometimes can occur and be mistaken for true nocturnal seizures, and it is important to differentiate these from true seizures because of difference in management.

Five patients were originally described with episodes of abnormal movements that were tonic and often violent during NREM sleep almost every night. Ictal and interictal EEGs were normal. Later, 12 patients were described with NREM sleep–related choreoathetotic, dystonic, and ballistic movements each night, often occurring many times during the night for many years. The term *NPD* was coined for this entity (Table 72.14). The patients all responded to carbamazepine, and the spells lasted less than a minute. It was suggested that these spells were a type of unusual nocturnal seizure. Later, cases of NPD showed EEG evidence of epileptiform abnormalities arising from the frontal lobes. A study comparing groups of patients with NPD and those with undisputed frontal lobe seizures supported the contention that NPD patients may have frontal lobe seizures

Table 72.14: Features of nocturnal paroxysmal dystonia

Onset: infancy to fifth decade
Usually sporadic; rarely familial
Sudden onset from non–rapid eye movement sleep
Two clinical types
 Common type is short-lasting (15 secs to <2 mins)
Semiology: ballismic, choreoathetotic, or dystonic movements
Often occurs in clusters
Electroencephalogram: generally normal
Short-duration attacks are most likely a type of frontal lobe seizure
Treatment: carbamazepine effective in patients with short-
 lasting attacks

Table 72.15: Features of frontal lobe seizures

Age of onset: infancy to middle age
Sporadic, occasionally familial (dominant)
Both diurnal and nocturnal spells, sometimes exclusively
 nocturnal
Sudden onset in non–rapid eye movement sleep with sudden
 termination
Duration: mostly less than 1 min, sometimes 1–2 mins with
 short postictal confusion
Often occurs in clusters
Semiology: tonic, clonic, bipedal, bimanual, and bicycling
 movements; motor and sexual automatisms; contralateral
 dystonic posturing or arm abduction with or without eye
 deviation
Ictal EEG may be normal; interictal EEG may show spikes;
 sometimes depth recording is needed

EEG = electroencephalogram.

(Hening et al. 1999). Therefore, short-duration NPD attacks may represent a form of frontal lobe seizures (Table 72.15) that are evoked specifically during sleep at night.

Autosomal Dominant Nocturnal Frontal Lobe Epilepsy

An autosomal dominant form of frontal lobe epilepsy usually starts in childhood and persists throughout adult life. Attacks are characterized by brief motor seizures in clusters during sleep. Neurological examination and neuroimaging are normal. Videotelemetry during the attacks confirms the epileptic nature, and the response to carbamazepine is excellent (Chokroverty and Quinto 1999).

Effect of Epilepsy on Sleep

Although the usefulness of sleep in the diagnosis of epilepsy was established, the altered sleep characteristics in epileptics are not well known. Most studies have been conducted in patients who have been on anticonvulsants, thus adding the confounding factors of the effect of anticonvulsants on sleep architecture. Additionally, there is a dearth of longitudinal studies to determine the effect of epilepsy on sleep in the early stage versus the late stage of illness. A general consensus has been reached, however, on the effects of epilepsy on sleep and sleep structure. These effects can be summarized as follows: an increase of sleep-onset latency; an increase in waking after sleep onset; a reduction in REM sleep; increased instability of sleep states, such as unclassifiable sleep epochs; an increase in NREM stages I and II; a decrease in NREM sleep stages III and IV; and a reduction in the density of sleep spindles.

Sleep Disorders Associated with Neuromuscular Disorders

Clinicians first became aware of sleep-related respiratory dysrhythmias in patients with neuromuscular diseases by observing hypoventilation in poliomyelitis. Sleep disturbances in neuromuscular diseases are generally secondary to respiratory dysrhythmias associated with these diseases.

In neuromuscular disorders, sleep disturbances are secondary to involvement of respiratory muscles, phrenic and intercostal nerves, or neuromuscular junctions of the respiratory and oropharyngeal muscles. The most common complaint is EDS resulting from transient nocturnal hypoxemia and hypoventilation, causing repeated arousals and sleep fragmentation. In addition to the sleep-related respiratory dysrhythmias, some patients, particularly those with painful polyneuropathies, muscle pain, muscle cramps, and immobility due to muscle weakness, may complain of insomnia. Patients with neuromuscular diseases often complain of breathlessness, particularly in the supine position.

Respiratory disturbances are generally noted in the advanced stage of primary muscle disorders or myopathies, but respiratory failure may appear in an early stage. Sleep complaints and sleep-related respiratory dysrhythmias are common in Duchenne's and limb-girdle muscular dystrophies as well as myopathies associated with acid maltase deficiency. They may also occur in other congenital or acquired myopathies, mitochondrial encephalomyopathy, and polymyositis.

Many patients with myotonic dystrophy have been described with central, mixed, and upper airway OSAs; alveolar hypoventilation; daytime fatigue; and hypersomnolence. Nocturnal oxygen desaturation accompanies alveolar hypoventilation and apneas and becomes worse during REM sleep. EDS in myotonic dystrophy often occurs in the absence of sleep apnea. An entity called *proximal myotonic myopathy (PROMM)* has been described. PROMM is a hereditary myotonic disorder that is differentiated from myotonic dystrophy by absence of the chromosome 19 CTG trinucleotide repeat that is associated with classic myotonic dystrophy. A brief report (Chokroverty et al. 1997) describes sleep disturbances in two patients consisting of difficulty initiating sleep, EDS, snoring, and frequent awakenings and movement during sleep. Overnight PSG study showed decreased sleep efficiency, increased number of arousals, and sleep architectural abnormalities. One patient had absent REM sleep; the other had dissociated REM sleep characterized by phasic REM bursts associated with EEG patterns showing sleep spindles and alpha intrusions. These sleep abnormalities in PROMM suggested involvement of the REM- and NREM-generating neurons as part of a multisystem membrane disorder.

In polyneuropathies, involvement of the nerves supplying the diaphragm and the intercostal and accessory muscle of respiration may cause breathlessness on exertion and other respiratory dysrhythmias. These may worsen during sleep, causing sleep fragmentation and daytime hypersomnolence. In painful polyneuropathies, patients may have insomnia.

Neuromuscular junctional disorders (e.g., myasthenia gravis, myasthenic syndrome, botulism, and tic paralysis) are characterized by easy fatigability of the muscles, including the bulbar and other respiratory muscles, as a result of nerve impulses of the neuromuscular junctions not being transmitted. Patients with myasthenia gravis may have central, obstructive, and mixed apneas and hypopneas accompanied by oxygen desaturation. A sensation of breathlessness on awakening in the middle of the night and early morning hours may indicate respiratory dysfunction. Sleep-related hypoventilation and sleep apnea in neuromuscular junctional disorders may be severe enough to require assisted ventilation.

Sleep and Spinal Cord Diseases

Sleep disturbances related to respiratory dysfunction can occur in some patients with high cervical spinal cord lesions. Patients with poliomyelitis, amyotrophic lateral sclerosis (ALS) affecting the phrenic and intercostal motor neurons in the spinal cord, spinal cord tumors, spinal trauma, spinal surgery (e.g., cervical cordotomy, anterior spinal surgery), and nonspecific or demyelinating myelitis may all have sleep disturbances. The most common symptom is hypersomnia secondary to sleep-related respiratory arrhythmias. Occasionally, patients with spinal cord diseases may complain of insomnia as a result of immobility, spasticity associated with flexor spasms, neck pain, and central pain syndrome.

Sleep Disturbances in Poliomyelitis and Postpolio Syndrome

Respiratory disturbances worsening during sleep may occur in many patients during the acute and convalescent stages of poliomyelitis. Some are left with the sequela of sleep-related apnea or hypoventilation requiring ventilatory support, especially at night. Another group of patients develops symptoms decades later that constitute postpolio syndrome, in which sleep disturbances and sleep apnea or hypoventilation have also been noted. Postpolio syndrome is manifested clinically by increasing weakness or wasting of the

previously affected muscles and by involvement of previously unaffected regions of the body, fatigue, aches and pains, and sometimes symptoms secondary to sleep-related hypoventilation (e.g., EDS and tiredness).

Sleep and Headache Syndromes

In day-to-day practice, headaches and sleep complaints are common. Sleep disturbance in OSAS may cause headache, and headache itself may cause sleep disturbance. The ICSD (1997) includes cluster headache, chronic paroxysmal hemicrania, and migraine under the heading of sleep-related headaches. PSG recordings in patients with chronic migraine and cluster headaches show a clear relationship between REM sleep and attacks of headache, although sometimes migraine headaches with arousals may occur out of both slow-wave and REM sleep. Cluster headaches are thought to be related to REM, but cluster headaches may sometimes be triggered by NREM sleep. Chronic paroxysmal hemicrania, which is probably a variant of cluster headache, is most commonly associated with REM sleep. Significant sleep disruption in the form of decreased total and REM sleep time, accompanied by an increased number of awakenings during REM sleep, has been described in patients with chronic paroxysmal hemicrania. PSG has documented sleep apnea in some patients with chronic recurring headache syndromes. The relationship between early morning headache and upper airway OSAS has been somewhat controversial, with contradictory reports.

A rare benign headache syndrome, called *hypnic headache syndrome*, is described in patients older than 60 years. The patients are awakened from sleep at a constant time each night. Hypnic headache syndrome is differentiated from chronic cluster headache by generalized distribution, age of onset, and lack of autonomic manifestation. These patients often respond to lithium treatment.

Exploding head syndrome is an unusual phenomenon that usually occurs in the transition from wake to sleep, abruptly arousing the patient with the sound of an explosion in the head, accompanied by bright light flashes. This is a benign condition and may represent a form of "sleep starts."

Kleine-Levin Syndrome

Kleine in 1925 and Levin in 1936 described an episodic disorder occurring mostly in adolescent boys (but also described later in girls) and characterized by periodic hypersomnolence and bulimia. The episodes usually last days to weeks. During sleep "attacks," the patient sleeps 16–18 hours a day or more and on awakening, eats voraciously. Other behavioral disturbances during the episode may include hypersexuality, confusion, hallucination, inattention, and memory impairment. The condition is generally self-limited and disappears by adulthood. PSG study shows normal sleep cycling, and MSLT shows pathological sleepiness without SOREM. The cause of the condition remains undetermined, although a limbic-hypothalamic dysfunction is suspected but not proved. Lithium treatment is effective, and valproic acid may also be useful.

Idiopathic Recurrent Stupor

Idiopathic recurrent stupor is a rare condition, later renamed *endozepine stupor* (Lugaresi et al. 1998), characterized by episodic loss of consciousness. The condition occurs predominantly, but not exclusively, in middle-aged men and is characterized by recurrent episodes of stupor in whom no metabolic, toxic, or structural brain dysfunction is found. The characteristic EEG finding is nonreactive, diffusely distributed fast rhythms (13–16 Hz). The frequency of the episodes of stupor varied between one to six per year to more than six per year; duration varied between 2 hours and 5 days. Benzodiazepinelike activity, identified as endozepine-4 in plasma and cerebrospinal fluid, was markedly elevated. Flumazenil (0.5–2.0 mg intravenously), a benzodiazepine-receptor antagonist, rapidly reversed the clinical manifestation and the EEG abnormalities to a normal state.

Fatal Familial Insomnia

Fatal familial insomnia (FFI) is a rare and rapidly progressive autosomal dominant prion disease with a mutation at codon 178 of the prion protein gene, *PrP*. FFI was originally described in a family with a progressive neurological illness characterized by insomnia and dysautonomia that terminated in death. Clinical manifestations are impaired control of the sleep-wake cycle, including circadian rhythms; autonomic and neuroendocrine dysfunction; and somatic neurological, cognitive, and behavioral manifestations. Profound sleep disturbances and, in particular, severe insomnia are noted from the very beginning of the illness. PSG study shows almost total absence of sleep pattern and only short episodes of REM sleep, lasting for a few seconds or minutes, without muscle atonia. This abnormal sleep pattern is associated with dream-enacting behavior in the form of complex gestures and motions and myoclonus. The terminal stage of the illness is characterized by progressive slowing of the EEG, with the patient drifting into coma. Autonomic function tests reveal evidence of sympathetic hyperactivity with preserved parasympathetic activity (Montagna et al. 1995). Neuroendocrine functions in FFI show a dysfunction of the pituitary-adrenal axis, as manifested by striking elevation of serum cortisol but normal adrenocorticotropic hormone, indicating abnormal feedback suppression of adrenocorticotropic hormone. Persistently elevated serum catecholamine levels associated with abnormal secretory patterns of growth hormone, prolactin, and melatonin are noted. The nocturnal secretory peaks of growth hormone are absent. Plasma melatonin levels progressively decrease, and in the most advanced stage of the illness, there is a complete abolition of melatonin rhythm. Somatic neurological manifestations consist of ataxia, evidence of pyramidal tract dysfunction, myoclonus, tremor, and bizarre astasia-abasia. Neuropsychological studies reveal impairment of attention, vigilance, and memory. The disease progresses rapidly and ends in coma and death.

The neuropathological hallmark of FFI is severe atrophy of the thalamus, particularly the anterior ventral and dorsomedial thalamic nuclei associated with variable involvement of the inferior olive, striatum, and cerebellum. There are no spongiform changes, except in those with the longest duration of symptoms, who show mild-to-moderate spongiform degeneration of the cerebral cortex. Severe hypometabolism of the thalamus and mild hypometabolism of the cingulate cortex are the main findings on PET study in FFI patients. Based on biochemical, genetic, and transmission studies, it has been concluded that FFI is a transmissible prion disease resulting from a mutation at codon 178 of *PrP*, associated with substitution of aspartic acid with asparagine along with the presence of methionine codon at position 129 of the mutant allele. All human prion diseases (e.g., Creutzfeldt-Jakob disease, Gerstmann-Sträussler-Scheinker disease) should be considered in the differential diagnosis. Approximately 10 families of patients with FFI have been identified so far. The study of FFI has rekindled investigation of the thalamus's role in sleep-wake regulation.

Stroke and Sleep Disturbances

Sleep disruption and sleep complaints resulting from sleep-related breathing dysrhythmias have been reported in many patients with cerebral hemispheric stroke. There is, however, a dearth of well-controlled studies establishing a relationship between sleep disorders and cerebrovascular disease. Sleep apnea, snoring, and stroke are intimately related. Sleep apnea may predispose to stroke, and stroke may predispose to sleep apnea. Based on case-controlled, epidemiological, and laboratory studies, there is increasing evidence that snoring and sleep apnea are risk factors for stroke. Several confounding variables are common risk factors for snoring, sleep apnea, and stroke, however, and these should be considered when attempting to establish a relationship between snoring, sleep apnea, and stroke. These variables include hypertension, cardiac disease, age, body mass index, smoking, and alcohol consumption. There is an increased frequency of sleep apnea in both infratentorial and supratentorial strokes. It is important to make a diagnosis of sleep apnea in stroke patients because this may adversely affect short-term and long-term outcomes in patients with stroke and because there is effective treatment for sleep apnea that can decrease the risk of future stroke. Other causes of sleep disruption causing insomnia may include associated depression, spasticity, and immobility.

Hypersomnolence has been described after bilateral paramedian thalamic infarcts. Several authors have described sleep disturbances in brainstem infarction. PSG findings generally consist of increased wakefulness after sleep onset and decreased REM and slow-wave sleep in these patients. EEG findings in several reports of patients with locked-in syndrome resulting from ventral pontine infarction generally showed reduced or absent REM sleep and variable changes in NREM sleep, including reduction of slow-wave sleep and total sleep time (Chokroverty 1999d).

Brainstem infarction may cause the syndrome of primary failure of automatic respiration, or Ondine's curse. Voluntary breathing control is intact, but metabolic control, which is the only respiratory control during sleep, is impaired. Therefore, the patients become apneic during sleep. Severinghaus and Mitchell named the condition. The syndrome of Ondine's curse is usually caused by bilateral lesions anywhere caudal to the fifth cranial nerve in the pons down to the upper cervical spinal cord in the ventrolateral region. Occasional patients with unilateral brainstem infarction have been described with loss of automatic respiratory control during sleep.

Traumatic Brain Injury and Sleep Disturbances

Traumatic brain injuries (TBIs) include concussion, contusion, laceration, hemorrhage, and cerebral edema. Insomnia, hypersomnia, and circadian rhythm sleep dysfunction may occur after TBI, but objective sleep studies in such patients documenting sleep disturbances have not been adequately performed. After a severe TBI, brainstem function is compromised and the patient becomes comatose. There have been many EEG studies in patients with coma after head trauma. However, no studies have adequately addressed the sleep-wake abnormalities in these patients after recovery from coma as well as in patients after minor brain injuries that did not result in coma. Many of these patients experience so-called postconcussion syndrome, which is characterized by a variety of behavioral disturbances, headache, and sleep-wake abnormalities. A few reports list subjective complaints of sleep disturbance but do not include formal sleep studies. In one report of patients with closed head injury, PSG studies documented sleep-maintenance insomnia with an increased number of awakenings and decreased night sleep. The mechanism of these sleep abnormalities is unknown. Post-traumatic hypersomnolence is listed in the ICSD (1997). TBI may cause central and upper airway OSA by inflicting functional or structural alterations on the brainstem respiratory control system. Many of these patients may, however, have had sleep apnea syndrome before sustaining TBI. Circadian rhythm sleep disturbances have been described in severely brain-damaged patients. There are two reports, one in a 13-year-old boy and another in a 48-year-old adult, of DSPS after TBI (Chokroverty 1999d).

Sleep and Multiple Sclerosis

Sleep-related breathing abnormalities and other sleep difficulties, including insomnia, EDS, and depression, have been described in patients with MS. Sleep disturbances in MS are thought to result from immobility, spasticity, urinary bladder sphincter disturbances, and sleep-related respiratory dysrhythmias due to affected respiratory muscles or impaired central control of breathing.

Sleep Disturbances in Neurodegenerative Diseases

Neurodegenerative diseases are traditionally defined as a group of heterogeneous diseases of the CNS for which no causal agent can be identified. The disorders generally affect one or more systems symmetrically and run an inexorably progressive course.

Sleep-wake–promoting neurons are involved in the process of diffuse degeneration, causing a variety of sleep disorders in these illnesses (Hening et al. 1999). Neurodegenerative diseases can be considered under two broad categories: degeneration of the somatic neurons and degeneration of the autonomic neurons. Somatic neuronal degeneration can be predominantly cortical (e.g., Alzheimer's disease [AD]); predominantly basal ganglia, or basal ganglia-plus syndromes (e.g., Parkinson's disease [PD], progressive supranuclear palsy [PSP], Huntington's chorea, torsion dystonia, and Tourette's syndrome); predominantly cerebellar or cerebellar-plus syndromes (spinocerebellar ataxias [SCAs], including olivopontocerebellar atrophy [OPCA]); or predominantly motor neurons of the cerebral cortex, brainstem, and spinal cord (ALS or motor neuron disease). Neurodegeneration of the autonomic neurons is responsible for multiple system atrophy (MSA), or Shy-Drager syndrome (Table 72.16).

Diseases of Somatic Neurons

Alzheimer's Disease

AD is the most common cerebral degenerative disorder causing dementia. Reports of sleep disturbances in AD have been contradictory. Sleep disorders may be related to the severity of dementia as well as to associated PLMS and sleep-related respiratory dysrhythmias. In addition, the artificial environment of the hospital and laboratory where the sleep disturbance is evaluated may be partly responsible for confusional episodes, including "sundowning" in AD patients. Insomnia, inversion of the sleep rhythm, and in some cases, EDS are the presenting complaints. Sleep disturbances in AD should be differentiated from those occurring in depression, which is common in elderly subjects. A reduction in the amount of REM sleep and reduced REM density are quite different from the reduced REM latency and increased REM density often seen in depressed patients.

Table 72.16: Salient clinical manifestations of multiple system atrophy

Autonomic features
  Cardiovascular
    Orthostatic hypotension
    Postprandial hypotension
    Postural syncope
    Postural dizziness, faint feelings, or blurring of vision
    Orthostatic intolerance
  Genitourinary
    Urinary bladder dysfunction (incontinence, hesitancy, frequency, nocturia)
    Impotence in men
  Sudomotor
    Hypohidrosis or anhidrosis
  Gastrointestinal
    Gastroparesis
    Intermittent diarrhea or constipation (intestinal or colonic dysmotility)
    Abnormal swallowing (esophageal dysmotility)
  Ocular
    Horner's syndrome
    Unequal pupils
Nonautonomic manifestations
  Parkinsonism
    Rigidity
    Bradykinesia or akinesia
    Postural instability
  Cerebellar dysfunction
    Ataxic gait
    Scanning speech
    Dysmetria
    Dysdiadochokinesia
    Intention tremor
  Upper motor neuron signs
    Extensor plantar responses
    Hyperreflexia
    Spasticity
  Lower motor neuron signs
    Muscle wasting
    Fasciculations
  Respiratory
    Sleep apnea-hypopnea
    Other respiratory dysrhythmias
  Normal mentation
  Normal sensation

Sleep-related respiratory dysrhythmia has been estimated to be present in 33–53% of AD patients. The questions remain somewhat controversial whether there is an increased prevalence of sleep apnea in AD and whether sleep apnea increases with the severity of the illness or more rapid progression of the disease. Sundowning is a major problem in many AD patients, causing nocturnal confusional episodes, often accompanied by partial or complete inversion of sleep schedule, with increased wakefulness at night and somnolence in the daytime. The exact relationship between sleep disruption, severe dementia, and sundowning is not clear. Several factors, singly or in combination, may be responsible for sleep

disturbances in AD. They are degeneration of the neurons of the SCN, of cholinergic neurons in the nucleus basalis of Meynert, of the PPT and LDT nuclei, and of noradrenergic neurons of the brainstem; associated depression or PLMS; medication effects; associated general medical diseases; and environmental factors.

Parkinson's Disease

Sleep difficulties have been noted in 70–90% of patients with PD. Common complaints include difficulties in initiating and maintaining sleep, inability to turn over during the night or on awakening, and inability to get out of bed unaided. Leg cramps and jerks, dystonic spasms of the limbs or face, back pain, and excessive nocturia are also common. A clear relationship has been noted between sleep disruption and disease progression.

Motor abnormalities during sleep in PD include persistence of tremor in the lighter stages of sleep or its re-emergence in the transition between sleep and wakefulness and on awakening, as well as decreased body movements and positional shifts. Other motor abnormalities in PD during sleep include rapid blinking at sleep onset, blepharospasm during onset of REMs, and intrusion of REMs into NREM sleep. Sleep benefit (early morning improvement of parkinsonian motor features, lasting 1–3 hours) may be noted mostly in mild PD.

Sleep in PD may be secondarily affected because of associated depression, dementia, sleep-related respiratory dysrhythmias, RLS, PLMS, RBD, and other parasomnias (sleepwalking and sleep talking) as well as circadian rhythm disturbances. RBD is a common occurrence in PD, and in some cases, this disorder appears even before parkinsonian symptoms are clinically evident. It is estimated that about 30% of PD patients may have PLMS, and this proportion increases in elderly patients.

Sleep-related respiratory dysrhythmias may be more common in PD patients than in age-matched controls. Obstructive, central, or mixed apneas have been described in PD patients, and such respiratory difficulties have been noted with increasing incidence in patients with autonomic dysfunction. Antiparkinsonian medications may cause respiratory and other dyskinesias, which could be peak-dose dyskinesia (mainly choreiform) or end-of-the-dose dyskinesia (mostly dystonic). These dyskinesias may cause sleep disruption or fragmentation of sleep. Vivid or frightening dreams (nightmares) can occur after long-standing dopaminergic treatment, causing sleep maintenance problems and EDS.

Other Basal Ganglia Disorders

A variety of sleep disturbances have been observed in other basal ganglia disorders, such as Huntington's chorea, PSP, and torsion dystonia. Insomnia with difficulty initiating and maintaining sleep is a common complaint in these conditions. Sleep disturbance is present in almost all cases of PSP.

A particular type of dystonia, called *hereditary progressive dystonia* with diurnal fluctuation, dopa-responsive dystonia, or Segawa variant, presents with parkinsonian-type masked facies, rigidity, and flexed posture. Patients with this dystonia may obtain significant symptomatic relief from sleep and show dramatic improvement with small doses of levodopa.

Predominantly Cerebellar or Cerebellar-Plus Syndromes

Sleep disturbances occur in many patients with OPCA and other types of SCAs. Although several genes (*SCA1, SCA2, SCA3*/Machado-Joseph disease, *SCA6, SCA7,* and dentatorubropallidoluysian atrophy) have been described with expanded CAG repeats responsible for autosomal dominant cerebellar ataxia, approximately 40% of dominant ataxias have not been identified at a genotypic level. Cases of recessive or sporadic OPCA are now classified under MSA. Central, obstructive, or mixed sleep apneas have been described in many patients with OPCA, but the apneas have been less frequent and less intense in this condition than in MSA. Typical features of RBD have been described in OPCA. Other complaints in SCAs, particularly in SCA3, consist of sleep initiation and maintenance problems.

Degenerative Disease of the Motor Neurons

The classic example of degenerative disease of motor neurons is ALS, also called *motor neuron disease.* The most common sleep complaint in ALS is daytime hypersomnolence as a result of repeated sleep-related apneas or hypopneas, hypoxemia, hypercapnia, and sleep fragmentation. Some patients may complain of insomnia. Sleep-related breathing disorders in ALS may result from weakness of upper airway, diaphragmatic, and intercostal muscles due to involvement of the bulbar, phrenic, and intercostal nerve nuclei. In addition, degeneration of the central respiratory neurons may occur, causing both CSA and OSA in this condition.

Sleep Disorders in Autonomic Diseases: Multiple System Atrophy (Shy-Drager Syndrome)

In a consensus conference (1996), the term *MSA* was suggested to replace the term Shy-Drager syndrome. MSA defines a sporadic adult-onset progressive disorder of multiple systems characterized by autonomic dysfunction, parkinsonism, and ataxia in various combinations (see Table 72.16). *Striatonigral degeneration* is the name used when the predominant feature is parkinsonism, whereas *OPCA* is used when the cerebellar features are the predominant manifestations. The term *Shy-Drager syndrome* is still used when the autonomic feature is the predominant feature. Some patients complain of insomnia, and many patients manifest RBD, which may occasionally be the presenting feature, but the most common sleep disturbance in patients with MSA results from respiratory dysrhythmias associated with repeated arousals and hypoxemia. Sleep-related respiratory dysrhythmias in MSA may include obstructive, central, or mixed apneas and hypopneas as well as Cheyne-Stokes breathing or a variant of Cheyne-Stokes breathing. Other breathing disorders in sleep in MSA consist of nocturnal inspiratory stridor, apneustic breathing, inspiratory gasping, or dysrhythmic breathing. Hypersomnia often results from nocturnal sleep disruption. Sudden nocturnal death in patients with MSA, presumably from cardiorespiratory arrest, has been reported.

Both direct and indirect mechanisms are responsible for the pathogenesis of sleep disruption in MSA. These may include one or more of the following: degeneration of the sleep-wake–generating neurons in the brainstem and hypothalamus; degeneration of the respiratory neurons in the brainstem or direct involvement of projections from the hypothalamus and central nucleus of amygdala to the respiratory neurons in the nucleus tractus solitarius and nucleus ambiguus; interference with the vagal inputs from the peripheral respiratory receptors to the central respiratory neurons; sympathetic denervation of the nasal mucosa; and alteration of the neurochemical environment.

SLEEP IN OTHER MEDICAL DISORDERS

A number of medical disorders other than neurological illnesses may cause severe disturbances of sleep and breathing that have important practical implications in terms of diagnosis, prognosis, and treatment (Chokroverty 1999e). Sleep disturbances may have adverse effects on the course of a medical illness. A vicious cycle may result from the effect of sleep disturbance on the medical illness and the effect of the medical illness on sleep architecture. Sleep architecture, sleep continuity, and sleep organization may be affected by a variety of medical illnesses. Patients may present with either insomnia or hypersomnolence, but most medical disorders present with insomnia. Some patients may have a mixture of insomnia and hypersomnolence (e.g., those with COPD or nocturnal asthma). The general features of insomnia and medical disorders causing insomnia have been briefly described (see Insomnia, earlier in this chapter). The general features of hypersomnolence and medical conditions presenting with hypersomnolence are briefly described in Chapter 6. PSG findings in those presenting with insomnia include prolonged sleep latency, reduction of REM and slow-wave sleep, more than 10 awakenings per night, frequent stage shifts, early-morning awakening, increased waking after sleep onset, and increased percentage of wakefulness and stage I NREM sleep. PSG findings in those presenting with hypersomnolence may consist of SDB, repeated arousals with oxygen desaturation at night, sleep fragmentation, sleep-stage shifts, reduced slow-wave sleep, shortened sleep-onset latency in MSLT, and sometimes REM sleep abnormalities. When a patient presents to a sleep specialist with a sleep disturbance, either with a complaint of insomnia or hypersomnia, an important step is to obtain a detailed medical history and other histories, followed by physical examination to uncover the cause of the sleep disturbance.

In an important epidemiological study by Gislason and Almqvist involving a random sample of 3,201 Swedish men, aged 30–69 years, difficulty initiating or maintaining sleep and too little sleep were the major sleep complaints, followed by EDS (Chokroverty 1999e). Sleep-maintenance problems were frequent with increasing age. The following conditions were associated with sleep complaints: systemic hypertension, bronchitis and bronchial asthma, musculoskeletal disorders, obesity, and diabetes mellitus. The authors suggested that the reported increased mortality among patients with sleep complaints might be related to the intercurrent somatic diseases.

Cardiovascular Disease and Sleep

Sleep disturbance is very common in patients with ischemic heart disease. Pain may awaken the patient frequently, thereby reducing sleep efficiency. Nocturnal angina is known to occur during both REM and NREM sleep. Epidemiologically, there is a clear relationship between increased cardiovascular morbidity and mortality and sleep disturbances associated with SDB. Patients with coronary artery disease and OSA may have an increased cardiac risk due to nocturnal myocardial ischemia triggered by apnea-associated oxygen desaturation. Increased mortality rates were found among patients with ischemic heart disease, stroke, and cancer who slept 4 hours or less, or more than 10 hours. An important finding in several reports is circadian susceptibility to myocardial infarction (attacks are most likely between midnight and 6:00 AM).

In patients with CHF, sleep disturbances, periodic breathing, and hypoxemia at night have been described. Multiple factors, including associated SDB and nocturnal oxygen desaturation, are responsible for increased morbidity and mortality in CHF. Cheyne-Stokes respiration, which is commonly associated with CHF, may result in hypoxemia, hypercapnia, sleep disruption due to repeated arousals, daytime somnolence, and impaired cognitive function. Thus, Cheyne-Stokes respiration and CHF may present as sleep apnea syndrome. Javaheri et al. (1995) reported an AHI higher than 20 in 45% of patients with stable heart failure without other comorbid factors. After treatment with nocturnal oxygen administration, CPAP titration, and medications such as theophylline, the patients improved. However, the role of CPAP in the maintenance treatment of CHF remains controversial.

A relationship between sleep and atrioventricular arrhythmia has been noted, but the reports are controversial. Contradictory results have also been noted in human studies of the effect of sleep on ventricular arrhythmia, but most studies show an antiarrhythmic effect of sleep on ventricular premature beats due to enhanced parasympathetic tone during sleep. An analysis of the time of sudden cardiac death in 2,023 individuals by Muller and associates revealed high incidence from 7:00 AM to 11:00 AM. Nonfatal myocardial infarction and myocardial ischemic episodes are also more likely to occur in the morning. It is known that sympathetic activity increases in the morning, causing increased myocardial electrical instability; thus, sudden cardiac death may result from a primary fatal arrhythmia.

Several studies reported a frequency of 20–48% of sleep apnea and related symptoms in patients with systemic hypertension, whereas the frequency of hypertension in patients with sleep apnea is approximately 50–90%. Some studies have confirmed that treatment of sleep apnea by nasal CPAP reduces blood pressure. In contrast, Stradling and Davies (1997) contended that there is no convincing evidence to support the notion that sleep apnea is a significant independent risk factor for sustained hypertension in humans. Others believe that even when the confounding factors are taken into consideration, OSA is an independent risk factor for hypertension and that treatment of OSA reduces daytime as well as nighttime blood pressure.

Sleep and Chronic Obstructive Pulmonary Disease

Disturbances in sleep architecture in patients with COPD have been reported by several authors and may be summarized as follows: a reduction of sleep efficiency, delayed sleep onset, increased wake time after sleep onset, frequent stage shifts, and frequent arousals. Factors that may be responsible for sleep disturbance in COPD include the use of drugs that have a sleep-reducing effect (e.g., methylxanthine); increased nocturnal cough, resulting from accumulated bronchial secretions; and associated hypoxemia and hypercapnia. Severe nocturnal hypoxemia in many patients with COPD may or may not be accompanied by sleep-related apnea, hypopnea or periodic breathing, and impairment of gas exchange. Repeated or prolonged oxygen desaturation at night may cause cardiac arrhythmias and may lead to pulmonary hypertension and cor pulmonale. Administration of supplemental oxygen at 2 liters per minute by nasal cannula during sleep is found to improve both oxygen saturation at night and sleep architecture by decreasing sleep latency and increasing all stages of sleep, including REM and slow-wave sleep.

Sleep Disturbances in Bronchial Asthma

A variety of sleep disturbances have been noted in patients with asthma, including early-morning awakenings, difficulty maintaining sleep, and EDS. Sleep disturbances in general consist of a combination of insomnia and hypersomnia. PSG studies may reveal disruption of sleep architecture as well as sleep apnea in some patients. Nocturnal exacerbation of symptoms during sleep is a frequent finding in asthmatic patients. There is also evidence of progressive bronchoconstriction and hypoxemia during sleep in patients with asthma. Several pathogenic mechanisms, including circadian factors, have been suggested for sleep disturbances and nocturnal exacerbation of asthma.

Gastrointestinal Diseases and Sleep

Sleep disturbances in peptic ulcer patients characteristically result from episodes of nocturnal epigastric pain. These symptoms cause arousals and repeated awakenings, thereby fragmenting and disturbing sleep considerably. With duodenal ulcers, there is increased nocturnal acid secretion, which can be abolished by vagotomy, thus improving healing of ulcers. Furthermore, duodenal ulcer patients do not have inhibition of gastric acid secretion during the first 2 hours after sleep onset. In light of evidence about the role of *Helicobacter pylori* infection and nonsteroidal anti-inflammatory drugs in the pathogenesis of gastroduodenal ulcers, the theory of hypersecretion of acid in peptic ulcer patients has been displaced.

Gastroesophageal reflux disease, which is preferable to the term *reflux esophagitis*, characteristically causes heartburn, which is described as retrosternal burning pain. This pain causes difficulty in initiating sleep, frequent awakenings, and fragmentation of sleep. Facilities for all-night PSG study and 24-hour esophageal pH monitoring have contributed to an understanding of the association between sleep and peptic ulcer diseases and esophageal reflux. Sleep adversely affects patients with gastroesophageal reflux disease by increasing the episodes of reflux and prolonging acid clearance time. Furthermore, repeated spontaneous reflux episodes adversely affect sleep by causing arousals, frequent awakenings, and sleep fragmentation.

Sleep and Endocrine Diseases

In patients with myxedema, upper airway OSA and CSA that disappear after thyroxine replacement therapy have been described. Mechanisms of SDB in this condition include deposition of mucopolysaccharides in the upper airway as well as impaired central respiratory drive, as evidenced by decreased hypercapnic and hypoxic ventilatory responses.

Patients with diabetes mellitus, particularly that associated with autonomic neuropathy, may have upper airway OSA and CSA. These sleep-related respiratory dysrhythmias may cause fragmentation of sleep, resulting in EDS.

CSA has been described in many patients with acromegaly. CSA has been generally associated with increased levels of growth hormone. The relationship between the growth hormone level and sleep apnea, however, has remained somewhat controversial. Octreotide, a long-acting somatostatin analogue, is an effective noninvasive treatment for sleep apnea in acromegaly.

Sleep Disturbances in Chronic Renal Failure

Sleep disturbances are common in patients with chronic renal failure (CRF) with or without dialysis, particularly in those with end-stage renal disease. Sleep complaints include insomnia, EDS, and day-night reversal or disturbed nocturnal sleep. PSG findings include reduced sleep efficiency, increased sleep fragmentation, frequent awakenings with difficulty maintaining sleep, decreased slow-wave sleep, and disorganization of sleep cycle. Many patients with CRF on and off dialysis have sleep apnea syndrome, mainly upper airway OSAS, and may have PLMS. A PSG study to establish the diagnosis of OSA should be performed in any patient with a history of EDS and disturbed night sleep because CPAP titration has been found to be an effective form of treatment in hemodialysis patients with OSA. Another important finding in patients with CRF is the presence of a secondary form of RLS. Uremic RLS and idiopathic RLS resemble each other and cannot be distinguished clinically. There has been one report of cure of this form of RLS after successful kidney transplantation.

Fibromyalgia Syndrome

Fibromyalgia syndrome (FMS) is characterized by diffuse muscle aches and pains not related to diseases of the joints, bones, or connective tissues. Specific diagnostic criteria for FMS have been established. Sleep disturbance is very common in FMS. The characteristic PSG finding is intermittent alpha activity during NREM sleep, giving rise to the characteristic alpha-delta or alpha-NREM sleep pattern in the recording. Another important association is the presence of PLMS on PSG examination. Alpha-NREM sleep pattern is not specific for this condition and has been noted in other rheumatic disorders, and even in normal individuals, as well as some psychiatric patients. The most common complaints in FMS patients include nonrestorative sleep associated with nonspecific PSG abnormalities of sleep fragmentation, increased awakenings, decreased sleep efficiency, and alpha-NREM sleep.

Sleep of Intensive Care Unit Patients

Patients in an intensive care unit (ICU) are generally admitted with acute medical, surgical, or neurological illnesses. All these conditions can be associated with sleep disturbances (insomnia, hypersomnia, and sleep-related respiratory dysrhythmia). The ICU environment itself is deleterious to normal sleep and conducive to sleep deprivation, with attendant complications, such as ICU psychosis. Noise, bright light, and constant activity by ICU personnel for monitoring and drug administration play a significant role

Table 72.17: Features of sleepwalking (somnambulism)

Onset: common between ages 5–12 yrs
High frequency of a positive family history
Abrupt onset of motor activity arising out of slow-wave sleep during the first one-third of the night
Duration: less than 10 mins
Injuries and violent activity: reported occasionally
Precipitating factors: sleep deprivation, fatigue, concurrent illness, sedatives
Treatment: precaution, benzodiazepines, imipramine

in disturbing the sleep of ICU patients. A variety of drugs in the ICU may aggravate sleep and sleep-related respiratory disturbances. ICU syndrome is a characteristic mental state defined as a reversible, confusional state developing 3–7 days after ICU admission; sleep deprivation has been cited as the major cause of ICU syndrome. ICU psychosis is more common in surgical than in medical ICUs. PSG findings to document disruption of sleep structure in the ICU consist of marked diminution of slow-wave sleep and REM sleep, frequent awakenings, sleep fragmentation, and reduced total sleep time. ICU patients often have EDS because of disturbed night sleep. It is important to be aware of various ICU factors contributing to the problem of sleep disturbances so that correct diagnosis and management of secondary complications can be implemented promptly.

Acquired Immunodeficiency Syndrome

Acquired immunodeficiency syndrome (AIDS) is a multisystem disorder caused by infection with HIV. Sleep disturbances have been reported in patients with AIDS, but adequate systematic PSG studies to document sleep disruption have not been undertaken. HIV infection can also cause SDB.

African Sleeping Sickness (Trypanosomiasis)

African sleeping sickness is caused by *Trypanosoma gambiense* or *T. rhodesiense* and is transmitted to humans by the bite of tsetse flies. CNS involvement is initially characterized by personality changes followed by delusions, hallucinations, and reversal of sleep-wake rhythm. The patient remains somnolent in the daytime and progresses gradually into the stages of stupor and coma. PSG studies document disruption of the circadian sleep-wake rhythm, which is proportional to the severity of the illness. Circadian disruption of plasma cortisol, prolactin, and sleep-wake rhythms is seen in the most advanced patients. These findings of circadian disruption suggest selective changes in the SCN. The diagnosis of trypanosomiasis is based on history as well as confirmation that the organism is in blood, bone marrow, cerebrospinal fluid, lymph node, aspirates, or a scraping from the chancre. The treatment of choice for patients in the meningo-encephalitic stage is arsenical melarsoprol.

SLEEP DISTURBANCES IN PSYCHIATRIC ILLNESS

Insomnia is more common than hypersomnia in psychiatric illnesses (see Insomnia, earlier in this chapter, for a brief review).

PARASOMNIAS

Parasomnias can be defined as abnormal movements or behavior intruding into sleep during the night intermittently or episodically without disturbing the sleep architecture. The *ICSD* classifies parasomnias into four groups (see Table 72.3): arousal disorders, sleep-wake transition disorders, REM-related parasomnias, and other parasomnias. This classification lists 24 distinct entities, several of which are very rare. Major parasomnias can also be classified into motor and behavioral parasomnias. Motor parasomnias are abnormal movements intruding into sleep and are classified into four categories: NREM sleep parasomnias; REM sleep parasomnias, sleep-wake transition disorders; and diffuse parasomnias (no stage preference). Several parasomnias occurring in NREM and REM sleep may be mistaken for seizures, particularly complex partial seizures. Somnambulism, night terror, confusional arousals, somniloquy, bruxism, head banging, nocturnal enuresis, RBD, and nightmares are some of the parasomnias that may be mistaken for seizures. RBD and nightmares are the only ones associated with REM sleep. Characteristic clinical features combined with EEG and PSG recordings are essential to differentiate these conditions.

Somnambulism (Sleepwalking)

Sleepwalking is common in children between 5 and 12 years of age (Table 72.17). Sometimes, it persists in adulthood or (rarely) begins in adults. Sleepwalking begins with abrupt motor activity arising out of slow-wave sleep during the first one-third of sleep. Episodes generally last less than 10 minutes. There is a high incidence of positive family history in sleepwalking. Injuries and violent actions have been reported during sleepwalking episodes, but generally, individuals can negotiate their way around the room. Sleep deprivation, fatigue, concurrent illness, and sedatives may act as precipitating factors.

Sleep Terrors

Sleep terrors, or pavor nocturnus, also occur during slow-wave sleep (Table 72.18). Peak onset is between 5 and 7 years of age. As with sleepwalking, there is a high frequency of familial cases in sleep terror. Episodes of sleep terrors are characterized by intense autonomic and motor symptoms, including a loud, piercing scream. Patients appear highly confused and fearful. Many patients also have a history of sleepwalking episodes. Precipitating factors are similar to those described with sleepwalking.

Table 72.18: Features of sleep terrors

Onset: peak is between ages 5–7 yrs
High frequency of familial cases
Abrupt arousal from slow-wave sleep during the first one-third of the night with a loud, piercing scream
Intense autonomic and motor components
Many patients also sleepwalk
Precipitating factors: stress, sleep deprivation, fever
Treatment: psychotherapy, benzodiazepines, tricyclics

Confusional Arousals

Confusional arousals occur mostly before the age of 5 years. As in sleepwalking and sleep terrors, these episodes arise out of slow-wave sleep with confusion. Patients may have some automatic and inappropriate behavior, but the majority of spells are benign, necessitating no treatment.

Hypnic Jerks

Hypnic jerks, or "sleep starts," occur at sleep onset in many normal individuals and are physiological phenomena without any pathological significance. The episodes are associated with sudden brief myoclonic jerks of the limbs or the whole body lasting for a few seconds. Sometimes these are accompanied by sensory phenomena, such as a sensation of falling. These may be triggered by stress, fatigue, or sleep deprivation. "Sleep starts" may occur in up to 70% of the general population.

Rhythmic Movement Disorder

Rhythmic movement disorder is noted mostly before 18 months of age and is occasionally associated with mental retardation. It is a sleep-wake transition disorder with three characteristic movements: head banging, head rolling, and body rocking. Rhythmic movement disorder is a benign condition, and the patient outgrows the episodes.

Nocturnal Leg Cramps

These are intensely painful sensations accompanied by muscle tightness that occur during sleep. The spasms usually last for a few seconds but sometimes persist for several minutes. Cramps during sleep are generally associated with awakening. Many normal individuals have nocturnal leg cramps; the cause remains unknown. Local massage or movement of the limbs usually relieves the cramps.

Nightmares (Dream Anxiety Attacks)

Nightmares are fearful, vivid, and often frightening dreams, mostly visual but sometimes auditory, seen during REM sleep. Nightmares may accompany sleep talking and body

Table 72.19: Features of rapid eye movement (REM) sleep behavior disorder

Onset: middle-aged or elderly men
Presents with violent dream-enacting behavior during sleep causing injury to self or bed partner
Often misdiagnosed as a psychiatric disorder or nocturnal seizure (partial complex seizure)
Etiology: 55% idiopathic, 45% causal association with structural central nervous system lesion or related to alcohol or drugs (sedatives-hypnotics, tricyclics, anticholinergics)
Polysomnography: REM sleep without muscle atonia
Experimental model: bilateral peri–locus ceruleus lesions
Treatment: 90% respond to clonazepam

movements. These most commonly occur during the middle to late part of sleep at night. Nightmares are mostly a normal phenomenon. Up to 50% of children, perhaps even more, have nightmares beginning at age 3–5 years. The frequency of nightmares continues to decrease as the child grows older, and the elderly have very few or no nightmares. Very frightening and recurring nightmares (e.g., one or more per week) are not common and may occur in a very small percentage (<1%) of individuals. Nightmares can also occur as side effects of certain medications, such as antiparkinsonian drugs (pergolide, L-dopa), anticholinergics, and antihypertensive drugs, particularly beta blockers. Nightmares are common after sudden withdrawal of REM-suppressant drugs (e.g., tricyclic antidepressants, selective serotonin reuptake inhibitors). Benzodiazepines (e.g., diazepam, clonazepam) often suppress nightmares, but withdrawal from these drugs may precipitate nightmares. Nightmares have also been reported after alcohol ingestion or sudden withdrawal from barbiturates. Nightmares may sometimes be the initial manifestation of schizophreniform psychosis along with severe sleep disturbance. Many people with a certain personality type have nightmares throughout life. Nightmares generally do not require any treatment except reassurance. In patients with recurring and fearful nightmares, however, combined behavioral or psychotherapy and REM-suppressant medications may be helpful.

Rapid Eye Movement Sleep Behavior Disorder

RBD is an important REM sleep parasomnia commonly seen in elderly persons (Table 72.19). A characteristic feature of RBD is intermittent loss of REM-related muscle hypotonia or atonia and the appearance of various abnormal motor activities during sleep. The patient experiences violent dream-enacting behavior during REM sleep, often causing self-injury or injury to the bed partner. The condition may be either idiopathic or secondary to a neurological illness (e.g., PD, MSA, OPCA, and other structural lesions of the brainstem). RBD is sometimes associated with alcoholism or ingestion of drugs (e.g., sedative-hypnotics, tricyclic antidepressants, and anticholinergics). The prominent finding in a PSG recording is REM sleep without muscle atonia. Multiple-muscle EMG from the upper and lower extremities should be obtained during the PSG recording in addition to the traditional tibialis anterior muscle EMG because absence of muscle atonia may not be seen in all muscles. In experiments, similar behavior was produced by a bilateral peri–locus ceruleus lesion in cats many years before discovery of human RBD.

Bruxism (Tooth Grinding)

Bruxism occurs most commonly between the ages of 10 and 20 years. It is also commonly noted in children with mental retardation or cerebral palsy. Bruxism is noted most prominently during NREM stages I and II and REM sleep. The episode is characterized by stereotypical tooth grinding and often precipitated by anxiety, stress, and dental disease. Occasionally, familial cases have been described.

Benign Neonatal Sleep Myoclonus

Benign neonatal sleep myoclonus occurs during the first few weeks of life and is generally seen in NREM sleep but sometimes during REM sleep. Episodes often occur in clusters involving arms, legs, and sometimes the trunk. The movements consist of jerky flexion, extension, abduction, and adduction. The condition is benign, needing no treatment.

Nocturnal Paroxysmal Dystonia

Although NPD (see Table 72.14) is classified under other parasomnias (see Table 72.3), most cases—particularly attacks of short duration—probably represent a type of frontal lobe seizure. These are described under Nocturnal Paroxysmal Dystonia, Paroxysmal Arousals and Awakenings, and Episodic Nocturnal Wanderings, earlier in this chapter.

PEDIATRIC SLEEP DISORDERS

Pediatric sleep disorders remain a neglected field despite a high frequency of sleep disturbance in children. Several recent surveys found that about 25% of children aged 1–5 years have some kind of sleep problem. Mentally handicapped children and those with attention-deficit/hyperactivity disorder have higher rates of sleep disorders than normal children do. Some of the common sleep problems in children include a variety of parasomnias, such as sleepwalking, nightmares, sleep talking, sleep enuresis, bruxism, sleep terrors, and rhythmic movement disorder; sleeplessness due to specific childhood-onset disorder or food allergy; EDS (e.g., narcolepsy, OSA); and DSPS or ASPS. Adjustment sleep disorder, limit-setting sleep disorder, sleep-onset association disorder, and nocturnal eating (or drinking) syndrome are some distinct sleep disorders causing insomnia in infants and children.

ICSD (1997) defines adjustment sleep disorder as a type of sleep disturbance that is temporally related to acute stress, conflict, or environmental change that causes emotional arousal. The disturbance in most cases is brief. Sleep-onset or maintenance insomnia or daytime sleepiness may be the presenting complaint, but insomnia is more common than sleepiness in children.

Limit-setting sleep disorder is exclusively a childhood sleep disorder characterized by stalling or refusing to go to sleep at an appropriate time as a result of inadequate enforcement of bedtime by the caregiver. The condition usually resolves as the child grows older.

Sleep-onset association disorder is a childhood sleep disorder characterized by an impairment of sleep onset because of absence of a certain object or set of circumstances (e.g., using a bottle, sucking on a pacifier, being rocked, watching television, or listening to the radio). Sleep is normal when the particular association is present.

ICSD (1997) defines nocturnal eating (drinking) syndrome as a condition characterized by recurrent awakenings with inability to return to sleep without eating or drinking. This condition is common in infancy and early childhood. Treatment involves gradual withdrawal from eating or drinking behavior.

OSAS occurs in children, but there are certain differences from adults. Children may present with EDS, but common symptoms include hyperactivity and behavioral problems during the daytime, impaired school performance, intellectual changes, increased motor activity, disturbed sleep at night, and nocturnal snoring for many months or years. An important cause in children is enlargement of tonsils and adenoids. If OSAS is suspected, an overnight PSG study is indicated for documenting OSA. In contrast to adults, removal of the tonsils and adenoids in children promotes symptomatic improvement. Some cases of sudden infant death syndrome are thought to be related to OSA, but the relationship remains unproved and controversial. The most important factor in sudden infant death syndrome is sleeping in the prone position, and every attempt must be made to keep the infant in the supine position.

Primary enuresis is a condition of persistent bed-wetting after age 5 years in the absence of urological, medical, psychiatric, or neurological disorders. Enuretic episodes occur during all stages of sleep but most commonly occur during the first one-third of the night. Treatment includes behavioral modification and, in some cases, tricyclic antidepressants (e.g., imipramine).

LABORATORY ASSESSMENT OF SLEEP DISORDERS

Laboratory investigation for sleep disorders should be considered an extension of the history and physical examination. First and foremost in the diagnosis of a sleep disorder is a detailed history, including sleep and other histories, as outlined earlier, under Approach to a Patient with Sleep Complaints. This should be followed by a careful physical examination to uncover any underlying medical, neurological, or other causes of sleep dysfunction. Laboratory tests should include diagnostic workup for the primary condition causing secondary sleep disturbance and workup for the sleep disturbance itself. The two most important laboratory tests for diagnosis of sleep disturbance are PSG and MSLT. Various other tests are important for assessment of a patient with sleep dysfunction.

Polysomnographic Study

An overnight PSG study is the single most important laboratory test for the diagnosis and treatment of patients with sleep disorders, particularly those associated with EDS. All-night PSG is required rather than a single-day nap study. A daytime single-nap study generally misses REM sleep, and most severe apheic episodes are noted during REM sleep. Maximum oxygen desaturation also occurs at this stage; therefore, a daytime study cannot assess severity of the symptoms. For CPAP titration, an all-night sleep study is essential. To determine the optimal level of pressure during CPAP titration, both REM and NREM sleep are required. In this section, PSG is described under three headings: technical considerations, indications for PSG, and characteristic PSG findings in various sleep disorders.

Technical Considerations

PSG includes simultaneous recording of various physiological characteristics, which allows assessment of sleep stages and wakefulness, respiration, cardiocirculatory functions, and body movements. Sleep staging is based on EEG, electro-oculogram, and EMG of some skeletal muscles, especially chin muscles. Multiple EEG channels of recordings are preferable to one or two channels for documenting focal and diffuse neurological lesions, accurately localizing epileptiform discharges in patients with seizure disorders, and more accurate determination of various sleep stages, awakenings, and transient events, such as microarousals. The Rechtschaffen and Kales (1968) technique of sleep scoring, despite limitations, remains the standard for sleep staging. Ideally, sleep scoring should be performed manually; computerized scoring is not reliable. For newborns and infants, the technique recommended by Anders and co-workers is the standard. The following terms are essential for sleep staging and scoring (Mitler et al. 1999):

1. Total sleep period: Time from sleep onset to final awakening
2. Total sleep time: Total time spent between sleep onset and final awakening, excluding time spent awake
3. Sleep latency: Time from lights-out to sleep onset
4. REM sleep latency: Time from sleep onset to the first REM sleep onset
5. Sleep efficiency: Ratio of total sleep time to total time in bed, expressed as a percentage
6. Sleep stages 1–4 NREM and REM sleep expressed as a percentage of total sleep time

7. Wake after sleep onset: Time spent awake during total sleep period
8. Number of sleep cycles, including REM cycles, during total sleep period:
9. Stage shifts:
10. Arousal index (based on guidelines proposed by the American Sleep Disorders Association): Number of arousals per hour of sleep

PSG should also include airflow, respiratory effort, electrocardiogram (ECG), oximetry, and limb muscle activity, particularly EMG of the tibialis anterior muscles bilaterally. It is advantageous to record snoring and body positions. Thermistors or thermocouples are used to record oronasal airflow qualitatively, but these are not reliable for accurate determination of hypopnea. Respiratory efforts can be recorded by use of strain gauges or inductance plethysmography. Inductance plethysmography or piezoelectric strain gauge is the preferred method; it can be used in a qualitative or semiquantitative fashion to monitor chest and abdominal movements. Intraesophageal balloon recording, an invasive method, accurately determines intrathoracic pressure swings and is essential for documentation of UARS. EMG of the intercostal muscles using surface electrodes may also be helpful in determining respiratory effort. SDB events are recorded as an AHI or RDI score, as defined previously. PLMS are recorded from tibialis EMGs. PLMS index is expressed as the number of PLMS per hour of sleep. The upper limit of the normal PLMS index is 5. Details on the technical aspects of PSG recording are beyond the scope of this chapter.

Indications for Polysomnography

Guidelines proposed by the American Sleep Disorders Association (1997) can be summarized as follows:

- PSG is routinely indicated for the diagnosis of sleep-related breathing disorders.
- PSG is indicated for CPAP titration in patients with sleep-related breathing disorders.
- PSG is indicated to evaluate for the presence of OSA in patients before they undergo laser-assisted uvulopalatopharyngoplasty (UPP).
- PSG is indicated for the assessment of treatment results after oral appliance used to push mandible and tongue forward and after surgical treatment of patients with moderately severe OSA, including those whose symptoms reappear despite an initial good response.
- A follow-up PSG is required when clinical response is inadequate or when symptoms reappear despite a good initial response after treatment with CPAP. It is also necessary after substantial weight loss or weight gain has occurred in patients previously treated with CPAP successfully.
- Overnight PSG followed by MSLT the day after PSG is routinely indicated in patients suspected of narcolepsy.

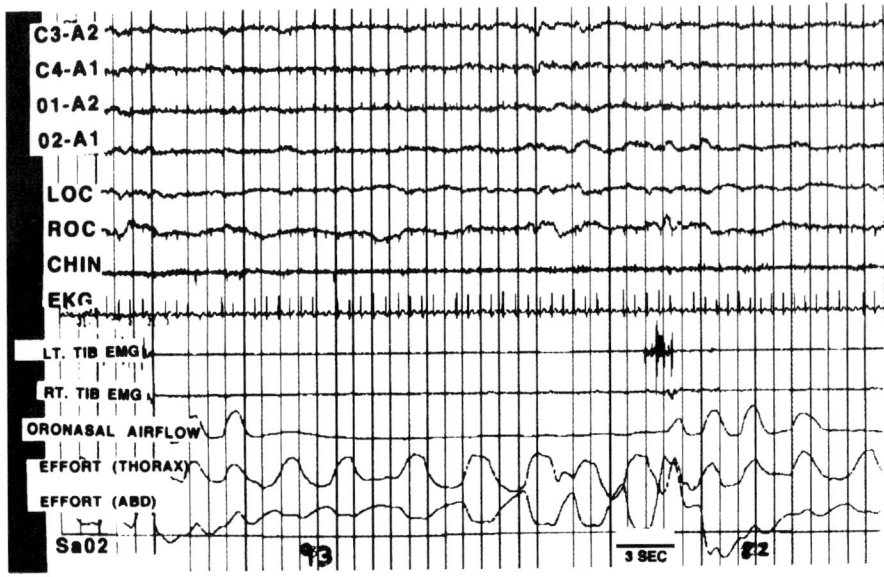

FIGURE 72.4 Polysomnographic recording of a patient with upper airway obstructive sleep apnea syndrome. Note absence of airflow for 23 seconds but continued effort and oxygen desaturation from 93% to 82% in stage II non–rapid eye movement sleep. (Top four channels = EEG; ABD = abdomen; chin = electromyogram of chin muscle; EKG = electrocardiogram; LOC = left electro-oculogram; LT. TIB EMG = left tibialis electromyogram; ROC = right electro-oculogram; SaO_2 = oxygen saturation; RT. TIB EMG = right tibialis electromyogram.)

- PSG is indicated in patients with parasomnias if these are unusual or atypical or the behaviors are violent or otherwise potentially injurious to the patient or others. PSG, however, is not routinely indicated in uncomplicated and typical parasomnias.
- PSG is indicated in patients suspected of nocturnal seizures.
- Overnight PSG is required in patients with suspected PLMS, but it is not performed routinely to diagnose RLS.
- PSG may be indicated for patients with insomnia who have not responded satisfactorily to a comprehensive behavioral or pharmacological treatment program for the management of insomnia. In patients with insomnia, however, if there is a strong suspicion of the presence of sleep-related breathing disorder or associated PLMS, PSG study is indicated.

Polysomnographic Findings in Sleep Disorders

Characteristic PSG findings in OSAS include recurrent episodes of apneas and hypopneas, which are mostly obstructive (Figure 72.4) or mixed, and few central apneas accompanied by oxygen desaturation and followed by arousals with resumption of breathing. An AHI or RDI of 5 or below is considered normal. RDI of more than 5–19 may be considered evidence of mild OSAS, 20–49 as evidence of moderate OSAS, and 50 or more as evidence of severe OSAS. Similarly, percentage oxygen saturation of 80–89 may be found in mild OSAS, whereas in moderate OSAS 70–79 is typical, and in severe cases, 69 and below are the usual findings. An arousal index of up to 10 is considered normal; 10–15 can be considered borderline. An arousal index above 15 is definitely abnormal. There are some sleep architectural changes in OSAS (reduction of slow-wave and REM sleep); most of the sleep is spent in stage II NREM sleep. Other findings include short latency, increased time spent awake after sleep onset, and excessive snoring. In patients with CSA syndrome, the apneas are all central.

Overnight PSG findings in patients with narcolepsy include short sleep latency, excessive disruption of sleep with frequent arousals, reduced total sleep time, excessive body movements, and reduced slow-wave sleep and SOREMs (seen in 40–50% of cases). Some narcoleptics may have associated sleep apneas (Figure 72.5), particularly central apneas. In approximately 9–59% of patients, PLMS have been noted, and in about 12% of narcoleptic patients, RBD has been described.

PSG findings in MSA or Shy-Drager syndrome show a reduction of slow-wave, REM, and total sleep time; increased sleep latency; increased number of awakenings during sleep; absence of muscle atonia in REM sleep in those with RBD; and a variety of respiratory dysrhythmias, as described previously. Similar but less intense findings have been reported in patients with OPCA.

In AD, the essential features of sleep architectural alterations are reduced total sleep time, decreased REM and slow-wave sleep, reduction of sleep spindles and K complexes, increased nighttime awakenings, and sleep fragmentation. There is a high frequency of sleep apnea in those with AD compared with age-matched controls.

In PD, PSG study shows a variety of sleep architectural changes: decreased sleep efficiency, increased awakenings, sleep fragmentation, decreased REM and slow-wave sleep and sleep spindles, disruption of NREM-REM sleep cycling, absence of muscle atonia, and presence of increasing EMG activities in those presenting with RBD.

The characteristic PSG findings in RBD consist of absence of muscle atonia and presence of increased EMG activities in the upper and lower limbs (Figure 72.6). It is important to record EMGs from both upper and lower limbs because in some patients with RBD, EMG activities are present in the upper limbs but not in the lower limbs.

FIGURE 72.5 Polysomnographic recording in a patient with narcolepsy and sleep apnea. (Top four channels = EEG; EOG = electro-oculogram; mentalis [MENT], submental [SUBMENT], orbicularis oris [ORIS], sternocleidomastoideus [SCM], scalenus anticus [SCAL], alae nasi, and intercostal [INT] electromyograms [EMG]; abdominal pneumogram [ABD PNEUMO].) Note central apnea during rapid eye movement sleep.

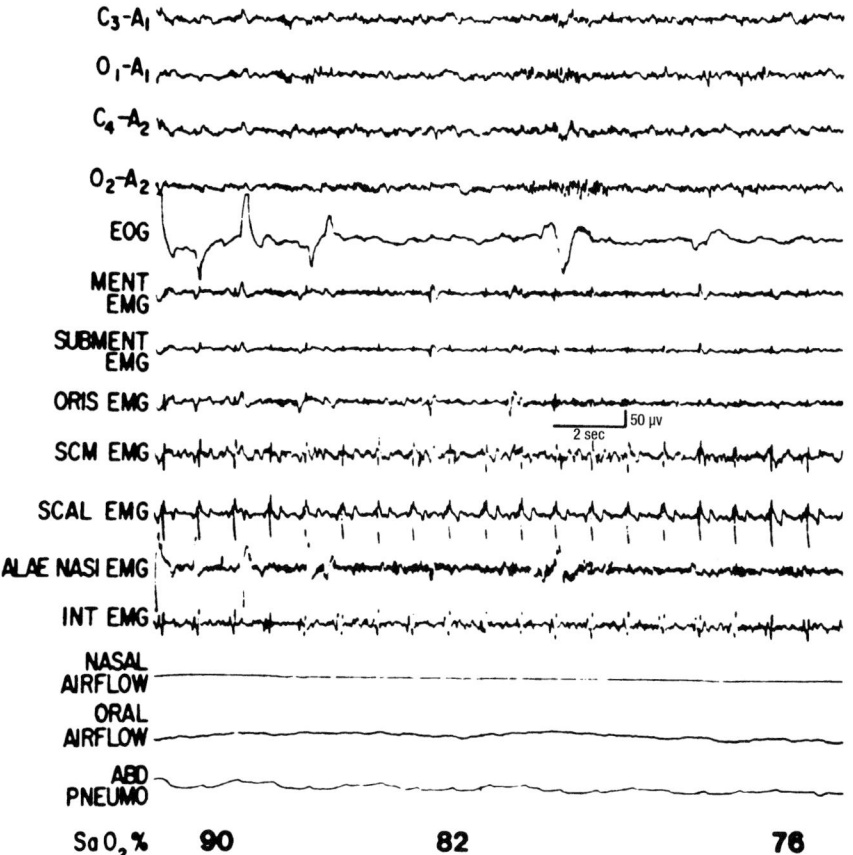

FIGURE 72.6 A portion of polysomnographic tracing in a 64-year-old man with rapid eye movement sleep behavior disorder. Electroencephalogram (C3-A2, C4-A1, O1-A2, O2-A1), shows mixed pattern with low-amplitude fast activities and theta activities. Chin electromyogram (EMG) as well as EMGs from left and right arms, left and right tibialis anterior muscles show tonic increase in muscle tone with superimposed phasic increase. (EKG = electrocardiogram.) (Reproduced with permission from R Broughton. Behavioral Parasomnias. In S Chokroverty [ed], Sleep Disorders Medicine: Basic Science, Technical Considerations, and Clinical Aspects. Boston: Butterworth–Heinemann, 1999. Courtesy of Drs. Carlos Schenck and Mark Mahowald.)

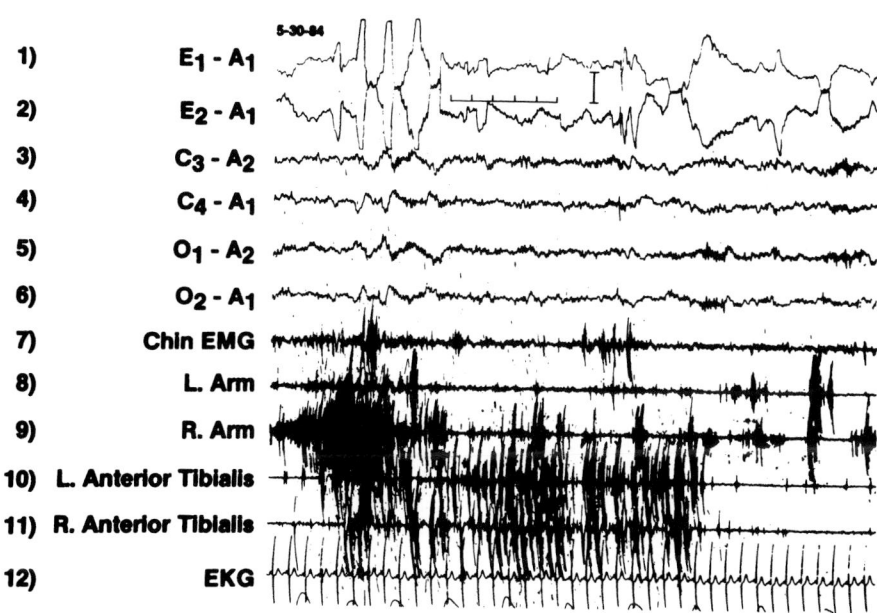

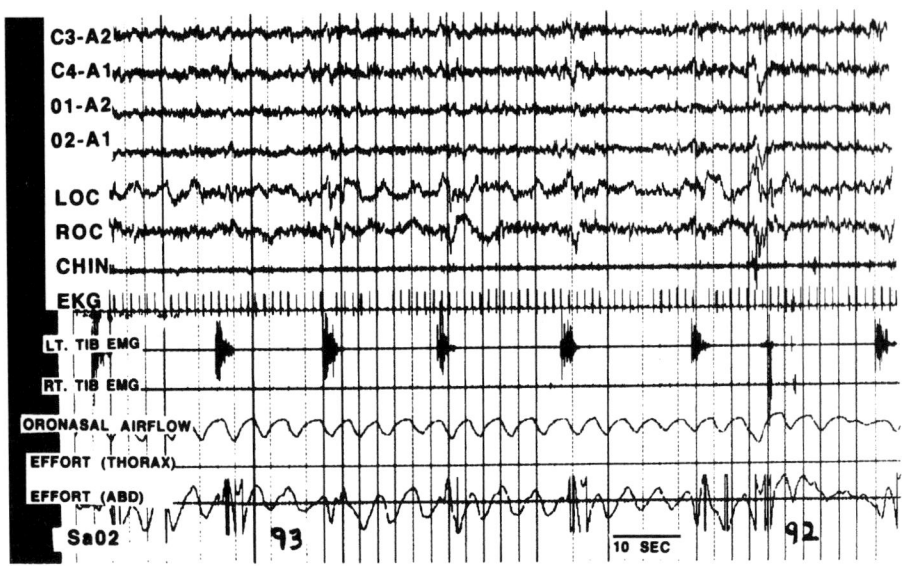

FIGURE 72.7 Polysomnographic study of a patient with restless legs syndrome showing periodic limb movements in sleep in the left tibialis electromyogram (LT. TIB EMG). (Top four channels = electroencephalogram [EEG]; ABD = abdomen; CHIN = electromyogram of the chin muscle, EKG = electrocardiogram; LOC = left electro-oculogram; RT. TIB EMG = right tibialis electromyogram; ROC = right electro-oculogram.)

In RLS, PSG documents sleep disturbance and PLMS (Figure 72.7), which is found in at least 80% of patients. Diagnosis of PLMD is based on the PLMS index (number of PLMS per hour of sleep); PLMS of up to 5 is considered normal. High PLMS index with arousal is more significant than the index without arousal.

PSG findings in myopathies, including Duchenne's and other muscular dystrophies as well as myotonic dystrophy, may include sleep fragmentation and disorganization; increased number of awakenings; reduced total sleep time; central, mixed, and upper airway OSAs or hypopneas associated with oxygen desaturation; and nonapneic oxygen desaturation becoming worse during REM sleep. Similar findings may be noted in polyneuropathies or neuromuscular junctional disorders. In addition, in painful polyneuropathies and in neuromuscular conditions associated with muscular pain and cramps, PSG may show sleep-onset insomnia and reduced sleep efficiency.

Multiple Sleep Latency Test

The MSLT is an important test for documenting excessive sleepiness objectively. The test has been standardized and is performed after an overnight PSG study. The test consists of four to five daytime recordings of EEG, EMG, and electro-oculogram at 2-hour intervals, each recording lasting for a maximum of 20 minutes. The test measures the average sleep-onset latency (timed to the first epoch of any sleep stage for the clinical purpose) and the presence of SOREM (timed from sleep onset to the first REM sleep). A mean sleep latency less than 5 minutes is consistent with pathological sleepiness. SOREM in two or more of the four to five recordings during MSLT suggests narcolepsy, although abnormalities of REM sleep-regulatory mechanism and circadian rhythm sleep disturbances also may lead to such findings. Pathological sleepiness is noted in all patients complaining of EDS (see Chapter

6). In approximately 85% of patients with narcolepsy-cataplexy syndrome, a mean sleep latency of less than 5 minutes and two or more SOREMs are both noted. Aldrich and coworkers (1997) documented that only in 61% of narcoleptics are both these findings present in the initial MSLT. Occasionally, narcoleptics may have normal mean sleep latency with one or more SOREMs. Rarely, MSLT may be entirely normal, particularly in narcoleptics who are very anxious. A large percentage of patients presenting with EDS and two or more SOREMs have a condition other than narcolepsy.

Maintenance of Wakefulness Test

The maintenance of wakefulness test (MWT) is a variant of the MSLT that measures the patient's ability to stay awake. MWT is performed at 2-hour intervals in a quiet, dark room; the patient adopts a semireclining position in a chair and is instructed to resist sleep. Four or five such tests are performed, each one lasting for 20 or 40 minutes. MWT may be important for monitoring the effect of treatment in narcolepsy, but it is not as good as MSLT for measuring daytime sleepiness.

Actigraphy

Actigraphy is a technique of motion detection that records activities during sleep and waking (Saadeh et al. 1995). It complements a sleep diary or sleep log data. The actigraphic instrument is a small device, slightly larger than a wristwatch, worn generally on the wrist but also on the ankle for 1–2 weeks. It is a cost-effective method for assessing a sleep-wake pattern. Actigraphy is very useful in the diagnosis of circadian rhythm sleep disorders (Figure 72.8), sleep-state misperception, and other types of insomnia. It can also be used to detect and quantify PLMS. It is not, however, suitable for assessment of SDB events.

FIGURE 72.8 Actigraphic recording in a 29-year-old man with delayed sleep-phase syndrome. The timing of the sleep period is delayed. Sleep typically occurs from 3:00 AM to about 10:00–11:00 AM (lighter areas). The dark areas represent the periods of activity.

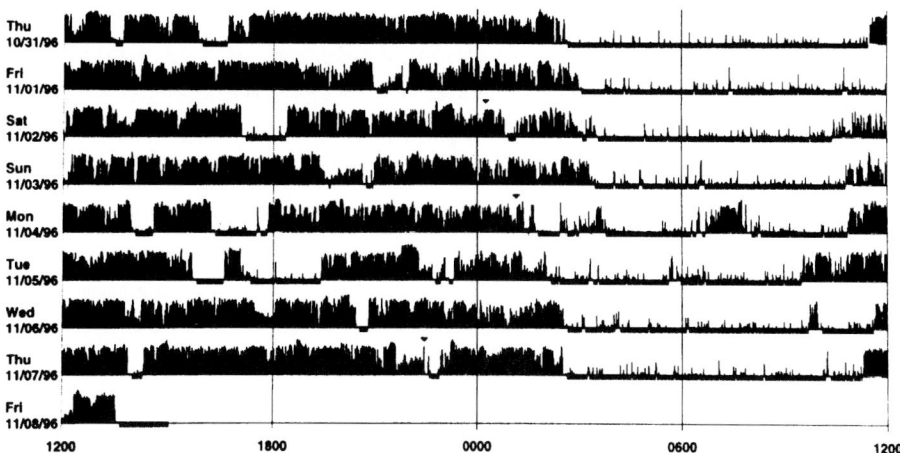

Video-Polysomnographic Study

Video-PSG study is important to document abnormal movements and behavior during sleep at night in patients with parasomnias, including RBD, nocturnal seizures (Figure 72.9), and other unusual movements occurring during sleep. Parasomnias are generally diagnosed on the basis of the clinical history, but sometimes video-PSG is required to document the condition. For nocturnal epilepsy, video-PSG using multiple-channel EEGs and multiple montages is required. Ideally, if sleep epilepsy is suspected, the video-PSG recording should be capable of EEG analysis at the standard EEG speed of 30 mm per second to identify epileptiform discharges.

Special Electroencephalographic Studies in Nocturnal Seizure

In addition to standard EEG recording, 24-hour ambulatory EEG recording and long-term video-EEG monitoring may be needed for documentation of seizures. If the results of the EEG, including long-term monitoring and neuroimaging, are discordant in localizing the focus, the patient should be referred to a specialized epilepsy center for intracranial recordings.

Neuroimaging Studies

Neuroimaging studies include anatomical and functional (physiological) studies. These studies are essential when a neurological illness is suspected of causing a sleep disturbance.

Cerebral angiography, including digital subtraction arteriography and magnetic resonance angiography, may be necessary to investigate for strokes in addition to computed tomography (CT) and MRI, which are important to detect structural lesions of the CNS (e.g., tumors, infarction, vascular malformations). CT and MRI are also helpful in patients with demyelinating and degenerative neurological disorders that may be responsible for disturbed sleep and sleep-related breathing dysrhythmias.

PET study dynamically measures cerebral blood flow, oxygen uptake, and glucose utilization and is helpful in the diagnosis of dementing, degenerative (e.g., PD, MSA), and seizure disorders. SPECT, which dynamically measures regional cerebral blood flow, may be useful for patients with cerebrovascular disease, AD, or seizure disorders. PET and SPECT can also be performed to investigate dopamine D_2-receptor changes in RLS-PLMS as well as narcolepsy. Functional MRI can be useful to study the generators and areas of activation in RLS-PLMS. Doppler ultrasonography is an important test for investigation of stroke due to extracranial vascular disease. Myelography other than CT and MRI is important for diagnosis of spinal cord diseases.

In selected patients, fiberoptic endoscopy may be performed to locate the site of collapse of the upper airway and cephalometric radiographs of the cranial base and facial bones to assess posterior airway space or maxillomandibular deficiency. These are important when surgical treatment is planned. For research investigations, cross-sectional areas of the upper airway during wakefulness may be measured by CT and MRI (Robinson and Guilleminault 1999).

Pulmonary Function Tests

Pulmonary function tests exclude intrinsic bronchopulmonary disease, which may affect sleep-related breathing disorders. Pulmonary function tests may include assessment of ventilatory functions (forced expiratory volume in 1 second [FEV_1], forced vital capacity [FVC], the FEV_1 to FVC ratio, peak expiratory flow rate, and forced expiratory flow rate); measurement of lung volumes (total lung capacity, residual volume, and functional residual capacity); gas distribution and gas transfer; and arterial blood gases (PO_2 and PCO_2). Respiratory muscle function of individuals with neuromuscular disorders should be specifically assessed, and it is important to measure the maximal static inspiratory and

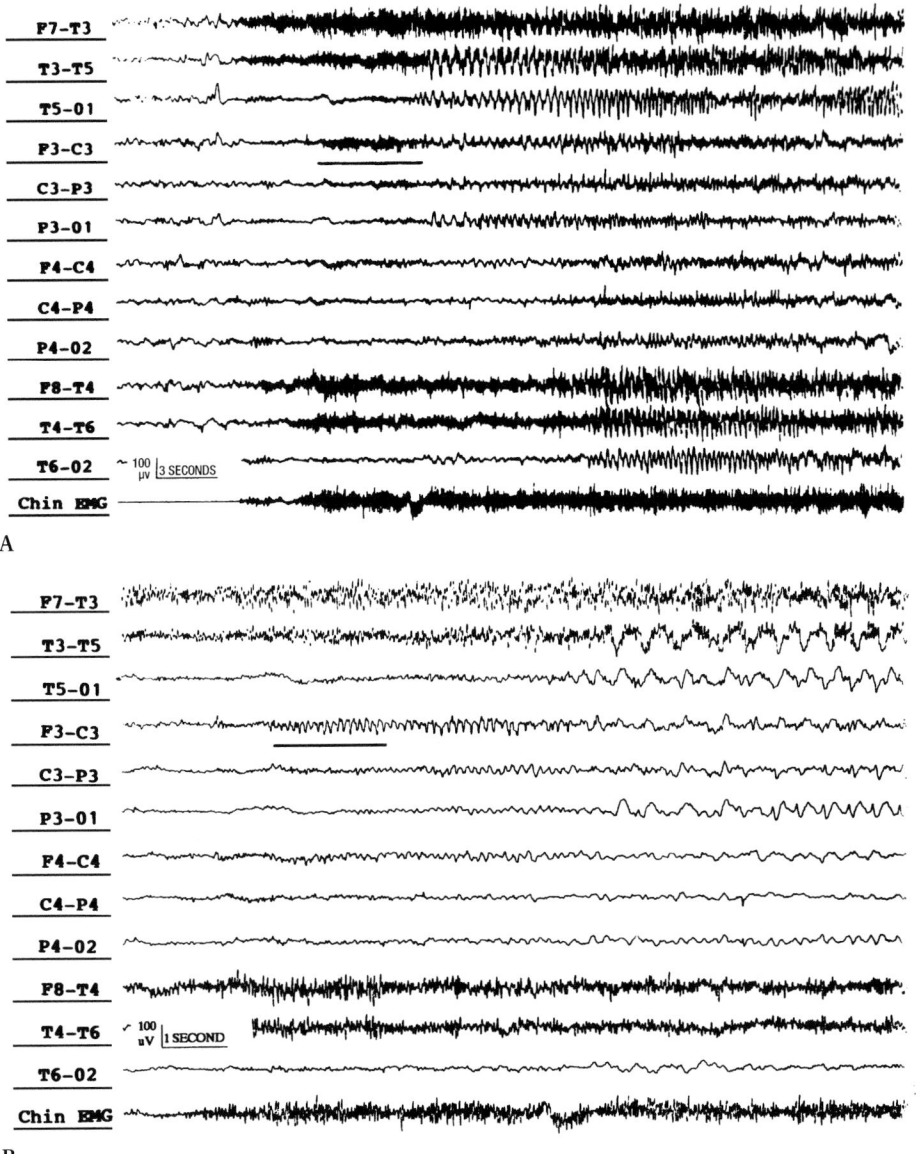

FIGURE 72.9 A portion of a polysomnographic recording showing the onset of a partial seizure using (A) 10-mm/second and (B) 30-mm/second paper speed. Twelve channels of electroencephalogram (International Ten-Twenty electrode placement) and chin electromyogram (EMG) are shown. The underlying activity represents rhythmic ictal discharges beginning at F3-C3 (left frontocentral) and spreading rapidly to the right hemisphere, and it is accompanied by clinical seizure. The underlying activity superficially resembles muscle artifacts at 10-mm/second paper speed (A) but it is obvious at 30-mm/second paper speed (B) that this activity is the beginning of the rhythmic epileptiform discharges in the electroencephalogram. (Reproduced with permission from M Aldrich, B Jahnke. Diagnostic value of video-EEG polysomnography. Neurology 1991;41:1060.)

expiratory pressures. Finally, chemical control of breathing (hypercapnic and hypoxic ventilatory responses) may be needed to assess respiratory functions and control systems in various neurological disorders causing dysfunction of the metabolic respiratory controllers as well as in patients with obesity-hypoventilation (pickwickian) syndrome.

Electrodiagnosis of the Respiratory Muscles

EMG of the upper airway and diaphragmatic and intercostal muscles may detect affection of these muscles in various neurological diseases. It is important to perform laryngeal EMG to detect laryngeal paresis in patients with MSA with laryngeal stridor. Phrenic nerve and intercostal nerve conduction study may detect phrenic and intercostal neuropathy, which may cause diaphragmatic and intercostal muscle affections in some patients with neurological disorders.

Other Laboratory Tests

Appropriate laboratory tests should always be performed to exclude any suspected medical disorders that may be the cause of patients' insomnia or hypersomnia. These tests may include blood and urinalysis, ECG, Holter ECG, chest radiography, and other investigations to rule out gastrointestinal, pulmonary, cardiovascular, endocrine, and renal disorders. In rare cases, when autonomic failure causes a sleep disturbance or sleep-related breathing disorder, autonomic function tests may be required for the diagnosis of the primary condition. In patients with narcolepsy, HLA typing may be performed as most of the patients with narcolepsy are positive for HLA, DR2 DQ1, and DQB1*0602 (Mignot 1998; Mignot 1999). In selected patients suspected of having a psychiatric cause of EDS, neuropsychiatric testing (e.g., Minnesota Multiphasic Personality Inventory) may be helpful.

In RLS patients, EMG and nerve conduction studies are important to exclude polyneuropathies or lumbosacral radiculopathies and other lower motor neuron disorders that may be associated with RLS or cause symptoms resembling idiopathic RLS. Other important laboratory tests in RLS include those necessary to obtain appropriate tests to exclude diabetes mellitus, uremia, anemia, and other associated conditions. It is particularly important to obtain levels of serum iron (including serum ferritin), serum folate levels, fasting blood glucose, blood urea, and creatinine. The role of nerve biopsy remains controversial. In the vast majority of cases, a nerve biopsy is not necessary, but it may be obtained for research purposes and when there is a strong suspicion of polyneuropathy.

MANAGEMENT OF SLEEP DISORDERS

It is important to determine a cause for sleep disturbance so that the primary condition can be adequately treated. Treatment of secondary sleep disturbances is unlikely to be successful unless the primary cause is properly diagnosed and treated. Treatment of an underlying cause may improve the sleep disturbance. If satisfactory treatment is not available for the primary condition or does not resolve the problem, however, treatment should be directed to the specific sleep disturbance. Certain general principles of treatment should apply to treatment of any sleep disorders. It is beyond the scope of this chapter to discuss management of various medical, psychiatric, and neurological disorders. General sleep hygiene measures are listed in Table 6.6 of Chapter 6.

Sleep Apnea Syndrome

The objective of management of sleep apnea syndrome is to improve the quality of life by improving the quality of sleep and to prevent life-threatening cardiac arrhythmias, pulmonary hypertension, and CHF, which are related to SDB. Treatment of sleep apnea syndrome includes (Table 72.20) general measures, pharmacological agents, mechanical devices, and surgical treatment (Robinson and Guilleminault 1999).

General measures include avoidance of sedative-hypnotics and alcohol, which can aggravate sleep-related breathing disorders, and reduction of body weight in obese patients.

Pharmacological Treatment

Pharmacological treatment has not been very helpful in OSAS. The agents that have shown partial success in treating mild sleep apnea-hypopnea syndrome are protriptyline and acetazolamide. Acetazolamide, a carbonic anhydrase inhibitor, produces metabolic acidosis, causing a shift in the CO_2 apnea threshold, and has been used with some success to treat central apnea at high altitude.

Table 72.20: Treatment of sleep apnea syndrome

General measures
  Avoid alcohol, particularly in the evening
  Avoid sedative-hypnotics
  Reduce body weight
Pharmacological treatment (in mild cases)
  Protriptyline
  Acetazolamide (central apnea at high altitude)
Mechanical devices
  Nasal continuous positive airway pressure for OSAS
  Bilevel positive airway pressure for OSAS
  Intermittent positive pressure ventilation for hypoventilation
    in neuromuscular disorders
  Dental appliances in some mild to moderate OSAS
  Tongue-retaining device for OSAS (unpredictable)
Surgical treatment
  Uvulopalatopharyngoplasty (UPP), including laser-assisted
    and radiofrequency UPP
  Major maxillofacial surgeries
  Tonsillectomy and adenoidectomy
  Diaphragm pacing (central sleep apnea)
  Tracheostomy (rarely performed nowadays)

OSAS = obstructive sleep apnea syndrome.

Mechanical Devices

Nasal CPAP is an important therapy for treating OSAS. CPAP opens up the upper airway passage so that obstructive apneas and hypopneas, hypoxemias, arousals, and sleep fragmentation are eliminated. The optimal CPAP pressure is first determined in the laboratory during overnight PSG, and the patient can purchase home units to use nightly during sleep. Instead of CPAP, some patients may require bilevel positive airway pressure, which delivers a higher pressure during inspiration and a lower pressure during expiration. It is important to follow up such patients for the purpose of compliance and to identify patients who did not have adequate benefit and may require repeat titration. All patients are not compliant with CPAP because of various problems, such as difficulty with the mask, claustrophobia, air leaks between the mask and face, and nasal congestion. The compliance varies from 60% to 70% of patients. Further study is needed to determine the factors for compliance and noncompliance and to understand the long-term effect on the natural history of patients with OSAS. The role of nasal CPAP in CSA syndrome is highly controversial. In a subgroup of patients with CSA who show narrowing or occlusion of the upper airway on fiberoptic scope, nasal CPAP may reverse the apneic episodes.

Surgical Treatment

In a few severe cases of OSAS in which CPAP therapy fails, UPP, including laser-assisted and radiofrequency UPP, has been tried with variable success. Significant improvement is noted in approximately 50% of patients, and many of

Table 72.21:   Drug treatment for narcolepsy syndrome

For sleep attacks
    Pemoline (Cylert): 18.75–37.50 mg/day, up to 150 mg/day
    Methylphenidate (Ritalin): 5 mg bid, 30 mins before meals
       to a maximum of 50 mg, rarely 100 mg/day
    Dextroamphetamine (Dexedrine): 5 mg qd or bid, up to
       50 mg/day
    Methamphetamine (Methedrine): 5 mg qd or bid, up to
       50 mg/day
    Mazindol: 2 mg qd or bid, up to 8 mg/day
    Modafinil: 200 mg/day
For cataplexy, sleep paralysis, and hypnagogic hallucinations
    Imipramine: 75–150 mg/day
    Clomipramine: 75–125 mg/day
    Fluoxetine: 20 mg qd, up to 80 mg/day
    Viloxazine: 150–200 mg/day

those who improve may still need CPAP for elimination of residual apneas. An overnight PSG study must always be performed before undertaking UPP because it may eliminate snoring without adequately relieving OSAs. Other surgical approaches may be needed in severe cases, including maxillofacial surgery, such as hyoid myotomy and suspension or mandibular osteotomy with genioglossus muscle advancement, although their role remains uncertain. Tracheostomy may still be needed in an occasional patient as an emergency measure during severe respiratory compromise or severe apnea associated with dangerous cardiac arrhythmias causing a life-threatening situation. Such patients may later be weaned. CPAP treatment has replaced tracheostomy for obstructive or mixed apneas. In patients with respiratory center involvement with CSA syndrome, diaphragm pacing or electrophrenic respiration has been used successfully, particularly for those who require ventilatory assistance during both day and night.

Other Ventilatory Supports

In patients with neuromuscular disorders, including those with ALS, poliomyelitis, and postpolio syndrome, ventilatory support is often needed with either negative pressure or positive pressure ventilators (Chokroverty 1999). Intermittent positive pressure ventilation (IPPV) can be administered through a nasal mask. Negative pressure ventilation can be delivered from a tank respirator or from a cuirass. With ventilatory support, patients with neuromuscular disorders often obtain relief of daytime hypersomnolence and show improvement of sleep architecture. A combination of a nasal mask and positive pressure ventilation may be needed. When OSA complicates sleep hypoventilation, IPPV through a nasal mask during sleep may be a better treatment than negative pressure ventilation and may obviate the need for tracheostomy or diaphragm pacing. Negative-pressure ventilation may improve these patients' nocturnal ventilation during NREM sleep but can produce upper airway obstructive apnea during REM sleep, causing severe

hypoxemia and hypercapnia. Patients with respiratory muscle weakness, including diaphragmatic muscle weakness, may require a combination of CPAP, cuirass, and later IPPV at night. Patients with motor neuron disease and associated sleep-related hypoventilation and apnea have been treated with cuirass ventilators, CPAP, and later IPPV at night with considerable symptomatic relief. Patients with poliomyelitis or postpolio syndrome who require ventilatory support to maintain respiratory homeostasis generally show improvement in sleep architecture and respiratory function after mechanical ventilation via nasal mask. Those with obstructive or mixed apneas respond to CPAP.

Other Treatment Modalities

Dental appliances can reduce snoring and help patients with mild sleep apnea, but at present, it is not possible to predict which patients will respond to such treatment. A tongue-retaining device is another unpredictable measure for treating sleep apnea.

Narcolepsy

The administration of stimulants, such as pemoline, methylphenidate, dextroamphetamine, or methamphetamine, is the treatment of choice (Table 72.21) for narcoleptic sleep attacks (Bassetti and Aldrich 1996). In 65–85% of patients, a significant improvement of EDS can be obtained. Methylphenidate is the drug most commonly used. In patients with mild-to-moderate sleepiness, however, an initial treatment with pemoline, starting with 18.75–37.50 mg in the morning, may be tried. Methylphenidate treatment may be started with 5–10 mg two to three times daily. To avoid insomnia, the last dose should not be taken after 4:00 PM. In patients who do not respond to methylphenidate, treatment with dextroamphetamine or methamphetamine can be administered, starting with 5–10 mg in the morning or twice a day. The maximum acceptable doses of stimulants for treatment of narcolepsy may include up to 150 mg daily for pemoline, 50 mg daily (rarely 100 mg) for methylphenidate, and 50 mg daily for both dextroamphetamine and methamphetamine. The most common side effects of the stimulants include nervousness, tremor, insomnia, irritability, palpitations, headache, and gastrointestinal symptoms. Another problem is the tolerance, which may be noted in up to 30% of patients, particularly with increasing doses. Modafinil, a novel wake-promoting agent, has been shown to be an effective treatment for EDS associated with narcolepsy in a recent 18-center, double-blinded, placebo-controlled trial in the United States. This will be an important option, and the dose is 200 mg daily..

The treatment of cataplexy and other auxiliary symptoms of narcolepsy (see Table 72.21) consists of administration of tricyclic antidepressants, such as protriptyline (starting with 5 mg/day), imipramine (25–200 mg/day), and clomipramine (10–200 mg/day). Specific serotonin reuptake inhibitors, such as fluoxetine (20–80 mg/day), have been used with success.

Nonpharmacological treatment of narcolepsy includes general sleep hygiene measures, short daytime naps, and joining narcolepsy support groups.

Idiopathic Hypersomnia

The treatment of idiopathic hypersomnia is unsatisfactory and is similar to the stimulant treatment for narcolepsy.

Parasomnias

No special treatment is needed for most of the parasomnias. The subjects with partial arousal disorders (e.g., sleepwalking, sleep terrors) must be protected from injury to self or others by arranging furniture, using a padded mattress, and paying particular attention to doors and windows. If attacks of sleepwalking or sleep terrors are frequent, treatment with an antidepressant (e.g., imipramine) or small doses of a benzodiazepine (e.g., clonazepam) may be tried for a short period.

Most cases of RBD respond dramatically to small doses of clonazepam (e.g., 1–2 mg at night).

Circadian Rhythm Sleep Disorders

Circadian rhythm sleep disorders may be profitably treated by the use of chronotherapy, phototherapy, or both. Chronotherapy refers to the intentional delay of sleep onset by 2–3 hours on successive days until the desired bedtime has been achieved. After this, the patient strictly enforces the sleep-wake schedule. One study reported a high success rate among patients with DSPS even when the disorder had been present for many years. After several months, however, the patient generally becomes less adherent to the schedule and begins to lapse into the original sleep habits.

Exposure to bright light on awakening is effective in altering sleep onset and in synchronizing body temperature rhythm in patients with DSPS. The patient sits in front of a 10,000-lux light for 30–40 minutes on awakening; in addition, room lighting must be markedly reduced in the evening to achieve the desired results. Response is generally evident after 2–3 weeks but frequently requires indefinite treatment to maintain. This treatment is still evolving, and no large-scale study with adequate follow-up has been conducted to assess the long-term effect of phototherapy in DSPS. In patients with ASPS, bright light exposure in the evening has been successful in delaying sleep onset.

Melatonin (0.5–7.5 mg/day), taken orally in the evening or at bedtime, has been reported to be effective in some blind people with hypernychthemeral syndrome.

Secondary circadian rhythm disorders (e.g., jet lag and shift work) may be treated with benzodiazepine or zolpidem. Phototherapy has been tried, but its effectiveness has

Table 72.22:   Drug treatment of restless legs syndrome

Major drugs
  Dopaminergic agents
    Carbidopa/L-dopa
    Pergolide
    Bromocriptine
    Pramipexole
    Ropinirole
  Benzodiazepines
    Clonazepam
    Temazepam
  Gabapentin
  Opiates
    Codeine
    Propoxyphene
    Oxycodone
    Methadone
Minor drugs
  Tramadol
  Baclofen
  Carbamazepine
  Clonidine
  Propranolol

not been determined. Melatonin is being evaluated for treatment of circadian rhythm disorders.

Restless Legs Syndrome and Periodic Limb Movements in Sleep

Four major groups of drugs have been used to treat RLS and PLMS (Table 72.22): dopaminergic agents, benzodiazepines, gabapentin, and opiates (Hening et al. 1999). The typical dose for carbidopa/L-dopa (Sinemet) is 25/100 mg to 100/400 mg taken in divided doses before bedtime and during the night. Pergolide can be started at 0.05 mg and gradually increased to 0.2–0.5 mg taken in divided doses. One dose is taken an hour before bedtime and, depending on severity, another dose may be needed earlier in the evening or during the middle of the night on awakening. Another dopamine agonist, bromocriptine, may be tried, beginning with 2.5 mg and gradually increasing to a maximum of 15 mg per day. Bromocriptine has not been found to be as useful as pergolide or carbidopa/L-dopa. Sometimes, a long-acting drug (e.g., Sinemet-CR) may be combined with short-acting carbidopa/L-dopa for maximum effect. Problems with the use of dopaminergic medications include abdominal pain, nausea, recurrence of RLS symptoms, poor sleep quality during the last part of the night, and the development of rebound or augmentation, consisting of symptoms of RLS-PLMS developing earlier in the day and more severely than before treatment. Nausea, vomiting, and headache also may occur after treatment with carbidopa/L-dopa, whereas nasal stuffiness, hypotension, and nightmares have been reported after pergolide. Two new dopamine agonists, pramipexole and ropinirole, have been approved by the U.S. Food and Drug Administration

Table 72.23:   Treatment of insomnia

Nonpharmacological treatment
    Relaxation therapy, including biofeedback
    Stimulus-control therapy
    Sleep-restriction therapy
    Sleep hygiene measures
    Chronotherapy (for circadian rhythm disorders)
    Phototherapy (for circadian rhythm disorders)
Pharmacological treatment
    Benzodiazepines
        Flurazepam: 15–30 mg
        Estazolam: 1–2 mg
        Clonazepam: 0.5–2.0 mg
        Lorazepam: 1–2 mg
        Temazepam: 15–30 mg
        Triazolam: 0.125–0.250 mg
    Nonbenzodiazepines
        Zolpidem: 5–10 mg
        Antihistamines
        Sedative antidepressants
        Melatonin

for the treatment of PD but have not undergone adequate study for treatment of RLS-PLMS. Preliminary study using pramipexole in RLS has been encouraging.

Clonazepam (0.5–2.0 mg/day at bedtime) or temazepam (15–30 mg at bedtime) may be useful in treating RLS-PLMS. Medications should be started with the lowest dose and gradually increased to obtain maximum benefit with minimal side effect. These agents may produce daytime sleepiness or confusional episodes, particularly in elderly patients.

Gabapentin is an anticonvulsant that has been found to be beneficial in mild-to-moderate cases of RLS-PLMS. Divided doses of 300–1,800 mg per day may be helpful but can produce somnolence, dizziness, ataxia, or fatigue in more than 10% of patients.

Opiates are effective for treating RLS-PLMS but a less desirable alternative because of their proclivity to produce constipation and their potential for addiction. Codeine, propoxyphene, oxycodone, and methadone have all been used for this purpose. Tramadol, a non-narcotic agent with activity at the opiate μ-receptor, also has been used with some success in patients with RLS-PLMS.

In mild-to-moderate cases, one may start with gabapentin. In moderate-to-severe cases, some physicians start with carbidopa/L-dopa, whereas others use clonazepam. In refractory cases, one may have to use a combination of two to three drugs. In summary, the principle of treatment of RLS-PLMS is to start with the lowest possible dose and then increase by 1 tablet every 5–6 days until a maximum therapeutic benefit is reached or the side effects are noted. The dose can be divided and given 2 hours before bedtime, at bedtime, and in the middle of the night. If necessary, and in some severe cases, a daytime dose may be needed.

Other minor drugs (see Table 72.22) that have been helpful in occasional patients with RLS-PLMS include baclofen (10–60 mg daily), carbamazepine (200–600 mg daily), and

clonidine, an adrenergic agent (0.1–0.9 mg daily), and propranolol (80–120 mg daily).

In secondary RLS, the primary condition should be treated and the deficiency states, including the iron deficiency, should be corrected. The patient should also follow general sleep hygiene measures. Finally, the patients should avoid certain medication and agents that might aggravate RLS, including neuroleptics, tricyclics, selective serotonin reuptake inhibitors, antidepressants, certain antinausea medications, calcium-channel blockers, caffeine, alcohol, and smoking.

Treatment of Insomnia

Insomnia is a syndrome and not a specific disorder, and therefore treatment depends on the underlying cause of the syndrome. Treatment of secondary insomnia is unlikely to be successful unless the primary cause of the disturbance is diagnosed and properly treated. Both nonpharmacological and pharmacological therapies may be useful in the management of insomnia (Kupfer and Reynolds 1997).

Nonpharmacological Treatment

The mainstay of treatment for patients with chronic insomnia consists of nonpharmacological measures in conjunction with the judicious, intermittent use of hypnotics. Nonpharmacological interventions include relaxation therapy and biofeedback; stimulus-control therapy; sleep restriction; and patient education about sleep hygiene, sleep habits, attitudes toward sleep, and the role of autonomic and cognitive arousals (Table 72.23). Sleep hygiene measures are listed in Table 6.6

Relaxation therapy involves progressive muscle relaxation and biofeedback to reduce somatic arousal. One small study of several relaxation procedures found a 42% improvement in self-reported sleep complaints after 1 year of relaxation therapy. Stimulus-control therapy may also be useful in patients with chronic insomnia. Bootzin's stimulus-control technique is directed at discouraging the learned association between the bedroom and wakefulness and re-establishing the bedroom as the major stimulus for sleep. These techniques have been reported to improve insomnia complaints in approximately 50% of individuals after 1 year. Sleep-restriction therapy may improve sleep efficiency by restricting the total time in bed for sleep. Once this has occurred, gradually increasing the time allocated to sleep may improve the level of daytime functioning and the overall quality of sleep. Roughly one-fourth of patients with insomnia may benefit from such a regimen. The relative efficacy of these various nonpharmacological approaches has not been well established. One meta-analysis involving 2,102 patients in 59 trials found that sleep-restriction and stimulus-control therapies were more effective than relaxation techniques used alone. Sleep hygiene measures alone did not show evidence of efficacy. The extent to which the concomitant use of nonpharmacological therapy augments the performance of pharmacological treatment is also unclear.

Pharmacological Therapy

Hypnotic medications have generally not been the treatment of first choice for chronic insomnia (see Table 72.23). When they are prescribed, they should be used intermittently and always combined with nonpharmacological therapies.

Judicious use of hypnotics may be helpful when treating transient or short-term, idiopathic, and psychophysiological insomnia, but their use should be restricted to less than 4 weeks' duration. Intermittent use of hypnotic medications (e.g., 1–2 nights/week) may be necessary in some patients with chronic idiopathic or psychophysiological insomnia who do not respond adequately to nonpharmacological treatment, although the drugs should not be the main component of therapy. Hypnotic medications are contraindicated in pregnancy because of data showing an increased risk of fetal malformations with diazepam or diazoxide if used during the first trimester. The drugs should also be avoided or used judiciously in patients with alcoholism or renal, hepatic, or pulmonary disease. A combination of alcohol and hypnotics is absolutely contraindicated. The drugs should also be avoided in patients with sleep apnea syndrome.

Benzodiazepine drugs (temazepam, flurazepam, triazolam, and estazolam) and one nonbenzodiazepine drug (zolpidem) are commonly used as hypnotics; two other benzodiazepine drugs—lorazepam and clonazepam—are also used frequently for this indication. Triazolam is no longer available in Great Britain because of reports of serious side effects, such as amnesia, rebound insomnia, and anxiety. The selection of a specific hypnotic agent should be based primarily on the elimination half-life. Short-acting drugs, such as temazepam, estazolam, triazolam, and zolpidem, are generally preferable because they produce less residual sleepiness the morning after use. However, these drugs, particularly triazolam, may have a high incidence of amnesia and rebound insomnia and should be used cautiously in patients with anxiety disorders. Adjustment in dosage may be necessary in patients who have prolonged drug elimination half-life due to age or impaired renal or hepatic function. Dependence and tolerance are the major disadvantages of long-term hypnotic use. The drugs should be discontinued gradually rather than abruptly to avoid precipitating symptoms of withdrawal.

Sedating antidepressants (e.g., amitriptyline, trazodone) are most useful in the management of patients in whom depression and insomnia coexist but are of limited usefulness in nondepressed patients because of rapidly developing tolerance to the sedative effects. Many over-the-counter sleep aids contain the sedating antihistamine diphenhydramine or doxylamine. These medications are generally not helpful in the management of chronic insomnia. Melatonin, a normal product of the pineal gland, is sold as a food supplement and an orphan drug in the United States, but over-the-counter sales are banned in the United Kingdom. Data on the efficacy and safety of melatonin are minimal, but the hormone does not appear to be a potent hypnotic for most patients with chronic insomnia. However, a subgroup of elderly patients with low melatonin levels have benefited from mela-tonin treatment, and it also is useful in some patients with jet lag, DSPS, and hypernychthemeral syndrome.

Sleep Disturbances in Neurological Illness

Treatment of neurological illnesses causing sleep-related dysrhythmias have been described (see Sleep Apnea Syndrome, earlier in this chapter).

Nocturnal seizures should be treated with standard anticonvulsant medications. Sleep disturbances in these patients often improve after effective therapy for seizures.

Treatment of acute confusional states associated with dementia should be directed toward the precipitating or causal factors for such episodes. Often, episodes are precipitated when the patient is transferred from home to an institution. As much as possible, the home environment of such patients should be preserved. The darkness of night often precipitates episodes, so a night-light is helpful. Medication that could have adverse effects on sleep and breathing should be reduced in dose or changed. Associated conditions that could interfere with sleep (e.g., pain due to arthritis and other causes) should be treated with analgesics. Depression is often an important feature in patients with AD, and a sedative antidepressant may be helpful. Frequency of urination in such patients may result from infection or enlarged prostate and may disturb sleep at night. Appropriate treatment should be directed toward such conditions. Patients should be encouraged to develop good sleep habits. They should be discouraged from taking daytime naps and should be encouraged to exercise (e.g., walking) during the day. They should not drink caffeine in the evening before bedtime. For sleeplessness, a trial with intermediate-acting benzodiazepines or zolpidem should be tried for a short period. For extreme agitation, patients should be tried with high-potency antipsychotics, such as haloperidol or thiothixene, in small doses. In some patients, appropriately timed exposure to bright light may be helpful.

Treatment of PD improves sleep inconsistently. In patients who have reactivation of parkinsonian symptoms during sleep at night, adjustment in the timing and choice of medication may be helpful. Some patients may benefit from an evening or bedtime dose. Longer-acting preparations of L-dopa also may help when taken near bedtime. Dopamine agonists (e.g., bromocriptine, pergolide) with their sustained actions may benefit sleep in some patients. Antihistamines such as diphenhydramine may promote sleep in addition to giving modest antiparkinsonian effect. A small dose of carbidopa/L-dopa, with a second dose later at night if the patient awakens, may sometimes help those with insomnia. In some patients, selegiline may improve sleep. Nocturnal dyskinesias related to L-dopa and causing insomnia may respond to a reduction in the dose of dopamine agonists or by addition of a small dose of benzodiazepine. In patients with nocturnal hallucinations and nightmares, including nocturnal vocalizations and RBD, clonazepam (0.5–1.0 mg) at bedtime may be beneficial. Nocturnal hallucinations and psychosis in PD patients have been treated successfully with clozapine or the newer drug olanzapine. During clozapine treatment, the usual precautions of monitoring blood count and testing liver function should be taken.

CONCLUSION

There has been an explosive growth in our understanding of sleep and its disorders. Sleep medicine is beginning to take its rightful place as a distinct subspecialty in medicine. Sleep disorders affect multiple systems and result from dysfunction of almost every system in our body. It is therefore important to have a basic understanding of the physiological changes during sleep and the clinical phenomenology of sleep disorders. In this review, I briefly summarize the essential physiological changes during sleep, which are quite different from those during wakefulness as well as circadian rhythms, the function of sleep, and neurobiology of sleep-wakefulness. Clinical manifestations of many primary and secondary sleep disorders, methods of laboratory investigation, and management are also briefly reviewed. Sleep is a function of the brain and neurological patients are particularly susceptible to disorders of sleep. Sleep adversely affects neurological illnesses, and neurological disorders in turn adversely affect the quality and quantity of sleep. Therefore, neurologists should be aware of the importance of understanding disorders of sleep as sleep dysfunction encroaches on almost every aspect of neurology.

REFERENCES

Aldrich MS. The clinical spectrum of narcolepsy and idiopathic hypersomnia. Neurology 1996;46:393–401.

Aldrich MS, Chervin RD, Malow BA. Value of the multiple sleep latency test (MSLT) for the diagnosis of narcolepsy. Sleep 1997;20:620–629.

American Sleep Disorders Association. Indications for Polysomnography Task Force, American Sleep Disorders Association Standards of Practice Committee. Practice parameters for the indication for polysomnography and related procedures. Sleep 1997;20:406–422.

Bassetti C, Aldrich MS. Idiopathic hypersomnia. A series of 42 patients. Brain 1997;120:1423–1435.

Bassetti C, Aldrich MS. Narcolepsy. Neurol Clin 1996;14:545–571.

Bearpark HM. Insomnia: Causes, Effects and Treatment. In R Cooper (ed), Sleep. London: Chapman & Hall, 1994;587–613.

Billiard M, et al. Family studies in narcolepsy. Sleep 1994;17:S54–S59.

Bonnett MH, Arand DL. We are chronically sleep-deprived. Sleep 1995;18:908–911.

Brzezinski A. Melatonin in humans. New Engl J Med 1997;336:186–195.

Chokroverty S. Insomnia. In S Rose (ed), UpToDate Medicine. Wellesley, MA: UpToDate, 1998.

Chokroverty S. An Overview of Sleep. In S Chokroverty (ed), Sleep Disorders Medicine: Basic Science, Technical Considerations and Clinical Aspects. Boston: Butterworth–Heinemann, 1999b;7–20.

Chokroverty S. Physiological Changes in Sleep. In S Chokroverty (ed), Sleep Disorders Medicine: Basic Science, Technical Con-

siderations, and Clinical Aspects. Boston: Butterworth–Heinemann, 1999c;95–126.

Chokroverty S. Sleep, Breathing and Neurological Disorders: In S Chokroverty (ed), Sleep Disorders Medicine: Basic Science, Technical Considerations, and Clinical Aspects. Boston: Butterworth–Heinemann, 1999d;509–571.

Chokroverty S. Sleep and degenerative neurologic disorders. Neurol Clin 1996;14:807–826.

Chokroverty S. Sleep Disorders Medicine: Basic Science, Technical Considerations, and Clinical Aspects. Boston: Butterworth–Heinemann, 1999a.

Chokroverty S. Sleep in Other Medical Disorders. In S Chokroverty (ed), Sleep Disorders Medicine: Basic Science, Technical Considerations, and Clinical Aspects. Boston: Butterworth–Heinemann, 1999e;587–617.

Chokroverty S, Quinto C. Sleep and Epilepsy. In S Chokroverty (ed), Sleep Disorders Medicine: Basic Science, Technical Considerations, and Clinical Aspects. Boston: Butterworth–Heinemann, 1999;697–727.

Chokroverty S, Sander HW, Tavoulareas GP, Quinto C. Insomnia with absent or disassociated REM sleep in proximal myotonic myopathy (abstract). Neurology 1997;48:256.

Coote JH. Sleep at High Altitude. In R Cooper (ed), Sleep. London: Chapman & Hall, 1994;243–264.

Crick F, Mitchison G. The function of dream sleep. Nature 1983;304:111–114.

Dinges DF. An overview of sleepiness and accidents. J Sleep Res 1995;4(Suppl. 2):4–14.

Douglas NJ, Polo O. Pathogenesis of obstructive sleep aphoe/hypopnoea syndrome. Lancet 1994;344:653–655.

Ellis CM, Simmons A, Lemmens G, et al. Proton spectroscopy in the narcoleptic syndrome. Is there evidence of a brainstem lesion? Neurology 1998;50(Suppl. 1):S23–S26.

Guilleminault C, Heinzer R, Mignot E, Black J. Investigations into the neurologic basis of narcolepsy. Neurology 1998;50(Suppl. 1):S8–S15.

Hening WA, Walters AS, Allen R, Chokroverty S. Motor Functions and Dysfunctions of Sleep. In S Chokroverty (ed), Sleep Disorders Medicine: Basic Science, Technical Considerations, and Clinical Aspects. Boston: Butterworth–Heinemann, 1999.

International Classification of Sleep Disorders (revised). Diagnostic and Coding Manual. Rochester, MN: American Sleep Disorders Association, 1997.

Javaheri S, Parker TJ, Wexler L, et al. Occult sleep-disordered breathing in stable congestive heart failure. Ann Intern Med 1995;122:487–.492

Kavanau JL. Memory, sleep and the evolution of mechanisms of synaptic efficacy maintenance. Neuroscience 1997;79:7–44.

Kilduff TS, Kushida CA. Circadian Regulation of Sleep. In S. Chokroverty (ed), Sleep Disorders Medicine: Basic Science, Technical Considerations, and Clinical Aspects. Boston: Butterworth–Heinemann 1999;135–147.

Krueger JM, Obal F Jr. Sleep Factors. In NA Saunders, Colin E. Sullivan (eds), Sleep and Breathing 1994;79–112.

Krueger JM, Obal F Jr, Kapas L, et al. Brain organization and sleep function. Behav Brain Res 1995;69:177–185

Kupfer DJ, Reynolds CF III. Management of insomnia. New Engl J Med 1997;337:341–346.

Lugaresi E, Montagna P, Tinuper P, et al. Endozepine stupor: recurrent stupor linked to endozepine-4 accumulation. Brain 1998;121:127–133.

Mahowald MW, Chokroverty S, Kader G, Schenck CH. Sleep Disorders. Baltimore: Williams and Wilkins, 1997.

McCarley RW. Sleep Neurophysiology: Basic Mechanism Underlying Control of Wakefulness and Sleep. In S Chokroverty (ed), Sleep Disorders Medicine: Basic Science, Technical Considerations, and Clinical Aspects. Boston: Butterworth–Heinemann, 1999;21–62.

Mignot E. Genetic and familial aspects of narcolepsy. Neurology 1998;50(Suppl. 1):S16–S22.

Mignot E. Genetics in Sleep Disorders. In S Chokroverty (ed), Sleep Disorders Medicine: Basic Science, Technical Considerations, and Clinical Aspects. Boston: Butterworth–Heinemann, 1999.

Mitler MM, Poceta JS, Bigby BG. Sleep Scoring Technique. In S Chokroverty (ed), Sleep Disorders Medicine: Basic Science, Technical Considerations, and Clinical Aspects. Boston: Butterworth–Heinemann, 1999;245–262.

Montagna P, Cortelli P, Gambetti P, Lugaresi E. Fatal familial insomnia: sleep, neuroendocrine and vegetative alterations. Adv Neuroimmunol 1995;5:13–21.

Pack AI. Obstructive sleep apnea. Adv Intern Med 1994;39:517–556.

Porkka-Heiskanen T, Strecker RE, Thakkar M, et al. Adenosine: a mediator of the sleep-inducing effects of prolonged wakefulness. Science 1997;276:1265–1267.

Robinson A, Guilleminault CG. Obstructive Sleep Apnea Syndrome. In S Chokroverty (ed), Sleep Disorders Medicine: Basic Science, Technical Considerations, and Clinical Aspects. Boston: Butterworth–Heinemann, 1999;331–354.

Saadeh A, Hauri P, Kripke DF, Lavie P. The role of actigraphy in the evaluation of sleep disorders. Sleep 1995;18:288–302.

Steriade M. Neurophysiologic Mechanisms of Non–Rapid Eye Movement (Resting) Sleep. In S Chokroverty (ed), Sleep Disorders Medicine: Basic Science, Technical Considerations, and Clinical Aspects. Boston: Butterworth–Heinemann, 1999;51–62.

Stradling J, Davies RJO. Sleep apnea and hypertension—what a mess! Sleep 1997;20:789–793.

Strollo PJ Jr, Rogers RM. Obstructive sleep apnea. N Engl J Med 1996;334:99–104.

Trenkwalder C, Walters AS, Hening W. Periodic limb movements and restless leg syndrome. Neurol Clin 1996;14:629–650.

Walters AS. The International Restless Legs Syndrome Study Group: toward a better definition of the restless legs syndrome. Mov Disord 1995;10:634–642.

Young T, Palta M, Dempsey J, et al. The occurrence of sleep-disordered breathing among middle-aged adults. N Engl J Med 1993;328:1230–1235.

Chapter 73
Headache and Other Craniofacial Pain

Jerry W. Swanson, David W. Dodick, and David J. Capobianco

Headache is one of humanity's most frequent afflictions. It has been estimated that one person in three experiences severe headaches at some stage of life. More than 13,000 tons of aspirin are consumed annually worldwide; a major part of it is taken for the relief of headache. Few symptoms lead to more self-treatment than does headache. Most people with a mild recurrent or isolated headache do not consult a physician, and therefore the true incidence is unknown. Population-based studies have estimated that the lifetime prevalence for any type of headache is in excess of 90% for men and 95% for women. A survey of 15,000 households in the United States by Stewart and co-workers (1992) revealed a prevalence of migraine of 17.6% in women and 5.7% in men. The result is 23 million Americans with migraine, with an economic cost of up to $17.2 billion in direct health care

The authors of this chapter acknowledge the efforts of the prior authors of this chapter (Drs. J. Keith Campbell and Richard Caselli) in the two previous editions of this book.

Table 73.1:   Classification of headache

Migraine
Tension-type headache
Cluster headache and chronic paroxysmal hemicrania
Headache associated with head trauma
Headache associated with vascular disorders
Headache associated with nonvascular intracranial disorders
Headache associated with substances and their withdrawal
Headache associated with noncephalic infection
Headache associated with metabolic abnormality
Headache or facial pain associated with disorders of cranium, neck, eyes, ears, nose, sinuses, teeth, mouth, or other facial or cranial structures
Cranial neuralgias, nerve trunk pain, and deafferentation pain
Other types of headache or facial pain
Headache not classifiable

Source: Data from Headache Classification Committee of the International Headache Society. Classification and diagnostic criteria for headache disorders, cranial neuralgias and facial pain. Cephalalgia 1988;8(Suppl. 7):1–96.

costs as well as the cost of lost productivity in the workplace (de Lissovoy and Lazarus 1994).

PAIN TRANSMISSION AND MODULATION AS RELATED TO HEADACHE

An understanding of the pathophysiology of headache must first start with a knowledge of which intracranial structures are pain sensitive. Ray and Wolfe reported on the pain-sensitive structures in the head and mapped the pattern of pain referral based on the structure stimulated from intracranial surgery performed during local anesthesia in the 1930s. The intracranial pain-sensitive structures include the arteries of the circle of Willis and the first few centimeters of their medium-sized branches, meningeal (dural) arteries, large veins and dural venous sinuses, and portions of the dura near blood vessels. Pain-sensitive structures that are external to the skull cavity include the external carotid artery and its branches, scalp and neck muscles, skin and cutaneous nerves, cervical nerves and nerve roots, mucosa of sinuses, and teeth. Pain from these structures is carried largely by cranial nerves V, VII, IX, and X.

Inflammation, traction, compression, malignant infiltration, and other disturbances of pain-sensitive structures lead to headache. Superficial structures tend to refer pain locally, whereas deeper-seated lesions may refer pain imprecisely to a distant part. A purulent maxillary sinus, for example, causes pain over the involved sinus, whereas within the cranial vault, nociceptive signals reach the central nervous system (CNS) largely by way of the first division of the trigeminal nerve, and therefore an occipital lobe tumor may refer pain to the frontal head region. Infratentorial lesions tend to refer pain posteriorly because this compartment is innervated by the second and third cervical nerve roots,

which also supply the back of the head. This rule can be broken when posterior lesions or cervical spine pathology produce frontal headache. This occurs because the caudal portion of the trigeminal nucleus extends down as far as the dorsal horn at the C3 level. Impulses arriving from C2-C3 converge on neurons within the trigeminal nucleus and may refer pain to the somatic distribution of cranial nerve V1.

Afferent pain impulses into the trigeminal nucleus are modified and modulated by descending facilitatory and inhibitory influences from critical brainstem structures, including the periaqueductal gray, rostral ventromedial medulla, and serotonergic and adrenergic nuclei. Opioids diminish the perception of pain by activating the inhibitory systems, whereas fear, anxiety, and overuse of analgesics may activate the facilitatory systems thereby aggravating the pain.

The trigeminovascular system is of critical importance in the understanding of how pain is generated and propagated centrally from peripheral pain-sensitive structures (Goadsby 1997).

CLASSIFICATION

In 1988, the Headache Classification Committee of the International Headache Society introduced detailed classification of headaches, which was also later reprinted (*ICD 10 Guide for Headaches* 1997). The 13 main headache types are shown in Table 73.1. Each headache type is further defined and subclassified according to criteria agreed to by several international subcommittees. Careful definition of the many types of migraine and other primary headache disorders is expected to free future research and clinical publications from the confusing and often poorly defined terminology of earlier work. Until the actual pathogenesis of primary headache syndromes is determined, it will not be possible to develop a unitary classification of head pain.

HEADACHE ASSOCIATED WITH NONVASCULAR INTRACRANIAL DISORDERS

Intracranial lesions that occupy space, often referred to as *mass lesions*, produce head pain by traction on or compression of pain-sensitive structures. The nature, location, and temporal profile of headache produced by an intracranial mass depend on many factors, including the location of the lesion, its rate of growth, its effect on the cerebrospinal fluid (CSF) pathways, and its tendency to cause cerebral edema. The intracranial mass lesion may be neoplastic, inflammatory, or cystic. Each type can result in either localized or generalized head pain. The type of headache is characteristic of raised intracranial pressure but is not diagnostic of a particular underlying disease.

Intracranial and intraparenchymal hematomas are also mass lesions and are responsible for traction headaches, but they are classified under vascular disorders causing headache.

Tumors

Approximately 50% of patients with brain tumors report having headaches, and in one-third to one-half of them it is considered the primary complaint. The headache can be a generalized cephalgia, but in approximately one-third of patients, it overlies the tumor and is referred to the position of the scalp nearest the lesion. Rapidly growing tumors are more likely to produce headache than are indolent lesions, but even the slowly enlarging lesions can eventually produce pain by compromising the ventricular system or exerting direct pressure on a pain-sensitive structure, such as the trigeminal nerve. Once the CSF circulation is partially obstructed, headache often becomes generalized and worse in the occipitonuchal area. This type of headache, which is a manifestation of raised intracranial pressure, is often worse on awakening, aggravated by coughing and straining, and sooner or later associated with nausea and vomiting. In children particularly, the vomiting may be precipitate and without nausea. This can lead to projectile vomiting because it occurs without warning. This rarely occurs in adults.

Large parenchymal tumors, such as gliomas and metastatic tumors, and small tumors that interfere with the CSF pathways can be associated with periodic increases in intracranial pressure. Monitoring reveals periods of increased pressure, the plateau waves of Lundberg, the beginning of which may be associated with increasing severity of headache and the peak of which may be associated with vomiting or other ictal events, such as a seizure or a change in respiration.

Supratentorial masses generally produce frontal or temporal head pain because of the trigeminal nerve supply to the anterior and middle cranial fossae. Because the superior surface of the tentorium cerebelli is supplied by the meningeal branches of the first division of the trigeminal cranial nerve, an occipital lesion can cause pain referred to the fronto-orbital region. Mass lesions of the posterior fossa generally cause occipitonuchal pain because the meningeal nerve supply is largely through the upper cervical nerves, which also supply the occipital and cervical dermatomes. Some sensory innervation of the posterior fossa is also carried through cranial nerves VII, IX, and X, and therefore pain referral can be more widespread. Posterior fossa tumors are more likely (in more than 80%) to result in headache earlier than their supratentorial counterparts because the greater likelihood of compromise of the ventricular system leads to rapidly developing hydrocephalus and raised intracranial pressure (Forsyth and Posner 1993).

Pituitary tumors and tumors around the optic chiasm commonly cause a frontotemporal headache, but they can also cause referred pain near the vertex.

Tumors growing in the ventricular system are rare, but they can present dramatically. The classic presentation of a colloid cyst of the third ventricle is a sudden headache of great severity, rapidly accompanied by nausea and vomiting and possibly by loss of consciousness. Intraventricular meningiomas, choroid plexus papillomas, and other intraventricular tumors can present in this abrupt way if they are mobile enough to suddenly obstruct the ventricular outflow pathways. A positional change may precipitate such an event; similarly, adoption of a different posture may rapidly relieve the headache and other symptoms. Colloid cysts of the third ventricle generally lead to slowly enlarging hydrocephalus that may result in a generalized, rather constant headache, superimposed on which may be episodes of catastrophic increases in headache. Obstruction of the egress of CSF from the ventricular system rapidly leads to increased intracranial pressure, which can exceed the capillary perfusion pressure of the brain, and hence lead to loss of consciousness secondary to cerebral ischemia. Headaches that have a rapid onset and are associated with loss of consciousness, amaurosis, or vomiting are obviously serious and should lead the examiner to consider conditions such as subarachnoid hemorrhage, brain tumor, or other mass lesions.

Headache, especially in the occipital region, that is brought on by exertion (e.g., coughing, sneezing, or lifting) should be taken seriously. A posterior fossa lesion, such as a cerebellar tumor or Chiari malformation, can lead to this clinical picture. In most patients with cough or exertional headache, however, no serious lesion is found.

Infiltrating tumors, such as gliomas, can reach considerable size without causing pain because they may not deform or stretch the pain-sensitive vessels and nerves. Such lesions are more likely to present as focal neurological deficits or with seizures than with headache. Sudden worsening of the neurological state due to hemorrhage into the tumor mass is, however, a potent cause of sudden headache. This may initially appear in the part of the skull overlying the tumor and then become generalized if intracranial pressure rises. Infarction of a tumor can cause edema and swelling that result in a similar dramatic onset of head pain and neurological deficit.

Tumors that are intracranial but extraparenchymal, such as meningioma, acoustic neuroma, pinealoma, and craniopharyngioma, can all produce headaches, but, as with the parenchymal lesions, there are no specific headache patterns. The headaches can be near the lesion, referred to a more distant site in the cranium, or generalized when intracranial pressure increases. Meningiomas and meningeal sarcomas can invade the skull and can even cause a mass externally by direct tumor spread or by overlying hyperostosis. Not surprisingly, such tumors are often associated with localized head pain. Meningeal carcinomatosis (carcinomatous meningitis) produces a headache in most subjects, but the associated cranial nerve involvement and other neurological symptoms are generally more striking.

The headache associated with other intracranial mass lesions, such as cerebral abscess and intracranial granuloma, is no more specific than that due to a cerebral neoplasm. The headache can be focal or generalized, and the temporal profile depends on the underlying abnormality.

In summary, the following features should serve as warnings that a patient's headaches may not be of benign origin and raise the possibility of an intracranial mass lesion:

1. Recent onset of headaches, especially in middle-aged and older patients. (Most primary headaches arise before middle age.)
2. Change in headache pattern, such as increased intensity of pain, increased frequency of attacks, development of new features, or decreased response to treatment.
3. Occurrence of other symptoms, particularly if present between attacks.
4. Abnormalities on neurological examination (Edmeads 1997).

Arachnoid Cysts

Cystic spaces bounded by arachnoid membranes can be found with computed tomography (CT) or magnetic resonance imaging (MRI) scans during the investigation of headaches. Rarely are these lesions responsible for the head pain. Uncommonly, an arachnoid cyst has a one-way valve-like structure in its wall, so that arterially induced pulsations of the CSF gradually pressurize the cyst and cause it to enlarge. Compression of cranial nerves, such as the trigeminal nerve, or distortion of the midline structures causes headaches that may be either generalized or localized. Serial CT scans reveal the cyst to be increasing in size, and this finding should lead to operative intervention. Enlargement of normal subarachnoid spaces, however, such as the cisterna magna and cisterna ambiens is not a cause for headache and should not lead to shunting or other surgical approaches.

Abnormalities of Cerebrospinal Fluid Circulation

Whether raised intracranial pressure, in the absence of a shift of intracranial structures, results in headache is uncertain. The rate at which the intracranial pressure is increased and the duration of the increase are probably factors that determine whether pain is produced.

Obstruction of the Cerebrospinal Fluid Pathways

Lesions that prevent free egress of CSF from the ventricular system result in obstructive hydrocephalus. If this occurs before closure of the cranial sutures, it results in enlargement of the skull, usually without producing headache. Ventricular obstruction after closure of the sutures leads to raised intracranial pressure and frequently to headache. The pain is often worse on awakening, occipital in distribution, and associated with neck stiffness. Vomiting, blurred vision, and transient obscuration of vision due to papilledema may follow as well as failing vision secondary to optic atrophy.

Rapidly developing obstruction due to a posterior fossa mass lesion or a ball-valve tumor, such as a third ventricular colloid cyst, can lead to a rapidly increasing headache followed by vomiting, impaired consciousness, and increasing neurological deterioration. Slowly developing hydrocephalus may result in massively dilated ventricles and may be associated with little or no headache.

Congenital obstruction of the foramina of the fourth ventricle, Dandy-Walker syndrome, can lead to ballooning of the ventricle and deformity of the cerebellum. Minor degrees of this malformation can remain asymptomatic until later in life and then present with obstructive hydrocephalus and headache. Similarly, the Chiari malformation in its various forms can obstruct the free circulation of CSF and lead to hydrocephalus and headache (Stovner 1993). This malformation can result in an occipital headache that is worsened or even initiated by Valsalva's maneuver during lifting, straining, or coughing. Thus, the Chiari malformation is one of the causes of an exertional or Valsalva's headache.

In communicating hydrocephalus, there is free communication between the ventricular system and the subarachnoid space but some impairment of CSF circulation or absorption. Obstruction in the basal cisterns or at the arachnoid granulations may follow subarachnoid hemorrhage, meningitis, and head injury. Venous sinus occlusion can impair absorption of CSF. Headache may be a prominent symptom of both obstructive and communicating hydrocephalus, except in the case of normal pressure hydrocephalus, which is generally painless (see Chapter 65).

Low Cerebrospinal Fluid Pressure Headache

The headache of lowered CSF pressure characteristically develops in the upright position and is rapidly relieved by recumbency. It most commonly occurs after a lumbar puncture, especially when this is performed as part of myelography. Loss of CSF volume, due in part to the removal of some CSF for diagnostic purposes and in part to later leakage through the hole in the arachnoid and dural layers, results in a traction headache. The brain normally floats in the intracranial CSF, loss of which allows the brain to sink and thereby exert traction on structures such as bridging veins and sensory nerves. Lying down removes the effect of gravity, and the traction headache is relieved. The headache that occurs after spinal tap usually resolves in a few days if the patient remains in bed with good hydration. Occasionally, the syndrome persists for days, weeks, or even months. Relief can usually be obtained by the application of a blood patch, in which 10–20 ml of the patient's own blood is injected into the epidural space close to the site of the original spinal tap. This technique prevents further leakage of CSF by exerting increased pressure in the epidural space and by coagulating the blood, thereby relieving the headache in a few hours. The injection of blood is associated with a small risk of causing cauda equina compression or subarachnoid hemorrhage, but it is unlikely if the blood volume is small and the blood is injected gently.

An identical syndrome of headache due to low CSF pressure can occur when there is a leak of fluid through the cribriform plate, through the petrous bones, or through any basal skull defect. CSF rhinorrhea and especially CSF otorrhea may not be obvious to the patient, whose complaint may be that of postoperative or post-traumatic headache. Leakage of CSF from the skull can occur spontaneously when intracranial pressure is raised or a tumor such as a basal meningioma erodes through the base of the skull. This occurs most often around the cribriform plate region, where the bone is especially thin. The CSF leak can be identified by radioisotope cisternography or by CSF studies using the dye fluorescein. Leakage of CSF through the nasal sinuses can be detected by placing numbered cotton pledgets in the nose next to the various ostia of the sinuses. Contamination of the pledgets by radioactivity or dye enables the sinus through which the fluid is leaking to be identified. CSF otorrhea is not easy to identify if the fluid is draining down the eustachian tube when the eardrum is intact. Scanning with a gamma camera after instillation of a radioactive tracer by lumbar puncture usually allows the leak to be identified. Treatment is usually surgical repair of the bony and meningeal defect.

A similar low CSF pressure headache can occur when a tear develops in the spinal theca. This is usually in the midthoracic region and may result from lifting or coughing or, at times, spontaneously. It can also occur with a crush injury to the chest or abdomen and in patients with overdraining CSF shunts. When it occurs without a significant history of trauma, it can be overlooked as a cause of daily headache. The history of a headache rapidly responding to recumbency should lead one to suspect the condition. However, in some patients whose headaches are long-standing, a persistent headache may be noted and the postural feature of the headache may become less prominent. Nausea or emesis, neck pain, dizziness, horizontal diplopia, changes in hearing, photophobia, upper limb paresthesias, vision blurring, and dysgeusia can also occur in some patients, particularly when the headache first develops. The diagnosis first requires a clinical index of suspicion followed by a determination of the opening CSF pressure. However, in only 50% of cases is the CSF pressure less than 40 mm of H_2O.

Often, these patients have a variable pleocytosis with up to 40 or more mononuclear cells per mm^3 and a mild-to-modest increase in CSF protein (Mokri 1997). MRI has become an invaluable diagnostic tool in this syndrome, with the cardinal features being diffuse pachymeningeal thickening with gadolinium enhancement, subdural collections of fluid, and evidence of brain descent (Figures 73.1–73.3). This evidence includes cerebellar tonsillar descent (resembling Chiari type I malformation); reduction in size or effacement of the prepontine, perichiasmatic, and subarachnoid cisterns; inferior displacement of the optic chiasm; and descent of the iter (the opening of the aqueduct of Sylvius as seen on midsagittal MRI).

In patients with the typical clinical and radiographic features of low CSF pressure headache, the patient may be managed conservatively with bed rest and hydration for 1–2 weeks. If this is either not practical or not effective, further diagnostic studies will be necessary to identify the site of the CSF leak, which in spontaneous cases usually occurs at the spinal level, especially at the level of the thoracic spine or the cervicothoracic junction. Myelography with CT of the spine is more sensitive than radioisotope cisternography or MRI of the spine, but the latter procedures may serve as guides for obtaining multiple CT images at the appropriate levels. An autologous blood patch may then be attempted and repeated in the event of a suboptimal response. Most patients respond to either conservative therapy or a blood patch, but in resistant cases, surgical intervention with repair of the dural tear may be necessary. Even after a protracted duration, surgical repair of the causative dural tear can be quite effective (Schievink et al. 1998).

Pseudotumor Cerebri

Headache, transient visual obscuration, pulsatile tinnitus, and diplopia are the most frequent presenting symptoms of pseudotumor cerebri. The headache is rather nonspecific but tends to be worse on awakening and to be aggravated by activity. The blurring and obscuring of vision are a direct result of raised intracranial pressure leading to papilledema. Once it has been determined by MRI that there is no intracranial mass, obstruction of the ventricular system, or thrombosis of a dural venous sinus, the high CSF pressure can be confirmed by lumbar puncture manometry. Removal of CSF to achieve a normal closing pressure relieves the headache and temporarily prevents visual obscuration. Long-term management of pseudotumor cerebri is discussed in Chapter 65.

Headache Due to Cranial and Intracranial Infection

Inflammation of any pain-sensitive structures in the cranial cavity can produce headache. Meningitis and meningoencephalitis both have headache as a major symptom. The characteristics of the head pain depend on whether the infection is acute or chronic. Acute meningitis produces a severe headache with neck stiffness and other signs of meningism, including photophobia and irritability. Pain is often retro-orbital and worsened by moving the eyes. Chronic meningitis due to fungal or tuberculous infection can also lead to headache that may be severe and unrelenting. The headache of intracranial infection is nonspecific but must be considered in the differential diagnosis, especially in those with compromised immune response from corticosteroids, chemotherapy, or acquired immunodeficiency syndrome. The diagnosis can be confirmed only by examination of the

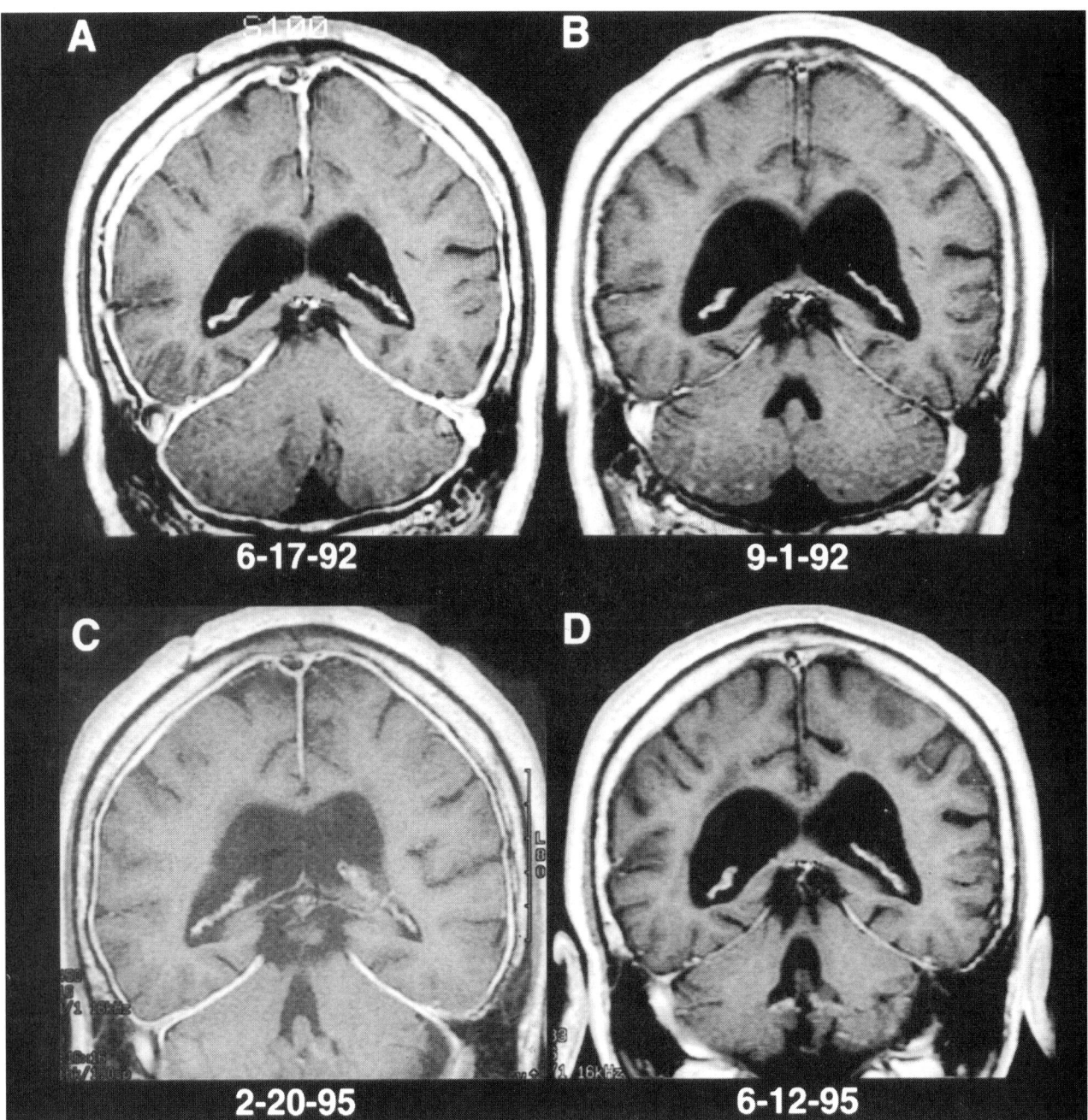

FIGURE 73.1   Coronal T1-weighted magnetic resonance images with gadolinium in a patient with an overdraining cerebrospinal fluid shunt and low-pressure headache demonstrate diffuse pachymeningeal thickening and enhancement (**A**) with resolution after shunt revision and resolution of headaches (**B**). Patient developed recurrent symptoms and imaging abnormalities after shunt revision (**C**) followed by resolution after another shunt revision (**D**). (Reprinted with permission from B Mokri, DG Piepgras, GM Miller. Syndrome of orthostatic headaches and diffuse pachymeningeal gadolinium enhancement. Mayo Clin Proc 1997;72:400–413.)

CSF. The chronic granulomatous meningitis of sarcoid may require biopsy of the basal meninges to confirm the diagnosis. Meningitis is discussed further in Chapter 59.

Sinusitis, mastoiditis, epidural or intraparenchymal abscess formation, and osteomyelitis of the skull can all cause focal and generalized headache. The diagnosis is usually suspected from the associated symptoms and signs.

After craniotomy, increasing pain and swelling in the operative site may be due to osteomyelitis of the bone flap. Plain skull roentgenograms reveal the typical mottled appearance of the infected bone. Removal of the flap is necessary.

Mollaret's meningitis is rare, recurrent, and sterile (see Chapter 77). The CSF cellular response includes large epithelioid cells (Mollaret's cells). The pathogenesis is

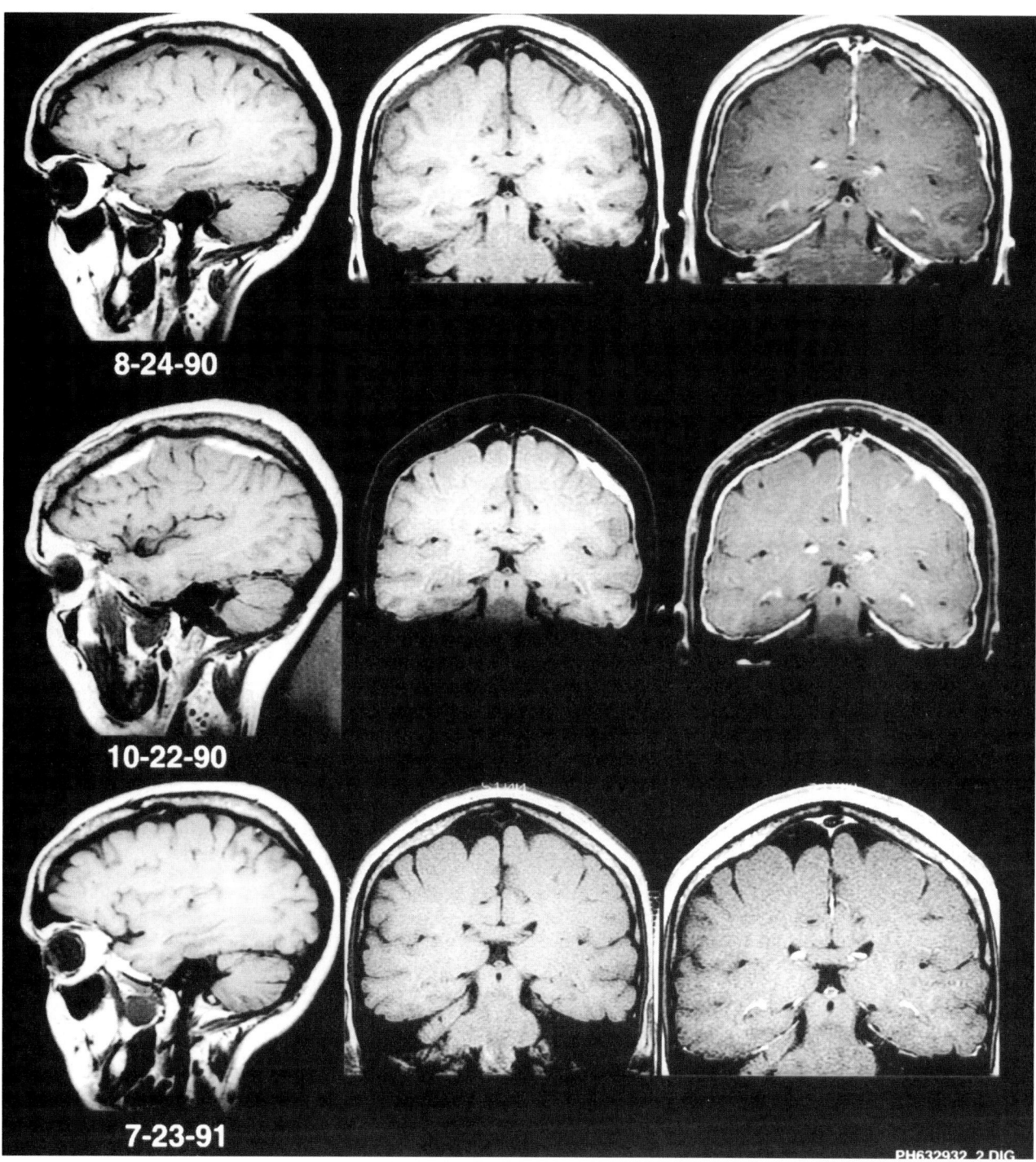

8-24-90

10-22-90

7-23-91

FIGURE 73.2   Sagittal and coronal T1-weighted magnetic resonance images with gadolinium of a patient with spontaneous low cerebrospinal fluid (CSF)-pressure headaches demonstrate subdural fluid collections and pachymeningeal enhancement (*top row*) with loculation and progression of subdural fluid collections (*middle row*). Bottom row demonstrates resolution of the fluid collections and meningeal enhancement after correction of the CSF leak and headache resolution. (Reprinted with permission from B Mokri, DG Piepgras, GM Miller. Syndrome of orthostatic headaches and diffuse pachymeningeal gadolinium enhancement. Mayo Clin Proc 1997;72:400–413.)

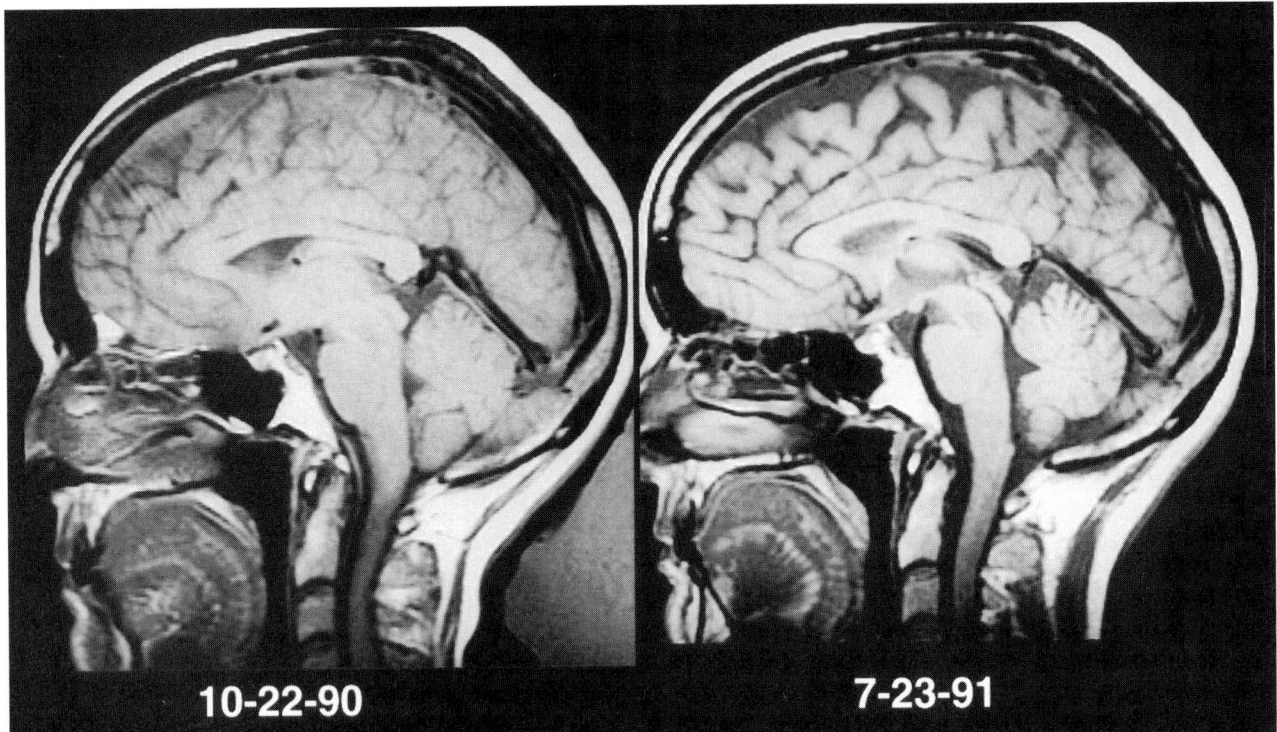

FIGURE 73.3   Sagittal T1-weighted magnetic resonance images (MRI) demonstrate cerebellar tonsillar descent and crowding of the posterior fossa in a patient with spontaneous low-pressure headaches. After symptomatic resolution, MRI of the posterior fossa returns to normal. (Reprinted with permission from B Mokri, DG Piepgras, GM Miller. Syndrome of orthostatic headaches and diffuse pachymeningeal gadolinium enhancement. Mayo Clin Proc 1997;72:400–413.)

unknown but may be related to the herpes simplex virus (Picard et al. 1993). The condition may recur every few days or every few weeks for months or years. Headache, signs of meningism, and low-grade fever accompany each attack. Treatment is mainly symptomatic.

Transient Syndrome of Headache with Neurological Deficits and Cerebrospinal Fluid Lymphocytosis

There is a transient syndrome characterized by recurrent episodes of headache accompanied by reversible neurological deficits and CSF pleocytosis, originally termed *migrainous syndrome with CSF pleocytosis*. Several reports of this syndrome used various terms, including headache with neurological deficits and CSF lymphocytosis (Berg and Williams 1995) and pseudomigraine with temporary neurological symptoms and lymphocytic pleocytosis (Gomez-Aranda et al. 1997). This self-limited syndrome consists of one to several episodes of variable neurological deficits accompanied by moderate-to-severe headache and sometimes fever. Each episode lasts hours, with total duration of the syndrome from 1 day to 70 days. CSF abnormalities have included a lymphocytic pleocytosis varying from 10 to more than 700 cells/mm^3, elevation of CSF protein, and in some cases, elevated opening pressure. MRI and CT scans are invariably normal, but EEG often shows focal or diffuse slowing. Microbiological studies have been negative. The etiology of the syndrome is unclear, although it has been speculated to be due to an immune response to a viral infection. No treatment has been shown to alter the self-limited course of this disorder.

HEADACHE ASSOCIATED WITH VASCULAR LESIONS OF THE HEAD AND NECK

Aneurysms and Arteriovenous Malformations and Thunderclap Headache

Intracranial aneurysms are rarely responsible for headache unless they rupture. Rapid enlargement of an aneurysm may produce local pain by pressure on a cranial nerve, especially the trigeminal nerve, or on other pain-sensitive structures. This is most common with aneurysms of the internal carotid and posterior communicating arteries. Enlargement of an aneurysm may occur shortly before rupture, and the local pain is therefore important but, unfortunately, is rarely recognized clinically. Cerebral aneurysms are not a cause of recurrent migrainelike headaches, even when the headache attacks are confined to one side. The incidence of migraine in patients with subarachnoid hemorrhage due to a ruptured aneurysm is similar to the incidence of migraine in the general population.

Parenchymal arteriovenous malformations (AVMs) rarely cause pain before rupture. Very large lesions can be associated with ipsilateral or bilateral throbbing cephalgia, but they rarely cause a migrainelike syndrome. Large AVMs can usually be suspected by the presence of a cranial bruit or of the classic triad of migraine, seizures, and focal neurological deficits. The incidence of headache in patients harboring AVMs is probably no higher than that in the general population.

The myth has developed that headaches of a migrainous type, if consistently on one side of the head, could be due to an aneurysm or an AVM. In the past, this belief led to many unnecessary arteriograms. The worry expressed by patients and physicians that a recurrent headache might be due to an aneurysm or AVM is now usually easily resolved by obtaining a cranial MRI or magnetic resonance angiogram (MRA). Any aneurysm or AVM responsible for a recurrent or persistent headache has a very high probability of being demonstrated. Both aneurysms and AVMs can bleed in such a way as to produce a less than catastrophic subarachnoid hemorrhage. These small warning leaks can result in one or more sentinel headaches. Each may be relatively mild and short-lived. They usually have a sudden, but not very dramatic, onset. Identification of the sentinel headache is important but is very difficult.

Patients who are not usually subject to headaches should be investigated whenever they report new onset of headaches or even a single episode if it is described as "the worst headache I've ever had," or if it was associated with neck stiffness or pain, transient neurological symptoms (e.g., extraocular nerve palsy), or fever. Patients in whom there is any suspicion of a sentinel bleed or who describe a recent thunderclap headache should be examined with CT scanning to detect blood in the subarachnoid cisterns. If the scan is negative, the continuing suspicion of a warning bleed should lead to an examination of the CSF. If the CSF is bloodstained or xanthochromic or if, despite the absence of positive findings on the lumbar puncture, there is still a suspicion of a sentinel hemorrhage, an MRA or cerebral angiography may be advisable.

The term *thunderclap headache* describes a severe headache of instantaneous onset, which may be a symptom of an expanded unruptured aneurysm. Several follow-up studies of patients with thunderclap headache and negative evaluations for subarachnoid hemorrhage have elucidated the often benign natural history of this peculiar headache disorder. Slivka and Philbrook (1995) reported four patients with thunderclap headache without subarachnoid hemorrhage, in three of whom angiography revealed diffuse segmental intracerebral arterial vasoconstriction. Resolution of the vasospasm was seen in the one case in which

Table 73.2: Diagnostic criteria for thunderclap headache

Thunderclap headache without neurological signs or symptoms
    Very severe pain intensity
    Hyperacute onset of pain (<30 secs)
    Headache lasts 1 hour to 10 days (may last up to 4 wks)*
    Headaches may recur over a 7-day period but do not recur regularly over subsequent weeks or month (may recur over subsequent months to years)*
    Associated with a normal cerebral vasculature or reversible segmental vasoconstriction
    May be clinically indistinguishable from thunderclap headache associated with intracranial disorder*
    May occur spontaneously or be precipitated by Valsalva's maneuver, sexual activity, exercise, or exertion
Thunderclap headache with neurological signs or symptoms
    Headache and angiographic features as described above
    Neurological signs or symptoms transient or result in minimal residual deficits
Thunderclap headache associated with intracranial disorder
    Associated conditions include subarachnoid hemorrhage (cerebral venous sinus thrombosis, pituitary apoplexy)*
    May have associated neurological or systemic signs or symptoms, depending on underlying disorder

*Modifications to diagnostic criteria. (Adapted with permission from DW Dodick, RD Brown, JW Britton, J Huston. Nonaneurysmal thunderclap headache with diffuse, multifocal, segmental, and reversible vasospasm. Cephalalgia 1999;19:118–123.)

angiography was repeated. We have seen two similar cases, and through this collective experience, a characteristic profile has begun to emerge (Table 73.2).

Thunderclap headache is a hyperintense pain of acute onset with peak pain intensity reached by 30 seconds. The headache can last from 1 hour to 10 days but may last up to 4 weeks. Thunderclap headaches may recur over a 7-day period but do not recur regularly over subsequent weeks to months. The headache may occur spontaneously or be precipitated by Valsalva's maneuver, sexual activity, or exercise. The headache may be associated with transient neurological signs or symptoms and reversible segmental vasoconstriction on angiography.

Primary thunderclap headache may be clinically indistinguishable from thunderclap headache associated with intracranial disorders, such as subarachnoid hemorrhage, cerebral venous sinus thrombosis (de Bruijn et al. 1996), or pituitary apoplexy (Dodick and Wijdicks 1998). These entities are associated with significant neurological morbidity and may be elusive on initial CT imaging, thus underscoring the need for MRI in this group if the initial workup is negative.

Subarachnoid Hemorrhage

Rupture of an intracranial aneurysm or AVM results in a subarachnoid hemorrhage, with or without extension into the parenchyma of the brain. The headache of a subarachnoid hemorrhage is characteristically explosive in onset and of overwhelming intensity. Subjects who survive occasionally relate that they thought they had been hit on the head. The headache rapidly generalizes and may quickly be accompanied by neck and back pain. Loss of consciousness may rapidly supervene, but many patients remain alert enough to complain of the excruciating headache. Vomiting is frequently present and aggravates the head pain. Intraventricular blood, the distortion of the midline structures, and the heavy contamination of the basal cisterns by blood can each contribute to the rapid development of hydrocephalus, which worsens the headache.

The diagnosis is easily suspected and can be confirmed by an unenhanced CT scan that reveals blood in the subarachnoid cisterns or within the parenchyma. Early hydrocephalus may also be seen. When a CT scan unequivocally shows blood in the subarachnoid spaces, it is not necessary or advisable to perform a lumbar puncture because the resultant reduction of CSF pressure may cause herniation of the brain or may remotely induce further bleeding from the aneurysm. Demonstration of subarachnoid hemorrhage generally indicates the need for cerebral angiography. The timing of this procedure and the subsequent mode of treatment are detailed in Chapter 57C.

Relief of the intense headache of subarachnoid hemorrhage generally requires parenteral analgesics. The need to provide pain relief must be balanced against the need to interfere as little as possible with the level of consciousness, respiration, and physical signs, such as pupil size and reaction. Parenteral codeine is often used, but meperidine is also useful. Sedation with phenobarbital may also be required if the patient is restless because of pain. The headache that occurs after a subarachnoid hemorrhage may be very persistent, lasting up to 7–10 days. In some cases, a chronic daily headache may persist for months to years.

The headache of subarachnoid hemorrhage is aggravated by movement and is associated with photophobia and phonophobia. Therefore, it is customary to nurse patients in a dark, quiet room and to disturb them as little as possible. Straining at stool, vomiting, and coughing should be prevented appropriately.

The hemorrhage and the headache that can result from a ruptured AVM have qualities and behavior that are essentially identical to those from a ruptured berry aneurysm of the circle of Willis.

Parenchymal Hemorrhage

Until the advent of CT scanning, it was widely believed that a stroke due to a cerebral hemorrhage was associated with severe headache and that an ischemic stroke was generally painless. However, modern imaging techniques have shown that cerebral infarction is often painful and that cerebral hemorrhage can be painless. These caveats notwithstanding, a hemorrhage into the cerebral or cerebellar tissue is a potent source of headache of rapid onset and of increasing severity. The intraparenchymal mass causes a traction headache by deforming and shifting the pain-sensitive vascular and meningeal and neural structures. As the hematoma enlarges, it may obstruct the CSF circulation through the ventricular system and lead to abrupt increases in intracranial pressure. Initially, the pain of a cerebral hemorrhage is ipsilateral, but it may generalize if hydrocephalus and raised intracranial pressure occur. Rupture of the hematoma into the subarachnoid space or leakage of the blood into the basal cisterns through the CSF pathways causes the headache to increase and be associated with neck stiffness and other signs of meningeal irritation.

Cerebral and cerebellar hemorrhage can be due to hypertension of any cause; to a bleeding diathesis, including the medical administration of anticoagulants; to an arteritis and amyloid angiopathy; or to an aneurysm or AVM, as discussed earlier. Bland cerebral infarcts, primary and secondary brain tumors, and areas of cerebritis, such as occur in herpes simplex encephalitis, can each be complicated by hemorrhage into the lesion. Headache may signal the presence of the lesion or a worsening of the clinical condition. Almost without exception, the headache of intraparenchymal hemorrhage is of acute or subacute onset and does not indicate the exact nature of the underlying disease. Headache associated with focal or generalized cerebral or cerebellar signs demands examination with an unenhanced CT scan.

Cerebellar hemorrhages, which account for about 10% of cases of intraparenchymal bleeding, can result in a catastrophic clinical picture. The available space in the posterior fossa is limited. An enlarging hematoma in the cerebellum rapidly compresses vital brainstem structures and obstructs the outflow of CSF from the ventricular system. This leads to occipital headache, which is rapidly followed by vomiting; impaired consciousness; and various combinations of brainstem, cerebellar, and cranial nerve dysfunction. Cerebellar hemorrhage is a neurological and neurosurgical emergency. A CT scan should be obtained as soon as possible. Evacuation of the hematoma with or without ventricular drainage may be the only chance of saving the patient.

The treatment of headache due to intraparenchymal bleeding is of secondary importance, but it should include suitable analgesics. The primary concern is to evacuate the hematoma if it is large and causing a major shift of the midline structures or one of the several herniation syndromes. Temporary measures that reduce intracranial pressure include administration of mannitol, urea, or glycerol. Ventricular drainage and monitoring of intracranial pressure may be useful. Sedation and narcotic analgesics must be used with care so as not to compromise respiration or mask the vital neurological functions needed to follow the state of the patient.

Subdural Hematoma

Bleeding into the subdural space is generally due to tearing of one or more of the bridging veins that cross the space to reach the venous sinuses, particularly the sagittal sinus. Most subdural hematomas occur over the convexity of the cerebral hemispheres, but they can occur in the posterior fossa or adjacent to the tentorium. Only 50–80% of patients give a history of head trauma to explain the development of the hematoma. Chronic subdural hematomas are an important cause of headache in that enlargement of the lesion may be very insidious and unaccompanied by serious neurological signs for a considerable time. Changes in personality, alterations in cognitive abilities, a subacute dementia, and nonspecific symptoms, such as dizziness and excessive sleepiness, may be present for weeks or months. Focal seizures, focal weakness, or sensory changes and, ultimately, decreasing levels of consciousness may occur. Symptoms of chronic subdural hematoma, including headache, may be fluctuating and intermittent. Transient ischemic attacks (TIAs) may be seen. Headache is the single most common symptom and often is a severe bitemporal pain. Headache secondary to subdural hematoma is more common in young people, in whom cerebral atrophy is less than in elderly patients. In the presence of atrophy, a larger hematoma can accumulate before stretching and deforming pain-sensitive structures. Subdural hematoma should be considered in an elderly person with recent onset of headaches. Once suspected, a subdural hematoma should be sought with a CT scan or MRI. Treatment of subdural hematomas is discussed in Chapter 56B. Once the lesion is drained or when it is spontaneously absorbed, headaches tend to resolve.

Cerebral Ischemia

Cerebral infarction, whether embolic or occlusive, frequently causes head pain (Arboix et al. 1994). The location of the pain is a poor predictor of the vascular territory involved. Similarly, the pain poorly correlates with mechanism of the stroke, whether embolic or thrombotic. It may be either steady or throbbing and is not as explosive or as severe as the headache of subarachnoid hemorrhage. The infarct responsible for the pain may be of a moderate size or very extensive. Even small ischemic events that clear in 24 hours, by definition TIAs, may be associated with transient head pain in up to 40% of patients. Carotid distribution ischemia leads to frontotemporal head pain, whereas vertebrobasilar ischemia leads to occipital headache.

Although most headaches that occur in association with stroke develop once the ischemic event has occurred, incipient cerebrovascular insufficiency can result in a headache before the ischemic event. The appearance of a new headache in a patient over the age of 50 years, particularly in the presence of atherosclerotic risk factors, should prompt consideration of a possible imminent cerebral ischemic event

because headaches may precede a TIA or ischemic stroke by days or weeks. The mechanism of these headaches is unclear, but it may be that amines liberated from platelet-fibrin thrombi cause a chemically mediated dilatation of blood vessels. The headaches may resemble either migraine or tension-type, so a high index of suspicion is needed.

If a large cerebral or cerebellar infarct produces a significant mass effect as a result of edema, headache may worsen. Obstruction of the ventricular system results in increasing hydrocephalus and further aggravation of the pain. Like all vascular headaches, the pain may be pulsatile and may be worsened by straining or by the head-low position. As the infarct lessens in size and the phase of hyperemia subsides, headache generally eases, although for some weeks there may be a recurrent tendency to focal headache over the site of the infarct. Evolution of a bland infarct into a hemorrhagic infarct is generally associated with worsening of headache.

Flashing lights, field defects, and other visual disturbances may represent symptoms of cerebrovascular disease. Similarly, migraine with aura can produce many different visual symptoms before the headache develops. Hence, it is not always possible to differentiate the visual disturbances of migraine from those of more serious cerebrovascular disease. The visual aura of migraine is usually an initially irritative phenomenon producing scintillating, often zigzag, visual hallucinations that can be seen with the eyes open or closed. This is described as a positive scotoma, having the effect of spontaneously producing the sensation of light or color. Visual disturbances due to serious visual pathway ischemia or retinal ischemia more often than not results in vision loss or a negative scotoma, which cannot be appreciated in the dark or with the eyes closed. Like many rules in medicine, this one is not absolute. An embolus to a retinal artery can result in showers of bright flashes, and calcarine ischemia can occasionally produce scintillating scotoma that resembles those of migraine. The migrainous aura tends to march across the visual field over the course of a few minutes and is generally followed by the headache after a latent interval. The headache of cerebrovascular insufficiency or occlusion has a more variable relationship to the visual disturbances.

Carotid and Vertebral Artery Occlusion and Dissection

Occlusion of the cervical portion of the carotid artery can result in headache in several ways. A consequent cerebral infarct may increase the intracranial pressure, as described previously. Ipsilateral headache may be due to vasodilatation of collateral vessels in and around the orbit. Headache due to carotid occlusion may be associated with a partial ipsilateral Horner's syndrome, in which facial sweating is not affected. The sympathetic hypofunction may be due to interference with the sympathetic fibers around the internal carotid artery as they ascend from the superior cervical ganglion to the intracranial structures. The combination of

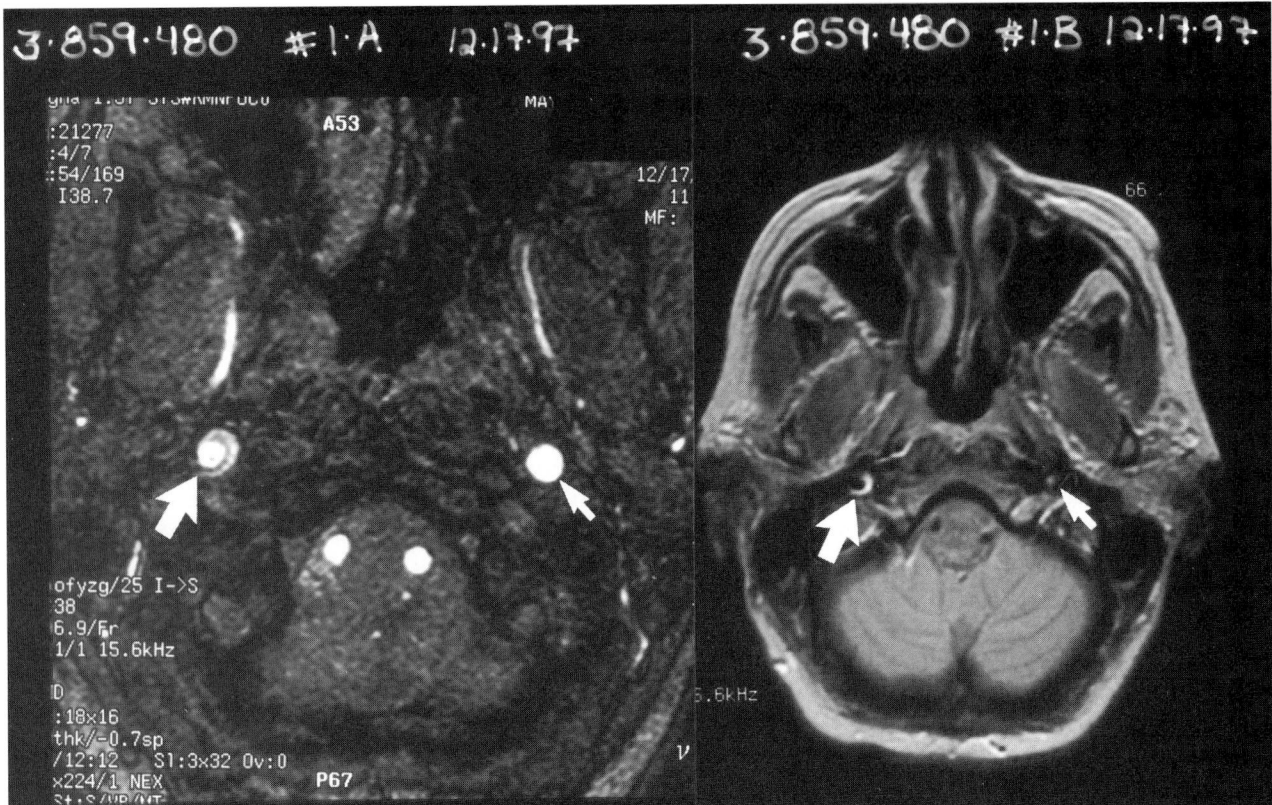

FIGURE 73.4   Magnetic resonance images of a patient with right internal carotid artery dissection. The large arrow in each figure points to the right internal carotid artery, which has a smaller flow void than that of the left internal carotid artery (*small arrows*), reflecting the narrowed lumen of the vessel. The region of the flow void is surrounded by a hyperintense crescent representing the intramural hematoma.

headache, ipsilateral Horner's syndrome, and contralateral hemiparesis is generally due to carotid occlusion.

Cervicocephalic arterial dissections result from penetration of the circulating blood through an intimal tear into the wall of an artery. The penetration of blood is usually within the media. A variety of results may occur with dissection, including formation of an intramural hematoma that pushes the lumen to one side, resulting in an elongated narrowing of the vessel lumen. Other results are compression of the lumen to cause an occlusion of the vessel; dissection of the intramural hematoma distally into the true lumen, with creation of two parallel channels; and expansion of the intramural hematoma toward the adventitia, resulting in an aneurysmal dilatation. The condition can result from intrinsic factors that predispose to dissection, including fibromuscular dysplasia, cystic medial necrosis, and in association with Marfan's syndrome and Ehlers-Danlos syndrome. Extrinsic factors, such as trivial trauma, may play a pathogenic role when superimposed on structurally abnormal arteries. Severe head and neck trauma may occasionally be the proximate cause of dissection.

In most patients, the initial manifestation of internal carotid dissection is pain (headache, face pain, or neck pain), which is typically ipsilateral to the dissection; in a minority, the pain may have a bilateral distribution. Cerebral or retinal ischemic symptoms are the initial manifestations in a lower percentage of patients. The common clinical syndromes with which patients present with carotid dissection include (1) hemicranial pain plus an ipsilateral oculosympathetic palsy, (2) hemicranial pain and delayed focal cerebral ischemic symptoms, or (3) lower cranial nerve palsies, usually with ipsilateral headache or face pain.

The most common symptom of vertebral dissection is headache and neck pain. The most frequent syndrome consists of headache, with or without neck pain, followed after delay by focal CNS ischemic symptoms.

MRI or MRA often can confirm the diagnosis. With the involved level, the lumen of the artery appears as a dark circle of flow void of smaller caliber than the original vessel, and the intracranial clot appears as a hyperintense and bright crescent or circle (in both T1 and T2 images) surrounding the flow void (Figure 73.4). Occasionally, catheter angiography is necessary to confirm the diagnosis (Mokri 1997).

The pain associated with cervicocephalic dissections is of variable duration and may require treatment with potent analgesics. Patients are usually treated with either antiplatelet agents or, if evidence of distal embolization has occurred, anticoagulation.

Giant Cell Arteritis

Giant cell arteritis is a vasculitis of late middle age and maturity that has gone by many other names, including temporal arteritis, cranial arteritis, granulomatous arteritis, polymyalgia arteritica, and Horton's syndrome. It is one of the most ominous causes of headache in elderly persons. When left unrecognized and untreated, it frequently leads to permanent blindness. The single most common reason patients with giant cell arteritis are seen by neurologists is headache of an unknown cause.

Clinical Symptoms

The clinical manifestations of giant cell arteritis result from inflammation of medium and large arteries. Table 73.3 summarizes the clinical symptoms in 166 patients examined at the Mayo Clinic between 1981 and 1983. Headache was the most common symptom, experienced by 72% of patients at some time, and was the initial symptom in 33%. The headache is most often throbbing, and many patients report scalp tenderness on combing their hair. Headache, though often generalized, is associated with striking focal tenderness of the affected superficial temporal or, less often, occipital artery. One-third of patients with headache may have no objective sign of superficial temporal artery inflammation.

More than one-half of patients with giant cell arteritis experience polymyalgia rheumatica, and it is the initial symptom in one-fourth. Polymyalgia rheumatica consists of aching in proximal and axial joints, proximal myalgias, and often significant morning stiffness. Fatigue, malaise, and a general loss of energy occur in 56% of patients and are the initial symptoms in 20%.

Jaw claudication occurs commonly and is the initial symptom in 4% of patients. Tongue claudication occurs rarely. A nonproductive cough or a sore throat, occasionally severe enough to produce dysphagia, can occur.

One of the most ominous symptoms to occur in giant cell arteritis is amaurosis fugax because 50% of affected patients, if left untreated, develop subsequent partial or total blindness. Ten percent of the patients in the Mayo Clinic series experienced amaurosis fugax, which was bilateral in 35%. Blindness occurred in 8%, was monocular in 86%, but was preceded by amaurosis fugax in only 14%. In untreated giant cell arteritis, the frequency of permanent vision loss approximates 40%. Diplopia can occur and may be horizontal or vertical.

Fourteen percent of patients have a neuropathy, which is a peripheral polyneuropathy in 48%, multiple mononeuropathies in 39%, and isolated mononeuropathy in 13%. Limb claudication occurs in 8% of patients and more frequently involves the upper limbs. TIAs and strokes occur in 7% of patients, and the ratio of carotid to vertebral events is 2 to 1. Vertigo and unilateral hearing loss can occur. An acute myelopathy, acute confusional state, or subacute stepwise cognitive deterioration are rare manifestations.

Table 73.3: Symptoms of giant cell arteritis in 166 patients*

Symptom	Patients with symptom (%)	Patients in whom it was initial symptom (%)
Headache	72	33
Polymyalgia rheumatica	58	25
Malaise, fatigue	56	20
Jaw claudication	40	4
Fever	35	11
Cough	17	8
Neuropathy	14	0
Sore throat, dysphagia	11	2
Amaurosis fugax	10	2
Permanent vision loss	8	3
Claudication of limbs	8	0
Transient ischemic attack/stroke	7	0
Neuro-otological disorder	7	0
Scintillating scotoma	5	0
Tongue claudication	4	0
Depression	3	0.6
Diplopia	2	0
Tongue numbness	2	0
Myelopathy	0.6	0

*Some patients had coincident onset of more than one symptom.
Source: Data from RJ Caselli, GG Hunder, JP Whisnant. Neurologic disease in biopsy-proven giant cell (temporal) arteritis. Neurology 1988;38:352–359.

Physical Findings

Signs on physical examination relate to involvement of various arteries and the end-organ damage sustained from vasculitis-induced tissue infarction.

Forty-nine percent of patients with histologically verified giant cell arteritis have physical signs of superficial temporal artery inflammation, including erythema, pain on palpation, nodularity, thickening, or reduced pulsation on the affected side. Eighteen percent of patients with signs of superficial temporal artery inflammation do not complain of headache. Although it is rare, ischemic necrosis of the scalp and tongue can occur.

Almost one-third of patients have large artery bruits or diminished pulses. The carotid artery is the most frequently affected vessel. The upper limb arteries are more frequently affected than are those in the lower limbs, and some patients have vasculitic involvement of the aorta or its major branches. Coronary arteritis with consequent myocardial infarction may also occur.

Ocular findings in giant cell arteritis may be striking. During amaurosis fugax, which may be orthostatically induced in rare patients, there is visible sludging of blood in the retinal arterioles. With infarction of the optic nerve, vision loss precedes the funduscopical signs of an anterior ischemic optic neuritis by up to 36 hours. During the acute stage there is papilledema. The disc appears pale, and the resulting visual field defect, when subtotal, tends to be alti-

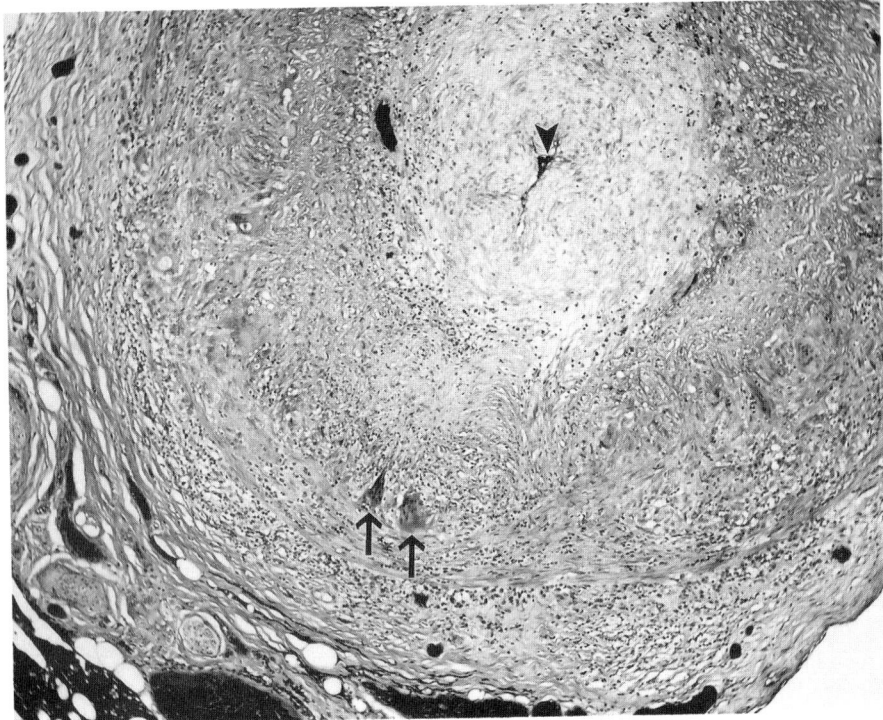

FIGURE 73.5 Transverse section of temporal artery showing narrowed lumen (*arrowhead*) and giant cells (*double arrows*) in relation to the elastic lamina (hematoxylin-eosin stain × 100). (Micrograph courtesy of R. Jean Campbell, M.B.Ch.B.)

tudinal. Papilledema is followed by the gradual development of optic atrophy.

Extraocular muscle palsies show daily fluctuations in the severity of specific extraocular muscle involvement. Oculosympathetic paresis (partial Horner's syndrome) may occasionally occur.

Laboratory Studies

The most often recognized laboratory abnormality in giant cell arteritis is elevation of the erythrocyte sedimentation rate (ESR) (mean, 85 ± 32 mm in 1 hour with the Westergren method), although it may be normal (<29 mm in 1 hour) in 3%. Patients are usually anemic (mean hemoglobin value, 11.7 ± 1.6 g/dl) and show a mild thrombocytosis (mean platelet count, 427 ± 116 × 10^3/µl). Mild elevation of plasma α_2-globulins, serum aspartate aminotransferase, and alkaline phosphatase may be present. All these findings are nonspecific, and the diagnosis rests on confirmatory temporal artery biopsy.

Angiography of the cerebral circulation may fortuitously demonstrate a vasculitis of the superficial temporal, vertebral, or carotid artery, although it is too insensitive to be reliable. The temporal artery shows alternating stenosis and dilatation over several-centimeter segments, often more pronounced distally. Angiography of the aortic arch vessels may show long segments of smoothly tapered stenosis and occlusions of subclavian, brachial, and axillary arteries.

Physiology

The symptoms and signs of giant cell arteritis result from systemic and local inflammatory processes leading to arterial stenosis and occlusion. End organs, such as the optic nerve, extraocular muscles, spinal cord, peripheral nerves, and brain, may be rendered transiently ischemic or infarcted. In amaurosis fugax, ischemia of the optic nerve and retina results from sludging of blood within the arterioles due to vasculitic involvement of the ophthalmic, posterior ciliary, and (less often) central retinal arteries.

Pathology

The histopathological features of the diagnostic arterial lesion include intimal proliferation with consequent luminal stenosis, disruption of the internal elastic membrane by a mononuclear cell infiltrate, invasion and necrosis of the media progressing to panarteritic involvement by mononuclear cells, giant cell formation with granulomata within the mononuclear cell infiltrate, and, variably, intravascular thrombosis (Figure 73.5). Involvement of an affected artery is patchy (skip lesions). Long segments of normal unaffected artery are flanked by vasculitic foci. Treatment with oral corticosteroids may change the histopathological findings within days, and a previously vasculitic focus may appear normal or show only intimal fibrosis. For these reasons, biopsy of the superficial temporal artery should be generous (4- to 6-cm–long specimens), multiple histological sections should be taken, and the biopsy may be bilateral if necessary. If the first two conditions are satisfied, 86% of cases of giant cell arteritis are correctly diagnosed by biopsy.

The term *temporal arteritis* can lead to a false sense of security that giant cell arteritis is largely a focal vasculitis affecting the relatively inconsequential superficial temporal artery. Up to one-third of patients, however, have clinically significant large artery disease. The most frequent causes of vasculitis-related death are cerebral and myocardial infarction. Rupture of the aorta occurs rarely. In fatal cases, vertebral, ophthalmic, and posterior ciliary arteries are as frequently and as severely involved as the superficial temporal arteries. Peripheral neuropathic syndromes occur, and in cases of acute mononeuropathies, ischemic infarction of peripheral nerves due to vasculitis has been demonstrated. Intracranial vascular involvement has been reported only rarely.

Immunology, Etiology, and Pathogenesis

Giant cell arteritis is considered an autoimmune disease of unknown cause. Although it is often a systemic vasculitis, giant cell arteritis usually occurs much more focally than polyarteritis nodosa and is characterized by a mononuclear cell infiltrate with giant cell formation, suggesting differences in immunopathogenesis. No distinctive antigen has been identified to explain the particular tropism of giant cell arteritis, although the possibility that the immune reaction is directed against the internal elastic lamina, which is absent from small cerebral vessels, has been suggested to explain the paucity of intracranial involvement. Lymphocytes sensitized to the purported antigen infiltrate the internal elastic lamina and release a host of lymphokines, which attract a mononuclear cell infiltrate. Activated macrophages release lysosomal proteases and may transform into epithelioid and multinucleate giant cells. T cells themselves, by antibody-dependent cell-mediated cytotoxicity or natural killer cell actions, may also mediate the angioclasis. Additionally, antibody and complement deposits have been demonstrated at the internal elastic lamina, which suggests that humoral mechanisms are involved.

Epidemiology

In a population-based study of Olmsted County, MN, the incidence of giant cell arteritis was found to increase over a 25-year period from 5.1 to 17.4 cases per 100,000 population per year in people aged 50 or older. This increase was attributed to greater clinical awareness and increased diagnosis. The prevalence was 133 cases per 100,000 population in people aged 50 or older on January 1, 1975. The female-to-male ratio was 3.7 to 1. The median age at onset was 75 years (range, 56–92 years).

Course and Prognosis

The clinical onset of giant cell arteritis may be acute (as in patients presenting with sudden transient or permanent vision loss), subacute, or chronic. The median duration of symptoms before diagnosis is 1 month, but exceptional patients may present with a history of up to several years of polymyalgia rheumatica.

On institution of corticosteroid treatment, reversible symptoms and ESR normalize within days. With tapering doses, relapses may occur at any time and may consist of prior symptoms or new symptoms. Neurological complications, including neuropathies and cerebrovascular events, are not always prevented by corticosteroid administration and have a median onset of 1 month after initiation of treatment. Similarly, large artery involvement can occur up to 7 months after initiation of treatment.

The occurrence of amaurosis fugax often brings a patient with undiagnosed giant cell arteritis to medical attention, but permanent loss of vision after initiation of treatment has been documented in rare instances. In patients with acute and incomplete loss of vision, some visual function may return with the immediate institution of corticosteroids, but this is exceptional.

Treatment and Management

Once the diagnosis is suspected, histological confirmation should be obtained and treatment started immediately. Treatment should not be withheld pending the result of temporal artery biopsy. Treatment consists of oral corticosteroids given initially in high doses and gradually tapered over months. Prednisone may be initiated at 40–60 mg per day and continued for 1 month, after which time a cautious taper of less than 10% of the daily dose per week may be started. If, at the time of presentation, ischemic complications are imminent or evolving, parenteral high-dose corticosteroids should be implemented until these complications stabilize. The adjunctive use of anticoagulants for ischemic cases may be tried, but their efficacy in this setting is unproved.

Disease activity must be monitored with both clinical assessment and determination of the ESR. A flare of symptoms accompanied by an increase in the ESR mandates increasing the corticosteroid dose at least to the last effective higher dose and, often, boosting it temporarily to a higher level. Relapses generally reflect too rapid a taper, and resumption of a more slowly tapering regimen is indicated after the relapse has stabilized. Some patients may require continuation of low-dose (7.5–10.0 mg/day) prednisone for several years, although complete withdrawal remains the goal.

Finally, the multitude of well-known adverse effects of exogenous corticosteroids necessarily influence management by prompting a more rapid taper and treatment of the side effects themselves. Three particularly difficult treatment complications include symptomatic vertebral body compression fractures (26% of patients), corticosteroid myopathy (11%), and corticosteroid-induced organic brain syndrome (3%). All may limit treatment by necessitating a more aggressive taper and thereby exposing the patient to the attendant risks of a relapse of the vasculitis.

HEADACHE CAUSED BY DISEASES OF THE EYES, EARS, NOSE, MOUTH, OR OTHER CRANIAL OR NECK STRUCTURES

Ocular Causes of Headache

In the absence of injection of the conjunctiva or other obvious signs of eye disease, headache and eye pain rarely have an ophthalmic cause. The maxim is that a white eye is not the cause of a painful eye. Acute angle-closure glaucoma is a rare but dramatic event. The patient may present with extreme eye and frontal head pain and vomiting and may be in early shock. The sclera is injected, the cornea steamy, the pupil fixed in midposition, and the globe stony hard. It is a true ophthalmological emergency.

Refractive errors, imbalance of external eye muscles, amblyopia, and (in the terminology used by many patients) eyestrain are not causes of headache in most instances. In children and teenagers, however, refractive errors, especially hyperopia, can produce dull frontal and orbital headaches from straining to achieve accommodation at school. Myopic children are unaffected.

Soon after initiation of miotic preparations such as pilocarpine, some patients with glaucoma complain of eye and frontal discomfort due to ciliary muscle spasm. This subsides with continued use of the drops.

Cluster headaches, migraine, dissection of the carotid artery, and many other varieties of headache cause orbital and retro-orbital pain. Each is discussed elsewhere in this chapter. Sharp jabs of pain through the eye lasting 1 second or longer can occur as part of the ice-pick headache or idiopathic stabbing headache. This condition is of unknown pathogenesis but is most commonly seen in migraineurs. The sharp eye pain, known by various names, including *ophthalmodynia periodica*, is occasionally felt in the ipsilateral occipital region simultaneously.

Nasal Causes of Headache and Facial Pain

Acute purulent sinusitis causes local and referred pain. The distribution of the pain depends on the sinuses involved. Maxillary sinusitis causes pain and tenderness over the cheek. Frontal sinus disease gives rise to frontal pain; sphenoid and ethmoidal sinusitis causes pain behind and between the eyes, and the pain may also be referred to the vertex. Purulent sinusitis may be associated with fever and other constitutional symptoms. The pain is worse on bending forward and is often relieved as soon as the infected material drains from the sinus. Chronic sinusitis is rarely a cause of headache in adults, but it can be in children. In any age group, a chronic mucocele of a frontal or sphenoid sinus gives rise to local pain and tenderness. Frontal sinusitis that spreads through the posterior wall of the sinus to produce an epidural abscess is a serious cause of local head pain. If neglected, the abscess may pass through the meningeal layers to produce meningitis or a brain abscess.

Malignant tumors of the sinuses and nasopharynx can produce deep-seated face and head pain before involving cranial nerves or otherwise becoming obvious. MRI scanning is the optimal imaging technique for the detection of these cryptic lesions. Bony abnormalities of the nose, particularly a deviated nasal septum that is impacted against a turbinate bone, can give rise to an episodic pain syndrome resembling chronic cluster headache. Swelling of the nasal mucosa during sleep leads to further impaction of the bones and results in nocturnal pain. Diagnosis and treatment are within the expertise of the otorhinolaryngologist.

Temporomandibular Joint Disorders

In 1934, Costen first drew attention to the temporomandibular (TM) joint as a cause of facial and head pain. Until recently, Costen's syndrome was rarely diagnosed. During the past two decades, however, interest has been increasing in disorders of the TM joint, the muscles of mastication, and the bite as they relate to headaches. Articles in the popular press and diagnoses by dentists have led many patients to believe that TM joint disorders are the most common cause of headache. Mechanical disorders of the joint, alterations in the way the upper and lower teeth relate, and congenital and acquired deformities of the jaw and mandible can all give rise to head and face pain and are very occasionally responsible for the episodic and chronic pain syndromes seen by neurologists.

For the neurologist evaluating a head or facial pain, the criteria for identification and localization of TM disorders listed in Table 73.4 should be helpful.

Bruxism, teeth clenching, and chronic gum chewing are important in the production of pain in the masseter and temporalis muscles. Arthritis and degenerative changes in the TM joint, loss of teeth, ill-fitting dentures or lack of dentures, and other dental conditions can all lead to the TM joint or myofascial pain dysfunction syndrome that manifests as facial and masticatory muscle pain. Head pain and facial pain, even when associated with the criteria listed in Table 73.4, require full evaluation, which should include a detailed history and examination, appropriate radiographs, and laboratory studies to exclude other more serious causes. If TM dysfunction is thought to be the source of the pain, further evaluation and treatment are in the province of the appropriate dental specialist. Even when TM dysfunction is believed to be responsible for facial or head pain, conservative management with analgesics, anti-inflammatory agents, application of local heat, and nonsurgical techniques to adjust the bite generally provide relief. Before surgical modalities are employed on the TM joint or mandibles, the diagnosis must be secure and other causes of head and face pain excluded by appropriate investigations.

Other Dental Causes of Craniofacial Pain

Pulpitis and root abscess generally give rise to dental pain that a patient can localize. The cracked tooth syndrome results from an incomplete tooth fracture, most frequently involving a lower molar. The initial pain is usually sharp and well localized, but thereafter the pain is often diffuse and hard to locate. After the initial fracture, the tooth is sensitive to cold. Pain may be felt in the head and face ipsilateral to the damaged tooth. With time, infection develops in the pulp, leading to extreme and well-localized pain. Confirmation of the diagnosis and treatment of the cracked tooth require the expertise of a dentist.

Headaches and the Cervical Spine

Degenerative joint disease and cervical disc herniation rarely give rise to headache in the absence of neck pain. Occipital headache and neck pain on awakening are not uncommon with arthritis of the cervical spine. With activity, the headache and associated stiffness of the neck subside. Similarly, holding the head in one position for hours while driving or working at a desk can cause an increase in neck and head pain in the presence of degenerative changes. The cervical myalgias can spread upward to produce a muscle contraction headache. Relief follows rest or simply adoption of a different position. For patients with severe degenerative changes in the cervical facet joints, exercise, heat, and the use of simple analgesics can help both the neck and the head pain. Surgical fusion or discectomy should be performed only if there is bony instability or spinal cord or nerve root compression. A cervical fusion for relief of headache in the absence of these indications is likely to be ineffective.

Cervicogenic headache is a controversial entity consisting of a strictly unilateral migrainelike head and face pain with associated neck pain and stiffness. Attacks of pain are often accompanied by ipsilateral autonomic phenomena, such as tearing and even erythema of the face, and can be precipitated by neck maneuvers. Tenderness on the side of the neck ipsilateral to the head pain is sometimes accompanied by triggering of the attacks by pressure over the C2 nerve root, the greater occipital nerve, or the transverse process of C4-C5. At present, the concept of cervicogenic headache remains controversial.

Table 73.4: Criteria for identification and localization of temporomandibular joint disorders

Temporomandibular pain	Temporomandibular dysfunction
The pain should relate directly to jaw movements and mastication	Interference with mandibular movement (clicking, incoordination, and crepitus)
Tenderness in the masticatory muscles or over the temporomandibular joint on palpation	Restriction of mandibular movement
Anesthetic blocking of the tender structures should confirm the presence and location of the pain source	Sudden change in the occlusal relationship of the teeth

MIGRAINE

Few medical conditions have been recognized as long as migraine has. Aretaeus of Cappadocia, who lived in the second century AD, described a paroxysmal headache often felt on one side of the head, often associated with nausea, and followed by pain-free intervals. Galen (130–200 AD) emphasized the unilateral nature of the attacks and introduced the term *hemicrania* (from the Greek *hemikranios*). The Romans translated the word to the Latin *hemicranium*, later corrupted to *hemigranea* and hence *migranea*. These terms were in turn modified to the Middle English *megrim*. The current name *migraine*, the French translation, gained acceptance in the eighteenth century and finally gave rise to the term *migraineur* for one who has this type of headache.

Definition and Classification

Until the cause of migraine is known, the classification must be based on descriptive terms. Several attempts have been made to develop sufficiently detailed definitions of migraine to allow clinicians, researchers, and others to discuss the condition without ambiguity. No entirely satisfactory nomenclature yet exists, and misunderstandings still occur.

Migraine is now classified according to the scheme devised by the Headache Classification Committee of the International Headache Society (*ICD 10 Guide for Headaches 1997*), as shown in Table 73.5.

Clinical Aspects

Migraine can begin at almost any age; most commonly, the initial attack occurs during the teenage years, and by 40 years of age, 90% of those with the condition have had their first attack. Although migraine can begin in older patients, it should be viewed with suspicion because a serious intracranial disorder could be masquerading as vascular headache.

Table 73.5: Classification of migraine

Migraine without aura
Migraine with aura
    Migraine with typical aura
    Migraine with prolonged aura
    Familial hemiplegic migraine
    Basilar migraine
    Migraine aura without headache
    Migraine with acute-onset aura
Ophthalmoplegic migraine
Retinal migraine
Childhood periodic syndromes that may be precursors to or be
    associated with migraine
    Benign paroxysmal vertigo of childhood
    Alternating hemiplegia of childhood
Complications of migraine
    Status migrainosus
    Migrainous infarction
Unclassifiable migrainelike disorder

Source: Data from Headache Classification Committee of the International Headache Society. Classification and diagnostic criteria for headache disorders, cranial neuralgias and facial pain. Cephalalgia 1988;8(Suppl. 7):1–96.

After puberty, migraine is more common in females, whereas in children there is a small preponderance of male subjects. A family history of migraine is present in up to 90% of patients. The prevalence of migraine has been assessed on numerous occasions with widely varying results. Several studies have shown the prevalence of migraine in women to be approximately 20% and in men approximately 6% whereas other large population studies have placed the prevalence somewhat lower. Once migraine has developed, it tends to recur with varying frequency throughout much of a patient's life. Attacks have a tendency to get milder and less frequent in later years.

Although migraine attacks have been classified into those with and those without an aura, they are not mutually exclusive, and many patients have separate attacks of the two types.

Migraine without Aura

Migraine without aura occurs episodically and is not preceded or accompanied by any easily identifiable aura due to focal cerebral or brainstem disturbances. Some subjects have a change in mood or energy level as long as 24 hours before the attack and may have a feeling of well-being or of extra energy the day before an episode of migraine. This prodromal phase often leads to working or playing harder than usual and then paying for it the next day. Other victims pass through a vague period of increased fatigue or actual depression lasting a few hours. Excessive yawning may herald the imminent attack. After these inconstant or premonitory warnings, the headache may occur the next day. The attack may awaken the subject during the night, but this is less common than finding that the attack has already started when the patient awakens at the normal time. At this stage, the pain may be unilateral and is usually supraorbital, but it may be holocephalic. An initial unilateral headache may progress to a generalized head pain, or it may switch to the contralateral side during the course of the attack. A common pattern is for the headache to migrate posteriorly and become an occipital and upper cervical pain. This process is probably due to the development of sustained contraction of the scalp and upper cervical paraspinal muscles. The opposite migration can also occur, in which the subject first develops upper cervical pain and stiffness, which then progresses to a migraine headache.

A migraine syndrome that is characterized by episodes of pain in the cheek, nose, ear, and neck has been called lower-half headache. It is not common, but it should be considered when pain in the lower part of the face is associated with nausea, vomiting, or photophobia. The condition is most easily diagnosed when the subject has been or is currently subject to the more typical cephalgia of migraine. Pain in the lateral portion of the neck with tenderness over the carotid artery may be found in lower-half headache. When the carotid pain and tenderness predominate, the term *carotidynia* is applicable. The management of this condition is similar to that of the more common cephalic forms of migraine.

The quality of the pain of migraine is frequently described as throbbing (pulsatile). Many patients, however, describe the pain as steady while they remain still. It tends to pulsate or throb at the heart rate with exertion, after Valsalva's maneuver, or during the head-low position. Strict insistence on obtaining a history of a throbbing pain in vascular headaches leads to many erroneous conclusions. The pain of migraine may vary during the attack and from episode to episode. Some attacks are mild and are no more than an inconvenience, whereas others are severe and incapacitating.

With all but mild-to-moderate attacks, the person remains still. Most patients try to lie down; in a few, however, assuming this position aggravates the pain and they prefer to recline at an angle or sit with the head resting on a table. Any increase in jugular venous pressure, such as occurs when lying down, may increase the pain. Any reduction in arterial pressure in the scalp and head vessels gives some relief of pain. Manual compression of the scalp vessels gives temporary relief. Some people even compress the ipsilateral carotid artery to obtain some respite. Release of the compressed artery is followed by a transient increase in the ipsilateral pain, which usually then throbs for a few seconds. Application of an ice pack to the scalp gives partial relief in some patients, whereas others prefer to apply heat to the painful part. Still others have discovered that a hot shower or bath provides some reduction in pain, possibly by producing widespread vasodilatation and a reduction in blood pressure.

Many symptoms are frequently associated with the pain of migraine. Photophobia and phonophobia are common. Many are pale, cold, and clammy during the attack, especially when nausea develops. The onset of nausea and vomiting in migraine can occur almost as soon as the pain develops, but it is more commonly delayed until the attack has been in progress for an hour or longer. Anorexia, even intolerance to the smell of food, is even more common than nausea. The gastrointestinal symptoms can include diarrhea. Intolerance of odors such as perfume is frequently described during migraine. Even inveterate smokers can rarely smoke during an attack.

The pain of an attack of migraine tends to build up to a peak over 30 minutes to several hours. Rarely the onset is described as being more explosive. The attack generally lasts several hours to a full day. Severe episodes can continue for several days and, if associated with vomiting, can lead to prostration and dehydration. Very prolonged attacks or a series of attacks with minimal relief between them is called *status migrainosus*, and it often warrants admission to the hospital for pain relief and correction of fluid and electrolyte imbalance. More commonly, the attack subsides within a day or after a night's sleep. The day after the intense pain, the patient feels tired and listless. The head is still heavy and hurts when shaken.

The frequency and severity of episodes of migraine without aura (common migraine) are extremely variable. The fortunate ones have one or two attacks in a lifetime. Most migraineurs are less fortunate, and the severely afflicted dread the next attack. For most victims, the frequency varies widely throughout life, depending on many identified and many unidentified factors. Recurrence of attacks one to four times per month is not uncommon, and attacks in relation to the menstrual cycle are a common pattern in women during the reproductive years. Attacks at less than weekly intervals are common in patients who attend neurology clinics and generally indicate that a chronic daily headache pattern is evolving (Silberstein 1993).

Blurred vision is a common complaint during all types of migraine. Lightheadedness is also common and may go on to actual syncope in a small percentage. Subconjunctival hemorrhages, orbital ecchymoses, and epistaxis have all been reported to accompany migraine. Fever, tachycardia, and paroxysmal atrial tachycardia are rare migraine-related symptoms, possibly due to associated disturbances of the autonomic nervous system. Sacks' 1992 monograph on migraine has a complete listing of the symptoms that have been described in migraine.

Migraine with Aura

This is a recurrent, periodic headache preceded or accompanied by an aura consisting of transient visual, sensory, motor, or other focal cerebral or brainstem symptoms. The head pain is identical to that of migraine without aura but is unilateral in a higher percentage of patients. Alterations in mood and other premonitory symptoms may precede the aura by several days.

The most common aura is the disturbance of vision known as a scintillating scotoma (teichopsia). This generally begins as a shimmering arc of white or colored lights in the homonymous part of the left or right visual field. The arc of light gradually enlarges and becomes more obvious. It may have a definite zigzag pattern. It may be a single band of light or may have a much more complex pattern. It has a shimmering or flickering quality, similar to that seen when a fluorescent light fixture is close to failure or a strobe light is just short of the flicker fusion frequency. Gradually, over the course of a few minutes, the scintillating pattern migrates across the visual field to approach the point of fixation. On occasion, the positive scotoma is preceded or followed by a spreading zone of vision loss (negative scotoma). Even if there is no identifiable area of vision loss, the disturbance of vision produced by the scintillating scotoma makes it difficult to read or drive. Often, a mild feeling of dizziness or even vertigo occurs during the visual disturbance. Even though the scotoma is believed to originate in the calcarine cortex of one cerebral hemisphere and should therefore be an essentially congruent homonymous field defect, it is often described as being seen in one eye only or as worse on one side than the other. Patients often describe the visual disturbance in vague terms, such as blurry vision, double vision, or jumpy vision. Close questioning or showing the patient an artist's representation of a scintillating scotoma generally clarifies the complaint.

There are many variations of migrainous teichopsia (subjective visual images). The zigzag appearance may be so pronounced as to justify the term *fortification spectrum* because of its fanciful resemblance to the ground plan of a fort. Occasionally, the scotoma is less complex and is simply described as a ball of light in the center of the visual fields, and it may obscure vision to a significant degree. This type of teichopsia may represent a bilateral calcarine disturbance. The scintillating and positive (bright) scotomata can still be seen with the eyes closed or while in the dark. This is not a feature of the negative scotomata (areas of darkness), which disappear in the dark.

The teichopsia of migraine may be more complex and formed than the usual lines and geometric patterns. Rarely, a complex scene is visible to the migraineur; it may be recognizable as an image from the patient's past experience, or it may be an unknown scene. Disturbances of this complex type may be due to dysfunction in the posterior temporal lobe. Changes in the perception of the shape or form of viewed objects, metamorphopsia, can lead to frightening and bizarre visual hallucinations. The story of Alice in Wonderland, in which the heroine perceived herself shrinking, is believed to have been based on Lewis Carroll's own experience of migrainous metamorphopsia. Migraineurs may describe leaving their own bodies during the aura phase and viewing themselves from above.

Visual disturbances due to retinal dysfunction are relatively uncommon in migraine and may take the form of unilateral flashes of light (photopsia), scattered areas of vision loss, altitudinal defects, or even transient unilateral vision loss. When such monocular visual disturbances are followed by a headache, the term *retinal migraine* is appropriate. When the photopsia, teichopsia, and other disturbances are seen in both visual fields simultaneously, they probably originate from the calcarine cortex. A homonymous visual aura is generally followed by a headache on the contralateral side of the head, but exceptions are not uncommon. In such patients, the headache is ipsilateral to the visual disturbance, or it is bilateral.

Paresthesias can occur as an aura, alone or in conjunction with one of the previously described visual symptoms. The numbness or tingling may be felt in almost any distribution, from a hemisensory disturbance to one that involves all four limbs or a much more restricted area, such as the lips, face, and tongue. The paresthesias can last from a few seconds to 20–30 minutes. Sensory symptoms ipsilateral to the subsequent headache may be due to a disturbance of the uncrossed autonomic system. The paresthesias of migraine aura seem to have a predilection for the face and hands. This may be due to the large representation of these structures in the sensory cortex or thalamus. The term *cheiro-oral migraine* is sometimes applied to cases involving a sensory disturbance of the fingers, lips, and tongue during the aura phase.

The rate of spread of a sensory aura is important to help distinguish it from a sensory seizure and the sensory disturbance of a TIA. Just as a visual aura spreads across the visual field slowly, taking as long as 20 minutes to reach maximum, the paresthesias may take 10–20 minutes to spread from the point at which they are first felt to reach their maximal distribution. This is slower than the spread or march of a sensory seizure and much slower than the spread of sensory symptoms of a TIA. A migrainous sensory aura generally resolves over the course of a few minutes. After the aura there is usually a latent period of a few minutes before the onset of the headache. In some subjects, the aura and the headache merge.

Weakness of the limbs or facial muscles on one side of the body occurs only rarely as a motor aura of migraine. Many patients describe a sense of heaviness in the limbs on one side before a headache, but examination during this phase rarely reveals any true weakness. If actual paresis does occur, it is usually detected in the upper limb and may be accompanied by mild dysphasia if the dominant hemisphere is involved. The weakness generally lasts 20–30 minutes.

A rare occurrence is for the motor aura of migraine apparently to precipitate a focal motor seizure. This may indicate an area of abnormal cortex that has a predisposition to act as a seizure focus. The seizure appears to be triggered by the cortical abnormality that occurs in the aura of migraine.

Dysphasia or aphasia can occur as the aura of migraine. Commonly, there is some associated dominant upper limb weakness or heaviness. The aphasia, which is usually mild and transient, can be either an expressive or a receptive type. Alexia and agraphia can also occur. All the disturbances of this type are rare. Each can be associated with mild confusion and difficulty concentrating. The ensuing headache generally resembles ones the patient has had in the past and that followed the more typical visual aura.

Episodes of vertigo, transient abdominal symptoms, periods of disturbed mentation, déjà vu experiences, and other bizarre symptoms have all been thought to be the aura of migraine with aura at various times. The number of patients involved has generally been so small that the true nature of the experiences remains in doubt when compared with the frequently encountered visual, sensory, and motor auras already described.

Migraine Aura without Headache or Migraine Equivalents

When a visual, sensory, motor, or psychic disturbance characteristic of migraine aura is not followed by headache, the episode is termed a *migraine equivalent* or *acephalic migraine*. Most commonly encountered in patients who have a past history of migraine with aura, the episodes can begin de novo, usually after age 40 years, but they can occur at almost any age.

Migraine equivalents are easily recognized when the attacks occur on a background of migraine with aura. In the absence of such a history, the transient disturbance may be difficult to distinguish from an episode of transient cerebral or brainstem ischemia. Cerebral angiography, echocardiography, and tests of hemostasis may be needed to exclude the more serious causes. The typical scintillating scotoma, with its slow spread and zigzag appearance in both visual fields, is almost invariably migrainous, whether or not it is followed by a headache. Under these circumstances, it is rarely necessary to perform invasive investigations. A contrast-enhanced CT or MRI scan is a reasonable compromise when there is doubt about the migrainous nature of the event.

Acute episodes of confusion can occur with migraine, usually representing the aura stage. Acute confusional or dysphrenic migraine occurs most often in children or adolescents, but it can occur later in life. In the absence of a long history of migraine with aura, the episodes are rarely suspected of being migrainous at first. In an elderly patient, the diagnosis is considered only after exclusion of more serious conditions, including transient ischemic events. As a migraine equivalent, the acute confusional state may be unaccompanied by headache. The term *dysphrenic migraine* has been used to describe severe confusional states progressing to partial or generalized seizure activity or coma in young patients. Transient global amnesia can occur as a migraine equivalent and may occur repetitively. The migrainous nature may be suspected from the past history of more typical migraine with aura.

Basilar Migraine

Basilar migraine is usually first encountered during childhood or the teenage years. It was initially thought to be primarily a disorder of women, but further case reports indicate that it occurs in men almost as commonly (Olesen et al. 1993). Basilar migraine is recognized only in the classic form because only the dramatic constellation of brainstem symptoms allows its recognition. The headache is occipital and usually severe. The aura, which lasts 10–45 minutes, usually begins with typical migrainous disturbances of vision, such as teichopsia, graying of vision, or actual temporary blindness. The visual symptoms are bilateral. Numbness and tingling of the lips, hands, and feet often occur bilaterally. Ataxia of gait and ataxic speech may lead to the suspicion of intoxication.

Involvement of the brainstem reticular formation can lead to impairment of consciousness, especially in young patients. This often occurs as the other symptoms of the aura are subsiding. The level of coma is never profound and can resemble sleep from which the patient can be temporarily aroused. Recovery usually coincides with onset of the severe throbbing occipital headache. The pain may generalize to the whole head and is frequently associated with prolonged vomiting. After sleep, the headache is usually gone. A basilar migraine equivalent occurs in which teenagers have the symptoms just described without the headache. This is a clinical picture that can be difficult to recognize. Certain investigations are needed for reassurance. Contrast-enhanced CT or MRI scanning and electroencephalography (EEG) usually suffice. Rarely, patients with otherwise typical basilar migraine can have seizures with the attacks of headache. Epileptiform EEG abnormalities have been recorded under these circumstances.

With increasing maturity of the nervous system, attacks of basilar migraine become less common and are generally replaced by migraine without aura. Basilar migraine can occur in later life, but its onset at that age should be viewed with suspicion because arteriosclerotic vertebrobasilar artery insufficiency is more common and can produce almost identical symptoms.

Ophthalmoplegic Migraine

Ophthalmoplegic migraine can occur for the first time on a background of common migraine or migraine with aura, but it may develop de novo. It has been reported in infancy, but onset in the fourth or fifth decade can occur. Recurrent attacks are the usual pattern. Each episode begins with a unilateral orbital and retro-orbital headache, often accompanied by vomiting, lasting 1–4 days. Either during the painful stage or occasionally as the headache subsides, ipsilateral ptosis occurs and, within a few hours, progresses to a complete paralysis of cranial nerve III. Rarely, cranial nerve VI and the ophthalmic division of the trigeminal nerve may be involved at the same time. The neural deficit can last from an hour to several months. The focal nature of the deficit has often led to major investigations, including angiography to rule out the presence of an internal carotid or posterior communicating artery aneurysm, but usually

no abnormality is found. Edema of the wall of the carotid artery in the region of the cavernous sinus is one possible explanation for the involvement of the cranial nerves in this region. The prognosis is favorable for recovery unless very frequent attacks occur.

Complications of Migraine

Attacks of migraine with associated hemiparesis can occur sporadically or, rarely, as a familial condition. Either form can occur singly or recurrently. The diagnosis can be considered only if the subject has a convincing past history of migraine with aura. The attack usually begins with a motor aura involving the limbs on one side, and facial involvement may be present. Unlike the common aura, however, this motor aura may involve quite profound weakness, which persists throughout the headache phase and for a variable period thereafter. The muscle weakness may last for hours, days, or even weeks in rare cases. Recovery is usually complete, except in patients in whom a dense hemiplegia develops and in whom a CT or MRI scan demonstrates an area of infarction. CSF pleocytosis can occur with hemiplegic migraine. The increased cell count is transient and is believed to occur in response to clinical or subclinical cerebral infarction. The sporadic form of hemiplegic migraine, if it is recurrent, can alternate sides. In the familial form, the involved side tends to be the same with each attack. Inheritance of this condition may be a dominant trait and is discussed further under Migraine Genetics, later in this chapter.

A facioplegic form of complicated migraine with recurrent episodes of upper and lower motor neuron facial palsy also occurs. Whether this state is separate from hemiplegic migraine is unclear.

Usually on a background of migraine with visual aura, an occasional patient reports the persistence of visual symptoms for long periods or even indefinitely. Most such patients are found to have a field defect. It can be congruous and due to a cerebral lesion, or rarely it can be uniocular and due to a retinal abnormality. CT scans have shown small infarcts in the occipital lobes or along the course of the central visual pathways in some patients. In those with retinal involvement, occlusion or spasm of the retinal arteries has been observed. A negative scotoma can persist, and scintillating scotomata can persist for long periods. The association between migraine and stroke is also discussed in Chapter 57A.

Physical Findings

Between attacks, the migraineur generally has a normal physical examination. During an attack of migraine, the scalp vessels may be distended and tender. The blood pressure is likely to be raised secondary to the pain. Many patients are pale and clammy during the attack, especially if nauseated. The patient is likely to object to the lights of the examination room and try to avoid the glare of the ophthalmoscope during the eye examination. Occasionally, there is some inequality of the pupils, with the one ipsilateral to the headache generally being larger. A fully developed ophthalmoplegic migraine reveals various degrees of a third cranial nerve deficit, with ptosis, a dilated pupil, and impaired medial and upward movement of the involved eye. Involvement of cranial nerve VI impairs lateral deviation of the globe. Subjective impairment of sensation of the ophthalmic division of the trigeminal nerve may be detected ipsilateral to the ophthalmoplegia.

Mild weakness, especially of the upper limbs, may be found during a motor aura, and various degrees of weakness up to hemiplegia may occur in complicated migraine.

Demonstration of impaired vision during the visual aura is difficult. Most often, a patient's visual complaints are purely subjective.

Laboratory Findings

No special investigations are useful for the clinical diagnosis of migraine. EEG, MRI, and CT scan abnormalities may be found during or shortly after an attack, but they are not specific for that condition and simply detect cortical or parenchymal changes that accompany the headache. The EEG changes can range from an area of focal slowing over the hemisphere ipsilateral to the headache to focal spikes, sharp waves, or the more generalized spike-wave discharges seen in idiopathic seizure disorders. Similar findings in basilar migraine may be seen. Even when such abnormalities are noted in migraine, there is no evidence that treatment with anticonvulsants is helpful or indicated for the headache.

Visual evoked potentials are slowed in some subjects with repeated attacks of migraine. This observation, though important for evaluation of the pathophysiology of the condition, is of little use clinically. CT and MRI scans can reveal large areas of decreased attenuation and signal changes over the hemisphere ipsilateral to the headache, especially if it is severe and prolonged. These changes, which are temporary and resolve in a few days, are believed to represent edema of the affected region. Complicated migraine, especially that leading to a permanent deficit, such as a hemiparesis or a visual field defect, shows an appropriate area of cerebral infarction. The relationship of antiphospholipid antibodies to migrainous infarction is unclear, although the presence of such antibodies is considered a separate risk factor for stroke even in the absence of migraine. Detection of antiphospholipid antibodies in a migraineur should lead to the administration of anticoagulants or antiplatelet agents.

Angiography may be necessary when the diagnosis of migraine is in doubt and the noninvasive techniques of CT scanning and MRI are not helpful. The most common indication for an angiogram in this setting is any question of a vascular lesion, such as an aneurysm or AVM, or of occlusive arterial disease. Finding a lesion such as an aneurysm does not always mean that the diagnosis of migraine was incorrect. It may simply mean that the patient has migraine and an incidental aneurysm as well. In other circumstances, the angiographic findings may negate the diagnosis of migraine entirely. The risk of angiography in migraineurs is probably no higher than in other persons of the same age.

Migraine Genetics

The prevalence of a family history of migraine has been recognized since the seventeenth century. Although prior familial migraine studies have shown no clear mendelian inheritance patterns, recent genetic epidemiological surveys and a twin study using a polygenic, multifactorial model support the hypothesis of a genetic contribution (Honkasalo et al. 1995). In 1993, a cerebral autosomal dominant arteriopathy with subcortical infarcts and leukoencephalopathy (CADASIL) was mapped to chromosome 19q12. In addition to dementia, seizures, and subcortical infarcts, migraine is a prominent feature of this disorder. The association of CADASIL and migraine inspired linkage studies of familial hemiplegic migraine (FHM) with chromosome 19 markers, which led to the mapping of FHM to chromosome 19p13 (Joutel 1993). About 50% of tested families show linkage to this genomic region. Mutations in a newly characterized brain-specific P/Q-type calcium channel α_1-subunit gene, CACNL1A4, located on chromosome 19p13, are also involved in some FHM pedigrees. Mutations in the same gene have been found in some pedigrees with hereditary paroxysmal cerebellar ataxia, indicating that these two disorders, which share several features, are allelic channelopathies. In support of the channelopathy theory of migraine pathogenesis, Gardner and colleagues (1997) discovered a new locus for FHM on chromosome 1q31 in a 39-member four-generation pedigree showing a clear FHM phenotype. This region on chromosome 1 is reported to contain a neuronal calcium channel α_{1E} subunit gene.

Although FHM is a rare genetic subtype of migraine with aura, the clinical similarities (with typical migraine, with and without aura) suggest at least the possibility of a shared pathophysiology. The discovery of a genetic locus for FHM has ignited considerable interest and prompted a large effort in the field of molecular genetics to find the fundamental defect in the more common forms of migraine. However, studies testing the 19p13 region for linkage to typical migraine have produced conflicting results. A recent study concluded that chromosome 19 mutations either in the CACNL1A4 gene or a closely linked gene are implicated in some pedigrees with familial typical migraine, and that the disorder is genetically heterogeneous (Nyholt et al. 1998). Further study will clearly be necessary to determine whether the more common types of migraine in the general population might be influenced by these FHM genes. This may then lead to the unraveling of the precise molecular defects that underlie this highly prevalent and disabling condition.

Pathophysiology

Genesis of the Migraine Syndrome

Clinical and experimental evidence supports the concept that there is abnormal intracranial and extracranial vascular reactivity in migraine and other vascular headaches. Dilatation of the scalp arteries causes increased scalp blood flow and large-amplitude pulsations during attacks of migraine. Radioactive xenon cerebral blood flow studies show significantly reduced regional flow through the cortex during the aura stage of migraine with aura. At first sight, these studies seem to support the long-held theory of cerebral vasoconstriction during the aura and increased external carotid flow during the headache phase. However, the vasoconstriction-vasodilatation model has several difficulties. First, there is some evidence that the phase of oligemia is preceded by a phase of focal hyperemia. Second, headache may begin while cortical blood flow is still reduced, thereby rendering obsolete the theory that vasodilatation is the sole mechanism of the pain. The oligemia that spreads across the cerebral cortex at a rate of 2–3 mm per minute does not conform to discrete vascular territories, making unlikely the theory that vasospasm of individual cerebral arteries with subsequent cerebral ischemia is the source of the aura. The headache after an aura is often on the inappropriate side. In other words, a right-sided visual field or somatosensory aura can be followed by an ipsilateral headache, despite the fact that the cerebral blood flow changes occurred in the opposite hemisphere. Finally, migraine is also associated with a prodromal phase in about 25% of patients, which would be incompatible with a vascular or ischemic hypothesis. This prodromal phase consists of mood changes, thirst, food cravings, excessive yawning, and drowsiness. It has been suggested that this periodic central disturbance can be generated by the hypothalamus. There is abundant neuroanatomical, morphometric, immunocytochemical, neurobiochemical, and clinical data to support the hypothesis that the suprachiasmatic nucleus, the central pacemaker in the hypothalamus, may be the site at which a migraine attack is generated (Zurak 1997).

The observations on spreading oligemia led to a resurgence of the central or neuronal theories of migraine. Briefly, the phase of oligemia demonstrated during the aura of migraine by the tomographic blood flow techniques begins in one occipital pole and spreads forward over the ipsilateral hemisphere at a rate of about 3–4 mm per minute. The area of reduced cerebral blood flow does not correspond to the distribution of any particular cerebral artery but crosses the areas perfused by the middle and posterior cerebral arteries while advancing with a distinct wave front until some major change in cortical cellular architecture is reached (e.g., at the central sulcus). Recently, the description of a patient with migraine without aura who had an attack during positron emission tomography placed beyond a doubt the phenomena of spreading oligemia (Woods 1994).

This study suggested the possibility that blood flow changes may occur in migraine with and without aura because this patient had only transient and mild visual blurring, a ubiquitous symptom in migraineurs. This slow, deliberate march of a wave of oligemia brings to mind two old observations. Lashley, in 1941, studying his own scintillating scotoma, postulated on purely theoretical grounds that it must have been due to a change spreading over his occipital cortex at about 3 mm per minute. In 1944, Leao, during his research on epilepsy, observed a wave of cortical electrical depression passing over the exposed brain of lower animals. Activating the posterior cortex of rats started a wave of electrical depression that moved out from the point of initiation at a rate of 3–4 mm per minute.

The spreading depression noted by Leao's and Lashley's observations led to the hypothesis that the aura of migraine is primarily a neuronal event that causes the cortical circulation to close down in response to decreased metabolic requirements (Olesen et al. 1993). Although spreading depression has not been documented to occur in human cortex, the physiological substrate may exist in human cortex to explain this phenomenon. There is growing evidence for a disturbance in energy metabolism both in the brain and extraneural tissues of migraine patients. Based on abnormalities identified in the mitochondrial respiratory chain and matrix enzyme activities from the muscle and platelets of patients with migraine, it has been proposed that the defect in brain energy metabolism is due to abnormal mitochondrial oxidative phosphorylation (Welch and Ramadan 1995). In support of these findings, interictal phosphorus-31 magnetic resonance spectroscopy (MRS) studies have shown reduced phosphocreatine and phosphorylation potential, and increased adenosine diphosphate in the occipital lobes of migraineurs. Phosphorus-31 MRS studies done during the ictal phase reveal depletion of high-energy phosphates without an accompanying change in intracellular pH, indicating that the energy failure results from defective aerobic metabolism rather than vasospasm with ischemia.

In addition, there is an increasing body of evidence to support the presence of both systemic and brain magnesium deficiency in migraineurs, particularly in the occipital lobes (Gallai 1993; Welch and Ramadan 1995). Magnesium normally maintains a strongly coupled state of mitochondrial oxidative phosphorylation. Magnesium also plays an important role in "gating" N-methyl-D-aspartate (NMDA) receptors. A magnesium deficit can therefore result in an abnormality of mitochondrial oxidative phosphorylation and lead to a gain in NMDA receptor function, thereby causing an instability of neuronal polarization because of a loss of ionic homeostasis. This would then lead to a state of neuronal hyperexcitability and a lower threshold for spontaneous depolarization.

Spreading depression might therefore be more aptly described as spreading activation, followed by a wave of spreading depression. This would support the clinical observation of "positive" visual "scintillations" followed by a "negative" visual scotoma or by the march of positive sensory (paresthesia) symptoms. This theory may also explain why spreading oligemia may be preceded by focal hyperemia. These findings taken together suggest that the changes in blood vessel caliber and blood flow may be secondary to a primary neuronal event, triggered by enhanced neuronal excitability and susceptibility to spontaneous depolarization, resulting in prolonged hypometabolism because of an impairment in energy metabolism secondary to mitochondrial dysfunction. This hypothesis has also been supported by the finding of increased interictal lactate levels in the occipital cortex of migraineurs using hydrogen-1 MRS (Watanabe et al. 1996).

The theory that the migraine aura is a primary neuronal event was further strengthened by a recent study, which demonstrated no change in the apparent diffusion coefficient on diffusion-weighted MRI despite a reduction of regional cerebral blood flow during spontaneous migraine aura. Because diffusion-weighted MRI is very sensitive to tissue ischemia, the authors concluded that the reduction in cerebral flow was not of sufficient magnitude to cause tissue ischemia (Cutrer et al. 1998).

Platelets and Serotonin

Platelets obtained from migraineurs are known to aggregate more readily than normal in response to exposure to several vasoactive amines, including serotonin (5-hydroxytryptamine), adenosine diphosphate, the catecholamines, and tyramine. It is also known that platelets contain most of the serotonin normally present in blood and that at the onset of an attack of migraine there is a significant rise in plasma serotonin followed by an increase in urinary 5-hydroxyindoleacetic acid, a breakdown product of the serotonin. Platelet aggregation is necessary for its release. The platelets of migraineurs, even between attacks of migraine, contain less monoamine oxidase than normal, and a further decrease occurs with an attack of headache.

Although the platelet may not have a direct role in the biochemical changes that appear to underlie the basic pathogenesis of migraine, it has been extensively studied by virtue of its similarities to serotonergic nerve terminals (de Belleroche et al. 1993).

The role of serotonin in migraine has yet to be fully defined. It constricts large arteries and is a dilator of arterioles and capillaries; also, perhaps of more importance, it is a neurotransmitter. Serotonin-containing neurons are especially concentrated in the brainstem raphe, the projections of which have a widespread distribution to other neuronal centers and cerebral microvessels. The importance of the brainstem in migraine is still uncertain. Its role is certainly highlighted by the presence of binding sites for specific antimigraine drugs and the demonstration of persistent brainstem activation during and after a migraine attack, as imaged by positron emission tomography (Weiller et al. 1995). Moreover, recurrent migraine headaches were pre-

cipitated in a nonmigraineur after a stereotactic procedure produced a lesion in the dorsal raphe and periaqueductal gray matter, which is part of the endogenous antinociceptive system. Welch has recently found evidence for simultaneous activation of red nucleus, substantia nigra, and occipital cortex during provoked attacks with a visual stimulation paradigm. This was demonstrated using functional MRI–blood-oxygen level dependent, which revealed hyperoxia in these regions. Furthermore, serotonergic circuits are believed to be involved in the modulation of sleep cycles, pain perception, and mood, all of which are important factors in migraine syndrome.

Interest in the role of serotonin in migraine and the recognition of multiple subtypes of serotonin (5-HT) receptors has led to the development of a number of agents having high affinities for specific receptors. This has revolutionized the field of migraine therapeutics (for more details, see Acute Menstrual Migraine Therapy, later in this chapter).

Mechanism of the Headache

Although the aforementioned data strongly suggest that the initiation of a migraine attack is centrally driven, this does not adequately explain the mechanism of the head pain. Pain-sensitive intracranial structures, including large cerebral blood vessels, pial vessels, dura mater, and large venous sinuses, are innervated by a plexus of largely unmyelinated fibers that arise from the ophthalmic branch of the trigeminal nerve. Once this trigeminal vascular system is activated, impulses are transmitted centrally toward the first synapse within lamina I and IIo of the trigeminal nucleus caudalis (TNC), which extends to the dorsal horn of C2-C3. Activation of neurons in the TNC is reflected in the increased expression of c-fos activity, an immediate early gene. From this point, nerve impulses travel rostrally to the cortex via thalamic relay centers.

In addition to central transmission, there is evidence that neuropeptide transmitters are antidromically released from the widely branching perivascular trigeminal axon nerve terminals. These neuropeptides, including substance P, calcitonin gene-related polypeptide, and neurokinin A, mediate a neurogenic inflammatory process that can activate nociceptive afferents resulting in the central transmission of pain impulses. Neurogenic inflammation consists of vasodilatation, vascular endothelial activation with formation of microvilli and vacuoles, increased leakage of plasma protein from dural vessels into surrounding tissue, increased platelet aggregation, mast cell degranulation, and activation of the local cellular immune response. A series of elegant experiments have suggested that the pain of migraine may be due to neurogenic inflammation, which would also explain the changes in serotonin and platelet serotonin reported in migraine (Moskowitz and Cutrer 1994).

The importance of neurogenic inflammation in the production of the pain of migraine is further underscored by the fact that medications that block neurogenic inflammation and mediate vasoconstriction are successfully used to abort a migraine attack. Neurogenic plasma extravasation can be inhibited by the ergot alkaloids, indomethacin, acetylsalicylic acid, valproic acid, and the new highly selective serotonin receptor (5HT-1) agonists, which are discussed in the section Symptomatic Treatment, later in this chapter. Ergotamine compounds and the "triptans" also act centrally to inhibit the activity of neurons within the TNC, which may be important in the termination of an attack.

Summary

A unified hypothesis for migraine pathogenesis is as yet unavailable. It appears that the susceptibility to migraine is hereditary and that the migrainous brain is qualitatively and quantitatively different from the nonmigrainous brain. These differences give rise to a threshold of susceptibility governed by factors that lead to neuronal hyperexcitability and a tendency toward spontaneous depolarization. These factors may include a deficit in mitochondrial oxidative phosphorylation, a gain in calcium-channel function, intracellular magnesium deficiency, or a combination thereof. Neuronal excitability may be responsible for the phenomena of spreading activation and depression, with subsequent changes in regional cerebral blood flow. In animal models, spreading depression can activate critical brainstem regions, including the TNC. This critical structure can generate neurogenic inflammation via the antidromic release of neuropeptides from the axon terminal of nociceptive trigeminal fibers that innervate meningeal blood vessels. The TNC also receives impulses from trigeminal vascular afferents, which are activated by sterile perivascular neurogenic inflammation. This two-way system could account for migraine headache that is triggered either from the vascular system by vasodilator substances or arteriography, or from the central mechanism of cortical spreading depression, or activation of hypothalamic-brainstem connections.

Treatment and Management

After a complete examination and appropriate investigations, the nature of migraine should be explained to the patient and reassurance given that it is a painful but generally benign condition that can, in most instances, be controlled or alleviated. The lack of a cure for migraine should be mentioned. It is important that patients be made to feel that the physician understands their complaint of headache and does not dismiss them as having a headache for psychological reasons. A normal CT or MRI scan offers considerable reassurance. Many patients are more interested in knowing that they do not have a brain tumor or other potentially lethal condition than they are in obtaining relief from the pain.

Avoidance of trigger factors is important in the management of migraine, but simply advising a patient to avoid stress and relax more is usually meaningless. Advice to reduce excessive caffeine intake, to stop smoking, and to reduce alcohol intake may be more useful. Current medication use should be reviewed and modified if necessary. The use of drugs known to cause headaches, such as reserpine, indomethacin, nifedipine, theophylline derivatives, caffeine, vasodilators (including the long-acting nitrates), and alcohol should be discontinued or other agents should be substituted if possible. Use of estrogens and oral contraceptives should be discontinued if they are suspected of contributing to the headaches.

Exercise programs to promote well-being, correction of dietary excesses, and avoidance of prolonged fasts and irregular sleeping habits can be helpful.

The topic of dietary factors in migraine is difficult. Many patients ask about special migraine diets that they have read about in newspapers or magazines. Radical alterations in the diet are rarely justified, but there are exceptions. Avoidance of foods containing nitrites, such as hot dogs and preserved cold cuts, and of prepared foods containing monosodium glutamate can be helpful. Avoiding monosodium glutamate can be difficult because it is a constituent of many canned and prepared foods and is widely used in restaurants, especially in the preparation of Chinese dishes. Ripened cheeses, fermented food items, red wine, chocolate, chicken liver, pork, and many other foods have been suspected of precipitating headaches. They mostly contain tyramine, phenylethylamine, and octopamine. An occasional patient identifies an offending foodstuff, but in our experience, dietary precipitation of migraine is uncommon. Other headache authorities and many allergists disagree. Some migraineurs have some of their attacks precipitated by strong odors, especially of the perfume or aromatic type. Avoiding the use of strong-smelling soaps, shampoos, perfumes, and other items (e.g., fabric softeners and after-shave lotions) can be helpful for some individuals.

Everyone is under stress at some time as part of living. People with migraine are not under more stress than any other group of the population, although their responses to stress may differ on the basis of personality and the effectiveness of their defense mechanisms. Many people react to stress by mechanisms that increase the blood pressure, increase the production of gastric acid, or produce symptoms of increased gastrointestinal motility. Others develop various dermatological conditions. The migraineur seems to react with the cerebral and cranial circulations by mechanisms that are far more complex than this statement would imply.

Helping the patient deal with or avoid stress is difficult. It may be helpful to use a minor tranquilizer or sedative if the response to stress is overwhelming and if the source of the stress is temporary. Long-term stress management requires the help of a psychologist or other appropriately trained professional. Many techniques are used, including biofeedback, relaxation training, and hypnosis. Evidence that these techniques are helpful is difficult to evaluate because double-blinded trials are impractical and the results reported

Table 73.6:   Ergot preparations available in the United States

Brand name	Route of administration	Ergotamine (mg)	Caffeine (mg)	Belladonna (mg)	Other (mg)
Ercaf	Oral	Ergotamine tartrate (1)	—	—	—
Wigraine	Oral	Ergotamine tartrate (1)	100	—	—
Bellergal-S	Oral	Ergotamine tartrate (0.6)	—	0.2	Phenobarbital (30)
Wigraine	Rectal	Ergotamine tartrate (1)	100	—	—
Cafergot	Rectal	Ergotamine tartrate (2)	100	—	—

often depend on the enthusiasm of the therapist as much as on the treatment itself.

Pain management programs that have gained popularity in the past few years are helpful for some headache patients, but the relapse rate is high and they are not helpful for most migraineurs. Simple relaxation methods, as taught by physical therapists, may be as useful as the more costly and time-consuming techniques of biofeedback.

Pharmacotherapy

Medical therapy can be administered prophylactically to prevent attacks of migraine or symptomatically to relieve the pain, nausea, and vomiting of an attack. Prophylactic therapy is rarely needed unless the frequency or duration of attacks seriously interferes with the patient's lifestyle. In general, a prophylactic program should be considered if attacks occur more frequently than several times each month.

Symptomatic Treatment

Symptomatic treatment should usually be started as early in the development of an attack as possible. If an aura is recognized, most medications should be taken during it rather than waiting for the pain to begin. One exception is sumatriptan, which is less effective if taken before the onset of the headache phase. Whether this holds for the other new 5-HT agonists is uncertain. It must be recalled, though, that once the attack is fully developed, oral preparations are almost always less effective because of decreased gastrointestinal motility and poor absorption. If vomiting develops, oral preparations are no longer appropriate.

For many patients, a simple oral analgesic, such as aspirin, acetaminophen, propoxyphene hydrochloride, naproxen, or ibuprofen, or an analgesic combination with caffeine, may be effective. Caffeine aids absorption, helps to induce vasoconstriction, and may reduce the firing of serotonergic brainstem neurons. The addition of 10 mg of metoclopramide by mouth may be helpful with any simple analgesic regimen. Rest in a dark, quiet room with an ice pack on the head allows the analgesic the best chance of relieving the pain. If sleep occurs, the patient often awakens headache-free. In some countries, walk-in headache clinics provide a patient with a simple analgesic, an antinausea agent, and a place to sleep for a few hours. In North America, both patients and physicians have come to expect a

quick fix; thus, stronger and stronger analgesics and other drugs have been given to those with a headache. Drug addiction is a major problem in some patients who are treated this way. Induction of sleep, control of nausea, simple analgesics, and other non-narcotic agents should be more widely used.

Although supplanted in some cases by newer agents, ergot preparations are important in the symptomatic treatment of migraine. The actions of ergotamine tartrate and other ergot preparations are complex. They are both vasoconstrictors and vasodilators, depending on the dose and the resting tone of the target vessels. Internal and external carotid vessels are believed to react differently to therapeutic doses of these preparations. The external carotid vessels are constricted by ergot preparations. There is no convincing evidence that the internal carotid vessels are similarly affected. The ergot preparations likely exert their effects on migraine via agonism at 5-HT receptors. The use of ergotamine tartrate in migraine necessitates intelligent administration by both patient and physician if it is to be effective and if side effects are to be minimized. Oral preparations are far less effective than those given rectally or parenterally.

It is important to know the amount of ergotamine in the various preparations and to be familiar with the dose limits and the signs and symptoms of ergotism. Table 73.6 shows the composition and strength of some ergotamine preparations available in the United States. Evidence for the efficacy of these agents in the treatment of migraine is largely based on uncontrolled clinical observations.

For the treatment of an acute attack of migraine, 2 mg of ergotamine tartrate should be administered by mouth as soon as the patient recognizes the symptoms. This dose can be combined with a simple oral analgesic-caffeine combination, and the ergot preparation can be repeated in 1 hour. Possibly a better regimen, but one that is inconvenient and unpleasant to some patients, is to administer ergotamine tartrate by rectal suppository. At the onset of the aura or pain, a 1- or 2-mg rectal suppository of ergotamine tartrate should be inserted and a simple analgesic taken orally. The ergot preparation can be repeated in 60 minutes. Experience in the course of several attacks can be used to determine the amount of ergotamine needed to obtain relief. With subsequent attacks, the entire dose can be taken at the onset. If nausea is troublesome, metoclopramide in doses of 10 mg orally aids absorption of the ergotamine tartrate and may prevent vomiting. In actual practice, we routinely have

Table 73.7: 5-HT agonists used in acute migraine treatment

Drug	Route(s)	Dose	May repeat doses if headache recurs	Maximum dose per 24 hrs
Dihydroergotamine (DHE-45)	IV	0.5–1.0 mg	1 hr	3 mg
	IM	0.5–1.0 mg	1 hr	3 mg
	SQ	0.5–1.0 mg	1 hr	3 mg
(Migranal)	Nasal spray	2 mg (0.5 mg/spray) one spray in each nostril, repeat in 15 mins	—	3 mg
Naratriptan (Amerge)	Oral	1 mg, 2.5 mg*	4 hrs	5 mg
Rizatriptan (Maxalt)	Oral	5 mg, 10 mg*	2 hrs	30 mg
Sumatriptan (Imitrex)	Oral	25 mg, 50 mg*	2 hrs	300 mg
	SQ	6 mg	2 hrs	12 mg
	Intranasal	5 mg, 20 mg*		40 mg
Zolmitriptan (Zomig)	Oral	2.5 mg*, 5 mg	2 hrs	10 mg

*These are the recommended starting dosages based on efficacy and tolerability.

patients take metoclopramide, 10 mg, with ergotamine orally to improve gastric emptying and absorption. For patients who are close to vomiting or who are vomiting, an antiemetic suppository, such as chlorpromazine (25–100 mg) or prochlorperazine (25 mg), can be helpful. Analgesics in rectal suppository form include aspirin, acetaminophen, and indomethacin, any of which may provide some relief.

With frequent attacks of common migraine, care must be taken to avoid entering a vicious cycle wherein ergotamine is used so frequently that the drug-induced vasoconstriction is almost continuous. If this occurs, a few hours of abstinence from ergotamine leads to relative vasodilatation and results in a withdrawal headache. Such patients frequently awaken with a vascular headache, obtain relief with a further dose of ergotamine, and thus perpetuate the vicious cycle. A similar phenomenon can occur with caffeine in people dependent on coffee or caffeine-containing soft drinks. If more than 6 mg of ergotamine is required per week, substitution of an alternative prophylactic program is preferable.

Ergotamine must be used cautiously in patients with hypertension and in those with peripheral vascular disease. It is contraindicated in patients with angina and those who are pregnant. Administration of ergotamine to patients in whom the aura is particularly prolonged or characterized by a major neurological deficit is also considered unwise. The fear of potentiating the vasospasm to the point of cerebral infarction may be unjustified, but the potential risk can be avoided by withholding potent vasoconstrictors. As an alternative to ergotamine in the symptomatic treatment of migraine, the sympathomimetic agent, isometheptene mucate, is useful. It is available in proprietary preparations combined with acetaminophen. It has the advantage of not increasing nausea and of being well tolerated, but it may fail to give relief with severe attacks.

Dihydroergotamine (DHE) has been used for treatment of migraine since the 1940s. Its poor oral bioavailability limits its administration to the parenteral and intranasal routes (Tables 73.7 and 73.8). Patients can be readily taught to self-administer this drug by each of these routes.

This medication should be considered when nausea and vomiting limit the use of oral medications or when other medications are ineffective. Although the effect of DHE is slower than sumatriptan (see Table 73.8), it does have similar efficacy after 2 hours, and it is associated with a lower recurrence of headache in 24 hours (Winner et al. 1996). It is associated with increased nausea in some patients, and it may need to be combined with an antiemetic agent. When given intravenously in an acute medical care setting, the use of an antiemetic is mandatory.

The development of sumatriptan heralded a new class of antimigraine agents that are highly selective at certain 5-HT (serotonin) receptors. These agents, sometimes called the *triptans*, together with the less selective ergots, have strong agonist activity at the 5-HT$_{1B}$ receptor, which mediates cranial vessel constriction, and at the 5-HT$_{1D}$ receptor, which leads to inhibition of the release of sensory neuropeptides from perivascular trigeminal afferents. The CNS is largely impermeable to sumatriptan, and hence its action is presumably in the periphery. However, it has been shown experimentally that activation of 5-HT$_{1B}$/5-HT$_{1D}$ receptors can also attenuate the excitability of cells in the TNC, which receives input from the trigeminal nerve. Accordingly, newer 5-HT$_{1B}$/5-HT$_{1D}$ agonists act at central as well as peripheral components of the trigeminal vascular system, and at least part of their clinical action may be centrally mediated (Martin 1997).

Sumatriptan can be administered orally, intranasally, and by subcutaneous injection (Table 73.9; see also Tables 73.7 and 73.8). Given as a 6-mg subcutaneous injection, either self-administered using the manufacturer's auto-injector device or by conventional subcutaneous injection, sumatriptan resulted in significant pain relief at 1- and 2-hour time points after drug administration (see Table 73.8). For subjects who had no significant pain relief after 1 hour, administration of a second dose of 6 mg provided little further benefit.

Associated symptoms, including nausea, photophobia, and phonophobia, are lessened by sumatriptan, which also

Table 73.8: Subcutaneous and intranasal 5-HT agonists

Drug	Dose	Headache response[a]			Recurrence of headache[b]
		1 hr	2 hrs	4 hrs	
Dihydroergotamine					
Subcutaneous	1 mg	57%	73%	85%	18%
Intranasal	2 mg	46%	47–61%	56–70%	14%
Sumatriptan					
Subcutaneous	6 mg	70%	75%	83%	35–40%
Intranasal	20 mg	55%	60%	NA	35–40%

NA = not available.
[a]Headache response is defined as a reduction of headache severity from moderate or severe pain to mild or no pain.
[b]Recurrence of headache within 24 hours after initial headache response.

Table 73.9: Oral 5-HT agonists

Drug	Dose	Headache response[a]			Recurrence of headache[b]
		1 hr	2 hrs	4 hrs	
Naratriptan	1.0 mg	19%	42%	51%	17–28%
	2.5 mg	21%	48%	67%	
Rizatriptan	5.0 mg	30%	60%	NA	30–35%
	10.0 mg	37%	67–77%	NA	
Sumatriptan	25 mg	NA	52%	68%	35–40%
	50 mg	NA	50%	70%	
	100 mg	NA	56%	75%	
Zolmitriptan	2.5 mg	38%	64%	75%	31%
	5.0 mg	44%	66%	77%	

NA = not available.
Note: Composite data from product information inserts and literature.
[a]Headache response is defined as a reduction in headache severity from moderate or severe pain to mild or no pain.
[b]Recurrence of headache within 24 hours after initial headache response.

improves the patient's ability to return to normal functioning. Possibly related to a short plasma half-life or rapid rate of dissociation of drug from the 5-HT receptors, recurrence of the migraine attack occurs in about 40% of those who initially have a good therapeutic response. This is similar to both intranasally and orally administered sumatriptan. Treatment of a same-day recurrence with another dose of sumatriptan usually successfully terminates the attack.

Side effects of sumatriptan by injection include local reaction at the injection site, usually of mild-to-moderate severity, and a transient tingling or flushed sensation that may be localized or generalized. A more unpleasant sense of heaviness or pressure in the neck or chest has also been described in a small percentage of recipients. It rarely lasts more than a few minutes and is generally not associated with electrocardiogram changes or other evidence of myocardial ischemia. However, as sumatriptan has been shown to produce a minor reduction in coronary artery diameter during coronary angiography, it should be used with caution in patients who have significant risk factors for coronary artery disease and should not be given to patients with any history suggestive of coronary insufficiency. It is also contraindicated in untreated hypertension, peripheral vascular disease, and in those using ergot preparations. It should not be given to women during pregnancy or lactation or to patients with hemiplegic or basilar migraine.

Oral sumatriptan is administered in 25- to 100-mg doses with a limit of 300 mg in 24 hours. It is rapidly absorbed and, provided vomiting has not started, the oral form of sumatriptan is effective, providing relief in two-thirds of subjects at 2 hours. Recurrence of the headache within 24 hours is about the same as after the injectable form, namely, 40%. Photophobia, nausea, and vomiting are also relieved. The systemic side effects of flushing, tingling, and chest heaviness are somewhat less frequent than with the subcutaneous form.

Intranasal sumatriptan is well absorbed via the nasal mucosa and is rapidly effective. Side effects are similar to the other routes of administration except that bad taste and nausea is more common.

Since the advent of sumatriptan, other selective 5-HT$_{1B}$/5-HT$_{1D}$ agonists (triptans) have been undergoing development. Three of these new agents, naratriptan, rizatriptan, and zolmitriptan, have been released in the United States. Each is available only as an oral preparation. Unlike sumatriptan, each of these agents has good CNS penetration, which may be of therapeutic importance. In addition to providing headache relief, each of these has also been shown to reduce the associated symptoms of a migraine attack, including nausea, photophobia, and phonophobia. Naratriptan, 1.0–2.5 mg, has a slower onset of action, although efficacy at 4 hours at the higher dose is quite good. This agent also has a side-effect profile that is similar to placebo and may be associated with slightly fewer headache recurrences than are other members of the group (see Table 73.9). Rizatriptan has the highest 1-hour response rate of these oral agents. The headache recurrence rate, though, is similar to that of sumatriptan. Zolmitriptan has a high 2-hour headache response rate for both the 2.5- and 5.0-mg doses, exceeding that reported for sumatriptan. The headache recurrence rate appears to be a bit lower than with sumatriptan (Gawel and Tepper 1998). In general, both the indications and contraindications for these newer 5-HT$_1$ agonists are the same as for sumatriptan. They have not been shown to be safe when administered within 24 hours of ergots or other members of the triptan class.

At this time, there is no evidence to allow an accurate prediction as to which of these agents will be most effective in a given patient. A few practical guidelines can be given based on the clinical situation and knowledge about available agents. If severe nausea or vomiting occur early in an attack, the parenteral or intranasal routes should be used. For individuals whose headaches peak rapidly, rizatriptan and zolmitriptan should be considered, given their early response rates. Some patients may prefer nasal or injectable routes (sumatriptan, dihydroergotamine). For patients with benign but intolerable side effects from this group of medications, naratriptan should be considered, given its favorable side-effect profile. Finally, if there is recurrence of headache after initial relief, DHE or naratriptan should be considered. If one agent is used and fails, it seems reasonable, barring major side effects, to try another agent in the class.

There is evidence that most of these agents have a lower oral bioavailability when taken during acute migraine attacks than when taken interictally. Accordingly, it is logical to consider combining these with metoclopramide to improve gastric emptying. Furthermore, experience would suggest that coadministration with a nonsteroidal anti-inflammatory drug (NSAID) might be helpful, especially in individuals who respond only partially or who tend to have a headache recurrence after initial relief (Peroutka 1998).

Symptomatic treatment of migraine with uncomplicated aura is essentially the same as that described previously. Although sumatriptan is not effective if taken during the aura phase, the new class of brain penetrating triptans are currently under investigation for this purpose. Modification of the aura is rarely possible or needed.

For many patients, an attack of migraine becomes a harrowing experience. After a variable period, they go to an emergency room or physician's office expecting relief. These patients pose a difficult problem for the physician. The simplest treatment, and generally what the patient wishes or demands, is injection of a combination of a narcotic, most

frequently meperidine (75–100 mg), and an agent for nausea, such as chlorpromazine (25–50 mg), promethazine hydrochloride (12.5–25.0 mg), or prochlorperazine (5–10 mg). This is an effective treatment and one that can be used if the physician is sure the patient genuinely has a headache of major proportions. Unfortunately, the complaint of headache is all too easy to simulate as a drug-seeking behavior. The decision to treat with a narcotic must be made in each case on the basis of the patient's behavior, the physician's knowledge of the previous history from emergency room records, and the local knowledge of the nursing and emergency room staff. Unfortunately, many patients with headache who report to emergency rooms are given less than adequate relief for fear of pandering to drug-seeking behavior. To avoid using narcotics, one can use neuroleptic agents acutely, with or without DHE. DHE, 0.5–1.0 mg, with metoclopramide, 10 mg by intravenous injection, is an effective treatment for acute headache and provides an alternative to the use of a narcotic. Similarly, prochlorperazine, 10 mg intravenously over 3–4 minutes alone or combined with DHE, can be effective. Sumatriptan, 6 mg subcutaneously, may provide relief of both the headache and the associated symptoms. Some evidence points to the possible role of magnesium deficiency in the pathogenesis of migraine, and intravenous infusion of 1 g of magnesium sulfate results in rapid relief of headache pain in patients with low serum ionized magnesium (Mauskop et al. 1996). Alternatively, chlorpromazine, 5 mg injected intravenously every 10 minutes to a maximum of 25 mg, is also an effective agent when used acutely. The latter agent frequently produces hypotension, and patients should first receive a bolus of 250–500 ml of D5 half-normal saline. (Dehydrated patients then should always receive appropriate intravenous hydration.) Some patients develop acute extrapyramidal symptoms after treatment with neuroleptic agents. These can be treated with parenteral diphenhydramine, 25–50 mg. The neuroleptic agents do produce sedation, and patients should be advised not to operate a motor vehicle after treatment. Injectable ketorolac, 60 mg given intramuscularly, is another alternative to the narcotic or sedative agents. Care is needed to avoid the use of this NSAID in the elderly, those who are dehydrated, or those having any history of renal insufficiency. A single dose of dexamethasone combined with parenteral meperidine and promazine has been used for the emergency room treatment of attacks of intractable migraine.

When a migraine has lasted for many days with little or no relief, the term *status migrainosus* has been used. Dehydration, tiredness due to lack of sleep, and continued pain may necessitate admission to a hospital to terminate the attack. Fluid replacement, correction of electrolyte imbalance, and suppression of vomiting with metoclopramide, chlorpromazine, or prochlorperazine generally result in improvement. DHE initially given intravenously and later subcutaneously every 8 hours may abort migraine status. It is effective, but increased nausea and vomiting may be a reason to switch to an alternative regimen. Administration of corticosteroids, such as dexamethasone or prednisolone, can be used. Prednisolone dosage in the range of 20 mg every 6 hours initially, followed by a rapidly tapering dose over 2–3 days may help abort status migrainosus. It is best to avoid narcotic and benzodiazepine agents when treating status migrainosus.

Prophylactic Treatment

When the attacks of migraine occur weekly or several times a month, or when they are less frequent but very prolonged and debilitating, a preventive program is appropriate. Attacks of migraine that occur in a predictable pattern can also respond to prophylactic medication. For example, menstrual migraine can be treated in this way (see Prophylactic Menstrual Migraine Therapy, later in this chapter).

β-Adrenergic blocking drugs are widely used for the prophylaxis of vascular headaches (Ziegler et al. 1993). Propranolol is effective in 55–93% of patients. These figures do not mean that the migraine attacks stopped but that the responding patients reported at least a 50% reduction in the frequency and severity of their attacks. In other studies, more than 50% of patients have responded favorably to a placebo.

Propranolol should be administered in doses of 80–240 mg per day and, if tolerated, should be given a 2- to 3-month trial. Compliance has increased since the development of a long-acting form of propranolol that can be given once daily. Side effects are not usually severe. Lethargy or depression is not uncommon and may be a reason for stopping use of the medication. Hypotension, bradycardia, impotence, insomnia, hair loss, and nightmares can all occur. As with all β-adrenergic blocking agents, administration of propranolol should be discontinued slowly to avoid cardiac complications. It is contraindicated in people with an asthmatic history and should be used with caution in patients using insulin or oral hypoglycemic agents because it may prevent the adrenergic corrective responses to hypoglycemia. The benefit of propranolol in migraine may be separate from its action as a β-adrenergic blocking agent, but exact mechanism of action is unknown.

Almost all the available β-adrenergic blocking agents have been tested for their potential use in migraine. Timolol, nadolol, atenolol, and metoprolol have each been shown to have approximately the same benefit in migraine as propranolol.

Amitriptyline and other tricyclic antidepressants can be helpful in migraine prophylaxis (Ziegler et al. 1993), just as they are useful in the prevention of muscle contraction (tension) headaches. The benefit seems to be independent of their antidepressant action. Blockade of noradrenaline uptake at catecholamine terminals and inhibition of serotonin reuptake may be related, but their action in migraine is unclear at present. Used in doses of 10–150 mg at night, amitriptyline, imipramine, desipramine, or nortriptyline may provide some protection against frequent attacks of migraine and especially against the chronic daily headache that may have evolved from more typical intermittent migraine. Side effects are rather troublesome. Morning drowsiness, dryness of the mouth, impotence, constipation, and weight gain are common. The anticholinergic side effects may decrease with time. If tolerated, the tricyclic agents should be given a trial of at least 3 months after a therapeutic blood level is reached. The optimal dose for migraine prophylaxis must be determined by titration of the dose.

The newer antidepressants of the selective serotonin reuptake–inhibiting type, such as fluoxetine and sertraline, have a relatively limited role in the prophylaxis of migraine. Headache is a common side effect of several of these recently developed antidepressants.

The use of the monoamine oxidase inhibitor phenelzine for migraine prophylaxis is based on the agent inhibiting the breakdown of serotonin, which would thereby continue to act as a constrictor of cranial vessels. Unfortunately, the dietary restrictions that must be carefully followed if a hypertensive crisis is to be avoided limit the widespread use of these inhibitors for prevention of migraine. For patients with particularly severe and intractable attacks, the monoamine oxidase inhibitors should be considered. The patient must be given a list of amine-containing foodstuffs to be avoided, such as strong cheese, red wine, beer, yeast products, cream, broad beans, fermented foods, yogurt, and many others. Dangerous drug interactions can occur with preparations such as sympathomimetic agents, L-dopa, central anticholinergics, tricyclic antidepressants, and narcotics, especially meperidine. Side effects of monoamine oxidase inhibitors include hypotension as well as hypertension, agitation, hallucinations, retention of urine, and inhibition of ejaculation.

The calcium-channel antagonists prevent spasm of arteries by inhibiting contraction of smooth muscle. Their use in migraine is based on their ability to prevent vasoconstriction and on their other actions, including prevention of platelet aggregation and alterations in release and reuptake of serotonin. Several clinical trials have indicated some benefit in preventing recurrent migraine. Currently, the calcium-channel blocking agents are nifedipine, verapamil, diltiazem, nimodipine, and flunarizine. Not all are available worldwide at present. Nifedipine seems to cause a generalized headache as a side effect and has little to add to migraine prophylaxis. Verapamil in doses of 80–120 mg three times a day reduces the frequency of migraine with aura, but it is not as useful in common migraine. Experience with diltiazem is too limited to permit an assessment of its value at this time.

Sodium valproate has been shown, in a triple-blind, placebo-controlled crossover study, to have a beneficial effect in the prophylactic treatment of migraine without aura (Jensen et al. 1994). Fifty percent of patients responded with a 50% or better reduction in migraine frequency.

Methysergide may be an effective prophylactic agent for all types of vascular headache. Unfortunately, its potential for producing serious complications, such as retroperitoneal, pulmonary, and heart valve fibrosis, seriously limits its use as a long-term prophylactic. It should be reserved for the most intractable migraine headaches and should be given for periods of only 6 months at a time. Between such courses, methysergide should be discontinued for 4 weeks. A clinical examination, urinalysis, and serum creatinine determination may be undertaken to detect any evidence of the fibrotic complications. Some authorities also advise obtaining a chest roentgenogram, serum creatinine level, and an abdominal CT or MRI scan. If there are no signs of side effects, treatment with the drug can be restarted and continued for another 6 months. The incidence of fibrotic complications is low, perhaps 1 in 1,000 patients. If fibrosis does develop, it may resolve if methysergide is immediately and permanently withdrawn, but this is not always the case.

Whenever methysergide is prescribed, it must be started very slowly. A fraction of a 2-mg tablet is the initial dose, followed by a gradual increase over 7–10 days to the minimal effective dose, generally in the range of 6–8 mg in three or four divided doses per day. Rapid introduction of the drug leads to nausea, abdominal cramps, pain in the legs (possibly due to venospasm), hallucinations, and agitation. Methysergide is a derivative of lysergic acid diethylamide (LSD), although it has no psychotropic action. It can act as a serotonin antagonist peripherally and as a serotonin agonist centrally, but its mode of action in vascular headaches is incompletely understood.

Cyproheptadine is also a peripheral serotonin antagonist. It also has weak antibradykinin activity and prevents platelet aggregation. In adults, it has a minor role in the prevention of migraine, but it is more effective in children. At all ages, it causes drowsiness and may cause significant weight gain.

Riboflavin administered orally in a dose of 400 mg per day has been shown to be effective in migraine prophylaxis in a prospective randomized controlled study that enrolled a relatively small number of subjects. The effect of the frequency of attacks was not statistically significant until the third month of the trial (Schoenen et al. 1998). There are minimal side effects associated with this treatment.

Oral magnesium supplementation has also been shown in double-blinded, placebo-controlled, randomized studies to be effective in migraine prophylaxis. Oral magnesium supplementation with 600 mg of a chelated or slow-release preparation is recommended. Magnesium-induced diarrhea and gastric irritation are the most common side effects (Mauskop and Altura 1998).

Aspirin, 325 mg taken every other day for the prevention of cardiovascular disease, reduces the frequency of migraine slightly. The NSAIDs have been tried for migraine prophylaxis, with some benefit. They are, however, helpful for providing analgesia during the acute attack.

Hormones and Migraine

Migraine occurs with equal frequency in both sexes before puberty, but it becomes three times more common in women after menarche. Approximately 25% of women have migraine during their reproductive years, with an average prevalence of 16%. The changing hormonal environment throughout a woman's life cycle, including menarche, menstruation, oral contraceptive use, pregnancy, menopause, and hormonal replacement therapy (HRT), can have a profound effect on the course of migraine.

Menstrual Migraine

Migraine attacks are associated with menses in one of three ways. The attacks may occur exclusively during menstruation and at no other time during the cycle. This association is referred to as *true menstrual migraine* (TMM), and it has recently been proposed that TMM be defined as attacks which occur between days −2 and +3 of the menstrual cycle (MacGregor 1996). The frequency of TMM according to this definition is approximately 7%. More commonly, migraine attacks occur throughout the cycle but increase in frequency or intensity at the time of menstruation. This association occurs in up to 60% of female migraineurs. Finally, premenstrual migraine can occur between days −7 and −3 before menstruation as part of premenstrual syndrome or late-luteal phase dysphoric disorder. This disorder is characterized by a cluster of symptoms in the luteal phase, including depression, irritability, fatigue, appetite changes, bloating, backache, breast tenderness, and nausea. These different relationships between migraine and the menstrual cycle can reliably be determined by reviewing headache diaries, and their distinction is important because pathophysiology may differ, as would the therapeutic approach.

Numerous mechanisms have been proposed to explain the pathogenesis of menstrual migraine, but there is as yet no unifying hypothesis. There is abundant clinical and experimental evidence to support the theory that estrogen withdrawal before menstruation is a trigger for migraine in some women. Estrogen withdrawal may modulate hypothalamic β-endorphin, dopamine, β-adrenergic, and serotonin receptors. This complex relationship causes significant downstream effects, such as a reduction in central opioid tone, dopamine-receptor hypersensitivity, increased trigeminal mechanoreceptor receptor fields, and increased cerebrovascular reactivity to serotonin. These changes, which occur during the luteal phase of the cycle, may be germane to menstrual migraine pathogenesis.

Several lines of investigation have implicated both prostaglandins and melatonin in the pathogenesis of menstrual migraine. Prostaglandins and melatonin are important mediators of nociception and analgesia, respectively, in the CNS. The concentration of prostaglandin F_2 and nocturnal melatonin secretion increase and decrease, respectively, during menstruation in female migraineurs. These observations are the basis for the clinical use of NSAIDs and melatonin for the prophylaxis of menstrual migraine.

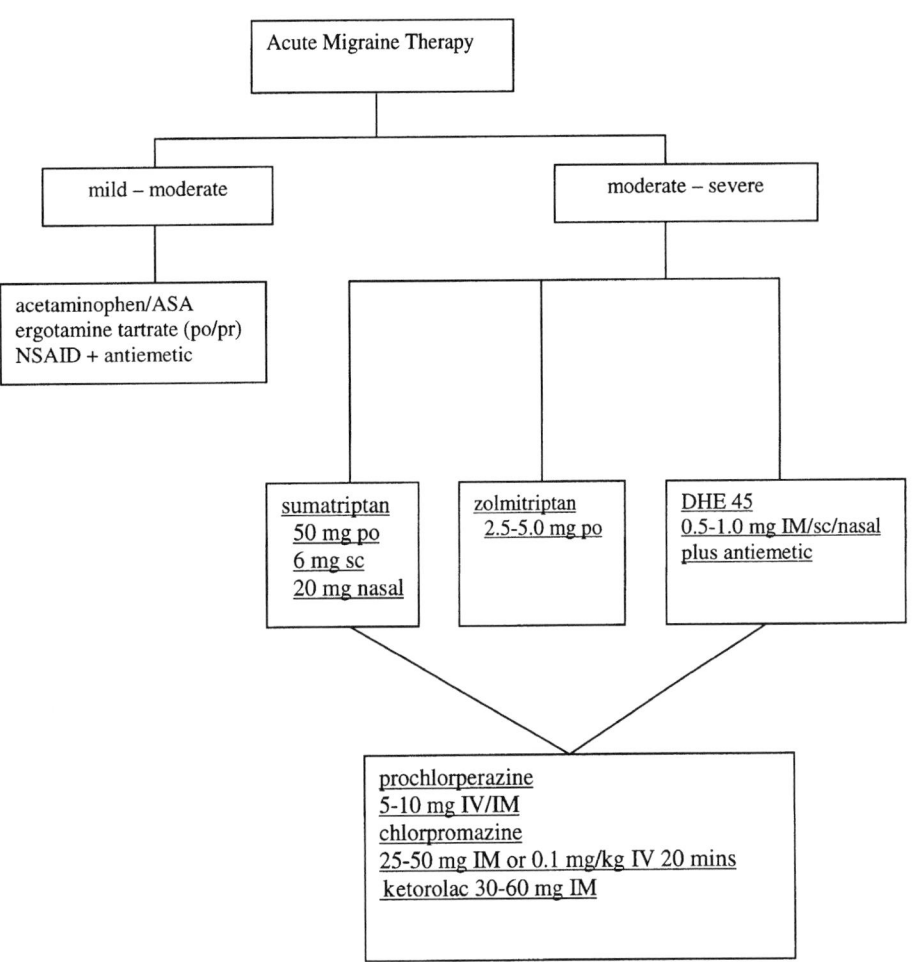

FIGURE 73.6 Algorithm for acute treatment of menstrual migraine. (ASA = acetosalicyclic acid; DHE = dihydroergotamine; NSAID = nonsteroidal anti-inflammatory drug.)

Management of Menstrual Migraine

A direct link between menstruation and headache attacks must be established by asking the patient to keep a diary card of their migraine attacks and menstrual periods for at least 3 consecutive months. The nature of this relationship determines subsequent therapy. For example, for patients who have both menstrual and nonmenstrual attacks (menstrual-associated migraine), a standard prophylactic medication might be employed throughout the cycle rather than the perimenstrual use of a prophylactic agent. The goals of therapy should be clearly outlined in addition to the dosages, benefits, and side-effect profile of each recommended medication. A headache diary should ideally be started in an effort to identify other nonhormonal triggers that may be important to eliminate. Biofeedback and relaxation therapy can be quite helpful in selected patients and should be used whenever possible. Lifestyle factors, such as regular meals, sufficient sleep, and regular aerobic exercise, are important items to emphasize. These simple efforts can have a significant impact on the patient's headache burden and may limit the frequency of attacks that require pharmacological intervention.

Acute Menstrual Migraine Therapy

The goal of acute menstrual migraine therapy is to decrease the severity and duration of pain as well as the associated symptoms of an individual migraine attack, including nausea, vomiting, photophobia, and phonophobia. Some women may control attacks of menstrual migraine quite adequately with abortive therapy only, thereby obviating the need for prophylaxis (Figure 73.6).

The acute management of menstrual migraine does not differ from the treatment of migraine not associated with menstruation. Mild attacks (which are relatively infrequent) can be managed with acetaminophen or NSAIDs. Moderate-to-severe attacks can be treated by using an oral triptan, such as sumatriptan or zolmitriptan. If there is significant nausea and vomiting, however, an alternate route of administration is necessary. In this setting, parenteral therapy with sumatriptan, DHE, ketorolac, or a neuroleptic, such as prochlorperazine, is appropriate. Alternatively, both sumatriptan and DHE are available in a nasal formulation and can be helpful in patients with significant gastrointestinal upset. The combination of an antiemetic with any of these

Table 73.10: Nonhormonal prophylaxis for menstrual migraine

Cyclic (perimenstrual) days –3 through +3
  Nonsteroidal anti-inflammatory drugs
    Naproxen sodium 550 mg bid
    Mefenamic acid 250 mg tid
    Ketoprofen 75 mg tid
    Ergotamine tartrate + caffeine (Wigraine) 1 mg qhs or bid
    Dihydroergotamine 0.5–1.0 mg (SQ, IM, or intranasal) bid
Noncyclic (throughout cycle)
  Tricyclic antidepressant
    Nortriptyline or amitriptyline 10–150 mg qhs
  Beta blocker
    Propranolol or nadolol 40–240 mg daily
  Calcium-channel blocker
    Verapamil 240–480 mg daily
  Anticonvulsant
    Divalproex 250–500 mg bid
  Dopamine agonists
    Bromocriptine 2.5–5.0 mg tid
  Other
    Magnesium 360–600 mg daily

Table 73.11: Hormonal prophylaxis for menstrual migraine

Static high-maintenance levels
  Transdermal estradiol (1 × 100 µg days –3/–1/+2)
  Combined oral contraceptive or transdermal patch (3–4 mos)
  Percutaneous estradiol (1.5 mg daily days –3 to +6)
Static low-maintenance levels
  Danazol 200–600 mg/day
  Tamoxifen 5–15 mg/day (days 7–14 luteal cycle)
  Goserelin (treatment limited to 6 mos)

medications may not only alleviate nausea and vomiting but may also potentiate the efficacy of these compounds.

Prophylactic Menstrual Migraine Therapy

Prophylaxis may either be perimenstrual (cyclic) or continuous (noncyclic) (Table 73.10). Many of the regimens suggested for perimenstrual migraine prophylaxis depend on regular menstruation. Perimenstrual prophylaxis commences a few days before the period is expected and is continued until the end of menstruation. In women whose cycles are difficult to predict, continuous prophylaxis with standard migraine prophylactic agents, such as tricyclic antidepressants and beta blockers, can be quite effective if taken continuously.

NSAIDs are considered to be a first-line agent for both acute and prophylactic therapy in patients with either menstrual-associated migraine or TMM when the timing of menstruation is predictable. Different classes of NSAIDs should be tried because response may vary in a given individual. Ergot derivatives in the form of ergotamine tartrate, ergonovine maleate, and DHE can also be effective when used as a symptomatic or prophylactic drug around the time of menstruation. Concerns about habituation or rebound headaches are minimal given the limited duration of treatment when used perimenstrually.

For those with TMM, attacks can also be prevented by stabilizing estrogen levels during the late luteal phase of the cycle. Estrogen levels can be stabilized by maintaining high levels with estrogen supplements or by maintaining low levels that result from a natural or medically induced menopause (Table 73.11).

Estradiol implants, percutaneous estradiol gel, and estrogen patches produce reasonably stable levels of estrogen and can be effective preventive strategies. If periods are less predictable, suppression of the ovulatory cycle with high, static estrogen levels can be accomplished with either a low-dose combined estrogen-progestin oral contraceptive pill taken continuously for 3–4 months, or with two 100-µg patches replaced every 3 days in combination with cyclic progestogens. Treatments that suppress the cycle by reducing estrogen levels (danazol), inducing a medical menopause (goserelin [Zoladex]), or modifying the effect of estrogen (tamoxifen) have also been anecdotally successful in the treatment of resistant menstrual migraine. They are not commonly employed in clinical practice, however, because the menopausal side effects of these medications can be unpleasant. Their use should be reserved for recalcitrant cases. Progesterone alone is ineffective in the treatment of menstrual migraine.

Bromocriptine, a dopamine (D_2)-receptor agonist, may decrease perimenstrual symptoms of breast engorgement, irritability, and headache when administered during the luteal phase of the cycle. Efficacy is enhanced, however, when the medication is used continuously throughout the cycle rather than perimenstrually (Herzog 1997).

The use of magnesium for the acute and prophylactic treatment of migraine and menstrual migraine has received considerable attention over the past few years. Low levels of systemic magnesium have been found in women with menstrual migraine, and MRS studies have demonstrated reduced levels of intracellular magnesium in the cerebral cortex of migraine sufferers. Low levels of intracellular magnesium may lead to neuronal hyperexcitability and spontaneous depolarization, which may be the central process by which a migraine attack is initiated. This has led some investigators to study the effect of magnesium on both the acute and prophylactic management of menstrual migraine (Mauskop and Altura 1998).

Some physicians still advocate the use of hysterectomy and oophorectomy in women with intractable PMS and menstrual migraine who respond to medical ovariectomy. There are no long-term follow-up or controlled studies to conclusively substantiate this position. Because no study is placebo controlled, the positive results seen in some studies may reflect the daily postoperative use of estrogen. Although two-thirds of women who have physiological menopause experience migraine relief, the opposite effect may occur with surgical menopause with bilateral oophorectomy. A retrospective study of 1,300 women also demonstrated the unfavorable effects of surgical menopause on migraine (Granella et al. 1993). Therefore, until convincing evidence demonstrates otherwise, hysterectomy with or without oophorectomy is *not* currently recommended for women with menstrual migraine.

Oral Contraception in Female Migraineurs

Migraine prevalence is highest in women during their reproductive years, the very population that uses oral contraceptive therapy. Oral contraceptives have a variable effect on migraine. Migraine may begin de novo after starting the pill, pre-existing migraine may worsen in severity or frequency, or the characteristics of the migraine attack may change. For example, aura symptoms may develop in a woman who for years may have had migraine without aura. On the other hand, migraine may improve after starting an oral contraceptive, particularly in women whose migraine attacks had a very close menstrual relationship. In the majority of women, however, the pattern of migraine does not change appreciably after starting an oral contraceptive, particularly with the lower dose of estrogen and progestin now found in most oral contraceptives.

The concern surrounding the use of synthetic estrogen in women with migraine pertains to the increased risk of ischemic stroke in this population, relative to age-matched women without migraine. There is now convincing evidence that female migraineurs have greater risk of experiencing ischemic stroke. Tzourio and colleagues (1995) found migraine to be strongly associated with the risk of ischemic stroke in young women (odds ratio 3.5), and this association was independent of other vascular risk factors. The risk of ischemic stroke was particularly increased in women with migraine who were using oral contraceptives (odds ratio 13.9), were heavy smokers (odds ratio 10.2), or who had migraine with aura (odds ratio 6.2). It has been estimated that the incidence of ischemic stroke in young women with migraine with aura who use oral contraceptives is 28 and 78 per 100,000 women aged 25–34 and 35–44, respectively. This is in contrast to the incidence of ischemic stroke of approximately 4 and 11 per 100,000 women in the general population in the same respective age groups (Becker 1997).

Although the relative risk of ischemic stroke is increased in this group, it is important to bear in mind that the absolute risks are still small. The decision to use oral contraceptives in women with migraine must therefore be individualized and the benefits and risks discussed with each patient and a joint decision made. It is important that the lowest possible dose of estrogen be used in women with migraine. Oral contraceptives should be discontinued if headaches worsen or neurological symptoms develop (e.g., visual scotoma or sensory symptoms). For women who either have migraine with aura or migraine with or without aura and other significant vascular risk factors, such as smoking or hypertension, the use of estrogen-containing oral contraceptives should be discouraged. Several progestin-only contraceptives are available in this setting.

Migraine and Pregnancy

Pregnancy has a variable effect on migraine. Although approximately 70% of women experience improvement or remission of migraine symptoms during pregnancy, the attacks can either remain unchanged or worsen. Moreover, migraine may even begin for the first time during pregnancy. Remission or improvement occurs more frequently in women with pre-existing menstrual migraine, whereas worsening is more common in those with a history of migraine with aura. In women who develop migraine during pregnancy, the majority have migraine with aura. Although there is a trend for improvement to occur in the second and third trimester, there is no significant correlation between improvement or worsening of migraine and a specific trimester.

If remission occurs during pregnancy, migraine often recurs in the postpartum period, particularly in those with a history of menstrual migraine or migraine associated with estrogen withdrawal. Postpartum migraine is most frequent 3–6 days after delivery. As with pregnancy itself, migraine may first begin in the postpartum period, although this is a very infrequent occurrence.

The use of medication to treat migraine during pregnancy should be limited. For most mild-to-moderate attacks, non-pharmacological treatment, including biofeedback, rest, and relaxation therapy, should be employed. Acetaminophen may be combined with codeine, but the indiscriminate use of codeine may present a risk to the fetus during the first or second trimester.

For patients with severe attacks or status migrainosus, the risk to the developing fetus may be greater than the judicious use of a limited repertoire of medications. The intravenous use of neuroleptics, supplemented with either intravenous narcotics or corticosteroids, is an effective strategy for these patients. Either chlorpromazine or prochlorperazine (10 mg) delivered in 4 ml of crystalloid or 50 ml normal saline as a bolus over 10–15 minutes can be very effective for both the headache as well as the nausea and vomiting associated with a severe attack. Methylprednisolone (50–250 mg) delivered intravenously can also be an effective method to terminate a severe acute migraine attack or status migraine during pregnancy. Methylprednisolone is preferred over dexamethasone because the latter more readily crosses the placenta.

Migraine in the Menopause

Just as with pregnancy, the effect of menopause on the course of migraine is somewhat unpredictable. Although two-thirds of women with a previous history of migraine improve with a physiological menopause, migraine can either regress or worsen at menopause (Neri et al. 1993), and in a minority of women, migraine or its functional equivalents may begin after menopause.

Women with menopausal symptoms resulting from erratic or diminished estrogen secretion may benefit from HRT. There is evidence that HRT reduces the risk of osteoporosis and coronary artery disease. Studies are ongoing to evaluate the preventative value of estrogen replacement in Alzheimer's disease and cerebrovascular disease. Few published studies have assessed the effects of HRT on migraine in perimenopausal women, but the evidence available appears to highlight the importance of both route and method of administration. With any preparation of estrogen, the lowest effective dose should be used. In general, parenteral or transdermal preparations provide a more physiological ratio of estradiol to estrone and a steady-state concentration of estrogen. They are also more suitable delivery systems for women with migraine or for those whose headaches are worsened by oral estrogen replacement therapy (Silberstein and Merriam 1997). Also, continuous rather than interrupted ERT may be more effective in female migraineurs, particularly if their headaches had been associated with estrogen withdrawal.

Migraine headaches may be worsened by the use of cyclic progestins. For hysterectomized women who require combined estrogen and progesterone therapy, a transdermal progestin usually circumvents this problem.

CLUSTER HEADACHE

Among the many painful conditions that affect the head and face, the one known by the most names is also unique in several other respects. Cluster headache, Horton's headache, histaminic cephalgia, or migrainous neuralgia, as the condition is variously known, is without doubt the most painful recurrent headache and the one that produces the most stereotyped attacks. Despite its readily recognizable features, the syndrome continues to be misdiagnosed as trigeminal neuralgia or sinus or dental disease, and therefore is ineffectually treated.

Classification and Terminology

In episodic cluster headache, attacks of pain occur daily for days, weeks, or months before an attack-free period of remission occurs. This respite may last from weeks to years before another cluster of attacks develops. In *chronic* cluster headache, attacks of pain occur for more than a year without a remission longer than 2 weeks (*ICD 10* Guide for Headaches 1997). This chronic form of the disease may develop de novo or may evolve from episodic cluster headache. Chronic cluster headache can therefore be divided into primary and secondary chronic types.

Clinical Features

Cluster headache is predominantly a disease of men. Onset typically begins in the third decade of life. Cluster headache has been described as early as 1 year of age and as late as the seventh decade.

Periodicity is a cardinal feature of cluster headache. In most patients, the first cluster of attacks, cluster period, persists on average 4–8 weeks, and is followed by a remission lasting months or even years. The duration of the cluster period is often strikingly consistent for a given patient. A frequently observed pattern is one or two cluster periods per year. With time, however, the clusters may become seasonal and then more frequent and longer lasting. During a cluster, the patient may experience from one to three or more attacks in 24 hours, and the attacks commonly occur at similar times throughout the 24 hours for many days. Onset during the night or 1–2 hours after falling asleep is common. In some patients, this may correspond to the onset of rapid eye movement sleep. At times, several attacks per night can result in sleep deprivation in chronic patients, particularly when they avoid sleep for fear of inducing a further attack. With increasing age, the distinct clustering pattern may be less recognizable. In some patients, perhaps as many as 10%, periods of relief become less common, and the condition enters the chronic phase in which attacks may occur daily for months or years. In these patients, the condition may persist into old age, but in nearly 50% the attacks eventually cease.

Whether the patient is in the episodic or the chronic phase, the attacks of pain are identical for all individuals. The pain is strictly unilateral and almost always remains on the same side of the head from cluster to cluster; rarely, it may switch to the opposite side in a subsequent cluster. The pain is generally felt in the retro-orbital and temporal region but may be maximal in the cheek or jaw (lower syndrome). It is usually described as steady or boring and of terrible intensity (so-called suicide headache). Graphic descriptions of feeling the eye being pushed out or an auger going through the eye are very common.

Onset is usually abrupt or preceded by a brief sensation of pressure in the soon-to-be-painful area. An occasional patient may describe tension and discomfort in the limbs and neck ipsilateral to the pain, either during the attack or just preceding it. The pain intensifies very rapidly, peaking in 5–10 minutes and then persisting for 45 minutes to 2 hours. Toward the end of this time, brief periods of relief are followed by several transient peaks of pain before the attack subsides over a few minutes. Occasionally, attacks last twice as long, or, even less commonly, the attacks may seem to merge together, producing 12 or more hours of pain. After the attack, the patient is then completely free from pain, but exhausted; however, the respite may be transient because another attack may occur shortly.

During the pain, patients are almost invariably unwilling to lie down because doing so increases the intensity of the pain. Unlike patients with migraine, they are restless and prefer to pace or sit during an attack. Some remain outdoors, even in freezing weather, for the duration of the attack. Otherwise rational persons may strike their heads against a wall or hurt themselves in some other way as a distraction from the intense head pain. Most patients prefer to be alone during the attack, possibly to withdraw from distressed relatives who are unable to give them comfort. Some apply ice to the painful region, others prefer hot applications; almost all press on the scalp or the eye to try to obtain temporary relief. During the pain, many patients consider suicide; a few attempt it. Even watching a patient during an attack of cluster headache is a harrowing experience.

During the pain of cluster headache, the nostril on the side of the pain is generally blocked; this blockage in turn leads to ipsilateral overflow of tears caused by blockage of the nasolacrimal duct. The conjunctiva is injected ipsilaterally, and the superficial temporal artery is visibly distended. Profuse sweating and facial flushing on the side of the headache have been described but are rare. Nasal drainage usually signals the end of the attack. Ptosis and miosis on the side of the pain are common. This partial Horner's syndrome may persist between the attacks and is believed to be due to compression of the sympathetic plexus secondary to vasodilatation or other changes in the region of the carotid siphon. Photophobia during the painful stage is less common than in migraine, but it may occur and may be accompanied by phonophobia. Nausea during the attack is uncommon and usually is due to the use of analgesics or ergotamine. Facial swelling, most often periorbital, may develop with repeated attacks. Infrequently, transient localized swellings of the palate ipsilateral to the pain can be observed. More commonly, the patient complains that the palate feels swollen, but no abnormality can be detected by the examiner, even during an attack.

Patients with cluster headaches have a high incidence of duodenal ulceration and elevated gastric acid levels that may approach those found in the Zollinger-Ellison syndrome. They also tend to have coarse facial skin of the *peau d'orange* type, deep nasolabial folds, and an increased incidence of hazel eye color. Many of the patients are heavy cigarette smokers and tend to use more alcohol than age- and sex-matched control subjects.

Investigations

In most patients, the diagnosis is so certain on clinical grounds that special neurological investigations are unnecessary. However, imaging studies are warranted in any patient presenting with an atypical episodic cluster headache or patients in the chronic phase. As part of the management, however, it may be advisable to obtain a contrast-enhanced CT or MRI scan to help reassure the patient and the relatives that the extremely painful attacks are not due to some major intracranial abnormality. On occasion, examination of the eyes should include measurement of the ocular tension to detect glaucoma. Tests of a general nature are needed to determine any contraindications to the use of various medications.

Pathophysiology

The pathogenesis of cluster headache is unknown. Although vasodilatation is generally believed to be responsible for the pain, the site of this increased blood flow is not fully known. The vascular changes during an attack are difficult to study, and conflicting findings have been reported. Several studies suggested dilatation of the ophthalmic (Waldenlind et al. 1993) and internal carotid arteries, whereas a radiographic study showed constriction of the carotid siphon during an attack. Blood flow studies showed increased hemispheric flow bilaterally during an attack, with the greatest flow contralateral to the pain. Thermographic studies have shown persistent cold spots in the forehead, ipsilateral to the pain, in the distribution of the supraorbital artery.

The belief that vasodilatation occurs at the time of the attack is supported by the observation that various vasodilators precipitate an attack within a few minutes when the patient is in the cluster phase. Nitroglycerin (1 mg sublingually), histamine (0.35 mg intravenously or subcutaneously), and oral alcohol are all effective and consistent with cluster precipitants. Nitroglycerin is a direct nitric oxide donor, and histamine causes the release of nitric oxide. This ubiquitous molecule has been implicated in the pathogenesis of migraine and other vascular headaches. Most patients discover very quickly that they cannot drink alcohol in any form as soon as a cluster develops; once a period of remission is entered, however, alcohol usually fails to precipitate an attack. Other evidence that vasodilatation causes the pain comes from the fact that drugs that produce vasoconstriction, such as norepinephrine, ergotamine tartrate, and DHE, give relief rapidly when administered by an appropriate route.

Moskowitz (1993) emphasized the role of the trigeminovascular connections and substance P in the pathogenesis of vascular head pain. Further evidence suggests activation of the trigeminovascular system as manifest by increased levels of calcitonin gene-related peptide in blood sampled from the external jugular vein ipsilateral to an acute spontaneous attack of cluster headache (Goadsby and Edvinsson 1994). Elevated levels of vasoactive intestinal polypeptide were similarly elevated in the cranial venous blood during a cluster attack, demonstrating activation of the cranial parasympathetic nervous system (Goadsby and Edvinsson 1994).

Several observations suggest that histamine may play a role in the cause of this condition. During painful attacks, increased histamine levels have been detected in the blood and urine, but whether this increase is a primary or secondary phenomenon remains unknown. Morphological studies of the increased number and abnormal distribution of mast cells in the forehead skin of patients with cluster headache support the theory that local release of histamine is involved in some way in this condition. Evidence to the contrary, however, comes from the observation that blockade of H_1- and H_2-histamine receptors by antihistamine drugs has no effect on the painful attacks.

There has been increased speculation of late, based on circumstantial evidence, that cluster headache may be the result of an inflammatory process in the region of the cavernous sinus and adjacent draining veins. Orbital phlebography has revealed total or partial occlusion of the cavernous sinus and adjacent draining veins and other venous abnormalities in a small number of patients in an active cluster period. Venous vasculitis in the region of the cavernous sinus may be an important factor in the cause of cluster headache (Hardebo and Moskowitz 1993).

Any explanation as to the etiology of cluster headache must account for the cyclically occurring attack-susceptible periods. The periodicity of cluster headache is likely related to hypothalamic dysfunction. Changes have been shown in the levels of melatonin, cortisol, prolactin, β-endorphin, and testosterone between cluster periods and remissions (Leona and Bussone 1993).

Although it is highly speculative, the possibility of a neuroimmunological mechanism has been suggested (Martelletti and Giacovazzo 1996). The response of cluster headache to lithium therapy may be related in part to the HLA makeup of the patients. Populations of monocytes and natural killer cells are increased in active cluster periods.

Epidemiology

Compared with tension headache and migraine, the syndrome of cluster headaches is uncommon. In many headache clinic populations, migraine is 10–50 times more common than cluster headache. In the general population, the comparative percentages vary somewhat because people with migraine do not always seek help, whereas the intensity of cluster headache can rarely be endured in silence. Estimates of the prevalence of the disorder have ranged from 0.4% for men to 0.08% for women. The male-to-female ratio is at least 5 to 1 and is probably higher. Inheritance does not seem to be a major factor, although a positive family history of cluster headache has been noted in 7% of cases (Russell 1997). The incidence of migraine in patients with cluster headache is no higher than that in the general population.

Differential Diagnosis

The diagnosis of cluster headache is essentially clinical and depends on obtaining an accurate history from the patient. It is helpful to have confirmation from the spouse or relatives of the periodicity, rapidity of onset and resolution, and presence of conjunctival injection, rhinorrhea, ptosis, and altered behavior during the attack. Despite the stereotyped nature of the attacks from episode to episode and from patient to patient, the diagnosis is often missed for several years. Conditions that cause episodic, unilateral head and face pain should be considered, but they are easy to exclude. Trigeminal neuralgia, sinusitis, dental disease, and glaucoma may superficially mimic the pain of cluster headache; however, in each, the temporal profile, lack of associated autonomic features, and past history allow easy differentiation. Similarly, migraine, temporal arteritis, and the headache of intracranial space-occupying lesions should give little cause for difficulty in reaching a diagnosis of cluster headache. Episodic headache due to pheochromocytoma or hypoglycemia produced by endogenous or exogenous insulin is likely to be bilateral and unaccompanied by tearing, nasal stuffiness, or ptosis. Orbital, retro-orbital, and frontal pain associated with an incomplete Horner's syndrome can result from ipsilateral dissection of the carotid artery; unlike the pain of cluster headache, however, it is not episodic and does not produce the restlessness so characteristic of this condition. The pain associated with Tolosa-Hunt syndrome and Raeder's paratrigeminal syndrome is accompanied by oculomotor or trigeminal nerve dysfunction, a feature that should easily prevent confusion with cluster headache. Similarly, compression of the third cranial nerve by an aneurysm should be easy to distinguish from cluster pain, especially when partial or complete third cranial nerve palsy is detected.

Treatment and Management

The patient and relatives must be reassured that the clinical pattern they describe is one that has been seen before. Care should be taken to reassure the patient that the syndrome, even though unbearably painful, is benign and not life-threatening. Pain reduction but not cure should be promised.

The frequency, severity, and brevity of individual attacks of cluster headache and their lack of response to many symptomatic measures necessitate the use of a prophylactic program for most patients. The choice of preparation is determined by several factors, including whether the phase of the disorder is episodic or chronic and the presence or absence of other disease states, such as hypertension and coronary or peripheral vascular insufficiency.

Pharmacological Management

During the initial cluster, or when the patient's past history suggests that a cluster will be of limited duration, relief can usually be obtained by administering a short course of corticosteroids. Several regimens are effective, such as 60 mg of prednisone as a single daily dose for 3–4 days followed by a 10-mg reduction after every third or fourth day to thereby taper the dose to zero over 18 or 24 days. Alternatively, an intramuscular injection of triamcinolone (80 mg) or methylprednisolone (80–120 mg) can be used to give a tapering corticosteroid blood level. Whichever program is used, the patient usually obtains relief from the headaches until the lower doses or blood levels of corticosteroids are approached. The course can be repeated several times, but thereafter the risk of side effects suggests that an alternative prophylactic program should be used if the cluster has not run its course.

Ergotamine tartrate can be given orally or by rectal suppository on retiring to prevent nocturnal attacks of headache. This approach may only postpone the attack until morning, when it may be more troublesome if it occurs when the patient is at work. Prophylactic use of ergotamine tartrate can nevertheless be most valuable, but great care must be taken to regulate the dose if chronic ergotism is to be avoided. Most patients with cluster headache can be given 2 mg of ergotamine tartrate daily for several weeks without adverse effects. Nausea and peripheral paresthesias are common side effects of ergot regardless of the route of administration. DHE is a well-tolerated ergot derivative that can be given in a dose of 0.5–1.0 mg every 6–8 hours in an attempt to prevent headaches, but this dose should be continued for only a few days to avoid ergotism.

The calcium-channel blockers, such as verapamil, are effective for the prevention of cluster headache in many patients. Few published accounts are available so far, but, on the basis of clinical experience, verapamil results in improvement in more than 50% of chronic patients. Doses in the range of 80–120 mg three times a day often results in a dramatic decrease in the frequency and intensity of attacks. Subsequent reduction in benefit can be overcome by an increase in dose or by a drug holiday, followed by reintroduction of the agent. The benefit of the calcium-channel blockers makes them a logical choice over the more toxic and troublesome agents, such as methysergide and lithium.

Methysergide in a dose ranging from 4 to 10 mg per day is effective for reducing or preventing cluster headache in about 60% of patients. The side effects, which include leg cramps, nausea, and fluid retention, are usually minor, and the drug seems to be better tolerated in patients with cluster headache than in those with migraine. The risk of retroperitoneal and other types of fibrosis is important only when methysergide must be taken for months or longer. For the episodic phase of cluster headache, this drug may be needed for only a few weeks; therefore, the risk of serious side effects is low. If methysergide gives relief, the lowest effective dose should be determined and the use of the preparation continued for 2–4 weeks after the last attack. It can be restarted if the headaches return after discontinuation. If the cluster period is very long or if the patient has chronic cluster headache, methysergide can be taken for 3–6 months. It should be discontinued for 4 weeks, during which time an abdominal CT scan or MRI, chest roentgenogram, and determination of serum creatinine level are recommended by some authorities. If the patient has no signs of fibrosis, treatment with methy-

sergide can be continued for a further 3–6 months, after which the drug should again be temporarily stopped.

For patients who have chronic cluster headache with attacks that occur daily for years, relief may be obtained with lithium. Lithium carbonate, 300 mg three times a day, can be given initially and the dose adjusted at 2 weeks to obtain a serum lithium level of about 1.0 mEq/liter. Side effects at this level include a mild tremor of the limbs, gastrointestinal distress, and increased thirst. The therapeutic range is very narrow, and blood levels of more than 1.5 mEq/liter are to be avoided. Nephrotoxicity, goiter formation, and a permanent diabetes insipidus–like state have been reported after lithium treatment. In chronic cluster headache, lithium should have a beneficial effect within a week; however, the response may be delayed for several weeks. Although attacks may recur after some months, a renewed response to lithium may occur if the drug is withdrawn and then reintroduced after a few weeks. In patients who respond to lithium, use of the drug should be discontinued every few months to determine whether the cluster headaches have subsided. While lithium is being given, it is necessary to monitor the blood level at regular intervals to avoid the development of serious side effects. Thiazide diuretics should not be used concurrently because they can cause a rapid elevation of blood levels to the toxic range.

Despite the available treatments, management of patients with chronic cluster headache can be extremely difficult because many of them do not respond, or respond only briefly, to the programs already described. In such patients, a combination of several drugs may give relief. The combination of verapamil and lithium is preferred. In particularly resistant cases, triple therapy may be necessary, consisting of a prophylactic ergot preparation with lithium and verapamil or methysergide. Corticosteroids can be useful in chronic cluster headache to provide brief remissions for fixed periods. Valproate may also be an effective prophylactic agent in patients with cluster headache.

Despite these drastic measures, chronic cluster headaches remain resistant to prophylactic measures in some patients. Other drugs that may be helpful in prophylaxis include chlorpromazine, indomethacin, cyproheptadine, clonidine, and intranasal capsaicin.

Many other treatments have been proposed for chronic cluster headache, but none has proved effective. Histamine desensitization, the administration of anticonvulsants, and estrogens are among those that have been abandoned.

Oral administration of drugs for symptomatic relief is generally ineffective in acute cluster headache because of the rapid onset and limited duration of the pain. Rectally administered ergotamine tartrate (1–2 mg) at the onset of an attack often shortens the painful episode. Dosage limitations must be stressed to minimize the risk of ergotism. DHE, 0.5–1.0 mg subcutaneously or intravenously, as well as the intranasal preparation, shortens an attack of cluster headache considerably. Unlike patients with migraine, those with cluster headache do not commonly develop ergot dependence or rebound headaches due to a temporary reduction in dosage.

Sumatriptan by subcutaneous injection in a dose of 6 mg is an effective means of aborting an individual cluster headache. The intranasal formulation holds similar promise.

Analgesics are essentially useless in cluster headache because the intensity of the pain is such that only a narcotic would give relief, and the recurrent nature of the attacks precludes the use of agents of this type. Inhalation of oxygen via a loosely applied face mask at a flow rate of 8–10 liters per minute can be dramatically effective for aborting a cluster headache. Oxygen is believed to help because of its vasoconstrictive properties. It is a harmless but inconvenient therapy, requiring that a bulky cylinder be available both at home and at work if the patient has attacks both day and night.

Surgical Treatment

Thirty to 50 years ago, injection of alcohol into the gasserian ganglion and trigeminal root section was used in the treatment of chronic migrainous neuralgia (cluster headache). These procedures did not gain widespread acceptance and were gradually abandoned because of the high incidence of complications, including neuroparalytic keratitis, postoperative herpes keratitis, and anesthesia dolorosa of the denervated area.

Recently, interest has been renewed in the surgical relief of this condition. Onofrio and Campbell reported their results in a series of 26 patients with intractable chronic cluster headaches treated surgically. Their patients had radiofrequency thermocoagulation of the gasserian ganglion or sensory root section of the trigeminal nerve through a posterior fossa approach. Approximately two-thirds of the patients obtained excellent-to-good relief of pain. Most of the remaining patients were not relieved of pain because of the production of incomplete first-division anesthesia, but in several subjects, pain persisted despite dense trigeminal sensory loss in all three divisions of the nerve. Keratitis and anesthesia dolorosa are serious complications of any destructive procedure on the trigeminal nerve. Thermocoagulation of the gasserian ganglion and injection of glycerol into Meckel's cave have been effective for providing pain relief in this condition. More recently, stereotactic radiosurgery with the gamma knife under local anesthesia has been used to treat patients with chronic cluster headache refractory to medical therapy (Ford et al. 1998).

INDOMETHACIN-RESPONSIVE HEADACHE SYNDROMES

Indomethacin-responsive headache syndromes (IRHSs) represent a unique group of primary headache disorders that are characterized by a prompt, absolute, and often permanent response to indomethacin. IRHSs can easily be confused with cluster headache because of the associated facial

autonomic features associated with individual headaches. In addition, attacks may occur during sleep and can be triggered by alcohol, also features that characterize cluster headache. However, IRHSs can be distinguished from cluster headache by their short duration, with the exception of hemicrania continua, and by the high frequency of attacks. Several other primary short-lasting headache syndromes respond either partially or entirely to indomethacin, although with less consistency. These include idiopathic stabbing headache and benign cough, exertional, and sexual headache, which are described later in this chapter.

Paroxysmal Hemicranias

The paroxysmal hemicranias are primarily a disorder of young adults, with typical onset in the second and third decades. The female-to-male ratio is approximately 3 to 1, which in addition to the differences in attack profile (frequency and duration), stands in contrast to cluster headache where there is an overwhelming male predominance. Chronic and episodic paroxysmal hemicrania differ predominantly in their temporal profile. Chronic paroxysmal hemicrania, as the name implies, occurs daily, with multiple discrete attacks occurring throughout a 24-hour period. Episodic paroxysmal hemicrania is characterized by discrete attack and remission phases. The headache phase can range from 1 week to 5 months, and remission periods can last 1–36 months. Both disorders are associated with daily attacks of severe, short-lived, unilateral pain, which is often maximally felt in the orbital-periorbital or temporal region, although extratrigeminal pain in the ear or occiput can occur. The attacks occur with an average frequency of 5 per day (range, 1–40/day). Each attack lasts approximately 20 minutes (range, 2–45 minutes). Similar to cluster headache, each paroxysm is accompanied by at least one robust ipsilateral autonomic feature, which may include lacrimation, ptosis, eyelid edema, conjunctival injection, nasal congestion, or rhinorrhea (Goadsby and Lipton 1997).

Hemicrania Continua

As the name implies, hemicrania continua is characterized by a continuous unilateral headache of moderate intensity that may involve the entire hemicranium or simply be confined to a focal area. The female-to-male ratio is approximately 2 to 1, and the average age of onset is 34 years (11–78 years). Although invariably continuous, this disorder may sometimes resemble a prolonged unilateral migraine attack lasting several days to weeks, with headache-free remissions. The continuous headache is often punctuated by painful unilateral exacerbations lasting 20 minutes to several days. Attacks may alternate sides, and unilateral attacks may rarely become bilateral. These periods of increasing pain intensity are often but not invariably accompanied by one or more autonomic features, which are usually more subtle than that seen in the paroxysmal hemicranias or cluster headache. Ice-pick head pains are often a feature of this disorder, usually on the ipsilateral side, and usually during a period of exacerbation. Because of its daily persistence, hemicrania continua may be seen in the context of medication overuse, which may alter the clinical features and affect the response to treatment. Therefore, a higher index of suspicion may be required in these cases (Newman et al. 1994).

Treatment

The response of IRHSs to indomethacin is often quite striking, although the mechanism is not yet understood. Despite this dramatic response, all patients require neuroimaging to exclude a structural cause because organic mimics have been described. Indomethacin is effective in dosages ranging from 25 to 250 mg daily. The usual starting dosage is 25 mg three times daily with meals. The dose is titrated according to the patient's response and the side-effect profile. A slow-release preparation or rectal suppository is available for patients with nocturnal breakthrough headaches and for those with gastric intolerance. A treatment response is usually seen within 48 hours. Tachyphylaxis is not a feature, but medication withdrawal is often met with recurrence of the headaches. Nevertheless, once an effective dose is achieved and maintained for several weeks, a tapering schedule is recommended in an effort to find the lowest effective dose possible, which often varies from patient to patient. If indomethacin is contraindicated, or in the rare circumstance where it is ineffective in treating CPH, other medications, with anecdotal reports of success, may be tried. These include the calcium-channel blockers (verapamil, nicardipine, flunarizine), NSAIDs (ibuprofen, aspirin, piroxicam), corticosteroids, acetazolamide, and lithium. The natural history of these disorders is not known, but long-term treatment appears to be required in the majority of patients.

OTHER TYPES OF HEADACHE AND FACIAL PAIN

Headache Associated with Metabolic Abnormalities

Carbon dioxide retention and exposure to carbon monoxide can both lead to a vascular headache. The presumed mechanism is vasodilatation. Chronic hypercapnia from chronic obstructive pulmonary disease can lead to chronic headaches and eventually to raised intracranial pressure with papilledema. Carbon dioxide retention and oxygen desaturation secondary to sleep apnea of both the primary and the obstructive type can result in nocturnal and early morning headaches that diminish with activity. Tissue anoxia secondary to anemia or lack of oxygen, as occurs at high altitude, can each produce a throbbing vascular headache. Similarly, the headache that follows a generalized seizure or prolonged syncopal spell results from carbon dioxide buildup and lack of oxygen. Hypoglycemia can cause a headache that has vascular features.

Hypertension is rarely the cause of headaches unless there is a rapid and major increase in blood pressure. The headache of a pheochromocytoma characteristically occurs with dramatic suddenness and is associated with a significant elevation in blood pressure. Occasionally, early-morning headache is a sign of sustained hypertension. Preeclampsia with the accompanying high blood pressure can lead to headaches during pregnancy. The onset of severe headache around the time of delivery may indicate the onset of eclampsia.

Tension-Type or Muscle Contraction Headache

Almost everyone has a headache at some time when stressed, overworked, or angry. Such headaches, which can also result from muscular strain due to working in a physiologically unsound position, rapidly subside with relaxation, sleep, or ingestion of simple analgesics. The prevalence of this type of headache is unknown because medical help is sought only when the condition becomes sufficiently frequent or chronic to interfere with the patient's lifestyle.

Chronic headaches that are not associated with focal neurological symptoms and do not have the gastrointestinal features of migraine are often diagnosed as tension headaches and have historically been ascribed to persistent contraction of the scalp, neck, and jaw muscles. The term *tension* has been tacitly taken to mean both emotional tension and muscle tension, thus implying both pathogenesis and pain mechanism. The International Headache Society classification of headache has instituted a small but important change in the terminology of tension or muscle contraction headache. The word *type* has been added after tension, thus the term *tension-type headache* is now employed to bring attention to the fact that actual muscle tension or sustained contraction may not be a key factor in the pathophysiology of this common head pain (*ICD 10 Guide for Headaches* 1997).

The concept of muscle contraction causing headache has been questioned in recent times, and the distinction between vascular headaches and tension-type headaches has become much less certain. Electromyographic (EMG) studies of neck and scalp muscles during headache do not show a difference between people with migraine headaches and those diagnosed clinically as having a muscle contraction headache. Pericranial muscle spasm and tenderness are as common in migraine as in muscle contraction headache. Provocation of headache by alcohol and nitroglycerin is almost as common in subjects with a history of tension-type headaches as in those with a history of migraine. Similarly, patients thought to have tension-type headaches may have a throbbing quality to the pain. The platelet serotonin concentration is low in patients prone to frequent tension-type headaches. Similar findings have been noted in migraine. Autogenic training and relaxation therapy are as helpful in migraine as in muscle contraction headaches. These observations and many others have led to the concept that muscle contraction headache and migraine may not be entirely different disorders but are the extreme ends of a continuum or spectrum of headache (Silberstein 1993). However, evidence in favor of tension-type headache and migraine being separate conditions comes from Schoenen (1993). Schoenen showed that exteroceptive suppression of voluntary contraction of the jaw muscles in response to electrical stimulation of the labial commissure is abnormal in subjects diagnosed as having tension-type headaches but not in those with migraine or other types of headache.

Many patients with chronic daily headaches have a history of episodic headaches of the common migraine type. The evolution or transformation of one type of headache to another may be associated with overuse of analgesics and ergot preparations (Silberstein 1993). Depression may also be an important factor.

Clinical Symptoms

Tension-type or muscle contraction headaches, which can begin at any age, are generally bilateral (commonly occipitonuchal, bitemporal, or bifrontal). They are often described as being like a tight band around the head, a sense of pressure, or a bursting sensation. The pain may wax and wane throughout the course of a day or may be described as being present and steady for days, weeks, or even years at a time. Despite the complaint of a constant headache, sleep may be undisturbed.

Physical Findings and Laboratory Studies

Physical examination in acute tension-type headache is generally unrevealing. Chronic tension-type headache may be associated with tenderness in the cervical paraspinal muscles, restricted neck motion, and tenderness over the temporalis muscles and in scattered areas over the scalp. Laboratory studies are unhelpful, except to rule out other conditions. The erythrocyte sedimentation rate should be determined in elderly patients with headache to help exclude temporal arteritis. The recent onset of headaches in any patient, even when the symptoms are clearly those of muscle contraction headache, warrants a CT or MRI scan of the head to look for intracranial disease. All manner of serious structural intracranial disease can mimic benign muscle contraction headache. Cervical spine films may be needed to detect bony and joint disease that can trigger sustained contraction of the cervical and scalp muscles leading to secondary tension headache.

Psychological Factors

Anxiety, depression, repressed resentment, anger, and hostility have all been identified as factors contributing to the production of tension-type headaches, but the prevalence of these emotions in the population without headaches is unknown. Although psychosocial stress, anxiety, and depression are important in patients with chronic headaches, it is uncertain whether they are always causative factors or are secondary to the chronic pain.

The somatoform disorders, including hypochondriasis, somatization disorder (previously called *hysteria*), and the somatoform pain disorder, can have headache as part of the clinical picture. Together with headaches as a manifestation of somatic delusions, these are now classified under tension-type headaches, with the recognition that scalp and neck muscle contraction is not a primary factor in the pathogenesis.

Pathogenesis

The long-held belief that emotional tension leads to muscle tension and hence headache is too simplistic. A growing number of authorities suspect that a far more complex central mechanism is responsible for the pain. Disturbances originating in the hypothalamus and spreading by way of the mamillothalamic tract to the upper brainstem and influencing the antinociceptive mechanisms have been suggested. Alterations in central pain modulation and changes in serotonin and endorphin levels are also likely to be important in chronic tension-type headache. The role of the descending tract and nucleus of the trigeminal nerve and its relationship to noxious input from the cervical spine via the upper cervical roots is currently being studied.

Course and Prognosis

Chronic tension-type headache, especially when it becomes a daily event, can persist for years. It is difficult to manage and rarely responds completely to any therapeutic regimen. Spontaneous remissions may occur, and in some patients the condition subsides with age. Secondary depression, drug addiction, and chronic pain behavior are frequently the result of chronic headaches.

Treatment and Management

An understanding, sympathetic physician who communicates an interest in the patient's headache will achieve far better results than one who dismisses the patient with the exhortation to relax more or the statement that the headache is all due to "nerves." Many patients are more interested in knowing that the headache is not due to a serious intracranial pathological condition than in obtaining relief of pain. Reassurance that the headache is not serious can be given only after a thorough examination and after appropriate investigations, including neuroimaging. Such reassurance may considerably relieve the patient's anxieties and thereby relieve the headaches.

Techniques to promote relaxation of the scalp and neck muscles can be helpful; these methods include stretching exercises, the application of heat and massage to the neck, biofeedback conditioning, and relaxation training. Although short-term results confirm the efficacy of these techniques, long-term beneficial effects are not so obvious. Many patients revert to their muscle-contracting habits unless the relaxation techniques are frequently reinforced.

For occasional mild tension-type headache, aspirin or acetaminophen may be sufficient treatment. More severe headaches usually require a prescription analgesic, but no specific preparation has been shown to be better than another. Aspirin or acetaminophen in combination with propoxyphene or butabarbital and caffeine is often effective for temporary relief but should be avoided for frequent, long-term use because of the risk of barbiturate addiction and paradoxical worsening of the headache related to analgesic rebound. NSAIDs, such as naproxen or ibuprofen, are often helpful. Preparations containing codeine or dihydrocodeine are often avoided because of the risk of addiction; however, these preparations are occasionally useful to carry patients through difficult periods when headaches are more frequent than usual. Muscle relaxants and the major and minor tranquilizers are generally ineffective for long-term management of tension-type headache but are useful for short-term relief.

The most effective prophylactic drug is amitriptyline. Controlled trials have shown an improvement of more than 50% in more than 65% of cases. The usual dose is 50–150 mg per day, but higher doses may be needed. The drug is better tolerated if given as a single bedtime dose. Side effects include weight gain, drowsiness, and anticholinergic effects, such as dryness of the mouth, urinary hesitancy, blurred vision, and constipation. Elderly patients may also be troubled by confusion and orthostatic faintness, but the latter side effect is minimized by the bedtime dose regimen. A satisfactory response does not depend on the presence of underlying depression.

Chronic tension-type headache can be the most difficult headache to treat. Transient improvement often follows introduction of any treatment, but most patients continue to complain until the headaches lessen or subside spontaneously. This improvement usually occurs with some change for the better in the subject's life or when a reaction to stress diminishes.

Many vascular headaches are associated with muscle contraction pain, thereby producing the so-called mixed or tension-vascular headache, although the International Headache Society classification of headache does not recognize a mixed headache. Both migraine and tension-type headache should be diagnosed. This condition is treated with all the methods used for the treatment of migraine and tension-type muscle contraction headaches when they occur separately. Tricyclic antidepressants, β-adrenergic blockers, NSAIDs, biofeedback, and psychotherapy are all used.

Post-Traumatic Headache

Headaches, dizziness, difficulty concentrating, irritability, decreased libido, and fatigue are common complaints after head injury (Haas 1993a). Serious head trauma, resulting in major brain damage, gives rise to post-traumatic headaches less often than do seemingly minor head injuries. This difference may be more apparent than real because the seriously injured patient may have so many symptoms that headache is of less importance than other complaints. Headache is far more common after industrial and traffic accidents than after trauma sustained in sporting activities or in circumstances in which litigation is not a factor. Despite this, few still hold to the postulates claiming the post-traumatic syndrome is a neurosis that persists until there is compensation settlement and that is not seen in professional and managerial people or after serious head trauma.

The headache that occurs as part of the post-traumatic (or postconcussive) syndrome can be generalized and resemble a tension-type headache, localized to the site of the head injury, or hemicranial and resemble migraine. The physical examination is often unrevealing, although scalp tenderness and decreased motion of the cervical spine are often found. Examination by CT scan rarely reveals any abnormalities, although unexpected subdural hematomas are occasionally found. Examination of head-injured patients with MRI has shown a higher than expected incidence of previously undetected small extracerebral hematomas, cortical contusions, and indeterminate changes in the cerebral parenchyma. Other observations to support the organic basis for the post-traumatic syndrome are that EEG is frequently abnormal and there are transient or long-lasting abnormalities in the visual evoked responses and brainstem evoked responses in some subjects.

Treatment of the post-traumatic syndrome and post-traumatic headache is difficult. Encouragement, reassurance, and a sympathetic attitude on the part of the physician are essential. All the treatments useful for tension-type headaches, migraine, occipital neuralgia, and neck sprains may be needed. Physical therapy, biofeedback, and psychotherapy each have a place in treatment. Drug treatment may require analgesics (non-narcotic), NSAIDs, and antidepressants. The tricyclic preparations can be particularly helpful.

Recovery from post-traumatic syndrome, including the headache, may be significantly delayed. Most patients who continue to have headaches for more than 2 months after the trauma continue to have them for 1–2 years (Haas 1993b). Treatment can be difficult and the results disappointing.

The post-traumatic syndrome may develop more commonly when patients believe that the evaluation shortly after the injury has been incomplete. Their initial fear and that of their relatives is that a skull fracture or brain injury has been overlooked. Physicians know that a skull fracture is generally unimportant unless it is depressed or results in a CSF leak, but any head injury or skull fracture has serious implications to the patient. Emergency room physicians and others caring for head-injured patients should therefore conduct a thorough examination, obtain whatever radiological investigations seem indicated, and then, if appropriate, reassure the patient that no serious damage has been caused. If the history included a period of unconsciousness or if there is a simple skull fracture, a limited period of bed rest followed by a graduated return to full activity should be advised. Cervical spine injuries should not be overlooked in the head-injured patient.

Post-traumatic dysautonomic cephalgia usually follows a neck injury, often blunt trauma. The patient develops a throbbing unilateral headache, ipsilateral mydriasis, and facial sweating. Overactivity of the cervical sympathetic system seems to be induced by the neck injury. This rare syndrome responds to treatment with propranolol. Minor head trauma, such as occurs when a soccer ball is headed, may be rapidly followed by a headache indistinguishable from migraine. This syndrome may occur repetitively with minor head trauma. A head injury can also be followed by recurring attacks of migraine, even in the absence of a history of similar headaches.

Cold-Stimulus Headache

Ice cream headache is so common as to be within almost everyone's experience. It occurs when an extremely cold substance comes into contact with the roof of the mouth and the upper incisors. The pain, which is most often felt midfrontally, begins within seconds of the cold stimulus, peaks in 20-60 seconds, and subsides in about the same time. It is less commonly felt bitemporally or even in the occipital region. The complaint is more common in migraineurs than in the general population. The pathogenesis is not completely understood, but reflex vasoconstriction may be involved. Accompanying the pain is a decrease in the skin temperature of the forehead of 1°C. The pain can be prevented by avoiding ice-cold food and drink.

Ice-Pick Headache

Persons subject to migraine may describe brief, extremely sharp twinges of pain that occur without warning and that can be felt anywhere in the head, including the orbit. The pains are graphically described as being like a spike being driven into the skull, hence the term *ice-pick headache*, but similar pains have been described under different terms by other authors. Similar jabbing pains may occur spontaneously (50%) or in association with another underlying headache disorder, such as cluster headache, cervicogenic headache, CPH, and tension-type headache (Pareja et al. 1996). Some patients report precipitants for this type of pain, including sudden postural changes, physical exertion, and transition from darkness to light. Because of the brevity of the pain, the sporadic nature of attacks, and frequent spontaneous remissions, treatment is not usually required and reassurance generally suffices. However, in cases of "ice-pick status" where stabs of pain occur frequently (hourly), the treatment of choice is indomethacin, administered in a regimen similar to that described for the paroxysmal hemicranias.

Neck-Tongue Syndrome

Pain and paresthesias in one-half of the tongue precipitated by neck movement are the cardinal features of the neck-tongue syndrome. The tongue discomfort has been accompanied by a variable constellation of other symptoms. Occipital pain, discomfort in the trapezius region, ipsilateral hand paresthesias, and neck pain have been described. All can be precipitated by neck movement. The exact mechanism is unknown. Atlantoaxial subluxation, cervical spondylosis, and various lesions of the cervical cord and the emerging cervical nerves have been suggested. Neural anastomosis between the glossopharyngeal nerve and the hypoglossal nerve via the pharyngeal plexus may explain the unusual syndrome. The condition is benign and has responded to temporary immobilization of the neck in a cervical collar.

Atypical Facial Pain

Atypical facial pain is a term far too readily applied to any obscure pain in the face. As Professor Neil Raskin advises, a more preferable term is *facial pain of unknown cause*. It is not appropriate to attribute all causes of idiopathic facial pain to psychogenic mechanisms.

The diagnosis of atypical facial pain should be considered only when all facial pains due to disturbances of anatomy and pathophysiology have been excluded. Exhaustive radiographic and other imaging techniques may be necessary to exclude conditions such as nasopharyngeal and sinus neoplasms, bony abnormalities of the base of the skull, and dental conditions, such as cryptic mandibular and maxillary microabscesses. The evaluation may also require a chest roentgenogram or chest CT if referred pain from lung cancer is suggested by the history (smoker) or examination (digital clubbing).

Patients in whom atypical facial pain is eventually diagnosed are usually middle-aged and predominantly female, and they complain of deep, poorly localized pain. Generally unilateral, but occasionally bilateral, the pain may be described in graphic terms, such as tearing, ripping, or crushing, or frequently as aching and boring. The pain is usually present all day and every day and gradually worsens with time. It is not influenced by factors such as alcohol consumption, heat, or cold or by factors that trigger trigeminal neuralgia. Local anesthetic blocks of the trigeminal nerve do not relieve the pain. Many patients have already undergone extensive dental, nasal, or sinus operations, to no avail. Depression is often present, and most patients are preoccupied with the pain, but there is no convincing evidence that the pain is due to the depression. Amitriptyline or a similar agent helps patients with atypical facial pain more than analgesics, which may perpetuate the syndrome by causing addiction.

Cough Headache

Cough headache is a bilateral headache of sudden onset that is precipitated by a brief, nonsustained Valsalva's maneuver, such as coughing, laughing, sneezing, and bending. The pain is usually described as bursting or explosive and lasts seconds to minutes. As a rule, the patient is pain-free between attacks, but benign cough headache with negative neuroimaging has rarely been described to last up to 24 hours. The headache is usually bilateral and often occipital or suboccipital. The mean age at onset of this headache syndrome is approximately 55 years (range, 19–77 years) with a 4-to-1 male predominance. The proportion of patients with an underlying structural cause is difficult to determine because many of the patients were reported in the pre-CT and MRI era. However, a recent study suggests that more than 50% of patients have an underlying structural cause (Pascual et al. 1996). Chiari type I malformation is the most common structural abnormality found, but other entities have been described, such as basilar invagination, platybasia, colloid cysts of the third ventricle, and other space-occupying lesions. All patients therefore require MRI before a diagnosis of benign cough headache is made. The treatment of choice is indomethacin, employed in a similar fashion to the regimen used in the paroxysmal hemicranias. The response to indomethacin is not absolute, however.

Exertional Headache

Exertional headache is a bilateral, throbbing headache that is precipitated by sustained physical exercise, such as weightlifting, dancing, running, bowling, and football. The headache is not explosive in onset but rather builds in intensity and lasts between 5 minutes to 24 hours, in contrast to the headache profile seen with cough headache. The headache can be prevented by avoiding excessive exertion, particularly in hot weather or at high altitude. Similar to cough headache, this disorder can be benign or symptomatic of an underlying cause. In one series, 12 of 28 patients with exertional headache were found to have underlying causes (Pascual et al. 1996). These patients, however, were older (mean age 42 versus 24), developed acute, severe, bilateral headaches lasting 1 day to 1 month, and developed accompanying symptoms of nausea, vomiting, photophobia, or diplopia. Well-described causes of symptomatic exertional headache include subarachnoid hemorrhage, cerebral metastases, pansinusitis, and pheochromocytoma. Appropriate investigations are therefore mandatory in each patient. Indomethacin, either given shortly before exercise or on a regular basis, is effective in the majority of benign exertional headaches. Other medications that may be effective include ergotamine before exercise or the regular administration of a beta blocker or calcium-channel blocker.

Headache Associated with Sexual Activity

The onset of a severe headache, usually in the occipitonuchal region, during intercourse or at orgasm is usually benign. The headache may be of two types. The more common is a cervical and occipital headache that builds up through intercourse and is believed to be due to sustained contraction of the cervical and scalp muscles. This headache rapidly resolves with rest. The more acute and frightening headache develops at the height of orgasm and may be very severe. It usually subsides in minutes, although it may persist for hours and may cause the subject to seek immediate medical attention. Both types of coital headache are more common in men than in women. They may occur as isolated events or may be recurrent. If the patient is examined during or soon after the headache, it is important to exclude a subarachnoid hemorrhage. A CT scan of the head should be obtained. If there is no sign of bleeding, a lumbar puncture should be undertaken to examine the CSF for the presence of erythrocytes or xanthochromia. Even if these examinations are negative, angiography may be necessary if the history and the physical examination suggest that a small subarachnoid hemorrhage or sentinel bleed may have occurred.

Recurrent orgasmic headache may be prevented in some patients by the use of indomethacin or ergotamine tartrate taken several hours before intercourse.

CRANIAL AND FACIAL NEURALGIAS

Trigeminal Neuralgia

One of the most severe pains known, trigeminal neuralgia was first described by John Fothergill in 1773.

Clinical Symptoms

The pain of trigeminal neuralgia is paroxysmal. It is felt within the distribution of one or more divisions of the trigeminal nerve. The pain is frequently triggered by a sensory stimulus to the skin, mucosa, or teeth innervated by the ipsilateral trigeminal nerve. The pain is described as electric shock–like, shooting, or lancinating. Each attack lasts only seconds, but the pain may be repetitive at short intervals so that the individual attacks blur into one another. After many attacks within a few hours, the subject may describe a residual lingering facial pain. Attacks of trigeminal neuralgia are most common in the second and third divisions of the nerve. Pain confined to the ophthalmic division is extremely rare. Although the tongue is supplied by the mandibular division of the nerve, it is uncommon for the pain to spread into the tongue, even when the lower lip and mandible are involved.

Physical Findings

In primary trigeminal neuralgia or tic douloureux, there is no sensory impairment and the motor division of the nerve is intact. Examination of the face may be difficult because the patient is reluctant to let the examiner stimulate the skin for fear of triggering an attack. Male patients occasionally present with one portion of the face, the trigger zone, unshaven. Initiation of the pain by chewing, brushing the teeth, and talking, and even by cold drafts striking the face, is commonly reported. Attacks of pain during sleep are rare. Weight loss, dehydration, and secondary depression can occur if the attacks are frequent.

When trigeminal neuralgia occurs as a result of a lesion involving the gasserian ganglion, main sensory root, or root entry zone in the pons (secondary trigeminal neuralgia), there may be associated physical signs. These include sensory loss in the fifth cranial nerve distribution, weakness and atrophy of the muscles of mastication, and involvement of adjacent cranial nerves. When tic douloureux occurs bilaterally, it is often due to multiple sclerosis.

Laboratory and Radiological Findings

In classic trigeminal neuralgia, there are no accompanying laboratory or radiographic abnormalities. EMG and nerve stimulation techniques, such as blink reflex studies, reveal normal responses. Trigeminal neuralgia due to structural lesions, such as a meningioma compressing the gasserian ganglion, a schwannoma of the nerve, or malignant infiltration of the skull base, is associated with the expected abnormalities on studies such as CT scans, MRI, and basal skull roentgenography. Enlargement of the foramen ovale or foramen rotundum can be seen on appropriate roentgenographic studies and may suggest a schwannoma of the trigeminal nerve.

Pathology

There are degenerative changes within the gasserian ganglion in patients with trigeminal neuralgia. Vacuolated neurons, segmental demyelination, vascular changes, and other abnormalities were more common in ganglia from patients with a history of tic douloureux than in control specimens. Demyelination of the axons in the main sensory root may be associated with compression by vascular loops.

Pathogenesis and Etiology

The cause of trigeminal neuralgia is probably multifactorial. Multiple sclerosis, cerebellopontine angle tumors, schwannomas, and other local lesions account for a very small proportion of cases. Most cases have long been called idiopathic. The work of Jannetta has revitalized Dandy's vascular loop-nerve compression theory. Jannetta has found arterial compression of the posterior root in 59% of patients and venous compression in 25%. Vascular compression is believed to increase with age and to result in changes in the trigeminal sensory root and root entry zone that give rise to prolongation of electrical impulses within the nerve and to re-excitement of the axons, leading to repetitive neuronal discharges. The vascular compression theory has, however, not found universal support.

Epidemiology

Trigeminal neuralgia begins after the age of 40 years in 90% of patients. It is slightly more common in women.

Course and Prognosis

Once trigeminal neuralgia has developed, it is likely to have an exacerbating and remitting course over many years. During exacerbations, the painful attacks may occur many times a day for weeks or months at a time. A spontaneous remission may occur at any time and last for months or years. The reasons for these fluctuations are unknown.

Treatment and Management

Treatment of tic douloureux due to some local lesion compressing the sensory root of the trigeminal nerve is surgical exploration and decompression of the nerve. Management of primary trigeminal neuralgia can be either medical or surgical.

Carbamazepine is the most effective drug for the treatment of trigeminal neuralgia. Approximately 75% of patients respond. Administration of the drug must be initiated with small doses of 50–100 mg and increased slowly as tolerated. Vertigo, drowsiness, and ataxia are common side effects, especially in elderly patients, if the preparation is introduced too quickly. Therapeutic doses generally range from 600 to 1,200 mg per day. A serum concentration ranging from 40 to 100 µg/ml should be achieved. Once the pain is controlled completely, the dose can be tapered every few weeks to determine whether a remission has developed. Regular blood counts should be obtained for the first few months and thereafter about once a year while carbamazepine is administered, in view of the earlier reports of agranulocytosis with this preparation.

Second-line options for the management of trigeminal neuralgia include phenytoin, baclofen, and valproate. Other drugs that have been used include gabapentin, clonazepam, and lamotrigine (Cheshire 1997). The above drugs are less effective than carbamazepine but should be considered for trial, alone or in combination, when carbamazepine is either not helpful or not tolerated.

On occasion, one may encounter a patient in the midst of a severe attack. A useful technique in this situation is the administration of intravenous fosphenytoin at a dose of 250 mg. A recently described technique of anesthetizing the ipsilateral conjunctival sac with the local ophthalmic anesthetic proparacaine has also proved most effective in providing relief from pain for several hours to days.

The simplest nonmedical therapy is an alcohol block of the peripheral branch of the division of the trigeminal nerve that is painful. The mental or mandibular nerve can be blocked with 0.50–0.75 ml of absolute alcohol to control mandibular division trigeminal neuralgia. The infraorbital and supraorbital nerves can also be injected for pain involving the second and first divisions. Relief of pain occurs in a high proportion of patients so treated, but relapse is likely in most after 6–18 months. The procedure can be repeated once or twice, but thereafter it is prudent to perform a more proximal and lasting procedure because the further injection of alcohol is likely to be ineffective. The advantages of a peripheral alcohol injection include the lack of morbidity and the temporary nature of the sensory loss. Preservation of corneal sensation is also an advantage. Avulsion or section of the peripheral branches has been used for control of pain but is now rarely used.

For many patients, especially those who are elderly or who have complicating medical conditions, percutaneous radiofrequency thermocoagulation of the trigeminal nerve sensory root as it leaves the gasserian ganglion is the procedure of choice. Authors have reported pain relief in up to 93% of patients. Recurrence rates vary with the period of follow-up. The procedure can be repeated when relapse occurs. Complications include damage to the carotid artery, the adjacent cranial nerves, and the trigeminal nerve motor root. Corneal sensory loss can lead to serious eye complications. *Anesthesia dolorosa*, a distressingly painful sensation in the numb area, occurs occasionally. Troublesome dysesthesias of the face are more commonly encountered.

Section of the sensory root of the trigeminal nerve via a middle fossa or posterior fossa approach is used for the treatment of trigeminal neuralgia less often than previously. This decline has largely been due to the increasing use of the technique of microvascular decompression advocated by Jannetta. In his 1991 series of 1,185 patients, 70% had persistent excellent relief of pain 10 years after the trigeminal nerve and the compressing vessel were separated (Barker et al. 1996). Relief of pain without the production of anesthesia is the major advantage of the procedure. The disadvantages include the need for a posterior fossa exploration, with a reported mortality of between 1% and 2%, and the risk of injury to other cranial nerves, most commonly IV, VII, and VIII. When no vascular loop is found at the time of operation, the options include performing a partial or complete sensory root section or subsequently performing a radiofrequency procedure.

For a young patient who does not respond to medical treatment, posterior fossa microvascular decompression should be considered. For an elderly or medically compromised patient, however, the ease of a radiofrequency thermocoagulation makes it the procedure of choice, possibly preceded by an alcohol block so that the sensation of facial numbness can be experienced before the more permanent procedure.

More recently, several new procedures have shown promise in patients with trigeminal neuralgia refractory to medical management. Percutaneous trigeminal nerve compression has been shown to be an effective and technically simple treatment (Brown et al. 1993). Stereotactic radiosurgery with the gamma knife has also been shown to be an effective therapy for trigeminal neuralgia (Young et al. 1997).

SUNCT

SUNCT (short-lasting, *u*nilateral, *n*euralgiform, headache attacks with *c*onjunctival injection, *t*earing, rhinorrhea, and forehead sweating) is a severe unilateral cephalalgia charac-

terized by neuralgiform pain of very short duration (15–120 seconds). These painful paroxysms are usually felt in or around the eye and can sometimes be triggered by cutaneous stimuli or neck movements. They occur with a frequency ranging from 1 or 2 per day, up to 30 per hour, but patients are typically pain-free between paroxysms. Unlike trigeminal neuralgia, the pain occurs exclusively in a cranial nerve V1 distribution, whereas the brevity and high frequency of attacks in SUNCT should make the distinction with cluster headache quite clear. In addition, the medications usually used to treat either trigeminal neuralgia or cluster are ineffective in patients with SUNCT. Although anecdotal reports of pain relief with corticosteroids, sumatriptan, and carbamazepine are available, no drug has shown consistent and lasting efficacy (Pareja and Sjaastad 1997).

Glossopharyngeal Neuralgia

The pain in neuralgia of the ninth cranial nerve is similar in quality and periodicity to that of trigeminal neuralgia. The pain is lancinating and episodic and may be severe. It is felt in the distribution of the glossopharyngeal nerve and the sensory distribution of the upper fibers of the vagus nerve. Pain in the throat, the tonsillar region, the posterior third of the tongue, the larynx, the nasopharynx, and the pinna of the ear is often described patients with this rare neuralgia. The pain is usually triggered by swallowing, chewing, speaking, laughing, or coughing. The pain is unilateral in most patients. Bilateral involvement does occur, but it is very rare. The age group involved is generally older than 40 years. Bradycardia and syncope can occur when the painful attack strikes.

Secondary glossopharyngeal neuralgia may be due to oropharyngeal malignancies, peritonsillar infections, and other lesions at the base of the skull. Most cases have been thought to be idiopathic, but vascular compression of the ninth cranial nerve has been described.

Carbamazepine and phenytoin have been administered with mixed success in glossopharyngeal neuralgia. Intracranial section of the glossopharyngeal and upper rootlets of the vagus nerve is almost always successful in giving complete pain relief. Microvascular decompression of the ninth cranial nerve root entry zone has also relieved the pain.

Geniculate Neuralgia (Nervus Intermedius Neuralgia of Hunt)

The sensory root of the geniculate ganglion, the nervus intermedius of Wrisberg, innervates the inner ear, the middle ear, the mastoid cells, the eustachian tube, and part of the pinna of the ear. A syndrome of pain in the ear, pinna, and auditory canal has been ascribed to neuralgia of the geniculate ganglion and nervus intermedius. There is no known pathological condition. Clinical features of this syndrome are not well defined. If one were to characterize geniculate neuralgia by paroxysmal pain of great intensity but short duration in the ear, pinna, or auditory canal, this syndrome must be exceedingly rare. Some would argue that geniculate neuralgia, unlike the neuralgias already described, need not be lancinating and episodic, but tends to be more prolonged. It may be sharp or burning. It occurs in middle-aged adults, more often in women than in men.

Treatment with carbamazepine is appropriate, but the rarity of the condition has prevented accumulation of any meaningful results. Excision of the nervus intermedius and the geniculate ganglion via a middle fossa approach has provided permanent relief (Lovely and Jannetta 1997).

Geniculate Herpes Zoster or Ramsay Hunt Syndrome

Presumed infection of the geniculate ganglion with herpes zoster virus results in ear pain with radiation to the tonsillar region ipsilaterally. Vesicles are found in the external auditory canal and on the pinna. Less often, they are also seen on the anterior pillar of the fauces. The infection may affect the chorda tympani, leading to loss of taste on the anterior two-thirds of the tongue. In almost all cases, the main trunk of the facial nerve is involved, causing facial paralysis. Adjacent nerves may also become involved, most commonly the eighth, which leads to hearing loss and vertigo. The exact site of the herpes infection is debated and may be within the brainstem rather than confined to the geniculate ganglion. Treatment is symptomatic. Recovery of facial nerve function tends to be less complete than after idiopathic Bell's palsy.

Occipital Neuralgia

A headache in the occipital region may be due to entrapment of the greater or lesser occipital nerves on one or both sides. The patient may have a history of trauma to the back of the head, but more commonly the condition develops spontaneously. Chronic contraction of the neck and posterior scalp muscles may be responsible for entrapment of the occipital nerves.

The pain is described as shooting from the nuchal region up to the vertex. In addition to the lancinating pains, dull occipital discomfort may be present. Percussion over the occipital nerves should reproduce the symptoms, and discrete tenderness should be evident in the area of the nerve low in the occipital region. Local anesthetic can be infiltrated around the nerve as a diagnostic procedure. While the area remains anesthetized, the spontaneous pain should be relieved, and pain should not be triggered by percussion over the nerve. A local corticosteroid preparation should then be injected. In many instances, this treatment results in long-term relief. Avulsion or nerve section should be avoided because these procedures often do not give complete relief and may lead to formation of a neuroma.

Postherpetic Neuralgia

Herpes zoster of the trigeminal nerve almost always involves the ophthalmic division. The typical eruption is strictly unilateral and involves the forehead and upper part of the eyelid. It may be accompanied by a keratitis that can permanently scar the cornea. Pain during the acute phase is severe and may require narcotic analgesics. In elderly patients, the acute phase may be followed by a terribly distressing, long-lasting, painful dysesthetic stage. Postherpetic neuralgia is not common, occurring in about 10% of patients with herpes zoster ophthalmicus.

The pain of the acute attack may merge into the postherpetic stage. The pain is constant, with superimposed lancinating pains. Terms such as *burning*, *stabbing*, and *tearing* are used to describe the pain. The site of the previous eruption may be either hypoesthetic or hyperesthetic.

Inflammatory changes and the results of such inflammation have been found throughout the peripheral and central trigeminal pathways, even as far caudal as the lower portion of the descending trigeminal tract in the cervical cord. Thus, the pain is a central phenomenon, which explains why peripheral surgical procedures to relieve postherpetic neuralgia are generally ineffective.

Once developed, postherpetic neuralgia sometimes persists indefinitely, although with time it may become less severe. Many elderly patients with this distressing pain become depressed, lose weight, and become withdrawn. During the acute phase, oral or systemic corticosteroids are thought to be helpful for reducing the pain and inflammation and may reduce the likelihood of postherpetic neuralgia developing. Oral acyclovir reduces acute pain and speeds healing of the lesions but does not prevent the development of neuralgia. Treatment of established postherpetic neuralgia is difficult and in many instances ineffective. Local massage, the use of a vibrator, and application of ultrasound are advised to desensitize the involved area. Carbamazepine and other anticonvulsants have not been helpful. Administration of amitriptyline may be useful. It can be given alone or in combination with a phenothiazine such as fluphenazine. Application of capsaicin as a 0.025% topical cream to the painful area three or four times daily can provide some relief.

Procedures to denervate the affected area of skin, trigeminal destructive procedures, and trigeminal tractotomy have been used for control of pain, but they are rarely used at present.

Other Neuralgias

Various painful syndromes of the head and neck have been described as neuralgias. Specific nerves have been incriminated with little to support the claim. Many of the syndromes have features resembling those of cluster headache. Similar temporal profiles, similar accompanying autonomic features, and similar response to treatment indicate that the mechanisms underlying these syndromes may be identical to those responsible for cluster headache. Examples include Sluder's sphenopalatine neuralgia, Vail's vidian neuralgia, Charlin's ciliary neuralgia, and Gardner's petrosal neuralgia. With the possible exception of the condition described by Sluder, there is little to be gained by adhering to the belief that specific painful syndromes are due to disturbances of these nerves.

HEADACHE IN CHILDREN

Almost everything in the previous sections of this chapter applies equally to children and adults. However, the approach to the diagnosis and treatment of headaches in children has some important differences.

Obtaining the child's history of head pain can be challenging because most subjects younger than 10 years are unable to give clear details on the temporal profile of the headache, its frequency, and its characteristics. The examiner is very dependent on the observations of the parents. It is important to understand the effect of the headache on the child's behavior. Does the youngster continue to play, want to go to bed, refuse food, refuse to go to school, and then appear to recover? It is also important to determine whether the headache is episodic and separated by periods of well-being, as occurs with migraine; chronic and progressive, as might occur with a brain tumor; or chronic and nonprogressive, as might occur with a psychogenic headache or depressive equivalent.

The neurological examination in a child should evaluate the same factors as in an older patient. In addition, the head size should be measured, the fontanelles examined, and the developmental markers checked.

Investigations are undertaken after a thorough history and physical examination of the child. In many subjects, the history is so characteristic that few investigations are needed. The child with acute episodes of headache relieved by sleep and not associated with any neurological findings does not require a CT scan or MRI of the head unless the story changes or unless the parents are so worried that reassurance by the neurologist will not suffice. The child with a progressive headache requires all the imaging techniques available until a diagnosis is reached. The child with a constant, nonprogressive headache may need a psychological evaluation, and the family dynamics may require full evaluation. Reports from teachers are of value in assessing the child's performance.

Migraine

Migraine is the most common cause of headaches in children referred to a neurologist. It can manifest all the features seen in older patients. However, migraine attacks in children are often shorter and less frequent than in adults, and unilateral location is not a specific feature of juvenile migraine (Guidetti 1997). It is triggered by similar factors at all ages, including stress, fever, head trauma, and dietary factors. In girls, the onset of migraine may coincide with menarche.

Nonpharmacological approaches to treatment include elimination of known triggers and training in biofeedback and relaxation techniques. Biofeedback and relaxation training may be of benefit in patients above the age of 9 years.

Pharmacological treatment of migraine in children relies on many of the agents used in adults, but the details depend on the age of the child. In children under age 6 years, modest doses of acetaminophen combined with rest in a dark quiet room works well. In older children, medications such as NSAIDs and butalbital-containing analgesic compounds may be used. The potential for analgesic-induced rebound headaches can be avoided so long as frequent long-term use is not undertaken. Narcotic medication should be avoided.

The results of treatment with oral preparations of 5-HT-1 agonists have been mixed in older children and adolescents. In some studies, the efficacy has not been as great as has been demonstrated in adults. Nevertheless, sumatriptan in doses of 25 mg and greater have been useful in some patients. Studies of newer agents will need to be undertaken to determine their efficacy and safety in this age group. Ergotamine tartrate with an analgesic can also be used but has a higher incidence of side effects, such as nausea.

Both suppository and oral forms of antiemetics are helpful in patients when migraine attacks are accompanied by significant nausea and vomiting. A 25- to 50-mg suppository of promethazine hydrochloride is often effective in children. Prochlorperazine and metoclopramide should be used with caution in children because of the potential of dystonic reactions.

For acute incapacitating headaches, parenteral DHE and sumatriptan have been effective. The intravenous form of DHE in a dose of 0.1–0.2 mg with 2 mg of metoclopramide has been an effective acute treatment. Subcutaneous injection of sumatriptan with a dose adjustment of 0.06 mg/kg to a maximum of 6 mg can be efficacious (Winner 1997).

For children with frequent migraine attacks (one a week or several prolonged attacks per month), prophylactic treatment should be considered. Propranolol in an initial dose of 0.5–1.0 mg/kg in two daily divided doses (to a maximum of 10 mg bid initially) can be gradually increased until a therapeutic response occurs or side effects preclude further increases. As in adults, a clinical response may not occur for several weeks. If a β-adrenergic blocking agent is ineffective or contraindicated, one of the calcium-channel antagonists may be tried, such as verapamil or nimodipine. Cyproheptadine, long known as an antihistamine and antiserotonin agent, is also a calcium-channel antagonist and may be helpful in migraine prophylaxis. It is effective in less than 50% of patients, though, and drowsiness and weight gain are common side effects. Tricyclic antidepressants, such as nortriptyline and amitriptyline, are sometimes effective prophylactic agents, although no controlled studies have been reported in children. Their side-effect profile (particularly cardiac) limits their use in children.

Tension-Type Headache

Chronic tension-type headaches in children are similar to the same condition in adults. Life stresses are often the underlying cause. Depression and anxiety may result from peer pressure, excessive parental expectations, conflict with teachers, and physical or sexual abuse. The headache is often diffuse, present to some degree almost continuously, and unaccompanied by any physical signs. School refusal and other secondary gain mechanisms may be obvious. Treatment is difficult and may require psychotherapy and family counseling. Temporary use of benzodiazepines and a tricyclic antidepressant may be needed.

Seizures and Headache

Episodic headaches in children may be a postictal symptom, and occasionally headache may be the only recognizable manifestation of a seizure disorder. An EEG is needed in the investigation of such children. If an epileptogenic abnormality is found, even in the absence of a history of clinical seizures, a trial of an anticonvulsant is warranted.

REFERENCES

Arboix A, Massons J, Oliveres M, et al. Headache in acute cerebrovascular disease—a prospective clinical study in 240 patients. Cephalalgia 1994;14:37–40.

Barker FG, Jannetta PJ, Bissonette DJ, et al. The long-term outcome of microvascular decompression for trigeminal neuralgia. N Engl J Med 1996;334:1077–1083.

Becker WJ. Migraine and oral contraceptives. Can J Neurol Sci 1997;24:16–21.

Berg MJ, Williams LS. The transient syndrome of headache with neurologic deficits and CSF lymphocytosis. Neurology 1995;45:1648–1654.

Brown JA, McDaniel MD, Weaver MT. Percutaneous trigeminal nerve compression for treatment of trigeminal neuralgia: results in 50 patients. Neurosurgery 1993;32:570–573.

Cheshire WP. Trigeminal neuralgia. A guide to drug choice. CNS Drugs 1997;7:98–110.

Cutrer FM, Sorensen AG, Weisskoff RM, et al. Perfusion-weighted imaging defects during spontaneous migrainous aura. Ann Neurol 1998;43:25–31.

de Belleroche J, Joseph R, D'Andrea G. Platelets and Migraine. In J Olesen, P Tfelt-Hansen, KMA Welch (eds), The Headaches. New York: Raven, 1993;185–191.

de Bruijn SFTM, Stam J, Kappelle LJ for the CVST Study Group. Thunderclap headache as the first symptom of cerebral venous sinus thrombosis. Lancet 1996;348:1623–1625.

de Lissovoy G, Lazarus SS. The economic cost of migraine. Present state of knowledge. Neurology 1994;44:S56–S62.

Dodick DW, Wijdicks EFM. Pituitary apoplexy presenting as thunderclap headache. Neurology 1998;50:1510–1511.

Edmeads J. Brain Tumors and Other Space-Occupying Lesions. In PJ Goadsby, SD Silberstein (eds), Headache. Boston: Butterworth–Heinemann, 1997;313–326.

Ford RG, Ford KT, Swaid S, et al. Gamma knife treatment of refractory cluster headache. Headache 1998;38:3–9.

Forsyth PA, Posner JB. Headaches in patients with brain tumors: a study of 111 patients. Neurology 1993;43:1678–1683.

Gallai V, Sarchielli P, Morucci P, Abbritti G. Red blood cell magnesium levels in migraine patients. Cephalalgia 1993;13:84–91.

Gardner K, Barmada MM, Ptacek LJ, Hoffman EP. A new locus for hemiplegic migraine maps to chromosome 1q31. Neurology 1997;49:1231–1238.

Gawel MJ, Tepper SJ. The Triptan Revolution. In AM Rapoport, FD Sheftell (eds), Seminars in Headache Management. Hamilton, Ontario: Decker, 1998;1–10.

Goadsby PJ. Current concepts of the pathophysiology of migraine. Neurol Clin 1997;15:27–42.

Goadsby PJ, Edvinsson L. Human in vivo evidence for trigeminovascular activation in cluster headache. Neuropeptide changes and effects of acute attack therapies. Brain 1994;117:427–434.

Goadsby PJ, Lipton RB. A review of paroxysmal hemicranias, SUNCT syndrome and other short-lasting headaches with autonomic feature, including new cases. Brain 1997;120:193–209.

Gomez-Aranda F, Canadillas F, Marti-Masso JF, et al. Pseudomigraine with temporary neurological symptoms and lymphocytic pleocytosis. A report of 50 cases. Brain 1997;120:1105–1113.

Granella F, Sances G, Zanferrari C, et al. Migraine without aura and reproductive life events: a clinical epidemiological study in 1300 women. Headache 1993;33:385–389.

Guidetti V. Headaches in Children. In AM Rapoport, FD Sheftell (eds), Seminars in Headache Management. Hamilton, Ontario: Decker, 1997;1–5.

Haas DC. Acute Posttraumatic Headache. In J Olesen, P Tfelt-Hansen, KMA Welch (eds), The Headaches. New York: Raven, 1993a;623–627.

Haas DC. Chronic Posttraumatic Headache. In J Olesen, P Tfelt-Hansen, KMA Welch (eds), The Headaches. New York: Raven, 1993b;629–637.

Hardebo JE, Moskowitz MA. Synthesis of Cluster Headache Pathophysiology. In J Olesen, P Tfelt-Hansen, KMA Welch (eds), The Headaches. New York: Raven, 1993;569–576.

Herzog AG. Continuous bromocriptine therapy in menstrual migraine. Neurology 1997;48:101–102.

Honkasalo ML, Kaprio J, Winter T, et al. Migraine and concomitant symptoms among 8167 adult twin pairs. Headache 1995;35:70–78.

ICD-10 Guide for Headaches. International headache classification committee. Cephalalgia 1997;17(Suppl. 19):1–82.

Jensen R, Brinck T, Olesen J. Sodium valproate has a prophylactic effect in migraine without aura. A triple-blind placebo-controlled crossover study. Neurology 1994;44:647–651.

Joutel A, Bousser MG, Biousse V, et al. A gene for familial hemiplegic migraine maps to chromosome 19. Nat Genet 1993;5:40–45.

Leona M, Bussone G. A review of hormonal findings in cluster headache. Evidence for hypothalamic involvement. Cephalalgia 1993;13:309–317.

Lovely TJ, Jannetta PJ. Surgical management of geniculate neuralgia. Am J Otol 1997;18:512–517.

MacGregor EA. "Menstrual" migraine: towards a definition. Cephalalgia 1996;16:11–26.

Martelletti P, Giacovazzo M. Putative neuroimmunological mechanisms in cluster headache. An integrated hypothesis. Headache 1996;36:312–315.

Martin G, Dixon R, Seaber E. Preclinical and Clinical Pharmacology of Zolmitriptan: A Novel Antimigraine Agent. In J Olesen, P Tfelt-Hansen (eds), Headache Treatment: Trial Methodology and New Drugs. Philadelphia: Lippincott-Raven, 1997.

Mauskop A, Altura BM. Role of magnesium in the pathogenesis and treatment of migraines. Clin Neurosci 1998;5:24–27.

Mauskop A, Altura BT, Cracco RQ, Altura BM. Intravenous magnesium sulfate rapidly alleviates headaches of various types. Headache 1996;36:154–160.

Mokri B. Headache in Spontaneous Carotid and Vertebral Artery Dissections. In PJ Goadsby, SD Silberstein (eds), Headache. Boston: Butterworth–Heinemann, 1997;327–354.

Mokri B, Piepgras DG, Miller GM. Syndrome of orthostatic headaches and diffuse pachymeningeal gadolinium enhancement. Mayo Clin Proc 1997;72:400–413.

Moskowitz MA. Neurogenic inflammation in the pathophysiology and treatment of migraine. Neurology 1993;43:S16–S20.

Moskowitz MA, Cutrer FM. Possible Importance of Neurogenic Inflammation within the Meninges to Migraine Headaches. In HI Fields, JC Liebeskind (eds), Progress in Pain Research and Management. Seattle: IASP Press, 1994.

Neri I, Granella F, Nappi R, et al. Characteristics of headache at menopause: a clinico-epidemiologic study. Naturitas 1993;17:31–37.

Newman LC, Lipton RB, Solomon S. Hemicrania continua: ten new cases and a review of the literature. Neurology 1994;44:2111–2114.

Nyholt DR, Lea RA, Goadsby PJ, et al. Familial typical migraine: linkage to chromosome 19p13 and evidence for genetic heterogeneity. Neurology 1998;50:1428–1432.

Olesen J, Tfelt-Hansen P, Welch KMA. The Headaches. New York: Raven, 1993.

Pareja JA, Ruiz J, de Isla C, et al. Idiopathic stabbing headache (jabs and jolts syndrome). Cephalalgia 1996;16:93–96.

Pareja JA, Sjaastad O. SUNCT syndrome. A clinical review. Headache 1997;37:195–202.

Pascual J, Iglesias F, Oterino A, et al. Cough, exertional, and sexual headaches: an analysis of 72 benign and symptomatic cases. Neurology 1996;46:1520–1524.

Peroutka SJ. Beyond monotherapy: rational polytherapy in migraine. Headache 1998;38:18–22.

Picard FJ, Dekafon GA, Silva J, Rice GPA. Mollaret's meningitis associated with herpes simplex type 2 infection. Neurology 1993;43:1722–1727.

Russell MB. Genetic epidemiology of migraine and cluster headache. Cephalalgia 1997;17:683–701.

Schievink WI, Morreale VM, Atkinson JL, et al. Surgical treatment of spontaneous spinal cerebrospinal fluid leaks. J Neurosurg 1998;88:243–246.

Schoenen J. Tension-Type Headache: Neurophysiology. In J Olesen, P Tfelt-Hansen, KMA Welch (eds), The Headaches. New York: Raven, 1993;463–470.

Schoenen J, Jacquy J, Lenaerts M. Effectiveness of high-dose riboflavin in migraine prophylaxis: a randomized controlled trial. Neurology 1998;50:466–470.

Silberstein SD. Tension-type and chronic daily headache. Neurology 1993;43:1644–1649.

Silberstein SD, Merriam GR. Sex Hormones and Headache. In PJ Goadsby, SD Silberstein (eds), Headache. Boston: Butterworth–Heinemann, 1997;143–147.

Slivka A, Philbrook B. Clinical and angiographic features of thunderclap headache. Headache 1995;35:1–6.

Stovner LJ. Headache associated with Chiari type 1 malformation. Headache 1993;33:175–181.

Tzourio C, Tehindrazanarivelo A, Iglesias S, et al. Case-control study of migraine and risk of ischaemic stroke in young women. BMJ 1995;310:830–833.

Waldenlind E, Ekbom K, Torhall J. MR-angiography during spontaneous attacks of cluster headache: a case report. Headache 1993;33:291–295.

Watanabe H, Kuwabara T, Ohkubo M, et al. Elevation of cerebral lactate detected by localized ^{1}H-magnetic resonance spectroscopy in migraine during the interictal period. Neurology 1996;47:1093–1095.

Weiller C, May A, Limmroth V, et al. Brain stem activation in spontaneous human migraine attacks. Nat Med 1995;1:658–660.

Welch KMA, Ramadan NM. Mitochondria, magnesium and migraine. J Neurol Sci 1995;134:9–14.

Winner PK. Treating Headache in Children. In V Guidetti (ed), Seminars in Headache Management. Hamilton, Ontario: Decker, 1997;12–13.

Winner P, Ricalde O, Le Force B, et al. A double-blind study of subcutaneous dihydroergotamine vs subcutaneous sumatriptan in the treatment of acute migraine. Arch Neurol 1996;53:180–184.

Woods RP, Iacoboni M, Mazziotta JC. Brief report: bilateral spreading hypoperfusion during spontaneous migraine headache. N Engl J Med 1994;331:1689–1692.

Young RF, Vermeulen SS, Grim P, et al. Gamma knife radiosurgery for treatment of trigeminal neuralgia. Idiopathic and tumor related. Neurology 1997;48:608–614.

Ziegler DK, Hurwitz A, Preskorn S, et al. Propranolol and amitriptyline compared in the prophylaxis of migraine. Arch Neurol 1993;50:825–830.

Zurak N. Role of the suprachiasmatic nucleus in the pathogenesis of migraine attacks. Cephalalgia 1997;17:723–778.

Chapter 74
Cranial Neuropathies

Mícheál P. Macken, Patrick J. Sweeney, and Maurice R. Hanson

OLFACTORY NERVE

For a discussion of the olfactory nerve, see Chapter 20.

OPTIC NERVE

See Chapters 15 and 41 for discussions of the optic nerve.

OCULOMOTOR NERVE

Neuroanatomy

Arising from paired nuclei in the dorsal midbrain, beneath the superior colliculus, the oculomotor cranial nerve (CN) components derive from individual cell groups that include parasympathetic fibers from the Edinger-Westphal nucleus. The fibers pursue a curved course through the tegmentum and cerebral peduncles of the midbrain, some traversing the red nucleus itself. Emerging from the side of the interpeduncular fossa, they pass forward through the lateral wall of the cavernous sinus into the orbit through the superior orbital fissure. Markinovic and Gibo (1994) provide an extensive review of the vascular supply of the oculomotor nerve (CN III).

Brainstem Syndromes

Dysfunction of the third CN can occur anywhere from its nuclear origins in the midbrain to its final terminations in the orbit. As the fascicles pass through the midbrain and exit from anteromedial aspects of the cerebral peduncles, well-defined syndromes can result, allowing anatomical localization of the problem. Thus, it is possible for a strategically located lesion to involve selectively both of the third CNs or even just a portion of their nuclear origins. Current neurology and neuro-ophthalmology texts differ somewhat in their descriptions of these named midbrain syndromes (Table 74.1).

Table 74.1: Terminology for midbrain syndromes

Syndrome	Miller (Walsh and Hoyt)	Glaser	Leigh and Zee	Original description
Benedikt's (1889)	Oculomotor palsy Contralateral chorea, tremor, ballismus, or athetosis LS: third nF, RN	Oculomotor palsy Contralateral ataxia and intention tremor LS: third nF, RN	Oculomotor palsy ? LS: third nF, RN, CP	Oculomotor palsy Contralateral hemiparesis Contralateral involuntary movements or tremor LS: third nF, CP, SN?, RN?
Claude's (1912)	Oculomotor palsy Contralateral asynergia, ataxia, dysmetria, dysdiadochokinesia LS: third nF, RN, BC	Not mentioned	Oculomotor palsy Contralateral ataxia and slow rubral tremor LS: third nF, RN	Oculomotor palsy Contralateral ataxia, asynergy, dysdiadochokinesia
Nothnagel's (1879)	Oculomotor palsy Ipsilateral ataxia LS: third nF, BC	Not mentioned	Oculomotor palsy with vertical gaze palsy LS: third nF and ?	± Trochlear palsy, ± sensory loss LS: third nF, RN, SCP (± fourth nerve, ML, MLF) Bilateral oculomotor palsies of varying degree and usually asymmetrical ± Nystagmus Gait ataxia LS: superior and inferior colliculi

BC = brachium conjunctivum; CP = cerebral peduncle; LS = lesion site; ML = medial lemniscus; MLF = medial longitudinal fasciculus; RN = red nucleus; SCP = superior cerebellar peduncle; SN = substantia nigra; third nF = third cranial nerve fascicle.
Source: GT Liu, CW Crenner, EL Logigian, et al. Midbrain syndromes of Benedikt, Claude and Nothnagel: setting the record straight. Neurology 1992;42:1820–1822.

Posterior circulation disturbances with infarction or hemorrhage are common causes of these rare syndromes. Less commonly, demyelinating disease and neoplasia, primary or metastatic, may be etiological factors. Symmetrical ptosis may be a sign of caudal midline nuclear involvement of the third CN. Silverman and colleagues (1995) provide a comprehensive review of brainstem syndromes and crossed paralysis. See also Chapter 23 for discussion of brainstem syndromes affecting the third CN.

Aneurysmal Involvement of the Oculomotor Nerve

After the fascicles of the oculomotor nerve exit the brainstem, they fuse in the interpeduncular fossa. Any extra-axial mass in this subarachnoid area could involve one or both oculomotor nerves. An aneurysm of the posterior communicating artery may produce internal ophthalmoplegia, with a dilated and relatively fixed pupil as its initial manifestation. Oculomotor dysfunction is also relatively common as a complication of surgery on a basilar bifurcation aneurysm. The palsy is likely due to retraction of the nerve during surgery. When it occurs in isolation, the prognosis for recovery is good, with resolution occurring over a period of several months. On the other hand, when the third CN dysfunction is accompanied by a hemiparesis, recovery is often incomplete.

Raised intracranial pressure, from whatever cause, may produce transtentorial uncal herniation with extrinsic compression of the third CN on the margin of the tentorium. Because of the peripheral location of the pupilloconstrictor fibers, or their vulnerability to compression, a unilateral pupillary enlargement on the side of the lesion may be the earliest sign of increased intracranial pressure (Hutchinson's pupil).

Trauma

The third CN in the subarachnoid space can be injured in head trauma. Even minor head trauma may produce a third CN palsy as the initial sign of parasellar or clival tumor, presumably because the oculomotor nerves are already stretched over the tumor, or partially encased and fixed by the tumor, and hence vulnerable to sudden mechanical stress. A third CN palsy triggered by mild head injury should prompt investigation for a basal tumor.

Cavernous Sinus Syndromes

As the third CN enters the cavernous sinus, it courses forward in the upper aspects of the lateral sinus wall, above the trochlear and trigeminal nerves. In this location, it is prone to compromise by a variety of pathological processes that may simultaneously compromise other cavernous sinus structures. Compression and dysfunction of the third, fourth, or sixth CNs in the cavernous sinus may be caused by a carotid artery enlarged by dissection, but the more likely cause of ocular motor palsies in spontaneous carotid dissection is interruption of the nutrient arteries supplying the nerves.

Thrombophlebitis of the cavernous sinus is a potentially life-threatening condition secondary to contiguous infection in the surrounding sinuses, eye, or nose. Involvement of the third CN, along with any other CNs or vascular structures traversing this cavity, can result in a clinical picture of a sick and septic patient with headache, varying degrees of ophthalmoplegia, chemosis, and proptosis. If the condition is untreated, the initial unilateral picture may become bilateral via spread through the circular sinus. In the immunosuppressed or poorly controlled diabetic in acidosis, mucormycosis must be considered in the differential diagnosis. This fungal infection, caused by either *Rhizopus* or *Mucor* species, often produces nasal turbinate necrosis and a serosanguinous nasal discharge. Surgical débridement of the area and intravenous amphotericin B may save the patient from otherwise certain death. Other fungal infections, such as *Aspergillus*, may produce similar manifestations.

Aneurysms of the carotid artery in the cavernous sinus, as well as primary and metastatic neoplasia, are important causes of third or sixth CN dysfunction. A coexisting involvement of both parasympathetic and sympathetic pupillary function suggests localization to this area.

Infarction of the third CN in the cavernous sinus involves the central core of the nerve, sparing peripheral pupilloconstrictor fibers, producing a characteristic painful, pupil-sparing palsy of CN III. In the past, this was offered as a reliable sign of noncompressive disease that obviated the need for invasive studies, such as angiography. Vascular versus compressive etiologies can often be predicted from how the iridoplegia and ophthalmoplegia evolve during the first 7 days of the illness.

Superior Orbital Fissure and Orbit

The third CN passes through the superior orbital fissure in its passage from the cavernous sinus into the orbit. It is often difficult to distinguish lesions of CN III in the orbit from those of the superior orbital fissure and those in the proximal orbit. Coexisting optic nerve dysfunction suggests orbital involvement. Involvement of maxillary division facial sensation suggests that the lesion extends at least as far back as the midcavernous sinus. Although the superior orbital fissure may be involved in almost any of the conditions mentioned previously, the Tolosa-Hunt syndrome merits special comment. Usually appearing in the fourth through sixth decades of life, this syndrome manifests over a period of several weeks as a steady, boring, unilateral orbital pain. Palsies of the third, fourth, or sixth CNs, in any combination, are possible. Optic nerve involvement is unusual. Although first-division trigeminal sensory involvement may occur, involvement of the maxillary division is uncommon. Both sexes are affected equally, and sponta-

neous remissions are reported. The entity is diagnosed by exclusion of other space-occupying lesions in the area of the superior orbital fissure and its contiguous parts. Corticosteroid responsiveness is the rule. Pathological examination reveals nonspecific inflammatory granulation tissue strangulating the involved arteries and structures.

Distal Branch Syndromes

As the oculomotor nerve enters the orbit, it subdivides into superior and inferior branches. The former, passing lateral to the optic nerve, supplies the superior rectus and levator palpebrae superioris muscle. The inferior branch, the larger of the two, supplies the inferior and medial rectus muscles and inferior oblique muscle. A twig of nerve passing to the inferior oblique also supplies, through the short ciliary nerves, the sphincter of the pupil and ciliary body. Selective paralysis of these terminal branches has multiple causes, including orbital trauma, but may be idiopathic.

Isolated superior branch oculomotor palsies produce a characteristic picture of unilateral ptosis, with weakness of the superior rectus and preserved pupillary, medial, and inferior rectus muscle function. The cause is frequently idiopathic and presumed to be viral, but internal carotid artery aneurysms, located either in the intracavernous portion or on the posterior communicating artery, may damage nerve fibers in the oculomotor nerve before division into its terminal superior and inferior branches. Myasthenia gravis may occasionally cause a similar picture.

Aberrant Regeneration Phenomena

Aberrant regeneration phenomena are oculomotor synkinesias that encompass a variety of signs, the most classic of which is lid retraction on adduction or depression (pseudo-Graefe's sign) of the ipsilateral eye. This type of phenomenon seldom occurs in ischemic, infarcted oculomotor nerves but rather suggests prior trauma or chronic compressive lesions, such as meningioma or aneurysm.

TROCHLEAR NERVE

Neuroanatomy

The trochlear or fourth CN is unique among the CNs in several ways. It originates from cells beneath the inferior colliculus just above the medial longitudinal fasciculus and caudal to the third CN complex. It is the only CN to exit on the dorsal aspect of the brainstem and is the only CN that is completely crossed. Thus, fibers from the right fourth CN nucleus cross in the anterior medullary velum to reach the left orbit, and vice versa. It is also the smallest of the CNs to the extraocular muscles and has only approximately

2,100 axons as compared with the oculomotor nerve, which has 15,000, and the abducens nerve, which has 3,500. The fourth CN travels forward in the lateral wall of the cavernous sinus beneath the third CN and above the trigeminal nerve to reach the orbit and ultimately the superior oblique muscle.

Congenital Versus Acquired Palsies

The diplopia in traumatic fourth CN palsies usually subsides in less than 1 year. When trauma is excluded, a small number of patients are found with congenital fourth CN palsies. Image tilting combined with vertical diplopia occurs only in acquired cases of recent onset, not in congenital fourth CN paralysis.

Etiology

Trauma is the most common cause of trochlear nerve palsy in adults. Twenty percent of traumatic cases are bilateral. Head impact at the time of trauma may produce disruption of the crossing fibers in the anterior medullary velum, perhaps by distention of the fourth ventricle. Transient ipsilateral trochlear nerve paresis may occur after anterior temporal lobectomy for intractable seizures (Jacobsen et al. 1995).

The etiology of a large number of palsies of CN IV remain undetermined. Vascular ischemic disease from hypertension, diabetes, and atherosclerosis accounts for approximately one-fifth of cases. On very rare occasions, aneurysm in such disparate locations as the cavernous sinus and the posterior fossa may produce a fourth CN paralysis. Myasthenia gravis must always be considered in the differential diagnosis of any ocular muscle palsy of nontraumatic origin. On rare occasions, fourth CN palsy may follow an attack of herpes zoster ophthalmicus, but its onset may be delayed up to 4 weeks after the rash.

In a child, fourth CN palsy prompts consideration of congenital origin, with head trauma being the second most common cause.

TRIGEMINAL NERVE

Neuroanatomy

The trigeminal or fifth CN is a mixed motor and sensory nerve. The larger lateral portion of the fifth CN transmits sensation from sharply defined cutaneous fields on the face, oral cavity, and nasal passages. The smaller motor branch provides motor function to the muscles of mastication and travels with the third division.

The ophthalmic, maxillary, and mandibular nerves enter the cranial cavity through the superior orbital fissure, foramen rotundum, and foramen ovale, respectively, to unite in the gasserian (semilunar) ganglion situated on the cerebral surface of the petrous bone.

Atrophy and fatty replacement of muscle mass can be visualized with magnetic resonance imaging (MRI) when the mandibular division of CN V has undergone motor denervation (Russo et al. 1997).

Trigeminal Sensory Neuropathy

Trigeminal sensory neuropathy presents with sensory disturbance in one or more divisions of the nerve. Patients with a benign form have no associated neurological defects and have preservation of the corneal reflex. The paresthesias may resolve completely in a matter of months, with only a small percentage of patients developing other conditions, such as trigeminal neuralgia. Sinister etiologies include infiltrating neoplasms or vasculitis. In this population, patients usually have other neurological signs associated with the facial numbness. If intraoral sensation is impaired sufficiently, there may be difficulty in chewing and swallowing. Perineural spread of facial skin cancer and nasopharyngeal carcinoma may occur months or years after excision of the malignancy (Catalano et al. 1995; Su and Lui 1996).

Trigeminal sensory neuropathy may be associated with scleroderma and other connective tissue disease. Distinguishing features of connective tissue disease are bilaterality, associated pain, and paresthesias that are not confined to individual nerve territories. Typically, the trigeminal motor pathway is spared. The site of involvement may be the cisternal portion of the nerve or gasserian ganglion, where motor and proprioceptive fibers bypass the sensory root (Föster et al. 1996).

Interferon-α, used in the treatment of a variety of malignancies, may produce intermittent or continuous sensory disturbance in the trigeminal distribution (Read et al. 1995).

Numb Chin and Cheek Syndromes

Numbness of the lower lip may be the initial manifestation of metastatic disease to the lower jaw, affecting primarily the inferior alveolar nerve. Metastatic lung and breast cancers are the most common primary tumors.

There are also neoplastic causes of numbness in the malar region. History of basal or squamous cell carcinomas of the face should be sought. There may be a spread of this type of tumor along regional nerves to the skull base and into the intracranial space, with meningeal involvement. As a result of mandibular bone atrophy from aging, the elderly may develop stenosis at the mental nerve foramen with paresthesias in the ipsilateral chin.

Trigeminal Neuralgia

See Chapter 73 for a discussion of trigeminal neuralgia.

Traumatic Neuropathies

Both cranial and facial trauma may affect the peripheral infraorbital and supraorbital branches of the trigeminal nerve. Cavernous sinus tumors may also involve the trigeminal nerve, but often there is associated contiguous CN involvement that localizes the site of the disease. Trigeminal nerve branch injury can rarely result from dental anesthetic injections.

Lingual nerve (a branch of the mandibular division of CN V) injury may occur after surgery on the third molar as well as after laryngeal mask airway placement (Laxton and Kipling 1996). These patients present with complaints of paresthesias on the ipsilateral tongue surface.

Herpes Virus Infections

Viral infection with herpes simplex and herpes zoster may occur. The recurring herpes simplex mucous membrane lesions that occur throughout an individual's lifetime are associated with lifelong residence of that virus in the trigeminal ganglia. Herpes zoster, which is the result of life-long varicella zoster virus residence in the ganglion, produces a much more fulminating infection, with disabling pain. Preherpetic neuralgia may precede the rash by several days and is followed by postherpetic neuralgia in about one-third of the cases. The ophthalmic division of the trigeminal nerve is most frequently affected.

ABDUCENS NERVE

Neuroanatomy

Of all the motor nuclei of the extraocular nerves, those of the abducens nuclei lie farthest from their muscles of termination and originate at the lowest level in the brainstem. They lie just below the floor of the fourth ventricle, close to the midline, in the caudal pons. In contrast to the trochlear nerve, but in common with the oculomotor fibers, the abducens or sixth CN fibers have a considerable intramedullary extent. The axons course ventrally and in a somewhat caudal direction through the brainstem parenchyma to emerge at the pontomedullary junction.

The nerve then makes a right-angle turn to pass upward along the face of the clivus; it turns anteriorly at Dorello's canal and passes into the medial aspect of the cavernous sinus, where it lies just beneath the internal carotid artery. The abducens nerve supplies the lateral rectus muscle.

Brainstem Syndromes

As with the other CNs, lesions at different foci in the brainstem produce distinct syndromes. This anatomy explains the rare combinations of ipsilateral sixth CN palsy, gaze palsy, and peripheral seventh CN weakness (Millard-Gubler syndrome) and of sixth CN palsy and contralateral hemiplegia (Foville's syndrome). Infarction in the territory of anterior inferior cerebellar artery is probably the most common cause of these syndromes. Foville's syndrome is often combined with varying degrees of ipsilateral Horner's syndrome, facial hypesthesia, and hearing loss. A characteristic disorder, referred to as *one-and-a-half syndrome*, consists of preservation of abduction in only one eye, which also exhibits jerk nystagmus in the abducted position, while the other eye lies fixed in midline for all attempts at lateral movement.

See Chapter 23 for a discussion of brainstem syndromes affecting the abducens nerve.

Extra-Axial Posterior Fossa Syndromes

It is possible for any cerebellopontine angle tumor to cause varying combinations of trigeminal, facial, and auditory nerve dysfunction. Chordomas of the clivus may selectively involve the sixth nerve in its climb along the clivus. In the preantibiotic era, medial extension of middle ear infection or mastoiditis resulted in osteitis of the petrous pyramid and paralysis of CN VI as it approached Dorello's canal and the petroclinoid ligament (Gradenigo's syndrome). Metastatic disease to the same area or primary neoplasia, such as cholesteatoma, may produce a similar painful sixth CN palsy. In the middle-aged to elderly adult with abducens nerve palsy and a combination of cervical lymphadenopathy, serous otitis media, and blood-tinged nasal discharge, evaluation must exclude a nasopharyngeal carcinoma. Both unilateral and bilateral abducens paresis may occur in the syndrome of spontaneous intracranial hypotension (Berlit et al. 1994).

For a discussion of cavernous sinus syndromes, see Oculomotor Nerve, earlier in this chapter.

Pathophysiology

Of all the ocular motor palsies, abducens nerve paresis is the one most frequently reported and, at the same time, most often indeterminate in cause. In the middle-aged to elderly adult population, especially if there is a history of hypertension or diabetes, small-vessel ischemic infarction of the nerve is the most likely cause. The microscopic neuroanatomy of the abducens nerve, as well as of the oculomotor and trochlear nerves, reveals that they are penetrated by small nutrient vessels, occlusion of which produces infarction. If the sixth CN palsy is bilateral, however, ischemia is seldom the cause, and neoplasia, demyelinating disease, subarachnoid hemorrhage, meningeal infection, and increased intracranial pressure must be considered.

Unilateral or bilateral abducens weakness is also encountered as part of Wernicke's disease in the nutritionally deprived alcoholic population. Myasthenia gravis may produce isolated weakness of abduction, mimicking abducens nerve palsy.

Abducens Nerve Palsy in Childhood

In children, abducens nerve palsies are most frequently due to neoplasia (13%) and trauma (40%). Often the neoplasm is a primary brainstem glioma, and abducens weakness may be the first sign of disease. In the newborn period, abducens nerve paresis may be a transitory and benign finding. Amblyopia may be a complication of sixth CN paresis in children, and close monitoring to prevent this complication is warranted (Aroichane and Repka 1995).

FACIAL NERVE

Neuroanatomy

The facial nerve (CN VII) is a mixed motor-sensory nerve supplying the muscles of facial expression, salivary and lacrimal glands, and mucous membranes of the oral and nasal cavities. CN VII also conveys taste sensation from the anterior two-thirds of the tongue via the lingual nerve and the chorda tympani.

Motor fibers to the facial muscles arise in the pons, sweep around the abducens nucleus, and pass through the brainstem to emerge from the caudal pons. Fibers for voluntary and reflexive facial movements are anatomically separate rostral to the lower pons (Urban et al. 1998). The motor fibers then join the nervus intermedius or sensory portion of the facial nerve to run with the eighth CN in the cerebellopontine angle and pass into the internal auditory canal. The facial nerve then enters the facial canal to unite with the geniculate ganglion. Branches go to the stapedius muscle, chorda tympani, posterior belly of the digastric, and stylohyoid muscles, with a small sensory twig to the posterior auricular area. Exiting the skull through the stylomastoid foramen, the nerve forms a plexus in the parotid gland and branches to supply the muscles of facial expression.

A large number of congenital and acquired disease states may damage the facial nerve anywhere along its course, from its brainstem nuclear origin to its peripheral terminations in the face.

Congenital Disorders

Congenital disorders of the facial nerve must be distinguished from traumatic damage to the facial nerve as a result of birth injury. Difficult forceps delivery, periauricular ecchymosis, hemotympanum, and swelling often provide clues to a traumatic cause, but many seem to have an uncomplicated birth history.

In contrast to infants with traumatic facial paralysis, newborns with congenital disorders of facial palsy have a poor prognosis for improvement in facial nerve function. Clues pointing to a congenital cause may be other birth defect stigmata, especially microtia and external auditory canal atresia. Congenital malformations elsewhere in the body, such as limb deformity or hypoplasia of the pectoral muscle, also suggest a congenital cause for the facial palsy. There are a number of well-recognized syndromes of congenital facial palsy, including cardiofacial syndrome and Möbius' syndrome. Cardiofacial syndrome comprises facial asymmetry when crying but not at rest and may result from isolated weakness of the depressor anguli oris and depressor labii inferioris muscles of the lower lip. It does not interfere with smiling or sucking and does not result in drooling, but it may be associated with congenital heart defects and other anomalies.

Möbius' syndrome consists of a spectrum of abnormalities; most cases occur on a sporadic or familial basis. The genes of one large family with dominantly inherited Möbius' syndrome were mapped to the long arm of chromosome 3. The most consistent features are congenital paresis of CNs VII and VIII with variable orofacial and limb malformation. Necroscopy has shown defects ranging from hypoplasia to agenesis of the respective CN nuclei.

Toxins

Peripheral facial paralysis may occur in thalidomide embryopathy. Medical and occupational exposure to the antiseptic solution chlorocresol, used in electrode paste and various dermatological skin creams, may produce transient facial paralysis. Ingestion of the antifreeze component ethylene glycol, either in a suicide attempt or for inebriation, may also cause bilateral peripheral facial weakness, either permanent or temporary.

Traumatic Facial Palsy

A peripheral facial paralysis occurring in the context of head trauma should always raise the possibility of basilar skull fracture. Basilar temporal bone fractures are generally categorized as either longitudinal (extending medially along the bony external canal) or transverse (crossing the long axis of the petrous pyramid). Both types of fracture may be accompanied by facial nerve palsy.

Transient facial palsy may occur in up to 20% of patients undergoing sphenoidal electrode insertion for prolonged video-electroencephalographic monitoring. The mechanism is likely related to the effect of local anesthesia on the peripheral branches of the facial nerve.

Bilateral Facial Palsy

Bilateral simultaneous peripheral facial weakness can be part of the clinical spectrum in several syndromes. Best known is the facial diplegia of varying intensity that accompanies the Guillain-Barré syndrome. Bilateral facial weakness in the presence of aseptic meningitis, or with a slightly erythematous indurated face resembling painless cellulitis, should raise the possibility of Lyme disease. The conjunction of Lyme aseptic meningitis and facial weakness is sometimes referred to as *Bannwarth's syndrome*. Recurrent bilateral facial palsy is also sometimes seen in sarcoidosis and at the time of seroconversion in human immunodeficiency virus infection.

Keane (1994) provided an authoritative review on the topic of bilateral facial palsy. In his extensive series, one-half of the 44 patients reported had self-limited causes, including Bell's palsy and Guillain-Barré syndrome.

Neoplasia

Tumor involvement of the facial nerve itself is not common, but it remains an important consideration in the differential diagnosis, particularly with slowly progressive (over many days to several weeks) peripheral facial weakness. Metastatic invasion of the temporal bone is the most common type. Breast, lung, and prostate are the most common primary tumors. Direct extension of regional tumors and primary schwannomas of the facial nerve also occur. In all these cases, the onset and course are slow and progressive. Parotid gland cysts and tumors, both benign and malignant, may involve terminal branches of the facial nerve that produce varying degrees of peripheral weakness. Obtaining a history of facial skin cancer in a patient presenting with a partial facial palsy or facial paresthesia is important because perineural spread of tumor can present long after "complete" excision of a skin malignancy (Catalano et al. 1995).

Bell's Palsy

The most common affliction of the facial nerve is the idiopathic variety, Bell's palsy. This disorder affects males and females of all ages and is believed to be of viral origin (most often herpes simplex). It often begins with pain in or behind the ipsilateral ear, suggesting an ear infection. Unilateral weakness invariably follows within several days and usually achieves a maximum paralysis within 48–72 hours. Patients may report tingling paresthesias on the involved side of the face early in the course, but this symptom is seldom prominent. Impairment of taste and hyperacusis (due to weakness of the stapedius muscle) is present in many cases. MRI shows contrast enhancement of the involved nerve (Sartoretti-Schefer et al. 1998).

Eighty percent to 85% of patients recover completely within 3 months of onset. Incomplete paralysis at the onset is perhaps the most favorable prognostic sign. Electrophysiological demonstration of lack of excitability of the facial nerve to electrical stimulation and electromyographic evidence of denervation of the involved facial muscles after 2–3 weeks establish severe axon loss. This implies a more

prolonged and probably incomplete recovery, with risk of aberrant regeneration of the facial nerve fibers. The prognosis is poorer in the syndrome of facial nerve palsy with geniculate herpes (Ramsay Hunt syndrome), which involves pain and vesicles in the external auditory canal or soft palate. Recurrent Bell's palsy may be associated with a deeply furrowed tongue (lingua plicata) and recurrent facial edema in Melkersson's syndrome; the prognosis is initially good, but permanent paralysis may eventually result.

Aberrant regeneration may have several variations, the most prominent being involuntary tearing of the eye on the involved side when eating ("crocodile tears") or synkinesis of the facial musculature when chewing. This often takes the form of a jaw-winking phenomenon, wherein the lid closes on the involved side when the jaw opens (Marin-Amat syndrome). The onset of Bell's palsy in an elderly person should prompt the physician to consider the possibility of diabetes or hypertension before the administration of prednisone, which is an often prescribed but controversial treatment.

Infections

Infection of the central nervous system by *Borrelia burgdorferi* (Lyme meningitis) is an increasingly recognized cause of peripheral nerve weakness in endemic areas. Leprosy also affects the facial nerve (see Chapter 59).

COCHLEAR-VESTIBULAR NERVE

For a discussion of the cochlear-vestibular nerve, or eighth CN, see Chapters 18, 19, and 42.

GLOSSOPHARYNGEAL NERVE

Neuroanatomy

Fibers of the glossopharyngeal nerve, or ninth CN, originate from several nuclear complexes (tractus solitarius [gustatory nucleus], nucleus ambiguus, and inferior salivatory nucleus) in the brainstem. They pass outward as several distinct subsets of fibers, to emerge from the medulla between the inferior olive and inferior cerebellar peduncle, caudal to the seventh CN and rostral to the tenth CN. CN IX exits the skull through the jugular foramen along with CNs X and XI and comes to lie between the internal jugular vein and the internal carotid artery. It ultimately reaches the lateral wall of the pharynx by tracking along the inferior border of the stylopharyngeus muscle.

Clinical Features

Isolated lesions of the glossopharyngeal nerve are extremely uncommon. Almost invariably, involvement of this nerve occurs in conjunction with that of the vagus, accessory, and hypoglossal nerves. Isolated paralysis of the glossopharyngeal nerve produces slight and usually transient difficulty in swallowing, due to involvement of the stylopharyngeus muscle, and temporary decrease in parotid gland secretions.

Peripheral dysfunction of the nerve may be due to blunt neck trauma, such as nonfatal suicidal hanging, diseases of the middle ear, and pharyngeal abscesses.

Glossopharyngeal Neuralgia

See Chapter 73 for a discussion of glossopharyngeal neuralgia.

Glomus Jugulare Tumors

Neoplasms, on rare occasion, may involve the glossopharyngeal nerve. These may include an isolated neurofibroma or a glomus jugulare tumor arising from the chemoreceptors of the jugular bulb. Glomus jugulare tumor is a highly vascular tumor that may involve the glossopharyngeal nerve as well as the other nerves running through the jugular foramen (vagus and accessory) and can enlarge sufficiently to damage the facial and hypoglossal nerves. The patient usually presents with pulsatile tinnitus followed by conductive hearing loss. Because the tumor partially or completely occludes the intravascular portion of the jugular vein, the patient may also present with increased intracranial pressure. Other symptoms encompass a spectrum of nonspecific dizziness, headache, and earache. Otological examination sometimes reveals the pulsating dark red lesion behind the eardrum. Biopsy of these tumors is contraindicated because of their hypervascularity. Treatment often consists of initial radiotherapy, followed, if necessary, by surgical removal of the tumor en bloc with the jugular bulb.

VAGUS NERVE

Neuroanatomy

The vagus nerve, or tenth CN, is the longest of all the CNs. In many respects, its origins and functions are similar to those of the glossopharyngeal nerve.

The motor fibers of the vagus arise from the nucleus ambiguus and the dorsal motor nucleus of the vagus. The sensory portions have cell bodies of origin in the jugular and nodose ganglia. Exiting the skull through the jugular foramen, the vagus travels within the carotid sheath between the internal jugular vein and carotid artery, giving off pharyngeal branches as well as superior and inferior (recurrent) laryngeal nerves. Spontaneous dissection of the internal carotid artery may present with an isolated vagal neuropathy (Moussouttas and Tuhrim 1998).

Brainstem Lesions

Supranuclear involvement of the vagus nerve is significant only when it is bilateral, producing a pseudobulbar-type syndrome with dysphagia and dysarthria. Nuclear involvement of the vagus nerve may be encountered as part of motor neuron disease in patients with progressive bulbar palsy. Poliomyelitis and primary brainstem neoplasms may also produce dysfunction at a nuclear level. See Chapter 23 for a fuller discussion of brainstem lesions affecting the vagus nerve.

Vascular lesions within the medulla may involve the vagus nerve. In this situation, Wallenberg's syndrome is the most common presentation, with the acute onset of singultus (hiccup), vertigo, and ataxia. On examination, an ipsilateral Horner's syndrome and crossed (ipsilateral face and contralateral body) loss of pain and temperature sensation with ipsilateral cerebellar tremor constitute the clinical picture.

Systemic Disorders

Vagal nerve dysfunction with vocal cord paresis is sometimes the initial manifestation of multisystem atrophy. The recurrent laryngeal branches of the vagus nerve may be damaged as a result of primary thoracic disease, the left more frequently than the right because it is longer. Of clinical value in localizing lesion sites in vagal disease is that the pharyngeal branches depart the vagus high in the neck; therefore, the absence of sensory changes in the pharynx suggests that the lesion is below this level. Tumors of the mediastinum and lung are the most frequent causes of an isolated vocal cord palsy. Cytomegalovirus infection of the laryngeal nerves with hoarseness may occur in patients with acquired immunodeficiency syndrome.

Neuralgia of the superior laryngeal branch of the vagus nerve resembles glossopharyngeal neuralgia. The pain in this instance, however, tends to be localized over the upper portion of the thyroid cartilage and is sometimes provoked by either yawning or sneezing. It may respond to carbamazepine.

SPINAL ACCESSORY NERVE

Neuroanatomy

The spinal accessory nerve, or eleventh CN, is entirely motor in function and composed of two portions: a smaller cranial part ("accessory" to the vagus) and the larger spinal portion (arising from the upper five cervical cord segments). The former, with the vagus and glossopharyngeal nerves, supplies the musculature of the pharynx and larynx, whereas the latter innervates the sternocleidomastoid and upper portions of the trapezius musculature.

The spinal portion emerges as a series of rootlets between the dentate ligament and dorsal horns of the spinal cord. Merging, they ascend and pass through the foramen magnum. Here they join the accessory rootlet originating from the

Table 74.2: Syndromes of the upper, middle, and lower cranial nerves

Syndromes	Cranial nerve involvement	Clinical abnormalities
Weber's	III	Oculomotor palsy with contralateral hemiplegia due to pyramidal tract involvement at the base of the midbrain.
Benedikt's	III	Oculomotor palsy with contralateral corticospinal signs, tremor, and cerebellar ataxia due to involvement of the red nucleus and the corticospinal tract.
Tolosa-Hunt	Varying combinations of III, IV, V (ophthalmic or maxillary), and VI	Multiple designated cranial nerve palsies with cavernous sinus lesions. Coexisting optic nerve dysfunction suggests a distal cavernous sinus, superior orbital fissure locus.
Millard-Gubler and Foville's	VI and VII	Combinations of abducens and peripheral facial palsies and contralateral hemiplegia from pontine lesion; sometimes a gaze palsy to the side of a lesion (Foville's).
Vernet's (jugular foramen)	IX, X, and XI	Loss of taste at the posterior one-third of tongue; paralysis of the VC, palate, and pharynx; paralysis of trapezius plus SCM.
Schmidt's	X and XI	Paralysis of the soft palate, pharynx, and larynx; ipsilateral weakness of the trapezius and SCM.
Tapia's	X and XII	Paralysis of the pharynx and larynx; paralysis and atrophy of the tongue.
Jackson's	X, XI, and XII	Paresis of the palate, pharynx, and larynx; paresis of the trapezius and SCM; paresis and atrophy of the tongue.
Collet-Sicard	IX, X, XI, and XII	Anesthesia of the palate; paresis of the VC and palate; weakness of the trapezius and SCM; paresis and atrophy of the tongue; hemianesthesia of the pharynx and larynx.
Villaret's	IX, X, XI, XII, and cervical sympathetic	Same as Collet-Sicard, plus Horner's syndrome.

SCM = sternocleidomastoid; VC = vocal cord.

nucleus ambiguus in the caudal medulla oblongata. These fused components then pass through the jugular foramen with CNs IX and X. After they exit the skull, a branch travels with the vagus, and the spinal accessory nerve proper continues, supplying the sternocleidomastoid and trapezius muscles.

Clinical Syndromes

Supranuclear involvement, as from stroke, usually causes only modest dysfunction of CN XI, manifested by some drooping of the shoulder and weakness of the upper portions of the trapezius muscle of the affected side. The sternocleidomastoid receives maximum input from the ipsilateral cerebral hemisphere (De Toledo and Dow 1998); thus, there is weakness of the head turning away from the hemiparetic limbs in patients with a hemispheric stroke. Nuclear involvement of CN XI occurs in motor neuron disease, syringobulbia, and syringomyelia and is associated with muscle paresis, atrophy, and fasciculations.

Spinal accessory nerve palsy, along with long thoracic nerve and C7 cervical radiculopathies, enters into the differential diagnosis of scapula winging. In spinal accessory nerve lesions, however, winging is accentuated by abduction of the arms from the sides (see Chapter 21), whereas in long thoracic nerve lesions, winging is increased by forward elevations of the arm.

A large group of named syndromes (Table 74.2) occurs with involvement of this nerve and other medullary structures. Isolated peripheral involvement of the spinal accessory nerve is uncommon and, as with central involvement, is usually attended by evidence of involvement of other structures as well. Causes include internal jugular vein cannulation, biting injuries to the neck, shoulder dislocation, unsuccessful attempts at suicidal hanging, and radical neck dissection. Selective trapezius involvement has occurred in patients undergoing carotid endarterectomy. Traction on the sternocleidomastoid muscle during surgery is believed to produce stretch injury to the branch to the trapezius. In myotonic dystrophy, atrophy of the sternocleidomastoid muscle, simulating selective spinal accessory nerve involvement, is prominent.

A benign self-limited isolated paralysis of the eleventh CN may be analogous to other types of spontaneous and restricted neuropathies, such as Bell's palsy or long thoracic nerve palsy. There is the abrupt onset of sharp pain localized to the posterior sternocleidomastoid region, followed by resolution of the pain and the typical features of an accessory nerve lesion, with winging of the scapula and drooping of the affected shoulder.

Matz and Barbaro (1996) and London and colleagues (1996) provide excellent reviews of the diagnosis and treatment of iatrogenic spinal accessory nerve injury.

HYPOGLOSSAL NERVE

Neuroanatomy

A purely motor nerve, the hypoglossal nerve (CN XII) supplies innervation to the extrinsic and intrinsic muscles of the tongue. Arising from the hypoglossal nucleus beneath the floor of the fourth ventricle in the caudal medulla, it courses anteriorly through the brainstem to exit between the pyramidal tract and the olivary eminence. The rootlets coalesce and pass through the hypoglossal canal to exit the skull. The nerve travels briefly with the ninth, tenth, and eleventh CNs before it separates at approximately mastoid level and passes on to the tongue musculature. Ipsilateral weakness and wasting of the tongue results from a lesion of one hypoglossal nerve.

Clinical Syndromes

Isolated dysfunction is rare but occasionally occurs in the context of inadvertent nerve trauma incurred at the time of carotid endarterectomy because of the proximity of CN XII to the carotid bifurcation. Dysfunction is usually temporary.

Keane's review (1996) of 100 cases of twelfth CN palsy provides an overview of common etiologies for dysfunction in this CN. Tumors, predominantly malignant, produced nearly one-half of the palsies (49 cases). Gunshot wounds made trauma the second most common cause (12) and stroke (6) the third.

Aneurysms or dissection of the carotid artery may selectively compress the twelfth CN (Lemmerling et al. 1996). Vertebrobasilar vascular disease may, on occasion, produce an ipsilateral hypoglossal paralysis (medial medullary syndrome) (see Chapter 23). In medial medullary syndrome, as a result of occlusion of either the vertebral artery or the anterior spinal artery high in the neck, there is ipsilateral paralysis of the tongue (nucleus or root fibers) with a contralateral corticospinal tract lesion causing paresis of the arm and leg. The syndrome also involves diminished proprioceptive and tactile sense due to medial lemniscus involvement.

Motor neuron disease may involve the hypoglossal nuclei, causing progressive tongue atrophy with fasciculations. Poliomyelitis may also involve the twelfth CN nucleus. Primary bony disease and malformation affecting the base of the skull (as seen with platybasia and Paget's disease) may produce mechanical damage to the hypoglossal nerve.

REFERENCES

Aroichane M, Repka MX. Outcome of sixth nerve palsy or paresis in young children. J Pediatr Ophthalmol Strabismus 1995;32:152–156.

Berlit P, Berg-Dammer E, Kuehne D. Abducens nerve palsy in spontaneous intracranial hypotension. Neurology 1994;44:1552.

Catalano PJ, Sen C, Biller HF. Cranial neuropathy secondary to perineural spread of cutaneous malignancies. Am J Otol 1995;16:772–777.

De Toledo JC, Dow R. Sternomastoid function during hemispheric suppression by Amytal: insights into the inputs to the spinal accessory nerve nucleus. Mov Disord 1998;13:809–812.

Förster C, Brandt T, Hund E, et al. Trigeminal sensory neuropathy in connective tissue disease: evidence for the site of the lesion. Neurology 1996;46:270–271.

Jacobsen DM, Warner JJ, Ruggles KH. Transient trochlear nerve palsies following anterior temporal lobectomy for epilepsy. Neurology 1995;45:1465–1468.

Keane JR. Bilateral seventh nerve palsy: analysis of 43 cases and review of the literature. Neurology 1994;44:1198–1202.

Keane JR. Twelfth nerve palsy. Analysis of 100 cases. Arch Neurol 1996;53:561–566.

Laxton CH, Kipling R. Lingual nerve paralysis following the use of the laryngeal mask airway. Anesthesia 1996;561:869–870.

Lemmerling M, Crevits L, Defreyne L, et al. Traumatic dissection of the internal carotid artery as an unusual cause of hypoglossal nerve dysfunction. Clin Neurol Neurosurg 1996;98:52–54.

London J, London NJ, Kay SP. Iatrogenic accessory nerve injury. Ann R Coll Surg Engl 1996;78:146–150.

Markinovic S, Gibo H. The neurovascular relationships and the blood supply of the oculomotor nerve: the microsurgical anatomy of its cisternal segment. Surg Neurol 1994;42:505–516.

Matz PE, Barbaro NM. Diagnosis and treatment of iatrogenic spinal accessory nerve injury. Am Surg 1996;62:682–685.

Moussouttas M, Tuhrim S. Spontaneous internal carotid artery dissection with isolated vagus nerve deficit. Neurology 1998;51:317–318.

Read SJ, Crawford DHE, Pender MP. Trigeminal sensory neuropathy induced by interferon alpha therapy. Aust N Z J Med 1995;25:54.

Russo CP, Smoker WR, Weissman JL. MR appearance of trigeminal and hypoglossal motor denervation. AJNR Am J Neuroradiol 1997;18:1375–1383.

Sartoretti-Schefer S, Kollias S, Wichmann W, Valavanis A. T2-weighted three-dimensional fast spin-echo MR in inflammatory peripheral facial nerve palsy. AJNR Am J Neuroradiol 1998;19:491–495.

Silverman IE, Lui GT, Galetta SL. The crossed paralyses. The original brain-stem syndromes of Miller-Gubler, Foville, Weber and Raymond-Cestan. Arch Neurol 1995;52:635–638.

Su CY, Lui CC. Perineural invasion of the trigeminal nerve in patients with nasopharyngeal carcinoma. Cancer 1996;78:2063–2069.

Urban PP, Wicht S, Marx J, et al. Isolated voluntary facial paresis due to pontine ischemia. Neurology 1998;50:1859–1862.

Chapter 75
Movement Disorders

David E. Riley and Anthony E. Lang

INTRODUCTION TO THE BASAL GANGLIA

The basal ganglia are a group of large nuclei that lie in the ventromedial cerebral hemispheres. Although there is no consensus regarding which structures should be included under this rubric, for the purpose of this discussion the basal ganglia consist of the striatum (caudate nucleus and putamen) and globus pallidus (or the pallidum), plus two related nuclei, the subthalamic nucleus and the substantia nigra.

Not all movement disorders covered in this chapter are related to disease in the basal ganglia; many are merely presumed to be on the basis of suggestive evidence. The correlation between basal ganglia disease and movement disorders is poor. The latter can be produced by lesions outside the basal ganglia, and asymptomatic lesions are often found within the basal ganglia on imaging studies (e.g., magnetic resonance imaging [MRI]) or at postmortem examination. The experimental correlation between basal ganglia lesions and movement disorders is also weak. Before the discovery that the toxin 1-methyl-4-phenyl-1,2,3,6-tetrahydropyridine (MPTP) produces parkinsonism in animals, the only reliable animal model of a human movement disorder resulting from damage to a basal ganglia structure was hemiballism caused by destruction of the subthalamic nucleus.

Nevertheless, a basic understanding of current knowledge about the basal ganglia is fundamental to formulating concepts regarding the diseases described in this chapter, because so many of them either have characteristic pathology involving these structures or clinically resemble others that do.

ANATOMY

The caudate nucleus courses along the lateral side of each lateral ventricle. It is contiguous with the putamen at each end. The putamen and globus pallidus sit in the middle of each cerebral hemisphere in a wedge-shaped configuration (the lenticular nucleus) in the horizontal and coronal planes, with the pallidum placed medially. The pallidum is composed of histologically identical lateral (GPl) and medial (GPm) portions (alternatively, the external [GPe] and internal [GPi] segments, respectively), which are distinguished by their projections. The subthalamic nucleus is a small structure on the border between the brainstem and cerebrum, lying lateral and inferior to the thalamus. The substantia nigra begins just below the subthalamic nucleus and runs the length of the midbrain on either side, dorsal to the cerebral peduncle. It consists of a densely cellular, heavily pigmented portion (the pars compacta, or SNc) and a relatively hypocellular zone (the pars reticulata, or SNr). Histological and electrophysiological studies suggest that the SNr is actually a portion of GPm that is divided by the internal capsule during development.

The basal ganglia have several prominent internuclear connections (Figure 75.1). The bulk of striatal outflow goes to the entire globus pallidus. The striatum and substantia nigra have major reciprocal pathways, as do the pallidum and subthalamic nucleus. Nigrostriatal fibers originate in the SNc, whereas striatonigral fibers terminate in the SNr. Pallidosubthalamic projections arise in the GPl. Subthala-

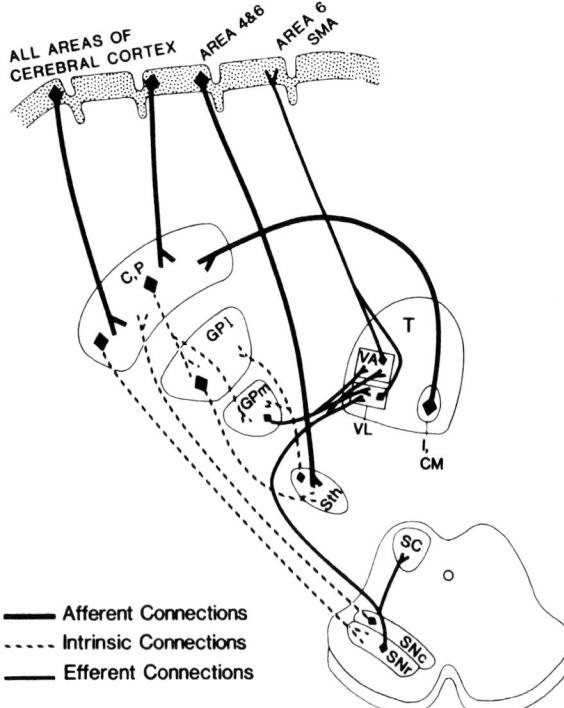

FIGURE 75.1   Major afferent, efferent, and internuclear pathways of the basal ganglia. Some pathways, including the subthalamonigral fibers and afferents from the locus ceruleus and the raphe nucleus, have been omitted for the sake of clarity. (C,P = caudate nucleus and putamen [striatum]; GP = globus pallidus [l = lateral; m = medial]; SC = superior colliculus; SMA = supplementary motor area of cortex; SN = substantia nigra [c = compacta; r = reticulata]; Sth = subthalamic nucleus; T = thalamus [nuclei: VA = ventral anterior; VL = ventrolateral; CM = centromedian; I = other intralaminar nuclei].)

Table 75.1:   Major neurotransmitters in the basal ganglia

Origin	Termination	Transmitters
Afferent connections		
Cortex	C+P, STh	Glutamate
Locus ceruleus	C+P, SN	Norepinephrine
Raphe nuclei	C+P, SN	Serotonin
Thalamus (intralaminar nuclei)	C+P	Acetylcholine (?) glutamate (?)
Intrinsic connections		
SNc	C+P	Dopamine, CCK
C+P	C+P (interneurons)	Acetylcholine, somatostatin, neuropeptide Y, nitric oxide, GABA, calretinin
C+P	SNr	GABA, dynorphin, substance P
C+P	GPl	GABA, enkephalin
C+P	GPm	GABA, substance P
GPl	STh	GABA
STh	GPm, SNr, GPl	Glutamate
Efferent connections		
GPm, SNr	Thalamus (see text)	GABA

CCK = cholecystokinin; C+P = caudate nucleus and putamen (striatum); GABA = γ-aminobutyric acid; GP = globus pallidus (l = lateral, m = medial); SN = substantia nigra (c = compacta, r = reticulata); STh = subthalamic nucleus.

BIOCHEMISTRY

Knowledge concerning the neurotransmitters of the basal ganglia pathways is continually expanding. To the classic transmitters (catecholamines, acetylcholine, amino acids) has been added a growing list of peptides. One or more peptides coexist in nerve endings with a catecholamine or amino acid transmitter (colocalization); cholinergic neurons do not appear to have an additional peptidergic function.

Multiple amino acid, amine, and peptide neurotransmitters exist within the complex of afferent, efferent, and intrinsic connections of the basal ganglia (Table 75.1). The best known neurotransmitter system is the dopaminergic nigrostriatal pathway. Striatopallidal, striatonigral, pallidothalamic, pallidosubthalamic, and nigrothalamic fibers all probably use the inhibitory transmitter γ-aminobutyric acid (GABA), as well as a variety of neuropeptides. Corticostriatal, corticosubthalamic, thalamocortical, and the subthalamopallidal projections likely use glutamate, an excitatory neurotransmitter. Thalamostriate fibers are probably cholinergic.

The striatum is a biochemically heterogeneous structure comprising up to six different neuronal types. Separate islands of cells, or striosomes, which stain weakly for acetylcholinesterase, are dispersed within a stronger staining matrix. Striosomal and matrix neurons receive distinct afferent input, use different neurotransmitters, and have different efferent projection sites.

mopallidal fibers project to both the GPl and the GPm-SNr complex. Intranuclear interneuronal connections are also extensive, particularly within the striatum.

Major afferent pathways to the basal ganglia arrive in the striatum from all areas of the cerebral cortex; smaller contributions come from the intralaminar nuclei of the thalamus and brainstem centers, such as the locus ceruleus and raphe nuclei. The subthalamic nucleus also receives a substantial projection from the frontal cortex. The most significant efferent connections arise in the GPm and SNr and project to the thalamus, as well as selected brainstem sites such as the pedunculopontine nucleus. Pallidothalamic fibers originate in the GPm and course via the ansa lenticularis and lenticular fasciculus to the ventral anterior, ventrolateral, and centromedian thalamic nuclei. Nigrothalamic fibers arise in the SNr and terminate in the ventral anterior, ventromedial, and mediodorsal nuclei; many send axon collaterals to the superior colliculus. The ventral anterior and ventrolateral nuclei project to the motor and premotor cortex, with the basal ganglia output directed mainly to the premotor and supplementary motor areas. All of these projections maintain distinct somatotopic relationships.

PHYSIOLOGY AND PROPOSED FUNCTION

Studies of the physiology of the basal ganglia using the classic techniques of experimental lesions and electrical stimulation have been plagued by inconsistent or conflicting results and a lack of correlation with the clinical phenomena of movement disorders. One important electrophysiological approach to the study of basal ganglia function has been microelectrode recording of the activity of single nerve cells in various locations in awake-behaving monkeys trained to perform specific tasks. The findings of these studies and resulting hypotheses of basal ganglia function are beyond the scope of this chapter.

The striatum serves as the major receiving area of the basal ganglia; most of its input comes from all areas of the cerebral cortex. The dopaminergic nigrostriatal pathway somehow modulates striatal output, which projects to the globus pallidus and the SNr. The GPm and SNr are the output stations of the basal ganglia, projecting to the cerebral cortex via the thalamus, to the superior colliculus, to the reticular formation, and to brainstem locomotor regions. The subthalamic nucleus somehow controls this output through a feedback circuit with the GP. Because the basal ganglia do not interact directly with spinal motor neurons, they exert their influence indirectly via corticospinal, tectospinal, and reticulospinal pathways.

Clinicopathological and microelectrode studies support the notion that the major function of the basal ganglia is related to motor behavior. The lack of a direct sensory pathway to the basal ganglia and of major efferent projections extending lower than the midbrain suggests that they act as modulators rather than executors of movement. The fact that the bulk of both afferent and efferent fibers project from and to (via the thalamus) the cerebral cortex implicates this as the likely route (the cortico-striato-pallido-thalamo-cortical circuit) by which the basal ganglia serve this function.

Knowledge is lacking regarding the actual manner in which this influence is exerted, as well as the precise role of individual nuclei. Some suggestive information may be garnered from clinical correlation of the most frequent syndromes arising from lesions in specific sites (Table 75.2), but this is a gross oversimplification. For instance, the strongest relationship exists between lesions of the subthalamic nucleus and ballism, yet it is clear that an identical clinical picture can be produced by lesions elsewhere within and outside of the basal ganglia.

Evidence is increasing that the function of the basal ganglia extends beyond simple or traditional concepts of motor control. Based on the origin and final destination of different connections, it has been suggested that the cortico-striato-pallido-thalamo-cortical circuit actually comprises several distinct and segregated loops, each with a different (albeit comparable) function. Within each loop there appear to be parallel pathways with antagonistic effects on the circuit outflow. These are known, respectively, as the *direct* (when a single neuron spans the distance between the striatum and GPm) and *indirect* (when there are intermediate

Table 75.2: Clinical correlation of basal ganglia lesions

Clinical syndrome	Most common location of pathological condition in basal ganglia
Parkinsonism	SNc (less often striatum, GP)
Chorea	Striatum, especially caudate nucleus (less often subthalamic nucleus)
Ballism	Subthalamic nucleus (less often striatum)
Dystonia	Striatum, especially putamen (less often thalamus GP, extra-BG sites)
Tremor	Variable, most types require disease outside BG
Tics	Unknown (ventral striatum?)
Myoclonus	Wide variety of sites, not limited to BG

BG = basal ganglia; GP = globus pallidus; SNc = substantia nigra compacta.

synapses in the GPl and subthalamic nucleus) pathways (Figure 75.2). The direct striatopallidal influence is inhibitory to the GPm neurons, which are themselves inhibitory to the thalamic outflow to the cortex. The net effect of direct pathway activity is to stimulate cortical activity. By contrast, the result of increased activity in the indirect pathway is excitatory to the GPm neurons, leading to an ultimately inhibitory effect on cortical activity. Knowledge of these circuits has led to an increased understanding of the pathophysiology underlying some movement disorders (Wichmann and DeLong 1997) (see Figure 75.2). It also has laid the foundation for development of more successful surgical approaches to treatment of basal ganglia diseases. However, our understanding of basal ganglia function remains rudimentary despite valiant efforts to explain these complex areas (Young and Penney 1998).

AKINETIC-RIGID SYNDROMES AND PARKINSONISM

Parkinson's Disease (Idiopathic Parkinsonism, Paralysis Agitans)

James Parkinson's *Essay on the Shaking Palsy* in 1817 marks the start of the history of movement disorders. This work was based entirely on personal interviews and visual observations, because it predated systematic neurological examination, and pathological findings were not presented. Thus, it is proper to speak of parkinsonism, a clinical syndrome that may be found in a number of different disease states (see Chapter 25, Table 25.1), many of which are detailed here. Parkinson's disease (PD), a chronic progressive condition with typical history and pathological features, is the most common cause of this syndrome.

Clinical Features

The symptoms of PD generally start insidiously. The major initial manifestations are tremor and slowness, stiffness or clumsiness, usually of an arm. Less common presenting com-

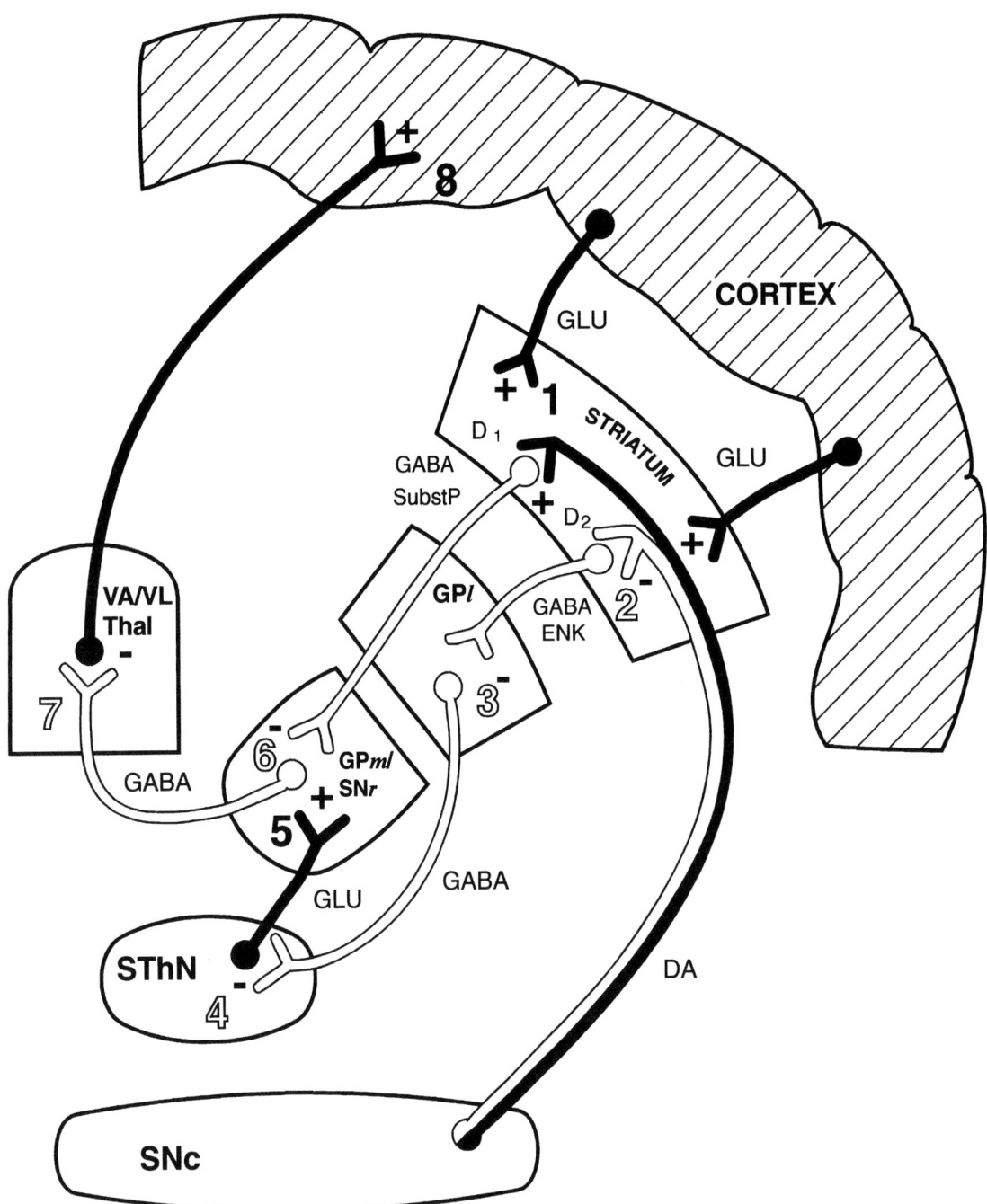

plaints are hypophonia (soft voice), dysarthria, hypomimia (expressionless face), gait difficulty, fatigue, and depression. One of these features may be present for months, or even years, before others develop.

Symptoms tend to be unilateral or asymmetrical at the outset, and this pattern may persist indefinitely. Usually, however, one can detect at least subtle dysfunction on the contralateral side with careful examination. The cardinal signs of parkinsonism are tremor, rigidity, akinesia, and disturbances of pos-

ture and equilibrium. A description of the motor examination related to these manifestations is provided in Chapter 25.

The most distinctive clinical feature of PD is the tremor; it is typically present with the limb in repose and most often affects the upper limbs. The legs or lower jaw also may be involved. Concentration on mental or physical tasks may be required to elicit it. A minority of patients have tremor predominating with sustained postures or with action, and little or none at rest. It is rare to find a patient with

◀ **FIGURE 75.2** Model of direct and indirect basal ganglia pathways. The direct striatopallidal pathway extends from the striatum to the medial globus pallidus (GP*m*) and the substantia nigra pars reticulata (SN*r*), ending at the inhibitory synapse (S) 6. The indirect striatopallidal pathway detours through the lateral globus pallidus (GP*l*) at S3 and subthalamic nucleus (SThN) at S4 before terminating in the excitatory S5 in the GP*m*-SN*r*. This model helps explain how basal ganglia disease can either reduce thalamocortical (excitatory) activity (S8), resulting in akinesia, or increase such activity, causing hyperkinesia.

In Parkinson's disease (PD), degeneration of the substantia nigra pars compacta (SNc) causes a loss of striatal dopaminergic influence, which is excitatory at S1 and inhibitory at S2. Through the direct pathway, there is reduced activity at S6, leading to an increase in the inhibitory output of GP*m*-SN*r*. In the indirect pathway, dopamine deficiency results in disinhibition of striatopallidal neurons synapsing in GP*l* (S3), which leads to reduced activity in the inhibitory pallidosubthalamic neurons (S4). This results in increased activity of subthalamic nuclear neurons and excess stimulation at S5, further enhancing the inhibitory output of GP*m*-SN*r*. The net effect via both pathways is to inhibit the ventral anterior (VA) and ventrolateral (VL) nuclei of the thalamus (Thal) at S7, thus reducing thalamocortical activity at S8. L-Dopa induces dyskinesias by increasing dopaminergic activity at S1 and S2 and reversing the sequences in both pathways.

In Huntington's disease (HD), chorea may result from predominant involvement of GABA-ENK striatal neurons in the indirect pathway projecting to GP*l*, reducing activity at S3. In turn, this causes increased inhibition of subthalamic neurons at S4, reduced stimulation of GP*m*-SN*r* at S5, decreased inhibition of VA/VL at S7, and increased thalamocortical outflow. The akinetic-rigid variant of HD may result from preferential involvement of direct pathway neurons, mimicking the effects of PD at S6, S7, and S8.

In hemiballism caused by a lesion of the SThN, reduced excitatory activity at S5 causes a reduction of inhibitory activity at S7 with a resulting increase in activity of thalamocortical neurons and more stimulation at S8.

1. Parkinson's disease
   $\downarrow 1 \rightarrow \downarrow 6$ ———
   $\downarrow 2 \rightarrow \uparrow 3 \rightarrow \downarrow 4 \rightarrow \uparrow 5$ ——— $\rightarrow \uparrow 7 \rightarrow \downarrow 8$

2. L-Dopa–induced dyskinesias
   $\uparrow 1 \rightarrow \uparrow 6$ ———
   $\uparrow 2 \rightarrow \downarrow 3 \rightarrow \uparrow 4 \rightarrow \downarrow 5$ ——— $\rightarrow \downarrow 7 \rightarrow \uparrow 8$

3. Huntington's disease
   a. Chorea
   $\downarrow 3 \rightarrow \uparrow 4 \rightarrow \downarrow 5 \rightarrow \downarrow 7 \rightarrow \uparrow 8$
   b. Akinetic-rigid variant
   $\downarrow 6 \rightarrow \uparrow 7 \rightarrow \downarrow 8$

4. Hemiballism
   $\downarrow 5 \rightarrow \downarrow 7 \rightarrow \uparrow 8$

Key to neurons, synapses, and neurotransmitters: Filled neurons = excitatory neurons; open neurons = inhibitory neurons; filled numbers = excitatory synapses; open numbers = inhibitory synapses; DA = dopamine; ENK = enkephalin; GABA = γ-aminobutyric acid; GLU = glutamate; SubstP = substance P.

untreated PD without some form of tremor, and its absence should prompt consideration of an alternative cause of the akinetic-rigid syndrome (see Chapter 25, Table 25.1). Other key points regarding the examination are the assessment of muscle tone and the observation of repetitive limb movements, gait, and handwriting (Figure 75.3).

In practice, the majority of patients with PD present no difficulty in diagnosis, showing some combination of tremor, rigidity, and akinesia. Abnormalities of posture may be found early or late, but loss of orthostatic stability (with falling) generally occurs only in advanced PD. Other manifestations that usually occur later in the course of the disease include

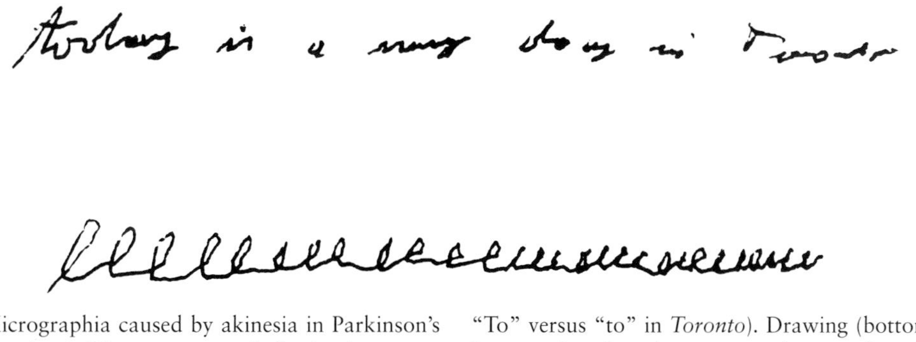

FIGURE 75.3 Micrographia caused by akinesia in Parkinson's disease. Handwriting (top): The sentence reads "today is a sunny day in Toronto." Note the progressive decrease in amplitude from the beginning to the end of the sentence (e.g., "to" in *today* versus the initial "To" in *Toronto*), as well as within a single word (e.g., "To" versus "to" in *Toronto*). Drawing (bottom): The patient is instructed to draw loops across the page from left to right. Note the progressive decline in the height and width of the loops, as well as in the interloop distance.

freezing episodes, dysphagia, and abnormalities of whole body movement including arising from a chair or turning over in bed.

Several clinical features exist whose relationship to PD is uncertain. Dementia is a particularly controversial topic, and estimates of its frequency and severity vary widely. Consensus on this issue is lacking largely because of deficient diagnostic precision for both PD and dementia. A commonly quoted figure for the incidence of dementia in PD is one in three patients, but true global dementia is probably less frequent. However, higher order cognitive disturbances suggestive of frontal lobe dysfunction are extremely common in nondemented patients with PD. Dementia is a major contributor to the increased mortality associated with PD (Lang and Lozano 1998). Autonomic disturbances, including orthostatic hypotension, intestinal motility disorders (often resulting in constipation), and bladder dysfunction, may develop in PD but are rarely disabling. Prominent and early autonomic disturbances should suggest an alternative diagnosis of multiple system atrophy (MSA) (see Striatonigral Degeneration and Multiple System Atrophy, later in this chapter). Study of both dementia and autonomic dysfunction in PD is hampered also by contamination from the side effects of antiparkinsonian medications. Ocular motor abnormalities also may form part of the clinical picture. However, these do not reach the magnitude usually seen in progressive supranuclear palsy (PSP) (see Progressive Supranuclear Palsy, later in this chapter). In general, all these features can be seen as late complications of PD, but their early appearance should lead one to suspect another diagnosis. Another common early or later feature of PD that is poorly understood is increased skin greasiness or seborrhea, especially over the forehead and face.

Investigations

Conventional laboratory studies do not contribute to the diagnosis or management of PD. Computed tomographic (CT) scans and MRI scans of the brain are normal or show only variable degrees of atrophy. Positron emission tomography (PET), using 6-[^{18}fluorine]-fluorolevodopa, shows reduced accumulation of radioisotope in the striata (especially the putamina), with a greater loss contralateral to the side most affected clinically (Plate 75.I). Single-photon emission CT using ligands, such as β-CIT, for the dopamine transporter reveal similar changes indicative of presynaptic nigral cell loss.

Pathology

Historically, pathologists have differed in their descriptions of the findings in PD, but it is now generally agreed that the major lesion involves degenerative changes in the zona compacta of the substantia nigra. This is seen grossly as a pallor of this region of the midbrain (Figure 75.4). Microscopically, there is depigmentation and loss of neurons, especially in the ventrolateral nigra; pigment granules are found extracellularly or within the cytoplasm of macrophages; and gliosis occurs. In some surviving neurons, there are cytoplasmic inclusion bodies with an eosinophilic core surrounded by a clear halo (Lewy bodies) (Plate 75.II). Similar abnormalities may be present in the locus ceruleus and dorsal motor nucleus of the vagus nerve, and other pigmented brainstem nuclei, as well as in the substantia innominata and the intermediolateral cell column of the spinal cord. The Lewy body is not entirely specific but is a highly sensitive marker for PD. When Lewy bodies occur diffusely in the cerebral cortex they may cause a condition known as dementia with Lewy bodies. Alzheimer's disease and dementia with Lewy bodies make up the main identifiable pathological substrates for dementia in PD, as they do for late-onset dementia without PD.

Depletion of the dopaminergic neurons of the substantia nigra results in reduction of striatal dopamine, which is thought to be the main biochemical abnormality in PD. However, the pathological and biochemical alterations are considerably more widespread (Table 75.3).

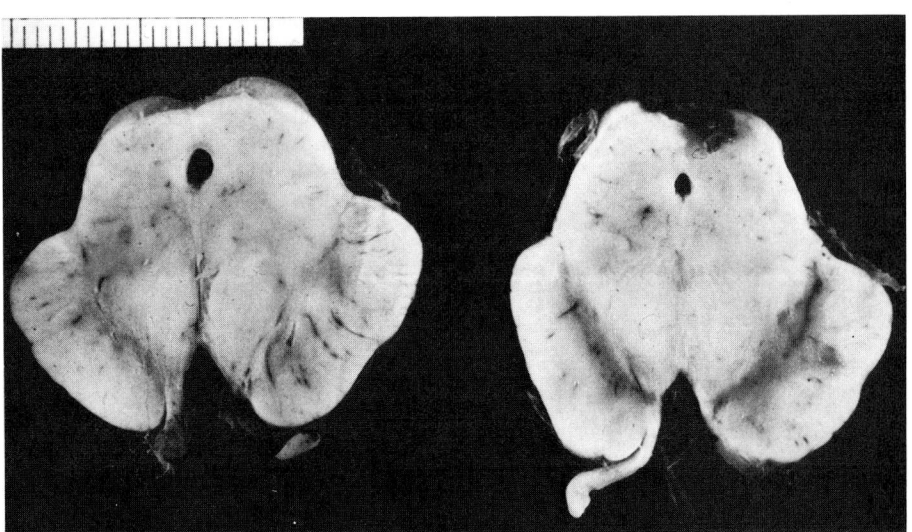

FIGURE 75.4 Depigmentation of the substantia nigra in Parkinson's disease (left). A comparable midbrain section from a normal individual of the same age is shown on the right. (Photograph courtesy of Dr. Lothar Resch.)

Table 75.3: Neurotransmitter disturbances in Parkinson's disease[a]

Neurotransmitter	Location	Severity of depletion (%)
Dopamine	Caudate, putamen	>80
	Nucleus accumbens, paraolfactory gyrus, cingulate and entorhinal cortex, hippocampus, olfactory tubercle	50–70
Norepinephrine	Neocortex, limbic forebrain	60
	Hypothalamus, nucleus intermedialis, striae terminalis	40–70
Serotonin	Frontal cortex, caudate, putamen, substantia nigra, hippocampus	50–60
Acetylcholine	Cerebral cortex, hippocampus	Variable[b]
Somatostatin	Cerebral cortex	Variable[c]
Cholecystokinin-8	Substantia nigra	30
Substance P	Substantia nigra, pallidum	30–40
Met-enkephalin	Substantia nigra, ventral tegmental area	70
	Putamen, pallidum	30–40
Leu-enkephalin	Pallidum, putamen	30–40

[a]For further details, see review by Y Agid, F Javoy-Agid, M Ruberg. Biochemistry of Neurotransmitters in Parkinson's Disease. In CD Marsden, S Fahn (eds), Movement Disorders (2nd ed). London: Butterworth–Heinemann, 1987;166–230.
[b]Most prominent in demented patients.
[c]Up to 60% in demented patients.

Etiology and Course

The cause of PD is unknown. The discovery of an acute and usually persistent illness that is caused by a toxic chemical (MPTP) and that mimics PD in nearly every detail has stimulated a search for environmental agents that might be implicated in the pathogenesis of PD. Support for an environmental cause also comes from prevalence studies that show PD crossing racial but not geographic boundaries and the lack of demonstrable genetic contribution in the majority of patients, including studies of monozygotic and dizygotic twins. However, concordance in twins may be increased in PD of younger onset. Furthermore, PD clearly is inherited in an autosomal dominant fashion in a small number of families, although most of these show atypical clinical features. Identification of a defective gene for alpha-synuclein on chromosome 4q in a few families, combined with the fact that this protein is found in abundance in all Lewy bodies studied to date in sporadic diseases (PD and dementia with Lewy bodies) as well, has opened a new avenue of research into the pathogenesis of PD. A second genetic locus on chromosome 2p is associated with more typical PD in a larger number of families. Rare pedigrees show an exclusively maternal inheritance pattern consistent with a defect in mitochondrial DNA. Whether hereditary or environmental influences are dominant, evidence exists for disturbances in oxidative phosphorylation in PD, particularly a reduction in the activity of complex I of the mitochondrial electron transport chain and increased levels of free iron, which may enhance the formation of toxic free radicals. As our understanding of these factors increases, further attempts could be made to slow or halt the progression of PD with drugs that interact or interfere with these mechanisms. Identification of a single etiology for PD may elude us because multiple endogenous and exogenous factors may contribute to the cause of PD, or PD may have entirely different etiologies in different patients.

PD mainly affects people in middle to late adult life; the mean age at onset is approximately 55–60 years. Cases beginning before 30 years of age are distinctly rare. Some studies have indicated that the age-specific incidence declines after 70 years, although this may be an artifact caused by ascertainment bias. The incidence of PD does not appear to be changing with time. Prevalence rates are significantly higher in the United States than in China or Nigeria, and American blacks have a prevalence much closer to that of American whites than to that of Nigerian blacks. A wide variety of epidemiological factors have been investigated in PD, but few consistent results have emerged. One of these is the low frequency of smoking among patients with PD. This may be caused by a protective effect of nicotine or may be an epiphenomenon caused by attrition of smokers before they can develop PD, or a long-standing personality trait in patients with PD making it less likely that they will take up the smoking habit.

The course of PD is variable, but mainly in terms of the rate rather than the mode of evolution. In most cases the disease progresses slowly but inexorably. At the ends of the spectrum there may be a benign course, with symptoms limited to one side for many years, or a rapidly progressive malignant course, with severe disability occurring over a few years. The greatest distinctions, in terms of disability, progression, and complicating factors, particularly dementia, have been drawn between patients who are predominantly akinetic and rigid with early postural instability and gait disturbances and those who suffer mainly from tremor, with the latter said to enjoy a better prognosis.

In the typical case, the illness begins with focal tremor or difficulty in using one limb. Patients may remain monosymptomatic for prolonged periods before the more full-blown syndrome develops. Eventually, the symptoms become more numerous and generalized, and the complaints change from inconvenience and embarrassment to true disability. Patients may present for medical assessment at any time, depending on the degree of symptom interference with occupation or other activities, or with self-image. Postural abnormalities enter the picture later, producing a festinating gait, retropulsion, or falls. Virtually everyone with PD has been treated with medication by the time they reach this stage, and the natural course of PD has been greatly altered by the advent of effective therapy.

Treatment

Treatment of PD remains purely symptomatic. Initially this consists of using one or more of a variety of medications; several surgical procedures may enhance later management. As with almost all movement disorders, the decision to treat PD is based largely on the degree of disability and discomfort that the patient is currently experiencing and, to a lesser extent, on the apparent rate of decline. Selection among available drugs depends on the patient's main complaint, which usually relates to tremor or akinesia.

Six types of medications are used commonly to treat PD. The oldest of these is the anticholinergic class of drugs, including trihexyphenidyl, benztropine, and ethopropazine. These are muscarinic receptor blockers, which penetrate the central nervous system (CNS) and presumably antagonize the transmission of acetylcholine by striatal interneurons. These are most effective in reducing tremor and rigidity, akinesia being little, if at all, improved. Side effects result from both central and peripheral cholinergic blockade. In the latter category are dry mouth, constipation, urinary retention, and visual blurring (from paralysis of accommodation). More disturbing are the adverse effects referable to the CNS, including lapses of memory and concentration, hallucinations, and confusion, to which elderly patients and those with previously precarious cognitive states are most vulnerable.

Amantadine was originally developed as an antiviral agent and was fortuitously found to have antiparkinsonian activity. Its mechanism of action is controversial. It is now believed that its predominant pharmacological effect is in blocking N-methyl-D-aspartate (NMDA). Its clinical effect is a relatively equal but limited relief of akinesia, rigidity, and tremor. Amantadine is the only antiparkinsonian drug that can decrease the severity of L-dopa–induced dyskinesias. Common side effects include lower extremity edema and livedo reticularis; amantadine may produce psychiatric complications similar to those caused by anticholinergic drugs.

The cornerstone of antiparkinsonian therapy is L-dopa, the immediate natural precursor of dopamine, which is converted to the deficient neurotransmitter by the enzyme aromatic amino acid decarboxylase. Initially, the use of this drug was associated with a high rate of side effects, particularly nausea and vomiting, caused by peripheral dopamine receptor stimulation. These are now largely obviated by the simultaneous administration of peripheral decarboxylase inhibitors, namely carbidopa and benserazide. L-Dopa is the most effective antiparkinsonian agent available, and it is equally beneficial for all symptoms.

Side effects are numerous, but the only common early adverse effect is nausea. This usually responds to ingestion of the drug with meals and an increase in the ratio of decarboxylase inhibitor to L-dopa, by changing from a 1 to 10 to a 1 to 4 formulation or by adding separate carbidopa to a combination carbidopa and L-dopa preparation. If this proves ineffective, pretreatment with domperidone, a peripherally acting dopamine receptor antagonist, may be necessary. Long-term (often higher dose) treatment is associated with three major categories of complications: fluctuations in the hourly "motoric" state; a wide variety of dyskinesias; and a number of psychiatric manifestations, especially hallucinations and confusion (Table 75.4). The mechanisms resulting in these difficulties are complex and incompletely understood in that they are frequently unrelated to the dosage timing and quantity. A simplified scheme of management of these and other problems associated with chronic treatment with L-dopa is provided in Table 75.5.

The direct dopamine agonists are analogues of dopamine that directly stimulate the receptors for the neurotransmitter. At least two general classes of dopamine receptor exist, one coupled to adenylate cyclase (D1) and another not so linked (D2). Most effective antiparkinsonian dopamine agonists stimulate D2 receptors predominantly. The importance of individual receptor types to normal and aberrant motor function is not fully understood.

Bromocriptine, pergolide, cabergoline, lisuride, pramipexole, ropinirole, and apomorphine are dopamine agonists. The spectrum of side effects is similar to that of L-dopa, with a lower occurrence of dyskinesias but a greater tendency to produce adverse mental reactions. Most of the dopamine agonists have comparable clinical benefit. Apomorphine may be administered by nasal spray, sublingually, subcutaneously, or by suppository, and thus may be particularly useful when rapid benefit is desired. The first four agonists in the previous list are ergot derivatives. Rarely, these are capable of inducing a pleuropulmonary reaction or retroperitoneal fibrosis.

Selegiline (deprenyl) is a selective inhibitor of monoamine oxidase B. By blocking the metabolism of central dopamine, this drug may improve a patient's response to L-dopa, especially in those with mild to moderate dose-related fluctuations or "wearing off." Some evidence exists that this agent also might have a neuroprotective effect; however, this remains controversial. A more effective method of blocking dopamine metabolism involves inhibition of the enzyme catechol-O-methyltransferase (COMT). Tolcapone and entacapone are COMT inhibitors that prolong the benefit of L-dopa by extending the life span of the dopamine to which it is converted. Tolcapone may cause severe hepatotoxicity and is the only drug for PD requiring regular laboratory monitoring. COMT inhibitors also may enhance

Table 75.4: Late-stage problems in L-dopa–treated Parkinson's disease

Drug-related
  Reduction in efficacy (simply related to progression of under-lying disease?)
  Dyskinesias
    Dystonia
      Morning dystonia (usually in feet)
      Off-period dystonia (when benefit of medication is exhausted)
      Peak dose dystonia (occurring at presumed time of maximum serum level)
    Chorea/athetosis
      Peak dose
      Square wave (present throughout duration of benefit from each dose)
      Beginning of dose, end of dose (occurring at onset and end of dose-related benefit, respectively; diphasic when both occur)
    Myoclonus
    Other (rare): includes asterixis, tics
  Fluctuations
    Wearing-off
      Morning akinesia
      End-of-dose akinesia (off symptoms sometimes more severe during initial wearing-off phase [super off])
    Increased latency to individual dose responses
    Periodic doses ineffective
    Sudden unpredictable fluctuations (the on-off phenomenon)
  Psychiatric disturbances
    Vivid dreams, nightmares, altered sleep patterns (including rapid eye movement behavior disorder)
    Benign (insight retained) hallucinations (usually visual)
    Paranoid psychosis
    Mania
    Toxic confusional state
Disease-related[a] (often resistant to therapy)
  Motor
    Postural instability with falls
    Severe freezing
    Speech disturbances
    Increasing parkinsonism
  Cognitive and affective
    Depression
    Bradyphrenia
    Dementia
  Sensory disturbances
    A variety of sensory complaints, including pain
    Akathisia
  Autonomic[b]
    Postural hypotension
    Urinary disturbances
    Gastrointestinal hypomotility
    Sexual dysfunction

[a]Several of these, such as depression and sensory complaints, are not limited to the later stages of the disease.
[b]Several of these disturbances are aggravated by antiparkinsonian therapy.

Table 75.5: Management of complications in L-dopa–treated Parkinson's disease

Complication	Management
Nausea	Administer drug with meals*
	Increase decarboxylase inhibitor to L-dopa ratio
	Domperidone before each dose*
Orthostatic hypotension	Increase salt intake*
	Elevate head of bed*
	Compressive stockings*
	Mineralocorticoids*
	Midodrine*
	Domperidone*
Dyskinesias	
Peak dose	Lower the dose
	Amantadine
	Try liquid preparation for more graded titration
Beginning of dose and/or end of dose	Increase the dose
	Shorten dose interval
	Add direct dopamine agonist
	Amantadine
Morning dystonia	Earlier morning dose of L-dopa
	Add direct dopamine agonist
	?Lithium, baclofen, amantadine
Nocturnal myoclonus	Eliminate evening L-dopa dose
	Clonazepam (also useful for rapid eye movement behavior disorder)
	?Methysergide, tricyclic antidepressant
Freezing episodes (not necessarily on L-dopa)	Low-obstacle visual cues
	Rhythmic routines
Fluctuations	
Predictable wearing off or unpredictable	Shorten the dose interval
	Increase the dose
	Catechol-O-methyltransferase inhibitor
	Add direct dopamine agonist or selegiline
	Low-protein diet
	Controlled-release L-dopa formulations
	Experimental therapies, such as duodenal infusion of L-dopa (via nasogastric or gastrostomy tube), or subcutaneous infusion of dopamine agonist (e.g., apomorphine, lisuride)
Ineffective or missed doses	If pills, crush before ingestion
	If pills, dissolve in carbonated beverage
	Avoid taking with meals
	Low-protein diet
Hallucinations or confusion	Withdraw anticholinergic drug
	Withdraw amantadine
	Withdraw selegiline
	Reduce or withdraw dopamine agonis
	Withdraw catechol-O-methyltransferase inhibitor
	Atypical, dopamine antagonist (e.g., clozapine, quetiapine, olanzapine)
	?Electroconvulsive therapy

*Also useful for bromocriptine-, pergolide-, pramipexole-, and ropinirole-treated patients.

Table 75.6:   Rank order in management choices for wearing-off fluctuations

Attribute	First order	Second order	Third order
Efficacy (high to low)	COMT inhibitors	CR L-dopa Dopamine agonists	Amantadine Seligiline Low-protein diet
Ease of use (high to low)	Amantadine Seligiline	COMT inhibitors	CR L-dopa Dopamine agonists Low-protein diet
Risk of dyskinesias (low to high)	Amantadine	Low-protein diet Seligiline Dopamine agonists	CR L-dopa COMT inhibitors
Risk of cognitive side effects (low to high)	None	CR L-dopa COMT inhibitors Seligiline Low-protein diet	Amantadine Dopamine agonists
Cost (low to high)	Amantadine	CR L-dopa COMT inhibitors Low-protein diet	Dopamine agonists Seligiline

COMT = catechol-O-methyltransferase; CR = controlled-release.

L-dopa–induced side effects, particularly dyskinesias, and a reduction in L-dopa dose is often necessary.

There is no consensus regarding the management of PD. A particularly thorny issue is the timing of initiating L-dopa therapy; conflicting views would have one believe that early L-dopa treatment is ultimately either beneficial to longevity or detrimental in the development of side effects. Some have advocated the simultaneous initiation of L-dopa and a dopamine agonist when therapy with either is indicated, based on studies showing a lower frequency of fluctuations and dyskinesias than are produced by monotherapy with L-dopa. However, this approach is not universally accepted (Factor and Weiner 1993). Many PD specialists now begin treatment with a dopamine agonist alone, adding L-dopa when disability is not adequately controlled.

Once symptoms reach the point of requiring therapy, a rational approach is to use anticholinergics and amantadine for minor isolated symptoms, but to start L-dopa and a peripheral decarboxylase inhibitor, or a dopamine agonist, with the first evidence of disability. The dose of L-dopa should be 300 mg to begin with, and increased to 400–600 mg if necessary. Sufficient dopa decarboxylase inhibitor must be given to block the peripheral enzyme completely. In the case of carbidopa (in Sinemet), this requires 75–150 mg or more per day in divided doses.

Where L-dopa–related fluctuations are concerned, there are a number of alternatives with many contrasting features to consider (Table 75.6). The variety of choices is a positive development for patients but makes it difficult to make blanket recommendations regarding the best approach to treatment. The decision about which option to pursue must be modified according to the patient's mental status, economic means, and experience with side effects from other medications. Certain attributes will be primary or secondary considerations, depending on the patient to be treated. For example, ease of use is a feature reflecting the properties of uniformity of dosing and the ability to reach a rapid conclusion regarding efficacy, which are particularly attractive in elderly or demented patients. Amantadine and selegiline are easy to use because they are manufactured in only one strength (although amantadine is also available as a syrup) and have little variation in dosing (amantadine, one capsule two or three times daily; selegiline, one tablet once or twice a day). Thus, they might be good choices for patients who have trouble following complicated medication schedules. Unfortunately, neither is frequently useful in reducing fluctuations. If the patient has existing problems with confusion or psychosis, either controlled-release L-dopa or a COMT inhibitor (always given with an L-dopa preparation) may be the preferred choice, but if the patient already has difficulty with dyskinesias, one may opt to try another agent first. Amantadine may merit first consideration in some patients because it is the only agent that may simultaneously improve parkinsonism and peak-dose dyskinesias. Tolcapone is the only antiparkinsonian drug requiring laboratory monitoring (for liver dysfunction). A protein-restriction diet is the cheapest alternative.

Increased understanding of physiological disturbances in the basal ganglia in PD, as well as technical improvements, have led to an increased tendency to apply surgical solutions to problems in PD management. Stereotaxic thalamotomy should be considered in patients with predominant tremor that is resistant to available pharmacological therapy. High-frequency thalamic stimulation is an effective alternative to thalamotomy, with fewer permanent complications. Rigidity may also improve, but akinesia, usually the most disabling feature of PD, remains unaltered by thalamic surgery. Medial pallidotomy and pallidal stimulation are highly effective in diminishing contralateral L-dopa–induced dyskinesias and frequently abolish tremor as well. They are also more beneficial than thalamic procedures for akinetic symptoms, but this effect is inconsistent. Subthalamic nucleus stimulation has shown the most improvement in akinesia and may ultimately prove to be the site of choice for stereotaxic lesioning if preliminary results hold true. Studies of brain implantation for PD, using fetal human or porcine substantia nigra, are progressing. Further research is required before the practical applicability of this and other experimental approaches is known.

Postencephalitic Parkinsonism

Between 1916 and 1927, a worldwide epidemic of encephalitis lethargica (sleeping sickness) took place, affecting as many as 750,000 people. Approximately one-third of them died acutely, another one-third recovered completely, and the remainder were left with chronic neurological deficits. Although previous outbreaks of the disease probably occurred in the seventeenth and eighteenth centuries, it was by studying the initial victims of the great epidemic of the early twentieth century that von Economo in 1917 first came to describe its neurological manifestations and sequelae.

Clinical Features

The great majority of patients with chronic postencephalitic complications exhibit parkinsonism, which could emerge at the time of the acute encephalitis, or any time until 20 years later or more. However, the latency was less than 5 years in 50% and less than 10 years in 85% of patients. Up to one-fourth of patients with typical manifestations of postencephalitic parkinsonism do not give a history of antecedent encephalitis.

Parkinsonism following encephalitis lethargica can be indistinguishable from the manifestations of PD, and the diagnosis is based on the associated historical details and additional abnormal signs. Most patients have a history of an acute febrile illness with extreme lethargy. Other notable features of the acute period include behavioral and mental disturbances, changes in sleep patterns, ocular motor dysfunction, and a wide spectrum of other movement disorders. The same clinical abnormalities, if persistent, help to distinguish chronic postencephalitic parkinsonism from the idiopathic variety. Oculogyric crises were a particularly common and unique phenomenon of the disease.

Once established, the neurological deficits show extremely slow progression, much slower than is observed in PD. Other clinical features seen in a significant proportion of these patients include various forms of dystonia, chorea (including buccolingual masticatory movements similar to those of tardive dyskinesia [TD]), myoclonus, assorted respiratory disturbances, tics, pyramidal tract signs, and a variety of behavioral changes. These patients tend to tolerate anticholinergic agents better (often in very high doses) and L-dopa less well (because of psychiatric disturbances and dyskinesias) than those with PD.

Pathogenesis and Epidemiology

Although a virus is presumed to have been the causative agent of encephalitis lethargica, none has ever been identified. Several acute viral encephalitides may be associated with transient or self-limited parkinsonism. However, whether other viral encephalitides can produce chronic parkinsonism is controversial. The only common laboratory abnormality is a mild lymphocytosis in the spinal fluid. The gross pathological findings in acute cases are normal, but microscopically, vascular engorgement with perivascular inflammation and neuronal necrosis are seen, affecting mainly the midbrain and basal ganglia. In chronic cases the substantia nigra is uniformly depigmented. Its neurons are greatly reduced in number, and many surviving nerve cells contain neurofibrillary tangles. Perivascular mononuclear infiltrations may persist. Similar microscopic changes may be found throughout the brainstem, basal ganglia, and cortex.

Encephalitis lethargica showed no age, race, or sex preference. During the epidemic, a much higher incidence was noted in the winter and early spring in Europe and North America, and in the summer in Japan. Although some clusters were recorded, the disease was not considered contagious.

There have been no reported epidemics of encephalitis lethargica since 1930. At its peak it was probably responsible for two-thirds of all cases of parkinsonism; today it is a diagnostic rarity. Nevertheless, there is little doubt that sporadic cases of postencephalitic parkinsonism continue to occur (Blunt et al. 1997). Some of these patients have demonstrated oligoclonal banding in the spinal fluid. The diagnosis should be suspected in any parkinsonian patient, particularly with a young onset, showing florid psychiatric disturbances, sleep-cycle alterations, or ocular motor deficits, with or without a history of encephalitis.

Progressive Supranuclear Palsy

In 1964, Steele, Richardson, and Olszewski reported the clinical and pathological findings in PSP. They described a progressive illness consisting of a vertical supranuclear ophthalmoplegia, pseudobulbar palsy, axial rigidity, and mild dementia with pathological features of neuronal loss, neurofibrillary tangles, gliosis, and granulovacuolar degeneration in the basal ganglia and upper brainstem neurons.

Clinical Features

The clinical manifestations begin in the sixth or seventh decade of life. The most common presenting symptoms are an unsteady gait with a propensity to sudden falls (Litvan 1998), particularly backward, dysarthria or dysphonia, intellectual or psychiatric deficits, and visual complaints. A wide-eyed stare with elevated eyebrows, furrowed forehead, lack of eye contact, and slow, slurred speech with a strained voice frequently suggest the diagnosis on meeting the patient. Other common findings include axial rigidity out of proportion to that in the limbs, brisk facial reflexes, akinesia, and a gait abnormality that is often difficult to characterize. Dementia is common but usually remains mild.

The most distinctive clinical feature, and the sine qua non for the premortem diagnosis of PSP, is a vertical supranuclear gaze palsy, usually affecting downward more than upward gaze (Figure 75.5). The supranuclear aspect of the ophthalmoplegia is demonstrated by the lack of voluntary movement of the eyes, even though the nuclear mechanisms for eye movements are preserved, as demonstrated by the presence of normal reflex eye movements. Saccades are the first movements affected. In the early stages this may be detectable only as a loss of the fast component of optokinetic nystagmus. Later, pursuit movements become involved. There is preservation of the vestibulo-ocular reflex, caloric responses (slow phases), and Bell's phenomenon, the last being more variable than the others. Eventually, these too may be abolished when the cranial nerve nuclei become affected. Horizontal eye movements may deteriorate in the same sequence. Other ocular motor and eyelid motor abnormalities are common in PSP. Cases without ocular motor abnormalities during life have been described.

Generally, this is a sporadic disorder, but more recently possible genetic factors have been emphasized with the description of autosomal dominant inheritance in a small number of families and a significant association between more typical sporadic cases and a homozygote state of the A0 allele of the *tau* gene.

Investigations

The major value of diagnostic investigations is to exclude other conditions that may produce similar manifestations, such as hydrocephalus or multiple infarctions. A CT or MRI scan may demonstrate cerebral atrophy, especially of the midbrain; however, the diagnosis of PSP remains purely clinical. The clinical picture is frequently mistaken for that of PD, especially if the eye movement abnormalities are not prominent. Helpful distinguishing features of PSP include early gait and speech disturbances and little or no tremor. Patients with a greater degree of asymmetry, including limb dystonia, may be mistaken for cortical-basal ganglionic degeneration (CBGD) (see Cortical-Basal Ganglionic Degeneration, later in this chapter).

Pathology

The gross pathology shows only a small midbrain and enlarged sylvian aqueduct and third ventricle. Microscopically, there is gliosis and neuronal loss with prominent neurofibrillary tangles (Figure 75.6) containing abnormally phosphorylated tau protein. Other pathological hallmarks include glial fibrillary tangles, neuropil threads, and granulovacuolar degeneration. The areas chiefly affected are the globus pallidus, subthalamic nucleus, substantia nigra, superior colliculi, pretectal nuclei, and periaqueductal gray matter. Degeneration of portions of the cerebral cortex is recognized increasingly. In keeping with the prominent substantia nigra lesions, the levels of dopamine and homovanillic acid in the caudate and putamen are greatly reduced in PSP. However, dopamine D2 receptors are also decreased in the striatum, suggesting that in PSP, unlike PD, striatal neurons including cholinergic interneurons are affected as well. This notion is supported by the reduction of choline acetyltransferase activity in the striatum. Ultrastructurally, the neurofibrillary tangles are predominantly straight filaments rather than the paired helical filaments found in Alzheimer's disease, but both types of tangles can be found in either condition and they appear to be antigenically identical. A comparative postmortem study of postencephalitic parkinsonism and PSP has suggested the possibility of an etiological relationship between the two disorders (Geddes et al. 1993).

Course and Treatment

PSP is relentlessly progressive, with a median survival from time of onset of less than 6 years; the cause of death is usually pneumonia. Treatment of the disease is largely unrewarding. In some patients the rigidity and akinesia may respond to antiparkinsonian agents, but the effect is usually transient. More often, there is little or no response to these agents, another feature that serves to distinguish PSP from PD. The additional basal ganglia pathology downstream from the nigrostriatal pathway probably explains the failure of direct dopamine agonists and anticholinergics, as well as L-dopa, to relieve the symptoms of PSP. Infrequent success has been noted with tricyclic antidepressants and amantadine. The most life-threatening complication of PSP is the dysphagia. Efforts to avoid aspiration may include diet alteration, cricopharyngeal myotomy, nasogastric intubation, or gastrostomy.

Striatonigral Degeneration and Multiple System Atrophy

The discovery of the oligodendroglial inclusion has provided conclusive evidence that three disorders, striatonigral degeneration, adult-onset sporadic olivopontocerebellar (OPCA), and Shy-Drager syndrome belong under the single rubric of MSA (Quinn 1994). The first descriptions of striatonigral degeneration came during the early 1960s, when Adams, van Bogaert, and Vander Ecken outlined the unusual pathological findings in a small number of patients clinically diagnosed as having PD. They found atrophy and discoloration in the putamina and depigmentation of the substantia nigra. Microscopically, severe neuronal loss and gliosis had occurred in these structures and, to a lesser extent, in the globus pallidus and the caudate and subthalamic nuclei. Lewy bodies were found in two of four cases. The distinction from PD was made on the basis of the striking striatal degeneration. In the past, the term *OPCA* has

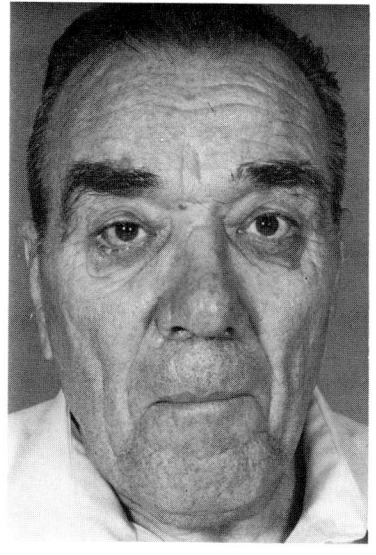

A

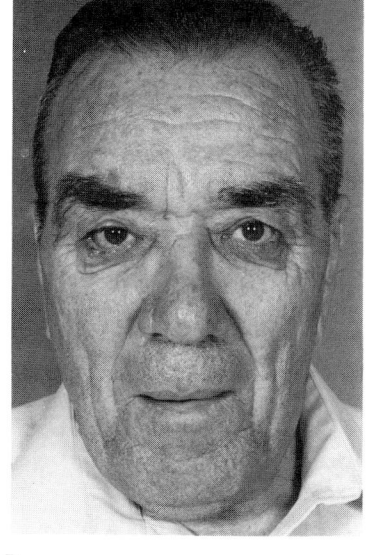

B

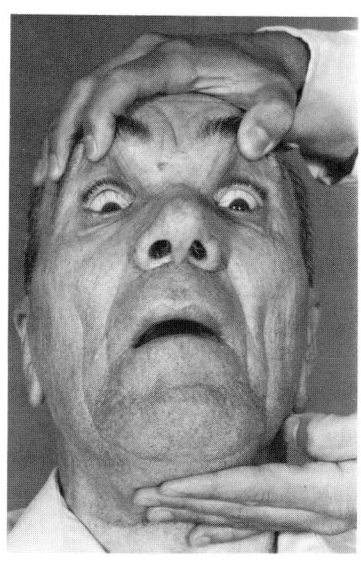

C

FIGURE 75.5 Facial appearance and supranuclear gaze palsy in progressive supranuclear palsy. (**A**) Patient looking straight at the camera. Note the characteristic wide-eyed stare (asymmetrical here) with furrowing of the forehead. There is also deepening of other facial creases, such as the nasolabial folds. (**B**) Attempted downward gaze (note descent of eyebrows). (**C**) Full downward gaze elicited with the vestibulo-ocular reflex. (**D**) Attempted upward gaze. (**E**) Much greater upgaze is achieved with the vestibulo-ocular reflex. (**F, G**) Voluntary horizontal eye movements are relatively less affected, but still slightly limited.

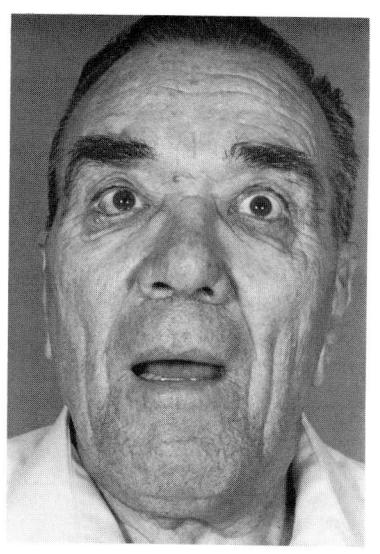

D

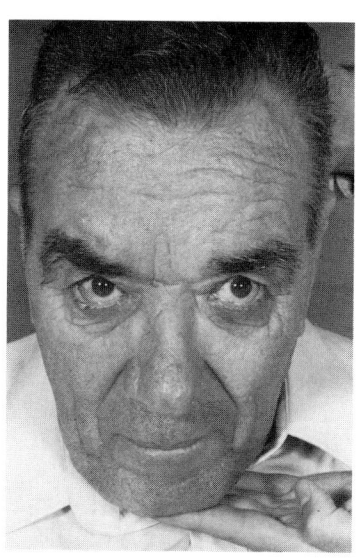

E

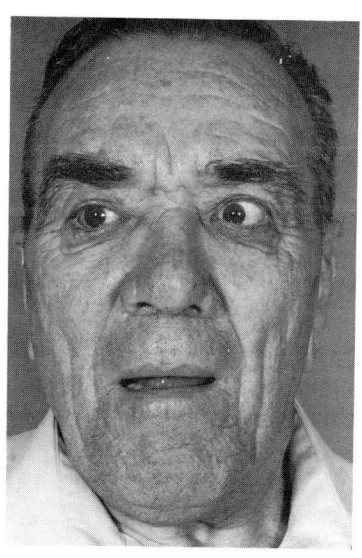

F

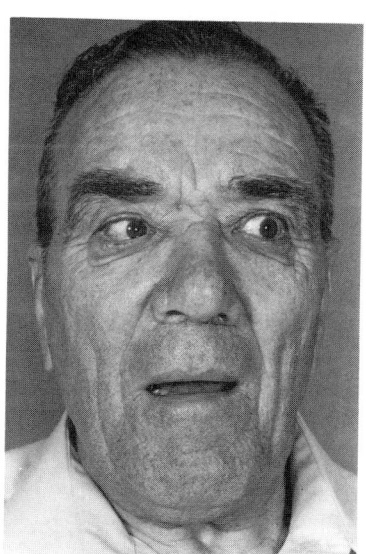

G

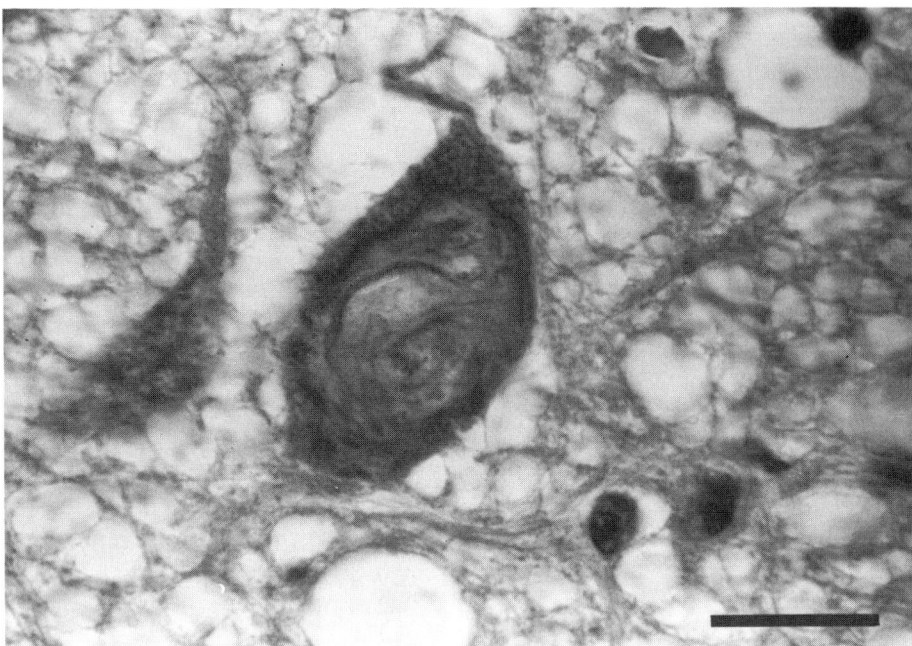

FIGURE 75.6 A typical globose neurofibrillary tangle present in a midbrain neuron of a patient with progressive supranuclear palsy (hematoxylin and eosin stain). (Courtesy of Dr. Lothar Resch.)

been applied to both sporadic and familial cases. Now, most inherited cases are classified as forms of spinocerebellar ataxia (see Chapter 76), whereas a large proportion of adult-onset sporadic cases are probably examples of MSA. Pathologically, these brains show variable degeneration in the inferior olives, ventral pontine nuclei, and cerebellar cortex, as well as a number of other areas including the substantia nigra and striatum. Finally, Shy and Drager, in 1960, first described a disease of adult onset characterized by the progressive development of autonomic deficits. The major pathological lesion was a striking degeneration of the sympathetic preganglionic neurons in the intermediolateral cell column of the thoracic and upper lumbar spinal cord (Figure 75.7), resulting in symptoms of orthostatic hypotension, impaired gastrointestinal motility, and urinary and sexual dysfunction. Even at the time of this first report, additional pathological features as are found in OPCA and striatonigral degeneration were described.

It is now recognized that dysautonomia (of varying degrees) is a nearly universal feature of patients with MSA.

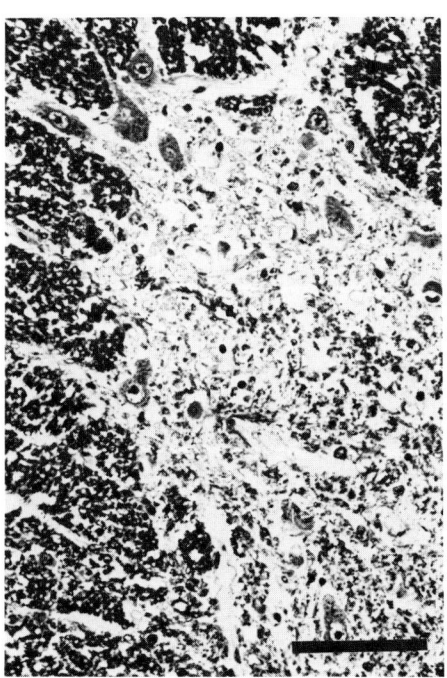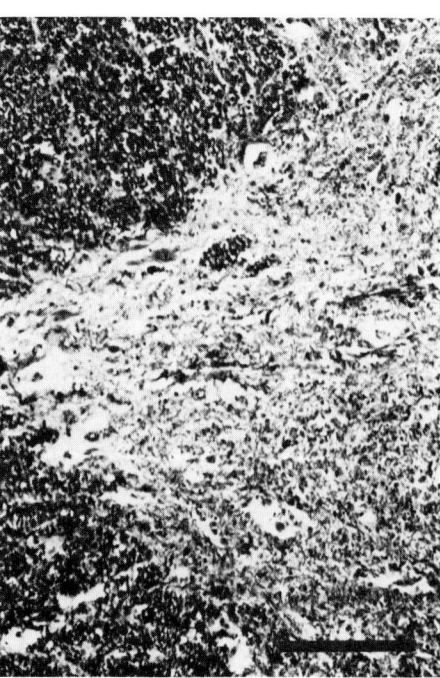

FIGURE 75.7 Microscopic spinal cord pathology of Shy-Drager syndrome. On the left is a section of the intermediolateral column from a normal thoracic spinal cord. On the right is a loss of volume and neuronal depletion in the intermediolateral column from a patient with Shy-Drager syndrome (Luxol fast blue and hematoxylin and eosin stains combined). (Courtesy of Dr. Lothar Resch.)

Thus the term *Shy-Drager syndrome* serves little purpose and is best avoided. In addition to dysautonomia, patients with MSA most often present with a predominantly parkinsonian form of the disorder (caused by striatonigral degeneration pathology) or a largely cerebellar form (caused by OPCA pathology). Acknowledging these symptom-predominant forms, the terms *MSA-P* (for parkinsonism; alternatively, the striatonigral degeneration form of MSA) and *MSA-C* (for cerebellar; alternatively, the OPCA form of MSA) have been proposed. Although most patients demonstrate one of these two forms, many have overlapping features, often with additional pyramidal tract deficits such as pathologically brisk deep tendon reflexes and extensor plantar responses.

Clinical and Pathological Features

No clinical features have emerged that distinguish pure striatonigral degeneration from PD. Tremor is said to be less prominent in the former, and the response to dopaminergic agents usually has been poor, but these cannot be used as reliable criteria for diagnosis in individual patients. The age and sex distribution is the same in the two conditions. The clinical state deteriorates progressively at a variable rate until death, much as in untreated or unresponsive PD. Proof of uncomplicated striatonigral degeneration requires an autopsy. The diagnosis is suggested antemortem by a progressive akinetic-rigid syndrome that is poorly responsive to antiparkinsonian therapy. Additional features of prominent dysautonomia (often predating the parkinsonism) and cerebellar ataxia strongly suggest the diagnosis of MSA. Stimulus-sensitive myoclonus of limbs and facial muscles, poor postural stability with the early need for a wheelchair, extreme anteroflexion of the neck, corticospinal tract signs, dusky discoloration of the extremities, slurred or scanning speech, dysphonia, stridor, and severe cranial dystonia in response to L-dopa are other clues to the diagnosis of MSA.

Heavily weighted T2 MRI may show low-intensity signal in the putamen (possibly caused by excessive iron deposition) equal to or greater than that normally present in the globus pallidus, and a linear hyperintensity lateral to the putamen (Figure 75.8) (also seen on proton density scans). MRI also shows pronounced atrophy of the putamen, especially the posterior part. In those with MSA-C (OPCA form), there may be cerebellar and pontine atrophy (Figure 75.9), often with altered signal in the middle cerebellar peduncles and basis pontis on MRI.

Pathological examination demonstrates neuronal loss and gliosis in a variety of sites, especially in the striatum (putamen more than caudate), substantia nigra, locus ceruleus, inferior olive, pontine nuclei, Purkinje's cells of the cerebellum, intermediolateral cell column of the thoracic spinal cord, and Onuf's nucleus. A hallmark of MSA is the widespread presence of argyrophilic oligodendroglial inclusions or glial cytoplasmic inclusions in suprasegmental motor systems and supraspinal autonomic systems, and in their target nuclei (Papp and Lantos 1994). It has been suggested

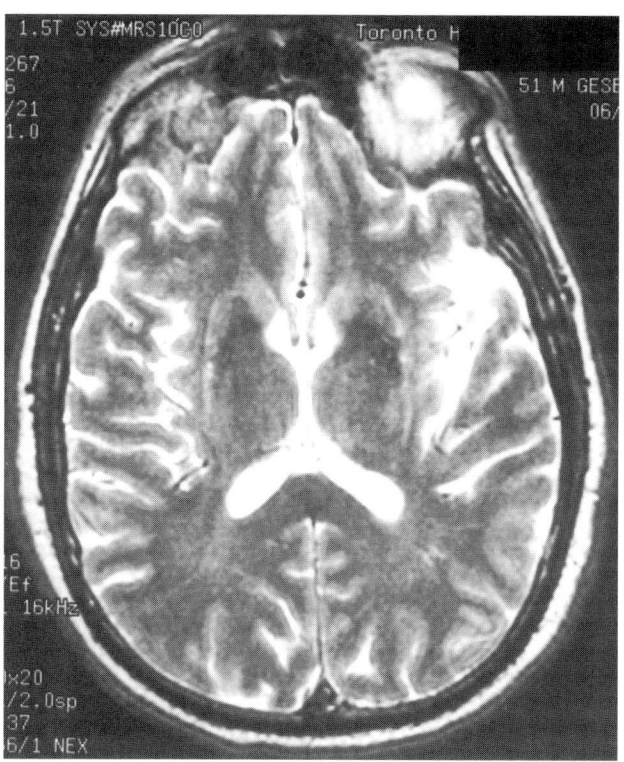

FIGURE 75.8 T2-weighted magnetic resonance imaging scan of a patient with multiple system atrophy demonstrating putaminal atrophy and linear hyperintensity at the lateral margin of the putamen.

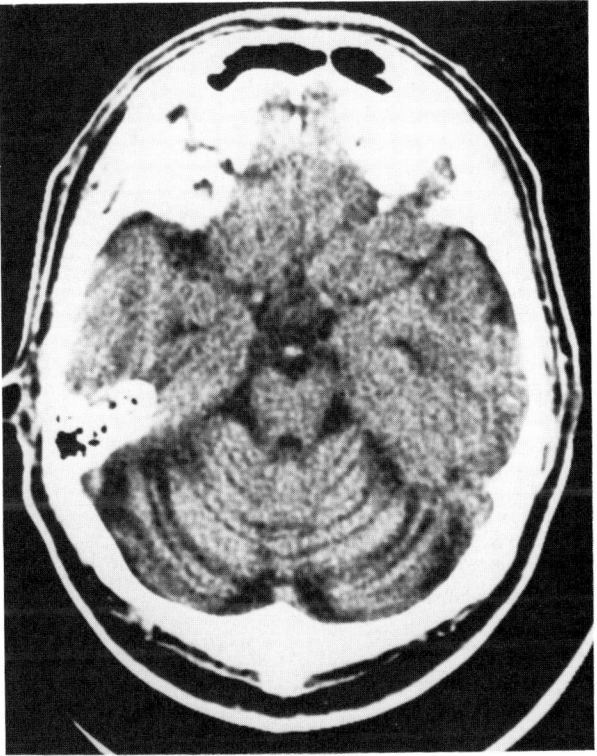

FIGURE 75.9 Computed tomographic scan in olivopontocerebellar atrophy, demonstrating severe atrophy of the cerebellum and brainstem.

that inclusion-bearing oligodendroglial degeneration may cause or contribute to the clinical manifestations even before neuronal alterations occur. However, glial cytoplasmic inclusions are not exclusive to MSA, and should be considered analogous to Lewy bodies in PD.

Treatment and Course

The management of patients with MSA is usually complex. Parkinsonism may respond markedly to L-dopa, especially early on, but the response is usually incomplete and short-lived. Autonomic side effects, particularly orthostatic hypotension, are extremely common and often provide the first clue to the diagnosis. Treatment of these autonomic disturbances can be quite problematic; however, opportunity for symptomatic treatment of hypotension, urinary retention or incontinence, impotence, and bowel dysfunction exists (see Chapter 81). The parkinsonism of MSA often progresses relatively rapidly compared with typical PD, with death occurring from the complications of severe neurological dysfunction within 4–10 years of onset.

Cortical-Basal Ganglionic Degeneration

CBGD encompasses features pointing to dysfunction in both the cerebral cortex and basal ganglia. Like PSP and striatonigral degeneration, it was first described in the 1960s. In recent years it has been recognized with increased frequency, and it is now a major consideration in the differential diagnosis of parkinsonism.

Clinical Features

The onset of symptoms occurs in the sixth decade or later. Typical basal ganglia manifestations include signs of parkinsonism (akinesia, rigidity, disequilibrium) and limb dystonia. A postural or action tremor and focal reflex myoclonus are also common. Cerebral cortical involvement is signaled by apraxia, cortical sensory loss, and the alien limb phenomenon. Other features may include athetosis, orolingual dyskinesias, frontal lobe reflexes, impaired ocular or eyelid motion, dysarthria, speech apraxia, dementia, hyperreflexia, and Babinski's signs. These findings may occur in any combination and in any chronological sequence, so a wide variety of possible clinical presentations exists. However, CBGD is typically highly asymmetrical at onset and throughout its course, and the summation of multiple motor disorders often produces a characteristic stiff, dystonic, jerky, useless arm.

Investigations

CT scan or MRI usually demonstrates some degree of cerebral atrophy, often more striking contralateral to the side where clinical manifestations are more severe. PET scanning may show asymmetrical reduction of cortical metabolism using fluorodeoxyglucose, and striatal tracer uptake using fluorolevodopa. However, these studies are normal in some patients, and there is no test that is especially sensitive or specific for CBGD. Electroencephalography, nerve conduction studies, electromyography, and evoked potential studies usually yield normal results.

Pathology

Cerebral atrophy can almost always be appreciated macroscopically, predominantly in the medial frontal and parietal lobes. Atrophy is usually asymmetrical, more prominent opposite the side of greater clinical impairment. Depigmentation of the substantia nigra is the other common gross finding. Microscopically, in the areas of cortical atrophy one sees neuronal loss, gliosis, and vacuolation, particularly in layers III and V. Surviving neurons may exhibit achromasia and immunoreactivity to phosphorylated neurofilament epitopes. Cortical plaques containing abnormal tau in distal astrocytic processes (astrocytic plaques) are a hallmark of the disorder (Feany and Dickson 1995). In the substantia nigra, neuronal loss, pigmentary incontinence, and gliosis occur. Surviving nigral cells may show weakly basophilic cytoplasmic inclusions. Degenerative changes also may be found in the subthalamic nucleus, red nucleus, lateral thalamic nuclei, globus pallidus, and elsewhere. When the same pathology has an anterior cortical predominance, the clinical presentation may simulate a frontotemporal dementia, whereas more lateral dominant hemisphere frontal lobe changes may result in a primary progressive aphasia rather than the classical CBGD syndrome described previously.

Course and Treatment

CBGD progresses in a gradual fashion. Abnormalities may remain limited to one limb for up to a few years, but inevitably there is spread to generalized involvement. New motor disorders may supplant others, or evolve from them, as myoclonus often develops from an irregular tremor. However, the trend is always one of further disability. The clinical manifestations of CBGD are notoriously resistant to symptomatic therapy. In particular, L-dopa does not produce any significant or sustained improvement. Clonazepam may help the myoclonus. Late-onset dysphagia poses the greatest threat to a patient's survival.

Parkinsonism-Dementia Complex of Guam

The recognition of a high incidence of parkinsonism, amyotrophic lateral sclerosis, and dementia among the Chamorro population of Guam suggests an endemic cause for these disorders. Other pockets of these diseases have been noted in West New Guinea and the Kii peninsula of Japan. In subsequent years the high incidence of these disorders significantly decreased.

The parkinsonism is similar to that of PD, with the exception that tremor is not often prominent. The most striking feature is that it is invariably accompanied by progressive dementia. The majority of patients also have clinical signs of motor neuron disease, and a small proportion may have features similar to those of PSP. Pathological findings include gross cerebral atrophy, with widespread neuronal loss in the cerebral cortex, basal ganglia, brainstem, and cerebellum. Abundant neurofibrillary tangles are present throughout these structures, although senile plaques and Lewy bodies are not present. The pathogenic similarity between this disorder, PSP, and postencephalitic parkinsonism suggests possible overlapping etiologic factors (Geddes et al. 1993).

The pathogenesis of this vanishing epidemiological curiosity is unknown. The strongest evidence seems to favor an environmental cause related to calcium and magnesium deprivation or to ingestion of toxic plant material, particularly cycads. Genetic factors also may contribute in some fashion to development of the disorder. The decrease of parkinsonism-dementia and amyotrophic lateral sclerosis in these hyperendemic foci has been attributed to exposure of isolated peoples to Western living and dietary customs.

Other Parkinsonian Syndromes

A number of other conditions may cause the clinical manifestations of parkinsonism. The most important consideration in this differential diagnosis is Wilson's disease (see later section). Among the degenerative diseases, progressive pallidal atrophy is characterized by the onset, usually in childhood, of parkinsonism and dystonia, with gradual progression to death over the course of 20 or more years. Several variants have been described. Parkinsonism also may complicate Alzheimer's disease and a number of less common degenerative disorders (see Chapter 25, Table 25.1).

The concept of vascular parkinsonism has enjoyed a resurgence in recent years. The pathological basis is usually multiple lacunar infarctions, probably involving the corpus striatum more often than the substantia nigra. Other vascular causes include parkinsonism contralateral to a single infarct, Binswanger's encephalopathy, dilatated perivascular spaces, vasculitides, and amyloid angiopathy. Vascular disease may account for cases of parkinsonism predominantly affecting the lower body, with severe gait disturbances and freezing but little or no upper limb dysfunction.

Parkinsonism is a rare sequela of head trauma, where it is probably related to midbrain hemorrhage. Such patients invariably show other evidence of brainstem dysfunction. Repetitive trauma as seen in boxers may result in progressive parkinsonism as well as dementia (dementia pugilistica). Here the disorder consists of diffuse neuronal loss and neurofibrillary tangle formation. Parkinsonism has been found in association with both obstructive and communicating hydrocephalus. Symptoms and signs may resolve with decompressive therapy and recur with blockage of the shunt. The pathophysiology is obscure, but patients may respond to L-dopa therapy, suggesting dysfunction of the nigrostriatal pathway, possibly on a compressive basis.

Side effects of neuroleptic drugs, including the psychotropics such as the phenothiazines and the butyrophenones, and the antiemetic metoclopramide, represent one of the most common causes of secondary parkinsonism (see Drug-Induced Movement Disorders, later in this chapter). A variety of other drugs also may produce parkinsonian manifestations (Riley 1998). Acute poisoning with carbon monoxide or cyanide and chronic exposure to manganese are among the toxic processes reported to cause parkinsonism. A striking example of neurotoxicity was demonstrated in the early 1980s when some intravenous drug abusers developed acute parkinsonism following injection of MPTP, an impurity formed during processing of synthetic narcotics. The ability of MPTP toxicity to mimic the clinical and pathological features of PD and to reproduce them in animals has led to an explosion of research into the mechanism of action of MPTP and the use of animal models of MPTP-induced parkinsonism.

All of the clinical features of parkinsonism may occur as a consequence of brain tumors. In most cases the site is supratentorial, meningiomas being the most common tumor type. The mechanism may be mass compression or invasion of the corpus striatum; a smaller number of cases are caused by involvement of the substantia nigra. The exact pathophysiology of parkinsonism induced by tumors not directly involving the basal ganglia is unknown, but many cases resolve with removal of the offending lesion, suggesting an underlying reversible metabolic process.

In rare cases parkinsonism may be a prominent feature of an infectious illness other than encephalitis lethargica. This list would include neurosyphilis, subacute spongiform encephalopathy (Creutzfeldt-Jakob disease), and acquired immunodeficiency syndrome.

Parkinsonism occurring during childhood or adolescence may have diverse causes (see Chapter 25, Table 25.1). Most patients presenting with pure juvenile parkinsonism of unknown cause beginning before age 21 years have a positive family history of a similar disorder. A subset of this group demonstrates marked diurnal variations and sensitivity to L-dopa, suggesting a link to dopa-responsive dystonia, discussed later in this chapter.

DYSKINESIA

Tremor

Essential Tremor

Clinical Features. Some of the major features of, and misconceptions about, essential tremor are revealed by its aliases: senile tremor, familial tremor, and benign essential tremor. The incidence increases with age, and the tremor

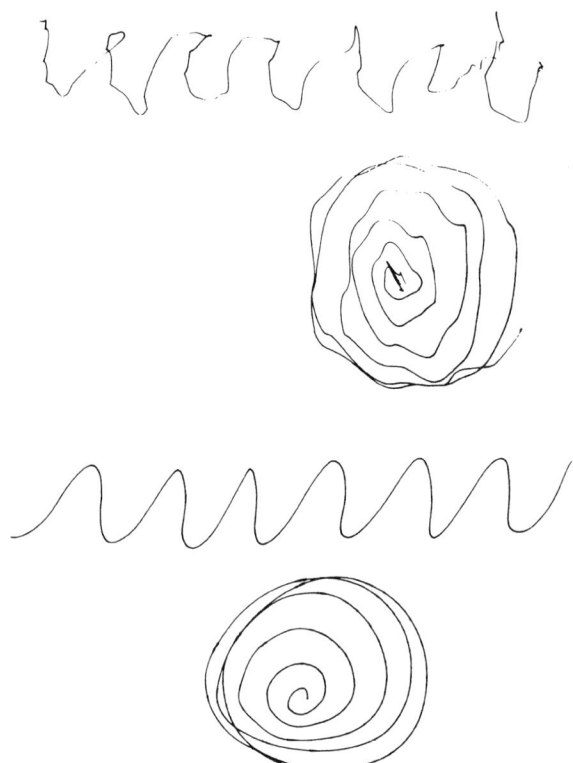

FIGURE 75.10   Essential tremor. The illustration shows two drawings useful in the clinical assessment of patients with movement disorders. Here a right-handed patient with mild essential tremor, primarily affecting the dominant side, has drawn the upper waveform and spiral with the right hand and the lower ones with the left; note the striking asymmetry of involvement.

often remains barely perceptible for many years; thus, most patients seek medical attention at a later age. However, the onset may occur at any time of life. The tremor is likely inherited, but one-third of those affected give no family history of tremor. The label *benign* is the most misleading, in that resultant functional incapacity may be severe. Admittedly, the tremor is rarely associated with other neurological deficits, and progression is usually slow, making this diagnosis less ominous than others associated with tremor.

Essential tremor is mainly an affliction of the distal upper limbs; it may be highly asymmetrical. Patients frequently complain of difficulty with handwriting (Figure 75.10), pouring a drink, holding a cup, or manipulating tools. The tremor is usually absent at rest, becoming evident with sustained postures or action. The head is also tremulous (titubation) in 50% of patients, more often in women. The muscles of speech and the chin, tongue, trunk, and lower extremities are involved less often. Patients may present with head or voice tremor that persists as an isolated finding. The legs are seldom affected, but older patients often have difficulty with tandem walking (Hubble et al. 1997). The neurological examination is otherwise normal, apart from the occasional patient who may show orofacial dys-

kinesias, an associated dystonia, or other mild extrapyramidal features.

One of the most striking characteristics of essential tremor, which often serves as a diagnostic criterion, is its responsiveness to low doses of alcohol. More than 60% of patients relate that one or two alcoholic drinks substantially dampens the amplitude of their tremor for several hours. Excitement, stress, and fatigue may worsen the symptoms.

Inheritance follows an autosomal dominant pattern in familial cases; penetrance is variable. The disorder is probably genetically heterogeneous. A gene for one large kindred with essential tremor maps to the short arm of chromosome 2, and linkage also has been reported on chromosome 3q in 16 Icelandic families. Although reported incidences in different populations vary widely, no consistent gender or race predilection has been identified. Progression of symptoms is usually slow, and patients' estimates of time of onset are often vague. In many cases the tremor remains mild; only approximately 10% of affected individuals seek medical help. However, the severity can be such that livelihood or routine daily activities are greatly hampered.

Investigation.   Classic neurological teaching maintained that electrophysiological studies in essential tremor demonstrate simultaneous contraction of antagonistic muscle groups, in contrast to an alternating pattern in PD. However, there are a sufficient number of exceptions in both groups of patients to thwart the diagnostic utility of these findings. Electromyography has demonstrated that the frequency of essential tremor (5–8 Hz) lies between that of parkinsonian rest tremor (4–5 Hz) and that of physiological tremor (8–12 Hz); the frequency tends to be inversely proportional to the amplitude of the tremor.

Pathogenesis.   The pathogenesis of essential tremor remains unknown. It is not even known whether it originates in the CNS. Neuropathological studies have found no consistent abnormalities. PET scan studies support a role of the cerebellum in the generation of essential tremor (Jenkins et al. 1993). The differential diagnosis includes a large number of causes for postural tremor (see Chapter 25, Table 25.3). Identical tremors can be found in a variety of peripheral neuropathies. A high incidence of a postural tremor clinically similar to essential tremor is found in patients with dystonias, particularly spasmodic torticollis, and essential myoclonus. An association has been claimed also between essential tremor and PD. In selected families there does seem to be a link between essential tremor and PD; however, in general there is little evidence for an association between the two.

Treatment.   The treatment of disabling essential tremor consists of drug therapy with either primidone or β-adrenergic antagonists. The anticonvulsant primidone may be useful in doses from 50–750 mg per day. Initial intolerance is frequently caused by nausea, dizziness, and sedation.

Treatment must begin with small doses, as little as 25 mg per day, with gradual increments.

Beta blockers are equally effective but carry the risk of aggravating or precipitating more serious side effects such as asthma or congestive heart failure. The site of action of these agents and the subclass of receptors involved in the therapeutic response are unknown, but evidence favors a major role for peripheral β_2-adrenoceptors. None of the newer beta blockers is more effective than propranolol. Usually, the dose must reach at least 80–120 mg per day before any benefit results; further increases to 240 or 320 mg per day for full therapeutic effect may be necessary. However, some patients respond to low doses and can even use it strictly as needed. Most patients improve to some extent, but the degree of responsiveness to primidone or propranolol varies greatly; rarely is the tremor completely abolished. A response in hand tremor is usually more evident than in head or voice tremor, in part because the former is more frequently disabling, and thus changes are more often obvious to the patient.

Sedatives such as the benzodiazepines or phenobarbital are occasionally helpful. Other agents said to provide benefit include the carbonic anhydrase inhibitors methazolamide and acetazolamide, gabapentin, nimodipine, and glutethimide. Clonazepam may help those with kinetic tremor out of proportion to postural tremor, or with orthostatic tremor. This reinforces the notion that essential tremor may include a number of variants with differing pathophysiological mechanisms.

In a patient with disabling involvement of the dominant hand refractory to medical therapy, thalamotomy and thalamic stimulation have earned a reputation as the most reliable means to abolish the tremor on the contralateral side. The value of these procedures is greatest in patients with severe tremors, which rarely respond to medication. Surgical complications are gratifyingly infrequent but potentially devastating, so the impact of the anticipated improvement on the patient's daily life should be assessed carefully before referral.

Not all patients require treatment. In many, the tremor is not disabling, and they need only be reassured that their symptoms do not represent evidence of a more serious underlying neurological condition, such as PD. Alternatively, because propranolol is effective even in a single dose, patients may choose to take 40–120 mg of propranolol in anticipation of specific stressful situations, such as public speaking. It is not uncommon for patients to use a drink of alcohol for this same purpose. There is some controversy over whether the incidence of chronic alcoholism is increased in patients with essential tremor.

Other Types of Tremor

Physiological tremor (see Chapter 25) may be enhanced in amplitude to a symptomatic level by various psychological and metabolic aggravating factors, such as anxiety, fatigue, alcohol withdrawal, and hyperthyroidism, or as a result of drugs or toxins. Caffeine is commonly blamed as a cause of enhanced physiological tremor. Physiological tremor is a result of the interaction of numerous mechanical and neuromuscular influences and appears to be mediated, at least in part, by peripheral β-adrenergic mechanisms.

Primary writing tremor involves only the affected upper extremity during the act of handwriting. It is of large amplitude, occurs at a frequency of 5–6 Hz, and produces mainly pronation and supination of the forearm. It shares the task specificity of an occupational dystonia and may be difficult to distinguish from writer's cramp or an essential tremor that is particularly aggravated by writing. Primary writing tremor may respond to anticholinergic therapy. Other task-specific tremors (e.g., with shaving or drumming) are occasionally seen.

Orthostatic tremor involves the legs and trunk and is present only when standing in one place or during other isometric leg muscle contractions. Electrophysiological studies usually yield a uniquely high frequency of 14- to 16-Hz contractions alternating between antagonists, found in a widespread distribution (trunk, arms, legs). Others have recorded 6- to 7-Hz activity synchronous in antagonistic muscles. The latter finding is consistent with the concept that some cases of orthostatic tremor represent variants of essential tremor. This is supported by the presence of upper limb postural and action tremors typical of essential tremor in some patients or members of their families. However, the tremor appears to respond more often to clonazepam than to primidone or propanolol.

Tremor commonly occurs secondary to disease of the cerebellum or its connections. Cerebellar tremors involving the limbs are typically absent during repose and in the initial stages of a movement, but are progressively evoked by the finer adjustments required for a precise projected movement. The dominant movement is a slow (approximately 3 Hz) oscillation in a horizontal plane. Tremor of the head and trunk (titubation) may be caused by midline cerebellar lesions. A peculiar type often referred to as *rubral tremor* may resemble parkinsonian rest tremor but is exacerbated by sustained postures and further amplified during active movement. The tremor was once attributed to lesions of the red nucleus but is more likely to be caused by interruption of fibers of the superior cerebellar peduncle carrying cerebellothalamic and cerebello-olivary projections in the midbrain contralateral to the affected limb. This form of tremor may be caused by any type of lesion arising in the appropriate location, including the ipsilateral cerebellar dentate nucleus and superior cerebellar peduncle (before its midbrain decussation). It occurs perhaps most often as a result of multiple sclerosis. Head injury and stroke are two other common causes. The term *Holmes's tremor* has been proposed for this form of tremor in order to replace the many confusing (and sometimes incorrect) designations.

Apart from the tremor commonly seen in drug withdrawal states, alcoholism is associated with postural tremor in a large proportion of individuals who are not actively using alcohol. The tremor is not severe, and functional disability is uncommon. Some of these patients may be turning to alcohol to suppress a pre-existing essential tremor. Alcoholic tremor can be distinguished from essential tremor by a higher frequency, a lack of family history of tremor, and a greater responsiveness to propranolol.

Dystonia

Primary Generalized Idiopathic Dystonia (Dystonia Musculorum Deformans, Idiopathic Torsion Dystonia)

The first case description of idiopathic torsion dystonia (ITD) was probably that of Destarac in 1901, although he thought that the torsion spasms he witnessed were psychogenic. It was Oppenheim in 1911 who first expressed the now-prevailing view that this was an organic illness. For many years generalized dystonia was considered to be merely a syndrome consequent to a number of identifiable neurological diseases, until Herz, in a series of articles in 1944, established the concept of a primary disease now known as ITD.

Clinical Features.   ITD usually begins in childhood with an action dystonia of one lower extremity. The ankle usually inverts and plantar flexes, causing the patient to walk on the toes. Symptoms progress in a characteristic manner from a highly focal dystonia produced by a specific action, such as walking forward but not running forward or walking backward, to involving other actions of the affected limb, and spreading to adjacent areas of the limb and later to the rest of the body. Dystonia of the trunk, pelvis, and legs results in a variety of peculiar disturbances of gait, which are frequently misdiagnosed as hysterical. Walking may become impossible, and patients are reduced to crawling or pulling themselves across the floor with their hands. Eventually dystonic movements and postures become present at all times in many body areas. The course is variable, but most patients develop their maximum manifestations within 5–10 years, with subsequent stabilization. Limited remissions may be seen. The majority of patients with generalized dystonia eventually become too disabled to work.

Other clinical presentations are possible. ITD may begin with upper limb, axial, cervical, or cranial focal dystonia. These are much more common in older patients. The likelihood of progression from focal to generalized dystonia is much greater in children. It follows, then, that the vast majority of patients with primary generalized dystonia have the onset of illness before the age of 15, with a peak between 6 and 12 years.

The physical findings in ITD are limited to observation of the movements. Despite the implications of the name, muscle tone is normal in dystonia unless there is active muscle contraction. Other abnormalities on examination should strongly suggest that one is not dealing with idiopathic dystonia.

Investigation.   Laboratory study results are unremarkable. Imaging studies, including PET scanning with fluorodeoxyglucose and fluorolevodopa, have been disappointingly unhelpful. Electromyographic evaluation of dystonic limbs reveals inappropriate tonic co-contraction of antagonistic muscles or muscle groups, and overflow into inappropriate ones, which experimental electrophysiological studies indicate may result from reduced activation of group 1a inhibitory interneurons in the brainstem and spinal cord. Complex tasks appear to pose particular difficulty in the transitions between individual components of the whole movement. Current evidence suggests that the fundamental mechanism underlying dystonia may be disordered striatal control of the pallidothalamic tract, resulting in dysfunction of cortical motor planning and execution areas (Berardelli et al. 1998).

Etiology.   Autopsy studies have failed to provide a reproducible pathological substrate for ITD. The lack of consistent pathological findings has led to a search for a biochemical basis for ITD. Limited studies of autopsied ITD patients found abnormalities related to noradrenergic and, to a lesser extent, serotonergic and dopaminergic systems.

A large proportion of juvenile-onset ITD cases are inherited, typically in an autosomal dominant pattern. ITD is genetically heterogeneous. There is a high incidence of familial ITD among Ashkenazi Jews, where penetrance is approximately 0.3–0.4, whereas among non-Jews there is a higher degree of penetrance. A mutation in a gene that codes for a previously unidentified protein called *torsinA* on chromosome 9 accounts for the majority of cases of juvenile, limb-onset ITD. Other phenotypes (e.g., craniocervical predominant) are caused by different genetic disorders that linkage studies have suggested are mutations in unidentified genes on chromosomes 18 and 8. Direct testing for the mutation in the torsinA gene (*DYT1*) is available.

Treatment.   As might be expected from the poor current understanding of the pathophysiology and biochemistry of ITD, the medical management of this condition is often ineffective. The best results have been obtained with high-dose anticholinergic therapy (trihexyphenidyl, 20–50 mg/day or more). Children tend to tolerate much higher doses than do adults; both peripheral and particularly central side effects (such as confusion and memory impairment) may limit the use of this therapy. Other drugs that may be of value in a minority of patients include baclofen, carbamazepine, and benzodiazepines as well as, paradoxically, both dopamine agonists and antagonists. All juvenile-onset dystonic patients deserve an initial trial of L-dopa in view of the excellent benefit obtained in a small group of dopa-responsive cases (see L-Dopa–Responsive Dystonia, later in this chapter). Botulinum toxin may be used for selected focal problems. Surgical procedures have shown inconsistent results and may be associated with severe complications, although some severely affected patients obtain benefit from stereotaxic thalamotomy. Bilateral pallidotomy has provided striking benefit in a few patients. Physiotherapy and occupational therapy are often invaluable adjuncts to management. Supportive counseling should be given to help patients cope with this extremely disabling condition.

Focal and Segmental Idiopathic Dystonias

In contrast to the primary generalized form, idiopathic dystonia that remains relatively localized is more likely to involve cranial, cervical, or upper limb muscles and to develop later in life. Most patients do not know of a family history of a similar disorder; however, careful direct evaluation of first-degree relatives often reveals other examples of dystonia or isolated postural tremor. This suggests that genetic factors play an important role in many cases of adult-onset focal dystonias.

The most common of the adult-onset focal dystonias is spasmodic torticollis, or cervical dystonia, in which dystonic movements of neck muscles cause deviation of the head from its natural position. These movements may be sustained or may have a jerky or tremulous appearance. The deviation may be in any plane or combination of planes, although there is usually some component of horizontal rotation (Dauer et al. 1998). In some cases the patient is unaware of the abnormal neck posture until a family member draws attention to it. Many patients note the onset as a sudden involuntary tendency for the head to pull in one direction and the need to return it voluntarily to the midline. Initially, this may occur only intermittently and infrequently, becoming more persistent later in the course. The peak incidence is in the fourth and fifth decades, with gradual progression over a number of years. Partial or full remissions occur in some patients, but these are almost always transient. Thus, patients may give a history of a similar short-lived problem several years earlier.

Torticollis, particularly early in its course, usually is relieved by sensory tricks (or gestes antagonistes) such as a light touch on the face or the back of the neck. A common observation is an improvement or resolution of the neck deviation while sitting with the head pressed against a wall or the back of a tall chair, or while lying in bed. To become less conspicuous, patients may hold a pipe or an object such as a pencil in their mouths, with a similar degree of relief. Activities such as walking, writing, and combing the hair can particularly aggravate the problem. Patients may experience discomfort in the neck, which varies from a mild aching in the active muscles to severe musculoskeletal or even radicular pain; this is more common after many months of resisting the turning of the head. Pain and tension may be the most prominent complaints. An associated upper limb tremor is a common finding.

Torticollis has been reported in association with a variety of lesions at several levels of the CNS, most often the basal ganglia and brainstem, but the few idiopathic cases studied to date have had no demonstrated neuropathological

abnormality. Experimental torticollis in primates is produced most commonly by lesions in the ventromedial midbrain tegmentum, but this is not an exact replica of the clinical condition found in humans.

The most effective treatment for torticollis is botulinum toxin injections. When proper techniques for administration are used, over 80% of patients enjoy relief of symptoms for 3–4 months or longer. Symptoms inevitably return, but reinjection can provide repeated benefit for an indefinite period. Some patients may become refractory to the effects of the toxin through the development of antibodies; the latter are associated with short treatment intervals (less than 3 months) or high doses. The long-term safety of botulinum toxin has not been fully established, but some patients have now been treated for well over a decade without any ill effects. The approach to drug treatment of torticollis is similar to that for ITD; the rate of success is similar. Surgical procedures for torticollis have been used extensively, yet results remain controversial. The most common of these operations combines bilateral anterior rhizotomy at several cervical levels with denervation of the dominant sternocleidomastoid muscle. A recent alternative causing fewer complications is a posterior ramisectomy at multiple cervical levels.

Involvement of lower axial muscles may occur in isolation or concomitant with torticollis. This can result in spasms of the trunk in any direction, which variably interfere with lying, sitting, standing, or walking. Continuous exercise such as walking may progressively worsen the situation to the extent that a patient who begins walking in a nearly upright position eventually is forced to stop because of severe twisting in one direction or the other.

Focal or segmental dystonia involving cranial muscles is known as cranial dystonia (Meige's syndrome) (Figure 75.11). The most common type is blepharospasm, which often begins as an increase in blinking frequency and progresses gradually to clonic and then tonic forced closure of the eyelids. There may be an accompanying local gritty discomfort or sensation of dry eyes. Like torticollis, blepharospasm frequently responds to diversionary tricks, in this case, talking, singing, or neck extension. A useful clinical point is that the bilateral spasm may be broken by a light touch to one eyelid early in the course, although vigorous prying may be required later. Symptoms are often aggravated by bright light, wind, and attempting to read or watch television. Patients may become functionally blind as a result of frequent or sustained eye closure; they may be unwilling to leave the house for fear of developing the problem in a dangerous situation, such as crossing the street.

Another major component of cranial dystonia is oromandibular dystonia, which may cause involuntary mouth opening or jaw clenching, tongue protrusion (Figure 75.12), dysarthria, and dysphagia. Manifestations may be minimal until a person attempts to eat or speak. The patient may find it helpful to place a finger on the teeth, chin, or elsewhere to lessen the involuntary jaw opening or closure. Damage to the teeth and oral soft tissues is common.

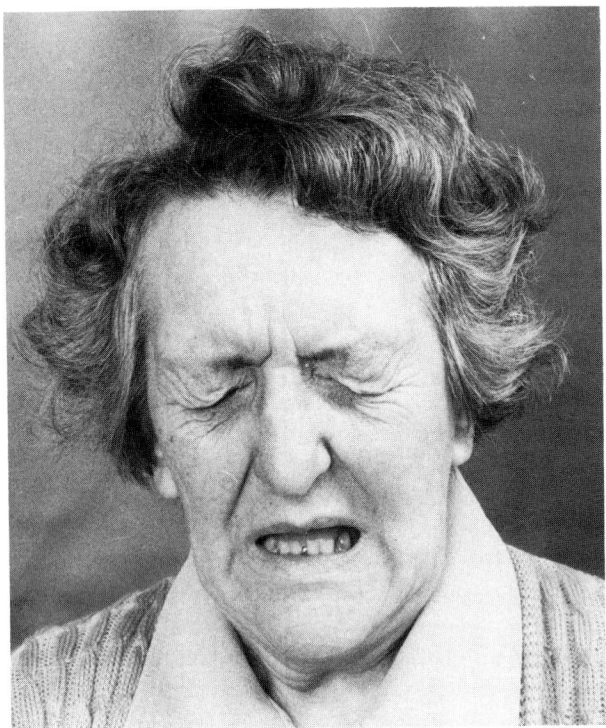

FIGURE 75.11   Cranial dystonia (Meige's syndrome). Note the extent of forced eyelid closure (blepharospasm) with depression of the eyebrows (Charcot's sign). Additional oromandibular dystonia with jaw opening and grimacing is also present.

Involvement of the laryngeal muscles is known as spasmodic dysphonia. This usually results in the voice becoming harsh, hoarse, and strained (because of hyperadduction of the vocal cords), or less often breathy and soft (caused by cord hyperabduction). As with many other forms of dystonia, frequently a superadded tremulous component exists. Occasionally, dystonia involves the pharyngeal muscles, resulting in pronounced difficulty swallowing. This must be distinguished from problems with chewing and propelling the bolus of food backward into the pharynx caused by the lower cranial dystonia described previously. All of these components of cranial dystonia may be seen in isolation or in any combination, often in association with torticollis. Cranial dystonia has a peak age of onset in the sixth decade and affects women more often than men.

The treatment of cranial dystonia has been revolutionized by the use of localized botulinum toxin injection therapy. The best results have been achieved with blepharospasm and adductor spasmodic dysphonia. The duration of improvement averages 3 months, and repeated treatments appear equally beneficial. In the case of eyelid injection, transient ptosis, diplopia, and incomplete eyelid closure are the only common side effects. Other forms of cranial dystonia also may respond to botulinum toxin injections, although with a lower success rate. If botulinum toxin therapy is unavailable or unsuccessful, medical management follows the same principles as for other forms of dystonia. Surgical

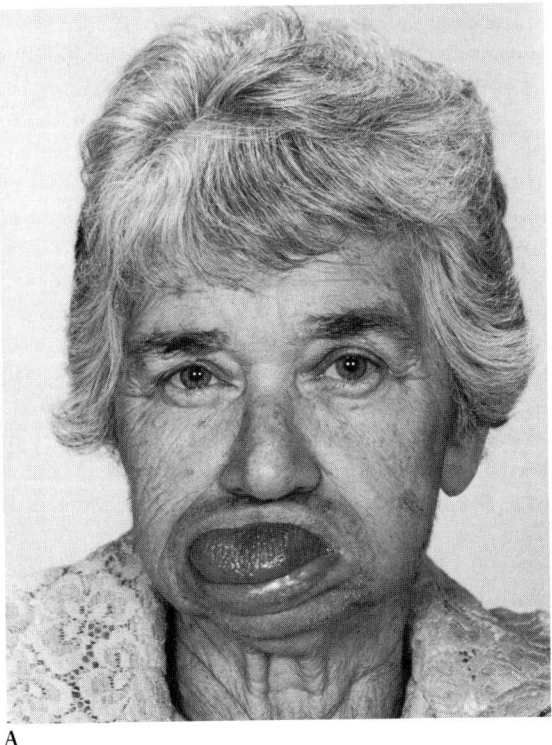

A

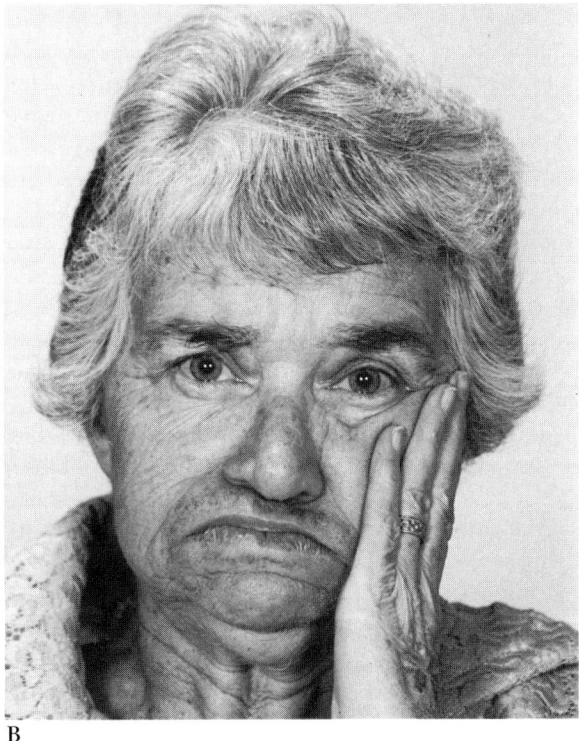

B

FIGURE 75.12   (A) Constant involuntary protrusion of the tongue in a patient with lingual and oromandibular dystonia. (B) With the aid of a sensory trick, in this case touching the side of her face, she was able to maintain her tongue retracted. She was obliged to keep her hand to her face to speak or eat.

approaches include eyelid muscle stripping or denervation of muscles of the lids and other areas of the upper face.

A number of dystonic conditions produced by specific actions occur in the upper extremities. They are closely related to skilled activities and thus are known as *occupational dystonias*. The best-known form is writer's cramp. This is a pure action dystonia in which abnormal tension or posturing develops in a hand or arm during the act of writing. The onset typically occurs in the second to fourth decades of life, and it frequently affects persons who write a great deal as part of their work. Initial symptoms may include clumsiness, sloppy writing, or excessive tension or tightness in the hand or forearm. Some patients complain of weakness, especially if the fingers splay away from the direction in which they were intended to go (Figure 75.13). Symptoms may progress to involve proximal muscles, producing shoulder elevation or arm retraction while writing, or to affect other actions using the same limb. Some relief may be afforded by adopting a different hand posture. Response to medical treatment is poor, and the best approach seems to be to use other strategies such as dictating, typing, using a writing device, or learning to write with the opposite hand, although a certain proportion develop comparable symptoms on the contralateral side. Similar action dystonias have been described in persons with professional skilled motor acts, such as musicians and typists. Electromyographically guided botulinum toxin injections have had some success in relieving these forms of dystonia.

L-Dopa–Responsive Dystonia

Segawa and colleagues, in 1976, described nine patients with the onset of progressive dystonia affecting the lower limbs initially and most severely. These cases were distinguished by marked diurnal variations in the disease manifestations, with progressive worsening during the day and amelioration with sleep, and by a universal response to low doses of L-dopa. Unexplained falls and a wide-based, stiff-legged gait, often misdiagnosed as spastic diplegia, may be among the presenting features. Diurnal fluctuations are noted in the majority of cases. Parkinsonism may develop later in the course of the illness; sometimes adult-onset parkinsonism is the presenting manifestation. Exertional and nocturnal leg cramps, precipitation of symptoms after trauma, and spontaneous remissions have been other features present in families we have studied.

The average age of onset is 6.1 years, and there is a 2 to 1 ratio of female to male subjects. Familial cases are consistent with an incompletely penetrant autosomal dominant mode of transmission. The disorder is usually caused by mutations in the gene coding for guanosine triphosphate cyclohydrolase 1 on chromosome 14. Mutations affecting other enzymes involved in tetrahydrobiopterin (BH4) synthesis may produce the same phenotype. BH4 is the cofactor for tyrosine hydroxylase, the rate-limiting enzyme in the synthesis of dopamine. Postmortem examination has shown

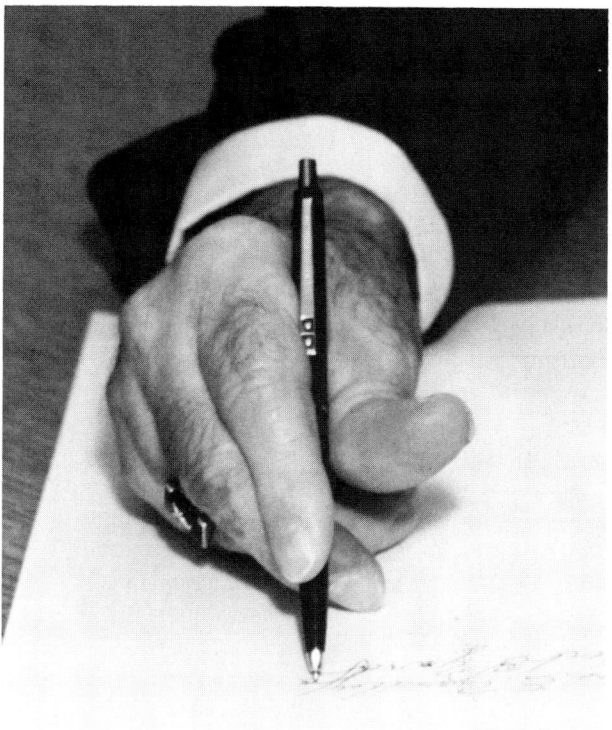

FIGURE 75.13   Writer's cramp. Involuntary extension of the thumb provoked by the act of writing. In this patient, the index finger also hyperextends, causing the pen to fall out of the hand. This same patient returned 5 years later with additional blepharospasm.

a normal number of neurons in the substantia nigra compacta (resulting in normal fluorodopa PET scan results), but these neurons are hypopigmented.

Low doses of L-dopa (100–300 mg/day in combination with carbidopa) are usually sufficient initially to obtain a good response, although with time subsequent increases in dose may be required. Anticholinergic drugs, in doses much lower than those required for cases of ITD, also may result in significant benefit. L-Dopa–responsive dystonia may account for up to 10% of cases presenting as juvenile-onset ITD. Given the poor response of the latter to therapy, a trial of L-dopa is indicated in all patients with idiopathic dystonia beginning in childhood, with the hope that they have the L-dopa–responsive disorder.

Selected Secondary Dystonias

As with many movement disorders, Wilson's disease (see Wilson's Disease, later in this chapter) is an important consideration in the differential diagnosis of dystonia. The syndrome of athetotic cerebral palsy is primarily a result of perinatal anoxia. Here, initial hypotonia is usually followed by delayed motor milestones and later by the development of a variety of abnormal movements. Choreoathetosis predominates, but prolonged dystonic posturing, ballism, and myoclonus all may occur. Vol-

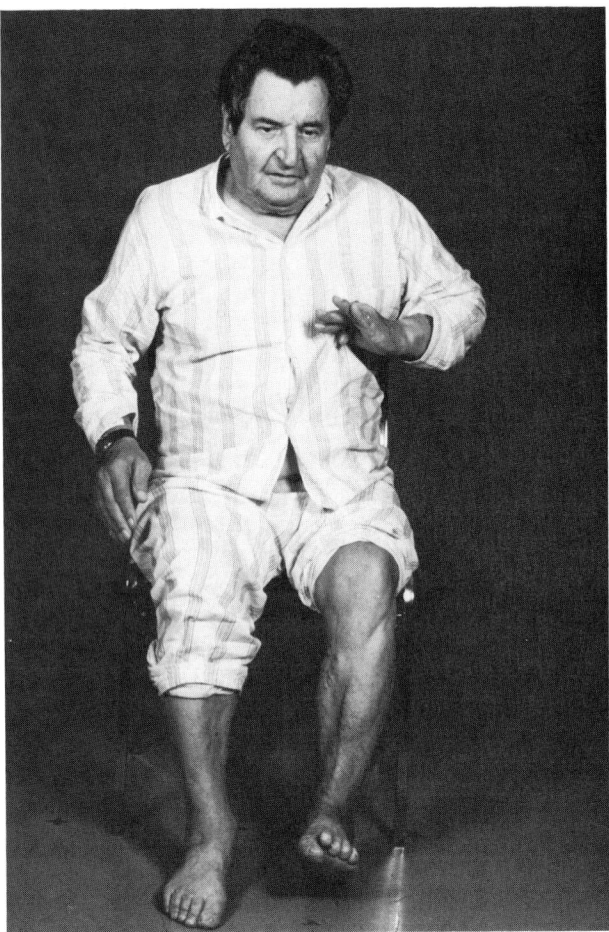

FIGURE 75.14 Hemidystonia. This patient is unusual in that his history and examination are otherwise typical of progressive supranuclear palsy.

Table 75.7: Causes of bilateral computed tomographic lucencies in the basal ganglia

Leigh disease*
Wilson's disease
Mitochondrial cytopathy*
Anoxia, prolonged hypotension
Carbon monoxide intoxication
Cyanide intoxication
Methanol intoxication
Familial holotopistic striatal necrosis
Infantile striatal necrosis
Biotin-responsive encephalopathy
Infections (such as influenza)
Hemolytic-uremic syndrome
Sickle cell disease
Wasp-sting encephalopathy
Organic acidemia (such as methylmalonic acidemia)
Head trauma
Dystonia with optic atrophy*

*Both Leigh disease and dystonia with optic atrophy and basal ganglia lucencies are probably forms of mitochondrial cytopathy.

untary goal-directed movement is additionally hampered by a defect in the normal patterned activation of muscles necessary for the smooth performance of the task. For example, attempted rapid abduction of the shoulder may result in initial inappropriate activation of shoulder adductors. Alternatively, the movement may begin with an excessively large agonist burst with little evidence for the well-organized triphasic pattern (agonist-antagonist-agonist), which normally accounts for all voluntary ballistic movements.

The severity of the movement disorder varies considerably from patient to patient. Mildly affected patients may note minimal clumsiness or dysarthria, whereas the most severely affected are completely dependent, chair-bound, and anarthric, gyrating wildly with any attempted movement. Despite their striking appearance, mentation is often completely preserved. In an individual case, the movement disorder may seem to progress or evolve well beyond the first decade and some patients note apparent progression even in midadult life. Pathological examination reveals hypermyelination (status marmoratus, *état marbré*), gliosis, and neuronal loss in the putamen, thalamus, and border zones of the cerebral cortex.

Kernicterus results in a similar clinical state, often with a greater risk of mental retardation. Deafness, ocular motor disturbances, limb rigidity, and spasticity also are seen. Neonatal jaundice, usually from erythroblastosis fetalis secondary to Rh- or ABO-blood-type incompatibilities, results in damage to the basal ganglia (especially the globus pallidus and the subthalamic nucleus), thalamus, brainstem (especially the nucleus of the oculomotor nerve and cochlear nuclei), and cerebellum. Fortunately, with improvements in obstetrical and perinatal care, the incidence of these previously common causes of childhood-onset choreoathetosis has been greatly reduced.

Although it has long been known that perinatal encephalopathies, especially anoxia and kernicterus, may cause generalized dystonia, this usually occurs within the first decade of life following a history of delayed motor development (athetotic cerebral palsy). In some patients, however, development is normal and dystonia may arise up to 20 years or more after the perinatal insult; this is referred to as *delayed onset dystonia*. A careful birth history may be necessary to distinguish this from ITD.

Focal cerebral lesions may cause unilateral dystonia, or hemidystonia (Figure 75.14). The lesion can be diagnosed with the help of imaging studies in most cases. The structures involved are the putamen or thalamus and less often the globus pallidus or caudate nucleus. The most common cause is cerebral infarction, in which case the dystonia evolves with resolution of a hemiparesis or after a variable delay of weeks to years. Other focal brain lesions also may cause hemidystonia.

With the widespread availability of neuroimaging studies, an increasing number of patients are being recognized with symmetrical bilateral basal ganglia lucencies (Table 75.7),

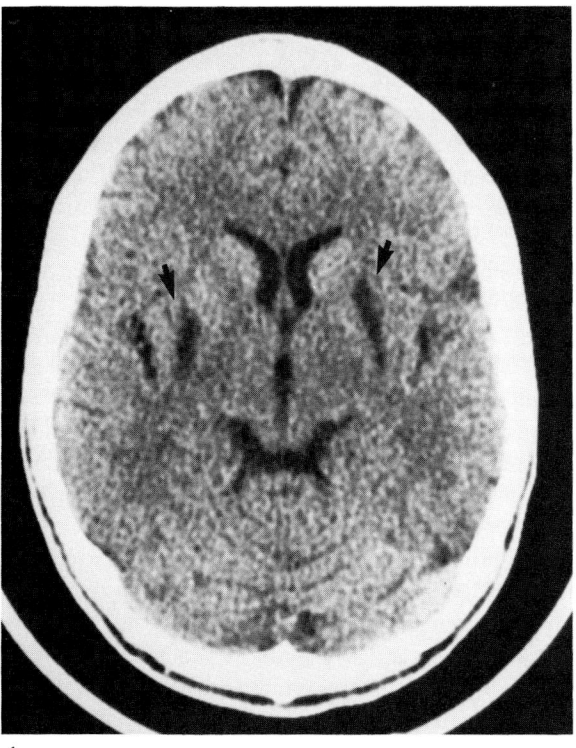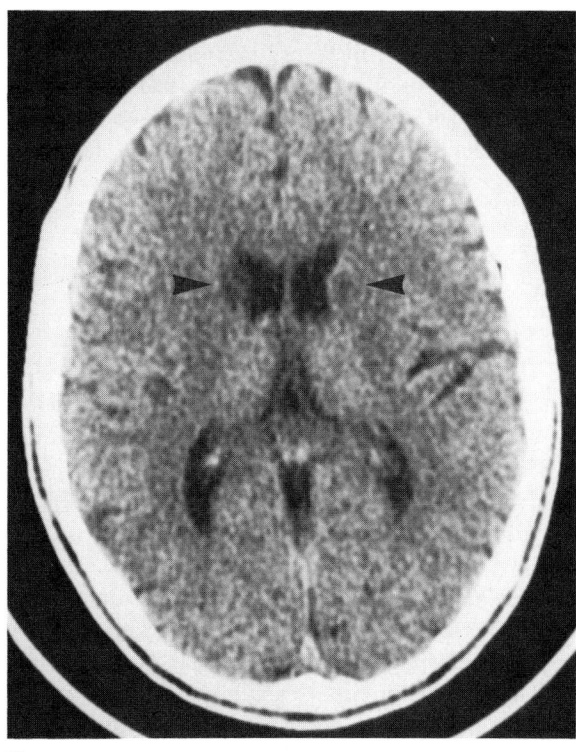

A   B

FIGURE 75.15   Bilateral striatal lucencies in a patient with generalized dystonia. (**A**) Lucencies in both putamina (*arrows*). (**B**) Lucencies in the heads of the caudate nuclei (*arrowheads*).

some of whom demonstrate a dystonic syndrome. One subgroup combines CT striatal lucencies with severe generalized dystonia as well as variable associated clinical findings such as cognitive impairment, optic neuropathy, corticospinal tract signs, and myopathic features. The radiological hypodensities (Figure 75.15) are presumed to be caused by necrotic lesions and may be linked to subacute necrotizing encephalomyelopathy (Leigh disease). There is evidence for maternal transmission in some patients, suggesting that this may represent a type of mitochondrial cytopathy. The phenotype of Leber's optic atrophy and dystonia with basal ganglia lucencies has been linked to mutations in mitochondrial DNA, most often at nucleotide pair 14459.

The term *dystonic lipidosis* has been applied to a condition characterized by dystonia, supranuclear gaze palsy, and splenomegaly. Foamy and sea-blue histiocytes are found in the bone marrow, as in some lysosomal lipid storage disorders. This disorder is now classified as a type of Niemann-Pick disease (type C), a cholesterol lipidosis distinct from the sphingomyelin lipidoses. Numerous neurodegenerative disorders including PD, PSP, MSA, CBGD, Huntington's disease (HD), and the pallidal degenerations also may result in dystonia. Another hereditary neurodegenerative disorder that results in a prominent dystonic syndrome is X-linked recessive dystonia-parkinsonism (lubag). This disorder is manifest almost exclusively in Filipino men as progressive dystonia and parkinsonism beginning in midlife. A mosaic

pattern of degeneration in the striatum (Waters et al. 1993) accounts for the clinical features and explains the resistance of the symptoms to most drug therapy, including L-dopa for the parkinsonism. Two other autosomal dominant hereditary dystonias that combine dystonia with other movement disorders are myoclonic dystonia and rapid-onset dystonia-parkinsonism. The former may be related to hereditary essential myoclonus (Quinn 1996). Both the myoclonus and dystonia may show a marked response to ethanol. Because drug therapy is often unsuccessful, alcoholism is a risk in these patients.

Chorea and Ballism

Rheumatic Chorea (Sydenham's Chorea)

The association between chorea of childhood and adolescence and rheumatic fever was pointed out by See in 1850. With the widespread availability of antibiotics for streptococcus A infections, rheumatic chorea has become extremely uncommon in developed countries.

Chorea differs from other manifestations of rheumatic fever in that it arises later (several months after the acute streptococcal infection) and usually affects only patients aged between 5 and 15 years, and girls more than boys. The distribution is most often generalized, but hemichorea may occur. The chorea develops insidiously, progresses in intensity over a matter of weeks, then gradually resolves spontaneously. Occasionally, there is no prior history of rheumatic fever, and the diagnosis is inferred from the characteristic history in an appropriately aged patient. One-fifth of patients may suffer a recurrent episode, usually within 2 years. Occasionally, patients experience multiple repeated bouts of chorea.

The pathogenesis of rheumatic chorea is thought to relate to the formation of antibodies that cross-react between the streptococcus and striatal neurons. A clinical and pathogenetic analogy between Sydenham's chorea and PANDAS (*p*ediatric *a*utoimmune *n*europsychiatric *d*isorders *a*ssociated with *s*treptococcal infection) has been drawn, although it is not believed that PANDAS is directly related to rheumatic fever. Patients exhibiting the B-cell alloantigen D8/17 are particularly susceptible to developing rheumatic chorea, and this may have diagnostic utility. MRI may demonstrate diffuse enlargement of the basal ganglia (Giedd et al. 1995). The chorea is frequently not disabling, but patients requiring treatment may respond to dopamine antagonists or possibly valproic acid. Severe cases may improve with immunosuppressant medication, plasmapheresis, or intravenous immunoglobulin. Drug treatment should be withdrawn after a short period, because remissions invariably occur.

Patients with a past history of rheumatic chorea are more susceptible to developing chorea that is drug-induced, for example, from oral contraceptives or phenytoin, or during pregnancy. A high incidence of late-onset chorea or action tremor has been found in patients examined more than a decade after their rheumatic chorea disappeared.

Huntington's Disease

In 1872, George Huntington described the variety of chorea that came to bear his name. His description contains all the essential features considered diagnostic of HD: a progressive disorder combining chorea and other movement disorders with behavioral disturbances and dementia, transmitted via an autosomal dominant inheritance pattern.

Clinical Features.   The disease may present with either neurological or psychiatric features, or both simultaneously. The movement disorder may be noted as twitching or jerking, or patients may complain of simple clumsiness or incoordination. Mental changes often take the form of a change in personality noted by family members, although other psychiatric syndromes such as depression or even a schizophreniform or paranoid psychosis may supervene; later, a progressive dementia emerges.

Neurological examination usually reveals generalized chorea, which becomes more obvious as the disease progresses. Impersistence of sustained movement, particularly tongue protrusion and hand grip (milkmaid grip), may be a prominent feature. Observation of the patient's gait is particularly helpful in that walking may elicit chorea in a case in which the signs are otherwise minimal. More severe gait disturbances include bizarre stuttering or dancing with ataxic features and even components of parkinsonism such as lack of arm swing. Another key aspect of the examination is oculomotor function. Common abnormalities include slow and hypometric saccades (more so in the vertical plane), saccadic pursuit, convergence paresis, and impersistence of gaze, which can be seen as difficulty suppressing saccades toward distracting stimuli. Patients may be unable to initiate saccades without head thrusts or blinking. Apraxia for orolingual movements (such as licking lips, sucking on an imaginary straw, or blowing air into cheeks) and manual dyspraxia also may compromise motor function in addition to the chorea and impersistence. Parkinsonian features, particularly bradykinesia, and dystonia become increasingly prominent as the disease progresses. Brisk reflexes and clonus are common, and Babinski's sign is occasionally present.

A small number of patients may present with a parkinsonian syndrome (the Westphal variant) instead of chorea; they are slow and rigid rather than hyperkinetic. Action tremor or myoclonus occasionally is prominent. Another group of patients demonstrates typical neurological features without psychiatric symptoms, or vice versa, for years. A family history compatible with HD is of paramount importance in diagnosing these clinical subgroups.

The majority of patients develop symptoms in their fourth or fifth decades, although onset at any age may be seen. Juvenile cases (onset before age 20) have a much higher incidence of the akinetic-rigid variant. No clear sex preponderance is evident. Low prevalence rates have been noted in Japan and among African and American blacks, and most patients are in fact of northern European ancestry.

Investigation.   The HD gene (*IT15*) resides in the short arm of chromosome 4 (The Huntington's Disease Collaborative Research Group 1993) at 4p16.3. Its mRNA codes for a protein known as *huntingtin*, which is widespread throughout CNS neurons. Its function is unknown. The gene contains an expanded trinucleotide (CAG) repeat sequence. Normally, fewer than 29 repeats occur, whereas HD patients usually have more than 35. The age of onset is significantly (but not constantly) related to the number of repeats, with juvenile-onset patients often having 50 or more. The discovery of this genetic abnormality has led to a reliable blood test for HD, which determines the size of the expanded CAG repeat using a polymerase chain reaction technique. This test confirms or excludes the diagnosis of HD with great accuracy in all but a small proportion of individuals who have an intermediate number of repeats (i.e., 29–35). Genes in this latter category are considered prone to further expansion, but probably not long enough to produce clinical manifestations (Ross et al. 1997).

A cornerstone of any diagnosis of HD is the family history. In most cases this is readily forthcoming in the form of a known diagnosis or a description of a deceased parent with typical manifestations. At times, however, the information available is sketchy, and the diagnosis must be inferred from suggestive evidence such as dying in an institution, suicide, inappropriate or socially deviant behavior such as abandoning the family, or fragments of chorea or motor impersistence. In some cases even this is lacking, but one of the parents will have died prematurely. A small number of patients do not have any of these features in their background. Correspondence with distant relatives or review of ancient medical records may be warranted.

The availability of a diagnostic blood test has made other investigations much less important. CT and MRI scanning may demonstrate atrophy of the caudate nucleus, which can be quantified by use of the bicaudate index. PET scans demonstrate hypometabolism of glucose in the striatum (Plate 75.III), even in patients with minimal clinical findings. However, none of these imaging findings is entirely specific.

Pathology.   At autopsy, the brain appears small with widened fissures and sulci, and brain weight is reduced. Coronal sections reveal striking shrinkage of the striata and especially the caudate nuclei (Figure 75.16). A less pronounced diffuse atrophy is present also. On light microscopy the striata show a marked depletion of neurons, with medium spiny cells affected out of proportion to medium and large aspiny neurons. There is a less prominent loss of glial cells, resulting in a relative increase of glia to neurons. The cerebral cortex exhibits milder neuronal loss, particularly in the sixth, fifth, and third layers. Surviving neurons in both the cerebral cortex and striatum contain intranuclear inclusion bodies, which react with antibodies to huntingtin or ubiquitin. Similar inclusion bodies are found in other diseases characterized by CAG triplet repeats, and it is believed that these may be important to the pathogenesis of cell death.

The neurons lost in HD are not members of a single neurotransmitter system. Numerous transmitters and the activities of related enzymes have been studied in HD, and many have been found to be either reduced or increased in amount. Although dopamine antagonists are the most effective drugs available for treating chorea, no consistent abnormalities in dopamine levels have been found. The most striking abnormalities have been reductions of GABA and acetylcholine levels and of the activities of glutamic acid decarboxylase and choline acetyltransferase. There is relative sparing of somatostatin-neuropeptide Y neurons in the striatum. These findings and the results of assessment of glutamate receptor subtypes support the current theory that neuronal degeneration in HD is caused by excitotoxicity via NMDA receptor stimulation. Peripheral energetic defects and oxidative damage in muscle have been demonstrated in the finding of multiple mitochondrial DNA deletions, most severely involving complex I.

Etiology.   Many of the genetic features of HD have been mentioned. Parents of either sex can transmit the gene to offspring of either sex. Penetrance is complete for alleles

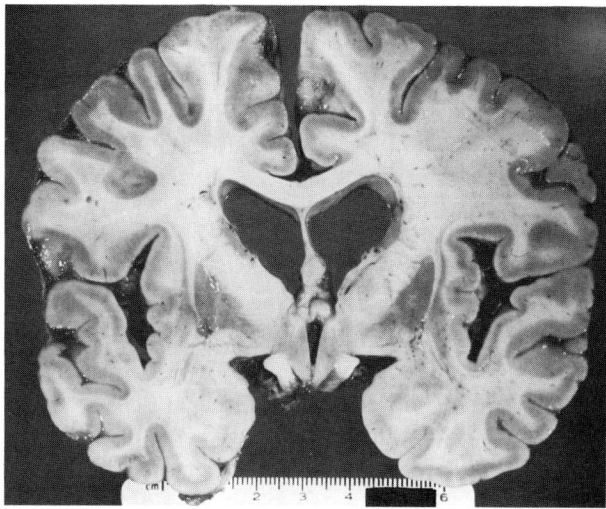

FIGURE 75.16   Transverse section of the brain of a patient with Huntington's disease, showing marked atrophy of the caudate nuclei. (Courtesy of Dr. Lothar Resch.)

with 42 or more triplets and incomplete when there are 36–41 repeats. The sex ratio of juvenile-onset patients is 1 to 1, but they are four times more likely to have inherited the HD gene from their father than from their mother. This is a result of trinucleotide repeat instability and a marked increase in the number of CAG triplets, which can occur at the time of spermatogenesis (Duyao et al. 1993). In a similar manner, spontaneous mutations arise from expansion of genes with an intermediate number of repeats. There may be a higher incidence of maternal inheritance in late-onset cases, suggesting maternal genetic factors also may have a modifying effect on clinical manifestations.

Course and Treatment.   Death most often results from dysphagia through aspiration pneumonia or suffocation, usually between 10 and 20 years after the onset of symptoms. Suicide is also a common cause of death. Juvenile-onset patients have a distinctly poorer prognosis than adults, with a high incidence of seizure disorders late in the course and a much shorter life expectancy. Conversely, onset of HD at a later age is associated with a slower progression of symptoms.

Until more definitive treatment of HD is available, considerable opportunity exists to provide patients with symptomatic relief. Chorea may respond to dopamine antagonists, both presynaptic (tetrabenazine or reserpine) and postsynaptic (neuroleptics such as haloperidol). The high incidence of serious adverse reactions to these agents limits their use to cases in which the dyskinesias are truly disabling. Atypical neuroleptics such as quetiapine or olanzapine, though less potent than haloperidol, may be tried first in hopes of reducing the risk of such side effects. Akinetic and rigid patients may benefit from antiparkinsonian drugs. Depression should be treated with conventional antidepressant agents. The dementia of HD is not currently treatable.

Perhaps more important in the management of HD is education of the patient and family about the disease and the implications of the diagnosis for other family members. Lay organizations are invaluable sources of information and support for HD families, as well as help with chronic care of patients.

The question of the propriety of presymptomatic testing of at-risk individuals has often been raised. Some consider it irresponsible to diagnose patients prematurely when no remedy is available. Others believe it is the individual's right to know and plan for the future. Support for the latter position comes from a study that demonstrated that individuals who were determined to be at high risk for HD by linkage analysis actually fared better psychologically than those whose fate remained unpredictable. The ethics of such a test and the manner in which to deal with a family given a positive result have yet to be fully resolved. Genetic counseling is recommended for all affected and at-risk families to ensure that all interested individuals are informed of the many issues surrounding HD testing. This discussion would become moot if successful protective therapy were developed.

Chronic Juvenile Hereditary Chorea (Benign Hereditary Chorea)

A small number of families have been reported in which chorea develops in affected members in early childhood, then remains static or improves gradually during their lifetime. Inheritance is usually autosomal dominant with incomplete penetrance. The initial manifestations are delayed walking or a disturbance of gait. Generalized chorea then develops and reaches maximum severity shortly after onset; rare cases of a progressive nature have been described. The chorea is often mild but may reach disabling proportions; it is typically poorly responsive to medications. Patients may show additional mild cognitive abnormalities, but the pronounced psychiatric and mental changes of HD are not seen. HD gene testing should be performed on at least one affected family member.

Spontaneous Orofacial Dyskinesia

Among the many movement disorders that can affect the face, a seemingly spontaneous orofacial dyskinesia (SOFD) is found among elderly patients. As described in Chapter 25, this consists of continuous mouthing or masticatory movements, which may be suppressed by having the patient hold the mouth open and tongue protruded. The estimated prevalence of SOFD varies from 1.5–37.0%, depending on the population studied. The most common source of misdiagnosis is confusion with cranial dystonia. Some patients may have cerebellar infarctions, and we have seen cases

with infarctions limited to the basal ganglia. It has been suggested that an edentulous state may be an important factor in the genesis of SOFD. Dyskinesias were present in 16% of edentulous patients, and in these patients no movement of the tongue with the mouth open, minimal functional disability, and no movements outside the oral region were found. Although other authors have not found the edentulous state to contribute to SOFD, a dental assessment is probably indicated before contemplating pharmacological treatment. As with all movement disorders, the decision to initiate drug therapy should be determined by the level of discomfort or disability in the patient. Antidopaminergics are the agents of choice.

Other Choreas

The differential diagnosis of chorea is lengthy (see Chapter 25, Table 25.4). A few choreic syndromes merit special mention.

Chorea, parkinsonism, dystonia, and tics may be found in patients with neuroacanthocytosis (see Neuroacanthocytosis, later in this chapter). Dentatorubropallidoluysian atrophy may present with a phenotype indistinguishable from HD. Chorea is increasingly recognized as the presenting symptom of systemic lupus erythematosus (SLE). An association has been suggested with the circulating antibody known as the *lupus anticoagulant*; in patients not meeting the diagnostic criteria for SLE, a history of recurrent vascular thromboses or spontaneous abortions should prompt a search for the characteristic clotting abnormality, including assay of anticardiolipin antibodies. The chorea may disappear after treatment with prednisone or aspirin. The chorea associated with SLE is not necessarily an indication for the aggressive treatment required in some other forms of CNS lupus. Chorea also may be a manifestation of hyperthyroidism, pregnancy (chorea gravidarum), or oral contraceptive therapy. Chorea gravidarum may also be a manifestation of SLE.

In older patients, one must give consideration to basal ganglia infarction and polycythemia rubra vera. Senile chorea is a sporadic, progressive, late-onset chorea without dementia; it is probably a syndrome caused by several pathological disorders, including HD. In all age groups a number of drugs may cause chorea, including some used to treat other movement disorders, such as dopamine agonists, neuroleptics (see Drug-Induced Movement Disorders, later in this chapter), and anticholinergics. Hemichorea prompts the same anatomical and etiological considerations as hemiballism.

Hemiballism

Hemiballism is included under the choreatic syndromes because a number of authors view chorea and ballism as points on a common spectrum distinguished only by severity and distribution. However, it has pathological implications that earn it consideration as a distinct condition. The majority of patients with hemiballism have a lesion of the contralateral subthalamic nucleus (Figure 75.17), although it is well documented that lesions elsewhere (most often the striatum) may produce identical movements. Virtually any focal pathological process can affect the subthalamic nucleus (see Chapter 25, Table 25.6), hemorrhage and infarction being by far the most common. Thus, it follows that the typical case of hemiballism is one of abrupt onset in a patient over 60 years old with one or more risk factors for cerebrovascular disease, most notably diabetes mellitus and hypertension. Occasionally, ballism is preceded by typical sensory or motor complaints indicative of a vascular event involving the upper midbrain or diencephalon. A slow progressive development of hemiballism later replaced by severe weakness and other neurological deficits might suggest an enlarging mass lesion. In most instances the movement disorder resolves in a matter of weeks to months. Even in self-limited cases, treatment is often indicated because the movements prove exhausting to the patient. The most effective agents are antidopaminergic, either dopamine depletors or neuroleptics. In rare persistent disabling cases, stereotaxic thalamotomy or pallidotomy may be considered.

Tic Syndromes

Tourette's Syndrome

Georges Gilles de la Tourette, in 1885, described a condition characterized by motor incoordination with involuntary vocalizations, echolalia, and echopraxia. Today we recognize this incoordination as the result of multiple motor tics. It is noteworthy that the syndrome was discovered during a deliberate attempt to uncover patients with a movement disorder; however, Gilles de la Tourette was not scouring the streets of Paris for *ticqueurs*, but for jumping Frenchmen of Maine (see Startle Syndromes, later in this chapter) such as had been described in North America.

Clinical Features.   Tourette's syndrome (TS) arises during childhood or early adolescence (usually around the age of 7), in boys four times as often as in girls. The most common initial symptoms are motor tics involving the cranial region, especially around the eyes. Subsequently, there develops a constellation of motor and vocal tics, of either a simple or a complex nature, which may span the entire range of human motion and expression (see Chapter 25, Table 25.8).

Two points about the course of TS are notable. One is the changing display of tics, and the other is the tendency toward periodic remissions and exacerbations. In those with a long history of TS, the assortment of tics typically varies with time. Many patients (or their families) also

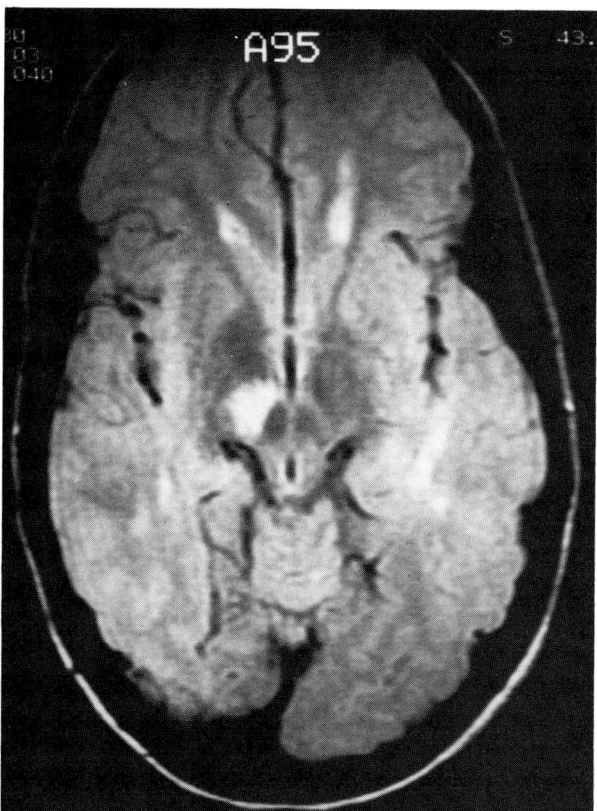

FIGURE 75.17   Magnetic resonance imaging scan showing the typical location of a lesion causing hemiballism. Here a demyelinative plaque involves the region of the subthalamic nucleus, in an unusual patient with multiple sclerosis complicated by hemiballism.

report that the severity and nature of manifestations seem to wax and wane, often in cycles lasting in the range of 6–10 weeks. Existing tics may subside altogether while others develop de novo or as a recurrence of previously experienced tics. A lesser number of patients show little change in distribution or with time. Despite its potential for striking variability, TS is recognized as a chronic disorder that generally reaches maximum expression during adolescence, then usually diminishes gradually during adulthood. A small proportion of otherwise typical patients obtain a complete and permanent remission during puberty.

A high frequency of various behavioral abnormalities attends TS, and these are often the most disabling aspects of the clinical picture. Given the usual age of onset, they may translate into poor school performance caused by disruptive activity and attentional difficulty; such patients may be relegated to special education classes. Learning disorders are extremely common in these children. Obsessive-compulsive disorder may be the most common behavioral feature, affecting as many as 50% of patients. Increasing evidence suggests that obsessive-compulsive disorder may be the only manifestation of the disorder, especially in girls. Attention-deficit hyperactivity disorder also is extremely common in patients with TS. Its relationship to the genetic disturbance of TS has not been established.

Although it has been reported that a majority of TS patients have subtle neurological deficits, such as clumsiness on rapid alternating movements, pronator drift, or mild alterations in tone or reflexes, in most authors' experience the neurological examination, apart from the tics, is normal. No laboratory tests of diagnostic value exist for TS.

Pathogenesis.   The pathophysiology of tics and TS is uncertain. Because of the observed response of symptoms to dopamine blockade, current thinking postulates a hyperactivity of central dopaminergic pathways as being a fundamental mechanism for the production of tics, but its anatomical and etiological basis is unknown. Quantitative three-dimensional reconstruction studies of the basal ganglia using MRI have shown that patients with TS lack the asymmetry with left-sided predominance found in normal controls (Singer et al. 1993). Neuropathological studies have been largely unrewarding. Postmortem biochemical studies have shown increased numbers of presynaptic dopamine reuptake sites, suggesting that patients with TS have a larger population of dopaminergic nerve terminals in the striatum than normal. Another intriguing finding has been a striking reduction in dynorphinlike immunoreactivity in the globus pallidus in four of five brains studied. Alterations in caudate D2 receptor binding predicted differences in phenotypic variability in a study of monozygotic twins who were discordant for symptom severity (Wolf et al. 1996).

There is a higher incidence of tics and obsessive-compulsive behavior in relatives of patients with TS. Some investigators believe that a single major gene contributes to the expression of the syndrome, with autosomal dominant inheritance and sex-specific penetrance. However, a gene for TS has not been identified, strengthening speculation that the inheritance of TS may be polygenic (Sadovnick and Kurlan 1997), with homozygosity at the major locus leading to higher penetrance and more severe symptoms. That many affected relatives of an individual with TS have mild tics of which they are unaware, or for which they have not sought medical attention, indicates that TS may be one of the most common movement disorders. Currently, quoted prevalence rates of 0.1–0.5 per 1,000 are probably underestimated, and some authors suggest lifetime figures in the range of 1–10 per 1,000.

Treatment.   Several options are available for the pharmacological treatment of TS. Assessment of the efficacy of any drug is hampered by the fluctuating nature of the manifestations of the disorder. Dopamine antagonists are generally the most successful agents against tics, and the original responses to haloperidol provided the impetus for defining the syndrome as an organic neurological disorder rather than a functional psychological one. However, dopamine antagonist use is fraught with complications, and satisfactory results may be achieved with less toxic therapy. A major concern in treating children with TS is sedation and impairment of learning performance. Clonazepam is a relatively weak but benign drug for tics that may provide just enough additional control for less seriously affected patients. Clonidine may be beneficial for both tics and behavioral problems. Of the postsynaptic dopamine receptor blockers, pimozide and fluphenazine may produce less sedation than haloperidol. Risperidone may be quite effective and entail less risk of extrapyramidal side effects, including TD. Other atypical antipsychotics such as olanzapine and quetiapine appear to confer an even lower risk of extrapyramidal side effects, although the efficacy of these agents is not proven. Presynaptic dopamine antagonists, such as tetrabenazine, lack any risk of TD, although they have not been proved as effective as the dopamine-receptor blockers. Low doses of the dopamine agonist pergolide have been reported to be effective in reducing tics, perhaps by stimulating presynaptic autoreceptors. For obsessive-compulsive disorder, clomipramine, fluoxetine, fluvoxamine, and other serotonin-specific reuptake inhibitors may all improve symptoms without affecting tic severity. Treating attention-deficit hyperactivity disorder in patients with TS may be problematic because of the reported tendency of stimulants to aggravate tics. Clonidine, guanfacine, and tricyclic antidepressants are alternatives to consider.

Before embarking on pharmacological treatment, the question of its necessity should be raised. As in other movement disorders, the disability and distress of the patient should dictate the drug treatment of TS. Management also should include education regarding the behavioral as well as neurological aspects of the illness. Young patients with TS can be difficult to raise and teach; parents and educators should be encouraged to obtain literature and support from local and national lay organizations.

Other Tic Disorders

Table 25.9 summarizes other disorders of this type. Current thought regards the chronic primary tic disorders as forming a spectrum of related conditions classified according to duration and severity. Chronic multiple motor tics are distinguished from TS only by the lack of vocalizations. Patients with a single tic persisting from childhood throughout life are said to have a chronic simple tic. Unless multiple motor and vocal tics are present to confirm a diagnosis of TS, prospective distinction among these categories of tic disorder may be difficult and even somewhat artificial. Strong support for the concept of a link between these tic disorders and TS is provided by the fact that family members of patients with TS may display simple tics, multiple motor tics, or even isolated obsessive-compulsive features without tics. A transient tic of childhood subsides within a year of onset; up to 15% of children may exhibit such movements.

Tics are less likely to have an identifiable cause than are other movement disorders. They have been recognized in the settings of infectious illnesses (particularly encephalitis lethargica), stroke, trauma, and many drugs. The symptomatic therapy for other tic disorders is similar to that for TS. Many cases of tic disorders may have an autoimmune basis. Cases with acute onset, or sudden exacerbations, of obsessive-compulsive disorder and tic disorder have shown a significant association with group A beta-hemolytic streptococcal infection; it has been suggested these patients represent a new syndrome known as *PANDAS*. Given that streptococcal pharyngitis and tics are both common in young people, much work remains to be completed before this concept can be fully embraced (Kurlan 1998).

Myoclonus

Essential Myoclonus

Essential myoclonus is a chronic condition with onset in the first two decades of life and little subsequent progression. Apart from the possible exceptions noted in the following discussion, other neurological deficits are absent. Electroencephalography is normal. When a positive family history is obtained, inheritance follows an autosomal-dominant pattern with variable penetrance. However, most cases are sporadic in occurrence.

Essential myoclonus is frequently induced or aggravated by action but may occur spontaneously and even be dampened by movement. The myoclonic jerks are often suppressed by alcohol and worsened by stress. The frequency is usually erratic, although rhythmic and oscillatory forms have been described. The distribution of muscles affected may be focal, segmental, generalized, or multifocal, but involvement of neck and proximal arm muscles is characteristic (Quinn 1996). Somatosensory evoked potentials, even during active jerking, do not show the large amplitude responses of cortical reflex myoclonus (see Chapter 25), suggesting a subcortical origin for essential myoclonus. No pathological studies have been reported.

There are families in which essential myoclonus and a postural tremor identical to isolated essential tremor are found both together and independently. Patients also may demonstrate dystonic features, which may respond also to alcohol.

The most effective treatment for essential myoclonus is clonazepam. Sometimes anticholinergic therapy is of benefit. Valproic acid tends to be less effective than in other forms of myoclonus.

Nocturnal Myoclonus

Under this rubric are included at least three different types of movement. Hypnic (or hypnagogic) jerks, or sleep starts, are the massive jerks experienced by most normal individuals on falling asleep or during light sleep. Less commonly, otherwise normal individuals or their spouses complain of rapid myoclonic jerks in the limbs, especially the legs, while asleep. Others experience a different type of dyskinesia,

which has been termed *periodic movements of sleep* (PMS). This syndrome is characterized by tonic and clonic movements of the lower extremities during stages I and II of sleep. Typically, this consists of single or several clonic jerks followed by tonic contractions of foot and toe dorsiflexors and hip and knee flexors, lasting up to 5 seconds. The distribution pattern varies among patients. A distinctive feature of this condition is the periodicity of the recurrence of these movements, at regular intervals less than 90 seconds long. One or both legs may be affected, usually asymmetrically and asynchronously. The occurrence of PMS is an age-related phenomenon, increasing in prevalence to a reported 29% in those over 50 years old. The site of origin of PMS is presumed to be in the CNS but remains unknown.

Because the activity occurs during sleep, PMS generally do not cause distress to patients; however, they can be disturbing to someone sharing the patient's bed. Patients are more apt to complain if their PMS are associated with the restless legs syndrome (RLS). The latter condition consists of restlessness and paresthesias or uncomfortable dysesthesias of the legs, which are most prominent while resting in the evening or at night and are relieved by activity, especially walking. Dyskinesias ranging from myoclonic to dystonic in appearance may be present during wakefulness but tend to be less regular than PMS. A family history consistent with autosomal dominant inheritance may be found.

The majority of patients with RLS have PMS, and their treatment is similar. A wide assortment of drugs have been claimed to be useful in RLS and PMS. L-Dopa is the most consistently successful agent, but may ultimately result in a rebound or augmentation phenomenon. Dopamine agonists, such as pergolide, pramipexole, or ropinirole, may produce equal benefit and sustain it for a longer time. Other effective treatments include benzodiazepines (especially clonazepam at bedtime), gabapentin, and opiates such as codeine. RLS patients treated successfully with opiates have not tended to abuse them.

Postanoxic Action Myoclonus

In 1963, Lance and Adams reported four patients who developed action myoclonus as the predominant manifestation of an anoxic encephalopathy. The myoclonus follows an episode of coma of variable duration, sometimes lasting less than a day. Any cause of cardiac or respiratory arrest may be the inciting event, with a high number associated with anesthesia and surgery. Most patients show generalized seizures and spontaneous myoclonus during the comatose period. There are no known factors in the past history or surrounding the anoxic event and coma that predispose patients to developing action myoclonus rather than the more common sequelae of anoxia.

Action myoclonus is present as the patient emerges from coma and may affect muscles of the limbs, face, pharynx, and trunk. In addition, various forms of sensory (including visual and auditory) stimulation may produce reflex myoclonus. The majority of patients have a persistent seizure disorder. Walking is often most severely involved by both myoclonic jerks and postural lapses (negative myoclonus). Severity varies, but most patients are unable to walk independently. Once established the syndrome persists, although symptoms may lessen over time and rare spontaneous remissions have been described.

The pathophysiology of postanoxic action myoclonus is almost certainly related to serotonin deficiency. The spinal fluid level of 5-hydroxyindoleacetic acid, the chief metabolite of serotonin, is reduced. More important, the myoclonus responds to drugs that enhance serotonin activity: L-5-hydroxytryptophan (L-5-HTP), the immediate synthetic precursor to serotonin; 5-hydroxytryptamine given with a monoamine oxidase inhibitor; or fluoxetine, an inhibitor of serotonin reuptake, is generally an effective treatment. Furthermore, methysergide, a serotonin antagonist, blocks the therapeutic effect of L-5-HTP. However, the actual abnormality affecting serotonin activity is not known, and these observations do not explain why other drugs that do not directly affect serotonergic pathways, such as valproic acid, can suppress postanoxic action myoclonus. Pathological findings have been highly variable, and occasionally only minor abnormalities are found, prompting the speculation that this syndrome is caused by a functional derangement of anatomically intact neurons.

Dramatic relief can be obtained from the use of L-5-HTP (1–4 g/day), in combination with carbidopa (75–150 mg/day) to prevent peripheral decarboxylation. More readily available agents such as valproic acid and clonazepam may be equally effective, and thus are generally considered the treatments of choice. Piracetam is a drug with few side effects that has proven especially beneficial in patients with electrophysiological features of cortical reflex myoclonus. A number of other agents also have been reported to be useful, and patients often require a combination of differently acting drugs to suppress the myoclonus. Pronounced postural lapses, possibly caused by negative myoclonus in muscles of the trunk and legs, may result in falls, which are particularly resistant to therapy. Despite striking responses to a variety of treatment options and a tendency to improve with time, most patients remain disabled to some degree (Werhahn et al. 1997).

Segmental Myoclonus

Segmental myoclonus refers to regular or irregular repetitive contraction of muscles innervated by single or contiguous levels of the brainstem or spinal cord. The frequency of the movement varies from patient to patient, being most commonly in the range of 1–3 Hz. Usually the movements are continuous; change little with posture, action, or sensory input; and persist in sleep, although this is less consistent in cases of spinal myoclonus.

Palatal myoclonus (PM) (also known as palatal nystagmus or palatal tremor) is a form of segmental myoclonus characterized by bilateral or unilateral, usually rhythmic, oscillations of the soft palate, often with synchronous involvement of other muscles including those of the pharynx, larynx, floor of the mouth, lower face, neck, eyes, and respiratory muscles. Occasionally, the other muscles listed may be affected without the soft palate, or the muscles of the trunk or limbs may be involved. When isolated to the palate, the disorder is commonly asymptomatic. However, an annoying rhythmic clicking may be heard by the patient caused by opening and closing of the eustachian tube. This may be audible to others nearby or to the examiner by placing a stethoscope in the patient's ears and listening through the bell.

PM has been correlated with a unique combination of hypertrophy and degeneration in the inferior olivary nucleus, which appears to be transsynaptic in origin. It is produced by a lesion involving the pathway connecting the inferior olive to the dentate nucleus via the ipsilateral superior cerebellar peduncle and the contralateral central tegmental tract. Any focal lesion in this area may cause PM, with pontine infarction being most common. Unilateral PM is caused by a lesion in the contralateral cerebellar pathway or the ipsilateral brainstem. When a precipitating clinical event can be identified, the palatal movements usually develop only after a latency of many weeks to months. Unilateral or bilateral high-signal abnormalities are often evident on proton-density or T2 MRI scans in these patients. The essential form of PM is typified by ear clicking caused by tensor veli palatini contractions. Ear clicking is rare in symptomatic cases, where levator veli palatini activity predominates. Eye and extremity muscles are never involved in essential PM and patients tend to be younger than those with secondary PM.

In spinal myoclonus, muscle groups from one or several adjacent spinal motor roots are involved, most often abdominal, axial, and lower limb muscles. The movements can usually be correlated with a lesion at the appropriate spinal cord level. The pathological process varies, but tumors and trauma are among the most common causes. Others include infectious and parainfectious conditions, ischemia, cervical spondylosis, disc herniation, demyelination, and syrinx. Another form of spinal myoclonus is propriospinal myoclonus (Brown et al. 1994). This usually results in irregular axial flexion movements that are often stimulus-sensitive. Conduction from one spinal segment to another is relatively slow, suggesting the involvement of the polysynaptic propriospinal pathway. The cause in most cases is uncertain, but it has been described with spinal cord injury and multiple sclerosis.

Once established, segmental myoclonus, especially of the palatal variety, tends to persist indefinitely. Clonazepam is the most established treatment. Success also has been reported with tetrabenazine, 5-HTP, trihexyphenidyl, and carbamazepine. PM responds less frequently than spinal myoclonus; fortunately, it is better tolerated, and treatment is often unnecessary, although the extrapalatal movements in secondary PM can be a major source of disability.

Startle Syndromes

Excessive startle responses are abnormal exaggerations of a normal human alerting reaction to sudden sensory stimuli. They can be seen as a secondary feature of many disorders (see Chapter 25, Table 25.12); they also are the most prominent manifestation of three syndromes: hyperekplexia, startle-automatic obedience syndromes, and startle epilepsy. Clinical and physiological differences between various syndromes manifesting startlelike behavior suggest that this grouping arose more out of convenience than as a result of pathophysiological similarities.

Hyperekplexia most often occurs as a hereditary disorder caused by a dominant mutation of the α1-subunit of the glycine receptor gene on the long arm of chromosome 5 (*GLRA1*). Families with autosomal recessive inheritance are recognized also. In nonhereditary cases hyperekplexia may result from brainstem lesions or arise sporadically. Patients respond to unexpected visual, auditory, or tactile stimuli with a sudden generalized myoclonic jerk followed by a momentary generalized stiffening, with or without a glottic sound, causing a fall like a log. Patients often adopt a peculiar hesitant gait as a result of the frequent falls. Transient hypertonia during infancy precipitated by handling (stiff baby syndrome) and hypnagogic or diurnal generalized myoclonic jerks also may occur. The examination may show hyperreflexia and an abnormal response to startle demonstrated simply by tapping on the forehead or nose. Some family members with milder affection may show only an exaggerated startle response without falling. Electrophysiological analysis suggests that impairment of spinal inhibitory pathways may be involved (Floeter et al. 1996). Clonazepam is the current treatment of choice, often resulting in excellent control of the sudden starts and falls and, consequently, a marked improvement in the gait.

A number of syndromes show excessive startle at times with violent results, automatic obedience, echolalia, and echopraxia. The best known of these in the English-speaking literature is that of the jumping Frenchmen of Maine, first delineated by Beard in 1878. Similar conditions, such as latah and myriachit, have been described in other locations around the world. Although these disorders were initially lumped with multiple tic syndromes by Gilles de la Tourette, it is now clear that there are distinct differences. Their tendency to affect unsophisticated people only in certain social circumstances has led some authors to conclude that they represent culturally determined behaviors rather than biological diseases. However, this does not explain similar disturbances in occasional isolated cases or as a sequel to physical illness.

Startle epilepsy is a condition associated with congenital focal cerebral lesions. A tonic spasm of the contralateral side in response to startle is followed by a complex partial seizure. Clonazepam is sometimes effective.

Table 75.8: Drug-induced movement disorders

Movement disorder	Common offending agents
Postural tremor	Lithium, sympathomimetics, tricyclic antidepressants, valproic acid
Parkinsonism	Antipsychotics, dopamine-depleting agents, metoclopramide
Chorea (including tardive dyskinesia)	L-Dopa, dopamine agonists (including amphetamines), antipsychotics, metoclopramide, phenytoin, estrogen preparations, anticholinergics, antihistamines
Dystonia	L-Dopa, dopamine agonists, antipsychotics, metoclopramide
Tics	Antipsychotics, amphetamines, L-dopa, dopamine agonists, carbamazepine
Akathisia	Antipsychotics, dopamine depletors, serotonin selective reuptake inhibitors
Myoclonus	Tricyclic antidepressants, L-dopa, dopamine agonists, many others in toxic doses
Asterixis	Phenytoin, other anticonvulsants

Drug-Induced Movement Disorders

A large number of drugs cause movement disorders as part of their toxic manifestations (Table 75.8). Some are discussed elsewhere in this chapter under the heading of the appropriate dyskinesia. The most common agents resulting in disturbances severe enough to warrant neurological evaluation are those that block dopamine receptors, such as the antipsychotics and metoclopramide. At normal therapeutic doses, these drugs produce movement disorders frequently enough to merit the detailed consideration that follows.

Acute Dystonic Reactions

Approximately 2–5% of patients develop dystonia within days (sometimes hours) of beginning therapy with neuroleptic agents. Young men are at higher risk than others. The cranial, nuchal, and axial muscles are most commonly affected, causing oculogyric crises, grimacing, fixation of the jaw, retrocollis, torticollis, or opisthotonic posturing. The limbs seem more resistant to this type of disturbance, especially in older patients. With the decline of postencephalitic parkinsonism, neuroleptic therapy is now the most common cause of oculogyric crises. All types of neuroleptics may cause acute dystonic reactions (ADR), including substituted benzamides such as metoclopramide, but those with stronger anticholinergic properties are less likely to do so. The risk of inducing a dystonic reaction increases with the size of the dose.

Untreated, ADR last from seconds to hours and may recur for up to 48 hours. Intravenous anticholinergic drugs (e.g., benztropine, 1 mg, or diphenhydramine, 50 mg) usually abort the dystonia within 15 minutes. Diazepam also may be effective. Oral anticholinergic therapy should continue for 2–3 days to prevent recurrences.

The pathophysiology of ADR is unknown. The low incidence rates suggest that predisposing factors may exist. Because the risk may be higher in relatives of patients with idiopathic generalized dystonia or previous ADR, this susceptibility may be genetic. More severe ADR also are said to occur in patients with underlying hypocalcemia. The response to treatment indicates that the mechanism producing ADR may involve excessive cholinergic activity. The status of the dopamine system in ADR is controversial.

Akathisia

Akathisia was first described as an unusual manifestation of PD. It now is recognized as the most common movement disorder induced by dopamine antagonists (both receptor blockers and presynaptic depletors).

Akathisia has two clinical components: a subjective inner restlessness and inability to remain still, and the objective motor manifestations resulting from attempts to satisfy the urge to move. Depending on the intensity of the former, the latter may cover the spectrum from distal limb movements (drumming fingers, tapping toes) to pacing or even running. Leg swinging and other movements of the lower extremities may be characteristic of akathisia.

The pathogenesis of akathisia is not fully understood. The occurrence after treatment with dopamine antagonists as well as in idiopathic and postencephalitic parkinsonism strongly suggests an interference with normal dopamine activity as a key factor. A reduction of dopamine activity in the mesocortical dopaminergic system may be important. Akathisia also may be caused by selective serotonin reuptake inhibitor antidepressants. This suggests a potential role for serotonergic systems.

Neuroleptic-induced akathisia is most often acute, in which case it develops within a few days of drug initiation and is dose related. There is no age or gender predisposition. It tends to continue as long as the medication is maintained and subside shortly after cessation. For patients in whom reduction of the medication is not feasible, akathisia has been reported to respond to many therapeutic agents, such as anticholinergics, amantadine, β-adrenergic antagonists, clonazepam, and opiate agonists. Akathisia may be resistant to therapy, and the discomfort caused by the symptom is a common cause of poor neuroleptic drug compliance. Newer atypical neuroleptics have a much lower incidence of akathisia, and switching to one of these is an important therapeutic option. Less often, akathisia develops late in the course of treatment (tardive akathisia), in which case it may persist despite withdrawal of the causative drug. Here, management is similar to other tardive syndromes (see following discussion).

Drug-Induced Parkinsonism

A clinical syndrome indistinguishable from that caused by PD may be induced by a wide variety of drugs that block dopamine receptors or deplete dopamine stores. Approximately 15% of patients taking neuroleptics on a chronic basis develop parkinsonism, usually 2–10 weeks after initiation of treatment. Older patients tend to be more susceptible to this complication. Akinesia is the most common presenting symptom. A rest tremor, though usually less prominent, may be as vigorous as in PD. Parkinsonism, infrequently in most cases, is also caused by many other drugs with less established effects on dopaminergic systems (Riley 1998).

Management of neuroleptic-induced parkinsonism should be instituted with the knowledge that the manifestations tend to dissipate gradually and spontaneously after several months despite continued use of the causative drug. If symptoms are disabling or sufficiently distressing, consideration should first be given to lowering the dose of the offending agent or substituting with atypical antipsychotics such as olanzapine, quetiapine, or clozapine. If antiparkinsonian medication is required, the drugs of choice are anticholinergics or amantadine. Withdrawal from antiparkinsonian medication should be undertaken after 3 months to reassess the need for therapy. The majority of neuroleptic-treated patients on concomitant anticholinergic therapy can be withdrawn (slowly) from the latter without adverse effect.

In almost all cases signs of parkinsonism disappear within weeks of withdrawal from the causative agent. In rare cases the manifestations persist for up to 18 months. Patients who do not experience resolution of parkinsonism may have had occult PD that became clinically apparent with the additional drug-induced insult to the dopamine system. Alternatively, some authors believe that neuroleptics are capable of causing a persistent form of parkinsonism (sometimes referred to as tardive parkinsonism).

Neuroleptic Malignant Syndrome

Neuroleptic malignant syndrome is a highly unpredictable consequence of neuroleptic therapy that may arise at any time during treatment, most often early or when doses are being increased quickly. It may result from use of a drug that was previously taken without incident. Reintroduction of the offending drug may not produce a recurrence, suggesting that neuroleptic use alone is insufficient to cause neuroleptic malignant syndrome. Pre-existing brain disease, exhaustion, and both dehydration and hyponatremia have been proposed as possible inciting factors. High-potency agents and long-acting depot preparations may cause neuroleptic malignant syndrome more frequently. Young patients, especially men, seem to be at greater risk than others, although this is a group of patients who tend to be treated aggressively with high-potency neuroleptics. An identical syndrome may develop during therapy with the presynaptic catecholamine depletor tetrabenazine, and after acute withdrawal of antiparkinsonian medication in PD.

Clinically, the neuroleptic malignant syndrome is characterized by extreme rigidity, fever and other autonomic disturbances, and a depressed or fluctuating level of consciousness, developing over a period of 1–3 days. Occasionally tremor, dystonia, or other dyskinesias are prominent. The diagnosis is supported by the finding of an elevated serum creatine kinase level, but this finding is highly nonspecific (Buckley and Hutchinson 1995).

Management consists of immediate withdrawal of the offending agent and provision of supportive care. Manifestations may persist up to 10 days after discontinuation of neuroleptics, and longer with depot preparations. Antiparkinsonian drugs (especially L-dopa and dopamine agonists), dantrolene, or both may result in a more rapid resolution of symptoms. Without specific treatment, death ensues in approximately 25% of cases. A high index of suspicion and the early initiation of therapy are critical in reducing mortality.

Tardive Dyskinesia

TD refers to the development of a movement disorder after chronic exposure to dopamine receptor antagonists. It was first observed in the 1950s, when antipsychotic therapy became widely available. Extensive clinical experience since then has permitted the delineation of several distinct tardive syndromes.

The original descriptions of TD referred to a syndrome characterized primarily by stereotyped orolingual and masticatory movements of a choreic nature taking the form of lip smacking and lip pursing, tongue protrusion, and licking and chewing movements. The muscles of the upper face are much less commonly involved. The truncal and limb musculature may be affected, giving rise to respiratory dyskinesias, pelvic thrusting, and chorea in the extremities; in rare cases, these are present without cranial involvement. As emphasized in Chapter 25, the movements tend to be repetitive and stereotypic in appearance and distribution, rather than random as in true chorea. One peculiarity of this syndrome is that the movements may not distress the patient, particularly if limited to the lingual and buccal muscles. Another typical feature is that voluntary movement of the affected area suppresses TD, whereas movement of other body parts may exacerbate it.

This remains by far the most common of the tardive drug-induced syndromes. Reported prevalences vary considerably, but estimates of 20% are readily acceptable. Older patients are at notably greater risk. One study of patients older than 55 years of age treated with typical neuroleptics found evidence of TD after 1, 2, and 3 years of treatment in one-fourth, one-third, and one-half of patients, respectively (Woerner et al. 1998). Whereas the vast majority of other drug-induced movement disorders resolve rapidly after discontinuation of the medication, TD may take months to years to remit. Women may have a higher rate of more severe and persistent TD. Many cases appear to be permanent, making this the most feared complication of chronic neuroleptic therapy.

There are many theories regarding the pathophysiology of classic TD. Denervation supersensitivity of striatal dopamine receptors remains the most attractive hypothesis. However, problems with this concept have encouraged alternative suggestions, for example, those primarily involving GABA mechanisms or free-radical toxicity of neuroleptics.

Prevention is of paramount importance in dealing with TD. The indication for long-term use of neuroleptic agents must be well established. Patients must be evaluated repetitively in hopes of early detection of TD. Once TD is present, the causative drug should be withdrawn if possible. Although the manifestations may emerge or worsen shortly after cessation of the drug (withdrawal dyskinesias), this effect is transient and no evidence exists that TD will progress without continued provocation. If the patient is not disabled by the dyskinesia, it is best not to treat but simply to observe and hope for a spontaneous recovery. In those with pronounced disability, treatment is difficult. A minor tranquilizer such as the benzodiazepine clonazepam may provide mild symptomatic relief. Occasional patients benefit from a trial of baclofen. In more severe or disabling cases, presynaptic dopamine blockade by reserpine or tetrabenazine may be used to control the dyskinesias after neuroleptic withdrawal. Clozapine as well as newer atypical antipsychotics, such as olanzapine and quetiapine, may not only not cause or aggravate TD, but may ultimately prove to be highly useful therapeutic agents. However, the long-term safety of these drugs is not fully established. The key step in management of TD is early detection to prevent the development of more severe manifestations. Based on evidence for the role of lipid peroxidation in the pathogenesis of TD, it has been suggested that high doses of vitamin E may have a role in both prevention and treatment of TD.

Another tardive phenomenon being recognized with increasing frequency is a dystonic syndrome (Kiriakakis et al. 1998). In affected patients a focal or segmental dystonia develops, usually involving cranial or cervical musculature or both. Retrocollis and partial opisthotonus seem particularly common. Tardive dystonia differs from classic TD somewhat in that there is no age predilection, and it appears to be induced by shorter courses of neuroleptic therapy. Unfortunately, the two syndromes share the property of persistence after neuroleptic withdrawal. Tardive dystonia may be particularly resistant to treatment. Presynaptic catecholamine depletors (reserpine, tetrabenazine) and high-dose anticholinergics yield the most favorable results. Tardive cranial and cervical dystonias often respond well to botulinum toxin, much like their idiopathic counterparts. In some cases clozapine has resulted in pronounced benefit; it is not clear if

Table 75.9:   Diagnostic tests in Wilson's disease

Test	Abnormal result
Slit-lamp examination	Kayser-Fleischer ring, sunflower cataract
Serum ceruloplasmin	<20 mg/dl
Serum copper	<90 mg/dl
Urine copper[a]	>100 mg/24 hrs
Liver copper[b]	>30 mg/g wet weight or >250 mg/g dry weight

[a]Collected in copper-free container.
[b]Using copper-free biopsy needle.

the effects have been directly antidystonic or simply allowed the dystonia to improve spontaneously while controlling the underlying psychosis.

Approximately one-half of schizophrenic children develop dyskinesias within 1 month of abrupt cessation of neuroleptic medication. This is known as the withdrawal-emergent syndrome; it differs from TD in that the movements are those of typical generalized chorea, which always resolve within a matter of a few weeks to months. This self-limited syndrome requires no treatment, unless the movements are disabling. In the latter event the neuroleptics should be reinstituted and withdrawn more slowly.

A much rarer complication of chronic neuroleptic therapy is the development of a tardive tic syndrome; both motor and vocal tics typical of TS may be present. Finally, a syndrome of tardive akathisia has been recognized. These patients have akathisia that is clinically identical to the usual neuroleptic-induced form but shares the pharmacological profile of TD, i.e., onset after prolonged exposure to neuroleptics, exacerbation on withdrawal or reduction of the offending medication, and alleviation by dosage increases or the use of dopamine depletors. Tardive akathisia and tardive dystonia are the two most disabling variants of TD.

Wilson's Disease

The description of familial progressive hepatolenticular degeneration by Kinnear Wilson in 1912 can be considered a landmark in the study of movement disorders, for it is here that Wilson first clearly delineated the concept of extrapyramidal motor manifestations of neurological illness.

Clinical Features

Wilson's disease is a systemic illness of protean presentation related to an abnormality of copper metabolism. During childhood, copper accumulates in the liver. Nearly one-half of patients at this stage develop overt manifestations of hepatitis, which may reach fulminant proportions. All those who remain untreated go on to develop cirrhosis.

A small number of patients present in unusual ways, such as with hemolytic anemia, bleeding from esophageal varices, hypersplenism with thrombocytopenia, or renal dysfunction. The rest go on to the insidious development of neurological abnormalities. These abnormalities usually become evident in adolescence or early adulthood, but cases with onset of neurological symptoms in the fifth or sixth decade have been recorded.

A wide spectrum of tremors has been seen in association with Wilson's disease. A fine action tremor is often present; rest tremor and the classic postural wing-beating tremor are less common. Incoordination of hands and gait is prominent and may be caused by a combination of ataxia, tremor, and akinesia. Dysarthria and dysphagia, often accompanied by profuse drooling, may be so striking as to lead to anarthria and a need for nasogastric intubation or percutaneous gastrostomy feeding. Facial muscles fixed in a smile may give patients an inappropriate grinning appearance. Dystonia is common and may result in muscular contractures; rigidity, bradykinesia, athetosis, and ataxia are often seen as well, whereas chorea and seizures are less common. Disturbances of primary sensation or special sensory modalities do not occur. Dementia may develop but is usually mild; the severity of the neurological abnormalities may make accurate assessment of intellectual function difficult.

These manifestations may be preceded or overshadowed by psychiatric disturbances of all sorts, including affective disorders, psychoses, personality changes, and behavioral abnormalities. Frequently, with onset at a young age, these are attributed to adjustment problems or the usual varieties of psychiatric illness, and the diagnosis may remain undiscovered until other features of Wilson's disease appear.

When cerebral dysfunction is present, patients almost invariably demonstrate copper deposition in Descemet's membrane of the cornea, the Kayser-Fleischer ring. Usually this is visible to the naked eye as a rusty brown clouding of the outer rim of the cornea, most prominent at the superior and inferior poles; examination with a slit lamp may be required for definitive diagnosis. Pigmented corneal depositions occur in association with cirrhosis due to other causes, but the Kayser-Fleischer ring should still be regarded as a highly sensitive and specific clinical sign of Wilson's disease.

Investigations

The diagnosis can be confirmed by finding low levels of serum ceruloplasmin (the major copper-containing protein in the blood) and elevated excretion of copper in the urine (Table 75.9). If these are not found, until recently the diagnosis could not be reliably excluded without a liver biopsy to measure copper content, which is elevated in Wilson's disease, and assessment by electron microscopy for pathognomonic ultrastructural changes. Abnormal routine liver function test results, aminoaciduria, hypouricemia, and demineralization of bone are other frequent investigational findings. In addition to the Kayser-Fleischer ring, ocular assessment should search for a sunflower cataract. Patients with neurological disturbances almost always show evidence of brain atrophy; putaminal, thalamic, or brainstem hypodensities on CT scans; or both; the lenticular lucencies may resolve with treatment. Similar abnormalities have been noted in some neurologically asymptomatic individuals. MRI scans may be more sensitive than CT scans in detecting basal ganglia or thalamic lesions and may demonstrate additional abnormalities in the brainstem and cerebral white matter.

Pathology and Pathogenesis

Pathologically, the brain may show varying degrees of gross enlargement of sulci, fissures, and ventricles. The lenticular nuclei may appear shrunken and discolored brown or may show evidence of cavitation. Microscopically, there is a diffuse hyperplasia of Alzheimer's type II astrocytes throughout the brain. The corpus striatum shows varying degrees of cell loss. So-called Opalski's cells, which are of unknown origin, and demyelination of white matter may be found.

Wilson's disease is inherited in an autosomal recessive fashion and is caused by mutations in a gene coding for a copper-transporting adenosine triphosphatase on chromosome 13q. Dozens of mutations in this gene are known, and most patients have different mutations in their two alleles. Unfortunately, this heterogeneity has prevented development of a genetic screening test.

Although the link to a defect in copper metabolism is indisputable, the actual pathogenesis of Wilson's disease is unclear. There is no correlation between clinical status and liver or brain pathological findings, and the liver toxicity is not related to accumulation of copper in a dose-dependent fashion. The clinical and particularly the pathological features of neurological impairment may be indistinguishable from those seen in conjunction with cirrhosis not associated with abnormalities of copper metabolism (acquired hepatolenticular degeneration). Thus, to view Wilson's disease as mere toxicity of copper caused by failure to incorporate it into a nontoxic form (ceruloplasmin) is simplistic, perhaps even erroneous. Yet the mainstays of successful therapy act by preventing copper absorption or removing it from body tissues and inducing hypercupriuria.

Treatment and Course

The treatment of Wilson's disease can be divided into acute and chronic stages. Initial treatment is usually begun with 250 mg of triethylene tetramine (trientine) or D-penicillamine four times daily on an empty stomach; immediate institution is warranted to minimize irreversible pathological changes. Pyridoxine supplements are also given. Adherence to a strict low-copper diet is no longer advocated, but patients should avoid foods with high copper content, such as nuts, shellfish, and liver. Determination of the serum free-copper concentration, which should be lowered, and the urinary excretion of copper, which should be raised initially, may be used as indices of the effectiveness of chelation therapy, because clinical response may be delayed for weeks or months following the start of treatment. Some patients improve but are left with severe neurological deficits or do not appear to respond at all. Early deterioration in neurological function after initiation of D-penicillamine occurs in 10% of patients; occasionally this is not readily reversible. Tetrathiomolybdate has been advocated as an alternative initial agent that is not associated with early worsening, but experience with this therapy is limited. The majority of patients treated with chelators experience a reversal of symptoms if properly treated, and even the most striking neurological features have the potential for recovery. The dose of trien or D-penicillamine may be raised to 1.5–2.0 g per day if necessary. Early allergic sensitivity may be sidestepped by reinstituting treatment at a reduced dose and using gradual increments.

Maintenance therapy aims to keep systemic copper levels low. Chelating agents may be continued indefinitely, although D-penicillamine causes a large number of serious toxic responses. Late reactions include various dermatopathies, the nephrotic syndrome, a lupuslike syndrome, thrombocytopenia, myasthenia gravis, and Goodpasture's syndrome. Trien is considerably less toxic and, given its equivalent efficacy, is preferred over penicillamine. Oral zinc salts can effectively lower body copper stores by preventing dietary copper absorption. Zinc acetate appears particularly well tolerated and is a suitable alternative to chelators for lifelong maintenance. Even with a striking resolution of neurological features, hepatic damage may be beyond repair, and death from liver failure may occur. Liver transplantation has been performed in this situation. There are also some claims that severe, seemingly irreversible neurological features may improve in response to orthotopic liver transplantation.

The rarity of this disease (30 patients per million population) and the wide variety of clinical manifestations ensure that no physician ever becomes familiar with the disease. Yet the need for specific therapy to be instituted as early as possible requires that the diagnosis be made promptly. Thus, it is imperative to maintain a conscious effort to suspect Wilson's disease in all young persons with neurological or psychiatric dysfunction for which a ready explanation is not available.

Paroxysmal Dyskinesias

A number of movement disorders are characterized by the intermittent nature of their manifestations (see Chapter 25, Table 25.12). Depending on the underlying cause, the neurological examination may be normal between attacks. Two well-defined idiopathic syndromes have been delineated. The more common, paroxysmal kinesigenic choreoathetosis, usually begins in childhood or early adolescence and affects boys four times as often as girls. In one-half of the cases there is a family history of a similar disorder, usually suggesting autosomal dominant inheritance. Paroxysms of chorea, dystonia, or a combination of the two are precipitated by rapid voluntary movements or startle and never last more than 5 minutes (usually <1 minute). They may involve either or both sides of the body during different episodes in the same patient.

Paroxysms may increase in frequency during adolescence, reaching a maximum of up to 100 times per day. After each episode there is typically a refractory period lasting several minutes during which the abnormal movements cannot be provoked. During adult life, the frequency may gradually decrease. The paroxysms are usually highly sensitive to anticonvulsants, especially phenytoin. Doses required for a satisfactory response are generally lower than those used in epilepsy. Investigations are unrevealing, and the interictal electroencephalogram is normal. Pathological studies have been unremarkable.

Paroxysmal nonkinesigenic choreoathetosis (PNKC) is distinguished from paroxysmal kinesigenic choreoathetosis by a number of clinical features. The onset is usually during infancy; boys are again more often affected but the ratio of boys to girls is only 3 to 2. The majority of these cases are familial with autosomal dominant transmission, but sporadic cases do occur. The gene for typical PNKC has been localized to chromosome 2q, whereas a form associated with spasticity has been assigned to chromosome 1p. The nature of the movement disorder is similar to that of paroxysmal kinesigenic choreoathetosis, but the duration is from 10 minutes to several hours; thus, PNKC is much more incapacitating. The frequency of PNKC is often only a few episodes per month, although individuals may suffer up to three paroxysms daily.

As the name implies, movement does not precipitate PNKC. However, fatigue, stress, or ingestion of alcohol or caffeine may induce paroxysms. PNKC does not respond to anticonvulsants, and medical therapy is often unrewarding. Limited success has been achieved with anticholinergics, L-dopa, acetazolamide, carbamazepine, haloperidol, gabapentin, and benzodiazepines, particularly clonazepam.

Families and sporadic cases have been described with an intermediate form consisting of dystonic spasms of both legs lasting 5–30 minutes and brought on by sustained exertion rather than sudden initiation of movement. Response to treatment is not striking.

A large proportion of patients with paroxysmal dyskinesias experience a prodrome of paresthesias, tightness, or some other vague premonitory sensory disturbance in the limbs to be affected, and some patients are able to suppress the paroxysms at this time using various techniques. Understanding of these paroxysmal dyskinesias and the related paroxysmal ataxias is advancing rapidly with the discovery of causative mutations in several genes coding for distinct ion channels (known as *channelopathies*).

Another paroxysmal movement disorder of uncertain classification is familial paroxysmal hypnogenic dystonia. This condition consists of brief, occasionally painful dystonic spasms occurring during non–rapid eye movement sleep. Age at onset and frequency of episodes are variable. Although anticonvulsants may be ineffective, there is considerable reason to believe that most, if not all, of these patients actually suffer from seizures originating in the frontal lobes, especially the supplementary motor area.

Stiff Man (Stiff Person) Syndrome

The stiff man syndrome is a disease of sporadic occurrence in adulthood. It develops insidiously as progressive stiffness, usually involving the lower back and legs. Triggered by movement, startle, or emotional distress, intermittent severe muscle spasms may be quite painful. The gait is particularly affected; it may appear slow, awkward, and robotic. Superimposed reflex action myoclonus may produce a jerking stiff man syndrome (Barker et al. 1998).

Pathological study results are usually normal, but electrophysiological investigations suggest the principal site of abnormality is spinal interneurons. The etiology is unknown. An autoimmune pathogenesis is suspected because of an association with diseases known to be autoimmune in nature (especially diabetes mellitus), and with the presence of antibodies to glutamic acid decarboxylase, each found in approximately 40% of patients. Additional evidence comes from the response of many patients to corticosteroid therapy, intravenous immunoglobulin, or plasmapheresis. Other useful treatments include diazepam, oral and intrathecal baclofen, valproate, vigabatrin, tizanidine, and botulinum toxin injections in paraspinal muscles.

Hallervorden-Spatz Disease

In 1922, Hallervorden and Spatz described the syndrome and pathological findings that characterize the disease that bears their names. Subsequent reports have strayed somewhat from the original description. The term *Hallervorden-Spatz disease* should probably be reserved for the pediatric neurodegenerative disorder (Halliday 1995). The majority of cases are familial, and the pattern of inheritance suggests autosomal recessive transmission, with demonstrated linkage to chromosome 20p.

The clinical manifestations begin insidiously in childhood or early adolescence with motor difficulties, especially with gait and speech. On examination, dystonia usually is present, often in conjunction with rigidity, tremor, or athetosis. Signs of corticospinal tract dysfunction are usually evident. Dementia is common. The motor abnormalities progress, and the combination of dystonia, rigidity, and spasticity leads to extreme stiffness and immobility of the limbs, particularly the legs. Seizures, retinitis pigmentosa, and optic atrophy have been recorded. Death usually ensues in early adulthood.

For the diagnosis to be made with any certainty, there must be pathological confirmation in the patient or a relative. Some authors have demonstrated increased radioactive iron uptake in globus pallidus antemortem. CT scanning findings have been variable and nonspecific; usually there is pronounced shrinkage of the whole brain and occasionally increased density in the globus pallidus, possibly indicative of iron deposition. T2-weighted MRI scans in patients suspected of having Hallervorden-Spatz disease have revealed a marked reduction in signal intensity in the pallidum and substantia nigra reticulata consistent with iron deposition, often with intermixed areas of increased signal in the pallidum (the eye-of-the-tiger sign).

Gross inspection of the brain at autopsy reveals brown discoloration of the globus pallidus and substantia nigra pars reticulata, reflecting a heavy accumulation of iron and other pigments in these areas. Microscopically (Figure 75.18), these nuclei show loss of neurons and myelinated fibers with gliosis and a large number of axonal swellings known as *spheroids*, which are found also in lesser numbers elsewhere in the brain and spinal cord. The presence of the latter structures suggests a common link with infantile neuroaxonal dystrophy.

Hallervorden-Spatz syndrome is a more nonspecific term encompassing a number of disorders, each having the triad of pallidal iron deposition, axonal spheroids, and gliosis (Halliday 1995). Speculation regarding the pathogenesis of these pathological changes has centered around abnormal peroxidation of lipofuscin to neuromelanin and deficient cysteine dioxygenase activity. Prompted by the cerebral depositions, attempts to define an abnormality of iron metabolism have been fruitless. Iron chelation therapy has not been rewarding, and no effective treatment for the disease is known. Dopaminergic agents and anticholinergics may lessen symptoms temporarily. Another autosomal recessive disorder associated with severe iron deposition in brain and visceral organs resulting in progressive dementia, dystonia, orofacial dyskinesias, tics, ataxia, and diabetes is hereditary ceruloplasmin deficiency with hemosiderosis.

Calcification of the Basal Ganglia

Cerebral deposition of calcium may follow numerous focal and diffuse pathological brain processes. In this section we are concerned with symmetrical calcium deposits in the basal ganglia, specifically the lenticular nuclei, which accumulate spontaneously (i.e., without a prior history of cerebral disease). Extensive calcification of other cerebral structures, including cortex, white matter, and cerebellum, may be present (Figure 75.19).

Calcification of the basal ganglia (CBG) may be found in three clinical situations: in association with hypoparathy-

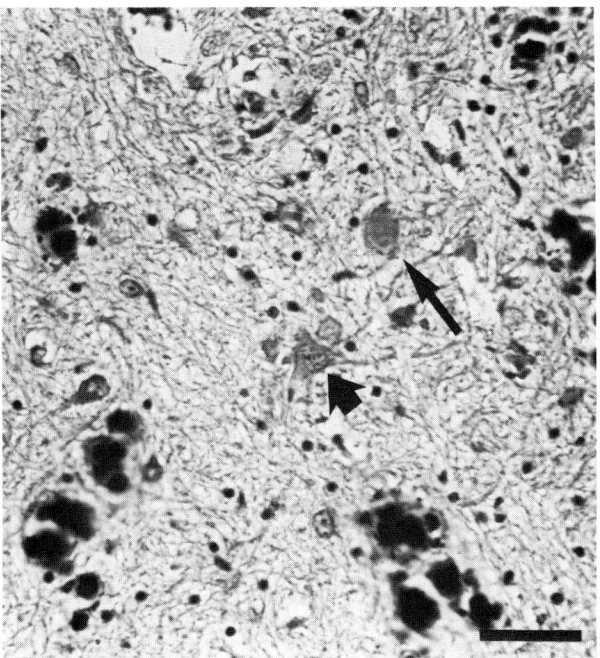

FIGURE 75.18 Microscopic pathology of Hallervorden-Spatz syndrome. This section from the globus pallidus shows iron concretions (*dark masses*), and axonal spheroid (*long arrow*), and a reactive astrocyte (*short arrow*) (hematoxylin and eosin stain). (Courtesy of Dr. Lothar Resch.)

roidism of any type or, rarely, with other metabolic diseases (e.g., mitochondrial cytopathies); as a familial trait (Kobari et al. 1997); and as a sporadic condition without abnormality of calcium metabolism. The advent of CT has revealed that the last situation is by far the most common, and up to 1.5% of all brain scans may demonstrate this finding. The vast majority of individuals have no corresponding clinical signs, leading one to question the significance of calcification in those few patients who are symptomatic. In otherwise healthy individuals CBG usually consists of small deposits in the medial segment of the globus pallidus, which increase in frequency with age. Symptomatic patients generally have more extensive calcification, but there is little correlation between the extent of CT or even pathological changes and the symptoms.

Many causes exist for CBG (Table 75.10), several without known disturbances of calcium metabolism. One uncommon form, familial idiopathic cerebral calcification, may be inherited as an autosomal dominant or recessive trait. The onset of symptoms is usually in the third or fourth decade. Symptoms and signs of this disorder, or of CBG associated with hypoparathyroidism, include movement disorders, such as parkinsonism, dystonia, or chorea; epilepsy; a variety of psychiatric disturbances; dementia; pyramidal tract signs; and ataxia. The cause of the calcium deposits is unknown, and the course is one of deterioration of neurological function over several years, with death

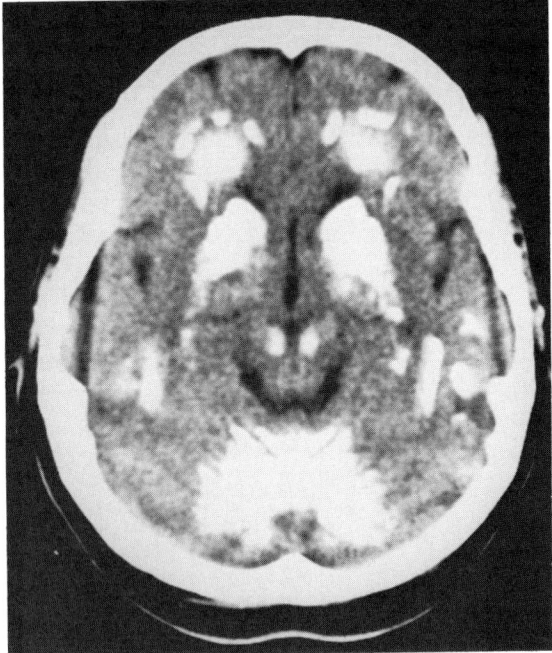 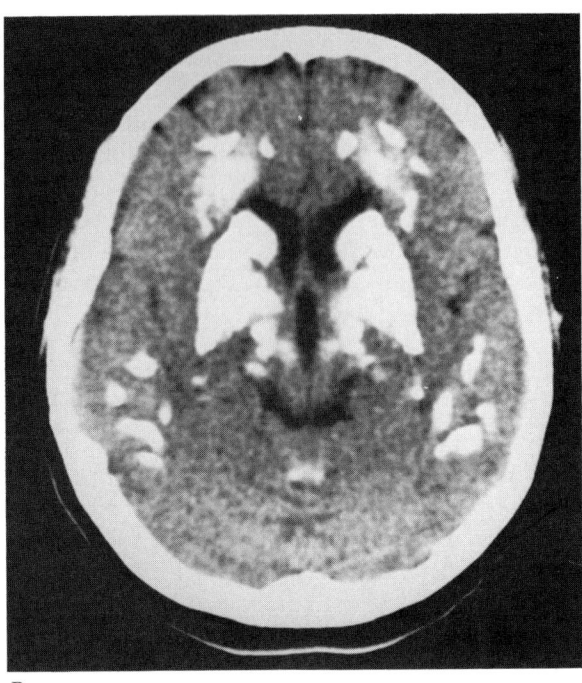

A   B

FIGURE 75.19   Extensive idiopathic calcification of the brain, including striatum, pallidum, cerebral white matter, and cerebellum, in computed tomographic scans without contrast enhancement. (Courtesy of Dr. Joseph Chu.)

occurring as a complication of seizures or secondary medical illness.

Doubt regarding the pathogenetic relevance of the calcium deposits to the clinical picture stems from both familial and hypoparathyroid patient groups. In autosomal dominant basal ganglia calcification and dystonia, each of these two features frequently is found in isolation in other members of the family. Complete resolution of parkinsonism in a patient with surgical hypoparathyroidism and CBG can occur within

2 days of correction of hypocalcemia; this is clearly insufficient time to permit resorption of the calcium deposits and suggests that the parkinsonism was related to the underlying metabolic defect. However, normalization of serum calcium does not always result in reversal of symptoms.

In summary, CBG is a finding of uncertain clinical significance. Its main value should be to prompt evaluation for an underlying metabolic abnormality and assessment of other family members.

Table 75.10:   Causes of symmetrical calcification of the basal ganglia

Physiological
Hypoparathyroidism (various causes including
   pseudohypoparathyroidism)
?Hyperparathyroidism
Familial idiopathic cerebral calcification (Fahr's syndrome)
Birth anoxia
Carbon monoxide intoxication
Lead poisoning
Tuberous sclerosis
Cockayne's syndrome
Postinfectious
Acquired immunodeficiency syndrome (especially in children)
Radiation therapy
Methotrexate therapy
Kearns-Sayre syndrome and other mitochondrial diseases
Familial encephalopathies
Down syndrome

Neuroacanthocytosis (Choreoacanthocytosis)

Acanthocytes are red blood cells with an appearance characterized by irregular stubby spines or projections from the cell surface. They are presumed to arise from a defect in membrane lipids. Their presence in the blood is correlated with a number of systemic abnormalities. In Bassen-Kornzweig disease, acanthocytosis is associated with abetalipoproteinemia, retinitis pigmentosa, and a progressive neurological deficit, mainly ataxia. Another related disorder with basal ganglia symptomatology, particularly orofacial dystonia, is the HARP syndrome (hypoprebetalipoproteinemia, acanthocytosis, retinitis pigmentosa, and pallidal degeneration).

A number of reports have described a movement disorder in association with acanthocytosis with characteristic clinical and laboratory manifestations. The disorder may be inherited in an autosomal recessive fashion, and genetic linkage has been established on chromosome 9q21. Rare cases related to McLeod's syndrome are X-linked. Clinically unaffected family members may have a higher than normal proportion of acanthocytes in their blood. The illness usually begins in the third or fourth decade of life with orofacial dyskinesias, which may produce mutilation of the lips and tongue. Some patients have pronounced difficulty eating as a result of lingual and oral action dystonia. Vocal and motor tics may be present. Additional features include generalized chorea with some dystonic features, cognitive changes, parkinsonism, a predominantly motor peripheral neuropathy with amyotrophy, and seizures.

Acanthocytes account for at least 10% of all peripheral red blood cells. These are best appreciated using a fresh blood smear (wet preparation). The serum creatine kinase is usually elevated, and electrodiagnostic studies confirm the presence of the motor neuropathy. The plasma lipid profile is normal. MRI may demonstrate atrophy of the caudate nucleus or T2-weighted hyperintensities in the striatum. PET scans have shown reduced striatal glucose metabolism.

Clearly, the clinical picture of chorea with cognitive changes may lead to a diagnosis of HD, and the imaging abnormalities noted previously are common to both HD and neuroacanthocytosis. It is imperative to perform a blood smear in all patients presenting with this syndrome. Other distinguishing features are peripheral neuropathy, self-mutilation, seizures (also common in juvenile-onset HD), and different inheritance patterns.

Biopsy material shows a mixed picture of axonal degeneration and demyelination in peripheral nerve and neurogenic atrophy in muscle. At autopsy, the CNS abnormalities are concentrated in the basal ganglia, comprising severe neuronal loss and gliosis in the striatum and, to a lesser degree, in the globus pallidus (Rinne et al. 1994).

Treatment is limited to symptomatic therapy for the movement disorder and seizures. In late stages the dyskinesias may be supplanted by typical parkinsonism. The rate of progression is highly variable; death may ensue within a few years, but survival for decades is known also.

Hemifacial Spasm

Hemifacial spasm is a focal movement disorder causing intermittent clonic and tonic contraction of the muscles innervated by the facial nerve. It most often begins insidiously in the orbicularis oculi muscle and, in the early stages, may be confused with benign fasciculations of the eyelid. Electromyography shows that the spasms are caused by brief bursts of normal motor units firing at high frequency. The disorder usually spreads slowly to involve the ipsilateral facial musculature. The distribution, rhythm, and amplitude of individual contractions are highly variable. Paroxysms of spasms may increase in frequency and intensity and climax in a sustained contraction lasting up to a minute; emotional upset and fatigue typically aggravate them. Spasms may be precipitated by active movement of any facial muscle. The movements cannot be suppressed voluntarily and may persist during sleep. Rare bilateral cases exist; here, the time of onset and the timing of individual spasms on each side are each independent of the other.

Hemifacial spasm almost always begins in adult life and is more common in women. There is usually no antecedent history, but occasionally it follows a Bell's palsy or trauma to the seventh cranial nerve. Even in cryptogenic cases there may be mild weakness of ipsilateral voluntary facial movements, but frequently weakness is more apparent than real. In long-standing cases synkinetic movements may be seen. Extended remissions lasting weeks to years have been noted in some cases, but for most patients the condition is permanent in the absence of treatment.

The safest and most successful treatment for hemifacial spasm is injection of botulinum toxin. Relief is usually prompt and lasts several months. Microsurgical decompression of the facial nerve is also effective but is much costlier and exposes patients to a much greater risk of severe complications. This procedure, which is often curative, commonly demonstrates mechanical compression of the facial nerve at the root exit zone by an arterial loop. The occurrence of rare "symptomatic" forms of hemifacial spasm caused by operable lesions, such as aneurysms and cerebellopontine angle tumors, encourages the need for investigation with MRI or contrast-enhanced CT scan. Medical treatment using the anticonvulsants carbamazepine, phenytoin, or gabapentin may occasionally control the facial spasms.

PSYCHOGENIC MOVEMENT DISORDERS

Specialists in movement disorders shied away from diagnoses of psychogenic illness when it became clear that dystonia was largely a neurological and not a psychiatric entity. More recently, the maturation of the subspecialty, in part because of familiarity with typical organic movement disorders after decades of study, has led to confidence in the ability to distinguish patients with psychogenic movement disorders. Although any formal discussion involves the listing of multiple diagnostic criteria (Fahn 1994), the presence of atypical clinical features is the most important factor suggesting that a movement disorder may have a psychological basis. Other highly suggestive findings include inconsistencies in the appearance of the movements, psychiatric abnormalities, and secondary gain.

The most common movement disorders to appear on a psychogenic basis are tremor, dystonia, myoclonus, and gait disorders. Psychogenic movements are often mixed in type or bizarre and difficult to characterize. Psychogenic parkinsonism also has been described. Women outnumber men in most studies. One-half of patients also suffer from a psychiatric illness, usually depression, and up to 10% have psychogenic dyskinesias superimposed on an organic neurological disorder. Considering the many ways harm can be done by mislabeling someone with a psychogenic illness, it is crucial that confirmation of such a diagnosis come from one experienced in every variety of movement disorder.

The treatment of psychogenic illness must naturally be tailored to each patient's personality, but certain guiding principles should be followed. The patient must be recognized as being as disabled as one with the same deficits occurring on an organic basis. The lack of evidence of permanent damage to the nervous system, and the chance for complete remission, should be emphasized. Routine psychiatric consultation is warranted because of the high frequency of depression and other treatable conditions. Unfortunately, in many cases, especially those with long-standing symptoms and without an obvious acute precipitant, prognosis for recovery is poor.

REFERENCES

Barker RA, Revesz T, Thom M, et al. Review of 23 patients affected by the stiff man syndrome: clinical subdivision into stiff trunk (man) syndrome, stiff limb syndrome, and progressive encephalomyelitis with rigidity. J Neurol Neurosurg Psychiatry 1998;65: 633–640.

Berardelli A, Rothwell JC, Hallett M, et al. The pathophysiology of primary dystonia. Brain 1998;121:1195–1212.

Blunt SB, Lane RJ, Turjanski N, Perkin GD. Clinical features and management of two cases of encephalitis lethargica. Mov Disord 1997;12:354–359.

Brown P, Rothwell JC, Thompson PD, Marsden CD. Propriospinal myoclonus: evidence for spinal "pattern" generators in humans. Mov Disord 1994;9:571–576.

Buckley PF, Hutchinson M. Neuroleptic malignant syndrome. J Neurol Neurosurg Psychiatry 1995;58:271–273.

Dauer WT, Burke RE, Greene P, Fahn S. Current concepts on the clinical features, aetiology and management of idiopathic cervical dystonia. Brain 1998;121:547–560.

Demirkiran M, Jankovic J. Paroxysmal dyskinesias: clinical features and classification. Ann Neurol 1995;38:571–579.

Duyao M, Ambrose C, Myers R, et al. Trinucleotide repeat length instability and age of onset in Huntington's disease. Nat Genet 1993;4:387–392.

Factor SA, Weiner WJ. Early combination therapy with bromocriptine and levodopa in Parkinson's disease. Mov Disord 1993; 8:257–262.

Fahn S. Psychogenic Movement Disorders. In CD Marsden, S Fahn (eds), Movement Disorders (3rd ed). London: Butterworth–Heinemann, 1994;359–372.

Feany MB, Dickson DW. Widespread cytoskeletal pathology characterizes corticobasal degeneration. Am J Pathol 1995;146: 1388–1396.

Floeter MK, Andermann F, Andermann E, et al. Physiological studies of spinal inhibitory pathways in patients with hereditary hyperexplexia. Neurology 1996;46:766–772.

Geddes JF, Hughes AJ, Lees AJ, et al. Pathological overlap in cases of parkinsonism associated with neurofibrillary tangles. Brain 1993;116:281–302.

Giedd JN, Rapoport JL, Kruesi MJ, et al. Sydenham's chorea: magnetic resonance imaging of the basal ganglia. Neurology 1995;45:2199–2202.

Halliday W. The nosology of Hallervorden-Spatz disease. J Neurol Sci 1995;134:84–91.

Hubble JP, Busenbark KL, Pahwa R, et al. Clinical expression of essential tremor: effects of gender and age. Mov Disord 1997; 12:969–972.

The Huntington's Disease Collaborative Research Group. A novel gene containing a trinucleotide repeat that is expanded and unstable on Huntington's disease chromosomes. Cell 1993;72:971–983.

Jenkins IH, Bain PG, Colebatch JG, et al. A positron emission tomography study of essential tremor: evidence for overactivity of cerebellar connections. Ann Neurol 1993;34:82–90.

Kiriakakis V, Bhatia KP, Quinn NP, Marsden CD. The natural history of tardive dystonia. A long-term follow-up study of 107 cases. Brain 1998;121:2053–2066.

Kobari M, Nogawa S, Sugimoto Y, Fukuuchi Y. Familial idiopathic brain calcification with autosomal dominant inheritance. Neurology 1997;48:645–649.

Kurlan R. Tourette's syndrome and "PANDAS": will the relation bear out? Neurology 1998;50:1530–1534.

Lang AE, Lozano AM. Parkinson's disease. N Engl J Med 1998;1044–1053, 1130–1143.

Litvan I. Progressive supranuclear palsy: staring into the past, moving into the future. The Neurologist 1998;4:13–20.

Papp MI, Lantos PL. The distribution of oligodendroglial inclusions in multiple system atrophy and its relevance to clinical symptomatology. Brain 1994;117:235–243.

The Parkinson Study Group. Effects of tocopherol and deprenyl on the progression of disability in early Parkinson's disease. N Engl J Med 1993;328:176–183.

Quinn N. Essential myoclonus and myoclonic dystonia. Mov Disord 1996;11:119–124.

Quinn N. Multiple System Atrophy. In CD Marsden, S Fahn (eds), Movement Disorders (3rd ed). Oxford: Butterworth–Heinemann, 1994;262–281.

Riley DE. Secondary Parkinsonism. In J Jankovic, E Tolosa (eds), Parkinson's Disease and Movement Disorders (3rd ed). Baltimore: Williams & Wilkins, 1998;317–339.

Rinne JO, Daniel SE, Scaravilli F, et al. The neuropathological features of neuroacanthocytosis. Mov Disord 1994;9:297–304.

Ross CA, Margolis RL, Rosenblatt A, et al. Huntington disease and the related disorder, dentatorubral-pallidoluysian atrophy (DRPLA). Medicine 1997;76:305–338.

Sadovnick D, Kurlan R. The increasingly complex genetics of Tourette's syndrome. Neurology 1997;48:801–802.

Singer HS, Reiss AL, Brown JE, et al. Volumetric MRI changes in basal ganglia of children with Tourette's syndrome. Neurology 1993;43:950–956.

Waters CH, Faust PL, Powers J, et al. Neuropathology of lubag (X-linked dystonia parkinsonism). Mov Disord 1993;8:387–390.

Werhahn KJ, Brown P, Thompson PD, Marsden CD. The clinical features and prognosis of chronic posthypoxic myoclonus. Mov Disord 1997;12:216–220.

Wichmann T, DeLong MR. Physiology of the Basal Ganglia and Pathophysiology of Movement Disorders of Basal Ganglia Origin. In RL Watts, WC Koller (eds), Movement Disorders: Neurologic Principles and Practice. New York: McGraw-Hill, 1997;87–97.

Woerner MG, Alvir JM, Saltz BL, et al. Prospective study of tardive dyskinesia in the elderly: rates and risk factors. Am J Psychiatry 1998;155:1521–1528.

Wolf SS, Jones DW, Knable MB, et al. Tourette syndrome: prediction of phenotypic variation in monozygotic twins by caudate nucleus D2 receptor binding. Science 1996;273:1225–1227.

Young AB, Penney JB. Biochemical and Functional Organization of the Basal Ganglia. In J Jankovic, E Tolosa (eds), Parkinson's Disease and Movement Disorders (3rd ed). Baltimore: Williams & Wilkins, 1998;1–13.

Chapter 76
Cerebellar and Spinocerebellar Disorders

Nicholas W. Wood and Anita E. Harding[†]

This chapter describes diseases affecting the cerebellum and its afferent projections from the spinal cord. Although these structures are involved in a wide variety of disorders, degenerative disease, either inherited or idiopathic, is the most common cause of progressive cerebellar or spinocerebellar syndromes. For this reason, and because many of the other causes of cerebellar dysfunction are discussed in detail elsewhere in this book, a large part of this chapter deals with degenerative ataxias.

DEVELOPMENTAL DISORDERS AFFECTING THE CEREBELLUM

The cerebellum has a long developmental period and is not fully mature until about 18 months of age. The length of this period renders the developing cerebellum susceptible to a large number of insults, including intrauterine infections, ischemic damage, and toxins. Some of these developmental anomalies, such as dysgenesis or agenesis of the vermis,

cerebellar hemispheres, or parts of the brainstem, give rise to congenital ataxia, usually associated with other features of neurological dysfunction. These are described in Chapter 66 and include the Chiari malformations and Dandy-Walker syndrome. By definition, the congenital ataxias are not progressive disorders, and in most cases, coordination improves with age. The majority of these nonspecific congenital ataxic disorders are difficult to label precisely on clinical grounds (Table 76.1). Postmortem examination most commonly shows ponto-neocerebellar hypoplasia or granule cell hypoplasia. Many patients are diagnosed as having ataxic cerebral palsy during life, especially if there are no similarly affected siblings. Affected sibling pairs are often reported, and about 50% of single cases of congenital cerebellar ataxia are recessively inherited. Autosomal dominant and X-linked pedigrees have also been described.

The clinical features of this group of disorders are variable. Rare but distinctive clinical syndromes exist in which maldevelopment of the cerebellum is associated with other features (see Table 76.1). For example, episodic abnormal eye movements and hyperpnea are seen in Joubert's syndrome, an autosomal recessive disorder in which there is

---

[†]Dr. Harding died before revision of the chapter.

Table 76.1: Congenital inherited ataxic disorders

Congenital ataxia with mental retardation and spasticity (includes ponto-neocerebellar and granule cell hypoplasia); autosomal recessive, autosomal dominant, and X-linked

Congenital ataxia with episodic hyperpnea, abnormal eye movements, and mental retardation (Joubert's syndrome; autosomal recessive)

Congenital ataxia with mental retardation and partial aniridia (Gillespie's syndrome; uncertain inheritance)

Disequilibrium syndrome (autosomal recessive)

X-linked recessive ataxia with spasticity, mental retardation, and microcephaly (Paine's syndrome)

Source: Adapted from AE Harding, JV Diengdoh, AJ Lees. Autosomal recessive late-onset multisystem disorder with cerebellar cortical atrophy at autopsy: report of a family. J Neurol Neurosurg Psychiatry 1984;47:853–856.

dysgenesis of the cerebellar vermis. Partial aniridia is a distinctive feature of Gillespie's syndrome, together with ataxia and mental retardation. The disequilibrium syndrome, described mainly in Scandinavia and transmitted as an autosomal recessive trait, is characterized by mental retardation, ataxia, and marked motor delay. Affected children do not walk until approximately 10 years of age. Carbohydrate-deficient glycoprotein syndrome produces a retinopathy, hypotonia, developmental delay, and, perhaps most distinctive of all, an unusual fat distribution. It is an autosomal recessive disorder, and one form of the disorder has been linked to chromosome 16p13. As the name suggests, a defect of glycoprotein metabolism has been demonstrated.

Patients with less severe developmental anomalies of the cerebellum and its connections often have nonspecific clinical features. Cerebellar dysfunction in an infant or young child may be overlooked because it often gives rise to relatively nonspecific abnormal motor development, such as delayed motor development and hypotonia. Later nystagmus, obvious incoordination on reaching for objects, and truncal ataxia when first attempting to sit are observed. Mental retardation is common; limb spasticity may occur.

INFECTIONS INVOLVING THE CEREBELLUM

Infections diffusely affecting the nervous system are described in Chapter 59. This section deals with infectious illnesses that give rise to prominent cerebellar dysfunction.

Infections Causing Progressive Ataxia with a Chronic or Subacute Course

Infectious causes of progressive ataxia are rare. In childhood, the chronic panencephalitis of congenital rubella infection can cause a progressive cerebellar syndrome, accompanied by dementia, optic atrophy, and occasionally multifocal myoclonus with onset between the ages of 8 and

19 years. This condition has many features in common with subacute sclerosing panencephalitis and sometimes follows childhood rubella infection. Ataxia has also been described in children with the acquired immunodeficiency syndrome and encephalopathy.

In adults, cerebellar dysfunction may dominate the clinical picture of the Creutzfeldt-Jakob disease phenotype of prion disease for several months, but other features of the disease, such as dementia and myoclonus, develop relatively quickly and are prominent in most cases. Patients with the Gerstmann-Sträussler phenotype (or kuru) often have marked cerebellar ataxia in the early phase of the disease (see Chapter 59). The so-called new variant Creutzfeldt-Jakob disease, first described in Britain in 1996, may also present with prominent cerebellar features and must be considered in the differential diagnosis of progressive cerebellar syndromes (Stewart et al. 1998). The role of tonsillar biopsy to establish the diagnosis is still under review (Collinge et al. 1998).

Infections Causing Ataxia with Acute or Subacute Onset

The most common cerebellar syndrome attributed to viral infection is acute cerebellar ataxia of childhood, although serological evidence of viral infection is lacking in most cases. It usually occurs in children aged 1–8 years, but older children and adults with a similar illness have been described. The neurological illness is often preceded by varicella but may also follow a trivial respiratory or gastrointestinal tract infection. A severe truncal ataxia with less prominent limb involvement occurs, and it is maximal at onset. There is often static and kinetic tremor of the head, trunk, and limbs. Recovery is usually complete but can take up to 6 months. A mild mononuclear cerebrospinal fluid (CSF) pleocytosis may be present. Other implicated viruses include echovirus, Coxsackie groups A and B, poliovirus, Epstein-Barr, and herpes simplex. This syndrome has also been described after some bacterial infections in childhood.

Patients with Bickerstaff's brainstem encephalitis may be ataxic, but the ataxia is usually overshadowed by other features of brainstem involvement, including ophthalmoplegia. This condition should be distinguished from the Miller-Fisher variant of acute inflammatory polyneuropathy (see Chapter 80).

Other Infections

Cerebellar involvement has been described in central nervous system (CNS) infection by *Mycoplasma pneumoniae*, *Legionella pneumoniae*, and *Toxoplasma gondii*, as well as in typhoid fever and tick paralysis. Cerebellar ataxia, combined with bilateral facial palsy and a lymphocytic CSF pleocytosis, has also been described in *Borrelia burgdorferi* infection (Lyme disease). A transient cerebellar syndrome lasting several weeks and resembling acute cerebellar ataxia of childhood has been reported after *Plasmodium falciparum* infection. Cerebellar signs, particularly gait ataxia, are common in the racemose form of cysticercosis. Bacterial cerebellar abscess usually gives rise to headache and other features of raised intracranial pressure, as well as ataxia. The same applies to CNS tuberculosis, in which ataxia may occur secondary to hydrocephalus or posterior fossa tuberculomas.

NEOPLASTIC DISORDERS: PARANEOPLASTIC CEREBELLAR DEGENERATION

Primary and secondary tumors involving the cerebellum are discussed in Chapters 58. In 1965, Brain and Wilkinson established in detail the occurrence of cerebellar degeneration as a nonmetastatic complication of malignancy. It has since become apparent that this syndrome is heterogeneous, consisting of several disorders that can be distinguished clinically and immunologically, differing in the types of associated malignancies.

Approximately one-half of patients with paraneoplastic cerebellar degeneration (PCD) have demonstrable antibodies directed against neurons in serum and CSF. These antibodies differ in their pattern of immunostaining and the size of antigen detected on Western blotting. They are not detected in patients with other cerebellar diseases.

The most common antibody seen in PCD is called *anti-Yo*. It specifically stains Purkinje's cell cytoplasm in a granular pattern corresponding to Nissl's substance and detects a 62-kD antigen on Western blots. It is found exclusively in women; one-half of them have ovarian cancer, and the rest have breast or other gynecological malignancies or adenocarcinoma of unknown source. Presentation with ataxia precedes diagnosis of the malignancy in 70% of cases and is usually subacute, progressing to severe disability over several months or even weeks and then stopping. Onset may be acute and is sometimes accompanied by vertigo, mimicking a vascular event. There is severe truncal, gait, and limb ataxia and dysarthria. Abnormal eye movements are common, with nystagmus, often downbeat, and occasionally opsoclonus. Opsoclonus may be combined with myoclonus, producing a disorder in adults similar to dancing eye syndrome of childhood, which is sometimes associated with neuroblastoma. Mild cognitive impairment, peripheral neuropathy, or both occur in a minority of patients.

The CSF usually shows a mild lymphocytic pleocytosis and contains oligoclonal immunoglobulin G (IgG). Imaging studies show cerebellar atrophy, but marked ataxia may predate these changes. Pathologically, there is depletion of Purkinje's cells with proliferation of Bergmann's astrocytes and minor inflammatory infiltration of the cerebellar leptomeninges. The underlying tumor tissue expresses the antigen recognized by anti-Yo antibodies. There is no evidence of a useful response to immunosuppressant therapy or to plasma exchange, but there are anecdotal reports of some improvement or stabilization after removal of the primary tumor. The best method of screening for the underlying malignancy is debated, but standard magnetic resonance imaging (MRI) may be complemented by whole-body positron emission tomography. Searching for primary tumor markers is also useful.

A different type of Purkinje's cell antibody is seen in about one-third of patients with PCD associated with Hodgkin's disease. It stains the cytoplasm diffusely and is not detectable on Western blot. PCD in Hodgkin's disease is more common in men with known lymphoma, although onset is not related to stage of disease; it may herald a relapse. The clinical features are very similar to those seen in patients with anti-Yo antibodies, but there is a slightly higher chance of spontaneous recovery.

Anti-Hu antibodies stain nuclei of cells throughout the CNS and are most commonly detected in patients with small-cell lung cancer and paraneoplastic sensory neuropathy or diffuse encephalomyelitis. Diffuse encephalomyelitis occasionally presents clinically as isolated PCD. A patient with breast cancer, PCD, and antineuronal antibodies who shared some, but not all, features of anti-Hu antibodies was reported to improve substantially after intravenous gamma globulin therapy (Moll et al. 1993).

Excluding those with Hodgkin's disease, PCD patients without detectable antineuronal antibodies are most likely to have breast or lung cancers. In the latter, PCD may be combined with Lambert-Eaton myasthenic syndrome (see Chapter 82). Significantly, the antibodies in Lambert-Eaton myasthenic syndrome are directed against a voltage-gated calcium channel. The CNS equivalent of this channel is mutated in hereditary episodic ataxia type 2 and spinocerebellar ataxia type 6 (SCA6) (see Episodic Ataxia type 2 and Late-Onset Inherited Ataxias, later in this chapter). The clinical and investigative features are similar to those described in association with anti-Yo antibodies, although progression may be slightly slower, with less severe involvement of speech and ocular movements. It seems that patients in this seronegative group are more likely to improve neurologically after treatment of their cancer.

The exact prevalence of PCD is hard to establish, but it probably occurs in less than 5% of patients with lung or ovarian cancer. It is not a common cause of slowly progressive degenerative cerebellar disease after age 40, as has been suggested in the past, but it probably accounts for at least 50% of cases of subacute cerebellar syndromes in this age group. Detection of antineuronal antibodies is of value diagnostically (although their absence does not exclude PCD) and may point to a specific occult malignancy, such as a gynecological lesion in the presence of anti-Yo antibodies.

VASCULAR DISEASES INVOLVING THE CEREBELLUM

Cerebrovascular disease is discussed in detail in Chapter 57 and is mentioned in terms of differential diagnosis in Chap-

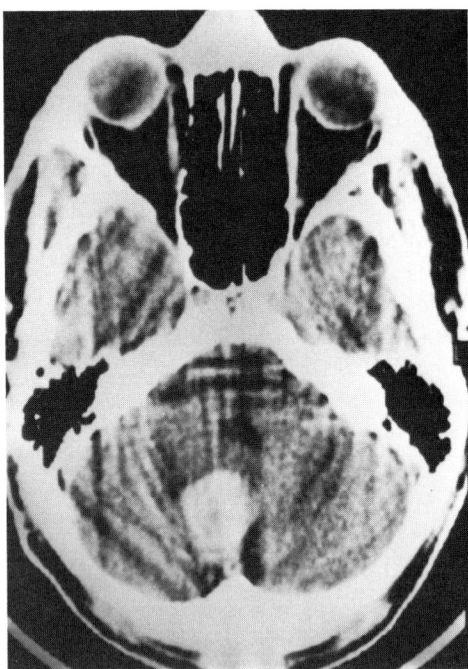

FIGURE 76.1 Computed tomographic scan showing cerebellar hemorrhage, particularly involving the left hemisphere and displacing the fourth ventricle.

Table 76.2: Inherited ataxic disorders with known metabolic defects

Intermittent ataxias
  With hyperammonemia: ornithine transcarbamylase deficiency, argininosuccinate synthetase deficiency (citrullinemia), argininosuccinase deficiency (argininosuccinicaciduria), arginase deficiency (hyperornithinemia)
  Aminoacidurias: Hartnup disease, intermittent branched-chain ketoaciduria, isovaleric acidemia
  Disorders of pyruvate and lactate metabolism: pyruvate dehydrogenase deficiency, pyruvate carboxylase deficiency, Leigh disease, multiple carboxylase deficiencies
Progressive ataxias
  Abeta- and hypobetalipoproteinemia
  Hexosaminidase deficiency*
  Cholestanolosis*
  Leukodystrophies*: metachromatic, late-onset globoid cell, adrenoleukomyeloneuropathy
  Mitochondrial encephalomyopathies*
  Partial hypoxanthine guanine phosphoribosyl transferase deficiency*
  Wilson's disease*
  Ceroid lipofuscinosis*
  Sialidosis
  Sphingomyelin storage disorders*
Disorders associated with defective DNA repair
  Ataxia telangiectasia
  Xeroderma pigmentosum*
  Cockayne's syndrome

*Ataxia may not be a prominent feature.
Source: Adapted from AE Harding, JV Diengdoh, AJ Lees. Autosomal-recessive late-onset multisystem disorder with cerebellar cortical atrophy at autopsy: report of a family. J Neurol Neurosurg Psychiatry 1984;47:853–856.

ter 24. Only aspects of vascular disease specific to cerebellar function are described in this chapter.

Transient ischemic attacks involving the vascular supply to the cerebellum rarely produce ataxia and dysarthria alone; associated symptoms of brainstem dysfunction, such as vertigo, diplopia, and blurring of vision, are usually more prominent. Cerebellar ataxia is hardly ever reported during the prodrome of an attack of migraine in adults, although it occurs in children.

Infarction and Hemorrhage

Cerebellar infarction (from embolus or, more commonly, vertebrobasilar occlusive disease) and hemorrhage (usually on a background of hypertension or, less commonly, secondary to a vascular malformation or tumor) are relatively rare. They are difficult to distinguish from each other on clinical grounds and are often misdiagnosed, unless imaging is performed early (Figure 76.1). Late diagnosis of cerebellar hemorrhage is associated with a poor prognosis, and approximately 20% of patients die before reaching medical attention. Both infarction and hemorrhage may be amenable to surgical therapy.

Superficial Siderosis

Superficial siderosis (or hemosiderosis) is a rare disorder that causes slowly progressive cerebellar ataxia, mainly of

gait, and often sensorineural deafness, corticospinal tract signs, dementia, bladder disturbance, anosmia, and sensory signs.

METABOLIC DISORDERS GIVING RISE TO CEREBELLAR DYSFUNCTION

Intermittent Metabolic Ataxias

A number of metabolic disorders with onset in infancy or early childhood, such as disorders of the urea cycle, some aminoacidurias, and disorders of pyruvate and lactate metabolism, give rise to intermittent ataxia, among other features (Table 76.2) (see Chapter 68). Hyperammonemia, usually caused by deficiencies of urea cycle enzymes (ornithine transcarbamylase [OTC], argininosuccinate synthetase, argininosuccinase, and arginase), is the most common metabolic abnormality associated with intermittent ataxia. These disorders have a similar clinical picture, comprising intermittent ataxia, dysarthria, vomiting, headache, ptosis, involuntary movements, seizures, and confusion, which develops in early childhood. Such episodes may be precipitated by high protein loads and intercurrent illness. A variable degree of mental retardation is associated. Brittle hair and dysmorphic features are common in children with argininosuccinicaciduria (argininosuccinase deficiency). Hyperornithinemia, which is not a urea cycle enzyme deficiency disorder, is also associated with hyperammonemia and an intermittant ataxia. Treatment consists of protein restriction and intravenous fluid administration during acute episodes of neurological dysfunction.

OTC deficiency is X-linked, but all other hyperammonemias have autosomal recessive inheritance. OTC deficiency is the most common urea cycle enzyme defect; affected males die in the neonatal period, but severity varies considerably in females, from severe neurological deficit to no symptoms apart from mild protein intolerance. Prenatal diagnosis is possible in OTC deficiency and some of the other hyperammonemias.

Some aminoacidurias, including intermittent branched-chain ketoaciduria and isovaleric acidemia, present in a similar way clinically to hyperammonemia. In Hartnup disease, renal and intestinal transport of monoamino-monocarboxylic acids is defective. The features of this disorder are intermittent ataxia, tremor, chorea, psychiatric disturbances, and mental retardation associated with a pellagralike rash in childhood. Inheritance is autosomal recessive. A high-protein diet and oral nicotinamide therapy may be of benefit.

Pyruvate dehydrogenase (PDH) deficiency is rare and probably heterogeneous, although the majority of cases are caused by mutations in the gene for the E1 α-subunit of the enzyme. This gene is on the X chromosome, and there is a high frequency of manifesting female heterozygotes with a wide spectrum of disease severity due to variable X chromosome inactivation. The disease either presents in infancy with severe lactic acidosis and early death or is dominated by neurological dysfunction and may run a more protracted course, occasionally with survival into adult life; the latter is more common in females. Although ataxia, sometimes episodic and related to lactic acidosis, is well recognized in PDH deficiency, it is not usually the major clinical feature. More commonly, the picture is dominated by seizures, severe mental retardation, and spasticity. Structural (dysplastic) abnormalities of the brain are common. The diagnosis is made most easily by assay of PDH activity in cultured fibroblasts.

Intermittent ataxia has been reported as a feature of multiple biotin-dependent carboxylase deficiencies. The neurological syndrome also comprises generalized seizures, myoclonus, nystagmus, and hypotonia. There are associated defects of humoral- and cell-mediated immunity. Biotin therapy may result in clinical improvement.

Progressive Metabolic Ataxias

Ataxia may be a minor feature of storage and other metabolic neurodegenerative disorders developing in early childhood (see Table 76.2). The proportion of patients with progressive ataxias of adolescent or early adult onset who are recognized to have demonstrable metabolic defects is gradually increasing. Some enzyme deficiencies that usually give rise to diffuse neurodegenerative disorders developing in infancy or early childhood, in which ataxia is usually a minor feature, have been identified in patients with predominantly ataxic disorders developing in late childhood or early adult life. These include the sphingomyelin lipidoses, metachromatic leukodystrophy, galactosylceramide lipidosis (Krabbe's disease), and the hexosaminidase deficiencies. Also in this group is adrenoleukomyeloneuropathy, a phenotypic variant of adrenoleukodystrophy. This is diagnosed by estimation of very-long-chain fatty acids. Although the disease is X-linked and hence predominantly affects males, approximately 8% of carrier females may manifest neurological abnormalities. The role of diet and dietary supplements (e.g., oleic acid and Lorenzo's oil) remains to be established.

Hexosaminidase deficiency results in a group of autosomal recessive disorders known as the GM_2 gangliosidoses. These are genetically heterogeneous; multiple gene loci are involved in the synthesis of hexosaminidase, and it is clear that the phenotypic expression of the numerous possible mutations is very variable. There are at least three hexosaminidase isoenzymes: A, B, and S. Infantile Tay-Sachs disease is associated with deficiencies of hexosaminidases A and S.

A progressive ataxic syndrome has also been described in patients with hexosaminidase A deficiency. Age of onset varies but was generally before 15 years. Intention tremor and dysarthria were prominent early features, along with limb and gait ataxia. Some patients had facial grimacing, defective upward gaze, and proximal neurogenic muscle weakness. There was distention of neurons with lamellar inclusions on rectal biopsy. We have seen two siblings with hexosaminidase A deficiency and a similar but even later-onset syndrome comprising ataxia, supranuclear ophthalmoplegia, and proximal neurogenic muscle weakness. There was striking selective atrophy of the cerebellum and brainstem on computed tomography (CT) scan (Figure 76.2).

Ataxia may be prominent in Niemann-Pick disease type C (juvenile dystonic lipidosis), combined with a supranuclear gaze palsy. Sphingomyelinase activity is normal, but foamy storage cells are found in the bone marrow.

Cholestanolosis (also called cerebrotendinous xanthomatosis) is a rare autosomal recessive disorder caused by defective bile salt metabolism resulting from a deficiency of mitochondrial sterol 27 hydroxylase. It gives rise to ataxia, dementia, spasticity, peripheral neuropathy, cataract, and tendon xanthomata in the second decade of life. The molecular cloning and characterization of the genomic structure of sterol 27 hydroxylase has led to the identification of several mutations, including mis-sense, nonsense, and frameshift changes (Leitersdorf et al. 1993).

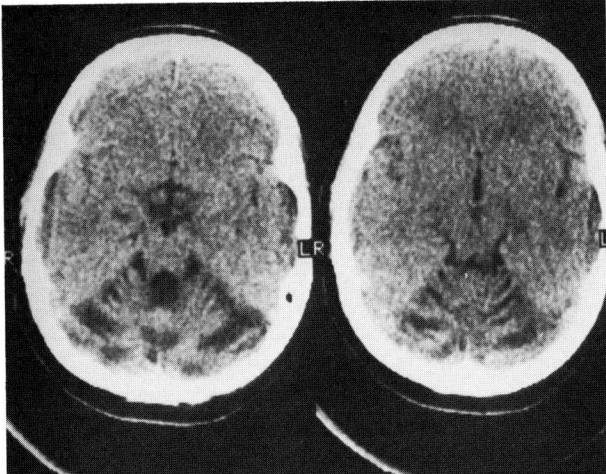

FIGURE 76.2 Computed tomographic scans showing striking cerebellar and brainstem atrophy in a patient with hexosaminidase A deficiency and late-onset ataxia, supranuclear ophthalmoplegia, and neurogenic proximal muscle weakness; there was no supratentorial atrophy. (Reprinted with permission from AE Harding, EP Young, F Schon. Adult onset supranuclear ophthalmoplegia, cerebellar ataxia, and neurogenic proximal muscle weakness in a brother and sister: another hexosaminidase A deficiency syndrome. J Neurol Neurosurg Psychiatry 1987;50:688.)

Treatment with chenodeoxycholic acid appears to improve neurological function.

Various phenotypes that are classifiable as hereditary ataxias have been described in the mitochondrial encephalomyopathies. These include late-onset ataxic disorders associated with such features as dementia, deafness, and peripheral neuropathy (Figures 76.3 and 76.4); Ramsay Hunt syndrome of ataxia and myoclonus; and Kearns-Sayre syndrome. Many of these disorders are associated with a defect of mitochondrial DNA (Table 76.3). Ramsay Hunt syndrome has a number of other causes, including ceroid lipofuscinosis and sialidosis; after intensive investigation, a number of cases remain for which no cause can be found.

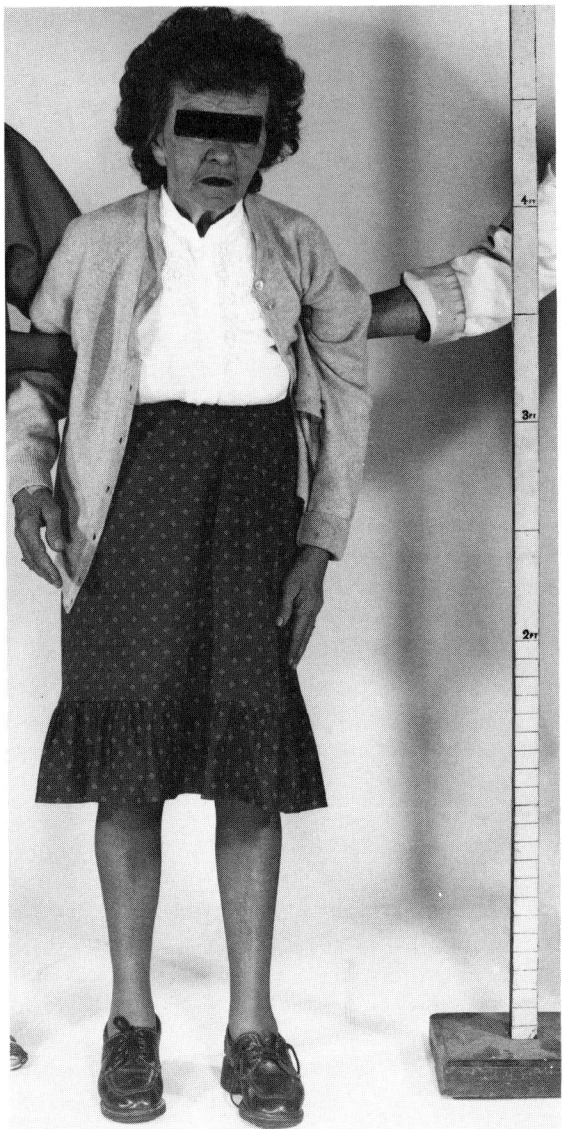

FIGURE 76.3 A 52-year-old woman with mitochondrial myopathy and complex I deficiency who presented with short stature and a 4-year history of ataxia and dementia. She had mild fatigable limb weakness but no ophthalmoplegia. (Courtesy of Dr. J. A. Morgan-Hughes.)

Acquired Metabolic and Endocrine Disorders Causing Cerebellar Dysfunction

Acquired metabolic and endocrine disorders causing cerebellar dysfunction, including hepatic encephalopathy, pontine and extrapontine myelinolysis related to hyponatremia, and hypothyroidism, are described in detail in Chapters 55 and 62. Hypothyroidism is only rarely a cause of a cerebellar syndrome in both children and adults, but because it is potentially treatable, it should always be considered. Symptoms of hypothyroidism precede loss of balance and clumsiness, and it is extremely rare to find subclinical hypothyroidism in patients presenting with a cerebellar syndrome. Ataxia affects

gait more commonly than it does the limbs, and dysarthria is rare; there may be an accompanying peripheral neuropathy. Neurological symptoms and signs usually resolve completely with thyroid replacement therapy.

ATAXIC DISORDERS ASSOCIATED WITH DEFECTIVE DNA REPAIR

Ataxia Telangiectasia

Ataxia telangiectasia (AT) is an autosomal recessive disorder with an average worldwide frequency of 1 in 40,000–100,000

FIGURE 76.4 Magnetic resonance image of a 55-year-old man with mitochondrial encephalomyopathy presenting with ataxia, dementia, and deafness. There is cerebral and cerebellar atrophy.

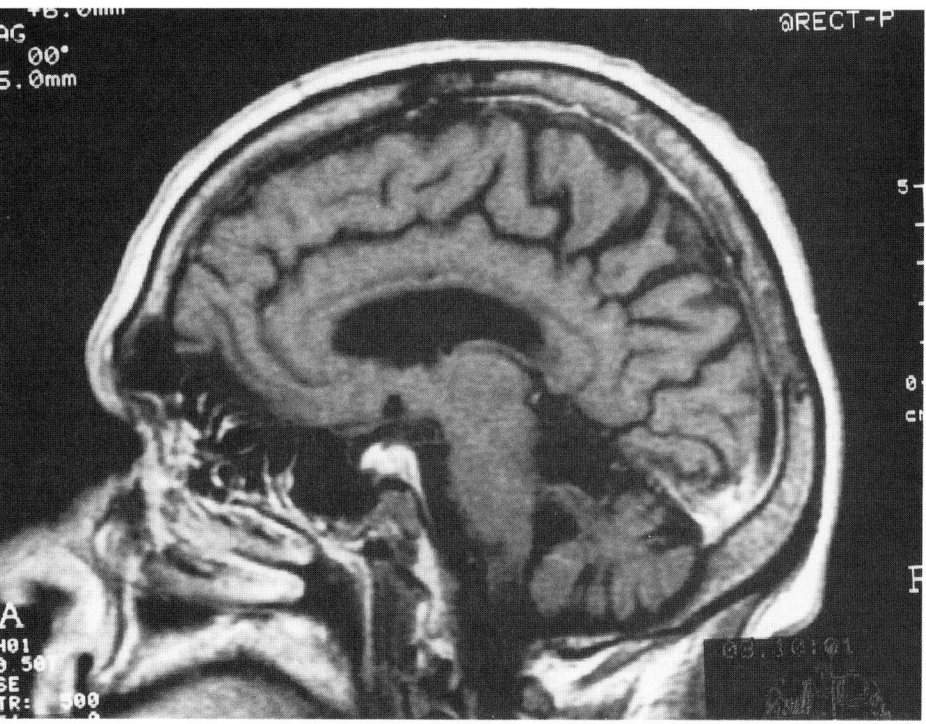

Table 76.3: Ataxia associated with mitochondrial DNA defects

Sporadic
   Kearns-Sayre syndrome (large deletion or duplication)
Maternally inherited in many cases
   MERRF (8344-bp mutation)
   Some patients with MELAS mutation (3243-bp mutation)
   Neurogenic muscle weakness, ataxia, and retinitis pigmentosa
      (8993-bp mutation)

MELAS = mitochondrial encephalopathy, lactic acidosis, and strokelike episodes; MERRF = myoclonus epilepsy with ragged-red fibers.

live births. Characteristically, motor development is often delayed and ataxia noted at the time of first walking. Growth retardation and delayed sexual development are frequent, and there is mild mental retardation in some cases. Patients with AT exhibit a characteristic eye movement disorder that includes oculomotor apraxia. Patients have impassive facies, a tendency to drool, and slow, slurred speech. Motor dysfunction is variable, often with a combination of ataxia, dystonia, and chorea. An associated peripheral axonal neuropathy is common, particularly in older patients. The cutaneous telangiectasia of AT may not be obvious at the time of presentation, and diagnosis is accordingly difficult. Telangiectases tend to develop on the conjunctivae (Figure 76.5) between the ages of 3 and 6 years, but occasionally they are inconspicuous or absent in adult life.

AT is associated with abnormalities of both humoral and cell-mediated immunity; most patients with early onset have recurrent respiratory and cutaneous infections from early childhood. Serum concentrations of immunoglobulin (Ig)A and IgG (particularly IgG2) are subnormal. About one-fifth of patients with AT develop malignancies, frequently of lymphoreticular origin, but solid tumors have also been reported. An increased incidence of malignancy has been described in known or presumptive AT heterozygotes. Patients' lymphocytes and fibroblasts demonstrate increased sensitivity to ultraviolet, gamma, and X-irradiation, and spontaneous chromosome breaks are frequent. Defective induction of damage-induced signal transduction pathways—most notably, cell-cycle checkpoints—has been reported (Shiloh 1995). Serum concentrations of α-fetoprotein are elevated in 90% of patients, and this can be a useful diagnostic test in clinical practice. Few patients are ambulant after puberty, and survival after the age of 30 is rare, although patients with a particularly protracted and relatively benign course without significant immunodeficiency are increasingly recognized. Autopsy shows striking loss of Purkinje's cells in the cerebellum, with less prominent degenerative changes in the granule cell layer, dentate and inferior olivary nuclei, and posterior columns.

The gene locus was mapped to chromosome 11q, and the gene has been cloned (Savitsky et al. 1995). The gene, called *ATM* (i.e., AT mutant), is large and contains 66 exons spanning approximately 150 kb of genomic DNA. It is now apparent that there are numerous different mutations, which limits direct mutation screening as a diagnostic tool or method of carrier identification. The vast majority of patients are homozygous or are compound heterozygotes for null alle-

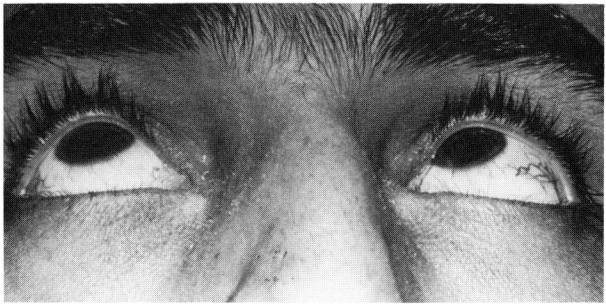

FIGURE 76.5   Conjunctival telangiectasia in a 19-year-old man with ataxia telangiectasia.

les. Mis-sense mutations are surprisingly rare. Brown and colleagues (1997) showed that the ATM protein is a single, high-molecular-weight (370-kD) protein predominantly confined to the nucleus of human fibroblasts. They also reported that truncated ATM protein was not detected in lymphoblasts from AT patients who were homozygous for mutations leading to premature protein termination. The exact function of the ATM protein remains unknown, but it is expressed and localized in the nucleus. The carboxy terminal region is homologous to the catalytic domain of the signal transduction enzyme phosphatidylinositol 3-kinase. These data are consistent with its potential role in choreographing appropriate cellular responses to genomic damage.

It is important to treat infections in AT patients as they arise, and postural drainage is indicated for bronchiectasis. The use of fresh frozen plasma infusions may reduce the frequency of infection. Repeated radiological examinations and radiotherapy should be avoided.

A disorder similar to AT, but without telangiectasia, elevated α-fetoprotein concentrations, immunodeficiency, or chromosomal instability, was reported by Aicardi and colleagues. Inheritance appeared to be autosomal recessive, and the main features were ataxia, oculomotor apraxia, chorea, hyporeflexia, and dystonia developing between the ages of 2 and 7 years. The oculomotor disorder was rather different from that seen in AT because it involved vertical as well as horizontal eye movements (This varient is genetically the same as AT).

Xeroderma Pigmentosum and Cockayne's Syndrome

Xeroderma pigmentosum is characterized by a reduced capacity to perform excision repair of DNA damaged by ultraviolet light and by some chemical carcinogens. It is genetically heterogeneous: Cell hybridization and complementation studies have identified eight types (A–G and a variant form). Even within these groups there is clinical heterogeneity, including xeroderma pigmentosum, Cockayne's syndrome, and trichothiodystrophy (reviewed by Bootsma et al. 1998). Inheritance is autosomal recessive. Several types are associated with neurological disease,

although these disorders primarily manifest as a skin disease with photosensitivity and skin malignancies. The associated neurological disorder is often complex, consisting of various combinations of choreoathetosis, seizures, mental retardation, dementia, deafness, cerebellar ataxia, spasticity, and large-fiber sensory peripheral neuropathy. Mental retardation, ataxia, and hyporeflexia are the most frequent manifestations. Neurological symptoms usually develop before the age of 30. Autopsy shows widespread neuronal loss in the cerebrum, cerebellum, and brainstem with degenerative changes in the long tracts of the spinal cord.

Cockayne's syndrome is another rare recessive disorder in which there is skin photosensitivity, mental retardation, short stature, ataxia, neuropathy, and progeric features. Trichothiodystrophy is characterized by brittle hair, an abnormality of sulfur content in the hair, mental retardation, and abnormal facies. Several genes have been shown to cause these diseases, and to confuse matters further, there is allelic heterogeneity (i.e., the gene for xeroderma pigmentosum type D can be responsible for all three phenotypes) (Bootsma et al. 1998).

DEFICIENCY DISORDERS AND ALCOHOLISM

Deficiency disorders and alcoholism are discussed in detail in Chapters 62 and 63.

Vitamin E Deficiency

There is good evidence that vitamin E (α-tocopherol), a highly hydrophobic, fat-soluble vitamin, is essential for normal neurological function. Patients are described with progressive spinocerebellar disorders who have isolated vitamin E deficiency but no evidence of malabsorption. The clinical features of this syndrome include progressive gait ataxia, incoordination of the limbs, areflexia, and large-fiber sensory loss. Onset of symptoms occurs between the ages of 3 and 13 years. Unlike Friedreich's ataxia (FA), which it resembles, sensory conduction in peripheral nerves is preserved relative to delay in the posterior columns, as demonstrated by somatosensory evoked potentials. These patients had an impaired ability to incorporate vitamin E (α-tocopherol) into very-low-density lipoproteins in the liver.

The gene was mapped to chromosome 8q (Ben Hamida et al. 1993), and mutations in a gene encoding α-tocopherol transfer protein were later demonstrated (Ouahchi et al. 1995). A number of mutations have been described. The α-tocopherol transfer protein is necessary to maintain the adequate circulation of α-tocopherol, and therefore inefficient recycling leads to a deficiency. Dietary supplementation with vitamin E can overcome the loss and may prevent or, in some cases, reverse further neurological damage. Onset of ataxia in the sixth decade has now been reported (Gotoda et al. 1995).

Table 76.4: Neurological features of vitamin E deficiency

	Abetalipoproteinemia	Cholestatic liver disease	Cystic fibrosis	Intestinal resection	Isolated deficiency (AVED)
Age of onset of symptoms (yrs)	5–20	3–18	10–19	17–52	3–13
Retinopathy	+++	+	+	++	—
Ophthalmoplegia	++	++	+++	++	—
Dysarthria	+	+	+	++	+
Muscle weakness	++	++	+	++	++
Ataxia	+++	+++	+++	+++	+++
Areflexia	+++	+++	+++	++	+++
Loss of position/vibration sense	+++	+++	+++	+++	+++
Loss of pain/touch sense	+	+	+	+	+
Abnormal peripheral sensory conduction	+	+	+++	++	—

— = not recorded; + = less than 25% of cases; ++ = 25–75% of cases; +++ = more than 75% of cases; AVED = vitamin A and vitamin E deficiency.
Source: Adapted from AE Harding, EP Young, F Schon. Adult onset supranuclear ophthalmoplegia, cerebellar ataxia, and neurogenic proximal muscle weakness in a brother and sister: another hexosaminidase A deficiency syndrome. J Neurol Neurosurg Psychiatry 1987;50:688.

The most severe vitamin E deficiency state occurring in humans is abetalipoproteinemia. Abetalipoproteinemia is an autosomal recessive syndrome caused by defects of the gene encoding the 97-kD subunit of a microsomal triglyceride transfer protein (Shoulders et al. 1993) and is associated with low levels of apoprotein B, which normally carries lipid from the intestinal cell to plasma. This condition results in very low levels of circulating lipids, particularly cholesterol, and severe malabsorption of the fat-soluble vitamins A, D, E, and K. Serum vitamin E concentrations are either low or undetectable from birth, and acanthocytes are usually present in the peripheral blood. Symptoms of fat malabsorption may be mild and overlooked; patients then present in the second decade of life with a progressive neurological syndrome reminiscent of FA, comprising ataxia, areflexia, and proprioceptive loss. In some cases there is a pigmentary retinopathy. Pathologically, there is degeneration of the posterior columns and spinocerebellar tracts in the spinal cord and loss of large myelinated fibers in peripheral nerves.

Hypobetalipoproteinemia is genetically distinct from abetalipoproteinemia. It is autosomal dominant and characterized by moderately reduced serum concentrations of cholesterol, triglyceride, and low-density lipoproteins. Most patients are asymptomatic. The plasma lipid profile in homozygous hypobetalipoproteinemia is identical to that of abetalipoproteinemia; the main distinction between the two disorders is that heterozygotes for abetalipoproteinemia have normal serum lipid concentrations. A neurological syndrome similar to that seen in abetalipoproteinemia has been described in homozygous hypobetalipoproteinemia, but it seems to be less severe.

A similar neurological syndrome has been described in patients with diseases affecting fat digestion in the gastrointestinal tract, including cholestatic liver disease, cystic fibrosis, and celiac disease, and after extensive intestinal resection (Table 76.4). Most reported cases have been children with congenital biliary atresia; adults with hepatic cholestasis do not tend to develop such severe vitamin E deficiency. Patients with cystic fibrosis do not usually develop neurological dysfunction associated with profound vitamin E deficiency unless they have hepatobiliary disease. A few patients have been reported with areflexia, ataxia, and proprioceptive loss developing many years after extensive small bowel resection (most commonly for Crohn's disease), which gives rise to virtually undetectable serum concentrations of vitamin E. The etiology of the retinopathy present in some of these syndromes is less clear; it may be due to both vitamin A and E deficiency (AVED). This retinopathy does not occur in cases of isolated vitamin E deficiency, which may support the suggestion of a synergistic effect of vitamin A deficiency in the retinopathy of abetalipoproteinemia.

Establishing the diagnosis of vitamin E deficiency is important because treatment with vitamin E can prevent progression of the neurological syndrome and can, in rare circumstances, lead to some improvement. It should be noted that dosage of vitamin E is a complex matter, and there are many different preparations. As a general rule, vitamin E deficiency due to malabsorption requires large, sometimes parenteral doses, whereas for AVED, more modest doses are adequate.

In autopsy studies of cases of biliary atresia and a progressive spinocerebellar syndrome, there was degeneration of the posterior columns, most marked rostrally, less prominent changes in the spinocerebellar tracts, and mild distal loss of large myelinated fibers in peripheral nerves. Similar changes have been observed in vitamin E–deficient monkeys, which demonstrates that vitamin E deficiency chiefly produces a dying-back neuropathy in sensory neurons, affecting centrally directed fibers more than peripheral ones.

Thiamine Deficiency and Alcoholism

Despite the well-known acute effects of alcohol on cerebellar function, there is convincing evidence that the more chronic cerebellar syndrome observed in alcoholics is caused by thiamine deficiency rather than toxicity from alcohol itself. Alcoholics with this syndrome are almost invariably malnourished, often giving a history of profound weight loss before developing neurological symptoms. Ataxia may develop during periods of abstinence, and identical cerebellar degeneration has been observed in nonalcoholic patients with severe malnutrition. Cerebellar ataxia is common in Wernicke-Korsakoff syndrome, and the pathological features of this syndrome and of cerebellar degeneration are frequently found together.

The neurological deficit often has a subacute onset, and some patients become severely ataxic over a period of weeks. There may be associated features of Wernicke-Korsakoff syndrome, such as confabulation and ophthalmoplegia. The cerebellar syndrome predominantly affects stance and gait, sometimes with truncal ataxia and titubation; dysarthria and upper limb ataxia are rare. Pathologically, degeneration is most pronounced in the anterior vermis, and loss of Purkinje's cells is striking.

With administration of thiamine, some improvement may occur in early cases of alcoholic cerebellar degeneration, but if the patient is already confined to a wheelchair, the response to treatment is limited. Treated patients with Wernicke's encephalopathy often have a residual gait disorder similar to that of alcoholic cerebellar degeneration (see also Chapter 63).

Other Deficiency Disorders

Trace metal deficiencies do not appear to give rise to cerebellar disease in most instances. However, dysarthria, limb and gait ataxia, tremor, altered taste, irritability, paranoia, and anorexia occurred in patients who were made zinc deficient by the administration of histidine. The neurological symptoms resolved promptly after oral zinc therapy.

TOXINS AND PHYSICAL AGENTS

Cerebellar dysfunction in humans occurs as a consequence of exposure to a wide range of toxins, including pharmaceutical products, solvents, and heavy metals (see Chapter 64).

Drugs

The most common cause of a cerebellar syndrome due to drug toxicity in neurological practice is that associated with anticonvulsant medication, particularly phenytoin. Transient ataxia, dysarthria, and nystagmus usually develop when serum concentrations of phenytoin, carbamazepine, or barbiturates exceed the therapeutic range; these symptoms remit when concentrations return to the therapeutic range. Chronic phenytoin toxicity may cause persistent cerebellar dysfunction, and this is associated pathologically with loss of Purkinje's cells.

A condition termed *worm wobble* is a reversible cerebellar syndrome that occurs in children taking piperazine for threadworm infestation. High-dose administration of 5-fluorouracil or cytosine arabinoside also causes reversible cerebellar ataxia. A persistent cerebellar deficit, with cerebellar atrophy on CT scan, dysarthria, and limb and gait ataxia, has been described as a sequel to the acute encephalopathy of lithium toxicity that is usually precipitated by fever or starvation. Serum lithium levels are not always elevated in such cases.

Solvents

Recreational or accidental exposure to a number of solvents, including carbon tetrachloride and toluene, causes cerebellar ataxia along with other neurological problems, including psychosis, cognitive impairment, and pyramidal signs in the case of toluene. The neurological deficit is potentially reversible but may persist after prolonged exposure in solvent abusers.

Heavy Metals

Inorganic mercury poisoning gives rise to tremor, but methyl mercury toxicity causes prominent cerebellar ataxia accompanied by distal paresthesias and cortical blindness. Cerebellar signs are also seen in thallium poisoning, although peripheral neuropathy and encephalopathy are usually more striking. Thallium poisoning is also associated with hair loss, which may occur some weeks after the acute event. Children with lead poisoning may have a staggering gait and tremor, but other neurological features tend to overshadow these.

Other Toxins

Acute ataxia has been reported in ciguatera-type tropical fish poisoning. Acrylamide poisoning may give rise to ataxia that is thought to be of cerebellar origin.

Physical Agents

The cerebellar Purkinje's cells are particularly sensitive to a wide variety of insults, and their loss is striking at autopsy after severe hypoxia and hyperthermia. However, specific signs of cerebellar dysfunction are usually overshadowed by the generalized cerebral dysfunction seen in survivors of

Table 76.5: Ataxic disorders of unknown etiology: autosomal recessive ataxias (onset usually before 20 years of age)

Friedreich's ataxia
Early-onset cerebellar ataxia with:
   Retained tendon reflexes
   Hypogonadism
   Myoclonus (progressive myoclonic ataxia, Ramsay Hunt syndrome)
   Childhood deafness
   Congenital deafness
   Optic atrophy with or without mental retardation (including Behr's syndrome)
   Cataract and mental retardation (Marinesco-Sjögren syndrome)
   Pigmentary retinopathy
Autosomal recessive late-onset ataxia

severe hypoxia. Cerebellar ataxia is a prominent part of the neurological sequelae of heat stroke.

HEREDITARY AND DEGENERATIVE DISORDERS

The degenerative cerebellar and spinocerebellar disorders are a complex group of diseases, most of which are genetically determined. In some, an underlying metabolic disorder exists, and diagnosis is crucial because there are important implications for treatment and genetic counseling. In the past few years, our knowledge of the genetic basis of many of the group referred to as cerebellar and spinocerebellar degenerations has grown rapidly. The next phase will be to understand how these genes and the abnormal proteins they produce cause cell-specific neu-

ropathology. Inherited ataxic disorders can be divided according to their mode of inheritance (Tables 76.5 and 76.6). Most autosomal recessive disorders are of early onset (before age 20), and autosomal dominant disorders are usually of later onset (after age 20).

AUTOSOMAL RECESSIVE ATAXIAS

Friedreich's Ataxia

FA is the most common of the autosomal recessive ataxias (see Table 76.5) and accounts for at least 50% of cases of hereditary ataxia in most large series reported from Europe and the United States. Its prevalence in these regions is similar (i.e., 1–2 per 100,000); prevalence appears to be slightly higher in Quebec.

Clinical Features

The age of onset, generally with gait ataxia, is usually between the ages of 8 and 15 years. Later onset also occurs (ages 20–30), with all other diagnostic criteria fulfilled. Since mutational analysis became available, the latest reported age at onset is 51 years (Durr et al. 1996). In addition to the ataxia, other variable features include dysarthria and pyramidal tract involvement. The initial pyramidal tract involvement may be mild, with extensor plantar responses only, but after 5 or more years, a pyramidal pattern of weakness in the legs is invariable, eventually leading to paralysis. Distal wasting, particularly in the legs, is seen in about one-half of patients. Muscle tone is usually decreased or normal, although flexor spasms are common. Significant weakness of the arms is rare before

Table 76.6: Ataxic disorders of unknown etiology: correlation of clinical and genetic classifications of autosomal dominant cerebellar ataxias (onset usually after 20 years of age)

Clinical classification	Locus	Normal repeat size	Disease repeat size
ADCA I: Ataxia with ophthalmoplegia, optic atrophy, dementia, or extrapyramidal features (including Machado-Joseph disease)	SCA1 (chr 6p)	6–38	39–80
	SCA2 (chr 12q)	16–30	36–52
	SCA3 (chr 14q)	14–40	60–85
	SCA4 (chr 16q)	Linkage only	N/A
ADCA II: Ataxia with pigmentary maculopathy with or without ophthalmoplegia or extrapyramidal features	SCA7	7–19	37–220[b]
ADCA III: "pure" ataxia	SCA5 (chr 11p)	Linkage only	N/A
	SCA6[a] (chr 19)	5–20	21–28
	SCA11 (chr 15q)	Linkage only	N/A
Periodic dominant ataxia	EA 1 (chr 12)	Potassium channel	Point mutations
	EA 2[a] (chr 19)	Calcium channel	Point mutations

ADCA = autosomal dominant cerebellar ataxia; chr = chromosome; EA = episodic ataxia; N/A = not available; SCA = spinocerebellar ataxia.
[a]SCA6 can also be classified as ADCA I because occasional additional features are found. Also the CAG repeat is in the 3' region of the calcium channel responsible also for EA 2 (see text).
[b]Intermediate allele 28–35 has been reported; these may expand in paternal transmission into the disease range.

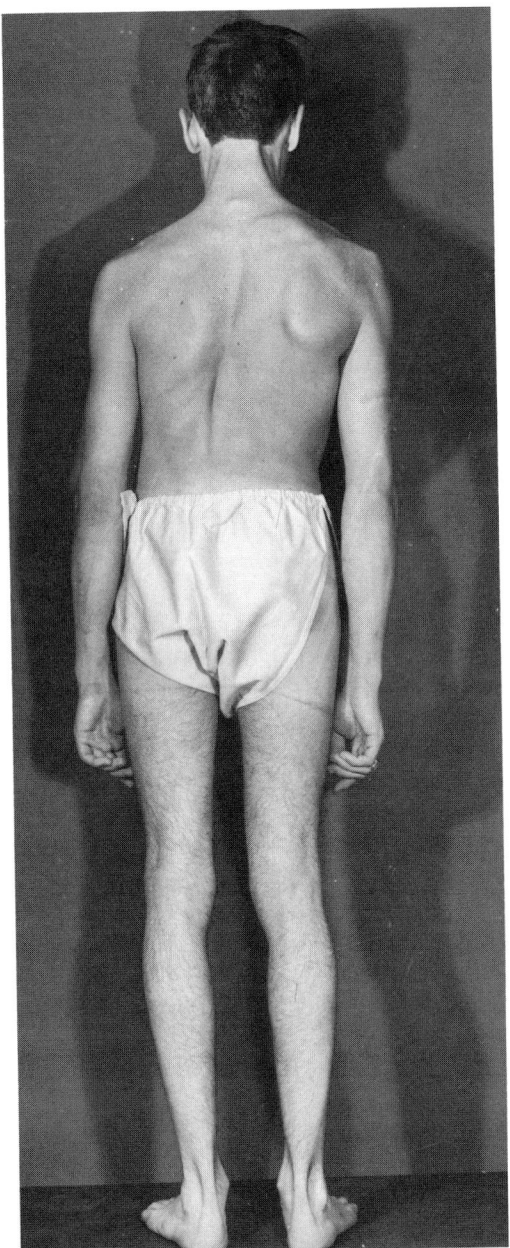

FIGURE 76.6   Scoliosis in a 28-year-old patient with Friedreich's ataxia.

the patient is virtually confined to bed. The association of extensor plantar responses (90%), absence of ankle reflexes, and a progressive course are core features. Additional signs include large-fiber sensory loss (distal loss of joint position and vibration sense) and skeletal abnormalities, including scoliosis (85%) (Figure 76.6) and foot deformities. Although pes cavus is the best known (50%), pes planus and equinovarus are also common. Amyotrophy of the lower leg and, rarely, the hands may also be found. Additional clinical features include optic atrophy (25%), but less than 5% of patients have major visual impairment. Deafness occurs in less than 10% of patients, but more have impairment of speech discrimination. Nystagmus is

seen in only approximately 20%, but the extraocular movements are nearly always abnormal, with broken-up pursuit, dysmetric saccades, square wave jerks, and no fixation suppression of the vestibulo-ocular reflex. Sphincter dysfunction, particularly urgency of micturition and constipation, occurs but is not usually severe.

Electrophysiological examination reveals evidence of an axonal sensory neuropathy. About 65% of patients with FA have an abnormal electrocardiogram (ECG). Widespread T-wave inversion is common, particularly in the inferior standard and lateral chest leads (Figure 76.7), along with ventricular hypertrophy. These changes may develop before the onset of neurological symptoms or up to 15 years later. Episodes of supraventricular arrhythmia and sinus arrest may be seen on ambulatory ECG monitoring. The most frequent echocardiographic abnormality in FA is symmetrical, concentric ventricular hypertrophy, although some patients have asymmetrical septal hypertrophy. Cardiac symptoms are relatively rare, apart from exertional dyspnea, which may be explicable on the basis of neurological disability. Palpitations and angina sometimes occur. There may be clinical evidence of ventricular hypertrophy, systolic ejection murmurs, and third or fourth heart sounds. Signs of heart failure occur late in the disease, often as a preterminal event. Severe scoliosis gives rise to increased cardiopulmonary morbidity.

Diabetes mellitus occurs in 10% of patients with FA, and an additional 10–20% have impaired glucose tolerance. Most diabetic patients require insulin therapy, but some achieve reasonable control with oral hypoglycemic drugs.

Investigations and Differential Diagnosis

Diagnostic testing has changed with identification of the gene and the availability of testing for the common mutation (see Genetics, later in this chapter). The diagnosis of FA is still essentially a clinical one, however, and using the above criteria, the accuracy is extremely high (Lamont et al. 1997). In the presence of all the typical features, the differential diagnosis is small, and in the past, there was a tendency to lump all early-onset ataxias under the rubric of FA or variants. The most common condition to be misdiagnosed as FA is hereditary motor and sensory neuropathy (HMSN) type I, which presents in childhood with clumsiness and areflexia but little in the way of distal muscle weakness and wasting. Distinction between the two disorders can be clinically difficult at a stage when a child with FA may not have developed dysarthria or extensor plantar responses. This issue is easily resolved with nerve conduction studies. Although sensory action potentials are small or absent in both disorders, upper limb motor nerve conduction velocity always exceeds 40 m per second in FA but is slower in HMSN type I. This distinction is important because the prognosis for HMSN type I is much better than that of FA and because inheritance is dominant, although de novo mutation can occur in HMSN type I.

FIGURE 76.7 Electrocardiographic abnormalities in Friedreich's ataxia. There is widespread T-wave inversion and left ventricular hypertrophy. (Leads I, II, II, avL, and avF above and V 1–6 below.)

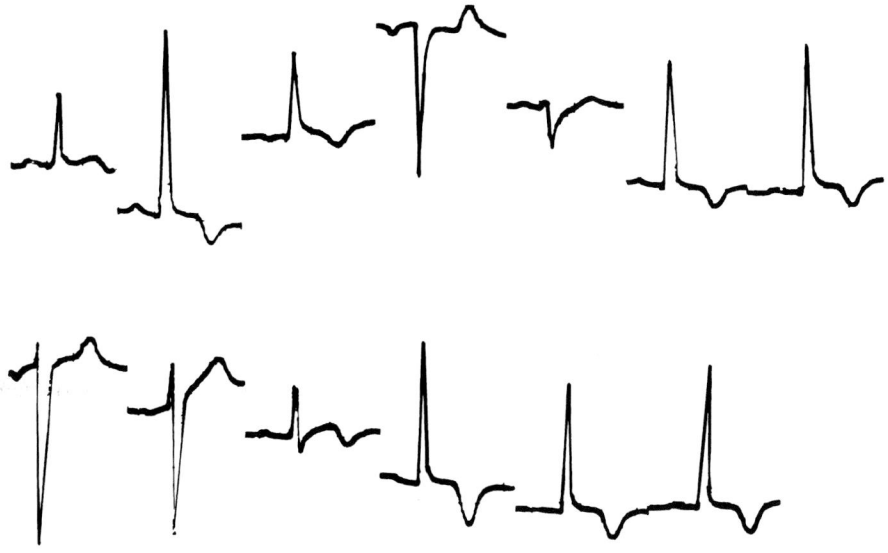

The other important diagnoses to be considered are those due to vitamin E deficiency, especially abetalipoproteinemia and AVED. These disorders resemble FA, but they are treatable. The ECG is a particularly valuable investigation in possible cases of FA because the widespread T-wave inversion, if present in this context, is virtually diagnostic of FA (see Figure 76.7). These changes are not found in any other hereditary ataxias. CT or MRI scans are either normal or show mild cerebellar atrophy (usually seen only late in the disease). The cervical spinal cord is often atrophied (Klockgether et al. 1998b).

Genetics

The gene for FA was mapped to chromosome 9q13 in 1988 by Chamberlain and colleagues. There then followed a competitive hunt for the gene and a refinement of the genetic locus. This enabled a re-evaluation of the strict clinical criteria described in the previous section, and it became apparent that onset of FA could be seen after age 20 and retention of reflexes was not an absolute exclusion. It was also shown that the milder variant of the disease described in the Acadian population also mapped to the same locus. After an international collaboration, an anonymous transcript called X25 was identified (Campuzano et al. 1996). Further work showed that the predominant mutation was a trinucleotide repeat (GAA) in intron 1 of this gene. Expansion of both alleles was found in more than 96% of patients. The translated protein was named *frataxin,* and initial messenger RNA (mRNA) studies reported a decrease in frataxin mRNA. The tissue-specific distribution of frataxin, including expression in the pancreas, heart, and dorsal spinal cord, mirrors that of the pathology of the disease.

FA was the first autosomal recessive condition found to be due to an unstable triplet repeat. Identification of the repeat has permitted the introduction of a specific and sensitive diagnostic test because it is a relatively simple matter to measure the repeat size. On normal chromosomes, the number of GAA repeats varies from 7 to 22 units, whereas on disease chromosomes, the range varies from approximately 100 to 2,000 repeats. This is in sharp contrast to the modest exonic repeat expansions seen in the dominant genetic ataxias. The polymerase chain reaction with nucleotide primers spanning the repeated region is used to amplify the DNA in intron 1; the products are then fractionated on an agarose or polyacrylamide gel. The rarity of point mutations means that it is extremely unlikely that a case of FA will have two point mutations; therefore, a normal-sized repeat length on both chromosomes argues strongly against a diagnosis of FA. The exact mechanism of action of this repeat in intron 1 is not known, but it is possible that this huge expansion disrupts normal splicesome binding and therefore exon 1 is not spliced correctly to exon 2. This results in a reduction in frataxin mRNA and protein levels accordingly.

Affected individuals have a risk of transmitting the disease to offspring of 1 in 220, based on the heterozygote frequency of 1 in 110. Thus, carrier testing is also possible, but currently only the expansion is generally looked for, and point mutations (<3%) are not excluded. About one-fifth of patients with FA do reproduce, and there is the occasional occurrence of pseudodominance—that is, an affected patient produces an affected child because of the partner's carrier status. There do not appear to be any specific problems associated with pregnancy, but the difficulties of child rearing caused by physical disability represent a greater problem.

Genotype-Phenotype Correlations

The identification of a diagnostic test has permitted a re-evaluation of the clinical phenotype. It has been confirmed that retained reflexes are seen in a small proportion of patients with FA. Although most patients present before age 25, onset can occur later. Studies of a large number of patients (Lamont et al. 1997) have shown a broad consensus: Length of repeat size is a determinant of age of onset and therefore to some degree influences the severity of the disease in that those with early onset tend to progress more rapidly. However, this correlation is applicable for populations of patients but is not useful for guiding an individual patient or family. The presence of cardiomyopathy is also linked to the length of the repeat, but further studies are needed to disentangle the exact relationship.

Pathology

Pathological studies in FA show degeneration of the posterior columns, which is most severe in the cervical region of the spinal cord, and extensive loss of larger cells in the dorsal root ganglia. Degeneration of the pyramidal tracts is most severe in the lumbar part of the spinal cord. These findings are reflected electrophysiologically by delayed, dispersed somatosensory evoked potentials recorded at the sensory cortex and abnormal central motor conduction. Degenerative changes are also seen in the spinocerebellar tracts. The brainstem, cerebellum, and cerebrum are relatively normal. There may be patchy loss of Purkinje's cells in the cerebellum and mild degenerative changes in the pontine and medullary nuclei and optic tracts. In the peripheral nerves, there is loss of large myelinated axons and scanty paranodal and segmental demyelination. It has been suggested that demyelination is secondary to axonal atrophy, although the evidence for this is not convincing. Loss of large myelinated fibers is seen in the sural nerves of very young children with FA; this increases with age and disease duration.

Pathogenesis and Etiology

There has been progress in our understanding of the location and potential role of frataxin. Babcock et al. (1997) have investigated a yeast analogue of the protein and shown it to be a mitochondrial iron transporter. There is preliminary evidence in human studies that frataxin is also mitochondrially located. If this is indeed the function of frataxin in humans, the corollary is that iron builds up inside the mitochondria with its relative diminution in the cytosol. The free iron may cause a number of problems of free radical regulation and oxidative phosphorylation. Clinically this fits: A syndrome of ataxia and neuropathy, in association with diabetes, cardiomyopathy, deafness, and optic atrophy, has the hallmarks of a mitochondrial disease.

Course and Prognosis

The rate of progression of FA is variable, but at least 95% of patients are confined to a wheelchair by the age of 45 years. On average, patients lose the ability to walk 15 years after onset of symptoms. Age at death is also rather variable: Reported mean ages have usually been in the mid-30s, although survival into the sixth and seventh decades is not unknown. If there is associated heart disease and diabetes, death usually occurs earlier.

Management

Attempts at treating ataxia in FA have been variable and largely disappointing. Many of the trials have been open and poorly controlled. In double-blinded, controlled trials, choline chloride and lecithin did not produce significant functional improvement. Suggestions have not been confirmed that physostigmine, γ-vinyl γ-aminobutyric acid, thyrotropin-releasing hormone, and 5-hydroxytryptophan with benserazide may be helpful in FA. It is hoped that after elucidation of the exact role of frataxin, a more rational approach will be possible. There is growing interest in the role of antioxidants and possible iron chelation therapy based on the data emerging about the mitochondrial location and action of frataxin. It is probable that a large multicenter study will be required to demonstrate an effect.

The management of diabetes has been mentioned; cardiac failure and arrhythmias should be treated as they arise. Surgery for foot deformity and scoliosis may be of benefit in carefully selected patients. It is essential that perioperative bed rest be minimized.

Early-Onset Cerebellar Ataxia with Retained Reflexes

Many patients with early-onset cerebellar ataxia with retained reflexes have mutations in the frataxin gene. The other early-onset ataxias listed in Table 76.5 are rare. The prognosis for this group is better than for classic FA, and the ability to walk is lost approximately 13 years later. It is genetically heterogeneous; inheritance is probably autosomal recessive in most cases. The age of onset of symptoms ranges between 2 and 20 years. Upper limb and knee reflexes are normal or increased, but ankle jerks may be absent. Optic atrophy, severe skeletal deformity, and cardiac involvement do not occur. Cerebellar atrophy is more frequently found on CT or MRI scans than in FA. The pathology is that of olivopontocerebellar atrophy (OPCA) in some cases.

Cerebellar Ataxia with Hypogonadism

The association of hypogonadotropic hypogonadism with progressive ataxia is rare and was first described by Holmes in 1907. Abnormal sexual development is obvious from the time of expected puberty. Neurological symptoms usually develop in the third decade, although the age range is 1–30 years. The disorder comprises dysarthria, nystagmus, and progressive limb and gait ataxia. Less frequent clinical features include mental retardation, dementia, deafness, distal weakness and wasting, choreoathetosis, retinopathy, and loss of vibration and joint position sense. Cerebello-olivary atrophy is found at autopsy. Inheritance appears to be autosomal recessive.

Cerebellar Ataxia with Myoclonus

Cerebellar ataxia in combination with myoclonus is often called Ramsay Hunt syndrome (dyssynergia cerebellaris myoclonica). It is a heterogeneous syndrome, not a disease, and thus has a differential diagnosis that overlaps that of progressive myoclonic epilepsy. This includes mitochondrial encephalomyopathy (myoclonus epilepsy with ragged-red fibers), sialidosis, and myoclonic epilepsy of Unverricht and Lundborg (Baltic myoclonus, EPM1). An underlying cause is more likely to be found in patients with prominent seizures than in those who can be described as having progressive myoclonic ataxia, which represents an amalgam of rare and heterogeneous conditions. A point mutation of mitochondrial DNA (see Table 76.3) exists in approximately 80% of cases of myoclonus epilepsy with ragged-red fibers, and blood screening is a useful diagnostic procedure.

Baltic myoclonus has been reported particularly often in Scandinavia, but it is also seen elsewhere. Stimulus-sensitive myoclonus or generalized seizures develop at the end of the first decade. Ataxia and dysarthria are evident for a few years later, often with pyramidal signs in the limbs. The myoclonic component of these disorders may respond to clonazepam, sodium valproate, or piracetam with substantial improvement in motor function. Inheritance is autosomal recessive, and the gene locus was mapped to chromosome 21 in families from Scandinavia and many other parts of the world (Cochius et al. 1993). Pennacchio and colleagues (1996) found several point mutations in a gene encoding cystatin B. Cystatin B is a small protein and a member of the superfamily of cysteine protease inhibitors. It is thought to act as a protector against the proteinases leaking from lysosomes. In view of the ubiquitous expression of this protein, it is not understood why mutation of the gene encoding cystatin B causes the symptoms of EPM1, an apparent tissue-specific phenotype. Lalioti and colleagues (1997) have presented evidence that the common mutation mechanism in EPM1 is expansion of the dodecamer repeat in the promoter region.

Other Autosomal Recessive Ataxias

Autosomal recessive early-onset ataxias with associated ocular and other features are rare. Pigmentary retinopathy and ataxia have been reported in combination with mental retardation, peripheral neuropathy, and deafness.

The combination of optic atrophy, spasticity, ataxia, and mental retardation is often referred to as *Behr's syndrome*;

there is sometimes an associated peripheral neuropathy. Optic atrophy and ataxia, with or without mental retardation and deafness, have been described as an autosomal recessive trait. Marinesco-Sjögren's syndrome comprises cataracts, mental retardation, short stature, delayed sexual development, and ataxia.

Early-onset cerebellar ataxia with mental retardation and deafness with onset in childhood has been reported, as has childhood-onset deafness followed by the development of cerebellar ataxia in midlife in siblings. Congenital deafness may also be associated with ataxia developing in the third decade of life. Cerebellar ataxia is sometimes observed, along with predominant extrapyramidal features, in pallidopyramidal degeneration. Autosomal recessive inheritance of late-onset cerebellar ataxia is very unusual.

X-linked inheritance is rare in the hereditary ataxias. In five families, the neurological syndrome had its onset in childhood or adolescence with a mild spastic paraparesis, followed by the development of upper limb ataxia and dysarthria. Another X-linked spastic-ataxic syndrome with later development of dementia has been reported. It is worth noting that X-linked inheritance is rare in the hereditary ataxias and therefore the chance of a singleton male case having an X-linked disorder is small unless the clinical picture conforms to that delineated here.

LATE-ONSET INHERITED ATAXIAS

Autosomal Dominant Ataxias

The classification of autosomal dominant cerebellar ataxias (ADCAs) has been controversial, with some authors preferring the pathological term *OPCA*. This clearly makes no sense at a clinical level. Moreover, OPCA is a nonspecific pathological syndrome that has been described in patients with different types of dominant ataxias, sporadic late-onset ataxias, and mitochondrial encephalomyopathy. The pathology is only rarely confined to atrophy of the inferior olivary and pontine nuclei and cerebellar cortex. Other features include spinal cord, basal ganglia, cerebral cortex, and peripheral nerves abnormalities. Finally, the pathological features may also vary between members of the same kindred, with the pons or olives being spared in some affected individuals but not in others.

An additional complexity in the classification of ADCAs is that disorders in this group have also been assigned genotypic numbering (e.g., SCA types 1–7) that does not follow the ADCA nomenclature (see Table 76.6). ADCA type I is characterized by a progressive cerebellar ataxia and is variably associated with other extracerebellar neurological features, such as ophthalmoplegia, optic atrophy, peripheral neuropathy, and pyramidal and extrapyramidal signs. The presence and severity of these signs depends partly on the duration of the disease. Mild or moderate dementia may occur, but it is usually not a prominent early feature. ADCA

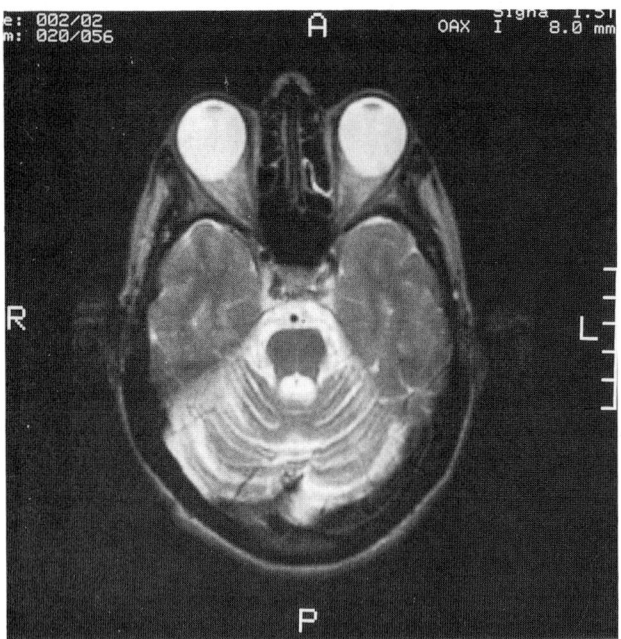

FIGURE 76.8 Magnetic resonance image of a 48-year-old woman with autosomal dominant cerebellar ataxia type I and the SCA1 mutation. There is cerebellar and brainstem atrophy.

type II is clinically distinguished from ADCA type I by the presence of pigmentary macular dystrophy (Enevoldson et al. 1994), whereas ADCA type III is a relatively pure cerebellar syndrome and generally starts at a later age. This clinical classification remains useful, despite the tremendous improvements in our understanding of the genetic basis of these disorders, because it provides a framework that can be used in the clinic and helps direct the genetic evaluation.

Autosomal Dominant Cerebellar Ataxia Type I

ADCA type I is the most common of the ADCAs, and at least five loci are independently responsible for this phenotype. The age of symptom onset ranges from 15 to 65 years; symptoms usually appear in the third or fourth decades in most families. Progressive ataxia of gait is the most frequent presenting symptom. It later involves the arms, when it is invariably associated with dysarthria. Patients usually have a pure cerebellar syndrome during the first few years of the illness, but associated features, particularly supranuclear ophthalmoplegia, are common in established cases. Nuclear and internuclear eye movement disorders have also been described, and slow saccades appear to be particularly common in Indian patients. Optic atrophy is sometimes found, but prominent vision loss is

rare. Cognitive impairment is also a feature in some of these patients. Extrapyramidal features, such as parkinsonism, chorea, and dystonia, also occur. There may be muscle wasting and fasciculation of the face and tongue. The tendon reflexes are often normal or brisk at presentation but tend to become depressed or absent as the disease progresses. Loss of proprioception and vibration sense and pyramidal weakness also increase in frequency with disease duration. Cerebellar and brainstem atrophy, sometimes with cerebral atrophy, are seen in CT or MRI scans (Figure 76.8). There is often electrophysiological evidence of peripheral neuropathy, which may not be clinically evident. Most patients lose the ability to walk within 20 years of onset, and life expectancy is shortened due to disability and bulbar dysfunction. Early onset generally predicts more rapidly progressive disability.

The identification of the mutations responsible for SCA1 and SCA3 has permitted detailed genotype-phenotype correlations (Giunti et al. 1995). Even this retrospective approach found no sign that reliably distinguished the two diseases. However, the group of patients who were negative for known mutations were clinically distinct from subjects with SCA1 and SCA3 in that their tendon reflexes were depressed or absent and saccades tended to be slow.

Depressed tendon relexes and slow saccades were shown in a large family of Italian origin that had shown linkage to the SCA2 locus (Giunti et al. 1994), and had clinical features reminiscent of Cuban families with SCA2 (Gispert et al. 1993). Three groups using different techniques have confirmed that the SCA2 mutation is an unstable trinucleotide (CAG) repeat in the coding region of the gene (Imbert et al. 1996). These patients have slow saccades and depressed reflexes. As with SCA1 and SCA3, the SCA2 phenotype appears to have high inter- and intrafamily variability, and anticipation is seen. Detailed volumetric MRI studies by Klockgether and colleagues (1998b) showed significant atrophy of the cerebellum and brainstem in all three SCA mutations compared with age- and sex-matched controls. Furthermore, comparison between SCA groups showed that cerebellar and brainstem atrophy was more severe in SCA2 than in SCA1 and SCA3. Putaminal and caudate volume was reduced only in SCA3 but not in SCA1 and SCA2. These findings fit the subtle clinical differences between these groups.

Machado-Joseph Disease

Machado-Joseph disease (MJD), initially reported in individuals of Azorean or Portuguese descent, is now known to be caused by a mutation in the *SCA3* gene. Clinically, it comes under the rubric of the ADCA type I group. MJD may therefore be thought of as one form of presentation of SCA3, and facial fasciculation and dystonia may be more common in MJD than in other families with ADCA type I.

FIGURE 76.9 Left fundus of a blind patient with autosomal dominant cerebellar ataxia type II. There is extensive retinal degeneration, particularly involving the macular region. (Courtesy of Mr. Michael Sanders.)

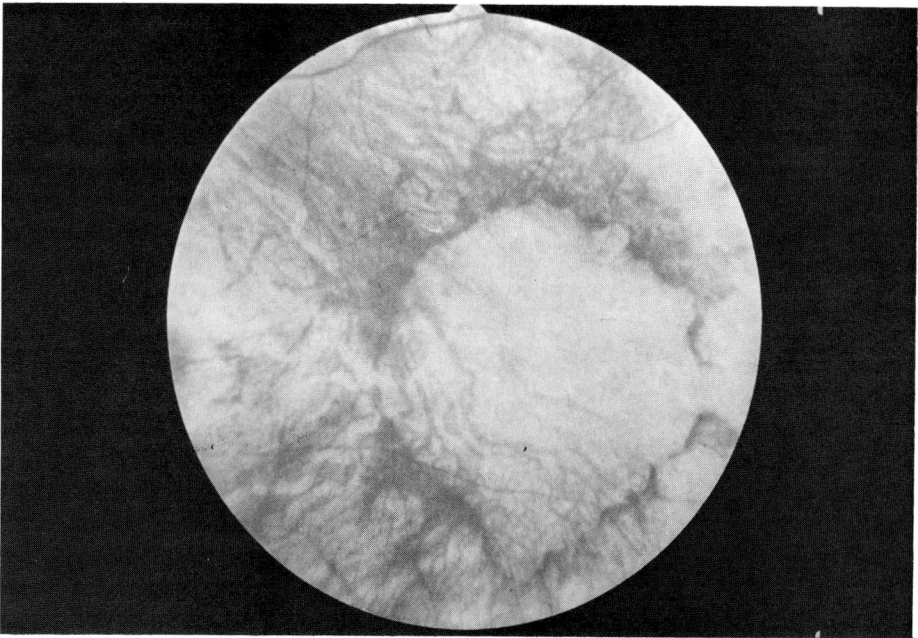

Autosomal Dominant Cerebellar Ataxia Type II

ADCA type II is clinically and genetically distinguished from ADCA type I by pigmentary maculopathy (Enevoldson et al. 1994). It may be associated with a variety of additional features similar to ADCA type I, but the vision impairment distinguishes it. Supranuclear ophthalmoplegia is found in the majority of patients, and associated dementia and extrapyramidal features have also been reported. Most patients are wheelchair-bound 15 years after onset. The range of age at onset of symptoms is wide (2–65 years), and onset may occur with ataxia or vision loss (Enevoldson et al. 1994). Retinopathy predominantly involves the macula and leads to blindness (Figure 76.9); it may then extend to the peripheral fundus. The early macular changes are subtle and only evident on indirect ophthalmoscopy. Early blue-yellow color disturbances can be noted. Unlike ADCA types I and III, this group is largely genetically homogeneous. The *SCA7* gene has recently been identified and the mutation confirmed to be a CAG expansion in the coding region of the gene, similar to that in other SCA diseases (David et al. 1997) (see Table 76.6).

Kindreds containing adult-onset cases and others with onset in early childhood and a rapidly progressive course have been described; such patients nearly always have affected fathers (i.e., as in SCA types 1–3, there is a paternal transmission effect [anticipation]). There are also occasional obligate gene carriers who do not develop symptoms of the disease, despite living until the age of 65 or more, which provides evidence of reduced penetrance in this disorder.

Autopsy data from these patients reveals retinal atrophy and cerebellar atrophy affecting the cerebellar cortex, spino-cerebellar and olivocerebellar tracts, and efferent cerebellar pathways. The pyramidal pathways and the motor neurons of the brainstem and spinal cord are also affected (Martin et al. 1994).

Autosomal Dominant Cerebellar Ataxia Type III

ADCA type III is a relatively pure cerebellar syndrome in which ocular or extrapyramidal features and peripheral neuropathy do not occur. It is also genetically heterogeneous: Of 23 families, 11 had consistently late onset (after age 40 in all patients, and at 50 years or later in all but three patients). In the other 12 families, onset was earlier, ranging from the second to fourth decade of life. In these 12 families, the disease course was only slowly progressive, with patients not losing the ability to walk until 30–40 years after onset (Giunti et al. 1994). An autopsy of one patient showed cerebellar cortical atrophy with loss of cells in the dentate nuclei. There are at least three genes responsible for this phenotype. *SCA5* was linked to chromosome 11 after evaluation of two branches of the descendants of Abraham Lincoln. This locus has not been found in other families. SCA type 6 is characterized by a pure later-onset (after age 40) ataxic disorder. It is caused by yet another CAG repeat in a calcium-channel subunit gene and is allelic to familial hemiplegic migraine and episodic ataxia type 2. In the United Kingdom, SCA type 6 accounts for approximately 50% of cases of ADCA type III. However, additional features, hyporeflexia, and extrapyramidal signs are seen occasionally, and therefore SCA type 6 should also be considered in the differential diagnosis of ADCA type I.

Dentatorubropallidoluysian Atrophy

Dentatorubropallidoluysian atrophy, a dominant disorder reported mainly in Japanese families, has a variable phenotype comprising various combinations of ataxia, dystonia, myoclonus, various types of seizure, dementia, and parkinsonism. Onset ranges from late childhood to late adult life. The pathological features are incorporated in the name of the disease. This disorder was mapped to chromosome 12p in Japan, and the disease mutation is another expanded CAG repeat (Nagafuchi et al. 1994). The same mutation has now been described in other populations, but it is still much rarer than Huntington's disease (HD) outside Japan.

Molecular Genetics of the Autosomal Dominant Cerebellar Ataxias

The classification of the ADCAs is potentially confusing. There is still a place for the clinical system described above, as it guides the neurologist in approaching the patient and deciding on the genetic tests required. The progress in our understanding of genes and mutations has led to an additional classification system; there are many common features between these disorders.

The first ADCA to be linked was labeled *SCA1*. This locus was localized to chromosome 6p. Thereafter, each new locus was given a new SCA number: SCA2 to chromosome 12q (Gispert et al. 1993), SCA3/MJD to chromosome 14q (Stevanin et al. 1994), SCA4 to chromosome 16 (Flanigan et al. 1996), SCA5 to chromosome 11, SCA6 to 19q, and SCA7 to 3p. Currently, only linkage data is available for SCAs 4 and 5. For all the others, the genes have been cloned and the causative mutations established. Table 76.6 lists these disorders and their mutations. They are all caused by an expansion of an exonic CAG repeat. The resultant proteins all possess an expanded polyglutamine tract, and there are now at least eight conditions caused by these expansions. Despite the length of this list of conditions, a few basic principles can be applied. All the CAG-repeat disorders so far described are the result of a relatively modest expansion in the coding region. Although the exact number of repeats on both normal and abnormal alleles varies between diseases (see Table 76.6), the usual normal range of repeats is in the 20s, whereas for the disease-carrying allele, it tends to be greater than 40. These diseases are predominantly adult-onset neurodegenerative disorders, and most show evidence of anticipation, particularly in paternal transmissions. The exact function of the polyglutamine tract remains unknown, but some data are emerging. It has now been shown that the repeat length is a major determinant of age of onset and probably also partly determines severity. This fact alone supports the view that it is the polyglutamine expansion that is directly pathogenic rather than being a mutational epiphenomenon. This is further supported by transgenic animal studies and cell culture systems, from which it is known that the CAG repeat is first made into equal amounts of mRNA

as the normal allele and equal amounts of protein. This strongly supports the hypothesis of a toxic gain of function.

Many questions remain. What is the explanation of the cellular specificity, given that these proteins (both wild type and mutant) are often widely expressed? What is the common link between an expanded polyglutamine tract and toxicity? The answers are still unknown; however, there are lessons to be learned from HD. There appear to be at least 14 other proteins that interact with the protein huntingtin, which is mutated in HD, and some or all of these may account for some or all of the neuronal specificity. An insight into the toxic pathway has begun to emerge. Davies and colleagues (1997) reported that mice transgenic for exon 1 of the human huntingtin gene carrying more than 100 CAG repeats developed abundant intranuclear inclusions. These pathological changes predated the neurological phenotype. These findings have been confirmed not only in HD but also in several other CAG repeat disorders. The search is now on to understand the structure and formation of the inclusions and to establish whether they are part of the pathogenic pathway or are bystander phenomena. The hope is to identify a common downstream pathway, which, if interrupted, might lead to a therapy for all of these disorders.

Treatment and Counseling

Despite the encouraging developments in molecular genetics, the late-onset inherited ataxias remain largely untreatable. The focus is on supportive care with input from physiotherapy, speech therapy, and social organizations. The author has seen a modest response to L-dopa in some patients with parkinsonism in association with their degenerative ataxia. The children of patients with the ADCAs face the same sort of difficult reproductive decisions as do those at risk for developing HD because of the late age of disease onset. Predictive testing is now possible in families with identified mutations, but it is essential that this be performed using the same careful counseling protocols as in HD.

Other Dominant Ataxias

Other types of ADCA (see Table 76.6) are rare. The May-White syndrome of deafness, late-onset cerebellar ataxia, myoclonus, and peripheral neuropathy may be a mitochondrial encephalopathy; it has been maternally transmitted in reported families. Some patients also had generalized tonic-clonic seizures. Autopsy studies showed atrophy of cerebellar white matter, loss of Purkinje's cells, and cell loss in the dentate nuclei. Other dominant ataxic syndromes include those associated with essential tremor, cataracts, deafness, parkinsonism, and peripheral neuropathy. Patients with Gerstmann-Sträussler syndrome have prominent ataxia in the early phase of the disease, although the accompanying dementia usually predominates later.

Autosomal Dominant Periodic Ataxia

Autosomal dominant periodic ataxia is characterized by childhood or adolescent onset of attacks of ataxia, dysarthria, vertigo, and nystagmus. Not all patients have affected relatives. There are at least two forms of this disorder.

Episodic Ataxia Type 1

In episodic ataxia type 1, the attacks tend to be relatively brief (minutes and occasionally hours), and clinically and electrophysiologically, myokymia may be seen. Mutations in a potassium channel have been found. These patients may benefit from acetazolamide, and phenytoin has also anecdotally been reported to be useful. Patients tend to be neurologically normal between attacks.

Episodic Ataxia Type 2

The attacks of episodic ataxia type 2 tend to be longer lasting (hours or even days). They are usually associated with vertigo and consequent nausea and vomiting. They tend to be more severe in childhood, with associated drowsiness, headache, and fever. Although when the disease begins, patients are well between attacks, an interictal nystagmus can be seen. As the years pass, a slowly progressive ataxia is seen. MRI may reveal cerebellar atrophy. These patients tend to respond better to acetazolamide therapy than do patients with episodic ataxia type 1. The locus had been mapped to chromosome 19q in the same region as familial hemiplegic migraine. Subsequently, point mutations in a large calcium-channel gene have been demonstrated in families with both disorders (i.e., they are allelic). As a general rule, mis-sense mutations give rise to familial hemiplegic migraine, and truncating mutations cause episodic ataxia type 2. The CAG repeat that causes SCA6 is found in the 3' region of the same gene.

IDIOPATHIC DEGENERATIVE LATE-ONSET ATAXIAS

The first reports of sporadic cases of late-onset cerebellar ataxia appeared at the same time as those of familial ones. Such patients have probably been relatively underreported in the literature compared with those with ADCA. About two-thirds of cases of degenerative ataxia developing after age 20 are singleton cases, and they represent a significant clinical problem; it is difficult even to know how to label them. I prefer to use the term *idiopathic late-onset cerebellar ataxia* rather than the more common label of *OPCA*. The pathological findings in these disorders are variable, including cerebello-olivary atrophy and cerebellar cortical atrophy, as well as OPCA, which is seen in at least one-half of sporadic cases (Figure 76.10).

Three broad groups of cases can be defined on clinical grounds. The most common is a syndrome similar to that described by Dejerine and Thomas in 1900. Onset of symptoms usually occurs between ages 35 and 55, and men are

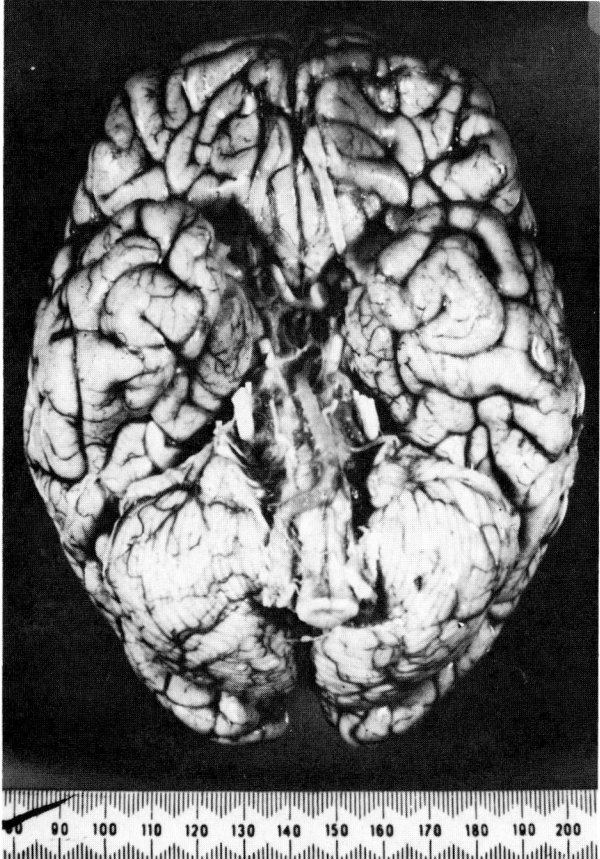

FIGURE 76.10   Undersurface of the brain of a 60-year-old man with olivopontocerebellar atrophy. The cerebellar hemispheres are slightly shrunken, and there is severe atrophy of the pons. (Courtesy of Dr. F. Scaravilli; reprinted with permission from AE Harding. The Hereditary Ataxias and Related Disorders. Edinburgh: Churchill Livingstone, 1984.)

affected more often than women are. Few patients have a pure cerebellar syndrome; dementia and peripheral neuropathy, giving rise to hyporeflexia and sensory loss, are common associated features, and supranuclear ophthalmoplegia is seen in some cases. Optic atrophy and pigmentary retinopathy are rare, in contrast to cases of ADCA.

A proportion of patients in this group, probably approximately 15%, progress to develop the features of multiple system atrophy (MSA). Facial impassivity and extrapyramidal rigidity are found in some, and others present with a cerebellar syndrome and then develop features of autonomic failure, such as postural hypotension, impotence, bladder dysfunction, and a fixed cardiac rate. A cerebellar presentation occurs in about 15% of patients with MSA (Quinn and Marsden 1993). Distinguishing idiopathic late-onset cerebellar ataxia from MSA may therefore be difficult clinically at presentation; a history of impotence or urinary urgency suggests MSA. Patients who are going to develop other features of MSA often have a rather unusual gait, with a narrow rather than a wide base. This may reflect early impairment of postural reflexes in the absence

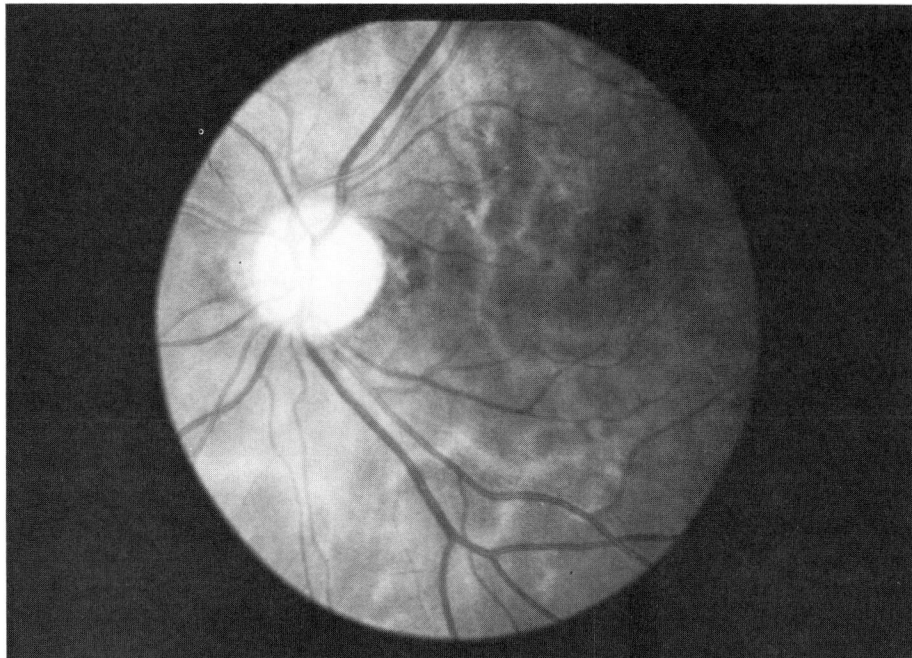

FIGURE 76.11 Patchy pigmentary macular degeneration in Kjellin's syndrome. (Courtesy of Mr. Michael Sanders; reprinted with permission of the author and publisher from AE Harding. The Hereditary Ataxias and Related Disorders. Edinburgh: Churchill Livingstone, 1984.)

of other features of parkinsonism. There is considerable pathological overlap between MSA and other degenerative late-onset ataxias in that many share the changes of OPCA.

Patients with late-onset degenerative ataxias who first develop symptoms after the age of 55 years often have a relatively pure midline cerebellar syndrome, with marked gait ataxia but only mild cerebellar dysfunction in the limbs. Dysarthria is mild or absent in most cases; dementia occurs in some. These cases are similar to those reported by Marie, Foix, and Alajouanine in 1922. Autopsy studies showed cerebellar atrophy, which was most marked in the vermis. There was also olivary atrophy, but the pons was normal; mild degenerative changes were seen in the long tracts of the spinal cord.

A third, rather smaller, group of patients has late-onset cerebellar ataxia associated with prominent resting or postural tremor and gross intention tremor. Onset usually occurs in the fifth and sixth decades of life. This disorder corresponds to the dyssynergia cerebellaris progressiva (not to be confused with dyssynergia cerebellaris myoclonica) of Ramsay Hunt.

Most patients with idiopathic late-onset cerebellar ataxia lose the ability to walk independently 5–20 years after onset, and life span is slightly shortened by immobility. Those who go on to develop MSA have a particularly poor prognosis (Klockgether et al. 1998a). Investigations, apart from those excluding acquired causes of cerebellar degeneration, such as malignancy and hypothyroidism, tend to be unhelpful. Electrophysiological evidence of a sensory peripheral neuropathy is found in approximately 50% of cases, which can be a useful pointer to the presence of a degenerative multisystem disorder. CT or MRI scan may show cerebellar and brainstem atrophy, or pure cerebellar atrophy. The prognosis is worse in patients with clinical

and radiological evidence of brainstem involvement than in those with a pure cerebellar syndrome and cerebellar atrophy alone on MRI, and this is so even if patients with MSA are excluded (Ormerod et al. 1994).

The cause of these disorders is unknown. Excluding patients with MSA that has not been convincingly reported in more than one member of a family, it is likely that a small proportion of cases represent new dominant mutations. The risk that offspring of patients will be similarly affected is estimated at 5–10%. Because autosomal recessive inheritance is so rare in late-onset ataxia, it seems unreasonable to suggest that many of these patients have a recessively inherited disorder. Treatment with cholinergic and other drugs has, with one or two exceptions, been disappointing.

HEREDITARY SPASTIC PARAPLEGIAS

Although most patients with hereditary spastic paraplegias have a disorder confined to dysfunction of the pyramidal tracts, at least clinically (these disorders are discussed in Chapter 79), there is some overlap with spinocerebellar syndromes. Hereditary spastic paraplegias can be divided into two groups, depending on whether the disorder is a pure spastic paraplegia or a more complex syndrome consisting of spastic paraplegia and other associated features. An autosomal recessive syndrome of cerebellar dysarthria, mild ataxia in the upper limbs with or without distal wasting, and spastic paraplegia is quite a common clinical problem, although it has rarely been documented. Some patients with this syndrome have mental retardation and a pigmentary macular degeneration (Kjellin's syndrome). The macular degeneration (Figure 76.11) may easily be overlooked because it does not usually give rise to vision loss. Dominantly inherited paraplegia with dysarthria and cerebellar signs in the upper limbs has also been described.

REFERENCES

Babcock M, de Silva D, Oaks R, et al. Regulation of the mitochondrial iron accumulation by Yfh1p, a putative homolog of frataxin. Science 1997;276:1709–1712.

Ben Hamida C, Doerflinger N, Belal S, et al. Localization of Friedreich ataxia phenotype with selective vitamin E deficiency to chromosome 8q by homozygosity mapping. Nat Genet 1993; 5:195–200.

Bootsma D, Kraemer KH, Cleaver J, Hoeijmakers JHJ. Nucleotide Excision Repair Syndromes: Xeroderma Pigmentosum, Cockayne Syndrome and Trichothiodystrophy. In CR Scriver, AL Beaudet, WS Sly, D Valle (eds), The Metabolic Basis of Inherited Disease (8th ed). New York: McGraw-Hill, 1998; 245–274.

Brown KD, Ziv Y, Sadanandan SN, et al. The ataxia-telangiectasia gene product, a constitutively expressed nuclear protein that is not up-regulated following genome damage. Proc Natl Acad Sci U S A 1997;94:1840–1845.

Campuzano V, Montermini L, Molto MD, et al. Friedreich's ataxia: autosomal recessive disease caused by an intronic GAA triplet repeat expansion. Science 1996;271:1423–1427.

Cochius JI, Figlewicz DA, Kalviainen R, et al. Unverricht-Lundborg disease: absence of nonallelic genetic heterogeneity. Ann Neurol 1993;34:739–741.

Collinge J, Rossor MN, Thomas D, et al. Diagnosis of Creutzfeldt-Jakob disease by measurement of S100 protein in serum. Tonsil biopsy helps diagnose new variant Creutzfeldt-Jakob disease. BMJ 1998;317:472–473.

David G, Abbas N, Stevanin G, et al. Cloning of the gene for autosomal dominant cerebellar ataxia with progressive macular dystrophy (SCA7) reveals a highly unstable CAG repeat expansion. Nat Genet 1997;17:65–70.

Davies SW, Turmaine M, Cozens B, et al. Formation of neuronal intranuclear inclusions underlies the neurological dysfunction in mice transgenic for the HD mutation. Cell 1997;90:537–548.

Durr A, Cossee M, Agid Y, et al. Clinical and genetic abnormalities in patients with Friedreich's ataxia. N Engl J Med 1996;335: 1169–1175.

Enevoldson PG, Sanders MD, Harding AE. Autosomal dominant cerebellar ataxia with pigmentary macular dystrophy: a clinical and genetic study of eight families. Brain 1994;117:445–460.

Fearnley JM, Stevens JM, Rudge P. Superficial siderosis of the central nervous system. Brain 1995;118:1051–1066.

Filla A, De Michele G, Cavalcanti F, et al. The relationship between trinucleotide (GAA) repeat length and clinical features in Friedreich ataxia. Am J Hum Genet 1996;59:554–560.

Flanigan K, Gardner K, Alderson K, et al. Autosomal dominant spinocerebellar ataxia with sensory axonal neuropathy (SCA4): clinical description and genetic localization to chromosome 16q22.1. Am J Hum Genet 1996;59:392–399.

Gispert S, Twells R, Orozco G, et al. Chromosomal assignment of the second (Cuban) locus for autosomal dominant cerebellar ataxia (SCA2) to human chromosome 12q23-24.1. Nat Genet 1993;4:295–299.

Giunti P, Spadaro M, Jodice C, et al. The trinucleotide repeat expansion on chromosome 6p (SCA1) in autosomal dominant cerebellar ataxias. Brain 1994;117:645–649.

Gotoda T, Arita M, Arai H, et al. Adult-onset spinocerebellar dys-

function caused by a mutation in the gene for the alpha-tocopherol transfer protein. N Engl J Med 1995;333:1313–1318.

Imbert G, Saudou F, Yvert G, et al. Cloning of the gene for spinocerebellar ataxia 2 reveals a locus with high sensitivity to expanded CAG/glutamine repeats. Nat Genet 1996;14:285–291.

Klockgether T, Ludtke R, Kramer B, et al. The natural history of degenerative ataxia: a retrospective study in 466 patients. Brain 1998a;121:589–600.

Klockgether T, Skalej M, Wedekind D, et al. Autosomal dominant cerebellar ataxia type I. MRI-based volumetry of posterior fossa structures and basal ganglia in spinocerebellar ataxia types 1, 2 and 3. Brain 1998b;121:1687–1693.

Lalioti MD, Scott HS, Buresi C, et al. Dodecamer repeat expansion in cystatin B gene in progressive myoclonus epilepsy. Nature 1997;386:847–851.

Lamont PJ, Davis MB, Wood NW. Identification and sizing of the GAA trinucleotide repeat expansion of Friedreich's ataxia in fifty-five patients: clinical and genetic correlates. Brain 1997;120:673–680.

Leitersdorf E, Reshef A, Meiner V, et al. Frameshift and splice-junction mutations in the sterol 27-hydroxylase gene causes cerebrotendinous xanthomatosis in Jews of Moroccan origin. J Clin Invest 1993;91:2488–2496.

Martin JJ, Van Regemorter N, Krols L, et al. On an autosomal dominant form of retino-cerebellar degeneration: an autopsy study of five patients in one family. Acta Neuropathol (Berl) 1994;88:277–286.

Moll JWB, Henzen-Logmans SC, van der Meche FGA, et al. Early diagnosis and intravenous immune globulin therapy in paraneoplastic cerebellar degeneration. J Neurol Neurosurg Psychiatry 1993;56:112.

Nagafuchi S, Yanagisawa H, Sato K, et al. Expansion of an unstable CAG trinucleotide on chromosome 12p in dentatorubral and pallidoluysian atrophy. Nat Genet 1994;6: 15–18.

Ormerod IEC, Harding AE, Miller DH, et al. Magnetic resonance imaging in degenerative ataxic disorders. J Neurol Neurosurg Psychiatry 1994;57:51–57.

Orr HT, Chung M, Banfi S, et al. Expansion of an unstable trinucleotide CAG repeat in spinocerebellar ataxia type 1. Nat Genet 1993;4:221–226.

Ouahchi K, Arita M, Kayden H, et al. Ataxia with isolated vitamin E deficiency is caused by mutations in the alpha-tocopherol transfer protein. Nat Genet 1995;9:141–145.

Pennacchio LA, Lehesjoki AE, Stone NE, et al. Mutations in the gene encoding cystatin B in progressive myoclonus epilepsy (EPM1). Science 1996;271:1731–1733.

Quinn NP, Marsden CD. The motor disorder of multiple system atrophy. J Neurol Neurosurg Psychiatry 1993;56:1239–1242.

Savitsky K, Bar-Shira A, Gilad S, et al. A single ataxia telangiectasia gene with a product similar to PI-3 kinase. Science 1995; 268:1749–1753.

Shiloh Y. Ataxia telangiectasia: closer to unravelling the mystery. Eur J Hum Genet 1995;33:116–138.

Shoulders CC, Brett DJ, Bayliss JD, et al. Abetalipoproteinaemia is caused by defects of the gene encoding the 97-kDa subunit of a microsomal triglyceride transfer protein. Hum Mol Genet 1993;2:2109–2116.

Stevanin G, Le Guern E, Ravise N, et al. A third locus for autosomal dominant cerebellar ataxia (ADCA) type I maps to chromosome 14q24.3-qter: evidence for the existence of a fourth locus. Am J Hum Genet 1994;54:11–20.

Stewart GE, Ironside JW. New variant Creutzfeldt-Jakob disease. Curr Opin Neurol 1998;11:259–262.

Chapter 77
Disorders of Bones, Joints, Ligaments, and Meninges

Richard B. Rosenbaum

Disorders of the bones, joints, ligaments, and meninges, because of their close proximity to the nervous system, can cause several different myelopathic and radiculopathic syndromes and can affect the cranial nerves and intracranial contents. This chapter considers many of these disorders, both congenital and acquired. Chapters of overlapping interest include Chapters 28, 56C, 57F, and 66.

CONGENITAL AND INHERITED SPINAL DISORDERS

Disorders of the craniocervical junction include bony abnormalities of the occiput and foramen magnum, dysfunction of connecting ligaments, hindbrain malformations, upper cervical skeletal deformities, and syringomyelia or syringobulbia. Many of these are congenital; their embryogenesis is discussed in Chapter 66. Magnetic resonance imaging (MRI) and computed tomographic (CT) scanning have improved the detection, understanding, and treatment of these anomalies.

Craniocervical Deformities

Occipitalization of the Atlas

Occipitalization of the atlas refers to congenital partial or complete fusion of the atlas (first cervical vertebra) to the occiput (Figure 77.1). The anterior arch of the atlas may fuse to the lower end of the clivus or the posterior arch of the atlas may fuse to the occiput. The anomaly is often asymptomatic until early adult life and may become symptomatic after trauma. The loss of movement between the occiput and atlas increases the stresses at the atlantoaxial joint, predisposing it to gradual degeneration or traumatic dislocation. Patients with occipitalization of the atlas may have associated anomalies, such as the Klippel-Feil anomaly, basilar impression, or Chiari malformation.

Basilar Impression

Basilar impression or *invagination* refers to abnormal cephalad position of the foramen magnum. Several radiological lines (Chamberlain's, McGregor's, McRae's, digastric) (Figure 77.2) and measurements can be used to make the diagnosis. Congenital basilar impression may occur in isolation or be associated with conditions such as achondroplasia, occipital dysplasia, Down syndrome, Hurler's syndrome, Klippel-Feil anomaly, and cleidocranial dysplasia. Some instances of basilar impression are familial. The skeletal anomaly is often accompanied by anomalies of the neuraxis, including Chiari I or II malformation and syringomyelia. Basilar impression can lead to compression of the brainstem (Figure 77.3) or cerebellum, or, rarely, to vertebral artery compression, leading to vertebrobasilar ischemia. It is often asymptomatic, particularly when mild and unaccompanied by other anomalies.

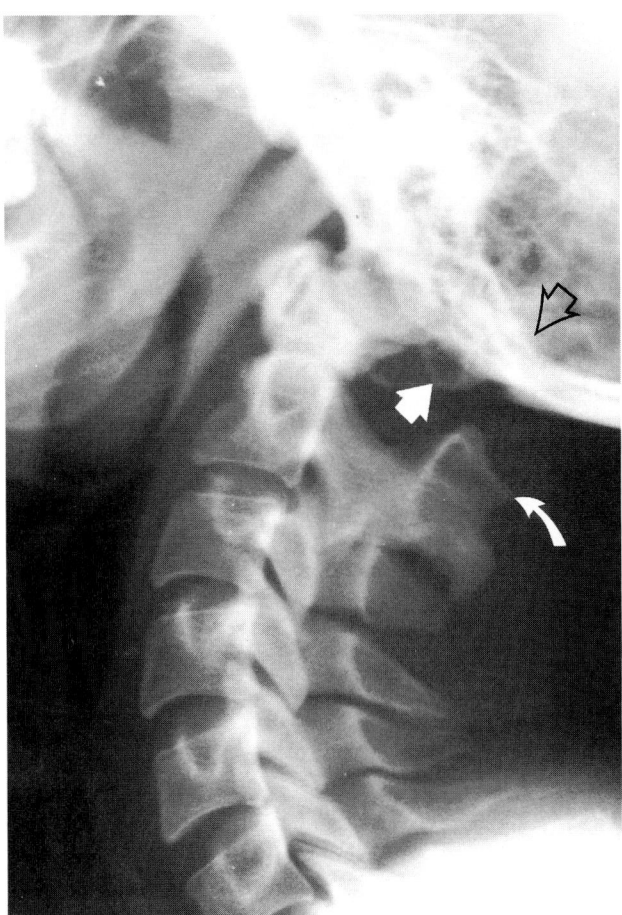

FIGURE 77.1 Occipitalization of the atlas. Radiograph shows fusion of the lamina of the atlas to the occiput (*open arrow*). The lamina contain the circular arcuate foramina (*arrow*), through which the vertebral arteries pass. The spinous process of the atlas (*curved arrow*) has fused with C2, making this a partial incorporation of C1 into the skull base. There is a broad spectrum of variations in this congenital anomaly. (Courtesy of Erik Gaensler, M.D.)

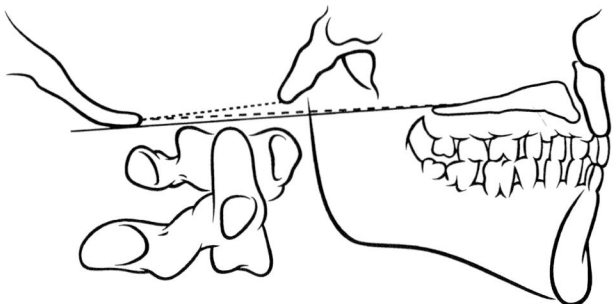

FIGURE 77.2 Chamberlain's line (*dashes*) extends from the roof of the hard palate to the posterior lip of the foramen magnum; McGregor's line (*solid*) extends from the roof of the hard palate to the most caudal portion of the occipital bone; McRae's line (*dots*) extends from the anterior lip of the foramen magnum to the posterior lip of the foramen magnum. The tip of the odontoid is normally not more than 5 mm above McGregor's line and not above Chamberlain's or McRae's lines. (Modified with permission from RB Rosenbaum, SM Campbell, JT Rosenbaum. Clinical Neurology of Rheumatic Diseases. Boston: Butterworth–Heinemann, 1996:187.)

Platybasia or *flattening of the skull* refers to straightening of the angle between the clivus and the floor of the anterior fossa. It infrequently accompanies basilar impression; it can occur also as an isolated radiographic finding without any adverse neurological consequences.

Acquired basilar impression is uncommon, accounting for less than 10% of the cases. The causes are generally diseases that lead to softening of bone such as Paget's disease, osteogenesis imperfecta, osteomalacia or rickets, or parathyroid dysfunction. It also can be caused by diseases causing vertical atlantoaxial subluxation such as rheumatoid arthritis (RA), neurofibromatosis, hypothyroidism, fibrous dysplasia, and gargoylism. Basilar impression is rarely traumatic.

Klippel-Feil Anomaly

Patients with the Klippel-Feil anomaly (congenital synostosis of the cervical vertebrae) (Figure 77.4) have short necks, low hairlines, and limitation of cervical motion. The diagnosis is confirmed by radiographic demonstration of fused cervical vertebrae. The condition is congenital, caused by failure of normal segmentation of the cervical vertebrae between the third and eighth weeks of fetal development. Although familial instances occur, most cases are isolated and idiopathic. Direct nerve root or cervical spinal cord compression may be caused by the anomaly. Congenital deafness is common. Mirror movements of the hands may occur in children with Klippel-Feil anomaly and is attributed to incomplete decussation of the pyramidal tracts. Patients with Klippel-Feil anomaly can have a wide variety of associated abnormalities of brain, spinal cord, or skeletal development, especially congenital scoliosis or Sprengel's deformity with unilateral shoulder elevation. Patients may develop hydrocephalus, syringomyelia, or syringobulbia. However, most patients with Klippel-Feil anomaly have no neurological symptoms or signs (Thomsen et al. 1997).

Atlantoaxial Dislocation

Various congenital or acquired conditions can disrupt the integrity of the atlantoaxial joint, leading to its dislocation (Stevens et al. 1994) (Table 77.1). In horizontal subluxation, C1 usually moves anteriorly to C2. The movement can be assessed by measuring the separation between the dens and the anterior arch of C1 on flexion radiographs; in adults the separation should not exceed 3.5 mm. Patients with horizontal atlantoaxial joint subluxation are likely to compress their spinal cords if the diameter of the spinal canal at the level of the dens is less than 14 mm, and unlikely to if the diameter is greater than 17 mm. The actual relationship between the cord and the subluxating

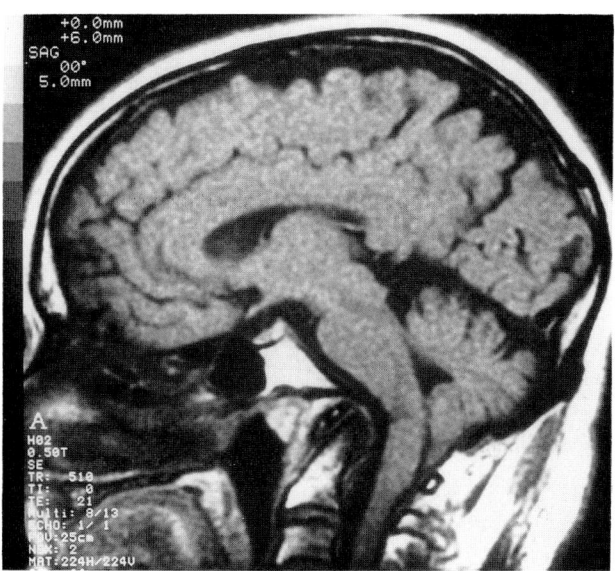

FIGURE 77.3   Magnetic resonance image of a patient with basilar impression showing angulation of the brainstem.

bones is best imaged with MRI or CT myelography, which should include flexion and extension views. In some patients, particularly those with acquired inflammatory disease, such as RA, inflamed adjacent soft tissue contributing to cord compression is best characterized by MRI.

Patients with congenital atlantoaxial dislocation may have associated abnormalities such as Chiari I malformation or diastematomyelia. They can develop secondary syringomyelia. Atlantoaxial subluxation in patients with long-standing RA is a prime example of acquired abnormality of the atlantoaxial joint and is discussed in more detail later in this chapter. Patients with atlantoaxial subluxation may be asymptomatic, particularly if their spinal canal diameter is generous. However, they are vulnerable to spinal cord trauma during intubation or other neck motion under anesthesia, or in relation to a whiplash injury. Patients at risk for atlantoaxial dislocation, such as those with Down syndrome or chronic RA, should have lateral flexion and extension cervical spine radiography performed before general anesthesia so that the anesthesiologist can plan appropriate care during intubation.

Arnold-Chiari Malformation and Syringomyelia

Arnold-Chiari Malformation

Chiari (1891, 1896) described four types of malformations with cerebellar tonsillar displacement (Anson et al. 1997). Cleland (1883) had previously written about them. Arnold (1894) reported a case of Chiari II malformation. In cur-

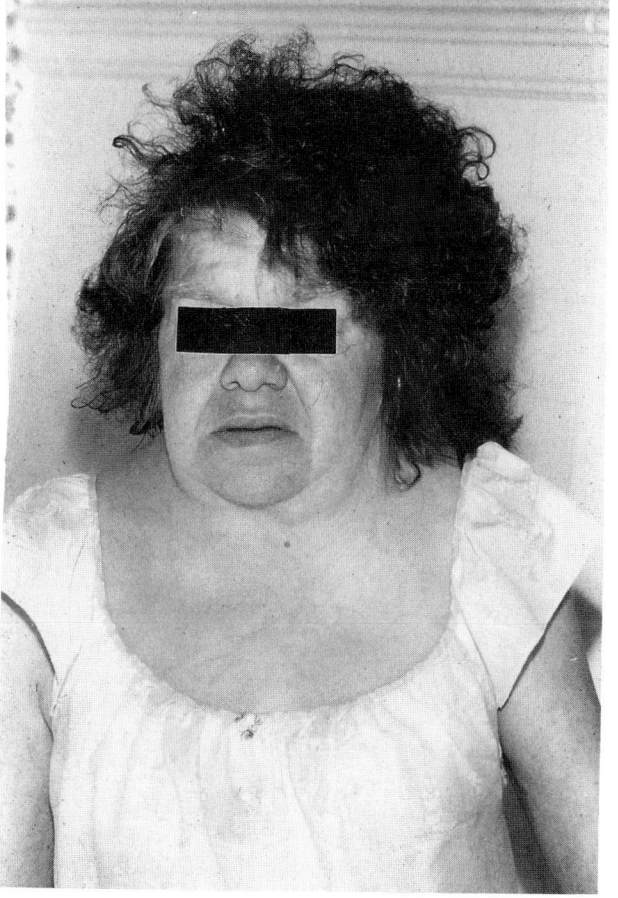

FIGURE 77.4   Patient with Klippel-Feil syndrome showing short neck.

Table 77.1:   Mechanisms of atlantoaxial dislocation

I. Congenital
 A. Os odontoideum (failure of the odontoid to fuse with the body of the axis)
  1. Isolated
  2. With connective tissue dysplasias (e.g., Down syndrome, pseudoachondroplasia, multiple epiphyseal dysplasia, spondyloepiphyseal dysplasia, Morquio's disease, Klippel-Feil anomaly, Conradi's syndrome)
 B. Hypoplastic dens
  1. With connective tissue dysplasia
  2. With incomplete segmentation (e.g., occipital assimilation of atlas, basilar invagination, incomplete segmentation of C2, C3, and so forth)
 C. Other anomalies of C2 (e.g., bifid dens, tripartite dens with os apicale, agenesis of all or part of dens)
 D. Laxity of the transverse atlantal ligament (e.g., Down syndrome)
II. Acquired
 E. Traumatic, acute or chronic ununited dens fracture
 F. Infectious
 G. Neoplastic (e.g., neurofibroma)
 H. Arthritic (e.g., in rheumatoid arthritis, ankylosing spondylitis)
 I. Bone disease (e.g., vitamin D resistant rickets and others associated with basilar invagination)

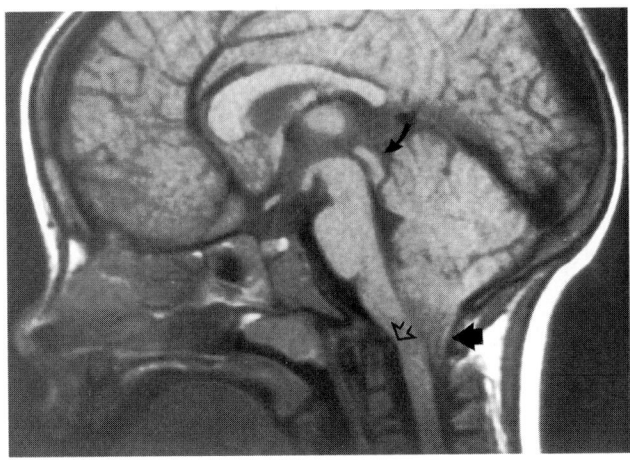

FIGURE 77.5   Sagittal magnetic resonance image of patient with Arnold-Chiari I malformation. This midline sagittal T1-weighted image demonstrates low cerebellar tonsils (*arrow*), which extend more than 1.5 cm through the foramen magnum, compressing the cervicomedullary junction. The lower medulla (*open arrow*) is mildly indented by the odontoid. The posterior fossa size is normal, and none of the supratentorial abnormalities of Chiari II malformation are present. Specifically, note the normal appearance of the tectum (*curved arrow*), which has a beaked appearance in the Chiari II malformation. (Courtesy of Erik Gaensler, M.D.)

rent usage the terms *Arnold-Chiari* and *Chiari malformation* are often used interchangeably for all four types.

Chiari I malformation (Figure 77.5) is characterized by abnormal extension of the cerebellar tonsils below the foramen magnum. Some rostral displacement or extension of the medulla may exist. Slight extension of the tonsils below the foramen is normal in childhood, and normal values decrease with increasing age (Table 77.2). Cerebellar tonsillar displacement below the foramen magnum can occur also as an acquired condition caused by downward herniation of the brain caused by mass lesions or sagging of the brain in patients with low intracranial pressure. Patients with Chiari malformations of all types often have hydrocephalus and syringomyelia or syringobulbia. The malformation is best seen on sagittal MRI of the brain and cervical spinal, which allows assessment for accompanying syrinx and for brainstem compression. Patients may have associated bony abnormalities such as basilar impression, occipitalization of the atlas, or C1 spina bifida. Chiari I malformations may be asymptomatic or may cause headache or neck ache. Clinical findings may be caused by brainstem compression or from a syrinx. Surgical treatment is aimed at brainstem decompression or drainage of the syrinx, depending on which element is the cause of symptoms (Bindal et al. 1995).

Chiari II malformation combines the features of Chiari I with caudal displacement of the medulla and fourth ventricle. The brainstem is elongated and distorted at the foramen magnum. Usually, patients have a lumbar myelomeningocele.

In Chiari III malformation the displaced cerebellar and brainstem tissue extends into an infratentorial meningoencephalocele.

Chiari type IV malformation is characterized by cerebellar and brainstem hypoplasia rather than displacement and is probably a variant of the Dandy-Walker malformation.

Hydromyelia, Syringomyelia, and Syringobulbia

Hydromyelia is an abnormal dilatation of the central spinal canal, which almost always communicates with the fourth ventricle. A syrinx is a cavity in the spinal cord (syringomyelia) or brainstem (syringobulbia) (Figures 77.6 through 77.8). The cavity may be connected with a dilatated central spinal canal or may be separate from the central canal. There are several different causes of syringomyelia.

Clinical Presentation.   The prototypical presentation of a syrinx is the combination of lower motor neuron signs at the level of the lesion (usually in the arms or lower cranial nerves), a dissociated sensory loss (impaired pain and temperature sensation but preserved light touch, vibration, and position sense in a cape or hemi-cape distribution on the arms and upper trunk), and spinal long tract dysfunction below the level of the lesion. However, few patients show this total picture, and the clinical features vary with the size,

Table 77.2: Suggested upper limits of normal for position of the cerebellar tonsils below the foramen magnum

Decade of life	Distance below the foramen magnum (mm)
First	6
Second or third	5
Fourth to eighth	4
Ninth	3

Source: Data from DJ Mikulis, O Diaz, TK Egglin, et al. Variance of the position of the cerebellar tonsils with age: preliminary report. Radiology 1992;183:725–728.

location, and shape of the cavity and with associated neurological conditions.

Pain is a prominent symptom in most patients with syringomyelia. Common complaints include neck ache, headache, back pain, radicular pain, and areas of segmental dysesthesia (Milhorat et al. 1996). Patients may have trophic changes corresponding to the segmental dysesthesia. Syringomyelia can cause neuropathic monoarthritis (Charcot's joints), most commonly in a shoulder or elbow.

The most common location of a syrinx is in the cervical spinal cord. Syringes developing from hydromyelia of the central canal are most likely to occur associated with Chiari I or II malformations, communicating hydrocephalus, or abnormalities at the craniocerebral junction. Hydromyelia and these associated syringes may be noted as asymptomatic abnormalities on MRI scans obtained to study the cranial problems. As the syrinx enlarges as an asymmetrical localized paracentral outpouching from the hydromyelia, particularly at its cranial or caudal ends or at its level of greatest axial cross section, the paracentral extensions often lead to local segmental signs such as cranial nerve dysfunction in patients with syringobulbia, and segmental lower motor neuron signs and dissociated sensory changes at the level of spinal involvement. Patients with eccentric cavities have some combination of long tract and segmental signs depending on the location of the cavity and of any associated cord pathology such as tumor, ischemia, or contusion. A syrinx associated with a spinal cord tumor can occur at any level of the spinal cord.

Causes. *Communicating and Noncommunicating Syringes.* The terms *communicating* and *noncommunicating syrinx* are used to indicate whether the syrinx is in communication with the cerebrospinal fluid (CSF) pathways. However, it is frequently difficult to determine this, even at autopsy, and hence these terms are mainly of use in discussions of etiology. It is better to classify syringomyelia according to its associations.

Abnormalities of the Cervicomedullary Junction. The exact mechanism of production of the syrinx in patients with abnormalities of the cervicomedullary junction and posterior fossa is controversial. The central canal of the

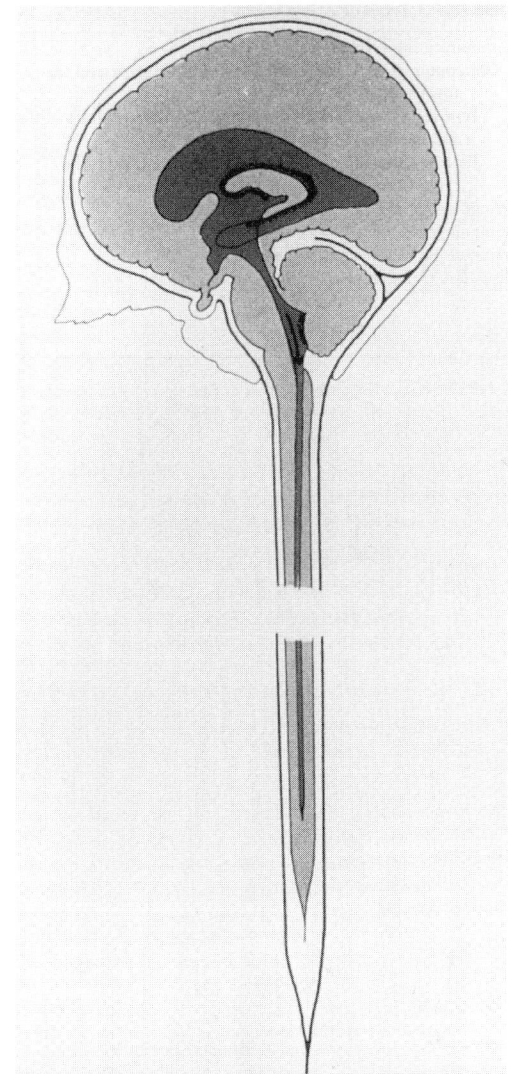

FIGURE 77.6 Diagrammatic representation of persistent central canal extending throughout the length of the spinal cord.

spinal cord is normally widely open during embryonic life, and becomes atretic after birth. It can be found occasionally to be patent in the adult (see Figure 77.6). It is more frequently dilatated (hydromyelia) when associated with abnormalities of the cervicomedullary junction, including Chiari anomalies types I and II, and the Dandy-Walker malformation. Syringes often arise in association with hydromyelia, and some evidence suggests that they are formed as outpouchings of the dilatated central canal (see Figures 77.7 and 77.8). One hypothesis is that the posterior fossa abnormalities interfere with the passage of CSF from the fourth ventricle through the foramina of Luschka and Magendie into the subarachnoid space. The consequence is transmission of bulk flow and of the various pressure waves of the CSF (arterial, venous, respiratory, and so forth) down the central canal of the spinal cord, leading to dissection of a syrinx into the

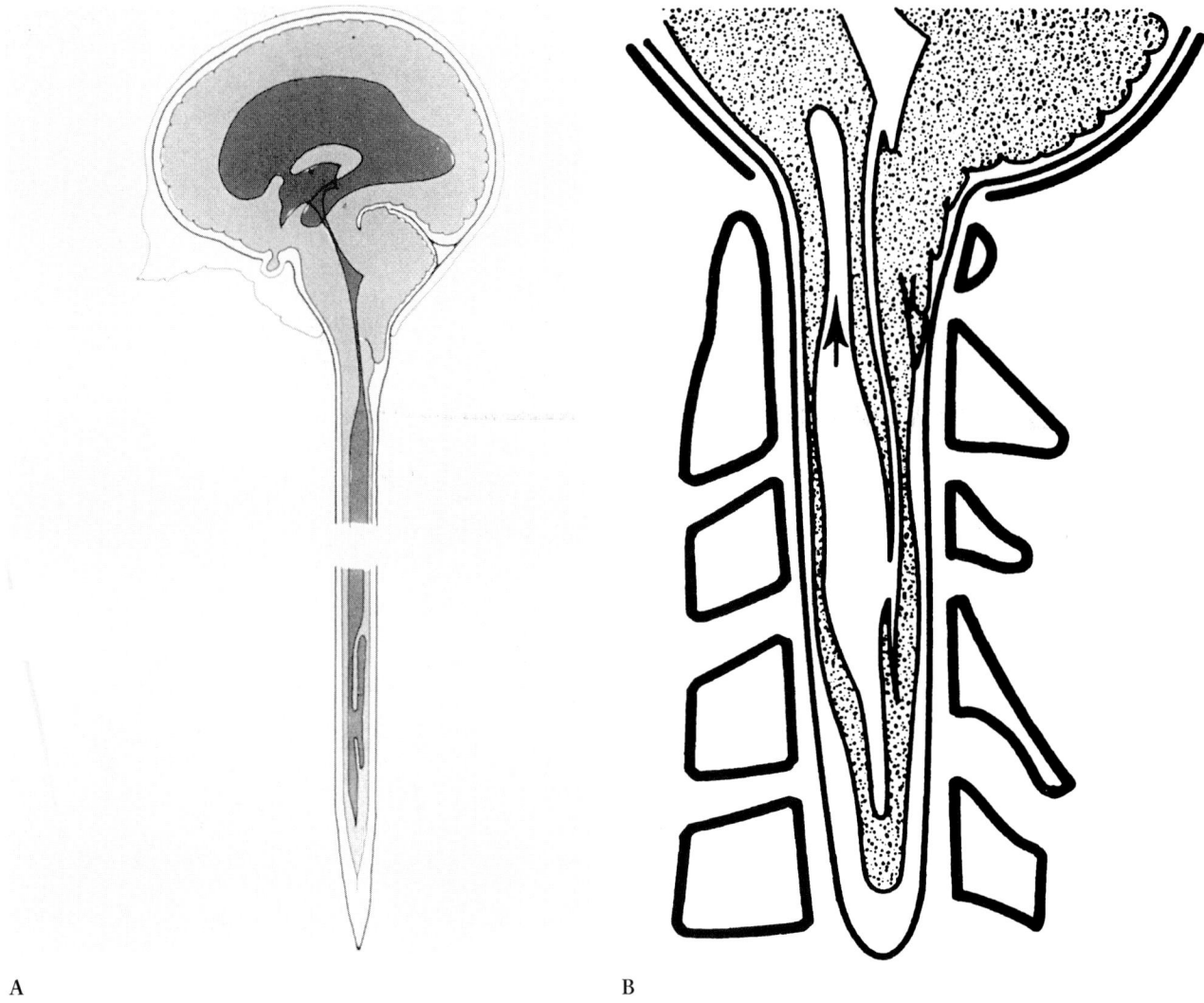

A   B

FIGURE 77.7   Diagrammatic representations of hydromyelic cavities with differing types of syringomyelic cavities. (A) Lumbosacral syrinx. (B) Syrinx tracking cephalad to produce syringobulbia.

substance of the spinal cord. Noncongenital abnormalities at the cervicomedullary junction that can at times cause syringomyelia include arachnoiditis and meningiomas.

Syrinx Associated with Spinal Cord Tumors. Syringomyelia accompanies 25–60% of intramedullary spinal tumors; conversely, 8–16% of syringes are caused by tumors (Samii and Klekamp 1994) (Figure 77.9). Intramedullary tumors in von Hippel–Lindau syndrome or neurofibromatosis are particularly likely to be accompanied by syringes. The syrinx extends from the tumor, more often rostrally than caudally.

Syrinx Associated with Spinal Cord Trauma. Syringes develop as late sequelae in perhaps 3% of cases of serious spinal cord trauma (el Masry and Biyani 1996; Schurch et al. 1996). Symptoms of long tract or segmental spinal cord dysfunction develop months or years after the acute traumatic myelopathy has stabilized, improved, or even become asymptomatic. Pain is often a prominent symptom. Findings usually evolve gradually, but occasionally worsen suddenly following events such as a cough or Valsalva's maneuver. The cavity is usually eccentric, arising from an area of post-traumatic myelomalacia, then spreading rostrally or caudally.

Syrinx Associated with Other Focal Spinal Cord Pathologies. Any illness causing arachnoid inflammation can lead to formation of a noncommunicating syrinx (Klekamp et al. 1997). Reported causes include meningitis, subarachnoid hemorrhage, spinal trauma, epidural infections, epidural anesthesia, myelography with oil-based dyes, and spinal surgery, but many cases of focal arachnoiditis are idiopathic. Syringes can develop as a complication of various intramedullary pathologies including trauma and tumors (see previous discussion), spinal ischemic or hemorrhagic strokes, radiation necrosis, or transverse myelitis.

Treatment. Indications for and approaches to surgical therapy for syringes are far from standardized. The cavity may be drained by simple myelotomy or by shunting to the sub-

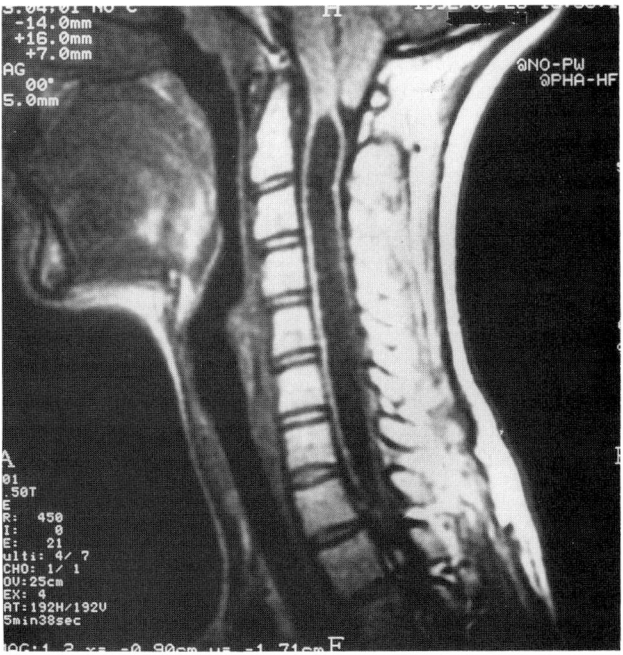

FIGURE 77.8 Magnetic resonance image demonstrates a large syringomyelic cavity in the cervical cord.

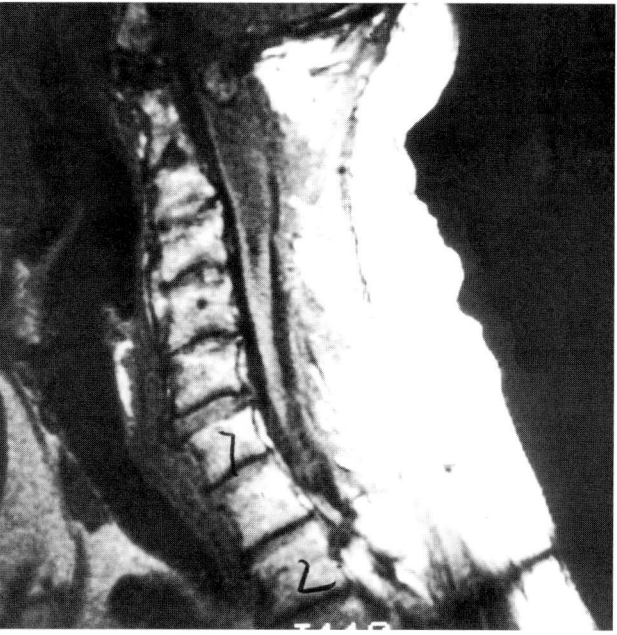

A

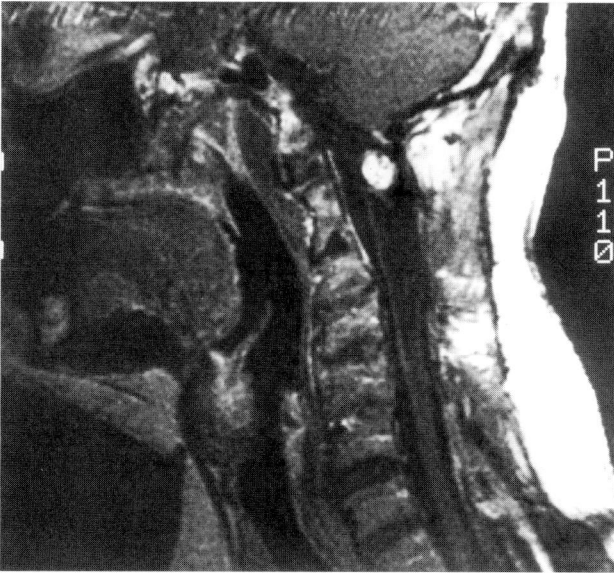

B

FIGURE 77.9 Magnetic resonance image demonstrates syrinx associated with spinal cord tumor (hemangioblastoma). (**A**) T1-weighted image shows enlargement has a nodule on the upper cervical cord caused by a low-signal central mass suggestive of a cyst. The upper border of the cyst has a nodular component. (**B**) Postgadolinium image shows that the nodule intensely enhances, which is classic for hemangioblastoma. (Courtesy of Erik Gaensler, M.D.)

arachnoid, peritoneal, or pleural cavities. In patients with Chiari I malformations, the syrinx may improve after decompression of the malformation with suboccipital craniectomy, upper cervical laminectomy, and dural grafting. When the syrinx extends from an intramedullary tumor, resection of the tumor often leads to regression of the syrinx, so that no specific surgical drainage of the cavity is needed. When the syrinx extends from an area of localized arachnoiditis, some surgeons report satisfactory results after resection of the arachnoiditis without shunting or entering the cavity.

Achondroplasia

Achondroplasia, the most common cause of abnormally short stature, is an autosomal dominant disorder of endochondral bone formation caused by a specific mutation of the fibroblast growth factor 3 gene. The mutant genotype has complete penetrance, and approximately three-fourths of cases occur because of spontaneous mutation. The diagnosis can be confirmed by pathognomonic radiographic changes or by DNA testing. Neurological complications of achondroplasia are common (Table 77.3). In early childhood children should be observed for complications such as hydrocephalus, compression at the foramen magnum, thoracolumbar kyphosis, and sleep apnea. Neurological complications of spinal stenosis tend to occur later in life.

Spinal Dysraphism

Spinal dysraphism is congenital failure of the neural tube to close during fetal development. In spina bifida occulta the vertebral elements fail to fuse, but the thecal and neural

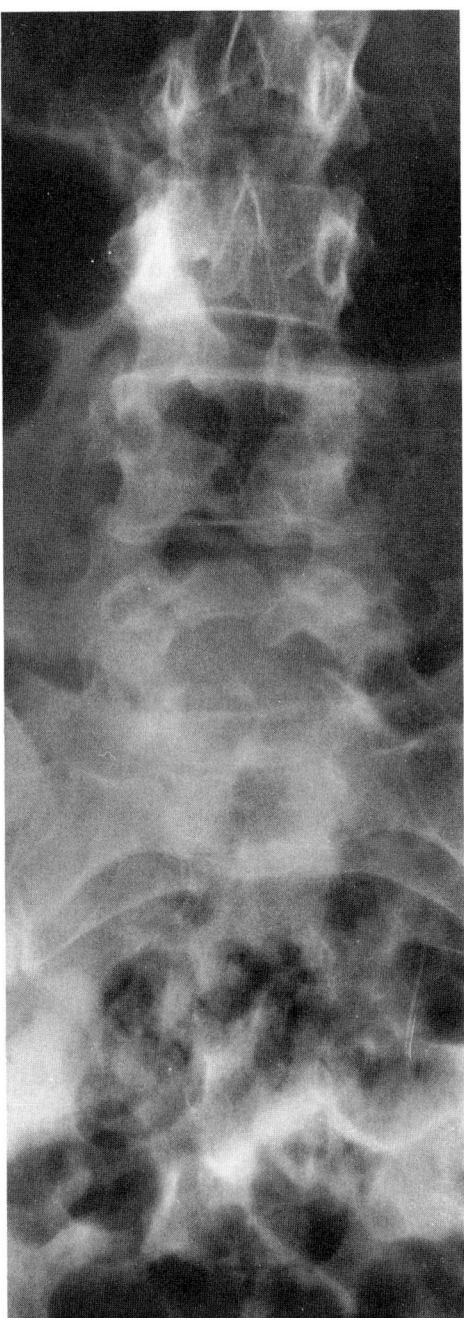

FIGURE 77.10 Lumbar spine radiograph shows spina bifida occulta.

Table 77.3: Neurological complications of achondroplasia

Macrocrania, with or without hydrocephalus
Foramen magnum abnormalities with cervicomedullary
    compression
Respiratory disturbances, including sleep apnea and sudden
    infant death syndrome
Syringomyelia, diastematomyelia
Spinal stenosis with spinal cord or nerve root compression
Infantile hypotonia
Cortical atrophy
Atlantoaxial subluxation
Psychomotor delay (most have normal intelligence)

Source: Adapted from M Ruiz-Garcia, A Tovar-Baudin, V Del Castillo-Ruiz, et al. Early detection of neurological manifetations in achondroplasia. Child Nerve Syst 1997;13:208.

Table 77.4: Dorsal midline skin findings associated with spina bifida occulta

Asymmetrical gluteal fold
Dermal sinus or dimple
Hairy tuft
Hemangioma
Lipoma
Nevus
Pilonidal sinus
Rudimentary tail
Spinal aplasia cutis

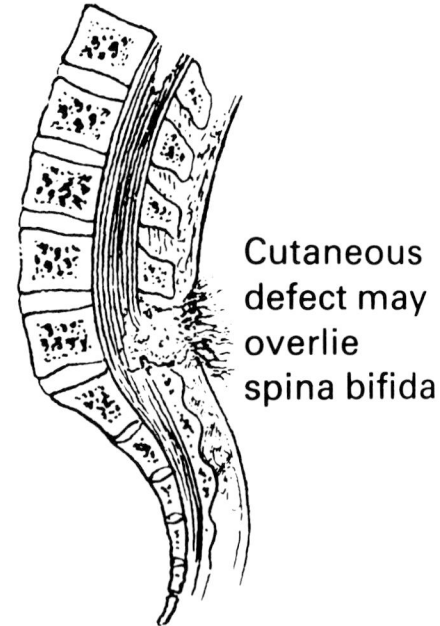

Cutaneous
defect may
overlie
spina bifida

FIGURE 77.11 Diagrammatic representation of spina bifida with minor cutaneous defect.

elements remain within the spinal canal. In spina bifida cystica (also called *spina bifida aperta*), the meninges protrude out of the spinal canal through the bony defect; neural elements may be contained within the protruding sac.

Spina Bifida Occulta

Spinal bifida occulta is usually asymptomatic. It is most common at posterior elements of L5-S1 and is usually noted as an incidental finding on spinal plain radiography (Figure 77.10). Cutaneous abnormalities may be associated (Table 77.4, Figure 77.11). Orthopedic foot deformities, urinary or rectal sphincter dysfunction, or focal neurological abnormalities can indicate that the spina bifida occulta is associated with compression or malformation of neural tissues or with spinal cord tethering.

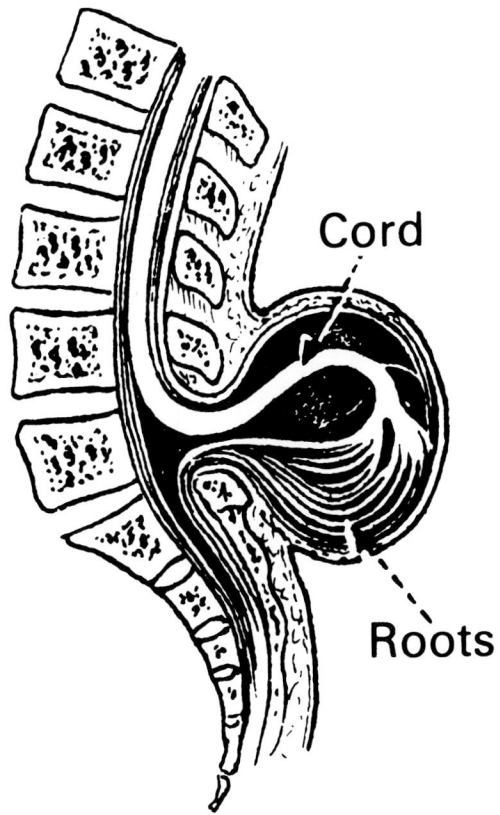

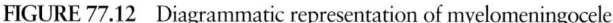

FIGURE 77.12   Diagrammatic representation of myelomeningocele.

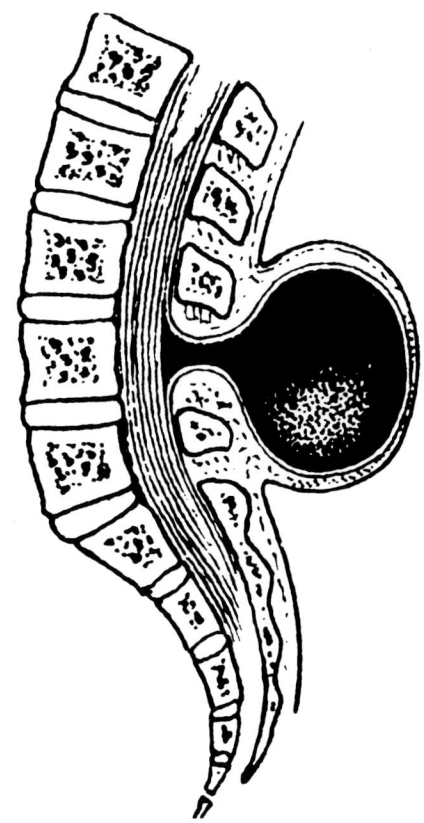

FIGURE 77.13   Diagrammatic representation of meningocele.

Myelomeningocele

Myelomeningocele and meningocele (spina bifida cystica) are congenital defects of spinal closure that, when present, are often visible on examination of the back of the newborn (Figures 77.12 and 77.13). When the skin and vertebral canal are unclosed, a sac of meninges is directly visible. The defect is most common in the lumbar region. If it contains nerve roots or spinal cord, it is a myelomeningocele; if neural elements are absent from the sac, it is a meningocele. It is often accompanied by hydrocephalus and may be accompanied by cerebellar tonsillar herniation (Chiari II malformation), syringomyelia, or cerebral malformations such as polymicrogyria. Initial surgical treatment in the neonatal period can provide cosmetic repair and decrease the risk of infection; hydrocephalus can be shunted. Any existing myelopathic or radiculopathic neurological deficit is likely to persist following surgery. The infants are at risk for later development of tethered cord syndrome (see Tethered Cord Syndromes, later in this chapter) or of spinal dermoid or epidermoid inclusion cysts.

Myelomeningocele is the most common major birth defect. An important cause is maternal folate deficiency, and most cases would be prevented if women with childbearing potential routinely took 0.4 mg of folic acid daily. Other risk factors include family history of neural closure defects, and maternal treatment with valproic acid. Pregnant women can be screened for serum α-fetoprotein levels, which are elevated when the fetus has neural closure defects. The defects also can be detected by fetal ultrasound.

Tethered Cord Syndromes

Congenital abnormalities of the spinal cord or cauda equina can prevent normal cephalad movement of the conus medullaris during early life (Table 77.5). The child or adult may develop progressive neurological dysfunction due to traction on the cord or nerve roots. The most common neurological finding is unilateral lower motor neuron dysfunction in one leg, but patients also may have sensory, upper motor neuron, or sphincter dysfunction. Children also may present with orthopedic foot deformities or scoliosis.

Table 77.5:   Causes of tethered cord syndrome

Myelomeningocele
Lipomyelomeningocele
Anterior sacral meningocele
Diastematomyelia
Hypertrophied filum terminale

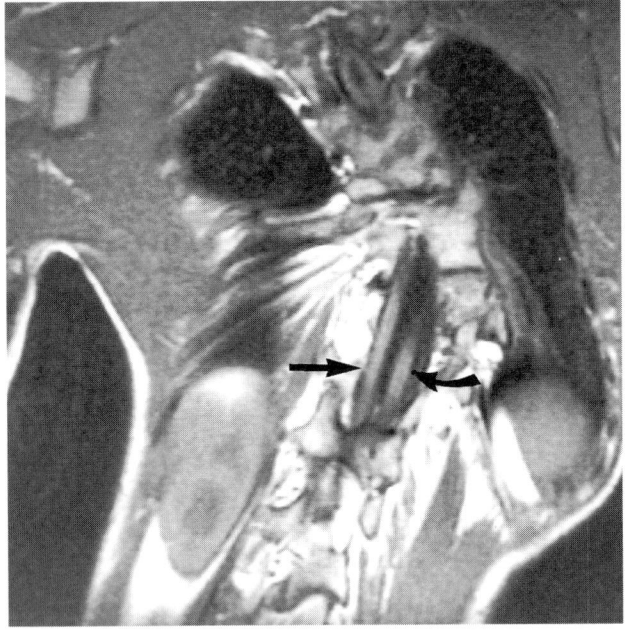

A

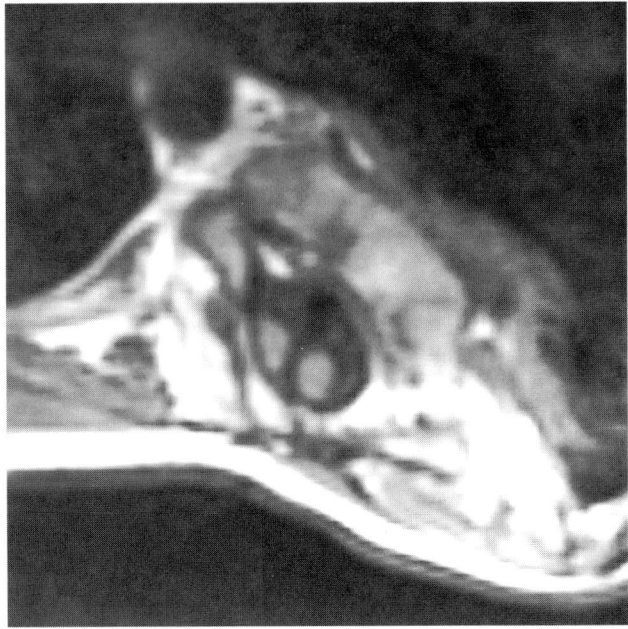

B

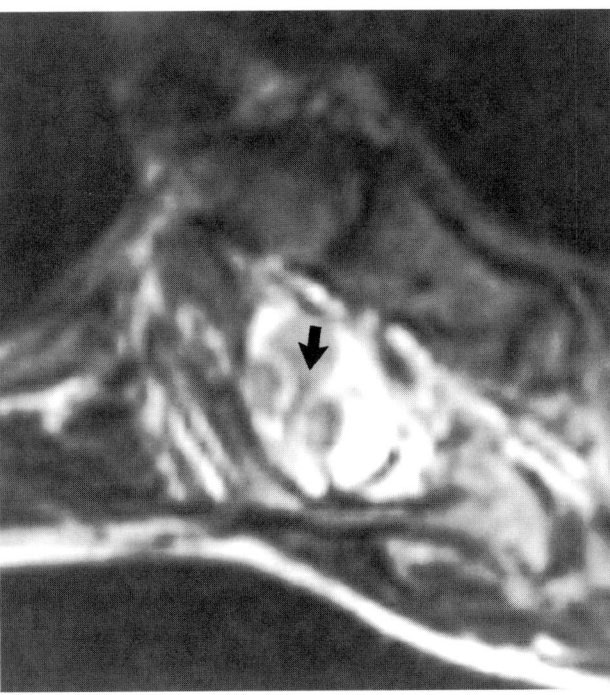

C

FIGURE 77.14   Magnetic resonance image of patient with diastematomyelia. (**A**) Sagittal T1-weighted image shows severe scoliosis and division of the spinal cord into right (*arrow*) and left (*curved arrow*) hemicords. (**B**) Axial T1-weighted image confirms the presence of two hemicords. (**C**) Axial gradient echo image demonstrates that there are two separate subarachnoid spaces divided by a central fibrous spur (*arrow*). (Courtesy of Erik Gaensler, M.D.)

Diastematomyelia (Figure 77.14) is a congenital malformation of the spinal cord characterized by sagittal division of a portion of the cord into two hemicords. In most instances the division is located in the lower thoracic or lumbar regions. It is classically, but not invariably, accompanied by a bony, cartilaginous, or fibrous spur and by dura in the cleft between the two portions of the cord. It is often accompanied by skin abnormalities, such as a tuft of hair at the level of the lesion. The spinal cord is usually tethered by the spur, leading to progressive neurological dysfunction during growth. The diagnosis can often be suspected on plain radiography, which shows widening of the interpeduncular distance and a posterior bony bridge at the level of the lesion. MRI scans or CT myelography can confirm the diagnosis. Surgical therapy consists of attempts to free all structures tethering the cord by removing the spurs and dura in the cleft and cutting the filum terminale if abnormal.

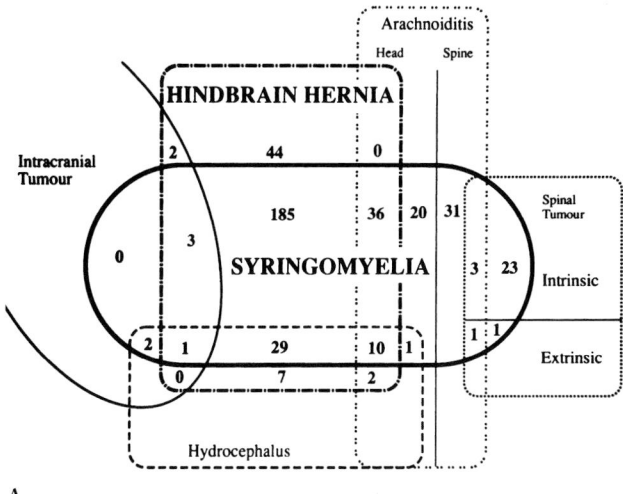

A

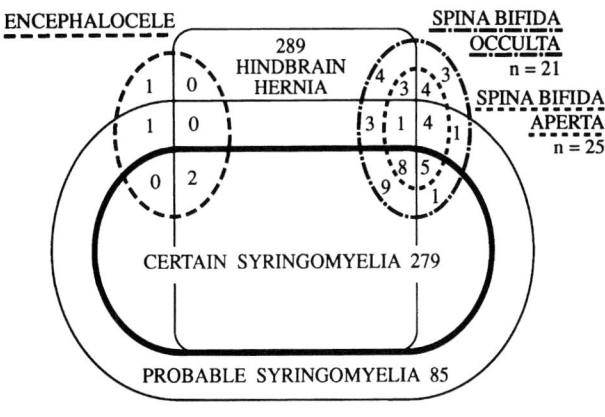

B

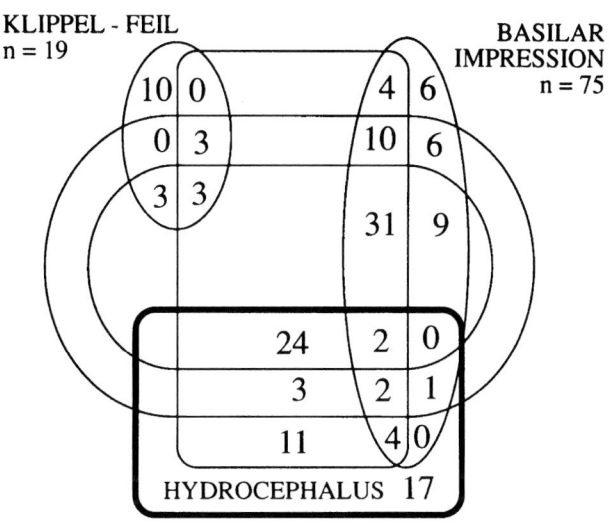

C

FIGURE 77.15   Venn diagrams shows the overlap of various craniospinal abnormalities from patients seen at a center specializing in syringomyelia. (A) Findings in 346 patients with syringomyelia and 304 patients with Chiari malformations (hindbrain hernia). (B) Findings in patients with dysraphism syndromes compared with patients with syringomyelia or Chiari malformations. (C) Findings in Klippel-Feil anomaly or basilar impression compared with patients with syringomyelia (ovals) or Chiari malformations (round rectangle). (Reprinted with permission from B Williams. Pathogenesis of Syringomyelia. In U Batzdorf [ed], Syringomyelia: Current Concepts in Diagnosis and Treatment. Baltimore: Williams & Wilkins, 1991;59–90.)

Clinical Correlations

A single patient often has more than one of the conditions discussed previously (Figure 77.15). Thus, a patient with one of the Chiari hindbrain malformations also may have some combination of bony abnormalities of the foramen magnum or cervical spine, syringomyelia, and meningomyelocele.

The clinical manifestations of craniocervical deformities are protean depending on which neural structures and associated anomalies are involved. When a patient has these problems, diagnosis and treatment starts by analyzing each component. MRI and CT imaging have greatly eased the analytic process. Many patients are asymptomatic or first present with neurological complaints in adult life. Patients may have short necks or abnormal neck posture or movement, particularly if there is an element of skeletal deformity (e.g., Klippel-Feil anomaly, occipitalization of the atlas). Findings attributable to the brainstem or cerebellum

may occur with Chiari malformations, compression of the brainstem (e.g., basilar impression or vertical displacement of the dens), or syringobulbia. Infrequently, atlantoaxial disease or basilar invagination can cause compromise of vertebrobasilar circulation, causing posterior circulation strokes or transient ischemic attacks. Specific findings suggestive of disease at the foramen magnum include downbeat nystagmus or the combination of long tract signs with lower motor neuron dysfunction in the lower cervical spinal cord; the lower motor neuron dysfunction has been attributed to impaired spinal venous drainage at the foramen magnum.

Spinal cord syndromes can be caused by syringomyelia or by extramedullary cord compression (e.g., by the dens with atlantoaxial dislocation or by spinal stenosis in Klippel-Feil anomaly). Additional neurological dysfunction can occur when the anomalies form part of more widespread developmental failure (e.g., lumbar effects of myelomeningocele in

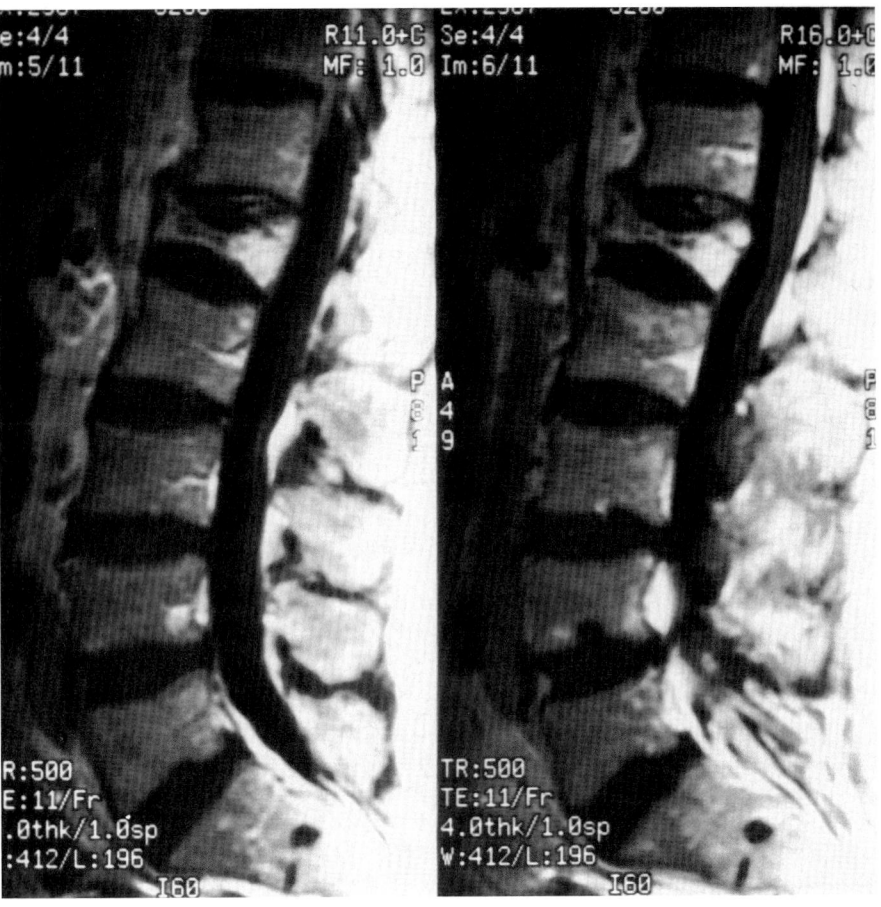

FIGURE 77.16 Spinal magnetic resonance image of patient with vertebral compression fracture secondary to osteoporosis. T1-weighted images of the lumbar spine show 70–80% loss of height of the mid-portion of the L1 vertebral body with relative preservation of the height of the posterior portion of the vertebral body. The bright appearance of the vertebra indicates preservation of the fat within the marrow compartment, which would be dark if replaced by tumor. (Courtesy of Erik Gaensler, M.D.)

Chiari II malformation or accompanying cerebral malformations in Klippel-Feil anomaly).

SPINAL DEFORMITIES AND METABOLIC BONE DISEASE

Osteoporosis

Osteoporotic vertebral compression fractures (Kanis 1994) occur most frequently in the thoracic and thoracolumbar spine (Figure 77.16). The majority occur in postmenopausal women. By age 75 years, nearly one-fourth of women have vertebral compression fractures; although these may lead to kyphosis and loss of body height, most are painless. In younger men and women, acute post-traumatic compression fractures are more likely to be painful. The pain usually is centered at the level of the compression and is accompanied by loss of spinal range of motion. Pain increases with activity, decreases with bed rest, and resolves slowly, sometimes incompletely. Benign compression fractures infrequently lead to spinal cord or nerve root compression, so that if a compression fracture is accompanied by a focal neurological compression syndrome, the possibility of a metastatic vertebral lesion should be considered. MRI features that favor a malignant cause of the compression fracture include decreased T1-weighted and increased T2-weighted signal in the vertebral body, pedicle involvement, and associated epidural or paravertebral mass (Rupp et al. 1995).

Osteogenesis Imperfecta

The various types of osteogenesis imperfecta are inherited connective tissue disorders manifested by brittle, osteopenic bones and recurrent fractures. Four types are known, with variations in severity and in associated findings such as short stature, blue sclera, hearing loss, scoliosis, and skeletal abnormalities. Potential neurological complications of osteogenesis imperfecta include communicating hydrocephalus, basilar invagination, macrocephaly, skull fractures, and seizure disorder (Charnas and Marini 1993). The basilar invagination can lead to brainstem compression. Spinal cord compression, syringomyelia, Chiari I malformation, Dandy-Walker cysts, leptomeningeal cysts, microcephalus, or central nervous system tumors are rarer associations.

Osteomalacia and Rickets

Osteomalacia and rickets are conditions of deficient bone mineralization. Usually long bones are more involved than the spine. Spinal pain, kyphosis, and compression frac-

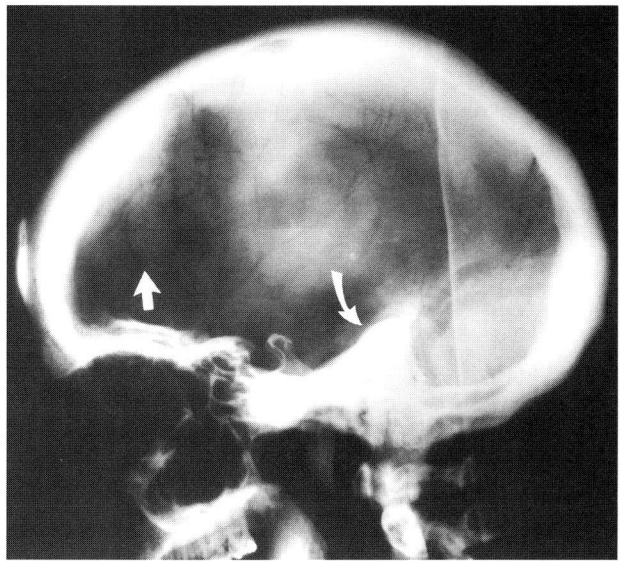

FIGURE 77.17   Radiograph of patient with osteopetrosis. The skull is extremely dense. The radiograph is slightly overexposed; note the darkness of the central areas (*arrow*). The bone of petrous apex (*curved arrow*) is particularly dense. (Courtesy of Erik Gaensler, M.D.)

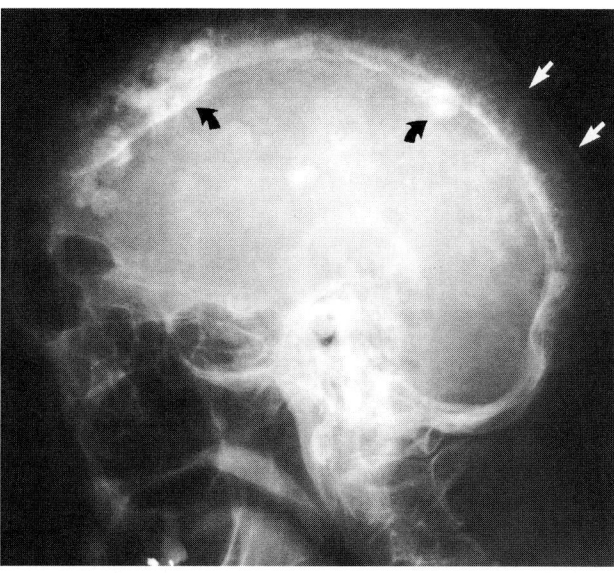

FIGURE 77.18   Radiograph of patient with Paget's disease of the skull. Note the thickening of the calvarium (*white arrows*) and the bony sclerosis with a cotton-wool appearance (*curved arrows*). The patient has basilar invagination; note the high position of the dens with respect to the clivus. (Courtesy of Erik Gaensler, M.D.)

tures can occur in osteomalacia, but compression of spinal cord or nerve roots is rare. Basilar impression can occur in patients with osteomalacia. The neuromuscular complications of osteomalacia are discussed in Chapter 83.

Osteopetrosis

Osteopetrosis is a rare disease characterized by increased bone density caused by impaired bone resorption (Figure 77.17). It may be inherited as an autosomal dominant or recessive disorder. Osteopetrosis of the skull can cause cranial neuropathies, basilar impression, hydrocephalus, or syringomyelia. Osteopetrosis of the spine can contribute to spinal canal stenosis with secondary compressive myelopathy.

Paget's Disease

Paget's disease is a focal metabolic bone disease of excessive osteoclastic bony destruction coupled with reactive osteoblastic activity (Delmas and Meunier 1997) (Figure 77.18). The incidence varies among ethnic groups, with a high incidence (nearly 5%) in whites of Northern European descent. Men are slightly more commonly affected. The current leading pathogenic hypothesis is that a chronic viral infection of osteoclasts causes the illness. The condition is usually asymptomatic and discovered only because of laboratory or radiographic abnormalities. However, it may cause symptoms by bone or joint distortion, fractures, compression of neurological tissue by calcification, hemorrhage, or focal ischemia caused by a vascular steal by the metabolically hyperactive bony tissue. Infrequently, osteogenic sarcoma can develop in pagetic bone.

Diagnosis

Paget's disease usually can be diagnosed by characteristic findings on radiography. Osteolytic activity can cause well-demarcated round patches of low bone density. Osteoblastic activity can lead to thickening of cortical bone, and then to general increase in bone density, often with distortion of normal organization. Osteolytic and osteoblastic findings are often present together.

Although most patients with Paget's disease have elevation of serum bone alkaline phosphatase and of markers of bone resorption, focal skeletal disease with neurological complications may occur in patients without laboratory abnormalities. Alkaline phosphatase levels, when elevated, are helpful not only in making the diagnosis but also in following response to treatment.

Cranial Neurological Complications

Paget's disease of the skull can lead to head enlargement. Patients often complain of headache. The most common focal neurological manifestation is hearing loss. Other cranial mononeuropathies, including optic neuropathy, trigeminal neuralgia, and hemifacial spasm, can occur. Distortion of the posterior fossa or basilar invagination can lead to brainstem or cerebellar compression, hydrocephalus, or syringomyelia. Patients with Paget's disease of the skull occasionally develop seizures. The pagetic skull is more vulnerable to bleeding from minor trauma, which can lead to epidural hematoma.

Spinal Neurological Complications

Symptomatic Paget's disease of the spine occurs most often in the lumbar region, where it can cause monoradiculopathies or a cauda equina syndrome. The disease may involve adjacent vertebral bodies and the intervening disc space or may cause root compression by extension from a single vertebral body. The differential diagnosis in patients with Paget's disease and neurological dysfunction in a single limb includes peripheral nerve entrapment by pagetic bone.

Paget's disease of the spine leading to myelopathy is more often thoracic than cervical. A variety of mechanisms are reported including extradural extension of pagetic bone, distortion of the spinal canal by vertebral compression fractures, spinal epidural hematoma, or sarcomatous degeneration leading to epidural tumor. In a few cases of myelopathy, imaging shows no evident cord compression, and vascular steal from the cord by hypermetabolic bone in the vertebral body is suggested. In support of this hypothesis, drug treatment of Paget's disease in these patients can lead to improved spinal cord function.

Treatment

The potent biphosphonates are the drugs of first choice for treatment of Paget's disease. Other treatment options include calcitonin, plicamycin, or gallium nitrate. Within 1–2 weeks of treatment, bone pain may improve, and serum alkaline phosphatase levels may decrease. Some patients experience significant neurological improvement following treatment, but improvement is often delayed 1–3 months (Wallace et al. 1995). In cases with severe cord compression, surgical decompression is indicated, but drug treatment before surgery decreases the risk of operative bone hemorrhage. Patients with cranial neuropathy have less impressive responses to drug therapy. Patients with hydrocephalus may benefit from ventricular shunting.

Juvenile Kyphosis

Juvenile kyphosis (Scheuermann's disease) manifests as thoracic or thoracolumbar kyphosis in adolescents. Spinal pain is more likely to accompany lumbar than thoracic disease. Spinal radiography shows anterior vertebral wedging. Neurological abnormalities are uncommon, but spinal cord compression can occur from thoracic disc herniation or direct effects of severe kyphosis.

Scoliosis

Scoliosis, with or without kyphosis, that develops as an idiopathic, painless condition in childhood and adolescence,

is usually not accompanied by neurological abnormalities (Lonstein et al. 1995). Most cases are idiopathic, but a minority have an accompanying syrinx or Chiari I malformation visible on MRI, even if the clinical neurological examination is normal (Evans et al. 1996). Spinal cord compression is a rare complication of idiopathic scoliosis and is particularly rare if no kyphosis is present. In each patient presenting with scoliosis and myelopathy, an important consideration is whether the myelopathy caused, rather than resulted from, the scoliosis.

Patients with congenital scoliosis, unlike those with idiopathic scoliosis, usually have anomalous vertebrae and may have other associated developmental problems such as Klippel-Feil anomaly or diastematomyelia. Scoliosis caused by skeletal disease, such as achondroplasia, is more likely than idiopathic scoliosis to lead to spinal cord compromise. Myelopathy can result also from spinal cord distraction during treatment of scoliosis with traction or surgery.

Scoliosis can be caused by various neurological diseases including cerebral palsy, spinocerebellar degenerations (e.g., Friedreich's ataxia), inherited neuropathies (e.g., Charcot-Marie-Tooth disease), myelopathies (e.g., syringomyelia), paralytic poliomyelitis, spinal muscular atrophy, dysautonomia (e.g., Riley-Day syndrome), and myopathies (e.g., Duchenne's muscular dystrophy). Scoliosis is the most common skeletal complication of neurofibromatosis type 1. Scoliosis that develops in adulthood can often be traced to an underlying cause such as trauma, osteoporotic fracture, degenerative spondylosis, or ankylosing spondylitis; it can result in local back pain, nerve root compression, or spinal canal stenosis.

Diffuse Idiopathic Skeletal Hyperostosis

Diffuse idiopathic skeletal hyperostosis (Forestier's disease, ankylosing hyperostosis) is a syndrome of excessive calcification that develops with aging, more often in men than in women. The diagnosis is made by spinal radiographs that show "flowing" calcifications along the anterior and lateral portion of vertebral bodies without loss of disc height and without typical radiographic findings of ankylosing spondylitis (Figure 77.19). Patients are often asymptomatic, but may have spinal pain or limited spinal motion. A rare complication is myelopathy caused by spinal stenosis if the calcifications are present also within the spinal canal. Like patients with ankylosing spondylitis, patients with diffuse idiopathic skeletal hyperostosis can develop spinal fractures after relatively minor trauma.

Ossification of the Posterior Longitudinal Ligaments or Ligamentum Flavum

Ossification of the posterior longitudinal ligament (Figure 77.20) and ossification of the ligamentum flavum are uncommon syndromes of acquired calcification within the spinal canal. The posterior longitudinal ligament extends the length of the spine, separating the posterior aspects of the discs and vertebral bodies from the thecal sac. The ligamentum flavum is in the dorsal portion of the spinal canal, attaching the laminae and extending to the capsules of the facet joints and the posterior aspects of the neuroforamina. Either ligament can ossify in later life, apparently independently of the usual processes of spondylosis and degenerative arthritis. Ossification of the posterior longitudinal ligament occurs more commonly in Asians than in whites. It is usually asymptomatic, but can be visible on lateral spinal radiography. It is better seen by CT scan, in which it is distinguished from osteophytes by favoring the middle of the vertebral bodies rather than concentrating at the endplates. Thickness of the calcification can range from 3–15 mm. Ossification of the posterior longitudinal ligament is most likely to be symptomatic in the cervical spine where it can contribute to cord compression if it is thick or if the canal is further narrowed by congenital and degenerative changes.

The ligamentum flavum can contribute by hypertrophy or ossification to spinal stenosis, most often in the lower thoracic or lumbar spine, affecting the cord or cauda equina. Risk factors for development of ossification of the ligamentum flavum are trauma, hemochromatosis, calcium pyrophosphate deposition disease, diffuse idiopathic skeletal hyperostosis, ankylosing spondylitis, or ossification of the posterior longitudinal ligament.

DEGENERATIVE DISEASE OF THE SPINE

Spinal Osteoarthritis and Spondylosis

Osteoarthritis of the spinal facet joints manifests radiographically as joint narrowing, sclerosis, and osteophyte formation. Spondylosis refers to degenerative disease of the intervertebral discs, visible on radiography as disc space narrowing, vertebral endplate sclerosis, and osteophyte development. Spinal osteoarthritis and spondylosis are inevitable consequences of aging that are visible on routine spinal radiography in over 90% of people by age 60 years. They are often asymptomatic, but may cause compression of the spinal cord or nerve roots in a minority of people. Nonetheless, they are the most common cause of compressive myelopathy or radiculopathy, accounting for far more neurological disease than all the other conditions discussed in this chapter combined.

In youth the intervertebral discs consist of a gelatinous central nucleus pulposus and a firm collagenous annulus fibrosus. The disc herniation syndromes occur when the nucleus pulposus bursts through a tear in the annulus fibrosus. This herniation can compress the nerve roots or spinal cord, depending on the spinal level involved. Rarely, disc material breaks into the thecal sac or a fragment rup-

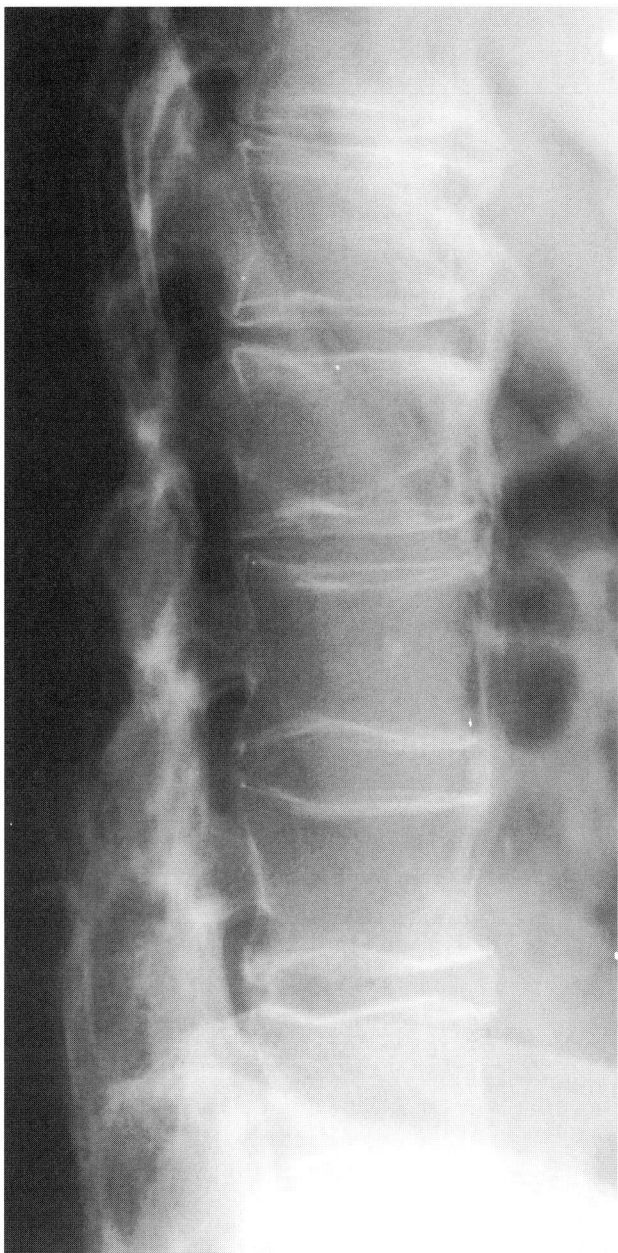

FIGURE 77.19 Lateral thoracic spinal radiograph shows diffuse idiopathic skeletal hyperostosis. Note the flowing calcification of the anterior osteophytes with preservation of disc heights. (Reprinted with permission from RB Rosenbaum, SM Campbell, JT Rosenbaum. Clinical Neurology of Rheumatic Disease. Boston: Butterworth–Heinemann, 1996:96.)

tures into an epidural vein. Disc herniation is most likely to occur in young adults.

By age 40 most adults have some disc degeneration with dehydration and shrinkage of the nucleus pulposus, necrosis and fibrosis of the annulus fibrosus, and sclerosis and microfractures of the subchondral bone at the vertebral endplate. Compression of neurological tissue can develop

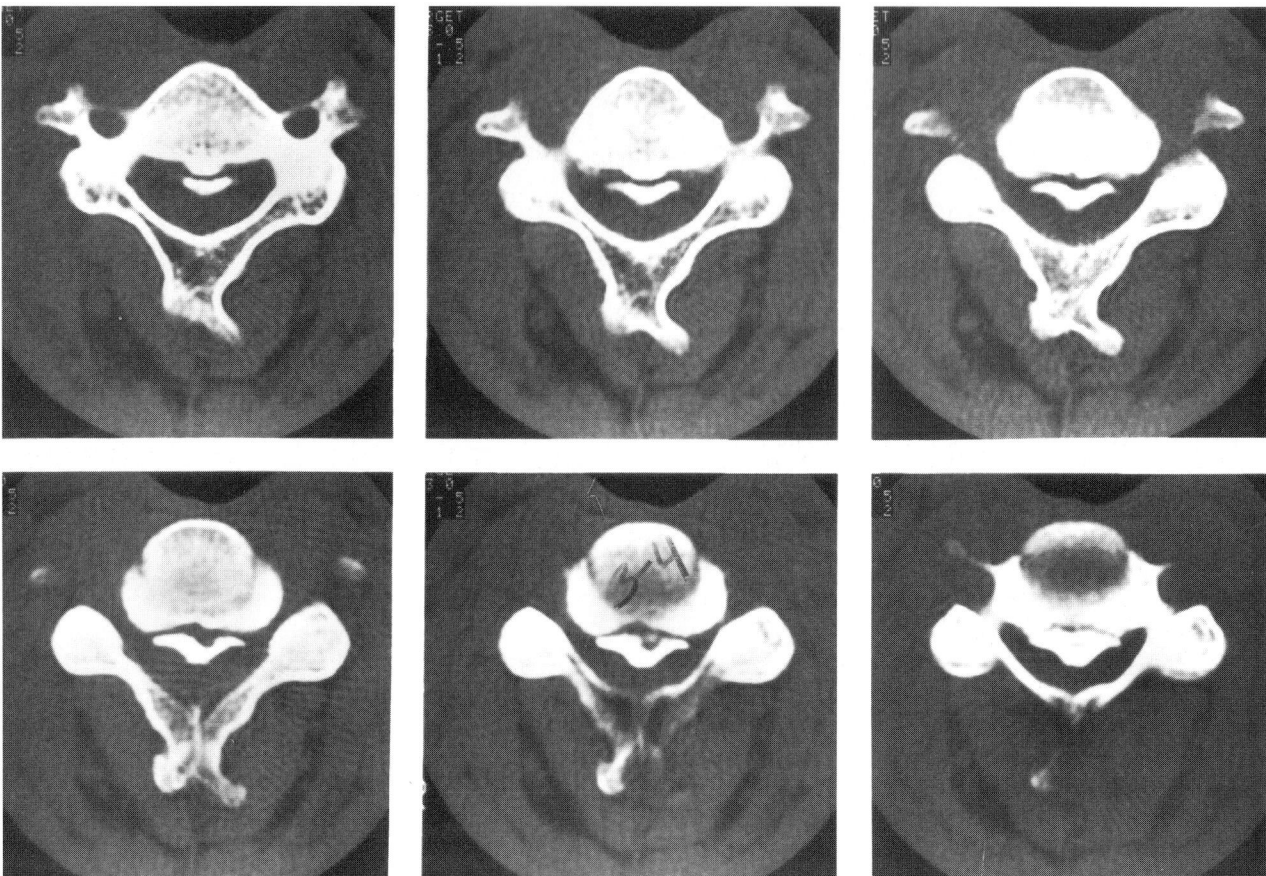

FIGURE 77.20   Computed tomographic scan of a patient with ossification of the posterior longitudinal ligament. Note the continuous bony ridge that is present at every level, not just at the disc space. In contrast to calcified degenerative spurs, these ligamentous calcifications are not connected to the vertebral bodies. (Courtesy of Erik Gaensler, M.D.)

from a combination of disc herniation, osteophyte formation, ligament hypertrophy, congenital stenosis of the spinal canal, low-grade synovitis, and deformity and misalignment of the spine.

Cervical Spondylosis

The cervical spinal column includes 37 joints that are continually in motion throughout life. Cervical osteoarthritis and spondylosis are ubiquitous with increasing age (Figure 77.21). These disorders can be attributed only rarely to specific activities or injuries. Patients with dystonia and other cervical movement disorders may be predisposed to premature cervical spinal degeneration. Because cervical osteoarthritis and spondylosis are so commonplace, it is usually difficult to ascertain their role in contributing to the pathogenesis of chronic neck pain or headache. Cervical spine surgery is rarely, if ever, indicated for treatment of headache or neck ache in the absence of cervical radiculopathy or myelopathy.

Cervical Radiculopathy

Clinical Presentation

The symptoms of cervical radiculopathy often appear relatively suddenly. Although disc herniation or nerve root contusion can be caused by acute trauma, many cases become symptomatic without an identifiable preceding traumatic event. Disc herniation is more likely to be the cause in patients under age 45 years; neural foraminal stenosis by degenerative changes becomes more likely with increasing age. Pain is usually in the neck with radiation to an arm; patients also may have headache. Radiculopathic arm pain may increase with cough or with Valsalva's maneuver. Arm pain may increase with neck rotation and flexion to the side of the pain (Spurling's sign).

Spondylosis, osteophytes, and disc herniations at the C4-C5 level can affect the C5 root, causing pain, paresthesias, and sometimes loss of sensation over the shoulder, with weakness of the deltoid, biceps, and brachioradialis muscles. The biceps and supinator reflexes

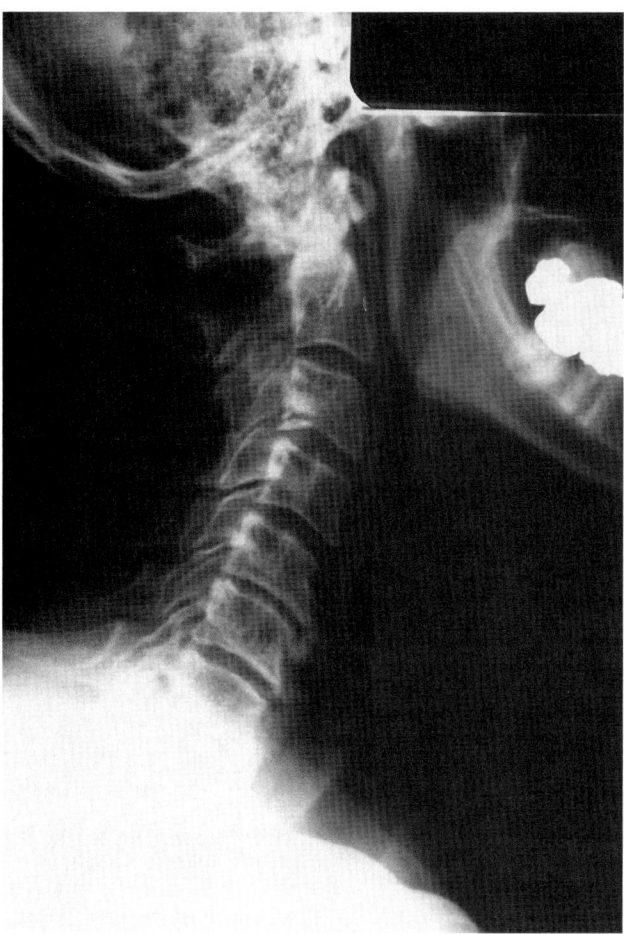

FIGURE 77.21   Lateral radiograph of the cervical spine shows typical changes of spondylosis and osteoarthritis. (Reprinted with permission from RB Rosenbaum, SM Campbell, JT Rosenbaum. Clinical Neurology of Rheumatic Disease. Boston: Butterworth–Heinemann, 1996:98.)

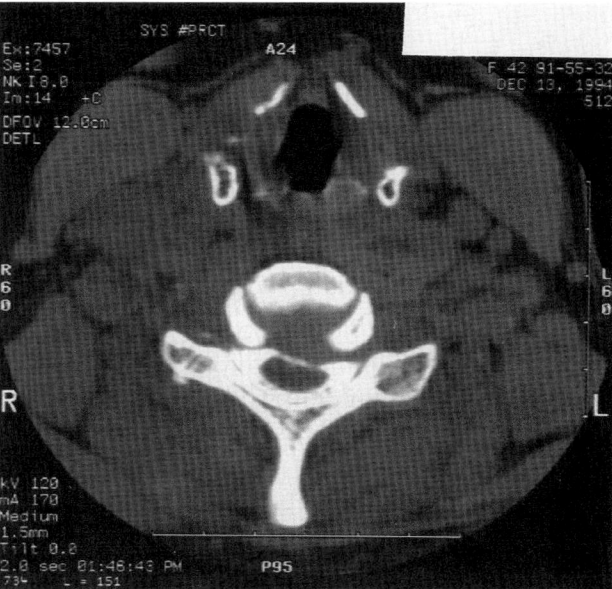

FIGURE 77.22   Computed tomographic scan of the cervical spine with intrathecal contrast shows herniated cervical disc. The spinal cord (gray) and thecal sac (white) are distorted on the left by the disc. (Reprinted with permission from RB Rosenbaum, SM Campbell, JT Rosenbaum. Clinical Neurology of Rheumatic Disease. Boston: Butterworth–Heinemann, 1996:100.)

may be lost, and the reflex may spread to the finger flexors (an inverted biceps reflex) and an increased triceps reflex, indicating the presence of a myelopathy at the C6 level. Spondylotic lesions at the C5-C6 level can affect the C6 cervical root and cause paresthesias in the thumb or lateral distal forearm and weakness in the brachioradialis, biceps, or triceps. The biceps and brachioradialis reflexes may be diminished. Lesions at the C6-C7 level, compressing the C7 root, cause paresthesias, usually in the index, middle, or ring fingers, and weakness in C7-innervated muscles, such as the triceps and pronators. The triceps tendon reflex may be diminished.

The C5, C6, and C7 roots are the ones most commonly involved in cervical spondylosis, because they are at the level of greatest mobility, where disc degeneration is greatest in the cervical spine. The relative frequency of root lesions in cervical spondylosis varies in different series (Radhakrishnan et al. 1994). Clinically evident compression of the C8 root or of roots above C5 is more rare.

Cervical radiography is of little value in diagnosing or excluding cervical radiculopathy. MRI scanning of the cervical spine is usually helpful in identifying nerve root compression in patients with cervical radiculopathy. Cervical myelography followed by CT scanning is sometimes more sensitive than MRI and may show nerve root compression that is invisible by MRI (Figure 77.22). However, cervical MRI, CT, and myelography must all be interpreted with caution because degenerative abnormalities are so commonly seen in the asymptomatic spine. Electromyography and nerve conduction studies can be useful in difficult diagnostic cases, both by identifying an affected myotome and by helping to exclude other diagnoses, such as brachial plexopathy or peripheral neuropathy.

Treatment

Most instances of cervical radiculopathy improve significantly over 4–8 weeks, regardless of treatment. Various treatments such as nonsteroidal anti-inflammatory drugs, use of a soft cervical collar, physical therapy, or cervical traction give similar results. Patients with a typical clinical presentation and little or no neurological deficit usually can be managed with these noninvasive approaches without radiography or electrodiagnostic studies. When patients have intractable weakness or pain or have not improved with nonoperative therapy, surgical nerve root

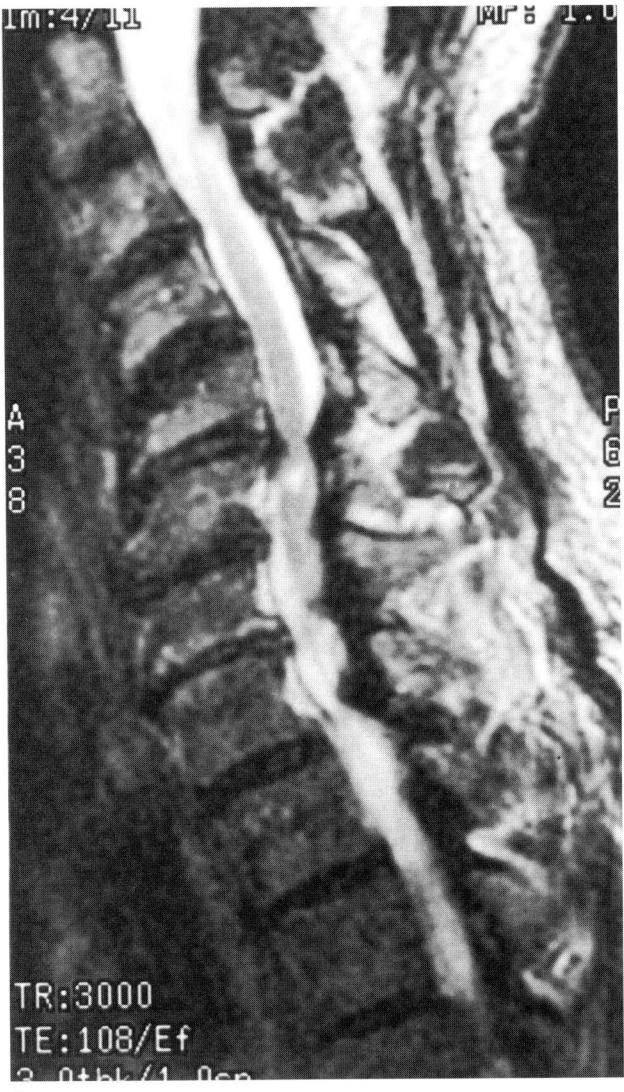

A

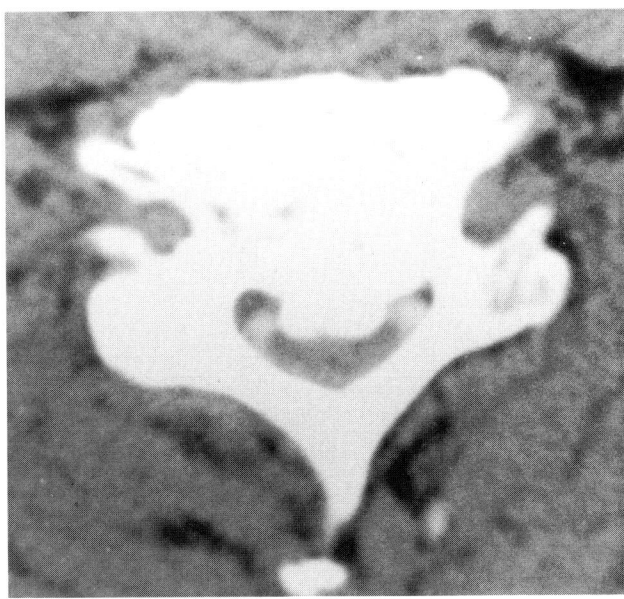

B

FIGURE 77.23 Cervical spondylotic myelopathy. (A) The sagittal T2-weighted magnetic resonance imaging scan shows maximal compression of the thecal sac and spinal cord at C5-C6. (B) The axial computed tomographic scan with intrathecal contrast at this level shows a large osteophyte arising from the posterior aspect of the vertebral body; the spinal cord at this level is compressed, and the thecal sac is so compressed that little of the white intrathecal contrast is visible. (Reprinted with permission from RB Rosenbaum, SM Campbell, JT Rosenbaum. Clinical Neurology of Rheumatic Disease. Boston: Butterworth–Heinemann, 1996:109.)

decompression is usually successful. Anterior cervical discectomy is used more widely than posterior cervical laminectomy.

Cervical Spondylotic Myelopathy

Myelopathy caused by compression of the cervical spinal cord by the changes of spondylosis and osteoarthritis usually develops insidiously, but it may be precipitated by trauma or progress in stepwise fashion. Typical findings are a combination of leg spasticity, upper extremity weakness or clumsiness, and sensory changes in the arms, legs, or trunk. Either spinothalamic tract–mediated or posterior column–mediated sensory modalities may be impaired. Sphincter dysfunction, if it occurs, usually is preceded by motor or sensory findings. Neck pain is often not a prominent symptom, and neck range of motion may or may not be impaired. Some patients experience leg or trunk paresthesia induced by neck flexion (Lhermitte's sign).

The anterior-posterior diameter of the cervical spinal cord is usually 10 mm or less. Patients rarely develop cervical spondylotic myelopathy if the congenital diameter of their spinal canal exceeds 16 mm. In congenitally narrow canals, disc protrusion, osteophytes, hypertrophy of the ligamentum flavum, ossification of the posterior longitudinal ligament, and vertebral body subluxations can combine to compress the spinal cord. The relation between the spinal canal and the spinal cord can be imaged by MRI or by CT myelography (Figure 77.23). MRI provides more intramedullary detail such as secondary cord edema or gliosis. CT provides better images of calcified tissues. Even with excellent cross-sectional imaging of the spinal canal, the clinical correlation between neurological deficit and cord compression is imperfect; dynamic changes in cord compression and vas-

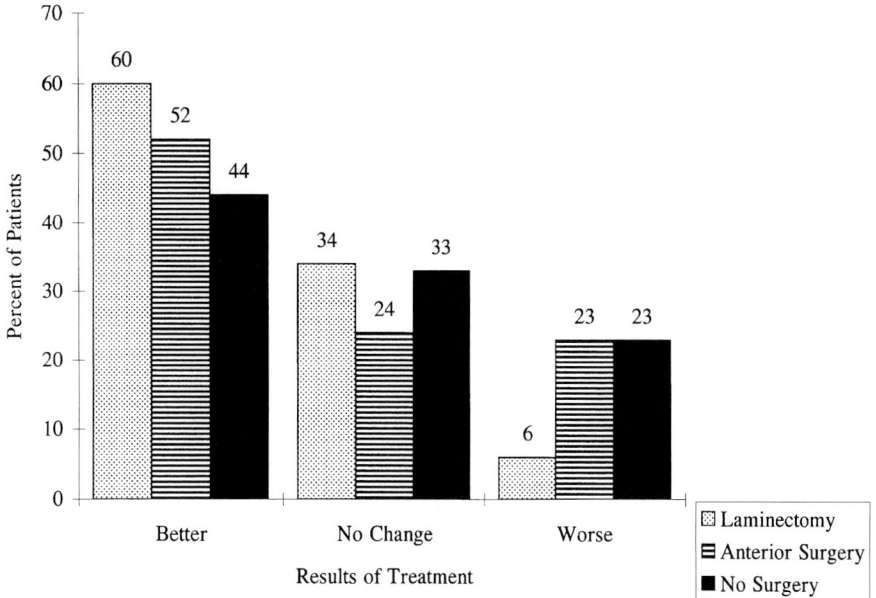

FIGURE 77.24 Results of treatment of cervical spondylotic myelopathy. (Reprinted with permission from RB Rosenbaum, SM Campbell, JT Rosenbaum. Clinical Neurology of Rheumatic Disease. Boston: Butterworth–Heinemann, 1996:112.)

cular perfusion undoubtedly contribute to the pathogenesis of cervical spondylotic myelopathy.

The natural history of cervical spondylotic myelopathy is variable. Some patients may have stable neurological deficit for many years without specific therapy, whereas other patients may have gradual or stepwise deterioration. Some patients improve with treatments such as bed rest, soft collars, or immobilizing collars, but these treatments have not been assessed in controlled trials. Many patients with cervical spondylotic myelopathy are treated by surgical decompression with variable surgical results (Figure 77.24). Surgical and nonsurgical treatment results are best when the neurological deficit is mild and present less than 6 months, and when the patient is younger than 70 years old. Anterior cervical discectomies are generally performed for spondylotic lesions at a limited number of levels, whereas posterior laminectomy, sometimes with an expanding laminoplasty, is generally performed for congenital spinal canal stenosis.

Vertebral Artery Stroke Caused by Cervical Osteoarthritis

Compression of a vertebral artery by an osteophyte is a rare cause of stroke in the vertebrobasilar circulation. The vertebral arteries pass through foramina in the transverse processes from C6-C2. Osteophytes from the uncinate joints can compress the arteries. The compression may only occur with head turning. However, the turning usually leaves the contralateral vertebral artery uncompressed, so ischemic symptoms are usually limited to those patients who have both osteophytic arterial compression on one side and a contralateral hypoplastic, absent, or occluded artery.

Thoracic Spondylosis

Degenerative changes are less common in the thoracic than in the lumbar or cervical spines. Thoracic osteophytes are more likely to develop on the anterior or lateral aspects of the vertebral bodies and infrequently cause clinical radiculopathy. Thoracic disc herniations are visible on MRI in many asymptomatic individuals (Wood et al. 1997). Thoracic disc herniations occur most frequently in the lower thoracic spine. These rarely cause cord compression and may regress spontaneously.

Thoracic myelopathy caused by disc herniation probably has an annual incidence of approximately 1 case per 1 million. Most cases occur between ages 30 and 60 years. Symptoms often develop insidiously, without identifiable preceding trauma. Back pain may or may not be present. Patients have some combination of motor and sensory findings of myelopathy; sphincter dysfunction is present in more severe cases. Thoracic MRI, CT, or myelography can confirm the diagnosis (Figure 77.25). The treatment is surgical decompression.

Lumbar Spondylosis

Low Back Pain

Approximately 80% of people experience episodes of acute low back pain, which usually resolve within a few days. These episodes often recur, and approximately 4% of people report chronic low back pain. Pain-sensitive structures in the lumbar region include the nerve roots, zygapophyseal joints, sacroiliac joints, intervertebral ligaments, mus-

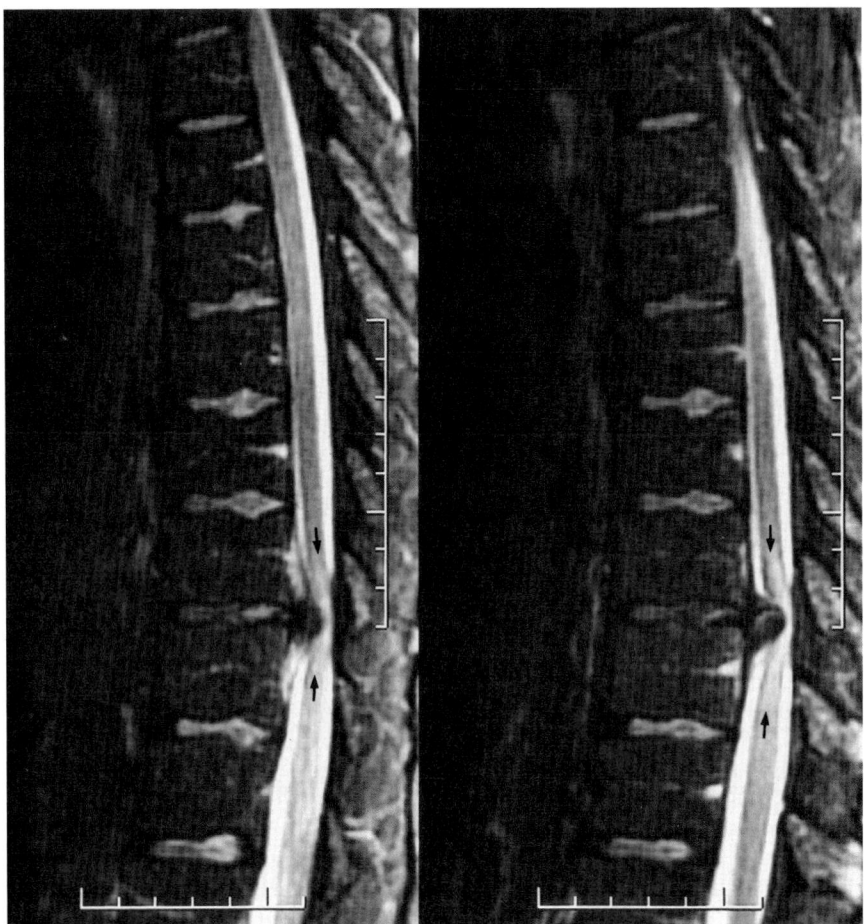

FIGURE 77.25 Thoracic magnetic resonance image of patient with thoracic disc herniation. This large acute disc herniation at T10-T11 consists of extrusion of most of the nucleus pulposus into the spinal canal. There is secondary narrowing of the disc space. There is spinal cord edema (*arrows*) above and below the level of spinal cord compression. (Courtesy of Erik Gaensler, M.D.)

cles, fascia, annulus fibrosis and circumferential portions of the discs, and vertebral periosteum. Controlled local anesthetic injection studies suggest that in some patients, the cause of low back pain can be localized to specific zygapophyseal joints or sacroiliac joints. In other patients, injection of contrast media into lumbar discs reproduces pain, suggesting that the lumbar disc is the source of pain in these patients. However, this localization cannot be achieved reliably by history or physical examination and, with current therapeutic techniques, invasive testing for localization is not valuable in planning therapy. Furthermore, localization of the source of pain is unsuccessful in many patients. Thus, in clinical practice, "nonspecific low back pain" is a commonly made diagnosis.

The findings of osteoarthritis and lumbar spondylosis on radiography (osteophytes, endplate sclerosis, disc space narrowing) appear gradually with increasing age and are rarely absent by age 60 years (Figure 77.26). The presence or absence of these findings does not correlate with symptoms and demonstrating them is of no diagnostic or therapeutic value. Therefore, radiography of the lumbar spine is indicated only when alternative diagnoses such as compression fractures, neoplasia, or infections are being seriously considered. The Agency for Health Care Policy and Research has recom-

mended that spinal radiography be reserved for patients with "red flags" for trauma, tumor, or infection (Table 77.6). Even limiting radiography to patients meeting these guidelines results in many needless radiographs. For example, back pain in a patient over age 50 years need not be an indication for imaging studies, unless other findings suggest a condition more serious than nonspecific low back pain.

Spondylolysis and Spondylolisthesis

Spondylolisthesis is movement of a lumbar vertebral body relative to an adjacent body. Some cases are caused by spondylolysis, a discontinuity in the vertebral pars interarticularis, that disrupts the normal stabilizing effect of the facet joints. Other causes of spondylolisthesis include congenital vertebral anomalies, degenerative spondylosis, and vertebral trauma. Spondylolysis occurs in 5–7% of the population and is usually asymptomatic. Spondylolisthesis is often painless or may cause low back pain that sometimes radiates to the buttocks. Spondylolytic spondylolisthesis is a common cause of back pain in adolescents. Occasionally, spondylolisthesis can advance to the point of compressing nerve roots in the neuroforamina or causing lumbar canal stenosis.

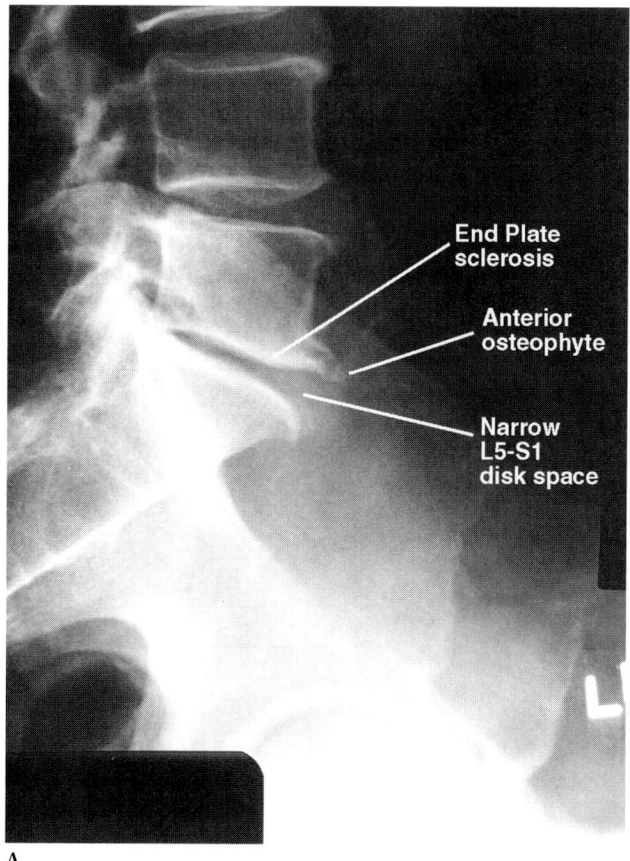
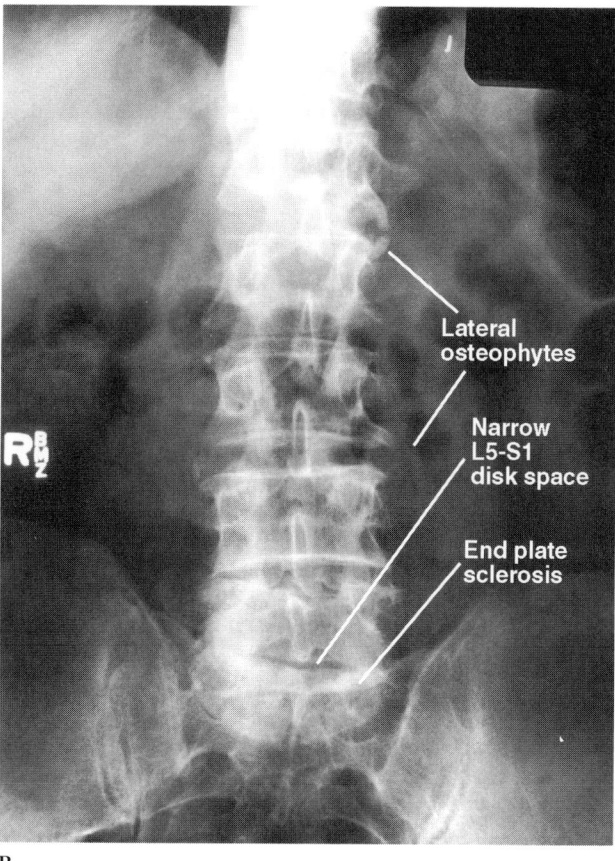

A   B

FIGURE 77.26   (A) Anteroposterior and (B) lateral radiographs of the lumbar spine showing osteophytes, disc space narrowing, and sclerosis of the vertebral body articular plates. (Reprinted with permission from RB Rosenbaum, SM Campbell, JT Rosenbaum. Clinical Neurology of Rheumatic Disease. Boston: Butterworth–Heinemann, 1996:121.)

Table 77.6:   Indications for lumbar spine radiography

Red flags for trauma
　Major trauma (e.g., motor vehicle accident, fall from height)
　Minor trauma or even strenuous lifting in older or
　　potentially osteoporotic patient
　Prolonged corticosteroid use
　Osteoporosis
　Age older than 70 years
Red flags for tumor or infection
　Age older than 50 years or younger than 20 years
　History of cancer
　Constitutional symptoms (e.g., fever, chills, weight loss)
　Risk factors for spinal infection (e.g., recent bacterial
　　infection, intravenous drug use, immunosuppression)
　Pain that is worse when supine or is severe at night

Source: Reprinted from Agency for Health Care Policy and Research. Acute Low Back Problems in Adults. Assessment and Treatment: Quick Reference Guide for Clinicians. Rockville, MD: U.S. Dept. of Health and Human Services, 1994.

Lumbar Radiculopathies

The back and leg neurological examination is key to decision making in patients with low back pain. Perhaps 1–2%

of patients with acute low back pain have significant lumbar nerve root compression. Three syndromes merit specific diagnostic consideration.

Monoradiculopathy

Clinical Presentation. Patients with an acute lumbar or lumbosacral monoradiculopathy caused by nerve root compression present with unilateral leg pain (sciatica) radiating into the buttock, lateroposterior thigh, and distally, sometimes with paresthesia. Patients usually also have low back pain. Pain may increase with movement, coughing, sneezing, or Valsalva's maneuver and decrease with rest. Pain often increases when the straightened ipsilateral leg is raised while the patient is supine (straight-leg–raising test, Laségue's sign) or when the leg is straightened at the knee while the patient is seated. The most commonly compressed nerve roots are L5, usually by L4-L5 disc herniation, or S1, usually by L5-S1 disc herniation. For L5 radiculopathy the findings are typically medial foot and hallux pain, paresthesia especially on the medial dorsal foot, and weakness in the extensor hallucis longus muscle, ankle dorsiflexors, and peroneal muscles. S1 nerve root compression can lead to lateral foot pain

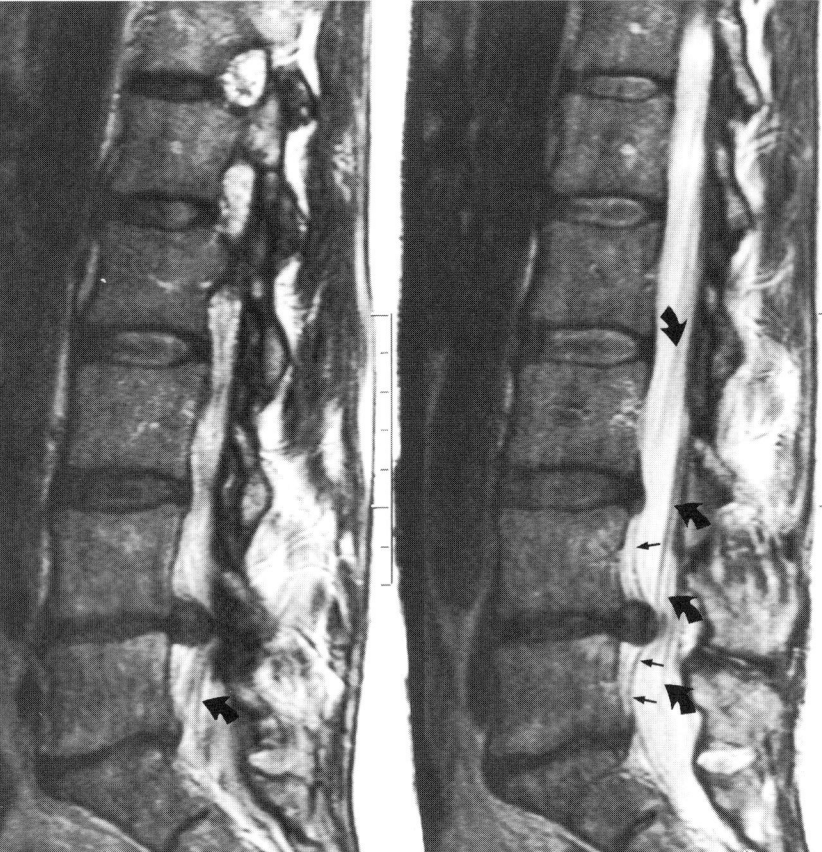

FIGURE 77.27 Lumbar magnetic resonance image of patient with lumbar disc herniation at L4-L5. The ventral dura is displaced (*straight arrows*) posteriorly. The roots of the cauda equina are compressed (*curved arrows*). (Courtesy of Erik Gaensler, M.D.)

and paresthesia, depressed ankle jerk, and weakness of peroneal muscles and less frequently of ankle plantar flexors. When the radiculopathy is mild, the patient may have no objective neurological deficit.

Diagnostic Studies. Disc herniations, osteophytes, spondylolysis and spondylolisthesis, facet joint hypertrophy, and hypertrophy or calcification of intraspinal ligaments can compress nerve roots of the cauda equina within the spinal canal or in the lateral recesses and neural foramina through which the roots exit the spinal canal. The anatomical relations between the nerve roots and the surrounding tissues are well visualized by lumbar MRI, CT, or myelography (Figure 77.27). Each technique has high sensitivity for demonstrating causes of nerve root compression. On occasion when a patient has strong clinical evidence of lumbar radiculopathy but initial imaging studies do not show the cause of the compression, a second complementary imaging study is indicated. For example, imaging with a lumbar MRI usually is sufficient for most clinical purposes, but occasionally a patient also needs CT myelography to clarify the anatomy. Unfortunately all spinal imaging modalities frequently show anatomical abnormalities that are not the cause of symptomatic nerve root dysfunction; all imaging results must be interpreted carefully in clinical context.

Electromyography can aid in neurological localization by demonstrating neuropathic abnormalities in specific myotomes. It is relatively insensitive because it only detects compression affecting motor roots severely enough to cause axonal interruption. However, in complex cases it is particularly helpful in separating monoradiculopathy from other conditions such as dysfunction of multiple roots, plexopathies, or peripheral neuropathy.

Treatment. Most sufferers of low back pain and sciatica recover within 6 weeks using simple, nonoperative therapies such as brief periods of bed rest, activity limitations as required by pain, simple analgesics, and physical or manipulative therapies. Evidence indicates that prolonged immobilization is detrimental, and that early mobilization results in more rapid recovery. Many patients with acute low back pain and sciatica can be managed at this stage based on clinical examination without spinal imaging studies. Patients who have progressive weakness or sensory loss, or who have severe pain that fails to improve after 6 weeks of nonoperative therapy, can be considered for surgical nerve root decompression. The patients least likely to benefit from lumbar nerve root surgery are those who lack objective neurological signs of nerve root dysfunction or who lack corresponding imaging evidence of nerve root compression.

A small fraction of patients develop a chronic low back pain syndrome or have repeated exacerbations of acute low back pain. Back strengthening exercises and the avoidance of maneuvers that put strain on the lower back, together with the judicious use of nonsteroidal anti-inflammatory drugs, generally improve such patients' pain. In some instances, the presence of ongoing litigation and compensation questions complicates and tends to perpetuate the chronic low back pain syndrome. When surgery is performed for lumbar nerve root compression, the surgical technique depends on the clinical details such as the cause of compression and the number of nerve roots compressed. In patients with sciatica caused by disc herniation, the most common surgical approach is microsurgical discectomy with minimal removal of the lamina. Perhaps 90% of patients report excellent relief of neuropathic pain following surgery. Many are able to return to physically strenuous work. However, a small proportion of patients postoperatively develop more severe chronic pain problems (*failed back syndrome*). These patients require careful neurological evaluation to consider such problems as surgery done at the wrong level, incomplete removal of extruded disc fragment or other matter compressing the nerve root, progression of spinal degeneration, postoperative arachnoiditis, and psychosocial issues interfering with recovery.

Acute Cauda Equina Syndrome

Acute cauda equina syndrome presents as low back and leg pain caused by compression of multiple lumbosacral nerve roots. Patients may have bilateral leg pain and neurological deficits in the distribution of multiple nerve roots. Particularly worrisome findings are sacral sensory loss or impaired function of the rectal and urinary sphincters. Acute cauda equina compression occurs in less than 1% of all patients who have lumbar or lumbosacral disc prolapses. The cause is usually a large midline disc herniation, most often at L4-L5 or L5-S1. When it occurs, the patient needs urgent spinal imaging and decompressive surgery, because a limited window of opportunity exists for restoration of neurological function.

Lumbar Canal Stenosis

Lumbar canal stenosis results from various anatomical changes that decrease the cross-sectional area of the spinal canal including congenitally small canal size, degenerative osteophytes, spondylolisthesis, facet joint hypertrophy, thickening of the ligamentum flavum, and disc herniation. It usually develops insidiously with aging and rarely becomes symptomatic before age 40. Men are more often affected than women. Stenosis is often asymptomatic. Patients often have some low back pain. The classic symptom of lumbar canal stenosis is neurogenic intermittent claudication: leg discomfort elicited by walking or by certain postures such as standing straight, which is relieved within minutes by stopping walking or changing posture. This is to be contrasted with the relief within seconds of stopping walking in vascular claudication. The pain may be anywhere in the legs or buttocks and may include numbness or paresthesia.

Patients sometimes can decrease their discomfort by bending forward while they walk and may be able to bicycle without difficulty. They may develop leg symptoms with sustained erect posture or after lying with their back straight. In contrast, vasogenic intermittent claudication may be elicited by almost any leg exercise and is not elicited by rest postures.

Most patients with neurogenic intermittent claudication do not have objective signs of nerve root dysfunction. However, occasionally a patient manifests progressive neurological deficits from chronic cauda equina compression. Some patients develop leg weakness or other abnormal neurological signs following exercise, and neurological examination before and after precipitation of the pain is an essential part of the evaluation of neurogenic claudication.

Diagnostic Studies. Spinal canal stenosis can be studied by MRI, CT, or myelography (Figure 77.28). MRI is best at demonstrating sagittal relationships, such as the role of spondylolisthesis in narrowing the canal. CT is best at studying calcified tissues. All three of the imaging modalities are imperfect at quantifying the extent of nerve root compression, and clinical correlations between symptoms and apparent reduction in size of the spinal canal are imperfect. In choosing which patients would benefit from decompressive surgery, one should rely more heavily on clinical findings than on the appearance of the canal on scans.

Treatment. Patients who have neurogenic intermittent claudication may have stable symptoms for many years without developing progressive neurological deficit. Some even note regression of symptoms after months of recurrent claudication. These patients may be managed with mild analgesics. Some describe decreased discomfort if they walk with a slight stoop or using a cane. Those patients with intractable leg pain or progressive neurological deficit can be treated with wide laminectomy of the stenosed spinal canal; most obtain improvement of claudication. Back pain is much less likely to improve following surgery. Those with severe or multilevel stenosis are least likely to benefit from surgery.

INFECTIOUS DISEASES OF THE SPINE

Pyogenic Vertebral Osteomyelitis and Epidural Abscess

Vertebral osteomyelitis (Calderone and Capen 1996) and spinal epidural abscess (see Chapter 59) are infrequent conditions that present with focal spinal pain and tenderness. Epidural abscesses in the anterior spinal canal are more likely than those in the posterior canal to be associated with osteomyelitis; in either location they can cause radiculopathic pain, compromise of nerve root function, or spinal cord compression. Some patients with spinal epidural abscess or with vertebral osteomyelitis are afebrile at presentation, but nearly all have an elevated sedimentation rate. Early in the infection, routine spinal radiography may be normal. If the diagnosis is being considered, an MRI scan (Figure 77.29) of the involved area is sensitive for detecting vertebral body abnormalities and particularly helpful to assess for epidural or

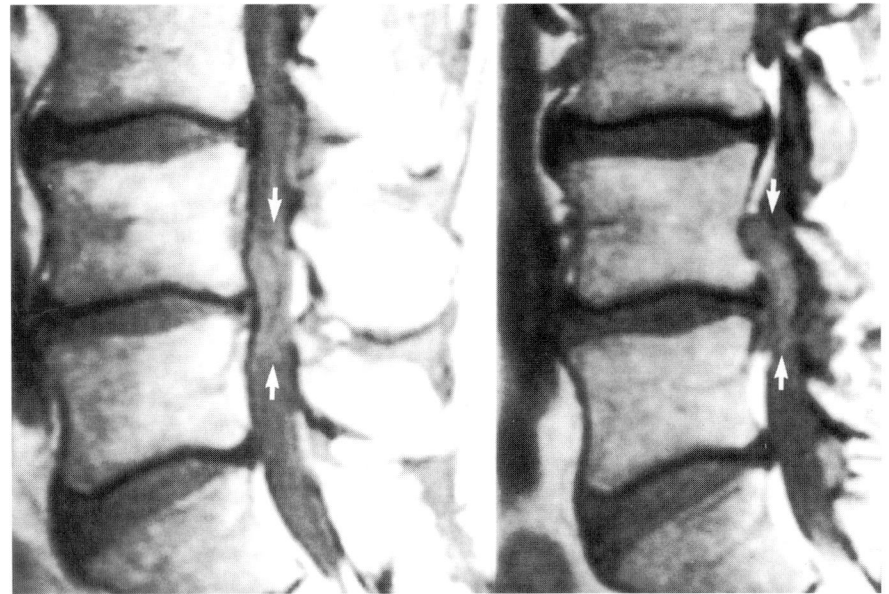

FIGURE 77.28 Magnetic resonance image of patient with lumbar spinal stenosis. (**A**) Midline and (**B**) parasagittal images of the lumbar spine show narrow anteroposterior dimensions of the spinal canal consistent with spinal canal stenosis (see normal dimensions in Figure 77.27). The L4-L5 disc herniation (*arrows*) that fills the entire spinal canal is actually much smaller than the herniation shown in Figure 77.27. (Courtesy of Erik Gaensler, M.D.)

A   B

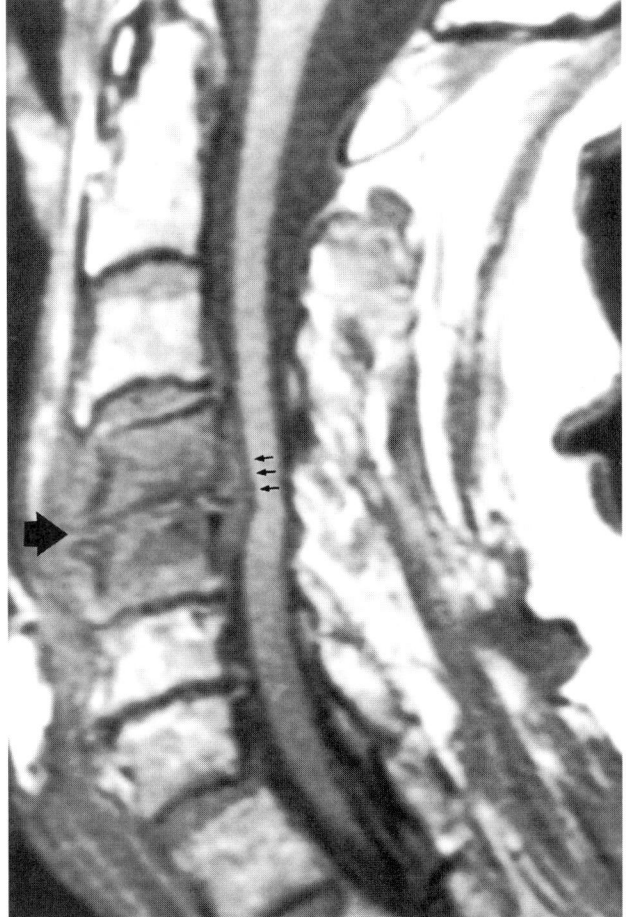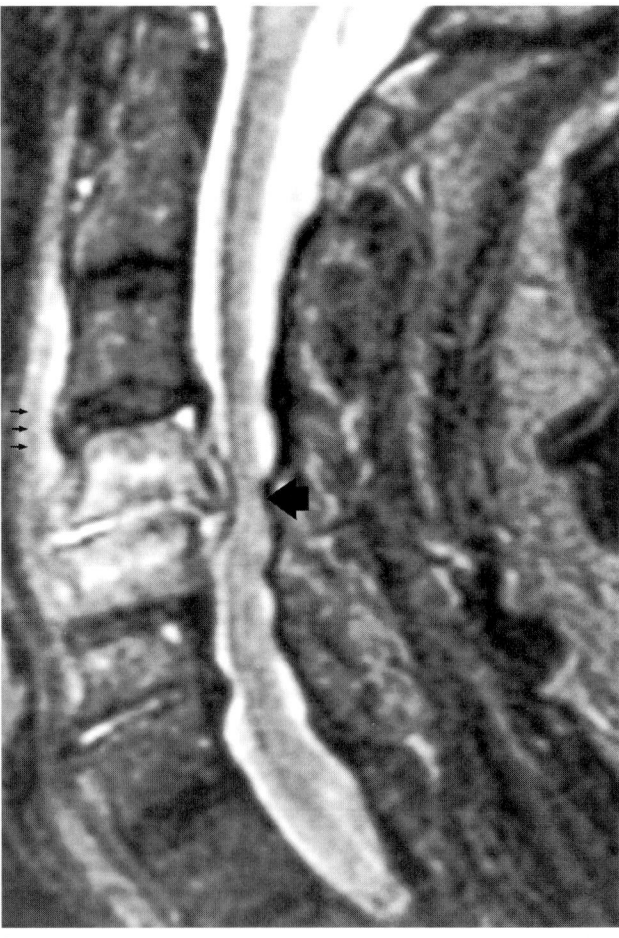

A   B

FIGURE 77.29 Magnetic resonance image of patient with pyogenic vertebral osteomyelitis. (**A**) T1 sagittal image shows replacement of the normal marrow fat of the C4 and C5 vertebrae with low signal intensity edema, with narrowing of the disc space (*arrow*) and thickening of the epidural soft tissue (*small arrows*).

(**B**) T2-weighted image shows mild spinal cord compression (*arrow*) and hyperintensity of the anterior longitudinal ligament, consistent with superior extension of the infectious process (*small arrows*). (Courtesy of Erik Gaensler, M.D.)

FIGURE 77.30   Magnetic resonance image of patient with tuberculous vertebral osteomyelitis. T2-weighted images show destruction of the posterior inferior portion of the T12 vertebra, with a soft tissue mass projecting posteriorly into the spinal canal, compressing the conus medullaris (*arrows*). Note that the T12 and L1 discs (*curved arrows*) are relatively well preserved, which is a distinguishing feature of spinal tuberculosis. (Courtesy of Erik Gaensler, M.D.)

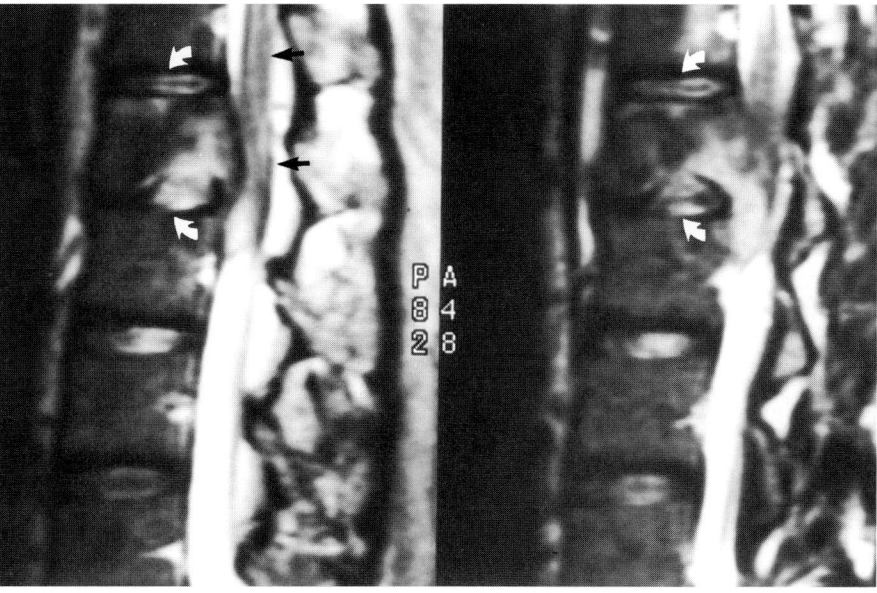

paravertebral infection. Spinal CT is useful if MRI is unavailable or contraindicated. Osteomyelitis may involve any vertebral body, but is least common in the cervical vertebrae. Often in pyogenic, but infrequently in granulomatous, osteomyelitis, the MRI shows involvement of the adjacent disc space. The most common causative organism is *Staphylococcus aureus*, but a wide variety of other bacteria can be responsible. Polymicrobial infection is uncommon after hematogenous infection but can occur when the source is open trauma or contiguous spread from other tissues. Osteomyelitis or spinal epidural abscess usually occurs by hematogenous spread and is more likely following septicemia. Diabetes, alcoholism, and other forms of immunosuppression increase the risk for its development. Other risk factors are intravenous drug use or spinal trauma. Cases may be iatrogenic following spinal surgery. When cases are diagnosed before development of spinal instability or compression of the spinal cord or nerve roots, long-term antibiotic therapy can be curative. Spinal instability may require surgical stabilization. Neurological compression is an indication for emergent surgical decompression.

Granulomatous Vertebral Osteomyelitis

Tuberculosis (TB) of the spine (Pott's disease) (Boachie-Adjei and Squillante 1996) is one of the more common forms of nonpulmonary TB and by far the most common granulomatous spinal infection. The risk is highest in regions or populations where TB is endemic. In the United States high-risk factors are immigration from an endemic area, human immunodeficiency virus infection, homelessness, and drug or alcohol abuse. Other organisms capable of causing granulomatous osteomyelitis include brucellosis, a variety of

fungi; *Nocardia*; and actinomyces. Granulomatous spinal infection typically presents with insidious progression of back pain. The patient often has symptoms of systemic infection such as weight loss, fever, night sweats, or malaise.

Pott's disease classically presents with destruction of vertebral bodies. Routine spine radiography results are usually abnormal by the time the diagnosis is made, and spinal deformity is a common complication. MRI or CT is needed to assess for contiguous abscess in the epidural or paraspinal spaces and to evaluate possible nerve root or spinal cord compression when the spine is deformed (Figure 77.30). Compression of spinal cord or nerve roots can occur in vertebral TB by vertebral deformity or collapse, epidural abscess, granulation tissue, or bony sequestrum. Patients may develop delayed neurological compromise after apparently successful treatment of the infection caused by infarction from endarteritis obliterans, delayed degenerative bony changes, or reactivation of infection. Neurological compression is most common with thoracic vertebral disease, hence the eponym *Pott's paraplegia*; cauda equina compression is uncommon in TB. Treatment of vertebral TB requires long-term multiple drug antituberculous therapy. Spinal surgery may be needed depending on the degree of spinal destruction or deformity and is often required in cases of neurological compression.

INFLAMMATORY JOINT DISEASE

Rheumatoid Arthritis

Systemic Presentation

RA is a chronic, inflammatory, symmetrical destructive immune-mediated polyarthritis. In population studies,

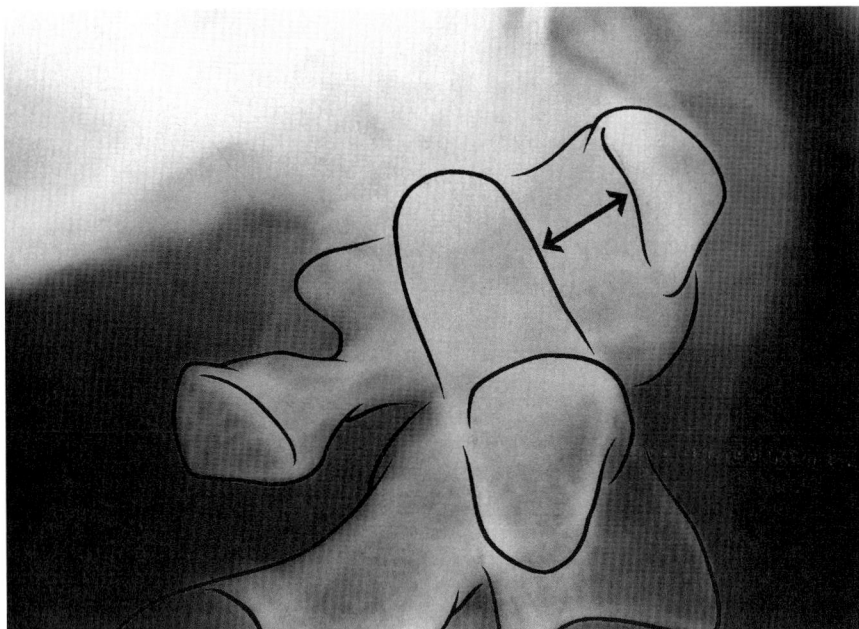

FIGURE 77.31 Lateral radiographs of the flexed neck of a patient with rheumatoid arthritis and anterior atlantoaxial subluxation. The odontoid and pedicle of C2 and the elements of the ring of C1 are outlined. The double arrow indicates the atlantoaxial separation. (Reprinted with permission from RB Rosenbaum, SM Campbell, JT Rosenbaum. Clinical Neurology of Rheumatic Disease. Boston: Butterworth–Heinemann, 1996:146.)

0.2–2.0% of the population is affected, women twice as often as men. The cause of RA is unknown, but genetic factors are evident in familial cases and susceptibility is linked to some HLA-DR types. The most commonly affected joints are the small joints of the hands and feet. The diagnosis is based primarily on characteristic clinical findings. Serological testing for rheumatoid factor can support the diagnosis. However, many patients have sero-negative RA, and, conversely, there are numerous other causes for elevation of rheumatoid factor. Radiography shows juxta-articular demineralization or characteristic joint erosions in advanced cases.

Pathogenesis

The immunopathogenesis of RA includes T- and B-cell activation, angiogenesis and cellular proliferation in the synovium, inflammation in soft tissue, and eventual destruction of cartilage and bone. Cytokine release, immune complex deposition, and vasculitis can all contribute to the inflammatory process. The inflamed proliferative rheumatoid synovium is called *pannus*. In the spine, pannus can disrupt stabilizing ligaments, particularly of the atlantoaxial joint, and thick pannus can add to compression of neurological tissue. Rheumatoid inflammatory tissue can form nodules in soft tissue; on the rare occasions that these nodules form in the dura, they can contribute to rheumatoid pachymeningitis.

Neurological Manifestations

Common neurological complications of RA (Rosenbaum et al. 1996) are carpal tunnel syndrome and other nerve entrapments, peripheral neuropathy, and myopathy; these are discussed in Chapters 55, 80, and 83. RA can evolve to

a rheumatoid vasculitis that, like other medium-sized vessel vasculitides, has the potential to cause ischemic mononeuritis, mononeuritis multiplex, or, rarely, stroke.

Headache and neck ache are common in patients with RA. These are often caused by rheumatoid disease of the cervical spine. Focal neurological dysfunction is a rarer and later manifestation of spinal RA. Patients with RA, of course, develop the ubiquitous changes of spinal osteoarthritis and spondylosis. In addition, early in RA cervical radiography may show rheumatoid changes such as erosions and sclerosis at vertebral endplates and apophyseal joints. Patients may have cervical subluxations. Disc space narrowing may occur at upper cervical discs, without associated osteophytosis. As the disease progresses, patients can develop subluxation at the atlantoaxial joint.

Lateral atlantoaxial joint subluxation rarely causes focal neurological dysfunction but can contribute to neck ache and headache. Horizontal atlantoaxial joint subluxation, often combined with adjoining soft tissue pannus, can cause myelopathy, especially in patients with smaller congenital canal diameter (Figure 77.31; see also Figure 56A.4). The earliest neurological sign is usually hyperreflexia; assessment of gait and strength in patients with advanced RA is often difficult because of their peripheral joint pain and deformity. Vertical subluxation can lead to spinal cord or brainstem compression, or rarely to vertebral artery compression or injury.

Choosing which patients will benefit from surgical stabilization of the subluxed joint is a clinical challenge. Findings of progressive myelopathy or brainstem dysfunction are usually indications for surgery if the general health of the patient permits. Neurological dysfunction caused by atlantoaxial subluxation usually occurs in patients who are already severely debilitated by their disease. Many patients do not regain neurological function after surgical stabilization of the subluxation; goals are limited to preventing deterioration. The 5-year survival of patients at this late stage of RA is perhaps 50%.

Patients with RA may also develop spinal subluxations, usually in the cervical spine, at levels caudal to the atlantoaxial joint. These subluxations can lead to spinal cord compression. Subaxial subluxations may progress after surgical stabilization of the atlantoaxial joint. A rare late manifestation of RA is rheumatoid pachymeningitis. The dura may develop either focal rheumatoid nodules or diffuse infiltration by inflammatory cells. In rare instances focal dural disease can lead to spinal cord, cauda equina, or cranial nerve compression or to focal cerebral complications such as seizures.

Inflammatory Spondyloarthropathies

Clinical Presentation

The inflammatory spondyloarthropathies include ankylosing spondylitis, Reiter's syndrome (reactive arthritis), psoriatic arthritis, and the arthritis of inflammatory bowel disease. Ankylosing spondylitis is characterized by inflammatory low back pain, loss of spinal range of motion, sacroiliitis, and, as it advances, radiographic evidence of sacroiliitis and spondylitis (Figure 77.32). The historic characteristics of inflammatory low back pain are insidious onset of low back (and sometimes buttock) pain, duration over 3 months, prominent morning stiffness, and improvement with activity. Most patients become symptomatic before age 40, and men are affected more commonly than women are. Other organ systems are affected commonly in patients with inflammatory spondyloarthropathies; manifestations include uveitis, mucocutaneous lesions, peripheral arthritis, gastrointestinal disease, cardiac disease, and enthesopathy. Entheses are sites of insertion of ligament or tendon to bone. The syndesmophytes that form where spinal ligaments joint vertebral bodies are one form of enthesopathy. Examples of other sites of enthesopathy are the foot (Achilles tendinitis, plantar fasciitis, heel pain), fingers or toes (dactylitis or sausage digits), symphysis pubis, clavicle, and ribs.

Reiter's syndrome or reactive arthritis is classically preceded by venereal or gastrointestinal infection. The triad of Reiter's syndrome is arthritis, conjunctivitis, and urethritis, but many patients do not have all three manifestations. Inflammatory low back pain is common in patients with Reiter's syndrome, and up to one-fourth of patients develop radiological evidence of sacroiliitis or spondylitis.

Pathogenesis

The inflammatory spondyloarthropathies are generated by a combination of genetic and environmental factors. In

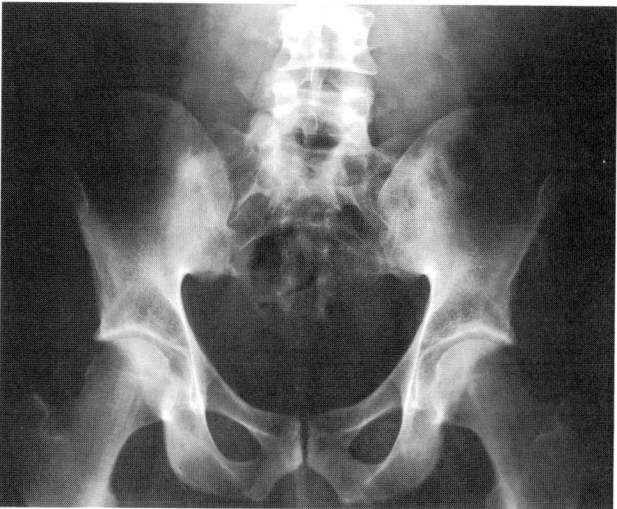

FIGURE 77.32   The anteroposterior radiograph of the sacroiliac joint shows sacroiliitis with some preservation of the left sacroiliac joint. (Reprinted with permission from RB Rosenbaum, SM Campbell, JT Rosenbaum. Clinical Neurology of Rheumatic Disease. Boston: Butterworth–Heinemann, 1996:183.)

ankylosing spondylitis the genetic factor is clearest, with perhaps 90% of patients expressing the gene for HLA-B27. However, only approximately 5% of people expressing this gene develop ankylosing spondylitis. In the other spondyloarthropathies, the prevalence of HLA-B27 positivity is lower. In Reiter's syndrome the environmental factors are clearest, with many patients experiencing a preceding gastrointestinal or genitourinary infection with organisms such as *Shigella*, *Salmonella*, *Yersinia*, *Campylobacter*, or *Chlamydia*. The inflammatory process is presumably mediated by autoimmune T cells with tissue specificity leading to inflammation at such sites as joints, entheses, and the eye.

Spinal Neurological Complications

The neurological complications of the inflammatory spondyloarthropathies generally do not occur until spinal disease is clinically advanced with loss of spinal range of motion and kyphosis and radiologically evident with vertebral body squaring and syndesmophytes. Spinal complications include atlantoaxial joint subluxation, spinal fractures, discovertebral destruction, spinal canal stenosis, and cauda equina syndrome caused by lumbar arachnoid diverticula (Table 77.7).

Subluxation of the atlantoaxial joint is a late and infrequent complication of inflammatory spondyloarthropathy. Diagnosis and management issues are the same as those for patients who develop atlantoaxial disease as part of RA. The fused spondylitic spine is particularly susceptible to fracture, especially in the midcervical region. The most frequent fracture site is C6, followed by C5 and C7. Following

Table 77.7:   Spinal complications of ankylosing spondylitis based on 105 hospitalized patients

	Anatomically abnormal	Neurologically abnormal
Spinal fracture	13	7
Discovertebral destruction	4	0
Atlantoaxial subluxation	1	0
Spinal canal stenosis	2	2

Source: Data from P Weinstein, RR Karpman, EP Gall, et al. Spinal injury, spinal fracture, and spinal stenosis in ankylosing spondylitis. J Neurosurg 1982;37:609–616. (Reprinted with permission from RB Rosenbaum, SM Campbell, JT Rosenbaum. Clinical Neurology of Rheumatic Disease. Boston: Butterworth–Heinemann, 1996:188.)

even minor trauma, the patient with advanced spondylitis needs radiographic assessment of the cervical spine to detect fractures, if possible, before myelopathic complications. Much more rarely, patients with spondylitic, rigid spines develop post-traumatic myelopathy caused by epidural hematomas or cord contusions.

Destruction of a disc, particularly in the low lumbar or high thoracic region, is a late complication of spondylitis (Figure 77.33). The adjacent vertebral bodies also may be involved. An initiating trauma is not always identified. The destruction may be asymptomatic or painful. The pain increases with movement and decreases at rest, in contrast to typical inflammatory low back pain. An epidural inflammatory response leading to cord compression can occur.

Cauda equina syndrome with insidious evolution of leg pain, sensory loss, leg weakness, and sphincter dysfunction is a late complication of inflammatory spondyloarthropathy. Imaging studies (MRI, CT, myelography) show posterior lumbosacral arachnoid diverticula (Figure 77.34).

Although arachnoiditis may play a role in development of this syndrome, the presence of the diverticula distinguishes it from most cases of chronic adhesive arachnoiditis.

Other unusual complications of spondyloarthropathy include lumbar monoradiculopathy secondary to disc herniation or osteophytes, spinal canal stenosis, and, from the era when spinal radiation was used to treat spondylitis, radiation-induced cauda equina sarcoma.

Nonspinal Neurological Complications

Unusual complications of inflammatory spondyloarthropathies include brachial plexopathy or tarsal tunnel syndrome. Proximal weakness and atrophy, sometimes with mild elevations of serum creatine kinase, often occur in advanced cases of spondylitis. In patients with psoriatic arthritis, the myopathy is occasionally painful. A number of case reports detail unusual neurological sequelae in patients with Reiter's syndrome (Table 77.8).

Laboratory Abnormalities

Patients with inflammatory spondyloarthropathies sometimes have mild elevations of CSF protein with normal glucose and cell counts. They can have unexplained abnormalities of visual, auditory, and somatosensory evoked responses.

Possible Associations with Multiple Sclerosis

Case reports and small series have reported the occurrence of multiple sclerosis and ankylosing spondylitis in the same patient, but insufficient data exist to determine if a true association exists between the two illnesses (Dolan

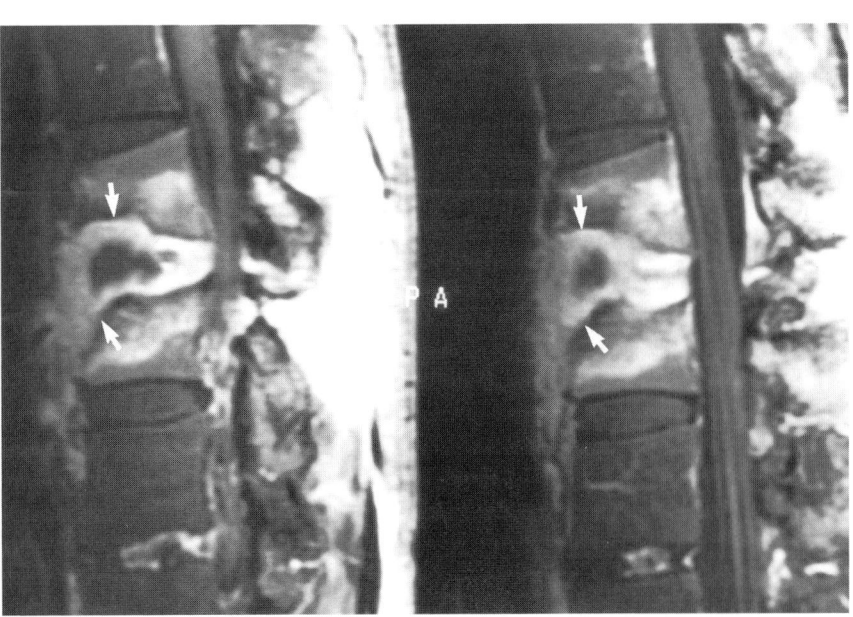

FIGURE 77.33 Magnetic resonance image shows discovertebral destruction (*arrows*) in a patient with ankylosing spondylitis. There is a chronic fracture in the lower thoracic spine, which is otherwise rigid because of bony fusion. Chronic hypermobility at this single nonfused segment has occurred, leading to exuberant fibrous tissue development. The fibrous tissue enhances on this postgadolinium T1-weighted image. This appearance can be mistaken for infectious spondylitis (see Figure 77.29) if the presence of a bamboo spine on plain films is overlooked. (Courtesy of Erik Gaensler, M.D.)

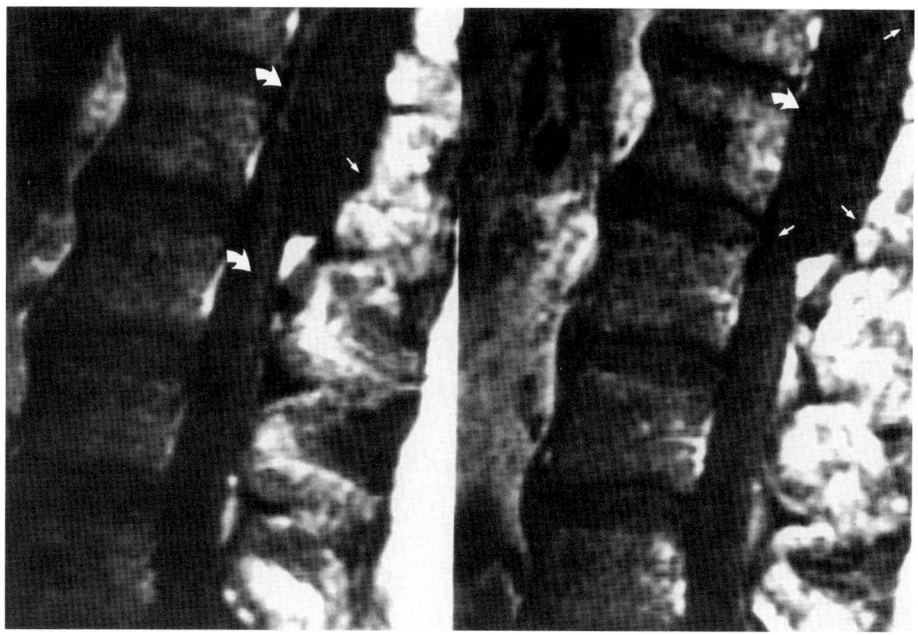

FIGURE 77.34 Magnetic resonance image of the lumbar spine shows a posterior lumbar arachnoid diverticulum in a patient with ankylosing spondylitis. The spinal canal is expanded at T12-L1 by a mass that shows signal intensity equivalent to cerebrospinal fluid on these T1-weighted images. Isointensity to cerebrospinal fluid suggests an arachnoid cyst, and the small arrows outline the internal margins of the cyst. The curved arrows show the nerves of the cauda equina, which have been displaced anteriorly. (Courtesy of Erik Gaensler, M.D.)

Table 77.8: Examples of neurological complications in Reiter's syndrome

Acute transverse myelitis
Brainstem dysfunction
Encephalitis
Neuralgic amyotrophy
Personality change
Seizures
Unilateral ascending motor neuropathy

Source: Reprinted with permission from RB Rosenbaum, SM Campbell, JT Rosenbaum. Clinical Neurology of Rheumatic Diseases. Boston: Butterworth–Heinemann, 1996:187.

and Gibson 1994). Evaluation is complicated because either condition might cause a myelopathy, transient vision loss (iritis versus optic neuritis), or evoked response abnormalities.

EPIDURAL LIPOMATOSIS

Epidural lipomatosis is a non-neoplastic accumulation of fatty tissue in the thoracic or lumbar epidural space that can occur as a complication of chronic corticosteroid therapy. Patients usually have been on corticosteroids for over 6 months and are obese and cushingoid; spinal radiography typically shows diffuse osteoporosis. The lipomatous tissue can compress nerve roots or spinal cord (Figure 77.35). The compressive tissue can regress when corticosteroid doses are decreased, but occasionally the compression of neurological tissue is severe enough to require laminectomy.

CHRONIC MENINGITIS

Most cases of chronic meningitis are caused by infection (Chapter 59), neoplasia (Chapter 58), or sarcoidosis (Chapter 55). Behçet's syndrome, isolated central nervous system angiitis (Chapter 57), systemic lupus erythematosus, Sjögren's syndrome, or Wegener's granulomatosis should be included in a comprehensive differential diagnosis. Some other chronic or recurring meningitic syndromes merit discussion.

Chronic Adhesive Arachnoiditis

Chronic focal or diffuse inflammation of the spinal theca can cause neurological symptoms caused by inflammation, adhesion, and distortion of nerve roots or spinal cord. This condition is termed *chronic spinal arachnoiditis* or *chronic adhesive arachnoiditis*. However, the process usually involves all layers of the meninges and in its chronic stages may be fibrotic rather than inflammatory. Calcification or the meninges (arachnoiditis ossificans) is an occasional late finding.

Adhesive arachnoiditis occurs as an occasional complication of a variety of violations or irritations of the thecal sac (Table 77.9). Focal arachnoiditis is most common in the cauda equina, following lumbar disc surgery or myelography, particularly if oil-based contrast has been used for the latter. The symptoms can include local or radicular pain, radicular paresthesia, and less commonly more severe findings of oligoradiculopathy such as motor loss or sphincter dysfunction. The diagnosis can usually be made by spinal MRI, which may show clumping of nerve roots, nodules in the subarachnoid space, loculation of spinal fluid, and local areas of enhancement. The nerve roots may clump at the periphery of the the-

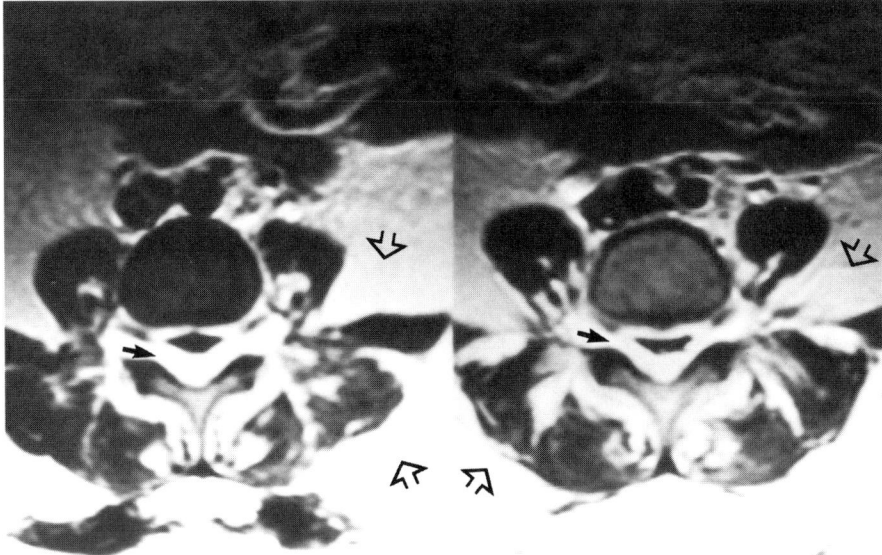

FIGURE 77.35   Magnetic resonance image shows epidural lipomatosis. T1-weighted axial images show markedly increased fat (*arrows*) within the spinal canal compressing the thecal sac, which is quite small. Note that the patient is quite obese, with large amounts of fat in the retroperitoneum and posterior paraspinous tissues (*open arrows*). (Courtesy of Erik Gaensler, M.D.)

Table 77.9:   Causes of adhesive arachnoiditis

Myelography, especially with oil-based dyes
Spinal surgery
Ankylosing spondylitis
Intrathecal or epidural chemical exposure, e.g., spinal
    anesthesia, corticosteroids
Granulomatous infection, e.g., tuberculosis
Ruptured dermoid or epidermoid cyst

cal sac, usually adjacent to an area of previous surgery, or in the center of the sac, usually in areas of spinal stenosis (Laitt et al. 1996). The extent of the MRI findings correlates poorly with the severity of the clinical nerve root dysfunction. Spinal fluid may show increased CSF protein and mild to moderate mononuclear pleocytosis. Surgical débridement of the arachnoiditis is sometimes attempted, but is usually unsuccessful and may lead to increased neurological deficit. Epidural or intrathecal corticosteroids are sometimes tried, but there is no proof of their efficacy, and there are reports of arachnoiditis caused by their use. Therefore, most treatment is aimed at symptomatic pain control, except in the unusual patient with progressive neurological deficits.

Arachnoiditis of the spinal cord is rarer than arachnoiditis of the cauda equina. It can occur after apparently successful treatment of granulomatous meningitis or of epidural or vertebral infection and can lead to myelopathy. Arachnoiditis, especially at the craniocervical junction, can cause syringomyelia.

Recurrent Meningitis

Patients with recurrent attacks of acute bacterial meningitis need to be screened for dural CSF leaks, parameningeal

infections, and immunodeficiency (see Chapter 59). Recurrent meningitis also can be caused by chemical irritation from leaking dermoid tumors or craniopharyngiomas. Drug-induced meningitis, most common as an idiosyncratic reaction to nonsteroidal anti-inflammatory drugs, can recur with repeated drug exposures. Rarely, recurrent meningitis can complicate systemic inflammatory diseases such as systemic lupus erythematosus, Sjögren's syndrome, Behçet's disease, Lyme disease, familial Mediterranean fever, or sarcoidosis.

Mollaret's meningitis is another form of recurrent aseptic meningitis. Attacks are self-limited, lasting a few days. The spinal fluid shows a mixed pleocytosis; sometimes large endothelial cells (Mollaret's cells) are present as well. Some cases may be caused by herpes virus infection, but usually a causative organism is not identified.

Uveo-Meningitic Syndromes

The combination of chronic or recurrent meningitis and uveitis has a specific differential diagnosis (Table 77.10). Often ophthalmological characterization of the uveitis can further limit the differential diagnosis. For example, the uveitis of Vogt-Koyanagi-Harada syndrome is bilateral and often causes retinal elevations and retinal pigmentary changes. Vogt-Koyanagi-Harada syndrome also causes skin and hair findings such as vitiligo, poliosis, or focal alopecia.

SUPERFICIAL HEMOSIDEROSIS

Superficial hemosiderosis is a rare disorder that causes slowly progressive cerebellar ataxia, mainly of gait, and sensorineural deafness, often combined with spasticity,

Table 77.10:   Causes of combined uveitis and meningitis

Acute multifocal placoid pigmentary epitheliopathy
Acute retinal necrosis
Behçet's syndrome
Human T-cell lymphotropic virus I infection
Infection in immunocompromised host
Isolated central nervous system angiitis
Lyme disease
Primary central nervous system lymphoma
Sarcoid
Syphilis
Systemic lupus erythematosus
Vogt-Koyanagi-Harada syndrome

Source: Reprinted with permission from RB Rosenbaum, SM Campbell, JT Rosenbaum. Clinical Neurology of Rheumatic Diseases. Boston: Butterworth–Heinemann, 1996:57.

brisk reflexes, and extensor plantar responses. Other features include dementia (24%), bladder disturbance (24%), anosmia (at least 17%), anisocoria (at least 10%), and sensory signs (13%). Less frequent features are extraocular motor palsies, neck or backache, bilateral sciatica, and lower motor neuron signs (5–10% each). Men are more often affected than women (3 to 1). The diagnosis may not be suspected clinically, but the neuroradiological abnormalities are striking. MRI shows a black rim around the posterior fossa structures and spinal cord, and less often the cerebral hemispheres, on T2-weighted images. These paramagnetic signal changes represent encrustation of the brain surfaces with hemosiderin. The adjacent neural tissue atrophies, with accumulation of ferritin in microglia and Bergmann's cells in the cerebellum. Superficial siderosis is most commonly secondary to chronic leaking of blood into the subarachnoid space, and it has been described after hemispherectomy and in association with chronically leaking intracranial aneurysms, arteriovenous malformations, spinal tumors, and dural injuries. However, the CSF may be normal, and not all patients have an identifiable source of bleeding. Treatment relies on identifying the source of bleeding; chelation therapy does not appear to be effective.

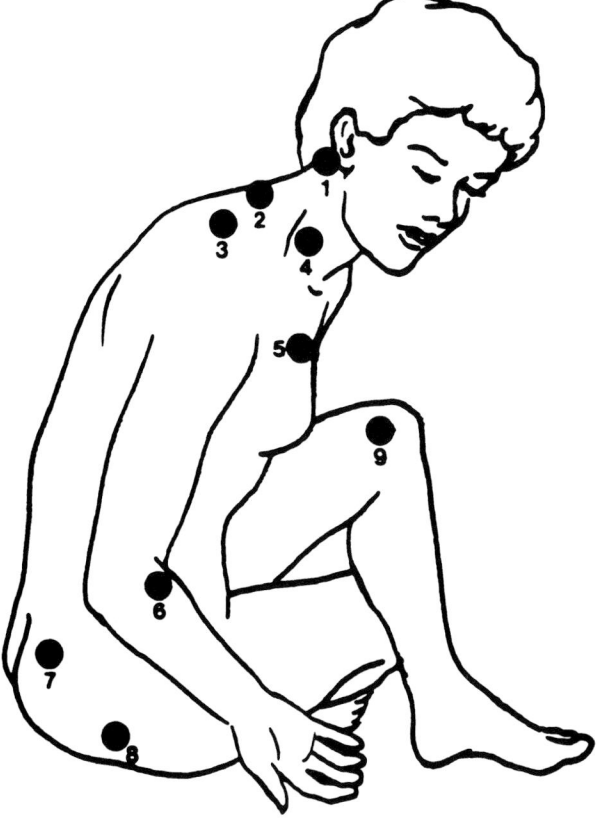

FIGURE 77.36   The tender point location of fibromyalgia. The nine paired tender points recommended by the 1990 American College of Rheumatology Criteria Committee for establishing a diagnosis of fibromyalgia are (1) insertion of the nuchal muscles into occiput; (2) upper border of the trapezius, midportion; (3) muscle attachments to upper medial border of scapula; (4) anterior aspects of the C5, C7 intertransverse spaces; (5) second rib space approximately 3 cm lateral to the sternal border; (6) muscle attachments to lateral epicondyle, approximately 2 cm below the bony prominence; (7) upper outer quadrant of gluteal muscles; (8) muscle attachments just posterior to the greater trochanter; and (9) medial fat pad of knee proximal to joint line. A total of 11 or more tender points in conjunction with a history of widespread pain is characteristic of the fibromyalgia syndrome. (Reprinted with permission from RM Bennett. The Fibromyalgia Syndrome: Myofascial Pain and the Chronic Fatigue Syndrome. In WN Kelley, ED Harris Jr, S Ruddy, et al. [eds], Textbook of Rheumatology [5th ed]. Philadelphia: Saunders, 1997;513.)

FIBROMYALGIA

Fibromyalgia enters the differential diagnosis of many patients with spinal pain. It is a syndrome defined by widespread musculoskeletal or soft tissue pain and multiple tender points. The American College of Rheumatology classification criteria for the diagnosis define pain as widespread when it is bilateral, above and below the waist, and axial. To meet the classification criteria, a patient must have tenderness to palpation at 11 or more of 18 specific points (Figure 77.36). The validity of these tender points as diagnostic criteria has been cogently questioned (Bohr 1996).

Typically, patients have multiple symptoms including fatigue, stiffness, nonrestorative sleep, headaches, and mood disorders. An acute version of the syndrome can be produced by sleep deprivation in normal volunteers. Patients may have many symptoms of neurological import such as weakness, paresthesia, and dizziness. Nonetheless, their neurological examinations are normal, unless they have a separate neurological illness. Neurological investigations such as brain imaging or electrodiagnostic studies are normal or show minor nonspecific abnormalities.

The cause of most cases of fibromyalgia is unknown. Despite investigations of muscle pathology, sleep physiology, spinal abnormalities, neuroendocrine function, and psychopathology, there are no widely accepted, objective diagnostic tests for fibromyalgia, and there is no established underlying pathophysiology (Goldenberg 1995). Some cases accompany an autoimmune disease, such as systemic lupus erythematosus, or other systemic illness, such as hypothyroidism. Focal trauma can cause localized, self-limited soft tissue myofascial pain, but data are lacking to suggest that trauma, on-the-job injury, or workplace stress can cause fibromyalgia (Wolfe 1996). Treatment includes a supportive doctor–patient relationship, tricyclic antidepressants, aerobic exercise, and avoiding inactivity.

REFERENCES

Anson JA, Benzel EC, Awad IA (eds). Syringomyelia and the Chiari Malformations. Park Ridge, IL: American Association of Neurological Surgeons, 1997.

Bindal AK, Dunsker SB, Tew JM Jr. Chiari I malformation: classification and management. Neurosurgery 1995;37:1069–1074.

Boachie-Adjei O, Squillante RG. Tuberculosis of the spine. Orthop Clin North Am 1996;27:95–103.

Bohr T. Problems with myofascial pain syndrome and fibromyalgia syndrome. Neurology 1996;46:593–597.

Calderone RR, Capen DA. Spinal infections. Orthop Clin North Am 1996;27:1–205.

Charnas LR, Marini JC. Communicating hydrocephalus, basilar invagination, and other neurological features in osteogenesis imperfecta. Neurology 1993;43:2603–2608.

Delmas PD, Meunier PJ. The management of Paget's disease of bone. N Engl J Med 1997;336:558–566.

Dolan AL, Gibson T. Intrinsic spinal cord lesions in 2 patients with ankylosing spondylitis. J Rheumatol 1994;21:1160–1161.

el Masry WS, Biyani A. Incidence, management, and outcome of post-traumatic syringomyelia. In memory of Mr. Bernard Williams. J Neurol Neurosurg Psychiatry 1996;60:141–146.

Evans SC, Edgar MA, Hall Craggs MA, et al. MRI of "idiopathic" juvenile scoliosis. A prospective study. J Bone Joint Surg 1996;78B:314–317.

Goldenberg DL. Fibromyalgia: why such controversy? Ann Rheum Dis 1995;54:3–5.

Hamamci N, Hawran S, Biering-Sfrensen F. Achondroplasia and spinal cord lesion. Three case reports. Paraplegia 1993;31: 375–379.

Kanis JA. Osteoporosis. London: Blackwell, 1994.

Klekamp J, Batzdorf U, Samii M, Bothe HW. Treatment of syringomyelia associated with arachnoid scarring caused by arachnoiditis or trauma. J Neurosurg 1997;86:233–240.

Laitt R, Jackson A, Isherwood I. Patterns of chronic adhesive arachnoiditis following Mydoil myelography: the significance of spinal canal stenosis and previous surgery. Br J Radiol 1996;69:693–698.

Lonstein JE, Bradford DS, Winter RB, Ogilvie JW (eds). Moe's Textbook of Scoliosis and Other Spinal Deformities (3rd ed). Philadelphia: Saunders, 1995.

Milhorat TH, Kotzen RM, Mu HT, et al. Dysesthetic pain in patients with syringomyelia. Neurosurgery 1996;38:940–946.

Radhakrishnan K, Litchy WJ, O'Fallon WM, et al. Epidemiology of cervical radiculopathy. A population-based study from Rochester, Minnesota, 1976 through 1990. Brain 1994;117: 325–335.

Rosenbaum RB, Campbell SM, Rosenbaum JT. Clinical Neurology of Rheumatic Diseases. Boston: Butterworth–Heinemann, 1996.

Rupp RE, Ebraheim NA, Coombs RJ. Magnetic resonance imaging differentiation of compression spine fractures or vertebral lesions caused by osteoporosis or tumor. Spine 1995;20: 2499–2504.

Samii M, Klekamp J. Surgical results of 100 intramedullary tumors in relation to accompanying syringomyelia. Neurosurgery 1994;35:865–873.

Schurch B, Wichmann W, Rossier AB. Post-traumatic syringomyelia (cystic myelopathy): a prospective study of 449 patients with spinal cord injury. J Neurol Neurosurg Psychiatry 1996;60: 61–67.

Stevens JM, Chong WK, Barber C, et al. A new appraisal of abnormalities of the odontoid process associated with atlanto-axial subluxation and neurological disability. Brain 1994;117:133–148.

Thomsen MN, Schneider U, Weber M, Johannisson R, Neithard FU. Scoliosis and congenital anomalies associated with Klippel-Feil syndromes types I–III. Spine 1997;22:396-401.

Wallace E, Wong J, Reid IR. Pamidronate treatment of the neurological sequelae of pagetic spinal stenosis. Arch Intern Med 1995;155:1813–1815.

Wolfe F. The fibromyalgia syndrome: a consensus report on fibromyalgia and disability. J Rheumatol 1996;23:534–539.

Wood KB, Blair JM, Aepple DM, et al. The natural history of asymptomatic thoracic disc herniations. Spine 1997;22:525–530.

Chapter 78
Disorders of Upper and Lower Motor Neurons

Hiroshi Mitsumoto

Recent progress in understanding motor neuron diseases has been rapid. Advances have been made in almost every aspect, undoubtedly because of simultaneous rapid progress in neuroscience and molecular biology. The molecular basis of several hereditary motor neuron diseases has been discovered, the pathogenesis of such diseases is better understood, diagnostic techniques have improved, some diseases are now treatable, and new approaches to treatment have been developed. This chapter reviews the causes, diagnosis, and treatment of motor neuron disease.

DISORDERS OF UPPER MOTOR NEURONS

Neuroanatomy of the Upper Motor Neurons

Lower motor neurons (LMNs) directly innervate the skeletal muscle, and upper motor neurons (UMNs) are responsible for conveying impulses for voluntary motor activity from the cerebral cortex to the LMNs. More broadly, the UMNs are the neurons rostral to the LMNs that send fibers to the LMNs, and that exert direct or indirect supranuclear control over the LMNs (Holstege 1995) (Table 78.1).

Motor Cortex

In the cerebral cortex, the UMNs are located in the primary motor cortex (Brodmann's area 4) and the premotor areas (Brodmann's area 6). The latter are subdivided into the supplementary motor area (sometimes called the *secondary motor cortex*) and the premotor cortex. Somatotopic organization and topographic specificity of the corticospinal projection appear to be far more complex and broader than the organization that has been previously mapped onto muscles. Betz's cells (giant pyramidal neurons) are a distinct group of neurons in layer 5 of the primary motor cortex and represent only a small proportion of the motor fibers in the corticospinal and corticobulbar tract, most of which derive from neurons that are smaller than Betz's cells. Individual motor neurons in the primary motor cortex initiate the contraction of small groups of skeletal muscles and control the force of contraction. The entire motor area of the cerebral cortex controls voluntary muscle movement, including motor planning and programming of muscle movement.

Corticospinal and Corticobulbar Tracts

Axons from the cortical motor areas form the corticospinal and corticobulbar tracts. Axons arising from neurons in the primary motor cortex constitute only about one-third of all the axons of the corticospinal and corticobulbar tracts. Betz's cell axons comprise 3–5% of the tract, and the remaining axons from the primary motor cortex arise from smaller neurons. Another one-third of the axons in these tracts derive from Brodmann's area 6, including the supplementary motor and lateral premotor cortex. The remaining

Table 78.1:   Upper motor neurons and their descending tracts

Motor areas
    Primary motor neurons (Betz's giant pyramidal cells and
        surrounding motor neurons)
    Premotor areas (the supplementary motor area and
        premotor cortex)
Corticospinal and corticobulbar tracts
    Lateral pyramidal tracts
    Ventral (uncrossed) pyramidal tracts
Brainstem control
    Vestibulospinal tracts
    Reticulospinal tracts
    Tectospinal tracts
Limbic motor control

one-third derive from the somatic sensory cortex (areas 1, 2, and 3) and the adjacent temporal lobe region.

The corticobulbar tract projects bilaterally to the motor neurons of cranial nerves V, VII, IX, X, and XII. Most corticospinal fibers (75–90%) decussate in the lower medulla (pyramidal decussation) and form the lateral corticospinal tract (the pyramidal tracts). The remaining fibers descend in the ipsilateral ventral corticospinal tract. The lateral corticospinal tract projects to ipsilateral motor neurons and their interneurons that control extremity muscle contraction, whereas the anterior corticospinal tract ends bilaterally on ventromedial motor neurons and interneurons, which control axial and postural muscles. These corticospinal axons provide direct and strong glutamatergic excitatory input to alpha motoneurons.

Basal Ganglia and Cerebellum

The basal ganglia and cerebellum have no direct input to the LMNs and thus are not considered part of the UMNs. However, the functional distinction between the pyramidal tracts (the principal UMN system) and the extrapyramidal system has become less distinct as knowledge of the functional neuroanatomy has increased. Although the basal ganglia and cerebellum traditionally do not belong to the UMN system, they closely modulate motor function in its entirety. The basal ganglia receive their input from the entire cerebral cortex and then create a feedback loop, sending output through the thalamus to the premotor and motor cortex and the associated prefrontal cortex. This indicates that the basal ganglia are modulating higher-order functions, which provide cognitive aspects of motor control, including the planning and execution of complex motor strategies. In contrast, the cerebellum directly regulates mechanical execution of movement because it receives input from the sensorimotor cortex and the spinal cord. The cerebellum (1) creates a feedback loop to the sensori-

motor cortex through the thalamus and (2) provides input indirectly to the LMNs via the vestibulospinal tracts.

Brainstem Control

Several brainstem nuclei can be considered part of the UMN system in a broad sense because they exert a supranuclear influence on the spinal cord LMNs. The projections from the brainstem to spinal cord LMNs are highly complex. The fibers originating in the medial and inferior vestibular nuclei in the medulla descend in the medial vestibulospinal tract and terminate on medial cervical and thoracic motor neurons and medial interneurons. These fibers excite the ipsilateral motor neurons and inhibit the contralateral motor neurons. The lateral vestibulospinal tracts originating in the lateral vestibular nucleus (Deiter's nucleus) activate the extensor motor neurons and inhibit the flexor motor neurons in the upper and lower extremities.

The brainstem reticular formation also strongly influences the spinal motor neurons, exerting widespread polysynaptic inhibitory inputs on extensor motor neurons and excitatory inputs on flexor motor neurons. The reticulospinal tracts modulate various reflex actions during ongoing movements. The brainstem reticular formation receives supranuclear control from the motor cortex via the corticoreticulospinal pathway, to act as a major inhibitor of spinal reflexes and activity. Therefore, a lesion of the corticoreticular pathway can disinhibit reticulospinal control of the LMNs. The tectospinal tract originates in the superior colliculus and controls eye and head movement. When the inhibitory effects on stretch reflexes (mediated by the dorsal reticulospinal tract) do not balance facilitatory effects on extensor spasticity (mediated by the medial reticulospinal tract and, to some extent, by the vestibulospinal tract), muscle tone is altered.

Limbic Motor Control

The limbic system is involved in emotional experience and expression and is associated with a wide variety of autonomic, visceral, and endocrine functions. It strongly influences the somatic motor neurons. The emotional status and experience of an individual determines overall somatic motor neuron activity. The limbic motor system also influences respiration, vomiting, swallowing, chewing, and licking (at least in animal studies). Furthermore, the generation of pseudobulbar signs in amyotrophic lateral sclerosis (ALS) is closely related to an abnormal limbic motor control, particularly in the periaqueductal gray matter and nucleus retroambiguus. The latter nucleus projects to the somatic motor neurons that innervate the pharynx, soft palate, intercostal, diaphragmatic, and abdominal muscles and probably the muscles of the larynx. Pseudobulbar symptoms may appear when UMN control over the periaqueductal gray matter and nucleus retroambiguus is impaired, and thus, limbic motor control is disinhibited (Holstege 1995).

Signs and Symptoms of Upper Motor Neuron Dysfunction

Loss of Dexterity

Loss of dexterity is one of the most characteristic signs of UMN impairment. Voluntary skillful movements require the integrated activation of many interneuron circuits in the spinal cord. Such integration is ultimately controlled by the corticospinal tract and thus by the UMNs. Loss of dexterity may be expressed as stiffness, slowness, and clumsiness in performing any skillful motor actions. In particular, rapid repetitive motions, such as foot or finger tapping, are impaired (Table 78.2).

Weakness

Although muscle strength is reduced, the degree of muscle weakness resulting from UMN dysfunction is generally mild. Extensor muscles of the upper extremities and flexor muscles of the lower extremities may become weaker than their antagonist muscles. This is because the UMN lesion disinhibits brainstem control of the vestibulospinal and reticulospinal tracts, which tend to increase contraction of the flexor muscle of the upper limbs and extensor muscles of the lower limbs.

Spasticity

Spasticity is the hallmark of UMN disease. The pathophysiology of spasticity is complex and controversial. Spasticity is a state of sustained increase in muscle tension when the muscle is lengthened. Clinically, spastic muscles lose their normal smooth stretching during passive movement, resulting in a sudden increase in resistance to further passive movement. This resistance is referred to as a *spastic catch*. However, when a sustained passive stretch is continued, spastic muscles quickly release the tension and relax, an event often described as the *clasp-knife phenomenon*. In severely spastic muscle, passive movement becomes very difficult and even impossible.

Pathological Hyperreflexia and Pathological Reflexes

Pathological hyperreflexia is a crucial clinical manifestation of UMN disease, as is the development of abnormal (pathological) reflexes. Babinski's sign (extensor plantar response) is the most important pathological reflex sign in the clinical neurological examination. It is characterized by extension of the great toe, often accompanied by fanning of the other

Table 78.2: Signs and symptoms of upper motor neuron dysfunction

Loss of dexterity
Slowed movements
Loss of muscle strength (weakness)
Spasticity
Pathological hyperreflexia
Pathological reflexes
Pseudobulbar (spastic bulbar) palsy

toes, in response to stroking the outer edge of the ipsilateral sole upward from the heel with a blunt object.

Pseudobulbar (Spastic Bulbar) Palsy

With dysfunction of the corticobulbar tracts that exert supranuclear control over the motor nuclei that control speech, mastication, and deglutition, pseudobulbar palsy (or spastic bulbar palsy) develops. The prefix *pseudo-* is used to distinguish this condition from bulbar palsy, in which there is a degeneration of only the LMNs of the brainstem motor nuclei. Articulation, mastication, and deglutition are affected in both pseudobulbar and bulbar palsies, but the degree of impairment in pseudobulbar palsy is generally milder. The key difference in symptoms is that pseudobulbar palsy is uniquely characterized by spontaneous or unmotivated crying and laughter. Any ordinary conversation or audiovisual materials about subjects with emotional content often trigger a highly stereotyped crying or laughter that is embarrassing to patients. The term *emotional incontinence* has been used to describe this symptom in spastic bulbar palsy.

Laboratory Evidence of Upper Motor Neuron Dysfunction

Neuroimaging

Brain magnetic resonance imaging (MRI) sometimes shows abnormal signal intensity in the corticospinal and corticobulbar tracts in the internal capsule. Normal subjects may occasionally have increased signal in the internal capsules in T2-weighted images, but abnormal signal intensity in these areas in both T2-weighted and proton density–weighted images appears to be a specific indicator of pyramidal tract involvement. However, the frequency of positive proton density–weighted MRI abnormalities in cases of pure UMN syndrome is only about 40% (true positives).

Magnetic Resonance Spectroscopy

A novel research technique potentially capable of objectively assessing UMN dysfunction in ALS is proton magnetic reso-

Table 78.3: Disorders of upper motor neurons and their key characteristics

Disorders	Key characteristics
Primary lateral sclerosis	A diagnosis of exclusion
Hereditary spastic paraplegia	Hereditary, usually autosomal dominant
HTLV-1–associated myelopathy	Slowly progressive myelopathy, endemic, and positive HTLV-1 test
Adrenomyeloneuropathy	X-linked recessive inheritance, myelopathy, increased serum very-long-chain fatty acids
Lathyrism	History of consumption of chickpeas

HTLV-1 = human T-cell leukemia virus–1.

nance spectroscopy. It is a noninvasive technique that combines the advantages of MRI with in vivo biochemical information. *N*-acetyl aspartate, a neuronal marker, is significantly reduced relative to creatine-phosphocreatine (used as an internal standard because all cells, including glial cells, contain creatine-phosphocreatine) in the sensorimotor cortices of patients with ALS who have UMN signs.

Transcranial Magnetic Stimulation

Another novel technique to measure UMN function is transcranial magnetic stimulation. Transcranial magnetic stimulation over the scalp at the region of the motor cortex induces motor evoked potentials that are recorded at the skeletal muscle. The response pattern of the motor evoked potential may correlate with UMN involvement.

Primary Lateral Sclerosis

Primary lateral sclerosis (PLS) is an uncommon motor neuron disease, constituting at most only a few percent of all cases of motor neuron diseases, including ALS (Table 78.3). Whether it is an independent disease entity or a variant of ALS remains to be determined.

Clinical Features and Diagnosis

Slowly progressive spastic paraparesis is the major clinical feature of PLS, leading to quadriparesis in some patients late in the disease course. Eventually, spastic bulbar palsy may evolve, leading to speech and swallowing problems and emotional lability, although many patients never reach this stage. The disease usually progresses very slowly, sometimes over decades.

The differential diagnosis of PLS is wide, and PLS is a diagnosis of exclusion. Evidence of LMN involvement that would indicate ALS must be excluded by performing thorough clinical and electromyographic (EMG) examinations. Other causes of this UMN syndrome include structural abnormali-

ties (Chiari malformation, spinal cord tumors, and extrinsic compressive lesions) and myelopathies, such as multiple sclerosis (MS), human immunodeficiency virus myelopathy, human T-cell leukemia virus–1 (HTLV-1) myelopathy, or adrenomyeloneuropathy. Cervical spondylotic myelopathy and MS are probably the most common causes of a progressive UMN syndrome that presents like PLS.

A positive family history should suggest familial spastic paraplegia or adrenomyeloneuropathy. Paraneoplastic syndromes and Sjögren's syndrome may clinically resemble PLS. The diagnosis of ALS cannot be excluded within 3 years of onset because LMN features may develop later. Thus, a careful follow-up examination is crucial before PLS is diagnosed with certainty. ALS can cause a pure UMN picture, which generally progresses more rapidly than PLS. Until a laboratory test allows definitive diagnoses of pure UMN-ALS and PLS, the question of these two conditions will remain controversial.

Treatment

No curative pharmacotherapy is available for this condition, but antispasticity drugs (baclofen and tizanidine by mouth, and intrathecal baclofen) are frequently beneficial.

Hereditary Spastic Paraplegia

The prevalence of hereditary spastic paraplegia (HSP) is estimated to be 0.5–11.9 in 100,000, but this may be an underestimate because of the benign nature of the disease in many families. The most common inheritance mode (approximately 70–85% of all cases) is autosomal dominant. The number of autosomal dominant cases may be underestimated if the parents of affected children are not fully examined. The remaining cases are transmitted as autosomal recessive or rare X-linked traits; both are often complicated by other central nervous system (CNS) involvement.

Recent genetic linkage studies have identified loci on at least three chromosomes that are responsible for autosomal dominant spastic paraplegia. The first region is on chromosome 14q (*FSP1*) in French or German families; this locus may overlap with the locus for autosomal dominant dopa-responsive dystonia. The second locus is on chromosome 15q (*FSP3*) and is seen in a large North American kindred of Irish descent. The third locus is on chromosome 2p (*FSP2*) found in Dutch and French kindreds. These three linkages account for about 50% of autosomal dominant families. In one family with an autosomal recessive form of pure spastic paraplegia, a linkage to the chromosome 8q12-q13 has been identified (Fink and Heineman-Patterson 1996).

Clinical Features

Autosomal dominant HSP is classified as type I or type II, based on age of onset, before or after age 35 years. In the more common type I, onset of symptoms usually occurs in childhood or young adulthood. Developmental motor milestones are usually abnormal. Delay in walking, toe-walking, difficulty in negotiating stairs, clumsiness, and noticeably poor athletic coordination in childhood are common clinical features. In some young children, spastic paraparesis is often obvious: Initially, the signs and symptoms of spasticity are limited to lower extremities, but gradually the upper extremities become involved. Pes cavus is seen in more than 50% of patients. When the disease has been present for more than 10 years, mild-to-moderate wasting of the distal upper extremity muscles may be seen. Other late features include loss of vibratory sensation in the legs and urinary urgency. Patients may have minor congenital malformations, such as short stature, an increased carrying angle of the elbows, and partial syndactyly of the second and third toes. The clinical characteristics of type II are very similar to those of type I, but the age of onset is later in adulthood, usually after age 35. The gene loci have not been identified in the type II form.

The less common autosomal recessive HSP is virtually indistinguishable from the autosomal dominant forms. In these families, consanguinity is often reported. Age of onset varies from early childhood to middle adulthood (45 years). The recessive form often has an earlier age of onset and more rapid progression than occurs in the autosomal dominant form. Rare forms include X-linked HSP and "complicated" HSP, which manifests more extensive CNS involvement. In all forms of HSP, there is degeneration of the corticospinal tracts and, to a lesser degree, of the posterior columns of the spinal cord (Harding 1993).

Diagnosis

The diagnosis of HSP is based on evidence of a family history, usually in an autosomal dominant mode in a patient with a slowly progressive paraplegia. When there is no family history, it is essential to exclude definable causes of spastic paraplegia. Differential diagnoses are the same as for PLS. Because there may be no clear family history in the recessive form, the diagnosis of autosomal recessive HSP is often missed.

Treatment

At present, treatment for HSP is limited to symptomatic interventions, supportive care to reduce spasticity, and assistive devices, such as canes, walkers, and wheelchairs. Antispasticity drugs, such as oral baclofen, tizanidine, or dantrolene, are often suboptimal. In patients with disabling spasticity, intrathecal baclofen may be more effective.

Human T-Cell Leukemia Virus Type 1–Associated Myelopathy or Tropical Spastic Paraparesis

HTLV-1 causes a chronic progressive myelopathy that is referred to as *tropical spastic paraparesis* (TSP) in the Caribbean and as *HTLV-1–associated myelopathy* (HAM) in Japan. This retrovirus, which is endemic in the Caribbean area, southern Japan, equatorial Africa, South Africa, and parts of Central and South America, produces a chronic, insidiously progressive myelopathy that typically begins after age 30. The clinical syndrome is characterized by spastic paraparesis, paresthesias and pain in the legs, and urinary bladder dysfunction. Sensory findings may be minor. Some patients may develop optic neuropathy, cerebellar ataxia, or polyneuropathy. Evidence of LMN involvement can be rare. The definitive diagnosis of TSP/HAM requires HTLV-1–positive serology in blood or cerebrospinal fluid (CSF). At present, no antiviral agents effectively treat TSP/HAM.

Adrenomyeloneuropathy

Adrenomyeloneuropathy is a variant of adrenoleukodystrophy, an X-linked recessive disorder (see Chapter 68). Adrenoleukodystrophy affects young boys, who develop severe adrenal insufficiency and progressive mental and psychological deterioration and progress to quadriparesis. In contrast, adrenomyeloneuropathy is milder, clinically characterized by slowly progressive spastic paraparesis and mild polyneuropathy in adult males, with or without sensory symptoms and sphincter disturbances. Adrenal insufficiency may also be very mild. It is important to know that adult female carriers may present with slowly progressive spastic paraparesis. Obtaining a detailed family history and appropriate testing are crucial. Electron micrographs of the sural nerve biopsy specimen may show characteristic crescentic empty lipid clefts in Schwann cell cytoplasm. Linkage studies have identified a locus at chromosome Xq28. The diagnostic test is the increased levels of very-long-chain fatty acids in the plasma.

Lathyrism

Lathyrism is a unique chronic neurological disease caused by long-term ingestion of large quantities of chickpeas (*Lathyrus sativus*). The responsible neurotoxin is β-N-oxalyl amino-L-alanine, which is an α-amino-3-hydroxyl-5-methyl-4-isoxazolepropionate (AMPA) glutamate receptor agonist. Chickpeas are relatively resistant to drought. Lathyrism occurs particularly in poorly nourished populations during periods of food shortage, when chickpeas become a more prominent dietary resource. The onset of clinical toxicity is either acute or chronic, manifesting as muscle spasms and leg weakness. The disease is characterized by spastic paraparesis with or without some sensory and bladder dysfunction. Leg motor neurons in the motor cortex and the corresponding pyramidal tracts are predominantly affected. Lathyrism has been found in the indigenous populations of Bangladesh, China, Ethiopia, India, Romania, and Spain; it also occurred in the concentration camps in Asia during World War II. Lathyrism is an important example of a disease in which a natural excitotoxin causes selective UMN impairment.

DISORDERS OF LOWER MOTOR NEURONS

Neuroanatomy of Lower Motor Neurons

Interneurons

The interneurons constitute the majority of neurons in the anterior horn of the spinal cord and determine the final output of the LMNs. The interneuron system receives supranuclear excitatory and inhibitory motor control from the brainstem descending tracts, corticospinal tracts, and limbic system. This system also receives afferent information, directly and indirectly, from the afferent peripheral nerves. The interneuron system forms intricate neuronal circuits involving the automatic and stereotyped spinal reflexes so as to coordinate and integrate the activation of synergist muscles and inhibition of antagonist muscles, the contralateral muscle, and sometimes even a distant motor pool. The same interneuron network that mediates such automatic and stereotyped reflex behavior is also known to act as the basic functional unit in highly skillful voluntary movements. Ultimately, all the interneuronal paths converge on the LMNs that innervate the skeletal muscles. Sherrington called this terminal path the *final common path*.

Lower Motor Neurons

The LMNs are located in the brainstem and spinal cord and send out motor axons that directly innervate skeletal muscle fibers. The spinal cord LMNs are also known as anterior horn cells. These motor neurons are clustered in nuclei, forming longitudinal columns; those innervating the distal muscles of the extremities are located in the dorsal anterior horn, whereas those innervating proximal muscles of the extremities are in the ventral anterior horn. The LMNs innervating the axial and truncal muscles are the most medially located. The normal cervical and lumbar enlargements of the spinal cord are the result of markedly enlarged lateral anterior horns, which contain the LMNs for arm and hand muscles (cervical) and leg muscles (lumbar).

Large spinal cord LMNs are called *alpha motoneurons*; they are the principal motor neurons innervating the muscle fibers. Medium-sized motor neurons (beta motoneurons) innervate both extrafusal muscle fibers and intrafusal (spindle muscle) fibers, and intermediate and small motor neurons (gamma motoneurons or fusimotor neurons) innervate only muscle spindle fibers. The rest of the small anterior horn cells are *interneurons*.

Alpha motoneurons are among the largest neurons of the nervous system, and each has a single axon that branches to innervate its many muscle fibers and a number of large dendrites to provide an extensive receptive field. One alpha motoneuron and its group of skeletal muscle fibers constitute the motor unit. The motor neuron determines the size and physiological function (e.g., fast, slow) of its motor unit.

Motor axons originate from LMN cell bodies (perikarya) and leave the CNS through the anterior (or ventral) spinal roots to become a part of the peripheral nervous system. Motor axons subsequently intermingle with sensory and autonomic nerve fibers and are reorganized into the individual peripheral nerves. All peripheral nerve fibers are ensheathed by Schwann cells, and all motor axons are myelinated. The environment of the peripheral nervous system is controlled by the blood-nerve barrier and perineurial sheath. Thus, the motor axon is exposed to the extracellular space only at the node of Ranvier and at the axon terminal. Macromolecules, such as neurotrophic factors, are believed to be taken up at the axon terminal, but other macromolecules (neurotoxins and viral particles) can also enter the motor axons at the terminal.

Signs and Symptoms of Lower Motor Neuron Dysfunction

Weakness

The loss of an LMN results in the denervation of its motor unit, whereas dysfunction of the LMN may lead to abnormal or impaired activation of the motor unit (Table 78.4). In either case, the number of fully functional motor units is decreased, which reduces overall muscle strength. In a disease causing chronic motor unit depletion, denervated muscle fibers may be reinnervated by neighboring axons belonging to healthy motor neurons. Hence, existing motor units are being continually modified. In this way, muscle strength is maintained as fully as possible. For example, in patients who recover from acute poliomyelitis, muscle that recovers to normal strength may lose 50% of its LMNs.

Muscle Atrophy and Hyporeflexia

Muscle fiber denervation causes muscle fiber atrophy and thus results in reduced muscle volume. Hyporeflexia tends to occur with LMN involvement, but the hyporeflexia is less than that seen in primary myopathy.

Muscle Hypotonicity or Flaccidity

Hypotonicity or flaccidity (the opposite of spasticity) refers to the decrease or complete loss of normal muscle resistance to passive manipulation.

Fasciculations

Fasciculations are spontaneous contractions of muscle fibers belonging to a single motor unit or some part

Table 78.4: Signs and symptoms of lower motor neuron involvement

Loss of muscle strength (weakness)
Muscle atrophy
Hyporeflexia
Muscle hypotonicity or flaccidity
Fasciculations
Muscle cramps

thereof. Clinically, fasciculations are seen through the skin as fine, rapid, flickering, and sometimes vermicular twitching contractions that occur irregularly in time and location. The impulse for the fasciculation appears to arise from hyperexcitable motor axons and is probably multifocal in origin. Fasciculations can occur in healthy individuals and in patients with LMN involvement, and thus fasciculations alone do not prove LMN disease (Blexrud et al. 1993).

In general, the larger the motor unit, the greater the size of the fasciculations. In tongue muscles, for example, fasciculations produce small vermicular movements on the tongue surface. Fasciculations usually do not cause any joint displacement, but when they occur in muscles with large reinnervated motor units, there may be tremor and movement of the fingers.

Muscle Cramps

A muscle cramp is clinically defined as an abrupt, involuntary, and painful shortening of the muscle accompanied by visible or palpable knotting, often with abnormal posture of the affected joint. Stretching or massaging can relieve muscle cramps (see Chapter 30). Muscle cramps are a common symptom of LMN involvement. The pathogenesis of cramps in LMN disease is poorly understood.

Laboratory Evidence of Lower Motor Neuron Dysfunction

In contrast to the limited techniques for the laboratory investigation of UMN involvement, LMN involvement is capable of precise investigation with EMG and muscle biopsy.

Electromyography

Peripheral electrophysiological studies consist of nerve conduction studies and EMG. When functional motor units are lost, the amplitude of the compound muscle action potentials elicited by a supramaximal electrical stimulation of the motor nerve is diminished. The greater the loss of functional motor units, the lower the amplitude of the compound muscle action potentials. When there is preferential loss of large motor axons, maximum motor nerve conduction velocity may be modestly diminished. Only when a demyelinating process affects nerve

fibers does the conduction velocity slow significantly (by 30% or more). A dispersion of compound muscle action potentials and focal conduction block may be found in acquired demyelinating motor neuropathy (see Chapter 37B). Sensory nerve conduction studies are normal in pure LMN disorders.

The needle electrode examination is crucial in obtaining electrophysiological evidence of abnormal motor units in LMN disorders (see Chapter 37B). Several electrophysiological techniques to estimate the number of functioning motor units are currently being investigated. Although the accuracy of these estimates is still uncertain, the methods may provide objective evidence of the existing number of motor units.

Muscle Biopsy

For assessing LMN involvement, the need for muscle biopsy has declined because the EMG needle electrode examination can provide sufficient evidence for LMN involvement. Muscle biopsy may reveal the earliest evidence of muscle fiber denervation, probably earlier than needle electrode examination (see Chapter 83). Denervated muscle fibers are small and angular and stain darkly by oxidative enzyme and nonspecific esterase stains. As the denervation process progresses, small groups of atrophied muscle fibers (group atrophy) may appear. In healthy individuals, the muscle fiber types seen with myosin adenosine-triphosphatase stain are randomly distributed. In chronic denervating disease, when the denervation and reinnervation processes are repeated, this random pattern is lost, and fiber type grouping develops.

Acute Poliomyelitis

Acute poliomyelitis is the prototypical disorder of acute LMN dysfunction. The disease is caused by poliovirus, which is a ribonucleic acid virus belonging to the genus *Enterovirus* and family *Picornavirus*. Immunization has eradicated the disease from the Western Hemisphere, and it is hoped that the Eastern Hemisphere will be free of polio shortly after the year 2000. In countries where wild disease has been eradicated, poliomyelitis is still encountered as a result of vaccine-associated illness from the live attenuated vaccine. Furthermore, an acute poliomyelitis syndrome can be caused by other enteroviruses. Most neurologists practicing today have not seen acute poliomyelitis, and it is important to be acquainted with the clinical features of the disease (Mitsumoto et al. 1997b).

Clinical Features

In an endemic region, almost all patients have asymptomatic exposure to poliovirus, as shown by antibody titers. Only a small proportion of people who are exposed to poliovirus develop either the minor illness (a gastrointestinal influenzalike illness) or the major illness several days after the infection. Clinically, the major illness resembles aseptic meningitis, and approximately 50% of patients progress to paralytic disease within 2–5 days of the initial symptom. The paralytic phase is characterized by localized fasciculations, severe myalgia, hyperesthesia, and usually fulminant focal and asymmetrical paralysis. Any muscles can be affected, but leg, arm, respiratory, and bulbar muscles are commonly involved; leg muscles are most frequently affected and bulbar muscles are least frequently affected. The risk of paralytic disease is relatively low in infancy and increases through childhood to adult ages. Most patients with paralytic disease eventually make significant recovery. Improvement may begin as early as the first week after onset of paralysis, and it has been estimated that 80% of recovery occurs by 6 months. Further improvement may be modest, but it may continue over the ensuing 18–24 months.

Laboratory Features

The CSF typically shows a pleocytosis, with polymorphonuclear cells predominating during the acute stages and lymphocytes predominating later in the disease. The CSF protein concentration shows a mild-to-moderate increase. The CSF poliovirus-specific immunoglobulin M (IgM) antibody test enables an accurate immunological diagnosis. Stool cultures are positive for poliovirus in nearly 90% of patients by the tenth day of illness. Traditionally, the diagnosis is established by documenting a fourfold or greater increase in poliovirus antibody titers in sera from the acute to the convalescent phase.

Differential Diagnosis

Acute paralytic disease caused by viruses other than poliovirus can be proved by an increase in neutralizing antibody titers of other viruses from acute to convalescent sera or by isolation of the virus by stool culture. Guillain-Barré syndrome may mimic acute poliomyelitis. Guillain-Barré syndrome often has sensory features. A dramatic or abrupt paralysis after severe pains and fasciculations is unusual in Guillain-Barré syndrome. A careful analysis of the CSF and EMG findings should differentiate these two diseases. Acute motor axonal neuropathy, or Chinese paralysis, should also be considered in the differential diagnosis. This motor neuropathy, which clinically resembles Guillain-Barré syndrome, usually presents with abrupt or rapidly progressive flaccid ascending paralysis without sensory symptoms. Serum antibody levels of anti-GM_1 antibody are elevated (see Chapter 80). Acute intermittent porphyria, which may mimic Guillain-Barré syndrome, must also be differentiated. Other diseases that may cause acute flaccid paralysis are myasthenia gravis, periodic paralysis, and acute rhabdomyolysis.

Treatment

The treatment for acute poliomyelitis consists mainly of general supportive care. Most patients require hospitalization in an intensive care unit to optimize close monitoring of respiratory muscle involvement. After the acute illness, rehabilitation is the main treatment, including assistive devices and corrective surgery, if necessary.

Vaccination

The trivalent oral polio vaccine (TOPV) had been widely used and was responsible for the eradication of wild-type poliomyelitis in the Western Hemisphere. It can cause vaccine-associated paralytic poliomyelitis in 1 of 2.5 million people who receive vaccination. In Western Europe, TOPV has been replaced by an enhanced inactivated vaccine, which is also replacing TOPV in the United States.

Progressive Postpoliomyelitis Muscular Atrophy

In the United States alone, it is estimated that 250,000–640,000 people survived acute poliomyelitis in the last epidemics in the 1940s and 1950s. Many years after the recovery from acute poliomyelitis, some patients experience progressive weakness, called *progressive postpoliomyelitis muscular atrophy* (PPMA), which is defined as a progressive weakness developing in a patient who has recovered from acute poliomyelitis and remained stable for at least 10 years after the recovery (Table 78.5). The reported incidence of PPMA ranges from 0 to 64%, which raises the concern about the identity of PPMA. In addition to the progressive LMN syndrome of PPMA, under the term of *postpolio syndrome* or *late effects of remote polio*, various neurological, orthopedic, musculoskeletal, and medical problems, including chronic fatigue, can influence neuromuscular function (Jubelt and Drucker 1993; Mitsumoto et al. 1997b).

Etiology

The etiology of PPMA has not been established. Chronic persistent poliovirus infection is a possibility, but numerous studies to identify poliovirus in PPMA have not provided convincing results. A persistent infection with defective poliovirus is also possible. Another hypothesis is a persistent immune-mediated mechanism, which would explain the presence of oligoclonal bands in the CSF and occasional lymphocytic infiltrates in muscle and spinal cord of patients with PPMA. The most widely held theory is that PPMA is a result of a kind of wear-and-tear process: The surviving LMNs have expanded motor unit territories as the result of reinnervation of once-denervated muscle fibers. This results in a long-standing high metabolic demand on the individual residual LMNs; unknown mechanisms (perhaps secondary to aging) then cause gradual dropout of the LMNs. Alternatively, the enlarged motor units may undergo gradual shrinkage (a type of dying-back phenomenon).

Clinical Features

Patients with PPMA experience progressive new muscle weakness and atrophy that follows a stable course for many years after the acute poliomyelitis infection. Progression usually occurs in the previously affected muscles (either with or without residual weakness) but it sometimes appears in muscles that were apparently not affected by the acute poliomyelitis. EMG reveals that many muscles that were not clinically affected by acute poliomyelitis often have clear evidence of previous disease.

Fatigue, either generalized or focal, is one of the most common features of this syndrome and occurs in the majority of patients. Global fatigue is often referred to as the *polio wall*. Dull and aching muscle pain is common in the involved muscles, and the pain appears to present with an overuse syndrome (i.e., muscle ache after exertion). Other musculoskeletal symptoms include joint pain. The progressive loss of previously maintained motor skills (i.e., new difficulty with arm or leg function, breathing, or bulbar function) is seriously alarming to these patients. Some patients develop sleep apnea, cold intolerance, and vasomotor instability. As patients realize that their motor function is becoming progressively impaired after lifelong compensation, they may become severely depressed.

The neurological examination reveals focal and asymmetrical muscle weakness and atrophy. It is often difficult, however, to determine what weakness and atrophy is new and progressive and what is old. Fasciculations are unusually coarse and large because the motor units in patients with remote polio are markedly enlarged.

Laboratory Features

Because EMG provides definitive evidence of remote poliomyelitis and can exclude diseases that mimic PPMA, it is an indispensable test when PPMA is suspected. EMG studies do not provide the diagnosis of PPMA, however. In patients with PPMA, the motor nerve conduction velocity may be abnormal when recorded from affected muscles. The needle electrode examination, particularly of affected weak muscles, typically shows a reduced number of motor units and chronic neurogenic motor unit potentials. Modest numbers of fibrillation potentials and occasional fasciculations may also be observed in muscles that are symptomatically worsening and in those that are statically weak.

The muscle biopsy specimen usually shows acute and chronic neurogenic atrophy (most often, marked fiber type grouping), which is evidence of a long-standing reinnervation process, but these findings are not specific.

Table 78.5: Characteristic features of progressive postpoliomyelitis muscular atrophy (PPMA)

Medical history
Recovery from acute poliomyelitis
A long, stable course, at least 10 yrs
Signs and symptoms
Progressive weakness, usually in previously affected muscles
Muscle pains and arthralgia accompanying over-use
Laboratory studies
EMG is helpful to identify evidence of previous polio infections
No test is specific for PPMA
Diagnosis
Exclusion of other treatable diseases
Treatment
Symptomatic and supportive care

EMG = electromyography.

Diagnosis

A history of clinical stability for at least 10 years after recovery from acute poliomyelitis is an absolute prerequisite for considering the diagnosis of PPMA. When this requirement is satisfied, PPMA is then a diagnosis of exclusion. All potential diseases causing progressive, focal, and asymmetrical weakness must be excluded. Cervical or lumbosacral radiculopathy, electrolyte abnormalities, endocrine diseases, diabetic amyotrophy, connective tissue disorders, entrapment neuropathies, inflammatory myositis, inflammatory neuropathy, and vasculitis are among the diseases to be ruled out by appropriate laboratory studies, including blood tests, neuroimaging, EMG, and lumbar puncture.

The diagnosis of ALS must be seriously considered in patients with PPMA. Although the full picture of ALS has both UMN and LMN involvement, the progressive focal muscle weakness and atrophy seen in PPMA raises the possibility of the progressive muscular atrophy (PMA) form of ALS. It is important to note that the occurrence of true ALS in patients with remote poliomyelitis is very uncommon, and UMN signs must be identified before a diagnosis of ALS is considered.

Treatment

No specific pharmacotherapy is available to treat PPMA. Thus, management must focus on general supportive measures that preserve function. The care plan should focus on avoiding fatiguing activities that aggravate symptoms; modifying activities to conserve energy, weight reduction for patients who are overweight; and treating underlying medical disorders that reduce overall well-being. Careful screening and treatment for possible sleep apnea and depression are important.

Physical therapy should focus on nonfatiguing aerobic exercise and modest isometric or isokinetic exercise. Stretch exercise is always important. In patients with more serious functional decline, appropriate assistive devices must be prescribed so that patients can maintain activities of daily living and ambulation. Those who develop respiratory

Table 78.6: Characteristic features of multifocal motor neuropathy

Signs and symptoms
    Slowly progressive, asymmetrical muscle weakness and
        atrophy
Laboratory features
    Multifocal conduction block in motor nerve conduction
        studies
    Elevated titers of serum anti-GM$_1$ antibodies
Differential diagnoses
    Benign focal amyotrophy
    Progressive muscular atrophy
    Spinal muscular atrophy
    Chronic inflammatory demyelinating neuropathy
Treatment
    Intravenous human immunoglobulin infusion
    Cyclophosphamide

insufficiency must be fully evaluated by pulmonologists for treatment of hidden pulmonary disease and for the use of noninvasive ventilators. Patients whose employment or lifestyle involves significant physical exertion may need to substantially modify their work duties and other activities.

Multifocal Motor Neuropathy

Multifocal motor neuropathy (MMN) is a treatable disease that resembles motor neuron disease. The term *motor neuron disease* indicates that the site of the disease is at the cell body, whereas *motor neuropathy* indicates that the disease is in the motor nerve fiber or axon. However, it is difficult to differentiate between neuronal cell body disease and axonal disease because the cell body and axon are components of the same neuron. Nevertheless, it is well established that MMN is characterized by a pure motor syndrome that develops in association with motor nerve fiber demyelination. Electrophysiologically, this particular motor neuropathy is associated with multifocal conduction block and elevated titers of antibodies against gangliosides. Clinically, patients develop slowly progressive multifocal muscle weakness and atrophy (Kornberg and Pestronk 1995; Mitsumoto et al. 1997b) (Table 78.6).

Etiology and Pathogenetic Mechanisms

The etiology of MMN is not established. However, anti-GM$_1$ ganglioside antibodies and evidence of conduction block in motor conduction studies strongly suggest an autoimmune disorder. Many experimental studies support this hypothesis. Rabbits immunized with GM$_1$ ganglioside develop a neuropathy resembling MMN. Intraneural injection of serum containing anti-GM$_1$ antibody can induce conduction block in the nerve. Furthermore, anti-GM$_1$ antibodies can bind to the node of Ranvier and anterior horn cells themselves. Physiologically, the antibody can alter K$^+$

and Na$^+$ currents in myelinated axons. The GM$_1$ ganglioside content is greater in motor nerve fibers than sensory nerve fibers. All these findings support the idea that MMN is an immune-mediated disease that predominantly affects motor nerve fibers.

Clinical Features

Clinically, MMN is characterized by asymmetrical, slowly progressive weakness that most commonly begins in the arms, particularly in the distal arm and hand. The relative preservation of muscle bulk despite marked weakness is often a clue to the demyelinating nature of the disease. The course often extends over several years. MMN may also affect the lower extremities, often with slowly progressive footdrop or focal leg weakness and atrophy. Age of onset is generally between 20 and 75 years. Men are affected slightly more often than women are. In affected muscles, the muscle stretch reflexes are diminished but often preserved, whereas regions with normal strength have normal reflexes. Fasciculations are not uncommon, which may suggest a motor neuron disease, such as ALS, but clear UMN signs and bulbar signs are conspicuously absent in MMN. Some patients may report paresthesias or reduced sensation, but sensory signs are usually absent or clinically insignificant. Rare optic neuritis, ophthalmoplegia, and sensory neuropathy also have been reported.

Laboratory Studies

A thorough peripheral electrophysiological study is imperative to establish the diagnosis of MMN. Patients with MMN have, by definition, focal conduction block along the motor nerve fibers. Conduction block is definite when a reduction in the compound muscle action potential amplitude or area under the curve at proximal sites exceeds 50% compared with distal sites of stimulation. Evidence of conduction block is most convincing when the change is found in a distal nerve segment, is focal, and is anatomically distinct from common entrapment sites. Motor conduction velocities and distal latencies are often unremarkable outside of the segments with conduction block. The EMG shows chronic neurogenic changes with evidence of modest or no acute denervation. Sensory nerve conduction studies are normal.

High titers of serum IgM anti-GM$_1$ antibodies occur in 40–60% of MMN cases. Modestly elevated titers of IgM anti-GM$_1$ antibodies also are seen in some patients with ALS or peripheral neuropathies. IgM anti-GM$_1$ antibodies at titers of 1:6,000 or greater are considered specific for immune-mediated motor neuropathies. Unusually elevated anti-GM$_1$ antibody titers (>1:40,000) are often associated with IgM monoclonal gammopathy. Immunofixation electrophoresis for serum and urine must be part of routine investigations when anti-GM$_1$ antibodies are elevated, to exclude monoclonal gammopathy.

Differential Diagnosis

Although focal and asymmetrical muscle weakness and atrophy occur in both ALS and MMN, the prominent UMN and bulbar findings of ALS are absent in MMN. It is important to note that the high titers of serum IgM anti-GM$_1$ antibodies seen in MMN occur in less than 5% of patients with typical ALS. A careful search for MMN is essential because it is improved with treatment, whereas ALS is not.

The PMA variant of ALS is a pure LMN syndrome that often presents with focal and asymmetrical weakness in the distal extremity muscles, mimicking MMN. Although a majority of patients with asymmetrical distal LMN syndrome do not respond to immunosuppressive or immunomodulating treatments, a small minority of the patients whose presentation is similar may have anti-asialo-GM$_1$ ganglioside antibodies or antibodies against NP-9 antigen with low binding to histone H3. Such rare patients may respond to aggressive immunotherapy, and thus detailed serum antibody studies may be justified (Pestronk et al. 1994).

Some patients develop progressive asymmetrical or symmetrical LMN syndromes with predominant early weakness in proximal musculature. These patients are likely to have PMA or adult spinal muscular atrophy (SMA). Nerve conduction studies and serum antibody studies should be able to distinguish these conditions from MMN and chronic inflammatory demyelinating polyradiculoneuropathy (CIDP). Benign focal amyotrophy or monomeric amyotrophy may mimic MMN because focal and asymmetrical weakness slowly progresses over several years. The paraneoplastic syndrome associated with lymphoproliferative disorders may resemble MMN, although it has a subacute progression. The identification of underlying lymphoma or leukemia is the key to differentiating it from MMN.

MMN and CIDP are both characterized by demyelination, and in fact, some consider MMN a variant of CIDP, but the two conditions differ significantly. MMN generally involves distal muscle in an asymmetrical fashion, whereas CIDP mainly involves proximal muscle in a symmetrical fashion. A remitting and relapsing course is common in CIDP but is uncommon in MMN. Although CIDP can manifest clinically as a predominantly LMN syndrome, sensory symptoms are the rule. In contrast, MMN rarely has sensory signs or symptoms or sensory nerve conduction abnormalities. Conduction block with normal conduction velocity is highly characteristic of MMN, whereas slow conduction velocities and abnormal distal latencies, as well as conduction block, are usual features in CIDP. In CSF studies, a high protein level is a cardinal sign in CIDP, but protein level is usually normal in MMN. CIDP responds well to prednisone, plasma exchange, or high-dose intravenous immunoglobulin (IVIG), whereas IVIG or high-dose cyclophosphamide is effective in MMN (Kornberg and Pestronk 1995).

Other immune-mediated demyelinating neuropathies, such as those associated with anti–myelin-associated glyco-protein antibodies or with monoclonal gammopathy, cause not only severe muscle weakness but also prominent sensory loss.

Treatment

Although MMN is considered an immune-mediated disease, prednisone treatment is generally ineffective and can actually worsen the condition. One of the two effective treatments for MMN is IVIG. A total dose of 2 g/kg, divided across 2–5 days, can improve strength in more than 50% of patients. The duration of benefit varies between patients, ranging from 2 weeks to 6 or more months. It is necessary to determine how long the benefits of the IVIG treatment last in each patient. Serum IgA should be checked before treatment: Those who have congenital IgA deficiency may develop severe allergic reactions, including an anaphylactic reaction, to the second or subsequent IVIG treatment because the IVIG preparation may contain IgA. Other side effects of IVIG include headaches and aseptic meningitis, allergic reactions (which can include acute renal failure), strokes, heart attacks, and fluid overload. IVIG treatment is expensive; therefore, objective documentation of improvement, including quantitative muscle strength testing and quantitative motor function testing, is important to prove efficacy.

Cyclophosphamide treatment is also effective and is the only immunosuppressive treatment that may induce a long-term benefit in more than 50% of patients with MMN. However, its potentially serious toxicity, including the increased risk of neoplasia with high cumulative lifetime doses (>75 g), requires a careful risk-to-benefit analysis in each patient. Cyclophosphamide is used only when the patient has a marked disability; with well-established MMN, clear evidence of conduction block, and high serum titer of specific IgM anti-GM$_1$ antibodies; when IVIG treatment cannot be used for any reason; or when the patient has a poor response to IVIG treatment. Pestronk recommends six monthly treatments with intravenous cyclophosphamide (1g/M^2), each preceded by two plasma exchanges. This regimen produces a sustained 60–80% reduction in serum anti-GM$_1$ antibody titer in two-thirds of patients, most of whom have a functional benefit with increased strength. Patients often do not improve when fewer than six monthly treatments are given. Improvement in strength after beginning therapy occurs late, often with a delay of 3–6 months. Remission usually lasts for 1–3 years, after which antibody titers often rise and weakness recurs. Retreatment may then be necessary.

Benign Focal Amyotrophy

The majority of diseases affecting the LMNs begin as muscle weakness in a focal area and in one extremity. In most cases, the disease steadily and rapidly spreads from one extremity to another. However, there is a condition in which weakness begins in a focal area and for the most part does not spread and, in most cases, involves a limited number of myotomes in one extremity. The terms *benign focal amyotrophy, monomelic amyotrophy,* and *juvenile muscular atrophy* are used to describe this intriguing entity (Donofrio 1994).

Etiology and Pathogenesis

The etiology is unknown. Autopsy studies have shown that the affected cervical spinal cord is flattened and the anterior horn is markedly atrophied and gliotic. The number of large and small motor neurons is reduced. Some believe that this disease is mechanically induced as the result of local compression during repeated neck flexion. Others believe that it is a segmental SMA, which is perhaps genetically determined. Rare familial occurrence has been reported. In one family, Werdnig-Hoffmann disease was found in a close relative of a patient who had benign focal amyotrophy.

Clinical Features

The disease often begins at age 20–30 years and has a male preponderance: More than 60% of patients are men. Painless weakness and atrophy in one hand or forearm is the most common initial manifestation, and the symptoms usually remain restricted to a limited number of myotomes. Sometime, muscle weakness causes a claw-hand deformity. The distribution of muscle weakness varies markedly from case to case. Tendon reflexes in the involved muscles are invariably hypoactive or absent. A small proportion of patients (approximately 20%) have hypesthesia to pinprick and touch. The cranial nerves, pyramidal tracts, and autonomic nervous system are spared. The muscle weakens, and atrophy may progress relatively rapidly for the first 2–3 years and more slowly thereafter. The arm is affected in approximately 75% of patients, whereas the leg is affected in the remaining 25%. The disease remains localized in about one-half of all patients; in the remaining patients, it becomes slowly multifocal and may spread to the contralateral extremity. In a few patients (approximately 5%), the disease becomes generalized.

Laboratory Studies

EMG studies are essential to define the disease process and make a diagnosis. Motor nerve conduction studies are either normal or reveal only slight reduction in the compound motor action potentials. No conduction block is identified in the motor nerve conduction studies. EMG examination shows fibrillation and fasciculation potentials and chronic neurogenic changes. The C5–T1 myotomes are most commonly involved when the arms are affected. Although benign focal amyotrophy involves only one side clinically, in approximately 70% of cases, EMG of the contralateral extremities often can identify involvement. In approximately one-third of cases, sensory nerve action potential amplitude is slightly abnormal.

There are no specific laboratory tests for this condition. Serum anti-GM_1 antibody levels are usually normal or only mildly elevated. Neuroimaging studies may reveal some abnormalities in patients with benign focal amyotrophy. Cervical MRI may show the spinal cord to be normal or to have bilateral atrophy or local unifocal atrophy corresponding to the location of amyotrophy, occasionally with T2-weighted changes of focal gliosis. Incidental spondylosis and spinal canal stenosis detected by MRI should be carefully evaluated before the diagnosis of benign focal amyotrophy is established.

Differential Diagnosis

Two diseases must be distinguished from benign focal amyotrophy: ALS and MMN. Patients with benign focal amyotrophy are sometimes initially diagnosed as having ALS. The age of onset is generally older in ALS than in benign focal amyotrophy, although in the latter, muscle stretch reflexes are usually absent or diminished, whereas the reflexes are abnormally brisk in classic ALS. EMG is helpful for identifying the widespread nature of motor neuron disease that is seen in ALS, but careful follow-up is required because differentiating benign focal amyotrophy from ALS may be impossible at the beginning.

Detailed motor nerve conduction studies and serum tests for elevated titers of anti-GM_1 antibodies can differentiate benign focal amyotrophy from MMN. Some cases that were previously diagnosed as benign focal amyotrophy may actually be MMN.

Other diseases that may mimic benign focal amyotrophy include cervical or lumbosacral radiculopathy, which is associated with radicular pains and sensory impairment, and brachial plexopathy, which may cause acute weakness and is usually accompanied by pain and sensory symptoms. Cervical syringomyelia or a benign tumor involving nerve roots or the spinal cord that causes progressive weakness can also mimic the disease, but there are usually long tract signs below the lesion in these patients. Careful EMG and neuroimaging studies should differentiate these diseases.

Treatment

The term *benign* in benign focal amyotrophy is used to distinguish it from "malignant" motor neuron disease, such as ALS. Although this condition is certainly not life threatening, it seriously impairs motor function in the involved extremity. Supportive care, consisting of physical and occupational therapy and effective use of assistive devices (splinting and braces), are the main treatment components. In selected patients with focal weakness in a muscle group whose function is crucial for certain activities, a tendon transfer using spared muscle tendons can be considered.

Table 78.7:   Childhood and adult spinal muscular atrophies

SMA type	Age of onset	Survival prognosis	Inheritance	Defective gene
Infantile SMA (Werdnig-Hoffmann)	Birth to 6 mos	Death by 2 yrs old	AR	SMN gene
Intermediate SMA	Before 18 mos	No walking, survive to childhood	AR	SMN gene
Juvenile (Kugelberg-Welander)	After 18 mos	Survive to adulthood	AR	SMN gene
Adult-onset SMA	After 20 yrs	Slow progression	AR	Unknown

AR = autosomal recessive; SMA = spinal muscular atrophy; SMN = survival motor neuron.

Infantile and Juvenile Spinal Muscular Atrophy

The incidence of infantile and juvenile SMA is estimated to be 1 in 6,000–20,000 births; SMA is one of the most common genetic causes of death and disability in childhood. It is inherited by autosomal recessive transmission, with a gene frequency in the general population of about 1 in 80. Autosomal dominant childhood SMA is rare and probably accounts for less than 2% of all childhood cases. Traditionally, SMA is classified into one of three types, based on age at onset: SMA type I (infantile SMA or Werdnig-Hoffmann disease), SMA type II (intermediate or "arrested" SMA), and SMA type III (juvenile SMA or Kugelberg-Welander disease) (Table 78.7).

Molecular Biology

All three types of childhood SMA have been mapped to the same telomeric region on chromosome 5, at 5q11.2 to 5q13.3. Two unrelated genes in this region have been identified as being responsible for SMA: the survival motor neuron (SMN) gene and the neuronal apoptosis inhibitory protein (NAIP) gene (Lefebvre et al. 1995; Roy et al. 1995). Additionally, these genes have adjacent centromeric copies, the function of which remains uncertain (Stewart et al. 1998).

The SMN gene is located at chromosome 5q13.3, consists of 8 exons, and encodes a protein of 294 amino acids. This protein has no homology to any known protein, however, and its function is unknown. More than 98% of patients with childhood SMA have a deletion involving exons 7 and 8. In the rest, the deletion involves only exon 7 or other types of mutation. The genotype-phenotype relationship is not clear in SMN gene abnormalities, but type I tends to be seen more frequently in patients with larger gene deletions.

The NAIP gene is located at chromosome region 5q13.1, contains at least 16 exons, and encodes a novel protein consisting of 1,232 amino acids that inhibits virus-induced insect cell apoptosis. The protein function of the NAIP gene in humans has not been determined, although its messenger RNA (mRNA) is expressed in various tissues, including the spinal cord. One of the difficulties involved in understanding the NAIP gene's role in SMA is that NAIP mutations are not consistently found in patients with SMA: Homozygous deletions in exons 5 and 6 were identified in 17 of 38 patients with type I SMA and in 13 of 72 with type II or type III SMA. Furthermore, a heterozygous or even homozygous deletion of this gene has been found in patients who have myotonic dystrophy, polycystic kidney disease, or cystic fibrosis but do not have SMA. Even more confusing is the finding that in two families in which a child was affected, the parents were unaffected, but each had a homozygous deletion of exons 5 and 6. Such findings suggest that an abnormal NAIP gene is not enough to cause the SMA phenotype. Large genomic deletions involving more than one gene (perhaps both SMN and NAIP genes) may be required for SMA phenotype expression; it may be that the greater the deletion, the more severe the phenotype. It is also possible that one of these genes is the disease-determining gene and the other is a disease modulator that, when defective, produces a more severe phenotype.

Clinical Features

Spinal Muscular Atrophy Type I, Infantile Form (Werdnig-Hoffmann Disease).   SMA type I begins between birth and 6 months of age. By definition, children with SMA type I are never able to sit without support. Death occurs before age 2 years. Although the pregnancy is usually normal, about one-third of mothers notice decreased fetal movements, usually toward the end of the pregnancy. The symptoms include severe hypotonia, a weak cry, and respiratory distress. Affected babies have no head control, as evidenced by an inability to lift the head when placed prone, and by severe head lag when the infant is pulled from a supine to a seated position (a "floppy" baby; Figure 78.1). The baby's posture at rest is a characteristic frog-leg position, with the thighs externally rotated and abducted and the knees flexed. Limb weakness is severe and generalized and is worse proximally. The infant is unable to sit and raise its arms or legs from the examining table, but there may be antigravity movements of the hands and flickering movements of the feet. Muscle stretch reflexes are usually absent. The sensory examination is normal. Contractures usually do not develop in the early phases but may develop when the long-standing immobilization occurs. Bulbar muscle weakness makes feeding laborious, causes a continuous gurgling, and eventually leads to airway aspiration and pneumonia. Fasciculation of the tongue is reported in about 50% of affected infants. In contrast to the bulbar and

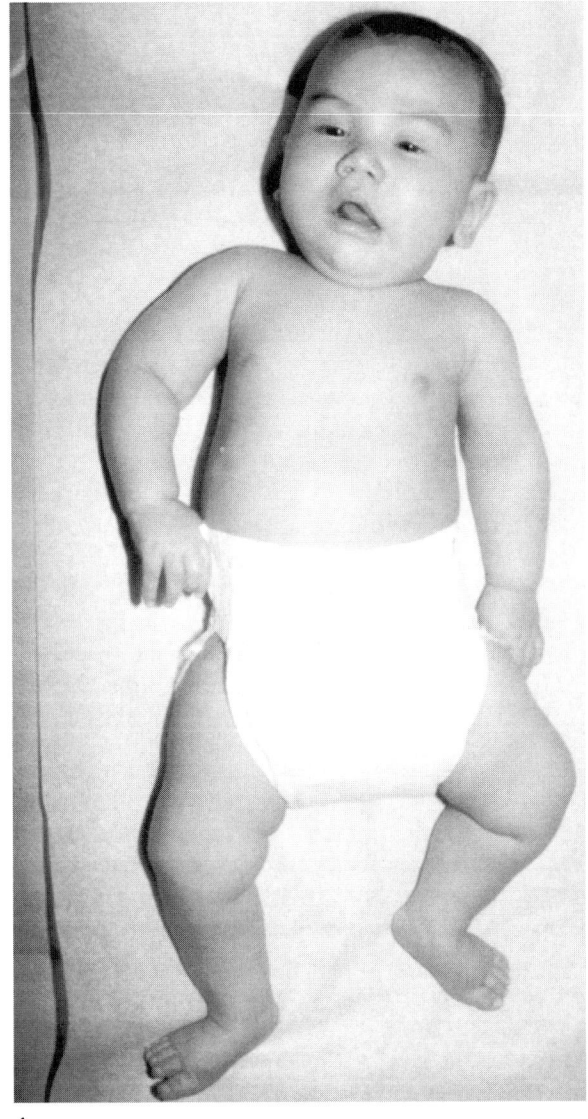

A

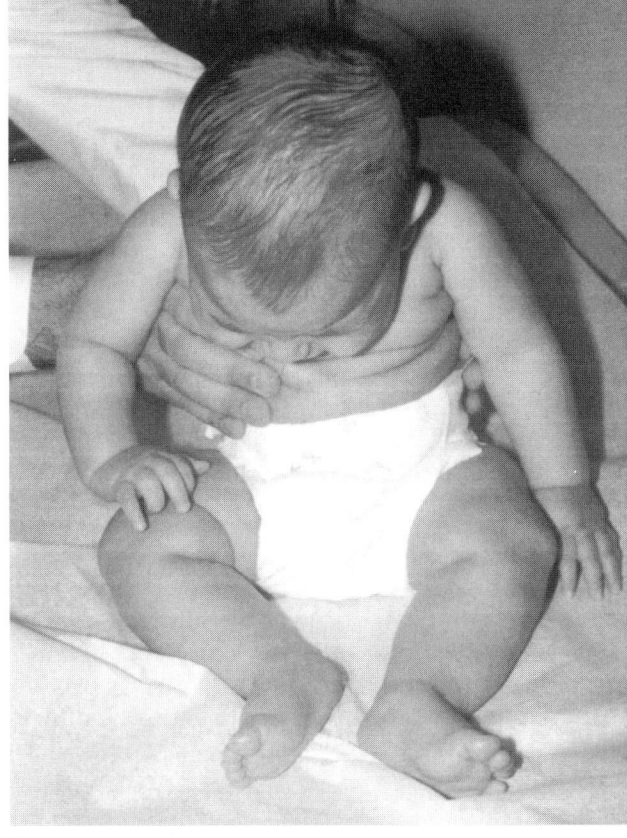

B

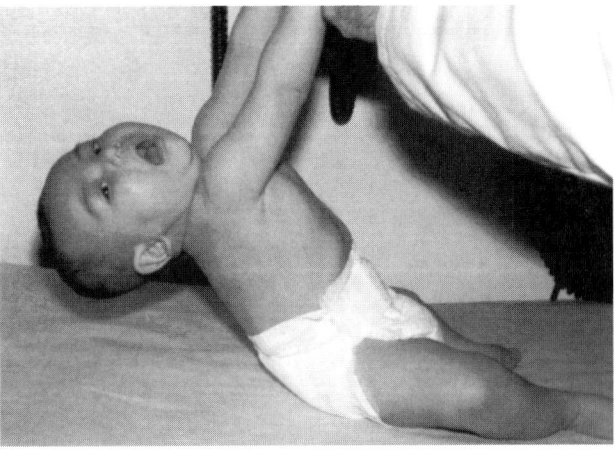

C

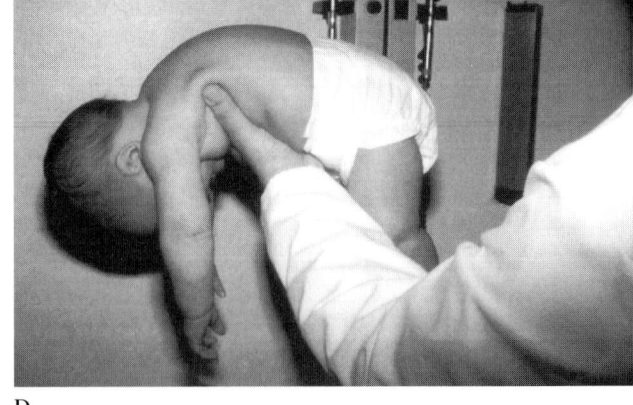

D

FIGURE 78.1 A 6-month-old baby with Werdnig-Hoffmann disease. (**A**) The baby has a typical "frog-leg" posture. The mouth is triangular, and the facial expression suggests facial weakness. (**B**) On sitting, the baby cannot sustain his head upright. (**C**) When the baby is pulled by the arms, the head falls back. (**D**) When the body is held supine, the head and extremities drop by force of gravity, and there is no active body motion. (Coutesy of Neil Fiedman, M.D., Cleveland Clinic Foundation.)

extremity muscles, the facial muscles are only mildly affected, if at all, giving these children an alert expression. Extraocular movements are always normal. The mechanism of the eventual respiratory failure is unique because the intercostal muscles are severely weakened but diaphragmatic strength is preserved.

Spinal Muscular Atrophy Type II (Intermediate or "Arrested" Form). The signs and symptoms of type II SMA usually begin before the age of 18 months. Although the symptoms may be present at birth, an insidious progressive weakness occurs during the first year of life. Delayed motor milestones are often the first clue to neurological impairment. A fine hand tremor is commonly observed by parents and physicians and suggests the diagnosis. The distribution, pattern, and progression of weakness are similar to that found in SMA type I, but the type II disease is quantitatively much milder and slower than type I.

Most children eventually are able to roll over and sit unsupported, but rarely do they achieve independent walking. In the sitting position, truncal muscle weakness produces a characteristic rounded kyphosis. As the shoulders weaken, the child becomes immobilized and wheelchair bound. Contractures of the hips and knees and disfiguring scoliosis eventually develop. Dislocation of the hips may also occur in the patient who has been wheelchair bound for many years. Some patients die in childhood because of respiratory failure, but many others survive into adulthood.

Spinal Muscular Atrophy Type III, Juvenile Form (Kugelberg-Welander Disease). The onset of the juvenile form of SMA typically occurs between the ages of 5 and 15 years. Difficulty in walking is the first manifestation in most cases. As weakness in hip-girdle muscles increases, the child develops trouble in climbing stairs. As the weakness progresses, the patient starts using Gowers' maneuver to rise from a supine position. Pseudohypertrophy of the calf muscles is sometimes reported, but this may be an illusion resulting from the preservation of the calf muscles compared with the severe wasting of the thigh muscles. Eventually, wasting and weakness of the neck, shoulders, and arms develops, but weakness in the lower extremity is nearly always more severe than in the upper extremities. Fasciculations are more often visible than in the other types. As in SMA type II, a fine action tremor is common. Reflexes are uniformly reduced or absent. The sensory examination is normal.

The clinical course of SMA type III is one of slowly progressive limb-girdle weakness. As in the intermediate form of SMA, there are long periods of stability, which may last for years, before progressive weakness develops. The eventual degree of disability is difficult to predict. Some patients remain ambulatory for as long as 30 years after the onset of illness. On the other hand, some patients are wheelchair bound before age 20. Usually, patients require a wheelchair by the time they reach their mid-30s (Mitsumoto et al. 1997b).

Laboratory Studies

Molecular genetic analysis to identify the *SMN* gene deletion is probably the most useful test (Stewart et al. 1998). Up to 95% of SMA type I patients have deletions of exons 7 and 8 of the telomeric *SMN* gene, and a smaller percentage of patients have deletions of the telomeric *NAIP* gene. The proportion of deletions is smaller in SMA types II and III, but nonetheless, the molecular genetic test is so frequently positive that it is the investigation of choice before invasive tests.

Of the invasive investigations, EMG study is also important, especially in SMA type I, but it provides evidence that is supportive rather than confirmatory of the diagnosis of infantile SMA. Compound muscle action potential amplitudes may be reduced, and the EMG may reveal evidence of acute denervation. Sensory nerve conduction studies are normal. The EMG study can be done under conscious sedation in young children. Muscle biopsy can confirm the diagnosis of infantile SMA because histologic changes are distinctive: Sheets of round, atrophic fibers of both type I and type II muscle fibers are present. Usually entire fascicles or groups of fascicles are atrophied, and other fascicles are composed of hypertrophied, mostly type I muscle fibers. In infantile SMA, when EMG and biopsy are done later, perhaps at several months of age, these tests may be more likely to reveal definite diagnostic abnormalities than when they are performed in a newborn.

In SMA type II, EMG and muscle biopsy changes are more fully developed, showing clear evidence of acute and chronic denervation.

In SMA type III, serum creatine kinase (CK) may be elevated by up to 10 times normal. Elevated CK levels usually are not seen in other SMA types. EMG studies reveal active and chronic denervation. Giant, polyphasic motor unit potentials reflect reinnervation and are more frequently seen in SMA type III than in other forms of the disease. Muscle biopsy reveals the typical features of denervation and reinnervation. Another prominent feature of this form of SMA is large and small group atrophy of both fiber types, along with type grouping. The muscle biopsy in long-standing denervating disorders, such as childhood SMA, can be complicated by secondary myopathic changes that include fiber size variability, fiber splitting, internal nuclei, and fibrosis.

Differential Diagnosis

For SMA type I, all causes of infantile hypotonia must be excluded. These include Pompe's disease, centronuclear myopathy, nemaline myopathy, congenital muscular dystrophy, central core disease, and congenital or infantile myotonic dystrophy. A positive *SMN* gene study establishes the diagnosis, but in its absence, the diagnosis can be established with muscle biopsy alone. For older children with suspected type II or III SMA, differential diagnoses of proximal weakness include myasthenia gravis, muscular dystrophies, inflammatory myopathies, and a variety of structural, metabolic, and endocrine myopathies. These disorders are usually distinguished easily by clinical, laboratory, and muscle biopsy features.

Treatment

Supportive and respiratory care constitute the main management goals in infantile SMA. Typical Werdnig-Hoffmann disease is almost uniformly fatal because respiratory failure or aspiration pneumonia usually occurs by age 2 years. However, some affected infants occasionally survive beyond infancy and live into childhood. Because one does not know which patients will survive infancy, aggressive management, including physiotherapy and respiratory therapy, is essential in all such infants.

The objective of management in young children with the intermediate form is twofold: (1) to maintain active mobility and independence as long as possible and (2) to prevent the development of contractures and kyphoscoliosis. Any device, even a scooter board, should be considered to maintain mobility. Patients should be fitted for an electric-powered wheelchair for independence. However, the timing of wheelchair use is critical because its use hastens the development of contractures and scoliosis. Stretching exercises in the major joints, such as the hips, knees, and ankles, should be part of the patient's daily routine.

Patients with SMA have normal or higher-than-normal intelligence. They attend school, often work outside the home in adulthood, and live independently. A well-coordinated, multidisciplinary approach is essential to optimize residual function, especially during periods of disease progression. Physical therapy with stretching exercises and chest clapping; occupational therapy for maintaining activities of daily living; an evaluation at a seating clinic to obtain the best wheelchair; and an orthopedic evaluation to delay or, if necessary, correct scoliosis are among the most important aspects of management. Also critical is emotional support, particularly while children with SMA are maturing. Maintaining an upright position delays the development of scoliosis. Thus, some advocate maintaining patients in an upright position by aggressive use of assistive devices. However, all patients inevitably lose the ability to stand and become wheelchair bound. Although a properly fitting wheelchair does not prevent scoliosis, a poorly fitting chair likely hastens it. A back brace may also potentially delay the development of scoliosis, but bracing in these patients is still controversial. Bracing may actually impair function in some patients by reducing spinal flexibility and vital capacity.

Progressive scoliosis eventually requires surgical correction in the majority of patients with juvenile SMA. In general, surgery should be delayed until growth ceases. In some patients who never ambulated or who lost ambulation early, surgical intervention for severe scoliosis may be considered even before growth has ceased. Improved esthetics, better balance for some patients, and greater comfort in seating are among the benefits. However, a rapid decline in muscle strength may occur with immobilization after surgery. Pros and cons for surgically treating scoliosis must be openly discussed with the patient, although for most, the benefits outweigh the disadvantages.

Genetic Counseling and Prenatal Diagnosis

SMA is one of the most devastating diseases of childhood. The parents of affected children and their relatives should receive genetic counseling, including determination of carrier status of *SMN* and *NAIP* genes. Appropriate family planning is important. For pregnant mothers of affected children, prenatal testing is available only if there is a demonstrated mutation of the *SMN* gene.

Other Forms of Childhood Spinal Muscular Atrophy

Childhood Autosomal Dominant Spinal Muscular Atrophy

Autosomal dominant SMA is rare, accounting for less than 2% of childhood cases of SMA, and because of its rarity, its natural history is not well defined. Typically, juvenile autosomal dominant SMA is a relatively benign disease.

Fazio-Londe Disease (Progressive Bulbar Paresis of Childhood)

Fazio-Londe disease is a rare form of progressive bulbar palsy that occurs between the ages of 21 months and 20 years. Affected children are normal at birth. The inheritance pattern is autosomal recessive or, rarely, autosomal dominant. Affected children develop progressive bulbar palsy and eventual respiratory failure. Neuronal systems other than those of the LMN may be affected in some patients. The differential diagnosis should include the possibilities of a structural brainstem lesion, myasthenia gravis, and the Miller Fisher variant of the Guillain-Barré syndrome. Accurate diagnosis is important because of the implications for prognosis and treatment.

Adult-Onset Spinal Muscular Atrophy

Adult-onset SMA is classified as SMA type IV. International collaborative studies that have analyzed the entire patient population with SMA have found that true adult onset comprises only a small proportion of patients with SMA, probably less than 10% of all SMA cases, with prevalence estimated at 0.32 in 100,000.

Inheritance and Genetic Abnormalities

Although autosomal recessive inheritance accounts for almost all (98%) of childhood SMA cases (types I, II, and

III), it constitutes only 70% of adult-onset SMA cases. The remaining 30% of adult-onset SMA cases are autosomal dominant. The homozygous microdeletions in the chromosome 5q12-13 region (*SMN* and *NAIP* genes) responsible for childhood SMA are rare in adult-onset SMA, which therefore appears to be a separate disease.

Clinical Features

By definition, the symptoms of adult-onset SMA must begin in patients older than age 20 years. The mean age of onset is the mid-30s. The course is relatively benign: Only a small proportion of patients become wheelchair bound in 20 years. Typically, there is slowly progressive limb-girdle weakness. Difficulty in walking, climbing stairs, and rising from a chair or the floor are the main problems in the early stages. Fasciculations occur in 75% of patients. Quadriceps muscle weakness is common and is often the predominant feature. Muscle cramps may occur but are not a prominent feature. Bulbar signs are rare, and respiratory muscles are generally not affected. In adult-onset SMA, bony deformity or scoliosis is rare. Although the distribution of muscle weakness is usually confined to the limb-girdle muscles (Figure 78.2), sometimes the weakness is generalized or distal in adult-onset SMA.

Laboratory Features

Serum CK and aldolase are mildly elevated, usually to less than 10 times the normal upper limits. Nerve conduction studies may reveal normal velocity and reduced compound muscle action potential amplitudes in involved muscles. EMG shows marked chronic neurogenic motor unit changes and modest, if any, evidence of acute denervation. Fasciculations are frequently found in involved muscles. Sensory nerve conduction studies are normal. Muscle biopsy typically shows evidence of a markedly chronic denervating disease process similar to that seen in type III SMA.

Although adult-onset SMA is generally not associated with microdeletions of the *SMN* and *NAIP* genes, these molecular genetic studies may need to be ordered, particularly when time of onset is unclear.

Differential Diagnosis

Limb-girdle muscular dystrophy is autosomal recessive, often has an adult onset, and affects predominantly the proximal muscles; therefore, it can be mistaken for adult-onset SMA. Muscle biopsy should show primary myopathy, and thus the differential diagnosis should be straightforward. On the other hand, muscle biopsy in patients with adult-onset SMA may also show secondary myopathic changes. Differential diagnosis may be difficult in such cases. In this situation, quantitative EMG or single-fiber EMG is necessary to differentiate the two conditions.

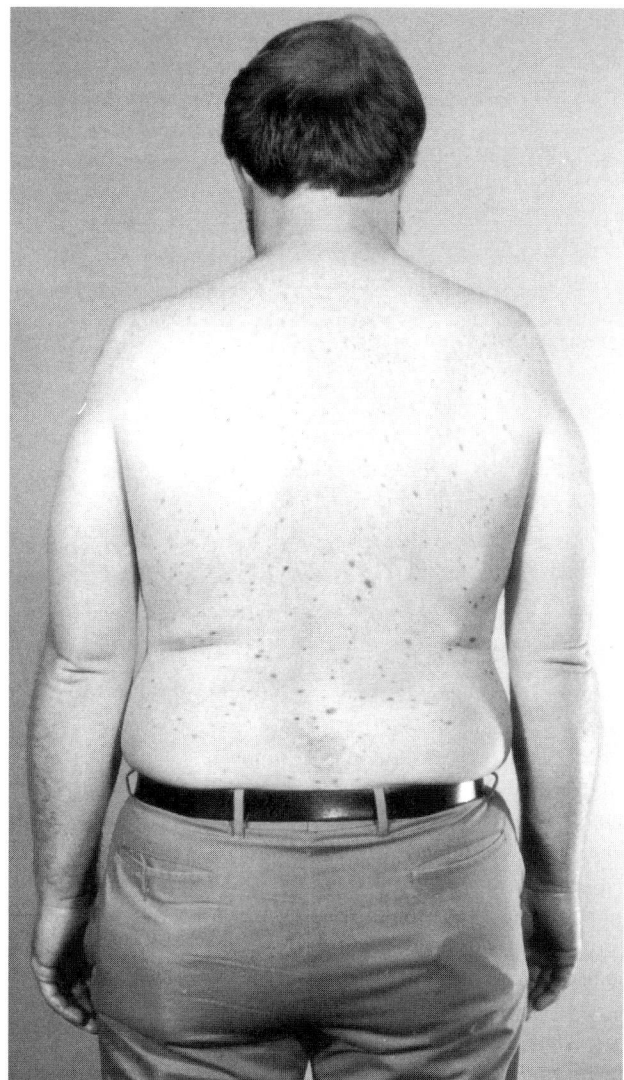

FIGURE 78.2 A patient with mild adult-onset proximal spinal muscular atrophy and marked shoulder girdle muscle atrophy. Note subluxation at both shoulder joints and marked deltoid muscle atrophy.

When molecular diagnoses become available for the several dystrophin-associated glycoproteins that are responsible for the various limb-girdle dystrophies, differential diagnosis will be easier. Other myopathies to be distinguished include polymyositis, adult-onset acid maltase-deficiency myopathy, and distal myopathy. Again, these diagnoses should be excluded by detailed electrodiagnostic tests and muscle biopsy, which reveal the features characteristic of each condition. CIDP may mimic SMA because of the chronic proximal muscle weakness. However, the underlying disease process is a demyelinating neuropathy, and CSF protein levels typically are increased. When adult-onset SMA presents with distal muscle weakness, Charcot-Marie-Tooth disease type II (a neuronal form of dominant hereditary sensorimotor polyneuropathy) must be differentiated. However,

Table 78.8: Characteristic features of Kennedy's disease

Pathogenesis
    X-linked recessive inheritance (only males affected)
    Abnormal CAG expansion in the gene encoding androgen
       receptor protein
Neurological manifestations
    Slowly progressive limb-girdle muscle weakness
    Slowly progressive moderate bulbar dysfunction
    Muscle cramps and prominent fasciculations
    Facial fasciculations
Systemic manifestations
    Gynecomastia (60–90%)
    Endocrine abnormalities (testicular atrophy, minor
       feminization, infertility)
    Diabetes mellitus
Laboratory studies
    Markedly abnormal sensory nerve conduction studies
    Elevated serum creatine kinase
    Abnormal sex hormone levels (often)
    Increased expansion of CAG repeats in the androgen
       receptor gene

hereditary neuropathy always involves the sensory system, so sensory nerve conduction studies and sural nerve biopsies are abnormal. Hexosaminidase-A deficiency in infants causes Tay-Sachs disease, a rapidly fatal gangliosidosis, whereas the same enzyme deficiency in adults (the type of mis-sense mutation differs from the infantile form) phenotypically causes a very different disease, similar to SMA. Although most reported cases of associated SMA have been in Ashkenazi Jews, adult forms of hexosaminidase-A deficiency clearly occur in other populations; therefore, the possibility should be considered.

One of the diseases most difficult to distinguish from adult-onset SMA is the ALS variant, PMA. When there is no family history of similar diseases (a common situation), the diagnosis of adult-onset SMA becomes quite difficult. It is nearly impossible to determine whether a recessive gene is expressed in only one member of the family or the disease is simply sporadic. Until the genetic marker is identified and a test is readily available, this question cannot be answered. However, several features distinguish these two conditions. Adult-onset SMA progresses very slowly, whereas PMA generally progresses at a rate similar to that of ALS. Adult-onset SMA generally shows marked denervation and reinnervation in both muscle biopsy and EMG, whereas PMA findings are consistent with acute denervation with only modest reinnervation.

Treatment

Supportive and symptomatic treatment is the primary treatment goal in adult-onset SMA. Generally, adult-onset SMA progresses very slowly, and patients learn to cope with the disease quite well. For patients who engage in physical work, appropriate vocational rehabilitation may help to accommodate eventual physical difficulties.

Kennedy's Disease (X-Linked Recessive Bulbospinal Neuronopathy)

Kennedy and colleagues reported a new X-linked recessive SMA with bulbar involvement and gynecomastia in 1968. The primary pathology was thought to be in the LMNs, but sensory system involvement was later recognized, which led to a new term, *bulbospinal neuronopathy*. Kennedy's disease, although rare, is more common than adult-onset SMA. Clinically, the disease is easily mistaken for ALS; thus, a clear understanding of Kennedy's disease is important (Table 78.8).

Pathogenesis

The gene abnormality responsible for Kennedy's disease is an abnormal increase in the trinucleotide cytosine-adenine-guanine (CAG) repeats in the region of the androgen receptor gene. In healthy individuals, the repeats range from 17 to 26, whereas in patients with Kennedy's disease, the repeat number ranges from 40 to 65.

There are two independent components to the symptoms of Kennedy's disease: one androgen dependent and the other androgen independent. Gynecomastia, seen in about two-thirds of patients, and occasional testicular atrophy may be associated with the classic function of the androgen receptor. Studies of cultured scrotal skin fibroblasts found that high-affinity dihydrotestosterone binding is decreased in some patients. The abnormal expansion of CAG repeats involves the first exon, an amino-terminal transactivating domain of the androgen receptor protein, and expansion of the CAG repeat causes a linear decrease in androgen receptor function. However, this expansion does not completely eliminate androgen receptor activity. The residual androgen receptor activity is sufficient to ensure normal development of male primary and secondary sexual characteristics, as evidenced by the fact that affected males are usually fertile and not feminized.

The LMN degeneration appears to be androgen independent. The trinucleotide expansion itself leads to neuronal dysfunction through a toxic gain of function. The increased number of CAG encodes an abnormally long polyglutamine tract in the androgen receptor protein. This may alter the normal protein, resulting in protein aggregation, particularly in the motor neuron nucleus, leading to abnormal intranuclear inclusions, ubiquitination, and eventual degeneration of the motor neurons. A similar process is seen in other diseases with expanded CAG repeats, such as Huntington's disease and spinocerebellar ataxia.

Clinical Features

Kennedy's disease affects only males, and patients usually become symptomatic after age 30 years. Prominent muscle cramps, muscle twitching, difficulty walking, and limb-girdle muscle weakness are the characteristic symptoms. Dysarthria and dysphagia occur in less than one-half of patients. Muscle weakness is typically LMN in type, involving the proximal shoulder girdle and hip muscles; the weakness is associated with decreased or absent reflexes and muscle atrophy. Kennedy's disease rarely causes respiratory muscle weakness. Hand and finger tremor is not unusual. Facial and particularly perioral fasciculation are highly characteristic, if not pathognomonic, of this disease, being present in more than 90% of patients. The tongue shows chronic atrophy, often as a longitudinal midline furrow. Although weakness in the facial and tongue muscles is nearly always present, bulbar symptoms are less often reported. Neurological examination of the sensory system shows only modest impairment.

Gynecomastia is a unique feature of Kennedy's disease and is found in 60–90% of patients (Figure 78.3). Endocrine abnormalities include occasional testicular atrophy, some degree of feminization, and infertility in approximately 40% of patients. Diabetes mellitus is also reported in 10–20% of patients.

The increase in the number of CAG repeats correlates inversely with age of onset: The greater the number of repeats, the younger the age of onset. However, the number of repeats has no correlation with other features, such as the severity of weakness, serum CK level, and presence or absence of gynecomastia, impotence, or sensory neuropathy. The phenotypic expression varies markedly within and among families. The course is one of slowly progressive LMN disease. If bulbar dysfunction is severe, the prognosis is less favorable (Mitsumoto et al. 1997b).

Laboratory Studies

To diagnose Kennedy's disease, molecular genetic testing is needed to identify the abnormal expansion of the CAG repeat in exon 1 of the androgen receptor gene on the X chromosome. Serum CK levels may be elevated as high as 10 times the upper limit of normal. Serum androgen levels are either normal or decreased, and estrogen levels are elevated in some patients. However, there is no consistent finding regarding sex hormone levels.

Peripheral electrophysiological and biopsy studies are useful when Kennedy's disease is suspected. Motor nerve conduction studies show the changes of a chronic LMN disorder, but in Kennedy's disease, sensory nerve conduction studies reveal a sensory polyneuropathy. Sural nerve biopsy usually reveals a significant loss of myelinated fibers.

Differential Diagnosis

The clinical features, such as progressive limb-girdle weakness, bulbar signs, muscle cramps, and prominent fasciculations, all resemble ALS, but a careful history and physical examination should provide sufficient clues to distinguish Kennedy's disease. Generally, ALS progresses more rapidly than Kennedy's disease. The EMG in Kennedy's disease shows abnormal sensory nerve conduc-

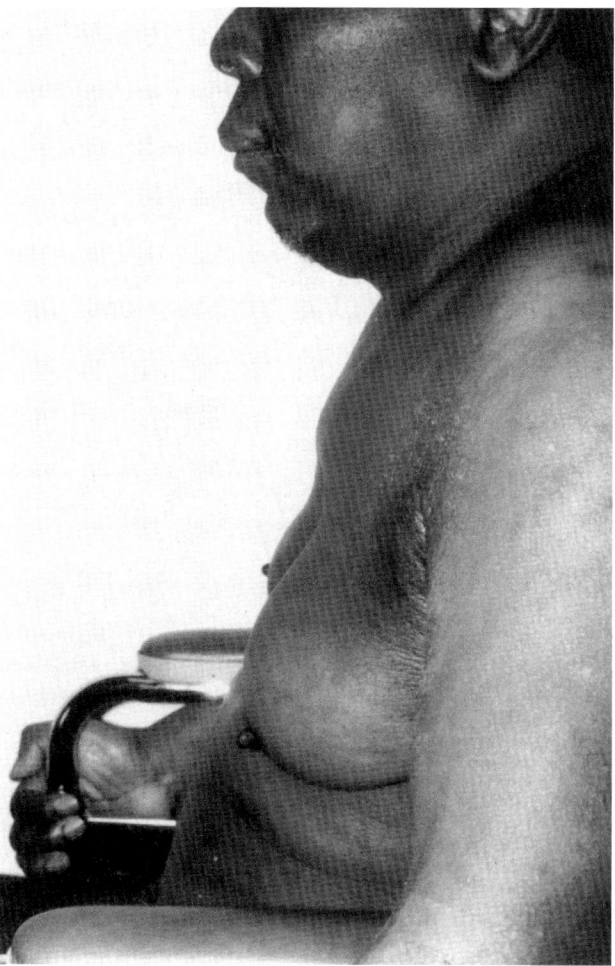

FIGURE 78.3   A man with X-linked recessive bulbospinal muscular atrophy (Kennedy's disease) showing gynecomastia.

tion studies. Kennedy's disease may also be mistaken for adult-onset SMA because of the slowly progressive limb-girdle weakness, but bulbar involvement is very unusual in SMA. Hereditary sensorimotor neuropathy, limb-girdle dystrophy, or facioscapulohumeral muscular dystrophy also may mimic Kennedy's disease. Careful EMG studies and muscle or nerve biopsy analyses should distinguish these disorders. The molecular genetic study to identify abnormal CAG repeats in the androgen receptor gene establishes the diagnosis.

Manifesting Female Carriers

The mother of an affected male patient is an obligate carrier. Female siblings of an affected patient have a 50% chance of carrying the mutant gene on one X chromosome. Female carriers may present with neuromuscular symptoms, such as exertional muscle pain and cramps. The EMG may detect mild chronic denervation in both upper and lower limb muscles.

Treatment

Supportive and symptomatic therapy are the key to treatment, as outlined in the section on adult-onset SMA. Muscle cramps may be problematic; quinine sulfate, baclofen, or vitamin E may alleviate the cramps.

In Kennedy's disease, dysarthria and dysphasia may cause marked disability. Although severe loss of bulbar function is rare in Kennedy's disease, speech therapy as well as appropriate communicative devices may help. Careful nutritional management is also important. Enteral feeding via a tube placed by percutaneous endoscopic gastroscopy (PEG) is the most effective and practical means to meet nutritional and fluid requirements. Genetic counseling is important for patients, potential carriers, and male siblings.

Progressive Muscular Atrophy

PMA is by definition a disease restricted to the LMNs during its entire clinical course. Although it has been questioned whether PMA is an independent disease or represents one end of the spectrum of ALS, the latter appears most likely from studies of familial ALS (FALS). In some families, the same gene mutation causes the phenotypes of PMA and ALS in different individuals. Autopsy studies show that the pyramidal tracts are often affected in patients who were clinically diagnosed as having PMA. Such findings strongly support the idea that PMA represents a form of ALS: PMA (LMN-onset ALS) is at one end of the ALS spectrum, PLS (UMN-onset ALS) is at the other end, and the typical ALS phenotype (UMN and LMN signs) falls in the middle. PMA comprises approximately 8–10% of all adult-onset motor neuron diseases. For clinical therapeutic research trials, PMA must clearly be distinguished from ALS, but for patient care purposes, PMA can be considered identical to ALS.

Etiology

All hypotheses about the cause of ALS are also applicable to PMA (see Etiology, under Amyotrophic Lateral Sclerosis, later in this chapter).

Clinical Features

By definition, the signs and symptoms of PMA remain restricted to the LMNs. During the early stages of the illness, however, it is uncertain whether the disease will evolve into the ALS phenotype. It is generally agreed that not until 3 years after the onset of the disease can one conclude that it will not spread to UMN involvement. Although PMA occurs in both sexes, males are slightly more often affected than females. PMA and ALS differ in several ways. The age of onset in PMA is younger than that in ALS. Also, deterioration in PMA occurs more slowly than in ALS, and thus, survival in PMA is longer than that in ALS.

Focal and asymmetrical muscle weakness in the distal extremities is a common presentation, and it gradually spreads to other contiguous muscles. The weakness and muscle atrophy is purely LMN in type and eventually involves both upper and lower extremities. Proximal muscle weakness can occur, although less commonly than distal weakness. Bulbar symptoms and respiratory involvement are less frequent in PMA than in ALS, but they can eventually cause death. The mean duration of the disease may range from 3 to 14 years.

Laboratory Studies

The serum CK level can be 10 times greater than normal upper limits, particularly when patients are physically active. In patients with PMA, high anti-GM_1 antibody titers should be absent. The peripheral electrophysiological studies can indicate whether LMN involvement is more widespread than clinically appreciated and can rule out other disease processes. Muscle biopsy should show denervation atrophy, but muscle biopsy is usually unnecessary unless the clinical features are unusual enough to cause one to suspect other diseases.

Differential Diagnosis

PMA is generally a fatal disease and has no cure. Therefore, the diagnosis of PMA should be made carefully after all treatable or definable diseases are excluded. MMN may present with focal and asymmetrical weakness, which closely resembles PMA. Detailed EMG analysis and serum tests for anti-ganglioside antibodies should distinguish the two conditions.

Inclusion body myositis (IBM) must also be differentiated from PMA; rare cases of IBM may respond to corticosteroid immunotherapy. Important clues that should lead one to suspect IBM are elevated serum CK levels (more than expected in typical PMA) and a selective weakness in the forearm flexor muscles and quadriceps muscles. The EMG in IBM shows evidence of a primary myopathy mixed with some neurogenic changes. Muscle biopsy is necessary to establish the correct diagnosis.

Other diseases that must be differentiated from PMA, although not treatable, are definable. Adult-onset SMA may mimic PMA, and sometimes, distinguishing between the two is quite difficult, as discussed in the section of adult-onset SMA. A marked chronicity of the disease, as revealed by the clinical history, EMG, and muscle biopsy, may support a diagnosis of adult-onset SMA. The main differential diagnosis of PMA is ALS. When a patient with ALS presents with only LMN signs initially (LMN-onset ALS), one cannot determine whether the patient's condition will evolve into ALS or remain purely LMN (as in PMA). Careful follow-up is therefore essential to make an appropriate diagnosis (Mitsumoto et al. 1997a).

Treatment

The treatment of PMA is identical to that for ALS (see Treatment, under Amyotrophic Lateral Sclerosis, later in this chapter).

Subacute Motor Neuronopathy in Lymphoproliferative Disorders

Rarely, a subacute, progressive, and painless LMN syndrome develops in patients who have lymphoproliferative disorders, particularly Hodgkin's or non-Hodgkin's lymphomas. Muscle weakness predominantly affects the lower extremities. Neuropathology shows a loss of anterior horn cells and ventral root nerve fibers without evidence of inflammation. The neurological disease may be relatively benign, the progression of muscle weakness tending to slow down after the initially rapid disease course. Some patients who develop this LMN syndrome have monoclonal gammopathy, increased CSF protein, or both, which suggests an autoimmune mechanism. Viral infection is another possible explanation for the cause of this paraneoplastic syndrome. UMN signs may develop in a small number of patients.

Postirradiation Lower Motor Neuron Syndrome

Radiation directed to the thoracolumbar paravertebral area for the treatment of para-aortic lymph node metastases from testicular cancer can cause a predominantly LMN syndrome in the legs. Symptoms begin 2–20 years after the irradiation. The disease usually progresses during the first few years after symptom onset but then becomes static. In some cases, it is a pure LMN syndrome, probably due to radiation-induced anterior horn cell degeneration. In others, sensory symptoms and signs as well as sphincter involvement suggest damage to the nerve roots of the cauda equina (Bowen et al. 1996).

DISORDERS OF BOTH UPPER AND LOWER MOTOR NEURONS

Amyotrophic Lateral Sclerosis

Jean Martin Charcot recognized the clinical and histological significance of UMN and LMN involvement occurring in the same patient, and in 1874, he established ALS as a separate disease. ALS is the most common form of adult motor neuron disease; it affects both UMNs and LMNs and has a fairly consistent clinical picture and outcome. The specific clinical features of UMN and LMN involvement define *classic ALS* in the sense that it was described by Charcot and stand in contrast to the ALS variants PLS, PMA, progressive bulbar palsy, and progressive pseudobulbar palsy. Whether ALS is a single disease or a syndrome caused by a number of different conditions remains to be determined.

The classification of ALS is shown in Table 78.9. ALS that presents with signs and symptoms that are exclusively limited to muscles innervated by the lower cranial nerves may be either bulbar-onset ALS or progressive bulbar palsy. The latter term indicates, by definition, that the disease begins and remains only in bulbar muscles throughout the

entire clinical course; however, such a situation is rare. Thus, progressive bulbar palsy is generally synonymous with bulbar-onset ALS.

ALS can be classified according to whether it is sporadic (nonfamilial) or familial. A few other conditions have a phenotypic expression similar to that of ALS, but their relationship to ALS is unclear. These include endemic ALS-parkinsonism-dementia complex and juvenile FALS.

The incidence of ALS is estimated at 1–3 per 100,000 population and is surprisingly uniform throughout the world. Several epidemiological studies have suggested that the incidence of ALS may have increased in the past two decades. Although improved diagnosis and better awareness of the disease may be the main reasons for such changes, the increase is thought to be real because it is independent of the health care, economic, and industrial levels of the countries studied. It is also important to note that the incidence of ALS is similar to that of MS. However, the prevalence of ALS is 4–10 per 100,000 population, which is significantly lower than that of MS, because disease duration in ALS is much shorter than in MS. Both genders are affected, but men are affected more often than women are by a ratio of approximately 1.5 to 1.0. ALS can occur as early as the second decade of life, but the peak incidence is usually in the late 50s to early 60s. Studies suggest that the age-specific incidence rates of ALS increase with age (Gutmann and Mitsumoto 1996; Mitsumoto et al. 1997a).

Etiology

In 1993, mutations of the gene for cytosolic copper-zinc superoxide dismutase (*SOD1*) were discovered in patients with FALS (Rosen et al. 1993). This mutation is responsible for approximately 20% of all cases of FALS and approximately 1–2% of all ALS cases because FALS accounts for 5–10% of all ALS cases. The discovery of the *SOD1* mutation resulted in a major breakthrough in understanding not only of FALS but also of the process of cell death of motor neurons in general (Brown 1996).

In the past few decades, extensive studies in ALS have suggested many plausible causal hypotheses, such as heavy metal intoxication, viral infections, environmental factors, immunological disease, DNA repair enzyme defects, calcium metabolism, and mitochondrial abnormalities. Although there is evidence to support these hypotheses, convincing evidence that one of the abnormalities is primary is still missing. It is possible that ALS is a syndrome caused by several independent factors or a multifactorial disease in which a combination of several factors leads to the disease. In the past several years, however, the mechanisms of motor neuron degeneration have been increasingly clarified, as has our understanding of the potential etiology of ALS. This chapter focuses on glutamate excitotoxicity and free radical injury in detail and considers autoimmune abnormalities briefly.

Glutamate Excitotoxicity and Free Radical Injury. Glutamate, which is the most abundant free amino acid in the

Table 78.9: A practical classification of amyotrophic lateral sclerosis (ALS)

Sporadic ALS
    Classic ALS
    Progressive muscular atrophy
    Primary lateral sclerosis
    Progressive bulbar palsy
    Progressive pseudobulbar palsy
Familial ALS
    Autosomal dominant
        Superoxide dismutase (*SOD1*) missense mutations
        Non-*SOD1* types
    Autosomal recessive
        SOD1 (Asp90→Ala) mutation
        Chronic juvenile ALS (Tunisia)
    X-linked
Western Pacific ALS-parkinsonism-dementia complex

CNS, is one of the major excitatory neurotransmitters, or excitatory amino acids (EAAs), which also include aspartate. Glutamate produces neuronal excitation and participates in many neuronal functions, including neuronal plasticity. In excess, it also causes neurotoxicity. There are two types of glutamate receptors: (1) ionotropic and (2) metabotropic. The former is an integral, cation-specific ion (particularly Ca^{2+}) channel, that is further grouped into two major subtypes, depending on receptor characteristics: *N*-methyl-D-aspartate (NMDA) receptors and non-NMDA receptors (AMPA-kainate receptor). The metabotropic receptor is coupled to the G protein and cyclic GMP, modulating the production of intracellular messengers and influencing ionotropic glutamate receptors. Recent studies in organotypic motor neuron cultures and in ALS spinal cord tissue show that motor neurons appear to receive the glutamate excitotoxic signal through non-NMDA receptors rather than through NMDA receptors.

The significance of glutamate excitotoxicity in neurodegeneration is strengthened by the observation that exogenous glutamate receptor agonists resulted in clinically observable neurotoxicity. Lathyrism (see Lathyrism, earlier in this chapter) is associated with neurotoxicity exerted by β-*N*-oxalyl amino-L-alanine, an AMPA glutamate receptor agonist. Another example is food poisoning associated with contaminated mussels, which presents with dementia and motor neuron disease. This particular food poisoning is caused by domoic acid, another potent non-NMDA receptor agonist. In patients with ALS, a series of endogenous glutamate abnormalities have been demonstrated; for example, glutamate is significantly increased in serum, plasma, and CSF. On the other hand, glutamate (and aspartate as well) and the ratio of glutamate to glutamine are significantly decreased in ALS CNS tissue. When glutamate metabolism is studied by loading with oral monosodium glutamate, plasma glutamate levels increase to a significantly greater degree in patients with ALS than in healthy patients. These studies clearly support the idea that glutamate excitotoxicity is involved in the pathogenesis of ALS, if it is not actually the cause.

Glutamate is normally released from presynaptic axon terminals to the synaptic cleft, where it binds to its receptors, causing signal transduction to occur. After signal transduction, interstitial glutamate must be reabsorbed into what is the main reservoir of glutamate, the surrounding astrocytic glial cells, and, to a degree, neurons themselves. This absorption process involves glutamate transporter or EAA transporter (EAAT) proteins. Four glutamate transporters have been found and are classified according to the CNS cells involved. Among these, the astrocytic glutamate transporter, termed EAAT2, is markedly reduced in patients with ALS, particularly in the motor cortex and spinal cord anterior horn. These findings would explain why interstitial or extracellular (including CSF and plasma) glutamate is increased in ALS. Rothstein and colleagues more recently found intriguing abnormalities in the mRNA processing for EAAT2, such as intron retention and exon skipping, that were associated with abnormal EAAT2 mRNA in more than 60% of patients with ALS. Such abnormalities in EAAT2 mRNA or EAAT2 protein itself may lead to the abnormal function of the glutamate transporter.

When glutamate transporter function is impaired, the amount of extracellular glutamate may increase and stimulate the glutamate receptor repeatedly, allowing excess calcium ions to enter the neuron. Excess calcium ions are usually buffered by intracellular calcium buffering proteins, such as parvalbumin or calbindin. Mitochondria may also function as an extra reservoir for excess intracellular calcium. However, when calcium ions exceed the buffering capacity of the neuron, calcium ions may catalyze activity in specific destructive enzymes that are not usually activated under normal conditions. These enzymes are related to excitotoxicity and include xanthine oxidase, phospholipase, and nitric oxide synthetase. All these produce free radicals, including reactive oxygen species.

These free radicals damage intracellular chemical components, including lipid cell membranes, proteins, and DNA. Superoxide (O_2^-), produced by xanthine oxidase, and nitric oxide (NO), produced by NO synthase, react to form peroxynitrite ($ONOO^-$), which is one of the most potent reactive nitrogen species. $ONOO^-$ causes nitration of tyrosine residues of intracellular proteins. Neurofilaments, various enzymes, and receptor proteins may be particularly vulnerable to tyrosine nitration because tyrosine residues are often associated with the active site on these proteins. Although the mechanisms are still unclear, free radical injury may also lead to apoptosis. It is still unclear, however, which process is the primary cause of cell injury in motor neuron degeneration. One theory is that free radical injury may be the primary cause of cell injury (the inciting event), and glutamate excitotoxicity may sustain this process (the maintenance event), whereas NO may promote injury to other cells (the propagating event) because it freely diffuses from one cell to another (Brown 1996; Rothstein et al. 1995; Rothstein 1996).

Immunological Abnormalities and Autoimmunity. A number of patients with ALS have a monoclonal gammopathy and, on rare occasions, a lymphoproliferative disorder; the prevalence in patients with ALS appears to be greater than that in the general population. This observation has led to a long-standing theory that an autoimmune disorder underlies ALS. More recently, serum antibodies to L-type voltage-gated calcium channels have been found in some patients with ALS. However, this particular antibody is apparently present in other autoimmune disorders. None of the currently available immunotherapies alters the course of ALS, which is a primary reason that autoimmune theory as currently proposed is not widely accepted.

Clinical Features

It is widely agreed that when the clinical symptoms of ALS first appear, the biological disease must have been developing for some time and is well into its course. Electrophysiological investigations in patients in the early stages of the disease suggest that significant remodeling of motor units has taken place by continuous denervation and reinnervation process before affected individuals can recognize muscle weakness. Therefore, an important preclinical, or asymptomatic, stage of ALS may precede the presentation of progressive muscle weakness.

Muscle weakness in ALS begins usually in a focal area, although sometimes the initial weakness is multifocal. The weakness invariably spreads to contiguous muscles in the same region (e.g., hand to arm and then to the leg on the same side). Onset in the upper extremities (hand or arm) is most common, and onset in the lower extremities is second in frequency. In 25% of patients, the weakness begins in muscles innervated by the lower cranial nerves to manifest as bulbar symptoms (bulbar-onset ALS). On rare occasions (1% or 2% of patients), the weakness starts in the respiratory muscles.

Symptoms of muscle weakness vary, depending on which motor function is impaired. For example, when LMN weakness begins in the hand and fingers, patients report difficulty in turning a key, buttoning, opening a bottle cap, or turning a doorknob (Figure 78.4). When LMN weakness begins in the lower leg, footdrop may be the first symptom (Figure 78.5). Awkward walking, imbalance, lack of coordination, or even fatigue may the first symptom when UMN signs develop in the lower extremities. When bulbar muscles are affected, the first symptoms may be slurred speech, hoarseness, or an inability to sing or shout, which may soon be followed by progressive dysphagia (Figure 78.6). Patients with bulbar-onset ALS often initially consult ear-nose-throat specialists. Progressive impairment in bulbar function during the disease course results in drooling (sialorrhea) and weight loss. In those who have a predominantly UMN-type bulbar involvement (pseudobulbar manifestation), inappropriate or

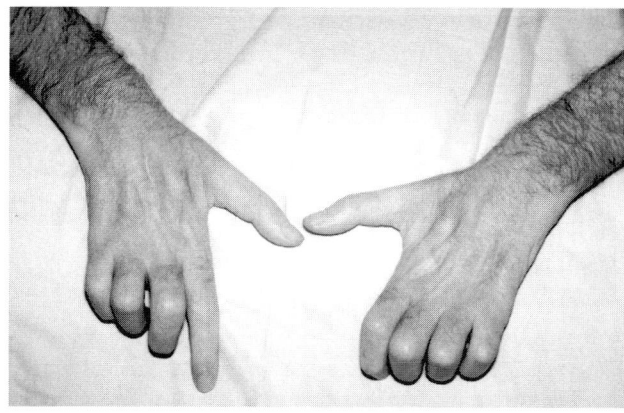

A

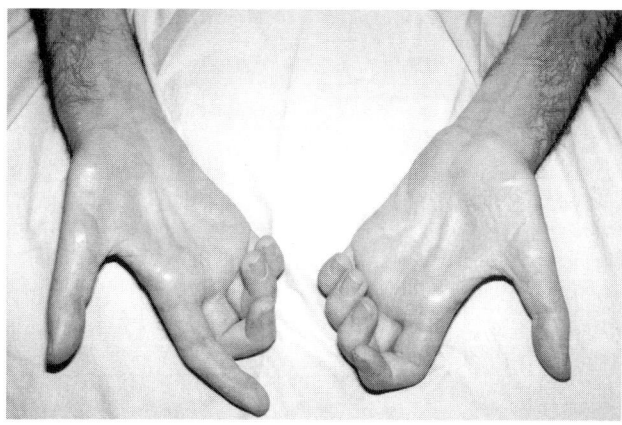

B

FIGURE 78.4   (A, B) Severe intrinsic hand muscle atrophy in a patient with amyotrophic lateral sclerosis. Note the "claw hand" and atrophy of muscles innervated by both ulnar and medial nerves.

forced crying or laughter may be the problems (see Signs and Symptoms of Upper Motor Neuron Dysfunction, earlier in the chapter). In the rare patient who presents with progressive respiratory muscle weakness, respiratory failure may lead to a pulmonary medicine consultation and an intensive care unit admission; the diagnosis of ALS is made when the neurologist sees the patient, who has repeatedly failed attempts to be weaned from the ventilator.

Head drop or droop, a distinctive feature in ALS, is caused by axial truncal muscle weakness, particularly upper thoracic and cervical paraspinous muscle weakness (myasthenia gravis and polymyositis are more common causes of this syndrome) (Figure 78.7). Patients may recognize muscle twitching or fasciculations, but it is more common for them to notice fasciculations only after a physician points them out. Fasciculations are a very important sign of ALS. Muscle cramps are one of the most common early symptoms in ALS. The cramps involve calf, thigh, abdomen, back, upper extremity, hand, neck, jaw, and even tongue muscles. Muscle cramps occurring in these uncommon sites should warn the clinician that the

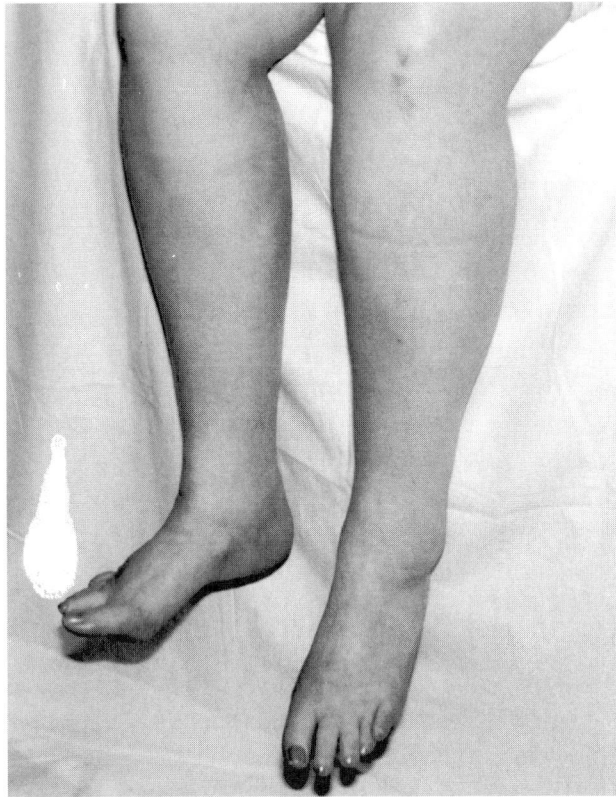

FIGURE 78.5   A typical left footdrop in a 45-year-old patient whose amyotrophic lateral sclerosis began 2.5 years earlier with bulbar symptoms. When she was asked to dorsiflex both feet, she was able to move her right foot only. The footdrop developed 6 months before the photo was taken, and the patient wears a left ankle-foot orthosis.

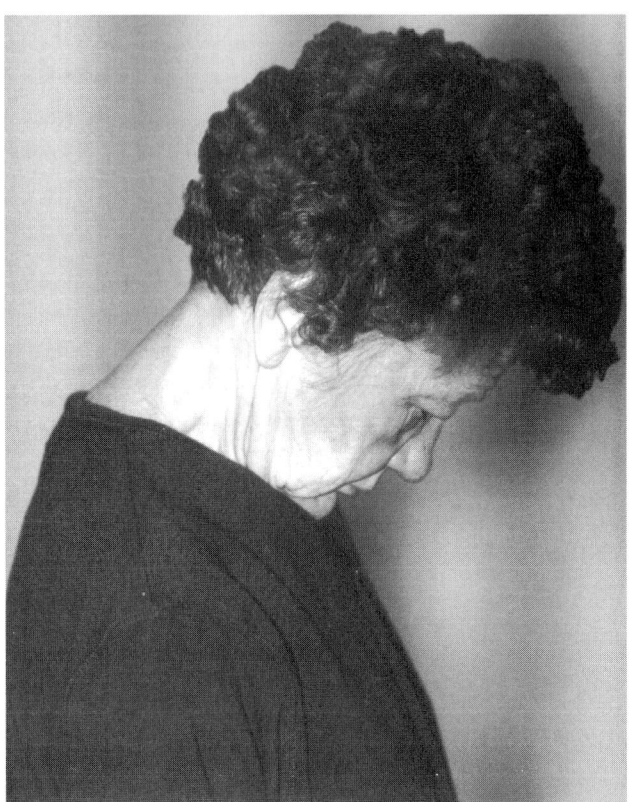

FIGURE 78.7   Patient with amyotrophic lateral sclerosis showing head droop caused by weakness of the thoracic and cervical paraspinal muscles.

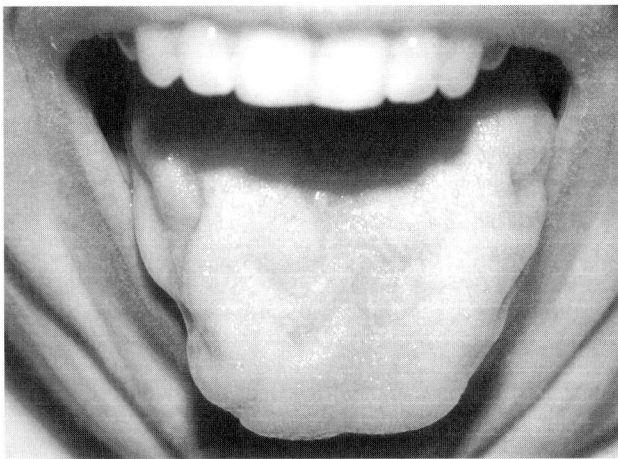

FIGURE 78.6   Atrophy of the tongue in amyotrophic lateral sclerosis.

disease may be ALS, although the cramps, like fasciculations, occur in otherwise healthy people.

Other signs and symptoms include marked fatigue that mimics myasthenia. Weight loss is often rapid and progres-sive. Loss of muscle mass and poor oral intake caused by dysphagia does not always explain the accelerated weight loss in some patients. Depression is a common and difficult problem that merits serious attention because, unless it is properly treated, it affects overall well-being and prognosis.

As the disease advances, motor function is progressively impaired, and activities of daily living (e.g., self-hygiene, bathing, dressing, eating, walking, and verbal communica-tion) become difficult. Accordingly, the patient's quality of life progressively deteriorates. Furthermore, dysphagia wors-ens, causing poor nutrition that accelerates muscle weak-ness. Aspiration of liquids, secretions, and food becomes a risk. Eventually, respiratory difficulty develops, causing the ultimate complex medical problem. At the beginning of res-piratory difficulty, patients may report only difficulty in sleeping when lying supine because of diaphragmatic weak-ness. Patients learn to use multiple pillows and to sleep on their side to compensate for this weakness. In more advanced stages, patients are unable to lie in bed because of frank orthopnea, and headaches are present on awakening in the morning. During the day, patients may have to breathe deeply frequently, mimicking sighs, and have exer-tional dyspnea and dyspnea even at rest.

Negative Features

Patients with ALS may report vague sensory symptoms, such as numbness or aching, but the sensory examination is negative. Other negative signs and symptoms for ALS include the absence of urinary and bowel sphincter dysfunction, higher cortical dysfunction, and impairment of external ocular movements. When patients have these signs, the diagnosis of ALS should not be made until all possible alternative diagnoses have been excluded. It is important to point out, however, that detailed and sophisticated investigations of the sensory and autonomic nervous systems, higher cortical function, and ocular motility may be abnormal in a small proportion of patients with ALS. In fact, approximately 5% of patients may have progressive frontotemporal dementia that appears different from that of Alzheimer's disease.

Natural History of the Disease

When the progression of ALS is analyzed according to the site of onset, the disease appears to spread anatomically. In patients with arm onset, the opposite arm is affected earlier than any other region, bulbar muscles are next affected, and lower extremity muscles are affected last. In patients with leg onset, however, the bulbar muscles are affected long after the arms. The pattern suggests that rostral-caudal progression is faster than caudal-rostral spread. Bulbaronset ALS occurs predominantly in women, but arm involvement after bulbar onset is more rapid in men than in women in the first 3 years of diagnosis, suggesting that gender might affect the pattern of neuronal degeneration. In the majority of patients with ALS, motor function declines linearly and somewhat symmetrically, but the rate of decline varies widely between patients. Occasionally, during the course of the disease, transient improvement, plateaus, or sudden worsening can occur. Spontaneous recovery has been reported, although such cases are rare.

Prognosis

The median duration of ALS, based on several epidemiological studies, ranges from 23 months to 52 months, the mean duration being 27–43 months. About 25% of patients survive for 5 years, and 8–16% of patients survive beyond 10 years. Factors influencing the prognosis of ALS include age of onset, clinical type, and duration from onset to the time of diagnosis. In general, the younger the patient or the longer the duration between onset and diagnosis, the better the prognosis. Pure UMN type, pure LMN type, or pseudobulbar palsy (bulbar signs due to pure UMN involvement) appear to have a better prognosis than classic ALS (mixed UMN and LMN type). Those who survive beyond 46 months and those who are psychologically well adjusted or not depressed seem to have a better prognosis. Those who have low-amplitude compound muscle action potentials, as revealed by motor nerve stimulation, appear to have a poorer prognosis. Low serum chloride levels are clearly associated with a poor prognosis because they reflect accumulation of bicarbonate due to respiratory decompensation.

Laboratory Studies

In some situations, investigations are almost superfluous because there is no alternative diagnosis besides ALS. The presence of hyperreflexia in a wasted arm, without sensory signs, is such a situation. However, most cases require laboratory investigations.

Peripheral electrophysiological studies are important for supporting the clinical diagnosis of ALS and excluding other disease processes. They provide evidence for acute denervation of the muscles that may be clinically undetected. A reduced number of motor units that fire rapidly in response to only modest contraction effort and remodeling of a motor unit that is produced by chronic denervation and reinnervation process are the other essential findings in electrodiagnostic tests. Fasciculation potentials are particularly important in patients who are suspected of having ALS. When no fasciculations are found on EMG, one must be cautious in making the diagnosis of ALS.

Neuroimaging studies are also important in most cases of suspected ALS. These tests are used to exclude structural diseases other than ALS that may cause UMN signs. The most common studies are MRI of the brain and spinal regions. Although the use of myelogram with or without CT scan has declined in recent years, patients with a cardiac pacemaker need such studies when cervical myelopathy must be excluded.

Blood tests should include blood chemistry (electrolytes, liver, thyroid, and kidney profiles), complete blood counts, serum CK, and immunofixation electrophoresis. When the disease appears to be typical of ALS, a test for serum anti-GM_1 antibodies is not useful or necessary. When the disease is atypical for ALS (e.g., the patient is markedly younger than is usual in ALS or laboratory tests are abnormal), lumbar puncture, muscle biopsy, and more elaborate blood tests must be ordered. When monoclonal gammopathy is found, radiological bone survey, bone scan, and bone marrow studies are indicated to rule out lymphoproliferative disorders. Generally, the earlier the disease stage in suspected ALS or the more uncertain the diagnosis, the more tests are required to exclude other possibilities.

A molecular genetic test for the SOD1 mutation is now available, although it is expensive. When ALS appears to be familial, the test should be ordered. It is not a routine diagnostic test when a suspected ALS case is obviously sporadic.

Diagnosis and Differential Diagnosis

As discussed earlier, the neurological examination of patients with ALS should reveal signs of UMN and LMN involvement in a widespread distribution. The World Federation of

Neurology Neuromuscular Diseases Subcommittee on Motor Neuron Disease (1994) established diagnostic criteria for ALS (the El Escorial criteria) for use in clinical therapeutic trials based on identification of signs according to four regions of motor neuron involvement: bulbar, cervical, thoracic, and lumbosacral. The UMN signs are identified by clinical examination alone, and LMN signs can be detected by clinical, EMG, or muscle biopsy findings. If UMN and LMN signs are detected independently in at least two of these regions, the diagnosis of ALS is established (or at least probable), but UMN signs must be in a region above (rostral to) the LMN signs. This particular requirement is important because spinal cord disease can produce UMN signs below (caudal to) the LMN involvement. However, effective use of neuroimaging should exclude such a possibility. The earliest points at which diagnosis of ALS (possible ALS) can be established is when clinical evidence of UMN and LMN involvement is detected in only one region; when neuroimaging, EMG, and laboratory studies clearly exclude any other diseases; or when UMN signs are detected in only one region but EMG or muscle biopsy confirm LMN involvement in at least two regions below the region in which the UMN signs are seen. Again, laboratory studies are crucial to exclude other diseases (Miller and Sufit 1997).

Because there are no specific diagnostic markers for ALS, differentiating all other motor neuron diseases that may produce signs and symptoms of UMN, LMN, or both UMN and LMN involvement is important for establishing the diagnosis of ALS. When UMN involvement is present, PLS, a progressive myelopathy, or HAM must be considered, whereas with LMN involvement, PMA, MMN, adult-onset SMA, and Kennedy's disease must be excluded. The previous sections on individual disorders of the UMN and LMN in this chapter discuss in detail the diseases that must be considered in the differential diagnosis; here the focus is on those that manifest with simultaneous UMN and LMN involvement. A combination of cervical (or rarely thoracic) myelopathy and spondylotic polyradiculopathy is the most important disease to differentiate from ALS because it is common, treatable, and, most important, carries a better prognosis. Pain, which is common in radiculopathy, and signs of myelopathy other than UMN involvement, such as a spastic bladder or posterior column signs, may be missing in some patients. Thus, EMG and neuroimaging tests are crucial to distinguish these two conditions. Other spinal cord conditions, such as an intrinsic or extrinsic cervical spinal cord tumor, can cause progressive UMN and LMN signs in the region of tumor involvement. Syringomyelia must be excluded because it can cause LMN signs at the level of the syrinx and UMN signs below the lesion.

MS may present with UMN signs, but on rare occasions LMN signs initially develop when the ventral root exit zones are affected by demyelinating plaques. Neuroimaging and lumbar puncture studies should distinguish the two conditions. CIDP may manifest as predominantly motor weakness (i.e., pure LMN involvement). A small propor-

tion of patients with CIDP also have CNS demyelinating lesions, which cause UMN signs.

When the disease presents with progressive bulbar palsy, several diseases must be differentiated. A foramen magnum tumor may cause brainstem signs and UMN signs below the lesion. Syringobulbia also causes both progressive bulbar signs and long tract signs (UMN signs and posterior column signs). A brain MRI is sufficient to exclude these conditions. The early stages of bulbar-onset ALS may mimic myasthenia gravis, and at times the differential diagnosis may be quite difficult because fatigability can be prominent in ALS. Unless there are clear signs of ALS (e.g., tongue atrophy, fasciculations, or pathological hyperreflexia [jaw clonus]) or, conversely, clear signs of myasthenia gravis (e.g., ptosis or ophthalmoplegia) bulbar-onset ALS and myasthenia gravis may be confused. Even EMG and testing for serum antibodies against acetylcholine receptor may be negative in cases of myasthenia gravis. Sometimes, patients must be treated for myasthenia gravis until the disease develops more fully, so that it can be clearly distinguished. Bulbar-onset ALS may also be mistaken for a brainstem stroke if the history suggests that the bulbar symptoms began suddenly; the progressive nature of bulbar symptoms and negative brain MRI indicates that the disease is bulbar-onset ALS.

On rare occasions, ALS may be confused with Parkinson's disease, probably because of generalized rigidity that is mistaken for spasticity. Patients may have dysarthria and extremity stiffness. However, a careful neurological examination and EMG studies should be able to distinguish ALS from Parkinson's disease. Multisystem atrophy may present with UMN signs along with LMN-type muscle weakness. Dysarthria and dysphagia may confuse the diagnosis further. However, in cases of multisystem atrophy, autonomic dysfunction and cerebellar ataxia may be present.

Other diseases that mimic ALS include adult hexosaminidase-A deficiency, which is an exceedingly rare cause of motor neuron disease; it can manifest with LMN signs, but UMN signs can develop, thus suggesting ALS. In hexosaminidase-A deficiency, one usually finds signs suggesting more widespread CNS involvement than occurs in ALS, including psychiatric disturbances, dementia, or cerebellar ataxia. In some patients with a paraneoplastic syndrome, broad CNS abnormalities, with UMN signs, ataxia, and chronic encephalopathy, may be present.

Treatment

Presentation of the Diagnosis of Amyotrophic Lateral Sclerosis. Presenting the diagnosis of ALS is the starting point in treating patients with ALS (Table 78.10). Physicians who present the diagnosis of ALS to their patients must be honest and straightforward but sensitive and compassionate because the patients are being given a diagnosis with devastating implications. It is important that the patient's spouse or other family members be involved in this process

Table 78.10: Comprehensive care and management for patients with amyotrophic lateral sclerosis (ALS)

Presentation of the diagnosis of ALS
Specific pharmacotherapy
Symptomatic treatment
Team approach at ALS clinic
Ethical and legal issues
Physical rehabilitation
Speech and communication management
Nutrition care
Respiratory care
Home care and hospice care

if they are available and the patient allows such involvement. Because ALS is well known to the public (widely known as *Lou Gehrig's disease* in the United States), physicians who disclose the diagnosis must be very familiar with the disease because patients may want a lot of information at the time the diagnosis is given. Providing as much general information on ALS as the patient desires at diagnosis is important. The physician must be kind and be sensitive to the needs of patients and their families. It is crucial that the physician strongly communicate his or her willingness and commitment to care for patients with ALS, which provides a sense of hope. Providing information on progress in research, newly available pharmacotherapies, and the possibility of active participation in clinical trials may increase hope for patients (Miller et al. 1999; Mitsumoto and Norris 1994; Mitsumoto et al. 1997a).

Specific Pharmacotherapy. Riluzole (Rilutek) was approved by the United States Food and Drug Administration as the first drug for the treatment of ALS in 1996. The studies that led to riluzole's approval showed that survival was longer in patients with ALS who took the medication, 50 mg/kg twice a day, compared with those that took a placebo (Miller and Sufit 1997). The drug may slow disease progression, but the effect is generally modest, and the majority of patients who take the medication may not see any improvement. The drug appears to be more effective at the beginning of treatment (within the first 16 months), which suggests that it should be started as soon as the diagnosis is established. The side effects of riluzole are relatively minor. Some patients notice fatigue, gastrointestinal upset, and dizziness. To minimize such side effects, we recommend 50 mg/day in the evening, and after a week or two, the patient can increase to the regular dose of 50 mg twice a day. The drug doses should be taken 90 minutes before food to maximize the blood level. Cost appears to be one of the factors affecting whether patients elect to take riluzole: A recent study at several ALS clinics in the United States showed that more than 60% of patients who took riluzole based their decision on the availability of insurance coverage.

Insulinlike growth factor–I (IGF-I [Myotrophin]) has been investigated for the treatment of ALS. Gabapentin, which was originally approved for treating epilepsy, is now widely used to treat various pain syndromes and has been tried for the treatment of ALS. Clinical trials with subcutaneous injections of ciliary neurotrophic factor and brain-derived neurotrophic factor (BDNF) showed no clinical benefit. In post hoc analyses, however, those who developed side effects from BDNF had a significantly better survival rate. These findings have encouraged further clinical trials of BDNF (BDNF Study Group 1999). Other clinical trials are investigating an oral agent that stimulates endogenous neurotrophic factors. Several other novel agents, such as oral non-NMDA receptor antagonist and other neuroprotective agents, are likely to come to clinical trials.

Aggressive Symptomatic Treatment. Although specific pharmacotherapy is still markedly limited for the treatment of ALS, symptomatic treatment can substantially improve a patient's symptoms and discomfort. Although ALS is considered incurable, this is not synonymous with *untreatable.* Providing aggressive symptomatic treatment is essential for managing the daily problems of patients with ALS. Table 78.11 summarizes specific medications that are helpful and nonpharmacological symptomatic treatments.

Team Approach at the Amyotrophic Lateral Sclerosis Clinic. The care for patients with ALS is especially challenging and differs from that for patients with other neurodegenerative disorders because of its rapid progression, impending respiratory difficulty, and unique loss of function, such as inability to communicate or eat. Treatment requires a strong commitment from everyone involved, including patient, family, and health care professionals; all must work together to provide the most appropriate treatment and to give meaning and value to the patients and caregivers. Such care and management appears to be most effective when provided in ALS clinics in which an experienced multidisciplinary team is available. The team often consists of neurologists, nurses, physical therapists, occupational therapists, dietitians, speech pathologists, and social workers. Pulmonary specialists and other health professionals should be available at least on an on-call basis. The team's goal is to make the patient independent as long as possible and to provide psychosocial support to patients and families using a holistic approach.

Ethical and Legal Issues. Several issues that are fundamental for the care of any patient require particular attention for patients with ALS. The patient should make all treatment decisions, and physicians must respect the patient's right to self-determination. In ALS, ethical and legal issues are particularly important in daily patient care because of the disease's progressive and terminal nature. Physicians

Table 78.11: Symptomatic treatment in amyotrophic lateral sclerosis

Symptoms	Pharmacotherapy	Other therapy
Fatigue	Pyridostigmine	Energy conservation
Antidepressants	Work modification	—
Amantadine	Assistive devices	—
Spasticity	Baclofen	Physical therapy
	Tizanidine	Range-of-motion exercises
	Dantrolene sodium	
	Diazepam	
Cramps	Quinine sulfate	Massage
	Baclofen	Physical therapy
	Vitamin E	
Fasciculations	Carbamazepine	Reassurance
Sialorrhea	Anticholinergic drugs	Mechanical clearing
	Tricyclic antidepressants	Aspiration devices
		Salivary gland radiation
Thick mucinous saliva	Beta blocker	Increased oral liquid intake
Pseudobulbar laughing and crying	Tricyclic antidepressants	None
	L-Dopa/carbidopa	
	Lithium	
Pulmonary secretion and expectoration	Dextromethorphan	Hydration
	Organidin	Moist air
		Aspiration devices
		In-exsufflator
Aspiration	Cisapride	Modified food consistency
		Tracheostomy with cuffed tube
		Modified laryngectomy and tracheal diversion
Joint pains	Anti-inflammatory drugs	Range-of-motion exercises
	Analgesics	Heat
Depression	Tricyclic antidepressants	Counseling
	SSRIs	Support group meetings
		Psychiatric consultation
Insomnia	Zolpidem tartrate	Hospital bed
	Lorazepam	Nocturnal BiPAP ventilator
	Opioids	
Anxiety	Buspirone hydrochloride	Counseling
	Alprazolam	
	Opioids	
Respiratory failure	Bronchodilators	Noninvasive ventilation
	Morphine sulfate	Permanent ventilation
Constipation	Metamucil	Increase oral liquid
	Bisacodyl suppositories	Exercise
	Lactulose and other laxatives	

BiPAP = bi-level positive airway pressure ventilator; SSRIs = selective serotonin reuptake inhibitors.

must educate the patient about the disease and treatment options in a way that is objective and nondirective, so patients can make their own decisions.

Physicians are also responsible for discussing advance directives with patients. At some point during the early stages of the disease, the physician (and sometimes, a nurse and social worker as well) must raise the issues of the living will and durable power of attorney for health care. Such a discussion should be initiated long before the patient begins to face the terminal stages of the disease. The advance directives are designed to protect and respect patients' wishes about care during the terminal stages, when any life-threatening events take place, or when they become physically or mentally unable to make decisions by themselves. It is difficult for anyone involved to initiate discussion of such issues, but the physician who offers kindness and compassion during the discussion makes this process less emotionally traumatic for everyone. It is also important to emphasize that the patient's decisions are not final. Periodically, and when significant changes are occurring, one should ask patients if they have changed their minds about these issues. One must also remember, however, that *not* making a decision is a type of decision making; thus, physicians must be forbearing with patients who find it impossible to make a decision.

Physical Rehabilitation. The main goal of rehabilitation for patients with ALS is to improve their ability to live with the disease. The treatment should keep the patient as active and independent as possible. Therefore, in all stages of the disease, rehabilitation is aimed at maintaining the patient at an optimal functioning level and preventing complications secondary to disuse of muscles and immobilization. In all aspects of rehabilitation, effective education of patients and caregivers is necessary.

Various types of exercise, including exercises that maintain or enhance strength, endurance, and range of motion, are critical in rehabilitating patients with ALS. Although the effects of strengthening and endurance exercises in patients with ALS are not well understood, excessive exercise appears to injure muscle fibers and may also injure the remaining functional motor neurons. The physiological basis of such events is not clear, nor is the mechanism of fatigue in ALS. Whether patients should avoid strengthening and endurance exercise is controversial, but strengthening exercises that stop short of fatigue, such as isometric exercise of unaffected muscles or accessory muscles, should be encouraged. Avoiding fatigue not only from exercise, but also from ordinary daily activities, is important. It is agreed that range-of-motion exercise is critically important for these patients throughout all stages of the disease. With proper education and monitoring by physical therapists, the patient and caregivers can effectively carry out an exercise program.

To maintain the patient's independence, assistive and adaptive equipment should be used judiciously and effectively. Arm and hand function is essential for many activities of daily living. Several orthoses, such as wrist extensor supports, mobile arm supports, and thumb shell splints, are highly effective for patients with hand and arm weakness. A wide array of modified tools that enhance daily function are available to patients.

Weakness of the neck extensor muscles causes head droop in patients with ALS and can be difficult to manage. For a mild head droop, a soft cervical collar is often effective; several types of rigid cervical orthoses are also available. As the problem becomes more pronounced, custom-made braces may be required, but they are not always effective. The ankle-foot orthosis is probably the most frequently used brace for patients with ALS, but some patients find it inconvenient because it prevents plantar flexion. For such patients, a two-piece plastic articulated orthosis is available.

During the early stages of gait difficulty, a cane is often helpful. When weakness progresses, the patient may require a walker. When independent walking becomes too fatiguing or impossible, a wheelchair becomes an essential adaptive device. Important considerations are whether the patient should have a manually operated or motorized wheelchair and the choice of special features and options for the wheelchair. Successful rehabilitation also includes an evaluation of the home environment. Home equipment can easily help preserve a patient's independence and safety.

Speech and Communication Management. Speech and communication dysfunction in the patient with ALS is probably one of the most serious factors reducing quality of life. An early and proactive approach is important. Ideally, speech pathologists should assess speech and communication function when impairment of function is first recognized. The goal of management is to help the patient maintain independent communication for as long as possible. To maximize communicative ability, I use a six-step approach as the disease progresses:

1. Maximize intelligibility strategies (e.g., teach the patient to speak slowly and face-to-face).
2. Introduce energy-conserving techniques.
3. Train the patient's main listener or communication partner.
4. Introduce an approach that includes nonverbal techniques (gestures and other body language).
5. Incorporate assistive devices (such as a palatal prosthesis) and augmentative communication devices and techniques.
6. Refer the patient for a complete augmentative and alternative communication evaluation by a speech pathologist.

Numerous communication devices are available that vary in sophistication and complexity. They range from simple and relatively inexpensive mechanical devices, such as alphabet or picture boards, to specialized and more expensive electronic devices, such as a voice synthesizer.

Nutritional Care. Bulbar-onset ALS, constituting approximately 25–30% of all cases of ALS, presents with progressive dysphagia. Even in patients with spinal-onset ALS, the majority eventually develop dysphagia sooner or later during the course of the disease. Oral intake progressively declines, which leads to accelerated weight loss and malnutrition, primarily secondary to energy loss (need for carbohydrate) but not protein loss. Malnutrition further aggravates disease progression in ALS.

Therefore, in every patient with ALS, nutritional status must be carefully evaluated at each visit. Two of the best indicators of a change in nutritional status is a change in body weight and a history of how the patient eats. In the history, one looks for the presence of cough or choking during swallowing, an increase in the time needed to finish a regular meal, and the patient's reasons for ending a meal (i.e., whether he or she has reached satiety or is too fatigued to continue eating). Although physicians can obtain such a history, evaluation by an experienced dietitian is often most helpful. Initially, patients should change the form and texture of their food and use a high-calorie food supplement, but eventually, such measures become insufficient to maintain the patient's weight, and enteral tube feeding becomes imperative.

A PEG is a standard, minor surgical procedure to effectively place an enteral tube and is performed by gastroenterologists or general surgeons. Although it is relatively simple surgery for otherwise healthy patients who have an isolated dysphagia, patients with ALS pose particular difficulties. By the time a PEG tube is needed, they often have impending respiratory failure that may complicate the procedure and even result in a poor outcome. Although every patient with progressive dysphagia should be advised to have a PEG tube placed, the timing of the procedure is critical. Generally, the earlier the procedure is done, the greater the benefits, because pulmonary complication is avoided. However, despite extensive education of patients and their families, patients are often very reluctant to consider PEG, viewing it as quite invasive. It is important to emphasize that those who receive a PEG tube can continue to eat by mouth. The purpose of enteral feeding is to provide calories and fluid but not to prevent aspiration. Aspiration found by the modified barium swallow test, therefore, may not be used as a laboratory indication for PEG. The enteral feeding tube should be placed in the stomach rather than the jejunum to avoid the symptoms of dumping syndrome. Jejunostomy should be reserved for patients with gastroparesis or incompetence of the cardiac sphincter, both of which are rare in ALS. After the PEG insertion, experienced dietitians must carefully assess the daily calorie and fluid requirements. Choking while eating and aspiration of saliva require consideration of a cuffed endotracheal tube to protect the airway and prevent aspiration pneumonia.

Relative contraindications for a PEG procedure include previous gastric surgery, major esophageal disease, and potentially severe respiratory failure. For patients with such contraindications, a nasogastric tube feeding is an alternative option. Patients often decline any type of feeding tube despite their impending inability to consume food and liquid orally. For such patients, sufficient palliative care should be instituted. It is important to remember, however, that patients who do not receive enteral feeding rarely report hunger because their nutritional requirements seem to be markedly reduced.

Respiratory Care. Except for rare patients who present with respiratory failure as the first manifestation of ALS, respiratory muscle weakness develops insidiously during the course of the disease. Respiratory failure is the cause of death in most patients with ALS. Currently, tracheostomy and mechanical ventilators easily prolong life in patients with ALS. However, issues of quality of life, psychological burdens experienced by patients and families, the staggering medical costs of mechanical ventilation, and other medical caregivers' expenses make the decision to use a mechanical ventilator very difficult. The recent advent of noninvasive positive pressure ventilation has changed this situation drastically. We vigorously support using this type of ventilation, particularly the bi-level positive airway pressure (BiPAP) ventilator, as an interim method of respiratory support before a major decision for a permanent ventilator is needed. Every patient with ALS who develops respiratory failure should try BiPAP. However, a number of patients, particularly those who have severe bulbar palsy, cannot tolerate a BiPAP ventilator. Also, those who have used BiPAP ventilation for some time, perhaps months or even years, may develop progressive respiratory inadequacy when BiPAP alone becomes insufficient. Thus, these patients eventually face the difficult decision of whether to use an invasive ventilator.

The physician is responsible for carefully assessing the patient's respiratory status. At every office visit, the slow or forced vital capacity should be measured. In the early stages of the disease, a pulmonologist should be consulted for a baseline pulmonary evaluation. It is crucial that the treating neurologist work with an experienced pulmonologist who has expertise and interest in pulmonary care for patients with ALS. Discouraging smoking and treating underlying pulmonary diseases, when possible, are also essential. Vaccination for pneumonia and influenza are part of routine respiratory care. Judicious use of antibiotics for impending pulmonary infection is advisable. Using an intermittent positive pressure breathing machine can expand the lung and reduce atelectasis in patients who have decreased breath sounds on examination (Miller et al. 1999).

When patients experience nocturnal respiratory difficulty, a home pulse oximeter should be ordered to monitor oxygen denaturation at night. If there is any evidence of oxygen denaturation, patients must be treated with a nocturnal BiPAP machine. Even during the day, BiPAP can be used effectively to alleviate respiratory muscle fatigue. Some patients have used BiPAP ventilation 24 hours a day and maintain an active life and relative independence. However, when all attempts to make the patient's life comfortable are unsuccessful, regardless of the use of a ventilator, compassionate and effective palliative care must be implemented. Judicious amounts of opioids, diazepam, and oxygen should be prescribed to allow patients to live their final days with dignity and in as much comfort as possible.

Home Care and Hospice Care. When the patient's condition deteriorates, home hospice care or admission to an alternative care site is required. Home care nurses are crucial for evaluating the home environment, the patient, and the family situation; they relay information to physicians for further recommendations, educate patients and caregivers, and even sometimes counsel patients and families. Close collaboration between patients, their caregivers, home care nurses and, ideally, the ALS clinic team ensures effective and satisfying home care. When a patient has no caregiver, a site other than the home should be chosen for extended care. In the terminal stages, hospice care should be started. The patient's primary physician must certify the patient's terminal medical status, but in situations such as ALS, hospice care should be used in earlier stages, before the patient develops respiratory failure. Hospice care provides highly effective palliative care to patients and their families. Just as important, hospice philosophy strongly affirms life, so that patients in the terminal stages of disease can maintain their independence and dignity to the greatest degree possible.

Amyotrophic Lateral Sclerosis with Dementia

Although it is rare, dementia can occur in patients who have otherwise typical ALS. Epidemiological data on concomitant dementia are scarce, but its frequency is reported to be less than 5% in patients with ALS. Mild dementia may not be detected, particularly in patients with bulbar palsy whose impaired ability to communicate verbally makes assessing mental status particularly difficult. In fact, dementia in ALS seems to be more common in those with bulbar palsy than in those with spinal-onset ALS. When dementia develops, confusion, forgetfulness, and poor memory are the usual early symptoms. Verbal and nonverbal fluency is also frequently impaired in these patients. However, behavioral changes and psychotic manifestations occur rarely. Care must be taken to exclude depression as a cause of "pseudodementia." Cognitive dysfunction and dementia in patients with ALS is closely associated with UMN involvement. Positron emission tomography and magnetic resonance spectroscopy analyses suggest that in patients with ALS with dementia, there is broader dysfunction than in uncomplicated ALS and that it affects the frontal and temporal lobes.

The dementia in ALS may be due to Alzheimer's disease in some patients. In most cases, the dementia in ALS is clearly distinct because neuronal degeneration and spongiform changes (status spongiosis) are present in the superficial layers of the frontotemporal cerebral cortices, and the substantia nigra is also frequently involved.

Autosomal Dominant Familial Amyotrophic Lateral Sclerosis and *SOD1* Mutation

In 5–10% of ALS patients, the disease is hereditary and the majority of cases have autosomal dominant inheritance. The frequency of these FALS cases may be higher than estimated: The affected individuals in the parents' generation may have died early, before the disease manifested. Occasionally, a parent develops the disease some years after the index son or daughter has developed ALS. In approximately 15–20% of patients with FALS, there is a mutation of the *SOD1* gene, located on chromosome 21q21 (Rosen et al. 1993). Although autosomal recessive or X-linked ALS has been identified in rare families, the genes responsible for the remaining 80% of all FALS cases still remain to be discovered.

Genetics and Protein Chemistry

The SOD enzyme detoxifies the superoxide anion (O_2^-) by proton H^+ to produce hydrogen peroxide and oxygen. There are three SOD enzymes: cytosolic Cu-Zn SOD (SOD1), mitochondrial Mn SOD (SOD2), and extracellular SOD (SOD3). The SOD1 protein is a monomer composed of 153 amino acids and weighing 16 kD. It contains one atom each of copper and zinc. The SOD1 form is coded by a gene consisting of 153 codons in five exons. The SOD1 enzyme is a dimer that is formed by strong hydrophobic interaction of two SOD1 monomers. The SOD1 active site contains the copper atom, and O_2^- is attracted at this site for the enzymatic reaction. SOD1 is abundant, accounting for as much as 1% of all protein in some neurons.

The majority of abnormalities in the *SOD1* gene are point mutations in which one nucleotide is substituted for another (missense mutation). This substitution usually results in the incorporation of a wrong amino acid in the protein. Other rare mutations include two splice-junction mutations, a dinucleotide deletion, and a premature stop codon. More than 60 distinct point mutations have been reported; mutation can occur in all five exons, although they are rare in exon 3.

Pathogenesis

Mutant SOD1 protein is often unstable, with the biological half-life reduced by an average of 30–70%. The activities of these mutant SOD1 enzymes also vary greatly, ranging from completely normal (aspartic acid replaced with alanine at codon 90) to entirely absent (glycine replaced with arginine at codon 85). Thus, the resulting cellular SOD1 activity in patients with FALS may be normal or reduced by up to 50%. In the latter case, the residual enzyme activity is maintained entirely by the normal SOD1 allele. Total SOD1 enzyme activity correlates poorly with the severity of the disease in FALS. Moreover, SOD1-knockout mice (animals genetically engineered to be born with no SOD1 proteins) have no motor neuron degeneration. Evidently, reduced enzyme activity cannot explain the mechanism of motor neuron degeneration in FALS with *SOD1* mutations.

An alternative hypothesis proposes that the mutated SOD1 protein might have new properties that are toxic to neurons; in other words, there is a "toxic gain of function" in mutated SOD1. Gained properties could include the following:

New toxic functions
Exposure to the cell environment of the toxic metal-ions (copper or zinc), which are normally surrounded by the SOD1 protein
Interference with the remaining normal SOD1 function by the abnormal SOD1 protein

The idea of new toxic functions for the mutant protein is supported by experiments in which multiple copies of the abnormal FALS *SOD1* gene are transferred to transgenic mice or cultured motor neurons. In these experiments, mutant SOD1 proteins are found to have structural abnormality, in which copper-related active site is exposed more to cytosolic environment and stimulates the production of hydroxy radicals. Therefore, mutant *SOD1* appears to produce excess reactive oxygen species, leading to free radical injury in motor neurons (Brown 1996).

Clinical Features

The gene in FALS has complete penetrance; thus, skipping a generation is unlikely. Phenotypic expression, however, may vary greatly between families and even among affected members of the same family. The clinical features of individual FALS patients with or without an *SOD1* gene mutation overlap those of patients with sporadic ALS. Generally, the diagnosis of FALS can be established only by the existence of other family members affected by ALS. However, there are some subtle differences between FALS and sporadic ALS. Lower-limb onset is more common in FALS. The age of onset for FALS is usually between 35 and 65 years and averages about 46 years of age, which is at least 10 years earlier than that of sporadic ALS. Another interesting difference is the male to female ratio: It is 1 to 1 in FALS but about 1.5 to 1.0 in sporadic ALS. Neuropathological analysis in FALS shows frequent posterior column involvement, although clinical signs of this pathological change are not usually apparent.

The rapidity of disease progression is the one feature that is often stereotypical within some families. For example, the two most common mutations, alanine replaced with valine at codon 4 in exon 1 and histidine replaced with arginine at codon 43 in exon 2, are associated with rapid progression, and most patients die within 1 year. In contrast, other mutations, such as histidine replaced with arginine at codon 46 in exon 2 and glycine replaced with arginine at codon 37 in exon 2, are associated with prolonged disease, with duration averaging more than 15 years. SOD1-linked FALS presenting with predominantly LMN signs is associated with a mutation in which valine replaces leucine at codon 84 in exon 4 (Cudkowicz et al. 1997; Juneja et al. 1997).

Autosomal Recessive SOD1 Mutation

Recessive patterns of inheritance may result from a few SOD1 mutations. Aspartic acid replaced with alanine at codon 90 in exon 4 has been reported in families, predominantly in Scandinavian countries. Only patients homozygous for this mutation develop ALS; those who are heterozygous are healthy. Patients often present with sensory symptoms, leg cramps, urinary urgency, decubitus ulcers, and posterior column dysfunction—features that are atypical in ALS. A patient with this mutation reported in the United States had ataxia in addition to the typical ALS symptoms. Most intriguingly, the same mutation also is a known cause of autosomal dominant FALS. Such observations obviously create a genetic conundrum. One possible explanation is that Scandinavian people may have genetic resistance to this mutation.

Autosomal Recessive Juvenile Familial Amyotrophic Lateral Sclerosis

Childhood-onset ALS is reported exclusively in the Tunisian population of northern Africa. This motor neuron disease is transmitted by an autosomal recessive gene and is characterized by pure motor dysfunction with both UMN and LMN involvement. Affected children develop spasticity, pathological hyperreflexia, generalized fasciculations, and bulbar and pseudobulbar palsy; sensory examination is normal. Besides the average age of onset of 12.1 years, it differs from autosomal-dominant FALS in that it progresses very slowly. The absence of sensory or non-UMN CNS abnormalities distinguishes childhood-onset FALS from adult-onset hexosaminidase-A deficiency and Machado-Joseph disease. The combination of UMN and LMN signs also distinguishes this condition from the spinal muscular atrophies. Childhood-onset FALS has been linked to chromosome locus 2q33-q35.

Paraneoplastic Motor Neuron Disease

Although a rare LMN syndrome occurring in patients with lymphoproliferative disorders is well recognized (see Subacute Motor Neuronopathy in Lymphoproliferative Disorders, earlier in the chapter), the relationship between cancer and ALS has been considered coincidental. However, there are rare patients with systemic cancer, particularly small cell lung cancer, who develop rapidly progressive LMN signs, occasionally with UMN signs (Graus et al. 1997). In these patients, other CNS manifestations or Lambert-Eaton syndrome may be identified. High titers of anti-Hu antibodies are found in the serum and CSF. Intensive immunotherapies are of no benefit in controlling weakness. Autopsy study shows a loss of anterior horn cells, marked gliosis, and findings consistent with paraneoplastic CNS lesions in the cerebellum and temporal lobes.

Another unusual condition has been reported in which UMN signs and symptoms that mimic PLS occur in patients with breast cancer. Although it is most likely coincidental, a slightly higher incidence of ALS has been noted in patients with cancer than in those without.

Amyotrophic Lateral Sclerosis–Parkinsonism-Dementia Complex

On the South Pacific Mariana Island of Guam and on the Kii peninsula of Japan, ALS is associated with parkinsonism and dementia, and prevalence was up to 100 times that in other parts of the world. Although this condition has been proved not to be hereditary, familial aggregation is common. In the past two decades, however, the incidence of this unique endemic disease has markedly dropped and now is only several times that of sporadic ALS in the rest of the world. The decline in incidence coincided with changes in water and food supply in these islands, which suggests that the disorder is related to environmental factors.

Clinically, about 5% of patients with parkinsonism-dementia complex in the Western Pacific develop ALS, whereas 38% of patients with ALS develop parkinsonism-dementia. Detailed neuropathological investigation in these patients showed that ALS seen in Guam (Guamanian ALS) and the parkinsonism-dementia complex are the same disease process. An extensive distribution of neurofibrillary tangles in the CNS is the characteristic feature of Guamanian ALS-parkinsonism-dementia complex. Most intriguing is that postmortem studies have shown that more than 70% of healthy native Guamanians have extensive neurofibrillary tangles, thereby suggesting either that neurofibrillary tangles may be a basic aging process in this population or that a substantial proportion of Chamorro people have subclinical or preclinical disease.

In the United States, the risk of dementia and the possibility of ALS in the relatives of patients with ALS is estimated to be twice that of normal controls. In pedigrees of patients with autosomal dominant ALS, dementia or parkinsonism have also been known to occur. Although it is rare, an autosomal recessive form of ALS-parkinsonism-dementia has been described. It is still unknown whether these apparently different neurological manifestations are part of a single neurodegenerative process (Qureshi et al. 1996).

Motor System Atrophy (Machado-Joseph Disease)

Machado-Joseph disease is an autosomal dominant syndrome with onset varying from the third to seventh decade of life (see Chapter 76). Although cerebellar ataxia is usually a predominant clinical feature, patients with an early onset (age 20–30) often present with generalized spasticity. There is often facial and tongue fasciculation. Therefore, Machado-Joseph disease may present in a fashion resembling ALS. Other characteristic findings include extrapyramidal signs, such as dystonia and rigidity, progressive external ophthalmoparesis, and bulging eyes. This disease is another example of a disease with expanded trinucleotide repeats. Affected patients have a two- to threefold expansion of CAG nucleotide repeats in a gene at chromosome 14q32.1.

Adult-Onset Hexosaminidase-A Deficiency

Late-onset GM_2 gangliosidosis, a rare autosomal recessive disorder, presents very differently from infantile GM_2 gangliosidosis (see Chapter 68). A common clinical presentation is slowly progressive weakness with UMN and LMN disease. Cramps may present in isolation, mimicking SMA. Usually, however, other signs, such as cerebellar ataxia, extrapyramidal signs, sensory impairment, intellectual decline, and psychosis, accompany the UMN and LMN signs. Generally, the features of such multisystem involvement are not mistaken for ALS. Late-onset GM_2 gangliosidosis differs from the infantile form because the disease is related to a partial deficiency in the activity of the lysosomal enzyme, hexosaminidase-A. This deficiency is caused by compound heterozygosity, in which each allele produces a protein with a small residual degree of activity (2–4%). It is unclear whether specific genotypes predispose patients to acquiring this selective motor disorder.

Disinhibition-Dementia-Parkinsonism-Amyotrophy

An autosomal dominant disease that is characterized clinically by progressive "childish" disinhibited behavior, dementia, parkinsonian manifestations, amyotrophy, and fasciculations has been reported. Autopsy studies showed widespread neuronal loss in the substantia nigra, cerebral cortex, and anterior horn of the spinal cord, and extensive spongy degeneration in the temporal and frontal lobes. The disease appears to be linked to chromosome 17q21-23.

Polyglucosan Body Disease

Polyglucosan body disease is probably an autosomal recessive disorder. Axons and neural sheath cells contain periodic acid-Schiff–positive polyglucosan bodies. These patients have progressive UMN and LMN signs, marked sensory loss, and neurogenic bladder dysfunction. No genetic analyses have been performed. The condition is rare and poorly understood. Two types of polyglucosan bodies may be seen in ALS: Lafora's bodies and corpora amylacea. Although Lafora's bodies are not a specific feature of ALS pathology, they have been identified in some patients. In a recessive form of FALS, autopsy study showed extensive Lafora's body–like inclusions in cortical motor neurons and other neurons. Corpora amylacea bodies were also markedly increased.

REFERENCES

BDNF Study Group (Phase III). A controlled trial of recombinant methionyl human BDNF in ALS. Neurology 1999;52:1427–1433.

Blexrud MD, Windebrank AJ, Daube JR. Long-term follow up of 121 patients with benign fasciculation. Ann Neurol 1993;34:622–625.

Bowen J, Gregory R, Squier M, et al. The post-irradiation lower motor neuron syndrome: neuronopathy or radiculopathy? Brain 1996;119:1429–1439.

Brown RH Jr. Superoxide dismutase and familial amyotrophic lateral sclerosis: new insights into mechanisms and treatments. Ann Neurol 1996;39:145–146.

Cudkowicz ME, McKenna-Yasek D, Sapp PE, et al. Epidemiology of mutations in superoxide dismutase in amyotrophic lateral sclerosis. Ann Neurol 1997;41:210–221.

Donofrio PD. AAEM Case report #28: monomelic amyotrophy. Muscle Nerve 1994;17:1129–1134.

Fink JK, Heineman-Patterson T. Hereditary spastic paraplegia: advances in genetic research. Neurology 1996;46:1507–1514.

Forsyth PA, Dalmau J, Graus F, et al. Motor neuron syndromes in cancer patients. Ann Neurol 1997;41:722–730.

Gutmann L, Mitsumoto H (eds). Advances in amyotrophic lateral sclerosis. Neurology 1996;47(Suppl. 2).

Harding AE. Hereditary spastic paraplegias. Semin Neurol 1993;13:333–336.

Holstege G. Somatic Motoneurons and Descending Motor Pathways. Limbic and Non-limbic Components. In PN Leigh, M Swash (eds), Motor Neuron Disease. Biology and Management. London: Springer, 1995;259–330.

Jubelt B, Drucker J. Post-polio syndrome: an update. Semin Neurol 1993;13:283–290.

Juneja T, Pericak-Vance MA, Laing NG, et al. Prognosis in familial ALS: progression and survival in patients with glu100gly and ala4val mutations in Cu,Zn superoxide dismutase. Neurology 1997;48:55–57.

Kornberg AJ, Pestronk A. Chronic motor neuropathies: diagnosis, therapy, and pathogenesis. Ann Neurol 1995;37(Suppl. 1):S43–S50.

Lefebvre S, et al. Identification and characterization of a spinal muscular atrophy-determining gene. Cell 1995;80:155–165.

Miller RG, Rosenberg JA, Gelinas DF, et al. Practice parameter: the care of the patient with amyotrophic lateral sclerosis (an evidence-based review). Neurology 1999;52:1311–1323.

Miller RG, Sufit R. New approaches to the treatment of ALS. Neurology 1997;48(Suppl. 4):S28–S32.

Mitsumoto H, Chad D, Pioro EP. Amyotrophic Lateral Sclerosis. Contemporary Neurology Series. Philadelphia: Davis, 1997a.

Mitsumoto H, Norris FT Jr (eds). Amyotrophic Lateral Sclerosis: Comprehensive Management and Treatment. New York: Demos, 1994.

Mitsumoto H, et al. Motor Neuron Diseases. In EL Mancall (ed), Continuum. Baltimore: Williams & Wilkins, 1997b.

Pestronk A, Lopate G, Kornberg AJ, et al. Distal lower motor neuron syndrome with high-titer serum IgM anti-GM$_1$ antibodies: improvement following immunotherapy with monthly plasma exchange and intravenous cyclophosphamide. Neurology 1994;44:2027–2031.

Qureshi AI, Wilmot G, Dihenia B, et al. Motor neuron disease with parkinsonism. Arch Neurol 1996;53:987–991.

Rosen DR. Mutations in Cu/Zn superoxide dismutase gene are associated with familial amyotrophic lateral sclerosis. Nature 1993;362:59–62.

Rothstein JD. Excitotoxicity hypothesis. Neurology 1996;47 (Suppl. 2):S19–S26.

Rothstein JD, Van Kammen M, Levey AI, et al. Selective loss of glial glutamate transporter GLT-1 in amyotrophic lateral sclerosis. Ann Neurol 1995;38:73–84.

Roy N, Mahadevan MS, McLean M, et al. The gene for neuronal apoptosis inhibitory protein is partially deleted in individuals with spinal muscular atrophy. Cell 1995;80:167–178.

Stewart H, Wallace A, McGaughran, et al. Molecular diagnosis of spinal muscular atrophy. Arch Dis Child 1998;78:531–535.

The World Federation of Neurology Research Group on Neuromuscular Diseases Subcommittee on Motor Neuron Disease. El Escorial World Federation of Neurology criteria for the diagnosis of amyotrophic lateral sclerosis. J Neurol Sci 1994;124(Suppl.):96–107.

Chapter 79
Disorders of Nerve Roots and Plexuses

David A. Chad

DISORDERS OF NERVE ROOTS

The nerve roots are susceptible to many of the disorders that affect the peripheral nerves. Although surrounded by a rigid bony canal, they are delicate structures subject to compression and stretching. Bathed by cerebrospinal fluid (CSF), they may be injured by infectious, inflammatory, and neoplastic processes that involve the leptomeninges. Separated from the blood by an incomplete blood-nerve barrier, their dorsal root ganglion (DRG) neurons may be injured by circulating neurotoxins.

In the clinical sphere, it is usually not difficult to recognize that a group of symptoms and signs is caused by a lesion of a nerve root. Radicular pain and paresthesias are accompanied by sensory loss in the dermatome, weakness in the myotome (defined as muscles innervated by the same spinal cord segment and nerve root), and diminished deep tendon reflex activity at a segmental level subserved by the nerve root in question. When many roots are involved by a disease process, however, as in a polyradicular syndrome, the clinical picture may resemble a disorder of the peripheral nerves, as in a polyneuropathy, or of the anterior horn cells, as in the progressive muscular atrophy form of amyotrophic lateral sclerosis (ALS). Diagnosis therefore may become more difficult. Clinicians then turn to laboratory studies for help in arriving at a diagnosis.

A disorder of the nerve roots is favored by abnormalities of the CSF (raised protein concentration and pleocytosis), of the paraspinal muscle needle electromyographic (EMG) examination (presence of positive sharp waves and fibrillation potentials), and of spinal cord magnetic resonance imaging (MRI) (compromise or contrast enhancement of the nerve roots *per se*).

The sections that follow cover some anatomical features relevant to an understanding of the pathological conditions that affect the nerve roots as well as specific nerve root disorders.

Anatomical Features

Each nerve root is attached to the spinal cord by four to eight rootlets, which are splayed out in a longitudinal direction (Stewart 1993). The dorsal roots are attached to the spinal cord at a well-defined posterolateral sulcus. The ventral rootlets are more widely separated and emerge over a greater area. At each spinal cord segment, a pair of dorsal and ventral roots unite just beyond the DRG to form a short mixed spinal nerve, which divides into a thin dorsal ramus and a thicker ventral ramus (Figure 79.1). The dorsal ramus innervates the deep posterior muscles of the neck and trunk (the paraspinal muscles) and the skin overlying these areas. The ventral ramus (the large anterior branch) contributes to the cervical, brachial, or lumbosacral plexus and thereby supplies the limb muscles.

The nerve roots lie freely in the subarachnoid space covered by a thin root sheath, which is a layer of flattened cells continuous with the pial and arachnoidal coverings of the spinal cord. They lack the epineurial and perineurial coverings found in peripheral nerves. Compared with spinal nerves, the roots have many fewer connective tissue cells in the endoneurium and considerably less collagen.

At the junction between root and mixed nerve, the thin root sheath becomes continuous with spinal nerve perineurium, and the dura mater that surrounds the roots becomes continuous with epineurium of the mixed nerve.

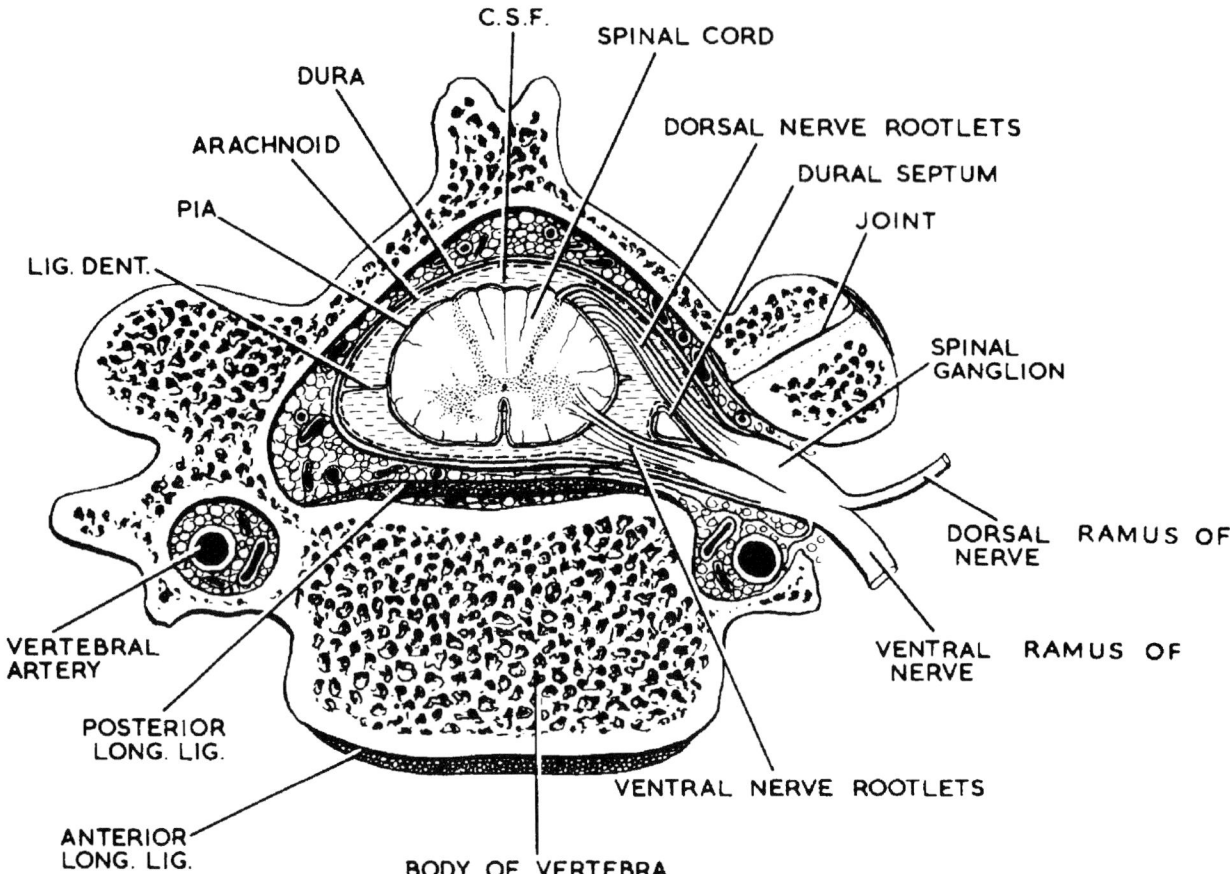

FIGURE 79.1 Relations of dura to bone and roots of nerve shown in an oblique transverse section. On the right, the relations between the emergent nerve and the synovial joint are seen, but the joint between the vertebral bodies is not in the plane of the section. The dorsal and ventral roots meet at the dorsal root ganglion in the intervertebral foramen to form the mixed spinal nerve. The small dorsal ramus is the most proximal branch of the mixed spinal nerve and serves the cervical paraspinal muscles (not shown). The dura becomes continuous with the epineurium of the mixed spinal nerve at the intervertebral foramen. The posterior longitudinal (Long.) ligament (Lig.) helps to contain the intervertebral disc (not shown), preventing protrusion into the spinal canal. (C.S.F. = cerebrospinal fluid; Lig. dent. = ligament dentate.) (Reprinted with permission from M Wilkinson. Cervical Spondylosis: Its Early Diagnosis and Treatment. Philadelphia: Saunders, 1971.)

At the intervertebral foramen, the root-DRG-spinal nerve complex is securely attached by a fibrous sheath to the transverse process of the vertebral body. Nerve fibers, together with their meningeal coverings, occupy 35–50% of the cross-sectional area of an intervertebral foramen. The remaining space is occupied by loose areolar connective tissue, fat, and blood vessels. On computed tomographic (CT) scans and MRI, the fat acts as an excellent natural contrast agent that defines the thecal sac and nerve roots, allowing detection of nerve root compression.

The dorsal roots contain sensory fibers that are central processes of the unipolar neurons of the DRG. On reaching the spinal cord, these fibers either synapse with other neurons of the posterior horn or pass directly into the posterior columns. In the ventral root, most fibers are essentially direct extensions of anterior horn motor neurons (alpha and gamma) or of neurons in the intermediolateral horn (preganglionic sympathetic neurons found in lower cervical and thoracic segments). In addition, ventral roots contain a population of unmyelinated and thinly myelinated axons, which come from sensory and sympathetic ganglia (Hildebrand et al. 1997).

Thirty-one pairs of spinal nerves run through the intervertebral foramina of the vertebral column: eight cervical, 12 thoracic, five lumbar, five sacral, and one coccygeal (Figure 79.2). A feature of clinical relevance is the pattern formed by the lumbar and sacral roots as they leave the spinal cord and make their way to their respective dorsal root ganglia to form spinal nerves (see Figure 79.2). In the adult, the spinal cord is much shorter than the spinal column, ending usually between L1 and L2. Therefore, the lumbar and sacral roots descend caudally from the spinal cord to reach the intervertebral foramina, forming the cauda equina; the concentration of so many nerve roots in a confined area makes this structure vulnerable to several pathological processes.

Traumatic Radiculopathies

Nerve Root Avulsion

The spinal roots have approximately one-tenth the tensile strength of the peripheral nerves because of lesser amounts of collagen and the absence of epineurial and perineurial sheaths in the roots. Therefore, the nerve roots are the weak link in the nerve root-spinal nerve-plexus complex, and nerve root avulsion from the spinal cord may result from a severe traction injury. Ventral roots are more vulnerable to avulsion than are dorsal roots, a consequence of the dorsal roots having the interposed DRG and a thicker dural sheath. In the vast majority of cases, root avulsion occurs in the cervical region. Lumbar and conus medullaris nerve root avulsions can occur with severe injuries to the legs and pelvis, but they are rare.

In most cases, avulsion at the level of the cervical roots results in two distinct clinical syndromes. One is Erb-Duchenne palsy, in which the arm hangs at the side internally rotated and extended at the elbow because of paralysis of C5- and C6-innervated muscles. The second is Dejerine-Klumpke palsy, in which there is weakness and wasting of the hand with a characteristic claw hand deformity because of paralysis of C8- and T1-innervated muscles. Injuries responsible for Erb-Duchenne palsy are those that cause a sudden and severe increase in the angle between the neck and shoulder, generating stresses that are readily transmitted in the direct line along the upper portion of the brachial plexus to the C5 and C6 roots. Today, motorcycle accidents are the most common causes of this injury, but the incidence of C5 and C6 root avulsions in the newborn during obstetrical procedures is increasing with the decline in the use of cesarean section. Brachial plexus injuries in the newborn are discussed in Chapter 84. The Dejerine-Klumpke palsy occurs when the limb is elevated beyond 90 degrees and tension falls directly on the lower trunk of the plexus, C8, and T1 roots. Such an injury may occur in a fall from a height in which the outstretched arm grasps an object to arrest the fall, leading to severe stretching of the C7, C8, and T1 roots.

Clinical Features and Diagnosis. At the onset of root avulsion, flaccid paralysis and complete anesthesia develop in the myotomes and dermatomes served by ventral and dorsal roots, respectively. Clinical features supplemented by electrophysiological and radiological studies help determine whether the cause of severe weakness and sensory loss is root avulsion or an extraspinal plexus lesion. For example, C5 root avulsion results in virtually complete paralysis of the rhomboids and spinatus muscles (innervated primarily by C5) and a varying degree of weakness of the deltoid, biceps, brachioradialis, and serratus anterior (which receive additional innervation from C6). A clinical sign of T1 root avulsion is an ipsilateral Horner's syndrome caused by damage to preganglionic sympathetic fibers as they traverse the ventral root to their destination in the superior cervical ganglion.

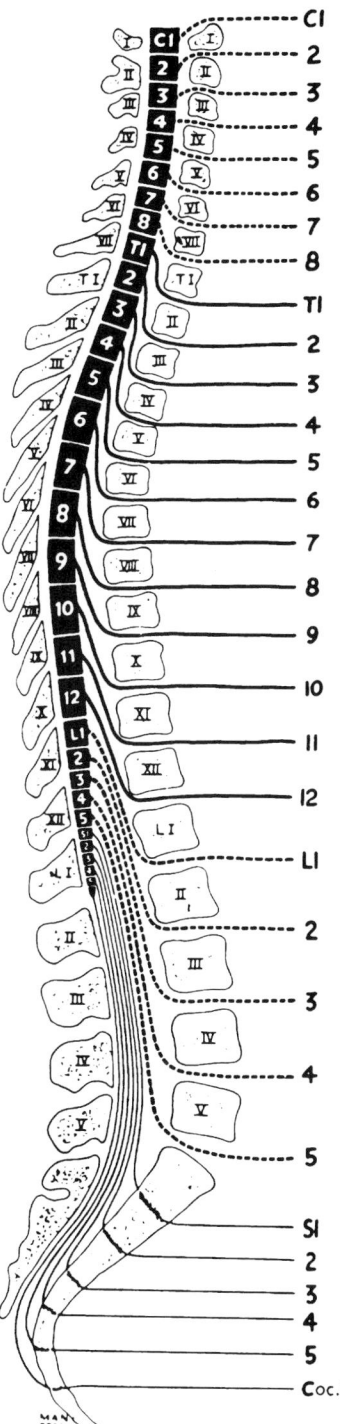

FIGURE 79.2   The relationship of spinal segments and nerve roots to the vertebral bodies and spinous processes in the adult. The cervical roots (except C8) exit through foramina above their respective vertebral bodies, and the other roots issue below these bodies. The spinal cord is much shorter than the spinal column, ending between vertebral bodies L1 and L2. The lumbar and sacral roots form the cauda equina and descend caudally, beside and below the spinal cord, to exit at the intervertebral foramina. (Reprinted with permission from W Haymaker, B Woodhall. Peripheral Nerve Injuries [2nd ed]. Philadelphia: Saunders, 1953.)

The electrophysiological tests include the measurement of a sensory nerve action potential (SNAP) and needle EMG examination of the cervical paraspinal muscles. In the setting of an isolated C5 root avulsion, the SNAP should be preserved, despite complete anesthesia in the dermatome because the peripheral axons and the DRG cell bodies remain intact. Needle EMG of the cervical paraspinal muscles permits separation of damage of the plexus and of ventral root fibers because the posterior primary ramus, which arises just beyond the DRG and proximal to the plexus as the first branch of the spinal nerve, innervates these muscles (see Figure 79.1). Thus, cervical paraspinal fibrillation potentials support the diagnosis of root avulsion. Radiological assessment uses postmyelographic CT or MRI, which usually demonstrate an outpouching of the dura filled with contrast or CSF at the level of the avulsed root. This post-traumatic meningocele results from tears in the dura and arachnoid sustained during root avulsion. Postmyelographic CT with 1- to 3-mm axial slices provides accurate diagnosis on the status of nerve roots in 85% of patients, compared to 52% for MRI (Carvalho et al. 1997).

In most cases these tests are helpful in ascertaining whether root avulsion has occurred. Sometimes, however, clinical assessment is difficult and results of testing are ambiguous. The physical examination may be limited because of severe pain. An absent SNAP indicates sensory axon loss distal to the DRG but does not exclude coexisting root avulsion. Even when this test of sensory function points to avulsion of the dorsal component of the root, the status of the ventral root may remain uncertain if paraspinal fibrillation potentials are not found. There are two reasons for their absence: First, they do not appear for 7–10 days after the onset of axonotmesis, and second, even if the timing of the needle EMG is right, they may not be seen because of innervation of the paraspinal muscles from multiple segmental levels. Finally, imaging studies are not always diagnostically accurate, at times disclosing classic post-traumatic meningoceles in patients without root avulsion (but only dural tear) or revealing normal findings in true root avulsion (de Verdier et al. 1993).

Treatment. Root avulsion produces an irreversible neurological deficit, and no intradural surgical procedure benefits the avulsed root. Treatment options are limited. When paralysis of the limb is complete, amputation may be indicated. With a less profound degree of injury, muscle and tendon transplants are sometimes used. In the case of a more restricted injury affecting only the low cervical roots and T1, early below-elbow amputation plus a below-elbow prosthesis has been recommended.

Disc Degeneration and Spondylosis

Beginning in the fourth or fifth decade of life, cervical and lumbar intervertebral discs are liable to herniate into the spinal canal or intervertebral foramina and impinge on the spinal cord, nerve roots, or both (see Chapter 77). Reinforcing the annulus fibrosus posteriorly is the posterior longitudinal ligament, which in the lumbar region has a dense, strong, central, and less well-developed lateral portion. Because of this anatomical feature, the direction of lumbar disc herniations tends to be posterolateral (paracentral), compressing the nerve roots in the lateral recess of the spinal canal. Less commonly, more lateral (foraminal) herniations compress the nerve root against the vertebral pedicle in the intervertebral foramen (Figure 79.3). On occasion, the degenerative process may be particularly severe. This leads to large rents in the annulus and posterior longitudinal ligament, thereby permitting disc material to herniate into the spinal canal as a free fragment with the potentially damaging capacity to migrate superiorly or inferiorly and compress two or more nerve roots of the cauda equina. Most cervical disc herniations are also paracentral or foraminal.

In the cervical and lumbar regions, disc degeneration is part of a larger condition, termed *spondylosis*, characterized by osteoarthritic degenerative changes in the joints of the spine, which include the disc itself and the Luschka (uncovertebral) and facet joints. Because it spawns osteophyte formation, this condition leads to compromise of the spinal cord in the spinal canal and the nerve roots in the intervertebral foramina. The restriction in the dimensions of these bony canals may be exacerbated by thickening and hypertrophy of the ligamentum flavum, which is especially detrimental in patients with congenital cervical or lumbar canal stenosis.

In the cervical region, nerve root compression is usually caused by disc herniation superimposed on chronic spondylotic changes. Isolated cervical disc herniation is uncommon and is found in younger people in the setting of neck trauma. In the lumbar region, isolated acute disc herniation is a common cause of lumbosacral radiculopathy in the younger patient (<40 years), whereas bony root entrapment with or without superimposed disc herniation is the usual cause of radiculopathy in the patient older than 50 years.

Clinical Features. Root compression from disc herniation gives rise to a distinctive clinical syndrome, which in its fully developed form comprises radicular pain, dermatomal sensory loss, weakness in the myotome, and reduction or loss of the deep tendon reflex subserved by the affected root. Nerve root pain is variably described as knifelike or aching and is widely distributed, projecting to the sclerotome (defined as deep structures, such as muscles and bones innervated by the root). Typically, root pain is aggravated by coughing, sneezing, and straining at stool (actions that produce Valsalva's maneuver and raise intraspinal pressure). Accompanying the pain are paresthesias referred to the specific dermatome, especially to the distal regions of the dermatomes; indeed, these sensations strongly suggest that the pain has its origins in compressed nerve roots rather than spondylotic facet joints. Sensory loss caused by

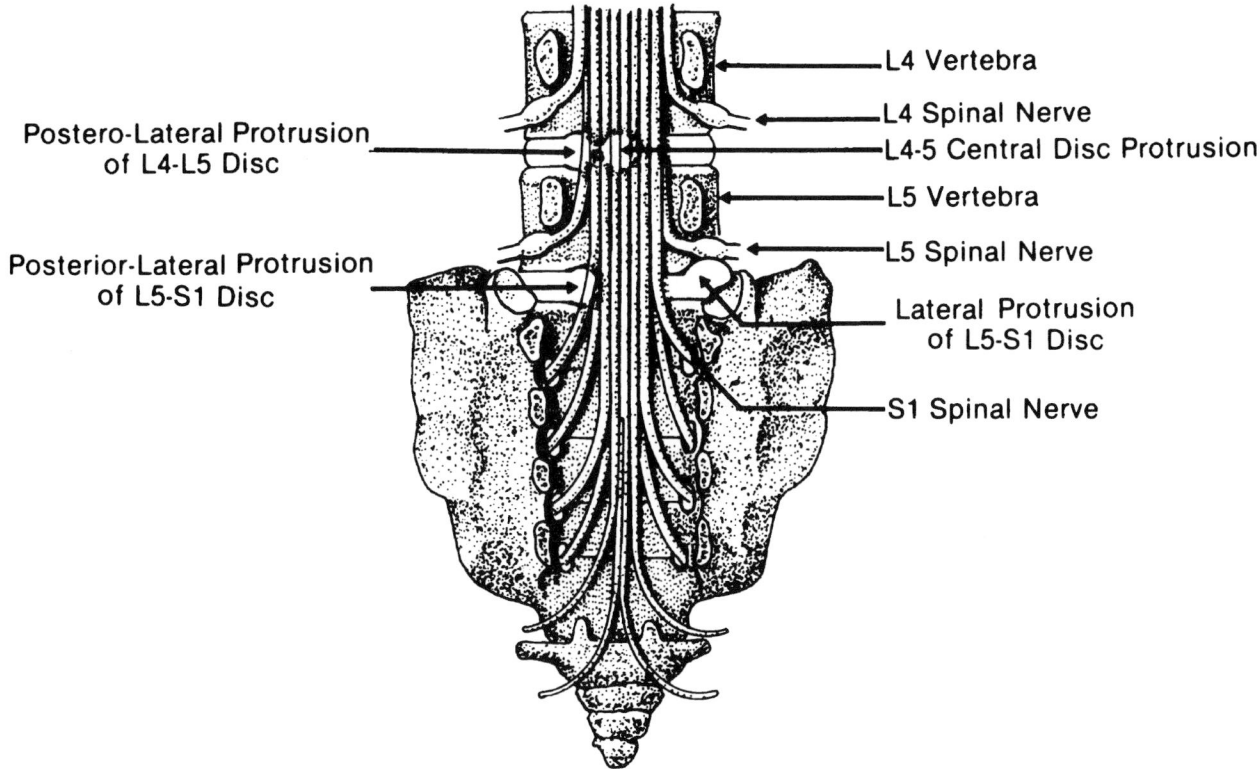

FIGURE 79.3   Dorsal view of the lower lumbar spine and sacrum, showing the different types of herniations and how different roots and the cauda equina can be compressed. (Reprinted with permission from JD Stewart. Focal Peripheral Neuropathies [2nd ed]. New York: Raven, 1993.)

the compromise of a single root may be difficult to ascertain because of the overlapping territories of adjacent roots, although loss of pain is usually more easily demonstrated than is loss of light touch (Figure 79.4).

Most radiculopathies occur in the lumbosacral region; compressive root lesions in this area account for 62–90% of all radiculopathies. Cervical radiculopathies are less common, comprising 5–36% of all radiculopathies encountered.

In the lumbosacral region, 95% of disc herniations occur at the L4-L5 or L5-S1 levels; L3-L4 and higher lumbar disc herniations are very uncommon (Stewart 1993). Knowing that the L4 root exits beneath the pedicle of L4 through the L4-L5 foramen and that L5 exits through the L5-S1 foramen, one might predict that disc herniation at these levels would generally compress the L4 and L5 roots, respectively (see Figure 79.3). In perhaps only 10% of cases of the disc herniating far laterally into the foramen is there compression of the exiting nerve root. More commonly, the posterolateral disc herniation compresses the nerve root passing through the foramen below that disc. Thus L4-L5 and L5-S1 herniations usually produce L5 and S1 radiculopathies, respectively.

In an S1 radiculopathy, pain radiates to the buttock and down the back of the leg (classic sciatica), often extending below the knee; paresthesias are generally felt in the lateral ankle and foot. The ankle jerk is generally diminished or

lost, and weakness may be detected in the plantar flexors and gluteus maximus. In an L5 radiculopathy, the distribution of pain is similar, but paresthesias are felt on the dorsum of the foot and the outer portion of the calf. The ankle reflex is typically normal, but there may be reduction of the medial hamstring reflex. Weakness may be found in L5-innervated muscles served by the peroneal nerve, including the extensor hallucis longus, tibialis anterior and peronei, as well as the tibialis posterior and the gluteus medius. Weakness may be restricted to the extensor hallucis longus. A positive straight-leg–raising test is a sensitive indicator of nerve root irritation. The test is deemed positive when the patient complains of pain radiating from the back into the buttock and thigh with leg elevation to less than 60 degrees. The test is positive in 95% of patients with a proven disc herniation at surgery. Less sensitive but highly specific is the crossed straight-leg–raising test, when the patient complains of radiating pain on the affected side with elevation of the contralateral leg. The less common L4 radiculopathy is characterized by pain and paresthesias along the medial aspect of the knee and lower leg. Knee jerk is diminished, and weakness may be noted in the quadriceps and hip adductors. When large herniations occur in the midline at either the L4-L5 or L5-S1 levels, all the nerve roots below that level may be compressed, producing the cauda equina syndrome of bilateral radicular pain, paresthesias, weakness, and attenuated reflexes below the disc level as well as

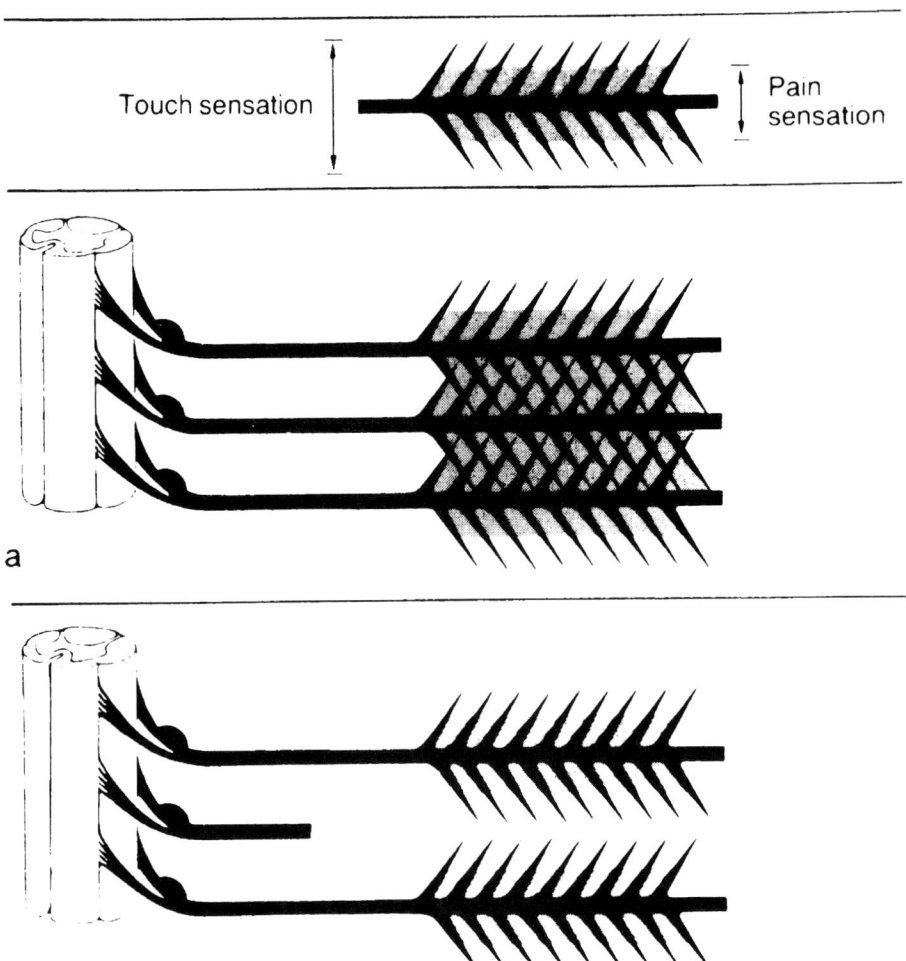

FIGURE 79.4 The zones of radicular touch and pain sensation. The area for touch sensation (hatched) supplied by one single root is wider than the area of pain sensation (gray). The areas of pain sensation do not overlap or at most overlap incompletely, whereas the areas of touch sensation of a single root are completely overlapped by those of the adjacent roots (**a**). Accordingly, monoradicular lesions (**b**) produce a hyperalgesic or analgesic zone while touch sensation remains intact or only minimally impaired. Only after two roots are involved is an anesthetic zone present. (Reprinted with permission from M Mumenthaler, H Schliack. Peripheral Nerve Lesions. Diagnosis and Therapy. New York: Thieme, 1991.)

urinary retention. This is a surgical emergency requiring urgent decompression.

In the cervical region, the greater mobility at levels C5-C6 and C6-C7 promotes the development of earlier and more extensive cervical disc degeneration and subsequent spondylosis at these levels. Cervical nerve roots emerge above the vertebra that shares the same numerical designation. Therefore, C7 exits between C6 and C7, and spondylotic changes with or without additional acute disc herniation would be expected to compress the C7 nerve root. Similarly, disc degeneration at C5-C6 and C7-T1 would compress the C6 and C8 roots, respectively. The most frequently encountered cervical radiculopathies occur at C6 and C7; compression of C5 and C8 are less common.

Involvement of C6 is associated with pain at the tip of the shoulder radiating into the upper part of the arm, lateral side of the forearm, and thumb. Paresthesias are felt in the thumb and index finger. The brachioradialis and biceps reflexes are attenuated or lost. Weakness may occur in the muscles of the C6 myotome supplied by several different nerves, including the biceps, deltoid, and pronator teres. The clinical features of C5 radiculopathies are similar, except that the rhomboids and spinatus muscles are more likely to be weak.

When the C7 root is compressed, pain radiates in a wide distribution to include the shoulder, chest, forearm, and hand. Paresthesias involve the dorsal surface of the middle finger. The triceps reflex is usually reduced or absent. A varying degree of weakness usually involves one or more muscles of the C7 myotome, especially the triceps and the flexor carpi radialis. Less common C8 root involvement presents a similar clinical picture with regard to pain. Paresthesias, however, are experienced in the fourth and fifth digits, and weakness, when it occurs, affects muscles innervated by several nerves, including finger extensors, hand interossei, and thenar muscles.

Diagnosis. Diagnosis is aided by a variety of imaging techniques, including plain radiography, myelography, CT-myelography, and MRI (see Chapter 38). Although plain radiography is not helpful in the identification of herniated disc *per se*, in both the cervical and lumbar areas it reveals spondylotic changes when present. It also may be useful in the identification of less common disorders that produce

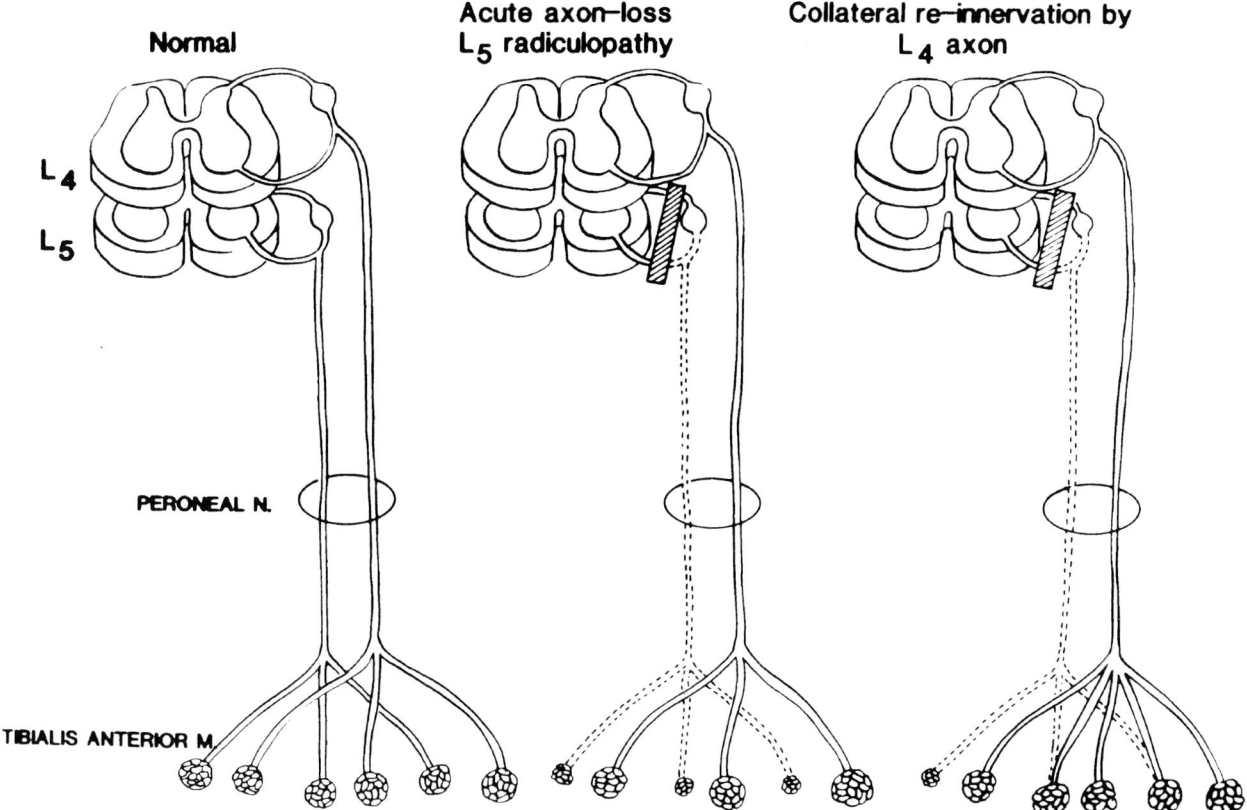

FIGURE 79.5   Diagram illustrating how muscle (M.) fibers denervated by a radiculopathy are reinnervated by collateral sprouting despite persisting root compression. (N. = nerve.) (Reprinted with permission from AJ Wilbourn, MJ Aminoff. The electrophysiologic examination in patients with radiculopathies. Muscle Nerve 1988;11:1099–1114.)

radicular symptoms and signs, such as bony metastases, infection, fracture, and spondylolisthesis.

In the cervical region, the best methods for assessing the relationship between neural structures (spinal cord and nerve root) and their fibro-osseous surroundings (disc, spinal canal, and foramen) are postmyelography CT (unenhanced CT reveals little more than the presence of bony changes) and MRI. MRI is equivalent in diagnostic capacity to postmyelography CT and therefore is preferred. In the lumbosacral region, CT is an effective method of evaluation of disc disease, but when available, MRI is considered the superior imaging study because of excellent resolution; multiplanar imaging; the ability to see the entire lumbar spine, including the conus; and the absence of ionizing radiation.

A variety of neurophysiological tests are used to assess patients with disc herniation, including motor and sensory nerve conduction studies, late responses, somatosensory evoked potentials, nerve root stimulation, and needle electrode examination. Customarily, radiculopathy is distinguished from plexopathy and peripheral nerve trunk lesions by preservation of SNAP, but in the specific instance of L5 radiculopathy, if intraspinal pathology is severe enough, compression of the L5 DRG may lead to loss of the superficial peroneal nerve SNAP (Levin 1998). Needle EMG is the most useful procedure in the diagnosis of suspected radiculopathy. A study is considered positive if abnormalities (fibrillation potentials) are present in two or more muscles that receive innervation from the same root, preferably via different peripheral nerves; no abnormalities should be detected in muscles innervated by the affected root's rostral and caudal neighbors. Motor unit potential abnormalities of reinnervation (high-amplitude, polyphasic potentials) are also sought by the needle electrode but are not as reliable as fibrillation potentials in establishing a definitive diagnosis of radiculopathy. Absence of fibrillation potentials does not, however, exclude the diagnosis of radiculopathy. Two main reasons for this exist. First, examination in the first 1–3 weeks after onset of nerve root compromise may be negative because it takes approximately 2 weeks for these potentials to appear. Second, fibrillation potentials disappear as denervated fibers are reinnervated by axons of the same or an adjacent myotome beginning 2–3 months after nerve root compression (Figure 79.5). The distribution of fibrillation potentials is relatively stereotyped for C5, C7, and C8 radiculopathies, whereas C6 radiculopathy has the most variable presentation; in one-half of patients, the findings are similar to C5 radiculopathy, whereas in the other half, findings are identical to C7 radiculopathy (Levin et al. 1996).

Treatment.   For cervical spondylotic radiculopathy, the mainstay of treatment is conservative management—a combination of reduced physical activity, soft cervical collar, and anti-inflammatory agents. Most patients improve, even those with mild-to-moderate motor deficits. However, a surgical approach may be warranted in certain instances: (1) if there are clinical and radiological signs of an accompanying myelopathy, (2) if there is unremitting pain despite an adequate trial of conservative management, or (3) if there is progressive weakness in the territory of the compromised nerve root.

In the lumbosacral region, disc herniation and spondylotic changes respond to conservative management in more than 90% of patients. Bed rest has been recommended in the past, but controlled trials have demonstrated that back-strengthening exercises, performed within the limits of the patient's pain, result in more rapid resolution of pain and return to normal function. Back-strengthening exercises should be done under the direction of a physical therapist. Follow-up MRI studies in conservatively managed patients indicate reduction in size or disappearance of herniated nucleus pulposus corresponding to improvement in clinical findings (Komori et al. 1996). Epidural corticosteroid injection may help to relieve pain but does not improve neurological function or reduce the need for surgery (Carette et al. 1997). Three situations occur, however, in which surgical referral is indicated: (1) in patients presenting with cauda equina syndrome (for which surgery may be required urgently), (2) if the neurological deficit is severe or progressing, or (3) if severe radicular pain continues after 4–6 weeks of conservative management.

Diabetic Polyradiculoneuropathy

Diabetic neuropathies can be classified anatomically into two major groups: symmetrical polyneuropathies and asymmetrical focal or multifocal disorders. Examples of the latter include the cranial mononeuropathies and the conditions covered in this section: thoracoabdominal and lumbosacral polyradiculoneuropathies. Although treated separately in the following paragraphs, they often coexist in an individual patient. Occasionally, a similar syndrome can occur in the cervical roots.

When there is predominant involvement of the thoracic roots, the presenting symptoms are generally pain and paresthesias of rapid onset in the abdominal and chest wall. The trunk pain may be severe, described variably as burning, sharp, aching, and throbbing. It may mimic the pain of acute cardiac or intra-abdominal medical emergencies and may also simulate disc disease, but the rarity of thoracic disc protrusions and the usual development of a myelopathy help to exclude this diagnosis. Findings of diabetic thoracoabdominal polyradiculoneuropathy include heightened sensitivity to light touch over affected regions; patches of sensory loss on the anterior, lateral, or posterior aspects of the trunk; and unilateral abdominal swelling owing to localized weakness of the abdominal wall muscles (Longstreth 1997).

Diabetic lumbosacral polyradiculoneuropathy involves the legs, especially the anterior thighs, with pain, dysesthesia, and weakness, reflecting the major involvement of upper lumbar roots. A variety of names have been used to describe it, including *diabetic amyotrophy, proximal diabetic neuropathy, diabetic lumbosacral plexopathy, diabetic femoral neuropathy,* and *Bruns-Garland syndrome.* Because it is likely that the brunt of nerve pathology falls on the nerve roots, it can be designated a diabetic polyradiculoneuropathy.

In most patients, onset is fairly abrupt, with symptoms developing over days to a couple of weeks. Early in the course of the condition, the clinical findings are usually unilateral and include weakness of muscles supplied by L2-L4 roots (iliopsoas, quadriceps, and hip adductors), reduced or absent patellar reflex, and mild impairment of sensation over the anterior thigh. As time passes, there may be *territorial spread,* a term used by Bastron and Thomas in 1981 to describe proximal, distal, or contralateral involvement as the polyradiculoneuropathy evolves. Worsening may occur in a steady or a stepwise fashion, and it may take several weeks to progress from onset to peak of the disease. At its peak, weakness varies in severity and extent from a mildly affected patient, with slight, unilateral thigh weakness, to a profound degree of bilateral leg weakness in the territory of the L2-S2 nerve roots. Rarely, the process of territorial spread is so extensive that it involves cervical roots and leads to profound generalized weakness, a condition designated *diabetic cachexia.* Rarely, an isolated diabetic cervical polyradiculoneuropathy may occur.

Diabetic polyradiculoneuropathy tends to affect patients in the sixth or seventh decade of life, who have often well-controlled diabetes of several years' duration. The condition occurs in diabetics, with or without treatment. The syndrome of painful polyradiculoneuropathy, whether referable to thoracic or lumbosacral roots, may be the presenting manifestation of diabetes. In 30–50% of patients, the disorder is preceded by substantial weight loss of 30–40 lb.

Laboratory studies disclose elevated fasting blood glucose in the vast majority of patients; when values are normal, they are found in treated diabetics. The erythrocyte sedimentation rate is usually normal, but in a subgroup of patients with diabetic lumbosacral polyradiculoneuropathy it is elevated, reflecting perhaps an immune-mediated disorder. In addition to abnormalities in paraspinal muscles seen on needle EMG, the neurodiagnostic studies disclose evidence for a diabetic distal polyneuropathy in approximately 75% of patients. The CSF protein is usually increased to an average of 120 mg/dl, but in some patients, values exceed 350 mg/dl; pleocytosis is not a feature of this condition. Biopsy of proximal nerve sensory branches reveals axon loss and demyelination; in more severely affected patients, inflammatory cell infiltration and vasculitis is found (Said et al. 1994). Imaging studies of the thoracic and lumbosacral spinal canal with CT, myelography, and MRI are normal.

The natural history of diabetic polyradiculoneuropathy is for improvement to occur in most patients, although the

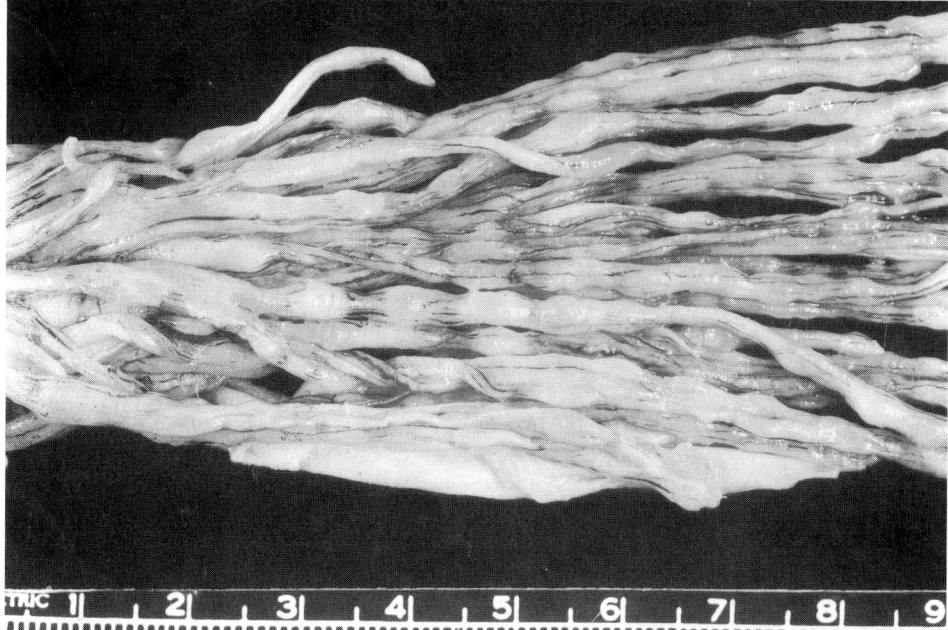

FIGURE 79.6 Cauda equina in leptomeningeal carcinomatosis. Seeding of multiple nerve roots by adenocarcinoma produces a nodular appearance. (Courtesy of Dr. T. W. Smith, Department of Pathology [Neuropathology], University of Massachusetts Medical Center, Worcester, MA.)

recovery phase is lengthy, ranging between 1 and 18 months with a mean of 6 months. Pain and dysesthesias improve or disappear entirely in 85% of patients; numbness improves or recovers in 50%; and strength is partially or completely restored in 70%. In some patients, episodes recur.

Therapy is usually directed toward ameliorating the severe pain of this condition. The tricyclics, especially desipramine (with a better side-effect profile than amitriptyline), selective serotonin reuptake inhibitors (such as sertraline and nefazodone hydrochloride [Serzone]), anticonvulsants (carbamazepine), clonazepam, baclofen, clonidine, mexiletine, intravenous (IV) lidocaine, and topical capsaicin may have a role separately or in combination.

The major differential diagnostic considerations are polyradiculoneuropathies related to degenerative disc disease and infectious, inflammatory, and neoplastic processes. These can usually be excluded by history, examination, and routine laboratory investigations, including CSF analysis. In our experience, however, the clinical presentation provoking the most anxiety is the frail elderly patient not known to be diabetic who has weight loss and the abrupt onset of lower extremity pain and weakness that progresses over months. In such a patient, the specter of neoplasia looms large, and thorough imaging studies of the nerve roots and plexuses are mandatory.

Neoplastic Polyradiculoneuropathy (Neoplastic Meningitis)

A wide variety of neoplasms are known to spread to the leptomeninges. These include solid tumors (carcinoma of the breast and lung and melanoma), non-Hodgkin's lymphomas, and leukemias. Although neoplastic polyradiculoneuropathy usually occurs in patients known to have an underlying neoplasm, meningeal symptoms may be the first manifestation of malignancy. The clinical features of neoplastic polyradiculoneuropathy include radicular pain, dermatomal sensory loss, areflexia, and weakness of the lower motor neuron type (Balm and Hammack 1996). Often, the distribution of the sensory and motor deficits is widespread and simulates a severe sensorimotor polyneuropathy. Often, associated clinical manifestations result from infiltration of the meninges, such as nuchal rigidity, confusion, and cranial polyneuropathies.

At postmortem examination, the cauda equina shows discrete nodules or focal granularity (Figure 79.6). Microscopy discloses spinal roots encased by tumor cells, which appear to infiltrate the root. It is presumed that disturbed nerve root function results from several mechanisms, including nerve fiber compression and ischemia.

The most revealing diagnostic procedure is lumbar puncture, which is almost always abnormal. A sensitive electrophysiological indicator of nerve root involvement is a change in the F wave. In the symptomatic cancer patient, prolonged F-wave latencies or absent F responses should raise the suspicion of leptomeningeal metastases. Postmyelography CT adds strong evidence in support of the diagnosis if it demonstrates multiple nodular defects on the nerve roots. Spinal MRI, especially with gadolinium enhancement, however, is the test of choice in the cancer patient in whom leptomeningeal involvement of the spine is suspected (Watanabe et al. 1993). Approximately 50% of patients with neoplastic meningitis and spinal symptoms have abnormalities on these studies. Gadolinium-enhanced MRI of the brain discloses abnormalities, including contrast enhancement of the basilar cisterns or cortical convexities, and hydrocephalus.

Standard therapy for neoplastic meningitis includes radiotherapy to sites of symptomatic disease, intrathecal chemotherapy (methotrexate, thiotepa, and Ara-C), and optimal treatment of the underlying malignancy.

Infectious Radiculopathy

Tabes Dorsalis

Tabes dorsalis, the most common form of neurosyphilis, begins as a spirochetal (*Treponema pallidum*) meningitis (see Chapter 59). After 10–20 years of persistent infection, damage to the dorsal roots is severe and extensive, producing a set of characteristic symptoms and signs. Symptoms are lightning pains, ataxia, and bladder disturbance; signs are Argyll Robertson pupils, areflexia, loss of proprioceptive sense, Charcot joints, and trophic ulcers. Lancinating or lightning pains are brief, sharp, and stabbing; they are more apt to occur in the legs than elsewhere. Sensory disturbances, such as coldness, numbness, and tingling, also occur and are associated with impairment of light touch, pain, and thermal sensation. Sudden visceral crises, characterized by the abrupt onset of epigastric pain that spreads around the body or up over the chest, occur in some 20% of patients.

Most of the features of tabes dorsalis can be explained by lesions of the posterior roots. Ataxia is caused by the destruction of proprioceptive fibers; insensitivity to pain is the result of partial loss of small myelinated and unmyelinated fibers; and bladder hypotonia with overflow incontinence, constipation, and impotence are the result of sacral root damage. Pathological study discloses thinning and grayness of the posterior roots, especially in the lumbosacral region, and the spinal cord shows degeneration of the posterior columns. A mild reduction of neurons in the DRG occurs, and there is little change in the peripheral nerves. Inflammation may occur all along the posterior root.

The CSF is abnormal in active cases. The opening pressure is elevated in 10% of patients. Fifty percent of patients have a mononuclear pleocytosis (5–165 cells/ml). More than 50% have mild protein elevation (45–100 mg/dl, with rare instances of values between 100 and 250 mg/dl), and 72% have positive CSF serology. In all cases of neurosyphilis, antibodies specific for *T. pallidum* are found, and the preferred treatment is aqueous penicillin G, 2–4 million units IV every 4 hours for 10–14 days, with careful CSF follow-up. CSF examination 6 months after treatment should demonstrate a normal cell count and falling protein content. If not, a second course of therapy is indicated. The CSF examination should be repeated every 6 months for 2 years, or until the fluid is normal.

Polyradiculoneuropathy in Human Immunodeficiency Virus–Infected Patients

Cytomegalovirus (CMV) polyradiculoneuropathy is a rapidly progressive, opportunistic infection that occurs late in the course of human immunodeficiency virus (HIV) infection, when the CD4 count is very low (<200/μl) and acquired immunodeficiency syndrome–defining infections are present. Patients often have evidence of systemic CMV infection (retinitis, gastroenteritis). The presentation is marked by the rapid onset of pain and paresthesias in the legs and perineal region, associated with urinary retention and progressive ascending weakness of the lower extremities. Examination discloses a flaccid paraparesis, absent deep tendon reflexes in the legs, reduced or absent sphincter tone, and variable loss of light touch, vibration, and joint position sense.

The CSF has an elevated protein, depressed glucose, and polymorphonuclear pleocytosis; CMV may be isolated from CSF cultures. The needle EMG discloses widespread fibrillation potentials in lower extremity muscles, and sensory conduction studies may reveal an associated distal sensory neuropathy that is common in the late stages of HIV infection. Imaging of the lumbosacral region is usually normal, but adhesive arachnoiditis has been described. The pathological features are marked inflammation and extensive necrosis of dorsal and ventral roots. Cytomegalic inclusions may be found in the nucleus and cytoplasm of endothelial and Schwann cells (Figure 79.7).

Untreated CMV polyradiculoneuropathy is rapidly fatal within approximately 6 weeks of onset. The antiviral nucleoside analogue ganciclovir may benefit some patients if treatment is instituted early; improvement occurs over weeks to months. Viral resistance to ganciclovir is suggested by persistent pleocytosis and depressed CSF glucose and should prompt consideration of an alternate antiviral agent, such as foscarnet; unlike ganciclovir, it does not require intracellular phosphorylation for its effect.

Other causes of rapidly progressive lumbosacral polyradiculoneuropathy in the HIV-infected patient are meningeal lymphomatosis, *Mycobacterium tuberculosis*, and axonal polyradiculoneuritis associated with HIV infection *per se* (Corral et al. 1997). Additionally, one must consider acute inflammatory demyelinating polyradiculoneuropathy. Syphilis has an accelerated course in the patient with acquired immunodeficiency syndrome, and syphilitic polyradiculoneuropathy may present with rapidly progressive pain, paraparesis, muscle wasting, and hyporeflexia. In addition to markedly elevated CSF protein, hypoglycorrhachia, and brisk pleocytosis, the CSF and serum VDRL serologies are positive. IV penicillin leads to prompt improvement. Other considerations include herpes simplex virus type 2 and varicella zoster virus infections that involve the lumbosacral nerve roots as well as the spinal cord, producing a radiculomyelitis. *Toxoplasma gondii* may also cause myelitis, presenting as a subacute conus medullaris syndrome that simulates the clinical features produced by CMV polyradiculoneuropathy. In the case of *T. gondii*, MRI may reveal abscess formation.

FIGURE 79.7 Cytomegalovirus polyradiculoneuropathy. Numerous mononuclear inflammatory cells are apparent, and the presence of myelin ovoids (*arrows*) reflects axon loss. (Hematoxylin-eosin stain, ×100 [original magnification].) Inset: A cytomegalic cell with intranuclear inclusion. (Hematoxylin-eosin stain, ×150 [original magnification].) (Courtesy of Dr. T. W. Smith, Department of Pathology [Neuropathology], University of Massachusetts Medical Center, Worcester, MA.)

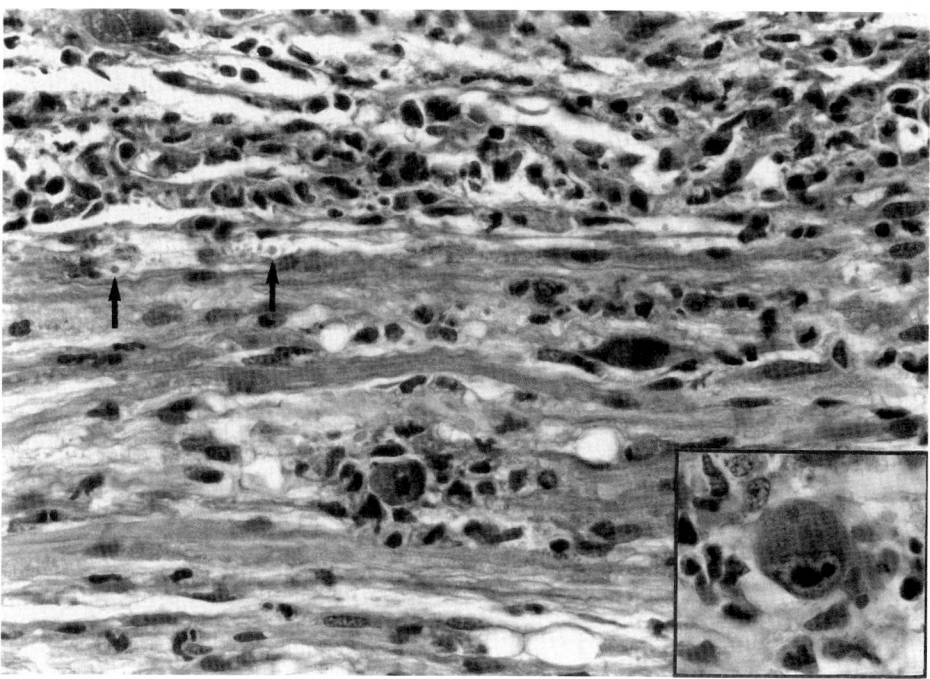

Lyme Radiculoneuropathy

Lyme disease is caused by the spirochete *Borrelia burgdorferi* transmitted by the tick *Ixodes dammini*. To help bring order to the understanding of this illness, it may be divided into three clinical stages. Stage 1 follows the tick bite and is marked by a characteristic skin rash, designated *erythema chronica migrans*, and fatigue, fever, headache, stiff neck, myalgias, and arthralgias. In stage 2, which develops weeks or months later, peripheral nerve and cardiac abnormalities may appear. Stage 3 emerges weeks to years after the tick bite and is associated with peripheral and central nervous system disturbances and arthritis. These divisions may, however, lack pathophysiological validity.

Nerve root and peripheral nerve abnormalities occur early (in stage 2) and late (in stage 3). In stage 2, a combination of aseptic meningitis, cranial neuropathy, radiculoneuropathy, and radiculoplexopathy (Sharma et al. 1993) occurs days to weeks after the onset of erythema chronica migrans. The clinical features of nerve root involvement include severe radicular pain, followed by weakness, sensory loss, and hyporeflexia in the territory of the involved roots. Nerve conduction studies provide evidence for an associated primarily axonal polyneuropathy. The CSF profile at this stage discloses protein elevation and mononuclear pleocytosis. Although this radiculopathy improves without treatment, antibiotics hasten recovery. In stage 3, the radiculoneuropathy is milder clinically than it is in stage 2; cranial nerve palsies and lymphocytic meningitis are unusual. Nerve root involvement is manifested by asymmetrical radicular pain in the cervical, cervicothoracic, thoracolumbar, and lumbosacral regions, but weakness is rare. The most frequent needle EMG finding is mild-to-moderate fibrillation potential activity in paraspinal, proximal, and distal muscles. The CSF is normal in patients with isolated radiculoneuropathy and abnormal when there is an associated encephalopathy. Clinical improvement occurs in 76% of patients treated with IV ceftriaxone.

Herpes Zoster

Herpes zoster, also known as *shingles*, is a common, painful, vesicular eruption occurring in a segmental or radicular distribution and caused by the varicella zoster virus (Arvin 1996) (see Chapter 59). It is most frequently seen in the thoracic dermatomes, less often in the cervical, and rarely in the lumbosacral segments. Zoster may also present in a division of the trigeminal nerve (e.g., herpes zoster ophthalmicus).

Zoster occurs during the lifetime of 10–20% of all people, with an incidence in the general population of approximately 3–5 per 1,000 per year. The incidence is low in young people and increases with age. Patients who are immunocompromised are at highest risk. During primary infection, the virus colonizes the DRG. There, the virus remains latent for many decades, until it is reactivated, either spontaneously or when cell-mediated immunity is impaired, and travels down sensory nerves. Pathological changes, which are characterized by lymphocytic infiltration and variable hemorrhage, are found in the DRG and spinal roots; involvement of the ventral roots and, on occasion, the spinal cord explains the development of motor signs in some patients (see below).

For several days before the onset of the rash, patients usually complain of radicular pain, sometimes accompanied by fever and malaise. The rash presents as grouped, clear vesicles on an erythematous base. These become pustules by 3–4 days and form crusts by 10 days. In the normal, immunocompetent host, lesions resolve in 2–3 weeks, often leaving a region of reduced sensation. Pain usually disappears as vesicles fade, but 20% of patients experience persisting, severe pain, termed *postherpetic neuralgia* (PHN). This complication is more likely to develop in the elderly, occurring in 50% of patients older than 60 years of age. In one-half of patients affected with PHN, the pain resolves within 2 months, and 70–80% of patients are pain free by 1 year. Rarely, pain persists for years. Ophthalmic zoster can cause ulcerations of the eyelids, conjunctivitis, keratitis, and uveitis.

In the immunologically normal host, dissemination of the virus is rare, occurring in less than 2% of patients. In the immunocompromised patient, however, dissemination occurs in 13–50% of patients. Most often, spread is to distant cutaneous sites, but involvement of the viscera (lung, gastrointestinal tract, and heart) and central nervous system may occur. A serious complication of herpes zoster ophthalmicus is delayed contralateral hemiparesis caused by cerebral angiitis. The syndrome usually develops 1 week to 6 months after the onset of zoster and occurs in patients of all ages, 50% of whom are immunologically impaired. The mortality from cerebrovascular complications is 25%, and only approximately 30% of survivors recover fully.

An uncommon complication of cutaneous herpes zoster is segmental motor weakness, which occurs in 3–5% of patients (Merchut and Gruener 1996). Segmental zoster paresis is approximately equally divided between the arms and legs, reflecting weakness in cervical and lumbar myotomes, respectively; abdominal muscles may be affected. The interval between skin eruption and paralysis is approximately 2 weeks, with a range of 1 day to 5 weeks. Weakness peaks within hours or days; spread to muscles served by unaffected segments does not usually occur. The prognosis for recovery is good, with 55% showing full recovery and another 30% showing significant improvement. One in 5 patients is left with severe and permanent residua.

The major goals of treatment are to relieve local discomfort, prevent dissemination, and reduce the severity of PHN. IV or high-dose oral acyclovir decreases the duration of viral shedding and new lesion formation, speeds healing, and lessens acute pain, all to a modest degree; there is less of an ameliorating effect, however, on PHN. In the immunocompromised patient with disseminated zoster, IV acyclovir (5 mg/kg q8h for 5 days) is the treatment of choice. Such an approach is also warranted for the seriously ill patient with herpes zoster ophthalmicus. Oral acyclovir (800 mg 5 times/day for 10 days) is indicated for the immunocompetent patient older than 50 years with herpes zoster because the antiviral agent speeds clearing of lesions and leads to immediate reduction in pain. In healthy patients older than 50 years, a course of prednisone (added to acyclovir) tapering over 3 weeks may improve quality of life.

The severe pain of PHN, described variably as continuous deep aching, burning, sharp, stabbing, and shooting, and triggered by light touch over the affected dermatomes, may be ameliorated by a number of agents. Singly or in combination, tricyclics (amitriptyline or desipramine), serotonin reuptake inhibitors (sertraline or nefazodone hydrochloride), anticonvulsants (carbamazepine), and topical capsaicin are helpful in 50–75% of patients.

Acquired Demyelinating Polyradiculoneuropathy

Acquired demyelinating polyradiculoneuropathy has two major clinical forms. One develops acutely and is known as *Guillain-Barré syndrome* (GBS); the other is chronic, progressive, or relapsing and remitting and is designated *chronic inflammatory demyelinating polyradiculoneuropathy* (CIDP). These disorders are described in detail in Chapter 80 but are mentioned here briefly because pathological changes may be pronounced in the spinal nerve roots, especially the ventral roots. There may be a dense mononuclear inflammatory infiltrate characterized by lymphocytes, monocytes, and plasma cells (Figure 79.8), and nerve fibers display segmental demyelination with relative sparing of axons. Neuroimaging with MRI discloses contrast enhancement of lumbosacral roots in both GBS and CIDP (Bertorini et al. 1995). The predilection for root involvement in these conditions helps to explain certain features, including the CSF formula, some neurophysiological findings, and disturbances in autonomic function that may be especially problematic in patients with the GBS.

A CSF profile of albuminocytological dissociation is characteristic of this syndrome. A high lumbar CSF protein concentration in the face of a normal cisternal protein level supports the hypothesis that increased CSF protein derives largely from capillaries of the spinal roots. Nerve conduction studies usually disclose slowed motor conduction velocities, dispersed motor responses, and partial conduction block, but additional abnormalities include delayed or unobtainable F-wave responses or H-reflexes, reflecting demyelination in nerve roots. Indeed, abnormalities of these late responses may be the sole finding in 10–20% of patients with GBS in the first few weeks of the illness. Last, a host of autonomic disturbances occur in GBS, some of which could be caused by involvement of preganglionic sympathetic fibers, which travel in the ventral roots en route to the paravertebral sympathetic ganglia.

Acquired Disorders of the Dorsal Root Ganglia

DRG may be selectively vulnerable to a variety of malignant and nonmalignant conditions. The resulting neurological disorder is a sensory neuronopathy syndrome whose clinical features are explained by the loss of large- and small-diameter DRG cells. Large cell dropout leads to

FIGURE 79.8 Cauda equina in the Guillain-Barré syndrome. A dense mononuclear infiltrate in the connective tissue surrounding the nerve roots is shown. (Hematoxylin-eosin stain.) (Courtesy of Dr. T. W. Smith, Department of Pathology [Neuropathology], University of Massachusetts Medical Center, Worcester, MA.)

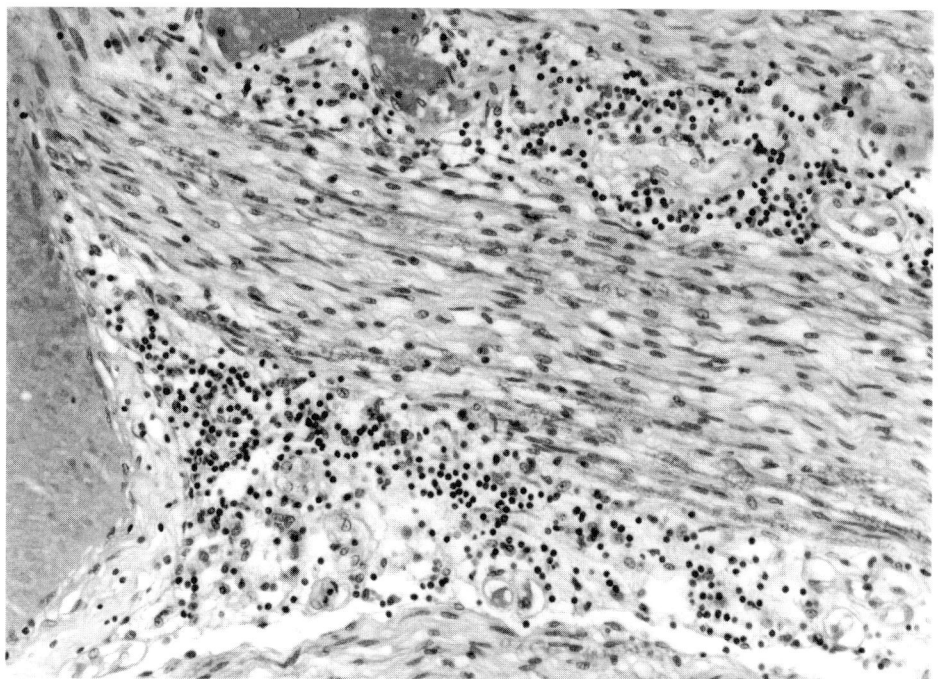

kinesthetic sensory impairment, poor coordination, loss of manual dexterity, ataxia, and areflexia; whereas small cell depletion contributes to a hyperalgesic state marked by burning pains and painful paresthesias.

Perhaps the best known of these uncommon conditions is paraneoplastic subacute sensory neuropathy (or neuronopathy), a disorder developing over weeks to months, characterized by ataxia and hyperalgesia while muscle strength is well preserved (Posner and Dalmau 1997). Some patients have clinical signs of brainstem and cerebral dysfunction, reflecting a more widespread encephalomyelitis. The neuropathy may antedate the diagnosis of cancer, usually small cell lung carcinoma, by months to years. The CSF profile discloses elevated protein concentration and a mild mononuclear cell pleocytosis. Nerve conduction studies reveal widespread loss of sensory potentials. Neuropathological features include inflammation and phagocytosis of the sensory neurons in the DRG. This condition is associated with the presence of specific antineuronal antibodies (anti-Hu), which are complement-fixing, polyclonal immunoglobulin G antibodies that react with the nuclei of the central nervous system and sensory ganglia but not with non-neuronal nuclei. The antigens recognized by the anti-Hu antibodies have been characterized as protein antigens with molecular weights of 35–40 kD. The presence of identical protein antigens in small cell lung cancer cells and neuronal nuclei supports the view that the pathogenesis of paraneoplastic subacute sensory neuropathy is immunologically mediated, with tumor antigens triggering the production of cross-reactive antibodies. Morphological studies provide evidence for both cytotoxic T cell–mediated attack and humoral mechanisms in the pathogenesis of this condition.

Other causes of DRG disorders include hereditary, toxic, and autoimmune disorders. Hereditary sensory neuropathies are usually marked by their chronicity, acrodystrophic ulcerations, fractures, bouts of osteomyelitis, and lack of paresthesias. Pyridoxine abuse and cisplatin neurotoxicity are generally easily recognized. Sjögren's syndrome may be accompanied by ataxia and kinesthetic sensory loss very similar to subacute sensory neuropathy. The presence of antibodies to extractable nuclear antigens, such as anti-Ro (SS-A) and anti-La (SS-B), help establish this diagnosis. A sensory neuronopathy syndrome has also been associated with elevated titers of anti-GD1b ganglioside antibody (O'Leary and Willison 1997).

Radiculopathies Simulating Motor Neuron Disease

Disorders of the motor roots may lead to clinical features that resemble those encountered in motor neuron disease. Detailed study of such motor neuron syndromes is important because it might provide clues to the pathogenesis of the most common form of motor neuron disease, ALS. Clinicians should consider the possibility of an ALS-mimic syndrome when a patient with clinical features of lower motor neuron involvement is found to have a monoclonal gammopathy. In that instance, investigations must vigorously pursue the possibility that physical findings stem from ventral root involvement rather than anterior horn cell degeneration. An elevated CSF protein along with a demyelinating process identified by nerve conduction studies suggests a potentially treatable motor polyradiculoneuropathy.

In some patients with a lower motor neuron syndrome, monoclonal gammopathy, raised CSF protein, and oligoclonal bands, an occult lymphoma is discovered during the course of evaluation. In fact, the association between lower motor neuron findings and lymphoma has been known since the 1960s and is designated *subacute motor neuronopathy*, but the site of major pathology is not certain and could be at a root as well as a neuronal level. It is characterized by subacute, progressive, painless, often patchy, and asymmetrical weakness of the lower motor neuron type, with greater involvement of the arms than the legs. The illness often progresses independently of the activity of the underlying lymphoma and tends to follow a relatively benign course, with some patients demonstrating spontaneous improvement.

A postradiation lower motor neuron syndrome affecting the lumbosacral region, probably a radiculopathy, has been described occurring 3–25 years after radiation therapy for testicular neoplasms. In some patients, MRI shows gadolinium enhancement. Neuropathological study discloses radiation-induced vasculopathy of proximal spinal roots with preserved motor neurons (Bowen et al. 1996). The course of the disorder is one of progression for several years and eventual stabilization.

DISORDERS OF THE BRACHIAL PLEXUS

Anatomical Features

The brachial plexus is formed by five ventral rami (C5-T1), each of which carries motor, sensory, and postganglionic sympathetic fibers to the upper limb. These five rami unite above the level of the clavicle to form the three trunks of the brachial plexus (Figure 79.9): C5 and C6 join to form the upper trunk; T1 and C8 unite to form the lower trunk; and C7, the largest of the five rami, continues as the middle trunk. Beneath the clavicle, each trunk divides into an anterior and posterior branch, leading to six divisions, which become the three cords of the brachial plexus, the lateral, medial, and posterior. The cords, which lie behind the pectoralis minor, take their names from their relationship to the subclavian artery. The lateral and medial cords carry motor fibers to the ventral muscles of the limb. The lateral cord is formed from anterior divisions of the upper and middle trunks; the medial cord from anterior division of the lower trunk. The posterior cord carries motor fibers to the dorsal muscles of the limb; it is formed from posterior divisions of the upper, middle, and lower trunks.

The major named nerves of the upper limb derive from the cords. After contributing a branch to the formation of the median nerve, the lateral cord continues as the musculocutaneous nerve. Similarly, after making its contribution to the median nerve, the medial cord continues as the ulnar nerve. The posterior cord divides into a smaller axillary nerve, which leaves the axilla via the quadrangular space to supply the deltoid and teres minor and the larger radial nerve. Also, from the level of the cords, branches are distributed to the pectoralis major and minor muscles (from the lateral and medial cords, respectively) and to the subscapularis, latissimus dorsi, and teres major muscles (from the posterior cord). In addition to these motor branches, sensory branches also arise at a cord level: The posterior cutaneous nerve of the arm arises from the posterior cord, and the medial cutaneous nerve of the arm and the medial cutaneous nerve of the forearm come from the medial cord.

Nerve branches to the serratus anterior, levator scapulae, rhomboids, and supra- and infraspinatus muscles derive from more proximal levels of the plexus. The first three muscles are supplied by branches of the anterior primary rami: the serratus anterior from C5, C6, and C7 (the long thoracic nerve) and the levator scapulae and rhomboids from branches of C5 (the dorsal scapular nerve). The supra- and infraspinatus muscles are supplied by the suprascapular nerve, a branch of the upper trunk of the plexus.

Clinical Features and Diagnosis

Neurological Examination

Patients with a brachial plexopathy present with a variety of patterns of weakness, reflex change, and sensory loss, depending on whether the whole or a portion of the plexus is disturbed. Most frequently encountered are three patterns resulting from involvement of the entire plexus, the upper trunk, and the lower trunk; less commonly seen are partial plexopathies caused by selective cord lesions.

In a pan-plexopathy, paralysis of muscles supplied by segments C5 through T1 occurs. The arm hangs lifelessly by the side, except that an intact trapezius allows shrugging of the shoulder. The limb is flaccid and areflexic, with complete sensory loss below a line extending from the shoulder diagonally downward and medially to the middle of the upper arm.

Lesions of the upper trunk produce weakness and sensory loss in a C5 and C6 distribution. Affected muscles include the supra- and infraspinati, biceps, brachialis, deltoid, and brachioradialis, so that the patient is unable to abduct the arm at the shoulder or flex at the elbow. If a lesion is so proximal as to involve the C5 ramus, the rhomboids and levator are also affected. The arm hangs at the side internally rotated at the shoulder, with the elbow extended and the forearm pronated in a "waiter's tip" posture. The biceps and brachioradialis reflexes are diminished or absent, and sensory loss is found over the lateral aspect of the arm, forearm, and thumb.

Lesions of the lower trunk produce weakness, sensory loss, and reflex changes in a C8 and T1 distribution. Weakness is present in both median- and ulnar-supplied intrinsic hand muscles and in the medial finger and wrist flexors. The finger flexion reflex is diminished or absent, and there

FIGURE 79.9   Brachial plexus. The components of the plexus have been separated and drawn out of scale. The five ventral rami (C5-T1) unite to form the upper, middle, and lower trunks of the plexus above the clavicle. Beneath the clavicle, each trunk divides into anterior (ant.) and posterior divisions. Three cords (lateral [Lat.], posterior [Post.], and medial [Med.]) lie below the pectoralis minor muscle (not shown). Major upper limb nerves (n's) originate from the cords. (cut. = cutaneous.) (Reprinted with permission of the author and publisher from W Haymaker, B Woodhall. Peripheral Nerve Injuries [2nd ed]. Philadelphia, Saunders, 1953.)

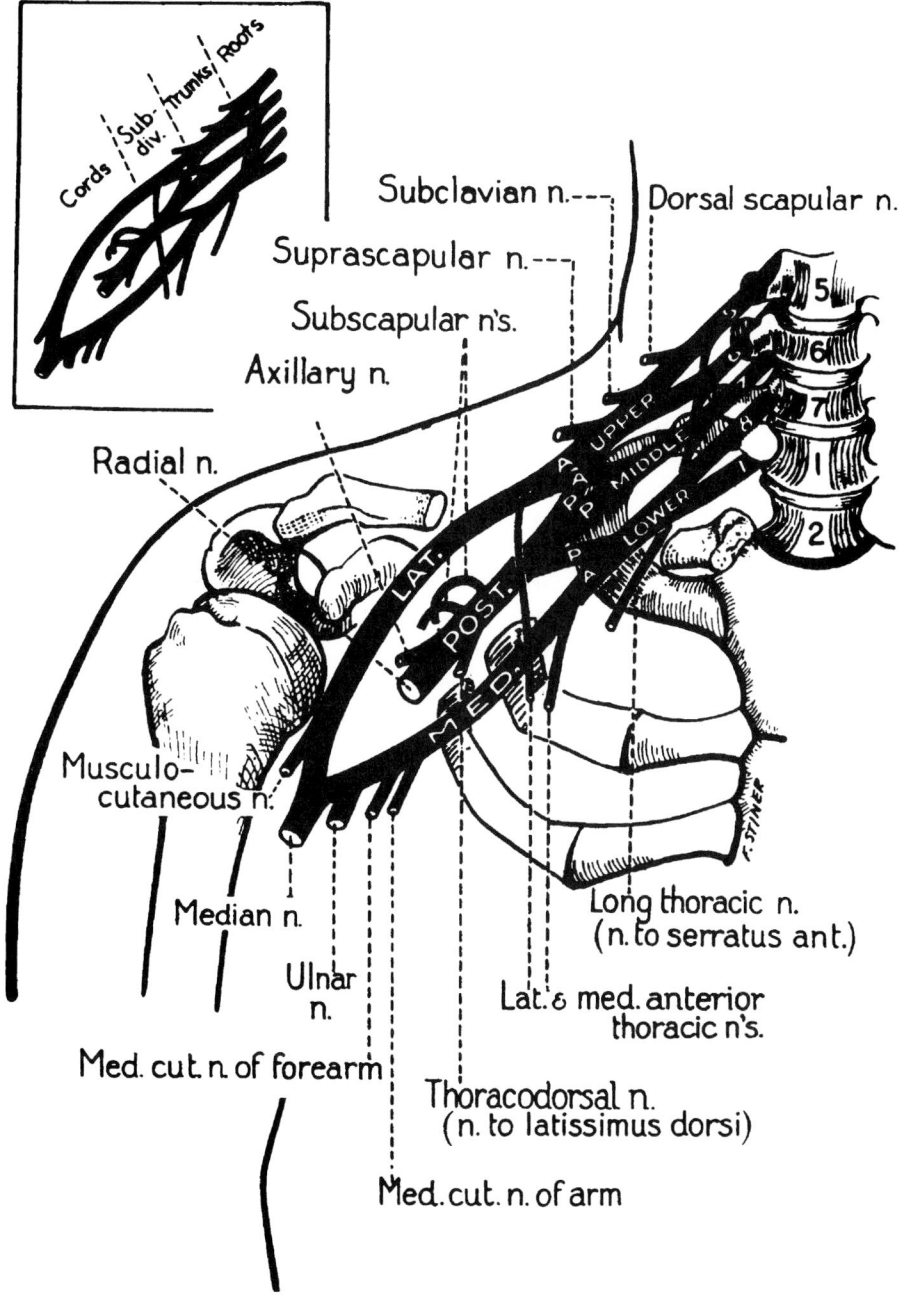

is sensory loss over the medial two fingers, the medial aspect of the hand, and the forearm.

Cord lesions are usually found in the setting of trauma. A posterior cord lesion produces weakness in the territory of muscles innervated by both radial and axillary nerves. Sensory loss occurs in the distributions of the posterior cutaneous nerve of the forearm and the radial and axillary nerves. This results in sensory loss over the posterior aspect of the arm, the dorsal surface of the lateral aspect of the hand, and a patch of skin over the lateral aspect of the arm. Lateral cord injuries produce weakness in muscles supplied by the musculocutaneous nerve as well as weakness in the

muscles of the median nerve supplied by the C6 and C7 roots (the pronator teres and flexor carpi radialis muscles). The median and ulnar nerve fibers originating from C8 and T1 segments are spared, and thus there is no intrinsic hand muscle weakness. In medial cord lesions, there is weakness in all ulnar nerve–supplied muscles and in the C8 and T1 median nerve–supplied muscles.

Electrodiagnostic Studies

The EMG is extremely helpful in confirming the diagnosis of brachial plexopathy. Evidence for a neurogenic lesion (fibrillation potentials, positive sharp waves, and reduced motor unit recruitment) in muscles innervated by at least two cervical segments involving at least two different peripheral nerves identifies the condition as a disorder of the plexus. Because the lesion in plexopathy is by definition distal to the origin of the dorsal primary rami, needle examination of the cervical paraspinal muscles is normal. In a plexopathy, numbness and sensory loss are associated with reduced or absent SNAPs because the lesion is located distal to the DRG. In contrast, in a radiculopathy, sensory loss is found in the face of a normal SNAP because the lesion is proximal to the DRG. In certain conditions, plexopathy and radiculopathy coexist, so that the EMG discloses paraspinal muscle fibrillation and absent sensory action potentials. This situation is encountered most commonly in patients with traumatic lesions that damage the plexus and injure or avulse nerve roots. It is also found in peripheral neuropathies, such as diabetes, and in malignant plexopathies, in which tumor not only injures the plexus but also infiltrates the nerve roots by tracking through the intervertebral foramina. Specific EMG changes are covered under individual disorders of the plexus, later in the chapter.

Radiological Studies

Plain films of the neck and chest are often very helpful in evaluating arm weakness that is thought to be caused by a disorder of the brachial plexus. The presence of a cervical rib or long transverse process of C7 may provide an explanation for hand weakness and numbness, as seen in thoracic outlet syndrome. A lesion in the pulmonary apex, erosion of the head of the first and second rib, or the transverse processes of C7 and T1 may reveal the cause of a lower brachial plexopathy, as found in cases of Pancoast's tumor. CT scanning and MRI of the brachial plexus are also useful in detecting mass lesions of the plexus and may allow early diagnosis and specific therapy (Bilbey et al. 1994). CT-guided biopsy can be used to obtain cytological or histological material for precise diagnosis.

Traumatic Plexopathy

Three general categories of brachial plexus injury exist: (1) direct trauma; (2) secondary injury from damage to structures around the shoulder and neck, such as fractures of the clavicle and first rib; and (3) iatrogenic injury, most commonly seen as a complication of the administration of nerve blocks. Direct injury may be either open (gunshot wounds and lacerations) or closed (stretch or traction). The main causes of brachial plexus palsies are traction and heavy impact. Injuries are usually secondary to motorcycle and snowmobile accidents, but sporting accidents in football, bicycling, skiing, and equestrian events are also important. Supraclavicular injuries are more common, more severe, and have a worse prognosis than do infraclavicular injuries (Midha 1997). Another form of brachial plexus traction is seen in rucksack paralysis. The straps of a rucksack or backpack pressed to the shoulders may exert heavy pressure in the region of the upper trunk of the brachial plexus and thus lead to weakness in the muscles supplied by the suprascapular and axillary nerves and sensory loss in the C5 and C6 distributions.

Early Management

The consequences of brachial plexus injury are weakness and sensory loss referable to a part or the whole of the plexus. The ultimate objective in management is to restore as much neurological function as possible with the hope of returning the limb to its preinjury status, but one must first ensure that the cardiovascular and respiratory systems are stable. In open injuries, there may be damage to great vessels in the neck and injury to the lung, so that immediate operative intervention is necessary to save the patient's life. At the time of this early, acute intervention, it is important to assess to what degree the various elements of the plexus have been injured. As far as possible, disrupted elements should be tagged for later repair. It may be difficult to suture damaged fascicles, and the formation of scar may prevent successful nerve regeneration. Most authors agree that nerve resection, grafting, and anastomosis are all very difficult in the acute situation because nerve continuity may be difficult to assess. If portions of a plexus have been sharply transected, however, primary repair should be carried out.

Long-Term Management

Once the patient's general condition has stabilized, a careful assessment of motor and sensory function should be made. At this stage, an important issue is whether there has been root avulsion. This is a critical determination, with implications for management, because there is no hope for return of motor and sensory function in territories supplied by avulsed roots. Root avulsion is determined as discussed in the section on Disorders of Nerve Roots, earlier in this chapter. If the plexus elements are in continuity and the nerve fibers have received a neuropraxic injury with minimal axonotmesis, then return of normal strength and sensation is expected. In the face of axonotmesis, the main factor limiting return of function is the distance the regenerating axon sprouts must traverse before making contact with end organs. Unless the muscles and sensory receptors are reinnervated within approximately 1 year, a good functional result is unlikely. Thus, recovery of proximal muscle strength from upper portions of the plexus is more likely than recovery of hand function when lower elements have been damaged.

Often, surgery must be performed to provide an exact intraoperative definition of the lesion's extent (see Chapter 56D; Berger and Becker 1994). Intraoperative motor evoked potentials are helpful in assessing the functional state of anterior motor roots and motor fibers. Depending on the findings, neurolysis, nerve grafting, or reneurotization is performed. Primary nerve reconstruction combined with joint fusion and tendon transfers provides a worthwhile return of function to many patients. The joint and tendon surgeries are best performed as secondary operations after a period of physiotherapy. Intensive physiotherapy and use of orthoses are often necessary to help restore maximum function. In general, the outcome after nerve grafting is relatively good for recovery of elbow flexors and extensors and for those of the shoulder girdle, but it is very poor for forearm and hand intrinsic muscles. Quality-of-life surveys after brachial plexus surgery indicate that 78% of patients report at least moderate satisfaction (Choi et al. 1997).

Neurogenic Thoracic Outlet Syndrome

Although it is frequently diagnosed, neurogenic thoracic outlet syndrome is a rare entity, seen only once or twice a year in busy EMG laboratories. The majority of patients are women. The mean age of onset is 32 years, but patients as young as 13 and as old as 73 have been reported. Pain is usually the first symptom, with either aching noted on the inner side of the arm or soreness felt diffusely throughout the limb. Tingling sensations accompany pain and are felt along the inner side of the forearm and in the hand. The majority of patients note slowly progressive wasting and weakness of the hand muscles. The physical examination discloses hand muscle weakness and atrophy, most marked in the lateral part of the thenar eminence. In a smaller number of patients, there is mild atrophy and weakness in the forearm muscles. Sensory loss is present along the inner side of the forearm. Except for the occasional Raynaud's-type episode, vascular symptoms and signs are uncommon.

In many cases, cervical spine roentgenograms disclose small, bilateral cervical ribs or enlarged down-curving C7 transverse processes. When not visualized in anteroposterior radiographs of the cervical spine, they can be seen on oblique views. MRI of the brachial plexus is a useful diagnostic method, revealing deviation or distortion of nerves or blood vessels and suggesting the presence of radiographically invisible bands (Panegyres et al. 1993). Electrodiagnostic studies on the affected side disclose a reduced median motor response with normal median sensory amplitudes along with a mildly reduced ulnar motor response and reduced ulnar sensory amplitude. The needle electrode examination typically discloses features of chronic axon loss with mild fibrillation potential activity in C8- and T1-innervated muscles. The clinical and electrophysiological findings point to a lesion of the lower trunk of the brachial plexus. In most patients, a fibrous band extending from the tip of a rudimentary cervical rib to the scalene tubercle of the first rib causes angulation of either the C8 and T1 roots or the lower trunk of the brachial plexus (Figure 79.10). Surgical division of the fibrous band can be expected to relieve pain and paresthesias and arrest muscle wasting and

weakness in the majority of patients; return of muscle bulk and strength, however, is unlikely.

Metastatic and Radiation-Induced Brachial Plexopathy in Patients with Cancer

Metastatic Plexopathy

Damage to the brachial plexus in patients with cancer is usually secondary to either metastatic plexopathy or radiation-induced injury. Lung and breast carcinoma are the tumors that most frequently metastasize to the brachial plexus; lymphoma, sarcoma, melanoma, and a variety of other types are less common. Tumor metastases spread via lymphatics, and the area most commonly involved is adjacent to the lateral group of axillary lymph nodes.

The hallmark of metastatic plexopathy is pain, which is often severe. It is generally located in the shoulder girdle and radiates to the elbow, medial portion of the forearm, and fourth and fifth digits of the hand. In many patients, the neurological examination discloses signs referable to the lower plexus and its divisions; more than one-half the patients have Horner's syndrome, whereas few have lymphedema of the affected limb. The predilection for involvement of the C8 and T1 spinal nerves and the lower trunk can be explained by the fact that the lateral group of axillary lymph nodes that drain the commonly located sites (breast and lung) are in close contact with the divisions of the lower trunk; the upper trunk and its divisions are remarkably free of lymph nodes. Some patients have signs indicating involvement of the entire plexus. In most of these patients, however, cervical CT myelography or MRI discloses epidural deposits that explain the upper plexus (C5 and C6 root) signs.

An important syndrome first described by Pancoast in 1932 is a superior pulmonary sulcus tumor, the vast majority of which are non–small cell bronchogenic carcinomas (Arcasoy and Jett 1997). The tumor arises near the pleural surface of the apex of the lung and grows into the paravertebral space and posterior chest wall, invading the C8 and T1 extraspinal roots, the sympathetic chain and stellate ganglion, the necks of the first three ribs, and the transverse processes and borders of the vertebral bodies of C7 through T3. The tumor may eventually invade the spinal canal and compress the spinal cord. Clinical features comprise a number of symptoms and signs: severe shoulder pain radiating to the head and neck, axilla, chest, and arm; pain and paresthesias of the medial aspect of the arm and digits IV and V; and weakness with atrophy of intrinsic hand muscles.

On occasion, metastatic brachial plexopathy may be difficult to distinguish from radiation plexopathy (see Radiation-Induced Plexopathy, later in this section). Imaging studies are usually informative. In patients with metastases, MRI can identify a mass adjacent to the brachial plexus and reveal

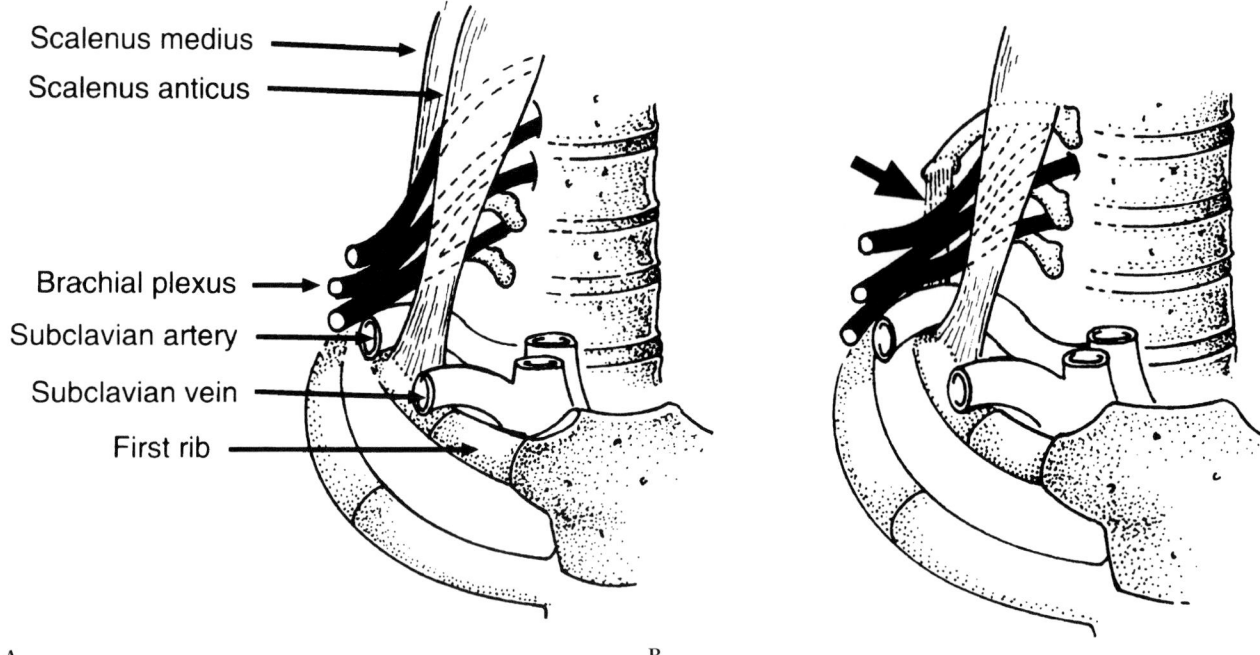

A   B

FIGURE 79.10   (A) The normal relationships of the subclavian artery and the brachial plexus as they course over the first rib between the scalenus medius and anterior muscles. (B) From the end of a short cervical rib arises a fibrous band (*arrow*), which attaches to the upper surface of the normal first rib. This stretches and angulates chiefly the lower trunk of the brachial plexus, causing neurogenic thoracic outlet syndrome. (Reprinted with permission from JD Stewart. Focal Peripheral Neuropathies [2nd ed]. New York: Raven, 1993.)

whether the tumor has encroached on the epidural space. CT remains a valued alternative investigation technique for this region because it provides good definition of the vertebral bodies. Nevertheless, sometimes exploration and biopsy by direct visualization may be the only definitive way to distinguish metastatic from radiation-induced plexopathy.

Results of the treatment of metastatic plexopathy are disappointing. Radiotherapy to the involved field and chemotherapy of the underlying tumor are the mainstays of treatment. Radiotherapy may relieve pain in 50% of patients but has little effect on return of muscle strength. A variety of procedures have been implemented to ameliorate the severe pain of this condition, including transcutaneous stimulation, paravertebral sympathetic blockade, and dorsal rhizotomies.

In the patient with Pancoast's tumor, preoperative radiotherapy followed by extended surgical resection is the most common treatment, with an overall 5-year survival rate of 20–35% (Arcasoy and Jett 1997).

Radiation-Induced Plexopathy

Radiation-induced plexopathy is unlikely to occur if the dose is less than 6,000 cGy. If more than 6,000 cGy is given, the interval between the end of radiation therapy and the onset of symptoms and signs of radiation plexopathy ranges from 3 months to 26 years, with a mean interval of approximately 6 years. The brachial plexus is more vulnerable to large fraction size, and thus fractions of 200 cGy or less are recommended. Cytotoxic therapy adds to the damaging effect of radiotherapy (Olsen et al. 1993).

Pain is usually a relatively minor aspect of the presenting symptom complex. Paresthesias and swelling, present in approximately one-half of patients, are more common than pain. Weakness is usually most prominent in muscles innervated by branches of the upper trunk, but involvement of the entire limb, from damage to the upper and lower portions of the plexus, has also been described.

The relative resistance of the lower trunk of the brachial plexus to radiation injury is perhaps explained by the protective effect of the clavicle and the relatively shorter course of the lower trunk and its divisions through the radiation port. The pathogenesis of radiation damage is thought to involve two factors: radiation-induced endoneurial and perineurial fibrosis with obliteration of blood vessels, and direct radiation-induced damage to myelin sheaths and axons. The natural history of radiation plexopathy is that of steadily increasing deterioration, although at times a plateau may be reached after 4–9 years of progression.

A diagnostic dilemma arises when symptoms and signs of brachial plexopathy develop in a patient who is known to have had cancer and radiation in the region of the brachial plexus. Some clinicians think that pain is the only feature that helps to separate the two forms of plexopathy (with severe pain favoring metastases). A painful lower trunk lesion with Horner's syndrome strongly suggests metastatic plexopathy, whereas a relatively painless upper trunk lesion with lymphedema is diagnostic of radiation-induced plexopathy. MRI is not always discriminating between metastatic and radiation because it may reveal an appearance of high signal intensity on T2-weighted images and contrast enhancement in cases of both radiation fibrosis and tumor infiltration (Wouter van Es et al. 1997). Needle EMG is helpful in separating radiation-induced plexopathy from neoplastic plexopathy by the presence of myokymic discharges in the former. These are spontaneously occurring grouped action potentials (triplets or multiplets) followed by a period of silence, with subsequent repetition of a grouped discharge of identical potentials in a semirhythmic manner. They appear to result from spontaneous activity in single axons induced by local membrane abnormalities. They have not been reported in cases of tumor plexopathy.

Idiopathic Brachial Plexopathy

Arm pain and weakness are the cardinal manifestations of idiopathic brachial plexopathy. It occurs in all age groups, but the majority of patients are distributed fairly evenly between the third and seventh decades. Men are affected two to three times more often than women; there appears to be a higher incidence among men engaged in vigorous athletic activities, such as weight lifting, wrestling, and gymnastics. Although one-half of the cases seem unrelated to any precipitating event, in others the neuropathy follows an upper respiratory tract infection, a flulike illness, an immunization, or prior surgery, or it occurs postpartum. Rare hereditary forms have also been described: a painless brachial plexopathy in patients with hereditary neuropathy with liability to pressure palsies, and a painful or painless hereditary neuralgic amyotrophy with predilection for the brachial plexus (Pellegrino et al. 1996).

Clinical Features

The illness begins with the abrupt onset of intense pain, described as sharp, stabbing, throbbing, or aching, located in a variety of sites, including the shoulder, scapular area, trapezius ridge, upper arm, forearm, and hand. The pain may last from hours to many weeks, and then it gradually abates. Lessening of pain is associated with the appearance of weakness. This may have been present during the painful period but was not appreciated because the pain prevented the patient from moving the limb. Weakness may progress for 2–3 weeks after the onset of pain. Although pain subsides in the majority of patients, it may continue for several weeks after weakness has reached its peak, and, rarely, it recurs episodically for a year or more. Paresthesias occur in approximately one-third of patients but do not correlate with the severity or extent of weakness.

On examination, approximately one-half of patients have weakness in muscles of the shoulder girdle, one-third have weakness referable to both upper and lower parts of the plexus, and approximately 15% have evidence of lower plexus involvement alone. Most appear to be incomplete because there is sparing of one or more muscles in the same root distribution. The patient may hold the arm in a characteristic posture, with flexion at the elbow and adduction at the shoulder, perhaps to reduce mechanical tension on the plexus.

Recognition is growing that the typical syndrome of brachial plexopathy need not always be associated with lesions of trunks or cords but can be caused by discrete lesions of individual peripheral nerves, including the suprascapular, axillary, long thoracic, median, and anterior interosseous. Thus, the term *brachial plexus neuropathy* may be appropriate. Sensory loss, found in two-thirds of patients, most commonly over the outer surface of the upper arm and the radial surface of the forearm, is usually less marked than is the motor deficit. One-third of cases are bilateral, but many fewer are symmetrical. In a small number of patients, unilateral or bilateral diaphragmatic paralysis occurs, and the combination of acute shoulder pain with respiratory symptoms should suggest the diagnosis of brachial plexus neuropathy.

Diagnosis

The major differential diagnostic consideration in a patient with acute arm pain and weakness is cervical radiculopathy related to cervicogenic disease. In this condition, however, pain is usually persistent, neck stiffness is invariable, and it is unusual for radicular pain to subside as weakness increases. Nonetheless, an upper trunk brachial plexopathy can simulate a C5 or C6 radiculopathy. The cervical paraspinal needle EMG done several weeks after the onset of pain should be normal in brachial plexus neuropathy but show increased insertional activity and fibrillation potentials in cervical radiculopathy. Another differential diagnostic consideration is neoplastic plexopathy, discussed earlier in this chapter. This entity is usually unremittingly painful, and neurological findings are most often referable to lower plexus elements. A third consideration might be a focal presentation of motor neuron disease, but pain is not a feature of this disease and sensation is always spared.

Electrodiagnostic testing is helpful in confirming the diagnosis and ruling out other conditions. Sensory studies are abnormal in one-third of patients; the most common abnormality is reduced amplitude of sensory action potentials of the median, ulnar, and radial nerves. Also helpful are musculocutaneous nerve conduction studies, which disclose significant reduction in the amplitude of the biceps compound muscle action potential. Needle EMG is helpful because it shows absence of fibrillation potentials in the cervical paraspinal muscles, thereby pointing to a pathological process distal to the DRG. Needle EMG is also helpful in sorting out the problems of localization, identifying lesions localized to the brachial plexus, individual peripheral nerves, or peripheral nerve branches. Finally, in a small number of patients, needle EMG is abnormal on the asymptomatic side as well as on the symptomatic side, indicating that brachial plexus neuropathy can sometimes be subclinical. Other laboratory studies are not helpful. In general, there are no specific immunological abnormalities, but syndromes resembling brachial plexus neuropathy have been found in association with systemic lupus erythematosus.

Pathophysiology and Etiology

The pathophysiology and pathogenesis of the disorder are not clear. An abrupt onset might suggest an ischemic mechanism; prior history of a viral syndrome or an immunization raises the possibility of an immune-mediated disorder. Complement-dependent, antibody-mediated demyelination may have participated in the peripheral nerve damage and nerve biopsy findings in four cases of brachial plexus neuropathy, which revealed florid multifocal mononuclear infiltrates, suggesting a cell-mediated component as well (Suarez et al. 1996). In some cases, rapid recovery bespeaks demyelination and remyelination; in others, a long recovery period is more in keeping with axonal degeneration followed by axonal regeneration. Indeed, a biopsy of a cutaneous radial branch in a severe case of plexopathy showed profound axonal degeneration. In most patients, electrophysiological abnormalities are restricted to the affected limb, whereas in a small number of cases, there is evidence of a more generalized polyneuropathy.

Treatment and Prognosis

In the acute stage of the disorder, narcotic analgesics are often required to control pain. A short, 10-day course of corticosteroids may be beneficial in a small number of patients. Arm and neck movements often aggravate pain; therefore, immobilization of the arm in a sling is helpful. With the onset of paralysis, range-of-motion exercises help to prevent contractures. In the small number of patients with significant permanent functional disability, orthotic devices may be helpful.

The natural history of brachial plexus neuropathy is benign; improvement occurs in the vast majority of patients, even in those with considerable muscle atrophy. Thirty-six percent have recovered by the end of 1 year, 75% by the end of 2 years, and 89% by the end of 3 years. Although some patients think they have made a full functional recovery, careful examination may disclose mild neurological abnormalities, such as isolated winging of the scapula, slight proximal or distal weakness, mild sensory loss, or reduced reflex activity. In two-thirds of patients, onset of improvement is noted in the first month after symptoms begin. Those who continue to be bothered by pain and lack any signs of improvement within the first 3 months of the illness take a longer time to recover.

DISORDERS OF THE LUMBOSACRAL PLEXUS

Anatomical Features

The lumbar plexus is formed within the psoas major muscle by the anterior primary rami of lumbar spinal nerves L1, L2, L3, and L4. It is connected to the sacral plexus in the true pelvis by the anterior division of L4 (Figure 79.11A). Branches of the lumbar plexus include the iliohypogastric and ilioinguinal nerves arising from L1 (with a contribution from T12), the lateral femoral cutaneous nerve of the thigh originating from the posterior divisions of L2 and L3, and the genitofemoral nerve arising from the anterior division of L1 and L2. Other branches are the femoral nerve, formed from the posterior divisions of L2, L3, and L4 within the substance of the psoas muscle, and the obturator nerve, formed by the anterior divisions of L2, L3, and L4.

The lumbar plexus communicates with the sacral plexus via the anterior division of L4, which joins with L5 to form the lumbosacral trunk at the medial border of the psoas at the ala of the sacrum. The trunk enters the pelvis and joins the sacral plexus in the piriformis fossa. The sacral plexus, derived from the anterior rami of spinal nerves L4, L5, S1, S2, and S3, forms in front of the sacroiliac joint (Figure 79.11B). Like the lumbar plexus, the sacral plexus has anterior and posterior divisions. The anterior division contributes to the tibial portion, and the posterior division contributes to the peroneal portion of the sciatic nerve, which leaves the pelvis through the greater sciatic notch. A number of important branches come from the sacral plexus in the pelvis; the superior and inferior gluteal nerves arise from posterior divisions of the sacral plexus and supply the gluteus medius and minimus muscles and the gluteus maximus, respectively. The posterior cutaneous nerve of the thigh is formed by the anterior divisions of S1, S2, and S3. It passes through the greater sciatic foramen into the buttock. The pudendal nerve originates from the undivided anterior primary rami of S2, S3, and S4 and extends into the gluteal region via the greater sciatic foramen.

Clinical Features

Neurological Examination

Lumbar plexopathy produces weakness, sensory loss, and reflex changes in segments L2 through L4, whereas sacral plexopathy leads to similar abnormalities in segments L5 through S3. Characteristic findings in lumbar plexopathy

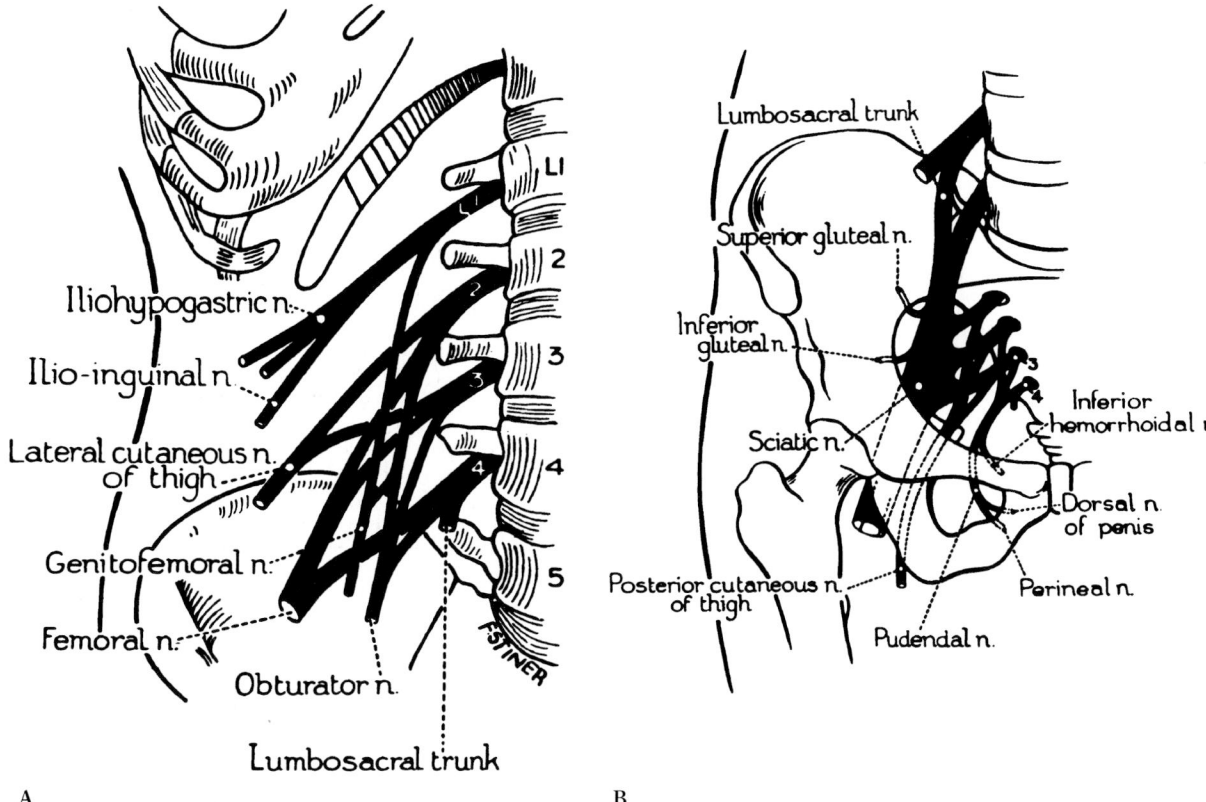

A   B

FIGURE 79.11 (A) The lumbar plexus is formed by anterior primary rami of lumbar spinal nerves (n's) L1, L2, L3, and L4. Note the branches that arise from the plexus. (B) The sacral plexus is connected to the lumbar plexus by the lumbosacral trunk. Note the branches that arise from the plexus in the pelvis. (Reprinted with permission of the author and publisher from W Haymaker, B Woodhall. Peripheral Nerve Injuries [2nd ed]. Philadelphia: Saunders, 1953.)

include weakness and sensory loss in both obturator- and femoral-innervated territories. Weakness of hip flexion, knee extension, and hip adduction, with sensory loss over the anteromedial aspect of the thigh, occurs; the knee jerk is absent or depressed. This combination of hip flexor and adductor weakness marks the disorder as either a plexopathy or radiculopathy. More precise localization depends on laboratory studies, including needle EMG, CT, and MRI.

Findings in sacral plexopathy include weakness and sensory loss in the territories of the gluteal (motor only), peroneal, and tibial nerves. Extensive leg weakness involving the hip extensors and abductors, knee flexors, and ankle plantar flexors and dorsiflexors exists. Sensory loss is found over the posterior aspect of the thigh, the anterolateral and posterior aspects of the leg below the knee, and the dorsolateral and plantar surfaces of the foot. Vasomotor and trophic changes may also be found in these areas. The ankle jerk is reduced or absent. Weakness of the gluteal muscles points to involvement of sacral plexus fibers proximal to the piriformis muscle in the true pelvis, or to a more proximal sacral root level. As in lumbar plexopathy, accurate diagnosis often depends on electrodiagnostic studies and neuroimaging procedures.

Electrodiagnostic Studies

Electrodiagnostic studies are performed for several reasons. First, the EMG is helpful in identifying a motor-sensory syndrome as a plexopathy and not a radiculopathy. The diagnosis of plexopathy is confirmed if the EMG discloses denervation (fibrillation potentials and positive sharp waves) and reduced recruitment (reduced numbers of motor units, firing rapidly) in muscles innervated by at least two lumbosacral segmental levels and involving at least two different peripheral nerves. An isolated plexopathy should not be associated with EMG abnormalities in paraspinal muscles. As will be seen, however, a number of pathological processes, including diabetes, radiation-induced changes, inflammation, vasculitis, and neoplasia may all involve the roots in addition to the plexus and produce a radiculoplexopathy. Second, EMG findings help to determine if a lumbosacral plexopathy is associated with a polyneuropathy. In the presence of the latter, signs of denervation and reinnervation are found bilaterally, especially in the distal muscles. Third, EMG findings may strongly suggest a particular type of plexopathy; for example, myokymic discharges point to the diagnosis of radiation plexopathy.

Table 79.1:   Clues to the nature of a plexopathy

Structural disorders
    History or presence of malignancy
    Hemophilia or treatment with an anticoagulant
    Pelvic trauma
    Known atherosclerotic vascular disease and hypertension
      (aneurysm)
    Pregnancy, labor, delivery
    Abdominal (pelvic) surgery
Nonstructural disorders
    Diabetes mellitus*
    Vasculitis
    Previous pelvic radiation

*Diabetics may develop a polyradiculoneuropathy that simulates a lumbosacral plexopathy.

Routine nerve conduction studies may help establish the diagnosis of plexopathy. Reduction in the amplitude of the sensory (sural and superficial peroneal) nerve action potentials indicates loss of axons distal to the DRG of S1 and L5, respectively. F responses are also sometimes useful in the diagnosis of a plexopathy. Prolongation in F-wave latency with normal motor nerve conduction studies distally suggests a proximal lesion, either at a root or plexus level. Finally, conduction across the lumbar and sacral plexuses with root stimulation in a plexopathy may show an increased latency across a particular portion of the plexus.

Neuroimaging Studies

Bone destruction found in plain radiographs of lumbar and sacral vertebrae and the pelvis provides evidence for a structural plexopathy. IV pyelography may demonstrate distortion of a ureter or the bladder. Barium enema may disclose displacement of the bowel. CT scanning of the abdomen and pelvis from a rostral point at the level of L1-L2 to a caudal point below the level of the symphysis pubis allows the regional anatomy of the entire lumbosacral plexus to be scrutinized (see Chapter 38).

The resolution of modern CT and MRI scanners allows identification of individual plexal components. The administration of oral or IV contrast is usually required to demonstrate the extent of structural abnormalities of the lumbosacral plexus, but it may not differentiate benign and malignant neoplasms, inflammatory masses, and hematoma. A normal MRI makes a structural plexopathy very unlikely. The CT may provide guidance for percutaneous needle biopsy of a lesion. Clues to the nature of a plexopathy are given in Table 79.1. An approach to evaluation of a plexopathy is summarized in Figure 79.12.

Differential Diagnosis

The differential diagnosis of lumbosacral plexopathy includes spinal root disorders, such as lumbosacral radiculopathy, polyradiculoneuropathy, cauda equina syndrome, anterior horn cell disorders, and myopathic conditions. Radiculopathies are usually painful, and the pain follows a predictable radicular distribution. Weakness is usually found in several muscles supplied by the same root, and the EMG usually demonstrates paraspinal muscle involvement. It is sometimes difficult to separate plexopathy from radiculopathy on clinical grounds alone, especially if several roots are involved.

Anterior horn cell disorders give rise to painless, progressive weakness with atrophy and fasciculation in the absence of sensory loss. When fully developed, such disorders should not be confused with lumbosacral plexopathy. In rare cases, however, a restricted anterior horn cell disorder, focal spinal muscular atrophy involving one leg, is seen. Absence of pain and sensory loss, normal imaging studies, and absence of diabetes and vasculitis all help point away from a disturbance of the lumbosacral plexus.

Myopathies are rarely confused with lumbosacral plexopathy. Myopathies with a focal, lower extremity onset can be distinguished from lumbosacral plexopathy by elevation of muscle enzymes, myopathic features on EMG (early recruitment of short duration, low-amplitude motor unit potentials), and muscle biopsy (variation in muscle fiber size, internalized nuclei, degeneration, regeneration, and inflammation).

Structural Lumbosacral Plexopathy

Hematoma

Patients with hemophilia and those receiving anticoagulants can develop hemorrhage in the iliopsoas muscle complex. It is important to recall that major components of the lumbar plexus, the femoral and obturator nerves, course from their origins in the lumbar paravertebral regions to their destinations in the thigh under cover of a tight layer of fascia. Over the iliac muscle, it is referred to as the *fascia iliaca*, and it becomes progressively thicker as it passes down, behind the inguinal ligament; at this site, it forms a dense and indistensible funnel enclosing the lower portions of iliacus and psoas.

Two major anatomical syndromes are associated with iliopsoas hematoma. In the first, the femoral nerve is the sole affected portion of the lumbar plexus. The hematoma arises in the iliacus and causes distention of the dense, overlying fascia above the inguinal ligament. In the second syndrome, hemorrhage arises in the psoas muscle or begins in the iliacus muscle and extends into the psoas. In this case, other components of the plexus, the obturator and lateral femoral cutaneous nerves, are involved.

Pain, often severe, is usually the first manifestation of a retroperitoneal hematoma. The pain is present in the groin and radiates to the thigh and leg. It is associated with gradually increasing paresthesias and weakness. When the femoral nerve is involved, weakness and sensory loss occur in its territory; when other components of the plexus are

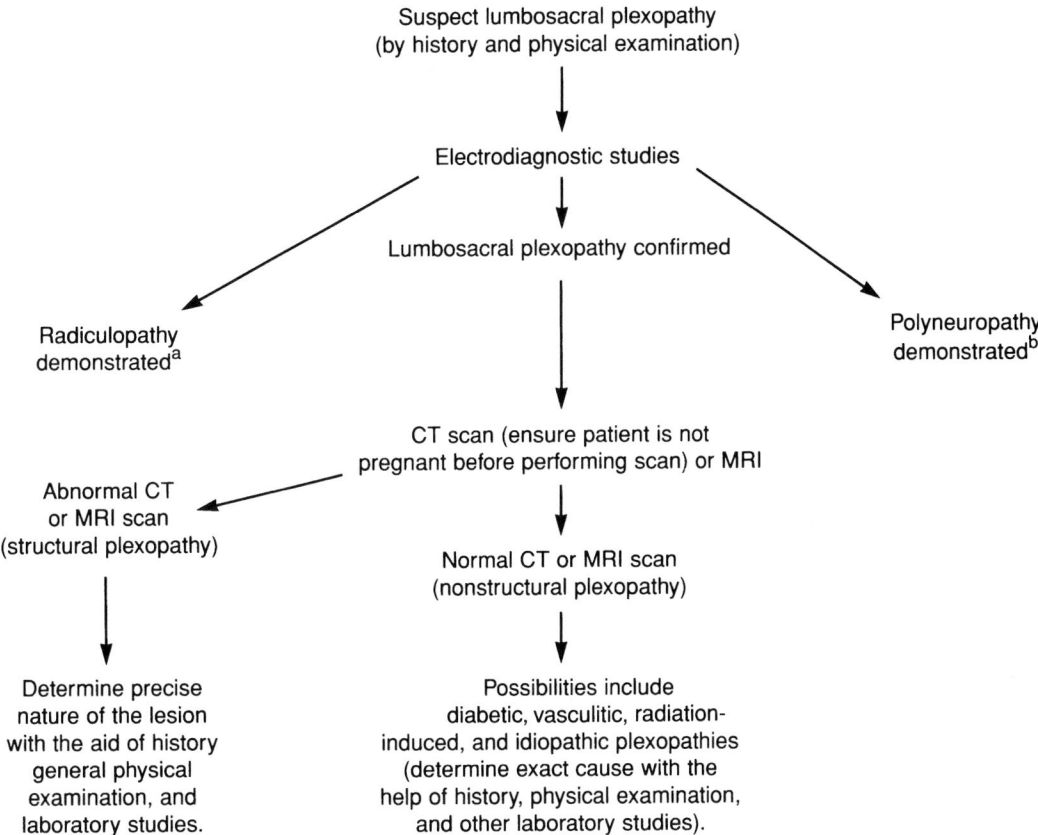

FIGURE 79.12   Approach to evaluation of lumbosacral plexopathy. (CT = computed tomography; MRI = magnetic resonance imaging.) [a]Radiculopathy is associated with plexopathy in diabetes, vasculitis, radiation, and malignancy. Electrophysiological identification of radiculopathy may require spinal CT myelogram or MRI for confirmation and precise diagnosis. [b]Polyneuropathy may accompany plexopathies due to diabetes, vasculitis, and certain malignancies (paraneoplastic neuropathies).

involved, changes are more extensive and conform to the territories supplied by the involved branches of the plexus. If the hemorrhage is large, a mass may develop in the lower abdominal quadrant. It typically arises from the lateral wall of the pelvis and can be seen in a CT scan to obscure the normal concavity of the inner aspect of the wing of the ilium (Figure 79.13). The patient usually lies in a characteristic posture with the hip flexed and laterally rotated because hip extension aggravates the pain. Several days after the onset of the hematoma, a bruise may appear in the inguinal area or femoral canal. In most patients, recovery is satisfactory, although 10–15% of patients show no improvement. Pain usually disappears within a week, and paresthesias and weakness resolve slowly.

Abscess

Psoas abscess was more common when tuberculosis was prevalent, but neurological complications, such as lumbar plexopathy and femoral neuropathy, were rare. This phenomenon was explained by the slow distention of the psoas sheath and by the fact that the abscess ruptured through the psoas fascia before the femoral nerve could be damaged

by raised intrapsoas compartment pressure. Similarly, acute nontuberculous psoas infection rarely produces nerve compression in cases of psoas abscess, presumably because the psoas fascia is distensible. Femoral neuropathy, however, does occur with iliacus muscle abscess because the fascia iliaca is relatively indistensible.

Aneurysm

Back and abdominal pain are often early manifestations of abdominal aortic aneurysms. Knowledge of abdominal and pelvic regional anatomy helps to explain the radiating characteristics of these pains. An expanding abdominal aortic aneurysm may compress the iliohypogastric or ilioinguinal nerve, leading to pain radiating into the lower abdomen and inguinal areas. Pressure on the genitofemoral nerve produces pain in the inguinal area, testicle, and anterior thigh. Compression of nerve trunks L5 through S2, which lie directly posterior to the hypogastric artery, may give rise to sciatica (Shields et al. 1997).

Hemorrhage from an abdominal aortic aneurysm may produce prominent neurological problems because of the retroperitoneal location of the hemorrhage or false

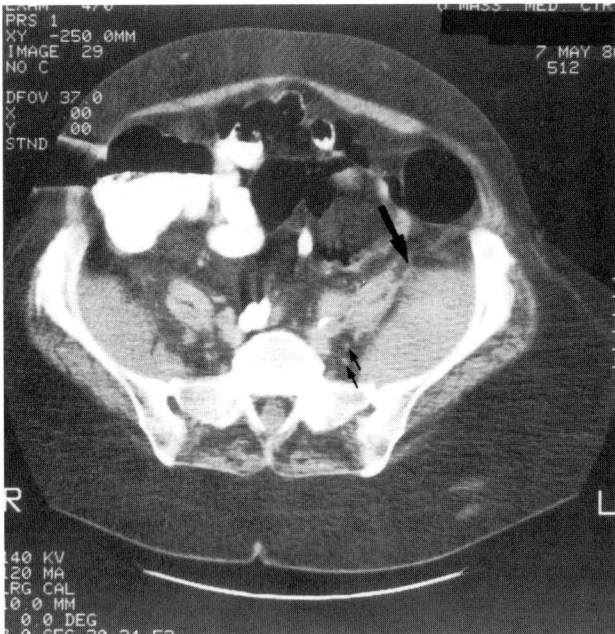

FIGURE 79.13 Hemorrhagic lumbosacral plexopathy. Computed tomographic scan at the L5-S1 level shows enlargement of the iliacus muscles, especially on the left side, owing to iliacus hematoma (*large arrow*). Small arrows indicate plexal elements. This large hematoma compresses the femoral and obturator nerves and the lumbosacral trunk.

aneurysm formation. In the case of an abdominal aortic aneurysm, a large retroperitoneal hematoma may injure the femoral and obturator nerves and even branches of the sacral plexus. Rupture of a hypogastric or common iliac artery aneurysm extends into the pelvis, compressing the L5 through S2 nerve trunk.

Ideally, the aneurysm should be diagnosed before rupture. Early recognition of an aneurysm is important because the mortality rate for operation on unruptured aneurysms is 5–7%, whereas that for symptomatic ruptured aneurysms is 35–40%. Unexplained back pain, leg pain, or pain radiating in the distribution of cutaneous nerves coming from the lumbar plexus should raise the suspicion of an aneurysm of the aorta or its major branches. A pulsatile mass felt while palpating the abdomen or, rarely, on rectal examination strongly suggests the presence of an aneurysm. Lumbosacral radiographs show a curvilinear calcific density, and abdominal sonography or CT scanning can confirm an aneurysm.

Trauma

Because of the relatively protected position of the lumbosacral plexus, traumatic lesions are not common. However, fracture of the pelvis, acetabulum, or femur or surgery on the proximal femur and hip joint may injure the lumbosacral plexus. Leg weakness is often incorrectly attrib-

uted to traumatic mononeuropathy involving the femoral or sciatic nerves rather than the lumbosacral plexopathy. The mechanism of post-traumatic paresis in lumbosacral plexopathies may involve a number of factors, including nerve crush caused by fractured bone fragments; retroperitoneal hemorrhage; and traction as a result of hyperextension, hyperflexion, or rotation around the hip joint. Conservative measures appear to be the most appropriate way to manage post-traumatic injuries. More than two-thirds of patients show good or moderate recovery of paresis after 18 months of follow-up after injury.

Pregnancy

The lumbosacral trunk may be compressed by the fetal head during the second stage of labor. This tends to occur in prolonged labor with midforceps rotation in a short, primigravida mother carrying a relatively large baby. A day or so after delivery, when the patient gets out of bed, she notes difficulty walking because of foot dorsiflexor weakness. Examination discloses weakness in dorsiflexion and inversion, with reduced sensation over the lateral aspect of the leg and dorsal surface of the foot. Nerve conduction studies disclose attenuation of the sural potential on the affected side, and EMG reveals denervation in muscles innervated by peroneal and tibial components of the sciatic nerve. The prognosis for recovery is very good. In subsequent pregnancies, a trial of labor can be allowed as long as there is no evidence of disproportion or malpresentation. If labor proceeds, forceps should be used with great caution. Midforceps use in a woman with a previous obstetrical lumbosacral trunk palsy invites danger. It is prudent to perform cesarean section if the trial of labor is unsuccessful or if the infant is very large.

Femoral neuropathy may occur in a thin patient during cesarean section in cases managed with self-retaining retractors (Alsever 1996). In the thin abdominal wall, a deep, lateral insertion of retractor blades exerts pressure on the psoas and may injure the femoral nerve. After surgery, the patient notes weakness and numbness in the territory of the femoral nerve. Recovery is usually rapid and full. The obturator nerve may be compressed by the fetal head or forceps near the pelvic brim. Patients note pain in the groin and anterior thigh as well as weakness and sensory loss in the territory of this nerve.

Neoplasia

The lumbosacral plexus may be damaged by tumors that invade the plexus either by direct extension from intra-abdominal neoplasm or by metastases. Most tumors involve the plexus by direct extension (73%), whereas metastases account for only one-fourth of cases. The primary tumors most frequently encountered are colorectal, cervical, and breast, as well as sarcoma and lymphoma. Three clinical syndromes occur: upper plexopathy with findings referable to the L1-L4 segments (31%); lower plexopathy with changes in the L4-S1 segments (51%); and pan-plexopathy with abnormalities in the L1-S3 distribution (18%). Neoplastic plexopathy typically has an insidious onset over weeks to months. Pain is a prominent early manifestation and is aching or cramping in quality. Weeks to months after pain begins, numbness, paresthesias, weakness, and leg edema develop. Incontinence or impotence occurs in fewer than 10% of patients. The most commonly encountered tumors are colorectal in upper plexopathy, sarcomas in lower plexopathy, and genitourinary tumors in pan-plexopathies. The majority of neoplastic plexopathies are unilateral, although bilateral plexopathies, caused usually by breast cancer, occur in approximately 25% of patients. The prognosis in lumbosacral plexopathy caused by neoplasm is poor, with a median survival of 5.5 months.

Three special syndromes do not fit easily into upper, lower, or pan-plexopathy categories. In the first, there are paresthesias or pain in the lower abdominal quadrant or groin, with little or no motor abnormality. These patients are found to have a tumor next to L1 leading to involvement of the ilioinguinal, iliohypogastric, or genitofemoral nerves. A second group has numbness over the dorsomedial portion of the foot and sole, with weakness of knee flexion, ankle dorsiflexion, and inversion. These patients have a lesion at the level of the sacral ala, with involvement of the lumbosacral trunk. A third group presents with perineal sensory loss and sphincter weakness and have neoplastic involvement of the coccygeal plexus, caused usually by rectal tumors.

Neuroimaging with CT or MRI usually establishes the diagnosis of neoplastic plexopathy, but MRI is probably more sensitive (Taylor et al. 1997). Because pelvic neoplasms may extend into the epidural space, most often below the conus medullaris, MRI of the lumbosacral spine is indicated in most patients. On occasion, a plexus neoplasm is difficult to discern by the best neuroimaging procedures. Two main explanations for this phenomenon exist. First, patients who have received previous radiotherapy may have developed tissue fibrosis that cannot be distinguished from recurrent tumor. Second, some tumors track along the plexus roots and do not produce an identifiable mass. In these instances, ancillary imaging tests (high-resolution MRI, bone scan, plain films, IV pyelogram), a biopsy of the plexus, or both may be required to determine the etiology.

Nonstructural Lumbosacral Plexopathy

Radiation Plexopathy

Radiation plexopathy usually produces slowly progressive, painless weakness. Pain develops in approximately one-half of patients with radiation plexopathy, but it is not usually a major problem. Most patients with radiation plexopathy eventually develop bilateral weakness, which is often asym-

metrical and affects predominantly the distal muscles in the L5-S1 distribution. In most patients, leg reflexes are absent, and superficial sensation is impaired. Symptoms referable to bowel or urinary tract are usually the result of proctitis or bladder fibrosis. The latent interval between radiation and the onset of neurological manifestations is between 1 and 31 years (median, 5 years), although very short latencies of less than 6 months have also been reported. No consistent relationship is evident between the duration of the symptom-free interval and the amount of radiation.

In most patients, radiation plexopathy is gradually progressive and results in significant or severe disability. CT and MRI of the abdomen and pelvis are normal. EMG discloses paraspinal fibrillation potentials in 50% of patients, suggesting that radiation damages the nerve roots in addition to the plexus; hence, a more appropriate designation is *radiation radiculoplexopathy*. In almost 60% of patients, the EMG discloses myokymic discharges, a feature that is only rarely seen in neoplastic plexopathy.

Vasculitis

Vasculitic neuropathy has generally been associated with the pattern of multiple mononeuropathy, but other neuropathic syndromes have also been described, including painful lumbosacral plexopathy. The portions of the peripheral nervous system most susceptible to vasculitis-induced ischemia are the segments of peripheral nerve located at the midhumerus and midfemur levels, regions of nerve that appear to be watershed zones between vascular territories of the vasa nervorum. Proximal nerve trunks and nerve roots may also be vulnerable to the vasculitic process.

When a lumbosacral plexopathy syndrome occurs in a patient known to have a vasculitis, such as polyarteritis nodosa or rheumatoid arthritis, vasculitic plexopathy is an obvious diagnosis. The clinical diagnosis is more difficult in the setting of a seemingly idiopathic polyneuropathy or plexopathy because the process may be monosystemic and restricted to the peripheral nervous system. In such a case, a nerve biopsy may be required to establish the correct diagnosis.

Idiopathic Lumbosacral Plexopathy

Lumbosacral plexopathy may occur in the absence of a recognizable underlying disorder. Thus, it can be considered a counterpart of idiopathic brachial plexus neuropathy (van Alfen and van Engelen 1997). It may begin suddenly with pain, followed by weakness, which progresses for days or sometimes many weeks. In many patients, the condition stabilizes, but in some, the course is chronic progressive or relapsing and remitting. Weakness is found in the distribution of upper and lower portions of the lumbosacral plexus in 50% of cases; major involvement occurs in the territory of the upper portion in 40% and in the lower portion in only 10% of patients. Most patients recover over a period of months to 2 years, although recovery is often incomplete. The EMG discloses a patchy pattern of denervation in the distribution of part or all of the lumbosacral plexus, but the paraspinal muscles are spared, indicating that the process does not affect the lumbosacral roots. The mechanism of plexopathy may be inflammation, but no confirmatory pathological studies are available. Some patients with the progressive disorder respond to high-dose IV immunoglobulin (Verma and Bradley 1994).

REFERENCES

Alsever JD. Lumbosacral plexopathy after gynecologic surgery: case report and review of the literature. Am J Obstet Gynecol 1996;174:1769–1778.

Arcasoy SM, Jett JR. Superior pulmonary sulcus tumors and Pancoast's syndrome. N Engl J Med 1997;337:1370–1376.

Arvin AM. Varicella-zoster virus: overview and clinical manifestations. Semin Dermatol 1996;15(2 Suppl.):4–7.

Balm M, Hammack J. Leptomeningeal carcinomatosis. Presenting features and prognostic factors. Arch Neurol 1996;53:626–632.

Berger A, Becker MH. Brachial plexus surgery: our concept of the last twelve years. Microsurgery 1994;15:760–767.

Bertorini T, Halford H, Lawrence J, et al. Contrast-enhanced magnetic resonance imaging of the lumbosacral roots in the dysimmune inflammatory polyneuropathies. J Neuroimaging 1995;5:9–15.

Bilbey JH, Lamond RG, Mattrey RF. MR imaging of disorders of the brachial plexus. J Magn Reson Imaging 1994;4:13–18.

Bowen J, Gregory R, Squier M, Donaghy M. The post-irradiation lower motor neuron syndrome: neuronopathy or radiculopathy. Brain 1996;119:1429–1439.

Carette S, Leclaire R, Marcoux S, et al. Epidural corticosteroid injections for sciatica due to herniated nucleus pulposus. N Engl J Med 1997;336:1634–1640.

Carvalho GA, Nikkhah G, Matthies C, et al. Diagnosis of root avulsions in traumatic brachial plexus injuries: value of computerized tomography myelography and magnetic resonance imaging. J Neurosurg 1997;86:69–76.

Choi PD, Novak CB, Mackinnon SE, Kline DG. Quality of life and functional outcome following brachial plexus injury. J Hand Surg (Am) 1997;22:605–612.

Corral I, Quereda C, Casado JL, et al. Acute polyradiculopathies in HIV-infected patients. J Neurol 1997;244:499–504.

de Verdier HJ, Colletti PM, Terk MR. MRI of the brachial plexus: a review of 51 cases. Comput Med Imaging Graph 1993;17:45–50.

Hildebrand C, Karlsson M, Risling M. Ganglionic axons in motor roots and pia mater. Prog Neurobiol 1997;51:89–128.

Komori H, Shinomiya K, Nakai O, et al. The natural history of herniated nucleus pulposus with radiculopathy. Spine 1996;21:225–229.

Levin KH. L5 radiculopathy with reduced superficial peroneal sensory responses: intraspinal and extraspinal causes. Muscle Nerve 1998;21:3–7.

Levin KH, Maggiano HJ, Wilbourn AJ. Cervical radiculopathies: comparison of surgical and EMG localization of single root lesions. Neurology 1996;46:1022–1025.

Longstreth GF. Diabetic thoracic polyradiculopathy: ten patients with abdominal pain. Am J Gastroenterol 1997;92:502–505.

Merchut MP, Gruener G. Segmental zoster paresis of limbs. Electromyogr Clin Neurophysiol 1996;36:369–375.

Midha R. Epidemiology of brachial plexus injuries in a multitrauma population. Neurosurgery 1997;40:1182–1188.

O'Leary CP, Willison HJ. Autoimmune ataxic neuropathies (sensory ganglionopathies). Curr Opin Neurol 1997;10:366–370.

Olsen NK, Pfeiffer P, Johannsen L, et al. Radiation-induced brachial plexopathy: neurological follow-up in 161 recurrence-free breast cancer patients. Int J Radiat Oncol Biol Phys 1993;26:43–49.

Panegyres PK, Moore N, Gibson R, et al. Thoracic outlet syndromes and magnetic resonance imaging. Brain 1993;116(Pt. 4):823–841.

Pellegrino JE, Rebbeck TR, Brown MJ, et al. Mapping of hereditary neuralgic amyotrophy (familial brachial plexus neuropathy) to distal chromosome 17q. Neurology 1996;46:1128–1132.

Posner JB, Dalmau JO. Paraneoplastic syndromes affecting the central nervous system. Annu Rev Med 1997;48:157–166.

Said G, Goulon-Goeau C, Lacroix C, Moulonguet A. Nerve biopsy findings in different patterns of proximal diabetic neuropathy. Ann Neurol 1994;35:559–569.

Sharma KR, Sriram S, Fries T, et al. Lumbosacral radiculoplexopathy as a manifestation of Epstein-Barr virus infection. Neurology 1993;43:2550–2554.

Shields RE, Aaron JO, Postel G, et al. A fatal illness presenting as an S1 radiculopathy. Vascular causes of lumbar radicular pain. J Ky Med Assoc 1997;95:268–270.

Stewart JD. Focal Peripheral Neuropathies (2nd ed). New York: Raven, 1993.

Suarez GA, Giannini C, Bosch EP, et al. Immune brachial plexus neuropathy: suggestive evidence for an inflammatory-immune pathogenesis. Neurology 1996;46:559–561.

Taylor BV, Kimmel DW, Krecke KN, Cascino TL. Magnetic resonance imaging in cancer-related lumbosacral plexopathy. Mayo Clin Proc 1997;72:823–829.

van Alfen N, van Engelen BGM. Lumbosacral plexus neuropathy: a case report and review of the literature. Clin Neurol Neurosurg 1997;99:138–141.

Verma A, Bradley WG. High-dose intravenous immunoglobulin therapy in chronic progressive lumbosacral plexopathy. Neurology 1994;44:248–250.

Watanabe M, Tanaka R, Takeda N. Correlation of MRI and clinical features in meningeal carcinomatosis. Neuroradiology 1993;35:512–515.

Wouter van Es H, Engelen AM, Witkamp TD, et al. Radiation-induced brachial plexopathy: MR imaging. Skeletal Radiol 1997;26:284–288.

Chapter 80
Disorders of Peripheral Nerves

E. Peter Bosch and Benn E. Smith

CLINICAL APPROACH TO DISORDERS OF PERIPHERAL NERVES

Peripheral neuropathies are caused by deranged function and structure of peripheral motor, sensory, and autonomic neurons. The main causes of neuropathy are entrapment, leprosy, diabetes, and other systemic diseases; inherited disorders; inflammatory demyelinating, ischemic, paraneoplastic conditions; deficiency states; and toxins. A logical systematic diagnostic approach consists of (1) a careful history, (2) a physical examination, and (3) electrophysiological studies, which not only confirm the presence of a peripheral nerve disorder but also may shorten the list of diagnostic possibilities. Further laboratory studies are often performed based on the outcome of the initial evaluation to arrive at a specific diagnosis. It is possible to establish a specific diagnosis in up to 75% of patients evaluated in tertiary referral centers by experts in neuromuscular disorders.

Pathological Processes Involving Peripheral Nerves

Despite the large number of causes of neuropathy, the peripheral nerve has a limited repertoire of pathological reactions to

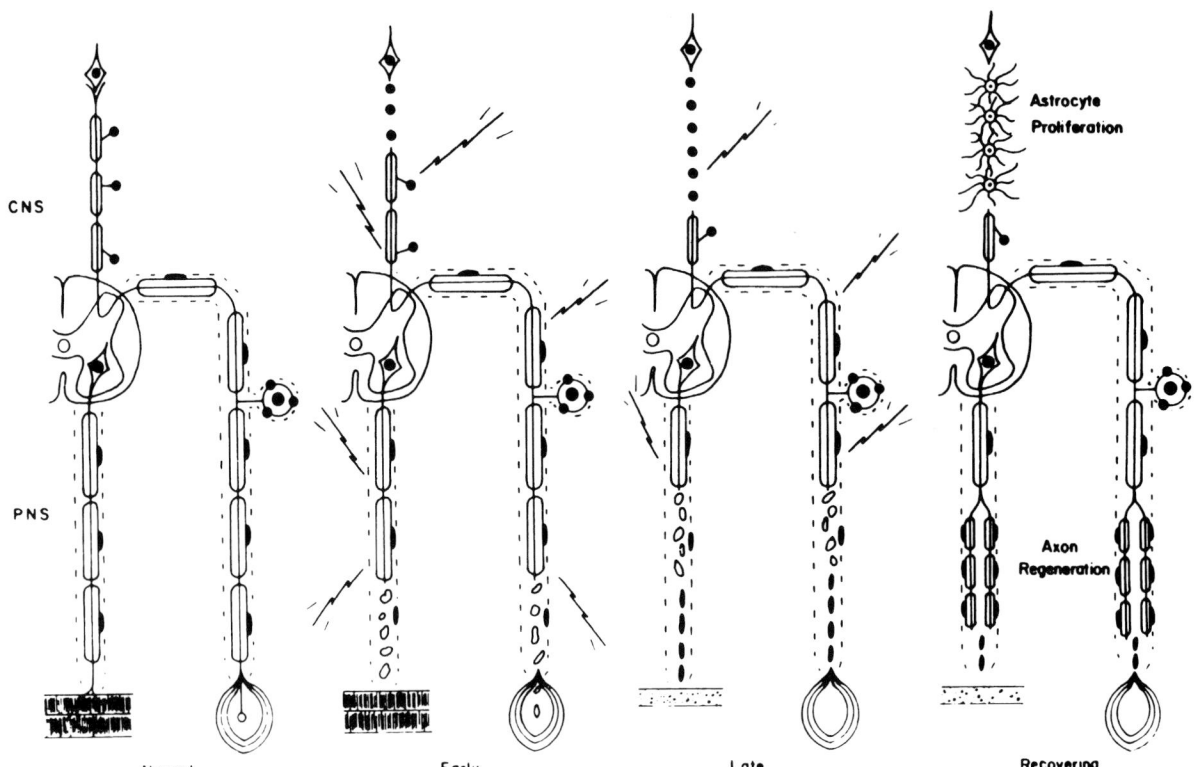

Normal   Early   Late   Recovering

FIGURE 80.1 A diagram of the main pathological events of distal axonal degeneration or axonopathy. The jagged lines indicate that either a toxin or a metabolic insult acts at multiple sites along motor and sensory axons in the peripheral nervous system (PNS) and central nervous system (CNS). Axonal degeneration begins at the most distal part of the nerve fiber and progresses proximally by the late stage. Recovery occurs by axonal regeneration but is impeded by astroglial proliferation in the CNS. (Reprinted with permission from HH Schaumburg, PS Spencer, PK Thomas. Disorders of Peripheral Nerves. Philadelphia: Davis, 1983.)

physical or metabolic insults. In general, these pathological reactions can be divided into four main categories: (1) wallerian degeneration, which is the response to axonal interruption; (2) axonal degeneration or axonopathy; (3) primary neuronal (perikaryal) degeneration or neuronopathy; and (4) segmental demyelination. The patient's symptoms, the type and pattern of distribution of signs, and the characteristics of nerve conduction study abnormalities provide information about the underlying pathological changes.

Any type of mechanical injury that causes interruption of axons leads to wallerian degeneration (degeneration of axons and their myelin sheaths) distal to the site of transection. Whereas motor weakness and sensory loss are immediate in the distribution of the damaged nerve, distal conduction failure does not occur until 3–9 days later as the distal nerve trunk becomes progressively inexcitable. Motor response amplitudes begin to decline by the third to fifth day after injury and excitability is lost by the seventh to ninth day. For sensory nerves the loss of evoked potentials is delayed a further 2–3 days. The temporal sequence of wallerian degeneration is length dependent, occurring earlier in shorter than in longer distal nerve stumps. Denervation potentials are seen in affected muscles 10–14 days after injury. Axonal interruption initiates morphological changes of the nerve cell body, termed *chromatolysis*, and produces a reduction in proximal

axonal caliber. Regeneration from the proximal stump begins as early as 24 hours following transection but proceeds slowly and is often incomplete. The quality of recovery depends on the degree of preservation of the Schwann cell–basal lamina tube and the nerve sheath and surrounding tissue, as well as the distance of the site of injury from the cell body, and the age of the individual.

Axonal degeneration, the most common pathological reaction of peripheral nerve, signifies distal axonal breakdown resembling wallerian degeneration, presumably caused by metabolic derangement within neurons (Figure 80.1). Systemic metabolic disorders, toxin exposure, and some inherited neuropathies are the usual causes of axonal degeneration. The myelin sheath breaks down concomitantly with the axon in a process that starts at the most distal part of the nerve fiber and progresses toward the nerve cell body, hence the term *dying-back neuropathy*. An identical sequence of events may occur simultaneously in centrally directed sensory axons, resulting in distal degeneration of rostral dorsal column fibers. The selective length-dependent vulnerability of distal axons could result from the failure of the perikaryon to synthesize enzymes or structural proteins, from alterations in axonal transport, or from regional disturbances of energy metabolism. In some axonopathies, alterations in axon caliber, either axonal atrophy or axonal swelling, may precede

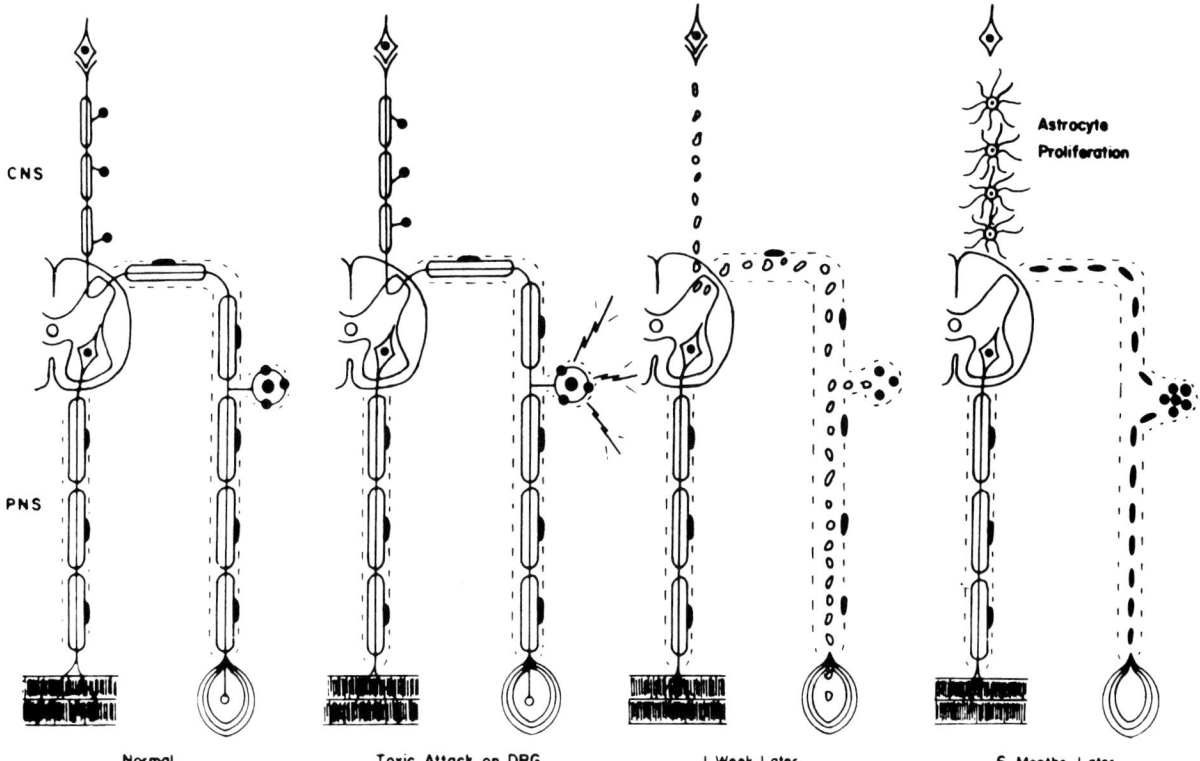

FIGURE 80.2 A diagram of the main pathological events of a sensory neuropathy or gangliopathy. A toxin, identified by the jagged lines, produces destruction of dorsal root ganglion (DRG) neurons, which results in degeneration of the peripheral-central axonal processes. Recovery is poor, as no axonal regeneration can take place. (CNS = central nervous system; PNS = peripheral nervous system.) (Reprinted with permission from HH Schaumburg, PS Spencer, PK Thomas. Disorders of Peripheral Nerves. Philadelphia: Davis, 1983.)

distal axonal degeneration. Clinically, dying-back neuropathy presents with symmetrical, distal loss of sensory and motor functions in the lower extremities and extends proximally in a graded manner. The result is sensory loss in a stockinglike pattern, distal muscle weakness and atrophy, and loss of ankle reflexes. Axonopathies result in low amplitude sensory nerve action potentials (SNAPs) and compound muscle action potentials (CMAPs), but they affect conduction velocities only slightly. Electromyography (EMG) of distal muscles shows acute, chronic, or both kinds of denervation changes (see Chapter 37B). Because axonal regeneration proceeds at a maximal rate of 2–3 mm per day, recovery may be delayed and is often incomplete.

Neuronopathy designates primary loss or destruction of nerve cell bodies with resultant degeneration of their entire peripheral and central axons (Figure 80.2). Either lower motor neurons or dorsal root ganglion cells may be affected. When anterior horn cells are affected as in anterior poliomyelitis or motor neuron disease, focal weakness without sensory loss is the result. *Sensory neuronopathy* or *polyganglionopathy* means damage to dorsal root ganglion neurons that results in inability to localize the limb in space, diffuse areflexia, and sensory ataxia. A number of toxins such as organic mercury compounds, doxorubicin, and megadoses of pyridoxine produce primary sensory neuronal degeneration. Immune-mediated inflammatory damage of dorsal root ganglion neurons occurs in paraneoplastic sensory neuronopathy and other conditions. It is often difficult to distinguish between neuronopathies and axonopathies on clinical grounds alone. Once the pathological processes are no longer active, sensory deficits become fixed and little or no recovery takes place.

The term *segmental demyelination* implies injury of either myelin sheath or Schwann cells, resulting in breakdown of myelin sheaths with sparing of axons (Figure 80.3). This occurs in immune-mediated demyelinating neuropathies and in hereditary disorders of Schwann cell–myelin metabolism. Primary myelin damage may be produced experimentally by myelinotoxic agents, such as diphtheria toxin, or mechanically by acute nerve compression. Demyelination also may occur secondary to alterations in axonal caliber, either atrophy or swelling, which may cause myelin remodeling over many consecutive internodes. Axonal atrophy and secondary demyelination are seen typically in uremic neuropathy. Remyelination of demyelinated segments usually occurs within weeks. The newly formed remyelinated segments have thinner than normal myelin sheaths and internodes of shortened length. Repeated episodes of demyelination and remyelination produce proliferation of multiple layers of Schwann cells around the axon, termed an *onion bulb*. The physiological consequence of acquired demyelination (i.e., inflammatory demyeli-

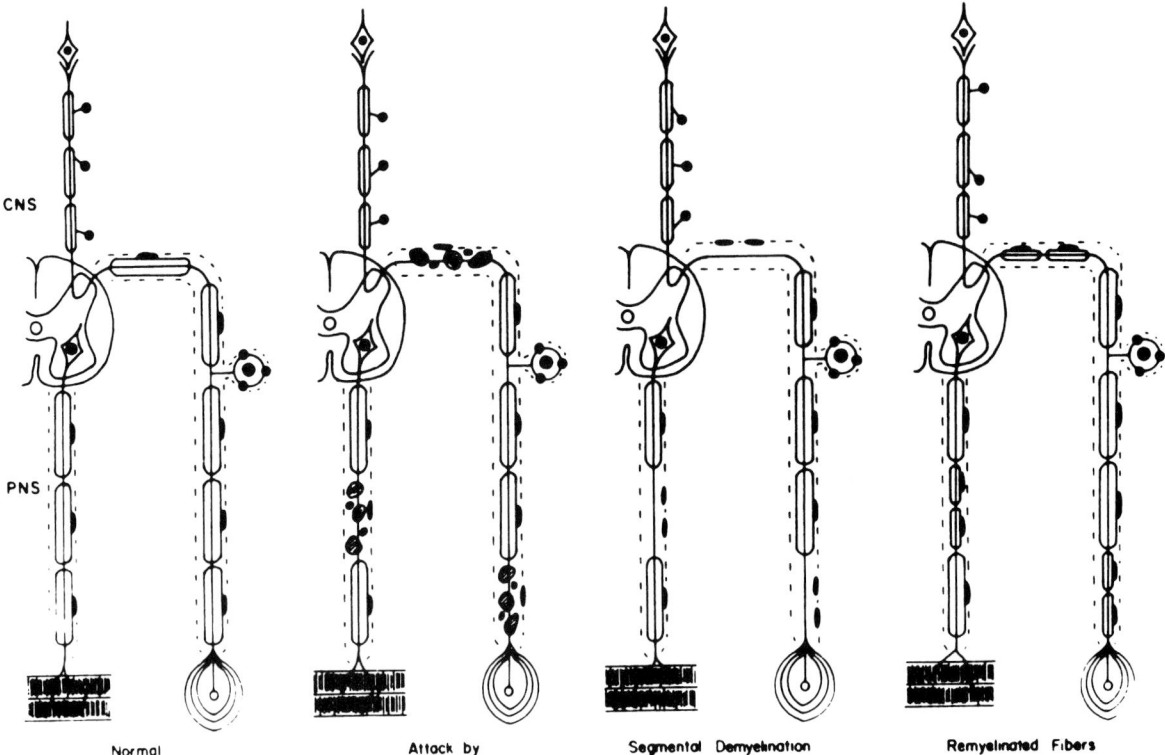

Normal   Attack by   Segmental Demyelination   Remyelinated Fibers
                Inflammatory Cells

FIGURE 80.3 A diagram of the main pathological events of primary segmental demyelination in immune-mediated inflammatory polyradiculoneuropathies. The attack by inflammatory cells causes multifocal demyelination along the entire length of nerve fibers but spares their axons. Recovery occurs by remyelination. The demyeli- nated segments become invested by several Schwann cells, resulting in a decrease in the internodal length of those areas. (CNS = central nervous system; PNS = peripheral nervous system.) (Reprinted with permission from HH Schaumburg, PS Spencer, PK Thomas. Disorders of Peripheral Nerves. Philadelphia: Davis, 1983.)

nation, but not hereditary myelinopathies) is conduction block, resulting in motor weakness. Relative sparing of temperature and pinprick sensation reflects preserved function of unmyeli- nated and small-diameter myelinated fibers. Early generalized loss of reflexes, disproportionately mild muscle atrophy in the presence of proximal and distal weakness, neuropathic tremor, and palpably enlarged nerves are all clinical clues that suggest demyelinating neuropathy. Nerve conduction studies or analy- sis of single teased nerve fibers can provide confirmation of demyelination. Demyelination is considered if motor and sen- sory nerve conduction velocities (NCVs) are reduced to less than 70% of the lower limits of normal. The presence of par- tial motor conduction block, temporal dispersion of CMAPs, and marked prolongation of distal motor and F-wave laten- cies are all features consistent with acquired demyelination (see Chapter 37B). Recovery depends on remyelination, and there- fore clinical improvement may occur within days to weeks. In many neuropathies, axonal degeneration and segmental demyelination coexist.

Diagnostic Clues from the History

The symptoms of neuropathic disorders fall under the gen- eral headings of motor, sensory, or autonomic disturbances. The inquiry should seek both negative and positive symp- toms. Muscle cramps, fasciculations, myokymia, or tremor are positive manifestations of motor nerve dysfunction. In polyneuropathies motor symptoms produce early distal toe and ankle extensor weakness, resulting in tripping on rugs or uneven ground. Complaints of difficulty walking do not distinguish muscle weakness from sensory, pyramidal, extrapyramidal, or cerebellar disturbance. If the fingers are weak, patients may complain of difficulty in opening jars or turning a key in a lock.

Positive sensory symptoms include prickling, searing, burning, and tight bandlike sensations. *Dysesthesia* is defined as an unpleasant, abnormal sensation in response to an ordinary, painless stimulus, whereas an unpleasant sensation arising spontaneously without apparent stimu- lus is called *paresthesia*. The presence of spontaneously reported paresthesias is helpful in distinguishing acquired (symptoms occurring in more than 60% of patients) from inherited (reported in only 17% of patients) neuropathies. Allodynia is the perception of nonpainful stimuli as painful. Neuropathic pain, the extreme example of a pos- itive symptom, is a cardinal feature of many neuropathies. Neuropathic pain often has a deep, burning, or drawing character that may be associated with jabbing or shoot- ing pains, and typically increases during periods of rest.

Autonomic dysfunction can be helpful in directing attention toward specific neuropathies that have prominent autonomic symptoms. It is important to ask about orthostatic lightheadedness, fainting spells, reduced or excessive sweating, and heat intolerance, as well as bladder, bowel, and sexual dysfunction. Anorexia, early satiety, and nausea are symptoms suggestive of gastroparesis. The degree of autonomic involvement can be documented by noninvasive autonomic function studies (Low 1993a) (see Chapter 81).

Historical information regarding onset, duration, and evolution of symptoms provides important clues to diagnosis. Knowledge about the tempo of disease (acute, subacute, or chronic) and the course (monophasic, progressive, or relapsing) narrows diagnostic possibilities. Guillain-Barré syndrome (GBS), acute porphyria, vasculitis, and some cases of toxic neuropathy have acute presentations. A relapsing course is found in chronic inflammatory demyelinating polyradiculoneuropathy (CIDP), acute porphyria, Refsum's disease, hereditary neuropathy with liability to pressure palsies (HNPP), familial brachial plexus neuropathy, and repeated episodes of toxin exposure.

In patients with a chronic indolent course over many years, inquiries about similar symptoms and foot deformities such as pes cavus in immediate relatives often point to a familial neuropathy. Inherited neuropathies are a major cause of undiagnosed neuropathy, accounting for 30–40% of patients referred to tertiary centers for diagnosis. The clinical and electrophysiological evaluation of relatives of patients with undiagnosed neuropathy may corroborate that the disorder is familial. Many neuropathies are caused by systemic disease. The presence of constitutional symptoms such as weight loss, malaise, and anorexia suggests an underlying systemic disorder. Inquiry should be made about preceding or concurrent associated medical conditions (diabetes mellitus, hypothyroidism, chronic renal failure, liver disease, intestinal malabsorption, malignancy, connective tissue diseases, human immunodeficiency virus [HIV] seropositivity), drug use, including over-the-counter vitamin preparations (vitamin B$_6$), alcohol and dietary habits, and exposure to solvents, pesticides, or heavy metals.

Diagnostic Clues from the Examination

The first step is to determine the anatomical pattern and localization of the disease process and the involvement of motor, sensory, or autonomic neurons inferred from the examination. Single root (monoradiculopathy) and brachial or lumbar plexopathies produce typical unilateral motor and sensory signs and symptoms (see Chapter 79).

Mononeuropathy means focal involvement of a single nerve and implies a local process. Direct trauma, compression or entrapment, vascular lesions, and neoplastic infiltration are the most common causes. Electrophysiological studies provide a more precise localization of the lesion

Table 80.1: Causes of multiple mononeuropathies

Axonal injury
Vasculitis (systemic, nonsystemic)
Diabetes mellitus
Sarcoidosis
Leprosy
Human immunodeficiency virus 1 infection
Demyelination/conduction block
Multifocal motor neuropathy
Multiple compression neuropathies (hypothyroidism, diabetes)
Hereditary neuropathy with liability to pressure palsies

than may be possible by clinical examination and can separate axonal loss from focal segmental demyelination. Nerve conduction studies may reveal widespread changes, indicating an underlying neuropathy that predisposes to nerve entrapment, such as diabetes mellitus, hypothyroidism, acromegaly, alcoholism, and HNPP.

Multiple mononeuropathy or mononeuropathy multiplex signifies simultaneous or sequential damage to multiple noncontiguous nerves. Confluent multiple mononeuropathies may give rise to motor weakness with sensory loss that can simulate a peripheral polyneuropathy. Electrodiagnostic studies ascertain whether the primary pathological process is axonal degeneration or segmental demyelination (Table 80.1). Approximately two-thirds of patients with multiple mononeuropathies display a picture of axonal damage. Ischemia caused by systemic or nonsystemic (peripheral nerve) vasculitis or microangiopathy in diabetes mellitus should be considered. Other less common causes are disorders affecting interstitial structures of nerve, namely infectious, granulomatous, leukemic, or neoplastic infiltration, including leprosy, sarcoidosis, and lymphomatoid granulomatosis. In the event that focal demyelination or motor conduction block leads to multiple mononeuropathies, hereditary liability to pressure palsies or multifocal motor neuropathy should be considered.

Polyneuropathy is characterized by symmetrical, distal motor and sensory deficits that have a graded increase in severity distally and by distal attenuation of reflexes. The sensory deficits produce a stocking-glove pattern. By the time sensory disturbances have reached the level of the knees, dysesthesias are noted in the tips of the fingers. When the sensory impairment reaches the midthigh, involvement of anterior intercostal and lumbar segmental nerves gives rise to a tent-shaped area of hypesthesia on the anterior chest and abdomen. Motor weakness is greater in extensor muscles than in corresponding flexors. For example, walking on heels is affected earlier than toe walking in most polyneuropathies. It is helpful to determine the relative extent of sensory, motor, and autonomic neuron involvement, although most polyneuropathies produce mixed sensorimotor deficits and some degree of autonomic dysfunction.

Table 80.2: Neuronopathies and neuropathies with predominantly motor manifestations

Motor neuron disease*
Multifocal motor neuropathy*
Guillain-Barré syndrome
Acute motor axonal neuropathy*
Porphyric neuropathy
Chronic inflammatory polyradiculoneuropathy
Osteosclerotic myeloma
Diabetic lumbar radiculoplexopathy
Hereditary motor sensory neuropathies (Charcot-Marie-Tooth
   disease)
Lead intoxication

*Pure motor syndromes with normal sensory nerve action
potentials.

Table 80.3: Neuropathies with facial nerve involvement

Guillain-Barré syndrome
Chronic inflammatory polyradiculoneuropathy (rare)
Lyme disease
Sarcoidosis
Human immunodeficiency virus 1 infection
Gelsolin familial amyloid neuropathy (Finnish)
Tangier disease

Table 80.4: Neuropathies with autonomic nervous system involvement

Acute
   Acute panautonomic neuropathy (idiopathic, paraneoplastic)
   Guillain-Barré syndrome
   Porphyria
   Toxic: vincristine, vacor
Chronic
   Diabetes mellitus
   Amyloid neuropathy (familial and primary)
   Paraneoplastic sensory neuronopathy (malignant
      inflammatory sensory polyganglionopathy)
   Human immunodeficiency virus–related autonomic
      neuropathy
   Hereditary sensory and autonomic neuropathy

Motor deficits tend to dominate the clinical picture in acute and chronic inflammatory demyelinating neuropathies, hereditary motor and sensory neuropathies, and in neuropathies associated with osteosclerotic myeloma, porphyria, lead or organophosphate intoxications, and hypoglycemia. Asymmetrical distal weakness without sensory loss suggests motor neuron disease or multifocal motor neuropathy with conduction block (Table 80.2). The distribution of weakness provides important information. The facial nerve can be affected in several peripheral nerve disorders (Table 80.3). In most polyneuropathies the legs are more severely affected than the arms. Notable exceptions to this rule are lead neuropathy, which frequently presents

with wrist drop, multifocal motor neuropathy with conduction block, familial amyloid neuropathy type 2, occasionally porphyria, and adult-onset Tangier disease. Polyradiculoneuropathies cause both proximal and distal muscle weakness. The nerve root involvement is confirmed by denervation in paraspinal muscles on needle EMG. For example, proximal and distal weakness is encountered in acute and chronic inflammatory demyelinating radiculoneuropathies, osteosclerotic myeloma, porphyria, and diabetic lumbar radiculoplexopathy.

Predominant sensory involvement may be a feature of neuropathies caused by diabetes, carcinoma, Sjögren's syndrome, dysproteinemia, acquired immunodeficiency syndrome (AIDS), vitamin B_{12} deficiency, intoxications with cisplatin or pyridoxine, and inherited and idiopathic sensory neuropathies.

Autonomic dysfunction of clinical importance is seen in association with specific acute (e.g., GBS) or chronic (e.g., familial amyloid neuropathy) sensorimotor polyneuropathies. Rarely, an idiopathic panautonomic neuropathy can be the exclusive manifestation of a peripheral nerve disorder without somatic nerve involvement (Table 80.4).

Loss of sensation in peripheral neuropathies usually involves all sensory modalities, but occasionally the impairment may be restricted to selective sensory modalities. The latter situation makes it possible to correlate the type of sensory loss with the pattern of afferent fiber loss according to fiber diameter size (Figure 80.4). Pain and temperature sensation are mediated by unmyelinated and small myelinated fibers, whereas vibratory sense, proprioception, and the afferent limb of the tendon reflex are subserved by large myelinated fibers. Light touch is mediated by both large and small myelinated fibers. Quantitative sensory testing assessing both vibratory and thermal detection thresholds has become a useful addition in controlled clinical trials to the bedside sensory examination. Its use in routine clinical practice remains limited because the test cannot overcome bias toward abnormality in individual patients. In polyneuropathies preferentially affecting small fibers, diminished pain and temperature sensation predominate, along with painful dysesthesias and autonomic dysfunction. Relative preservation of tendon reflexes, balance, and motor strength exist, and hence few objective neurological signs exist on examination. Because routine sensory conduction studies assess only large myelinated fibers, such studies may be entirely normal in selective small fiber neuropathies. Quantitative thermal sensory threshold testing, tests of autonomic function, and skin or nerve biopsy with morphometric studies of small and unmyelinated fibers may be necessary for confirmation. Sweating mediated by unmyelinated sympathetic cholinergic fibers is often involved. Impaired distal sweating can be assessed by the quantitative sudomotor axon reflex test. Relatively few disorders cause selective small fiber neuropathies (Table 80.5).

Selective large fiber sensory loss is characterized by areflexia, sensory ataxia, pseudoathetosis (involuntary move-

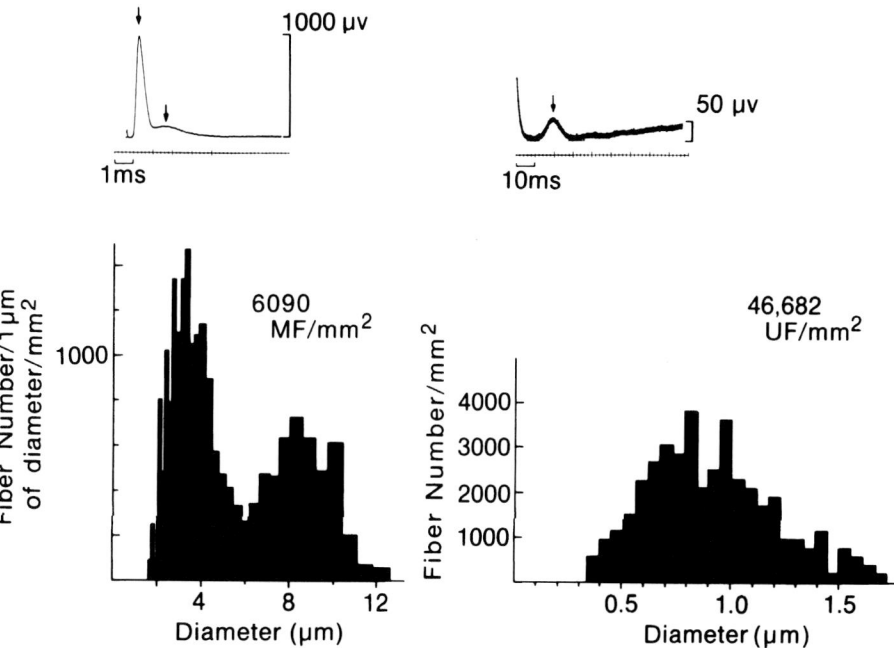

FIGURE 80.4 Myelinated fiber (MF) and unmyelinated fiber (UF) size-frequency histograms of a normal sural nerve. Fiber size distribution is bimodal for MF but unimodal for UF. The MF density in normal sural nerve ranges from 6,000 to 10,000 fibers/mm² of fascicular area. The number of UFs is normally approximately four times that of MFs. The corresponding compound nerve action potential recorded from the sural nerve in vitro is shown at top. Three distinct peaks indicated by arrows are, from left to right, Aα, Aδ, and C-potentials, which correspond to large MF, small MF, and UF peaks, respectively.

Table 80.5: Small fiber neuropathies

Amyloid neuropathy (familial and primary)
Diabetes mellitus (rare)
Idiopathic
Hereditary sensory and autonomic neuropathies
Fabry's disease
Tangier disease

Table 80.6: Sensory ataxic neuropathies

Sensory neuronopathies (polyganglionopathies)
   Paraneoplastic sensory neuronopathy (malignant inflammatory sensory polyganglionopathy)
   Sjögren's syndrome
   Idiopathic
Toxic polyneuropathies
   Cisplatin and analogues
   Vitamin B$_6$ excess
Demyelinating polyradiculoneuropathies
   Guillain-Barré syndrome (Miller Fisher variant)
   Immunoglobulin M monoclonal gammopathy of undetermined significance

Table 80.7: Neuropathies with skin, nail, or hair manifestations

Disease	Skin, nail, or hair manifestations
Vasculitis	Purpura, livedo reticularis
Cryoglobulinemia	Purpura
Fabry's disease	Angiokeratomas
Leprosy	Skin hypopigmentation
Osteosclerotic myeloma (POEMS syndrome)	Skin hyperpigmentation
Variegate porphyria	Bullous lesions
Refsum's disease	Ichthyosis
Arsenic or thallium intoxication	Mees' lines
Thallium poisoning	Alopecia
Giant axonal neuropathy	Curled hair

POEMS = *p*olyneuropathy, *o*rganomegaly, *e*ndocrinopathy, *m*onoclonal gammopathy, and *s*kin changes.

ments of fingers and hands when the arms are outstretched and the eyes are closed), and loss of joint position and vibration sense. A feature of sensory ataxia is a positive Romberg's sign, meaning disproportionate loss of balance with eyes closed compared with eyes open. Striking sensory ataxia together with inability to localize the limb in space or asymmetrical truncal or facial sensory loss directs attention to a primary disorder of sensory neurons or polyganglionopathies. The differential diagnosis of ataxic sensory neuropathies is limited (Table 80.6).

Palpation of peripheral nerves is an important part of the examination. Hypertrophy of a single nerve trunk suggests either a neoplastic process (neurofibroma, Schwannoma, or malignant nerve sheath tumor) or localized hypertrophic neuropathy. Generalized or multifocal nerve hypertrophy is found in a limited number of peripheral nerve disorders including leprosy, neurofibromatosis, Charcot-Marie-Tooth (CMT) disease types 1 and 3, acromegaly, Refsum's disease, and rarely CIDP.

Certain tell-tale signs of the skin and its appendages may direct the experienced examiner to a specific diagnosis (Table 80.7): Alopecia is seen in thallium poisoning; tightly curled hair in giant axonal neuropathy; white transverse nail bands termed *Mees' lines* in arsenic or thallium intoxications; telangiectasias over the abdomen and buttocks in Fabry's disease; purpuric skin eruptions of the legs in cryoglobulinemia and

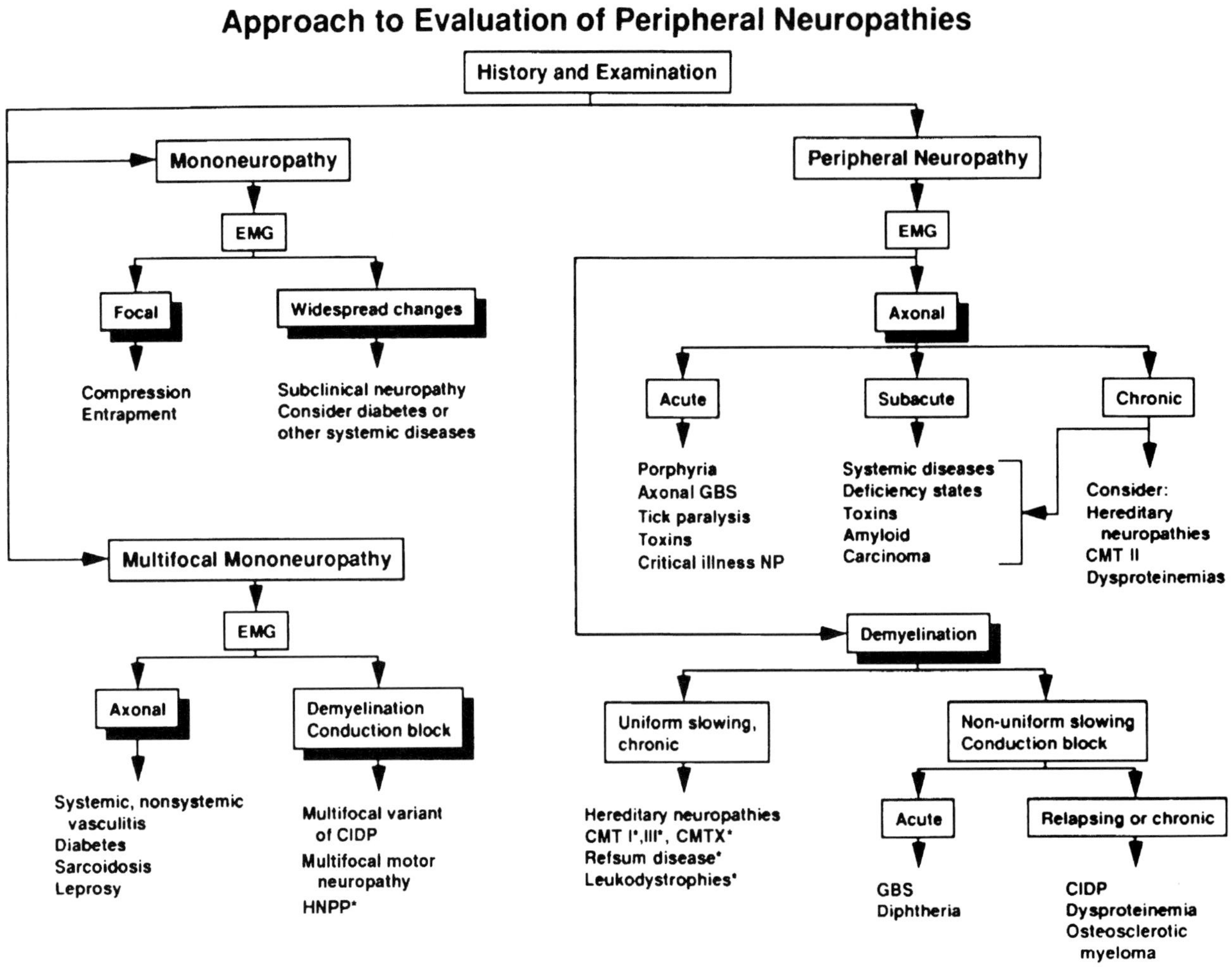

Approach to Evaluation of Peripheral Neuropathies

FIGURE 80.5 Diagnostic approach to the evaluation of a patient with peripheral neuropathy. Electromyography (EMG) denotes electrodiagnostic studies. DNA diagnostic testing or specific biochemical tests are available for those conditions marked with asterisks. (CIDP = chronic inflammatory demyelinating polyradiculoneuropathy; CMT = Charcot-Marie-Tooth disease; CMTX = Charcot-Marie-Tooth disease X-linked; GBS = Guillain-Barré syndrome; HNPP = hereditary liability to pressure palsies; NP = neuropathy.)

some vasculitides; skin hyperpigmentation or hypertrichosis in POEMS syndrome (characterized by *p*olyneuropathy, *o*rganomegaly, *e*ndocrinopathy, *m*onoclonal gammopathy, and *s*kin changes); enlarged yellow-orange tonsils in Tangier disease; pes cavus and hammer toes in CMT disease; and overriding toes and ichthyosis in Refsum's disease.

Electrodiagnostic Studies

It is helpful to follow a decision-making pathway initially based on the overall pattern of distribution of deficits, followed by the electrophysiological findings, and finally the clinical course (Figure 80.5). Electrodiagnostic studies, carefully performed and adapted to the particular clinical situation, play a key role in the evaluation by (1) confirming the presence of neuropathy, (2) providing precise localization of focal nerve lesions, and (3) giving information as to the nature of the underlying nerve pathology (see Chapter 37B).

Nerve Biopsy

Nerve biopsy should be performed only in centers with established experience with the technique; otherwise little useful information is likely to be obtained. The sural nerve is selected most commonly for biopsy because the resultant sensory deficit is restricted to a small area over the heel and dorsolateral aspect of the foot, and because its morphology has been well characterized in health and disease. The superficial peroneal nerve represents an alternative lower extremity cutaneous nerve suitable for biopsy and has the advantage of allowing simultaneous access to the peroneus brevis muscle through the same incision. This combined nerve and muscle biopsy procedure significantly increases the yield of identifying suspected vasculitis. Nerve biopsy has proved to be particularly informative when techniques such as single teased fiber preparations, semithin sections, ultrastructural studies, and morphometry are applied to quantitate the nerve fiber pathology. Relatively few disor-

Table 80.8: Indications for nerve biopsy

Nerve biopsy results show diagnostic abnormalities
   Vasculitis*
   Amyloidosis*
   Sarcoidosis*
   Leprosy
   Hereditary neuropathy with liability to pressure palsies
      (tomaculous neuropathy)
   Paraproteinemic neuropathy (immunoglobulin M monoclonal
      gammopathy with anti–myelin-associated glycoprotein
      antibody)
   Metachromatic leukodystrophy
   Giant axonal neuropathy
   Polyglucosan body disease
   Tumor infiltration
Nerve biopsy results show suggestive abnormalities
   Charcot-Marie-Tooth disease types 1 and 3
   Refsum's disease
   Chronic inflammatory demyelinating polyradiculoneuropathy
   Small fiber neuropathies

*Consider combined nerve and muscle biopsies.

Table 80.9: Neuropathies associated with serum autoantibodies

Autoantibody	Disease (% positive)
Antibodies against gangliosides	
GM$_1$ (polyclonal IgM)	Multifocal motor neuropathy (70%)
GM$_1$, GD1a (polyclonal IgG)	Guillain-Barré syndrome (30%)
GQ1b (polyclonal IgG)	Miller Fisher variant (>95%)
Antibodies against glycoproteins	
Myelin-associated glyco-protein (monoclonal IgM)	IgM monoclonal gammopathy of undetermined significance neuropathy (50%)
Antibodies against RNA-binding proteins	
Anti-Hu, antineuronal nuclear antibody 1	Malignant inflammatory polyganglionopathy (>95%)

Ig = immunoglobulin.

ders exist in which a nerve biopsy is essential for diagnosis (Table 80.8). In general, nerve biopsy is most useful in suspected vasculitis and amyloid neuropathy. It is helpful in the recognition of CIDP, inherited disorders of myelin, and some rare axonopathies in which there are distinctive axonal changes such as giant axonal neuropathy and polyglucosan body disease. The availability of molecular genetic tests for CMT type 1A, hereditary liability to pressure palsies, and familial transthyretin amyloidosis has decreased the necessity for nerve biopsy in these conditions. Nerve biopsy is an invasive procedure and is associated with a 15% complication rate. Minor wound infections, wound dehiscence, and stump neuromas may occur. Approximately one-third of patients (particularly those without much sensory loss initially) report unpleasant sensory symptoms at the biopsy site after 1 year. The area of the original sensory deficit declines by 90% after 18 months caused by collateral reinnervation (Theriault et al. 1998).

Punch skin biopsy is a promising, minimally invasive technique to evaluate cutaneous innervation in sensory neuropathies. Intraepidermal networks of unmyelinated nerve fibers can be demonstrated by immunostaining with the panaxonal marker protein gene product 9.5 and the use of confocal microscopy. The density of intraepidermal nerve fibers has been found to be reduced in skin obtained from patients with idiopathic, HIV-associated, and diabetic sensory neuropathies (Holland et al. 1997).

Other Laboratory Tests

The clinical neuropathic patterns and the results of electrodiagnostic studies guide the experienced clinician to select the most appropriate laboratory tests. A few laboratory tests should be obtained routinely in all patients with peripheral neuropathy. These include complete cell blood count, sedimentation rate, chemistry profile, fasting blood sugar, thyroid studies, vitamin B$_{12}$ level, and serum protein electrophoresis with immunofixation electrophoresis. It is important to screen for monoclonal proteins in all patients with chronic undiagnosed neuropathy, particularly those over 60 years of age, because 10% of such patients have a monoclonal gammopathy. Several serum autoantibodies with reactivity to various components of peripheral nerve have been associated with peripheral neuropathy syndromes, and reference laboratories offer panels of nerve antibodies for sensory, sensorimotor, and motor neuropathies. It must be emphasized that the clinical relevance of most autoantibodies has not been established for the management of patients, and that their use is not cost-effective. Those of greatest clinical utility are listed in Table 80.9 (Kissel 1998).

Cerebrospinal fluid (CSF) examination is helpful in the evaluation of suspected demyelinating neuropathies and polyradiculopathies related to meningeal carcinomatosis or lymphomatosis.

Outcome of Diagnostic Evaluations in Patients with Peripheral Neuropathy of Unknown Cause

In two large unselected series of patients with initially undiagnosed peripheral neuropathy referred to specialized centers, a definite diagnosis could be made in 76–87%. Inherited neuropathies, CIDP, and neuropathies associated with other diseases accounted for most diagnoses. The improved diagnostic rate was in large measure because of detailed clinical and laboratory evaluations and study of relatives of patients with undiagnosed neuropathy. Despite all efforts, a group of acquired neuropathies remains idiopathic. Acquired chronic sensorimotor and sensory neuropathies are common in individuals older than 55 years, with an estimated prevalence of more than 3%. Chronic idiopathic neuropathy commonly afflicts patients in the fifth or sixth decade and has either mixed sensorimotor or pure sensory features. Nerve conduction and nerve biopsy studies are compatible with a length-dependent axonal neuropathy. The sensorimotor neuropathies tend to pursue a slowly progressive course, whereas pure sensory neuropathies frequently reach a stable plateau. Independent ambulation is almost always maintained in both (Wolfe and Barohn 1998). Idiopathic distal painful axonal neuropathy presents with painful, burning feet, with or without numbness. The condition typically occurs in older patients without any associated systemic diseases or exposure to identifiable toxins. Most patients have elevated thresholds on sensory examination, reduced or absent SNAPs, and impaired distal sweating, measured by the quantitative sudomotor axon reflex test. Reduced intraepidermal nerve fibers on punch skin biopsy provide objective evidence of distal small fiber neuropathy in these patients.

PAIN IN PERIPHERAL NEUROPATHY

Pain is one of the cardinal symptoms of peripheral nerve disorders. In this section we describe the mechanisms of pain perception, list peripheral neuropathies that frequently cause pain, and present treatment strategies.

Pain Mechanisms

The sensation of pain in peripheral neuropathies is generated by nerve impulses triggered when free nerve endings (nociceptors) in sensitive tissues, particularly the skin, respond to noxious or painful stimuli. Pain may be either spontaneous or induced by normally nonpainful stimuli, for which the term *allodynia* is used. A number of neurophysiological studies have determined that both small myelinated Aδ fibers, and unmyelinated C fibers, mediate the afferent impulse of pain stimuli. A study using intraneural microstimulation of human sensory nerves showed that stimulating Aδ nociceptors evokes an acute sensation of sharp, well-localized pain that ceases during selective myelinated fiber block. In contrast, the stimulation of polymodal C nociceptors evokes a sensation of delayed, more diffuse burning pain. During the evolution of painful neuropathies most patients have both types of pain. Nociceptive stimulation that activates C fibers triggers a local tissue response known as neurogenic inflammation. The reaction consists of vasodilatation, increased capillary permeability and local release of neuropeptides such as substance P and calcitonin gene-related peptide, and activation of adjacent nociceptors producing pain at a distance from the original site of injury.

Pain normally arises from cognitive decoding of input generated at nociceptive receptors after conduction along specific afferent pathways. The second-order nociceptive neurons with their cell bodies in the dorsal horn and their axon terminations in the thalamus are mainly of two types: wide dynamic range neurons responding to both Aδ and C fiber afferents, and nociceptive-specific neurons responding only to noxious stimuli. Axons of both neuronal populations cross in the anterior white commissure and ascend the spinal cord in the anterolateral quadrant. Some axons terminate in the reticular formation of the brainstem whereas others project to the lateral and median nuclei of the thalamus. Third-order neurons from the lateral thalamic nuclei project to the primary somatosensory cortex and allow conscious localization and characterization of noxious stimuli. Neurons from intralaminar and median thalamic nuclei project to the anterior cingulate gyrus and other locations and are thought to be related to the suffering and emotional reaction to pain. A segmental modulating system in the spinal cord and a descending modulating system from the cortex, diencephalon, and brainstem have inhibitory effects on dorsal horn neurons. Both serotonin and norepinephrine play an important role in these descending pain-modulating pathways by inhibiting dorsal horn nociceptive neurons.

The specific pathological lesions responsible for neuropathic pain are not clear. For example, clinicopathological studies in diabetic neuropathy have failed to document distinct morphological differences between painful and nonpainful cases. Currently, the most accepted hypothesis suggests that ectopic spontaneous impulses result in neuropathic pain (Ochoa 1993). Abnormal ectopic discharges may arise from dysfunctional nerve fibers, regenerating sprouts from small myelinating and unmyelinated fibers, or dorsal root ganglia neurons. Microneurography has confirmed ectopic impulse generation in myelinated sensory fibers. Hyperalgesia (exaggerated pain from noxious stimuli) or allodynia (pain induced by non-noxious stimuli) may result from sensitization of nociceptors or abnormal ephaptic cross-excitation between primary afferent fibers. In chronic pain syndromes the central nervous system (CNS) reacts to and changes in response to peripheral nervous system (PNS) injury. Following nerve injury second-order dorsal horn neurons become sensitized and expand their receptive fields, which may enhance and maintain the perception of pain. In addition to the effects of neuroplasticity at the spinal cord level, psychological factors may further complicate the emotional reaction to pain.

Neuropathic pain can be a prominent presenting symptom in a great number of peripheral neuropathies (Table 80.10). Pain is characteristic of neuropathies with predominant small fiber involvement, but even in large fiber neuropathies a sufficient number of small fibers may be damaged to cause pain. The poor clinical correlation between morphological changes seen in nerve biopsy specimens and pain is not surprising, if one considers that ectopic impulses may arise from regenerating axonal sprouts or dysfunctional fibers at more proximal or distal sites than the nerve segment examined at biopsy. Neuropathic pain usually affects distal skin and subcutaneous structures, may be constant or intermittent (stabbing, electrical jolts), may often have a temporal pattern of worsening at periods of rest or bedtime, and is described with words such as *searing*, *burning*, or *icy-cold*. Sensory examination should use techniques to elicit abnormal positive sensory phenomena. Allodynia can be elicited by light touch or nonpainful cold stimuli using tuning forks kept in a refrigerator. When testing for hyperpathia, single and repeated pinpricks are used. Patients with hyperpathia may often complain of summation (pain perception increases with repeated stimulation) and aftersensations (pain continues after stimulation has ceased). Nerve trunk pain, a second type of neuropathic pain, is a deep-seated, sharp, knifelike proximal pain along nerve roots or trunks that improves with rest or optimal position, whereas it is aggravated by movement. Nerve trunk pain seems to be mediated by spontaneous impulses arising from nervi nervorum innervating nerve sheaths of affected nerve roots or trunks. Muscle pain and tenderness may develop with acutely evolving denervation of muscle as it occurs in GBS or acute poliomyelitis.

Management of Neuropathic Pain

Regardless of the underlying cause, the management to alleviate neuropathic pain is identical for all painful neuropathies. Symptomatic treatment of neuropathic pain rarely provides complete relief. Initially, simple analgesics (aspirin, acetaminophen, and certain nonsteroidal anti-inflammatory drugs) may be beneficial. However, most patients require additional pharmacotherapy. Several different pharmacological classes have been shown to be safe and effective in alleviating neuropathic pain. These including tricyclic antidepressants, anticonvulsants, and sodium-channel blockers. Opioid analgesics result in pain relief for most patients, but should be limited for pain of short duration or chronic pain unresponsive to any other agents following strict guidelines. Topical agents such as capsaicin or analgesic creams may be helpful in patients with distal painful neuropathies and have the advantage of producing no systemic side effects (Galer 1995). In general, once an agent is selected for treatment, the medication is started at the lowest possible dosage and slowly titrated by increasing the dose every 3–7 days until significant pain relief or intolerable side effects occur. Many treatment failures can be attributed to insufficient dosing or intolerance caused by rapid dose escalations.

The tricyclic antidepressants have been established to reduce pain in diabetic neuropathy independent of their effect on mood. The proposed mechanism of action of tricyclic antidepressants depends on their ability to block the reuptake of norepinephrine and serotonin, two neurotransmitters that are implicated in nociceptive modulation. Treatment should be initiated with low-dose (10–25 mg) amitriptyline, desipramine, or nortriptyline given at bedtime and increased by similar increments no more than

twice weekly. Pain relief may occur within 1 week after reaching a particular dose, although commonly the delay is similar to that seen for the effects on mood, namely 3 weeks. Most studies have shown that doses of tricyclics of 75–150 mg are required for pain suppression. At such high-dose levels, sedation, confusion, anticholinergic effects, urinary retention, and orthostatic hypotension are common side effects, particularly in elderly patients. Desipramine causes less sedation and has fewer anticholinergic effects than amitriptyline, and nortriptyline causes less orthostatic hypotension. Selective serotonin reuptake inhibitors alone are less effective than tricyclics alone in relieving neuropathic pain, but a combination of the two can be effective.

Anticonvulsants (carbamazepine and gabapentin) are considered second-line agents compared with antidepressants, but are frequently given to suppress shooting or stabbing pains. It is important to initiate treatment with carbamazepine at a low dose (100 mg twice daily) and increase slowly to avoid initial symptoms of nausea, disequilibrium, and memory impairment. Gabapentin has been effective in a variety of pain syndromes and is currently used with increasing frequency because of its favorable side-effect profile. In an open label comparison study, gabapentin was better than amitriptyline in reducing pain, with less frequent side effects in elderly patients with diabetic neuropathy. Recommended starting doses are 100 mg twice daily, and escalating every third day; if pain relief is not obtained, the dose can be increased to 3,600 mg per day given in three divided doses.

Mexiletine, a close structural analogue of lidocaine, has been shown to relieve both lancinating and constant pain in a controlled study of painful diabetic neuropathy. Its pain-relieving effect is attributed to the blocking of sodium channels, thereby inhibiting spontaneous activity in dysfunctional nerve fibers. To minimize side effects, most com-

Table 80.10: Peripheral neuropathies frequently associated with pain

Diabetic neuropathies
   Painful symmetrical polyneuropathy
   Asymmetrical polyradiculoplexopathy
   Truncal mononeuropathy
Idiopathic distal small-fiber neuropathy
Guillain-Barré syndrome
Vasculitic neuropathy
Toxic neuropathies
   Arsenic, thallium
   Alcohol
   Vincristine, cisplatin
   Didioxynucleosides
Amyloid neuropathies: primary and familial
Paraneoplastic sensory neuronopathy
Human immunodeficiency virus–related distal
   symmetrical polyneuropathy
Fabry's disease

monly nausea and tremor, mexiletine is started at 150 or 200 mg once or twice a day and gradually increased to 10 mg/kg per day. Mexiletine may exacerbate some cardiac arrhythmias and should be used with caution in patients with symptomatic heart disease.

If the previously mentioned approaches are unsuccessful, alternate agents should be considered. Tramadol, a non-narcotic centrally acting analgesic has been proved effective in painful diabetic neuropathy in a well-designed clinical trial in doses ranging from 200 to 400 mg per day (Harati et al. 1998). Low-affinity binding to μ-opioid receptors and inhibition of norepinephrine and serotonin uptake contribute to its analgesic action. High-dose dextromethorphan, a low-affinity N-methyl-D-aspartate (NMDA)-channel blocker provided partial relief in painful diabetic neuropathy but was associated with significant sedation and ataxia. Clonidine, an α_2-receptor agonist has shown partial effect in a subpopulation of patients with diabetic neuropathy. Opioid analgesics should be limited to patients who have failed adequate trials of first- to third-line agents. Specific guidelines for chronic opioid therapy in neuropathic pain have been published and should be followed. The opinion that neuropathic pain is opioid-unresponsive is incorrect, as indicated by the clinical benefit of oxycodone in patients with postherpetic neuralgia. In many such patients, tachyphylaxis to the opioids does not occur.

Topical agents that act through local skin absorption have the advantage of minimal or no systemic side effects and may be useful in patients with painful, burning feet. Capsaicin, an extract of chili peppers, presumably produces relief of pain through the depletion of substance P in unmyelinated nociceptive fibers. Capsaicin cream (0.025% or 0.075%) is applied to the affected area of skin three to four times a day. An initial intense burning frequently occurs after its application before any improvement is seen. Its use should be continued for at least 4 weeks before rejecting its effectiveness. Topical local anesthetics such as EMLA, a *e*utectic *m*ixture of *l*ocal *a*nesthetics (lidocaine 2.5% and prilocaine 2.5%) designed to penetrate intact skin and produce anesthesia, may provide relief from burning feet. Nonpharmacological treatments including physical therapy, low-intensity transcutaneous electrical nerve stimulation, acupuncture, medical hypnosis, and meditation may reduce the perception of pain and suffering. A comprehensive pain management program should be considered for patients with chronic refractory neuropathic pain.

ENTRAPMENT NEUROPATHIES

Entrapment neuropathy is defined as a focal neuropathy caused by restriction or mechanical distortion of a nerve within a fibrous or fibro-osseous tunnel. Compression, constriction, angulation, or stretching are important mechanisms that produce nerve injury at certain vulnerable anatomical sites (Tables 80.11 and 80.12). The term *entrapment* is a useful one in that it implies that compression occurs at particu-

lar sites where surgical intervention is often required to release the entrapped nerve, such as in the case of the median nerve at the wrist in moderate to severe carpal tunnel syndrome. Overuse has been implicated as the cause of entrapment neuropathies in certain occupations, including the playing of musical instruments by professional musicians.

In chronic entrapment, mechanical distortion of the nerve fibers leads to focal demyelination or, in severe cases, to wallerian degeneration. Morphological studies show a combination of active demyelination, remyelination, wallerian degeneration, and axonal regeneration at the site of entrapment. Endoneurial swelling, collagen proliferation, and thickening of perineurial sheaths accompany the nerve fiber changes. Ischemia is not a significant contributing factor to nerve fiber damage in chronic compression. In contrast, ischemia plays a more significant role in nerve injury associated with acute compression secondary to space-occupying lesions such as hematoma or the compartment syndromes.

The characteristic feature of entrapment neuropathy is either short segment conduction delay or conduction block across the site of entrapment (see Chapter 37B). In severe cases, wallerian degeneration gives rise to extensive denervation in affected muscles. Nerve conduction study measurements together with EMG are essential for diagnosis and reliable documentation of the site and severity of nerve entrapment. Although plain radiography, computed tomography (CT), or magnetic resonance imaging (MRI) may be of occasional value in identifying rare structural abnormalities, these imaging procedures are not required for routine diagnosis.

Double Crush Syndrome

When a sizable cohort of patients with electrodiagnostic evidence of distal upper limb entrapment neuropathies was found to have either electrophysiological or radiological and clinical evidence of cervical radiculopathy, Upton and McComas proposed that focal compression of single nerve fibers proximally might so alter axoplasmic transport as to render the distal nerve more susceptible to symptomatic entrapment neuropathy, resulting in a double crush syndrome. Although the concept of double crush syndrome has since been invoked in a wide variety of entrapment neuropathies, often as an explanation for failed decompressive surgeries of the neck or limb or as a rationale to decompress a nerve in multiple proximal to distal sites along its course, this phenomenon is of uncertain validity (Wilbourn and Gilliatt 1997).

Upper Extremities

Median Nerve Entrapment at the Wrist (Carpal Tunnel Syndrome)

Carpal tunnel syndrome is by far the most common entrapment neuropathy. This entrapment occurs in the tun-

Table 80.11: Entrapment neuropathies of upper limbs

Nerve	Site of compression	Predisposing factors	Major clinical features
Median	Wrist (carpal tunnel syndrome)	Tenosynovitis, etc.	Sensory loss, thenar atrophy
	Anterior interosseous	Strenuous exercise, trauma	Abnormal pinch sign, normal sensation
	Elbow (pronator teres syndrome)	Repetitive elbow motions	Tenderness of pronator teres, sensory loss
Ulnar	Elbow (cubital tunnel syndrome)	Elbow leaning, trauma	Clawing and sensory loss of fourth and fifth fingers
	Guyon's canal	Mechanics, cyclists	Hypothenar atrophy, variable sensory loss
Radial	Axilla	Crutches	Wrist drop, triceps involved, sensory loss
	Spiral groove	Abnormal sleep postures	Wrist drop, sensory loss
	Posterior interosseous	Elbow synovitis	Paresis of finger extensors, radial wrist deviation
	Superficial sensory branch (cheiralgia paresthetica)	Wrist bands, handcuffs	Paresthesias in dorsum of hand
Suprascapular	Suprascapular notch	Blunt trauma	Atrophy of supraspinatus and infraspinatus muscles
Dorsal scapular	Scalene muscle	Trauma	Winging of scapula on arm abduction
Lower trunk of the brachial plexus or C8/T1 roots	Thoracic outlet	Cervical rib, enlarged C7 transverse process	Atrophy of intrinsic hand muscles, paresthesias of hand and forearm

Table 80.12: Entrapment neuropathies of lower limbs

Nerve	Site of compression	Predisposing factors	Major clinical features
Sciatic	Sciatic notch	Endometriosis, intramuscular injections	Pain down thigh, footdrop, absent ankle jerk
	Hip	Fracture dislocations	
	Piriformis muscle	—	
	Popliteal fossa	Popliteal Baker's cyst	
Fibular	Fibular neck	Leg crossing, squatting	Footdrop, weak evertors, sensory loss in dorsum of foot
	Anterior compartment	Muscle edema	Footdrop
Posterior tibial	Medial malleolus (tarsal tunnel syndrome)	Ankle fracture, tenosynovitis	Sensory loss over sole of foot
Femoral	Inguinal ligament	Lithotomy position	Weak knee extension, absent knee jerk
Lateral femoral cutaneous	Inguinal ligament (meralgia paresthetica)	Tight clothing, weight gain, utility belts	Sensory loss in lateral thigh
Ilioinguinal	Abdominal wall	Trauma, surgical incision	Direct hernia, sensory loss in the iliac crest, crural area
Obturator	Obturator canal	Pelvic fracture, tumor	Sensory loss in medial thigh, weak hip adduction

nel through which the median nerve passes accompanied by the flexor digitorum tendons. Because the transverse carpal ligament is an unyielding fibrous structure forming the roof of the tunnel, tenosynovitis in this area often produces pressure on the median nerve.

Symptoms consist of nocturnal paresthesias, most often confined to the thumb, index, and middle fingers. Patients complain of tingling numbness and burning sensations, often awakening them from sleep. Referred pain may radi-

ate to the forearm and even as high as the shoulder. Symptoms are often worse after excessive use of the hand or wrist. Objective sensory changes may be found in the distribution of the median nerve, most often impaired two-point discrimination, pinprick and light touch sensation, or occasionally hyperesthesia, with sparing of the thenar eminence. Thenar (abductor pollicis brevis muscle) weakness and atrophy may be present with prolonged entrapment (Figure 80.6). The syndrome is frequently bilateral and usu-

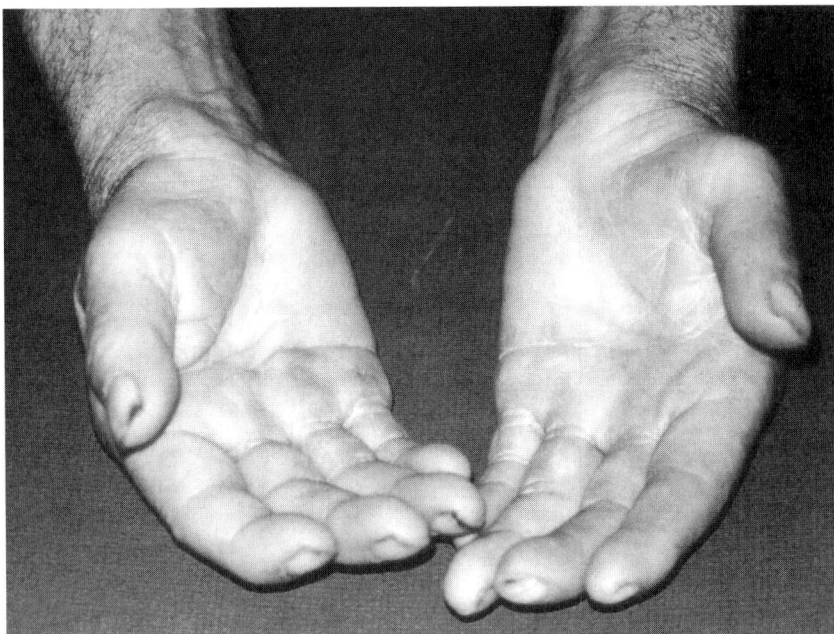

FIGURE 80.6   Thenar atrophy in chronic bilateral carpal tunnel syndrome.

ally of greater intensity in the dominant hand. A positive Tinel's sign, in which percussion of the nerve at the carpal tunnel causes paresthesias in the distribution of the median nerve, is present in approximately 60% of affected patients, but is not specific for carpal tunnel syndrome. Flexing the patient's hand at the wrist for 1 minute (Phalen's maneuver) or hyperextension of the wrist (a reversed Phalen's maneuver) can reproduce the symptoms.

Work-related wrist and hand symptoms (repetitive motion injury) from cumulative trauma in the workplace have received increasing attention by the general public in recent years. Although a proportion of these cases have bona fide carpal tunnel syndrome, longitudinal natural history data suggest that the majority of industrial workers do not develop symptoms of carpal tunnel syndrome (Nathan et al. 1998). Carpal tunnel syndrome appears to occur in work settings that include repetitive forceful grasping or pinching, awkward positions of the hand and wrist, direct pressure over the carpal tunnel, and the use of hand-held vibrating tools. Increased risk for the syndrome has been found in meat packers, garment workers, butchers, grocery checkers, electronic assembly workers, keyboard operators, musicians, and housekeepers. The highest reported incidence of work-related carpal tunnel syndrome based on the number of carpal tunnel surgeries performed was 15% among a group of meat packers (Dawson 1993).

The most sensitive electrodiagnostic test for carpal tunnel syndrome is the median nerve sensory conduction study, which exhibits a delayed sensory latency across the wrist in 70–90% of patients. Recording the latency at short distances over the course of the median nerve from palm to wrist and comparing this latency with the latency for the ulnar nerve at the same distance (palmar nerve conduction

studies) can increase the sensitivity of sensory conduction studies (Stevens 1997). Most cases with moderate to severe involvement have prolonged median nerve distal motor latency. Some patients with carpal tunnel syndrome have significantly narrower than average carpal canals.

Diseases and conditions that have been found to predispose to the development of carpal tunnel syndrome include pregnancy, diabetes, obesity, rheumatoid arthritis, hypothyroidism, amyloidosis, gout, acromegaly, certain mucopolysaccharidoses, arteriovenous shunts for hemodialysis, old fractures at the wrist, and inflammatory diseases involving tendons or connective tissues at the wrist level. On rare occasions, carpal tunnel syndrome may be familial.

Mild carpal tunnel syndrome must be distinguished from early median nerve involvement in polyneuropathy; occasionally the two conditions coexist. In cases with only mild sensory symptoms, treatment with splints in neutral position, nonsteroidal anti-inflammatory agents, and local corticosteroid injection often suffice. Evidence for the use of oral pyridoxine for carpal tunnel syndrome is conflicting at best and comes with the risk of toxic sensory polyganglionopathy (see Toxic Neuropathies, later in this chapter). Severe sensory loss and thenar atrophy suggest the need for surgical carpal tunnel release. Surgical sectioning of the volar carpal ligament is now usually performed with fiberoptic techniques, and results in more than 90% of patients having prompt resolution of pain and paresthesias (Mirza and King 1996). Improvement in distal latencies may lag behind the relief of symptoms. Rarely, symptoms persist after operation. Poor surgical results usually are associated with incomplete sectioning of the transverse ligament, surgical damage of the palmar cutaneous branch of the median nerve by an improperly placed skin incision, or scarring within the carpal tunnel. In such cases surgical re-exploration may be required.

Other Entrapment Syndromes of the Median Nerve

Anterior Interosseous Nerve Syndrome. The anterior interosseous nerve is a pure motor branch of the median nerve that supplies the flexor pollicis longus, pronator quadratus, and flexor digitorum profundus muscles of the index and middle fingers. In this relatively rare syndrome, the nerve may be compressed by fibrous bands attached to the flexor digitorum superficialis muscle. Isolated involvement of this nerve more often occurs spontaneously in the context of a partial idiopathic brachial plexus neuropathy (Parsonage-Turner syndrome) or less commonly as a restricted form of multifocal motor neuropathy with conduction block. Patients often complain of pain in the forearm or elbow. The clinical manifestations of an anterior interosseous nerve lesion include the inability to flex the distal phalanges of the thumb and index finger. This makes it impossible to form a circle with those fingers. Nerve conduction study results of the median nerve are normal, but the motor latency from elbow to the pronator quadratus muscle is often prolonged. EMG is necessary to document denervation in muscles innervated by the anterior interosseous nerve.

Spontaneous recovery usually occurs, and therefore, surgery may not be necessary unless penetrating injury, fracture, or significant entrapment is detected.

Pronator Teres Syndrome. In the pronator teres syndrome, the median nerve is compressed in the proximal forearm between the two heads of the pronator teres muscle, a fibrous arcade of the flexor digitorum superficialis muscle, or the lacertus fibrosus. This entrapment may develop in individuals engaged in repetitive pronating movements of the forearm. Patients complain of paresthesias and numbness of the radial fingers, as well as pain and tenderness in the proximal forearm that is increased by resistance to pronation. Weakness of the flexor pollicis longus and abductor pollicis brevis is demonstrated, whereas pronation of the forearm is normal. Nerve conduction study results of the median nerve may sometimes show slowing in the elbow-wrist segment. In contrast to the carpal tunnel syndrome, the distal median motor and sensory latencies at the wrist are normal. Injection of corticosteroids into the pronator teres muscle and immobilization often provide relief of symptoms, but on occasion surgery may be necessary.

Median Nerve Entrapment at the Ligament of Struthers. A supracondylar spur of the humerus is present in a small proportion of normal individuals. A fibrous band, the ligament of Struthers, extends from this spur to the medial epicondyle and may compromise the median nerve along with the brachial artery. Clinical symptoms resemble the pronator teres syndrome, but the radial pulse diminishes when the forearm is fully extended in supination because of the concomitant entrapment of the brachial artery. Electrodiagnostic studies may allow differentiation from the pronator teres syndrome, because the ligament of Struthers syndrome involves the pronator teres muscle.

Ulnar Nerve Entrapment

Ulnar Nerve Entrapment at the Elbow. Ulnar mononeuropathy is the second most common entrapment or compression mononeuropathy, although it is considerably less frequent than carpal tunnel syndrome. Ulnar neuropathies at the elbow are caused by direct compression in the retrocondylar groove or entrapment as the nerve passes through the cubital tunnel, a fibro-osseous canal, the floor of which is formed by the medial ligament of the elbow joint, and the roof by the aponeurosis of the flexor carpi ulnaris muscle (Khoo et al. 1996). The term *tardy ulnar palsy* is applied to an ulnar nerve lesion developing years after elbow trauma. Other possible sources of injury of the ulnar nerve at the elbow include direct compression during general anesthesia or periods of unconsciousness, repetitive chronic trauma, and arthritis of the elbow joint, although symptoms and signs sometimes attributed to ulnar neuropathy after coronary bypass surgery are most often the result of stretch injury to the lower trunk of the brachial plexus. Ulnar nerve lesions at the elbow cause weakness of the flexor carpi ulnaris, flexor digitorum profundus of the ring and little fingers, and the intrinsic hand muscles. Pinch strength is reduced by weakness of adductor pollicis, flexor pollicis brevis, and first dorsal interosseous muscles. As a compensatory maneuver during attempted pinch of the thumb and index fingers, the flexor pollicis longus, a median nerve–innervated muscle, is used involuntarily and flexes the distal phalanx of the thumb (Froment's sign). Weakness of the interossei muscles results in inability to produce a forceful extension of the interphalangeal joints as used in finger-flicking movements. Prominent atrophy of the first dorsal interosseous muscle ensues, together with clawing of the fourth and fifth fingers, the result of lumbrical weakness with secondary hyperextension of the metacarpophalangeal joints. The small muscles of the hand are always more severely involved than the forearm muscles. Sensory loss or hypesthesia involves the fifth finger, part of the fourth finger, and hypothenar eminence, and extends to the dorsum of the hand. Electrodiagnostic tests are useful in localizing the entrapment at the elbow. Focal slowing or localized reduction in the CMAP amplitude may be found in the elbow segment in approximately 50% of cases. In the remaining patients localization is less precise because of predominant axonal loss.

Conservative treatment should be attempted in patients with mild symptoms or in those with symptoms brought on by occupational causes. Avoidance of repetitive elbow flexion and extension or direct pressure on the elbow may alleviate the symptoms. Elbow protectors are helpful in patients with a history of excessive elbow leaning. Conservative treatment should be continued for at least 3 months before surgery is considered. Surgical approaches to the ulnar nerve lesion at the elbow include simple release of the flexor carpi ulnaris aponeurosis, anterior transposition of the nerve trunk, and resection of the medial epicondyle. The choice of procedure should be tailored to the specific lesion found at surgery. Only approximately 60% of patients benefit from surgery, and some experience worsening of symptoms.

Ulnar Nerve Entrapment at the Wrist in the Ulnar Tunnel (Guyon's Canal). Distal to the wrist, the ulnar nerve enters Guyon's canal, which is formed between the pisiform bone and the hook of the hamate, covered by the volar carpal ligament and the palmaris brevis muscle. Within Guyon's canal the ulnar nerve divides into its terminal deep and superficial branches. Depending on the exact location of entrapment, motor or sensory impairment may occur alone or in combination. Because the palmar cutaneous branch leaves the ulnar nerve proximal to the wrist and does not enter Guyon's canal, sensory loss is confined to the palmar surface of the ulnar-innervated fingers. Ulnar nerve entrapment in Guyon's canal occurs much less frequently than at the elbow. The usual cause is chronic or repeated external pressure by tools, bicycle handlebars, the handles of canes, or excessive push-ups. Compression also may be caused by degenerative wrist joint ganglia, rheumatoid arthritis, or distal vascular anomalies. The diagnosis is confirmed with prolonged distal motor latencies to the first dorsal interosseous or abductor digiti minimi muscles and when denervation is documented in ulnar-innervated hand muscles. MRI through Guyon's canal may demonstrate a structural lesion if compressive trauma is not the cause; in such cases surgical exploration may be required.

Radial Nerve Entrapment

Radial nerve compression in the axilla may result from crutches or from the weight of a sleeping partner's head (honeymoon palsy) or may occur at the spinal groove during drunken sleep wherein the arm is draped over a chair (Saturday night palsy). Lesions at the axilla are characterized by weakness of the triceps brachii, brachioradialis, supinator, and extensor muscles of the wrist and fingers. If compression occurs in the spiral groove of the mid-upper arm, the triceps brachii is spared, resulting in weakness confined to the brachioradialis, wrist, and finger extensors. Minimal sensory abnormalities may occur over the dorsum of the hand, thumb, index finger, and middle finger. Radial nerve lesions caused by pressure usually improve in 6–8 weeks. This compression neuropathy must be differentiated from radial nerve injury caused by fractures of the humerus. The radial nerve is often involved in isolation or in combination with other single nerves in multifocal motor neuropathy with conduction block.

Posterior Interosseous Nerve Syndrome. The posterior interosseous nerve, or deep radial nerve, is a pure motor branch of the radial nerve in the forearm. Before entering the supinator muscle, the radial nerve supplies the brachioradialis, extensor carpi radialis longus and brevis, and supinator muscles. The rest of the extensor muscles, including the extensor carpi ulnaris, are innervated by the posterior interosseous nerve. The nerve appears most vulnerable to entrapment at the level of the supinator muscle. This uncommon syndrome occurs in association with rheumatoid arthritis, trauma, fracture, soft tissue masses, or strenuous use of the arm. The clinical manifestations of a posterior interosseous nerve lesion are an inability to extend the fingers at the metacarpophalangeal joints as well as radial deviation of the wrist on wrist extension caused by the weakness of the extensor carpi ulnaris muscle. EMG confirms the diagnosis by demonstrating denervation in the muscles supplied by the posterior interosseous nerve with sparing of more proximal radial-innervated muscles.

In rheumatoid arthritis, local injection of corticosteroids may be helpful. If the syndrome is progressive, surgical exploration, including synovectomy or decompression of the posterior interosseous nerve, may become necessary.

Cheiralgia Paresthetica. A mononeuropathy of the superficial dorsal sensory branch of the radial nerve occurs as a result of trauma from tight wristbands or handcuffs and is called cheiralgia paresthetica. Paresthesias and pain in the distribution of the superficial sensory branch of the radial nerve characterize this benign, self-limiting condition. The symptoms can be aggravated by ulnar flexion of the hyperpronated forearm. A small area of hypesthesia in the dorsoradial aspect of the hand is frequently identified. Nerve conduction study results can show a low amplitude or absent dorsal radial SNAP.

Musculocutaneous Nerve Entrapment

The musculocutaneous nerve arises from the upper and middle trunks of the brachial plexus, penetrates the coracobrachialis muscle, and courses down the anterior aspect of the upper arm between the two muscles it innervates, the biceps brachii and brachialis. Although most often involved in idiopathic brachial plexus neuropathy, this nerve also may be damaged with shoulder dislocations, following general anesthesia, or with vigorous exercise such as weight lifting. In carpet carrier's palsy, the nerve is compressed by repetitive carrying of heavy objects on the shoulder held in place by the arm (Sander et al. 1997). The differential diagnosis includes C6 radiculopathy, restricted brachial plexopathy, and rupture of the biceps tendon.

Clinically, patients with musculocutaneous mononeuropathy present with weakness and atrophy of the biceps brachii and brachialis muscles, diminished biceps brachii reflex, and sensory loss over the lateral aspect of the forearm anteriorly. EMG demonstrates denervation limited to the biceps brachii and brachialis muscles. Nerve conduction studies show a reduced musculocutaneous biceps

CMAP and a low-amplitude lateral antebrachial cutaneous sensory response.

Spontaneous recovery is the rule. Local corticosteroid injection may provide some relief of pain. Surgical decompression is contemplated if no improvement occurs.

Suprascapular Nerve Entrapment

The suprascapular nerve is a pure motor branch of the upper trunk of the brachial plexus, which passes through the suprascapular notch to innervate the supraspinatus and infraspinatus muscles. Entrapment occurs after repetitive forward traction of the shoulders. This nerve also may be involved in a restricted form of idiopathic brachial plexus neuropathy. Diffuse aching pain in the posterior aspect of the shoulder is a cardinal symptom. Atrophy and weakness are confined to the infraspinatus and supraspinatus muscles. Slow and steady abduction of the arm starting from a vertical position alongside the chest is not possible with a severe lesion of the suprascapular nerve. Tendon ruptures of the rotator cuff need to be considered in the differential diagnosis. EMG shows denervation restricted to the supraspinatus and infraspinatus muscles. Local injection of corticosteroids may give temporary relief of pain.

Intercostobrachial Nerve Syndrome

The intercostobrachial nerve is a cutaneous sensory nerve derived from the second and third thoracic nerve roots and supplies the skin on the medial surface of the upper arm and axilla as well as the adjacent chest wall. It may be injured in modified radical mastectomy and other surgical procedures involving the axilla and lateral pectoral region (Wallace et al. 1996).

Neurogenic Thoracic Outlet Syndrome

Neurogenic thoracic outlet syndrome with objective neurological deficits is very rare.

Lower Extremities

Entrapment neuropathies of lower limbs are shown in Table 80.12.

Sciatic Nerve Lesions

The sciatic nerve consists of two distinct nerves, the posterior tibial and the common fibular (peroneal) nerves, which share a common sheath from the pelvis to the popliteal fossa. The sciatic nerve is occasionally vulnerable to entrapment as it crosses over the sciatic notch in leaving the pelvis. Most sciatic nerve lesions result from trauma, such as fracture dislocations, hematomas in the posterior thigh compartment, intramuscular injections, and complications of hip replacement surgery.

Recurrent sciatic mononeuropathy may be caused by endometriosis involving the nerve at the sciatic notch. Direct compression of the sciatic nerve is rare but occasionally occurs during coma, anesthesia, or prolonged sitting on a hard surface (toilet seat palsy). Either division of the nerve may be compressed by a Baker's cyst in the popliteal fossa.

A complete sciatic nerve lesion results in weakness of knee flexors and all the muscles below the knee, and sensory loss of the entire foot except for the small region supplied by the saphenous nerve over the medial malleolus. The fibular division is more commonly involved than the posterior tibial in proximal lesions of the sciatic nerve and may mimic a common fibular neuropathy. In such patients, evidence of denervation in the short head of the biceps femoris and posterior tibialis muscles and abnormal sural or medial plantar SNAPs helps localize partial proximal sciatic nerve lesions.

On rare occasions, the piriformis muscle may entrap the sciatic nerve trunk as it passes through or over the piriformis muscle (the piriformis syndrome). However, this clinical picture is almost always the result of lumbosacral root, sacral plexus, or sciatic nerve damage at other locations.

Common Fibular (Peroneal) Nerve Entrapment

Entrapment of the common fibular (peroneal) nerve is the most frequent entrapment neuropathy in the leg. Because of confusion between the terms *peroneal* and *perineal*, the Federative Committee on Anatomic Terminology has renamed the peroneal nerve the *fibular nerve*.

This nerve is particularly vulnerable in the region of the fibular neck as it passes through the origin of the fibularis (peroneus) longus muscle. Near this opening, the nerve divides into three main terminal divisions: the superficial, deep, and accessory fibular nerves. A common fibular nerve lesion leads to weakness of foot and toe extension and foot eversion, with a footdrop and steppage gait. Sensory impairment is found over the lateral aspect of the lower leg and the dorsum of the foot. Direct pressure to the fibular head area, habitual leg crossing, weight loss, or a recurrent stretch injury as a result of an unstable ankle causing excessive foot inversion may result in fibular neuropathy. Improperly applied plaster casts or unrecognized pressure on the nerve in debilitated or unconscious patients may be responsible for this nerve injury.

Fibular mononeuropathy needs to be differentiated from the anterior tibial compartment syndrome, in which the deep fibular nerve is compressed by muscle swelling within the anterior compartment, caused by injury, heavy exercise, trauma, or ischemia. This results in an acute syndrome of severe lower leg pain, swelling, and weakness of foot and toe extensors. The anterior tibial compartment must be decompressed rapidly by fasciotomy to prevent irreversible nerve and muscle damage.

Electrodiagnostic studies are useful for localizing lesions and may provide clues to the underlying cause and a guide to prognosis. Although it is often possible by nerve conduction studies to demonstrate focal conduction block or localized slowing in the region of the fibular head, contrary to common belief, the most frequent pathophysiological process is axonal loss regardless of the cause. EMG is important to exclude other sites of injury such as the sciatic nerve, lumbosacral plexus, and L5 nerve root.

The prognosis is uniformly good in cases of acute compression, whereas recovery is delayed in those with stretch injuries. Bracing with a custom-made plastic ankle-foot orthosis is necessary to improve the gait in the presence of severe footdrop. The few patients who do not improve spontaneously after 3 months, or those who have pain or a slowly progressive fibular nerve lesion, may require MRI studies and surgical exploration (Kim and Kline 1996).

Posterior Tibial Nerve Entrapment (Tarsal Tunnel Syndrome)

Entrapment of the posterior tibial nerve occurs behind and immediately below the medial malleolus. In this region, the laciniate ligament covers the tarsal tunnel through which the nerve passes together with the tendons of the tibialis posterior, flexor digitorum longus, and flexor hallucis longus muscles, as well as the posterior tibial artery and veins. Burning pain occurs in the toes and the sole of the foot. If the calcaneal sensory branches are involved, pain occurs at the heel. Examination usually reveals plantar sensory impairment and wasting of the intrinsic foot muscles. Percussion at the site of nerve compression or eversion of the foot may elicit pain and paresthesia. Electrodiagnostic study results should confirm the entrapment of the posterior tibial nerve at the tarsal tunnel by demonstrating involvement of motor fibers to the abductor digiti minimi and abductor hallucis muscles as well as involvement of the medial and lateral plantar sensory fibers with sparing of the sural nerve. EMG is important to exclude involvement of muscles proximal to the foot such as the gastrocnemius muscle. The majority of suspected cases of tarsal tunnel syndrome turn out to have generalized peripheral neuropathy, S1 radiculopathy, or non-neurological foot pain. Electrodiagnostic findings are sometimes complicated by previous failed surgical procedures in the foot that may have injured the nerves of interest.

Local injection with corticosteroids underneath the laciniate ligament may temporarily relieve the symptoms. Surgical decompression is needed for permanent results in those rare cases in which objective evidence of this syndrome exists.

Sural Nerve Lesions

Although the vast majority of sural nerve lesions are iatrogenic as the result of diagnostic sural nerve biopsy, mononeuropathy of the sural nerve has been reported with a number of other conditions including lower limb vein stripping surgery, Baker's cyst surgery, local trauma, tightly laced high-topped footwear such as ski boots or ice skates, and rarely as the initial presentation of vasculitic mononeuritis multiplex.

Femoral Nerve Lesions

Femoral mononeuropathy is rare but may occur as the result of direct trauma or acute compression rather than from chronic entrapment.

Lateral Femoral Cutaneous Nerve Entrapment (Meralgia Paresthetica)

The lateral femoral cutaneous nerve, which is a pure sensory nerve, passes medial to the anterior superior iliac spine under the inguinal ligament to enter the thigh under the fascia lata and supplies the skin of the anterolateral part of the thigh. The site of entrapment is usually at the level of the inguinal ligament. Rarely, the nerve can be affected in its proximal segment by retroperitoneal tumors or be injured during appendectomy. The disorder is most often seen in association with obesity, but may occur with enlargement of the quadriceps muscles from increased exercise and from pregnancy, ascites, or other conditions that increase intra-abdominal pressure. Direct compression by a belt or corset, fracture of the anterior portion of the ilium, or pelvic tilt causing undue stresses on the abdominal musculature are other causes. Patients develop numbness, painful burning, and itching over the anterolateral thigh. Pressure at the inguinal ligament medial to the anterior superior iliac spine elicits referred pain and dysesthesias.

Electrophysiological study results of the femoral nerve and quadriceps femoris muscle are normal, which helps to exclude lumbar radiculopathies.

A local anesthetic nerve block may have diagnostic value. Treatment consists of symptomatic measures such as rest, analgesics, and weight loss. Postural abnormalities should be corrected. Neurolysis is rarely beneficial.

Ilioinguinal Nerve

The ilioinguinal nerve is analogous to an intercostal nerve. Muscle branches innervate the lower portion of the transverse abdominal and internal oblique muscles. The cutaneous sensory nerve supplies the skin over the inguinal ligament and the base of the scrotum or labia. As the nerve takes a zigzag course, passing through the transverse abdominal and internal oblique muscles, it is subject to mechanical irritation. Pain is referred to the groin, and weakness of the lower abdominal wall may result in the formation of a direct inguinal hernia. Trauma, surgical procedures, and scar tissue are frequently responsible. Increased abdominal muscle tone, caused by abnormal posture as seen in chronic back pain or Parkinson's disease, also can result in this neuropathy.

Conservative treatment includes rest and nonsteroidal anti-inflammatory agents. Neurolysis may be required in refractory cases when a mechanical lesion is suspected.

Obturator Nerve

The obturator nerve is vulnerable to entrapment as it passes through the obturator canal, for instance, by an obturator hernia or osteitis pubis. The entrapment produces radiating pain from the groin down the inner aspect of the thigh. There is weakness of hip adduction and sensory impairment in the upper medial thigh. Interestingly, isolated painless weakness of the thigh adductors without sensory symptoms can be the initial manifestation of the myopathy of acid maltase deficiency. Obturator neuropathy may present as the first manifestation of primary or metastatic pelvic tumors. CT or MRI scanning is helpful in finding such lesions (Figure 80.7; Rogers et al. 1993).

This entrapment neuropathy is treated conservatively. If such treatment fails, or if symptoms progress to involve other nerves in the region, careful search for occult pelvic and retroperitoneal malignancy must be pursued.

Localized Perineurial Hypertrophic Mononeuropathy

A slowly progressive painless mononeuropathy that cannot be localized to entrapment sites and is caused by a focal fusiform enlargement of the affected nerve, termed *localized hypertrophic neuropathy*, may develop in young adults (Suarez et al. 1994). The fusiform enlargement is mainly composed of onion bulb–like whorls, formed by layers of perineurial cells (Figure 80.7B). The cause of the perineurial cell proliferation is not known, but it is considered reactive rather than neoplastic. The condition may involve any major nerve trunk but is seen more frequently in the upper limbs, particularly the posterior interosseous nerve. Sensory symptoms are minor, although sensory nerve fibers are obviously involved. Electrodiagnostic study results show an axonal mononeuropathy and help in the precise localization of the focal nerve lesion. MRI shows a focal enlargement of the affected nerve (Figure 80.7A).

Surgical exploration and a fascicular biopsy by a surgeon experienced in peripheral nerve microsurgery confirms the diagnosis and excludes malignant peripheral nerve sheath tumors, which can be difficult to exclude on clinical grounds alone. Surgical resection of the mass should be avoided as long as there is residual function.

HEREDITARY NEUROPATHIES

The hereditary neuropathies constitute a complex, heterogeneous group of diseases, which frequently share insidious onset and indolent course over years to decades. The number of such disorders in which the metabolic defect is known, such as in familial amyloid neuropathies, Refsum's disease, Fabry's disease, porphyria, hypolipoproteinemias, and some of the forms of CMT disease, is increasing rapidly. For other inherited neuropathies classification still depends on clinical phenotype, mode of inheritance, and class of neurons predominantly affected. These conditions include hereditary motor neuropathy or spinal muscular atrophy (see Chapter 78), hereditary motor and sensory neuropathy, and hereditary sensory and autonomic neuropathy (HSAN). Major advances in understanding the molecular basis of inherited neuropathies have come from identifying chromosomal loci or genes for a given disease phenotype through positional cloning. These investigations have led to the discovery of three genes, each of which codes for a specific gene product (PMP-22, myelin protein zero [P_0], and connexin-32), which are essential to myelin function (Lupski 1998).

Hereditary neuropathies are common disorders, the hereditary nature of which may remain unrecognized in a surprisingly large percentage of patients. Eliciting historical evidence of long-standing neuromuscular complaints, obtaining detailed family histories, looking for skeletal abnormalities such as hammer toes or high arches, and performing neurological evaluations in relatives are means of identifying previously unsuspected inherited neuropathy. Spontaneously reported paresthesia is three times more common in acquired than in inherited neuropathies. The possibility of an inherited neuropathy cannot be dismissed even in the face of a truly negative family history. Such a situation may arise in cases of early death of one or both parents, few blood relatives, or autosomal recessive disease. Available diagnostic DNA testing shows that isolated cases also may result from de novo gene mutations.

Charcot-Marie-Tooth Disease (Hereditary Motor and Sensory Neuropathy)

The syndrome of peroneal muscular atrophy or CMT disease was first described in the second half of the nineteenth century by Charcot and Marie in Paris, and Tooth in London. CMT disease is the most common inherited neuropathy, with an estimated prevalence of 1 in 2,500 in the United States. Clinical studies combined with electrophysiological and sural nerve biopsy investigations of a large number of families with peroneal muscular atrophy allowed a separation into two main groups: (1) the hypertrophic or demyelinating form of CMT disease or CMT1, also referred to as hereditary motor and sensory neuropathy type I, in which there is marked reduction in motor NCVs and nerve biopsy findings of demyelination and onion bulb formation; and (2) the neuronal form of CMT disease (CMT2), or hereditary motor and sensory neuropathy type II, in which motor NCVs are normal or near

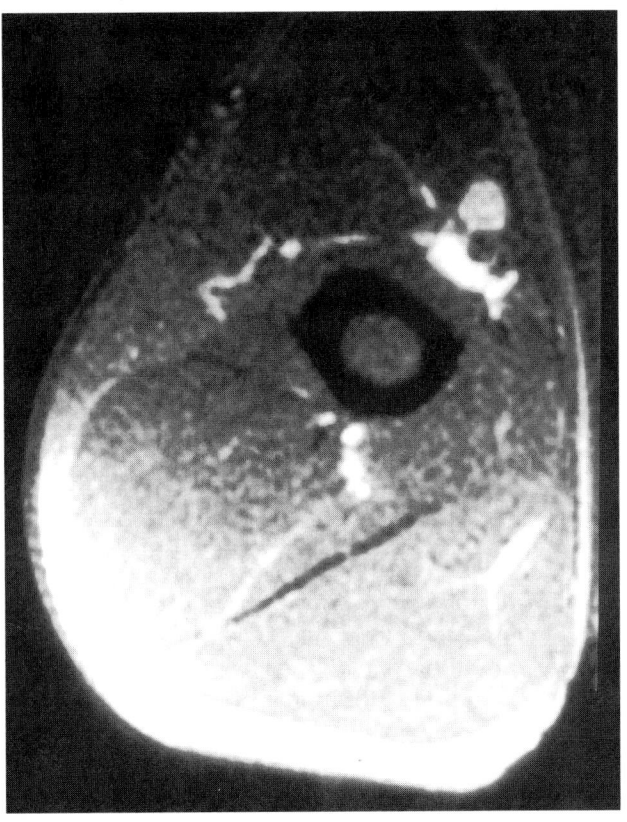

A

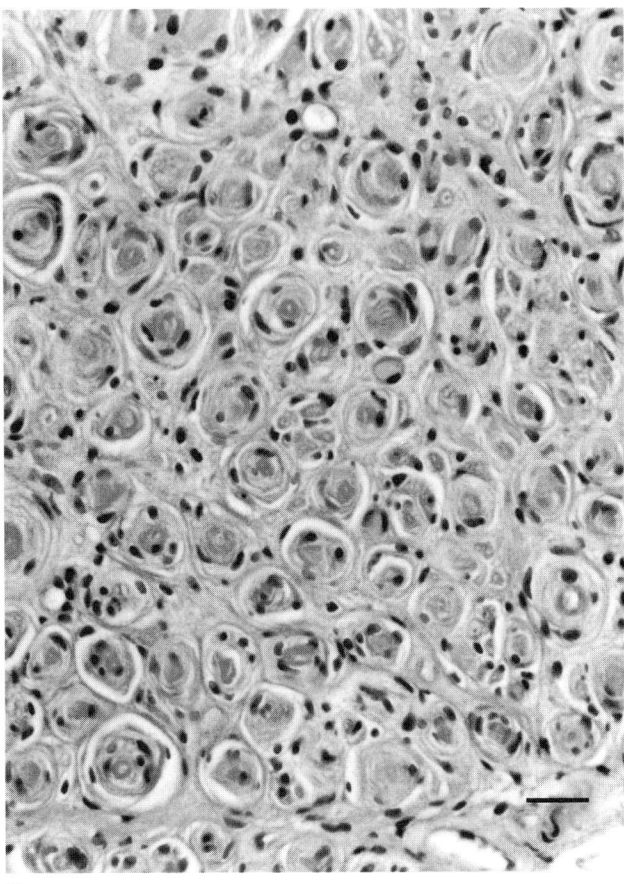

B

FIGURE 80.7   (A) Axial magnetic resonance imaging of the right upper arm 10 cm proximal to the epicondyles demonstrates a focal enhancing enlargement of the median nerve after gadolinium administration. The fusiform enlargement of the nerve extended approximately 4 cm in length and measured 7 mm in diameter at its greatest thickness on serial axial cuts. (B) Fascicular biopsy spec-imens of the enlarged median nerve segment shows numerous onion bulb structures. By immunochemistry, the onion bulbs consist of epithelial membrane antigen-positive cells, confirming their perineurial cell origin. (Hematoxylin and eosin; original magnification ×80; bar = 20 μm.) (Courtesy of Dr. P. J. Dyck, Mayo Clinic, Rochester, MN.)

normal, with nerve biopsy findings of axonal loss without demyelination (Harding 1995). The peroneal muscular atrophy phenotype without sensory involvement on either clinical or electrophysiological examination has been classified as hereditary distal spinal muscular atrophy. In addition to CMT types 1 and 2, there are rare cases of severe demyelinating neuropathy with onset in early childhood that are referred to as CMT type 3 or Dejerine-Sottas disease.

Both CMT1 and CMT2 display autosomal dominant inheritance. A minority of cases occur sporadically or in siblings only and have therefore been attributed to autosomal recessive inheritance or to de novo mutation. Because a great variability in clinical expression exists among affected kin in the dominant disorders, a recessive inheritance can only be accepted after clinical and electrophysiological examinations of both parents have proved to be normal; even then nonparental conception and new mutations have to be considered. CMT with X-linked inheritance (CMTX) phenotypically resembles CMT1.

Charcot-Marie-Tooth Disease 1

In CMT1, symptoms often begin during the first or second decade of life. Presenting symptoms include foot deformity and difficulties in running or walking. Symmetrical weakness and wasting is found in intrinsic foot, peroneal, and anterior tibial muscles. Similar distal involvement of the upper limbs develops later in two-thirds of patients. Inspection reveals pes cavus and hammer toes in nearly 75% of adult patients; mild kyphosis in approximately 10%; and enlarged, hypertrophic peripheral nerves in as many as 25% (Figure 80.8). Absent ankle jerks are universal and frequently are associated with absent or

FIGURE 80.8 Leg atrophy, pes cavus, and enlarged great auricular nerve (*arrow*) are evident in a patient with Charcot-Marie-Tooth type 1 disease.

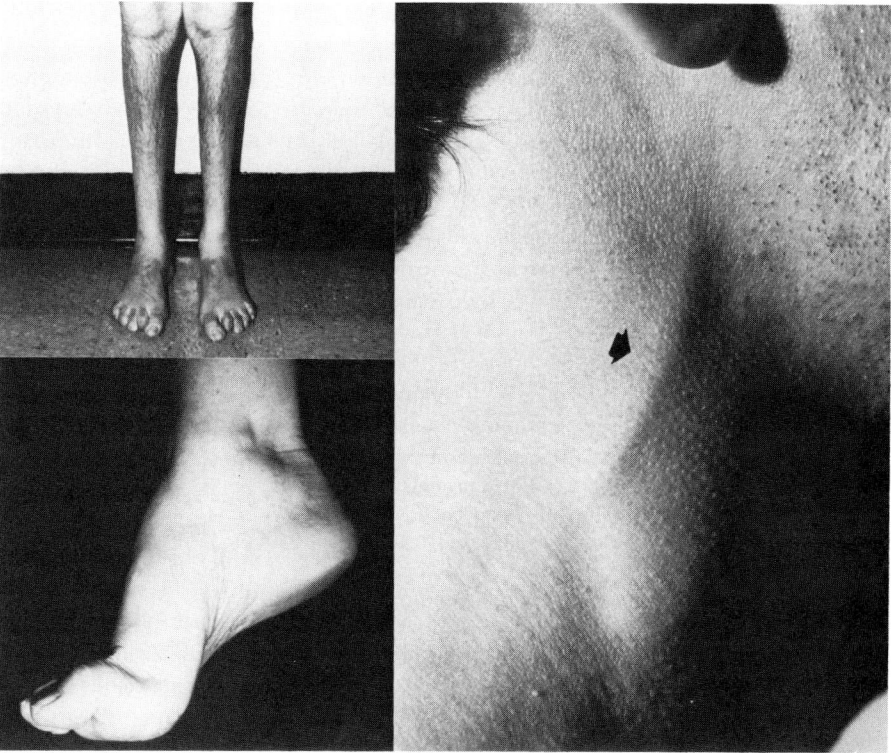

reduced knee and upper limb reflexes. Some degree of distal sensory impairment (diminished vibration sense and light touch in feet and hands) is usually found by examination, but rarely gives rise to symptoms. Occasionally, patients have an essential or postural upper limb tremor. Such cases have been referred to as *Roussy-Lévy syndrome*, although convincing evidence suggests that this is not a separate clinical or genetic syndrome. Severity in affected kin varies considerably. Approximately 10% of patients are asymptomatic but have slowing of NCVs. At the other end of the clinical spectrum, there are patients with severe neurological deficits who may become wheelchair dependent.

Motor nerve conduction studies show uniform slowing by more than 25% of the lower limits of normal in all nerves. Motor conduction of upper limb nerves proves more useful than studies of lower limb extremity nerves because distal fiber degeneration in the legs is often complete. A conduction velocity below 38 m per second in the forearm segment of the median nerve is proposed as a cutoff value to distinguish between CMT disease types 1 and 2. In a prospective study of CMT1A, the median motor NCV was slowed to less than 43 m per second in all subjects with documented chromosome 17p11.2-12 duplications (Kaku et al. 1993). Sensory conductions are similarly abnormal. SNAPs are usually absent with surface recordings. Motor nerve conduction studies provide an early,

age-independent, easily accessible marker for clinical involvement. Routine hematological, biochemical, and CSF studies provide normal results. Sural nerve biopsy typically shows the changes of a hypertrophic neuropathy characterized by onion bulb formation, increased frequency of fibers with demyelinated and remyelinated segments, an increase in endoneurial area, and loss of large myelinated fibers (Figure 80.9).

Charcot-Marie-Tooth Disease 2

CMT2 constitutes one-third of all autosomal dominant CMT disease. Clinical symptoms begin later than in CMT1, most commonly in the second decade, but may be delayed until middle age or beyond. Foot and spinal deformities tend to be less prominent in CMT2. The clinical features closely resemble those of CMT1 but differ in that peripheral nerves are not enlarged and upper limb involvement, tremor, and general areflexia occur less frequently. However, in individual cases it is often impossible to determine the type of CMT disease on the basis of clinical findings alone. Approximately 20% of patients are asymptomatic. A distinct subgroup of severely affected patients, designated CMT2C, develop vocal cord, intercostal, and diaphragmatic muscle weakness. Because of respiratory failure, life expectancy is shortened in these patients (Dyck et al. 1994).

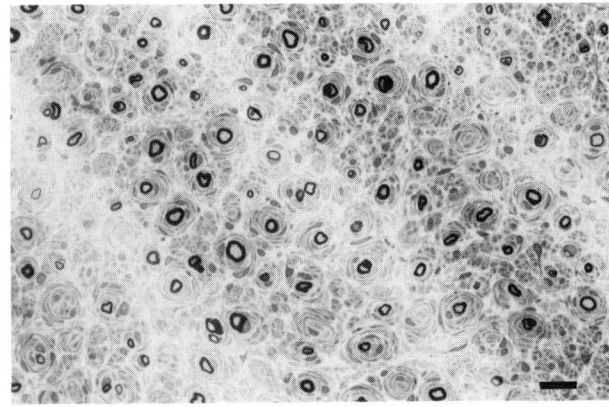

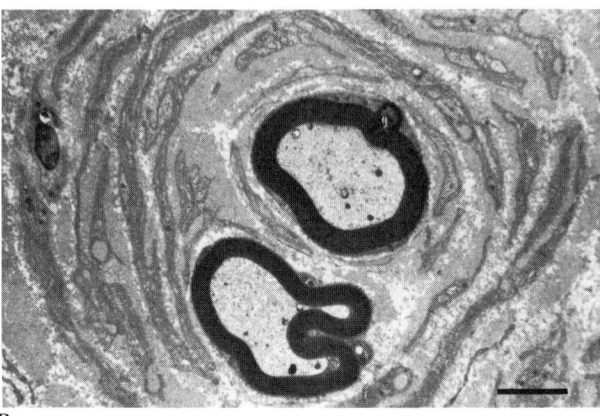

FIGURE 80.9 Charcot-Marie-Tooth disease type 1. **(A)** Semithin transverse section of sural nerve showing numerous onion bulbs. (Toluidine blue; bar = 20 μm.) **(B)** Electron micrograph of an onion bulb formation. Two small myelinated fibers are surrounded by multiple layers of Schwann cell processes. (Bar = 0.5 μm.)

Motor NCV may be normal or mildly reduced. SNAPs are either absent or reduced in amplitude. Sural nerve biopsy specimens show preferential loss of large myelinated fibers without significant demyelination; there may be clusters of regenerating myelinated fibers.

Linkage studies to identify the genes for CMT2 indicate that the disorder is genetically heterogeneous. CMT2 has been mapped to chromosomes 1 (1p35-36, designated CMT2A), 3 (3q13-22, CMT2B), and 7 (7p14, CMT2D), but the specific genes at these loci are yet to be identified (Saito et al. 1997). The CMT2C families have not been linked to any known loci.

X-linked Dominant Charcot-Marie-Tooth Disease

CMTX is phenotypically similar to CMT1. Male subjects tend to be more severely affected, whereas female subjects may have a mild neuropathy or be asymptomatic. No male-to-male transmission occurs. NCVs in men show significant slowing, whereas in women the slowing parallels the loss of CMAP amplitude.

Charcot-Marie-Tooth Disease 3 or Dejerine-Sottas Disease

CMT3, or Dejerine-Sottas disease, is an uncommon progressive hypertrophic neuropathy with onset in childhood. Motor development is delayed; proximal weakness, global areflexia, enlarged peripheral nerves, and severe disability are the rule. Although originally the disorder was thought to be autosomal recessive, the majority of cases are sporadic, and in some instances have been shown to result from a new dominant mutation.

Motor conduction velocities are severely slowed, often to less than 10 m per second. The CSF protein is frequently increased. Pathologically, pronounced onion bulb changes are associated with hypomyelination and myelinated fiber loss. Defective myelination is confirmed by an increased axon to fiber diameter ratio. Cases of congenital hypomyelination neuropathy probably represent a variant of CMT3 at the far end of a spectrum of defective myelination.

Charcot-Marie-Tooth Disease 4

CMT4 is an autosomal recessive neuropathy characterized by onset in early childhood and progressive weakness, leading to inability to walk in adolescence. NCV studies are slowed (20–30 m per second); CSF protein is normal. Nerve biopsy shows loss of myelinated fibers, hypomyelination, and onion bulbs. Affected families of ethnic Tunisian background are linked to chromosome 8 (8q13-21.1) and designated CMT4A (Othmane et al. 1993).

Complex Forms of Charcot-Marie-Tooth Disease

A number of families with peroneal muscular atrophy exhibit additional features such as optic atrophy, pigmentary retinal degeneration, deafness, and spastic paraparesis. Cardiac involvement is encountered in occasional patients, but prospective family studies find no association between cardiomyopathy and CMT disease. A syndrome of CIDP responding to prednisone and immunosuppression has been reported in patients with inherited CMT disease, providing evidence that nongenetic factors may play a role in clinical expression of the mutant gene.

Molecular Genetic Advances in the Study of Charcot-Marie-Tooth Disease

A classification of CMT disease based on the current molecular genetic advances is provided in Table 80.13 (Figure

Table 80.13: Molecular genetic classification of Charcot-Marie-Tooth disease and related disorders

Disease	Inheritance	Linkage	Gene product	Mechanisms
CMT1A	AD	C 17p11.2-12	PMP-22	Duplication (3 copies); point mutations
CMT1B	AD	C 1q22-23	P_0	Point mutations
CMT1C	AD	?	?	?
CMT2A	AD	C 1p36	?	?
CMT2B	AD	C 3q-22	?	?
CMT2C	AD	?	?	?
CMT3A	AR/AD	C 17p11.2-12	PMP-22	Homozygous duplication (4 copies); point mutations
CMT3B		C 1q22-23	P_0	
CMT4	AR	C 8q13-21.1	?	?
CMTX	X-linked dominant	Xq13.3	Connexin-32	Point mutations
HNPP A	AD	C 17p11.2-12	PMP-22	Deletion (1 copy)
HNPP B	AD	?	?	?

AD = autosomal dominant; AR = autosomal recessive; C = chromosome; CMT = Charcot-Marie-Tooth disease; CMTX = X-linked CMT; HNPP = hereditary neuropathy with liability to pressure palsies; P_0 = myelin protein zero; PMP-22 = peripheral myelin protein-22.

80.10; Lupski 1998). The clinical phenotype of CMT1 represents more than two distinct autosomal disorders. The most common form, referred to as CMT1A, localizes to chromosome 17. The majority of CMT1A patients have a DNA duplication at 17p11.2-12. The CMT1A duplication is a tandem repeat of 1.5 megabases that arises from unequal crossover during germ cell meiosis. The human peripheral myelin protein-22 (PMP-22) gene lies within the duplicated region on chromosome 17p. PMP-22 is a membrane glycoprotein that represents approximately 5% of the total protein found in peripheral myelin, where its expression is restricted to compact myelin. The CMT1A duplication is found in 70% of both autosomal dominant and isolated CMT1 cases. The disease phenotype in patients with the CMT1A duplication is related to a gene dosage effect caused by three copies of the normal PMP-22 gene (trisomic overexpression) (Gabriel et al. 1997). A small proportion of CMT1A patients have missense mutations of the PMP-22 gene, similar to the mouse mutants trembler and trembler-J that have a severe hypomyelinating neuropathy.

Families of CMT1B are linked to the Duffy blood group locus on the proximal long arm of chromosome 1 and make up 20% of CMT1 patients. P_0, a major structural glycoprotein of peripheral myelin, maps to the site associated with the CMT1B locus (C1q22-23). Point mutations of the P_0 gene were found to be responsible for the CMT1B phenotype (Hayasaka et al. 1993). P_0 plays a major role as an adhesion molecule in the formation and compaction of peripheral myelin. Different P_0 mutations have resulted in divergent morphological effects on myelin sheaths consist-

ing of uncompacted myelin or focal myelin foldings (Gabreëls-Festen et al. 1996).

The designation CMT1C is reserved for autosomal dominant CMT1 families not linked to either chromosome 17 or chromosome 1, suggesting involvement of as yet unidentified autosomal loci. Linkage studies in CMTX families have localized the gene to Xq13.1. The gene for connexin-32, a gap junction protein, lies within this region. More than 50 point mutations of the connexin-32 gene have been identified in affected members of CMTX families (Bergoffen et al. 1993). Connexin-32 is a gap junction protein involved in cell to cell communication. It localizes to the nodes of Ranvier and the Schmidt-Lanterman incisures by immunofluorescent staining and may play a role in the transfer of ions and nutrients to the innermost myelin layers and the axon.

Dejerine-Sottas disease or CMT3 can arise from different genetic mechanisms. Dominant point mutations of either the PMP-22 (CMT3A) or the P_0 (CMT3B) gene cause the disorder. Several reported cases of CMT3 result from the homozygous expression of the CMT1A duplication.

Treatment and Management

The rates of progression of CMT1 and CMT2 are slow, disability occurs relatively late, and life span may be normal. Management is mainly supportive. Patients should be instructed in proper foot care and advised to wear broad, well-fitting shoes. Insoles may be used to distribute body weight more evenly in patients with foot deformity. Ankle-foot braces or orthopedic procedures are indicated for severe footdrop.

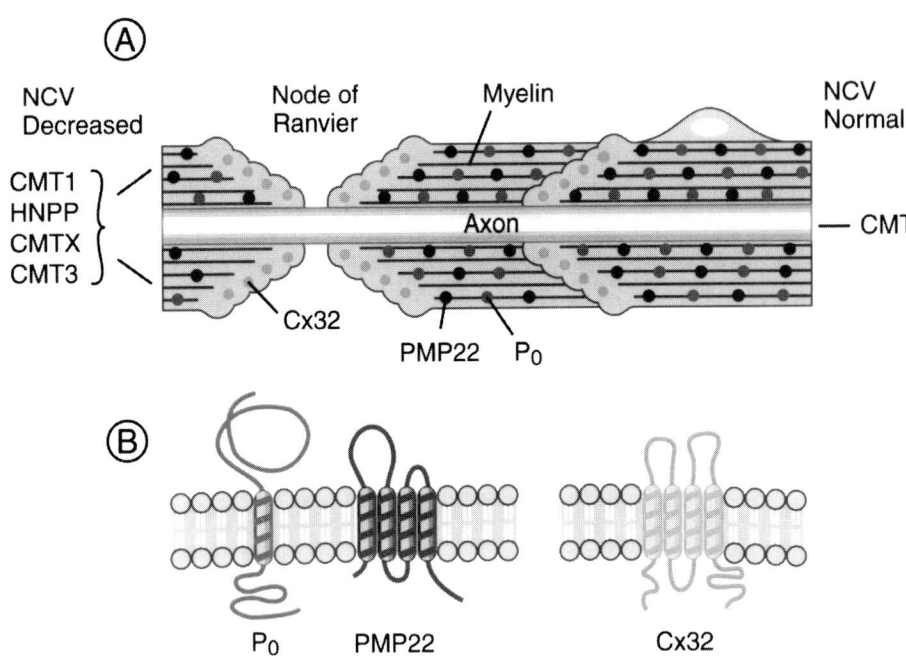

FIGURE 80.10 **(A)** Charcot-Marie-Tooth disease (CMT) and related disorders: CMT1, CMT with X-linked inheritance (CMTX), hereditary neuropathy with liability to pressure palsies (HNPP), and CMT3 are inherited disorders of myelin. CMT2 is a primary neuronal disorder. Alterations in dosage of peripheral myelin protein-22 (PMP-22) gene account for the majority of patients with CMT1A and HNPP. **(B)** Point mutations (connexin-32 [Cx32] > myelin protein zero [P_0] > PMP-22) of these gene products result in CMTX, CMT1B, and CMT3. (NCV = nerve conduction velocity.) (Adapted with permission from JR Lupski. Molecular Genetics of Peripheral Neuropathies. In JD Martin (ed), Molecular Neurology. New York: Scientific American, 1998. All rights reserved.)

Patients should be warned to avoid neurotoxic drugs because of greater susceptibility to agents such as vincristine.

Genetic counseling should be based on the inheritance pattern or the specific molecular lesion detected. DNA diagnostic testing is available for the CMT1A duplication and connexin-32 mutations. CMT1A duplication testing should be considered in chronic demyelinating neuropathy, even in the absence of a positive family history, given the high spontaneous mutation rate. In families known to have the CMT1A duplication, DNA testing can be used for presymptomatic screening. CMT1 patients who do not have the CMT1A duplication should be screened for connexin-32 mutations, which are the next most common cause of CMT1, accounting for 5–10% of patients. Screening tests for PMP-22 and P_0 point mutations are not routinely available but should be considered in childhood cases of severe demyelinating neuropathy suggestive of Dejerine-Sottas disease.

Hereditary Neuropathy with Liability to Pressure Palsies

HNPP is an autosomal dominant disorder of peripheral nerves leading to increased susceptibility to mechanical traction or compression. Patients present with recurrent episodes of isolated mononeuropathies, typically affecting, in order of decreasing frequency, the common peroneal, ulnar, radial, and median nerves. Painless brachial plexus neuropathy is seen in up to one-third of patients. The lack of dysmorphic features such as hypertelorism distinguishes the brachial plexus neuropathy of HNPP from familial brachial plexus neuropathy. Most patients experience the initial episode in the second or third decade of life. Attacks usually are provoked by compression, slight traction, or other minor trauma. Most attacks are of sudden onset, painless, and usually followed by complete recovery. Mild generalized neuropathy may be present in older individuals. Some patients have pes cavus and hammer toes.

Electrophysiological study results demonstrate diffuse polyneuropathy with motor and sensory conduction abnormalities in both clinically affected and unaffected nerves. Persistent motor conduction block or profound slowing of motor conduction velocities at one or more entrapment sites, or disproportionately prolonged distal motor latencies, are helpful clues to the diagnosis. Sural nerve biopsy specimens demonstrate distinctive, focal sausagelike thickenings of myelin termed *tomacula* (Figure 80.11), as well as segmental demyelination.

Linkage studies show a 1.5-megabase deletion of chromosome 17p11.2-12 that includes the PMP-22 gene and corresponds to the duplicated region in CMT1A in most affected patients with HNPP. Some families lack the 17p deletion and are labeled HNPPB. Substantial evidence supports the contention that the PMP-22 gene is a dosage-sensitive gene that causes HNPP when only one copy is present and CMT1A when present in three copies. These findings indicate that HNPP and CMT1A are caused by a reciprocal recombination event that generates a duplication on one chromosome and a deletion on the other. These reciprocal syndromes represent products of unequal crossover during meiosis (Chance et al. 1993). Molecular diagnosis of the 17p11.2 deletion is commercially available in reference laboratories and should be considered regardless of family history in any patient presenting with painless multiple mononeuropathies, brachial plexopathy, or recurrent demyelinating neuropathy (Tyson et al. 1996). The primary treatment strategy is to prevent nerve injury by avoiding pressure damage.

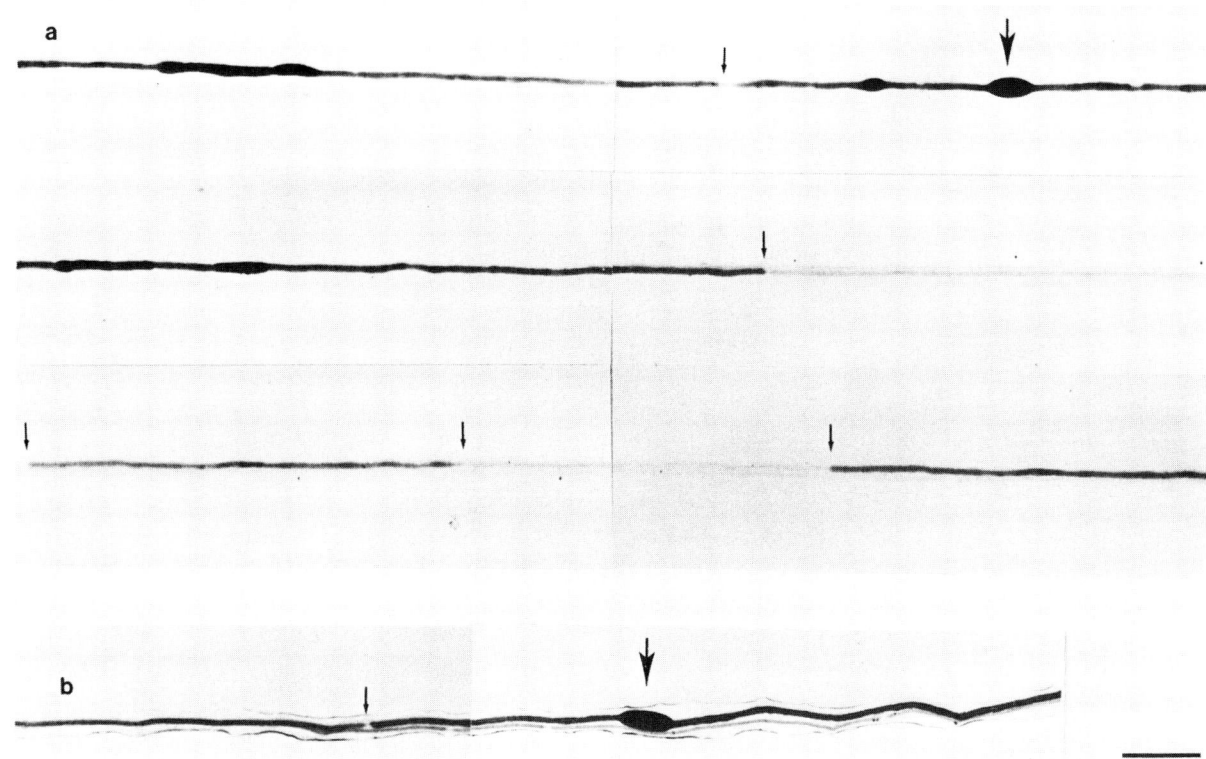

FIGURE 80.11   Single teased nerve fibers from a patient with hereditary liability to pressure palsies, showing examples of focal sausage-shaped enlargements of the myelin sheath (*large arrows*) in two fibers (a, b). Fiber a shows thinly remyelinated internodes. Successive nodes of Ranvier (*thin arrows*) can be followed from left to right. (Bar = 100 μm.) (Reprinted with permission from EP Bosch, HC Chui, MA Martin, et al. Brachial plexus involvement in familial pressure-sensitive neuropathy: electrophysiologic and morphologic findings. Ann Neurol 1980;8:620–624.)

Hereditary Sensory and Autonomic Neuropathy

HSAN are characterized by prominent sensory loss with autonomic features but without corresponding motor involvement. Currently, these neuropathies are divided into five main groups based on inheritance, clinical features, and populations of sensory neurons affected (Table 80.14). These neuropathies are distinctly rare compared with CMT. Genetic linkage studies have led to successful gene localization in some types. Sensory loss in HSAN predisposes to unnoticed, recurrent trauma that may lead to neuropathic (Charcot) joints, nonhealing ulcers, infections, and osteomyelitis resulting in acral mutilations (acrodystrophic neuropathy). These complications are preventable by avoiding trauma to the insensitive distal limb segments.

Hereditary Sensory and Autonomic Neuropathy Type I

HSAN type I is an autosomal dominant disorder that is the most common familial sensory neuropathy. Symptoms begin in the second or later decades with sensory loss and subsequent tissue injury mainly affecting the feet and legs. Sensory loss initially affects pain and temperature discrimination more than touch-pressure sensation, but includes all modalities as the disease progresses. Patients present with calluses on the soles, painless stress fractures, neuropathic foot and ankle joints, and recurrent plantar ulcers. If ulcers are neglected and become infected, severe acromutilations may result (Figure 80.12). Lancinating pains are often present. Some degree of distal motor involvement, variable neural hearing loss, or, rarely, spastic paraparesis may be seen. The dissociated sensory loss of the lower limbs was mistakenly diagnosed as lumbosacral syringomyelia until Denny-Brown demonstrated primary degeneration of dorsal root ganglia at autopsy.

The absence of SNAPs provides further evidence of a peripheral nerve disorder. Sural nerve biopsy confirms a severe loss of unmyelinated and small myelinated axons and to a lesser degree loss of large myelinated fiber (Figure 80.13). HSAN type I has been mapped to chromosome 9q22.1-22.3.

Hereditary Sensory and Autonomic Neuropathy Type II

HSAN type II is recessively inherited and begins in infancy, rarely later. All sensory modalities are affected and involve

Table 80.14:   Hereditary sensory and autonomic neuropathies

Disease	Inheritance	Age of onset	Clinical features	Biopsy findings	Chromosome
HSAN I	AD	Second decade or later	Feet and legs pain > touch	Loss of UF greater than MF	C 9q22.1-q22.3
HSAN II	AR	Infancy	UE and LE; pansensory loss	Absent MF	?
HSAN III (familial dysauto-nomia)	AR	Birth	Absent tongue papillae	Reduced UF	C 9q31-q33
HSAN IV	AR	Birth	Anhidrosis nl SNAP	Absent UF	C 1q21-q22
HSAN V	AR	Birth	Anhidrosis nl SNAP	Absent small MF	?
SCD Friedreich's ataxia	AR	Second decade	Areflexia; JPS and vibration impaired	Loss of large MF	C 9q13–q21; GAA; triplet repeat; gene product: frataxin

AD = autosomal dominant; AR = autosomal recessive; GAA = expanded GAA triplet repeat in intron of frataxin gene; HSAN = hereditary sensory and autonomic neuropathies; JPS = joint position sense; LE = lower extremity; MF = myelinated fibers; nl SNAP = normal sensory nerve action potential; SCD = spinocerebellar degenerations; UE = upper extremity; UF = unmyelinated fibers.

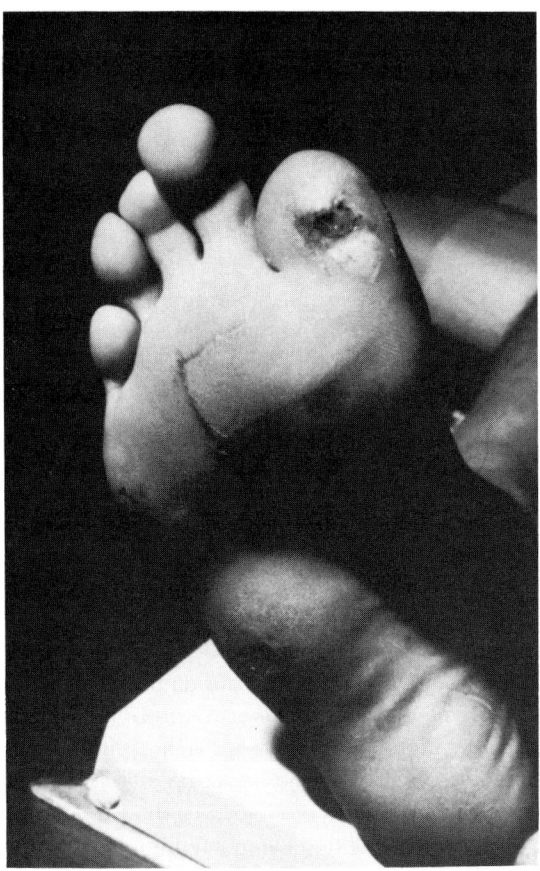

FIGURE 80.12   Nonhealing foot ulcer in a 33-year-old man with hereditary sensory and autonomic neuropathy type I. In his kinship, 10 individuals are affected in three generations.

distal upper and lower limbs more than trunk and face. The hands, feet, lips, and tongue are at risk for mutilation because of generalized pansensory loss. Autonomic symptoms include bladder dysfunction and impotence. Associations with spastic paraplegia, retinitis pigmentosa, motor weakness, or neurotrophic keratitis have been described. The clinical course is slowly progressive, with progressive axonal loss. SNAPs are absent. Sural nerve biopsy specimens show almost complete absence of myelinated fibers and reduced unmyelinated fiber populations (Figure 80.14). No chromosomal linkage has been identified in this group of patients.

Hereditary Sensory and Autonomic Neuropathy Type III

HSAN type III (familial dysautonomia or the Riley-Day syndrome) is an autosomal recessively inherited sensory neuropathy affecting mostly children of Ashkenazi Jewish extraction with prominent autonomic manifestations. Symptoms begin at birth and include poor feeding, episodes of vomiting, frequent pulmonary infections, and attacks of fever. Emotional stimuli provoke episodic hypertension, profuse sweating, and marked skin blotching caused by defective autonomic control. Later in childhood, hyporeflexia and insensitivity to pain, stunted growth, and scoliosis become apparent. Defective lacrimation and absence of fungiform papillae on the tongue are tell-tale signs. Ophthalmological examination is helpful to detect characteristic signs of postganglionic parasympathetic denervation supersensitivity of the pupil, shown by a positive miotic response to 0.1% pilocarpine or 2.5% methacholine, corneal insensitivity, and absence of tears. Patients are at risk to develop profound hypoxia following anesthesia or with high-altitude travel as a result of diminished respiratory response to hypercapnia and hypoxia.

Motor NCVs are generally normal, whereas SNAP amplitudes are frequently reduced. A marked reduction in

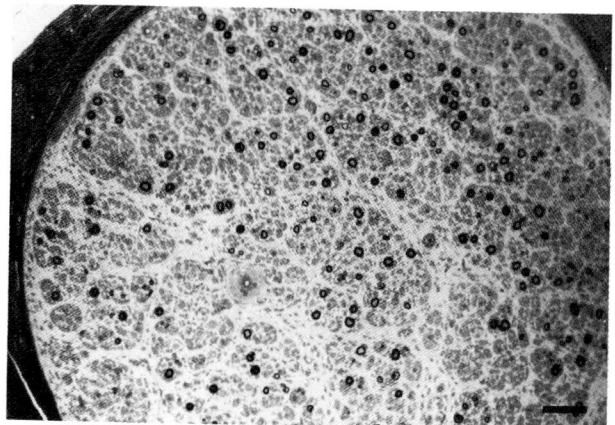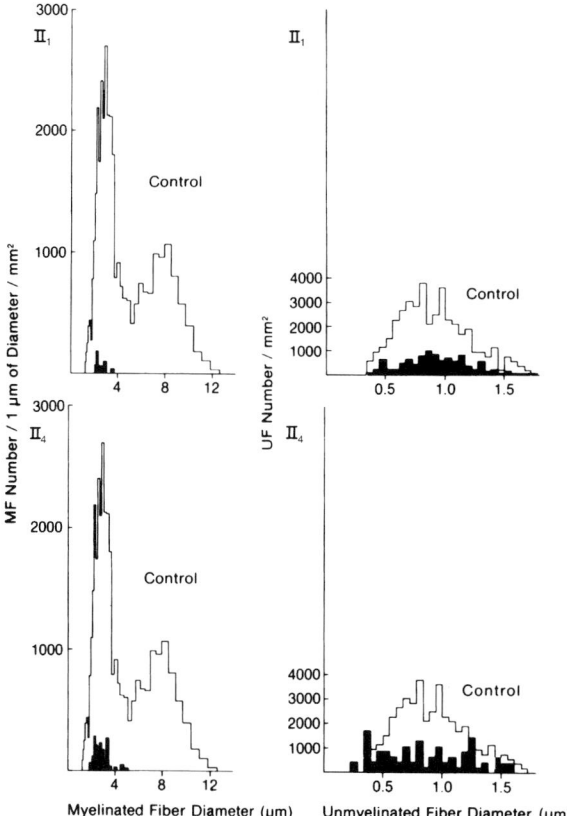

FIGURE 80.13 Semithin transverse section of sural nerve from a patient with hereditary sensory and autonomic neuropathy type I. Note loss of large and small myelinated fibers. (Toluidine blue; bar = 50 μm.)

FIGURE 80.14 Sural nerve fiber size-frequency histograms of myelinated fibers (MF) (left) and unmyelinated fibers (UF) (right) of two affected siblings with hereditary sensory and autonomic neuropathy type II (*black bars*) and control nerve (*white bars*). In the patients, the number of myelinated fibers was less than 500/mm² and that of the unmyelinated fibers less than 10,000/mm².

the density of unmyelinated axons is seen in sural nerve biopsy specimens. The number of neurons in the sympathetic, parasympathetic, and spinal ganglia is reduced. Linkage studies have mapped the gene locus responsible for HSAN type III to chromosome 9q31-q33.

Hereditary Sensory and Autonomic Neuropathy Type IV

HSAN type IV is a rare autosomal recessive disorder characterized by congenital insensitivity to pain, anhidrosis, defective temperature control, and mild mental retardation. Cutaneous sensory nerves show selective loss of unmyelinated axons and small myelinated fibers. Clinically similar cases with selective loss of only small myelinated fibers have been designated HSAN type V. In HSAN type IV, which selectively affects unmyelinated and small myelinated fibers, tendon reflexes and SNAPs are preserved. Confirmation of a neuropathic abnormality in cases of congenital indifference to pain without apparent neurological signs therefore depends on the morphometric study of unmyelinated and myelinated fiber populations in nerve biopsy specimens and the quantitative sudomotor axon-reflex test. The latter depends on an axon reflex mediated by postganglionic sympathetic fibers and becomes abnormal with small fiber involvement. The gene locus for HSAN type IV maps to chromosome 1q21-22. Mutations in the trkA gene encoding the tyrosine kinase receptor for nerve growth factor (NGF) have been described in a few patients with HSAN type IV. These findings indicate that the NGF-trkA system plays a crucial role in the development of unmyelinated nociceptive and sudomotor fibers.

Treatment and Management

The prevention of stress fractures and plantar ulcers is of utmost importance. This can be achieved by meticulous foot care, avoiding barefoot walking, daily inspection of feet and shoes, and proper skin care with moisturizing lotions. Whenever plantar ulcers develop, weight bearing should be discontinued until the ulcers heal.

Neuropathy Associated with Spinocerebellar Ataxia

In Friedreich's ataxia the PNS is affected consistently. Even in the early stages of the disease, examination reveals lower limb areflexia and impaired joint position and vibration sense, with preserved pain and temperature appreciation. Pes cavus and hammer toes occur in approximately 90% of cases.

Motor NCVs are normal or slightly reduced, and SNAPs are invariably reduced or absent. A selective loss of large myelinated fibers occurs in the sural nerve. For the early detection of affected children at risk in families with Friedreich's ataxia, nerve conduction studies and quantitative sensory examinations are useful investigations. Friedreich's

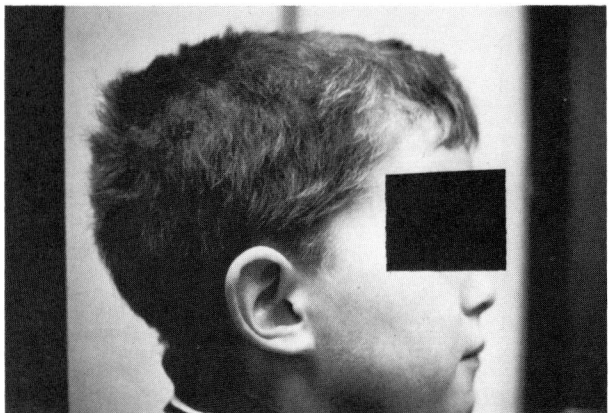

FIGURE 80.15 Tightly curled hair in a young child with giant axonal neuropathy.

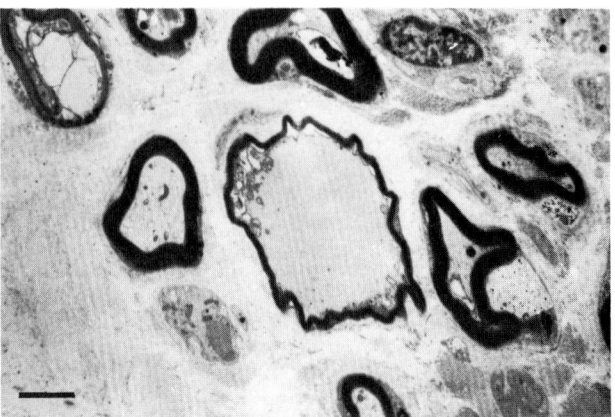

FIGURE 80.16 Giant axonal neuropathy. Electron micrograph of a giant axon filled with neurofilaments. Its myelin sheath is attenuated. (Bar = 1 μm.)

ataxia is an autosomal recessive triplet repeat disorder on chromosome 9q13-q21.1 leading to loss of frataxin expression (see Chapter 76). Peripheral nerve involvement has been found in association with other spinocerebellar ataxias, most notably spinocerebellar atxia type 4 (SCA4).

Giant Axonal Neuropathy

Giant axonal neuropathy is a rare sporadic or autosomal recessive disorder. The condition is characterized by a slowly progressive sensorimotor neuropathy of early childhood onset. Most affected children have tightly curled hair and distal leg weakness and develop a peculiar gait disturbance with a tendency to walk on the inner edges of the feet (Figure 80.15). With disease progression, evidence of CNS involvement occurs, including optic atrophy, nystagmus, cerebellar ataxia, and intellectual decline, as well as abnormal visual, auditory, and somatosensory evoked potentials. Sural nerve biopsy demonstrates the pathognomonic changes of large focal axonal swellings that contain densely packed disorganized neurofilaments (Figure 80.16). Further studies indicate that this neuropathy is a generalized disorder of intermediate filament organization affecting a variety of cells, including axons and glial cells of both the PNS and CNS. The gene responsible for giant axonal neuropathy has been mapped to chromosome 16q24 (Flanigan et al. 1998).

Familial Amyloid Polyneuropathy

Familial amyloid polyneuropathy (FAP) is a group of autosomal dominant disorders characterized by the extracellular deposition of amyloid in peripheral nerves and other organs. Amyloid is a fibrillar protein characterized by (1) green birefringence of Congo red–stained sections viewed in polarized light; (2) the presence of nonbranched 10-nm amyloid fibrils on electron microscopy; and (3) a β-pleated sheet structure on x-ray diffraction. Many different proteins can be deposited as amyloid in tissues. In FAP one of three aberrant proteins (transthyretin, apolipoprotein A1, or gelsolin [Falk et al. 1997]) can be found in the peripheral nerves. In acquired, primary systemic amyloidosis, polypeptides of immunoglobulin light chain origin are deposited in tissues as amyloid, which is referred to as *AL amyloid* (see Primary Systemic Amyloidosis, later in this chapter).

The classification of FAP was traditionally based on clinical presentation. Progress in understanding the protein composition and molecular genetics of these disorders justifies a different approach (Table 80.15).

Transthyretin Amyloidosis (Familial Amyloid Polyneuropathy Types I and II)

The majority of patients with FAP have mutations of the plasma protein transthyretin (TTR). This is a transport protein for thyroxin and retinol-binding protein, is predominantly synthesized in the liver, and consists of a single polypeptide chain of 127 amino acid residues. The gene for transthyretin is located on chromosome 18q11.2-q12.1. Mutations of the transthyretin gene result in transcriptions of aberrant proteins with predisposition toward amyloid formation and deposition in peripheral nerve, heart, kidney, and eye.

TTR-related amyloid polyneuropathies demonstrate two disparate clinical phenotypes. The original cases described by Andrade in Portugal are referred to as FAP type I. This is the most common form of FAP and has been observed in many ethnic groups. The neuropathy begins insidiously in the third and fourth decades with dissociated sensory impairment (loss of pain and thermal sense) in the lower extremities, often associated with lancinating pain and paresthesia. Autonomic dysfunction commonly includes impotence, postural hypotension, bladder dysfunction, distal anhidrosis, and abnormal pupils

Table 80.15: Familial amyloid neuropathies

Aberrant protein	Type	Decade of onset	Neuropathy	Associated lesions
TTR	FAP I	Third through fifth	Sensorimotor neuropathy, autonomic neuropathy	Heart, kidney
TTR	FAP II	Fourth through fifth	Carpal tunnel syndrome	Heart
Apolipoprotein A-1	FAP III	Third through fourth	Sensorimotor neuropathy	Kidney, peptic ulcers
Gelsolin	FAP IV	Third	Cranial	Corneal lattice dystrophy

FAP = familial amyloid polyneuropathy; TTR = transthyretin.

with scalloped margins. Gastrointestinal symptoms characterized by diarrhea and weight loss may be prominent. Eventually pansensory loss, distal wasting, weakness, and areflexia develop. Systemically, amyloid is deposited in the ocular vitreous, heart, and kidneys. The disorder is relentlessly progressive. Patients usually die of cardiac or renal failure or malnutrition 10–15 years after onset.

Electrophysiological studies reveal a distal axonal neuropathy that affects sensory fibers earlier and more prominently than motor fibers. Early changes include low-amplitude or absent SNAPs, mild reduction in CMAP amplitudes, and preserved motor conduction velocities. Evidence of denervation is found in distal leg muscles. Until specific biochemical and genetic studies became available, the diagnosis was confirmed by the presence of amyloid in tissue biopsy specimens. In early cases, sural nerve biopsy specimens show a predominant loss of unmyelinated and small myelinated fibers. Amyloid deposits are usually seen within the endoneurium or around vasa nervorum. Immunostaining with antibodies to transthyretin can frequently identify the specific type of amyloid. The pattern of myocardial involvement varies according to specific TTR mutations. Many but not all mutations have myocardial infiltration on echocardiography. The mechanisms of nerve fiber injury and their relationship to amyloid deposits are incompletely understood. It has been proposed that the preferential deposition of amyloid in sensory and autonomic ganglia interferes with neuronal function, leading to length-dependent axonal degeneration. An alternative theory suggests that endoneurial edema associated with amyloid deposition in blood vessels and the endoneurium results in ischemic nerve fiber injury.

Rukavina and colleagues described a more restricted form of the disease, referred to as FAP type II, which presents with carpal tunnel syndrome in the fourth or fifth decade and slowly progresses to peripheral polyneuropathy. Autonomic manifestations are absent. Vitreous opacities are common and cardiac involvement may develop. Surgical decompression of the carpal tunnel provides symptomatic relief. Demonstration of amyloid infiltration of the flexor retinaculum obtained at surgery establishes the diagnosis.

More than 50 different amino acid substitutions of the transthyretin protein have been identified as causing the clinical phenotypes, referred to as FAP I and II. The most common mutation is a methionine 30 substitution usually associated with the syndrome described by Andrade in Portuguese families. Other transthyretin variants, including isoleucine 33, alanine 60, and tyrosine 77 substitutions, have similar features of generalized polyneuropathy with varying degrees of autonomic involvement. A serine substitution at position 84 and histidine at position 58 are the two transthyretin mutations seen most commonly in FAP type II, beginning in the upper limbs with carpal tunnel syndrome.

Apolipoprotein A1 Amyloidosis (Familial Amyloid Polyneuropathy Type III, Van Allen)

The clinical manifestations of this variant have much in common with those of type I except for early renal involvement and a high incidence of duodenal ulcers among affected individuals. Uremia is the most common cause of death, typically occurring 12–15 years after the onset of neuropathy. An aberrant fragment of apolipoprotein A1 with a substitution of arginine for glycine accumulates in the tissues in FAP type III.

Gelsolin Amyloidosis (Familial Amyloid Polyneuropathy Type IV, Meretoja)

Gelsolin amyloidosis was first described in Finland, but subsequently isolated cases have been reported elsewhere. Symptoms begin in the third decade with corneal clouding caused by a fine network of amyloid filaments, referred to as *lattice corneal dystrophy*. This is followed in the fifth decade by progressive cranial neuropathies with prominent facial palsy and skin changes producing a typical baggy skin over the atrophic face. Other bulbar signs may develop together with mild peripheral neuropathy without autonomic dysfunction.

Gelsolin, the amyloid protein isolated from tissues of FAP type IV, is an actin-binding protein found in plasma, leukocytes, and other cell types. The gelsolin gene maps to chromosome 9. Amino acid substitutions (asparagine or tyrosine at position 187) result in amyloid-forming mutant gelsolin.

DNA Diagnosis of Familial Amyloid Polyneuropathy

The diagnosis of FAP requires several steps. Initially, the diagnosis is established by confirming the presence of amyloid in nerve and muscle biopsies or a sample of subcutaneous abdominal fat. Immunostaining using specific antibodies against one of the three aberrant proteins may identify the responsible protein. In sporadic cases, the more common AL amyloidosis should be excluded by a search for clonal plasma cell dyscrasia (see Primary Systemic Amyloidosis, later in this chapter). If no evidence of plasma cell dyscrasia exists, transthyretin can be identified by isoelectric focusing of the serum, which separates variant and wild-type transthyretin. The finding of a variant transthyretin should prompt genetic testing. DNA isolated from peripheral leukocytes or tissue can be amplified with the polymerase chain reaction and specific oligonucleotide primers used to amplify regions of the gene of interest, thereby demonstrating specific point mutations. DNA testing for the most common TTR mutations (Met-30, Ile-33, Ala-60, Tyr-77, Ser-84) is currently available in reference laboratories.

Treatment

The prognosis of TTR amyloidosis varies with the specific mutation, age of onset, and organ involvement. Supportive measures are essential for both the neuropathy and specific organ system involved, including cardiac pacing, dialysis, parenteral nutrition, and physical therapy. Because transthyretin is mainly synthesized in the liver, liver transplantation has been proposed as definite therapy for this disorder. Transplantation results in rapid clearance of the variant TTR from serum; there may be regression of amyloid deposits in tissues and partial improvement of the neuropathy, but in approximately one-half of the cases the disease progresses, presumably related to the total body amyloid load (Bergethon et al. 1996).

Porphyric Neuropathy

Hepatic porphyrias are caused by hereditary enzyme defects that affect the heme biosynthetic pathway, resulting in excess accumulation and excretion of porphyrins and their precursors. These dominantly inherited disorders include acute intermittent porphyria (AIP), variegate porphyria (VP), and hereditary coproporphyria (HCP). A fourth disorder referred to as *plumboporphyria* is inherited as an autosomal recessive trait and is caused by a deficiency of δ-aminolevulinic acid (ALA) dehydratase (Table 80.16). These partial enzyme defects remain latent until precipitating factors trigger acute attacks with neuropsychiatric manifestations. Precipitating factors include certain inducing drugs, alcohol, hormones, and a negative caloric balance either during intentional fasting or during an intercurrent illness. Precipitating factors share the ability to induce

hepatic δ-ALA synthase, the rate-limiting enzyme in heme biosynthesis, which leads to the overproduction and overexcretion of porphobilinogen (PBG) and δ-ALA.

Clinical Features of the Acute Porphyric Attack

The manifestations of the acute attack are identical regardless of the specific type of hepatic porphyria. All clinical symptoms can be explained by dysfunction of the autonomic nervous system, PNS, and CNS. Characteristically, porphyric attacks first occur during the third and fourth decades of life and are more common and severe in women. The most frequent presenting symptoms are abdominal pain, nausea, vomiting, and severe constipation. Other autonomic manifestations are tachycardia, labile hypertension, orthostatic hypotension, and difficulty with micturition. Only a few patients progress to develop the more ominous motor neuropathy or CNS involvement. Onset of the predominantly motor neuropathy is subacute, with generalized, proximal, or asymmetrical muscle weakness developing over days or weeks. The arms rather than the legs may be affected first, and proximal muscles may be preferentially involved. Muscular activity before onset of symptoms may influence the pattern of weakness. Cranial nerve involvement is common. In severe cases, flaccid quadriplegia with respiratory failure ensues. Rapidly progressive muscle wasting is a striking feature. Tendon reflexes are diminished or absent, but paradoxically ankle jerks may be retained. Sensory impairment may occur in a distal stocking-glove distribution or may affect the trunk and proximal limbs in an unusual bathing suit pattern. The rate of improvement is variable. Some patients rapidly recover function, suggesting a reversible acute toxic-metabolic neuronal injury. Those with fixed weakness caused by axonal degeneration improve slowly (mean recovery, 10.6 months for proximal muscles and nearly twice as long for distal muscles). The protean CNS manifestations during severe attacks include anxiety, confusion, delirium, seizures, and coma.

Patients with VP and HCP may develop cutaneous photosensitivity during adult life. The skin manifestations consist of blisters, hyperpigmentation, hypertrichosis, and increased skin fragility. AIP occurs in all ethnic groups, but is most common in individuals of Scandinavian or English descent. VP is common among the white population of South Africa.

Laboratory Studies

The biochemical hallmark of the porphyric attack is the marked elevation of ALA and PBG in blood and urine. Rapid screening tests for urinary PBG are the Watson-Schwartz and Hoesch tests, which give positive test results during virtually all acute attacks. A positive screening test result must be confirmed with quantitative urinary determinations of PBG and ALA. Levels of urinary ALA and PBG may decrease rapidly after an attack of VP or HCP,

Table 80.16:   Porphyric neuropathies

	Acute intermittent porphyria	Variegate porphyria	Hereditary coproporphyria	Plumboporphyria
Enzyme defect	PBG deaminase	Protoporphyrinogen oxidase	Coproporphyrinogen oxidase	ALA dehydratase
Inheritance	AD	AD	AD	AR
Photosensitive eruption	None	Present	Present	None
Porphyrin excretion				
Urine				
PBG	+++	+++	+++	0
ALA	+++	+++	+++	+++
Uro	+	+	+	Negative
Copro	Negative	++	+++	+
Feces				
Copro	Negative	+	+++	Negative
Proto	Negative	+++	+	+

AD = autosomal dominant; ALA = aminolevulinic acid; AR = autosomal recessive; copro = coproporphyrin; PBG = porphobilinogen; proto = protoporphyrin; uro = uroporphyrin; +++, ++, + = a relative indication of quantity excreted.

but remain elevated in AIP. Subsequently, stool assays for protoporphyrins and coproporphyrins are necessary to distinguish VP and HCP from AIP. The diagnosis of δ-ALA dehydratase deficiency is supported by increased urinary excretion of ALA without accompanying PBG elevation. Certain medications and disorders other than porphyrias are associated with increased urinary porphyrins, including lead poisoning, liver disease, alcoholism, chronic renal failure during hemodialysis, and certain medications (Tefferi et al. 1994). CSF is normal. Hyponatremia related to inappropriate antidiuretic hormone release is frequent.

Electrophysiological studies in patients with porphyric neuropathy reveal low-amplitude CMAPs, but normal or borderline slow motor conduction velocities. SNAPs are reduced in amplitude or absent. EMG obtained early in the course reveals poor recruitment of normal motor unit potentials. Denervation changes appear later, first in the paraspinal and proximal muscles and subsequently in distal muscles. Morphological study results support length-dependent axonal degeneration and preferential loss of large myelinated axons (Suarez et al. 1994).

Pathogenesis

The hepatic porphyrias have a lifelong genetic defect in hepatic heme synthesis. In AIP, a partial defect of PBG deaminase activity can be demonstrated in erythrocytes, fibroblasts, and hepatocytes. Carriers of AIP can be identified readily by measuring red cell PBG deaminase. In HCP, the block is more distal, involving coproporphyrinogen oxidase, whereas in VP it involves protoporphyrinogen oxidase, with resultant excessive fecal excretion of coproporphyrin and protoporphyrin, respectively. Assays for the latter two enzymes in skin fibroblasts are limited to research laboratories.

The mechanism of the neuronal axonal injury remains uncertain. The two leading hypotheses implicate neuronal heme deficiency with impaired energy metabolism or direct neurotoxicity of ALA.

Treatment and Management

The treatment of patients with acute hepatic porphyria involves three important steps: (1) prevention of attacks; (2) attempts to repress hepatic δ-ALA synthase activity, thereby reducing porphyrin production; and (3) supportive care. Ideally, attacks should be prevented by avoiding inducing drugs and circumstances. Among the inducing drugs, barbiturates are the most common precipitants, followed by sulfonamides, analgesics, nonbarbiturate hypnotics, anticonvulsants, and female sex hormones (see Bosch and Pierach 1987 for a complete list of inducing drugs). Intentional fasting and alcohol consumption should be avoided. Luteinizing hormone-releasing hormone analogues may benefit women with recurrent attacks related to the menstrual cycle. The attack must be treated promptly, as outlined in Figure 80.17. First, all offending drugs are removed and any intercurrent infection is treated. The administration of a high-carbohydrate diet (at least 400 g daily, or the equivalence of glucose or levulose infusions) results in reduced porphyrin precursor production. Persistent symptoms or neurological deficits that progress for 24 hours after carbohydrate loading are indications for treatment with hematin (a hydroxide of heme), which represses the activity of hepatic δ-ALA synthase and may restore cytochrome functions by replenishing an endogenous heme deficit. Hematin therapy, at the recommended dose of six infusions of 4 mg/kg body weight at 12-hour intervals, has resulted in consistent reduction of porphyrin precursors in serum and urine, and clinical improvement in more than 80% of attacks. Early administration of hematin is advocated to correct the metabolic insult before neuronal damage becomes irreparable.

Supportive treatment consists of the correction of fluid imbalance, close attention to respiratory function, and

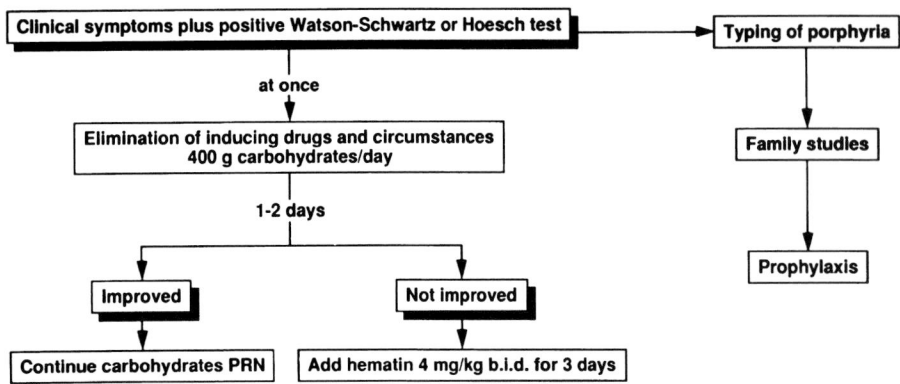

FIGURE 80.17   Management of acute porphyric attack. (PRN = as needed.) (Reprinted with permission from EP Bosch, CA Pierach. Acute Hepatic Porphyria. In RT Johnson [ed], Current Therapy in Neurologic Disease. Toronto: Decker, 1987;2: 293–297.)

physical therapy. Abdominal pain can often be controlled with simple analgesics, but may require narcotics. The treatment of seizures poses a difficult therapeutic problem because most anticonvulsants may exacerbate the disease. Intravenous diazepam or parental magnesium sulfate are both effective and safe for immediate seizure control.

Fabry's Disease

Fabry's disease is an X-linked recessive disorder in which there is deficiency of the lysosomal enzyme α-galactosidase, causing the accumulation of the glycolipid ceramide-tri-hexoside in the endothelial and smooth muscle cells of the blood vessels. Deposition of glycolipid in vascular structures leads to severe vascular disease affecting the heart, kidneys, and brain (Brady 1993). Skin involvement gives rise to the typical angiokeratomas, which are dark red telangiectases found mainly over the lower part of the trunk, buttocks, and scrotum (Figure 80.18). A painful small fiber neuropathy develops in childhood or adolescence. Distal paresthesia and lancinating pain are intensified by exertion, fever, or hot environments. Autonomic dysfunction includes diminished sweating, impaired tear and saliva formation, and decreased intestinal motility. Except for impairment of temperature sensation, overt neurological signs are absent frequently. Female carriers often show clinical involvement, but rarely develop the renal failure, which is characteristic of affected men.

NCVs are mildly reduced in two-thirds of patients. Deposition of glycolipid in small neurons of sensory and peripheral autonomic ganglia results in neuronal degeneration and selective loss of small myelinated and unmyelinated fibers in sural nerve biopsy specimens. Ultrastructurally, perineurial, endothelial, and perithelial cells contain typical lamellated glycolipid inclusions. Leukocyte preparations or skin fibroblasts are used for the diagnostic α-galactosidase assay.

Analgesics, phenytoin, or carbamazepine, along with avoidance of aggravating factors, are effective for pain relief. Kidney transplantation provides relief from renal failure and may improve the neuropathy.

Leukodystrophies with Neuropathy

The leukodystrophies result from inherited abnormalities of myelin metabolism that may affect both the CNS and PNS (see Chapter 68). Peripheral nerve involvement is seen in metachromatic leukodystrophy (MLD), Krabbe's disease, adrenomyeloneuropathy, and Cockayne's syndrome. Recognition of an associated neuropathy may be helpful in the differential diagnosis of the underlying leukodystrophy. Missense mutations in proteolipid protein, a major component of central myelin, cause a spectrum of X-linked CNS disorders without peripheral neuropathy, including Pelizaeus-Merzbacher disease and hereditary spastic paraparesis. Proteolipid protein is expressed also in Schwann cells and compact peripheral myelin. Absence of proteolipid protein expression caused by a frameshift mutation has been reported to produce a demyelinating neuropathy with less severe CNS manifestations (Gabern et al. 1997).

Metachromatic Leukodystrophy

MLD is an autosomal recessive disorder of sulfatide metabolism caused by deficiency of the lysosomal enzyme aryl-sulfatase-A, and subsequent accumulation of sulfatide in brain, peripheral nerve, and other tissues. The storage of sulfatide affects central and peripheral myelin, leading to progressive demyelination. The genetic defect has been localized to chromosome 22. Some mutations in the gene encoding for arylsulfatase-A have been correlated with different clinical phenotypes.

Three main clinical forms have been divided by age of onset: (1) late infantile (6 months to 2 years), (2) juvenile (3–16 years), and (3) adult. Peripheral nerve involvement characterized by a progressive gait disorder, hypotonia, and lower limb areflexia, is an early manifestation that frequently precedes CNS involvement in late infantile and early juvenile MLD. In contrast, behavioral abnormalities and progressive dementia predominate over subtle neuropathic signs in adult-onset MLD. Marked diffuse slowing of nerve conduction is seen in late infantile and juvenile cases. Reduced NCVs and delayed visual and somatosensory evoked potential latencies are present in most adult cases. Extensive segmental demyelination and abnormally thin myelin sheaths are seen in nerve biopsy specimens of all MLD variants, along with metachromatic inclusions within Schwann cells and macrophages. Peripheral nerve biopsy therefore offers a means of confirming the diagnosis, although this is rarely needed now. The diagnosis of MLD is supported by neuroimaging studies and confirmed by an increased urinary sulfatide excretion and abnormal arylsulfatase-A enzyme assays in leukocytes or fibroblasts.

Bone marrow transplantation may increase brain levels of arylsulfatase-A sufficiently to stop disease progression.

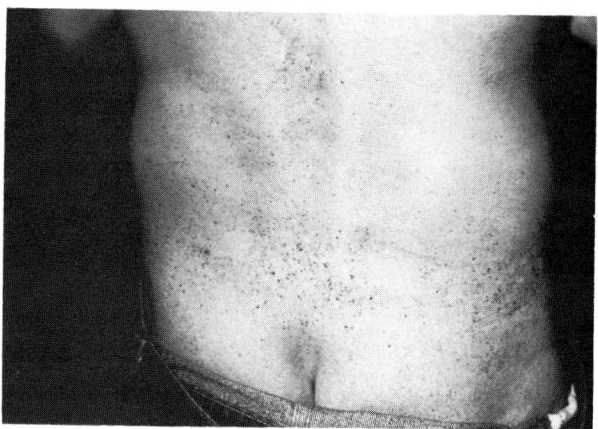

FIGURE 80.18   Fabry's disease. Typical angiokeratomas are clustered over the lower part of the trunk.

Globoid Cell Leukodystrophy

Globoid cell leukodystrophy, or Krabbe's disease, is an autosomal recessive disease caused by an inherited deficiency of the lysosomal enzyme galactocerebroside β-galactosidase. The gene for Krabbe's disease has been localized to chromosome 14. The disorder is characterized by extensive CNS and peripheral nerve demyelination and the presence of multinucleated macrophages (globoid cells) in the cerebral white matter. The classic presentation in early infancy consists of rapidly progressive deterioration in intellectual and motor development, accompanied by hypertonicity, opisthotonic posture, optic atrophy, and seizures. In the late-onset form, peripheral neuropathy and spasticity may be the only manifestations. Peripheral nerve involvement is demonstrated by marked slowing of motor conduction velocities. Segmental demyelination, together with ultrastructurally characteristic tubular or crystalloid inclusions within Schwann cells and macrophages, is seen in sural nerve. Bone marrow transplantation has provided early encouraging results.

Adrenomyeloneuropathy

Adrenomyeloneuropathy, the adult phenotype of adrenoleukodystrophy, is an X-linked recessive disorder of fatty acid metabolism characterized by adrenal insufficiency, progressive myelopathy, and peripheral neuropathy. A defect in beta-oxidation of saturated very-long-chain fatty acids (VLCFA) in peroxisomes leads to the accumulation of tetracosanoic (C24:0) and hexacosanoic (C26:0) acid in tissues and body fluids in affected patients. A significant increase of VLCFA levels in plasma, fibroblasts, or both, allows reliable detection in patients and heterozygote carriers. The defective gene is located in the region Xq28 and codes for a peroxisomal membrane protein referred to as ALDP (Moser 1995). Adrenomyeloneuropathy presents in the second to third decades with progressive spastic paraparesis, distal muscle weakness, sensory loss, and sphincter disturbances. Neurological features frequently are preceded by clinical or laboratory evidence of hypoadrenalism. Approximately 10% of patients have primary adrenal insufficiency without evidence of nervous system involvement. At least 20% of female carriers develop spastic paraparesis similar to that in men, but less severe and later in onset.

Electrophysiological studies are helpful in identifying peripheral nerve involvement that may escape clinical detection because of prominent upper motor neuron signs. Nerve conduction studies demonstrate a mixture of axonal loss and multifocal demyelination. Sural nerve biopsy shows loss of myelinated fibers, occasional small onion bulbs, and curvilinear lamellar lipid inclusions in Schwann cells. Brain MRI scan results are abnormal, demonstrating white matter changes in one-half of patients with adrenomyeloneuropathy at some time in the course of their disease.

Dietary restriction of VLCFA combined with the administration of oleic and erucic acids (Lorenzo's oil) lower plasma levels of VLCFA, but have no effect on the rate of neurological progression. Adrenal insufficiency responds to corticosteroid replacement.

Phytanic Acid Storage Disease (Refsum's Disease)

Refsum's disease, heredopathia atactica polyneuritiformis, is a rare autosomal recessive disorder of phytanic acid metabolism. The gene defect has been localized to chromosome 10 and encodes the peroxisomal enzyme phytanoyl-CoA-hydroxylase. The defect in the enzyme that initiates the alpha-oxidation pathway of β-methyl substituted fatty acids leads to phytanic acid accumulation in serum and tissues. Phytanic acid is derived exclusively from dietary sources, mainly chlorophyll, dairy products, meats, and fish oils. Clinical onset spans from childhood to the third decade of life. The cardinal manifestations include pigmentary retinal degeneration, with night blindness or visual field constriction, chronic hypertrophic neuropathy, ataxia, and other cerebellar signs such as nystagmus and intention tremor. Initially, the neuropathy affects the lower limbs with distal leg atrophy, weakness, areflexia, large fiber sensory impairment, and sometimes palpably enlarged nerves. Weakness becomes generalized later in the illness. In addition to pes cavus, overriding toes caused by symmetrically short fourth metatarsals are a helpful sign for Refsum's disease. Progressive sensorineural hearing loss, anosmia, cardiomyopathy, and ichthyosis are frequent. The course may be either progressive or fluctuating with exacerbations and remissions. Exacerbations are frequently precipitated by fasting, which mobilizes phytanic acid from endogenous fat stores.

Motor conduction velocities are markedly slowed, and SNAPs are reduced or absent. CSF protein is increased in the range of 100–700 mg/dl. Sural nerve biopsy reveals a hypertrophic neuropathy with prominent onion bulb formation. The diagnosis is confirmed by elevated serum levels of phytanic acid.

Chronic dietary treatment by restricting the exogenous sources of phytanic acid (<10 mg/day) and its precursor phytol results in reduction of serum phytanic acid levels and clinical improvement. The diet should provide sufficient calories to avoid weight loss. Plasma exchange has been used to lower toxic serum phytanic acid levels more rapidly in critically ill patients.

Tangier Disease

Tangier disease is an autosomal recessive disorder named after Tangier Island, VA, the origin of the first described cases. It is characterized by severe deficiency of plasma alpha or high-density lipoproteins, resulting in the deposition of cholesterol esters in many tissues, including the reticuloendothelial system and peripheral nerves. The accumulation of lipids leads to enlarged yellow-orange tonsils, which may provide a clue to the diagnosis. In adolescence or adult life, approximately one-half of the affected patients develop one of two distinct neuropathic syndromes. The first is a progressive symmetrical neuropathy, with dissociated loss of pain and temperature sensation in the face, arms, and upper trunk combined with faciobrachial muscle wasting and weakness. These findings bear a superficial resemblance to syringomyelia. The second syndrome consists of relapsing multifocal mononeuropathies involving the cranial, trunk, or limb nerves.

High-density lipoprotein and serum cholesterol are markedly reduced, whereas triglyceride concentrations are elevated. A neuropathic disorder is confirmed by absent or low-amplitude SNAPs and reduced conduction velocities. Nerve biopsy specimens from patients with the multiple mononeuropathy variant have shown segmental demyelination and remyelination. By contrast, a preferential loss of small myelinated and unmyelinated axons is found in the syringomyelialike variant. Typically, abundant lipid vacuoles in Schwann cells are present in both. No specific treatment is known.

Abetalipoproteinemia (Bassen-Kornzweig Syndrome)

Abetalipoproteinemia is a rare autosomal recessive disorder of lipoprotein metabolism. The condition is associated with gene defects coding for the microsomal triglyceride transfer protein, resulting in abnormal very-low-density lipoprotein secretion. Fat malabsorption is present from birth and results in a severe deficiency of the fat-soluble vitamins A, E, and K. Steatorrhea, hypocholesterolemia, and abnormally spiky red cells (acanthocytes) are present from birth. Most untreated patients develop retinitis pigmentosa, peripheral neuropathy, and spinocerebellar degeneration during the first two decades of life. A progressive, mainly large fiber sensory neuropathy occurs, with gait ataxia, areflexia, impaired proprioceptive sensation, and modest distal weakness. Patients have absence of serum β-lipoproteins and very low levels of vitamin E.

The neurological complications of abetalipoproteinemia have been linked to chronic vitamin E deficiency. Dietary fat restriction and large oral doses of vitamin E (100 mg/kg/day) can prevent the onset of symptoms or arrest their progression.

Mitochondrial Cytopathies and Polyneuropathy

The molecular basis has been established for several mitochondrial cytopathies, including Kearns-Sayre syndrome, MELAS (mitochondrial myopathy, encephalopathy, lactic acidosis, and stroke), and MERRF (myoclonus epilepsy with ragged-red fibers; see Chapter 83). In these syndromes, myopathy is the predominant neuromuscular manifestation, although a mild, often asymptomatic, sensory polyneuropathy is detected commonly by systematic electrophysiological and pathological studies. Peripheral neuropathy is a presenting clinical feature in three mitochondrial syndromes: neurogenic weakness, ataxia, and retinitis pigmentosa syndrome; mitochondrial neurogastrointestinal encephalomyelopathy; and sensory ataxic neuropathy associated with dysarthria and chronic progressive external ophthalmoplegia. The last subgroup of patients presents with a familial, disabling ataxic sensory neuropathy and progressive ophthalmoparesis that is associated with multiple mitochondrial DNA deletions (Fadic et al. 1997).

INFLAMMATORY DEMYELINATING POLYRADICULONEUROPATHIES

Inflammatory demyelinating polyradiculoneuropathies are acquired and immunologically mediated. These neuropathies can be classified by their clinical course into two major groups: an acute inflammatory demyelinating polyradiculoneuropathy (AIDP) called Guillain-Barré syndrome and chronic inflammatory demyelinating polyradiculoneuropathy (CIDP). In GBS, the maximal deficits develop over days, followed by a plateau phase and gradual recovery. Chronic forms pursue either a slowly progressive or a relapsing course.

Acute Inflammatory Demyelinating Polyradiculoneuropathy (Guillain-Barré Syndrome)

In 1916, Guillain, Barré, and Strohl emphasized the main clinical features of the syndrome: motor weakness, areflexia, paresthesias with slight sensory loss, and increased protein in CSF with absence of cells (albuminocytological dissociation). Our current understanding of the pathology was greatly enhanced when Asbury and coworkers described multifocal inflammatory demyelination of spinal roots and peripheral nerves. The frequent finding of motor conduction block and reduced NCVs provided electrophysiological confirmation of widespread demyelination. Improvement in modern critical care has dramatically changed outcomes in GBS. The mortality has fallen from 33% before introduction of positive pressure ventilation to the current rate of approximately 5–10%. The diagnosis of GBS depends on clinical criteria supported by electrophysiological studies and CSF findings (Table 80.17). These diagnostic criteria define AIDP, which is the most common form of GBS in Europe and North America. Observations have confirmed that axonal immune-mediated injury may produce similar clinical presentations of GBS. Feasby and colleagues first called attention to axonal GBS, noteworthy for its severity and poor recovery. This axonal variant is called *acute motor sensory axonal neuropathy* (AMSAN) because of involvement of both motor and sensory fibers. A second, pure motor axonal form called *acute motor axonal neuropathy* (AMAN) has been described in northern China where it occurs in summer epidemics in children and young adults. A tentative classification of GBS subtypes has been proposed based on variant clinical expressions and different electrophysiological and pathological findings (Table 80.18; Griffin et al. 1996).

Clinical Features

GBS is a nonseasonal illness that affects persons of all ages. With the decline of acute anterior poliomyelitis, GBS is the most common acute paralytic disease in Western countries. The mean annual incidence is 1.8 per 100,000 population. Incidence rates increase with age from 0.8 in those younger than 18 years to 3.2 for those 60 years and older.

Approximately two-thirds of patients report a preceding event, most frequently an upper respiratory or gastrointestinal infection, surgery, or immunization 1–4 weeks before the onset of neurological symptoms (Italian Guillain-Barré Study Group 1996; Table 80.19). The agent responsible for the prodromal illness frequently remains

Table 80.17: Diagnostic criteria for Guillain-Barré syndrome

Features required for diagnosis
  Progressive weakness of both legs and arms
  Areflexia
Clinical features supportive of diagnosis
  Progression over days to 4 wks
  Relative symmetry of signs
  Mild sensory symptoms or signs
  Cranial nerve involvement (bifacial palsies)
  Recovery beginning 2–4 wks after progression ceases
  Autonomic dysfunction
  Absence of fever at onset
Laboratory features supportive of diagnosis
  Elevated cerebrospinal fluid protein with <10 cells/μl
  Electrodiagnostic features of nerve conduction slowing or block*

*Features supporting an axonal process are seen in acute motor axonal neuropathy and acute motor sensory axonal neuropathy. *Source*: Adapted from AK Asbury, DR Cornblath. Assessment of current diagnostic criteria for Guillain-Barré syndrome. Ann Neurol 1990;27(Suppl.):S21–S24.

Table 80.18: Classification of Guillain-Barré syndromes

Acute inflammatory demyelinating polyradiculoneuropathy
Acute motor axonal neuropathy
Acute motor sensory axonal neuropathy
Miller Fisher syndrome
Acute pandysautonomia

Table 80.19: Antecedent events of Guillain-Barré syndrome (70% in large series)

Antecedent event	Percentage
Respiratory illness	58
Gastrointestinal illness	22
Respiratory and gastrointestinal illness	10
Surgery	5
Vaccination	3
Other	2
Serological evidence of specific infectious agents	
Campylobacter jejuni	26*
Cytomegalovirus	15*
Human immunodeficiency virus 1	?
Epstein-Barr virus	8
Mycoplasma pneumoniae	10

? = variable depending on patient population. Eight percent in retrospective study from large urban medical center.
*Percentages according to case-controlled prospective studies.

unidentified. Specific infections linked to GBS include cytomegalovirus (CMV), Epstein-Barr virus, varicella zoster virus, hepatitis A and B, HIV, and *Mycoplasma*. The most common identifiable bacterial organism linked to GBS and particularly its axonal forms is *Campylobacter jejuni*, a curved gram-negative rod that is a frequent cause of bacterial enteritis worldwide. Evidence of *C. jejuni* infection from stool cultures or serological tests was found in 26% of patients with GBS admitted to hospitals in the United Kingdom, compared with 2% of case controls (Rees et al. 1995). Retrospective studies from the United States, Holland, Germany, and Australia report serological evidence of recent *C. jejuni* infection ranging from 17–39% of patients with GBS. *C. jejuni* infection may play an even greater role in northern China where infection rates of 76% in patients with AMAN and 42% in patients with AIDP were found (Ho et al. 1995). Epidemiological data suggested a slight increase in cases of GBS following the 1976 A/New Jersey influenza vaccine, although no excess risk of developing GBS was seen with subsequent influenza vaccines. Other vaccines (notably tetanus and diphtheria toxoids, rabies, and oral polio vaccines); drugs, including streptokinase, suramin, gangliosides, and heroin; and Hymenoptera stings have been associated in a few cases. Several cases have occurred in immunocompromised hosts with Hodgkin's lymphoma or in pharmacologically immunosuppressed patients after solid organ or bone marrow transplantation.

Patients may initially present with paresthesias, sensory symptoms with weakness, or weakness alone. The fairly symmetrical weakness of the lower limbs ascends proximally over hours to several days to involve arm, facial, and oropharyngeal muscles, and in severe cases respiratory muscles. Less often, weakness may begin in proximal or cranial nerve innervated muscles. Its severity varies from mild involvement, in which patients are still capable of walking unassisted, to quadriplegia. Hyporeflexia or areflexia are invariable features. By definition progression ends by 1–4 weeks into the illness; if it continues longer, the condition is termed either *subacute inflammatory demyelinating polyradiculoneuropathy* if progression continues for 4–10 weeks or *CIDP* if there is chronic progression or multiple relapses. Cranial nerve involvement ranges from 45–75% in different series. Facial paresis, usually bilateral, is found in at least one-half of patients. Involvement of extraocular muscles and lower cranial nerves is seen less often. Pseudotumor cerebri with papilledema occurs as a rare complication and is almost always caused by chronically elevated intracranial pressure. The proportion of patients developing respiratory failure and requiring assisted ventilation seems to increase with age and ranges from 12% in epidemiological series to 23% in hospital-based series. Sensory loss is not a prominent feature and is limited frequently to distal impairment of vibration sense. Moderate to severe pain occurs in 85% of patients on admission to the hospital. Interscapular or low back pain with radiation into the legs is most common. Dysesthetic extremity pain described as burning or tingling is present in approximately one-half of patients, whereas myalgic limb pain associated with joint stiffness is less common (Moulin et al. 1997). Unusual clinical variants with restricted patterns of weakness may cause diagnostic difficulties. Isolated weakness of the face, oropharynx, neck, and arms without involving the legs is a distinctive feature of the pharyngeal-cervical-brachial variant. Rarely, weakness remains confined to the lower limbs, resembling a cauda equina lesion. Autonomic dysfunction of various degrees has been reported in 65% of patients admitted to the hospital (Zochodne 1994). Its manifestations may be related to either decreased sympathetic (orthostatic hypotension, anhidrosis) or decreased parasympathetic (urinary retention, gastrointestinal atony, or iridoplegia) function. Signs of excessive sympathetic activity include episodic or sustained hypertension, sinus tachycardia, tachyarrhythmias, episodic diaphoresis, and acral vasoconstriction. Excessive vagal activity accounts for sudden episodes of bradycardia, heart block, and asystole. These vagal spells may occur spontaneously or may be triggered by tracheal suctioning. Serious cardiac arrhythmias with hemodynamic instability tend to be more frequent in patients with severe quadriparesis and respiratory failure. Autonomic dysfunction can result in electrocardiographical changes including T-wave abnormalities, ST-segment depression, QRS widening, QT prolongation, and various forms of heart block.

Guillain-Barré Syndrome Variants

Several variations from this typical presentation have been described. Their link to GBS is supported by preceding infectious episodes, diminished reflexes, elevated CSF protein levels, and immune-mediated etiologies.

The Miller Fisher syndrome, which accounts for 5% of cases, is characterized by ophthalmoplegia, ataxia, and areflexia. Patients present with diplopia followed by gait and limb ataxia. Ocular signs range from complete ophthalmoplegia, including unreactive pupils, to external ophthalmoparesis with or without ptosis. Cranial nerves other than ocular motor nerves may be affected. Motor strength is characteristically preserved, although overlap with GBS seems to occur when some patients develop quadriparesis. The ataxia is attributed to a peripheral mismatch between proprioceptive input from muscle spindles and kinesthetic information from joint receptors. Patients presenting with rapid onset of symmetrical, multiple cranial nerve palsies, most notably bilateral facial palsy (polyneuritis cranialis) may be a forme fruste of this syndrome. Electrodiagnostic studies demonstrate an axonal process affecting predominantly sensory fibers with only mild motor conduction abnormalities. SNAP amplitudes are reduced or absent. Motor conduction studies, including F-wave latencies, are usually normal. Most patients have increased CSF protein without pleocytosis 1 week after onset. Neuroimaging studies do not demonstrate brainstem or cerebellar lesions. Gadolinium enhancement of ocular motor nerves has been reported. Serum IgG antibodies to the ganglioside GQ1b are found in acute phase sera of most patients with Miller Fisher syndrome and GBS with ophthalmoplegia, which suggests that the antibodies are disease-specific and related to the pathogenesis (Chiba et al. 1993). Miller Fisher syndrome has a benign prognosis, with recovery after a mean of 10 weeks.

Acute pandysautonomia is characterized by the rapid onset of combined sympathetic and parasympathetic failure without somatic sensory and motor involvement, although reflexes are usually lost during the course of the illness. These patients develop severe orthostatic hypotension, anhidrosis, dry eyes and mouth, fixed pupils, invariant heart rate, and disturbances of bowel and bladder function.

Feasby and coworkers drew attention to cases of fulminant GBS with poor prognosis for recovery (AMSAN). All patients had a hyperacute course progressing to a peak deficit in less than 7 days, developed profound quadriparesis with severe muscle wasting, and required prolonged respiratory support. Electrodiagnostic studies showed markedly reduced or absent CMAPs with distal supramaximal stimulation without conduction delay and absent SNAPs. The subsequent appearance of abundant fibrillation potentials on needle EMG, together with persistently inexcitable motor nerves, and poor recovery, suggested a primary axonopathy as the underlying disease process. Extensive wallerian axonal degeneration without significant inflammation or demyelination has been described in ventral and dorsal roots and in peripheral nerves at autopsy (Griffin et al. 1996).

Sporadic cases of a pure motor variant presenting with acute flaccid paralysis without clinical or electrophysiological involvement of sensory nerves have been observed among large series of patients with GBS. These case descriptions are similar to AMAN occurring in epidemic proportions among children and young adults in northern China during summer months (McKhann et al. 1993). AMAN differs from GBS by electrophysiological study results that demonstrate reduced compound muscle potential amplitudes but normal motor distal latencies and conduction velocities. Autopsy studies have shown noninflammatory wallerianlike degeneration of ventral roots and motor axons in mixed nerves. Most patients with AMAN recover as rapidly as patients with AIDP (Ho et al. 1997). The rapid clinical recovery rates and the paucity of pathological findings in some fatal cases could be explained by either conduction block of motor axons at nodes of Ranvier or by axonal degeneration of motor nerve terminals. Extensive axonal degeneration of motor nerve terminals was confirmed by motor point biopsy in a patient with AMAN. Antecedent *C. jejuni* infection was found by using serological tests in 76% of AMAN patients from northern China, which suggests that this organism plays a major role in the pathogenesis.

Laboratory Studies

CSF examination and serial electrophysiological studies are critical for confirming the diagnosis of GBS. Other laboratory studies are of limited value. Mild transient liver enzyme elevations without obvious cause are found in approximately one-third of patients. Hyponatremia is seen most frequently in ventilated patients because of inappropriate secretion of antidiuretic hormone. Deposition of immune complexes may rarely lead to glomerulonephritis and result in microscopic hematuria and proteinuria. In the

first week of neurological symptoms the CSF protein may be normal but then becomes elevated on subsequent examinations. In approximately 10% of cases, the CSF protein remains normal throughout the illness. Transient oligoclonal IgG bands and elevated myelin basic protein levels may be detected in some patients. Moderate CSF pleocytosis is a distinctive feature of GBS associated with HIV infection. Abnormalities of electrophysiological studies are found in approximately 90% of established cases and reflect an evolving picture of multifocal demyelination associated with secondary axonal degeneration. The most common electrophysiological abnormalities include prolonged distal motor and F-wave latencies, absent or impersistent F waves, conduction block, reduction in distal CMAP amplitudes with or without temporal dispersion, and slowing of motor conduction velocities (Cros and Triggs 1996). Conduction block of motor axons is the electrophysiological correlate to clinical weakness and is recognized by a decrease of greater than 30% in CMAP amplitude from distal to proximal stimulation in the absence of temporal dispersion. Early in the course of the disease, the F-wave latencies are prolonged or absent, and EMG shows decreased motor unit recruitment. Subsequently, if any amount of axonal degeneration occurs, fibrillation potentials appear 2–4 weeks after onset. Electrodiagnostic studies performed in the patients enrolled in the North American GBS Study found abnormalities of distal motor latencies and F-wave latencies in approximately one-half of patients studied within 30 days of onset. Partial motor conduction block (30%), slowing of motor conduction velocity (24%), and reduced distal CMAP amplitudes (20%) were less frequent. In cases with axonal degeneration, reduced CMAP and SNAP amplitudes are found. Such patients tend to have a slower and less complete recovery than those whose weakness is related primarily to conduction block. Electrodiagnostic parameters are the most reliable indicators of prognosis. A distal CMAP amplitude of less than 20% of the lower limit of normal was associated with poor outcome in the North American GBS Study.

Lumbosacral spinal MRI may demonstrate gadolinium enhancement of lumbar roots. The value of specific serological tests in the diagnosis of GBS is limited. Elevated serum antibodies to *Mycoplasma*, CMV, or *C. jejuni* can pinpoint the preceding infection. Serologic tests for *C. jejuni* infection are difficult both to perform and interpret. The proportion of GBS cases associated with *Campylobacter* infection remains uncertain but seems to range from 17–76% in various parts of the world. Preceding *Campylobacter* infection has been linked to axonal variants, worse outcome, and high titers of anti-GM_1, -GD_{1b}, and -GD_{1a} ganglioside antibodies of the IgG class (Jacobs et al. 1996). Other studies confirmed the presence of IgG antiglycolipid antibodies in 10–40% of patients with GBS but failed to show a correlation with *Campylobacter* infection (Ho et al. 1995). Elevated anti-GQ_{1b} ganglioside antibodies are consistently found in the Miller Fisher syndrome. Complement

Table 80.20:   Differential diagnostic considerations in Guillain-Barré syndrome

I.   Acute neuropathies
     Hepatic porphyrias
     Critical illness neuropathy
     Diphtheria
     Toxins
        Arsenic, thallium, organophosphates, lead
        Neurotoxic fish and shellfish poisoning (ciguatoxin, tetrodotoxin, saxitoxin)
        Buckthorn
        Tick paralysis
     Vasculitis
     Inflammatory meningoradiculopathies
        Lyme disease, cytomegalovirus lumbosacral radiculo-myelopathy
II. Disorders of neuromuscular junction
     Botulism, myasthenia gravis
III. Myopathies
     Hypokalemia, hypophosphatemia
     Rhabdomyolysis
     Polymyositis
     Intensive care myopathy
IV. Central nervous system disorders
     Poliomyelitis, rabies
     Transverse myelitis
     Basilar artery thrombosis

fixing antibodies to peripheral nerve myelin are present in most patients during the acute phase of GBS.

Differential Diagnosis

Care should be taken to distinguish GBS from other conditions leading to subacute motor weakness (Table 80.20). Among the neuropathies with acute onset, acute porphyria, diphtheria, and occasional toxic neuropathies (arsenic, thallium, buckthorn, acrylamide, organophosphorous compounds, and N-hexane) must be considered. Flaccid general weakness and failure to wean from the ventilator are common features of critical illness neuropathy that develops in patients confined to the intensive care unit with multiorgan diseases. Electrodiagnostic features of an axonal neuropathy and normal CSF findings distinguish critical illness neuropathy from GBS. A related syndrome, the acute myopathy of intensive care, follows the use of neuromuscular junction blocking agents in combination with intravenous corticosteroids. Metabolic disturbances (severe hypophosphatemia, hypokalemia, hypermagnesemia), myopathies, disorders of neuromuscular transmission, and tick paralysis should be considered also. Botulism develops after the consumption of contaminated foods, with symptoms of ophthalmoparesis and facial and bulbar weakness. Nerve conduction studies reveal low-amplitude compound muscle potentials. High-frequency repetitive nerve stimulation or maximal voluntary contraction leads to an incremental response that is typical for presynaptic neuro-

muscular transmission defects. Acute brainstem infarcts, spinal cord compression, or postinfectious transverse myelitis may present diagnostic difficulties before upper motor neuron signs develop and before results of electrodiagnostic and CSF studies become available. Among other signs, early urinary retention and a sharply demarcated sensory level on the trunk suggest spinal cord disease and call for spinal MRI. CSF pleocytosis (>50 cells per μl) casts doubt on the diagnosis of uncomplicated GBS and suggests inflammatory meningoradiculopathies caused by Lyme disease, HIV infection, or CMV in acquired immunodeficiency syndrome. Anterior poliomyelitis causes rapidly evolving asymmetrical weakness accompanied by fever and pleocytosis. A common pitfall to avoid is misdiagnosis of early GBS as hysterical weakness.

Pathology

Classic pathological studies of AIDP have demonstrated endoneurial perivascular mononuclear cell infiltration together with multifocal demyelination. The peripheral nerves may be affected at all levels from the roots to distal intramuscular motor nerve endings, although the brunt of the lesions frequently falls on the ventral roots, proximal spinal nerves, and lower cranial nerves. Intense inflammation may lead to axonal degeneration as a consequence of a toxic bystander effect. Ultrastructural studies have shown that macrophages play a major role in demyelination by stripping off myelin lamellae from its axon. The inflammatory infiltrates consist mainly of class II-positive monocytes and macrophages and T lymphocytes. The expression of class II antigen is increased in Schwann cells, raising the possibility that Schwann cells may present the antigen to autoreactive T cells and activate the destruction of myelin. Extensive primary wallerianlike degeneration of motor and sensory roots and nerves without significant inflammation or demyelination is found in cases of AMSAN.

Pathogenesis

A considerable body of evidence points to an organ-specific autoimmune disorder mediated by autoreactive T cells and humoral antibodies to still incompletely characterized peripheral nerve antigens (Hartung et al. 1995). A preceding infection may trigger an autoimmune response through molecular mimicry in which the host generates an immune response against an infectious organism that shares epitopes with the host's peripheral nerves. At the onset of disease, activated T cells play a major role in opening the blood-nerve barrier to allow circulating antibodies to gain access to peripheral nerve antigens. T-cell activation markers (interleukin-6, interleukin-2, soluble interleukin-2 receptor, and interferon-γ) and tumor necrosis factor-α, a proinflammatory cytokine released by T cells and macrophages, are increased in serum of patients. Additionally, adhesion molecules are critically involved in facilitating recruitment and transmigration of activated T cells and monocytes through the blood-nerve barrier. Soluble E-selectin, an adhesion molecule produced by endothelial cells, is increased in patients with GBS during the early stages of disease. A cell-mediated immune reaction against myelin components is supported by experimental allergic neuritis, the accepted animal model for AIDP. Experimental allergic neuritis can be produced by the injection of peripheral nerve myelin or PNS-specific myelin basic protein P2.

Several observations indicate that humoral factors participate in the autoimmune attack on peripheral nerve myelin: (1) immunoglobulins and complement can be demonstrated on myelinated fibers of affected patients by immunostaining; (2) intraneural injection of GBS serum into rat sciatic nerve produces in vivo demyelination and conduction block; (3) complement C1-fixing antiperipheral nerve myelin antibody can be detected in the serum of patients during the acute phase of GBS; and (4) plasmapheresis results in clinical improvement. The titer of the antiperipheral nerve myelin antibody correlates with the clinical course, declining with cessation of progression and during improvement.

Understanding of the immune mechanisms of GBS and its axonal variants was enhanced by the detailed immunohistochemical and ultrastructural studies of clinically well-defined, autopsied cases from northern China. The earliest changes seen in AIDP within days of onset consisted of deposition of complement activation products and membrane attack complex on the outermost Schwann cell surface followed by vesicular myelin changes at the outermost myelin lamellae with subsequent recruitment of macrophages and progressive demyelination (Hafer-Macko et al. 1996). Previously, the role of complement has been suspected by finding increased levels of complement activation products in CSF and soluble terminal complement complexes in serum of patients with AIDP. The immune attack in AIDP appears to begin with binding of autoantibodies to specific epitopes on the outermost Schwann cell membrane with consequent activation of complement (Figure 80.19). The nature of the epitope in AIDP, although still uncertain, is likely a glycolipid. Pathological studies of early cases of AMAN found deposition of activated complement components and immunoglobulins at nodal axolemma. This was followed by disruption of the paranodal space, allowing the entry of complement and immunoglobulins along the axolemma, with subsequent recruitment of macrophages to affected nodes. Finally, macrophages were shown to invade the periaxonal space leading to wallerian-like degeneration of motor fibers (Hafer-Macko et al. 1996; Figure 80.20). These findings suggest that AMAN is caused by an antibody- and complement-mediated attack on axolemmal epitopes of motor fibers. The most attractive candidate targets are GM_1- and asialo-GM_1-like gangliosides, which are present in nodal and internodal membranes of motor fibers. Certain Campylobacter strains associated with axonal GBS variants contain GM_1-like epitopes in their polysaccharide coats. Anti-GM_1 antibodies that cross-react to these lipopolysaccharide epitopes are found in a high proportion of AMAN and some GBS patients. These observations have led to the concept of molecular mimicry in which epitopes of the infectious agent elicit antibodies that cross-react with shared epitopes on axons. The nerve fibers thereby become the inadvertent targets of an immune response directed against an enteric organism. AMSAN may be caused by a more severe immune injury triggered by axonal epitopes because similar pathological changes affecting motor and sensory fibers have been observed in cases of AMSAN.

Treatment

Patients with rapidly worsening acute GBS should be observed in the hospital until the maximum extent of progression has been established. The reduction in mortality to less than 5% reflects improvements in modern critical care. Supportive care in intensive care units and the prevention of complications, of which respiratory failure and autonomic dysfunction are the most important, provide the best chance for a favorable outcome (Bosch 1998). Respiratory and bulbar function, the ability to handle secretions, heart rate, and blood pressure should be closely monitored during the progressive phase. An increased respiratory rate, inability to count on one breath to 20, the use of accessory respiratory muscles, paradoxical inward movements of the abdomen during inspirations, and decreased cough are clinical signs of diaphragmatic and respiratory muscle weakness. Signs of impending respiratory failure include deterioration in forced vital capacity (FVC), declining maximal respiratory pressures, and hypoxemia caused by atelectasis. Initially, it may be necessary to monitor FVC and negative inspiratory pressure every 4 hours while awake. Patients with FVCs that are rapidly declining or who have cardiovascular dysautonomia and associated medical disorders should be monitored in the intensive care unit. Elective intubation for ventilatory assistance should be performed when FVC falls below 12–15 ml/kg or below 18 ml/kg in patients with severe oropharyngeal weakness, or arterial PO_2 values fall below 70 mm Hg with inspired room air. When respiratory assistance is needed for longer than 2 weeks, a tracheostomy should be performed.

In the event of cardiac arrhythmias or marked fluctuations of blood pressure, continuous electrocardiographical and blood pressure monitoring allow early detection of life-threatening situations that require prompt treatment. Antihypertensive and vasoactive drugs must be used with extreme caution in the presence of autonomic instability. Tracheal suctioning may trigger sudden episodes of hypotension or bradyarrhythmia. Back and radicular pain often responds to nonsteroidal anti-inflammatory drugs. At times oral or parenteral opioids are required for adequate pain control. Increased metabolic requirements together with negative caloric intake caused by impaired swallow-

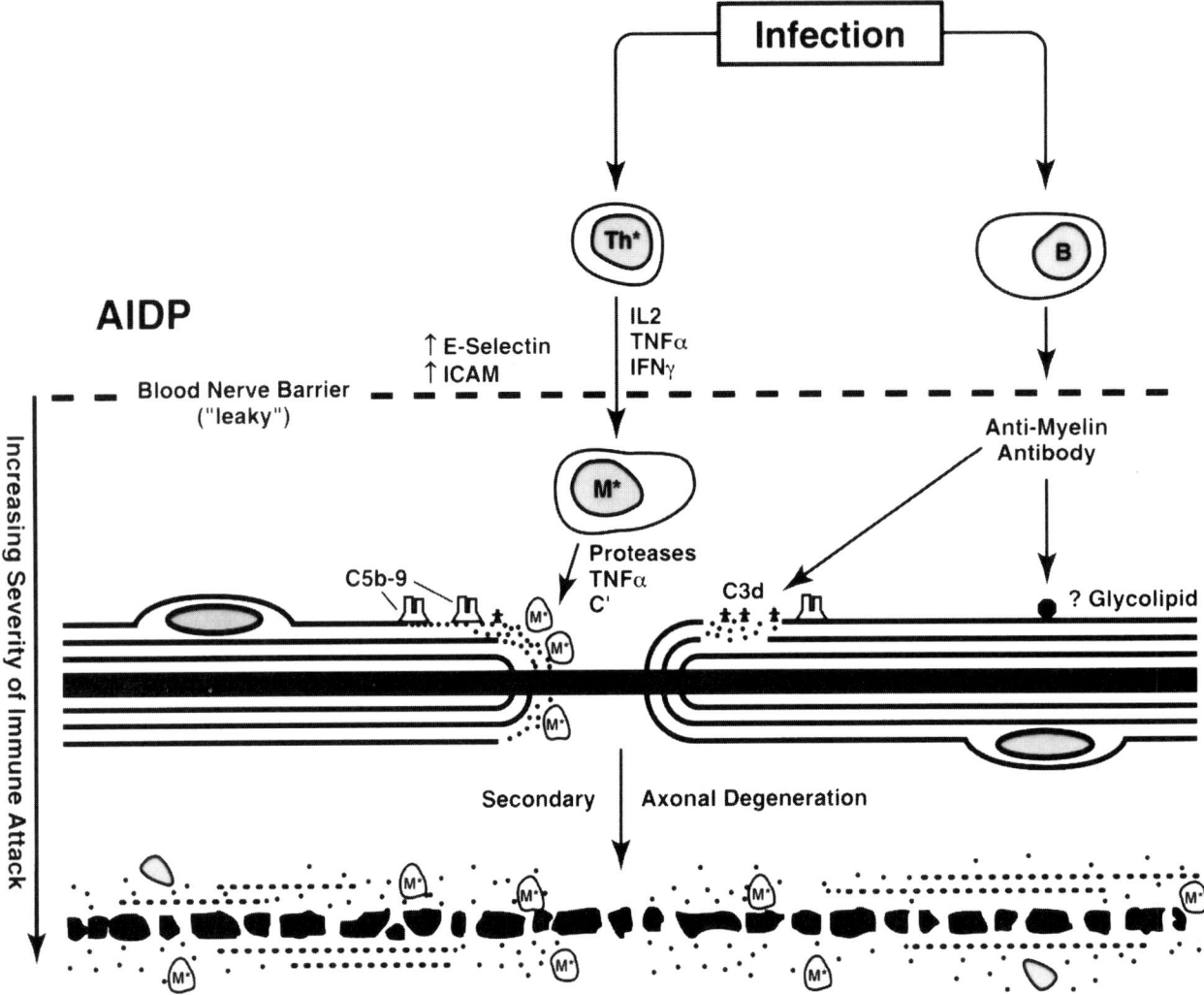

FIGURE 80.19 Immune injury to nerve fibers in acute inflammatory demyelinating polyradiculoneuropathy (AIDP). A preceding infection may trigger the formation of antimyelin autoantibodies and activated T-helper cells (Th*). Proinflammatory cytokines (tumor necrosis factor–α [TNFα], interferon-γ [INFγ]) and upregulation of adhesion molecules (E-selectin, intercellular adhesion molecule [ICAM]) facilitate the breakdown of the blood-nerve barrier to activated T cells, macrophages, and antimyelin antibodies. Antimyelin antibodies react with epitopes on the abaxonal Schwann cell membrane with consequent activation of complement. Deposition of complement activation products (C3d) and membrane attack complex (C5b-9) on the outermost Schwann cell membrane leads to vesicular myelin changes, followed by recruitment of macrophages (M*) and progressive demyelination. Intense inflammation may lead to secondary axonal degeneration. (B = B cell; IL2 = interleukin 2.) (Reprinted with permission from EP Bosch. Guillain-Barré syndrome: an update of acute immune-mediated polyradiculoneuropathies. Neurologist 1998;4:211–226.)

ing may lead to a state of relative starvation in severely affected patients. Nutritional requirements should be met by providing a high-caloric protein diet or by beginning enteral feedings as early as possible.

Subcutaneous heparin or low-molecular-weight heparin together with thigh-high thromboembolic deterrent stockings should be ordered routinely in immobilized patients to lower the risks of venous thrombosis and pulmonary embolism. Infections of the lung and urinary tract develop in almost one in four patients with GBS in the intensive care unit. Prevention and prompt treatment of nosocomial infections are important aspects of care. Chest physiother-apy and frequent oral suctioning aid in preventing atelectasis in patients with impaired cough and sigh. Skillful nursing care with regular turning and attention to skin, eyes, mouth, bowel, and bladder are essential. Exposure keratitis is avoided in cases of facial diplegia by using artificial tears and by taping the eyelids closed at night. Pressure-induced ulnar or fibular nerve palsies are prevented by proper positioning and padding. Physical therapy is started early because it helps prevent contractures, joint immobilization, and venous stasis. Psychological support and constant reassurance about the potential for recovery are important for the morale of patients and family members.

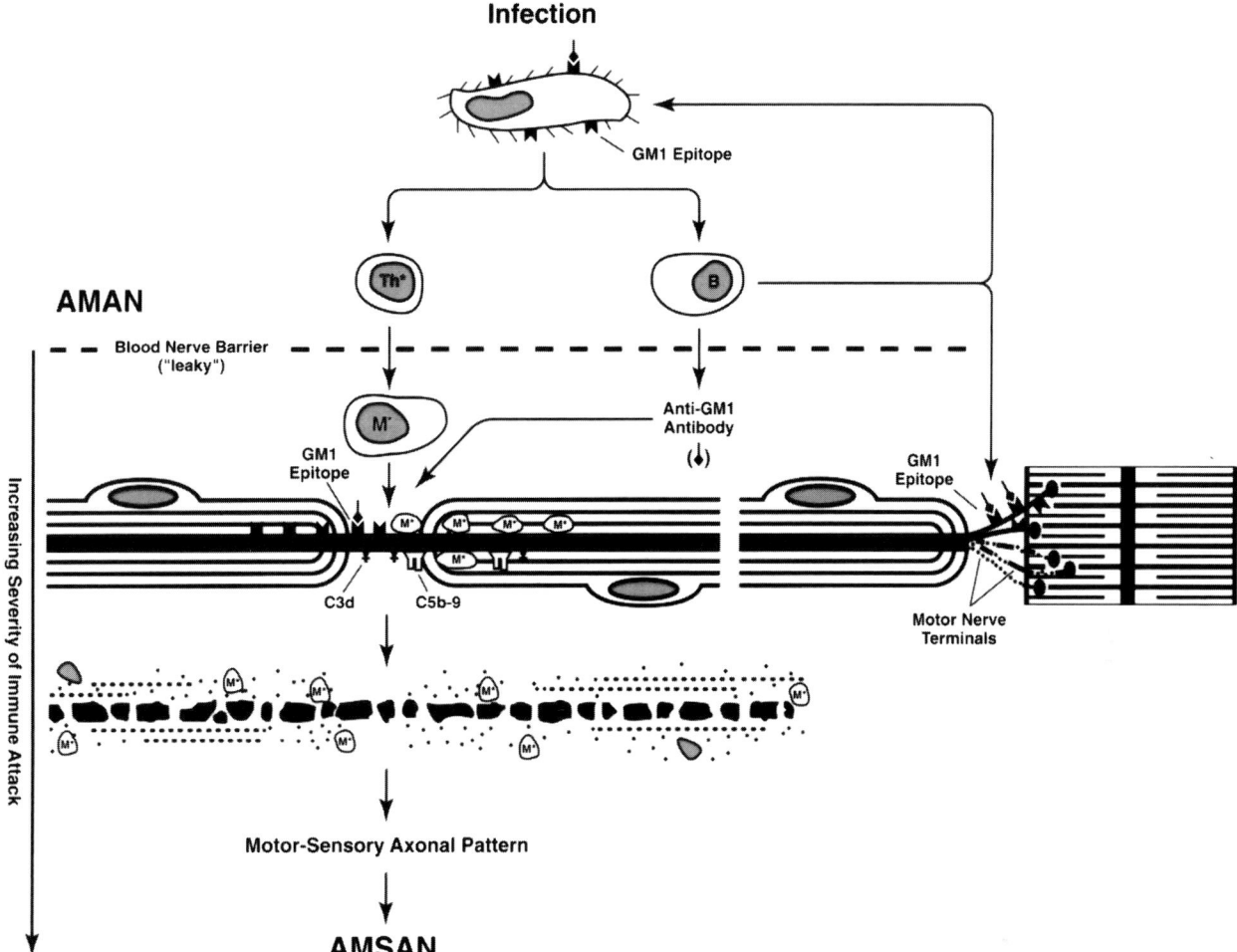

FIGURE 80.20   Immune injury to nerve fibers in acute motor axonal neuropathy (AMAN). Molecular mimicry of GM_1-like epitopes common to both lipopolysaccharide coats of certain *Campylobacter jejuni* strains and axonal membranes may cause an autoimmune response. Activated complement components (C3d, C5b-9) and immunoglobulins are found at nodes of Ranvier and along axolemma of motor fibers. Macrophages (M*) are recruited to the targeted nodes and invade the periaxonal space, leading to wallerian degeneration. The lack of blood-nerve barrier at motor nerve terminals may make these distal axons vulnerable to circulating GM_1 antibodies. (AMSAN = acute motor sensory axonal neuropathy; B = B cell.) (Reprinted with permission from EP Bosch. Guillain-Barré syndrome: an update of acute immune-mediated polyradiculoneuropathies. Neurologist 1998;4:211–226.)

In the recovery phase, skillful physical therapy and rehabilitation hastens recovery.

Among specific therapeutic interventions aimed at mitigating the harmful effects of autoantibodies, plasma exchange and high-dose intravenous immune globulin (IVIG) have been shown to be equally effective. Three large randomized, controlled trials involving more than 500 patients have established the benefit of plasma exchange in acute GBS by shortening the recovery time. Therapeutic plasma exchange is recommended for patients with moderate to severe weakness (defined as the ability to walk only with support or worse). Benefits are clearest when plasma exchange is begun within 2 weeks of onset. The recommended plasmapheresis schedule entails a series of five exchanges (40–50 ml/kg) with a continuous flow machine on alternate days using saline and albumin as replacement fluid. The effect of plasma exchange in mildly affected patients and the optimal number of exchanges were investigated by the French Cooperative Group on Plasma Exchange (1997). Even mildly affected patients benefited from two exchanges. Four exchanges were optimal for moderate and severe cases. Treatment-related relapses tend to occur in approximately 10% of patients within 3 weeks after treatment. Plasmapheresis should be performed only in centers with experience in exchange techniques in critically ill patients. Most serious complications are linked to venous access problems including hematoma formation at puncture sites, pneumothorax after insertion of central lines, and catheter-related septicemia. Septicemia, active bleeding, and severe cardiovascular instability are contraindications for plasmapheresis.

Two prospective randomized trials comparing IVIG with plasma exchange demonstrated the benefit of five daily

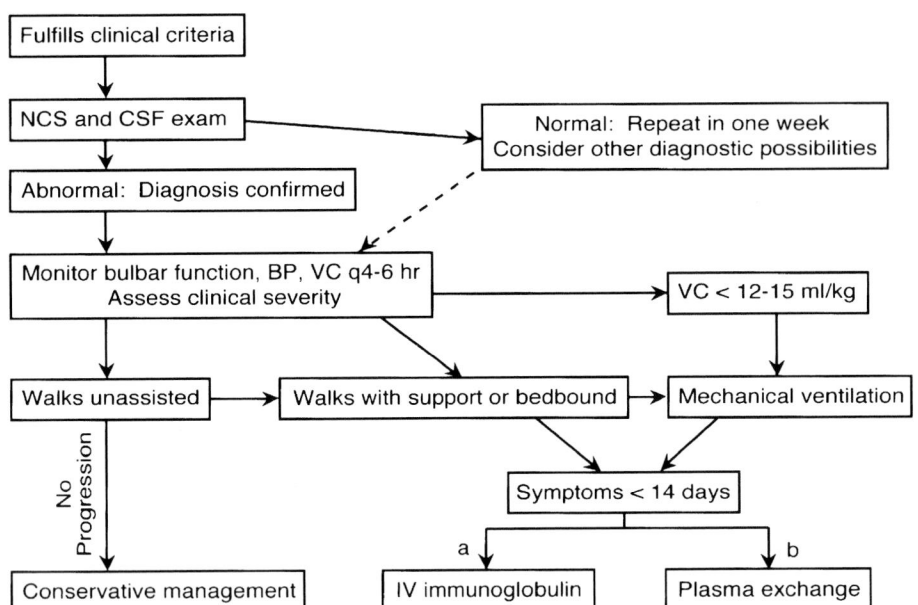

FIGURE 80.21 Decision-making pathway in the management of Guillain-Barré syndrome. Both treatment options, intravenous (IV) immune globulin (a) and plasma exchange (b), are equally efficacious. IV immune globulin is preferred because of its ease of administration. (BP = blood pressure; CSF = cerebrospinal fluid; NCS = nerve conduction studies; VC = forced vital capacity.) (Reprinted with permission from EP Bosch. Guillain-Barré syndrome: an update of acute immune-mediated polyradiculoneuropathies. Neurologist 1998;4:211–226.)

infusions of immune globulin (0.4 g/kg) given in the first 2 weeks of the disease (Plasma Exchange/Sandoglobulin Guillain-Barré Syndrome Trial Group 1997). Both treatment modalities were equally effective. There was no advantage of using both together. Anecdotal reports suggested a higher treatment-related relapse rate with IVIG infusions that was not confirmed in the controlled trials. Anti-idiotypic suppression of autoantibodies, global down-regulation of immunoglobulin production, blockade of Fc receptors, and nonspecific binding of activated complement are the proposed modes of action of immune globulin infusions. Minor side effects such as headaches, myalgias and arthralgias, flulike symptoms, fever, and vasomotor reactions are observed when infusion flow rates are excessive. More serious complications, such as anaphylaxis in IgA-deficient individuals, who develop anti-IgA antibodies after the first course of IgA-containing IVIG infusions, congestive heart failure, thrombotic complications (strokes and myocardial infarction), and transient renal failure, have rarely been reported (Brannagan et al. 1996). IVIG has become the preferred treatment for acute GBS because of ease of administration (Figure 80.21). In patients with hyperviscosity, congestive heart failure, chronic renal failure, or congenital IgA deficiency plasma exchange is preferred.

Corticosteroids have been advocated in the treatment of GBS but cannot be justified, because two randomized, controlled trials, one using conventional doses of prednisolone and the other using high-dose intravenous methylprednisolone, have found no benefit (Guillain-Barré Syndrome Steroid Trial Group 1993). The combination of IVIG with methylprednisolone is being evaluated in ongoing trials.

Course and Prognosis

By definition, patients should reach their maximum deficit within 4 weeks of onset; if the disease progresses for longer, it is classified as subacute or CIDP. Approximately 10–20% of patients develop respiratory insufficiency requiring assisted ventilation, and between 2% and 5% die of complications. After progression stops, patients enter a plateau phase lasting 2–4 weeks or longer before recovery begins. Although most patients recover functionally, 20% still have residual motor weakness 1 year later. Approximately 70% of patients complete their recovery in 12 months and 82% in 24 months. Approximately 3% of patients may have a recurrence following recovery. The North American Guillain-Barré Syndrome Study Group found that older age (>60 years), ventilatory support, rapid progression reaching maximum deficit in less than 7 days, and low amplitudes of distal CMAPs (20% of lower limit of normal or less) were poor prognostic factors that were associated with a less than 20% probability of walking independently at 6 months. Plasma exchange beneficially influences outcome in addition to these factors.

Chronic Inflammatory Demyelinating Polyradiculoneuropathy

Many similarities exist between CIDP and the acute form, GBS. Both disorders have similar clinical features and share the CSF albuminocytological dissociation and the pathological abnormalities of multifocal inflammatory demyelination, with nerve conduction features reflecting demyelination. An autoimmune basis is suspected for both disorders. On the other hand, CIDP has a more protracted clinical course, is rarely associated with preceding infections, has an association with human lymphocyte antigens, and responds to corticosteroid therapy. Two patterns of temporal evolution of CIDP can be seen. More than 60% of patients show a continuous or stepwise progressive course over months to years, whereas one-third have a relapsing course with partial or complete recovery between recurrences. The age of onset may influence the course of the disease. In one large series, the age of onset was younger (mean, 29 years) in those who had a relapsing course than in those pursuing a chronic progressive course (mean, 51 years). A history of preceding infection is found in less than 10%. In contrast, pregnancy is associated with a significant number of relapses, occurring mainly in the third trimester and the immediate postpartum period. Human lymphocyte antigen–linked genetic factors may influence susceptibility to CIDP.

Although precise prevalence figures are not available, CIDP represents approximately 20% of all initially undiagnosed neuropathies referred to specialized neuromuscular centers.

Clinical Features

The disease is seen at all ages, with peak incidence in the fifth and sixth decades. The majority of patients have symmetrical motor and sensory involvement, although occasional cases with predominantly motor involvement may be seen. To fulfill diagnostic criteria for CIDP, weakness must be present for at least 2 months. Proximal limb weakness is almost as severe as distal limb weakness. In fact, the presence of proximal muscle weakness sets this neuropathy apart from most others. Both upper and lower limbs are affected, although the legs are often more severely involved. Muscle wasting is rarely pronounced. These signs provide helpful clinical clues to separate CIDP patients from those with axonal neuropathies. Generalized hyporeflexia or areflexia are the rule. Sensory symptoms in a stocking-glove distribution (numbness or tingling) implicating large fiber involvement occur frequently, whereas pain is uncommon. Children differ from adults by a more precipitous onset and more prominent gait abnormalities. Additional findings, listed in decreasing order of frequency, are postural tremor of the arms, enlargement of peripheral nerves, papilledema, and facial and bulbar weakness. Massive nerve root enlargement causing myelopathy or symptomatic lumbar stenosis, or vision loss caused by progressive pseudotumor cerebri are unusual clinical features (Midroni and Dyck 1996).

In a small number of patients the findings are so asymmetrical and focal as to resemble multiple mononeuropathies. Electrophysiological studies demonstrating focal conduction block or severe slowing of nerve conduction distinguish this multifocal demyelinating neuropathy from the more common vasculitic multiple mononeuropathies.

CIDP may be associated occasionally with a relapsing multifocal demyelinating CNS disorder resembling multiple sclerosis, with CNS demyelination confirmed by abnormal visual and somatosensory evoked potentials and brain MRI. A CIDP-like syndrome may develop in cases of inherited neuropathy. These patients typically have a positive family history of affected kin and bony abnormalities such as pes cavus and hammer toes from an early age, but subsequently develop subacute deterioration with proximal muscle weakness and increased CSF protein. It is important to recognize this subgroup of patients because the newly acquired symptoms may respond to corticosteroid therapy, hence the term *prednisone-responsive hereditary motor and sensory neuropathy.*

Acquired demyelinating polyradiculoneuropathies meeting the diagnostic criteria for CIDP may be associated with HIV infection, systemic lupus erythematosus, monoclonal gammopathy of undetermined significance (MGUS) and plasma cell dyscrasias (macroglobulinemia, osteosclerotic myeloma, POEMS syndrome, Castleman's disease, chronic active hepatitis, inflammatory bowel disease, and Hodgkin's lymphoma). Compared with idiopathic CIDP, the patients with CIDP with a monoclonal gammopathy tend to be older, have a more protracted course but less severe functional impairment at presentation, and seem to respond less well to immunomodulatory therapy (Simmons et al. 1993). Appropriate laboratory studies are necessary to separate these polyradiculoneuropathies from idiopathic CIDP without concurrent disease.

Laboratory Studies

The diagnosis of CIDP is supported by a laboratory profile including electrophysiological, CSF, and nerve biopsy findings (Table 80.21). There is a pattern of nerve conduction changes that strongly supports acquired multifocal demyelination. This includes (1) nonuniform reduction in motor conduction velocities below 70% of normal in at least two motor nerves; (2) partial conduction block or abnormal temporal dispersion in at least one motor nerve; (3) prolonged distal latencies in at least two motor nerves; and (4) absent F waves or prolonged F-wave latencies in at least two motor nerves. On the other hand, familial demyelinating neuropathies characteristically have uniform slowing of nerve conduction. CSF protein values in excess of 45 mg/dl are found in 95% of cases and levels above 100 mg/dl are common. CSF pleocytosis is rare except in HIV-associated CIDP. Serum antibodies to tubulin have been reported to be elevated in 60% of patients with CIDP but are rarely elevated in other neuropathies. MRI scanning may demonstrate gadolinium enhancement of lumbar roots, providing radiological evidence of an abnormal blood-nerve barrier (Bertorini et al. 1995).

Blood cell counts, sedimentation rate, and biochemical screening tests are important to exclude systemic disorders. Serum and urine immunoelectrophoresis, a skeletal bone

Table 80.21: Diagnostic criteria for chronic inflammatory demyelinating polyradiculoneuropathy

I. Mandatory clinical criteria
   Progressive or relapsing muscle weakness for 2 mos or longer
   Symmetrical proximal and distal weakness in upper or lower extremities
   Hyporeflexia or areflexia
II. Mandatory laboratory criteria
   Nerve conduction studies with features of demyelination (motor nerve conduction <70% of lower limit of normal)
   Cerebrospinal fluid protein level >45 mg/dl, cell count <10/μl
   Sural nerve biopsy with features of demyelination and remyelination including myelinated fiber loss and perivascular inflammation
III. Mandatory exclusion criteria
   Evidence of relevant systemic disease or toxic exposure
   Family history of neuropathy
   Nerve biopsy findings incompatible with diagnosis
IV. Diagnostic categories
   A. Definite: Mandatory inclusion and exclusion criteria and all laboratory criteria
   B. Probable: Mandatory inclusion and exclusion criteria and 2 of 3 laboratory criteria
   C. Possible: Mandatory inclusion and exclusion criteria and 1 of 3 laboratory criteria

Source: Adapted from DR Cornblath, AK Asbury, JW Albers, et al. Research criteria for diagnosis of chronic inflammatory demyelinating polyneuropathy (CIDP). Neurology 1991;41:617–618.

survey, or both are required to look for an associated monoclonal gammopathy or underlying osteosclerotic myeloma.

The changes in sural nerve biopsy specimens do not fully represent the pathological process taking place in motor roots or more proximal nerve segments. In one large series of biopsies, demyelinating features were seen in only 48%, 21% had predominantly axonal changes, 13% had mixed demyelinating and axonal changes, and 18% were normal. Nevertheless, sural nerve biopsy is helpful in support of the diagnosis and in excluding other causes of neuropathy. Typically, moderate reduction in myelinated fibers, endoneurial and subperineurial edema, and segmental demyelination and remyelination occur. Onion bulb formations, a sign of repeated episodes of segmental demyelination and remyelination, may be absent or abundant, depending on chronicity. Endoneurial and epineurial mononuclear inflammatory cells are a helpful diagnostic sign when present. Using immunocytochemical markers the presence of inflammatory infiltrates can be highlighted. One study demonstrated epineurial T cells in perivascular clusters and endoneurial infiltration of macrophages and T cells (Schmidt et al. 1996).

Diagnostic criteria based on clinical features, electrodiagnostic studies, CSF examination, and results from nerve biopsy have been recommended by an American Academy of Neurology Subcommittee.

Treatment

Prednisone, plasmapheresis, and IVIG are all effective in CIDP and are the mainstays of treatment.

Daily single-dose prednisone is started at 60–80 mg (1.0–1.5 mg/kg for children). Improvement can be anticipated within 2 months; by 3 months 88% improve. Following improvement, the dose is converted to an alternate-day single-dose schedule. The initial daily dose is tapered to alternate-day prednisone by reducing the even-day dose by 10 mg per week; high-dose, alternate-day prednisone is maintained until a remission or plateau phase is achieved. More than 50% of patients reach this point by 6 months. After attaining maximum benefit, a slow taper of prednisone (e.g., 10 mg/month followed by 5-mg decrements at doses below 50 mg on alternate days) can then begin. The individual patient's clinical improvement and side-effect profile serve as guides to the rapidity of the taper. Some patients are exquisitely sensitive to reduction in corticosteroid dosage, this must be reduced slowly to avoid producing a severe relapse. Patients may need alternate-day prednisone (10–30 mg) for years to suppress disease activity. Side effects from prolonged prednisone use are significant. Osteoporosis causing vertebral compression fractures and cataracts are the most common long-term complications. Patients should be followed for the development of cataracts, increased intraocular pressure, hypertension, truncal obesity, hyperglycemia, aseptic necrosis of bone, peptic ulcer disease, and susceptibility to infection. Precautions taken to diminish complications include a low-sodium (2 g) and low-carbohydrate diet, and H_2-receptor antagonists for patients with peptic ulcer diathesis. Calcium and vitamin D supplements should be considered, and bone density should be monitored in an effort to limit osteoporosis. In patients with coexisting osteoporosis, nasal calcitonin or alendronate may be beneficial.

Two controlled studies have confirmed the benefit of therapeutic plasma exchange for CIDP of both chronic progressive and relapsing course. Ten plasma exchanges performed over 4 weeks resulted in substantial but transient improvement in 80% of patients (Hahn et al. 1996a). Improvement began within days of starting therapy, yet 70% of responders relapsed within 14 days after plasma exchange was stopped. The optimal schedule for plasma exchanges has not been established. A common approach employs three exchanges (50 ml/kg) weekly for the first 2 weeks, followed by two exchanges per week from the third through the sixth week. Then the treatment frequency is repeated according to clinical response. Plasma exchange is remarkably free of serious complications but can only be performed in medical centers with special expertise in apheresis and requires secure vascular access. Venous access problems may be overcome by placement of central venous catheters, although this approach carries the risk of serious infection. Plasmapheresis may be maintained for months and even years. The majority of patients needing prolonged

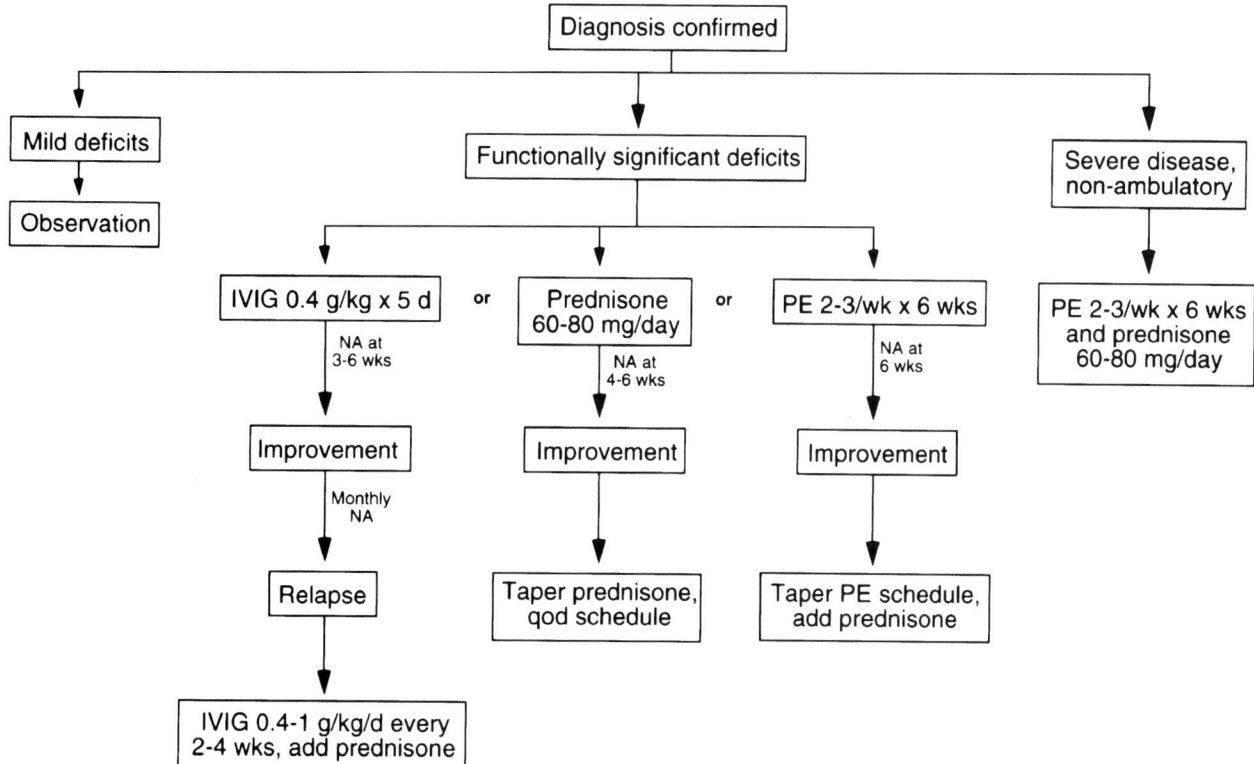

FIGURE 80.22   Decision-making pathway in the management of chronic inflammatory demyelinating polyradiculoneuropathy. (IVIG = intravenous immune globulin; NA = neurological assessment; PE = plasma exchange.)

plasmapheresis require the addition of prednisone for lasting benefit and stabilization.

Both open-label studies and a single double-blind study have demonstrated the benefit of high-dose IVIG in CIDP (Hahn et al. 1996b). The double-blind, sham-controlled trial of IVIG using 0.4 g/kg on 5 consecutive days resulted in significant improvement of 63% of patients with both chronic progressive and relapsing disease. Improvement was seen as early as the first week of treatment, whereas maximal benefit was reached at 6 weeks. Those patients who respond to the initial series of infusions may need maintenance infusions in single doses of 0.4–1.0 g/kg at intervals dependent on the disease response. The beneficial effect of IVIG was confirmed in a prospective study comparing IVIG (0.4 g/kg once a week for 3 weeks, followed by 0.2 g/kg weekly for the next 3 weeks) with plasmapheresis (Dyck et al. 1994). Both treatments were equally efficacious but short-lived, and most patients required continued intermittent treatment for sustained improvement. The risks and side effects of IVIG are mentioned earlier in this chapter, under Treatment for GBS.

In clinical practice, treatment with IVIG, plasma exchange, or prednisone should be limited to those patients with neuropathic deficits of sufficient magnitude to justify the risks and expense of treatment (Figure 80.22). There is an increas-

ing trend to use either IVIG or plasma exchange as primary treatment modalities, thereby avoiding the toxicity of chronic immunosuppression. As both treatments are equally expensive, IVIG is preferred because of its ease of administration. The best IVIG dosage schedule in patients with CIDP has not been established. Most patients receive an initial course of IVIG of 0.4 g/kg per day for 5 consecutive days. An essential aspect of the management of CIDP is the assessment of patients at baseline and at follow-up visits after treatment using objective and validated means of determining the severity of the neuropathic deficits. Following the initial post-treatment period of 3–6 weeks, responders are monitored at monthly intervals. When secondary deterioration occurs, patients are re-treated with single IVIG infusions (0.4–1.0 g/kg), depending on the severity of the relapse. The interval of repeat infusions is determined by the expected duration of the clinical benefit. For patients with residual deficits, small to moderate doses of prednisone may provide additional benefit. Patients who fail to respond to IVIG are treated either with plasma exchange or high-dose prednisone. Plasma exchange is combined with prednisone for severely affected, nonambulatory patients because of the slightly higher response rates of these treatments. The absence of any therapeutic response from these immune-modulating therapies should lead to a reappraisal of the diagnosis.

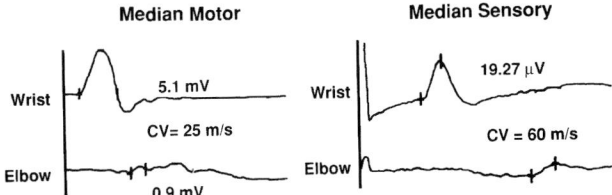

FIGURE 80.23 Partial motor conduction block of the median nerve. The compound muscle action potential (CMAP) was recorded from the abductor pollicis brevis. Supramaximal stimulation at the elbow produced an 80% drop in the amplitude of the median CMAP compared with stimulation at the wrist. Sensory conduction along the same nerve segment was preserved. (CV = conduction velocity.) (Courtesy of Dr. J. C. Stevens.)

Alternative forms of immunosuppressive treatment should be considered for patients with CIDP who are refractory to prednisone, plasma exchange, and IVIG. None of the alternative agents, however, have proven efficacy in controlled trials. Azathioprine (2–3 mg/kg/day) is used frequently as a corticosteroid-sparing, adjunctive agent in long-term management. Its use should be limited to patients with inadequate response to corticosteroids or those who require high corticosteroid maintenance doses with unacceptable side effects. Patients require monitoring of white blood cell count, platelets, and liver functions while on azathioprine. Approximately 10% of patients develop an early idiosyncratic reaction characterized by fever, myalgias, anorexia, and nausea that requires discontinuation of the drug. Other immune interventions include cyclosporine A (5 mg/kg in two divided doses per day), cyclophosphamide (2 mg/kg/day), and interferon-α (3 million IU subcutaneously three times a week for 6 weeks; Gorson et al. 1998). A small proportion of patients remain unresponsive or have significant residual deficits despite all efforts.

Prognosis

In contrast to the good prognosis in GBS, CIDP tends to be associated with prolonged neurological disability and is less likely to have spontaneous remissions. Although 95% of patients with CIDP show initial improvement following immunosuppressive therapy, the relapse rate is high and the degree of improvement modest. Despite the initial responsiveness, only 40% of patients in one series remained in partial or complete remission while receiving no medication. In one series of 53 patients followed for an average of 7.5 years, 4% recovered, 60% were employed and remained ambulatory, 28% were confined to a wheelchair or bed, and 11% died of complications of the disease.

Multifocal Motor Neuropathy with Conduction Block

Multifocal motor neuropathy has received much attention in recent years because it is a treatable demyelinating con-

dition that bears a superficial clinical resemblance to motor neuron disease. Whether multifocal motor neuropathy is a distinct nosological entity or simply a multifocal motor variant of CIDP is not established.

Clinical Features

The disorder is more common in men and mainly affects young adults, two-thirds being 45 years or younger. Progressive, asymmetrical, predominantly distal limb weakness and, to a lesser extent, atrophy develop over months to years. The upper extremities are more frequently affected than the lower. Wrist drop, grip weakness, or footdrop are the most common presenting features. Muscle cramps and fasciculations are common. Profound weakness in muscles with normal bulk or focal weakness in the distribution of individual nerves rather than in a spinal segmental pattern are clues that should alert the clinician to suspect this disorder. Cranial nerve involvement is unusual. Tendon reflexes are depressed or absent. Upper motor neuron signs are absent. Minor transient paresthesias are commonly reported by patients, but objective sensory deficits are usually absent. The course is slowly or less often stepwise progressive over months to years (Chaudhry 1998).

Laboratory Studies

The diagnosis depends on electrophysiological studies demonstrating persistent focal motor conduction block in one or more motor nerves at sites not prone to compression (see Chapter 37B). Additional features of multifocal motor demyelination are frequently present in nerve segments without conduction block, including motor conduction slowing, temporal dispersion, and prolonged F-wave and distal motor latencies (Katz et al. 1997). What makes multifocal neuropathy unique is that the block is confined to motor axons. SNAPs and sensory conduction are preserved (Figure 80.23). Abnormal amplitude reduction with proximal stimulation may be seen occasionally in other disorders; transient conduction block may occur in vasculitic neuropathy during the early stage of wallerian degeneration. There is no satisfactory explanation for the selective vulnerability of motor fibers. Kaji and colleagues (1993) reported a patient with pure motor weakness of the arm and proximal conduction block who underwent biopsy of a motor nerve branch adjacent to the site of focal conduction block that revealed scattered demyelinated axons and small onion bulbs without inflammatory changes. Needle EMG shows signs of denervation almost invariably confined to muscles that are clinically weak. Fasciculations are common, and myokymia may be seen. The spinal fluid protein is usually normal. The sural nerve frequently shows subtle pathological changes of demyelination and remyelination quite similar to those in CIDP but of lesser degree. These morphological abnormalities indicate that sensory nerves are involved in this disorder despite the lack of clinical or

Table 80.22: Differential diagnosis of multifocal motor neuropathy

Features	Multifocal motor neuropathy	CIDP	Amyotrophic lateral sclerosis
Lower motor neuron weakness	Distal, asymmetrical	Proximal and distal	Progressive
Upper motor neuron signs	Absent	Absent	Present
Sensory loss	Absent	Present	Absent
Motor conduction block	100%	Frequent	Rare and transient
Sensory conduction	Normal SNAP	Low to absent SNAP	Normal SNAP
Cerebrospinal fluid protein	Normal	Elevated	Normal
Anti-GM$_1$ antibodies	80%	Absent	<15 %

CIDP = chronic inflammatory demyelinating polyradiculoneuropathy; SNAP = sensory nerve action potential.

electrophysiological findings. MRI of the brachial or lumbosacral plexus may be helpful demonstrating focal enlargement and increased signal intensities of affected nerve trunks (van Es et al. 1997).

Attention has focused on a possible relationship between antiganglioside antibodies and acquired lower motor neuron syndromes. Among the gangliosides, GM$_1$ is abundantly found on the outer surface of neuronal membranes where potential binding sites could serve as antigenic targets. High titers of IgM anti-GM$_1$ antibodies can be found in 80% of patients with multifocal motor neuropathy and conduction block. High titers are occasionally (<15%) seen in amyotrophic lateral sclerosis and GBS variants including AMAN and the axonal form of GBS associated with *C. jejuni* infection, but rarely (<5%) in other peripheral neuropathies and non-neurological autoimmune disorders. Thus, anti-GM$_1$ antibodies are neither specific nor required for the diagnosis of multifocal motor neuropathy, but can be considered a marker for the disease.

The differential diagnosis of progressive limb weakness and atrophy without sensory symptoms is mainly restricted to motor neuron disease, including amyotrophic lateral sclerosis and its lower motor neuron form, progressive muscular atrophy, CIDP, and multifocal motor neuropathy (Table 80.22). Other conditions to be considered include postpolio syndrome, lead- or dapsone-induced motor neuropathies, the hereditary motor neuronopathies or spinal muscular atrophies, and hexosaminidase-A deficiency.

Treatment

Identifying patients with multifocal motor neuropathy is important because many such patients can be treated. High-dose intravenous cyclophosphamide (3 g/m^2 of body surface given in five divided doses over 8 days), followed by oral maintenance therapy (2 mg/kg/day), has been reported to be beneficial in an open uncontrolled study that resulted in meaningful improvement within 3–6 months. IVIG (0.4 g/kg body weight for 5 consecutive days) has been reported to benefit 94% of patients in open uncontrolled and small double-blind, placebo-controlled trials (Van den Berg et al. 1998). Improvement begins within days of treatment but lasts only for weeks to months. Most patients require maintenance infusions for years. Based on such observations, it is appropriate to initiate treatment with IVIG and continue maintenance infusions in patients who have a functionally meaningful response. Dose and frequency of repeated IVIG administration must be individualized for each patient, giving another dose just before the anticipated time of relapse. IVIG combined with oral cyclophosphamide (1–3 mg/kg/day) may reduce the frequency and therefore the high cost of frequent infusions. For nonresponders, intravenous cyclophosphamide is indicated depending on the degree of disability and the patient's understanding of the seriousness of potential side effects such as bone marrow depression, gonadal damage, hemorrhagic cystitis, and a long-term increased risk of cancer. Pestronk and colleagues (1994) suggested that monthly intravenous cyclophosphamide (1 g/m^2) for 6–8 months preceded on each occasion by two plasma exchanges may be an effective treatment with fewer adverse effects. Only occasional patients respond to prednisone and plasma exchange.

PERIPHERAL NEUROPATHIES ASSOCIATED WITH MONOCLONAL PROTEINS

Patients undergoing evaluation for chronic peripheral neuropathy of unknown cause should be screened for the presence of a monoclonal protein (M protein). A monoclonal protein is produced by a single clone of plasma cells and usually composed of four polypeptides: two identical heavy chains and two light chains. The M protein is named according to the class of heavy chain (IgG, IgM, IgA, IgD, IgE) and type of light chain, κ or λ. Approximately 10% of patients with idiopathic peripheral neuropathy have an associated monoclonal gammopathy, which represents a sixfold increase over the general population. The pathophysiological relationship between the M protein and the neuropathy is often obscure but some M proteins have antibody properties directed against components of myelin or axolemma. Finding an M protein among patients with neuropathy may lead to the discovery of underlying disorders such as primary systemic amyloidosis, multiple or osteosclerotic myeloma, macroglobulinemia, cryoglobulinemia, Castelman's disease, lymphoma, or malignant lymphoproliferative disease. In two-thirds of patients with a monoclonal protein, no detectable underlying disease is found, and they are described as having a *monoclonal gammopathy of undetermined significance* (MGUS). MGUS has replaced the

Table 80.23: Characteristic findings in monoclonal gammopathy of undetermined significance

Common monoclonal type	IgM, IgG, IgA
Common light chain	κ
Quantity	<3 g/dl
Urine light chains	Rare
Marrow—plasma cells	<5%
Skeletal lesions	Absent
Complete blood cell count	Normal
Organomegaly, lymphadenopathy	Absent

Ig = immunoglobulin.

term *benign monoclonal gammopathy* because up to one-fourth of patients develop malignant plasma cell dyscrasias after long-term follow-up. The characteristic features distinguishing MGUS from other plasma cell dyscrasias are listed in Table 80.23.

Routine serum protein electrophoresis frequently lacks the sensitivity required to detect small M proteins. Immuno-electrophoresis or immunofixation is required to detect small amounts of M proteins, confirm the monoclonal nature, and characterize the heavy- and light-chain types. Urine studies detect excretion of light chains (Bence Jones protein) that often accompany multiple myeloma or primary amyloidosis. All patients with neuropathy and associated M protein, as well as patients suspected of amyloidosis or myeloma should have a 24-hour urine collection for detection of Bence Jones protein. Following discovery of an M protein, a complete blood cell count with differential is necessary, immunoglobulins should be quantitated, and a radiological skeletal bone survey is indicated to detect lytic or sclerotic bone lesions of myeloma. A bone marrow aspirate and biopsy differentiate a malignant plasma cell dyscrasia from MGUS. Rectal, fat, or cutaneous nerve biopsies may be required to confirm a suspected diagnosis of amyloidosis (Kissel and Mendell 1995).

Monoclonal Gammopathy of Undetermined Significance

Approximately 5% of patients with MGUS have an associated polyneuropathy. The frequency of monoclonal IgM is overrepresented in patients with neuropathy (60% IgM, 30% IgG, and 10% IgA) compared with patients with only MGUS. The light-chain class is usually κ in contrast to patients with osteosclerotic myeloma or amyloidosis (Ropper and Gorson 1998).

Clinical Features

The clinical presentation of the neuropathies associated with different heavy-chain classes are generally indistinguishable from each other. Symptoms begin in later life with the median age of onset in the sixth decade, appear insidiously, and progress slowly over months to years. There is a male predominance. The most common presen-tation is a distal symmetrical sensorimotor polyneuropathy. Cranial nerves and autonomic functions are preserved. Sensory impairment can be prominent with variable involvement of light touch, pinprick, vibration, and position sense. Muscle stretch reflexes are universally diminished or absent. The lower limbs are involved earlier and to a greater extent than the upper. In approximately one-half of the patients, a polyradiculoneuropathy occurs that shares the clinical and laboratory features with CIDP. The CIDP patients with MGUS tend to be older and have a more indolent course with fewer motor than sensory findings, but poorer long-term functional outcome than the idiopathic CIDP group without M protein (Simmons et al. 1995). A predominantly sensory neuropathy may be seen in up to 20% of patients. Gait ataxia and upper limb postural tremor can be prominent, particularly in patients with IgM MGUS.

Laboratory Features

Electrophysiological studies show evidence of demyelination or more often both demyelination and axonal degeneration. Slow motor conduction velocities in the demyelinating range are more common in patients with IgM MGUS in which there is a predilection for distal demyelination. SNAPs are reduced in amplitude or unobtainable. EMG shows denervation. A small number of patients, usually with IgG MGUS, have electrophysiological features of a pure axonal neuropathy. When the frequency of MGUS in older patients is considered, the relationship between MGUS and neuropathy may be coincidental in these patients (Notermans et al. 1996a). Elevation of CSF protein is common, sometimes in excess of 100 mg/dl.

In at least 50% of patients with IgM MGUS neuropathy, the IgM monoclonal protein has reactivity against myelin-associated glycoprotein (MAG). MAG is a glycoprotein that makes up only 1% of peripheral nerve myelin. It is concentrated in periaxonal Schwann cell membranes, paranodal loops of myelin, and areas of non-compacted myelin, where it plays a role as an adhesion molecule for interactions between Schwann cells and axons. Anti-MAG antibodies cross-react with other components of peripheral nerve including several complex gly-cosphingolipids, PMP-22, and the main P_0 protein of myelin. Which of these reactivities relates to the neuropathy is unclear. Antibody activity to MAG can be detected by Western blot and enzyme-linked immunosorbent assay and can be demonstrated by immunocytochemical staining of nerves. Immunofluorescence studies show that IgM with anti-MAG activity binds to the periphery and peri-axonal regions of myelinated fibers that correspond to the distribution of MAG. Ultrastructurally, the myelin lamellae show a widened periodicity (myelin splitting), which is considered the pathological hallmark of anti-MAG antibodies (Figure 80.24). No consistent binding of monoclonal proteins to myelinated fibers is seen in nerve biopsy specimens from patients with IgG and IgA MGUS. Sural nerve biopsy findings of patients with M proteins of all three immunoglobulin classes show nerve fiber loss, segmental demyelination, and axonal degeneration.

The underlying mechanism of nerve fiber damage in MGUS neuropathy remains unknown, although an immune-mediated etiology is suspected (Tatum 1993). The case for pathogenic activity of IgM antibodies directed against MAG and other glycosphingolipids is better established than that for other antigens or for IgG and IgA antibodies. On the other hand, the lack of correlation between the deposition of anti-MAG antibody and the degree of pathological nerve damage, and the poor correlation between the amount of M protein in serum and the severity of neuropathy raise questions about causal linkage.

Treatment

The optimal treatment of MGUS neuropathy has not been established, and there are few prospective trials on which to base treatment decisions. The decision to treat depends on the severity of the neuropathy. Patients with minor deficits and indolent course are best followed without treatment. The more closely the neuropathy fulfills the criteria for CIDP, the more likely the patient will respond to immunomodulatory therapies. Patients have been treated with plasmapheresis, IVIG, and prednisone, often in combination with immunosuppressants, with good response in some but not all. In 1991, Dyck and colleagues confirmed the short-term benefit of plasmapheresis in a prospective, randomized, controlled trial. We generally begin with plasma exchange twice a week for 3–6 weeks. Subsequent intervals are dictated by the individual clinical response. If plasmapheresis cannot be performed and the patient fulfills criteria for CIDP, we treat with either IVIG (0.4 g/kg body weight for 5 consecutive days) or prednisone.

Patients with progressive, disabling neuropathy caused by IgM MGUS with or without anti-MAG reactivity may respond to aggressive immune interventions aimed at lowering the IgM level. This may be achieved by intermittent courses of oral cyclophosphamide (300 mg/m^2 body surface daily for 4 days) combined with prednisone (40 mg/m^2 body surface daily for 5 days) given at 4-week intervals for 6 months, or combination treatment with two plasma exchanges followed by intravenous cyclophosphamide given monthly for 5–7 months (Notermans et al. 1996b). A prospective open treatment trial found recombinant interferon-α (3 MU/m^2 body surface subcutaneously three times weekly) more effective than IVIG (Mariette et al. 1997). An algorithm for the treatment of MGUS neuropathy is proposed in Figure 80.25. Patients with rapid clinical deterioration of their neuropathy despite treatment should be re-evaluated for the development of underlying malignant lymphoproliferative disorders or amyloidosis.

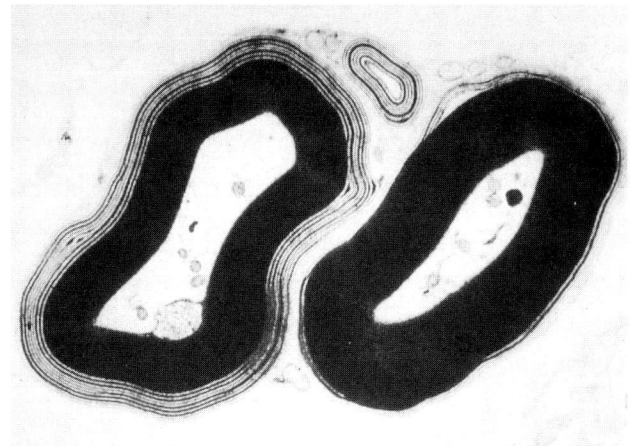
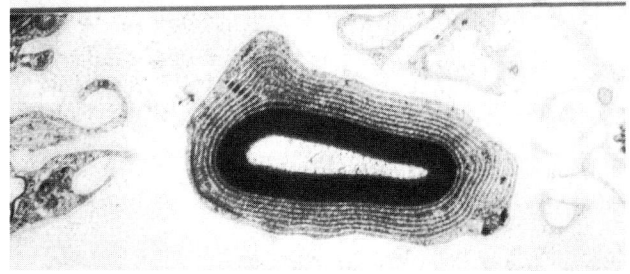

FIGURE 80.24 Electron micrographs showing fibers with myelin splitting. In the upper panel, the myelinating fiber on the left shows splitting of the myelin lamellae at the intraperiod line, whereas the nerve fiber on the right has normal compact myelin (×15,000). The lower panel illustrates similar myelin splitting (×20,000). The findings are characteristic of antimyelin-associated glycoprotein antibody deposits in the myelin sheath. (Reprinted with permission from JR Mendell, RJ Barohn, EP Bosch, et al. Continuum-peripheral neuropathy. Am Acad Neurol 1994; 1:1–103.)

Waldenström's Macroglobulinemia

Waldenström's macroglobulinemia (WM) is characterized by proliferation of malignant lymphocytoid cells in bone marrow and lymph nodes that secrete an IgM monoclonal spike of more than 3 g/dl. WM typically affects elderly men; systemic symptoms of fatigue, anemia, bleeding, and hyperviscosity dominate. Peripheral neuropathy occurs in approximately one-third of patients with WM and is a chronic symmetrical, predominantly sensory polyneuropathy similar to that associated with nonmalignant IgM M proteins. Other presentations include pure sensory or pure motor neuropathies, multiple mononeuropathies associated with cryoglobulins, and typical amyloid neuropathy. Anti-MAG reactivity is found in approximately 50% of WM patients with neuropathy. Patients with positive anti-MAG antibodies have slowed motor NCVs and prolonged distal latencies consistent with demyelination. Nerve biopsy findings are indistinguishable from those seen in IgM MGUS neuropathy. Patients with demyelinating polyneuropathy

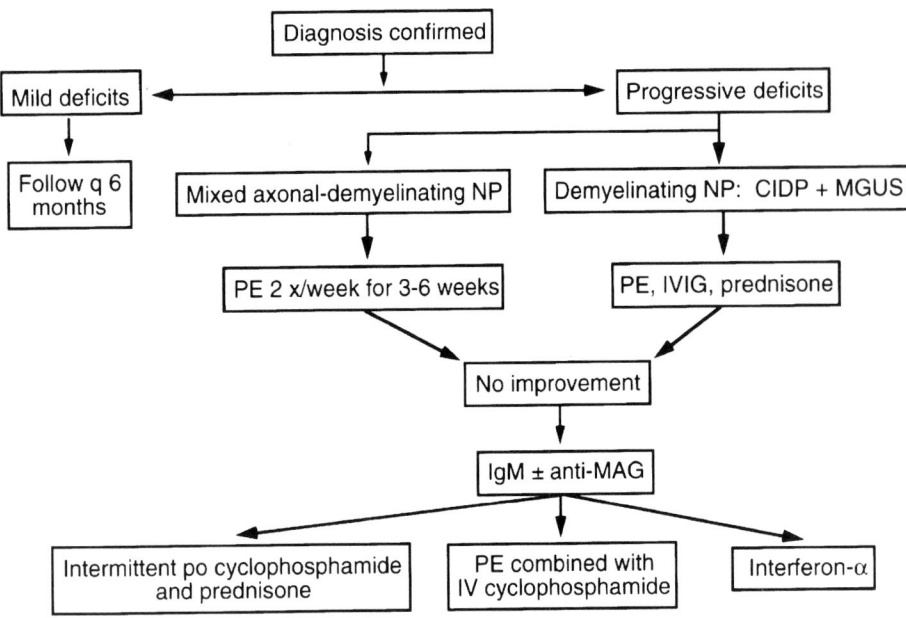

FIGURE 80.25 Decision-making pathway in the management of peripheral neuropathy with monoclonal gammopathy of undetermined significance (MGUS). (CIDP = chronic demyelinating polyradiculoneuropathy; IVIG = intravenous immune globulin; MAG = myelin-associated glycoprotein; NP = neuropathy; PE = plasma exchange.)

may respond to chemotherapy, plasmapheresis, or both, but the response appears to be less consistent than in IgM MGUS-related neuropathy.

Multiple Myeloma

Polyneuropathy occurs in approximately 5% of patients with multiple myeloma. One-third of patients are found to have abnormalities on careful electrophysiological studies. The most common neurological complications of multiple myeloma are related to cord and root compression from lytic vertebral lesions. Diffuse bone or radicular pain resulting from vertebral body involvement, concurrent anemia, renal insufficiency, and hypercalcemia may provide clues as to the underlying disorder. The clinical manifestations of myeloma neuropathy are heterogeneous. Most patients present with mild distal sensorimotor polyneuropathy. Less frequently, a pure sensory neuropathy is seen. Furthermore, AL amyloidosis complicates multiple myeloma in 30–40% of cases, and these patients have a high likelihood of death within the next 2 years. Painful dysesthesias, preferential involvement of small fiber sensory modalities, autonomic dysfunction, and carpal tunnel syndrome are suggestive of amyloid neuropathy. Rectal, abdominal fat, or sural nerve biopsy specimens should be obtained in all patients with progressive myeloma neuropathy in order to identify the patients with amyloidosis.

Nerve conduction and sural nerve biopsy studies are consistent with an axonal process with loss of myelinated fibers. Treatment of the underlying myeloma may sometimes improve the neuropathy.

Osteosclerotic Myeloma and POEMS Syndrome

Osteosclerotic myeloma occurs in less than 3% of all patients with myeloma but 85% of these patients present with an associated peripheral neuropathy. In this disorder, the plasma cell proliferation occurs as single or multiple plasmacytomas that manifest as sclerotic bone lesions. The neuropathy of osteosclerotic myeloma is different from that associated with multiple myeloma in several aspects: It occurs at an earlier age and mostly in men; it is a demyelinating, predominantly motor neuropathy with slow motor NCVs and elevated CSF protein levels, usually in excess of 100 mg/dl; an M protein is found in 90% of cases and virtually always composed of λ light chains associated with IgG and IgA heavy chains; it responds to irradiation or excision of the isolated plasmacytoma; and it is associated with systemic manifestations referred to as Crow-Fukase or POEMS syndrome. To reiterate, POEMS is the acronym for *p*olyneuropathy, *o*rganomegaly, *e*ndocrinopathy, *M* protein, and *s*kin changes, facilitating recognition of the most constant features of this multisystem syndrome.

The neuropathy of osteosclerotic myeloma bears a striking resemblance to CIDP with symmetrical proximal and distal weakness with variable sensory loss. Cranial nerves are spared except for occasional cases of papilledema. The clinical and electrophysiological similarities between this condition and CIDP emphasize the need to screen for an occult M protein and sclerotic bone lesions in all adult patients presenting with an acquired demyelinating neuropathy.

The skeletal lesions can be single or multiple and tend to involve the axial skeleton, the majority being in the spine, pelvis, and ribs. Their radiographical appearance varies from dense ivory to mixed sclerotic and lytic lesions with a

FIGURE 80.26 Radiography of the pelvis showing a dense sclerotic area in the upper sacrum and two smaller focal sclerotic lesions in the right pubic bone and the left femoral neck. Biopsy of one accessible lesion confirmed osteosclerotic myeloma.

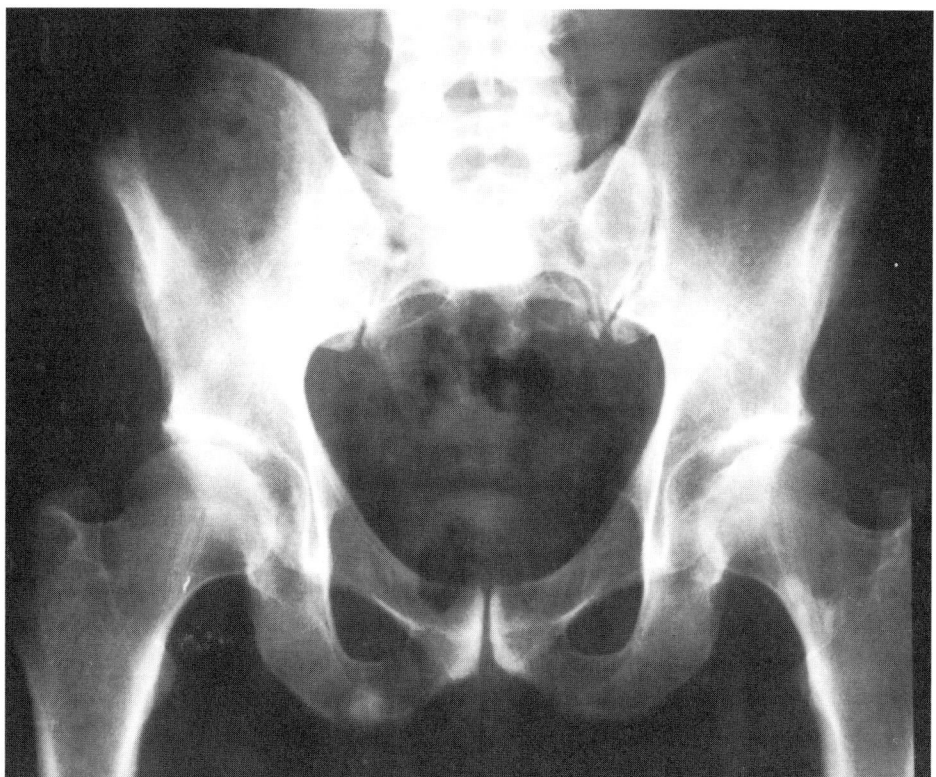

sclerotic rim (Figure 80.26). Radioisotope scans are less sensitive than radiographical skeletal surveys in detecting the lesions. Open biopsy is usually necessary to confirm the presence of an isolated plasmacytoma.

Most patients develop one or more of the multisystem manifestations of the POEMS syndrome. Hepatosplenomegaly is often encountered. Gynecomastia and impotence in men, secondary amenorrhea in women, diabetes mellitus, and hypothyroidism are the most common endocrinopathies. Hyperpigmentation, hypertrichosis, diffuse skin thickening, hemangiomas, and white nail beds are dermatological features. Pitting edema of the lower limbs, ascites, pleural effusions, and clubbing of the fingers are other signs. Approximately one-fourth of patients with POEMS syndrome have no associated bone lesions. Some of these patients have Castleman's syndrome (a nonmalignant form of angiofollicular lymphadenopathy), others have a plasma cell dyscrasia restricted to the lymphoreticular system.

The pathogenesis of this multiorgan disorder is poorly understood. The associated plasma cell dyscrasia seems to play a crucial role, as clinical improvement follows the disappearance of the monoclonal proteins. Elevated levels of proinflammatory cytokines, such as tumor necrosis factor–α have been implicated in the multisystem manifestations (Gherardi et al. 1994).

The importance of recognizing this rare syndrome lies in its potential for treatment. Patients with solitary lesions are treated with tumoricidal irradiation, complete surgical extirpation, or both. Patients with multiple bone lesions receive radiation combined with prednisone and melphalan. Substantial improvement of both neurological and systemic features is seen in one-half of the patients, but the response may take many months.

Cryoglobulinemia

Cryoglobulins are immunoglobulins that precipitate on cooling and redissolve on warming to body temperature. Cryoglobulins are classified into three groups: type I are monoclonal immunoglobulins that are associated with myeloma, macroglobulinemia, and other lymphoproliferative disorders; type II consists of a mixture of a monoclonal protein, usually IgM-κ with antirheumatoid factor activity, and polyclonal IgG; and type III are polyclonal IgM and IgG immunoglobulins. Mixed cryoglobulinemia may occur as a primary condition without any apparent underlying process, termed *essential mixed cryoglobulinemia*, or may be secondary to autoimmune diseases, infections, and chronic liver injury. Hepatitis C viral infection appears to be the most common cause of type II cryoglobulinemia. The frequency of peripheral neuropathy in essential mixed cryoglobulinemia ranges from 10% to 57%. Patients present with arthralgias, glomerulonephritis, Raynaud's phenomenon, hepatosplenomegaly, and recurrent purpura of the lower legs, often precipitated by cold temperatures. Neurological symptoms occur in the form of either multiple mononeuropathy or a painful sensorimotor polyneuropathy.

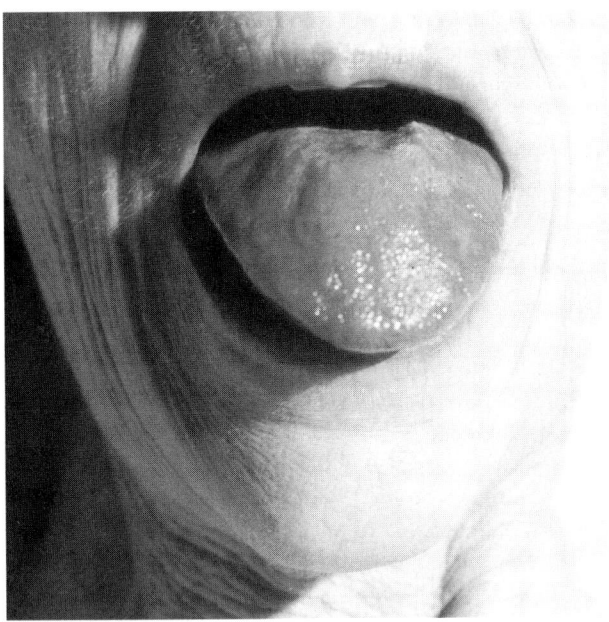

FIGURE 80.27   Macroglossia in AL amyloidosis. Tongue enlargement may be found in 20% of patients with AL amyloidosis. (AL = amyloid light chain.)

Electrodiagnostic studies show axonal changes with denervation, particularly in distal leg muscles. In most cases the sural nerve biopsy shows myelinated fiber loss, axonal degeneration, and necrotizing vasculitis of epineurial vessels. In other cases, occlusion of vasa nervorum by precipitating cryoglobulins may result in ischemic axonal damage.

Corticosteroids, cyclophosphamide, and plasma exchange are the major modes of treatment. Interferon-α has shown promise in hepatitis C virus–associated cryoglobulinemia (Khella et al. 1995).

Primary Systemic Amyloidosis

Primary systemic amyloidosis is a multisystem disorder characterized by extracellular deposition of fibrillar proteins arranged in a β-pleated sheet conformation in organs and tissues throughout the body. The β-pleated sheet configuration seems to be responsible for the typical staining properties with Congo red stain, appearing red microscopically under normal light, but apple-green in polarized light. In both primary systemic amyloidosis and amyloidosis complicating multiple myeloma or WM, amyloid is composed of fragments of immunoglobulin light chains from the amino-terminal variable regions, or less commonly the complete immunoglobulin light chain, and is designated *AL* for amyloid light chain (Falk et al. 1997). In primary systemic amyloidosis clonal populations of nonproliferative plasma cells synthesize light chain polypeptides that are deposited in tissues as amyloid. AL amyloidosis also occurs in association with multiple myeloma and WM, but is distinguished from primary systemic amyloidosis by the number and morphology of plasma cells in the bone marrow and the amount of M protein in the serum. Amyloid fibrils from patients with familial amyloid neuropathies are composed of one of three aberrant proteins caused by genetic mutations (see Familial Amyloid Polyneuropathy, earlier in this chapter). Immunohistochemical techniques using specific antibodies can distinguish the different types of amyloidogenic proteins on biopsy material.

Clinical Features

Primary amyloidosis usually occurs after age 40, with a median age of onset of 65 years. Men are twice as likely to be affected. The initial symptoms are frequently fatigue and weight loss followed by symptoms and signs related to specific organ involvement. The organs most commonly affected, either individually or together, are the kidney, heart, and PNS. Peripheral neuropathy occurs in 15–35% of patients and is the presenting manifestation in 10%. The majority have renal or cardiac presentations with peripheral neuropathy as a later manifestation. The neuropathy begins with painful dysesthesias in the legs and follows a chronic progressive course. Pain and temperature sensation are lost before light touch or vibratory sensation. Distal symmetrical weakness and a pansensory loss evolves later in the course of disease. Most patients develop features of autonomic dysfunction, including postural hypotension, impotence, gastrointestinal disturbances, impaired sweating, and loss of bladder control. Nearly 25% of patients develop a superimposed carpal tunnel syndrome caused by amyloid infiltration of the flexor retinaculum at the wrist. The constellation of painful dysesthesias, autonomic dysfunction, and a history of carpal tunnel syndrome should alert the clinician to the possibility of amyloidosis. Pitting edema related to hypoalbuminemia; spontaneous periorbital purpura caused by vascular infiltration; macroglossia, a sign occurring in 20% of patients (Figure 80.27); and hepatomegaly are typical findings on examination. Amyloid deposition between muscle fibers may cause pseudohypertrophy of muscles. Renal amyloidosis usually manifests as proteinuria and renal failure. Rapidly progressive congestive heart failure caused by cardiac infiltration is seen in one-third of patients.

Laboratory Features

Electrodiagnostic studies show changes of axonal neuropathy, with low-amplitude or absent SNAPs, low-amplitude CMAPs, but preserved motor conduction velocities. Distal median motor latencies are prolonged in patients with carpal tunnel syndrome. EMG frequently provides evidence of active denervation. A monoclonal protein or light chains are detected in 90% of patients by means of immunofixation electrophoresis of serum or urine. Monoclonal λ light chains are more common than κ light chains (ratio of λ to κ, 3 to 1). Bone marrow examination reveals slightly increased plasma cells and clonal dominance of a light chain isotype by immunohistochemical staining.

The diagnosis is established by the histological demonstration of amyloid deposition in tissues. Abdominal fat aspiration, bone marrow aspirate, or rectal biopsy are convenient procedures that provide approximately an 80% yield of positive results. In patients with suspected amyloid neuropathy, combined muscle and sural nerve biopsy is the most sensitive technique that provides confirmation in more than 90% of cases. Patients with apparent AL amyloidosis who do not have light chains in serum or urine pose a diagnostic problem to distinguish them from familial amyloidosis. In most of these patients, a clonal dominance of plasma cells can be identified by immunocytochemical staining of a bone marrow specimen, or positive identification of AL amyloid can be achieved in tissue samples by immunohistochemical staining using labeled antibodies specific for human light chains. If no evidence of plasma cell dyscrasia exists, familial amyloidosis should be considered even in the absence of a positive family history. In these patients molecular genetic testing to identify transthyretin mutations is indicated (see Familial Amyloid Neuropathy, earlier in this chapter). Results of sural nerve biopsy show amyloid deposition around blood vessels and within the endoneurial space (Figure 80.28), severe loss of myelinated and unmyelinated fibers, and active axonal degeneration. The pathogenetic mechanism of nerve fiber damage remains uncertain.

The prognosis in primary amyloidosis is poor, with a median survival of approximately 20 months. Death is commonly caused by progressive congestive heart failure or renal insufficiency. Patients with amyloid neuropathy without cardiac or renal involvement have a more favorable prognosis, with a median survival of 40 months. Intermittent oral melphalan and prednisone are reported to slow progression of renal and cardiac amyloidosis, but the treatment has no effect on the neuropathy. High-dose intravenous melphalan with autologous blood stem cell support has shown promising results with improvement of neurological deficits in a few selected patients.

NEUROPATHIES ASSOCIATED WITH SYSTEMIC DISORDERS

Diabetic Neuropathies

Diabetes mellitus is said to afflict more than 5 million people in the United States and to be growing at a rate of 5% per year. It is estimated that 5–65% of diabetics have some form of peripheral neuropathy. The wide range in estimated prevalences of diabetic neuropathy is a result of differences in case definitions, disparate methods of ascertainment, and a paucity of true population-based epidemiological investigations. The diagnosis of diabetic neuropathy should be based on clinical symptoms, objective neurological signs, and electrodiagnostic confirmation (Thomas 1997). The risk of developing symptomatic neuropathy in patients without neuropathic symptoms or signs at the time of initial diagnosis of diabetes is approximately 4–10% by 5 years and up to 15% by 20 years (Martyn and Hughes 1997). Factors predisposing to development of diabetic neuropathy appear to include longer duration of diabetes, male gender, and hypertension in patients with insulin-dependent diabetes mellitus.

Pathophysiology

Many mechanisms have been advanced for the pathogenesis of diabetic neuropathy, including (1) metabolic processes directly affecting nerve fibers, (2) endoneurial microvascular disease, (3) autoimmune inflammation, and (4) deranged neurotrophic support.

The metabolic hypothesis is in large measure derived from studies of nerve blood flow and derangements of the polyol pathway. Hyperglycemia generates rheological changes that increase endoneurial vascular resistance and reduce nerve blood flow. Animal models of diabetes suggest that the polyol pathway plays a significant role in the generation of nerve damage, with hyperglycemia causing depletion of nerve myoinositol through a competitive uptake mechanism. Persistent hyperglycemia activates the polyol pathway in nerve tissue through the enzyme aldose reductase, which leads to the accumulation of sorbitol and fructose in nerve and also induces nonenzymatic glycosylation of structural nerve proteins. These metabolic changes are likely to cause abnormal neuronal and axonal metabolism and subsequently to impair axonal transport. Findings in human diabetic sural nerve biopsy preparations, however, have not fully substantiated this mechanism, and controlled clinical trials of aldose reductase inhibitors have fallen short of demonstrating clinically meaningful benefits.

According to the microvascular hypothesis, endoneurial hypoxia is produced by decreased blood flow to the nerve and increased endoneurial vascular resistance. Once hypoxia is established, a vicious cycle of further capillary damage is set in motion that escalates hypoxia. Endoneurial hypoxia is thought to inhibit axonal transport and reduce nerve sodium-potassium ATPase activity. The impairment of these functions causes axonal atrophy, leading to reduced NCVs. Endoneurial hypoxia appears to play a more substantial role in noninsulin-dependent diabetes mellitus than in insulin-dependent diabetes mellitus. Although the mechanisms leading to capillary abnormalities that initiate hypoxia are unknown, the microvascular hypothesis provides a framework for further research into the pathogenesis of diabetic neuropathy.

In support of neurogenic inflammation as a mechanism of nerve damage in diabetes, a number of workers have demonstrated inflammatory infiltrates in nerves of diabetic patients with either polyneuropathy or asymmetrical lumbosacral radiculoplexopathy. Diabetic polyneuropathy may in part result from deficiency of specific neurotrophic factors. Early in the course of disease NGF-associated small-

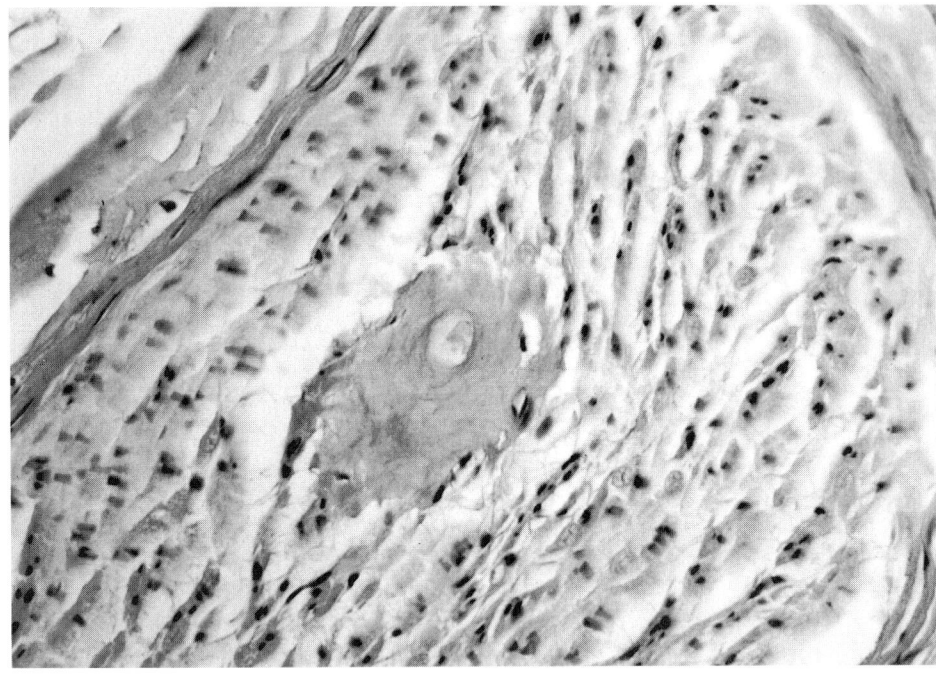

A

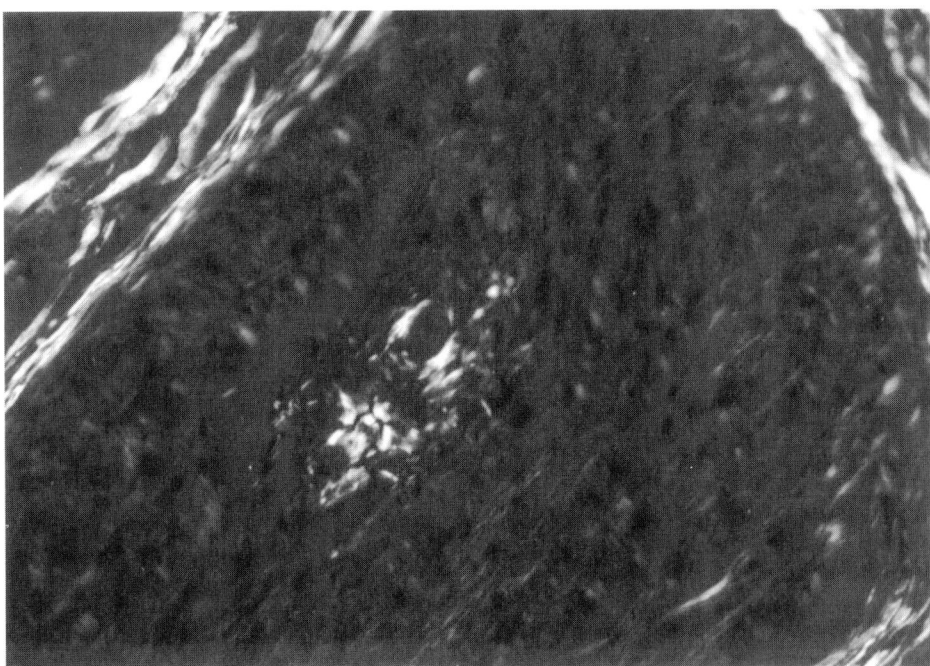

B

FIGURE 80.28   Amyloid neuropathy. (A) Sural nerve biopsy shows deposition of amyloid in the wall of an endoneurial vessel and loss of myelinated fibers. (B) Under polarized light the Congo red–positive area shows apple-green birefringent deposits typical of amyloid. (Congo red, original magnification ×250.)

diameter sensory fibers are affected before involvement of either sympathetic, large-diameter sensory, or motor fibers; when the condition progresses, levels of the neuropeptide calcitonin gene-related polypeptide fall as large-diameter sensory nerve fibers become involved (Anand 1996).

Pathology

The underlying pathological processes differ in the various types of diabetic neuropathy. Cranial and limb mononeu-

ropathy and multiple mononeuropathies are thought to be caused by small vessel occlusive disease. The precise location of the primary pathological process in diabetic asymmetrical proximal neuropathy remains unsettled. Postmortem examination of the obturator nerve in a single case of proximal neuropathy showed multiple infarcts caused by the occlusion of vasa nervorum. However, lumbar nerve roots were not examined. Whether ischemic lesions in multiple lumbar roots, plexus, or proximal nerve segments are responsible for this particular neuropathy still remains to be proven.

FIGURE 80.29   (A) Sural nerve biopsy from patient with diabetic lumbar radiculoplexopathy. Perivascular lymphocytic inflammation involves two epineurial arterioles. (Hematoxylin and eosin; original magnification ×25.) (B) In the same patient, semithin transverse section illustrates selective involvement of one fascicle with marked loss of myelinated fibers, a pattern highly suggestive of nerve ischemia. (Paraphenylenediamine-stained semithin epoxy section; original magnification ×80.) (Courtesy of Dr. P. J. Dyck, Mayo Clinic, Rochester, MN.)

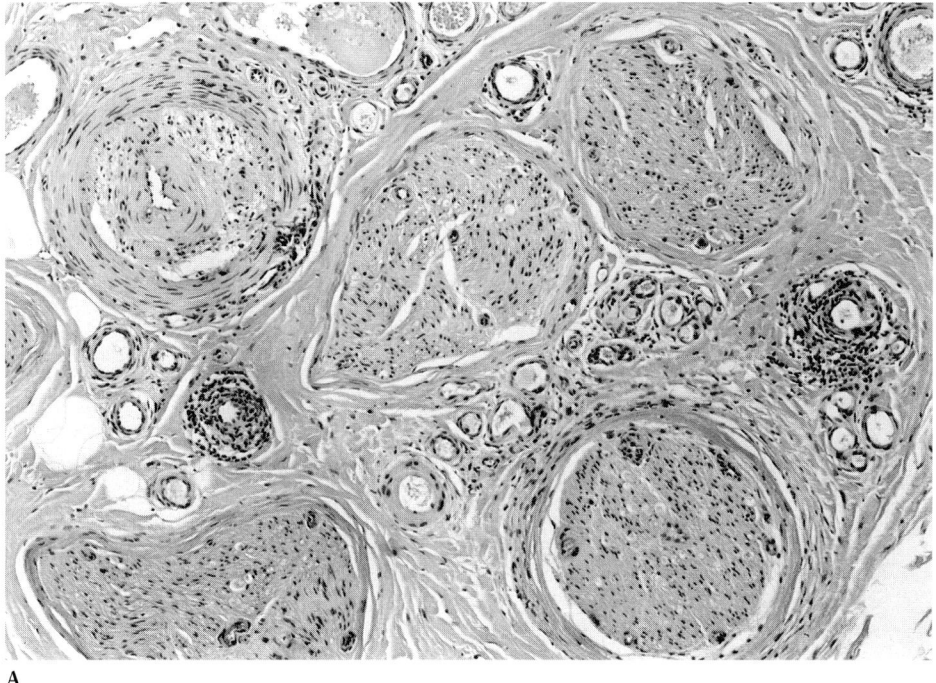

A

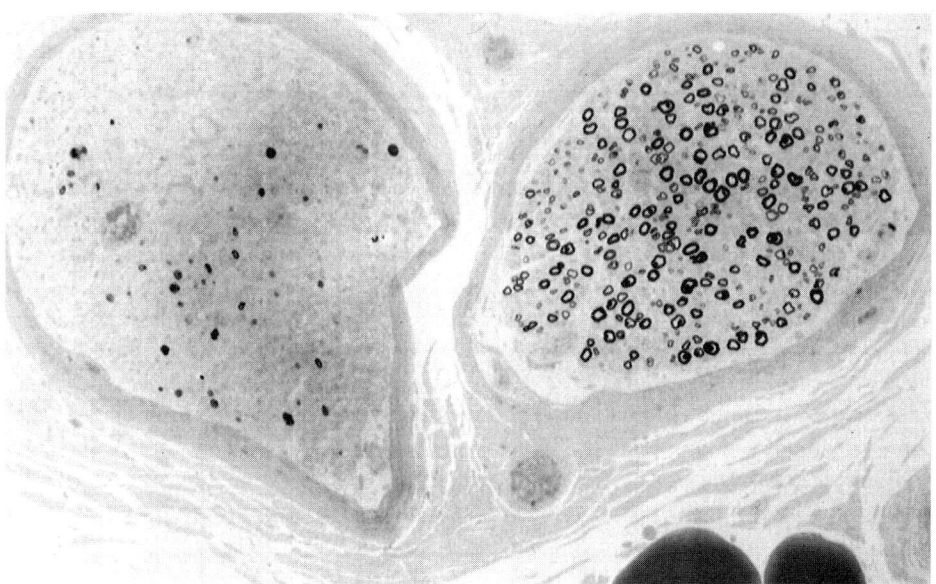

B

The pathological lesions of symmetrical distal polyneuropathy have been investigated extensively (Dyck and Giannini 1997). The sural nerve shows loss of myelinated fibers, acute axonal degeneration, some degree of demyelination, and, almost invariably, evidence of vasculopathy. The latter is characterized by narrowing or closure of the endoneurial capillary lumen, thickening of the capillary wall, and marked redundancy of basement membranes. Axonal degeneration has been shown to result from a dying-back centripetal degeneration of peripheral axons. Painless distal polyneuropathy affects predominantly the large nerve fiber populations, whereas painful distal dia-

betic polyneuropathy shows marked depletion of small myelinated and unmyelinated fibers. The demyelinating process in diabetes is interpreted as the result of primary progressive axonal atrophy. Extensive histometric studies of sural nerves demonstrate that the nerve fiber loss in diabetic neuropathy is distributed multifocally between and within different fascicles (Figure 80.29B). The pattern of such multifocal nerve fiber loss is similar to that reproduced in experimental microsphere occlusion studies. Three-dimensional studies from nerves along proximodistal segments indicate increasing nerve fiber depletion in distal nerve segments. This finding correlates with electrophysio-

Table 80.24:   Classification of diabetic neuropathies

Symmetrical polyneuropathies
  Distal sensory or sensorimotor polyneuropathy
  Small fiber neuropathy
  Autonomic neuropathy
  Large fiber neuropathy
Asymmetrical neuropathies
  Cranial neuropathy (single or multiple)
  Truncal neuropathy (thoracic radiculopathy)
  Limb mononeuropathy (single or multiple)
  Lumbosacral radiculoplexopathy (asymmetrical
    proximal motor neuropathy)
  Entrapment neuropathy
Combinations
  Polyradiculoneuropathy
  Diabetic neuropathic cachexia

logical studies demonstrating a diffuse abnormality of NCVs with proximal-distal gradients. Current investigations point to microvascular abnormalities contributing significantly to the development of both multifocal neuropathies and symmetrical polyneuropathies.

Patterns of Diabetic Neuropathy

Peripheral nerve involvement in diabetes mellitus may present in any of a number of distinct syndromes, each with a characteristic mode of onset and natural history. It is helpful to classify diabetic neuropathies into symmetrical and asymmetrical syndromes, although in any given patient there may be overlap and even multiple different forms of diabetic neuropathy (Table 80.24).

Symmetrical Polyneuropathies. Of the symmetrical diabetic neuropathies, distal symmetrical polyneuropathy, a predominantly axonal, length-dependent neuropathy is most prevalent. A common misconception is that the term *diabetic neuropathy* is synonymous with *distal symmetrical polyneuropathy*, perhaps in part because the latter accounts for nearly three-fourths of all diabetic neuropathies. This type of neuropathy characteristically begins with distal lower limb sensory disturbances, often beginning in the toes and ascending slowly over months. Often when the sensory symptoms have reached knee level, the finger and hand become affected. In longstanding cases the anterior abdomen and chest may lose sensation, often in a symmetrical diamond-shaped region centered at or above the umbilicus. The majority of patients have little if any motor involvement at onset, although motor involvement may increase as the deficits worsen. Generally autonomic involvement parallels the severity of the neuropathy. Neuropathic arthropathies or Charcot joints are complications seen in diabetics, who often have foot ulcers and autonomic impairment. Unlike the Charcot joints seen in syphilis, diabetic arthropathy tends to involve the small joints in the feet.

Small Fiber Neuropathy. Although the majority of individuals with diabetic polyneuropathy have roughly equivalent involvement of large diameter sensory fibers, small diameter sensory fibers, and autonomic fibers, and somewhat lesser deterioration of motor axons, the proportionate dysfunction of each of these fiber subtypes varies. One somewhat frequently encountered subset is the distal symmetrical diabetic neuropathies predominantly affecting small diameter axons, typically Aδ and C fibers. These may present with "burning feet" or even less often as a painful neuropathy with prominent autonomic features.

Large Fiber Neuropathy. So-called diabetic pseudotabes is a rare, relatively painless ataxic sensory polyneuropathy that results from disproportionate involvement of large-diameter sensory fibers. In the early stages, large-diameter sensory deficits are asymptomatic but often detectable by careful neurological examination.

Diabetic Autonomic Neuropathy. Still rarer in neurological practice is pure autonomic neuropathy. The spectrum of autonomic involvement in diabetic polyneuropathy, however, ranges from subclinical impairment of cardiovascular reflexes and sudomotor function, to severe cardiovascular, gastrointestinal, or genitourinary dysfunction. Orthostatic hypotension, resting tachycardia, or a heart rate that does not vary with respiration are the hallmarks of diabetic autonomic neuropathy. Significant orthostatic hypotension occurs mainly because of failure of the sympathetic nervous system to increase systemic vascular resistance in the erect posture, with impairment of compensatory cardiac acceleration. It is crucial to exclude confounding effects of medications or coexisting hypovolemia when diagnosing neurogenic postural hypotension. Vagal denervation of the heart results in a high resting pulse rate and loss of sinus arrhythmia. An increased incidence of painless or silent myocardial infarction is reported in diabetic patients with autonomic neuropathy. Gastrointestinal motility abnormalities and fecal incontinence may occur. Delayed gastric emptying leads to nausea, early satiety, and postprandial bloating. Diabetic diarrhea, caused by small intestine involvement, typically occurs at night, and is explosive and paroxysmal. Associated weight loss or malabsorption is rare. Bacterial overgrowth in the gut may occur and can often be treated successfully with small doses of tetracycline (250–500 mg/day in a single dose given at the onset of a diarrheal attack). Colonic atony produces constipation. Bladder atony leads to prolonged intervals between voiding, gradually increasing urinary retention, and finally overflow incontinence. The symptoms develop insidiously and progress slowly. Diabetics with neurogenic bladder should be encouraged to void routinely every few hours to prevent urinary retention. Impotence is often the first manifestation of autonomic neuropathy in diabetic men, occurring in 30–60% and causing serious emotional distress. Autonomic dysfunction involves both erectile failure and retrograde ejaculation. The majority of male diabetics with impotence have some evidence of associated distal symmetrical polyneuropathy. Sudomotor abnormalities produce distal anhidrosis, causing compensatory facial and truncal sweating and heat intolerance. A peculiar hyperhidrosis called gustatory sweating is characterized by profuse sweating in the face and forehead immediately following food intake. Pupillary abnormalities include constricted pupils with sluggish light reaction. A blunted autonomic response to hypoglycemia produces an unawareness of hypoglycemia that may seriously complicate intensive insulin treatment.

Asymmetrical Neuropathies. The asymmetrical diabetic neuropathy syndromes include single or multiple cranial mononeuropathies, single or multiple somatic mononeuropathies, asymmetrical lumbosacral radiculoplexopathy, and single or multiple monoradiculopathies.

Cranial Mononeuropathy. The most common diabetic cranial neuropathy syndrome is acute to subacute onset of painful ocular mononeuropathy (cranial nerve III, IV, or VI), which is followed typically by complete or partial recovery over weeks to a few months (see Chapter 74). A painful pupil-sparing third nerve palsy is characteristic of diabetic cranial mononeuropathy, reflecting injury to centrifascicular axons but sparing the peripherally situated pupillary motor fibers of the oculomotor nerve. Other established syndromes include facial neuropathy, and, less commonly, single or multiple cranial neuropathies associated with serious infection (Smith 1998). Rhinocerebral mucormycosis is a disorder often occurring in individuals with poorly controlled diabetes mellitus, frequently in the setting of ketoacidosis, which most often presents with abrupt onset of fever, headache, and malaise, followed by periorbital pain, swelling, and induration. Nasal mucosal necrosis gives rise to the characteristic black turbinate. Cranial nerves III, IV, VI, and V_1 may be affected, resulting in vision loss, total ophthalmoplegia, and upper hemifacial sensory loss. Left untreated, occlusion of the internal carotid artery ensues, which may be followed rapidly by meningeal extension, obtundation, and death. Treatment consists of surgical excision of affected tissues and intravenous amphotericin B therapy. Despite early recognition and aggressive intervention, the mortality of this disorder remains close to 50%. Malignant external otitis also occurs almost exclusively in diabetes mellitus. Most often presenting with ear pain, neurological manifestations occur 1–3 months after onset and may consist of facial palsy or other cranial neuropathies. Otoscopy typically shows lobulated erythematous granulation tissue in an edematous inflamed external canal, while cultures almost invariably grow *Pseudomonas aeruginosa.* Treatment involves intravenous antibiotics and débridement of necrotic tissues in the external ear.

Limb Mononeuropathy. Involvement of single nerves in diabetes mellitus may occur either from infarction or entrapment. Nerve infarction presents as acute focal pain, followed by weakness, atrophy, and variable sensory loss. With axonal degeneration recovery is often slow and incomplete. The median, ulnar, and fibular nerves are involved most often. Entrapment neuropathies of the median and ulnar nerves occur with greater frequency in diabetics. These include both the carpal tunnel syndrome (median neuropathy at the wrist) and the cubital tunnel syndrome (ulnar neuropathy at the elbow). In these neuropathies the underlying mechanism is primarily focal segmental demyelination, explaining the more rapid recovery profile.

Thoracic Radiculopathy or Truncal Neuropathy. Diabetic thoracic radiculopathy or truncal neuropathy involving the T4-T12 roots causes pain or dysesthesias in areas of the chest or abdomen. Bulging of the abdominal wall as a result of weakness of abdominal muscles may occur. This unique truncal pain syndrome is most often seen in older patients with noninsulin-dependent diabetes mellitus and may occur either in isolation or together with the typical lumbosacral radiculoplexopathy. The regions of sensory loss or dysesthesia involve the trunk in a highly variable pattern affecting either the entire dermatomal distribution of adjacent spinal nerves or, more often, restricted areas limited to the distribution of the posterior or anterior primary rami of spinal nerves. Patients describe burning, stabbing, boring, or beltlike pain. Contact with clothing or bedclothes can be unpleasant. The onset may be either abrupt or gradual. The clinical picture can mimic intra-abdominal, intrathoracic, and intraspinal diseases as well as dermatomal zoster with vesicles or zoster sine herpete, requiring careful differential diagnostic considerations. Neurological findings are limited to hypesthesia or hyperpathia over the thorax or abdomen. The symptoms may persist for several months before gradually subsiding.

Lumbosacral Radiculoplexopathy or Asymmetrical Proximal Diabetic Neuropathy. The term *diabetic amyotrophy*, coined by Garland, is an acute, painful, asymmetrical proximal lower limb syndrome developing over a few days, or less commonly, a more symmetrical proximal lower limb paraparesis developing over weeks to months in older diabetic patients (Pascoe et al. 1997). Although many terms have been used to describe this condition, it may be considered one of the manifestations of diabetic polyradiculopathy along with truncal monoradiculopathy and diffuse lower limb predominant polyradiculopathy. Although lumbosacral radiculoplexopathy most often occurs in diabetics over the age of 50, most have non–insulin-dependent diabetes mellitus, even though the onset does not appear to be correlated to the duration of glucose intolerance. Typically, severe unilateral pain in the lower back, hip, and anterior thigh heralds the onset. Weakness ensues over days to weeks, affecting proximal and distal lower extremity muscles (iliopsoas, gluteus, thigh adductor, quadriceps, hamstring, and anterior tibial muscles). In some cases, the opposite leg becomes affected after days to months. Reduction or absence of knee and ankle reflexes is the rule. Numbness or paresthesias are minor complaints. Weight loss occurs in more than one-half of the patients. The progression may be steady or stepwise and may continue for many months. The result is often a debilitating, painful, asymmetrical predominantly motor neuropathy with profound atrophy of proximal leg muscles. Pain usually recedes spontaneously long before motor strength begins to improve. Recovery continues as long as 24 months, because of the slow rate of axonal regeneration. In many cases mild to moderate weakness persists indefinitely. Overlap with distal symmetrical polyneuropathy is noted in up to 60% of patients. Those with polyneuropathy more frequently have gradual onset of symptoms, bilateral findings, significant weight loss, and diffuse paraspinal muscle denervation. The typical electrophysiological findings include prominent fibrillation potentials in thoracic and lumbar paraspinal muscles, neurogenic motor unit potential alterations in affected muscles, and prolongation of femoral nerve motor latencies. MRI studies of the lumbar spine, lumbosacral plexus, or both should be considered when lumbar root lesions, cauda equina disorders, or structural lumbosacral plexopathies are suspected (see Chapter 79). A vascular pathogenesis of this proximal neuropathy was documented by autopsy showing infarcts of the proximal nerve trunks and lumbosacral plexus, whereas biopsies of distal and proximal nerves suggest inflammation may be involved in at least a subset of cases (see Figure 80.29). Whether the brunt of pathological lesions affects the lumbar roots, the lumbosacral plexus, or proximal peripheral nerve trunks is uncertain.

Combinations. The symmetrical and asymmetrical categories are bridged by diabetic polyradiculoneuropathy. In this entity, symptoms often begin gradually with a distal symmetrical polyneuropathy. As the endocrinopathy progresses, first one root, perhaps in the middle or lower thoracic region, and then another at a different level becomes involved, eventually leading to confluent denervation in multiple bilateral sacral, lumbar, thoracic, and less commonly cervical root segments.

Diabetic neuropathic cachexia is an unusual syndrome in which adult patients, typically men with non–insulin-dependent diabetes, lose massive body weight, sometimes in excess of 40–50 kg, often in association with a painful symmetrical polyneuropathy or polyradiculoneuropathy, depression, insomnia, and impotence.

One danger of having diabetes mellitus is that when confronted by unexplained pain, weakness, or sensory loss, many physicians are quick to ascribe all neurological symptoms to new onset or worsening diabetic neuropathy or radiculoplexopathy. Appropriate evaluation for concomitant treatable neurological disease related or unrelated to the diabetes must be considered. Noteworthy combinations include diabetic polyneuropathy with superimposed carpal tunnel syndrome mimicking worsening polyneuropathy, compressive lumbar radiculopathy or pelvic malignancy masquerading as diabetic lumbosacral radiculoplexopathy, and painful oculomotor palsy with an unsuspected circle of Willis berry aneurysm in a diabetic patient.

Laboratory Findings

To establish the diagnosis of diabetes mellitus, blood sugar determinations are essential. Fasting plasma glucose levels greater than 126 mg/dl on more than one occasion, any plasma glucose greater than 200 mg/dl, or sustained postprandial plasma glucose of 200 mg/dl or greater at and before 2 hours after a 75-g oral glucose load confirms diabetes mellitus. Glycosylated hemoglobin (hemoglobin A1c) is a useful indicator of the long-term control of hyperglycemia. NCVs are significantly slower in diabetic patients than in healthy subjects. Abnormalities occur more commonly in sensory than in motor fibers, in the legs more than in the arms, and in distal more than in proximal nerve segments.

Treatment

The cornerstone in the treatment of diabetes and its complications remains optimal glucose control. There is considerable evidence that good diabetic control is associated with less frequent and less severe peripheral nerve complications. The Diabetes Control and Complication Trial (1995) showed that intensive glucose management by insulin pump or by three or more daily insulin injections in patients with insulin-dependent diabetes mellitus reduces the development of neuropathy by 64% at 5 years compared with conventional therapy. Successful pancreatic transplantation is beneficial in preventing the progression of diabetic neuropathy but the effect is not sustained in long-term follow-up. Attempts to treat diabetic neuropathy by manipulating nerve metabolism have been disappointing. Clinical trials of myoinositol supplementation have shown conflicting results. Studies of aldose reductase inhibitors have failed to produce convincing clinical improvement, although modest changes in nerve conduction and nerve pathology occurred. The longitudinal use of objective reproducible measures is critical to judge the course of diabetic neuropathy and especially response to therapy (Dyck et al. 1997). Use of high-dose IVIG for diabetic lumbosacral radiculoplexopathy has been reported to benefit patients with progressive deficits and biopsy evidence of inflammation in uncontrolled studies (Krendel et al. 1995).

Symptomatic treatment for pain, autonomic manifestations, and the complications of sensory loss can be offered to lessen the effect of neuropathic symptoms. Various oral medications including antidepressants (e.g., tricyclic agents and maprotiline), anticonvulsants (e.g., gabapentin and low-dose carbamazepine), mexiletine, tramadol, and sympatholytic agents, as well as topical preparations of capsaicin and anesthetics have been used with variable success in the management of neuropathic pain in diabetes mellitus. It is preferable to use one agent at a time, increase the dose slowly, allow an adequate treatment period of at least 3–4 weeks, and document the degree of response or lack of response carefully in the medical record for each medication used. Pain management is reviewed earlier in this chapter.

Several therapeutic interventions may reduce the symptoms of autonomic dysfunction. Patients with symptomatic orthostatic hypotension are advised to sleep with the head of the bed elevated 6–10 inches. The head-up tilt prevents salt and water losses during the night and combats supine hypertension. Practical suggestions include drinking two cups of strong coffee or tea with meals, eating more frequent small meals rather than a few large meals, and increasing the daily fluid intake (>20 oz/day) and salt ingestion (10–20 g/day). Elastic body stockings may be beneficial by reducing the venous capacitance bed, but are poorly tolerated by many patients. Plasma volume expansion can be achieved by fludrocortisone (0.1–0.6 mg daily). By increasing vasomotor and venomotor tone, the alpha-agonist midodrine is effective in increasing standing systolic blood pressure and reducing symptoms of lightheadedness in neurogenic orthostatic hypotension (Low et al. 1997). Nonsteroidal anti-inflammatory drugs, which inhibit prostaglandin synthesis, represent the next class of drugs to be considered; ibuprofen, 400 mg four times a day, is better tolerated than indomethacin. Phenylpropanolamine (25–50 mg three times a day), a direct-acting alpha-agonist, may be used next. A sustained-release form of phenylpropanolamine can be obtained over the counter (Dexatrim). Delayed gastric emptying is often relieved with metoclopramide; because it is a dopamine antagonist, extrapyramidal symptoms may occur at higher doses. Diabetic diarrhea may be treated with short courses of tetracycline or erythromycin. In some cases, clonidine has been reported to reduce the troublesome diarrhea. Genitourinary complications of diabetic autonomic neuropathy require close collaboration with a urologist. Patients with a neurogenic bladder should be encouraged to adhere to a frequent voiding schedule during the day, which helps diminish the amount of residual urine. For more severe involvement, manual abdominal compression or intermittent self-catheterization may be needed. Treatment of erectile impotence should be directed by a urologist, who can counsel the patient regarding the options of oral sildenafil, direct vasodilator injections into the corpora cavernosa, or penile implant surgery.

Sensory loss makes diabetic patients susceptible to repetitive, often painless injuries that set the stage for foot ulcers and distal joint destruction (acrodystrophic neuropathy). Chronic foot ulceration is one of the more severe complications of diabetes mellitus, caused by a combination of unnoticed, traumatic tissue damage, vascular insufficiency, and secondary infection. Prevention is better than treatment. Proper skin care in diabetics with cutaneous sensory loss, impaired sweating, and vascular disease is extremely important in order to prevent foot ulceration. This includes daily inspection of the feet, regular pedicure, and prompt attention to seemingly trivial injuries and infections.

Future Directions

Advances in the treatment of diabetic neuropathy are focusing on at least four areas: neuropeptide manipulation, antioxidant treatment, NMDA antagonist therapy, and essential fatty acid supplementation. NGF is critical for the development and support of small-diameter sensory and autonomic axons known to be affected in diabetic polyneuropathy. Although a trial with recombinant human NGF showed preliminary efficacy in patients with symptomatic symmetrical diabetic neuropathy (Apfel et al. 1998), a subsequent pivotal trial was negative. Antioxidant therapy with agents such as alpha lipoic acid have shown promise in reducing diabetic neuropathic symptoms in preliminary randomized controlled clinical trials (Ziegler and Gries 1997). Similar improvement is suggested by a randomized, double-blind, crossover study of the NMDA antagonist dextromethorphan in painful diabetic neuropathy (Nelson et al. 1997). As to the role of essential fatty acid in diabetic neuropathy, experimental evidence suggesting that the conversion of linoleic to gamma linoleic acid is impaired in human diabetes motivated two multicenter controlled clinical trials. Gamma linoleic acid seemed to improve clinical, electrophysiological, and quantitative sensory measures in diabetic neuropathy (Horrobin 1997).

Peripheral Neuropathy in Malignancies

Advances in the diagnosis and management of malignancy have accelerated in recent years, leading to novel chemotherapeutic strategies and prolonged survival rates for many cancers. With these welcome improvements come an increasing awareness of peripheral nerve complications in patients with various forms of neoplasm. Although rigorous epidemiological data regarding the incidence of neuropathy in cancer are rare, Lin et al. (1993) found that 2–3% of more than 500 Taiwanese cancer patients had neuropathies attributable to their cancer.

Neuropathy may result from one or more mechanisms related to cancer or its treatment. These include (1) compression or destruction of nerve trunks by direct extension of primary tumor; (2) metastasis to single or multiple sites in bone, soft tissues, or meninges with involvement of adjacent or transiting nerve fibers; (3) autoimmune paraneoplasia with generation of antineuronal antibodies; (4) entrapment neuropathies in individuals with profound cachexia and resultant loss of normal muscle and other soft tissue cushioning around nerve trunks; and (5) iatrogenic processes such as neurotoxic chemotherapy, radiation, and surgical procedures. Reviews by Hughes et al. (1994) and Amato and Collins (1998) provide detailed accounts of these neuropathies.

Mechanisms

Compression. Apart from head and neck tumors invading cranial and cervical peripheral nerves, focal neuropathies from primary neoplasms are uncommon. Salivary gland cancers are known to affect the facial and other cranial nerves, often growing insidiously by perineurial spread, thereby eluding early detection even by sophisticated imaging procedures. Nasopharyngeal carcinomas, meningiomas, and skull base tumors may interrupt cranial nerve fibers directly. Primary or recurrent neoplasms of the breast or lung apex in particular may invade the brachial plexus. Similar primary or recurrent pelvic or retroperitoneal cancers may involve the lumbosacral plexus (these conditions are discussed in Chapter 79).

Metastasis. Discrete single metastatic lesions may rarely cause cranial or somatic mononeuropathy. More commonly widespread metastases arise in the leptomeninges from carcinoma or lymphoma leading to leptomeningeal carcinomatosis or lymphomatosis, respectively.

Paraneoplasia. Particularly in patients with small cell carcinoma of the lung, antibodies to dorsal root ganglion and CNS neurons may develop, resulting in characteristic neurological syndromes that may antedate discovery of the primary neoplasm (see following discussion).

Entrapment. Individuals who lose substantial body mass, particularly over short periods of time, are subject to fibular (peroneal) neuropathy and perhaps other entrapment and compression neuropathies. This phenomenon has been documented in nutritionally deprived prisoners of war, in profound weight loss associated with malignancy, and in rapid weight loss with dieting.

Iatrogenic. Neurotoxic chemotherapeutic agents are discussed in the section on toxic neuropathy. The neurological complications of radiation, including radiation plexopathy, are discussed in Chapters 64 and 79. Surgical resection of bulky cancers may result in trauma to peripheral nerves, which may be unavoidable because of inextricable adherence or transit of nerve fibers through the tumor mass.

Carcinoma

The prevalence of clinical peripheral neuropathy in patients with carcinoma is estimated to be 2–3%, but increases to 37–50% if electrodiagnostic abnormalities are included in the criteria for diagnosis. Peripheral neuropathies associated with carcinoma are classified into three main clinical types: (1) malignant inflammatory sensory polyganglionopathy; (2) sensorimotor polyneuropathy (either axonal or demyelinating types); and (3) single or multiple mononeuropathy.

Malignant Inflammatory Sensory Polyganglionopathy. In 1948, Denny-Brown recognized the association between sensory neuropathy and cancer when he described two cases with rapidly progressive severe sensory loss and ataxia without weakness, as a remote effect of bronchogenic carcinoma. Subsequently, an increasing number of neurological syndromes have been identified as paraneoplastic complications or remote effects of cancer affecting different sites of the CNS or PNS. Distinct autoantibodies associated with spe-

cific syndromes have been identified providing important clues to assist in diagnosis. Paraneoplastic syndromes affect only a small minority of cancer patients, occurring less commonly than direct tumor invasion or neurotoxic complications of chemotherapy. The terms *subacute sensory neuropathy, carcinomatous sensory neuropathy, paraneoplastic sensory neuronopathy,* or *malignant inflammatory sensory polyganglionopathy* are synonyms to describe the distinct sensory neuropathy associated with cancer. The term *malignant inflammatory sensory polyganglionopathy* is preferred because it emphasizes the sensory ganglion cell as the primary site of injury, while recognizing that other neurons including autonomic ganglia and CNS nerve cells are often involved as well. The presence of an autoantibody directed against a nuclear protein that is shared by neuronal nuclei and tumor antigens, and the intense inflammatory response found in affected dorsal root ganglia, support an immune-mediated mechanism for this condition.

Clinical Features. The patients are middle-aged or older, and many are heavy smokers. Women are affected twice as often as men are. The most common underlying neoplasm is small cell cancer of the lung (approximately 90%), followed in decreasing order of frequency by breast carcinoma, ovarian cancer, and lymphoma. In 9 of 10 cases neurological symptoms are the presenting features and precede the discovery of the tumor by several months. The median interval from onset of neuropathic symptoms to diagnosis of the underlying neoplasm is 5 months. Symptoms may develop fulminantly within days or more gradually over months. Numbness, painful paresthesia, and lancinating pain often begin in one limb and progress to involve all four limbs. Occasionally, the trunk, face, or scalp are affected in somatotopic regions highly suggestive of neuronopathies. There is global loss of all sensory modalities with a striking loss of proprioception and the ability to localize the limb in space, leading to sensory ataxia and pseudoathetosis of the upper extremities. Tendon reflexes are globally reduced or absent. Muscle strength is preserved or only mildly decreased, although patients are often severely disabled and unable to walk because of their sensory deficits.

Approximately one-half of the patients have symptoms and signs reflecting more widespread involvement of myenteric plexus neurons, autonomic ganglia, spinal cord, brainstem, cerebellum, and limbic cortex. These patients display varying degrees of gastrointestinal dysmotility, autonomic dysfunction, myelopathy, cerebellar signs, brainstem findings, confusion, and dementia. Intestinal pseudo-obstruction presenting with abdominal pain, nausea, vomiting, and severe constipation may occur with subtle or no sensory deficits in association with small cell lung cancer.

Laboratory Features. The CSF is frequently abnormal with either mild pleocytosis or elevated protein. Nerve conduction studies show low-amplitude or absent SNAPs with relatively preserved amplitudes of CMAPs. EMGs may demonstrate minor abnormalities. The sural nerve frequently shows a combined loss of myelinated and unmyelinated fibers, axonal

Table 80.25: Differential diagnosis of sensory neuronopathies

Features	Paraneoplastic	Idiopathic	Sjögren's syndrome
Sex ratio (male to female)	1:3	0.5:1.0	1:9
Course	Subacute	Acute to chronic	Acute to chronic
Sensory loss	Global	Kinesthetic, large fiber	Kinesthetic, large fiber
Other	Gastrointestinal dysmotility	—	—
	Encephalomyelitis	None	Sicca syndrome
Autoantibodies	ANNA–type I	None	ENA (SS-A, SS-B)
Spinal fluid	Elevated protein	Normal	Normal
Schirmer's test	Normal (>5 mm)	Normal	<5 mm
Systemic disease	Small cell cancer of lung	None	Inflammation of salivary glands

ANNA = antineuronal nuclear antibody; ENA = extractable nuclear antigen.

degeneration, and minimal axonal regeneration, sometimes with mononuclear inflammatory cells around epineurial vessels. The principal neuropathological features first identified by Denny-Brown include degeneration of dorsal root ganglion cells with intense mononuclear cell inflammation, subsequent loss of sensory axons, and degeneration of the posterior roots, peripheral sensory nerves, and the posterior columns of the spinal cord. Many patients have pathological evidence of a more generalized encephalomyelitis characterized by inflammatory infiltrates and neuronal loss in hippocampus, brainstem, and spinal cord.

Patients presenting with sensory neuronopathy, encephalomyelitis, or gastrointestinal dysmotility associated with small cell lung cancer harbor characteristic antibodies in their serum and spinal fluid called type I antineuronal nuclear antibodies (ANNA-I) or anti-Hu. The antibodies react with 35- to 40-kD nuclear proteins expressed in the nuclei of most neurons of the CNS, dorsal root ganglia, myenteric plexus, and in most small cell lung cancers. Over 90% of patients with sensory neuronopathy associated with small cell lung cancer have significantly elevated titers of ANNA-I antibodies by immunohistochemistry or Western blot analysis; low titers have been found in 16% of patients with small cell lung cancer without neurological disease. In contrast, all patients with idiopathic sensory neuronopathy without cancer or sensory neuronopathy associated with Sjögren's syndrome are seronegative for ANNA-I antibodies. These results highlight the value of serological testing for ANNA-I antibodies as an aid in the differential diagnosis of ataxic sensory neuronopathies. Seropositive patients should have chest CT or MRI because the tumor may go undetected by chest roentgenography.

Differential Diagnosis. The diagnostic possibilities of acquired sensory neuronopathies include malignant inflammatory sensory polyganglionopathy, the ataxic sensory neuronopathy associated with Sjögren's syndrome, and idiopathic sensory neuronopathies (Table 80.25). These conditions share similar pathological lesions characterized by an inflammatory ganglionopathy. The toxic sensory neuronopathies caused by megadoses of pyridoxine or following chemotherapy with cisplatinum are readily excluded by history. Although it can be difficult to distinguish patients with malignant inflammatory sensory polyganglionopathy from those with other causes of sensory neuropathy, (1) discovery of prominent dysautonomia, (2) neurological signs suggesting disease outside the dorsal root ganglion (and particularly CNS deficits), or (3) ANNA-I antibodies should prompt a careful search for malignancy, and especially small cell carcinoma of the lung.

Prognosis. The outlook for patients with paraneoplastic sensory neuronopathy is poor. At best, successful treatment of the underlying neoplasm may be associated with stabilization in some cases, but more often the neuronopathy pursues a relentless, independent course, despite treatment with corticosteroids, immunosuppressive agents, and plasmapheresis. Minor modifications of the clinical course were observed in some patients receiving high-dose IVIG in an open-label study (Uchuya et al. 1996).

Polyneuropathy. It is far more common for cancer patients to have distal symmetrical sensorimotor polyneuropathy than malignant inflammatory sensory polyganglionopathy. Clinically, these more frequently encountered length-dependent neuropathies are often of slow onset, progress gradually, and are indistinguishable from distal axonal neuropathies in individuals without malignancy. Sites of neoplasm reported in association with this nondescript polyneuropathy, in decreasing order of frequency, include lung, stomach, breast, colon, pancreas, and testis. Whether these neuropathies are paraneoplastic remains to be proven.

A subset of sensorimotor neuropathy associated with cancer is the group with a clinical syndrome resembling either acute GBS or CIDP. These individuals are often found to have elevated CSF protein values in excess of 100 mg/dl, marked slowing of motor NCVs, and small mononuclear cell infiltrates on sural nerve biopsy.

Mononeuropathy and Multiple Mononeuropathies. Mononeuropathy and multiple mononeuropathies have been associated on rare occasions with cancer and lymphoproliferative disorders, especially hairy cell leukemia, possibly caused by vasculitis. Paraneoplastic vasculitic neuropathy is clinically indistinguishable from the more common multiple mononeuropathies caused by the systemic vasculitis.

Table 80.26: Classification of vasculitides affecting the peripheral nervous system*

Systemic necrotizing vasculitis
Classic polyarteritis nodosa (22%)
Allergic angiitis (Churg-Strauss syndrome)
Wegener's granulomatosis (1%)
Vasculitis associated with connective tissue disease (21%)
Rheumatoid vasculitis (18%)
Polyangiitis overlap syndrome (11%)
Hypersensitivity vasculitis
Giant cell arteritis
Temporal arteritis
Localized vasculitis (organ-specific)
Nonsystemic neuropathic vasculitis (34%)

*Relative frequency is based on more than 200 patients, with biopsy-proven vasculitis pooled from six neuromuscular centers.
Source: Adapted from RK Olney. Neuropathies associated with connective tissue disease. Semin Neurol 1998;18:63–72.

Lymphoma, Neurolymphomatosis, Leukemia, and Polycythemia Vera

Peripheral neuropathy is found in approximately 5% of patients with lymphoma (Hughes et al. 1994). Both chronic and subacute sensorimotor neuropathies have been reported. Acute polyneuropathy of the GBS type is more common in association with lymphomas, particularly Hodgkin's disease, than with other malignancies; however, malignant infiltration of nerve roots must be excluded. Some patients may develop a subacute lower motor neuron syndrome with muscle weakness as a remote effect of malignant lymphoma. Pathologically, the primary lesion appears to be a motor neuronopathy restricted to the anterior horn cells and their roots. In other lymphoreticular neoplasms such as leukemia and non-Hodgkin's lymphoma, peripheral neuropathies are encountered rarely.

Neurolymphomatosis is a rare condition with diffuse infiltration of peripheral and cranial nerves by lymphoma cells. Patients present with acute to subacute progressive sensorimotor deficits resembling GBS or with a progressive cauda equina syndrome. The diagnosis is confirmed by positive CSF cytology result or lymphomatous infiltration of nerves as seen by cutaneous nerve biopsy.

Although distal paresthesias are common in polycythemia vera, overt clinical polyneuropathy of a predominantly sensory type is a rare complication.

Neuropathy in Connective Tissue Diseases

Peripheral nerves, including cranial nerves, are affected frequently in connective tissue disorders (Olney 1998). Peripheral nerve manifestations may develop in patients with well-established disease or may be the initial manifestation of an undiagnosed connective tissue disease. Neuropathy may occur as part of the multisystem disease process itself.

It may be secondary to complications of other organ involvement (e.g., uremic neuropathy, nerve entrapment as a result of joint deformities, or iatrogenic drug toxicity). Finally, neuropathy may be coincidental and unrelated to the underlying disease. The pathogenesis of peripheral neuropathy in connective tissue disorders is complex and may vary with the specific disorder. Circulating immune complexes detected in a variety of connective tissue disorders may play a significant role. Vascular lesions are found in all types of connective tissue disorders. In some there is occlusion of the small vasa nervorum, whereas in others epineurial arterioles and small arteries are involved by necrotizing vasculitis, producing multiple nerve infarcts.

Peripheral Nerve Vasculitis

Peripheral neuropathy may be the presenting manifestation of a potentially life-threatening disorder, systemic necrotizing vasculitis, or be the only manifestation of a more indolent condition, nonsystemic (or monosystemic) vasculitic neuropathy. The vasculitides represent a clinicopathological spectrum of disorders characterized by inflammation and necrosis of blood vessel walls, leading to luminal occlusion and ischemia in the distribution of the damaged vessels. Multiple or isolated organ systems may be involved in the vasculitic process. PNS involvement is common, occurring in up to 75% of patients with systemic necrotizing vasculitis (Kissel 1994). There are four groups of vasculitides that may affect the PNS (Table 80.26). Systemic necrotizing vasculitis refers to a diverse group of diseases affecting multiple organ systems including the PNS and CNS. These vasculitides typically involve small and medium-sized vessels.

Polyarteritis nodosa, by far the most common vasculitis in this group, is characterized by necrotizing inflammation of medium-sized or small arteries affecting kidney, skeletal muscle, bowel, skin, PNS, and CNS. Peripheral nerve involvement occurs in 50–75% of patients. Hepatitis B surface antigen is found in one-third of the cases. Allergic angiitis or Churg-Strauss syndrome typically presents with asthma, eosinophilia, and pulmonary infiltrates and is associated with disseminated vasculitis of small and medium-sized vessels. The frequency of peripheral nerve involvement is similar to that seen in polyarteritis nodosa (Sehgal et al. 1995). Wegener's granulomatosis affects the upper and lower respiratory tract accompanied by glomerulonephritis and necrotizing vasculitis. The PNS is involved in 10–20% of cases. Cranial nerve involvement and external ophthalmoplegia occurs in 11% of patients as a result of granulomatous infiltration of the orbit or cavernous sinus (Nishino et al. 1993).

When vasculitis develops in association with connective tissue disorders, the clinical and pathological features resemble polyarteritis nodosa. Among the connective tissue disorders, rheumatoid vasculitis is by far the most common cause of vasculitic neuropathy. Approximately

15–30% of patients cannot be categorized and are classified as having an overlap syndrome or undifferentiated connective tissue disease. In the hypersensitivity vasculitides, cutaneous manifestations dominate the clinical picture, although peripheral nerves may be involved. Peripheral nerve lesions may complicate giant cell arteritis in 14% of cases. Giant cell arteritis affects large and medium-sized arteries. When the vasculitis includes the nutrient arteries of peripheral nerves, ischemic mononeuropathies or multiple mononeuropathies may result. More than 10% of patients with vasculitic neuropathy present in the setting of malignancies, most commonly myeloproliferative or lymphoproliferative disorders, and infections including HIV and hepatitis C virus. One-third of patients with biopsy-proven vasculitic neuropathy lack evidence of systemic disease or a definable connective tissue disease (see following section, Nonsystemic Vasculitic Neuropathy).

Nonsystemic Vasculitic Neuropathy

A restricted necrotizing vasculitis affecting only peripheral nerves and skeletal muscle is the most common cause of vasculitic neuropathy in patients presenting to a neurologist. Multiple mononeuropathies are the most common clinical presentation, followed by asymmetrical neuropathy or distal polyneuropathy. There are generally no constitutional symptoms or serological abnormalities, because joints, visceral organs, and skin are unaffected. The severity of symptoms and deficits varies considerably. The disease course is indolent and protracted over years without ever becoming life-threatening. The diagnosis depends exclusively on results of nerve and muscle biopsy. The pathological features are identical to those seen in classic polyarteritis nodosa affecting small and medium-sized arteries in muscle and nerve.

Pathogenesis

The precise immunological events leading to vessel injury in vasculitis is not well understood. Immune complex deposition within vessel walls and T cell–dependent, cell-mediated cytotoxic reactions are the two basic immunopathogenetic mechanisms causing destruction of vessel walls. Vascular endothelial cells may serve as antigen-presenting cells and have important functions initiating the cell-mediated immune process. Although drugs and certain infectious agents, including HIV and hepatitis B and hepatitis C viruses, have been implicated as triggers of the immune responses, in most instances an etiological agent cannot be identified. The final common pathway of vasculitic neuropathy is the extensive occlusion of vasa nervorum at the level of epineurial arterioles of 50–300 μm diameter leading to nerve ischemia. Nerve ischemia results in axonal degeneration. Because of the random, focal nature of vasculitis, axonal degeneration typically shows a pattern of asymmetrical, patchy involvement both between and within nerve fascicles. The ischemia is most pronounced in proximal nerves, such as the fibular division of the sciatic nerve at the midthigh or the ulnar nerve at the mid-upper arm, in watershed areas between the distributions of major nutrient arteries. The extensive branching and intermixing of nerve fibers may result in a more homogeneous nerve fiber loss in distal sensory nerves, which are suitable for biopsy. Large myelinated fibers appear to be more susceptible to ischemia than unmyelinated fibers.

Clinical Features

In systemic vasculitis, there are multisystem signs together with fever, malaise, and weight loss. The majority of patients with PNS involvement present with peripheral neuropathy as the initial manifestation of disease. Irrespective of the underlying vasculitic syndrome, the clinical features of vasculitic peripheral neuropathy are similar and depend on the extent, distribution, and temporal progression of ischemia. Three types of peripheral nerve involvement can be distinguished, although considerable overlap occurs between types (Figure 80.30): (1) multiple mononeuropathies with motor and sensory deficits restricted to the distribution of individual nerves (10–15%); (2) overlapping or confluent multiple mononeuropathies obscuring individual nerve involvement (60–70%) with severe flaccid weakness and pansensory loss in one or more extremities; and (3) subacute symmetrical, distal sensorimotor neuropathy caused by extensive widespread vasculitis (approximately 30%). This presentation of vasculitic neuropathy can be difficult to distinguish from other types of distal axonopathies and requires a high index of clinical suspicion. A detailed history may indicate that the neuropathy began focally and then followed a course of step-wise progression of deficits before becoming generalized. Initially, acute onset of deep-seated proximal pain in the affected limb is common. Burning pain, sensory loss, and weakness in the distribution of affected nerves develop over several days. However, a more chronic and indolent course with progressive deficits is not infrequent.

Laboratory Features

The laboratory evaluation of patients with suspected vasculitis should be directed toward identifying an underlying disorder or documenting serological abnormalities that may point to a specific vasculitic syndrome. These studies should include sedimentation rate, complete blood count with total eosinophil count, renal function, urinalysis, hepatic enzymes, rheumatoid factor, antinuclear antibody, extractable nuclear antigens, serum complements, antineutrophilic cytoplasmic antibodies, cryoglobulins, hepatitis B antigen and antibody, and hepatitis C antibody. Antineutrophilic cytoplasmic antibody is helpful (elevated in >80%) in the diagnosis of Wegener's granulomatosis, Churg-Strauss syndrome, and microscopic polyangiitis.

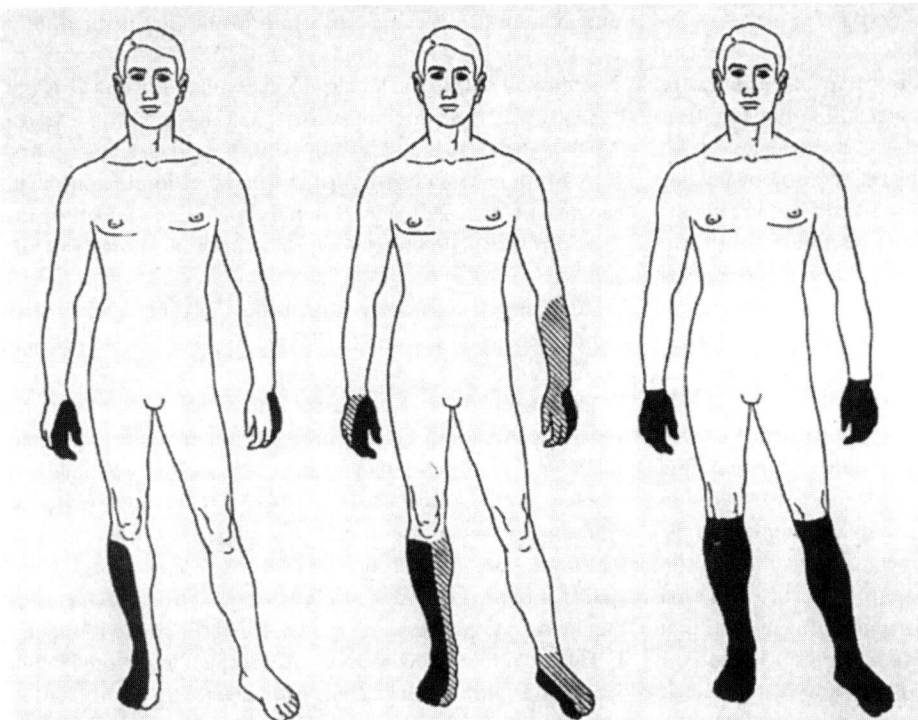

FIGURE 80.30   Clinical patterns of neuropathic involvement in vasculitic neuropathy. The left figure illustrates multiple mononeuropathies or mononeuritis multiplex; the middle figure illustrates overlapping multiple mononeuropathies obscuring individual nerve involvement; the right figure illustrates symmetrical sensorimotor polyneuropathy resulting from extensive proximal ischemic nerve lesions. (Reprinted with permission from JR Mendell, RJ Barohn, EP Bosch, et al. Continuum-peripheral neuropathy. Am Acad Neurol 1994;1:1–103.)

Electrodiagnostic studies are helpful in establishing the pattern of involvement and in documenting axonal nerve damage. Careful study may reveal that what clinically appeared to be a symmetrical polyneuropathy may in fact be an asymmetrical neuropathy, resulting from overlapping mononeuropathies. Nerve conduction studies reveal low-amplitude SNAPs and CMAPs in a multifocal distribution with normal or minimally reduced conduction velocities. Partial motor conduction block may be seen transiently with acute nerve infarcts. EMG demonstrates more widespread denervation than anticipated clinically. A definite diagnosis of vasculitis depends on confirmation of vascular lesions in nerve or muscle biopsies. Combined muscle and cutaneous nerve biopsy specimens often reveal the presence of vasculitis. Of the cutaneous nerves suitable for biopsy, the superficial fibular nerve is preferred because a simultaneous fibularis brevis muscle biopsy can be obtained through the same incision. In several pathological series in which both nerve and muscle specimens were examined, muscle has demonstrated vasculitis more frequently than has nerve. A pathological diagnosis of vasculitis requires the presence of transmural mononuclear inflammatory cells and vessel wall necrosis (Figure 80.31). Cellular infiltrates are composed predominantly of T cells and macrophages. Vascular deposits of immunoglobulins and complement including membrane attack complex can be demonstrated by immunostaining in over 80% of cases. The nerve itself characteristically shows selective fascicular involvement with extensive fiber loss or multifocal subfascicular or central fascicular loss of fibers with acute axonal degeneration. Osmicated teased fiber preparations demonstrate fibers at various stages of axonal degeneration.

Treatment

In systemic necrotizing vasculitis, disease activity must be suppressed rapidly to limit ongoing organ and nerve damage. Such patients are treated with a combination of prednisone and a cytostatic agent (usually cyclophosphamide). Treatment is started with oral cyclophosphamide at 2 mg/kg of body weight per day, together with daily prednisone (1.5 mg/kg/day). In fulminant cases, corticosteroids may be initiated by giving intravenous methylprednisolone (500–1,000 mg) daily for 3 days followed by oral prednisone. The role of plasmapheresis in the management of severe vasculitis remains controversial but may provide additional benefit in patients with life-threatening disease (Allen and Bressler 1997). From the onset of treatment, complete blood cell counts should be monitored frequently. The dose of cyclophosphamide should be adjusted frequently to maintain the total absolute lymphocyte count approximately 750 per µl, while maintaining the total leukocyte count above 3,000 per µl, and the total neutrophil count greater than 1,500 per µl. Maintenance of total leukocyte and neutrophil counts above these levels is critical because life-threatening infections tend to occur at lower levels. Platelet and red cell counts also should be monitored to ensure they do not fall to dangerous levels. Liberal fluid intake and frequent voiding may lessen

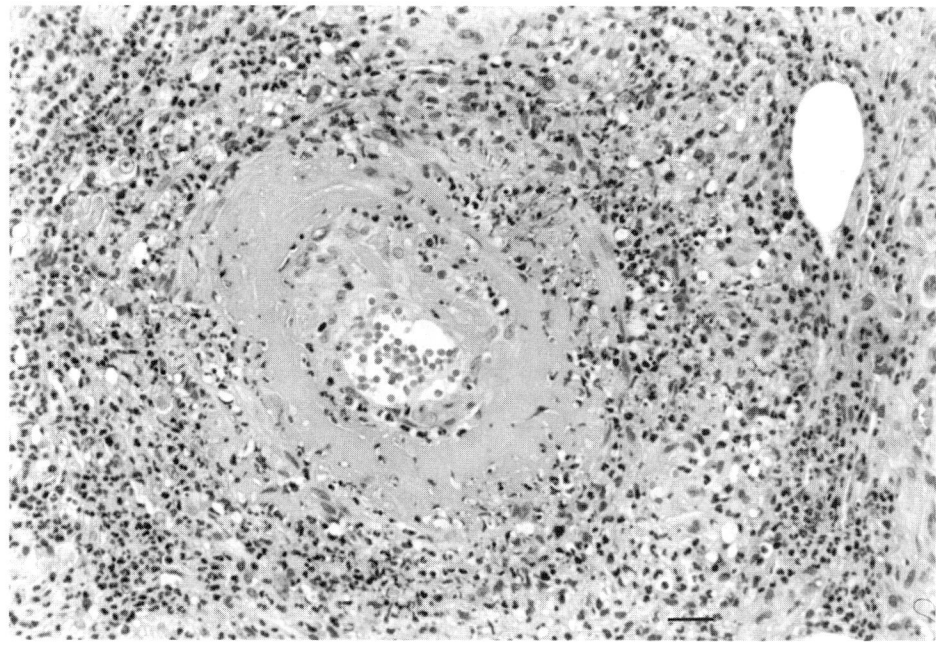

FIGURE 80.31 Sural nerve biopsy from patient with systemic vasculitis. A medium-sized epineurial blood vessel with fibrinoid necrosis of its wall and perivascular and transmural mononuclear cell infiltration is shown. (Hematoxylin and eosin, ×75; bar = 25 μm.)

the risk of hemorrhagic cystitis, which develops in approximately 15% of patients on oral cyclophosphamide. Urine should be monitored for the presence of microscopic hematuria. As surveillance for bladder cancer, urine cytology should be obtained every 6 months. Once clinical remission is achieved, prednisone can be tapered over a period of 4–6 weeks to a dosage of 1 mg/kg every other day. Patients are kept on both drugs until significant improvement occurs, at which time prednisone is gradually tapered. Cyclophosphamide is maintained for 1 year after the disappearance of all traces of disease activity. Combination immunosuppressive therapy results in an 80–90% remission rate in Wegener's granulomatosis and systemic necrotizing vasculitis. Death attributed to the underlying systemic necrotizing vasculitis has been reduced dramatically since cyclophosphamide was added to the treatment regime. Slow recovery from the neurological deficits is likely in survivors. Physical and occupational therapy is indicated to optimize activities of daily living. Meaningful recovery has been reported in 60% at 6 months and 86% of patients at 1 year. Patients with nonsystemic vasculitic neuropathy or giant cell arteritis may be treated initially with prednisone alone.

Rheumatoid Arthritis

Peripheral neuropathy occurs in 1–10% of patients with rheumatoid arthritis. At least four distinct types of peripheral neuropathies are seen in association with rheumatoid arthritis: (1) compression neuropathies, often found with early disease and caused by periarticular inflammation and fibrosis; (2) a distal, symmetrical, sensory polyneuropathy, possibly related to occlusive vasculopathy; (3) mononeuropathy or multiple mononeuropathies; and (4) a severe fulminating sensorimotor polyneuropathy, both caused by rheumatoid vasculitis.

Compression neuropathies in rheumatoid arthritis occur as a result of joint deformity or, on rare occasions, rheumatoid nodules. Treatment includes splint applications, local corticosteroid injection, or surgical decompression.

A symmetrical, predominantly sensory polyneuropathy causes dysesthesias, paresthesias, and loss of sensation in a patchy, stocking-glove distribution. It is not associated with severe active rheumatoid arthritis; most patients recover partially or completely. The pathogenesis is poorly understood. Ischemia caused by occlusive vasculopathy or low-grade vasculitis have been suggested as possible mechanisms. Because the prognosis is generally good, no specific treatment is recommended.

Systemic vasculitis develops in the setting of severe chronic rheumatoid arthritis, characterized by severe joint deformities, rheumatoid nodules, and cutaneous vasculitic lesions such as digital ulcerations, purpura, and livedo. Rheumatoid vasculitis is the second most frequently identified cause of vasculitic neuropathy, because rheumatoid arthritis is a common disorder affecting 2–5% of the general population. Acute mononeuropathy, mononeuropathy multiplex, and a distal symmetrical sensorimotor polyneuropathy develop as a result of widespread vasculitis. In contrast to other connective tissue disorders, cranial nerve involvement is rare.

The sedimentation rate and rheumatoid factor titer are always elevated. The C4 complement level is frequently low. Cutaneous nerve or muscle biopsy demonstrate a necrotizing vasculitis. The development of systemic vasculitis confers a poor prognosis in rheumatoid arthritis, with a reported 5-

year survival rate of 60% (Puéchal et al. 1995). Treatment should be started with high-dose prednisone and oral cyclophosphamide. Early aggressive intervention may arrest the progression of neuropathy.

Systemic Lupus Erythematosus

CNS manifestations are more prevalent than those of the PNS in systemic lupus erythematosus. Peripheral neuropathy develops in 6–21% of patients; the higher frequency is found by using quantitative sensory testing combined with extensive nerve conduction studies. A symmetrical, subacute, or chronic axonal polyneuropathy with predominant sensory symptoms is most common. Mononeuropathies of limb or cranial nerves, brachial plexopathy, and GBS or CIDP have occasionally been described in association with systemic lupus erythematosus. The basis for such associations is unknown but specific autoantibodies against peripheral nerve antigens or an immune-mediated vasculitis are proposed pathogenetic mechanisms.

On sural nerve biopsy specimens perivascular inflammatory cell infiltration is seen around epineurial vessels, but only occasionally definite vasculitis. Immune complex deposition leading to vasculitis is the presumed cause of nerve damage.

If the polyneuropathy associated with systemic lupus erythematosus results in significant disability, immunosuppressive treatment should be considered. In patients with proven vasculitis, treatment with plasmapheresis, prednisone, and cyclophosphamide has led to improvement.

Systemic Sclerosis

Systemic sclerosis (scleroderma) is a connective tissue disease characterized by excessive deposition of collagen. It affects the skin, gastrointestinal tract, lungs, heart, and kidneys. Neurological complications are uncommon, consisting mainly of myopathies. Peripheral nerve involvement unexplained by gastrointestinal or renal complications is rare. Peripheral sensorimotor neuropathy, isolated trigeminal neuropathy, and mononeuropathy related to carpal and cubital tunnel syndromes have been reported. Multiple mononeuropathies are seen with greater frequency in CREST (calcinosis, Raynaud's phenomenon, esophageal dysmotility, sclerodactyly, and telangiectasia) syndrome than in control subjects. Frank vasculitis, perivascular inflammation, and multifocal fiber loss is found in sural nerve biopsy specimens of CREST patients with multiple mononeuropathies (Dyck et al. 1997).

Sjögren's Syndrome

Sjögren's syndrome is an autoimmune disorder of exocrine glands characterized by diminished lacrimal and salivary gland secretion resulting in dry eyes and dry mouth (sicca complex). The sicca complex is related to lymphocytic and plasma cell infiltration and destruction of lacrimal and salivary glands. Sjögren's syndrome occurs as a primary or secondary disorder in association with other connective tissue disorders. Peripheral nerve involvement occurs in 10–32% of patients with primary Sjögren's syndrome and has a strong predilection for women (9 to 1). Neuropathic symptoms often precede and overshadow the sicca symptoms and may be the major presenting complaint (Grant et al. 1997). A distal symmetrical sensory neuropathy with mixed large and small fiber deficits is the most common presentation. Less common patterns of nerve involvement include sensorimotor neuropathy, polyradiculoneuropathy, multiple mononeuropathies, and trigeminal sensory neuropathy. A distinct subgroup of patients with sensory neuropathy presents with loss of kinesthesia and proprioception caused by an inflammatory sensory polyganglionopathy (Figure 80.32). For a differential diagnosis of sensory ataxic neuronopathies see Table 80.25.

Elevated sedimentation rate, rheumatoid factor, and hypergammaglobulinemia may be present. Antibodies to extractable nuclear antigens (SS-A) are seldom found in patients with neuropathy. The diagnosis depends on specific inquiry about sicca symptoms and confirmation of eye involvement with rose Bengal staining of the cornea or by Schirmer test (<5 mm wetting of a paper strip at 5 minutes). When an abnormal test result is found, a minor salivary gland biopsy of the lower lip showing chronic lymphocytic infiltrates is necessary for confirmation. Sural nerve biopsy frequently shows nonspecific perivascular lymphocytic (T cell) infiltrates together with diffuse decrease in myelinated fibers. Vasculitis is rarely found in patients with multiple mononeuropathies.

The role of immunosuppressive therapy is uncertain. Few patients respond to prednisone alone.

Trigeminal Sensory Neuropathy

This slowly progressive trigeminal sensory neuropathy is characterized by advancing unilateral or bilateral facial numbness. An association has been reported with several connective tissue diseases, including systemic sclerosis, mixed or undifferentiated connective tissue disease, Sjögren's syndrome, systemic lupus erythematosus, rheumatoid arthritis, and dermatomyositis. Sensory loss begins in perioral and cheek areas and is often associated with painful paresthesia. The frequent bilateral involvement (70%), sparing of muscles of mastication, and negative neuroimaging study results help to distinguish this condition from other causes of facial numbness. Disfiguring neuropathic ulceration of the nares may occur. The trigeminal blink reflex study confirms an afferent lesion that is detected by delayed or absent ipsilateral R1 and bilateral R2 responses in 50% of patients. The precise etiology of this presumed immune-mediated cranial sensory ganglionopathy remains unclear. Immunosuppressive therapy is not recommended in isolated trigeminal sensory neuropathy.

Other causes of trigeminal neuropathy are acute toxic reactions to trichloroethylene and the "numb chin" syndrome associated with a carcinoma or vasculitis (see Chapter 74).

Sarcoidosis

Sarcoidosis is a multisystem granulomatous disorder involving lung, lymph nodes, skin, and eyes. Neurological involvement (neurosarcoidosis) occurs in approximately 5% of patients, and 6–18% of neurological manifestations are caused by various forms of peripheral neuropathy (Scott 1993). Cranial neuropathies, particularly facial nerve palsy, are the most common neurological manifestations (73%). PNS involvement includes multiple mononeuropathies, bilateral phrenic nerve palsies, truncal sensory mononeuropathies, acute polyradiculoneuropathy resembling GBS, cauda equina syndrome, and chronic symmetrical sensorimotor neuropathy. The latter can produce severe wrist extensor and foot dorsiflexor weakness, and distal sensory loss in the legs. Neurological manifestations may be the presenting feature in more than 50% of cases or may develop at a time when there is little evidence of systemic sarcoidosis.

Electrodiagnostic studies show evidence of axonal degeneration. Sarcoid granulomas may be seen in muscle and sural nerve biopsy specimens. The nerve damage has been attributed to granulomas and angiitis of vasa nervorum producing axonal degeneration. If there are inflammatory changes in the CSF (such as pleocytosis, increased protein level, elevated IgG index, and occasionally hypoglycorrhachia), this implies granulomatous leptomeningeal involvement. Gallium scanning is often useful in the search for systemic involvement. An elevated serum angiotensin-converting enzyme level may suggest active systemic sarcoidosis. Biopsies of lymph nodes, muscle, or conjunctiva or bronchoalveolar lavage may be helpful in obtaining tissue for histological confirmation.

The response to corticosteroid therapy in sarcoid neuropathy is generally favorable. In patients refractory to corticosteroids, cyclosporine, cyclophosphamide, or azathioprine may be used as adjunctive therapy (Agbogu et al. 1995).

Alcoholic Neuropathy and Nutritional Deficiencies

Alcoholic Neuropathy

Alcoholic neuropathy is one of the most common peripheral neuropathies seen in general practice. Covert alcoholism may only be uncovered by a focused history provided by family members. A close association between alcoholic neuropathy and nutritional deficiency is well established.

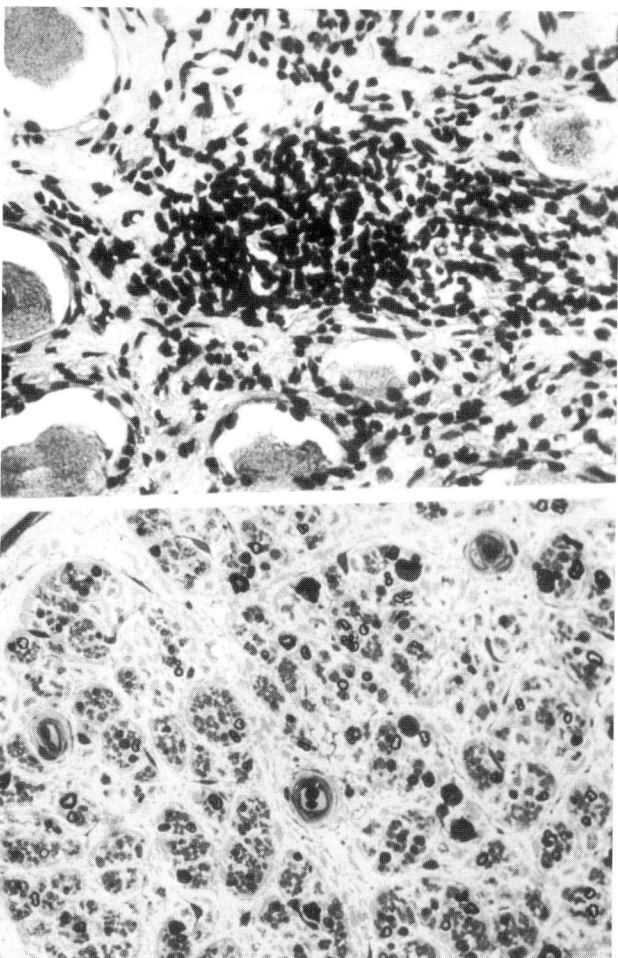

FIGURE 80.32   Thoracic dorsal root ganglion and sural nerve biopsies from patient with Sjögren's syndrome and nonmalignant inflammatory sensory polyganglionopathy. In the upper panel, a prominent mononuclear cell infiltrate is seen adjacent to neuronal cell bodies. (Hematoxylin and eosin; ×25.) The lower panel illustrates the sural nerve in the same patient showing marked decrease in fiber density and abnormality in size distribution of myelinated fibers. (Paraphenylenediamine-stained semithin epoxy section; ×25.) (Reprinted with permission from BE Smith. Inflammatory sensory polyganglionopathies. Neurol Clin 1992;10:735–759.)

Clinical Features. The symptoms of alcoholic neuropathy begin insidiously and progress slowly. Muscle weakness begins distally and spreads to more proximal muscles. Gait difficulty, weakness, and muscle cramps are common. Sensory loss and burning paresthesia are frequent. Hyperpathia and dysesthesia are troublesome in many patients. The legs are always more affected than the arms. Distal muscle wasting, loss of tendon reflexes, and sensory loss of all modalities in a stocking-glove distribution are common. In advanced cases, sensory ataxia caused by loss of joint position sense may coexist with alcoholic cerebellar ataxia.

Electrodiagnostic studies show a predominantly axonal sensorimotor polyneuropathy. NCVs are only slightly diminished. Low-amplitude or absent SNAPs are common. EMG shows active denervation with chronic reinnervation in distal muscles. Sural nerve biopsy specimens demonstrate loss of nerve fibers of all sizes. Acute axonal degeneration is particularly common in patients after binge drinking, whereas axonal regeneration is frequently seen in chronic alcoholism.

Etiology. Deficiency of thiamine and other B vitamins, caused by inadequate dietary intake, impaired absorption, and greater demand for thiamine to catalyze the metabolism of the alcohol, are the major causes of polyneuropathy in alcoholic patients.

Treatment. Abstinence from alcohol, expert counseling, and a nutritionally balanced diet constitute the principal therapy. Supplementation with thiamine and other B vitamins is important. In patients with significant gastrointestinal symptoms, parenteral vitamin treatment is initially required. Improvement in the polyneuropathy may be very slow, because it requires axonal regeneration. For the management of painful alcoholic neuropathy, see the earlier section on neuropathic pain.

Pellagra Neuropathy

Dietary deficiency of nicotinic acid (niacin) produces the syndrome of pellagra. Pellagra affects the gastrointestinal tract, skin, and nervous system resulting in the triad of dermatitis, diarrhea, and dementia. A distal sensorimotor polyneuropathy develops in 40–56% of patients with pellagra, and if diarrhea and skin changes are absent, is clinically indistinguishable from thiamine-deficiency neuropathy. Nonendemic pellagra rarely occurs in patients with alcoholism or malabsorption. Oral nicotinic acid is sufficient to treat symptomatic patients.

Pyridoxine (Vitamin B_6) Deficiency

The regular diet of most adults is adequate for the daily requirement of 1.5–2.0 mg of vitamin B_6. Isolated pyridoxine deficiency, however, may occur during treatment with isoniazid (INH), hydralazine, or, rarely, penicillamine. These drugs structurally resemble vitamin B_6 and interfere with pyridoxine coenzyme activity. Vitamin B_6-deficient peripheral neuropathy is characterized by distal sensory and motor deficits of insidious onset. When using INH, supplementary pyridoxine (100 mg daily) is recommended. Paradoxically, megadoses (500 mg/day and greater) of pyridoxine may cause a predominantly sensory polyneuropathy (see Toxic Neuropathies, later in this chapter).

Folate Deficiency Polyneuropathy

Folate deficiency may cause an axonal sensory polyneuropathy, characterized clinically by loss of joint position and vibratory sense and absent tendon reflexes. Addition-

ally, there may be evidence of spinal cord involvement, with spasticity of the legs and extensor plantar responses. In severe cases, encephalopathic symptoms may predominate. Macrocytic anemia is an important clue to either folate or vitamin B_{12} deficiency. Coexisting vitamin B_{12} deficiency must be excluded because folate therapy without cobalamin replacement may exacerbate neurological manifestations. Patients have been reported with neurological disease indistinguishable from subacute combined degeneration who rapidly responded to folate replacement.

Vitamin B_{12} Deficiency Polyneuropathy: Subacute Combined Degeneration

Cobalamin (vitamin B_{12}) and folate are essential vitamins necessary for effective DNA synthesis. Animal products (meat, poultry, fish, and dairy products) are the primary dietary source of cobalamin. The average Western diet provides an excess of the vitamin (daily requirement, 3–9 μg), which is stored in the liver. Within the acid environment of the stomach cobalamin is released from dietary proteins. Free cobalamin initially binds to gastric glycoproteins known as R-binders. In the duodenum the cobalamin-R-binder complexes are degraded by pancreatic enzymes. The released cobalamin then binds avidly to intrinsic factor, a 60-kD glycoprotein produced by gastric parietal cells. The vitamin B_{12}–intrinsic factor complex is absorbed by means of binding to intrinsic factor receptors in the terminal ileum. Malabsorption of cobalamin in patients with pernicious anemia is caused by intrinsic factor deficiency caused by progressive autoimmune destruction of parietal cells from the gastric mucosa. Acquired malabsorption of vitamin B_{12} may occur also following gastric and ileal resection and in the setting of a wide range of gastrointestinal disorders. Unusual causes include dietary insufficiency in strict vegetarians and fish tapeworms. Intraoperative use or recreational abuse of nitrous oxide, which inactivates cobalamin-dependent enzymes, may cause neurological manifestations, particularly in patients with marginal cobalamin stores. Intracellularly, cobalamin is converted into two coenzymes required for the formation of methionine and succinyl-CoA synthesis. Reduced methionine synthesis may be responsible for the neurological manifestations of cobalamin deficiency.

Population surveys estimate that 2% of persons 60 years and older have undiagnosed pernicious anemia. The disease is especially common in Northern Europeans and African Americans. The full-blown clinical picture of vitamin B_{12} deficiency consists of macrocytic anemia, atrophic glossitis, and neurological complications (Toh et al. 1997). The latter include peripheral neuropathy and optic atrophy, as well as lesions in the posterior and lateral columns of the spinal cord (subacute combined degeneration) and in the brain. The peripheral neuropathy results in paresthesias and large fiber modality sensory loss (vibration and proprioception). The spinal cord manifestations consist of posterior column damage, which may include a sensory level, and upper motor neuron defects causing limb weakness, spasticity, and extensor plantar responses. Cerebral involvement ranges from subtle behavioral changes and forgetfulness to dementia or stupor. An unsteady gait and positive Romberg's sign reflecting a sensory ataxia, and diffuse hyperreflexia and absent ankle jerks should raise the suspicion of cobalamin deficiency.

Nerve conduction studies show low-amplitude or absent SNAPs. Conduction velocities are normal. CNS involvement is suggested by abnormal visual and somatosensory evoked potential study results and is occasionally documented by confluent white matter abnormalities on brain MRI. Evidence of axonal degeneration is found in sural nerve biopsy specimens. The diagnosis is confirmed by low serum vitamin B_{12} levels (<170 pg/ml) and normal serum folate concentration. Approximately 30–40% of patients with neurological symptoms caused by vitamin B_{12} deficiency have borderline low levels of 150–200 pg/ml. In as many as 30% of patients, megaloblastic anemia with elevated red cell mean corpuscular volume (>94 fl) may be absent. Elevated serum methylmalonic acid and homocysteine levels, which are the substrates for cobalamin-dependent enzymes, are helpful when there is diagnostic uncertainty (Chanarin and Metz 1997). The two-part Schilling tests confirm that vitamin B_{12} deficiency is the result of intestinal malabsorption and caused by intrinsic factor deficiency. Antibodies to intrinsic factor are found in 70% of patients with pernicious anemia; antiparietal cell antibodies are more sensitive (90%) but lack specificity.

Initial treatment consists of daily intramuscular injections of 1 mg of cyanocobalamin or hydroxocobalamin in the first week, followed by weekly injections, until a series of 12 doses is completed. Then maintenance schedules of monthly injections of 100 μg or 1,000 μg every 3 months has been found satisfactory in preventing relapses (Savage and Lindenbaum 1995). This treatment corrects the anemia and may reverse the neurological complications completely if given soon after their onset. Major neurological improvement can be expected to occur during the first 3–6 months of therapy. For maintenance therapy, oral administration of vitamin B_{12} is feasible in compliant patients, because 1% of vitamin B_{12} is absorbed without intrinsic factor mediation. The initial severity of neurological deficits, duration of symptoms, and hemoglobin level before treatment correlate with neurological outcome. The inverse correlation between degree of anemia and neurological damage is not understood.

Vitamin E Deficiency

Significant vitamin E deficiency is seen in children and young adults with chronic severe intestinal fat malabsorption, as occurs in cholestatic liver disease, cystic fibrosis, celiac disease, following extensive intestinal resections, and in the inherited disorder of abetalipoproteinemia (see Hereditary Neuropathies, previously in this chapter). Rarely, vitamin E deficiency develops in the absence of fat malabsorption (Jackson et al. 1996). Isolated vitamin E deficiency is an autosomal recessive disorder in which mutations in the α-tocopherol transfer protein gene on chromosome 8q13 have been identified. Many years are required before neuromuscular symptoms develop in chronic vitamin E deficiency. A spinocerebellar syndrome similar to Friedreich's ataxia occurs, with a large fiber sensory neuropathy, weakness, ataxia, proprioceptive loss, areflexia, ophthalmoplegia, and pigmentary retinopathy. Myopathy and peripheral nerve disease may predominate in some cases.

The clinical syndrome of vitamin E deficiency is caused by a distal central-peripheral axonopathy of large-caliber axons affecting peripheral nerves and the posterior columns of the spinal cord, probably part of a multisystem degeneration caused by vitamin E deficiency. Lipofuscinlike accumulations are found in Schmidt-Lantermann clefts in sural nerve biopsy specimens. Impaired antioxidant protection may account for neurological and retinal lesions in longstanding deficiency. Electrophysiological study results show normal NCVs and low-amplitude or absent SNAPs. Vitamin E deficiency is established by low fasting plasma levels of vitamin E (<5 μg/ml). Laboratory studies used to confirm fat malabsorption include 72-hour fecal fat determination, vitamin A and D levels, amylase, liver function tests, peripheral blood smear to search for acanthocytes, and apolipoprotein B level.

Vitamin E supplementation is indicated regardless of etiology in all patients with low serum vitamin E levels. Oral supplementation with vitamin E in large doses (initially 400 mg twice daily and up to 100 mg/kg/day) may result in neurological improvement or cessation of further deterioration. If no absorption can be documented after a large oral loading dose of vitamin E, intramuscular therapy in doses of 100 mg per week is recommended.

Neuropathy Associated with Malabsorption Syndromes

Intestinal malabsorption may lead to myopathy or peripheral neuropathy. A careful search for occult malabsorption is important in patients with neuromuscular disease of unknown cause. Celiac disease or gluten enteropathy is rarely (5–8%) associated with varied neurological complications including a predominantly sensory axonal neuropathy, multiple mononeuropathies, ataxia, myelopathy, and encephalopathy. The cause of PNS involvement is poorly understood. Most studies have implicated vitamin deficiencies (B_{12}, E, D, folic acid, or pyridoxine). However, vitamin replacement rarely improves neurological deficits. Immunological factors have been proposed in patients without vitamin deficiencies.

Severe sensorimotor or predominantly sensory neuropathies with ataxia or burning feet may occur in starvation. After gastric partitioning procedures for morbid obesity, the patients at risk for developing neurological complications are those with accelerated weight loss and frequent vomiting in the postoperative period.

Uremic Neuropathy

Peripheral neuropathy develops in 80% of patients with end-stage renal failure who require chronic dialysis. Because chronic renal failure is now effectively treated with dialysis or renal transplantation, severe uremic neuropathy has become less frequent.

Uremic neuropathy is inexplicably more common in men than in women. The clinical features are those of a slowly progressive, predominantly sensory polyneuropathy. Severe pains are unusual, but cramps, unpleasant dysesthesias, and the restless legs syndrome occur. Muscle weakness involves mostly distal foot muscles. There is a graded loss of vibratory and joint position sense to a much greater extent than superficial pain and temperature sensations. The Achilles reflexes are absent. On rare occasions, uremic neuropathy develops abruptly in the initial few weeks of dialysis, mimicking GBS. The combination of uremic and diabetic neuropathies can produce an unusually severe polyneuropathy. A subacute predominantly motor polyneuropathy may develop in diabetic patients in end-stage renal failure on dialysis. An unusual feature of these cases is the relative absence of denervation potentials in clinically weak muscles on needle EMG. Some patients have improved by switching from conventional to high-flux hemodialysis, possibly related to enhanced removal of advanced glycosylation products (Bolton et al. 1997).

Compression neuropathies of the ulnar nerve at the elbow or the peroneal nerve at the fibular head may occur in cachectic patients recumbent for long periods. Carpal tunnel syndrome may be related to the presence of vascular shunts, or develop because of the deposition of β_2-microglobulin–associated amyloid in the carpal ligament in patients on long-term hemodialysis. Ischemic monomelic neuropathy is another serious complication of arteriovenous shunt placement that occurs almost exclusively in uremic diabetic patients with concomitant atherosclerotic vascular disease. The onset is abrupt and painful, and prompt surgical closure of the fistula is required to avoid permanent neurological deficits.

The diagnosis of uremic polyneuropathy should only be made in the context of chronic end-stage renal failure (creatinine clearance <10 ml/minute) of at least several months' duration. Drug toxicity or other systemic diseases, such as diabetes mellitus, vasculitis, or amyloidosis that may affect both kidneys and peripheral nerves, must first be excluded. Nitrofurantoin is a common cause of severe neuropathy in renal insufficiency.

CSF protein is often elevated, but rarely beyond 100 mg/dl. Generalized slowing of motor and sensory NCVs is common, and distal latencies are prolonged. Late responses (H-reflex and F-wave latencies) become abnormally prolonged early in the course of chronic renal failure at a time when motor conduction velocities are still normal. EMG examination shows evidence of active denervation in distal foot muscles. Regular hemodialysis rarely improves impaired conduction velocities in patients despite clinical improvement. Sural nerve biopsy shows axonal loss of large myelinated fibers and segmental demyelination. Morphometric investigations indicate that associated segmental demyelination is secondary to primary axonal atrophy.

The pathogenesis of uremic neuropathy is most likely secondary to the accumulation of systemic toxins, although no specific toxic factors have been isolated. Ethylene oxide has been proposed as a neurotoxin in patients on hemodialysis.

Treatment

The neuropathy usually remains stable or improves with chronic dialysis. If the neuropathy worsens during hemodialysis, it may be necessary to increase the frequency and duration of dialysis. There is little difference between hemodialysis and peritoneal dialysis in their effect on nerve function. Renal transplantation provides more significant improvement.

Peripheral Neuropathy in Liver Disease

Several neuropathic syndromes have been associated with acute and chronic liver disease. Acute GBS may sometimes develop as a complication of viral hepatitis A, usually occurring after the onset of jaundice. Hepatitis B has been linked with both acute and chronic demyelinating neuropathies. Hepatitis B antigenemia is found in one-third of the patients with polyarteritis nodosa. Most patients with mixed cryoglobulinemic vasculitis have an associated infection with hepatitis C virus.

In chronic cirrhosis, although a clinically overt neuropathy is uncommon, electrodiagnostic study results are frequently abnormal. The most common clinical features include paresthesia and dysesthesia in a stocking-glove distribution, loss of vibratory sense, and diminished tendon reflexes. Histological studies of the sural nerve show evidence of demyelination and remyelination.

Patients with primary biliary cirrhosis may develop a sensory polyneuropathy or dorsal root ganglionopathy. In some patients xanthomatous infiltration of cutaneous nerves has been found but in others an autoimmune process affecting dorsal root ganglia is suspected. The prevalence of associated autoimmune diseases is high in primary biliary cirrhosis, most notably Sjögren's syndrome, which in turn is linked to predominantly sensory neuropathies. Large fiber sensory neuropathies develop in children and young adults with chronic cholestatic liver disease and secondary vitamin E deficiency.

Endocrine Disorders Associated with Peripheral Neuropathy

Hypothyroid Neuropathy

Carpal tunnel syndrome is the most common peripheral nerve complication of hypothyroidism. One-third of patients with hypothyroidism may have clinical evidence of general polyneuropathy, which is predominantly sensory with paresthesias and muscle pain, distal sensory loss, and incoordination. Nerve conduction studies show absent or decreased SNAPs and slow motor conduction velocities. Sural nerve biopsy demonstrates demyelination and remyelination and increased glycogen and lysosomes in axonal and Schwann cell cytoplasm. Thyroid hormone replacement usually improves the neuropathy. Thyroid function studies should be checked in all patients presenting with carpal tunnel syndrome or a sensory polyneuropathy.

Acromegaly

Carpal tunnel syndrome is a well-recognized complication of acromegaly, but a generalized neuropathy also may develop independent of concomitant diabetes mellitus. Approximately one-half of patients have distal paresthesia, sensory loss in a stocking-glove distribution, diminished muscle stretch reflexes, and distal muscle weakness. SNAPs are diminished and motor NCVs are slightly to moderately reduced. Nerve biopsy shows enlargement of nerve fascicles because of an increase in endoneurial and subperineurial tissue and a reduced number of myelinated and unmyelinated fibers.

Hypoglycemic Amyotrophy

Primary hypoglycemia caused by insulinoma may cause slowly progressive distal muscle atrophy and weakness. Painful paresthesias are common, but there are usually no objective signs of sensory loss. The amyotrophy may precede the onset of typical recurrent hypoglycemic episodes by a few years. Electrodiagnostic studies show evidence of acute denervation and reinnervation.

Ischemic Monomelic Neuropathy

Ischemia caused by acute thromboembolic occlusion of major limb arteries or proximal arteriovenous shunt placement infrequently causes multiple axonal mononeuropathies that develop distally in the ischemic limb (ischemic monomelic neuropathy). Abrupt lightning or burning pains affect the involved extremity. Sensory examination shows a graded impairment of all modalities, particularly those mediated by large-diameter fibers. Muscle strength is usually maintained, although distal weakness may develop in severe cases. Tendon reflexes may be preserved.

Electrodiagnostic studies provide evidence of multiple axonal mononeuropathies in the involved ischemic limb. SNAPs are either absent or markedly reduced in amplitude, and motor conduction velocities are slowed. Acute denervation is limited to very distal extremity muscles. Both large and small fibers appear to be affected equally.

Surgical endarterectomy or bypass surgery may result in recovery of neurological deficits in a period of several months, even in long-standing ischemic neuropathy. Ischemic monomelic mononeuropathy following shunt placement demands immediate surgical closure of the arteriovenous fistula.

Severe aortoiliac occlusive disease or prolonged use of an intra-aortic balloon pump may occasionally lead to proximal sciatic and femoral nerve lesions, and also lumbosacral plexus lesions, caused by nerve infarcts in watershed areas between the distributions of major feeding arteries.

Peripheral Neuropathy in Chronic Obstructive Lung Disease

Approximately 20% of patients with chronic obstructive lung disease may develop a mild, distal sensorimotor polyneuropathy that appears to be correlated with severe hypoxemia.

Critical Illness Polyneuropathy

Critical illness polyneuropathy is a relatively common problem in intensive care units. When prospectively investigated, 50% of critically ill patients admitted to intensive care units with sepsis and multiple organ failure have electrodiagnostic features of an axonal neuropathy. This neuropathy is a major cause of difficulty in weaning patients from the respirator after cardiac and pulmonary causes have been excluded. Clinical evaluation of neuromuscular weakness acquired in the intensive care unit may be difficult because patients are often encephalopathic or sedated. Most have generalized flaccid weakness with depressed tendon reflexes. Pain or paresthesias are not major features of critical illness neuropathy.

Electrodiagnostic studies are necessary to establish the diagnosis. Nerve conduction studies reveal a distal axonal neuropathy with reduced CMAP and SNAP amplitudes, in conjunction with fibrillation potentials and decreased motor unit potentials on EMG. CSF is almost always normal. Primary axonal degeneration, more severe distally than proximally, is seen at autopsy. The neuropathy is thought to be a complication of the systemic inflammatory response syndrome that is triggered by sepsis, severe trauma, or burns. The pathophysiology of this syndrome is currently under intense investigation. Infection or trauma appears to initiate a series of events that ultimately lead to impaired microcirculation and multiple organ dysfunction

(Bolton 1995). In the setting of critical illness, an acute myopathy may develop also. This complication usually occurs in patients with asthma receiving high doses of intravenous corticosteroids and neuromuscular blocking agents. Plasma creatine kinase levels are transiently elevated. Muscle biopsy shows many fibers with loss of thick filaments (Lacomis et al. 1996). The presence of normal sensory conduction studies and small, short-duration, polyphasic motor unit potentials on EMG help to distinguish critical illness myopathy from its neuropathic counterpart. Repetitive nerve stimulation studies should be performed to exclude a defect of neuromuscular transmission caused by defective clearance of neuromuscular blocking agents.

Survivors slowly recover in 3–6 months following discharge from the intensive care unit.

Neuropathy Associated with Bone Marrow and Organ Transplantation

Peripheral neuropathy may complicate bone marrow or solid organ transplantation as a result of direct neurotoxic effects of chemotherapeutic or immunosuppressive agents, critical illness, or autoimmune responses cross-reacting with peripheral nerve. In some bone marrow transplant patients peripheral neuropathies resembling GBS or CIDP may develop in association with graft-versus-host disease. The clinical features consist of generalized polyneuropathy affecting proximal and distal muscles, hyporeflexia, and variable sensory loss. Increased CSF protein without pleocytosis is usually present. Electrodiagnostic studies may not meet strict criteria for demyelination. Patients improve with resolution of the underlying graft-versus-host disease (Amato et al. 1993).

TOXIC NEUROPATHIES

Peripheral neuropathy is one of the most common reactions of the nervous system to toxic chemicals. Industrial, environmental and biological agents, heavy metals, and pharmaceutical agents are known to cause toxic neuropathies (see Chapter 64). Drugs, most notably anticancer drugs, are the most common offenders in clinical practice today. Neurotoxic agents may produce distal axonal degeneration (axonopathy), nerve cell body degeneration (neuronopathy), or primary demyelination (myelinopathy) (see Pathological Processes Involving Peripheral Nerves, earlier in this chapter). The biochemical pathogenesis of toxic neuropathies remains, in many instances, poorly understood.

Most toxins produce symmetrical axonal degeneration in a dying-back pattern, beginning in the distal segments of long, large-caliber PNS fibers, which eventually spreads proximally with continued exposure. Many toxic axonopathies also affect the CNS with concurrent distal degeneration of dorsal column central projections of sensory neurons, and optic nerves; this contributes to incomplete recovery. Agents, such as n-hexane or organophosphates, causing simultaneous degeneration of corticospinal pathways may cause spasticity, which becomes apparent following the recovery from the peripheral axonopathy. Electrophysiological studies usually disclose evidence of axonal dysfunction.

The second type of toxin-induced axonal degeneration follows a neuronopathy or ganglionopathy. Methyl-mercury compounds, megadoses of pyridoxine, and doxorubicin are examples of toxins that produce neuronal degeneration. The neuronal loss limits functional recovery.

Primary demyelination is a less frequent mechanism; it occurs with diphtheria, buckthorn toxin, perhexiline, amiodarone, and suramin. Secondary demyelination is seen in hexacarbon neuropathy. In these situations, considerable reduction in NCV is found.

To establish a causal link between a potential neurotoxin and neuropathy, the following clinical criteria should be met:

- Exposure must be verified and temporally related to the onset of clinical symptoms. Neuropathic symptoms usually occur concurrently with the exposure or following a variable latency of up to several months.
- There must be subjective symptoms, neurological signs, and abnormal electrodiagnostic study results.
- Susceptibility factors such as pre-existing neuropathy, simultaneous use of other neurotoxic drugs, or metabolic dysfunction interfering with drug metabolism may increase the risk of developing a severe toxic neuropathy.
- Removal from the exposure results in cessation of progression and improvement, although in certain axonopathies cessation of exposure may be followed by a worsening of symptoms for weeks (coasting) before recovery begins.

A focused history probing for a background of occupational, environmental, or drug exposure is important. Most toxic neuropathies present clinically with length-dependent sensorimotor or purely sensory deficits. Autonomic dysfunction is rarely a prominent feature; exceptions include acrylamide, cisplatin, and *Vinca* alkaloids. Predominantly motor toxic neuropathy is rare, being limited to dapsone, lead, and organophosphate-induced delayed polyneuropathy. Rarely do typical pathological features such as neurofilamentous axonal swellings in hexacarbon neuropathy, or lamellar Schwann cell inclusions in amiodarone and perhexiline allow specific pathological identification of the cause.

The most important steps in treatment involve recognition of the offending agent and elimination of exposure.

Industrial and Environmental Toxins

Industrial and environmental agents that cause toxic neuropathies are discussed in Chapter 64 (Schaumburg and Kaplan 1995).

Table 80.27: Neuropathies caused by drugs

Drugs	Clinical and pathological features	Comment
Antineoplastic		
Cisplatin	S, DA, N	Binds to DNA; disrupts axonal transport?
Suramin	SM, DA, SD	DA: inhibits binding of growth factors; SD: immuno-modulating effects?
Taxoids (paclitaxel, docetaxel)	S, DA	Promote microtubule assembly; disrupt axonal transport
Vincristine	S>M, M, DA	Interferes with microtubule assembly; disrupts axonal transport
Antimicrobial		
Chloroquinine	SM, DA	Myopathy
Dapsone	M, DA	Optic atrophy
Isoniazid	SM, DA	Pyridoxine antagonist
Metronidazole	S, DA	
Nitrofurantoin	SM, DA	
Antiviral		
Dideoxynucleosides (dideoxycytidine, dideoxyinosine, stavudine)	S, DA	
Cardiovascular		
Amiodarone	SM, SD	Lysosomal lamellar inclusions, myopathy
Hydralazine	SM, DA	Pyridoxine antagonist
Perhexiline	SM, SD	Lipid inclusions
CNS		
Nitrous oxide	S, DA	Inhibits vitamin B_{12}–dependent methionine synthase; myelopathy
Thalidomide	S, N	
Other		
Colchicine	SM, DA	Myopathy, raised creatine kinase levels
Disulfiram	SM, DA	
Gold	SM, DA	Myokymia
Phenytoin	SM, DA	Asymptomatic in most
Pyridoxine	S, N, DA	Megadoses >300 mg/day
L-Tryptophan	SM, DA	Eosinophilia-myalgia syndrome

CNS = central nervous system–active drugs; DA = distal axonopathy; M = motor; N = neuronopathy; S = sensory; SD = segmental demyelination; SM = sensorimotor neuropathy.

Drug-Induced Neuropathies

Many pharmaceutical agents can cause peripheral neuropathy, which is generally reversible when the offending drug is discontinued. With the concomitant use of neurotrophins it may be possible in the future to blunt or prevent the dose-limiting neurotoxic effects of anticancer drugs. The neurotrophins are naturally occurring polypeptide growth factors (e.g., NGF, neurotrophin-3, brain-derived nerve growth factor, and insulinlike growth factor–I) that play a role in nerve regeneration and demonstrate neuroprotective properties in experimental studies. If the causal relationship between a potentially neurotoxic drug and neuropathy is established, unnecessary investigations to search for alternative etiologies can be avoided. Most drugs produce a length-dependent sensorimotor axonal neuropathy or pure sensory neuropathy or ganglionopathy. The selective vulnerability of Schwann cells and myelin to perhexiline maleate, amiodarone, and suramin results in primary demyelinating neuropathies. Furthermore, some drugs may cause additional damage to skeletal muscle, involve the CNS with distal degeneration in the corticospinal tracts and dorsal columns, or both.

Awareness of the possibility of drug-induced peripheral nerve damage is important. A careful drug history including over-the-counter vitamin preparations should be obtained in every patient with polyneuropathy. Some of the drugs that consistently produce peripheral neuropathy are listed in Table 80.27. Many anecdotal reports of neuropathy possibly induced by other drugs may represent coincidental occurrences.

Amiodarone

Amiodarone is a class III antiarrhythmic drug used in the management of refractory ventricular arrhythmias. Adverse effects include thyroid abnormalities, photosensitivity dermatitis, corneal microdeposits, hepatic dysfunction, pulmonary fibrosis, and a dose-dependent polyneuropathy. Sensorimotor polyneuropathy may develop in patients receiving long-term amiodarone (400 mg/day) therapy. There is moderate sensory impairment and distal and sometimes proximal muscle weakness. Electrophysiological studies show mild slowing of NCVs along with distal denervation. Nerve biopsy demonstrates loss of myelinated and unmyelinated fibers and axonal degeneration coexistent with segmental demyelination. A distinctive feature is the presence of lysosomal lamellar inclusions in Schwann cells, fibroblasts, and endothelial cells resulting from inactivation of the lysosomal enzyme sphingomyelinase.

Amphetamines

Abusers of amphetamines may develop multiple mononeuropathies caused by necrotizing hypersensitivity angiitis.

Chloramphenicol

Chloramphenicol can produce a peripheral and optic neuropathy following prolonged, high-dose therapy.

Chloroquine

Chloroquine is an antimalarial drug that is used also in the treatment of connective tissue disorders. Typically, a painful vacuolar myopathy with increased serum muscle enzymes develops after prolonged therapy. Chloroquine produces only mild neuropathy. Muscle and sural nerve biopsies show lamellar inclusions in muscle fibers and Schwann cells.

Cisplatin

Cisplatin is used widely in the treatment of ovarian, bladder, and testicular malignancies and squamous cell carcinomas. Cisplatin exerts its chemotherapeutic effects by cross-linking DNA and disrupting cell division. Peripheral neuropathy is the dose-limiting side effect. Cisplatin causes a dose-dependent, predominantly large fiber sensory polyneuropathy. Ototoxicity is common, manifested by tinnitus and high-frequency hearing loss. Paresthesias, Lhermitte's sign, loss of tendon reflexes, prominent proprioceptive loss, and sensory ataxia usually occur when cumulative doses exceed 400 mg/m^2. Autonomic symptoms, especially gastroparesis and vomiting, are frequent. The neuropathy may develop as late as 4 months after the drug has been stopped (coasting). Nerve conduction studies show reduced or absent SNAPs. Nerve biopsy reveals loss of large myelinated fibers and acute axonal degeneration. Most patients receiving cumulative doses below 500 mg/m^2 improve following cessation of therapy. Neurotrophins are currently under investigation to prevent or ameliorate the neurotoxicity of cisplatin.

Colchicine

Colchicine is used for the treatment of gout. Subacute proximal weakness and an associated mild distal axonal neuropathy may occur in patients with mild renal insufficiency receiving conventional doses of colchicine. Markedly elevated serum creatine kinase levels and electrodiagnostic findings of a neuromyopathic process occur. Both weakness and creatine kinase elevations remit after the drug is discontinued.

Dapsone

Dapsone is used in the management of leprosy and other skin disorders. High doses may cause a predominantly motor neuropathy characterized by weakness and atrophy of distal muscles, particularly intrinsic hand muscles. Severe optic neuropathy may occur also. Reduction of motor NCV is slight, even in the presence of severe denervation, suggesting an axonal neuropathy. Recovery is slow after the drug is discontinued.

Dideoxynucleosides

The nucleosides zalcitabine (dideoxycytidine or ddC), didanosine (dideoxyinosine), and stavudine are inhibitors of reverse transcriptase used to treat HIV-1 infection. These agents cause a dose-limiting dysesthetic sensory neuropathy (Berger et al. 1993). High doses of ddC produce an acute painful sensory neuropathy that may progress for 3 weeks after treatment is stopped. Lower doses cause a less painful, sensory neuropathy in 10–30% of patients. Preexisting neuropathy, diabetes mellitus, heavy alcohol consumption, and low serum cobalamin levels are risk factors that predispose to nucleoside neuropathy. Partial reversal of symptoms following withdrawal of drug allows the ddC neuropathy to be distinguished from the clinically similar HIV-1–associated distal sensory polyneuropathy.

Disulfiram

Disulfiram is used in the treatment of alcoholism. The incidence of neuropathy is dose related, as most patients receiving daily doses of 500 mg or more develop nerve damage after 6 months. The clinical manifestations are initial distal sensory impairment and later progressive weakness. Nerve conduction studies and EMG indicate an axonal neuropathy. Acute axonal degeneration and loss of myelinated fibers are seen in sural nerve biopsy specimens. After the drug is stopped improvement takes place over a period of months.

Ethambutol

Ethambutol is an antituberculous drug that causes peripheral sensory and optic neuropathy after prolonged administration at doses above 20 mg/kg per day.

Etoposide

Etoposide is a semisynthetic derivative of podophyllotoxin with established antineoplastic activity in small cell lung cancer and lymphoma. Distal sensory axonal neuropathy develops in approximately 10% of patients after high-dose etoposide therapy.

Gold

Organic gold salts are sometimes used in the treatment of rheumatoid arthritis. Although toxic allergic reactions involving skin, kidneys, and blood are well known, neurotoxic complications are uncommon. A dose-related, distal axonal polyneuropathy may develop in patients receiving gold therapy. Many have the distinctive features of profound myokymia, muscle aches, insomnia, and autonomic dysfunction such as sweating and labile hypertension. After the drug is discontinued improvement is the rule. Isolated case reports suggest that gold therapy may precipitate GBS with rapidly ascending limb weakness, sensory paresthesia, and elevated CSF protein. In these cases, nerve conduction studies show evidence of demyelinating neuropathy.

Heroin

Nontraumatic plexopathies in the brachial and lumbosacral distributions have been reported in heroin addicts. On resumption of heroin use after a period of abstinence the symptoms recur in one-third of patients. Intense pain is a common clinical presentation, whereas weakness and sensory impairment are less prominent. Spontaneous recovery occurs slowly over weeks or months. The mechanism of these plexopathies is unclear.

Hydralazine

Hydralazine is an antihypertensive drug that rarely produces a predominantly sensory polyneuropathy. Distal tingling in the extremities without overt clinical signs may develop in 15% of patients on hydralazine. The neuropathy may be caused by pyridoxine deficiency by a mechanism similar to that associated with INH. Symptoms improve after withdrawal of the drug or with vitamin B_6 supplementation.

Isoniazid

INH is an effective antituberculous drug that interferes with vitamin B_6-dependent coenzymes and thus leads to pyridoxine deficiency. INH is acetylated in the liver by the enzyme acetyltransferase. Individuals unable to acetylate at a normal rate (slow acetylators) maintain high blood levels of free INH for a longer time than do rapid acetylators and are therefore more susceptible to toxic neuropathy. The slow acetylation is inherited as an autosomal recessive trait. INH polyneuropathy occurs in approximately 2% of patients receiving conventional doses (3–5 mg/kg/day), and its incidence increases with higher doses. Typically 6 months pass before neuropathic symptoms of paresthesia, impaired sensation in the distal lower extremities, and weakness begin. The primary pathological process is axonal degeneration

affecting both myelinated and unmyelinated fibers, with prominent axonal regeneration. Unless recognition of this complication is delayed, recovery is rapid. Coadministration of vitamin B_6 (100 mg daily) prevents the neuropathy.

Metronidazole and Misonidazole

Metronidazole is used for the treatment of protozoal and anaerobic bacterial infections as well as inflammatory bowel disease. It may produce a predominantly sensory polyneuropathy following cumulative doses exceeding 30 g. Axonal degeneration of both myelinated and unmyelinated fibers can occur, with slow improvement after the agent is stopped. Misonidazole, a related compound used as an experimental radiation-sensitizing agent, causes a similar sensory neuropathy.

Nitrofurantoin

Nitrofurantoin is a broad-spectrum antibiotic used to treat urinary tract infections. A sensorimotor polyneuropathy of the distal axonal type may develop weeks to months after beginning therapy. Distal numbness, paresthesia, and weakness are common. Renal insufficiency predisposes patients to the development of neuropathy because of excessive tissue concentrations of nitrofurantoin, which is normally excreted by the kidneys. Electrophysiological studies show the typical changes of distal axonopathy. Improvement occurs after the medication is discontinued.

Nitrous Oxide

A predominantly sensory neuropathy and associated myelopathy develop in individuals heavily exposed to nitrous oxide, an inhalation anesthetic agent that is also used in the food industry as whipping cream propellant. Neurological symptoms occur following intentional abuse or rarely through contamination in operating rooms. Sharp radicular pains are common symptoms, along with numbness and distal sensory loss. A reverse Lhermitte's sign (neck flexion induces an electrical shock sensation traveling from the feet upward), increased reflexes, and extensor plantar signs may be present. Nerve conduction studies show decreased SNAP amplitudes. Nitrous oxide inhibits the vitamin B_{12}–dependent enzyme methionine synthase, producing a clinical syndrome indistinguishable from vitamin B_{12} deficiency. Nitrous oxide anesthesia may even precipitate subacute combined degeneration in patients with unrecognized cobalamin deficiency. Prognosis following cessation of exposure is good.

Perhexiline

Perhexiline maleate, previously used to treat angina pectoris, may cause hyperglycemia, abnormalities of liver function, and polyneuropathy. Mild to severe sensorimotor polyneuropathy commonly develops in patients treated with perhexiline (300–400 mg/day) for several months. Painful paresthesias, weakness, frequently involving proximal as well as distal muscles, and loss of reflexes occur, occasionally accompanied by orthostatic hypotension and papilledema. CSF protein is commonly elevated. Marked slowing of conduction velocities is characteristic. Sural nerve biopsy specimens show segmental demyelination and lamellar Schwann cell inclusions. Recovery occurs if the medication is stopped.

Phenytoin

Phenytoin, a widely used antiepileptic drug, may cause mild or asymptomatic polyneuropathy after many years of exposure. Typical manifestations are confined to lower extremity areflexia, distal sensory loss, and mildly reduced motor conduction velocities. The degree of abnormality is generally proportional to the duration of phenytoin treatment. Folate deficiency, which may develop during phenytoin therapy, is not related to the onset of neuropathy.

Pyridoxine

Megadoses of pyridoxine (vitamin B_6, 600–3,000 mg/day) cause a severe sensory neuropathy. Painful paresthesia, sensory ataxia, and Lhermitte's sign are common features. Nerve conduction studies show low-amplitude or absent SNAPs. Severe depletion of myelinated fibers and acute axonal degeneration are found in sural nerve biopsy specimens. Pyridoxine use should be queried in all patients with sensory neuropathy. In experimental studies, high doses of pyridoxine (300 mg/kg) produce widespread dorsal root ganglion degeneration. The fact that most clinical cases gradually recover suggests that a distal axonopathy is the predominant lesion in humans.

Sodium Cyanate

Sodium cyanate was used to treat sickle cell anemia. An insidious sensorimotor polyneuropathy may develop following prolonged therapy.

Suramin

Originally introduced as an antiparasitic agent, suramin is used currently as an investigational antineoplastic drug for refractory malignancies. It acts by inhibiting DNA polymerase activity and displacing several growth factors from their respective receptors. Suramin neurotoxicity is the dose-limiting side effect leading to two distinct patterns of neuropathy, one a length-dependent axonal polyneuropathy and the other a subacute demyelinating polyradiculoneuropathy (Chaudhry et al. 1996). The distal sensorimotor neuropathy that occurs in 30–55% of patients presents with paresthesias and mild distal leg weakness. In vitro experiments suggest that NGF inhibition by suramin may be an important neu-

rotoxic mechanism. Approximately 15% of patients develop a subacutely evolving, demyelinating polyradiculoneuropathy. Severe generalized flaccid weakness with bulbar and respiratory involvement, nerve conduction studies consistent with demyelination, increased CSF protein levels, and perivascular inflammation on sural nerve biopsy are typical features making this neuropathy virtually indistinguishable from GBS. The severe neuropathy occurs predominantly at peak plasma suramin concentrations above 350 µg/ml. Suramin may induce inflammatory demyelination by its many immunomodulatory effects. Patients improve after drug discontinuation and with plasmapheresis.

Tacrolimus

Tacrolimus, an immunosuppressive agent used in organ transplantation, may trigger an immune-mediated neuropathy by its complex actions on T cells. The few patients who developed a subacute, multifocal demyelinating polyneuropathy resembling CIDP after initiation of tacrolimus improved following plasmapheresis or intravenous immunoglobulin (Wilson et al. 1994).

Taxoids

Paclitaxel (Taxol), a plant alkaloid isolated from the bark of the western yew, is used for the treatment of ovarian cancer and other solid neoplasms. Taxol and its semisynthetic analogue docetaxel bind to tubulin and promote irreversible microtubule assembly, thereby forming bundles of disordered microtubules and disrupting axonal transport. A dose-related sensory neuropathy results with doses above 200 mg/m^2 body surface area. Burning paresthesia, sensory loss affecting all sensory modalities, and areflexia are followed by sensory ataxia and mild distal weakness. Disabling weakness is rare except in the presence of additional risk factors such as pre-existing diabetic neuropathy or combination therapy with other neurotoxic chemotherapeutic agents such as cisplatin. Neurotrophins have prevented paclitaxel neurotoxicity in animal models.

Docetaxel (Taxotere) is used in metastatic breast and ovarian cancer causing a dose-dependent sensory polyneuropathy similar to its parent compound. Motor symptoms are present only in the most severely affected patients (New et al. 1996).

Thalidomide

Thalidomide was introduced as a sedative-hypnotic agent in the 1950s, but was taken off the market when its disastrous teratogenic properties became evident. The drug is still in use to treat certain forms of leprosy reactions, other rare skin conditions, and graft-versus-host disease. Thalidomide causes dorsal root ganglion degeneration with selective involvement of large-diameter sensory neurons. Painful distal paresthesia and numbness occur with palmar erythema and brittle nails as prominent signs. In most patients the neuropathy is dose related, occurring after high doses or chronic administration for more than 6 months. After discontinuation of the drug, symptoms and signs improve very little. Glutethimide, a structurally related hypnotic compound, may produce a similar sensory polyneuronopathy in patients taking high doses for many months.

L-Tryptophan

An unusual syndrome called eosinophilia-myalgia syndrome was recognized in 1989 in individuals taking preparations containing L-tryptophan. By 1992, more than 1,500 patients had been diagnosed in the United States. A contaminated L-tryptophan source originating from a single manufacturer was responsible for the epidemic. One of the chemical impurities associated with eosinophilia-myalgia syndrome, designated *peak E*, is an unusual dimeric form of L-tryptophan. This abnormal tryptophan metabolite may activate eosinophils and trigger immune-mediated mononuclear cell infiltrates in connective tissues of many organs. Eosinophilia-myalgia syndrome is a systemic illness characterized by myalgias, fatigue, arthralgias, skin rash, swelling, and induration of the limbs and an elevation of the blood eosinophil count (>1,000 cells/µl). Many patients develop florid inflammatory myopathy. The onset of eosinophilia-myalgia syndrome may be delayed for months after L-tryptophan use, and clinical deterioration may peak months after stopping the medication. A severe axonal sensorimotor polyneuropathy may be a prominent feature in some patients. Electrodiagnostic studies are in keeping with an axonal process. EMG may show neurogenic and myopathic motor unit potential alterations. Pathological studies demonstrate acute axonal degeneration, epineurial and perineurial inflammatory infiltrates, and associated inflammatory vasculopathy in sural nerves. Inflammation is observed also in biopsy specimens of muscle, skin, and subcutaneous tissues. The clinical and pathological findings resemble those of the Spanish toxic oil syndrome, which was caused by denatured rapeseed oil. In general, clinical severity of the neuropathy seems to be positively related to the total dose ingested. Prednisone is not of benefit.

Vinca Alkaloids

Vincristine, the *Vinca* alkaloid most used in chemotherapeutic regimens, has length-dependent sensorimotor polyneuropathy as its dose-limiting side effect. Vinblastine and two semisynthetic derivatives, vindesine and vinorelbine, are less neurotoxic. *Vinca* alkaloids function as mitotic spindle inhibitors. Their neurotoxicity is related to tubulin binding, which interferes with axonal microtubule assembly, thereby impairing axonal transport.

Vincristine produces a mild polyneuropathy in virtually all patients treated with conventional doses (1.4 mg/m²/week). Paresthesias, often starting in the fingers before the feet, and loss of ankle jerks are common initial findings. Distal muscle

weakness and sensory impairment follow. Autonomic dysfunction, particularly gastroparesis, constipation, occasionally paralytic ileus, and urinary retention, is an early manifestation. Weakness, often accompanied by muscle pains, may evolve rapidly to severe motor impairment. Occasionally, isolated mononeuropathies have been reported. Cranial nerve involvement occurs infrequently and includes trigeminal sensory loss, ocular motility disorders, facial weakness, and recurrent laryngeal nerve palsies.

Electrophysiological studies reflect the degeneration of distal axons. SNAPs are reduced in amplitude, whereas NCVs are preserved. EMG shows denervation in distal muscles. The predominant pathological features are axonal degeneration and myopathic changes with spheromembranous inclusions. Reduction in dose or withdrawal from therapy at an early stage usually leads to complete recovery. Coadministration of glutamic acid or ORG 2766, an adrenocorticotropic hormone–derived synthetic peptide, has been reported to reduce the frequency and severity of vincristine neuropathy in small clinical trials. Neurotrophins have neuroprotective effects in experimental studies.

NEUROPATHIES ASSOCIATED WITH INFECTIONS

Peripheral neuropathy occurs in a number of infectious diseases including viral, prion, bacterial, and parasitic infections.

Viral Infections and Neuropathy

Human Immunodeficiency Virus Type 1

HIV-1 infection is associated with a wide variety of peripheral neuropathy syndromes, with onset from the time of seroconversion to the late stages of AIDS (Table 80.28; see Chapter 59). These are divided into neuropathies occurring early and late in the course of disease. The CD4 count inversely parallels the frequency of neuropathy, with normal counts in inflammatory demyelinating neuropathies and low counts in distal symmetrical polyneuropathies and lumbosacral polyradiculopathy. The estimated prevalence of peripheral neuropathy in patients with HIV-1 infection ranges from 15–30% based on clinical findings and increases substantially if electrophysiological variables are used for inclusion. More than 75% of patients with AIDS have pathological evidence of peripheral nerve involvement at autopsy.

Acute and Chronic Inflammatory Demyelinating Polyradiculoneuropathies. Of the neuropathies that occur in HIV-1 infection, AIDP and CIDP predominate during seroconversion and the early stages of disease.

An acute inflammatory demyelinating neuropathy clinically and electrophysiologically indistinguishable from GBS is seen in individuals who have positive test results for HIV-1. Its clinical course, spontaneous recovery, or response to

Table 80.28:   Neuropathies associated with human immunodeficiency virus infection

Neuropathies	Clinical features	Human immunodeficiency virus 1 stage
Distal symmetrical polyneuropathy	Pain, sensory loss	Late: CDC IV, AIDS, ARC
Autonomic neuropathy		
Treatment-induced	ddC, ddI, d4T	
Lumbosacral polyradiculoneuropathy	Cauda equina syndrome	Late: CDC IV, AIDS
CMV radiculopathy	CSF pleocytosis (polymorphonuclear cells)	
Lymphoma	CSF cytology (malignant cells)	
Diffuse infiltrative lymphocytosis syndrome	CD8 lymphocytosis	
Multiple mononeuropathies	Limited to extensive mononeuropathies	CDC III–IV; ARC, AIDS
Vasculitis		
CMV		
Lymphoma		
Inflammatory demyelinating polyneuropathies	Guillain-Barré syndrome or chronic inflammatory demyelinating polyradiculoneuropathy; cerebrospinal fluid pleocytosis	Early: CDC I–III
Cranial mononeuropathy	Facial palsy	Early: CDC I–III
Sensory neuronopathy	Sensory ataxia	Early: CDC I–III
Herpes zoster radiculitis	Dermatomal vesicular eruption	Early and late

AIDS = acquired immunodeficiency syndrome; ARC = AIDS-related complex; CDC I–IV = Centers for Disease Control and Prevention classification system for human immunodeficiency virus infection stages I–IV; CMV = cytomegalovirus; ddC, ddI, d4T = dideoxycytidine, dideoxyinosine, stavudine.

plasmapheresis or intravenous immunoglobulin therapy are similar to non–HIV-1 related GBS. CSF protein is elevated (>100 mg/dl), and pathologically demyelination with prominent inflammation in nerves and roots occurs. This acute polyradiculoneuropathy differs from non–HIV-1 related GBS by a CSF pleocytosis ranging from 10 to 50 cells/μl and by HIV-1 seropositivity.

Similar to HIV-1 seronegative patients, CIDP may be seen in association with HIV-1 infection. CSF pleocytosis and prominent inflammatory infiltrates consisting primarily of cytotoxic-suppressor T lymphocytes and macrophages in sural nerve biopsy specimens separate these patients from those with seronegative CIDP. It is advisable to test for the presence of HIV-1 antibodies in those patients with acquired demyelinating neuropathies who have conceivable HIV-1 risk factors or suspicious laboratory results, such as CSF pleocytosis, positive hepatitis B serology, or polyclonal hypergammaglobulinemia. In one series from a large urban center, 8% of patients with inflammatory demyelinating neuropathies tested HIV-1 seropositive. Plasmapheresis or IVIG is the preferred treatment for both acute and chronic inflammatory demyelinating polyneuropathies if the illness is sufficiently severe to warrant intervention.

Mononeuropathy and Multiple Mononeuropathies. Although isolated involvement of single cranial nerves, and particularly the facial nerve, may occur in the asymptomatic or early stages of symptomatic HIV-1 infection, multiple mononeuropathies associated with HIV-1 disease more frequently occur late in the course of illness. These may be associated with superimposed infection (including herpes zoster, CMV, hepatitis C, and syphilis), lymphomatous infiltration, or necrotizing vasculitis.

Unilateral or bilateral facial neuropathy may accompany HIV-1 seroconversion. Patients with involvement of one or two cranial or spinal nerves in association with CD4 counts greater than 200/μl often have a good prognosis, and many recover spontaneously. Multiple mononeuropathies with severe deficits, on the other hand, are more likely to occur in immunocompromised AIDS patients with CD4 counts below 200/μl; these patients should be investigated for CMV infection. If CMV cannot be demonstrated, peripheral nerve vasculitis is the most likely etiology. Peripheral nerve biopsy in multiple mononeuropathies demonstrates multifocal decreased density of myelinated fibers, degenerating fibers, and interstitial abnormalities dominated by epineurial mononuclear cell infiltrates and vessel wall necrosis.

When CMV is confirmed or even suspected clinically, treatment should begin immediately with ganciclovir. Other therapies that have been noted in case reports as being effective include corticosteroids, plasmapheresis, IVIG, and foscarnet. Use of corticosteroids might theoretically be risky, but is surprisingly well tolerated.

Distal Symmetrical Polyneuropathy. The most common neuropathy related to HIV-1 infection is painful distal symmetrical polyneuropathy. The onset occurs often with burning feet, painful paresthesia, and distal sensory loss, combined with mild distal weakness and autonomic dysfunction. In patients with symptomatic distal symmetrical polyneuropathy, nerve conduction studies show borderline to low amplitude sensory and motor responses, often accompanied by denervation changes in distal muscles. Electrophysiological evaluations of patients with HIV-1 infection demonstrate that as many as two-thirds may have peripheral nerve involvement. Sural nerve biopsy shows loss of myelinated fibers and unmyelinated fibers with no distinctive interstitial abnormalities.

Although the cause of distal symmetrical polyneuropathy in HIV-1 infection is unknown, direct infection of peripheral nerve is thought to be unlikely. Although low levels of HIV-1 in dorsal root ganglia macrophages may play a role, inflammatory cell infiltration and the release of cytokines appears to be the primary cause of the neuronal degeneration. A significant proportion of patients with HIV-1–related distal symmetrical polyneuropathy have antibodies to human T-cell lymphotropic virus 2, suggesting coinfection (Zehender et al 1995). Other factors that have been implicated include nutritional deficiencies (chiefly vitamin B_{12} and folate deficiencies) and toxic drugs (including vincristine, dapsone, INH, ddC, dideoxyinosine, and stavudine). A subset of HIV-1–positive patients with distal symmetrical polyneuropathy have been found to have necrotizing vasculitis (Bradley and Verma 1996).

Lumbosacral Polyradiculoneuropathy. Even though uncommon, acute lumbosacral polyradiculoneuropathy often associated with CMV infection is among the most devastating neurological complications in AIDS. The usual presentation is rapidly progressive flaccid paraparesis, sphincter dysfunction, perineal sensory loss, and lower limb areflexia (So and Olney 1994).

Electrophysiological studies show low-amplitude CMAPs and prolonged or absent F-wave latencies. Reduced or absent SNAPs are attributed to concomitant polyneuropathy. Within a few weeks of onset, EMG signs of active denervation become apparent. CSF examination in CMV-related lumbosacral polyradiculoneuropathy shows pleocytosis (>50 per µl; typically with more than 40% polymorphonuclear cells), elevated protein levels, and low glucose concentrations. With this CSF profile, a presumptive diagnosis of CMV polyradiculoneuropathy can be made, leading to empiric therapy, even before the demonstration of positive CSF culture results. MRI with gadolinium may demonstrate enhancement of cauda equina nerve roots. Other rare causes of lumbosacral polyradiculoneuropathy in AIDS include syphilis, mycobacterial infections, toxoplasmosis, and leptomeningeal lymphomatosis. Another condition associated with HIV-1 infection, diffuse infiltrative lymphocytosis syndrome, is a nonmalignant CD8 lymphocytosis that may affect multiple viscera as well as peripheral nerve and may respond to either corticosteroid or antiretroviral treatment (Gherardi et al 1998).

Empiric treatment with intravenous ganciclovir should be started promptly in AIDS patients with polymorphonuclear CSF pleocytosis and progressive flaccid paraparesis. Foscarnet alone or in combination with ganciclovir may be an alternative for patients who develop this syndrome during ganciclovir treatment for systemic CMV infection. Although early antiviral therapy may preserve neurological function, long-term prognosis is poor.

Herpes zoster radiculitis occurs in perhaps 10% of HIV-1 infected patients. Early in the course of HIV-1 infection, often at seroconversion or during the asymptomatic phase, ataxic sensory polyganglionopathy may develop; it remains unclear whether this syndrome or the associated degeneration of the gracile tract are related directly to HIV-1 infection.

Cytomegalovirus

CMV commonly causes an asymptomatic infection. In immunocompromised individuals, however, a life-threatening disseminated illness may result, often with fatal meningoencephalitis. Antecedent CMV infection has been associated with AIDP. In patients infected with the HIV-1 virus, severe painful lumbosacral polyradiculoneuropathy is known to occur (see Lumbosacral Polyradiculoneuropathy, earlier in this chapter).

Epstein-Barr Virus

Although most well known as the chief cause of infectious mononucleosis, the Epstein-Barr virus is associated with a variety of neurological complications. Those with peripheral nerve manifestations include rhombencephalitis with cranial nerve involvement, myelitis with spread to adjacent nerve roots, multiple mononeuropathies, and brachial as well as lumbosacral plexopathy.

Herpes Simplex Virus

Herpes simplex virus is a group of neurotropic DNA viruses that colonize primary sensory neurons. In the case of herpes simplex virus 1, the gasserian ganglion is most often affected, and repeated eruption of oral and labial ulceration ensues. With herpes simplex virus 2, a sexually transmitted disease, sacral dorsal root ganglion cells are the site of infection, leading to the periodic appearance of genital ulcers. Although segmental recurrence is most common, more widespread disease may result in disseminated eruptions in immunocompromised hosts. Antiviral treatment with acyclovir (200 mg five times daily for 10 days) or famciclovir (125 mg twice a day for 5 days) can reduce the duration of eruption and prolong the time to subsequent outbreak.

Herpes Zoster Virus

The most common symptomatic peripheral nerve viral infection is with the neurotropic varicella zoster (herpes) virus. It has been estimated that over the age of 70 years, the lifetime percent probability of segmental varicella zoster virus infection approximates years of life. The spectrum of peripheral neurological involvement in varicella zoster virus includes cranial zoster (chiefly affecting the trigeminal or less often the geniculate ganglion), radicular zoster (also called segmental zoster, zoster radiculopathy, or shingles), and polyradiculoneuropathy. Although sensory pathways are most affected, in cases with radicular zoster affecting one or two spinal root levels, there is an approximate 5% probability of significant motor involvement, leading to the designation segmental zoster paresis. Careful EMG study results show as many as 50% of segmental zoster patients may have subtle motor involvement (Haanpää et al. 1997). Occasional patients present with painful unilateral dermatomal pain and CSF evidence of varicella zoster virus DNA, but no cutaneous vesicular eruption (zoster sine herpete). Treatment with famciclovir (500 mg three times a day for 7 days) or acyclovir (800 mg five times daily for 10 days) is indicated at the onset of symptoms.

Hepatitis Viruses

Hepatitis B virus infection has been reported in association with demyelinating GBS and with multiple mononeuropathies and cutaneous vasculitis.

Infection with hepatitis C virus is transmitted by sexual contact, through blood transfusion, or via other means and may be particularly common in urban populations. Hepatitis C virus has been associated with essential cryoglobulinemia and may be its most common cause. The syndrome of hepatitis C virus infection, cryoglobulinemia, and vasculitic neuropathy has been recognized as a previously overlooked cause of multiple mononeuropathies. Although no controlled clinical trials have been carried out, individual patients have been observed to respond to interferon-α or plasma exchange.

Human T-Cell Lymphotropic Virus Type 1

Although the majority of patients infected by human T-cell lymphotropic virus type 1 present with a spinal cord syndrome and spastic paraparesis, sphincter disturbances, and impotence, many affected have dysesthesia and mild distal sensory loss, implicating additional involvement of peripheral nerve and dorsal column pathways. Because the syndrome is much more common in tropical regions, the term *tropical spastic paraparesis* has been used. CSF examination is essentially normal, but may show a mild lymphocytic pleocytosis. Somatosensory evoked potential studies are said to be abnormal in more than one-half of patients. NCVs are minimally slowed in approximately one-third of those studied. Progression is slow, although most patients eventually become severely disabled 10 years or more after onset of symptoms.

Tropical Ataxic Neuropathy

Tropical ataxic neuropathy is a predominantly sensory syndrome occurring in middle age that presents with burning feet, distal sensory loss, gait ataxia, and lower limb areflexia. Mild distal lower motor neuron signs, optic atrophy, and sensorineural hearing loss may be present also. Although nutritional, toxic, and infectious etiologies have been considered, some evidence suggests that infection with human T-cell lymphotropic virus 2 may play a significant role.

Peripheral Neuropathy in Creutzfeldt-Jakob Disease

Creutzfeldt-Jakob disease is a transmissible neurodegenerative disorder caused by prions, proteinaceous infectious particles (see Chapter 59). Prions interact with an abnormal host protein to produce clinical Creutzfeldt-Jakob disease. Although the CNS is the main target of Creutzfeldt-Jakob disease, a number of patients have been described with a demyelinating peripheral neuropathy that may precede cognitive and intellectual deterioration (Antoine et al. 1996).

Bacterial Infections and Neuropathy

Neuropathy Associated with Mycobacterium leprae

Hansen's disease (leprosy) is a major cause of neuropathy worldwide, especially in tropical and subtropical regions. As improvements in public health and use of multidrug therapy have advanced, the prevalence of Hansen's disease, as measured by registered cases, has dropped from 5.4 million in 1991 to 0.9 million in 1996. The Centers for Disease Control and Prevention reports that in the United States there were 144 new cases in 1995, whereas the total number of reported U.S. cases was 7,500. Of new cases, approximately 20% originate in this country (mainly Hawaii, Florida, Louisiana, and southern Texas), with the balance immigrating mainly from Asia or the South Pacific, and to a lesser extent from Mexico, India, and other parts of the world.

Mycobacterium leprae is thought to be transmitted through the upper respiratory tract. Once the nasal mucosa is colonized, the organism spreads slowly to other regions, with an estimated incubation time of 3–10 years. Particularly vulnerable tissue are those with mean daily temperatures in the 27° to 30°C range, as this promotes more rapid bacterial growth. The skin and superficial nerve trunks are particularly vulnerable, leading to cutaneous lesions, anesthesia, and paralysis of face and limb muscles. The disease is classified by host reaction to infection into two polar forms, tuberculoid and lepromatous, with three intermediate forms termed *borderline tuberculoid, intermediate borderline*, and *borderline lepromatous*.

The vigor of host cell–mediated immunity appears to dictate the course of events. Tuberculoid Hansen's disease is characterized by active cell–mediated immunity, intense delayed hypersensitivity response to lepra antigens such as lepromin, localized destruction of infected nerves by intense inflammatory lesions, and rare organisms detected in skin and nerve. Lepromatous Hansen's disease, on the other hand, is typified by unopposed proliferation of organisms, complete anergy to lepra antigens, and disseminated skin and nerve lesions with minimal inflammatory response. Intermediate forms share features of the two extremes. A comprehensive review of Hansen's disease neuropathy by Walters and Jacobs (1996) is recommended.

Clinical Features. The unique propensity of *M. leprae* to invade cutaneous nerves causes the cardinal symptom of sensory loss. In tuberculoid Hansen's disease sensory loss, initially affecting pinprick and temperature sensation, is detected within sharply demarcated hypopigmented skin lesions. Adjacent cutaneous nerves or mixed nerve trunks are apt to become involved. The associated intense inflammatory response can affect underlying nerve trunks and cause a mononeuropathy in the distribution of those nerves, which may become indurated and palpable because of fusiform swelling. Attention should be paid to the palpation of peripheral nerves that course close to the skin surface, including the great auricular, ulnar, radial, common fibular, and sural nerves, in order to detect nerve enlargement. The predominant sensory loss, particularly for pain, can lead to painless trauma with acrodystrophic deformities and autoamputations.

Lepromatous Hansen's disease is characterized by symmetrical bacillary infiltration of the skin with a predilection for cooler areas of the body, avoiding the scalp, palms, soles, and midline of the back. The skin may have multiple nodules, papules, macules, and ulcerations, or there may be diffuse cutaneous involvement with a waxy, myxedemalike appearance. Similarly, the distribution of sensory loss is related to the local skin temperature, the coolest parts such as the pinna of the ear; the tip of the nose; malar areas of the face; dorsal surfaces of the hands, forearms, and feet; and dorsolateral surfaces of the lower legs being affected first. Because of the minimal inflammatory response, nerve trunk involvement occurs late in this form. Commonly affected nerves include the ulnar, common peroneal, and superficial branches of the facial and median nerves, in that order. The selective involvement of small branches of the facial nerve leads to the typical patchy nature of facial paralysis with early weakness of medial forehead elevators. Preserved tendon reflexes are an important differential diagnostic sign, in contrast to the loss of reflexes seen in most polyneuropathies.

Either spontaneously or during the course of treatment, acute leprosy reactions may complicate the insidious course because of a sudden alteration in the host-immune response. In the reversal reaction, which is usually seen in the borderline-lepromatous stage, patients develop an increase in cell-mediated immunity. This reaction is identified clinically by swelling and exacerbations of existing skin and nerve lesions. Marked reversal reactions can be associated with intensely painful nerve trunks, and total loss of sensory and motor functions may develop within hours because of the pronounced inflammatory reaction of the affected nerves. These acute reactions appear most commonly during the first year of therapy and require immediate treatment with systemic corticosteroids or other anti-inflammatory agents to prevent further nerve damage.

Nerve conduction studies show reduced amplitudes of CMAPs and SNAPs, together with focal conduction slowing at sites of nerve enlargement. For diagnosis and accurate classification, a skin punch biopsy is necessary and should be taken from the active borders of the lesions. The architecture of cutaneous nerves is destroyed by an intense granulomatous inflammation in tuberculoid Hansen's disease (Figure 80.33). In lepromatous disease, multiple acid-fast organisms are found in Schwann cells, foamy macrophages, and axons of involved nerves, together with recurrent demyelination and progressive nerve fiber loss.

Treatment. Management consists of specific chemotherapy and prevention and treatment of deformities. The current recommendation for paucibacillary infections (those classified as indeterminate, tuberculoid, or borderline tuberculoid Hansen's disease) is the combination of dapsone, 100 mg per day, and rifampin, 600 mg per day for at least 6 months, followed by dapsone monotherapy for 3–5 years. Patients with multibacillary infections (borderline or lepromatous leprosy) receive the same combination therapy, with the addition of clofazimine (50 mg daily). Treatment is continued for a minimum of 2 years or until skin smear results are negative. For dapsone-resistant strains or patients with glucose-6-phosphate dehydrogenase deficiency, clofazimine and rifampin are used together, with consideration of a third agent, either ofloxacin (400 mg daily), clarithromycin (250 mg twice a day), or minocycline (100 mg daily).

Diphtheritic Neuropathy

Diphtheria is a localized infection of the upper respiratory tract or skin produced by *Corynebacterium diphtheriae*. The organism elaborates a protein exotoxin responsible for the delayed systemic manifestations, including cardiomyopathy and segmental demyelination of nerve roots and peripheral nerves. Diphtheria toxin is used as an experimental model of PNS demyelination. Local injection of the toxin produces focal demyelination of nerve fibers without inflammation.

The disease is now rare except in poor socioeconomic conditions where immunization is inadequate. It begins with a pharyngeal infection associated with a characteristic grayish-white exudate. Approximately 20% of cases develop a focal palatal neuropathy 4–30 days after the primary infection. Neurological symptoms begin with paralysis of the soft palate, impaired pharyngeal sensation, and paralysis of pupillary accommodation. Rarely, the diaphragm becomes weak at this stage. A local limb neuropathy may appear adjacent to cutaneous diphtheria. The focal palatal-pharyngeal neuropathy may progress 3–15 weeks after the infection to a generalized mixed sensorimotor polyneuropathy or less frequently to a sensory polyneuropathy presenting with ataxia in approximately 10% of patients (McDonald and Kocen 1993).

Culture of *C. diphtheriae* from the pharynx or the cutaneous ulcer establishes the diagnosis. CSF protein may be normal or elevated to more than 100 mg/dl. Mildly increased distal motor latencies and decreased NCVs are

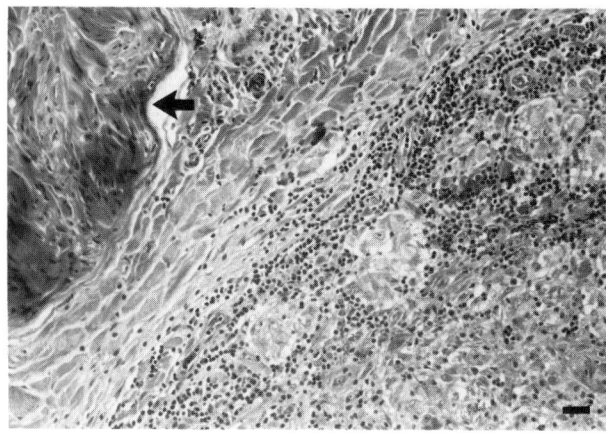

FIGURE 80.33 Tuberculoid leprosy. Biopsy of enlarged sural nerve demonstrates extensive epineurial inflammatory granuloma consisting of epithelioid and mononuclear inflammatory cells. The adjacent nerve fascicle (*arrow*) is devoid of myelinated fibers. (Hematoxylin and eosin; bar = 300 μm.)

seen in most patients 2 weeks after the onset of neurological symptoms. However, maximal slowing, with conduction velocities ranging from 15–35 m per second tends to occur later when clinical recovery has already begun. The brunt of the pathological changes, segmental demyelination with sparing of axons, is seen in the dorsal root ganglia and nerve roots, which have an ineffective blood-nerve barrier to the toxin because of fenestrated capillaries.

Prompt administration of antitoxin within 48 hours of the onset of the primary infection reduces the incidence and severity of neuropathy. Respiratory support may be needed for severe cases. Recovery takes place over a period of weeks and is usually complete.

Peripheral Manifestations of Lyme Borreliosis

Lyme disease is a multisystem illness caused by the tick-borne spirochete *Borrelia burgdorferi sensu lato*, with characteristic early and late neurological manifestations. Most cases (97%) in the United States have been reported from nine states in the Northeast, upper Midwest, and Pacific coastal regions. Endemic foci occur in northern and central Europe. It is now recognized that Lyme disease is distributed widely in temperate zones worldwide (see Chapter 59).

From the initial appearance of the pathognomonic skin lesion, known as *erythema migrans*, a distinctive early neurological syndrome results in approximately 15% of patients. This consists of cranial neuropathy (usually facial palsy), radiculoneuropathy, or lymphocytic meningitis, often in combination. These conditions usually abate without intervention over weeks to months and improve more rapidly with appropriate antibiotic treatment. Months to years after the initial infection, a late neurological syndrome may emerge. This consists of a predominantly sen-

sory polyradiculoneuropathy that may present with distal sensory symptoms or proximal radicular pain and does not often resolve on its own, but rather regresses only after use of efficacious antibiotics (Logigian 1997).

Laboratory investigations helpful in the diagnosis of early Lyme disease include CSF analysis, which shows a lymphocytic pleocytosis and mild elevation of the total protein. Intrathecal production of anti–*B. burgdorferi sensu lato* antibodies can usually be documented in these cases. Electrodiagnostic study results in patients with chronic Lyme polyradiculoneuropathy confirm a multifocal or widespread axonal process, with borderline to low amplitude distal responses, greater involvement of sensory than motor fibers, and little or no slowing of NCVs. EMG often shows signs of chronic partial denervation in distal and proximal muscles, including fibrillation potentials and neurogenic motor unit potential changes. Sural nerve biopsy confirms axonal degeneration as well as interstitial alterations with perivascular and perineurial mononuclear inflammation. Serological confirmation of Lyme disease documents prior exposure, although seropositivity alone is not sufficient to establish a causal relationship, because in endemic areas at least 10% of asymptomatic individuals are seropositive. The diagnosis must depend on appropriate exposure in endemic regions and a plausible clinical context. High titers of anti–*B. burgdorferi sensu lato* antibody in CSF are helpful to link the peripheral neurological manifestations to Lyme disease. Polymerase chain reaction assays to identify spirochetal DNA in CSF are promising techniques (Schmidt 1997).

The majority of patients treated with intravenous ceftriaxone, 2 g daily for 2–4 weeks, improve slowly over 3–6 months. Oral antibiotic therapy with doxycycline or amoxicillin may be effective in mild cases without CSF abnormalities.

Parasitic Infections Associated with Peripheral Neuropathy

American Trypanosomiasis (Chagas' disease)

American trypanosomiasis (Chagas' disease) occurs from the southern United States to southern Argentina and is known to have affected 17 million individuals, of whom approximately 5 million develop clinical symptoms attributed to the disorder. Chagas' disease is a parasitic infection caused by the flagellate protozoan *Trypanosoma cruzi*. The parasite is transmitted to humans by reduvid bugs of the order Hemiptera when the proboscides (sucking mouth parts) pierce the skin of their host to feed. The microorganism is not introduced with the insect bite, but rather it is passively deposited in reduvid feces and subsequently penetrates the bite wound into the bloodstream.

Once the protozoan gains access to the host circulation three stages of disease ensue. The acute phase is marked variably by either no symptoms or alternatively by malaise, local inflammation, gastrointestinal symptoms, and lymphadenopathy. The second phase, typically occurring approximately 3 months after initial inoculation, may last for years and is an asymptomatic period. During this time serological test results for trypanosomiasis become positive. The third or chronic stage affects approximately one-third of patients, and usually begins 10–20 years following the original reduvid bite. This phase is characterized by gastrointestinal, cardiac, and neurological manifestations. Approximately 10% of patients with chronic Chagas' disease develop a predominately sensory neuropathy.

Most patients with neuropathy complain of paresthesia in the distal lower limbs. On examination, distal hypesthesia and hyporeflexia are found, usually limited to the lower limbs, occasionally involving all four extremities, and rarely only in the distal upper limbs. Electrophysiological findings include low-amplitude sensory and motor responses, reduced NCVs, and distal neurogenic motor unit potential changes by EMG. Sural nerve biopsy demonstrates decreased density of large and small myelinated fibers, axonal clusters indicating regeneration, and on teased fiber preparations, paranodal and segmental demyelination (Sica et al. 1995).

REFERENCES

Agbogu BN, Stern BJ, Sewell C, et al. Therapeutic considerations in patients with refractory neurosarcoidosis. Arch Neurol 1995;52:875–879.

Allen NB, Bressler PB. Diagnosis and treatment of the systemic and cutaneous necrotizing vasculitis syndromes. Med Clin North Am 1997;81:243–259.

Amato AA, Barohn RJ, Sahenk Z, et al. Polyneuropathy complicating bone marrow and solid organ transplantation. Neurology 1993;43:1513–1518.

Amato AA, Collins MP. Neuropathies associated with malignancy. Semin Neurol 1998;18:125–144.

Anand P. Neurotrophins and peripheral neuropathy. Phil Trans R Soc London 1996;351:449–454.

Antoine JC, Laplanche JL, Mosnier JF, et al. Demyelinating peripheral neuropathy with Creutzfeld-Jakob disease and mutation at codon 200 of the prion protein gene. Neurology 1996;46:1123–1127.

Apfel SC, Kessler JA, Adornato BT, et al. Recombinant human nerve growth factor in the treatment of diabetic polyneuropathy. Neurology 1998;51:695–702.

Barohn RJ, Gronseth GS, LeForce BR, et al. Peripheral nervous system involvement in a large cohort of human immunodeficiency virus-infected individuals. Arch Neurol 1993;50:167–171.

Berger AR, Arezzo JC, Schaumburg HH, et al. 2'-3'-Dideoxycytidine (ddC) toxic neuropathy: a study of 52 patients. Neurology 1993;43:358–362.

Bergethon PR, Sabin TD, Lewis D, et al. Improvement in the polyneuropathy associated with familial amyloid polyneuropathy after liver transplantation. Neurology 1996;47:944–951.

Bergoffen J, Scherer SS, Wang S, et al. Connexin mutations in X-linked Charcot-Marie-Tooth disease. Science 1993;262:2039–2042.

Bertorini T, Halford H, Lawrence J, et al. Contrast-enhanced magnetic resonance imaging of the lumbosacral roots in the dysimmune inflammatory polyneuropathies. J Neuroimaging 1995;5:9–15.

Bolton CF. Critical Illness Polyneuropathy. In AK Asbury, PK Thomas (eds), Peripheral Nerve Disorders 2. Oxford: Butterworth–Heinemann, 1995;262–280.

Bolton CF, McKeown MJ, Chen R, et al. Subacute uremic and diabetic polyneuropathy. Muscle Nerve 1997;20:59–64.

Bosch EP. Guillain-Barré syndrome: An update of acute immune-mediated polyradiculoneuropathies. The Neurologist 1998;4:211–226.

Bradley WG, Verma A. Painful vasculitic neuropathy in HIV-1 infection: relief of pain with prednisone therapy. Neurology 1996;47:1446–1451.

Brady OR. Fabry Disease. In PJ Dyck, PK Thomas, JW Griffin, et al. (eds), Peripheral Neuropathy (3rd ed). Philadelphia: Saunders, 1993;1169–1178.

Brannagan III TH, Nagke KJ, Lange DJ, et al. Complications of intravenous immune globulin treatment in neurologic disease. Neurology 1996;47:674–677.

Chanarin I, Metz J. Diagnosis of Cobalamin Deficiency: The Old and the New. Br J Hematol 1997;97:695–700.

Chance PF, Alderson MK, Leppig KA, et al. DNA deletion associated with hereditary neuropathy with liability to pressure palsies. Cell 1993;72:143–151.

Chaudhry V. Multifocal motor neuropathy. Semin Neurol 1998;18:73–81.

Chaudhry V, Eisenberger MA, Sinibaldi VJ, et al. A prospective study of suramin-induced peripheral neuropathy. Brain 1996;119:2039–2052.

Chiba A, Kusonoki S, Obata H, et al. Serum anti-GQ1b IgG antibody is associated with ophthalmoplegia in Miller Fisher syndrome and Guillain-Barré syndrome: clinical and immuno-histochemical studies. Neurology 1993;43:1911–1917.

Cros D, Triggs WJ. Guillain-Barré syndrome: clinical neurophysiologic studies. Rev Neurol (Paris) 1996;152:339–343.

Dawson DM. Entrapment neuropathies of the upper extremities. N Engl J Med 1993;329:2013–2018.

Diabetes Control and Complication Trial Research Group. The effect of intensive diabetes therapy on the development and progression of neuropathy. Ann Intern Med 1995;122:561–568.

Dyck PJ, Chance PF, Lebo RV, et al. Hereditary Motor and Sensory Neuropathies. In PJ Dyck, PK Thomas, JW Griffin, et al. (eds), Peripheral Neuropathy (3rd ed). Philadelphia: Saunders, 1993;1094–1136.

Dyck PJ, Giannini C. Pathologic alterations in the diabetic neuropathies of humans: a review. J Neuropathol Exp Neurol 1997;55:1181–1193.

Dyck PJ, Kratz KM, Karnes JL, et al. The prevalence by staged severity of various types of diabetic neuropathy, retinopathy, and nephropathy in a population-based cohort: The Rochester Diabetic Neuropathy study. Neurology 1993;43:817–824.

Dyck PJ, Litchy WJ, Kratz KM. A plasma exchange versus immune globulin infusion trial in chronic inflammatory demyelinating polyradiculo-neuropathy. Ann Neurol 1994;36:838–845.

Dyck PJB, Hunder GG, Dyck PJ. A case-control and nerve biopsy study of CREST multiple mononeuropathy. Neurology 1997;49:1641–1645.

Fadic R, Russell JA, Vedanarayanan VV, et al. Sensory ataxic neuropathy as the presenting feature of a novel mitochondrial disease. Neurology 1997;49:239–245.

Falk RH, Comenzo RL, Skinner M. The systemic amyloidosis. N Engl Med J 1997;337:898–909.

Flanigan KM, Crawford TO, Griffin JW, et al. Localization of the giant axonal neuropathy gene to chromosome 16q24. Ann Neurol 1998;43:143–148.

Flaster M, Bradley W. Amyloidotic Polyneuropathy: A Review of Recent Molecular Genetic Advances. In G Serratrice, J-F Pellissier, J Pouget, et al. (eds), Système Nerveux, Muscles et Maladies Systémiques—Acquisitions Récentes. Paris: Expansion Scientifique Francaise, 1993;307–323.

The French Cooperative Group on Plasma Exchange in Guillain-Barré syndrome. Appropriate number of plasma exchanges in Guillain-Barré syndrome. Ann Neurol 1997;41:298–306.

Gabern JY, Cambi F, Tang X-M, et al. Proteolipid protein is necessary in peripheral as well as central myelin. Neuron 1997;19:205–218.

Gabreëls-Festen AAWM, Hoogendijk JE, Meijerink PHS, et al. Two divergent types of nerve pathology in patients with different Po mutations in Charcot-Marie-Tooth disease. Neurology 1996;47:761–765.

Gabriel JM, Erne B, Pareyson D, et al. Gene dosage effect in hereditary peripheral neuropathy. Expression of peripheral myelin protein 22 in Charcot-Marie-Tooth disease type 1A and hereditary neuropathy with liability to pressure palsies nerve biopsies. Neurology 1997;49:1635–1640.

Galer BS. Neuropathic pain of peripheral origin: advances in pharmacologic treatment. Neurology 1995;45(Suppl. 9):S17–S25.

Gherardi RK, Chouaib S, Malapert, et al. Early weight loss and high serum tumor necrosis factor alpha levels in polyneuropathy, organomegaly, M protein, skin changes syndrome. Ann Neurol 1994;35:501–505.

Gherardi RK, Chrétien F, Delfau-Larue M-H, et al. Neuropathy in diffuse infiltrative lymphocytosis syndrome. An HIV neuropathy, not a lymphoma. Neurology 1998;50:1041–1044.

Gorson KC, Ropper AH, Clark BD, et al. Treatment of chronic inflammatory demyelinating polyneuropathy with interferon-alpha 2a. Neurology 1998;50:84–87.

Grant IA, Hunder GG, Homburger HA, et al. Peripheral neuropathy associated with sicca complex. Neurology 1997;48:855–862.

Griffin JW, Li CY, Ho TW, et al. Pathology of the motor-sensory axonal Guillain-Barré syndrome. Ann Neurol 1996;39:17–28.

Guillain-Barré Syndrome Steroid Trial Group. Double-blind trial of intravenous methyl prednisolone in Guillain-Barré syndrome. Lancet 1993;341:586–590.

Haanpää M, Häkkinen V, Nurmikko T. Motor involvement in acute herpes zoster. Muscle Nerve 1997;20:1433–1438.

Hafer-Macko CE, Sheikh KA, Li CY, et al. Immune attack on the Schwann cell surface in acute inflammatory demyelinating polyneuropathy. Ann Neurol 1996;39:625–635.

Hahn AF, Bolton CF, Pillay N, et al. Plasma-exchange therapy in chronic inflammatory demyelinating polyneuropathy. A double-blind, sham-controlled, cross-over study. Brain 1996a;119:1055–1066.

Hahn AF, Bolton CF, Zochodne D, et al. Intravenous immunoglobulin treatment in chronic inflammatory demyelinating polyneuropathy. A double-blind, placebo-controlled, cross-over study. Brain 1996b;119:1067–1077.

Harati Y, Gooch C, Swenson M, et al. Double-blind randomized trial of tramadol for the treatment of the pain of diabetic neuropathy. Neurology 1998;50:1842–1846.

Harding AE. From the syndrome of Charcot, Marie and Tooth to disorders of peripheral myelin proteins. Brain 1995; 118:809–818.

Hartung HP, Pollard JD, Harvey GK, Toyka KV. Immunopathogenesis and treatment of Guillain-Barré syndrome—Part I. Muscle Nerve 1995;18:137–153.

Hayasaka K, Himoro M, Sato W, et al. Charcot-Marie-Tooth neuropathy type 1B is associated with mutations of the myelin Po gene. Nat Genet 1993;5:31–34.

Ho TW, Li CY, Cornblath DR, et al. Patterns of recovery in Guillain-Barré syndromes. Neurology 1997;48:695–700.

Ho TW, Mishu B, Li CY, et al. Guillain-Barré syndrome in northern China: relationship to *campylobacter jejuni* infection and anti-glycolipid antibodies. Brain 1995;118:597–605.

Holland NR, Stocks A, Hauer P, et al. Intraepidermal nerve fiber density in patients with painful sensory neuropathy. Neurology 1997;48:708–711.

Horrobin DF. Essential fatty acids in the management of impaired nerve function in diabetes. Diabetes 1997;46(Suppl. 2):S90–S93.

Hughes RAC, Britton T, Richards M. Effects of lymphoma on the nervous system. J R Soc Med 1994;87:526–530.

The Italian Guillain-Barré study group. The prognosis and main prognostic indicators of Guillain-Barré syndrome: a multicenter prospective study of 297 patients. Brain 1996;119:2053–2061.

Jackson CE, Amato AA, Barohn RJ. Isolated vitamin E deficiency. Muscle Nerve 1996;19:1161–1165.

Jacobs BC, van Doorn PA, Schmitz PIM. Campylobacter jejuni infections and anti-GM$_1$ antibodies in Guillain-Barré syndrome. Ann Neurol 1996;40:181–187.

Kaji R, Oka N, Tsuji T, et al. Pathological findings at the site of conduction block in multifocal motor neuropathy. Ann Neurol 1993;33:152–158.

Kaku DA, Parry GJ, Malamut A, et al. Nerve conduction studies in Charcot-Marie-Tooth polyneuropathy associated with a segmental duplication of chromosome 17. Neurology 1993;43:1806–1808.

Katz JS, Wolfe GI, Bryan WW, et al. Electrophysiologic findings in multifocal motor neuropathy. Neurology 1997;48:700–707.

Khella SL, Frost S, Hermann GA, et al. Hepatitis C infection, cryoglobulinemia, and vasculitic neuropathy. Treatment with interferon alfa: case report and literature review. Neurology 1995;45:407–411.

Khoo D, Carmichael SW, Spinner RJ. Ulnar nerve anatomy and compression. Orthop Clin North Am 1996;27:317–338.

Kim DH, Kline DG. Management and results of peroneal nerve lesions. Neurosurgery 1996;39:312–320.

Kissel JT. Autoantibody testing in the evaluation of peripheral neuropathy. Semin Neurol 1998;18:83–94.

Kissel JT. Vasculitis of the peripheral nervous system. Semin Neurol 1994;14:361–369.

Kissel JT, Mendell JR. Neuropathies associated with monoclonal gammopathies. Neuromuscul Disord 1995;6:3–18.

Krendel DA, Costigan DA, Hopkins LC. Successful treatment of neuropathies in patients with diabetes mellitus. Arch Neurol 1995;52:1053–1061.

Lacomis D, Giuliani MJ, Van Cott A, Kramer DJ. Acute myopathy of intensive care: clinical, electromyographic, and pathological aspects. Ann Neurol 1996;40:645–654.

Lin KP, Kwan SY, Chen SY, et al. Generalized neuropathy in Taiwan: an etiologic survey. Neuroepidemiology 1993;12:257–261.

Logigian EL. Peripheral nervous system Lyme borreliosis. Semin Neurol 1997;17:25–30.

Low PA. Laboratory Evaluation of Autonomic Failure. In PA Low (ed), Clinical Autonomic Disorders. Boston: Little, Brown, 1993a;169–195.

Low PA. Neurogenic Orthostatic Hypotension. In RT Johnson, JW Griffin (eds), Current Therapy in Neurologic Disease (4th ed). St. Louis: Mosby–Year Book, 1993b;369–373.

Low PA, Gilden JL, Freeman R, et al. Efficacy of midodrine vs. placebo in neurogenic orthostatic hypotension. A randomized, double-blind multicenter study. Midodrine study group. JAMA 1997;277:1046–1051.

Lupski JR. Molecular Genetics of Peripheral Neuropathies. In JD Martin (ed), Molecular Neurology. New York: Scientific American, 1998;239–256.

Lupski JR, Chance PF, Garcia CA. Inherited primary peripheral neuropathies: molecular genetics and clinical implications of CMT1A and HNPP. JAMA 1993;270:2326–2330.

Mariette X, Chastang C, Clavelou P, et al. A randomised clinical trial comparing interferon-alpha and intravenous immunoglobulin in polyneuropathy associated with monoclonal IgM. J Neurol Neurosurg Psychiatry 1997;63:28–34.

Martyn CN, Hughes RA. Epidemiology of peripheral neuropathy. J Neurol Neurosurgery Psychiatry 1997;62:310–318.

McDonald WI, Kocen RS. Diphtheritic Neuropathy. In PJ Dyck, PK Thomas, JW Griffin, et al. (eds), Peripheral Neuropathy (2nd ed). Philadelphia: Saunders, 1993;1412–1417.

McKhann GM, Cornblath DR, Griffin JW, et al. Acute motor axonal neuropathy. A frequent cause of acute flaccid paralysis in China. Ann Neurol 1993;33:333–342.

Mendell JR, Barohn RJ, Bosch EP, Kissel JT. Continuum-Peripheral Neuropathy, Part A, Vol. I. Minneapolis, MN: American Academy of Neurology, 1994;1:1–103.

Midroni G, Dyck PJ. Chronic inflammatory demyelinating polyradiculoneuropathy: unusual clinical features and therapeutic responses. Neurology 1996;46:1202–1212.

Mirza MA, King ET. Newer techniques of carpal tunnel release. Orthop Clin North Am 1996;27:355–371.

Moser HW. Clinical and therapeutic aspects of adrenoleukodystrophy and adrenomyeloneuropathy. J Neuropathol Exp Neurol 1995;54:740–745.

Moulin DE, Hagen N, Feasby TE, et al. Pain in Guillain-Barré syndrome. Neurology 1997;48:328–331.

Nathan DM. Long-term complications of diabetes mellitus. N Engl J Med 1993;328:1676–1684.

Nathan PA, Keniston RC, Myers LD, et al. Natural history of median nerve conduction in industry: relationship to symptoms and carpal tunnel syndrome in 558 hands over 11 years. Muscle Nerve 1998;21:711–721.

Nelson KA, Park KM, Robinovitz E, et al. High-dose oral dextromethorphan versus placebo in painful diabetic neuropathy and postherpetic neuralgia. Neurology 1997;48:1212–1218.

New PZ, Jackson CE, Rinaldi D, et al. Peripheral neuropathy secondary to docetaxel (Taxotere). Neurology 1996;46:108–111.

Nishino H, Rubino FA, DeRemee RA, et al. Neurological involvement in Wegener's granulomatosis: an analysis of 324 consecutive patients at the Mayo Clinic. Ann Neurol 1993;33:4–9.

Notermans NC, Lokhorst HM, Franssen H, et al. Intermittent cyclophosphamide and prednisone treatment or polyneuropathy associated with monoclonal gammopathy of undetermined significance. Neurology 1996b;47:1227–1233.

Notermans NC, Wokke JHJ, van den Berg LH, et al. Chronic idiopathic axonal polyneuropathy. Comparison of patients with and without monoclonal gammopathy. Brain 1996a;119:421–427.

Ochoa JL. The human sensory unit and pain: new concepts, syndromes, and tests. Muscle Nerve 1993;16:1009–1016.

Olney RK. Neuropathies associated with connective tissue disease. Semin Neurol 1998;18:63–72.

Othmane BK, Hentati F, Lennon F, et al. Linkage of a locus (CMT4A) for autosomal recessive Charcot-Marie-Tooth disease to chromosome 8q. Hum Mol Genet 1993;2:1625–1628.

Pascoe MK, Low PA, Windebank AJ, Litchy WJ. Subacute diabetic proximal neuropathy. Mayo Clin Proc 1997;72:1123–1132.

Pestronk A, Lopate G, Kornberg AJ, et al. Distal lower motor neuron syndrome with high-titer serum IgM anti-GM_1 antibodies: improvement following immunotherapy with monthly plasma exchange and intravenous cyclophosphamide. Neurology 1994;44:2027–2031.

Plasma Exchange/Sandoglobulin Guillain-Barré Syndrome Trial Group. Randomized trial of plasma exchange, intravenous immunoglobulin, and combined treatments in Guillain-Barré syndrome. Lancet 1997;349:225–230.

Puéchal X, Said G, Hilliquin P, et al. Peripheral neuropathy with necrotizing vasculitis in rheumatoid arthritis. Arthritis Rheum 1995;38:1618–1629.

Rees J, Gregson NA, Hughes RAC. Anti-ganglioside GM_1 antibodies in Guillain-Barré syndrome and their relationship to campylobacter jejuni infection. Ann Neurol 1995;38:809–816.

Rogers LR, Borkowski GP, Albers JW, et al. Obturator mononeuropathy caused by pelvic cancer: six cases. Neurology 1993;43:1489–1492.

Ropper AH, Gorson KC. Neuropathies associated with paraproteinemia. N Engl J Med 1998;338:1601–1607.

Sadler M, Nelson M. Peripheral neuropathy in HIV. Int J STD AIDS 1997;8:16–22.

Saito M, Hayashi Y, Suzuki T, et al. Linkage mapping of the gene for Charcot-Marie-Tooth disease type 2 to chromosome 1p (CMT2A) and the clinical features of CMT2A. Neurology 1997;49:1630–1635.

Sander HW, Quinto CM, Elinzano H, Chokroverty S. Carpet carrier's palsy: musculocutaneous neuropathy. Neurology 1997;48:1731–1732.

Savage DG, Lindenbaum J. Neurological complications of acquired cobalamin deficiency: clinical aspects. Bailliere Clin Haematol 1995;8:657–678.

Schaumburg HH, Kaplan JG. Toxic Peripheral Neuropathies. In AK Asbury, PK Thomas (eds), Peripheral Nerve Disorders 2. Oxford: Butterworth–Heinemann, 1995;238–261.

Schmidt B, Toyka KV, Kiefer R, et al. Inflammatory infiltrates in sural nerve biopsies in Guillain-Barré syndrome and chronic inflammatory demyelinating neuropathy. Muscle Nerve 1996;19:474–487.

Schmidt BL. PCR in laboratory diagnosis of human *Borrelia burgdorferi* infections. Clin Microbiol Rev 1997;10:185–201.

Scott TF. Neurosarcoidosis: progress and clinical aspects. Neurology 1993;43:8–12.

Sehgal M, Swanson JW, DeRemee RA, et al. Neurologic manifestations of Churg-Strauss syndrome. Mayo Clin Proc 1995;70:337–341.

Sica REP, Gonzalez Cappa SM, Sanz OP, Mirkin G. Peripheral nervous system involvement in human and experimental chronic American trypanosomiasis. Bull Soc Pathol Exot 1995;88:156–163.

Simmons Z, Albers JW, Bromberg M, et al. Long-term follow-up of patients with chronic inflammatory demyelinating polyradiculoneuropathy, without and with monoclonal gammopathy. Brain 1995;118:359–358.

Simmons Z, Albers JW, Bromberg MB, et al. Presentation and initial clinical course in patients with chronic inflammatory demyelinating polyradiculoneuropathy: comparison of patients without and with monoclonal gammopathy. Neurology 1993;43:2202–2209.

Skinner M, Lewis WD, Jones LA, et al. Liver transplantation as a treatment for familial amyloidotic polyneuropathy. Ann Intern Med 1994;120:133–134.

Smith BE. Cranial Neuropathy in Diabetes Mellitus. In PJ Dyck, PK Thomas (eds): Diabetic Neuropathy. Philadelphia: Saunders, 1998;457–467.

So YT, Olney RK. Acute lumbosacral polyradiculopathy in acquired immunodeficiency syndrome: experience in 23 patients. Ann Neurol 1994;35:53–58.

Stevens JC. The electrodiagnosis of carpal tunnel syndrome. Muscle Nerve 1997;20:1477–1486.

Suarez GA, Cohen ML, Larkin J, et al. Acute intermittent porphyria: clinicopathologic correlation. Report of a case and review of the literature. Neurology 1997;48:1678–1683.

Suarez GA, Giannini C, Smith BE, et al. Localized hypertrophic neuropathy. Mayo Clin Proc 1994;69:747–748.

Tatum AH. Experimental paraprotein neuropathy, demyelination by passive transfer of human IgM anti-myelin-associated glycoprotein. Ann Neurol 1993;33:502–506.

Tefferi A, Solberg Jr. LA, Ellefson RD. Porphyrias: clinical evaluation and interpretation of laboratory tests. Mayo Clin Proc 1994;69:289–290.

Theriault M, Dort J, Sutherland G, et al. A prospective quantitative study of sensory deficits after whole sural nerve biopsies in diabetic and nondiabetic patients. Surgical approach and the role of collateral sprouting. Neurology 1998;50:480–484.

Thomas PK. Classification, differential diagnosis, and staging of diabetic neuropathy. Diabetes 1997;46(Suppl. 2):S54–S57.

Thornton CA, Ballow M. Safety of intravenous immunoglobulin. Arch Neurol 1993;50:135–136.

Toh BH, Van Driel IR, Gleeson PA. Pernicious anemia. N Engl J Med 1997;337:1441–1448.

Tyson J, Malcom S, Thomas PK, Harding AE. Deletions of chromosome 17p11.2 in multifocal neuropathies. Ann Neurol 1996;39:180–186.

Uchuya M, Graus F, Vega F, et al. Intravenous immunoglobulin treatment in paraneoplastic neurologic syndromes with anti-neuronal antibodies. J Neurol Neurosurg Psychiatry 1996;60:388–392.

Van den Berg LH, Franssen H, Wokke JHJ. The long-term effect of intravenous immunoglobulin treatment in multifocal motor neuropathy. Brain 1998;121:421–428.

Van Es HW, Van den Berg LH, Franssen H, et al. Magnetic resonance imaging of the brachial plexus in patients with multifocal motor neuropathy. Neurology 1997;48:1218–1224.

Wallace MS, Wallace AM, Lee J, Dodke MK. Pain after breast surgery: a survey of 282 women. Pain 1996;66:195–205.

Walters MFR, Jacobs J. Leprous neuropathies. Baillieres Clin Neurol 1996;5:171–197.

Wilbourn AJ, Gilliatt RW. Double crush syndrome: a critical analysis. Neurology 1997;49:21–29.

Wilson JR, Conwitt RA, Eidelman BH, et al. Sensorimotor neuropathy resembling CIDP in patients receiving FK506. Muscle Nerve 1994;17:528–532.

Wolfe GI, Barohn RJ. Cryptogenic sensory and sensorimotor polyneuropathies. Semin Neurol 1998;18:105–111.

Yoshioka M, Shapshak P, Srivastava AK, et al. Expression of HIV-1 and interleukin-6 in lumbosacral dorsal root ganglia of patients with AIDS. Ann Neurol 1994;44:1120–1130.

Zehender G, DeMaddalena C, Osio M, et al. High prevalence of human T cell lymphotropic virus type II infection in patients affected by human immunodeficiency virus type I–associated predominantly sensory neuropathy. J Infect Dis 1995;172:1595–1598.

Ziegler D, Gries FA. Alpha-lipoic acid in the treatment of diabetic peripheral and cardiac autonomic neuropathy. Diabetes 1997;46(Suppl. 2):S62–S66.

Zochodne DW. Autonomic involvement in Guillain-Barré syndrome: a review. Muscle Nerve 1994;17:1145–1155.

Chapter 81
Disorders of the Autonomic Nervous System

Christopher J. Mathias

The autonomic nervous system supplies and influences virtually every organ in the body (Figure 81.1). Its effector (efferent) component consists of two major divisions, the sympathetic and parasympathetic nervous systems, whose activity is influenced by several factors: afferent signals from different parts of the body, neurons in the spinal cord, and cerebral centers, mainly in the hypothalamus and brainstem. Autonomic dysfunction may result from lesions in one or more areas of the central or peripheral nervous system. This may result in a generalized disorder, either restricted to the autonomic nervous system (as in primary autonomic failure [PAF]) or involving other neurological systems (as in multiple system atrophy [MSA] or Shy-Drager syndrome). Autonomic impairment may complicate disease processes affecting multiple organs (as in diabetes mellitus or systemic amyloidosis) or may be localized. The latter may cause varying effects: minimal symptoms (in Horner's syndrome); considerable discomfort, which may be socially unacceptable (as in gustatory sweating); and even life-threatening episodes (in carotid sinus hypersensitivity). The clinical problems in autonomic disorders, although often caused by failure, may result from the reverse, that is, the increased activity of hyperhidrosis or hypertension, which may occur in tetanus, Guillain-Barré syndrome, or high spinal cord lesions.

BASIC NEUROANATOMICAL, NEUROPHYSIOLOGICAL, AND NEUROCHEMICAL PRINCIPLES

The afferent pathways influencing the autonomic nervous system consist of virtually every sensory pathway (Figure 81.2), as observed in the autonomic control of blood pressure. The major baroreceptor afferents in the carotid sinus and aortic arch relay information to the brain through cranial nerves IX (glossopharyngeal) and X (vagal). Receptors in the heart and lungs (cardiopulmonary baroreceptors), skin, muscle, and viscera also influence blood pressure. Their role may be unmasked in tetraplegic patients with cervical cord transection above the spinal sympathetic outflow, where the peripheral sympathetic and cranial parasympathetic nervous systems function independently of the brain.

The major cerebral centers concerned with autonomic regulation are in the hypothalamus, midbrain (Edinger-Westphal nucleus and locus ceruleus), and brainstem (nucleus tractus solitarius and vagal nuclei), although many other cerebral areas may influence the autonomic outflow.

The parasympathetic outflow consists of cranial and sacral efferents. Cranial efferents accompany cranial nerves III, VI, IX, and X and supply the eye, lacrimal and salivary glands, heart and lungs, and gastrointestinal tract with associated

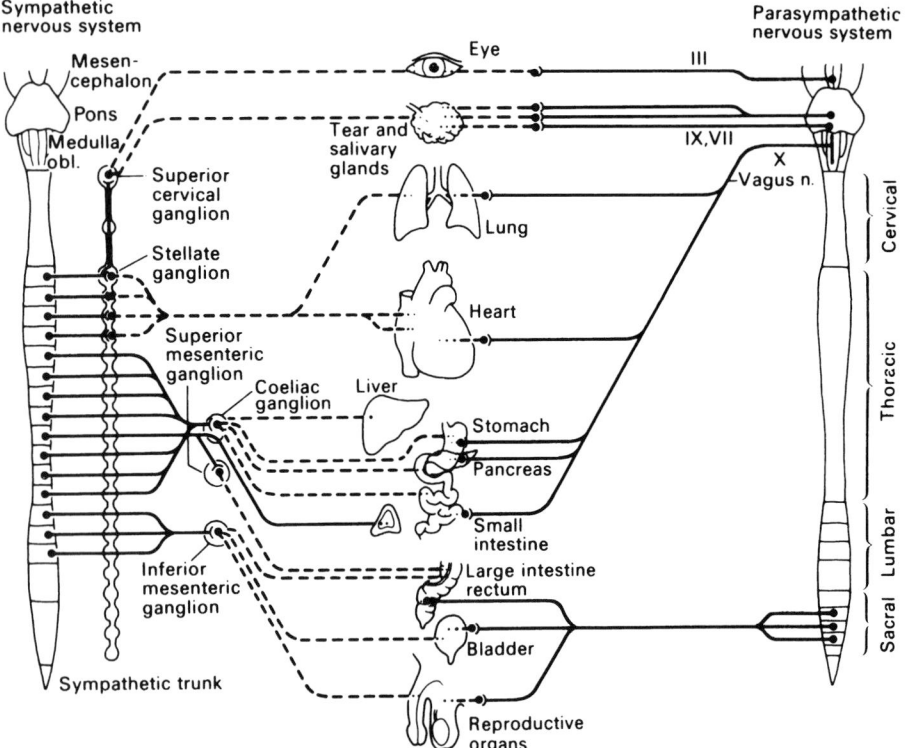

FIGURE 81.1 Parasympathetic and sympathetic innervation of major organs. (n. = nerve; obl. = oblongata.) (Reprinted with permission from W Janig. Autonomic Nervous System. In RF Schmidt, G Thews [eds], Human Physiology [2nd ed]. Berlin: Springer, 1987;333.)

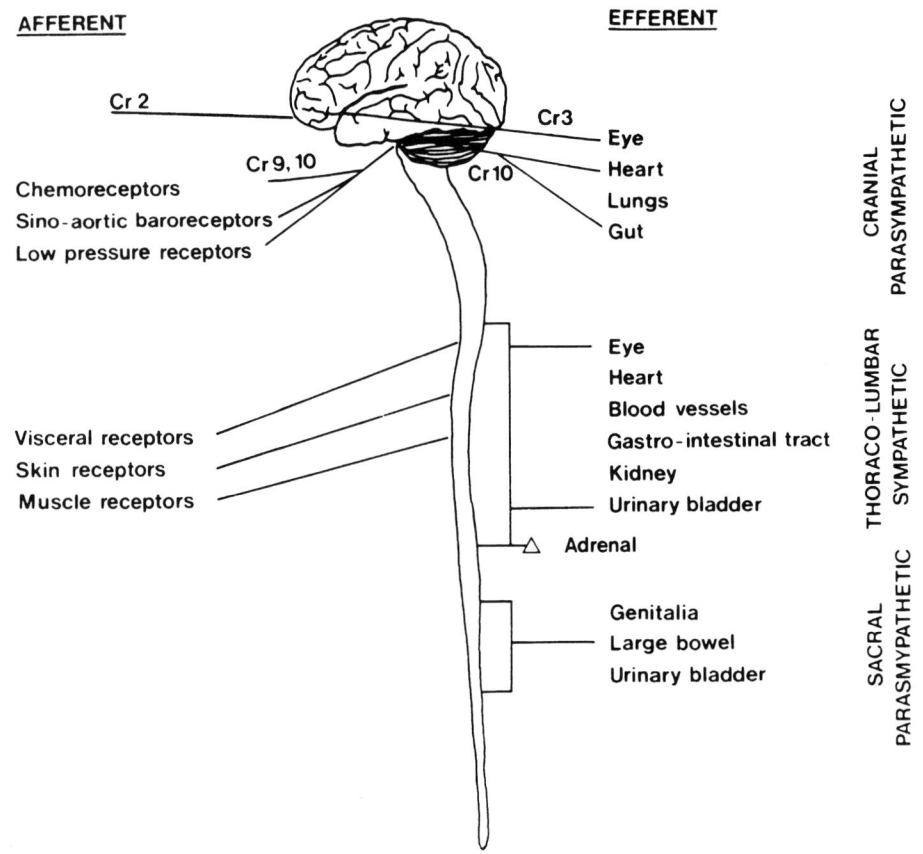

FIGURE 81.2 Schema to indicate the major afferent components that influence parasympathetic and sympathetic afferent activity. (Cr = cranial nerve.) (Reprinted with permission from W Janig. Autonomic Nervous System. In RF Schmidt, G Thews [eds], Human Physiology [2nd ed]. Berlin: Springer, 1987;333.)

structures, down to the level of the colon. The sacral outflow supplies the urinary tract and bladder, the large bowel, and the reproductive system. Cerebral and spinal parasympathetic nuclei have specific control, for example, the Edinger-Westphal nucleus in pupillary control and Onuf's nucleus in the second and third sacral segments in urinary sphincter function. Most parasympathetic ganglia are close to target organs, and acetylcholine is the major transmitter at the ganglia and at postganglionic sites (Figure 81.3).

The sympathetic outflow is connected with major nuclei in the hypothalamus, midbrain, and brainstem and descends through the cervical spinal cord, where axons synapse in the intermediolateral cell mass. From the thoracic and upper lumbar spinal segments, myelinated axons emerge in the white rami and synapse in the paravertebral ganglia, which are some distance from the target organs. The major ganglionic transmitter is acetylcholine. Postganglionic fibers, which are unmyelinated, rejoin the mixed nerve through the gray rami and innervate target organs except for the adrenal medulla, which has only a preganglionic supply. The neurotransmitter at postganglionic sites is predominantly noradrenaline, although sympathetic cholinergic fibers (with acetylcholine as the transmitter) supply sweat glands.

There are complex pathways in neurotransmitter formation, release, and function, as illustrated with the catecholamines (Figure 81.4). Many neurons have multiple neurotransmitters, which may be nonadrenergic and noncholinergic. For example, vasoactive intestinal polypeptide is cosecreted with acetylcholine, which explains the inability of atropine to block all the effects of parasympathetic stimulation, whereas neuropeptide Y may be released with noradrenaline, thus accounting for the fact that α-adrenoceptor blockers may not completely prevent the effects of sympathetic neural stimulation. The availability of specific agonists and antagonists should help dissect the interactions of numerous peptides, amino acids, and amines at multiple sites in response to different stimuli. Despite the multiplicity of neurotransmitters and neuromodulators, however, the autonomic nervous system selectively controls responses in specific regional vascular territories and organs, making it a highly complex but precisely regulated and integrated system.

CLASSIFICATION

Autonomic disorders can be broadly divided into primary, in which no cause has been determined, and secondary (Table 81.1), which are due to specific diseases (such as diabetes mellitus) or where there are strong associations, as with Holmes-Adie syndrome or aging. Drugs are a major cause of autonomic dysfunction, acting at single or multiple sites (Table 81.2). In neurally mediated syncope, there is an intermittent autonomic abnormality, as occurs in vasovagal syncope and carotid sinus hypersensitivity. Table 81.3 pro-

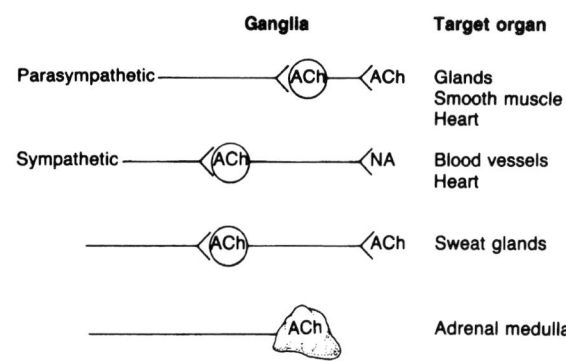

FIGURE 81.3 Outline of the major transmitters at autonomic ganglia and postganglionic sites on target organs. Ganglionic blockade at nicotinic receptors with hexamethonium prevents both parasympathetic and sympathetic activation. Atropine, however, only acts on muscarinic receptors at postganglionic parasympathetic and sympathetic cholinergic sites. (ACh = acetylcholine; NA = noradrenaline.)

vides examples of autonomic disorders in which localized deficits affect specific organs.

Primary Autonomic Failure

Disorders of primary autonomic failure are those in which autonomic failure is of unknown etiology. Most are chronic autonomic failure syndromes.

Chronic Autonomic Failure

These patients often have both sympathetic and parasympathetic failure (Table 81.4). Clinically they fall into three major categories (Figure 81.5). Patients with autonomic failure alone, and no other neurological features, have PAF. This group encompasses *idiopathic orthostatic hypotension* (without other neurological defects), a term that does not indicate the possible autonomic involvement of sweat glands, pupils, and urinary bladder, bowel, and sexual function. When primary chronic autonomic failure is associated with other neurological abnormalities and without a defined cause or association, the term *Shy-Drager syndrome* was used after the first neuropathological description and linkage between orthostatic hypotension and neurological abnormalities. *MSA* is often used synonymously with *Shy-Drager syndrome*; some have felt that MSA implies but does not necessarily include autonomic failure, unlike Shy-Drager syndrome. At a consensus meeting of international experts, MSA was defined as "a sporadic, progressive disorder characterized by autonomic dysfunction, parkinsonism, and ataxia in any combination" (Consensus Statement 1996). There are three major clinical forms of MSA, based on the additional neurological features. The presence of parkinsonian features is probably associated with striatonigral degeneration and loss of pig-

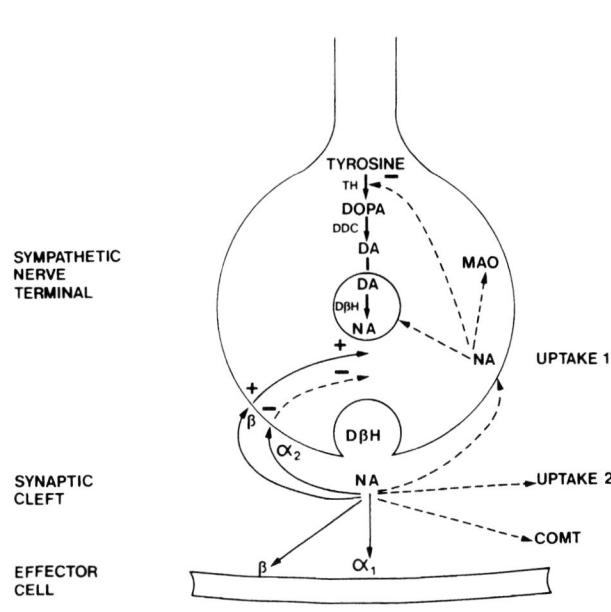

A

TYROSINE

DOPA

DOPAMINE

NORADRENALINE

ADRENALINE

B

FIGURE 81.4 (A) Outline of biosynthetic stages and enzymes involved in the formation of noradrenaline and adrenaline from tyrosine. (B) Schema of some pathways in the formation, release, and metabolism of noradrenaline from sympathetic nerve terminals. Tyrosine is converted into dihydroxyphenylalanine (DOPA) by tyrosine hydroxylase (TH). DOPA is converted into dopamine (DA) by dopa decarboxylase (DDC). In the vesicles, DA is converted into noradrenaline (NA) by dopamine β-hydroxylase (DβH). Nerve impulses release both DβH and NA into the synaptic cleft by exocytosis. NA acts predominantly on α₁-adrenoceptors but has actions on β-adrenoceptors on the effector cell of target organs. It also has

presynaptic adrenoceptor effects. Those acting on α₂-adrenoceptors inhibit NA release; those on β-adrenoceptors stimulate NA release. NA may be taken up by a neuronal process (uptake 1) into the cytosol, where it may inhibit further formation of DOPA through the rate-limiting enzyme TH. NA may be taken into vesicles or metabolized by monoamine oxidase (MAO) in the mitochondria. NA may be taken up by a higher-capacity but lower-affinity extraneuronal process (uptake 2) into peripheral tissues, such as vascular and cardiac muscle and certain glands. NA is also metabolized by catechol-O-methyl transferase (COMT). Thus, NA measured in plasma is the overspill not affected by these numerous processes.

mented cells in the substantia nigra and locus ceruleus; this is called the *parkinsonian* or *striatonigral degeneration form*. There may be cerebellar manifestations, with or without pyramidal signs, and an association with atrophy of the cerebellum, olives, and pons (called the *cerebellar* or *olivopontocerebellar atrophy form*). Many patients, especially as the disease progresses, have a combination of extrapyramidal, cerebellar, and pyramidal manifestations (called the *mixed* or *multiple form*). In our autonomic unit, which serves as a national referral center, approximately 20% of patients have the parkinsonian form, 20% have the cerebellar form, and 60% have the multiple form. This distribution probably varies depending on referral patterns, the special interests of the hospital, early consideration of the diagnosis, and the presence of an autonomic unit.

The extrapyramidal features may predate autonomic failure in the parkinsonian form of MSA and may be difficult to differentiate from idiopathic Parkinson's disease, especially in the early stages. This has been highlighted in postmortem studies, in which 7–22% of patients who were thought to have idiopathic Parkinson's disease actually had MSA. Separating the two disorders is important because the

prognosis is considerably poorer in MSA, and the frequency and nature of complications and the management of the conditions differ (Mathias and Williams 1994; Wenning et al. 1994). There are some differences in the extrapyramidal features between MSA and Parkinson's disease (Quinn and Marsden 1993), but these may not be clinically valuable, especially in individual subjects in the early stages. Although many MSA patients do not respond favorably to L-dopa or experience substantial side effects, such as postural hypotension, a proportion with the parkinsonian form benefit, especially in the early stages (Colosimo et al. 1995), as do the majority with idiopathic Parkinson's disease. Differentiation of the two groups is important in relation to drug trials and interventional studies (e.g., as with substantia nigra implantation) because those with MSA are unlikely to respond favorably.

There is a group with apparent idiopathic Parkinson's disease in whom autonomic failure may occur, often as a late complication. These patients usually are elderly and have been successfully treated with L-dopa and other antiparkinsonian drugs for many years. They thus differ clinically from those who have the parkinsonian forms of MSA. It is not

Table 81.1: Classification of disorders resulting in autonomic dysfunction

Primary (etiology unknown)
  Acute and subacute dysautonomias
    Pure cholinergic dysautonomia
    Pure pandysautonomia
    Pandysautonomia with neurological features
  Chronic autonomic failure syndromes
    Pure autonomic failure
    Multiple system atrophy (Shy-Drager syndrome)
    Autonomic failure with Parkinson's disease
Secondary
  Congenital
    Nerve growth factor deficiency
  Hereditary
    Autosomal dominant trait
      Familial amyloid neuropathy
      Porphyria
    Autosomal recessive trait
      Familial dysautonomia (Riley-Day syndrome)
      Dopamine β-hydroxylase deficiency
      Aromatic L-amino acid decarboxylase deficiency
    X-linked recessive
      Fabry's disease
  Metabolic diseases
    Diabetes mellitus
    Chronic renal failure
    Chronic liver disease
    Vitamin B_{12} deficiency
    Alcohol-induced
  Inflammatory
    Guillain-Barré syndrome
    Transverse myelitis
  Infections
    Bacterial: tetanus
    Viral: human immunodeficiency virus
    Parasitic: *Trypanosoma cruzi*; Chagas' disease
    Prion: fatal familial insomnia
  Neoplasia
    Brain tumors, especially of third ventricle or posterior fossa
    Paraneoplastic, to include adenocarcinomas: lung, pancreas, and Lambert-Eaton syndrome
  Connective tissue disorders
    Rheumatoid arthritis
    Systemic lupus erythematosus
    Mixed connective tissue disease
  Surgery
    Regional sympathectomy: upper limb and splanchnic denervation
    Vagotomy and drainage procedures: "dumping" syndrome
    Organ transplantation: heart, kidney
  Trauma
    Spinal cord transection
  Miscellaneous
    Subarachnoid hemorrhage
    Syringobulbia and syringomyelia
Neurally mediated syncope
  Vasovagal syncope
  Carotid sinus hypersensitivity
  Micturition syncope
  Cough syncope
  Swallow syncope
  Associated with glossopharyngeal neuralgia

Table 81.2: Drugs, chemicals, poisons, and toxins causing autonomic dysfunction

Decreasing sympathetic activity
  Centrally acting
    Clonidine
    Methyldopa
    Moxonidine
    Reserpine
    Barbiturates
    Anesthetics
  Peripherally acting
    Sympathetic nerve ending (guanethidine, bethanidine)
    α-Adrenoceptor blockade (phenoxybenzamine)
    β-Adrenoceptor blockade (propranolol)
Increasing sympathetic activity
  Amphetamines
  Releasing noradrenaline (tyramine)
  Uptake blockers (imipramine)
  Monoamine oxidase inhibitors (tranylcypromine)
  β-Adrenoceptor stimulants (isoprenaline)
Decreasing parasympathetic activity
  Antidepressants (imipramine)
  Tranquilizers (phenothiazines)
  Antidysrhythmics (disopyramide)
  Anticholinergics (atropine, probanthine, benztropine)
  Toxins (botulinum)
Increasing parasympathetic activity
  Cholinomimetics (carbachol, bethanechol, pilocarpine, mushroom poisoning)
  Anticholinesterases
    Reversible carbamate inhibitors (pyridostigmine, neostigmine)
    Organophosphorous inhibitors (parathion, sarin)
Miscellaneous
  Alcohol, thiamine (vitamin B_1) deficiency
  Vincristine, perhexiline maleate
  Thallium, arsenic, mercury
  Mercury poisoning (pink disease)
  Ciguatera toxicity
  Jellyfish and marine animal venoms
  First dose of certain drugs (prazosin, captopril)
  Withdrawal of chronically used drugs (clonidine, opiates, alcohol)

clear if they are a special group with idiopathic Parkinson's disease who are vulnerable to autonomic degeneration or their autonomic failure is associated with old age, chronic drug therapy, or a combination of such factors.

In chronic primary autonomic failure syndromes, a common feature accounting for sympathetic dysfunction is loss of small sympathetic cells in the intermediolateral cell column of the thoracic and lumbar spinal cord (Figure 81.6). In PAF, for which limited neuropathological data are available, there also is substantial neuronal cell loss in the paravertebral sympathetic ganglia (Matthews 1999). Some of the surviving ganglionic neurones in the paravertebral ganglia show Lewy bodies that are not found in MSA; these include "eosinophilic bodies" of bizarre serpiginous form, now regarded as intraneuritic Lewy bodies. The absence of additional neurological features, and the available biochemical

Table 81.3:   Examples of localized autonomic disorders

Horner's syndrome
Holmes-Adie pupil
Crocodile tears (Bogorad's syndrome)
Gustatory sweating (Frey's syndrome)
Reflex sympathetic dystrophy
Idiopathic palmar or axillary hyperhidrosis
Chagas' disease (*Trypanosomiasis cruzi*)[a]
Surgical procedures[b]
    Sympathectomy (regional)
    Vagotomy and gastric drainage procedures in "dumping" syndrome
    Organ transplantation (heart, lungs)

[a]Listed here because it specifically targets intrinsic cholinergic plexuses in the heart and gut.
[b]Surgery also may cause other localized disorders, such as Frey's syndrome, after parotid surgery.

Table 81.4:   Some of the clinical manifestations in primary chronic autonomic failure.

Cardiovascular: postural (orthostatic) hypotension
Sudomotor: anhidrosis, heat intolerance
Gastrointestinal: constipation, occasionally diarrhea, oropharyngeal dysphagia
Renal and urinary bladder: nocturia, frequency, urgency, retention, incontinence
Sexual: erectile and ejaculatory failure in the male
Ocular: anisocoria, Horner's syndrome
Respiratory: stridor, involuntary inspiratory gasps, apneic episodes
Other neurological deficits: parkinsonian and cerebellar or pyramidal features

and hormonal evidence which excludes central cerebral involvement (Kimber et al. 1997b; Mathias and Polinsky 1999), are consistent with a peripheral sympathetic lesion in PAF. In MSA, the evidence points to predominantly cerebral autonomic lesions. In addition, there is cell loss in the intermediolateral cell column of the thoracic and lumbar spinal cord. An additional feature is the involvement of neurons in the margins of the ventral horn of the second and third sacral segments (Onuf's nucleus), which innervate the voluntary sphincters of the urinary bladder and anus. These nuclei are spared in motor neuron diseases, which suggests that they are more likely to be parasympathetic than somatic neurons. It is not known if these cell groups are affected in PAF. In MSA, neurons of sympathetic ganglia are not in general severely reduced and do not exhibit major abnormalities, apart from a relative lack of Nissl material, that suggest partial denervation atrophy of long-standing duration.

In MSA, neuropathological studies indicate widespread abnormalities in the brain (Daniel 1999). In the parkinsonian form, the proportion of brainstem and cerebellum to whole brain is normal, unlike the cerebellar form. In the parkinsonian form, the putamen is shrunken with gray-green discoloration, and in severe forms, there is a cribriform appearance. Atrophy and discoloration of the caudate nucleus and pallidum are less common. The substantia nigra shows decreased pigmentation. There is pallor of the locus ceruleus. In the cerebellar form, the pons and the middle cerebellar peduncles are reduced, with atrophy of the folia. On microscopy, there is cell loss and gliosis in the parkinsonian forms, particularly in the putamen, and especially in the posterior two-thirds and dorsolateral regions, although this may be more widespread. Similar changes also occur in the caudate nucleus and globus pallidus but to a lesser extent than in the putamen. In the zona compacta of the substantia nigra, there is degeneration of pigmented nerve cells, as in the locus ceruleus. In the cerebellar

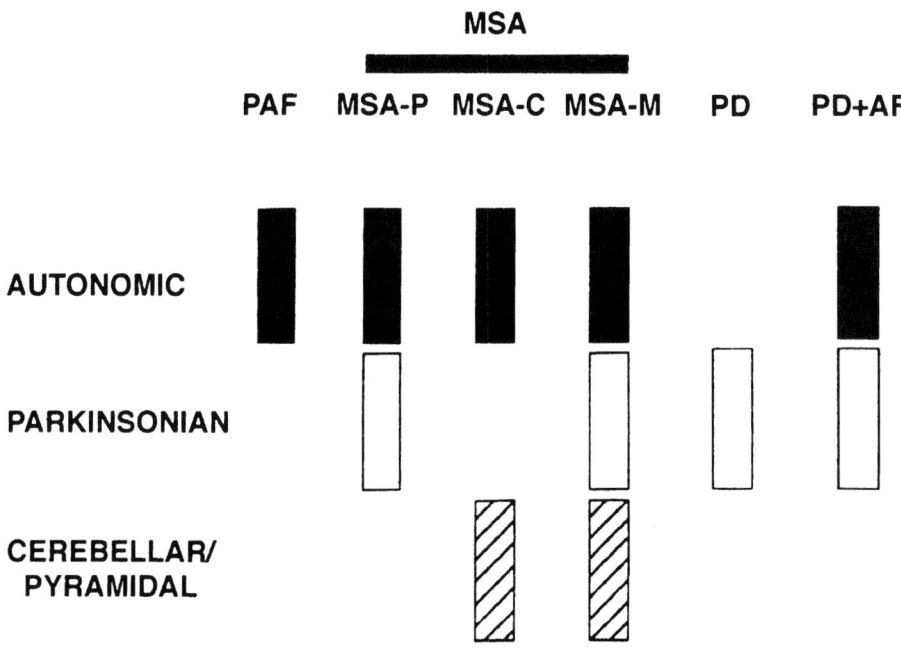

FIGURE 81.5 Schematic representation of the major clinical features of primary chronic autonomic failure syndromes. These include pure autonomic failure (PAF) and the three major neurological forms of multiple system atrophy (MSA): the parkinsonian form (MSA-P, synonymous with striatonigral degeneration), the cerebellar form (MSA-C, synonymous with olivopontocerebellar atrophy), and the mixed form (MSA-M, with both features). Also included are Parkinson's disease (PD) and the rarer subgroup with Parkinson's disease and autonomic failure (PD+AF). (Modified with permission from CJ Mathias. Autonomic disorders and their recognition. N Engl J Med 1997;10:721.)

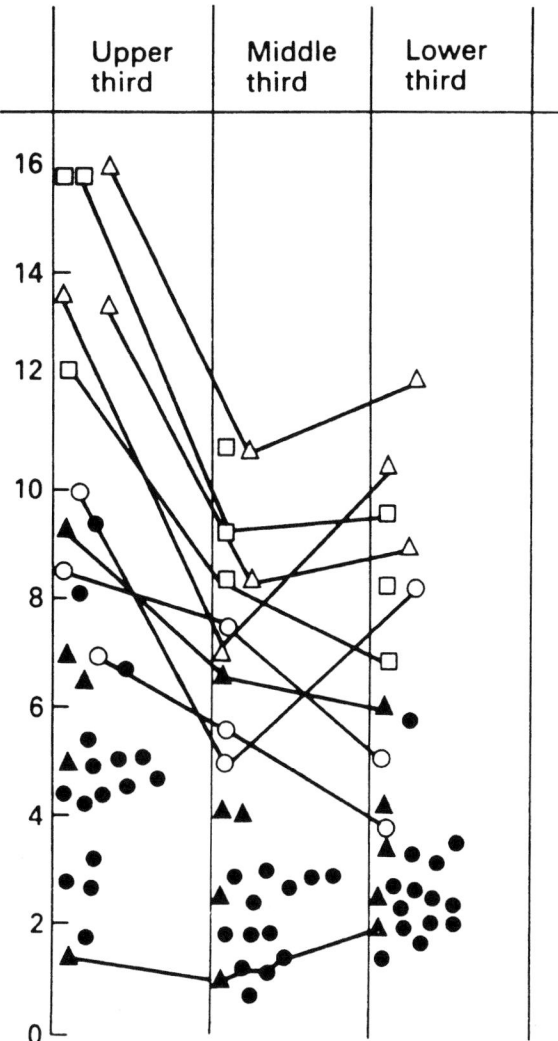

FIGURE 81.6   Cell counts in intermediolateral horns of upper, middle, and lower thoracic spinal cord. Figures indicate mean number of cells in a single lateral horn and 20-mm sections in controls. These include three patients with Parkinson's disease without autonomic failure (△), three patients with multiple system atrophy without autonomic failure (○), and 16 patients with autonomic failure (●), and five patients with autonomic failure showing Lewy bodies in the brainstem (▲). (Reprinted with permission from DR Oppenheimer et al. Lateral horn cells in progressive autonomic failure. J Neurol Sci 1980;46:393–404.)

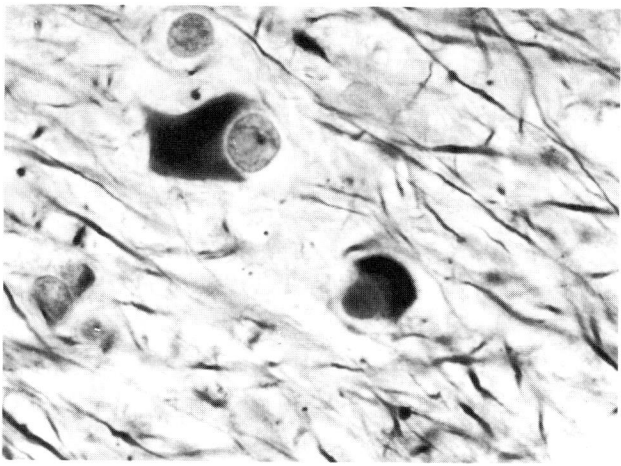

FIGURE 81.7   Photomicrograph showing appearance of oligodendrocyte glial cytoplasmic inclusions with modified Bielschowsky's silver impregnation and immunocytochemistry for alpha tubulin (frontal cortex, ×1250). (Reprinted with permission from SE Daniel. The Neuropathology and Neurochemistry of Multiple System Atrophy. In CJ Mathias, R Bannister [eds], Autonomic Failure. A Textbook of Clinical Disorders of the Autonomic Nervous System [4th ed]. Oxford: Oxford University Press, 1999;321–328.)

form, the neuropathology may be indistinguishable from familial forms of olivopontocerebellar atrophy. There is cell loss in the cerebellum, olives, and pons. Purkinje's cell nerve loss is often focal, rarely complete, and not accompanied by basket cell loss and thus different from cerebellar anoxic damage, in which both cell groups are vulnerable.

The parkinsonian forms, therefore, show features indicative of striatonigral degeneration, while those with the less common cerebellar form show olivopontocerebellar degeneration. Despite characteristic pathology in one or the other system in the two forms, there is often widespread involvement neuropathologically, consistent with in vivo findings using positron emission tomography (PET) (Rinne et al. 1995). As

the disease progresses, there is likely to be an increasing degree of cell loss and gliosis, which probably accounts for the varying pathological descriptions provided over the years.

A key feature in MSA has been the presence of glial intraneuronal cytoplasmic nuclei inclusions (Papp and Lantos 1994) (Figure 81.7). These stain with antibodies against ubiquitin, alpha and beta tubulin, and tau, thereby indicating a site of origin from cytoskeletal proteins. In MSA, they are present in large numbers and provide a pathological hallmark for the definition of the condition (Daniel 1999). They are also present in previously considered unaffected areas of the brain. Similar inclusions to those in MSA have been described in progressive supranuclear palsy, corticobasal degeneration, and familial olivopontocerebellar atrophy. However, in these conditions they are infrequent, require careful search, and have distinct differences in tau profile.

In MSA, a number of additional sites may be involved. These include degeneration of the thalamus and vestibular complex. There is a reduction of Edinger-Westphal neurons. Cell loss in the hypothalamus is minimal but with an apparent depletion of various catecholamines and neurotransmitters, which may account for the neuroendocrine abnormalities and impairment of hypothalamic function reported. There often is atrophy of the dorsal motor nucleus of the vagus. Despite laryngeal dysfunction being common, cell loss has not been documented in the nucleus ambiguus, which suggests a central biochemical deficit or more peripheral involvement, or both.

In summary, in PAF, the evidence favors a distal lesion involving the intermediolateral cell mass in the thoracolumbar regions and the paravertebral ganglia. The disorder usually is not progressive. It is probable that further classification will occur in those clinically considered to have PAF as precise deficits or etiological factors are recognized.

In MSA, there are varying clinical presentations and the disorder is progressive. Whether this is one or several diseases has been debated. Current data on the clinical course, with overlapping features in most patients together with in vivo neuroimaging data (Rinne et al. 1995) and neuropathological data, seem to indicate a single disorder. The reasons for selective involvement (at least initially in some patients), sparing of certain areas, and possible interaction with genetic and environmental factors remain to be determined.

Acute and Subacute Dysautonomias

Acute and subacute dysautonomias are rarer causes of primary autonomic failure that present either acutely or subacutely. The precise causes are unclear and may include viral infections, with immunological damage as a contributory factor. Two case reports have indicated a beneficial response to the intravenous administration of immunoglobulin, which favors an immunological etiology (Heafield et al. 1996; Smit et al. 1997). There are three clinical forms. In pure cholinergic dysautonomia, parasympathetic and sympathetic cholinergic pathways are impaired, resulting in alacrima, xerostomia, dysphagia, large bowel atony, detrusor muscle dysfunction, and, in men, erectile failure; anhidrosis also occurs. Thus, only the cholinergic system is affected. There is a response to cholinomimetic agents, such as bethanechol, indicating preservation of postsynaptic cholinergic receptor function and suggesting a presynaptic lesion. In the other forms with pandysautonomia, the parasympathetic and sympathetic nervous systems are impaired. In some, there are no other neurological features, whereas in others, there may be additional neurological lesions, often involving peripheral nerves. These lesions have been demonstrated on sural nerve biopsy, which shows a reduction in both myelinated and unmyelinated fibers.

Secondary Autonomic Dysfunction

The pathological changes of secondary autonomic dysfunction depend on the causative or associated disease or disorder. A brief description of some of the changes is provided in the following sections, based on the probable site of lesion within the nervous system.

Cerebral

Autonomic failure may result from specific lesions, especially in the brainstem. Posterior fossa tumors and syringobulbia may cause postural hypotension by ischemia or destruction of brainstem cardiovascular centers. Demyelination or plaque formation in multiple sclerosis may cause a variety of autonomic defects of cerebral origin (Thomaides et al. 1993), although it is difficult to exclude a spinal contribution. Autonomic failure in the elderly may be largely central, due to widespread neuronal degeneration, although peripheral neural and target organ deficits may contribute.

Certain cerebral disorders cause a pathological increase in autonomic activity. In bulbar poliomyelitis, hypertension has been associated with damage to the lateral medulla. In cerebral tumors, distortion or ischemia of specific pressor areas, which have been defined experimentally and termed *Cushing-sensitive areas*, may raise blood pressure by increasing sympathetic activity. This may account for the symptoms in a patient of Penfield, who had a tumor of the third ventricle and was thought to have diencephalic autonomic epilepsy. Similar mechanisms may also account for increased sympathetic activity, hypertension, and cardiac dysrhythmias associated with subarachnoid hemorrhage, although the local effects of various chemicals from extravasated blood also may influence cerebral centers. In tetanus, hypertension may result from increased sensitivity of brainstem centers through retrograde spread of tetanus toxin along the nerve fibers. In fatal familial insomnia, a prion disease predominantly involving the thalamus, there are abnormalities of autonomic function. These include an increase in blood pressure, heart rate, lacrimation, salivation, sweating, and body temperature, along with altered hormonal circadian rhythms in the presence of intact target organ function (Cortelli et al. 1997).

Spinal Cord

Damage to the spinal cord by trauma, transverse myelitis, syringomyelia, or spinal cord tumors may disturb or sever connections between the brain and the thoracolumbar sympathetic and sacral parasympathetic outflow. Spinal reflexes through unaffected areas in the cord below the lesion may be activated, resulting in abnormal peripheral autonomic activity.

Peripheral

Peripheral autonomic dysfunction is associated with a wide range of diseases and syndromes. It may involve a specific afferent pathway, as in carotid sinus hypersensitivity. The lesion may involve efferent pathways only, as in dopamine β-hydroxylase (DBH) deficiency, which selectively causes deficiency of noradrenaline and adrenaline, with elevation of the precursor dopamine and preservation of other transmitters in sympathetic nerve terminals (Mathias and Bannister 1999a). In a brother and sister with this disorder, genetic studies indicate an autosomal recessive transmission. DBH genes have been identified on chromosome 9, linked to 9q34, and do not have any obvious deletions in this disorder, thus raising the likelihood of point mutations. In Eaton-Lambert syndrome, the cholinergic system is primarily affected. In diabetes mellitus, different autonomic pathways may be affected as the disease progresses: The cardiac parasympathetic is often involved first, with sympathetic dysfunction occurring later. There may be associated involvement of specific components of peripheral nerves in certain disorders. One of these is nerve growth factor deficiency, which results in the deficiency of DBH, the sensory neuropeptides, substance P, and calcitonin gene-related peptide. Another such disorder is Riley-Day syndrome (familial dysautonomia), in which pathological changes occur in both dorsal root and sympathetic ganglia. In amyloidosis, deposits in the heart, blood vessels, and adrenal glands (causing adrenocortical deficiency) may compound autonomic dysfunction and thus increase the severity of orthostatic hypotension.

Autonomic dysfunction may complicate malignancies, including paraneoplastic syndrome, in which it is often not possible to determine the site of the lesion. Acquired immunodeficiency syndrome is associated with several autonomic abnormalities. Pheochromocytoma occasionally may be part of multiple endocrine neoplasia (such as Sipple's syndrome) or may be associated with neurofibromatosis and other neuroectodermal syndromes (tuberous sclerosis, von Hippel–Lindau disease, and Sturge-Weber syndrome). Carotid body tumors, ganglioneuromas, and neuroblastomas also arise from neuroectodermal tissue but are less likely to result in abnormal catecholamine secretion.

Neurally Mediated Syncope

Neurally mediated syncope is a disorder in which there is intermittent dysfunction affecting the autonomic nervous system. This dysfunction results in bradycardia due to increased parasympathetic cardiac activity and hypotension due to withdrawal of sympathetic vasoconstrictor tone. In the young, a common cause is vasovagal syncope. In the elderly, carotid sinus hypersensitivity is increasingly recognized; there may be rarer causes, some of which may be associated with neoplasia affecting the glossopharyngeal nerve.

Drugs, Chemicals, and Toxins

Drugs, chemicals, and toxins may act by interfering with, or stimulating, sympathetic or parasympathetic activity (see Table 81.2). A minor side effect of a drug may unmask or worsen autonomic deficiency; an example is postural hypotension, which is usually enhanced by L-dopa in the parkinsonian and mixed forms of MSA. Drugs administered locally, such as the beta blocker timolol (ocular drops), the α_2-agonist xylometazoline, and the α-agonist phenylephrine (intranasally), may enter the systemic circulation and have deleterious effects.

Alcohol may impair autonomic function either directly, by causing a neuropathy, or through associated deficiencies, such as that of vitamin B_1 (thiamine). The withdrawal of drugs, such as alcohol, opiates, and clonidine, especially when used in high doses chronically, may result in the reverse (sympathetic overactivity), with increased sweating, hypertension, and piloerection.

Vincristine is directly neurotoxic and may cause an associated autonomic neuropathy, as with perhexiline maleate, an antianginal agent. The latter is mainly associated with a metabolic deficit, which slows its degradation. Thallium, arsenic, and mercury increase autonomic activity by mechanisms that are unclear. Botulism mainly results in cholinergic deficits, but there may be associated sympathetic involvement in severe cases. Consumption of reef fish containing ciguatera toxin may cause bradycardia through increased vagal tone, which can be reversed by atropine.

Localized Autonomic Disorders

In Horner's syndrome (see Table 81.3), the sympathetic fibers to the pupil, upper eyelid (the nonstriated portion of the levator palpebrae superioris, or Müller's muscle), facial sweat glands, and facial blood vessels are affected by lesions that could be in the brain (hemorrhage), spinal cord (trauma), or periphery (neoplasms affecting the cervical ganglia, as in Pancoast's syndrome). When only the eye is involved, the lesion lies within the distribution of the internal carotid artery because the sympathetic nerves accompanying the external carotid artery are intact, thus sparing the facial sweat glands and vessels (Raeder's syndrome).

Holmes-Adie pupil is a benign condition, usually seen in women, and is characterized by a dilated pupil that is sluggishly responsive to light. The iris musculature is supersensitive to locally applied cholinomimetics, such as dilute methacholine or pilocarpine. The pathology is thought to involve the parasympathetic ciliary ganglia. When associated with absent tendon reflexes, the term *Holmes-Adie syndrome* is used. The lesion is thought to involve the dorsal root ganglia, which accounts for the absent H on electrophysiological testing. Some patients have sudomotor abnormalities (Ross's syndrome), cardiovascular autonomic deficits, diarrhea, or a dry, chronic cough (Kimber et al. 1998).

In the chronic form of Chagas' disease (after infection with *Trypanosoma cruzi*), fibrosis in the heart causes damage to the sinus node and conducting system. The esophagus and colon are often involved after ganglionitis and destruction of Meissner's and Auerbach's plexuses, thus causing dilatation of the esophagus, stomach, or large bowel. In congenital megacolon (Hirschsprung's disease), parasympathetic ganglion cells from the intramural (Auerbach's) plexus are absent in localized segments of the rectum and sigmoid colon, often with sympathetic aplasia, and cause colonic narrowing with proximal distention.

Increased lacrimation due to an abnormal gustolacrimal reflex (crocodile tears or Bogorad's syndrome) results from cross-innervation of the lacrimal and salivary glands. It may be acquired after Bell's palsy (with the lesion at, or proximal, to the geniculate ganglion) or after surgery to the greater superficial petrosal nerve (which contains fibers to the lacrimal gland and the submandibular and sublingual salivary glands). It may also occur after damage to the lesser superficial petrosal nerve, which supplies the parotid glands. If bilateral, the disorder is usually congenital. A similar situation may occur in gustatory sweating, in which parasympathetic fibers to the salivary glands reinnervate the sweat glands that normally have a sympathetic cholinergic supply (auriculotemporal or Frey's syndrome).

Sympathetic nerve damage may occur with limb or brachial plexus injuries and be either pre- or postganglionic.

Table 81.5: Symptoms that result from postural (orthostatic) hypotension and impaired perfusion of organs

Cerebral hypoperfusion
  Dizziness
  Vision disturbances
  Blurred vision, color defects, scotoma, tunnel, graying out,
    blacking out
  Loss of consciousness
  Impaired cognition
Muscle hypoperfusion
  Paracervical and suboccipital ("coat-hanger") ache
  Lower back or buttock ache
  Calf claudication
Cardiac hypoperfusion: angina pectoris
Spinal cord hypoperfusion
Renal hypoperfusion: oliguria
Nonspecific: weakness, lethargy, fatigue, falls

Source: Adapted with permission from CJ Mathias. Orthostatic hypotension—causes, mechanisms and influencing factors. Neurology 1995;45(Suppl. 5):S6–S11.

Table 81.6: Factors influencing postural (orthostatic) hypotension

Speed of positional change
Time of day (worse in the morning)
Prolonged recumbency
Warm environment (hot weather, central heating, hot bath)
Raising intrathoracic pressure by micturition, defecation, or
  coughing
Food and alcohol ingestion
Physical exertion
Maneuvers and positions (bending forward, abdominal com-
  pression, leg crossing, squatting, activating calf muscle pump)*
Drugs with vasoactive properties (including dopaminergic
  agents)

*These maneuvers usually reduce the postural fall in blood pressure, unlike the others.

If incomplete, severe pain (causalgia) may result from abnormal synaptic connections between the efferent sympathetic nerves and somatosensory afferent nerves. Similar changes may occur in post-traumatic reflex sympathetic dystrophy (Sudeck's atrophy). The precise role of the sympathetic nervous system in such disorders is unclear (Kimber et al. 1997a) and is relevant to their management (Schott 1998).

Transplantation of organs such as the heart and kidneys leaves them bereft of their autonomic nervous supply. After cardiac transplantation, upregulation of β-adrenoceptors may increase sensitivity to endogenous or exogenous catecholamines and could increase the risk from cardiac dysrhythmia. Renal function after transplantation does not appear to be impaired, although nocturnal polyuria may be attributed to lack of sympathetic control of tubular function. Reinnervation may occur, especially in the kidney.

CLINICAL FEATURES

Patients with primary chronic autonomic failure are usually middle-aged or elderly. There is a male predominance. Increased awareness of such disorders and earlier referral for autonomic investigation have resulted in recognition of a number of younger subjects, some in their mid-30s. A family history is unusual. Only two families with autonomic failure and additional neurological abnormalities have been reported, although from the descriptions available they were unlikely to have MSA. In MSA, there is no evidence that genetic, environmental, or occupational risk factors may contribute.

In secondary autonomic failure, the age of onset depends on the associated or causative disorder. Some may present at birth, as in Riley-Day syndrome (familial dysautonomia), which is transmitted as an autosomal recessive trait and usually affects siblings rather than successive generations. Riley-

Day syndrome occurs mainly in Ashkenazi Jews, in whom there is a high frequency of consanguinity. Patients with DBH deficiency syndrome have autonomic problems from childhood. In familial amyloid polyneuropathy, the presenting features usually occur in adulthood. Insulin-dependent diabetics of long duration may develop an autonomic neuropathy.

Cardiovascular System

Hypotension

The symptoms from postural (orthostatic) hypotension often provide the first clue and are usually the reason for requesting medical advice. They mainly result from cerebral hypoperfusion (Table 81.5). Dizziness and visual disturbances (such as blurred vision, graying out, blacking out, or tunnel vision) may precede loss of consciousness. These occur on assuming the upright posture, especially when getting out of bed in the morning (Table 81.6). Food, alcohol, exercise, and a raised environmental temperature usually enhance symptoms. Straining during micturition and bowel movements, which often are affected in autonomic disorders, may induce attacks. Many recognize the association between postural change and the early symptoms of cerebral hypoperfusion and either sit down, lie flat, or assume curious postures, such as squatting or stooping. Occasionally, the blood pressure may fall precipitously, and syncope may occur rapidly, as in a drop attack. Loss of consciousness may result in injury. Seizures may occur in some due to cerebral anoxia. Postural hypotension can be considerably aggravated by drugs (such as L-dopa) that normally cause minimal or no change in blood pressure. In diabetics with an autonomic neuropathy, administration of insulin, either by reducing blood volume through increasing transcapillary albumin escape or by vasodilatatory effects, occasionally may exacerbate postural hypotension.

The fall in blood pressure and symptoms during postural change may vary considerably (Figures 81.8 and 81.9). Many patients tolerate an extremely low cerebral perfusion

FIGURE 81.8   Blood pressure and heart rate measured by a noninvasive technique (with a Finapres [Ohneda, BOC Health Care, UK]) in two patients with autonomic failure before, during, and after head-up tilt. (A) Blood pressure falls to low levels, but the patient could maintain head-up tilt with a low blood pressure for 20 minutes with few symptoms. This patient had autonomic failure for many years and could tolerate such levels, unlike the patient in (B), who had to be put back to the horizontal fairly quickly. She developed severe postural hypotension soon after surgery. (Reprinted with permission from CJ Mathias. Disorders affecting autonomic function in parkinsonian patients. Adv Neurol 1996; 69:383.)

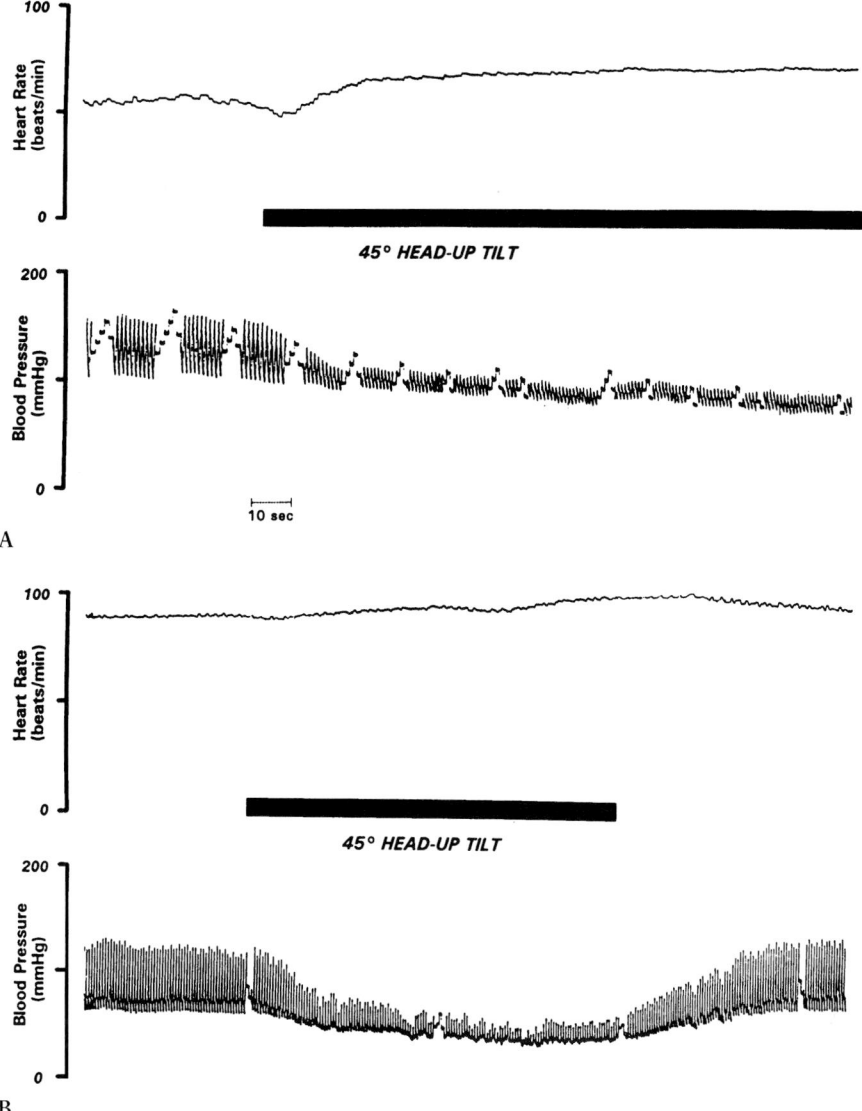

pressure without symptoms, presumably because of improved cerebrovascular autoregulation. This may explain why some patients are at their worst in the early stages of their disorder, as in those with high spinal cord injuries, who later tolerate head-up postural change despite a similar fall in blood pressure. Some may hyperventilate, which should be discouraged because it further reduces cerebral perfusion through cerebral vasoconstriction. Symptomatic tolerance appears to develop with repeated head-up tilt and exposure to hypotension. Patients with spinal injuries soon learn that activation of skeletal muscle spasms or urinary bladder contraction triggers spinal reflexes, and they use this to help reduce the postural fall in blood pressure. In the elderly, a relatively small fall in blood pressure may induce cerebral ischemia, especially in the presence of cerebrovascular insufficiency due to atheroma and stenosis.

Postural hypotension, especially when severe, may be accompanied by symptoms of hypoperfusion in other organs. Neck and shoulder ache in a "coat-hanger" distribution specifically related to a postural fall in blood pressure is common; the mechanisms are unclear. Angina pectoris may occasionally occur, even in the young with apparently normal coronary arteries. There may be symptoms suggestive of spinal cord ischemia during standing.

Hypotension and syncope may occur during events unrelated to postural change, as in neurally mediated syncope. A common cause, especially in young and otherwise healthy individuals with apparently normal autonomic reflexes, is vasovagal syncope, when both heart rate and blood pressure fall rapidly (Figure 81.10) because of increased vagal activity and sympathetic withdrawal. Fear, sometimes induced by venipuncture, and assumption of the upright position, especially on a tilt table, may provoke such a response. A variant, more common in wartime, is DaCosta's syndrome (soldier's heart, or neurocirculatory asthenia), in which dizziness and syncope on effort are accompanied by exhaustion, dyspnea, headache, palpitations, and pain over the heart. These symptoms resemble

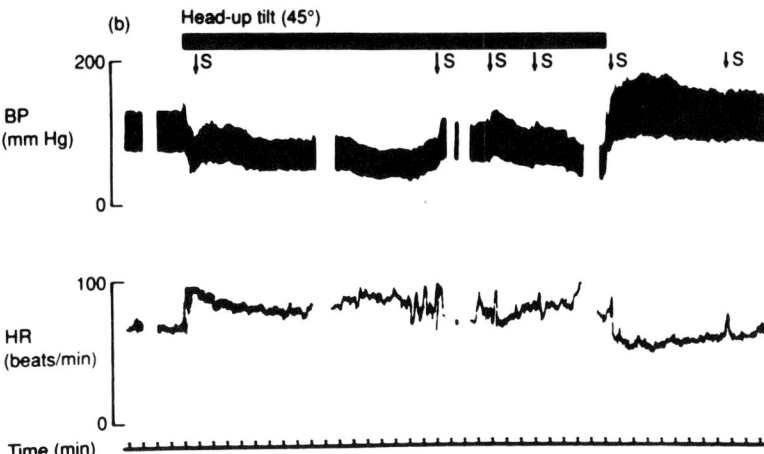

FIGURE 81.9 Intra-arterial recording of blood pressure (BP) and heart rate (HR) in a tetraplegic patient with a complete cervical spinal cord transection above the sympathetic outflow. There is an immediate fall in BP after head-up tilt, followed by a rise in BP during spontaneous skeletal muscle spasms (S). The slow recovery in BP may have been related to the release of renin and the subsequent formation of angiotensin II (measured at breaks in the record) because there is minimal or no change in plasma noradrenaline and adrenaline levels. On return to the horizontal, there is a BP overshoot. During tilt, heart rate rises due to an intact vagal efferent outflow. (Reprinted with permission from CJ Mathias, HL Frankel. Cardiovascular control in spinal man. Annu Rev Physiol 1988;50:577.)

orthostatic intolerance and syncope that may occur in chronic fatigue syndrome (De Lorenzo et al. 1997).

An increasingly recognized disorder is orthostatic intolerance with tachycardia on postural challenge, often not accompanied by a fall in blood pressure. It often occurs in young women. The cause is unknown, but there may be a relationship to hyperventilation and panic attacks, and there often is improvement with beta blockers. It is probably a heterogeneous disorder (Khurana 1995). These disorders differ from carotid sinus hypersensitivity, in which pressure over the carotid sinus due to turning the head or tightening of the collar may induce an attack. This disorder is being increasingly recognized in the elderly, especially those who present with falls of otherwise unknown etiology (McIntosh et al. 1993). Maintenance of heart rate alone, by a cardiac demand pacemaker or atropine, may not prevent hypotension in such patients. Paroxysms of coughing may induce syncope, especially in patients with chronic obstructive airway disease. Micturition syncope usually is not accompanied by a detectable autonomic lesion. Hypotension appears to result from the combination of vasodilatation due to warmth or alcohol and straining during micturition. These actions raise intrathoracic pressure and induce Valsalva's maneuver while standing, which is compounded by release of the pressor stimulus arising from a distended bladder.

Hypertension

Hypertension may be sustained in cerebral tumors, subarachnoid hemorrhage, or bulbar poliomyelitis, whereas lability of blood pressure occurs in certain autonomic disorders. Supine hypertension often occurs in primary chronic autonomic failure. The mechanisms are unclear but include impaired baroreflex activity, adrenoceptor supersensitivity, an increase in central blood volume because of a shift from the periphery, and the effects of drugs used to prevent postural hypotension. Headache may occur. Papilledema, cerebral hemorrhage, aortic dissection, myocardial ischemia, and heart failure are possible but infrequently reported complications.

Paroxysmal hypertension may occur in Guillain-Barré syndrome, porphyria, posterior fossa tumors, and pheochromocytoma, often without a precipitating cause. Hypertension in pheochromocytoma is usually associated with autonomous release of catecholamines, with or without other pressor substances from the tumor. In tetanus, hypertension may be precipitated by specific events, such as muscle spasms or tracheal suction. In high spinal cord lesions, contraction of the urinary bladder, irritation of the large bowel, noxious cutaneous stimulation, or skeletal muscle spasms can cause severe hypertension as part of autonomic dysreflexia, with an uninhibited increase in spinal sympathetic nervous activity (Figure 81.11). This is often accompanied by a throbbing or pounding headache, bradycardia, sweating and flushing over the face and neck, and cold peripheral limbs due to vasoconstriction.

Increased sympathetic nervous activity may initiate or maintain hypertension in renovascular disease (such as renal artery stenosis), in transplant recipients who receive cyclosporine as immunosuppressive therapy, and in preeclamptic toxemia (Schobel et al. 1996).

Cardiac Dysrhythmias

Tachycardia due to increased sympathetic discharge may occur with hypertension in the Guillain-Barré syndrome and in tetanus. In pheochromocytoma, it results from catecholamine release and β-adrenoceptor stimulation.

Bradycardia (with hypertension) may occur in cerebral tumors and during autonomic dysreflexia in high spinal cord injuries. In the latter, the afferent and vagal efferent components of the baroreflex arc are intact, and the heart slows in an attempt to control the rise in blood pressure. In pheochromocytoma, bradycardia with escape rhythms and atrioventricular dissociation may occur in response to a rapid rise in pressure.

Severe bradycardia can occasionally be a problem if the vagi are intact when there is an inability to increase severe sympathetic activity, as in patients with high cervical cord

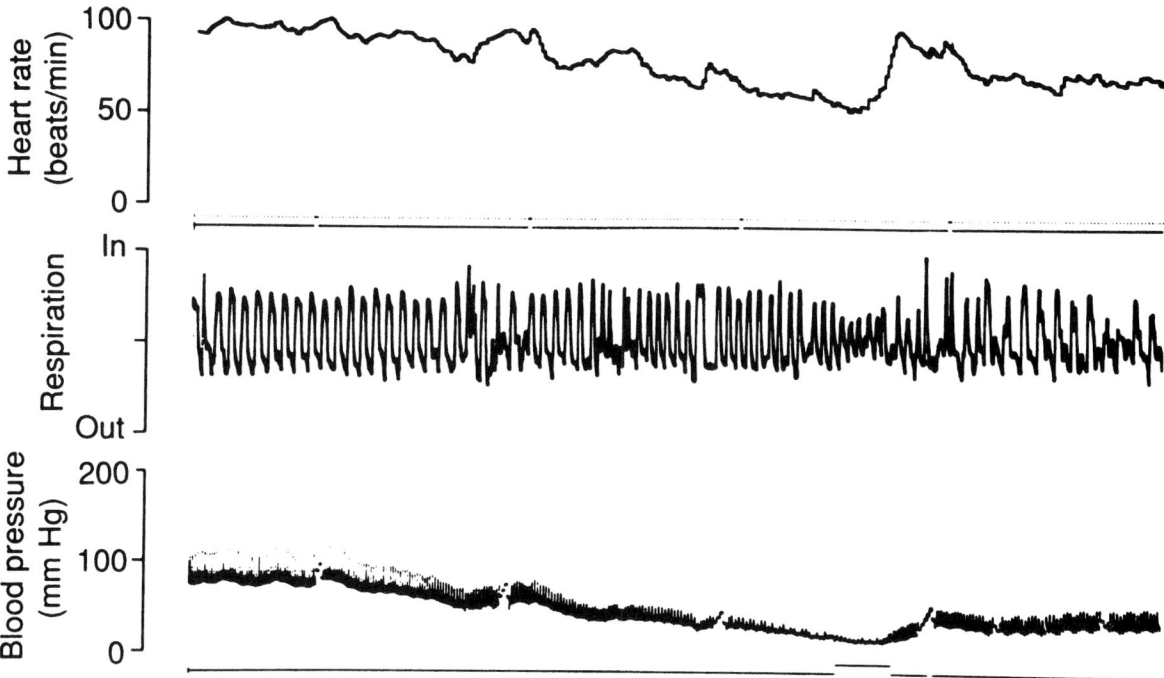

FIGURE 81.10   Blood pressure changes toward the end of a period of head-up tilt in a patient with recurrent episodes of vasovagal syncope. Blood pressure that was previously maintained begins to fall. There is also a fall in heart rate. There are relatively minor changes in respiratory rate, which can be derived from the time signal above it. Each minor dot indicates a second and the bolder mark indicates a minute. The patient was about to faint and was put back to the horizontal (indicated by the elevated time signal below), and then needed 5 degrees of head-down tilt. Blood pressure and heart rate recovered but still remained lower than previously. This patient had no other autonomic abnormalities on detailed testing. Blood pressure was measured noninvasively by the Finapres. (Reprinted with permission from CJ Mathias, R Bannister. Investigation of Autonomic Disorders. In CJ Mathias, R Bannister [eds], Autonomic Failure. A Textbook of Clinical Disorders of the Autonomic Nervous System [4th ed]. Oxford: Oxford University Press, 1999;169–195.)

transection who have diaphragmatic paralysis and need artificial respiration (Table 81.7). The intact vagi are sensitive to hypoxia, and stimuli such as tracheal suction can induce bradycardia and cardiac arrest (Figure 81.12). Cardiac arrest may also occur in chronically injured tetraplegic patients during general anesthesia, especially when muscle paralysis followed by intubation is performed without parasympathetic blockade.

In carotid sinus hypersensitivity, bradycardia and syncope may be difficult to distinguish from Stokes-Adams attacks. A cardiac demand pacemaker alone in some may not be of benefit because vasodilatation, hypotension, and syncope may occur despite preservation of heart rate.

In diabetes mellitus, the tendency toward cardiac vagal neuropathy appears to increase the incidence of cardiorespiratory arrest during anesthesia, for reasons that are unclear. Disorders of cardiac conduction are common in Chagas' disease and may occur in amyloidosis.

Facial Vascular Changes

In autonomic failure, facial pallor usually occurs as blood pressure falls, with prompt restoration of color on assuming the supine position, when blood pressure rises. Facial pallor may occur during an attack in pheochromocytoma and is usually accompanied by sweating, headache, and hypertension. In the acute phase of high spinal cord lesions, facial vasodilatation may be accompanied by nasal congestion (Guttmann's sign). The latter also may occur in patients on α-adrenoceptor blockers or sympatholytics, such as phenoxybenzamine, guanethidine, and reserpine. In chronic tetraplegia, hypertension during autonomic dysreflexia is often accompanied by flushing and sweating over the face and neck. The mechanisms are unknown. In Harlequin syndrome, there is vasodilatation and anhidrosis on one side of the face due to sympathetic impairment, with apparent sparing of the pupils, although abnormalities may be unmasked with pharmacological testing (Drummond 1994). The signs favor a lesion that spares the first thoracic segment (from which oculomotor fibers often leave), and involves preganglionic fibers of the second and third thoracic roots, although the lesion usually is not identified.

Sweating

Anhidrosis or hypohidrosis is common in primary autonomic failure and is usually noticed during exposure to warm temperatures. The eccrine glands, which are mainly

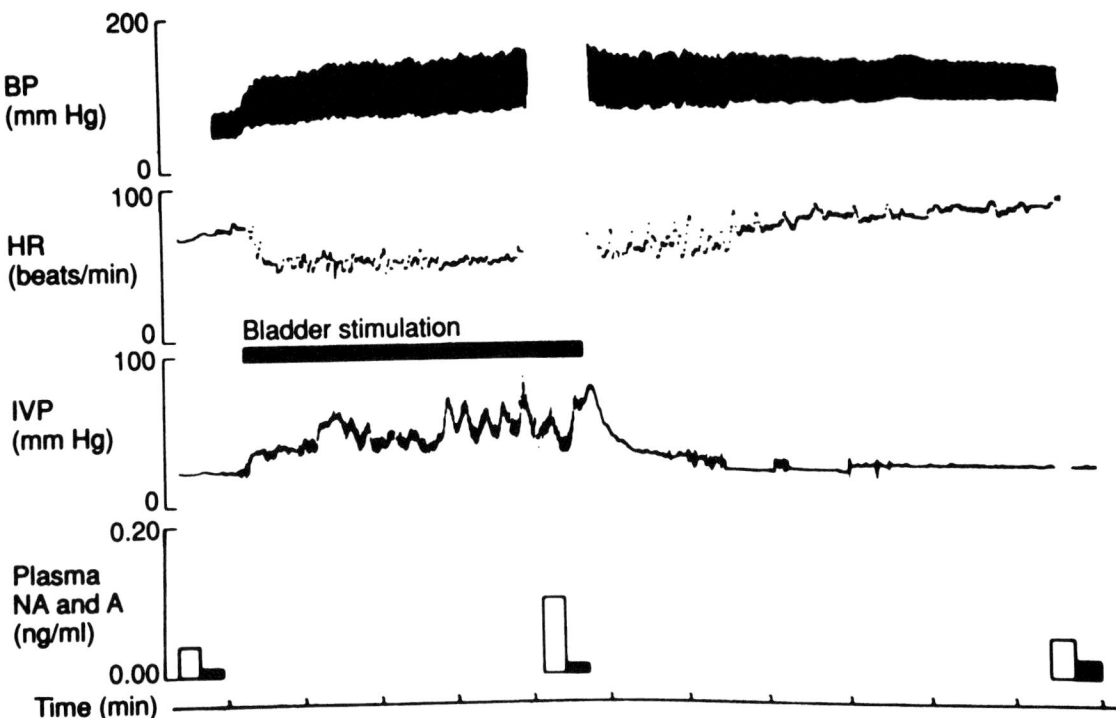

FIGURE 81.11   Blood pressure (BP), heart rate (HR), intravesical pressure (IVP), and plasma noradrenaline (NA, empty histogram) and adrenaline (A, filled histogram) in a tetraplegic patient before, during, and after bladder stimulation (BS) induced by suprapubic percussion of the anterior abdominal wall. A rapid rise in BP accompanies a fall in HR, which indicates increased cardiac vagal activity in response to the rise in BP. There is a rise in levels of plasma NA but not of adrenaline, which suggests sympathetic neural but not adrenomedullary activation. (Reprinted with permission from CJ Mathias, HL Frankel. The neurological and hormonal control of blood vessels and heart in spinal man. J Auton Nerv Syst 1986; [Suppl.]:457–464.)

Table 81.7:   Some of the mechanisms accounting for bradycardia and cardiac arrest in tetraplegic patients with high cervical lesions on artificial respiration, and the therapeutic interventions utilized

	Hypoxia	*Tracheal Suction*
Normal Subjects	Primary response is bradycardia opposed by pulmonary (inflation) vagal reflex, which causes tachycardia.	Increases sympathetic nervous activity, causing tachycardia and raising blood pressure.
Tetraplegic patients	Only causes the primary response, bradycardia, as disconnection from respirator eliminates pulmonary (inflation) reflex.	Sympathetic nervous activity is severely impaired, even at a spinal level in the early stages. Vagal afferent stimulation may lead to unopposed vagal efferent activity.

Increased vagal cardiac activity

Bradycardia and cardiac arrest

Oxygenation   Reconnection to respirator   Atropine   Demand pacemaker

FIGURE 81.12   (A) The effect of disconnecting the respirator (as required for aspirating the airways) on blood pressure (BP) and heart rate (HR) of a recently injured tetraplegic patient (C4-C5 lesion) in spinal shock, 6 hours after the last dose of intravenous atropine. Sinus bradycardia and cardiac arrest (also observed on the electrocardiograph) were reversed by reconnection, intravenous atropine, and external cardiac massage. (Reprinted with permission from HL Frankel, CJ Mathias, JMK Spalding. Mechanisms of reflex cardiac arrest in tetraplegic patients. Lancet 1975;ii:1183.) (B) The effect of tracheal suction 20 minutes after atropine. Disconnection from the respirator and tracheal suction did not lower either HR or BP. (Reprinted with permission from CJ Mathias. Bradycardia and cardiac arrest during tracheal suction—mechanisms in tetraplegic patients. Eur J Intensive Care Med 1976;2:147.)

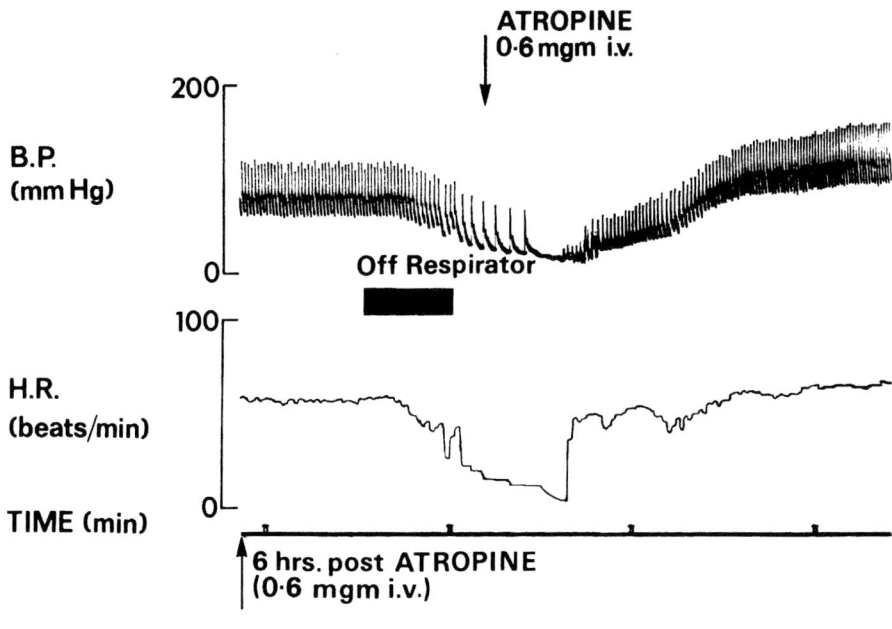

A

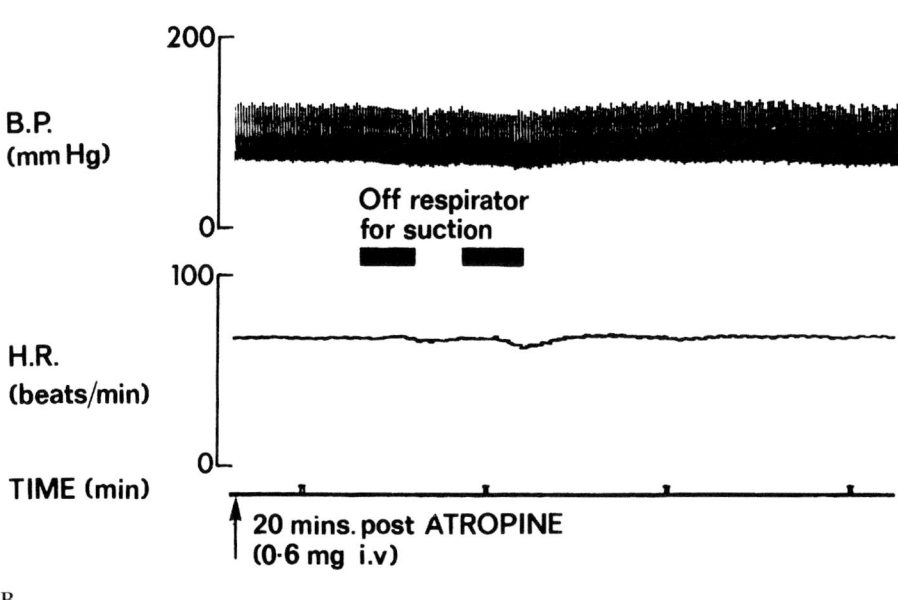

B

concerned with temperature regulation, are predominantly involved, whereas the apocrine glands, which are on the palms and soles and are influenced by circulating substances, including catecholamines, may remain functional. Occasionally, localized hyperhidrosis may occur, which is probably a compensatory response to diminished activity elsewhere rather than a response to denervation hypersensitivity in an incomplete lesion. Localized or generalized anhidrosis, sometimes with hyperhidrosis, may be associated with Holmes-Adie syndrome (Ross's syndrome).

A band of hyperhidrosis above the lesion often occurs in spinal cord injuries, with anhidrosis below the lesion. During autonomic dysreflexia in such patients, however, sweating usually occurs, but mainly over the face and neck. Facial and truncal hyperhidrosis may occur in Parkinson's disease. Hyperhidrosis may occur intermittently in pheochromocytoma. Generalized hyperhidrosis may accompany hypertension in tetanus, and may be the major manifestation in infants with mercury poisoning (acrodynia or pink disease).

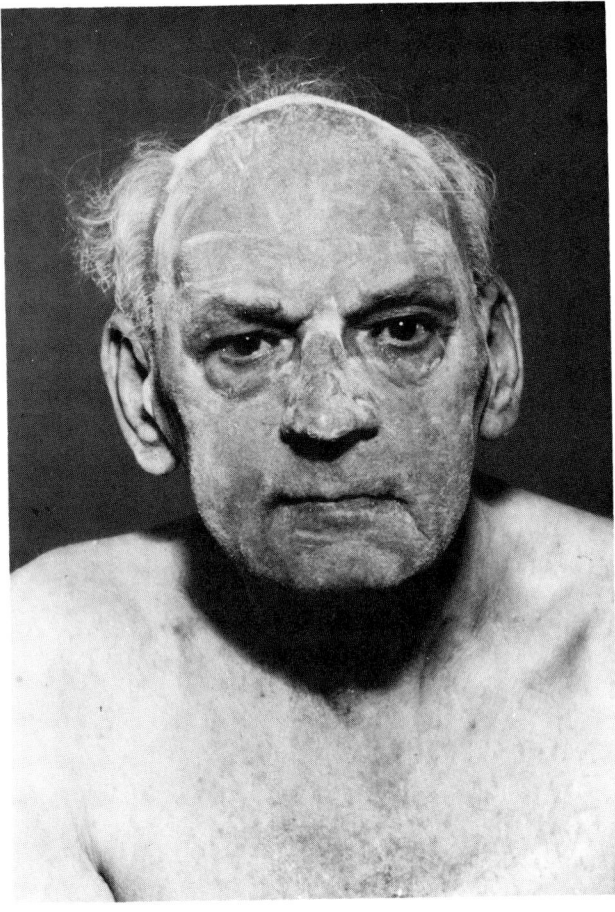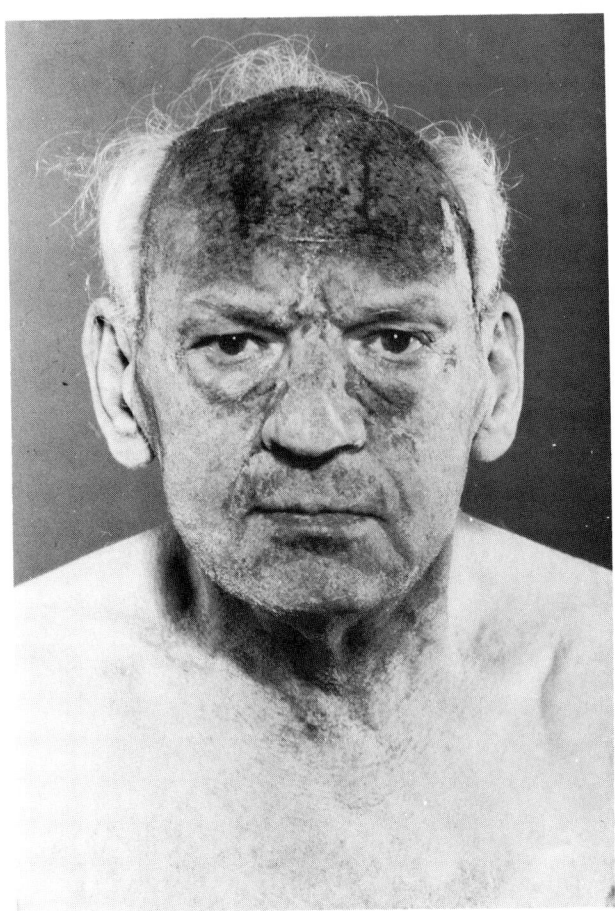

A   B

FIGURE 81.13   Sequential photographs showing the effects of quinazarin red (pale powder) before (**A**) and after (**B**) gustatory sweating induced by a cheese sandwich. There was profound sweating over the head and face.

Localized hyperhidrosis caused by food (gustatory sweating) can be socially distressing and may occur in diabetes mellitus or after trauma or surgery, as a result of aberrant connections between nerve fibers supplying the salivary and sweat glands (Figure 81.13).

Minimally invasive thoracic endoscopic techniques for sympathectomy are being increasingly used because of their success in reducing axillary and palmar hyperhidrosis, but may be complicated by abnormalities of sweating in other sites. Approximately one-half of patients may develop compensatory hyperhidrosis, usually of the trunk and lower limbs; the mechanisms are unclear.

Temperature Regulation

Hypothermia may occur in hypothalamic disorders, and in the elderly, in whom such lesions have been postulated. It usually is not a problem in primary autonomic failure. In patients with high spinal injuries, especially in the early phases, the combination of absent shivering thermogenesis and the inability to vasoconstrict and thus prevent heat loss can readily result in hypothermia. Hypothermia may be missed if only oral temperature is recorded without a low-reading thermometer (Figure 81.14).

Hyperpyrexia may be a problem in patients with anhidrosis who are exposed to high temperatures. Heat also increases vasodilatation and often enhances postural hypotension.

Gastrointestinal System

Xerostomia usually occurs in acute dysautonomias and especially in pure cholinergic dysautonomia. Dysphagia may be present due to impairment of esophageal function because the lower two-thirds of the esophagus contains smooth muscle with an autonomic innervation. Large bowel atony may occur. A barium meal should be avoided because it may solidify in the colon and require surgical removal. Dysphagia is unusual in PAF. It often occurs in the later stages of MSA. In primary autonomic failure, constipation is common. In secondary autonomic disorders, a wide variety of gastrointestinal manifestations may occur. The esophagus is often involved in Chagas' disease, with achalasia and megaesophagus causing vomiting. Gastroparesis in diabetes mellitus and amyloidosis may cause food stasis and vomiting. The reverse, increased gastric motility, is common in primary autonomic failure, but the relationship between postprandial hypotension and "dumping" is unclear. Paralytic ileus usually occurs in the early phases after spinal cord lesions and can cause abdominal distention and meteorism, which reduces mobility of the diaphragm, the major respiratory muscle in those with high lesions. In such patients, the vagus is intact and probably hyperactive, which may account for the tendency to increased gastric acid production, peptic ulceration, and gastrointestinal bleeding.

Constipation usually occurs in patients with sacral parasympathetic impairment. Diarrhea may occur, as in diabetes mellitus, for reasons that are often unclear and include incomplete digestion, altered bowel flora, or abnormal motility.

Kidneys and Urinary Tract

Nocturia is common in primary autonomic failure and probably is the result of recumbency itself rather than abnormal circadian rhythms. Factors such as redistribution of blood from the peripheral into the central compartment, alteration in release of hormones that influence salt and water handling (e.g., renin, aldosterone, and atrial natriuretic peptide), and postural changes in renal hemodynamics may contribute. Nocturia may cause an overnight weight loss greater than 1 kg, resulting in a reduction in extracellular fluid volume, a lower morning blood pressure, and an increased tendency to postural symptoms.

Involvement of the urinary bladder may result in frequency, urgency, incontinence, or retention. Loss of sacral parasympathetic function, as in the early phase of spinal cord injury, causes an atonic bladder with urinary retention, whereas recovery of isolated spinal cord function results in a neurogenic bladder. With training, there is often controlled bladder emptying. Dyssynergia, however, with detrusor contraction but not sphincter relaxation, may cause episodes of autonomic dysreflexia resulting in hypertension and, at times, urinary reflux that predisposes to renal damage, especially in the presence of a urinary tract infection. In older patients with primary autonomic failure, urinary symptoms initially may be attributed to prostatic hypertrophy in men or to pelvic muscle weakness, especially in multiparous women. Surgery usually is of no benefit. The use of drugs with anticholinergic effects may unmask urinary bladder dysfunction in autonomic failure.

Urinary infection is common when the bladder is involved. Some patients, including those with spinal injuries, are prone to urinary calculi, especially when immobility increases calcium excretion.

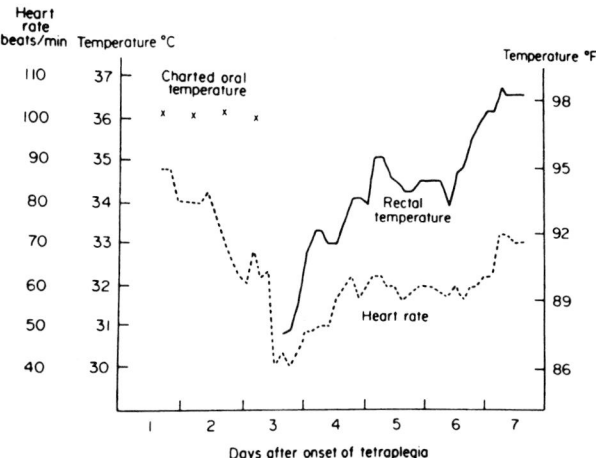

FIGURE 81.14 Fall in central temperature (measured as rectal temperature, *continuous line*) and heart rate (*interrupted line*) in a recently injured tetraplegic patient in a temperate climate. Measurements of oral temperature missed the hypothermia, which should be measured by a low-reading rectal thermometer. The impairment of shivering thermogenesis and the inability to vasoconstrict adequately predispose these patients to hypothermia. (Reprinted with permission from G Pledger. Disorders of temperature regulation in acute traumatic paraplegia. J Bone Joint Surg Br 1962;44:110.)

Reproductive System

Impotence is a common complaint in autonomic failure and may result from failure of erection, which appears to depend mainly on the parasympathetic system, and difficulty in or lack of ejaculation, which appears to be controlled largely by the sympathetic system. Retrograde ejaculation may occur, especially if there are urinary sphincter abnormalities. It may be difficult to dissociate the effects of increasing age, systemic illness, and depression from organic causes of impotence. Drugs normally not considered to have autonomic side effects, such as thiazides used in the treatment of hypertension, may cause impotence. Priapism due to abnormal spinal reflexes may occur in patients with spinal cord lesions.

In women, autonomic impairment itself does not directly affect reproductive function. Menstrual disorders, if present, are usually secondary to an underlying disorder. Conception and successful vaginal delivery have been recorded in high spinal cord transection and in patients with primary autonomic failure.

Eye and Lacrimal Glands

The nonstriated component of the levator palpebra superioris (Müller's muscle) is innervated by sympathetic fibers, and mild ptosis is part of Horner's syndrome. If the lesion is bilateral, as in high spinal cord transection, this is difficult to detect.

A variety of pupillary abnormalities may occur: miosis in Horner's syndrome, dilated myotonic pupils in Holmes-Adie syndrome, and small, irregular pupils in Argyll-Robertson syndrome due to syphilitic (*Treponema pallidum*) infection. Symptoms directly relating to the eye are usually minimal in such disorders. Drugs with anticholinergic effects may cause blurred vision due to cycloplegia; they also may raise intraocular pressure and cause glaucoma.

Impaired lacrimal production occasionally occurs in primary autonomic failure, sometimes as part of the sicca or Sjögren's syndrome, along with diminished salivary secretion. Excessive and inappropriate lacrimation occurs in crocodile tears syndrome (gustolacrimal reflex).

Respiratory System

In MSA, episodes of apnea may occur in the later stages of the disorder. These are probably due to involvement of brainstem respiratory centers. Inspiratory stridor and snoring may result from weakness of the cricoarytenoid muscles, the main laryngeal abductors. In certain disorders, reflexes from the respiratory tract may cause profound cardiovascular disturbances. Tracheal suction in curarized tetanus patients on respirators may result in severe hypertension and tachycardia, whereas in patients with high cervical cord transection, bradycardia and cardiac arrest may occur.

Additional Neurological Involvement

In the parkinsonian and mixed forms of MSA, extrapyramidal manifestations consist mainly of bradykinesia and rigidity with minimal tremor; this causes difficulties in mobility, especially while turning in bed and changing direction. Speech may become slurred. Facial expression is affected to a lesser degree than in Parkinson's disease. In idiopathic Parkinson's disease with autonomic failure, extrapyramidal features often have been present for a long period and remain responsive to L-dopa therapy even after the additional features of autonomic dysfunction occur.

In the cerebellar form of MSA, cerebellar features predominate, with an ataxic gait, an intention tremor, cerebellar speech, and nystagmus. Ataxia may be difficult to separate from, or may be compounded by, the unsteadiness caused by postural hypotension. There also may be pyramidal involvement, with increased tone and exaggerated tendon reflexes with extensor plantar responses. A varying combination of extrapyramidal, cerebellar, and pyramidal features occurs in the mixed form of MSA. Sensory deficits are uncommon in MSA, although nerve conduction studies indicate a mixed sensorimotor axonal neuropathy (Pramstaller et al. 1995).

Patients with secondary autonomic failure have the neurological features that are part of, or a complication of, the primary disease. In diabetes mellitus, a somatic neuropathy often coexists with, or precedes, the autonomic neuropathy.

Psychological and Psychiatric Disturbances

In primary autonomic failure, dementia is unusual. In patients with MSA, detailed testing of cognitive function shows deficits in visuospatial organization and visuomotor ability that are similar to observations in Parkinson's disease (Monza et al. 1997; Pillon et al. 1995). Most patients with MSA are not depressed, despite their disabilities and the probable deficit in central catecholamine levels; overall they have a normal affective state, especially when comparisons are made with patients with Parkinson's disease (Pillon et al. 1995). Anxiety and tremulousness may occur in secondary disorders, as in pheochromocytoma. Psychological factors may contribute to vasovagal syncope and essential hyperhidrosis. Frank psychiatric disturbances may complicate other conditions, such as porphyria.

INVESTIGATION

Investigation depends on the presenting problem and the primary or secondary disorder. The major aims of investigation are as follows:

1. To determine if autonomic function is normal or abnormal. Screening investigations often are restricted to a particular system, such as the cardiovascular system.
2. To assess (if an abnormality has been observed), the degree of autonomic dysfunction, with an emphasis on the site of the lesion and the functional deficit.
3. To ascertain if the abnormalities are of the primary or secondary variety because further investigations, prognosis, and management depend on the diagnostic category. In some disorders, as in generalized autonomic dysfunction, extensive investigation of various systems may be required (Table 81.8) (Mathias and Bannister 1999b).

The cardiovascular system provides an example of how investigations have been specifically designed to determine and elucidate the deficit, the site of the lesion, and the extent to which associated hormonal abnormalities contribute. As in the investigation of other systems, there has been an emphasis on developing noninvasive techniques that are safe and reliable and can be used for screening and repeated testing as well as determining disease progression and the effects of therapy. Different autonomic laboratories are unlikely to have similar equipment and an identical set of procedures, despite attempts to standardize such approaches. High specificity and sensitivity of the tests, although desirable, may not be practical in a global setting, especially because the findings often must be considered in the context of a wide variety of factors, including the patient's ability to cooperate in testing. The effect of drugs is another confounding factor. Significantly, the results must be linked with the relevant clinical symptoms and signs. These difficulties mainly arise in mild or moderate cases with questionable autonomic involvement, however, and are not usually relevant in patients with definite abnormalities.

Cardiovascular System

A postural fall in blood pressure, especially if consistently more than 20 mm Hg systolic, or less in the presence of symptoms, warrants further investigation. Head-up tilt is often used as the postural stimulus, especially when the neurological deficit or severe hypotension makes it difficult for the patient to stand. In some patients, postural hypotension initially may be unmasked by exercise (Smith et al. 1993) because vasodilatation in skeletal muscle is not appropriately counteracted by autonomic reflexes (Figure 81.15). Food ingestion also may be a provoking factor, presumably as a result of splanchnic vasodilatation not compensated for in other regions (Figure 81.16). There may be considerable variability in the basal supine levels and the postural fall in blood pressure; the greatest changes often occur in the morning and after a meal and physical exertion. Other, non-neurogenic causes of postural hypotension must be considered (Table 81.9). The same may occur with drugs that cause vasodilatation, even if this is only a side effect of the agent.

Both blood pressure and heart rate can be accurately measured using noninvasive techniques, many of which are automated and provide a printout at preset intervals. Intermittent ambulatory blood pressure and heart rate recordings over a 24-hour period using small computerized devices are of particular value, especially at home, in determining the effects of various stimuli in daily life (Figure 81.17). They may be of value in determining the beneficial effects of therapy in different situations. Beat-by-beat measurement of blood pressure and heart rate is essential in neurally mediated syncope (see Figure 81.14). This is especially so during carotid sinus massage, when the changes in blood pressure often are rapid, would be missed because of the slow response time of most noninvasive sphygmomanometers, and may be independent of changes in heart rate (Figure 81.18). The Finapres enables noninvasive blood pressure and heart rate recording with a finger cuff, provides beat-by-beat changes, and is a reliable measure of changes in blood pressure.

Screening investigations help determine the site and extent of the cardiovascular autonomic abnormality. The responses to Valsalva's maneuver, during which intrathoracic pressure is raised, depend on the integrity of the entire baroreflex pathway (Figure 81.19). Changes in heart rate alone, even in the absence of intra-arterial recording, provide a useful guide. Some patients may, however, raise mouth pressure without necessarily raising intrathoracic pressure, resulting in a falsely abnormal response. Stimuli that raise blood pressure, such as isometric exercise (by sustained hand grip for 3 minutes), the cold pressor test (immersing the hand in ice slush for 90 seconds), and men-

Table 81.8: Outline of investigations in autonomic failure

Cardiovascular
  Physiological
  Head-up tilt (45 degrees); standing; Valsalva's maneuver
  Pressor stimuli (isometric exercise, cold pressor, mental arithmetic)
  Heart rate responses
  Deep breathing, hyperventilation, standing, head-up tilt, 30:15 R-R interval ratio
  Liquid meal challenge
  Exercise testing
  Carotid sinus massage
  Biochemical: plasma noradrenaline: supine and head-up tilt or standing; urinary catecholamines; plasma renin activity and aldosterone
  Pharmacological
    Noradrenaline: α-adrenoceptors, vascular
    Isoprenaline: β-adrenoceptors, vascular and cardiac
    Tyramine: pressor and noradrenaline response
    Edrophonium: noradrenaline response
    Atropine: parasympathetic cardiac blockade
Sudomotor
  Central regulation thermoregulatory sweat test
  Sweat gland response to intradermal acetylcholine, quantitative sudomotor axon reflex test (Q-SART), localized sweat test
  Sympathetic skin response
Gastrointestinal: barium studies, video-cine-fluoroscopy, endoscopy, gastric emptying studies
Renal function and urinary tract
  Day and night urine volumes and sodium/potassium excretion
  Urodynamic studies, intravenous urography, ultrasound examination, sphincter electromyography
Sexual function
  Penile plethysmography
  Intracavernosal papaverine
Respiratory
  Laryngoscopy
  Sleep studies to assess apnea and oxygen desaturation
Eye
  Schirmer's test
  Pupil function, pharmacological and physiological

Source: Adapted with permission from CJ Mathias, R Bannister. Investigation of Autonomic Disorders. In R Bannister, CJ Mathias (eds), Autonomic Failure. A Textbook of Disorders of the Autonomic Nervous System (4th ed). Oxford: Oxford University Press, 1999.

tal arithmetic (using serial-7 or -17 subtraction), activate different afferent or central pathways, which then stimulate the sympathetic outflow. The heart rate responses to postural change, deep breathing (sinus arrhythmia), and hyperventilation provide further evidence of the integrity of cardiac vagal efferent pathways. Additional investigations may be needed to determine factors causing or contributing to postural hypotension and syncope. These include determining the responses to carotid sinus massage, food ingestion, and exercise. In suspected carotid sinus hypersensitivity, resuscitation facilities should be available

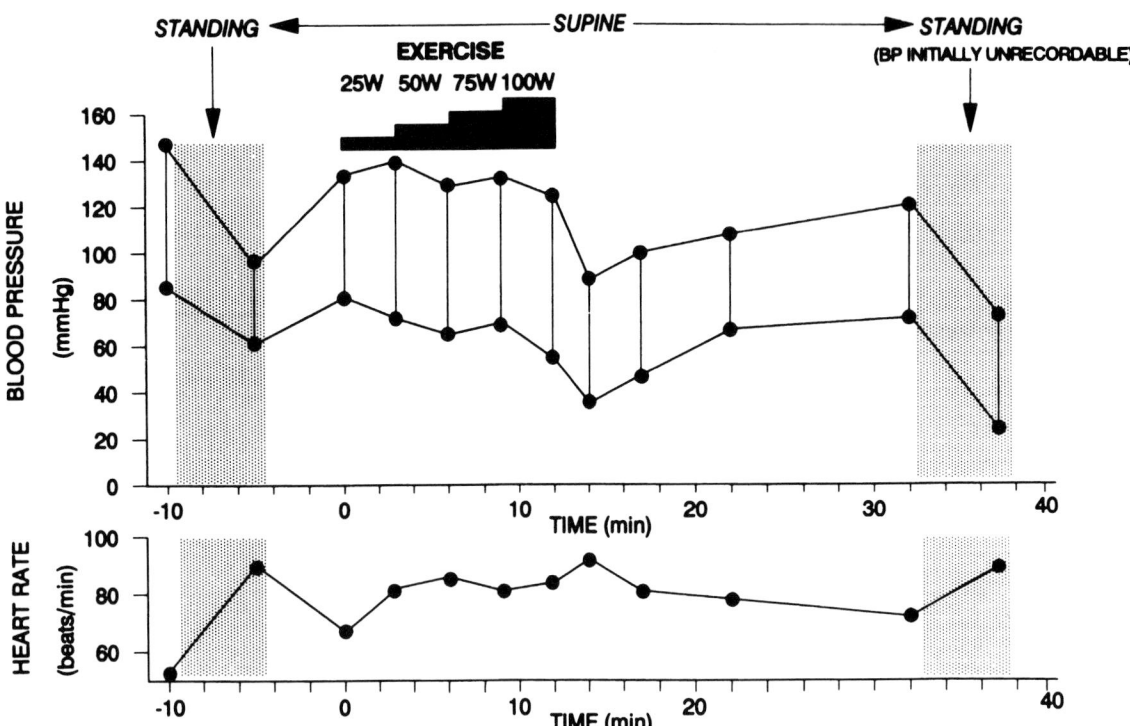

FIGURE 81.15 Blood pressure (BP) and heart rate responses in a patient with pure autonomic failure while lying and standing, before and after exercise. The stippled area indicates the periods of standing. There was a fall in blood pressure on standing. Exercise was performed on a bicycle ergometer in the supine position, and unlike normal subjects, in whom there is a rise in blood pressure, there was little or no change. On stopping exercise, blood pressure fell even while supine; after standing 20 minutes later, the blood pressure was initially unrecordable and the patient was near syncope. The observations were consistent with the patient's symptoms because he felt faint not during exercise but on stopping exercise. (Reprinted with permission from GDP Smith, R Bannister, CJ Mathias. Post-exercise dizziness as the sole presenting symptom of autonomic failure. Br Heart J 1993;69:359.)

because carotid massage may cause profound bradycardia or cardiac arrest with hypotension. Hypotension only may occur with the subject upright, presumably because of the greater dependence on sympathetic tone, which is withdrawn after carotid sinus stimulation. To assess postprandial hypotension, the cardiovascular responses to a balanced liquid meal containing carbohydrate, protein, and fat are determined while supine, with comparisons of the blood pressure response to head-up tilt before the meal and 45 minutes later. To evaluate exercise-induced hypotension, responses are obtained during graded incremental supine exercise using a bicycle ergometer with measurement of postural responses before and after exercise (see Figure 81.15).

In patients with PAF, the supine basal level of plasma noradrenaline is low (suggesting a distal lesion) compared with those with MSA, in whom supine levels are often within the normal range (Figure 81.20). The reasons for the normal supine levels in MSA are unclear and may include the central nature of the disorder and impairment of noradrenaline clearance mechanisms in the periphery. In both groups, however, there is an attenuation or lack of rise in plasma noradrenaline during head-up tilt, which indicates impairment of sympathetic neural activity. In high spinal cord lesions, basal plasma noradrenaline and adrenaline levels are low and do not rise with postural change. There is, however, a rise (but only moderately above the basal levels of normal subjects) during severe hypertension accompanying autonomic dysreflexia, which differentiates these patients from those with paroxysmal hypertension due to a pheochromocytoma, in which plasma noradrenaline or adrenaline levels are usually greatly elevated.

Extremely low or undetectable levels of plasma noradrenaline and adrenaline with elevated plasma dopamine levels occur in sympathetic failure caused by deficiency of the enzyme DBH, which converts dopamine into noradrenaline. Plasma levels of this enzyme are undetectable, but this may occur in 10% of normal individuals and is not diagnostic of the disorder. Immunohistochemical studies confirm the absence of the enzyme in tissues such as skin.

Measurement of plasma renin activity and plasma aldosterone levels is useful in certain cases. In Addison's disease and adrenocortical failure, basal plasma renin levels are markedly elevated, whereas plasma aldosterone is low or absent. In diabetic autonomic neuropathy, there may be low levels of both plasma renin and aldosterone, which contribute to hyperkalemia.

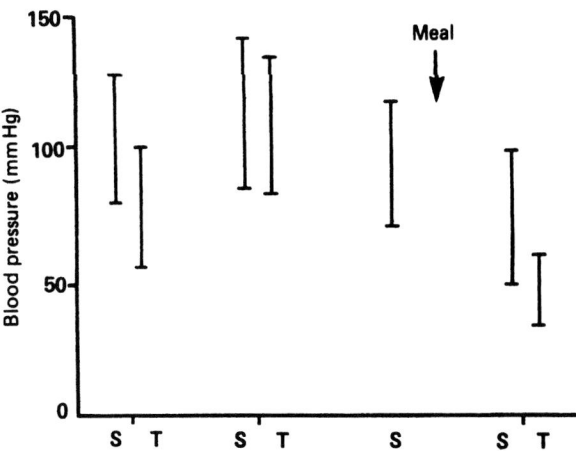

FIGURE 81.16 Systolic and diastolic blood pressure in a patient with multiple system atrophy while supine (S) and after 45-degree head-up tilt (T) on three occasions. On the first two, food intake was not controlled. The patient had not eaten on the second occasion, however, when the postural blood pressure fall was negligible. On the third, supine blood pressure was measured while fasting and 45 minutes after the meal. Postprandial tilt caused a considerable fall in blood pressure, and the patient had to be returned to the horizontal within 3 minutes. (From CJ Mathias, E Holly, E Armstrong, et al. The influence of food on postural hypotension in three groups with chronic autonomic failure: clinical and therapeutic implications. J Neurol Neurosurg Psychiatry 1991;54:726.)

Table 81.9: Examples of non-neurogenic causes of postural hypotension

Low intravascular volume	
Blood/plasma loss	Hemorrhage
	Burns
	Hemodialysis
Fluid/electrolyte loss	Inadequate intake (anorexia nervosa)
	Vomiting
	Diarrhea (including losses from ileostomy)
	Renal/endocrine
	Salt-losing nephropathy
	Adrenal insufficiency (Addison's disease)
	Diabetes insipidus
	Diuretics
Vasodilatation	Drugs (glyceryl trinitrate)
	Alcohol
	Heat
	Pyrexia
	Hyperbradykinism
	Systemic mastocytosis
	Extensive varicose veins
	Systemic mastocytosis
Cardiac impairment	
Myocardial	Cardiomyopathy
Impaired ventricular filling	Atrial myxoma
	Constrictive pericarditis
Impaired output	Aortic stenosis

Note: In patients with autonomic failure or on drugs impairing autonomic function, these associated disorders enhance postural hypotension considerably.

Muscle and skin sympathetic nervous activity can be recorded directly by percutaneous insertion of tungsten microelectrodes into the peroneal or median nerves. Muscle sympathetic activity is closely linked to the baroreceptor reflex, with a clear relationship to changes in blood pressure and discharge frequency. In patients with high spinal cord transection, there is reduced neural activity in the basal state compared to normal subjects. This is consistent with their low plasma noradrenaline and blood pressure levels, presumably because of the lack of transmission of tonic brainstem sympathetic activity. Increased firing occurs in patients with Guillain-Barré syndrome, in association with hypertension and tachycardia. These microneurographic approaches have aided our understanding of the pathophysiological processes but are of limited clinical application, especially in the investigation of autonomic failure.

Pharmacological approaches help in determining the degree of sensitivity of different receptors and the functional integrity of sympathetic nerves and the cardiac vagi. The pressor response to infusion of noradrenaline provides a measure of α-adrenoceptor sensitivity; it is usually greater in patients with postganglionic sympathetic lesions. The hypotensive response to isoprenaline is related to β_2-adrenoreceptor–mediated vasodilatation and is greater in the absence of corrective sympathetic reflexes. The heart rate response provides an indicator of β_1-adrenoceptor sensitivity, although the fall in blood pressure may increase heart rate through withdrawal of vagal tone, if intact. A rise in heart rate with atropine (usually up to 105 beats per minute with 1,800 mg intravenously) indicates preservation of cardiac parasympathetic activity. In primary autonomic failure, there is usually an impaired or absent response. The pressor and noradrenaline responses to infused tyramine provide a measure of the store of noradrenaline in sympathetic nerve endings.

Certain pharmacological challenges, as with the α_2-adrenoceptor agonist clonidine, can provide information in different disorders. In some patients, basal plasma noradrenaline levels may be elevated due to stress and other factors; in these situations, the central sympatholytic actions of this agent result in a reduction in plasma noradrenaline levels. This suppression does not occur when autonomous secretion occurs, as in pheochromocytoma (Figure 81.21). Another central action of clonidine, through the hypothalamus and anterior pituitary, is stimulation of growth hormone release. The rise in serum growth hormone levels that occurs in normal subjects is also observed in patients with PAF who have distal autonomic lesions (Figure 81.22A). There is no response in patients with MSA, however, in whom the lesions are central (Kimber et al. 1997b); thus the growth hormone response to neuropharmacological challenge with clonidine separates these two disorders. The

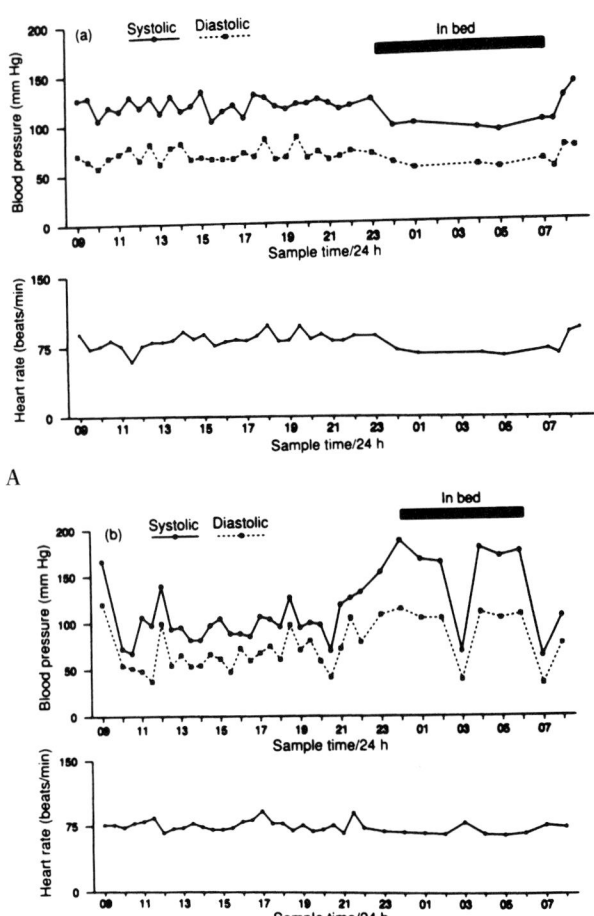

A

B

C

FIGURE 81.17   Twenty-four–hour noninvasive ambulatory blood pressure profile showing systolic and diastolic blood pressure and heart rate at intervals throughout the day and night. (**A**) Changes in a normal subject who did not have postural hypotension; there was a fall in blood pressure on sleeping. (**B**) Marked fluctuations in blood pressure in a patient with pure autonomic failure. The marked falls were usually the result of postural changes, either sitting or standing. Supine blood pressure, particularly at night, was elevated. Rising to micturate caused a marked fall in blood pressure (at 0300 hours). There was a reversal of the normal diurnal change in blood pressure. There were relatively small changes in heart rate considering the marked fluctuations in blood pressure. (Reprinted with permission from CJ Mathias, R Bannister. Investigation of Autonomic Disorders. In CJ Mathias, R Bannister [eds], Autonomic Failure. A Textbook of Clinical Disorders of the Autonomic Nervous System [4th ed]. Oxford: Oxford University Press, 1999;169–195.) (**C**) Changes in a patient with the Riley-Day syndrome (familial dysautonomia). The profile emphasizes the marked variability in blood pressure, with both hypotension and, at times, extreme hypertension. (Reprinted with permission from CJ Mathias. Disorders of the Autonomic Nervous System in Childhood. In B Berg [ed], Principles of Child Neurology. New York: McGraw-Hill, 1996;413.)

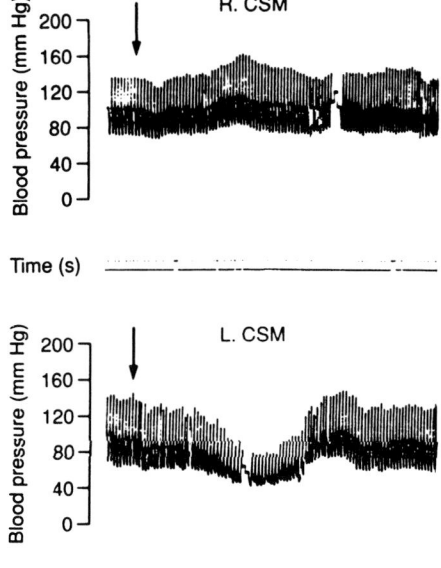

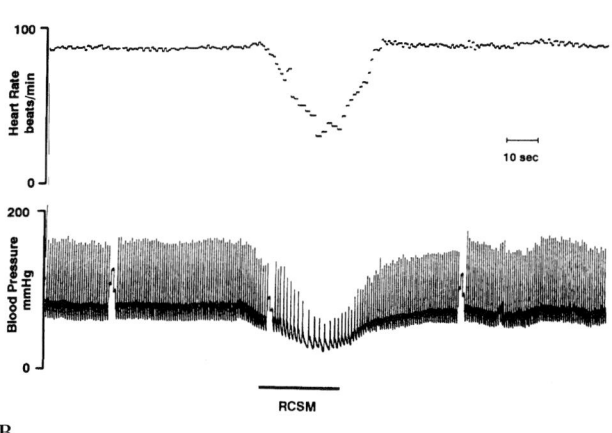

A   B

FIGURE 81.18 (**A**) Continuous noninvasive recording of finger arterial blood pressure (Finapres) before, during, and after carotid sinus massage on the right (R. CSM) and left (L. CSM). The fine dots indicate the time marker in seconds. The arrow indicates when stimulation began. Stimulation on the right for 10 seconds did not lower blood pressure and heart rate. On the left, carotid sinus massage caused a substantial fall in both systolic and diastolic blood pressure, during which the patient felt lightheaded and had graying out of vision. There was only a modest fall in heart rate. The syncopal attacks were abolished by left carotid sinus denervation. (Reprinted with permission from CJ Mathias, E Armstrong, N Browse, et al. Value of non-invasive continuous blood pressure monitoring in the detection of carotid sinus hypersensitivity. Clin Auton Res 1991;2:157.) (**B**) Continuous blood pressure and heart rate measured noninvasively (by Finapres) in a patient with falls of unknown etiology. Left carotid sinus massage caused a fall in both heart rate and blood pressure. The findings indicate the mixed (cardio-inhibitory and vasodepressor) form of carotid sinus hypersensitivity. (Reprinted with permission from CJ Mathias. Autonomic Dysfunction and the Elderly. In J Grimley-Evans [ed], Oxford Textbook of Geriatric Medicine [2nd ed]. Oxford: Oxford University Press, In press.)

FIGURE 81.19 Blood pressure (BP) and heart rate (HR) before and during Valsalva's maneuver. In the upper trace, the expiratory pressure is maintained at 40 mm Hg in a subject with intact sympathetic reflexes. The fall in BP is accompanied by a rise in HR. The fall in BP is due to the reduction in venous return, which then stimulates sympathetic activity. BP then partially recovers. After release of intrathoracic pressure, there is a BP overshoot and the HR falls below the pre-Valsalva level. In the lower trace, in a patient with impaired autonomic function, raising intrathoracic pressure lowered BP substantially, with no BP recovery. Note that the HR scale differs from normal subject. After release of intrathoracic pressure, there was no BP overshoot or immediate fall in HR below basal levels. BP slowly returned BP to pre-Valsalva levels. (Reprinted with permission from CJ Mathias, R Bannister. Investigation of Autonomic Disorders. In CJ Mathias, R Bannister [eds], Autonomic Failure. A Textbook of Clinical Disorders of the Autonomic Nervous System [4th ed]. Oxford: Oxford University Press, 1999.)

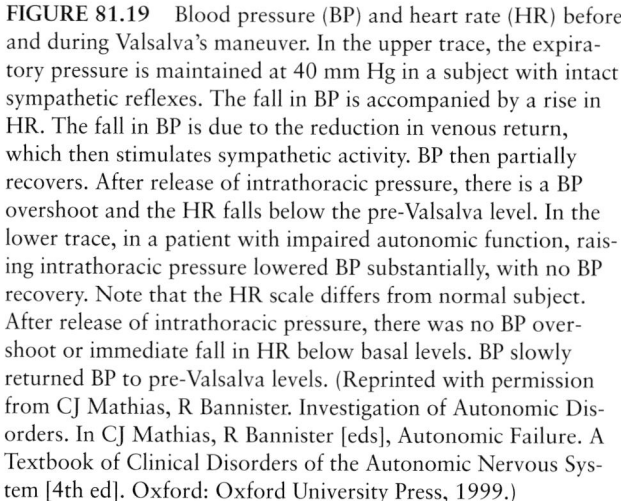

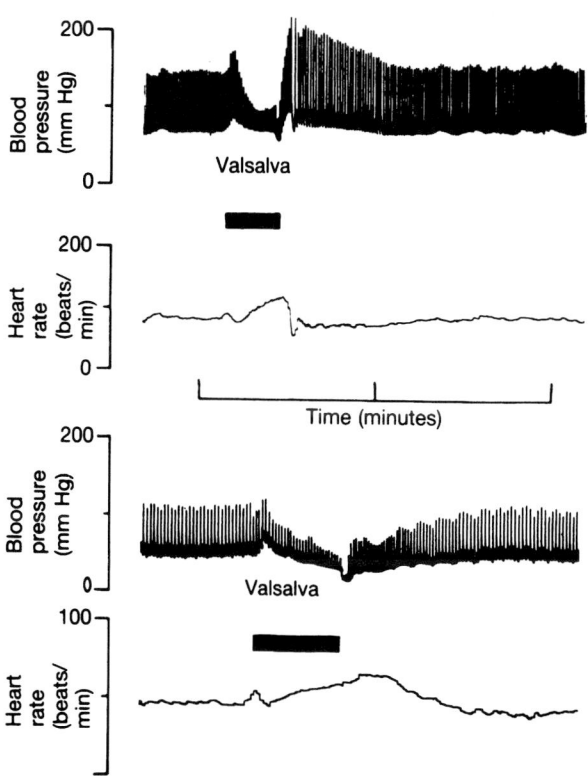

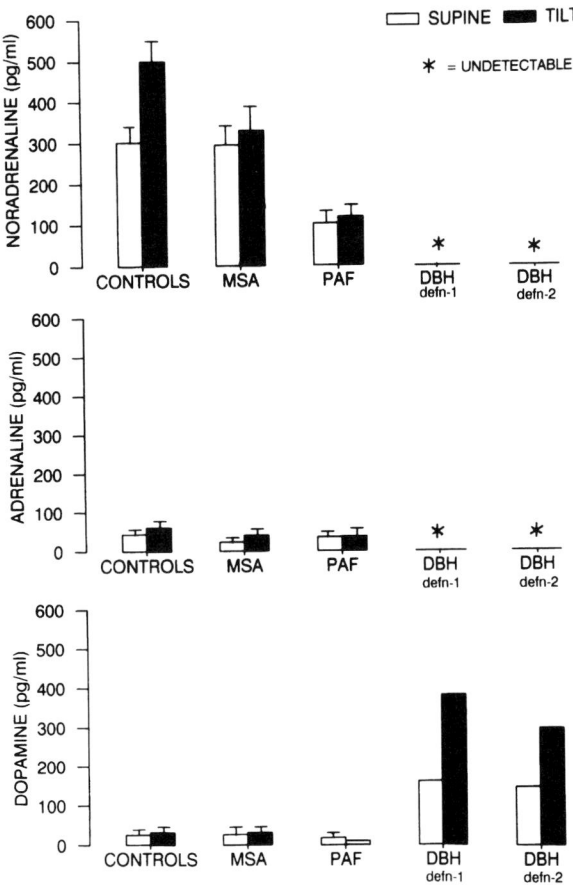

FIGURE 81.20   Plasma noradrenaline, adrenaline, and dopamine levels (measured by high-pressure liquid chromatography) in normal subjects (controls) and patients with multiple system atrophy (MSA, Shy-Drager syndrome) and pure autonomic failure (PAF), along with two patients with dopamine β-hydroxylase deficiency (DBH). Measurements were taken while patients were supine and after head-up tilt to 45 degrees for 10 minutes. The asterisk indicates levels below the detection limit, which are less than 5 pg/ml for noradrenaline and adrenaline and less than 20 pg/ml for dopamine. Bars indicate ± standard error of means. (Reprinted with permission from CJ Mathias, R Bannister. Investigation of Autonomic Disorders. In CJ Mathias, R Bannister [eds], Autonomic Failure. A Textbook of Clinical Disorders of the Autonomic Nervous System [4th ed]. Oxford: Oxford University Press, 1999;169–195.)

clonidine–growth hormone test may also aid distinction of parkinsonian forms of MSA from idiopathic Parkinson's disease (Figure 81.22B) (Kimber et al. 1997b).

Many techniques use the advances of modern technology and are being applied to the study of cardiovascular autonomic function in humans. These include techniques for the noninvasive measurement of cardiac function and blood flow in various regions (Puvi-Rajasingham et al. 1997). A variety of computer and spectral analytic techniques assess cardiovascular function (Parati et al. 1999)

and measure total body and regional noradrenaline spillover in regions such as the heart, splanchnic, and renal circulations and the brain (Lambert et al. 1997). Radionuclide 123-metaiodobenzylguanidine is used to image sympathetic nerves in the heart (Mantysaari et al. 1996), and PET scanning (using 6-[^{18}F] fluorodopamine) is employed to visualize sympathetic innervation of cardiac tissue (Goldstein et al. 1997). These techniques have a role in the clinical research setting, and in due course some of them may be applied to the routine investigation of cardiovascular autonomic function.

In the majority of autonomic disorders affecting the circulation, physiological testing using head-up postural challenge, a series of pressor tests, Valsalva's maneuver, deep breathing, and hyperventilation is often adequate for screening purposes. Depending on the disorder, additional tests may be needed, such as food and exercise challenge, carotid sinus massage, and appropriate biochemical and pharmacological studies.

Sweating

The thermoregulatory sweating response is tested by elevating body temperature by 10°C, with either a heat cradle or hot water bottles and a space blanket. This tests the integrity of central pathways, from the hypothalamus to the sweat glands. Sweating is assessed using powders, such as quinazarine or Ponceau red, which turn a vivid red on exposure to moisture. In autonomic failure, the thermoregulatory sweating response is lost, and additional tests are needed to distinguish between central and peripheral lesions. In postganglionic lesions, the sudomotor and pilomotor response to intradermal acetylcholine is lost. Various measures can be used, including the quantitative sudomotor axon reflex test. Intradermal pilocarpine assesses the function of sweat glands directly. In DBH deficiency syndrome, sympathetic cholinergic function and sweating is preserved, providing a clue to selective impairment of sympathetic noradrenergic function. In gustatory sweating, spicy foods, cheese, or substances containing tyramine are ingested to provoke sweating.

The sympathetic skin response (SSR) measures electrical potentials from electrodes on the foot and hand and may provide a measure of sympathetic cholinergic activity to sweat glands. The SSR can be induced by stimuli that are physiological (inspiratory gasps, loud noise, or touch) or electrical (median nerve stimulation). The response is usually absent in axonal neuropathies but present in demyelinating disorders. Despite numerous reports on the SSR in various disorders, there have been limited observations on influencing factors and few studies in adequate numbers of patients with clearly defined autonomic disorders. In peripheral disorders, such as PAF and pure cholinergic dysautonomia (Figure 81.23), the SSR is a reliable marker of sympathetic cholinergic function. However, this reliability depends on the use of presence or absence of the response, rather than latency and amplitude, which are highly variable (Magnifico et al. 1998). The value of the SSR in central autonomic disorders requires further definition. In MSA with confirmed sympathetic adrenergic failure, up to one-third of patients with the parkinsonian or cerebellar forms had a recordable SSR (see Figure 81.23C). This makes it unlikely that the SSR would be a valuable discriminatory test in separating MSA from idiopathic Parkinson's disease (without autonomic failure), especially in the early stages (Magnifico et al. 1997).

Gastrointestinal Tract

Video-cine-fluoroscopy is of value in assessing swallowing and the presence of oropharyngeal dysphagia (Figure 81.24). This is especially useful in patients with MSA, who in the later stages develop difficulties in deglutition, which appear to enhance the tendency to aspiration pneumonia. A barium swallow, meal, and follow-through are helpful in suspected upper gastrointestinal disorders, although alternative investigation by endoscopy provides the opportunity for biopsy. Esophageal manometry is of value in disorders of motility and esophagogastric function. Several methods (radioisotope methods and scintigraphic scanning) are available to determine gastric motility noninvasively. When bacterial overgrowth is a suspected cause of diarrhea, a therapeutic trial with broad-spectrum antibiotics, such as neomycin or tetracycline, may be used along with investigations such as jejunal aspiration and the C14 glycocholate test. Small bowel manometry and telemetric devices are of value in separating myopathic from neuropathic disorders of the gut. The measurement of transit time and proctological function tests are used to investigate lower bowel disorders causing diarrhea, constipation, and fecal incontinence.

Urinary Tract

Nocturnal polyuria can be assessed by separate day and night measurement of urine volume. Measurements of urine osmolarity and the concentration of sodium and potassium may be helpful. When the urinary bladder is involved, an intravenous pyelogram and micturating cystometrogram may be needed. Urodynamic measurements are valuable in defining the function of the bladder musculature and sphincter mechanisms. They may differentiate idiopathic Parkinson's disease from MSA; in the former, detrusor hyperreflexia may be present, whereas in MSA, there is usually a combination of both detrusor hyperreflexia and stress incontinence due to a weak urethral sphincter. Measurement of postmicturition residual volume (e.g., by ultra-

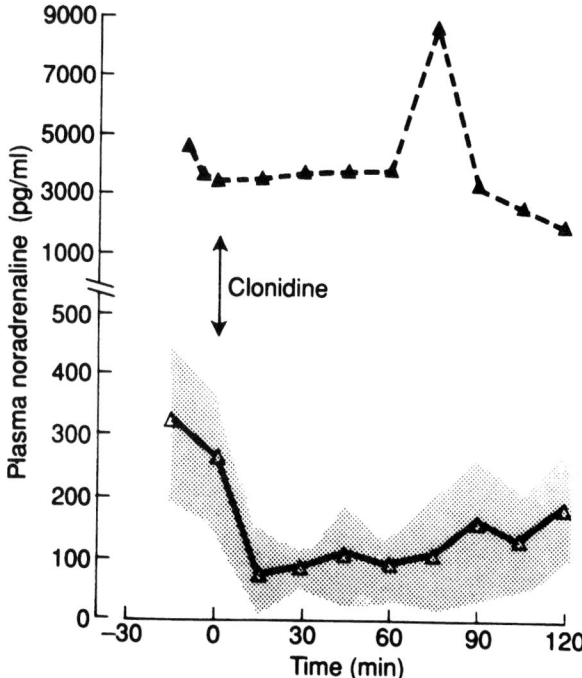

FIGURE 81.21   Plasma noradrenaline levels in a patient with a pheochromocytoma and in a group of patients with essential hypertension before and after intravenous clonidine, administration of which is indicated by an arrow (2 mg/kg over 10 minutes). Plasma noradrenaline levels fell rapidly in the essential hypertensives after clonidine and remained low over the period of observation. The stippled area indicates the ± standard error of means. Plasma noradrenaline levels are considerably higher in the pheochromocytoma patient and are not affected by clonidine. (Reprinted with permission from CJ Mathias, R Bannister. Investigation of Autonomic Disorders. In CJ Mathias, R Bannister [eds], Autonomic Failure. A Textbook of Clinical Disorders of the Autonomic Nervous System [4th ed]. Oxford: Oxford University Press, 1999;169–195.)

sound) is of particular importance. It may be high when the bladder is involved, as in MSA, and may result in urinary infection, which should be detected early and promptly treated. There are some groups, such as patients with spinal cord lesions, to whom particular care must be provided because recurrent infections, along with calculi, may result in renal failure.

Urethral sphincter electromyography provides an analysis of motor units affected when there is neuronal degeneration of Onuf's nucleus in the sacral cord. This results in sphincter denervation with subsequent reinnervation. Electromyography indicates an increase in amplitude and duration of individual motor units, which are often polyphasic. This combination of denervation and reinnervation is often present in the various forms of MSA, unlike idiopathic Parkinson's disease (without autonomic involvement). Similar changes occur in the anal sphincter (Beck et al. 1994).

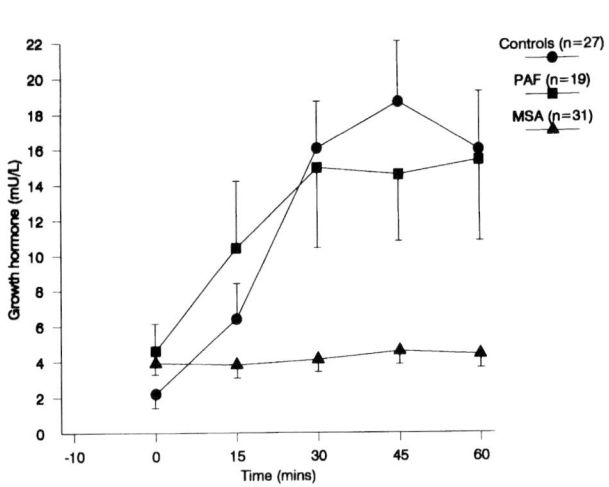

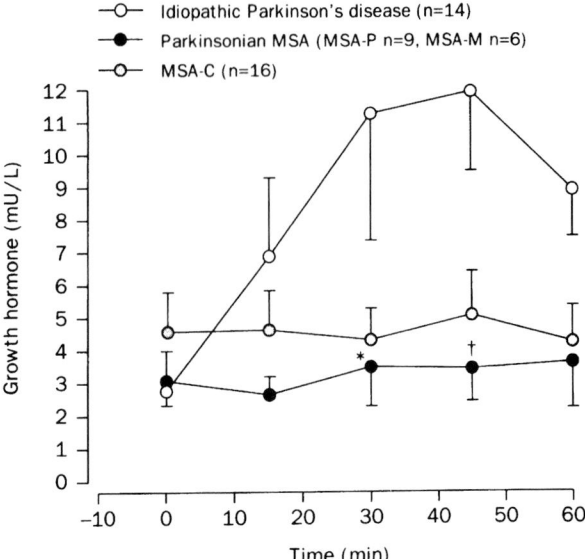

A

B

FIGURE 81.22 (A) Serum growth hormone (GH) concentrations before (0) and at 15-minute intervals for 60 minutes after clonidine (2 μg/kg/minute) in normal subjects (controls) and in patients with pure autonomic failure (PAF) and multiple system atrophy (MSA). GH concentrations rise in controls and in patients with PAF with a peripheral lesion; there is no rise in patients with MSA with a central lesion. (B) Lack of serum GH response to clonidine in the two forms of MSA (the cerebellar form [MSA-C] and the parkinsonian form [MSA-P]) in contrast to patients with idiopathic Parkinson's disease with no autonomic deficit, in whom there is a significant rise in GH levels. (MSA-M = mixed form.) (Reprinted with permission from JR Kimber, L Watson, CJ Mathias. Distinction of idiopathic Parkinson's disease from multiple system atrophy by stimulation of growth hormone release with clonidine. Lancet 1997;349:1877.)

Respiratory System

Respiratory rate and arterial blood gases should be measured to determine the degree of hypoxia, especially during sleep in patients with apneic episodes. Indirect and direct laryngoscopy detect laryngeal abductor paresis.

Eye

Various pharmacological preparations administered locally help determine the degree of sympathetic or parasympathetic involvement of pupils. Lacrimal secretion can be tested by Schirmer's test, and damage from deficient secretion can be assessed using rose bengal instillation followed by slit-lamp examination.

Miscellaneous

A range of additional investigations may be needed to determine the cause of the disorder or associated complications. Computed tomographic scans and magnetic resonance imaging (MRI) of the brain help in assessing basal ganglia and cerebellar involvement in primary autonomic failure. MRI scanning is of considerable value in identifying

brainstem causes of autonomic dysfunction. PET scanning has provided valuable information in central disorders, such as MSA (Gilman et al. 1996; Rinne et al. 1995). Brainstem auditory evoked responses are often abnormal in MSA but normal in PAF. In suspected peripheral nerve involvement, electrophysiological studies together with sural nerve biopsy are indicated. In amyloidosis, a rectal or renal biopsy may be diagnostic; the latter is indicated if there is renal involvement. To exclude adrenal insufficiency, a short or long Synacthen test should be performed.

In patients with localized lesions, specific investigations to determine the cause may be warranted. In Horner's syndrome, for example, this may include a computed tomographic scan or MRI of the brain to exclude a midbrain or medullary hemorrhage, bronchoscopy and radiography to exclude an apical bronchial neoplasm, and carotid artery angiography to assess lesions of the internal carotid artery.

PROGNOSIS

In primary autonomic failure, the prognosis depends on the diagnostic category, the degree of autonomic impairment, and the ability to prevent complications. In acute and subacute dysautonomias, complete recovery may occur, although mild or substantial residual autonomic deficits

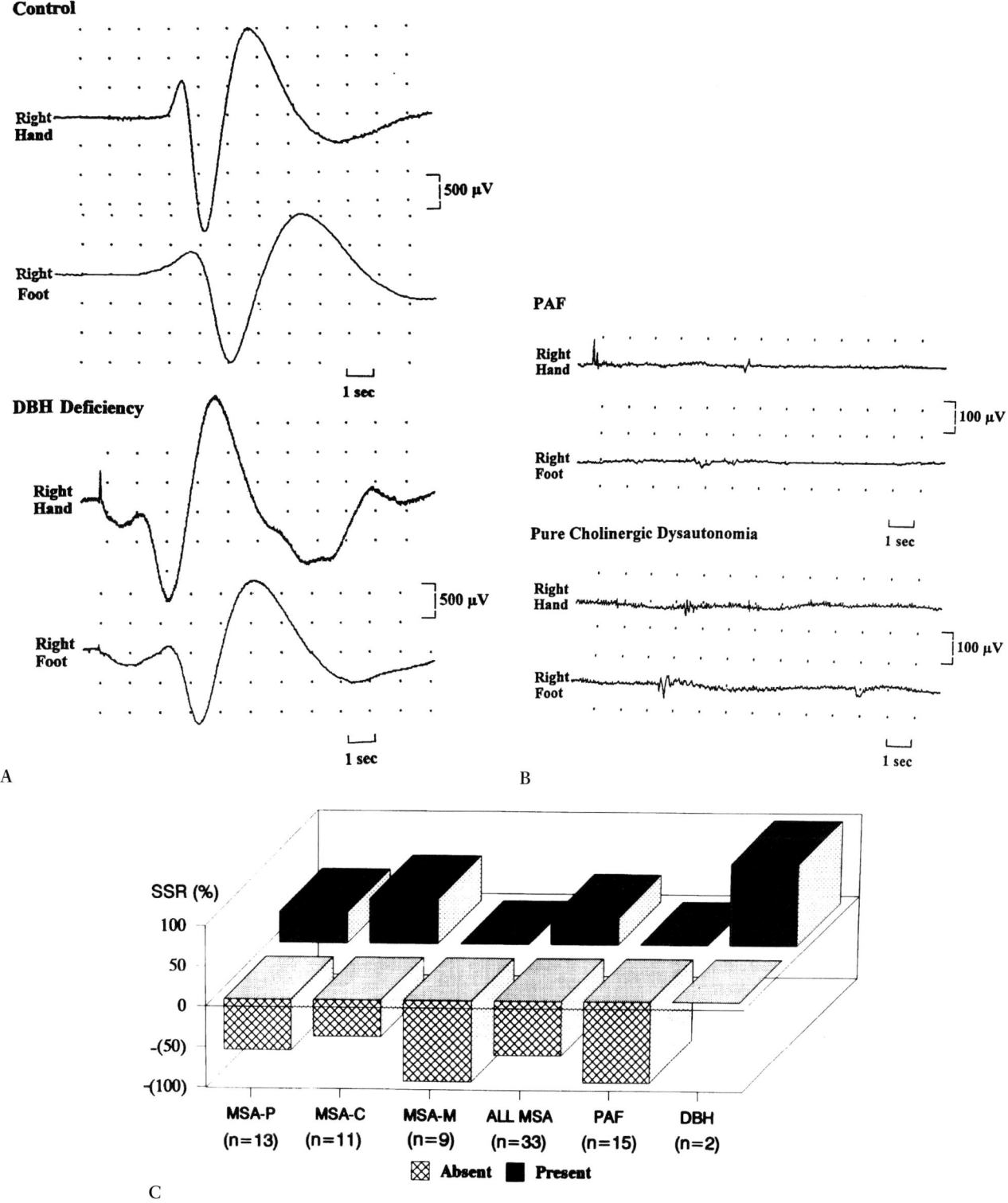

FIGURE 81.23 (**A**) The sympathetic skin response (in microvolts) from the right hand and right foot of a normal subject (control) and a patient with dopamine β-hydroxylase (DBH) deficiency. (**B**) The sympathetic skin response could not be recorded in two patients, one with pure autonomic failure (PAF) and the other with pure cholinergic dysautonomia. (Reprinted with permission from F Magnifico, VP Misra, NMF Murray, CJ Mathias. The sympathetic skin response in peripheral autonomic failure—evaluation in pure autonomic failure, pure cholinergic dysautonomia and dopamine-beta-hydroxylase deficiency. Clin Auton Res 1998;8:133–138). (**C**) Presence or absence of the sympathetic skin response (SSR) in 33 patients with multiple system atrophy (MSA), 15 patients with PAF, and two siblings with DBH deficiency. The SSR (as occurs in normal subjects) was present in the two patients with DBH deficiency who had adrenergic failure but preserved cholinergic function; it was absent in all patients with PAF with a peripheral sympathetic lesion. A proportion of patients (up to 30%) with the parkinsonian (MSA-P) and cerebellar (MSA-C) forms had preservation of the SSR despite postural hypotension and definite sympathetic adrenergic failure. (MSA-M = mixed form.) (Data from F Magnifico, VP Misra, NMF Murray, CJ Mathias. The laboratory detection of autonomic dysfunction in multiple system atrophy—the role of the sympathetic skin response. Neurology 1997;48[Suppl.]:A190.)

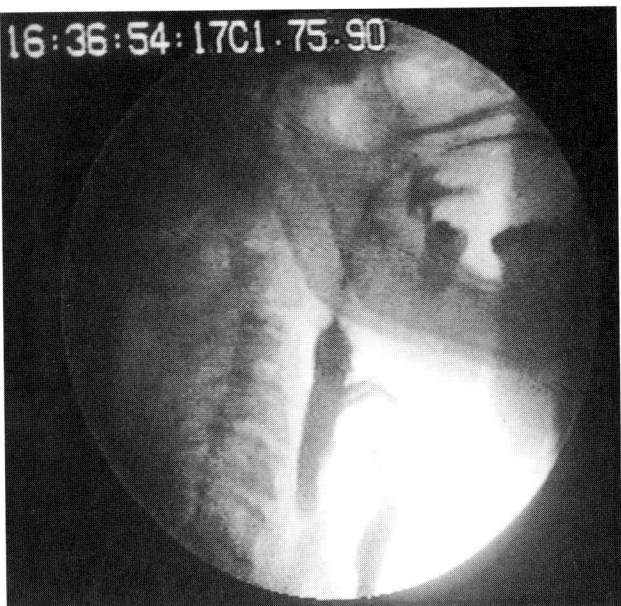

FIGURE 81.24   Still frame from video-cine-fluoroscopic examination in a patient with oropharyngeal dysphagia shows penetration of the larynx by contrast medium, indicating the potential to lead tracheal aspiration. (Reprinted with permission from CJ Mathias. Gastrointestinal dysfunction in multiple system atrophy. Semin Neurol 1996;16:251.)

often persist. In chronic autonomic failure syndromes, there are differences in prognosis. Subjects with PAF survive for many years, often with a virtually normal life expectancy, despite the disabilities resulting from autonomic failure. The disorder is usually not progressive, but dysfunction may increase with age, with coincidental illnesses (such as diarrhea), or with use of drugs with vasodilator properties. In MSA, the prognosis is poorer, with a mean life expectancy of around 9 years (Wenning et al. 1994), although there is considerable individual variation. Factors such as respiratory complications, difficulties with swallowing, and increasing motor deficits contribute to mortality. With improved awareness of these complications and the ability to prevent life-threatening events, survival in MSA is likely to increase.

In patients with secondary autonomic dysfunction, the prognosis depends largely on the associated disorder. With some (e.g., subarachnoid hemorrhage and brain tumors), the primary pathological process often dominates the outcome. In other disorders, such as tetanus, the complications arising from autonomic dysfunction may play a key role in determining morbidity and mortality. In conditions such as diabetes mellitus and familial amyloid polyneuropathy, autonomic impairment worsens the overall prognosis.

In the rarer subgroups with isolated disorders, there are considerable differences in prognosis. Patients with specific acetylcholine receptor abnormalities may have severe complications, whereas those with DBH deficiency seem to manage despite severe postural hypotension.

In certain localized disorders, such as Horner's syndrome, the prognosis depends on the initiating cause; in others, such as Chagas' disease, the outcome is determined by complications, such as those arising from cardiac involvement.

MANAGEMENT

Management depends on the autonomic abnormalities and their functional deficits, the associated clinical condition, and the degree of disability. This section discusses major principles of management relating to autonomic deficits.

Cardiovascular System

Postural Hypotension

Postural hypotension may cause considerable disability, with the potential risk of serious injury. Blood pressure maintenance is dependent, especially in the absence of sympathetic control, on the output of the heart; on tone in resistance and capacitance vessels, which is influenced by various pressor and depressor hormones present systemically or locally; and on intravascular fluid volume. Because no single drug can effectively mimic the actions of the sympathetic nervous system, a multipronged approach combining nonpharmacological and pharmacological measures is needed (Table 81.10).

Many factors other than postural change are now recognized as lowering blood pressure, and increasing patient awareness of these factors is important. Rapid postural change, especially in the morning when getting out of bed, should be avoided because the supine blood pressure often is lowest at this time, probably because nocturnal polyuria reduces extracellular fluid volume. Head-up tilt at night is beneficial and appears to reduce salt and water loss by stimulating the renin-angiotensin-aldosterone system or by activating other hormonal, neural, or local renal hemodynamic mechanisms, which reduce recumbency-induced diuresis. In some, head-up tilt may be impractical or the degree of tilt achieved inadequate. In these patients, nocturnal polyuria can be more effectively reduced with the antidiuretic agent desmopressin. Straining during micturition and bowel movement can lower blood pressure further by inducing Valsalva's maneuver. In toilets in small enclosed areas, this is dangerous because the person cannot fall to the floor and thereby recover blood pressure and consciousness. In hot weather, the elevation of body temperature because of impairment of thermoregulatory mechanisms, such as sweating, may increase

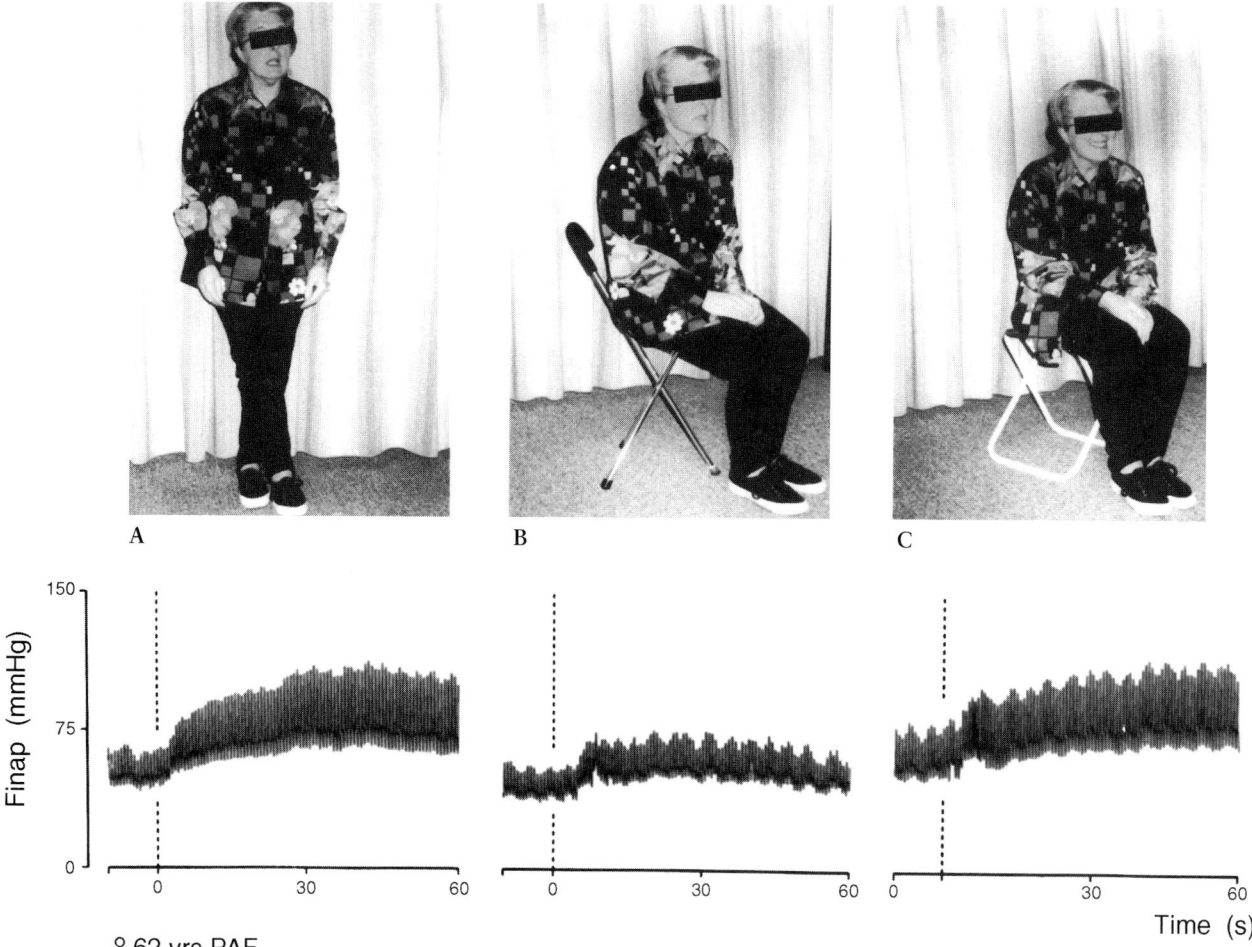

♀ 62 yrs PAF

FIGURE 81.25 The effect of standing in a crossed-leg position with leg muscle contraction (**A**), sitting on a derby chair (**B**), and fishing chair (**C**) on finger arterial blood pressure in a patient with postural hypotension. Postural symptoms were present while standing and disappeared while crossing legs. Sitting on a derby chair did not completely relieve the patient's symptoms. Note the greater increment in blood pressure while standing with crossed legs and leg muscle contractions, or sitting on the fishing chair, compared with sitting on a derby chair. (Reprinted with permission from AAJ Smit, MA Hardjowijono, W Wieling. Are portable folding chairs useful to combat orthostatic hypotension? Ann Neurol 1997;42:975–978.)

vasodilatation and worsen postural hypotension. Ingestion of alcohol or large meals, especially those containing a high carbohydrate content, may cause postprandial hypotension and aggravate postural hypotension. Various physical maneuvers (Wieling et al. 1993), such as leg crossing, squatting, sitting in the knee-chest position, and abdominal compression, are of value in reducing postural hypotension (Figure 81.25).

A number of devices aimed at preventing venous pooling during standing have been used. These include elastic stockings for the lower limbs, abdominal binders, and, in extreme cases, positive-gravity suits. Each has its limitations and may increase susceptibility to postural hypotension when not in use. In patients with amyloidosis and accompanying hypoalbuminemia, positive-gravity suits may be the last resort because it is virtually impossible to maintain intravascular volume in these patients without causing tissue edema.

Drugs often are needed to help sustain blood pressure (Table 81.11). The major mechanisms by which they act include constricting blood vessels, increasing cardiac output, preventing vasodilatation, and retaining salt and water. It should be recognized that enhanced responses usually occur to pressor and vasodepressor agents; the former may result in severe hypertension, especially when supine, but vasodepressors may cause marked hypotension. There are exceptions; patients with infiltration of blood vessels due to amyloidosis may not exhibit supersensitivity, despite a peripheral autonomic neuropathy. With increasing awareness of the precise biochemical deficit in some patients, agents can be given that bypass deficient enzyme systems and result in appropriate neurotransmitter replacement

Table 81.10: Summary outline of nonpharmacological and pharmacological measures in the management of postural hypotension due to neurogenic failure*

Nonpharmacological measures
   To be avoided
      Sudden head-up postural change (especially on waking)
      Prolonged recumbency
      Straining during micturition and defecation
      High environmental temperature (including hot baths)
      Severe exertion
      Large meals (especially with refined carbohydrate)
      Alcohol
      Drugs with vasodepressor properties
   To be introduced
      Head-up tilt during sleep
      Small frequent meals
      High salt intake
      Judicious exercise (including swimming)
      Body positions and maneuvers
   To be considered
      Elastic stockings
      Abdominal binders
Pharmacological
   Starter drug: fludrocortisone
   Sympathomimetics: ephedrine or midodrine
   Specific targeting: octreotide, desmopressin, or erythropoietin

*It should be emphasized that non-neurogenic factors (such as fluid loss due to vomiting or diarrhea) may substantially worsen postural hypotension. (Adapted with permission from CJ Mathias, JR Kimber. Treatment of postural hypotension. J Neurol Neurosurg Psychiatry 1998;65:285–289.

(Figure 81.26). An example is in DBH deficiency, in which the amino acid L-threo-3, 4-dihydroxyphenylserine is directly converted by dopa-decarboxylase into noradrenaline (Figure 81.27). Whether this occurs intra- or extraneuronally (or both) is unclear. Its potential value in the management of postural hypotension primary chronic autonomic failure remains to be determined (Kaufmann 1996).

A valuable starter drug, especially in mild postural hypotension, is fludrocortisone in a dose of 0.1 or 0.2 mg at night. There is no evidence of a mineralocorticoid deficiency in primary autonomic failure, and low-dose fludrocortisone probably acts by reducing the inability to retain salt and water, especially when recumbent, and by increasing the sensitivity of blood vessels to pressor substances. In the doses used, it is less likely to induce side effects such as ankle edema and hypokalemia. If nocturnal polyuria is not reduced by head-up tilt, fludrocortisone can be effectively combined with desmopressin, a vasopressin-2 receptor agonist with potent antidiuretic but minimal direct pressor activity. Five to 40 mg intranasally or 100–400 mg orally at night reduces the diuresis but, when used without fludrocortisone, does not prevent nocturnal natriuresis. These trials have been performed mainly in patients with primary chronic autonomic failure. Patients with PAF require smaller doses (usually 5–10 mg only) because they appear to be more sensitive to the drug than are patients with MSA. Plasma sodium must be monitored to exclude hyponatremia and water intoxication. These can be reversed by stopping the drug and withholding water,

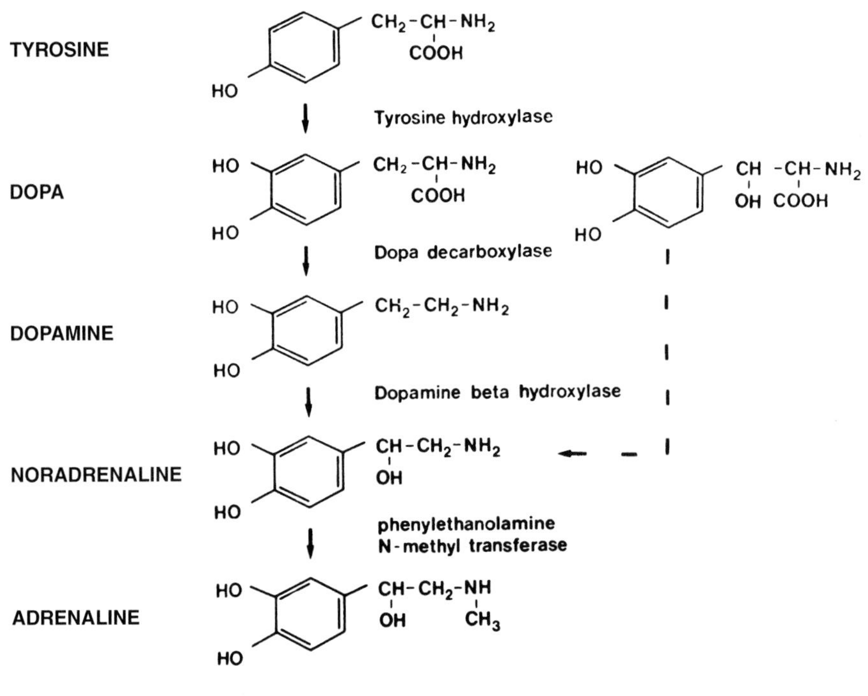

FIGURE 81.26 Biosynthetic pathway for noradrenaline synthesis and the structure of L-threo-3,4-dihydroxyphenylserine alongside. The enzyme dopa-decarboxylase, which is present both intra- and extraneuronally, converts it to noradrenaline, thus bypassing the hydroxylation step, which depends on dopamine β-hydroxylase.

but a diuresis then ensues, which may enhance postural hypotension.

A number of drugs that mimic the activity of noradrenaline, either directly or indirectly, have been used. Ephedrine acts both directly and indirectly and is of value in central and incomplete autonomic lesions, including MSA. In severe peripheral sympathetic lesions (as in PAF), it may have minimal or no effects. A dose of 15 mg three times daily initially, with an increase to 30 or 45 mg three times daily, can be used, although central side effects limit use of the higher doses. Drugs that act directly on α-adrenoceptors are of value, especially in peripheral lesions. These drugs often act mainly on resistance vessels, with the potential risk of deleterious arterial constriction, especially in the elderly and those with peripheral vascular disease. A well-studied example is midodrine, which is converted to the active metabolite, desglymidodrine (Low et al. 1997). The ergot alkaloid dihydroergotamine acts predominantly on venous capacitance vessels, but its effects are limited by its poor absorption; high oral doses (5–10 mg three times daily) may be needed.

Other therapeutic attempts to raise blood pressure have concentrated on pre- and postsynaptic α_2-adrenoceptor mechanisms. They have limited application in practice. Clonidine is mainly an α_2-adrenoceptor agonist, which predominantly lowers blood pressure through its central effects by reducing sympathetic outflow. It also has peripheral actions on postsynaptic α-adrenoceptors, which may raise blood pressure in the presence of pressor supersensitivity. These peripheral vasoconstrictor effects probably account for its modest success in severe, distal sympathetic lesions. Yohimbine blocks presynaptic α_2-adrenoceptors, which normally suppress release of noradrenaline and should theoretically be of benefit in incomplete sympathetic lesions, as observed in single-dose studies.

Supine hypertension is not uncommon in autonomic failure and may be worsened by treatment. It may occasionally result in cerebral hemorrhage, aortic dissection, myocardial ischemia, or cardiac failure. This may be a greater problem with certain drug combinations, such as tyramine (which releases noradrenaline) and monoamine oxidase inhibitors (such as tranylcypromine and moclobemide), which prolong its actions. Supine hypertension may increase symptoms of cerebral ischemia during subsequent postural change, probably through an unfavorable resetting of cerebral autoregulatory mechanisms. To prevent these problems, head-up tilt, omission of the evening dose of vasopressor agents, a prebedtime snack to induce postprandial hypotension, and even nocturnal use of short-acting vasodilatators have been suggested.

One approach to overcoming the problems with blood pressure variability is to use a subcutaneous infusion pump, as in the control of hyperglycemia with insulin in diabetes mellitus, and a short-acting but effective vasoconstrictor, such as noradrenaline. A pilot study with such a device had

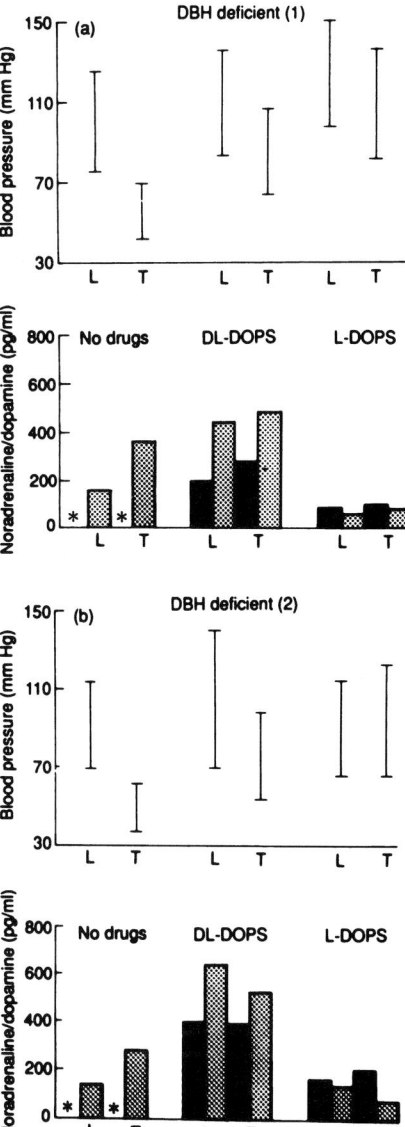

FIGURE 81.27   Blood pressure (systolic and diastolic) while lying flat (L) and during head-up tilt (T) in two siblings with dopamine β-hydroxylase (DBH) deficiency (1 and 2) before and during treatment with DL-dihydroxyphenylserine (DL-DOPS) and L-DOPS. Plasma noradrenaline (*histogram*) and dopamine (*stippled histogram*) levels are indicated before and during head-up tilt. Plasma noradrenaline was undetectable (asterisk <5 pg/ml) in both while off drugs. (Reprinted with permission from CJ Mathias, R Bannister, P Cortelli, et al. Clinical autonomic and therapeutic observations in two siblings with postural hypotension and sympathetic failure due to an inability to synthesize noradrenaline from dopamine because of a deficiency of dopamine beta-hydroxylase. QJM 1990;n.s. 75, 278:617.)

been successful, but there were a number of practical problems, including the accurate monitoring of blood pressure without an intra-arterial catheter. It is hoped that in due course these problems will be overcome, so as to benefit the

Table 81.11:   Outline of the major actions by which a variety of drugs may reduce postural hypotension

Reducing salt loss or plasma volume expansion: mineralocorticoids (fludrocortisone)
Reducing nocturnal polyuria: V_2-receptor agonists (desmopressin)
Vasoconstriction, sympathetic
   Directly
      On resistance vessels (midodrine, phenylephrine, noradrenaline, clonidine)
      On capacitance vessels (dihydroergotamine)
   Indirectly (ephedrine, tyramine with monoamine oxidase inhibitors, yohimbine)
   Prodrug (L-dihydroxyphenylserine)
Vasoconstrictor, nonsympathomimetic: V_1-receptor agents (terlipressin)
Preventing vasodilatation
   Prostaglandin synthetase inhibitors (indomethacin, flurbiprofen)
   Dopamine receptor blockade (metoclopramide, domperidone)
   β_2-Adrenoceptor blockade (propranolol)
Preventing postprandial hypotension
   Adenosine receptor blockade (caffeine)
   Peptide release inhibitors (somatostatin analogue: octreotide)
Increasing cardiac output
   Beta blockers with intrinsic sympathomimetic activity (pindolol, xamoterol)
   Dopamine agonist (ibopamine)
Increasing red cell mass: erythropoietin

severely hypotensive patient who is refractory to the combination of nonpharmacological and drug therapy.

Other therapeutic approaches in postural hypotension include prevention of vasodilatation. Prostaglandin synthetase inhibitors, such as indomethacin and flurbiprofen, have had some success and may act by blocking vasodilatory prostaglandins, by causing salt and water retention through their renal effects, or both. They have potentially serious side effects, however, such as gastrointestinal ulceration and hemorrhage. The dopamine antagonists metoclopramide and domperidone are occasionally of value when an excess of dopamine is contributory. β-Adrenoceptor blockers, such as propranolol, may be successful when postural hypotension accompanies tachycardia; the combination of blocking β_2-adrenoceptor vasodilatation and β_1-adrenoceptor–induced tachycardia may account for the benefit.

Certain β-adrenoceptor blockers, such as pindolol, with a high degree of intrinsic sympathomimetic activity, may increase cardiac output and through this, or other less well-understood mechanisms, raise blood pressure. Complications such as cardiac failure may occur. Another agent with similar properties, xamoterol, has had limited success and has been withdrawn because of deleterious effects. The dopamine agonist ibopamine has been used in a few patients only with varying success.

Various therapeutic approaches have been used to reduce severe postprandial hypotension. Caffeine has been advo-

cated and may act by blocking vasodilatory adenosine receptors. A dose of 250 mg, present in 2 cups of coffee, may be of benefit. The prodrug L-dihydroxyphenylserine (L-DOPS), presumably through adrenoceptor-induced vasoconstriction, reduces postprandial hypotension in primary autonomic failure (Freeman et al. 1996). The somatostatin analogue octreotide, which inhibits release of a variety of gastrointestinal tract peptides, including those with vasodilatory properties, has been successfully used to prevent postprandial hypotension; it also may partly reduce postural and exercise-induced hypotension (Smith and Mathias 1995). The need for subcutaneous administration is a drawback. It does not appear to enhance nocturnal (supine) hypotension (Alam et al. 1995). The development of an oral preparation will be a substantial advance in therapy.

Other strategies must be used in patients with specific disorders causing syncope. In carotid sinus hypersensitivity, a cardiac demand pacemaker may be of benefit in the cardioinhibitory form; in the mixed and vasodepressor forms, the use of vasopressor drugs and even carotid sinus denervation may be necessary. Bradycardia in patients with high spinal cord injuries who are on respirators may require a combination of atropine, oxygen, and, if necessary, a temporary demand pacemaker. Tachypacing with an implanted cardiac pacemaker is of no benefit in the management of postural hypotension (except in the rare situation when bradycardia also occurs), because raising the heart rate without increasing venous return (which is impaired because of pooling due to sympathetic vasoconstrictor failure) does not elevate cardiac output and therefore does not raise blood pressure.

Hypertension

Hypertension due to increased sympathetic nervous activity occurs in patients with tetanus, Guillain-Barré syndrome, porphyria, certain cerebral tumors, and subarachnoid hemorrhage. It usually responds to propranolol and other sympatholytic and antihypertensive agents. In patients with high spinal cord injuries, it is important to look for the precipitating cause of autonomic dysreflexia (Table 81.12) and rectify it. A range of drugs, based on knowledge of the pathophysiological mechanisms, has been used to prevent or reduce hypertension in these patients (Table 81.13).

Sweating Disorders

In idiopathic hyperhidrosis, pharmacological approaches may be beneficial. In hyperhidrosis over the palms and soles, local astringents containing glutaraldehyde and antiperspirants containing aluminum salts may reduce sweating. Anticholinergics, such as propantheline bromide and topical applications of hyoscine hydrobromide, may help. Low-dose clonidine may be of benefit, especially in those in whom there

Table 81.12: Some causes of autonomic dysreflexia in patients with high spinal cord injuries

Cutaneous
    Pressure sores
    Burns
    Infected ingrowing toenails
Skeletal muscle
    Spasms, especially in limbs with contractures
Abdominal viscera
    Ureter
        Calculus
    Urinary bladder
        Distention by blocked catheter
        Infection
        Discoordinated contraction
        Irritation by catheter, calculus, or bladder washout
    Rectum/anus
        Fecal retention
        Anal fissure
        Enemata
    Uterus
        Contraction during pregnancy
        Menstruation occasionally
    Gastrointestinal organs
        Gastric ulceration
        Appendicitis
        Cholecystitis, cholelithiasis
Miscellaneous
    Fractures of bones
    Urethral abscess
    Vaginal dilation
    Ejaculation
    Intrathecal neostigmine or electrical stimulation to
        induce ejaculation

Table 81.13: Drugs used in autonomic dysreflexia with their major site of action

Afferent: Topical lignocaine
Spinal cord
    Clonidine
    Reserpine
    Spinal anesthetics
Sympathetic efferent
    Ganglia: hexamethonium
    Nerve terminals: guanethidine
    α-Adrenoceptors: phenoxybenzamine
Target organ
    Blood vessels: glyceryl trinitrate
    Sweat glands: probanthine

Note: Drugs such as clonidine may act at multiple sites. Some must be given at specific sites, such as lignocaine into the bladder, if this is the source of the stimulus causing autonomic dysreflexia.

is a central or emotional component; in some patients, behavioral psychotherapy may provide relief. Minimally invasive (thoracic endoscopic) sympathectomy often is successful in reducing or abolishing palmar hyperhidrosis, but there is a high incidence of compensatory hyperhidrosis (Adar 1997), which in some may be more distressing than the original symptoms. In gustatory sweating, avoidance of foods that induce attacks may help. Recently, botulinum toxin has been used to treat both gustatory (Schulze-Bonhage et al. 1996) and palmar (Naumann et al. 1997) hyperhidrosis.

Thermoregulation

In hypothermia, the standard management of slowly warming patients, preferably with a space blanket and warm drinks, is recommended. In hyperpyrexia, cold drinks, tepid sponging, a fan to increase heat loss by convection, and, if possible, an air-conditioned environment are helpful, with immersion in ice-cold water occasionally necessary.

Gastrointestinal System

Xerostomia may be helped by artificial saliva. Achalasia of the esophagus may require surgery or dilatation. Patients with MSA who have oropharyngeal dysphagia need advice on the type and quantity of food to be ingested; if there is severe dysfunction and a risk of tracheal aspiration, a feeding gastrostomy may be necessary. Metoclopramide and domperidone increase gastric emptying and may be useful in gastroparesis. The prokinetic drug cisapride, which acts through intrinsic cholinergic plexuses, and the macrolide erythromycin, which stimulates motilin receptors, may be of value. In paralytic ileus, nasogastric suction with intravenous feeding is necessary. Peptic ulceration, as occurs in the early stages after high spinal cord injury, can be prevented by the prophylactic use of histamine$_2$-antagonists (such as cimetidine and ranitidine) or proton-pump inhibitors (such as omeprazole). In those with diarrhea, broad-spectrum antibiotics (neomycin or tetracycline) may be the initial step before using codeine phosphate or other opiate-based antidiarrheal agents. The somatostatin analogue, octreotide, may reduce diarrhea in some patients with amyloidosis and diabetic autonomic neuropathy. Aperients and laxatives, together with a high-fiber diet, are often needed in constipation.

Urinary Tract

In outflow tract obstruction, procedures that include prostatectomy, transurethral resection, or sphincterotomy may be needed. Surgical procedures often worsen incontinence in MSA. Bladder dysfunction may be helped by drugs that influence detrusor muscle activity (such as the anticholinergic, oxybutynin) or sphincter malfunction (e.g., alpha blockers phenoxybenzamine and prazosin). Side effects may be enhanced in patients with generalized autonomic failure. Intermittent or indwelling catheterization may be necessary. The urine should be checked frequently to detect infection. Nocturnal polyuria in chronic primary autonomic failure is often helped by desmopressin; it is also of value in other disorders, such as multiple sclerosis, in which nocturia may occur. Women often have difficulties with urinary drainage, even by catheterization, and the use of urinary diversion procedures, such as an ileal conduit, is occasionally necessary.

Reproductive System

Erectile failure in men may be helped by suction devices, an implanted prosthesis, or a variety of pharmacological approaches, including local instillation (intracavernosal or urethral) or orally administered drugs (sildenafil). In DBH deficiency, difficulty in ejaculation is improved by treatment with L-DOPS. In patients with spinal cord injuries, electroejaculatory procedures followed by artificial insemination have been successful. Pregnant women with high spinal injuries may develop severe hypertension with cardiac dysrhythmias and eclampsia during uterine contractions and delivery. This is best managed by spinal anesthesia, which reduces spinal sympathetic discharge and permits a normal delivery.

Respiratory System

A tracheostomy may be necessary if inspiratory stridor is due to laryngeal abductor paresis and there is evidence of oxygen desaturation, especially at night (Harcourt et al. 1996). In those with periodic apneic episodes, timed or triggered bilevel positive airway pressure ventilation may be useful.

Eye

In alacrima, tear substitutes such as hypromellose eye drops are of value.

Neurological Deficits

In the parkinsonian forms of MSA, a trial of L-dopa is indicated because some patients are responsive, especially in the early stages of the disease. It may, however, cause or enhance postural hypotension. The monoamine oxidase-B inhibitor, selegiline, has been used in combination with L-dopa, although there is no evidence that it delays progression of MSA; it may worsen postural hypotension. Postural hypotension also may occur with selegiline treatment in patients with idiopathic Parkinson's disease who do not have autonomic failure; the mechanisms that lower blood pressure may include the central effects of its metabolites, methyl-amphetamine (Churchyard et al. 1997). There is no

effective pharmacotherapy for cerebellar deficits in MSA. Supportive therapy using disability aids must be provided. The family and community must be involved in overall care. There is limited evidence that transplantation of the pancreas in diabetes mellitus, and of the liver in familial amyloid neuropathy, may favorably influence the neuropathy in these otherwise relentlessly progressive disorders.

REFERENCES

Adar R. Compensatory hyperhidrosis after thoracic sympathectomy. Lancet 1997;351:231–232.

Alam M, Smith GDP, Bleasdale-Barr K, et al. Effects of the peptide release inhibitor, octreotide, on daytime hypotension and on nocturnal hypertension in primary autonomic failure. J Hypertens 1995;13:1664–1669.

Beck RO, Fowler CJ, Mathias CJ. Genito-Urinary Dysfunction in Disorders of the Autonomic Nervous System. In D Rushton (ed), Handbook of Neuro-Urology. New York: Marcel Dekker, 1994;281–301.

Churchyard A, Mathias CJ, Boonkongchuen P, Lees AJ. Autonomic effects of selegiline: possible cardiovascular toxicity in Parkinson's disease. J Neurol Neurosurg Psychiatry 1997;63:228–234.

Colosimo C, Albanese A, Hughes AJ, et al. Some specific clinical features differentiate multiple system atrophy (striatonigral variety) from Parkinson's disease. Arch Neurol 1995;52:294–298.

Consensus Statement on the definition of orthostatic hypotension, pure autonomic failure and multiple system atrophy. Clin Auton Res 1996;6:125–126.

Cortelli P, Perani D, Parchi P, et al. Cerebral metabolism in fatal familial insomnia: relation to duration, neuropathology, and distribution of protease-resistant prion protein. Neurology 1997;49:126–133.

Daniel SE. The Neuropathology and Neurochemistry of Multiple System Atrophy. In R Bannister, CJ Mathias (eds), Autonomic Failure. A Textbook of Clinical Disorders of the Autonomic Nervous System (4th ed). Oxford: Oxford University Press, 1999;321–328.

De Lorenzo F, Hargreaves J, Kakkar VV. Pathogenesis and management of delayed orthostatic hypotension in patients with chronic fatigue syndrome. Clin Auton Res 1997;7:185–190.

Drummond PD. Sweating and vascular responses in the face: normal regulation and dysfunction in migraine, cluster headache and harlequin syndrome. Clin Auton Res 1994;4:273–285.

Freeman R, Young J, Landsbert L, et al. The treatment of postprandial hypotension in autonomic failure with 3,4-DL-threo dihydroxyphenyserine. Neurology 1999;47:1414–1420.

Gilman S, Frey KA, Koeppe RA, et al. Decreased striatal monoaminergic terminals in olivopontocerebellar atrophy and multiple system atrophy demonstrated with positron emission tomography. Ann Neurol 1996;40:885–892.

Goldstein DS, Holmes C, Cannon RO III, et al. Sympathethic cardioneuropathy in dysautonomias. N Engl J Med 1997;336:696–702.

Harcourt J, Spraggs P, Mathias C, Brookes G. Sleep-related breathing disorders in the Shy-Drager syndrome. Observations on investigation and management. Eur J Neurol 1996;3:186–190.

Heafield MT, Gammage MD, Nightingale S, Williams AC. Idiopathic dysautonomia treated with intravenous gammaglobulin. Lancet 1996;347:28–29.

Kaufmann H. Could treatmetn with L-DOPS do for autonomic failure what DOPA did for Parkinson's disease? Neurology 1996;47:1370–1371.

Khurana RK. Orthostatic intolerance and orthostatic tachycardia: a heterogeneous disorder. Clin Auton Res 1995;5:12–18.

Kimber J, Smith GDP, Mathias CJ. Reflex sympathetic dystrophy in a patient with peripheral sympathetic denervation. Eur J Neurol 1997a;4:315–317.

Kimber JR, Mitchell D, Mathias CJ. Chronic cough in the Holmes-Adie syndrome. A report in 5 cases with autonomic dysfunction. J Neurol Neurosurg Psychiatry 1998;65:583–586.

Kimber JR, Watson L, Mathias CJ. Distinction of idiopathic Parkinson's disease from multiple system atrophy by stimulation of growth hormone release with clonidine. Lancet 1997b; 349:1877–1881.

Lambert GW, Thompson JM, Turner AG, et al. Cerebral noradrenaline spillover and its relation to muscle sympathetic nervous activity in healthy human subjects. J Auton Nerv Syst 1997;64:57–64.

Low PA, Gilden JL, Freeman R, et al. Efficacy of midodrine vs. placebo in neurogenic orthostatic hypotension. A randomized, double-blind multicenter study. JAMA 1997;277:1046–1051.

Magnifico F, Misra VP, Murray NMF, Mathias CJ. The sympathetic skin response in peripheral autonomic failure—evaluation in pure autonomic failure, pure cholinergic dysautonomia and dopamine-beta-hydroxylase deficiency. Clin Auton Res 1998;8:133–138.

Magnifico F, Misra VP, Murray NMF, Mathias CJ. The laboratory detection of autonomic dysfunction in multiple system atrophy—the role of the sympathetic skin response. Neurology 1997;48(Suppl.):A190.

Mantysaari M, Kuikka J, Mustonem J, et al. Measurement of myocardial accumulation of 123-metaiodobenzylguanidine for studying cardiac autonomic neuropathy in diabetes mellitus. Clin Auton Res 1996;6:163–169.

Mathias CJ. Autonomic disorders and their recognition. N Engl J Med 1997;10:721–724.

Mathias CJ. Orthostatic hypotension—causes, mechanisms and influencing factors. Neurology 1995;45(Suppl. 5):S6–S11.

Mathias CJ, Bannister R. Dopamine-Beta-Hydroxylase Deficiency and Other Genetically Determined Autonomic Disorders. In R Bannister, CJ Mathias (eds), Autonomic Failure. A Textbook of Clinical Disorders of the Autonomic Nervous System (4th ed). Oxford: Oxford University Press, 1999a;9:387–401.

Mathias CJ, Bannister R. Investigation of Autonomic Disorders. In R Bannister, CJ Mathias (eds), Autonomic Failure. A Textbook of Clinical Disorders of the Autonomic Nervous System (4th ed). Oxford: Oxford University Press, 1999;329–339.

Mathias CJ, Kimber JR. Treatment of postural hypotension. J Neurol Neurosurg Psychiatry 1998;65:258–289.

Mathias CJ, Polinsky RJ. Separating the Primary Autonomic Failure Syndromes, Multiple System Atrophy and Pure Autonomic Failure from Parkinson's Disease. In G Stern (ed), Advances in Neurology. Philadelphia: Lippincott–Raven, 1999, In press.

Mathias CJ, Williams AC. The Shy Drager syndrome (and multiple system atrophy). In DB Calne, Neurodegenerative Diseases, 1st ed. Philadelphia: Saunders, 1994;473–768.

Matthews MR. Autonomic Ganglia in Multiple System Atrophy and Pure Autonomic Failure. In R Bannister, CJ Mathias (eds), Autonomic Failure. A Textbook of Disorders of the Autonomic Nervous System (4th ed). Oxford: Oxford University Press, 1998.

McIntosh SJ, Lawson J, Kenny RA. Clinical characteristics of vasodepressor, cardioinhibitory and mixed carotid sinus syndrome in the elderly. Am J Med 1993;95:203–208.

Monza D, Soliveri P, Radice D, et al. Cognitive dysfunction and impaired organization of complex motility in degenerative parkinsonian syndroms. Arch Neurol 1998;55:372–378.

Naumann M, Flachenecker P, Brocker E-B, et al. Botulinum toxin for palmar hyperhidrosis. Lancet 1997;349:252.

Owen-Reece H, Elwell CE, Smith M, Goldstone JC. Near infrared spectroscopy. Br J Anaesth 1999;82:418–426.

Papp MI, Lantos PL. The distribution of oligodendroglial inclusions in multiple system atrophy and its relevance to clinical symptomatology. Brain 1994;117:235–243.

Parati G, Di Rienzo M, Omboni S, Mancia G. Computer Analysis of Blood Pressure and Heart Rate Variability in Subjects with Normal and Abnormal Autonomic Cardiovascular Control. In R Bannister, CJ Mathias (eds), Autonomic Failure. A Textbook of Disorders of the Autonomic Nervous System (4th ed). Oxford: Oxford University Press, 1999;197–223

Pillon B, Gouider-Khouja N, Deweer B, et al. Neuropsychological pattern of striatonigral degeneration: comparison with Parkinson's disease and progressive supranuclear palsy. J Neurol Neurosurg Psychiatry 1995;58:174–179.

Pramstaller PP, Wenning GK, Smith SJ, et al. Nerve conduction studies, skeletal muscle EMG and sphincter EMG in multiple system atrophy. J Neurol Neurosurg Psychiatry 1995;58: 618–621.

Puvi-Rajasingham S, Smith GDP, Akinola A, Mathias CJ. Abnormal regional blood flow responses during and after exercise in human sympathetic denervation. J Physiol 1997;505:481–489.

Quinn NP, Marsden CD. The motor disorder of multiple system atrophy [Editorial]. J Neurol Neurosurg Psychiatry 1993;56: 1239–1242.

Rinne JO, Burn DJ, Mathias CJ, et al. Positron emission tomography studies on the dopaminergic system and striatal opioid binding in the olivopontocerebellar atrophy variant of multiple system atrophy. Ann Neurol 1995;37:568–573.

Schobel HP, Fischer T, Henszer K, et al. Pre-eclampsia—a state of sympathetic overactivity. N Engl J Med 1996;335:1480–1485.

Schott GD. Interrupting the sympathetic outflow in causalgia and reflex sympathetic dystrophy. A futile procedure for many patients. BMJ 1998;316:792–793.

Schulze-Bonhage A, Schroder M, Ferbert A. Botulinum toxin in the therapy of gustatory sweating. J Neurol 1996;243:143–146.

Smit AAJ, Vermeulen M, Koelman JHTM, Wieling W. Unusual recovery from acute panautonomic neuropathy after immunoglobulin therapy. Mayo Clin Proc 1997;72:333–335.

Smith GDP, Bannister R, Mathias CJ. Post-exercise dizziness as the sole presenting symptom of autonomic failure. Br Heart J 1993;69:359–361.

Smith GDP, Mathias CJ. Postural hypotension enhanced by exercise in patients with chronic autonomic failure. QJM 1995;88: 251–256.

Wenning GK, Ben Shlomo Y, Magalhães M, et al. Clinical features and natural history of multiple system atrophy. Brain 1994;117: 835–845.

Wieling W, van Lieshout JJ, van Leeuwen AM. Physical maneuvers that reduce postural hypotension in autonomic failure. Clin Auton Res 1993;3:57–66.

Library
Stepping Hill Hospital
Poplar Grove
Stockport SK2 7JE

Chapter 82
Disorders of Neuromuscular Transmission

Donald B. Sanders and James F. Howard, Jr.

MYASTHENIA GRAVIS

Myasthenia gravis (MG) is the most common primary disorder of neuromuscular transmission. The usual cause is an acquired immunological abnormality, but some cases result from genetic abnormalities at the neuromuscular junction. Much has been learned about the pathophysiology and immunopathology of MG during the past 20 years. What was once a relatively obscure condition of interest primarily to neurologists is now the best characterized and understood autoimmune disease. A wide range of potentially effective treatments are available, many of which have implications for the treatment of other autoimmune disorders. This chapter is based on the authors' experience with more than 1,100 patients with MG seen with our colleagues over a period of 20 years.

History

In 1672, Willis described a disease with fluctuating weakness that varied throughout the day and could render patients "mute as a fish." Erb described the classic signs of MG in three patients in 1879 and recognized that the fluctuating weakness differed from that seen in other diseases. In 1893, Goldflam provided a comprehensive description of the disease, and 2 years later, Jolly used the term *myasthenia gravis pseudoparalytica* to describe the condition in a 14-year-old boy. Jolly also showed that the visible twitch of muscle induced by electrical stimulation decreased with repetition.

An association between the thymus gland and MG was first suggested by Weigert in 1901, when he described a thymoma in a patient with MG. The association of thymic hyperplasia and MG was reported 4 years later by Buzzard. In 1913, Schumacher and Roth described the first thymectomy, performed 2 years earlier by Sauerbruch. In 1934, Mary B. Walker treated a 56-year-old woman with physostigmine, an acetylcholinesterase inhibitor, and noted a striking improvement in the patient's strength. Remen had tried neostigmine in MG, and it became the first accepted medical treatment after Walker reported its use in 1935.

Lindsley reported variation in the amplitude of single motor unit potentials in patients with MG in 1935. Harvey and Masland confirmed these findings in 1941 and described the decremental muscle response to repetitive nerve stimulation (RNS) that is the basis for the most commonly used electrodiagnostic test for the disease.

In 1960, Simpson noted a frequent association of MG with diseases that have a presumed autoimmune cause and postulated that MG resulted from an immunologically mediated attack on the muscle endplate. In 1964, Elmqvist and coworkers demonstrated a reduction in the amplitude of miniature endplate potentials, and in 1976, Albuquerque and co-workers showed that this was caused by reduced postjunctional sensitivity to acetylcholine.

Hormonal therapy of MG with anterior pituitary extract was first tried by Simon in 1935. Kjaer was the first to report successful therapy with prednisone, in 1971.

In 1973, Patrick and Lindstrom noted fluctuating, neostigmine-responsive weakness in rabbits immunized with acetyl-

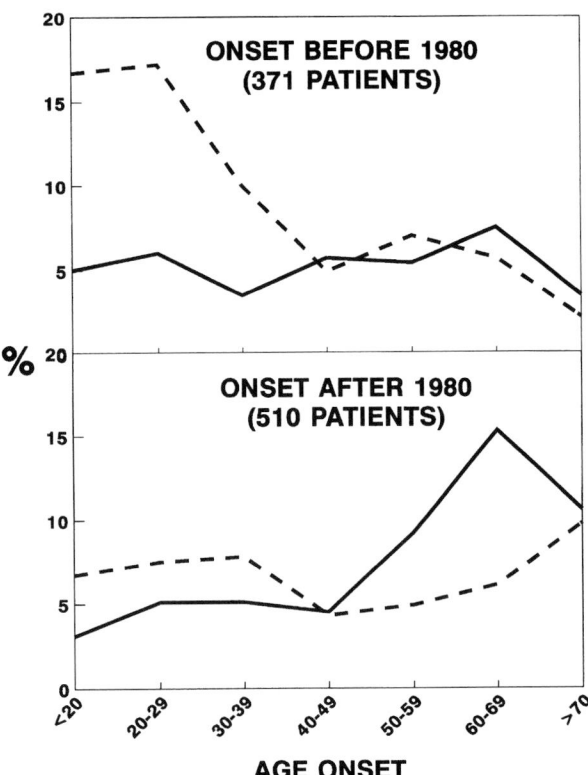

—MALES --FEMALES

**ONSET BEFORE 1980
(371 PATIENTS)**

**ONSET AFTER 1980
(510 PATIENTS)**

%

AGE ONSET

FIGURE 82.1 Age at onset of myasthenic symptoms in 944 patients with acquired myasthenia gravis whose disease began before or after 1980, demonstrating how the age and gender distribution has changed as the population has grown older (DB Sanders, JM Massey, JF Howard, unpublished observations). Data indicate the percentage of the total number of patients seen during each time period. More than 60% of patients diagnosed before 1980 were female; after that date, more than 50% were male.

choline receptor (AChR) protein. The similarity of this condition to MG, demonstration of antibodies to AChR in the serum of patients with MG by Lindstrom and colleagues in 1976, and demonstration of immune complexes on the postsynaptic muscle membrane by Engel and colleagues in 1977 were the seminal observations that ultimately led to the current understanding of the immune-mediated basis of MG.

Epidemiology

The prevalence of MG in the United States is estimated at 14 per 100,000 population—approximately 36,000 cases (Phillips and Torner 1996). However, MG is probably underdiagnosed, and the prevalence is probably higher. Previous studies showed that women were affected more often than men. The most common age at onset was the second and third decades in women and the seventh and eighth decades in men. As the population ages, the average age at onset has increased correspondingly, and now men are

more often affected than women, and the onset of symptoms is usually after age 50 (Figure 82.1).

Clinical Presentation

Patients with MG come to the physician complaining of specific muscle weakness and not of generalized fatigue. Ocular motor disturbances, ptosis, or diplopia were the initial symptom of MG in two-thirds of our patients; almost all had both symptoms within 2 years. Oropharyngeal muscle weakness and difficulty chewing, swallowing, or talking was the initial symptom in one-sixth of patients, and limb weakness in only 10%. Initial weakness was rarely limited to single muscle groups, such as neck or finger extensors or hip flexors.

The severity of weakness fluctuates during the day, usually being least severe in the morning and worse as the day progresses, especially after prolonged use of affected muscles. Ocular symptoms typically become worse while reading, watching television, or driving, especially in bright sunlight. Many patients find that dark glasses reduce diplopia and also hide drooping eyelids. Jaw muscle weakness typically becomes worse during prolonged chewing, especially tough meats or chewy candy.

Careful questioning often reveals evidence of earlier, unrecognized myasthenic features; frequent purchases of new eyeglasses to correct blurry vision, avoidance of foods that became difficult to chew or swallow, or cessation of activities that require prolonged use of specific muscles. Friends may have noted a sleepy or sad facial appearance caused by ptosis or facial weakness. The course of disease is variable but usually progressive. Weakness is restricted to the ocular muscles in approximately 10% of cases. The rest have progressive weakness during the first 2 years that involves oropharyngeal and limb muscles. Maximum weakness occurs during the first year in two-thirds of patients. In the era before corticosteroids were used for treatment, approximately one-third of patients improved spontaneously, one-third became worse, and one-third died of the disease. Spontaneous improvement frequently occurred early in the course. Symptoms fluctuated over a relatively short period and then became more severe for several years (active stage). The active stage was followed by an inactive stage, in which fluctuations in strength still occurred but were attributable to fatigue, intercurrent illness, or other identifiable factors. After 15–20 years, weakness becomes fixed, and the most severely involved muscles are frequently atrophic (burnt-out stage). Factors that worsen myasthenic symptoms are emotional upset, systemic illness (especially viral respiratory infections), hypothyroidism or hyperthyroidism, pregnancy, the menstrual cycle, drugs affecting neuromuscular transmission (see Drugs That Adversely Affect Myasthenia Gravis and Lambert-Eaton Myasthenic Syndrome, later in this chapter), and increases in body temperature.

The unusual distribution and fluctuating weakness of MG often suggests psychiatric illness. Conversely, ptosis and diplopia suggest increased intracranial pressure and often lead to unnecessary cranial imaging studies or arteriography.

Physical Findings

When examining patients with known or suspected MG, the examination must be modified to show variable weakness in specific muscle groups. Strength should be assessed repetitively during maximum effort and again after brief periods of rest. Performance on such tests fluctuates in diseases other than MG, especially if testing causes pain. The strength fluctuations of MG are best shown by tests of ocular and oropharyngeal muscle function because these are less likely to be affected by other factors.

Ocular Muscles

Most patients with MG have weakness of ocular muscles. Asymmetrical weakness of several muscles in both eyes is typical. The pattern of weakness is not characteristic of lesions of one or more nerves, and the pupillary responses are normal. In our experience, weakness is most frequent and most severe in the medial rectus muscles. Ptosis is usually asymmetrical and varies during sustained activity. To compensate for ptosis, the frontalis muscle may be chronically contracted, producing a worried or surprised look. Unilateral frontalis contraction is a clue that the lid elevators are weak on that side. This also may be the only visible evidence of facial weakness. Patients with ocular muscle weakness usually have weakness of eye closure.

Oropharyngeal Muscles

Oropharyngeal muscle weakness causes changes in the voice, difficulty chewing and swallowing, inadequate maintenance of the upper airway, and altered facial appearance. The voice may be nasal, especially after prolonged talking, and liquids may escape through the nose when swallowing because of palatal muscle weakness. Weakness of the laryngeal muscles causes hoarseness. This can also be shown by asking the patient to make a high-pitched "*eeeee*" sound. Difficulty chewing and swallowing is detected by a history of frequent choking or clearing of the throat or coughing after eating.

Myasthenic patients, particularly those with severe or long-standing disease, may have a characteristic facial appearance, as demonstrated in Figure 82.2. At rest, the corners of the mouth droop downward, making the patient appear depressed. Attempts to smile often produce contraction of the medial portion of the upper lip and a horizontal contraction of the corners of the mouth without the natural upward curling, which gives the appearance of a snarl.

Jaw weakness can be shown by manually opening the jaw against resistance, which is not possible in normal people. A frequent sign of jaw weakness is that the patient holds the jaw closed with the thumb under the chin, the middle finger curled under the nose or lower lip and the index finger extended up the cheek, producing a studious or attentive appearance.

The strength of eye closure is usually diminished in patients with MG and may be the only weakness that remains after treatment.

Limb Muscles

Any trunk or limb muscle can be weak, but some are more often affected than are others. Neck flexors are usually weaker than neck extensors, and the deltoids, triceps, and extensors of the wrist and fingers are frequently weaker than other limb muscles.

Inheritance of Myasthenia Gravis

MG is not transmitted by mendelian inheritance, but family members of patients are approximately 1,000 times more likely to develop the disease than is the general population. Increased jitter on single-fiber electromyography (SFEMG) is found in 33–45% of asymptomatic first-degree relatives, and AChR antibodies are slightly elevated in up to 50%. These observations suggest that there is a genetically determined predisposition to develop MG.

Pathophysiology of Myasthenia Gravis

The normal neuromuscular junction releases ACh from the motor nerve terminal in discrete packages (quanta). The ACh quanta diffuse across the synaptic cleft and bind to receptors on the folded muscle endplate membrane (Figure 82.3). Stimulation of the motor nerve releases many ACh quanta that depolarize the muscle endplate region and then the muscle membrane, causing muscle contraction.

In acquired MG, the postsynaptic muscle membrane is distorted and simplified, having lost its normal folded shape (see Figure 82.3). The concentration of AChRs on the muscle endplate membrane is reduced, and antibodies are attached to the membrane. ACh is released normally, but its effect on the postsynaptic membrane is reduced. The postjunctional membrane is less sensitive to applied ACh, and the probability that any nerve impulse will cause a muscle action potential is reduced.

The following observations support the concept that MG is an immune-mediated disease of the AChR complex:

1. Patients with MG have an increased incidence of other presumed or known immune-mediated diseases, such as rheumatoid arthritis.
2. A transitory neonatal form of the disease occurs in myasthenia and other immune-mediated diseases.
3. The HLA haplotypes that are common in patients with MG are also common in other autoimmune diseases.

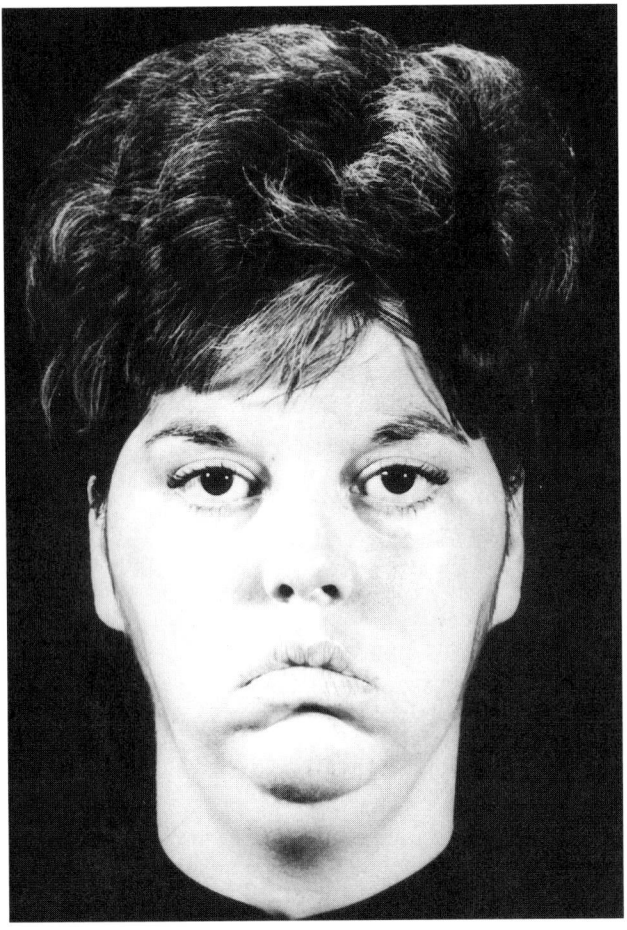

A

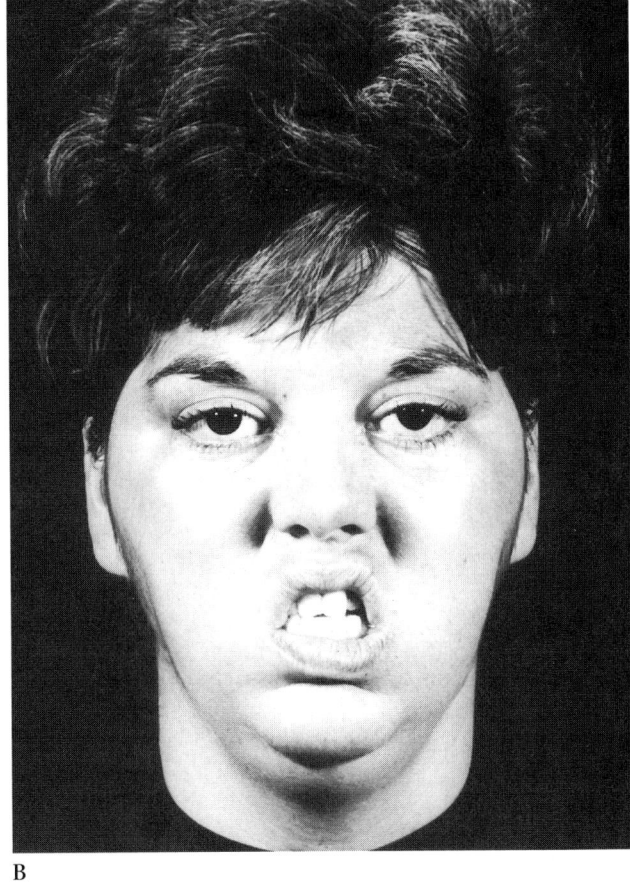

B

FIGURE 82.2 The characteristic facial appearance of a woman with moderately severe myasthenia gravis. (**A**) At rest: Note the bilateral lid ptosis and downward curve of the corners of the mouth, giving the patient a sad appearance. (**B**) Smiling: The "myasthenic snarl" that results from an upward movement of the medial portion of the upper lip and a horizontal contraction of the corners of the mouth rather than a normal upward turn of the corners of the mouth. This gives the patient an angry appearance and may be seen even when the patient is attempting to laugh.

4. The weakness in MG improves after removal of lymph by thoracic duct drainage and worsens after reinfusion of a high-molecular-weight protein fraction from the lymph, probably immunoglobulin G (IgG).

5. Immunosuppressive treatment, including plasma exchange, produces improvement in most patients with MG.

6. An animal model of MG can be produced by immunization with purified AChR protein.

7. Antibodies against human AChR are found in the serum of most patients with MG.

8. IgG and complement components are attached to the postsynaptic endplate membrane in myasthenic muscle.

9. Myasthenic serum or IgG produces a defect of neuromuscular transmission when injected into animals.

The role of serum antibodies against AChR in the pathophysiology of the disease is not fully understood. Although antibody levels are usually higher in patients with more severe disease, these values vary widely among patients, and as many as 25% are seronegative. Even seronegative patients may improve after plasma exchange, and the neuromuscular abnormality can be transferred to animals by injecting serum from seronegative patients. The antibodies responsible for the neuromuscular abnormality may not always be those that are measured, and the serum antibody level may not reflect the amount of antibody attached to the muscle endplate.

It is hypothesized that the predominant involvement of ocular muscles in MG is due to the presence of antibodies specific for the γ-subunit of the AChR (which is found in adult extraocular muscle). However, the levator palpebrae, which has a different AChR subunit composition, is as involved clinically as other ocular muscles, and γ-subunits have been found even in normal limb muscle.

Although T lymphocytes do not play a role in the damage to antigenic determinants at the neuromuscular junction, they do play a crucial role in the pathogenesis of the

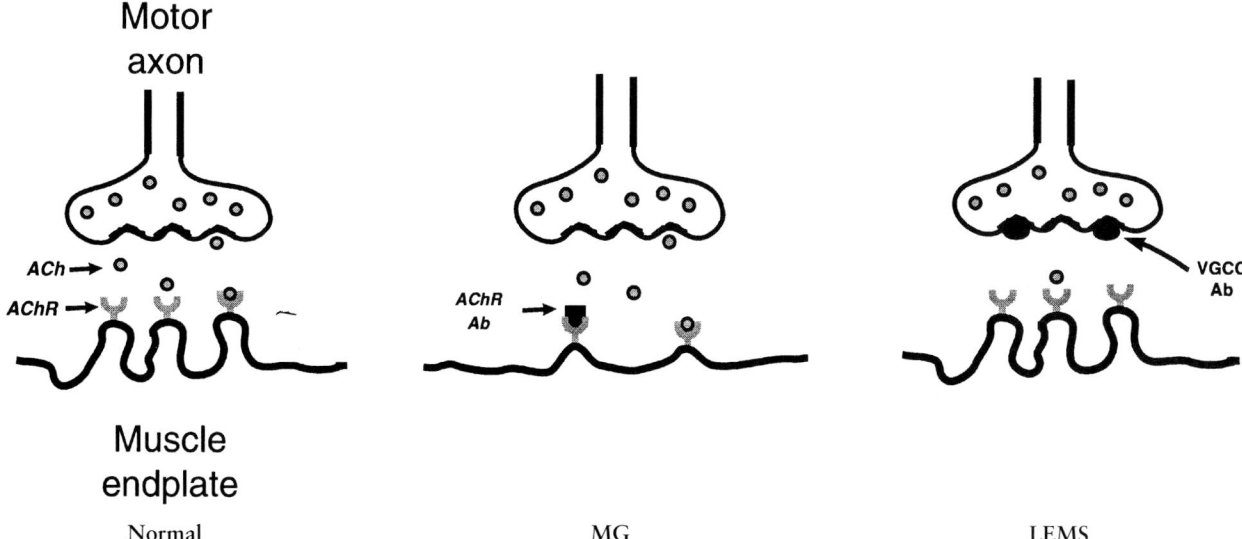

FIGURE 82.3   The neuromuscular junction. In acquired myasthenia gravis (MG), the muscle endplate membrane is simplified and the normal folded pattern is lost. Acetylcholine receptors (AChR) are lost from the tips of the folds and antibodies (AChR Ab) are attached to the postsynaptic membrane. In Lambert-Eaton myasthenic syndrome (LEMS), antibodies against the voltage-gated calcium channel (VGCC Ab) on the nerve terminal interfere with release of ACh.

disease. Several lines of evidence exist for such statements. The presence of high-affinity IgG anti-AChR antibodies in the serum and bound to the endplate region of myasthenic patients suggests that T cells have switched to synthesizing of the IgG isotype by anti-AChR B cells. T cell–independent antibody formation produces IgM antibodies only. In addition, anti-AChR reactive CD4+ T cells are found in the serum and thymus glands of myasthenic patients. These can be propagated in vitro and express T helper functions. Thymectomy, a common treatment for MG, results in a reduction in the anti-AChR reactivity of circulating T cells. Finally, synthesis of human anti-AChR antibodies and clinical myasthenic symptoms can be transferred to SCID mice after engraftment of the blood lymphocytes from myasthenic patients if they have not been depleted of CD4+ cells.

The Thymus in Myasthenia Gravis

Thymic abnormalities are clearly associated with MG, but the nature of the association is uncertain. Ten percent of patients with MG have a thymic tumor, and 70% have hyperplastic changes (germinal centers) that indicate an active immune response. These are areas within lymphoid tissue where B cells interact with helper T cells to produce antibodies. Because the thymus is the central organ for immunological self-tolerance, it is reasonable to suspect that thymic abnormalities cause the breakdown in tolerance that causes an immune-mediated attack on AChR in MG. The thymus contains all the necessary elements for the pathogenesis of MG: myoid cells that express the AChR antigen, antigen-presenting cells, and immunocompetent T cells. Thymus tissue from patients with MG produces AChR antibodies when implanted into immunodeficient mice. However, still uncertain is whether the role of the thymus in the pathogenesis of MG is primary or secondary.

Most thymic tumors in patients with MG are benign, well-differentiated, and encapsulated and can be removed completely at surgery. It is unlikely that thymomas result from chronic thymic hyperactivity because MG can develop years after thymoma removal, and the HLA haplotypes that predominate in patients with thymic hyperplasia are different from those with thymomas.

In our experience, patients with thymoma usually have more severe disease, higher levels of AChR antibodies, and more severe EMG abnormalities than do patients without thymoma. Almost 20% of our patients with MG whose symptoms began between the ages of 30 and 60 years have thymoma; the frequency of thymoma is much lower when symptoms began after age 60.

Diagnostic Procedures

The Edrophonium Chloride (Tensilon) Test

Weakness caused by abnormal neuromuscular transmission characteristically improves after intravenous administration of edrophonium chloride. With the exception of ocular and pharyngeal muscles, the examiner must rely on the patient

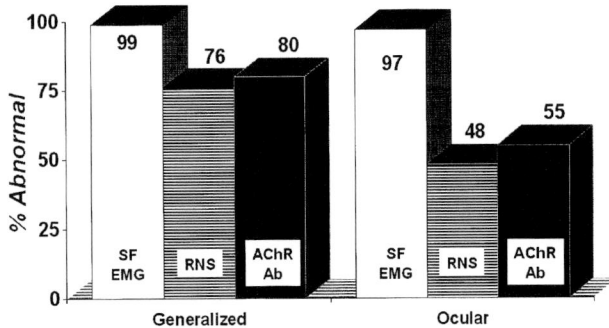

FIGURE 82.4 Comparison of abnormalities demonstrated by single-fiber electromyography (SF EMG), repetitive nerve stimulation of hand and shoulder muscles (RNS), and serum acetylcholine receptor antibody levels (AChR Ab) in 550 patients with acquired generalized or ocular myasthenia gravis (DB Sanders, JM Massey, JF Howard, unpublished observations).

to exert maximum effort before and after drug administration to assess its effect. For this reason, the test is most reliable when the patient has ptosis, discernible limitation of eye movements, or nasal speech.

We have found the edrophonium chloride test to be positive in more than 90% of patients with MG. However, improved strength after edrophonium chloride is not unique to MG. It may also be seen in motor neuron disease, where neuromuscular transmission is abnormal because of rapidly progressive denervation. We have also seen improved eye movements after edrophonium chloride in patients with lesions of the oculomotor nerves.

The ideal dose of edrophonium chloride cannot be predetermined. A single fixed dose, such as 10 mg, may be too much in some patients and cause increased weakness. An incremental dosing schedule is recommended. Two milligrams are injected intravenously and the response monitored for 60 seconds. Subsequent injections are 3 and 5 mg. If improvement is seen within 60 seconds after any dose, no further injections are given. Ten milligrams of edrophonium does not weaken normal muscle, and the occurrence of weakness after its injection indicates a neuromuscular transmission defect. The total dose of edrophonium chloride in children is 0.15 mg/kg administered incrementally. Subcutaneous administration can be used in newborns and infants, but the response may be delayed for 2–5 minutes.

Some clinicians administer edrophonium chloride in a blinded or double-blinded fashion to improve objectivity. This method has questionable value and is not needed when the end point is well defined, such as relief of ptosis.

Some patients who do not respond to intravenous edrophonium chloride may respond to intramuscular neostigmine because of its longer duration of action. Intramuscular neostigmine is particularly useful in infants and children whose response to intravenous edrophonium chloride may be too brief for adequate observation. In some patients, a therapeutic trial of oral pyridostigmine for several days may

produce improvement that cannot be appreciated after a single dose of edrophonium chloride or neostigmine.

Techniques that show a more objective effect of cholinesterase (ChE) inhibitors on ocular muscles are EMG of the ocular muscles, tonometry, oculography, and Lancaster red-green tests of ocular motility. These tests increase sensitivity to detect a neuromuscular abnormality but are nonspecific and may yield false-positive results.

Antibodies against Acetylcholine Receptors

Eighty percent of our patients with acquired generalized myasthenia and 55% with ocular myasthenia have serum antibodies that bind human AChR (Figure 82.4). The serum concentration of AChR antibody varies widely among patients with similar degrees of weakness and cannot predict the severity of disease in individual patients. Approximately 10% of patients who lack binding antibodies have other antibodies that modulate the turnover of AChR in tissue culture. The concentration of binding antibodies may be low at symptom onset and rise later. Repeat studies are appropriate when initial values are normal. AChR-binding antibody concentrations are rarely elevated in patients with systemic lupus erythematosus, inflammatory neuropathy, amyotrophic lateral sclerosis (ALS), rheumatoid arthritis taking D-penicillamine, thymoma without MG, and in normal relatives of patients with MG. In general, an elevated concentration of AChR-binding antibodies in a patient with compatible clinical features confirms the diagnosis of MG, but normal antibody levels do not exclude the diagnosis.

Virtually all patients with MG and thymoma have elevated AChR-binding antibodies, and many have high concentrations of AChR-modulating and anti–striated muscle antibodies. However, many patients with MG without thymoma also have high concentrations of these antibodies, and thus these serological findings cannot be used to predict the presence of thymoma.

Electromyography

Repetitive Nerve Stimulation. The amplitude of the compound muscle action potential (CMAP) elicited by nerve stimulation is normal or only slightly reduced in MG. Abnormal neuromuscular transmission is demonstrated when the amplitude of the fourth or fifth response to a train of low-frequency nerve stimuli falls at least 10% from the initial value. This decrementing response to RNS is seen more often in proximal muscles, such as the facial muscles, biceps, deltoid, and trapezius, than in hand muscles. We have found a significant decrement to RNS in either a hand or shoulder muscle in 61% of patients with MG.

Needle Electromyography. Needle-electrode EMG is performed to exclude other diseases that either resemble or occur concomitantly with MG, such as myositis or thyroid myopathy. Abnormal neuromuscular transmission may cause variability in the shape or amplitude of motor unit action potentials.

SFEMG (see Chapter 37B) is the most sensitive clinical test of neuromuscular transmission and shows increased jitter in some muscles in almost all patients with MG (Sanders and Stålberg 1996). Jitter is greatest in weak muscles but may be abnormal even in muscles with normal strength. Patients with mild or purely ocular muscle weakness may have increased jitter only in facial muscles.

Increased jitter is a nonspecific sign of abnormal neuromuscular transmission and can be seen in other motor unit diseases. Therefore, when jitter increases, EMG should be performed to exclude neuronopathy, neuropathy, and myopathy. Normal jitter in a weak muscle excludes abnormal neuromuscular transmission as the cause of weakness.

Comparison of Diagnostic Techniques. Intravenous edrophonium chloride is often diagnostic in patients with ptosis or ophthalmoparesis, but it is less useful when other muscles are weak. Elevated serum AChR-binding antibody virtually ensures the diagnosis of MG, but a normal level does not exclude it. RNS confirms impaired neuromuscular transmission but is not specific to MG and is frequently normal in patients with mild or purely ocular disease.

The measurement of jitter by SFEMG is the most sensitive clinical test of neuromuscular transmission and is abnormal in almost all patients with MG. A normal test in a weak muscle excludes the diagnosis of MG, but an abnormal test can occur when other motor unit disorders cause defects in neuromuscular transmission.

Treatment

There are few controlled clinical trials for any medical or surgical modality used to treat MG. All recommended regimens are empirical, and experts disagree on treatments of choice. Treatment decisions should be based on knowledge of the natural history of disease in each patient and the predicted response to a specific form of therapy. Treatment goals must be individualized according to the severity of disease, the patient's age and gender, and degree of functional impairment. The response to any form of treatment is difficult to assess because the severity of symptoms fluctuates. Spontaneous improvement occurs without specific therapy, especially during the early stages of the disease. Successful treatment of MG requires close medical supervision and long-term follow-up. Return of any weakness after a period of improvement should be taken as heralding further progression. This requires reassessment of current treatment and evaluation for underlying systemic disease or thymoma.

Cholinesterase Inhibitors

ChE inhibitors (Table 82.1) retard the enzymatic hydrolysis of ACh at cholinergic synapses so that ACh accumulates at

Table 82.1:   Cholinesterase inhibitors in myasthenia gravis

Advantages
  Produce symptomatic improvement in the majority of patients
  No proven chronic side effects
  Physician familiarity
Disadvantages
  Produce only temporary improvement
  Require close medical supervision
  Prone to over- and underdosage
  Frequent side effects, even at therapeutic levels
  Usually produce less than complete response
  Usually become less effective with time
Major role
  As a diagnostic test
  Early symptomatic treatment in most patients
  May be satisfactory chronic treatment in some patients
  Adjunctive therapy in the majority of patients
    undergoing more definitive therapy

the neuromuscular junction and its effect is prolonged. ChE inhibitors cause considerable improvement in some patients and little to none in others. Strength rarely returns to normal.

Pyridostigmine bromide (Mestinon) and neostigmine bromide (Prostigmin) are the most commonly used ChE inhibitors. Pyridostigmine is generally preferred because it has a lower frequency of gastrointestinal side effects. The initial oral dose in adults is 30–60 mg every 4–8 hours. The equivalent dose of neostigmine is 7.5–15.0 mg. In infants and children, the initial oral dose of pyridostigmine is 1.0 mg/kg and of neostigmine is 0.3 mg/kg. Equivalent dosages of these drugs are listed in Table 82.2. Pyridostigmine is available as a syrup (60 mg/5 ml) for children or for nasogastric tube administration in patients with impaired swallowing. A timed-release tablet of pyridostigmine (Mestinon Timespan, 180 mg) is useful as a bedtime dose for patients who are too weak to swallow in the morning. Its absorption is erratic, leading to possible overdosage and underdosage, and it should not be used during waking hours. Even at night, it is sometimes preferable for the patient to awaken at the appropriate dosing interval and take the regular tablet.

No fixed dosage schedule suits all patients. The need for ACh inhibitors varies from day to day and during the same day in response to infection, menstruation, emotional stress, and hot weather. Different muscles respond differently; with any dose, certain muscles get stronger, others do not change, and still others become weaker. The drug schedule should be titrated to produce an optimal response in muscles causing the greatest disability. Patients with oropharyngeal weakness need doses timed to provide optimal strength during meals. Ideally, the effect of each dose should last until time for the next, without significant underdosing or overdosing at any time. In practice, this is not possible. Attempts to eliminate all weakness by increasing the dose or shortening the interval causes overdose at the time of peak effect. Our goal is to keep the dose low enough to provide definite improvement 30–45 minutes later, and we

Table 82.2: Equivalent doses of anticholinesterase drugs

	Route and dose (mg)			
	Oral	Intramuscular	Intravenous	Syrup
Neostigmine bromide (Prostigmin Bromide)	15	—	—	—
Neostigmine methylsulfate (Prostigmin Methylsulfate)	—	1.5	0.5	—
Pyridostigmine bromide (Mestinon Bromide)	60	2.0	0.7	60 mg/5 ml
Mestinon Timespan	90–180	—	—	—
Ambenonium chloride (Mytelase Chloride)	5	—	—	—

Note: These values are approximations only. Appropriate doses should be determined for each patient based on the clinical response.

expect the effect to wear off before the next one is given. This minimizes the possibility that the dose will be increased to the point of causing cholinergic weakness. The practice of giving edrophonium at the time when pyridostigmine has its maximal effect, to determine if the patient will respond to greater dosages of ChE inhibitors, is dangerous. Acute overdosage may cause cholinergic weakness of respiratory muscles and apnea.

Adverse effects of ChE inhibitors may result from ACh accumulation at muscarinic receptors on smooth muscle and autonomic glands and at nicotinic receptors of skeletal muscle. Central nervous system side effects are rarely seen with the doses used to treat MG. Gastrointestinal complaints are common: queasiness, loose stools, nausea, vomiting, abdominal cramps, and diarrhea. Increased bronchial and oral secretions are a serious problem in patients with swallowing or respiratory insufficiency. Symptoms of muscarinic overdosage may indicate that nicotinic overdose (weakness) is also occurring. Gastrointestinal side effects can be suppressed with loperamide hydrochloride (Imodium), propantheline bromide (Pro-Banthine), glycopyrrolate (Robinul), and diphenoxylate hydrochloride with atropine (Lomotil). Some of these drugs produce weakness at high dosages.

Bromism, presenting as acute psychosis, is a rare complication in patients taking large amounts of pyridostigmine bromide. The diagnosis of bromide intoxication can be confirmed by direct measurement of the serum bromide level. Some patients are allergic to bromide and develop a rash even at modest doses. Neostigmine and pyridostigmine can be administered by nasal spray or nebulizer to patients who cannot tolerate or swallow oral medications.

Thymectomy

Thymectomy is recommended for most patients with MG. Most reports do not correlate the severity of weakness before surgery and the timing or degree of improvement after thymectomy. The maximal favorable response generally occurs 2–5 years after surgery. The response is relatively unpredictable, however, and significant impairment may continue for months or years after surgery (Table 82.3). Sometimes, improvement is only appreciated in retrospect. The best responses to thymectomy are in young people early in the course of their disease, but improvement

can occur even after 30 years of symptoms. In our experience, patients with disease onset after the age of 60 rarely show substantial improvement from thymectomy. Patients with thymomas do not respond to thymectomy as well as patients without thymoma do. Although thymectomy is not generally recommended for patients with purely ocular myasthenia, we have seen dramatic improvement after thymectomy in several such patients and do consider using this treatment in certain circumstances, particularly in young patients with relatively recent onset of myasthenia.

The preferred surgical approach is transthoracic; the sternum is split and the anterior mediastinum explored. Transcervical and endoscopic approaches have less postoperative morbidity but do not allow sufficient exposure for total thymic removal. In our experience, the operative morbidity from transthoracic thymectomy is very low when patients are optimally prepared with plasma exchange or immunosuppression and skilled postoperative management is provided. Extubation is usually accomplished within hours after surgery, and patients may be discharged home as early as the third or fourth postoperative day.

Repeat thymectomy provides significant improvement in some patients with chronic, refractory disease and should be considered when there is concern that all thymic tissue was not removed at prior surgery and when a good response to the original surgery is followed by later relapse.

Thymectomy may be followed by improvement, even in seronegative patients. We do not base the decision to perform thymectomy on the presence or level of AChR antibodies.

Table 82.3: Thymectomy in myasthenia gravis

Advantages
  Can produce long-lasting improvement in the majority
    of patients
  No known chronic side effects
  Excludes or removes thymomas
Disadvantages
  Operative morbidity and mortality
  Frequent long delay before improvement
  Total remission is rare
Major role
  Potentially beneficial in all patients with life expectancy of
    more than 10 yrs or in whom a thymoma is suspected

Table 82.4:   Corticosteroids in myasthenia gravis

Advantages
    Produce rapid improvement in most patients
    Produce total remission or marked improvement in more than
        75% of patients (high-dose, daily corticosteroids)
    Predictable time of response
    Relatively simple drug schedule
    Reduce the morbidity and mortality of subsequent
        thymectomy
Disadvantages
    Corticosteroid side effects
    Exacerbation of weakness after initiation
    Require chronic administration for maximum benefit
Major role
    As initial definitive therapy, producing rapid, virtually
        complete improvement in the majority of patients, permit-
        ting subsequent thymectomy to be performed with greater
        safety
    As secondary treatment in most patients who do not
        respond to thymectomy or other immunosuppressive
        therapy

Corticosteroids

Marked improvement or complete relief of symptoms occurs in more than 75% of patients treated with prednisone, and some improvement occurs in most of the rest (Table 82.4). Much of the improvement occurs in the first 6–8 weeks, but strength may increase to total remission in the months that follow. The best responses occur in patients with recent onset of symptoms, but patients with chronic disease also may respond. The severity of disease does not predict the ultimate improvement. Patients with thymoma have an excellent response to prednisone before or after removal of the tumor.

We have found that the most predictable response to prednisone occurs when treatment begins with a daily dose of 1.5–2.0 mg/kg per day. This dose is given until sustained improvement occurs, which is usually within 2 weeks, and is then changed to an alternate-day schedule, beginning with 100–120 mg. This dose is gradually decreased over many months to the lowest dose necessary to maintain improvement, which is usually less than 20 mg every other day. The rate of decrease must be individualized: Patients who have a prompt, complete response to prednisone can reduce the alternate-day dose by 20 mg each month until the dose is 60 mg. They can then reduce the dose by 10 mg each month until it is 20 mg and then by 5 mg every 3 months to a minimal dose of 10 mg every other day. If any weakness returns as the prednisone dose is reduced, further reductions are usually followed by even greater weakness. At this point, the prednisone dose should be increased, another immunosuppressant should be added, or both. Most patients who respond well to prednisone become weak if the drug is stopped but maintain strength on very low dosages (5–10 mg every other day). For this reason, we do not reduce the

dose further than this unless another immunosuppressant is also being given. Others recommend discontinuing prednisone if the patient is doing well after 2 years. In our experience, weakness ultimately returns if this is done.

Approximately one-third of patients become weaker temporarily after starting prednisone, usually within the first 7–10 days, and lasting for up to 6 days. This worsening usually can be managed with ChE inhibitors. In patients with oropharyngeal weakness or respiratory insufficiency, we use plasma exchange before beginning prednisone to prevent or reduce the severity of steroid-induced exacerbations and to produce a more rapid response. Because high-dose prednisone may exacerbate weakness, patients with oropharyngeal or respiratory involvement should be hospitalized to start this treatment. Once improvement begins, further exacerbations are unusual. Treatment can be started at a low dosage to minimize exacerbations; the dosage is then slowly increased until improvement occurs. Exacerbations may also occur with this approach, and the response is less predictable.

The preceding prednisone regimen can be used for both generalized and purely ocular myasthenia. An alternative approach in treating ocular myasthenia is to begin with 5 or 10 mg of daily prednisone and increase the dose by 5 mg every 3–4 weeks until improvement begins. The dosage is then kept constant until maximum improvement is achieved, whereupon it is tapered over 4–6 months to a maintenance dose of 5–10 mg every other day. Most patients with ocular myasthenia achieve complete resolution of ocular symptoms after treatment with prednisone; early immunotherapy also may reduce the proportion of patients who develop generalized MG (Sommer et al. 1997).

The major disadvantages of chronic corticosteroid therapy are the side effects. Hypercorticism occurs in approximately one-half the patients treated with the suggested regimen. The severity and frequency of adverse reactions increase when high daily doses are continued for more than 1 month. Fortunately, this is rarely necessary, especially if plasma exchange is begun at the same time as prednisone. Most side effects begin resolving as prednisone is tapered and become minimal at doses of less than 20 mg every other day. Side effects are minimized when patients use a low-fat, low-sodium diet and take supplemental calcium. Postmenopausal women should also take supplementary vitamin D. Patients with peptic ulcer disease or symptoms of gastritis need H_2 antagonists. Prednisone should not be given to people who have untreated tuberculosis.

Prednisone may be given with azathioprine if either drug is ineffective alone (see next section, Immunosuppressant Drugs).

Immunosuppressant Drugs

Several immunosuppressant drugs are effective in MG (Table 82.5). Azathioprine reverses symptoms in most patients, but the effect is delayed by 4–8 months. The initial dose is 50 mg daily, which is increased in 50-mg-per-day

Table 82.5:   Immunosuppressant drugs in myasthenia gravis

Advantages
    Produce marked, sustained improvement in most patients
Disadvantages
    Long delay before improvement
    Serious side effects
Major role
    As initial definitive therapy in patients with late-onset
        myasthenia gravis or in whom corticosteroids are
        contraindicated
    As secondary treatment in patients who do not respond to
        corticosteroids or thymectomy
    In combination with prednisone to enhance the response or
        to permit more rapid reduction of prednisone dose

increments every 7 days to a total of 150–200 mg per day. Once improvement begins, it is maintained for as long as the drug is given, but symptoms recur 2–3 months after the drug is discontinued or the dose is reduced below therapeutic levels. Patients who do not improve on corticosteroids may respond to azathioprine, and the reverse is also true. Some respond better to treatment with both drugs than to either alone. Because the response to azathioprine is delayed, both drugs may be started simultaneously with the intent of rapidly tapering prednisone when azathioprine becomes effective.

A severe allergic reaction, with flulike symptoms and possibly a rash, may occur within 2 weeks after starting azathioprine; this reaction requires that the drug be stopped. Patients may have mild, dose-dependent side effects that may require dose reductions but do not require stopping treatment. Gastrointestinal irritation can be minimized by using divided doses after meals or by dose reduction. Leukopenia and even pancytopenia can occur any time during treatment. The blood count must be monitored every week during the first month, each month for a year and every 3–6 months thereafter. If the peripheral white blood cell (WBC) count falls below 3,500 cells/mm^3, the dose should be temporarily reduced and then gradually increased after the WBC count rises above 3,500 cells/mm^3. Counts below 1,000 WBC/mm^3 require that the drug be temporarily discontinued. Serum transaminase concentrations may be slightly elevated, but clinical liver toxicity is rare. We discontinue treatment if transaminase concentrations exceed twice the upper limit of normal and restart the drug at lower doses when normal values are obtained. Rare cases of azathioprine-induced pancreatitis are reported, but the cost-effectiveness of monitoring serum amylase concentrations is not established. Because azathioprine is potentially mutagenic, women of childbearing age should practice adequate contraception.

Cyclosporine inhibits predominantly T lymphocyte–dependent immune responses and is sometimes beneficial in treating MG. We begin treatment with 5–6 mg/kg per day, in two divided doses taken 12 hours apart. Serum levels of cyclosporine and creatinine should be measured monthly until the dose has been adjusted to produce a trough serum cyclosporine concentration of 75–150 ng/ml and a serum creatinine level of less than 150% of pretreatment values. The needed dose decreases after tissue saturation is achieved, and it may take several months until the optimal dose has been determined for each patient. Thereafter, serum creatinine should be measured at least every 2–3 months and more frequently after any new medications are begun (Table 82.6). We usually give 10–20 mg prednisone every other day with cyclosporine to maximize the response.

Most patients with MG improve 1–2 months after starting cyclosporine, and improvement is maintained as long as therapeutic doses are given. Maximum improvement is achieved 6 months or longer after starting treatment. After achieving the maximal response, the dose is gradually reduced to the minimum that maintains improvement.

Renal toxicity and hypertension, the important adverse reactions of cyclosporine, are usually avoided or managed using the regimen provided. Many drugs are known to interfere with cyclosporine metabolism; these should be avoided or used with caution (see Table 82.6). However, when any new medication is begun, it is advisable to monitor the serum creatinine and cyclosporine levels monthly for several months.

Cyclophosphamide has been used intravenously and orally for the treatment of MG. The intravenous dose is 200 mg per day for 5 days; the oral dose is 150–200 mg per day, to a total of 5–10 g, as required to relieve symptoms. More than one-half of patients become asymptomatic after 1 year. Alopecia is the rule. Leukopenia, nausea, vomiting, anorexia, and discoloration of the nails and skin occur less frequently.

Life-threatening infections are an important risk in immunosuppressed patients, but in our experience, this risk is limited to patients with invasive thymoma. The long-term risk of malignancy is not established, but there are no reports of an increased incidence of malignancy in patients with MG receiving immunosuppression.

Plasma Exchange

Plasma exchange is used as a short-term intervention for patients with sudden worsening of myasthenic symptoms for any reason, to rapidly improve strength before surgery, and as a chronic intermittent treatment for patients who are refractory to all other treatments. The need for plasma exchange and its frequency of use is determined by the clinical response in the individual patient.

Almost all patients with acquired MG improve temporarily after plasma exchange (Table 82.7). A typical protocol of plasma exchange is to remove 2–3 liters of plasma 3 times a week until improvement plateaus, usually after 5–6 exchanges. Improvement begins within 48 hours of the first exchange. Maximum improvement may be reached as early as after the first exchange or as late as

Table 82.6:   Drugs to use with caution with cyclosporine

Drugs that may cause kidney damage when combined with
    cyclosporine:
  Antibiotics
    Gentamicin
    Tobramycin
    Vancomycin
    Trimethoprim (Bactrim, Septra)
    Ciprofloxacin (Cipro)
  Antifungals
    Amphotericin B (Fungizone)
    Ketoconazole (Nizoral)
  Antivirals
    Acyclovir (Zovirax)
  Antiulcer
    Cimetidine (Tagamet)
    Ranitidine (Zantac)
  Nonsteroidal
    Diclofenac (Voltaren)
    Ibuprofen (Advil, Motrin, Nuprin)
    Piroxicam (Feldene)
    Indomethacin (Indocin)
  Chemotherapy
    Melphalan (Alkeran)
    Etoposide (VePesid)
  Cardiac/blood pressure
    Captopril (Capoten)
    Acetazolamide (Diamox)
    Furosemide (Lasix)
    Disopyramide (Norpace)
Drugs that may raise blood cyclosporine levels:
  Antibiotics
    Erythromycin
  Antifungals
    Ketoconazole (Nizoral)
    Difluconazole (Diflucan)
    Iatroconazole

  Stomach/ulcer
    Metoclopramide (Reglan)
    Cimetidine (Tagamet)
  Cardiac/blood pressure
    Diltiazem (Cardiazem, Dilacor)
    Nicardipine (Cardene)
    Verapamil (Calan, Isoptin, Verelan)
  Hormones
    Danazol (Danocrine)
    Oral contraceptives
    Methylprednisolone
  Miscellaneous
    Bromocriptine (Parlodel)
Drugs that may decrease blood cyclosporine levels:
  Antibiotics
    Rifampin (Rifadin, Rifamate)
    Imipenem (Primaxin)
    Nafcillin (Unipen)
    Trimethoprim (Bactrim, Septra)
  Anticonvulsants
    Phenytoin (Dilantin)
    Phenobarbital
    Carbamazepine (Tegretol)
Drugs that may accumulate in the blood when taken with
    cyclosporine:
  Steroids
    Prednisolone
  Cardiac
    Digoxin (Lanoxin)
Other reactions:
  Cholesterol-lowering agents
    Lovastatin (Mevacor) may cause muscle damage
  Cardiac/blood pressure
    Angiotensin-converting enzyme inhibitors (Accupril, Altace,
      Capoten, Lotensin, Monopril, Prinivil, Vasotec, Zestril)
      may cause increased serum potassium

---

the fourteenth. Improvement lasts for weeks or months and then the effect is lost unless the exchange is followed by thymectomy or immunosuppressive therapy. Most patients who respond to the first plasma exchange respond again to subsequent courses. Repeated exchanges do not have a cumulative benefit.

Adverse reactions to plasma exchange include transitory cardiac arrhythmias, nausea, lightheadedness, chills, obscured vision, and pedal edema. Other reactions occur in specific situations: thromboses, thrombophlebitis, and subacute bacterial endocarditis when arteriovenous shunts or grafts are placed for vascular access; an influenzalike illness in patients with reduced immunoglobulin levels; and severe bacterial and systemic cytomegalovirus infections in patients being treated with cyclophosphamide.

Intravenous Immunoglobulin

Many groups have reported a favorable response to high-dose (2 g/kg infused over 2–5 days) intravenous immunoglobulin (IVIG). Possible mechanisms of action include downregulation of antibodies directed against AChR and the introduction of anti-idiotypic antibodies (Dalakas 1997).

Improvement occurs in 50–100% of patients, usually beginning within 1 week and lasting for several weeks or months. The common adverse effects of IVIG are related to the rate of infusion and include headaches, chills, and fever. These reactions can be reduced by giving acetaminophen or aspirin with diphenhydramine (Benadryl) before each infusion.

Severe reactions, such as alopecia, aseptic meningitis, leukopenia, and retinal necrosis, are rare but have been reported in patients receiving IVIG for diseases other than MG. Renal failure may occur in patients with impaired renal function. Vascular-type headaches are often sufficiently severe to limit the use of IVIG, but we find that these headaches can be managed by giving intravenous dihydroergotamine before and immediately after the IVIG infusion. IVIG is contraindicated in patients with selective IgA deficiency because they may develop anaphylaxis to the IgA

Table 82.7: Plasma exchange or intravenous immunoglobulin in myasthenia gravis

Advantages
    Produces rapid improvement in most patients
    No known chronic side effects
Disadvantages
    Expensive
    Requires concomitant immunosuppression, corticosteroids,
        or thymectomy for long-lasting benefit
Major role
    Adjunctive therapy, most useful in:
        Producing rapid improvement before thymectomy or
            other surgery or in myasthenic crisis
        Initiating improvement that may be maintained by other
            forms of immunotherapy
        Patients who have not responded to other forms of
            treatment

in Ig preparations. Ig levels are obtained in all patients before starting IVIG therapy to detect this condition. Human immunodeficiency virus is not known to be transmitted by IVIG, but the transmission of non-A, non-B hepatitis by IVIG has been reported. Although contamination of human blood products by donors having Creutzfeldt-Jakob disease has been reported, there is no reported case of transmission of this disease by blood products.

The indications for IVIG are similar to those for plasma exchange. IVIG is an effective alternative to plasma exchange, especially in patients with poor vascular access or when plasma exchange is not available (Gajdos et al. 1997).

Miscellaneous Treatments

Splenectomy, splenic radiation, and total body irradiation have been used in a small number of patients who did not improve with all other forms of immunotherapy. Aminopyridines facilitate transmitter release at central and peripheral synapses. 4-Aminopyridine produces significant and sometimes dramatic improvement in acquired MG, congenital myasthenia, Lambert-Eaton myasthenic syndrome, and botulism, especially when given with pyridostigmine. Confusion and seizures are the side effects that limit its use. 3,4-Diaminopyridine (DAP) has similar peripheral effects with less central toxicity but is not commercially available (see Treatment of Lambert-Eaton Myasthenic Syndrome, later in this chapter).

Ephedrine can be useful in patients with congenital myasthenia and in patients with acquired myasthenia in whom ChE inhibitors alone are not effective.

Association of Myasthenia Gravis with Other Diseases

MG is often associated with other immune-mediated diseases, especially hyperthyroidism and rheumatoid arthritis (Christensen et al. 1995). Seizures have been reported to

occur with increased incidence in children with MG. One-fifth of our myasthenic patients have another disease: 7% have diabetes mellitus before corticosteroid treatment, 6% have thyroid disease, 3% have nonthymus neoplasm, and less than 2% have rheumatoid arthritis. Cases of MG related to human immunodeficiency virus (Authier et al. 1995) and after allogeneic bone marrow transplantation (Mackey et al. 1997) suggest that there may be more than a coincidental relationship.

Treatment of Associated Diseases

The effect of concomitant diseases and their treatment on myasthenic symptoms is an important consideration. Thyroid disease should be vigorously treated; both hypo- and hyperthyroidism adversely affect myasthenic weakness. Intercurrent infections require immediate attention because they exacerbate MG and can be life threatening in patients who are immunosuppressed.

Drugs that cause neuromuscular blockade must be used with caution. Many antibiotics fall into that category. Ophthalmic preparations of beta blockers and aminoglycoside antibiotics may cause worsening of ocular symptoms (Khella and Kozart 1997). D-Penicillamine should not be used. If corticosteroids are needed to treat concomitant illness, the potential adverse and beneficial effects on MG must be anticipated and explained to the patient.

Annual immunization against influenza is recommended for all patients with MG, and immunization against pneumococcus is recommended before starting prednisone or other immunosuppressive drugs. Inactivated polio vaccine rather than attenuated live oral polio vaccine should be used in people who are immunocompromised or in children who have household contacts with immunocompromised individuals. The Centers for Disease Control and Prevention reports that those taking less than 2 mg/kg per day of prednisone or every-other-day prednisone are not at risk.

Treatment Plan

We use the following protocols to treat patients with MG.

Ocular Myasthenia

Most patients are started on ChE inhibitors. If the response is unsatisfactory, prednisone is added, either in incrementing or high daily doses. Thymectomy may be considered in young patients with relatively recent onset of ocular weakness that persists despite ChE inhibitors, in an effort to reduce the possibility that the disease will become generalized and ultimately require long-term medications. The development of weakness in muscles other than the ocular or periocular muscles moves patients with ocular myasthenia to the generalized myasthenia protocol.

Generalized Myasthenia, Onset before Age 60

Thymectomy is offered to all patients. High-dose daily prednisone or plasma exchange is used preoperatively in patients with oropharyngeal or respiratory muscle weakness to minimize the risks of surgery. If disabling weakness recurs or persists after thymectomy, or if there is not continual improvement 12 months after surgery, immunosuppression with high-dose daily prednisone, azathioprine, or cyclosporine is recommended (see Corticosteroids and Immunosupressant Drugs, earlier in this chapter.

Generalized Myasthenia, Onset after Age 60

Life expectancy and concurrent illness are important considerations in developing a treatment plan. The initial treatment is usually ChE inhibitors. If the response is unsatisfactory, we add azathioprine in patients who can tolerate a delay before responding. If treatment with azathioprine is unsatisfactory, high-dose daily prednisone is added or cyclosporine is substituted for azathioprine. We use high-dose daily prednisone as the first drug, with or without plasma exchange, in patients who need a rapid response. Azathioprine is added to prednisone if the response to prednisone alone is not satisfactory or unacceptable weakness develops as the prednisone dose is reduced.

Thymoma

Thymectomy is indicated in all patients with thymoma. The patients are pretreated with high-dose daily prednisone, with or without plasma exchange, until maximal improvement is attained.

Postoperative radiation is used if tumor resection is incomplete or if the tumor has spread beyond the thymic capsule. Medical treatment is then the same as for patients without thymoma.

Elderly patients with small tumors, who are not good candidates for surgery because of other health problems may be managed medically while tumor size is monitored radiologically.

Juvenile Myasthenia Gravis

The onset of immune-mediated MG before age 20 is referred to as *juvenile MG*. The pathophysiology is the same in children and adults.

In our experience, 20% of children with juvenile MG and almost 50% of those with onset before puberty are seronegative (see Seronegative Myasthenia Gravis, in the next section).Thymomas are rare in this age group, but the few that we have seen were malignant.

The female to male ratio in children is 3 to 1, as compared to almost 1 to 1 in adult-onset disease. When myasthenic symptoms begin in childhood, it is important to determine if the patient has acquired autoimmune MG or a

genetic form that does not respond to immunotherapy (see Genetic Myasthenic Syndromes, later in this chapter). Because the absence of AChR antibodies does not distinguish these conditions, a therapeutic trial of plasma exchange or IVIG is indicated. Those who definitely improve are candidates for thymectomy or immunotherapy, but no response does not exclude autoimmune MG.

Treatment decisions in children with autoimmune MG are made more difficult because the rate of spontaneous remission is high, but the response to early thymectomy in the first year of symptoms is good. We recommend ChE inhibitors alone in prepubertal children who are not disabled by weakness. If these drugs do not prevent disability or progressive weakness, we proceed to thymectomy. Removal of the thymus in infants or children does not have a deleterious effect on subsequent immunological development.

Children with postpubertal onset of disease are treated the same as adults.

Seronegative Myasthenia Gravis

One-fourth of patients with acquired, presumably immune-mediated MG do not have detectable serum antibodies against AChR-Ab (Sanders et al. 1997). Seronegative patients are more likely than seropositive patients to be male and to have milder disease, ocular MG, fewer thymomas, less frequent thymic hyperplasia, and more frequent thymic atrophy. In seronegative patients, the diagnosis is based on the clinical presentation, the response to ChE inhibitors, and EMG findings. Genetic myasthenia must be considered in all childhood-onset seronegative MG. The treatment of seronegative acquired MG is the same as for seropositive patients. The absence of AChR antibodies does not necessarily mean that an unsatisfactory response to immunosuppression, plasma exchange, or thymectomy is expected.

Special Situations

Myasthenic or Cholinergic Crisis. Myasthenic crisis is respiratory failure from disease. Patients in myasthenic crisis who previously had well-compensated respiratory function usually have a definable precipitating event, such as infection, surgery, or rapid tapering of immunosuppression.

Cholinergic crisis is respiratory failure from overdose of ChE inhibitors. It was more common before the introduction of immunosuppressive therapy, when very large dosages of ChE inhibitors were used. Respiratory failure of any cause is a medical emergency and requires prompt intubation and ventilatory support.

In theory, it should be easy to determine if a patient is weak because of too little or too much ChE inhibitor, but in practice this is often difficult. Administration of edrophonium chloride should distinguish overdose from underdose, but its use in crisis is dangerous unless the patient is already intubated and ventilated, and an apprehensive patient cannot cooperate with the test. Further, edrophonium chloride may make some muscles stronger and others weaker. Serial measurements of forced vital capacity and blood gases do not predict which MG patients will need mechanical ventilation (Rieder et al. 1995). The safest approach to crisis is to admit the patient to an intensive care unit, discontinue all ChE inhibitors, and ventilate the patient. ChE inhibitors should be resumed at low doses and slowly increased as needed.

Respiratory assistance is needed when the patient cannot maintain an inspiratory force of more than –20 cm H_2O, when tidal volume is 4–5 cc/kg body weight and maximum breathing capacity is three times the tidal volume, or when the forced vital capacity is less than 15 cc/kg body weight. A mask and breathing bag can be used in an emergency situation, but tracheal intubation should quickly be done with a low-pressure, high-compliance cuffed endotracheal tube. A volume-controlled respirator set to provide tidal volumes of 400–500 cc and automatic sighing every 10–15 minutes is preferred. The pressure of the tube cuff should be checked frequently and the tube position verified daily by chest radiographs. Assisted respiration is used when the patient's own respiratory efforts can trigger the respirator. An oxygen-enriched atmosphere is used only when arterial blood oxygen values fall below 70 mm Hg. The inspired gas must be humidified to at least 80% at 37°C to prevent drying of the tracheo-bronchial tree. Tracheal secretions should be removed periodically using aseptic aspiration techniques. Low-pressure, high-compliance endotracheal tubes may be tolerated for long periods and usually obviate the need for tracheostomy. When respiratory strength improves, weaning from the respirator should be started for 2 or 3 minutes at a time and increased as tolerated. Extubation should be considered when the patient has an inspiratory pressure greater than –20 cm H_2O and an expiratory pressure greater than 35–40 cm H_2O. The tidal volume should exceed 5 cc/kg, which usually corresponds to a vital capacity of at least 1,000 cc. If the patient complains of fatigue or shortness of breath, extubation should be deferred even if these values and the results of blood gas measurements are normal.

Prevention and aggressive treatment of medical complications offer the best opportunity to improve the outcome of myasthenic crisis (Thomas et al. 1997).

Anesthetic Management. The stress of surgery and some drugs used perioperatively may worsen myasthenic weakness. As a rule, local or spinal anesthesia is preferred over inhalation anesthesia. Neuromuscular blocking agents should be used sparingly, if at all. Adequate muscle relaxation usually can be produced by inhalation anesthetic agents alone. The required dose of depolarizing blocking agents may be greater than that needed in nonmyasthenic patients, but low doses of nondepolarizing agents cause pronounced and long-lasting blockade that require prolonged postoperative assisted respiration.

Pregnancy. Myasthenic women may improve, worsen, or remain unchanged during pregnancy. Worsening during the first trimester is more common in first pregnancies, whereas third-trimester worsening and postpartum exacerbations are more common in subsequent pregnancies. Therapeutic abortion is rarely, if ever, needed because of MG. The use of intravenous ChE inhibitors is contraindicated during pregnancy because they may produce uterine contractions. Although pregnancy is not usually recommended in patients treated with corticosteroids, adverse outcomes in children born to myasthenic mothers taking even high doses throughout pregnancy are not reported. We do not use cytotoxic drugs during pregnancy because of their potential mutagenic effects.

Labor and delivery are usually normal, and cesarean section is needed only for obstetrical indications. Regional anesthesia is preferred for delivery or cesarean section. Magnesium sulfate should not be used to manage pre-eclampsia because of its neuromuscular blocking effects. Barbiturates usually provide adequate treatment. In our experience, breast-feeding is not a problem, despite the theoretical risk of passing maternal AChR antibodies to the newborn.

The serum concentration of AChR antibodies in the mother and her newborn are similar. It is also likely that the fetus of an affected mother has an elevated concentration of AChR antibodies. Decreased fetal movement suggests the diagnosis of intrauterine myasthenia. Affected newborns may have arthrogryposis multiplex congenita because of decreased intrauterine movement, and decreased fetal movement is considered an indication for plasmapheresis or IVIG.

Transitory Neonatal Myasthenia. A transitory form of MG affects 10–20% of newborns whose mothers have immune-mediated MG. The severity of symptoms in the newborn does not correlate with the severity of symptoms in the mother. Affected newborns are hypotonic and feed poorly during the first 3 days. Symptoms usually last less than 2 weeks but may continue for as long as 12 weeks. Myasthenia does not recur later on.

Neonatal antibodies have a half-life of 2–3 weeks and are not detected after 5 months. This time course is consistent with the duration of clinical weakness. Passive transfer of maternal antibodies to the newborn does not fully explain the clinical syndrome of transitory neonatal myasthenia. The mechanism by which some newborns develop this syndrome and others, with equally high antibody concentrations do not, is uncertain.

All children of myasthenic mothers should be assessed for transitory neonatal MG. The diagnosis is established by edrophonium chloride or RNS. Affected newborns require symptomatic treatment with ChE inhibitors if swallowing or breathing is impaired. Plasma exchange should be considered in newborns with respiratory weakness.

D-Penicillamine–Induced Myasthenia Gravis. D-Penicillamine is used to treat rheumatoid arthritis, Wilson's disease, and cystinuria. Patients treated with D-penicillamine for several months may develop a myasthenic syndrome that disappears when the drug is stopped. D-Penicillamine–induced myasthenia is usually mild and often restricted to the ocular muscles. The diagnosis is often difficult because weakness may not be recognized when there is severe arthritis. The diagnosis is established by the response to ChE inhibitors, characteristic EMG abnormalities, and an elevated concentration of serum AChR antibodies. It is likely that D-penicillamine stimulates or enhances an immunological reaction against the neuromuscular junction. The myasthenic response induced by D-penicillamine usually remits 1 year after the drug is stopped. ChE inhibitors usually relieve the symptoms. If myasthenic symptoms persist after D-penicillamine is stopped, the patient should be treated for acquired MG.

GENETIC MYASTHENIC SYNDROMES

Genetic forms of myasthenia are not immune mediated. They are a heterogeneous group of disorders caused by several abnormalities of neuromuscular transmission (Engel 1994). Some have characteristic physiological or histological features. Symptoms are typically present at birth or early childhood but can be delayed until young adult life. Abnormal neuromuscular transmission is confirmed by the response to edrophonium chloride, characteristic EMG findings, or both.

The onset of myasthenic symptoms at birth is always genetic, with the exception of the transitory neonatal form. All genetic forms of myasthenia are known or presumed to be transmitted by autosomal recessive inheritance, except slow-channel syndrome, which is transmitted by autosomal dominant inheritance. Myasthenia that begins in infancy or childhood may be genetic or acquired.

Congenital Myasthenia

Congenital myasthenia is a clinical term that encompasses several genetic neuromuscular defects. Overall, there is a 2-to-1 male predominance. Children with congenital myasthenia develop ophthalmoparesis and ptosis during infancy. Mild facial paresis may be present as well. Ophthalmoplegia is often incomplete at onset but progresses to complete paralysis during infancy or childhood. Some children develop generalized fatigue and weakness, but limb weak-

ness is usually mild compared to ophthalmoplegia, and respiratory distress is unusual.

Congenital myasthenia should be suspected in any newborn or infant with ptosis or ophthalmoparesis. Subcutaneous injection of edrophonium chloride usually produces a transitory improvement in ocular motility. A decremental response to RNS occurs in some limb muscles, but it may be necessary to test proximal or facial muscles if hand muscles show a normal response. SFEMG shows increased jitter.

ChE inhibitors improve limb muscle weakness in many forms of congenital genetic myasthenia and may be effective even when edrophonium chloride is not. Ocular muscle weakness is less responsive to ChE inhibitors. The weakness in some children responds to DAP (Anlar et al. 1996), but this drug is not commercially available in the United States (see Treatment of Lambert-Eaton Myastenic Syndrome, later in this chapter).

Familial Infantile Myasthenia

Familial infantile myasthenia has characteristic clinical and electrophysiological features that differ from congenital myasthenic syndromes. Generalized hypotonia is present at birth, and the neonatal course is complicated by repeated episodes of life-threatening apnea and feeding difficulty. Assisted ventilation is often required. Arthrogryposis may be present. Ocular muscle function is usually normal. Within weeks after birth, the child becomes stronger and ultimately breathes unassisted. However, episodes of life-threatening apnea occur repeatedly throughout infancy and childhood, even into adult life. There is often a history of sudden infant death syndrome in siblings, and the correct diagnosis may not be suspected until a second affected child is born.

Edrophonium chloride usually improves both weakness and respiratory distress. A decremental response to RNS is usually present in weak muscles but may be present in strong muscles only after exhausting the muscle by several minutes of RNS. Abnormal resynthesis and repackaging of ACh in the motor nerve has been shown in some patients.

ChE inhibitors improve strength in most affected children, but sudden episodes of respiratory distress occur with intercurrent illness. As the patients get older, weakness improves, attacks of respiratory distress become less frequent, and the need for medication decreases.

Slow-Channel Syndrome

Slow-channel syndrome may be difficult to distinguish from acquired MG because the onset of symptoms may be delayed until adult life. The disease is transmitted by autosomal dominant inheritance, and a family history of similar illness often is obtained.

Slow-channel syndrome is rare. Onset of symptoms always occurs after infancy and may present as late as the third decade. Slowly progressive weakness selectively involves the arm, leg, neck, and facial muscles. Unlike other myasthenic syndromes, atrophy of symptomatic muscles is expected.

RNS shows a decremental response. Repetitive discharges are seen after nerve stimulation, similar to those seen in ChE inhibitor toxicity or congenital deficiency of endplate acetylcholinesterase. The underlying defect is a prolonged open time of the ACh channel.

ChE inhibitors, thymectomy, and immunosuppression are not effective treatment. Some investigations indicate that quinidine sulfate may improve strength in this condition (Harper and Engel 1998).

The Future

The future of MG lies in the elucidation of the molecular immunology of the anti-AChR response, with the goal of developing a rational treatment that will cure the abnormality in the immune system. Six broad categories of treatment strategies must be explored:

1. Treatments that target antigen-specific B cells
2. Treatments that target the antigen-specific CD4+ T cells
3. Treatments that interfere with the costimulatory response for antigen presentation
4. Treatments aimed at inducing tolerance or anergy of the CD4+ T cell to the autoantigen or CD4+ epitopes
5. Treatments designed to stimulate the immunological circuits that activate CD8+ cells specific for the activation antigens expressed by CD4+ cells
6. Treatments that affect cytokine function and discourage autoimmune-mediated inflammatory responses

Lambert-Eaton Myasthenic Syndrome

LEMS is a presynaptic abnormality of ACh release that was first described in association with malignancy, usually small cell lung cancer (SCLC). The probable mechanism in most, if not all patients, is an immune-mediated process directed against the voltage-gated calcium channels (VGCC) on nerve terminals (see Figure 82.3). LEMS usually begins after age 40, but it has been reported in children. Males and females are equally affected. Approximately one-half the patients with LEMS have an underlying malignancy; 80% of these have SCLC (Tim et al. 1998).

The cancer may be discovered years before or after the symptoms of LEMS begin. Weakness of proximal muscles, especially in the legs, is the major symptom. The weak muscles may ache and are occasionally tender. Oropharyngeal and ocular muscles may be mildly affected but not to the degree seen in MG. The weakness demonstrated on examination is usually relatively mild compared to the severity of symptoms. Strength may improve initially after exercise and then weaken with sustained activity. Edrophonium chloride does not improve strength to the degree seen in MG. Tendon reflexes are reduced or absent but are frequently enhanced by repeated muscle contraction or repeated tapping of the tendon. Dry mouth is a common symptom of autonomic dysfunction; other features are impotence and postural hypotension.

LEMS may be first discovered when prolonged paralysis follows the use of neuromuscular blocking agents during surgery. Clinical worsening has been described after administration of aminoglycoside antibiotics, magnesium, calcium-channel blockers, and iodinated intravenous contrast agents.

Although LEMS and MG are both immune-mediated disorders of neuromuscular transmission, their clinical features usually are quite distinct. The weakness in LEMS is not usually life threatening and more closely resembles cachexia, polymyositis, or a paraneoplastic neuromuscular disease.

Diagnostic Procedures

The diagnosis of LEMS is confirmed by EMG (see Chapter 37B). The characteristic findings are decreased size of CMAPs with further size reduction in response to RNS at frequencies between 1 and 5 Hz, doubling of CMAP size in response to repetitive stimulation at 20–50 Hz, and a transitory increase in CMAP size after brief maximum voluntary contraction. Virtually all patients with LEMS have a decrementing response to 3-Hz stimulation in a hand or foot muscle, and almost all have low-amplitude CMAPs in some muscle. Facilitation more than 100% is not seen in all muscles; thus, it may be necessary to examine several muscles to demonstrate this important finding (Tim et al. 1998). Abnormalities of these measurements may be partially masked by low muscle temperature; thus, hand and foot muscles should be warmed. In proximal muscles, the CMAP amplitude is normal, there is usually a decrementing pattern, and the amount of facilitation is variable.

When LEMS and MG are difficult to distinguish by clinical features and electrophysiology, the presence of elevated concentrations of AChR antibodies or lung cancer clarifies the diagnosis. Sometimes, the diagnosis is defined only by the response to treatment or the course of disease.

Immunopathology of Lambert-Eaton Myasthenic Syndrome

Patients with LEMS, like those with MG, have an increased risk of other immune-mediated diseases. LEMS patients who do not have cancer frequently have serum organ-specific autoantibodies, further confirming that LEMS is immune mediated. In LEMS, the motor nerve terminal active zone particles, which probably represent the VGCC, are disorganized in appearance and reduced in number. Similar changes are seen in recipient mice who are injected with IgG from LEMS patients. The mechanism is probably from cross-linking of the VGCC by antibodies.

SCLC cells are of neuroectodermal origin and contain high concentrations of VGCC. Calcium influx into these cells is inhibited by LEMS IgG, and antibodies to the VGCC are found in the sera of approximately 75% of LEMS patients with SCLC, 50% of those without cancer, and 10% of those with SCLC who do not have LEMS (Lennon et al. 1995). VGCC antibody titers do not correlate with disease severity among individuals, but the antibody levels may fall as the disease improves in patients receiving immunosuppression. These observations suggest that SCLC cells induce VGCC antibodies that react with the VGCC of peripheral nerves and cause LEMS. In LEMS patients who do not have SCLC, the VGCC antibodies may be produced as part of a more general immune-mediated disease.

Treatment of Lambert-Eaton Myasthenic Syndrome

Once the diagnosis of LEMS is established, an extensive search for underlying malignancy, especially SCLC, is mandatory. Chronic smokers should undergo bronchoscopy even if chest imaging studies are normal. Initial treatment is directed at the underlying malignancy, and weakness may improve after effective cancer therapy. In some patients, no further treatment is needed for the neuromuscular defect. If tumor is not found, the search for occult malignancy should be repeated periodically, especially during the first 2 years after onset of symptoms. The frequency of re-evaluation is determined by the patient's cancer risk factors.

Therapy is tailored to the individual based on the severity of weakness, underlying disease, life expectancy, and response to previous treatment. The following treatment plan is a general guide that should be modified to suit specific situations.

ChE inhibitors may relieve weakness in occasional LEMS patients. Pyridostigmine, 30–60 mg every 6 hours, should be tried for several days. In some patients, the major benefit is relief of dry mouth.

Guanidine hydrochloride increases the release of ACh and produces temporary improvement in strength in many LEMS patients. Guanidine is started at an oral dose of 5–10 mg/kg daily, divided into three doses 4–6 hours apart, and may be increased to a maximum of 30 mg/kg per day. Bone marrow depression may occur with doses as low as 500 mg per day. The dose should not be increased more often than every 3 days because the maximum response may be delayed for 2–3 days. The therapeutic response is enhanced by giving pyridostigmine (30–60 mg every 4–6 hours). In addition to bone marrow

depression, side effects seen at higher doses include renal tubular acidosis, chronic interstitial nephritis, cardiac arrhythmia, hepatic toxicity, pancreatic dysfunction, paresthesias, ataxia, confusion, and alterations of mood. Monthly blood counts are recommended for any patient receiving guanidine.

Oral DAP, 5–25 mg three to four times a day, improves strength and autonomic symptoms in most patients with LEMS (Sanders 1998). Like guanidine, DAP facilitates release of ACh from motor nerve terminals. The response to DAP is enhanced by the concomitant use of pyridostigmine, 30–60 mg, three or four times a day. Side effects usually are negligible: Transient perioral and digital paresthesias occur when DAP dosages exceed 10–15 mg, but doses of 100 mg per day may cause seizures. Cramps and diarrhea may occur when DAP is combined with pyridostigmine and can be minimized by reducing the dose of pyridostigmine. DAP promises to be a safe and effective treatment for LEMS but is not yet available for general clinical use in the United States. DAP can be obtained on a compassionate use basis for individual patients with LEMS. Information on the application process can be obtained from Jacobus Pharmaceutical Co., Inc., Princeton, NJ, Fax No. 609-799-1176.

If these treatments are not effective, it must be determined if the patient's weakness is sufficiently severe to warrant immunotherapy with prednisone, azathioprine, or cyclosporine, which are given as for MG.

Both plasma exchange and IVIG provide transitory improvement in some patients with LEMS (Rich et al. 1997; Tim et al. 1998), but the results are usually not as good as in MG. In patients with severe weakness, plasma exchange or IVIG may be used first and prednisone and azathioprine added after improvement begins. Repeated courses of treatment may be needed to maintain improvement.

The weakness of LEMS may be worse when the ambient temperature is elevated or when the patient is febrile. Patients should avoid hot showers or baths. Systemic illness of any sort may cause transient worsening of weakness in patients with LEMS.

Drugs That Adversely Affect Myasthenia Gravis and Lambert-Eaton Myasthenic Syndrome

Drugs that compromise neuromuscular transmission make patients with MG or LEMS weaker. The effects of competitive neuromuscular blocking agents, such as D-tubocurarine and pancuronium, are exaggerated and prolonged in these patients. Depolarizing agents, such as succinylcholine, also must be used with caution. Some antibiotics, particularly aminoglycosides, antiarrhythmics (quinine, quinidine, and procainamide), and β-adrenergic blocking drugs block neuromuscular transmission and increase weakness. Iodinated contrast agents have been reported to produce transitory worsening in patients with MG and LEMS, possibly because of the calcium-chelating

Table 82.8:   Drug alert for patients with myasthenia gravis or Lambert-Eaton myasthenic syndrome

1. D-Penicillamine should never be used in myasthenic patients.
2. The following drugs produce worsening of myasthenic weakness in most patients who receive them. Use with caution and monitor patient for exacerbation of myasthenic symptoms.

   Succinylcholine, D-tubocurarine, or other neuromuscular-blocking agents

   Quinine, quinidine, and procainamide

   Aminoglycoside antibiotics, particularly gentamicin, kanamycin, neomycin, and streptomycin

   Beta blockers: propranolol, timolol maleate eyedrops

   Calcium-channel blockers

   Magnesium salts (including laxatives and antacids with high Mg^{2+} concentrations)

   Iodinated contrast agents
3. Many other drugs are reported to exacerbate the weakness in some patients with myasthenia gravis. All patients with myasthenia gravis should be observed for increased weakness whenever a new medication is started.

effects of these agents. Ophthalmic solutions of timolol, betaxolol, and tobramycin may unmask or exacerbate myasthenic weakness. Many other drugs increase myasthenic weakness in isolated cases, and all patients with MG and LEMS should be observed for clinical worsening after any new medication is started.

Although avoidance of drugs that are known to impair neuromuscular transmission is desirable, this is not always possible. We find it useful to place a list of potentially hazardous drugs on the front of the hospital chart of patients with MG and LEMS (Table 82.8).

BOTULISM

Botulism is caused by a toxin produced by the anaerobic bacterium, *Clostridium botulinum*, that blocks the release of ACh from the motor nerve terminal. The result is a long-lasting, severe muscle paralysis. Of eight types of botulinum toxins, types A and B cause most cases of botulism in the United States. Type E is transmitted in seafood. Intoxication usually follows ingestion of foods that were contaminated by inadequate sterilization. Neuromuscular symptoms usually begin 12–36 hours after ingestion of contaminated food that contains botulinum toxin. Not all people who ingest contaminated food become symptomatic. Nausea and vomiting are the first symptoms of food-borne botulism, and the neuromuscular symptoms begin 12–36 hours after exposure.

The most common form of botulism in the United States now is wound botulism, which occurs predominantly in drug abusers after subcutaneous injection of heroin (MMWR 1995). *Clostridium* bacteria colonize the injection site and release toxin that produces local and patchy systemic weakness.

The major symptoms of botulism are blurred vision, dysphagia, and dysarthria. Pupillary responses to light are impaired, and tendon reflexes are variably reduced. The weakness progresses for several days and then reaches a plateau. Fatal respiratory paralysis may occur rapidly. Most patients have evidence of autonomic dysfunction, such as dry mouth, constipation, or urinary retention. In patients who survive, recovery may take many months but usually is complete. The edrophonium test is positive in only approximately one-third of patients and does not distinguish botulism from other causes of neuromuscular blockade (Burningham et al. 1994). The diagnosis of wound botulism is confirmed by wound cultures and serum assay for botulinum toxin.

Infant botulism results from the growth of *C. botulinum* in the infant gastrointestinal tract and the elaboration of small quantities of toxin over a prolonged period (Midura 1996). Symptoms of constipation, lethargy, poor suck, and weak cry usually begin at approximately 4 months of age. Examination reveals weakness of the limb and oropharyngeal muscles, poorly reactive pupils, and hypoactive tendon reflexes. Most patients require ventilatory support. The diagnosis of infant botulism is confirmed by demonstrating botulinum toxin in the stool or by isolating *C. botulinum* from stool culture.

Electromyographic Findings in Botulism

Electrophysiological abnormalities in botulism tend to evolve with time and may not be present early in the disease. The EMG findings in botulism include the following (Gutierrez et al. 1994):

1. Reduced CMAP amplitude in at least two muscles
2. At least 20% facilitation of CMAP amplitude during tetanic stimulation
3. Persistence of facilitation for at least 2 minutes after activation
4. No postactivation exhaustion

Not all patients with botulism meet the first criterion. If none of these criteria are met, the diagnosis of botulism is unlikely. If all four are met, only hypermagnesemia is in the differential diagnosis.

SFEMG demonstrates markedly increased jitter and blocking and has been abnormal in all reported cases with food-borne or wound botulism. Jitter and blocking may decrease as the firing rate increases, but this is not a consistent finding (Mandler and Maselli 1996).

Treatment consists of bivalent (type A and B) or trivalent (A, B, and E) antitoxin. Antibiotic therapy is not effective because the symptoms are caused by the ingestion of toxin rather than organisms. Otherwise, treatment is supportive; respiratory assistance is given when necessary. ChE inhibitors are not beneficial; guanidine or DAP may improve strength but not respiratory function. Recovery takes many months but usually is complete.

The use of botulinum A toxin for the treatment of focal dystonia has resulted in focal or regional weakness after injection of the toxin. Such adverse events have included diplopia, dysphagia, urinary incontinence, focal weakness, brachial plexopathy, and the unmasking of neuromuscular weakness due to LEMS and ALS. SFEMG has demonstrated abnormal neuromuscular transmission in muscles remote from the site of injection.

Other Causes of Abnormal Neuromuscular Transmission

Neuromuscular transmission may be abnormal in diseases of the motor unit that do not primarily affect the neuromuscular junction. Patients with ALS may have fluctuating weakness that responds to ChE inhibitors, an abnormal decremental response to RNS, and increased jitter and blocking. Features that can be attributed to abnormal neuromuscular transmission also are reported in syringomyelia, poliomyelitis, peripheral neuropathy, and inflammatory myopathy.

Several animal venoms contain neurotoxins that block neuromuscular transmission. The clinical features of venom inoculation resemble myasthenic crisis. Cobra venom causes a long-lasting nondepolarizing AChR blockade. α-Bungarotoxin, a component of the venom from the *Bungarus* species of kraits, produces irreversible postsynaptic AChR blockade. Another component of *Bungarus* venom (β-bungarotoxin) blocks ACh release. Many animal venoms contain multiple toxins that affect several organs; neuromuscular transmission may be affected, but paralysis is not a feature. Examples are the venoms of sea snakes, rattlesnakes, black widow spiders, and scorpions.

Abnormal neuromuscular transmission is suspected when initial ocular or oropharyngeal weakness progresses to limb muscles, especially when pupillary responses are normal, sensation and sensorium are intact, and tendon reflexes are hypoactive. The suspicion is confirmed if weakness responds to administration of edrophonium chloride and RNS produces a decremental response.

REFERENCES

Anlar B, Varli K, Ozdimir E, Ertan M. 3,4-Diaminopyridine in childhood myasthenia: double-blind, placebo-controlled trial. J Child Neurol 1996;11:458–461.

Authier FJ, De Grissac N, Degos JD, Gherardi RK. Transient myasthenia gravis during HIV infection. Muscle Nerve 1995;18:914–916.

Burningham MD, Walter FG, Mechem C, et al. Wound botulism. Ann Emerg Med 1994;24:1184–1187.

Christensen PB, Jensen TS, Tsiropoulos I, et al. Associated autoimmune diseases in myasthenia gravis. A population-based study. Acta Neurol Scand 1995;91:192–195.

Dalakas MC. Intravenous immune globulin therapy for neurologic diseases. Ann Intern Med 1997;126:721–730.

Engel AG. Congenital myasthenic syndromes. Neurol Clin N Am 1994;12:401–437.

Gajdos P, Chevret S, Clair B, et al. Clinical trial of plasma exchange and high-dose intravenous immunoglobulin in myasthenia gravis. Myasthenia Gravis Clinical Study Group. Ann Neurol 1997;41:789–796.

Gutierrez AR, Bodensteiner J, Gutmann L. Electrodiagnosis of infantile botulism. J Child Neurol 1994;9:362–365.

Harper CM, Engel AG. Quinidine sulfate therapy for the slow-channel congenital myasthenic syndrome. Ann Neurol 1998;43:480–484.

Khella SL, Kozart D. Unmasking and exacerbation of myasthenia gravis by ophthalmic solutions—betaxolol, tobramycin and dexamethasone—a case report. Muscle Nerve 1997;20:631.

Lennon VA, Kryzer TJ, Griesmann GE, et al. Calcium-channel antibodies in the Lambert-Eaton syndrome and other paraneoplastic syndromes. N Engl J Med 1995;332:1467–1474.

Mackey JR, Desai S, Larratt L, et al. Myasthenia gravis in association with allogeneic bone marrow transplantation—clinical observations, therapeutic implications and review of literature. Bone Marrow Transplant 1997;19:939–942.

Mandler RN, Maselli RA. Stimulated single-fiber electromyography in wound botulism. Muscle Nerve 1996;19:1171–1173.

Midura TF. Update: infant botulism. Clin Microbiol Rev 1996;9:119–125.

MMWR. Wound botulism—California, 1995. MMWR Morb Mortal Wkly Rep 1995;44:889–892.

Phillips LH II, Torner JC. Epidemiologic evidence for a changing natural history of myasthenia gravis. Neurology 1996;47:1233–1238.

Rich MM, Teener JW, Bird SJ. Treatment of Lambert-Eaton syndrome with intravenous immunoglobulin. Muscle Nerve 1997;20:614–615.

Rieder P, Louis M, Jolliet P, Chevrolet JC. The repeated measurement of vital capacity is a poor predictor of the need for mechanical ventilation in myasthenia gravis. Intensive Care Med 1995;21:663–668.

Sanders DB. 3,4-Diaminopyridine (DAP) in the treatment of Lambert-Eaton myasthenic syndrome (LEMS). Ann N Y Acad Sci 1998;841:811–816.

Sanders DB, Andrews PI, Howard JF, Massey JM. Seronegative myasthenia gravis. Neurology 1997;48(Suppl. 5):S40–S45.

Sanders DB, Stålberg EV. AAEM Minimonograph #25: Single-fiber electromyography. Muscle Nerve 1996;19:1069–1083.

Sommer N, Sigg B, Melms A, et al. Ocular myasthenia gravis: response to long-term immunosuppressive treatment. J Neurol Neurosurg Psychiatry 1997;62:156–162.

Thomas CE, Mayer SA, Gungor Y, et al. Myasthenic crisis: clinical features, mortality, complications, and risk factors for prolonged intubation. Neurology 1997;48:1253–1260.

Tim RW, Massey JM, Sanders DB. Lambert-Eaton myasthenic syndrome (LEMS). Clinical and electrodiagnostic features and response to therapy in 59 patients. Ann N Y Acad Sci 1998;841:823–826.

Chapter 83
Disorders of Skeletal Muscle

Michael H. Brooke

Disorders of skeletal muscle include a wide variety of illnesses that cause weakness, pain, and fatigue in any combination. They vary from the protean symptoms of aches, cramps, and pains that often defy any explanation to the muscular dystrophies, which can be instantly recognized on clinical grounds. The disorders with primary involvement of the anterior horn cells (amyotrophic lateral sclerosis and the spinal muscular atrophies) cause similar symptoms and may be difficult to differentiate on clinical grounds from primary disorders of muscle. These disorders are discussed in Chapter 78.

Some definitions are worth reviewing. *Myopathy* simply refers to an abnormality of the muscle and has no other connotation. *Muscular dystrophies* are genetic myopathies, usually caused by a disturbance of a structural protein. *Myositis* implies an inflammatory disorder and is usually reserved for disorders in which the muscle histology shows an inflammatory response. The *myotonias* are diseases in which the normal contractile process is distorted by the occurrence of involuntary, persistent muscle activity accompanied by abnormal repetitive electrical discharges, which may occur after percussion or voluntary contraction. *Meta-*

bolic myopathies, in this context, refers mainly to abnormalities of muscle biochemistry that impair the resynthesis of adenosine triphosphate (ATP) or cause an abnormal storage of material in the cell. In a general medical context, *metabolic myopathy* is often synonymous with *endocrine myopathy*. *Congenital myopathies* are a group of illnesses that occur in young children; many of these illnesses are relatively nonprogressive.

Striated muscle is the tissue that converts chemical energy into mechanical energy. The component processes include (1) excitation and contraction occurring in the muscle membranes, (2) the contractile mechanism itself, (3) various structural supporting elements that allow the muscle to withstand the mechanical stresses, and (4) the energy system that supports the activity and integrity of the other three systems. Logically, myopathies should be categorized according to the part of the system involved. Until recently, this was impossible because the molecular basis of muscle activity was unknown. With the advances since the 1980s, it is now possible to attempt a classification along these lines.

Abnormalities in the membrane ion channels involved in muscle excitation are referred to as *channelopathies* and

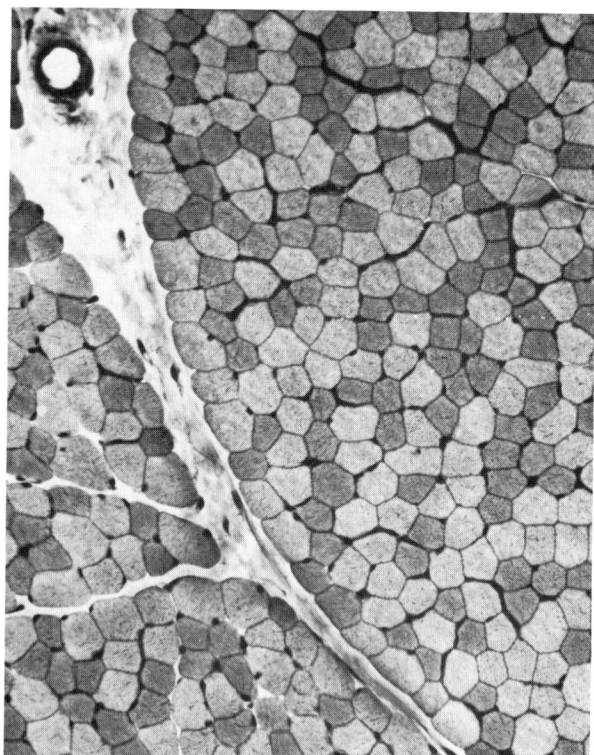

FIGURE 83.1 Normal muscle biopsy. The fibers are roughly equal in size, the nuclei are peripherally situated, and the fibers are tightly apposed to each other with no fibrous tissue separating them. (Verhoeff-Van Gieson stain.)

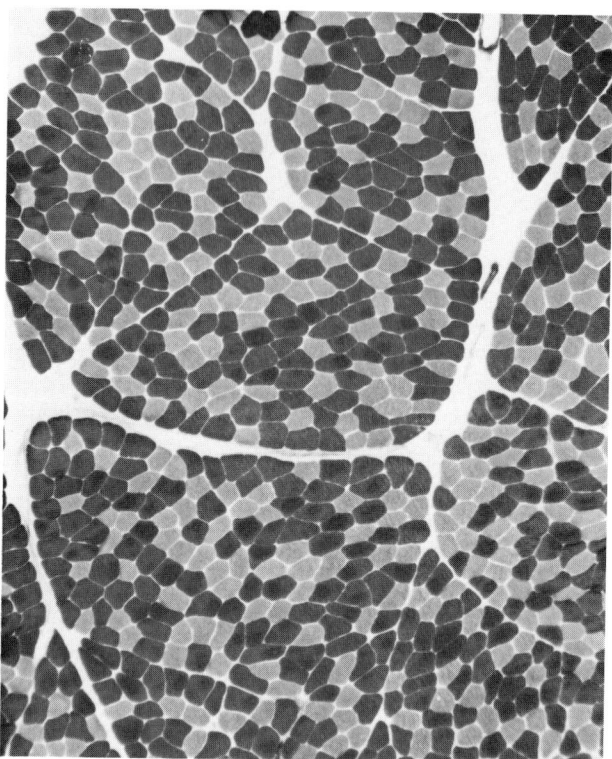

FIGURE 83.2 Normal muscle biopsy. Myosin adenosine triphosphatase stain at pH 9.4 demonstrates the relative proportions in the size of type 1 (light) and type 2 (dark) fibers.

cause various forms of myotonia and periodic paralysis. The complex of proteins, which include dystrophin, the sarcoglycans, and laminin, constitute a vital structural mechanism linking the contractile proteins with the extracellular supporting structures. Defects in these proteins are found in many forms of muscular dystrophy. Although our knowledge is still incomplete, it seems reasonable to modify the classic description of the myopathies to incorporate the new information. For this reason, in the sections that follow, the diseases are described under the heading of their known molecular defect, where possible; the classic appellation appears parenthetically.

Before the description of the illnesses themselves is undertaken, the techniques used in the clinical evaluation of these patients are briefly reviewed.

MUSCLE BIOPSY

The technique of muscle biopsy is not difficult. Under local anesthesia, a small incision is made over the muscle, and with careful dissection, a small strip of muscle is removed. Needle biopsies may also be used in some situations. Histochemical studies of frozen sections are essential for proper interpretation. A transverse section of normal muscle shows fibers that are roughly of equal size and average approxi-

mately 60 mm transverse diameter (Figure 83.1). The muscle fibers of infants and young children are proportionately smaller. Each fiber consists of hundreds of myofibrils separated by an intermyofibrillar network containing aqueous sarcoplasm, mitochondria, and the sarcoplasmic reticulum with the associated transverse tubular system. Each muscle fiber is surrounded by a thin layer of connective tissue (the endomysium). The fibers are grouped into a fascicle by strands of connective tissue and separated from each other by the perimysium. Groups of fascicles are collected into muscle bellies surrounded by epimysium.

Situated at the periphery of the fibers are the sarcolemmal nuclei. The fibers are of different types. The simplest division is into type 1 and type 2 fibers, best demonstrated with the histochemical reaction for myosin ATPase (Figure 83.2). The type 1 and type 2 fibers are roughly equivalent to slow and fast fibers or to oxidative and glycolytic fibers in human muscle. The intermyofibrillar network pattern is best demonstrated with the histochemical reactions for oxidative enzymes, such as reduced nicotinamide adenine dinucleotide dehydrogenase. A regular network is seen extending across the whole fiber. In addition to the routine stains with hematoxylin and eosin, myosin ATPase, and nicotinamide adenine dinucleotide dehydrogenase, other special stains may be used to demonstrate fat (Sudan black or oil red 0), complex carbohydrates (periodic acid–Schiff), or specific

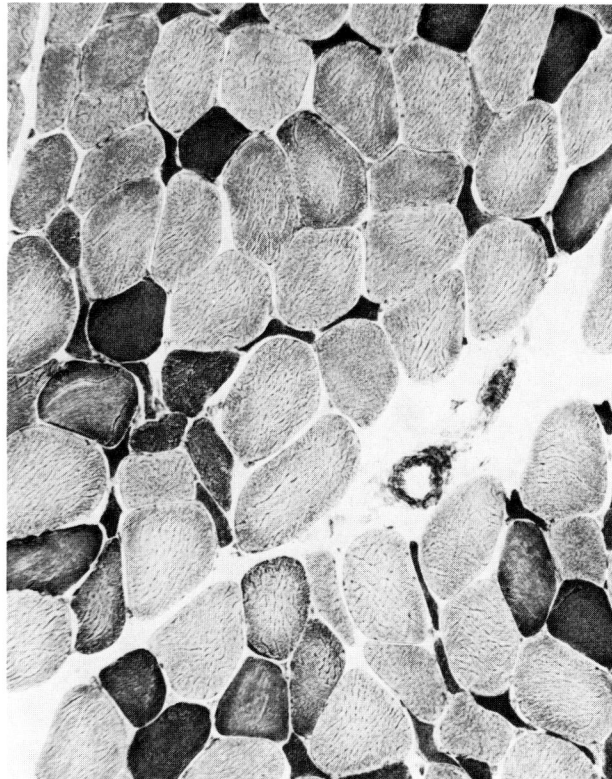

FIGURE 83.3   Denervation. Notice the small, dark, angulated fibers demonstrated with this oxidative enzyme reaction. (Nicotinamide adenine dinucleotide dehydrogenase stain.)

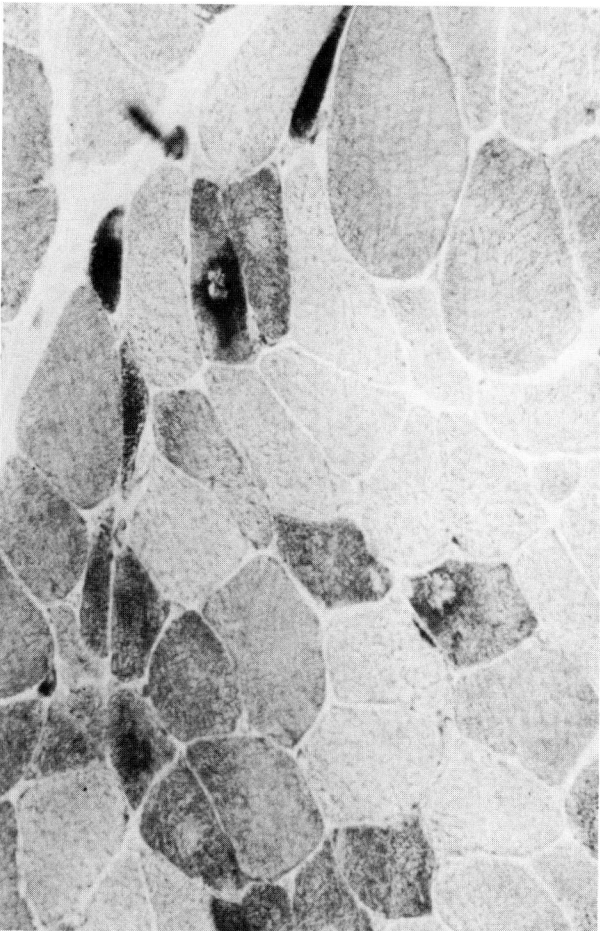

FIGURE 83.4   Denervation. Target fibers. (Nicotinamide adenine dinucleotide dehydrogenase stain.)

enzymes (e.g., phosphorylase, lactate dehydrogenase [LDH], and cytochrome oxidase). Immunocytochemical techniques are used to demonstrate the location and integrity of structural proteins, such as dystrophin, or to characterize the cell types in biopsies with inflammatory changes.

The muscle fibers belonging to one motor unit innervated by the same anterior horn cell are uniform in type, implying that there are fast and slow anterior horn cells. In addition, subsets of fiber types have been described, namely types 2A, 2B, and 2C. The metabolism of type 2A fibers is more oxidative than that of type 2B. The type 2C fiber is present in fetal muscle.

Changes of Denervation

When the muscle loses its nerve supply, the muscle fiber atrophies, often resulting in the fiber's being squeezed into the spaces between normal fibers and assuming an angulated appearance (Figure 83.3). Scattered angulated fibers are seen early in denervation. Sometimes, picturesque changes in the intermyofibrillar network occur, as in the target fiber, which characterizes denervation and reinnervation. This is a three-zone fiber, on which the intermediate zone stains more darkly and the central "bull's eye" stains much lighter than normal tissue (Figure 83.4). Often, a dener-

vated fiber may be reinnervated by a neighboring nerve twig, which results in two or more contiguous fibers being supplied from the same anterior horn cell. If that nerve twig then undergoes degeneration, instead of one small, angulated fiber being produced, a small group of atrophic fibers are produced. Small-group atrophy suggests denervation (Figure 83.5). When the process continues, large-group or geographical atrophy occurs, in which entire fascicles may be rendered atrophic. In addition to the change in size, there is also a redistribution of the fiber types. Normally, there is a random distribution of type 1 and 2 muscle fiber types, sometimes incorrectly called a *checkerboard* or *mosaic pattern*. The same process of denervation and reinnervation results in larger and larger groups of contiguous fibers being supplied by the same nerve. Because all fibers supplied by the same nerve are of the same fiber type, the normal mosaic pattern is replaced by groups of type 1 fibers next to groups of type 2 fibers. This fiber type grouping is pathognomonic of reinnervation (Figure 83.6). When longstanding denervation is present, the atrophic muscle fibers almost disappear, leaving small clumps of pyknotic nuclei in their place.

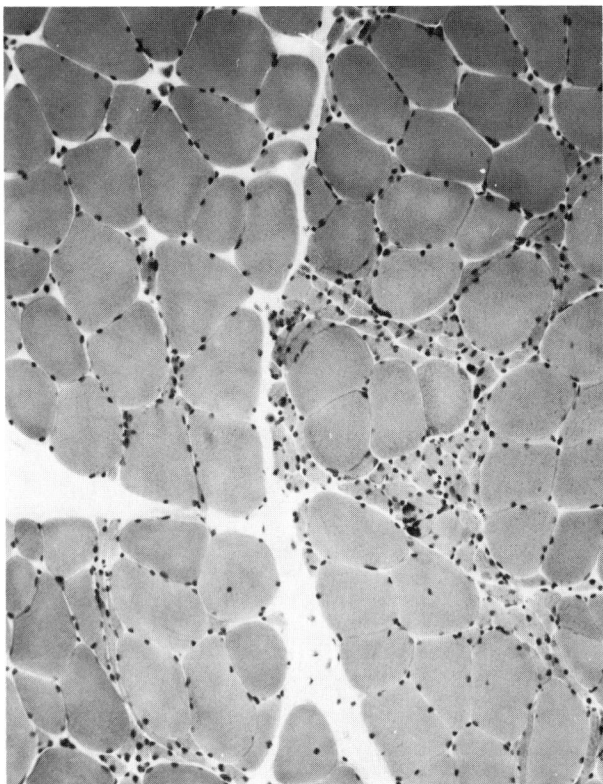

FIGURE 83.5   Denervation. Small groups of atrophic fibers are scattered throughout the biopsy. (Hematoxylin-eosin stain.)

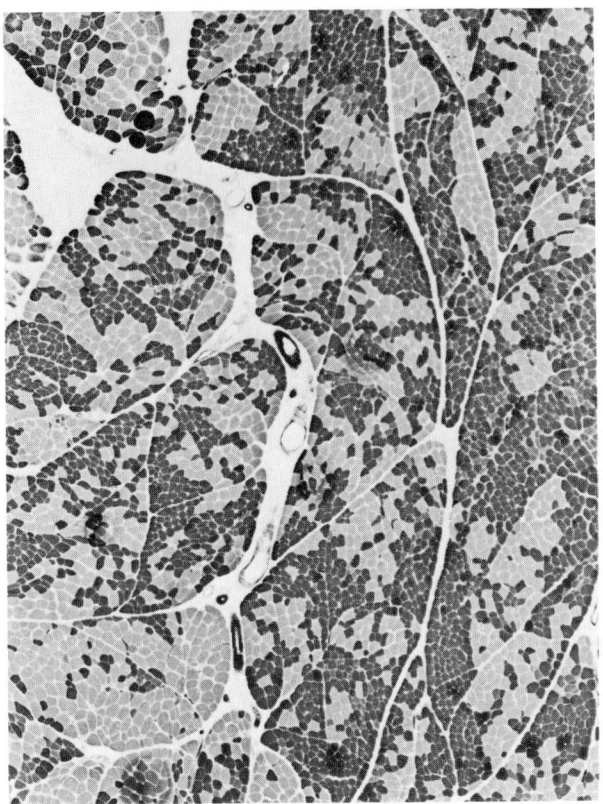

FIGURE 83.6   Chronic denervation and reinnervation. Instead of the usual mosaic pattern of the two fiber types, the fibers are clumped together, groups of one type appearing next to groups of the other type. (Myosin adenosine triphosphatase stain, pH 9.4.)

Myopathic Changes

Primary diseases of the muscle cause much greater variation in pathological changes than does denervation. The type of change that occurs depends on the type of muscle disease. The normal peripherally placed nuclei may migrate toward the center of the fiber. Occasional central nuclei may be seen in normal muscle (up to 2% of fibers), but when they are numerous, they usually indicate a myopathic, often dystrophic, disease. In myotonic dystrophy and limb-girdle muscular dystrophies (LGMDs), numerous internal nuclei are seen. Occasionally, internal nuclei are seen in some of the chronic denervating conditions (e.g., juvenile spinal muscular atrophy). Necrosis of muscle fibers, in which the fiber appears liquefied and later presents as a focus of phagocytosis, is seen in many of the myopathies. These changes almost always represent a relatively acute process. They often are seen in myoglobinuria, metabolic myopathies, and some of the more acute dystrophic conditions. Fiber-size variation may occur in primary diseases of muscle, with large fibers and small fibers intermingling in a random pattern. It is sometimes the only indication of the pathological process. Fiber splitting often accompanies muscle fiber hypertrophy. In transverse section, these split fibers can be recognized because of a thin fibrous septum, often associated with a nucleus that crosses part of the way but not all

the way across the fiber. A detailed study of serial transverse section may reveal more split fibers than in a single section. Fiber splitting is particularly visible in dystrophic conditions, such as LGMD. It usually is not seen in Duchenne's muscular dystrophy (DMD), Becker's muscular dystrophy (BMD), or acquired myopathies, such as polymyositis.

Many illnesses are characterized by degeneration and regeneration of fibers. When this occurs, the regenerating fibers often become basophilic as a result of the accumulation of RNA needed for protein synthesis. Fiber basophilia is a sign of an active myopathy. It is particularly characteristic of DMD, in which small basophilic groups of fibers may be prominent. Cellular responses include frank inflammatory reactions around blood vessels, which characterize the collagen vascular diseases, dermatomyositis, and polymyositis. In some of the adult-onset dystrophies and in facioscapulohumeral dystrophy (FSHD), inflammatory cellular responses may be quite pronounced, but they are associated with muscle fibers rather than with blood vessels.

Another reactive change in muscle is fibrosis. Normally, a very thin layer of connective tissue separates the muscle fibers. In dystrophic conditions, this layer thickens, and muscle fibrosis may be quite pronounced. In DMD, muscle fibrosis gives the muscle a hard, gritty texture; however,

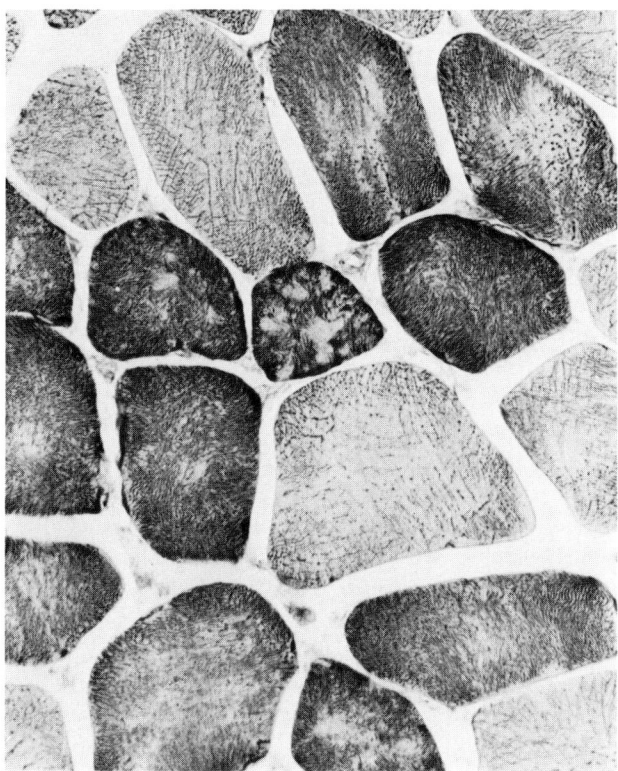

FIGURE 83.7   Myopathy. Moth-eaten, whorled fibers. The intermyofibrillar network pattern is distorted, and some areas lack the proper stain. (Nicotinamide adenine dinucleotide dehydrogenase stain.)

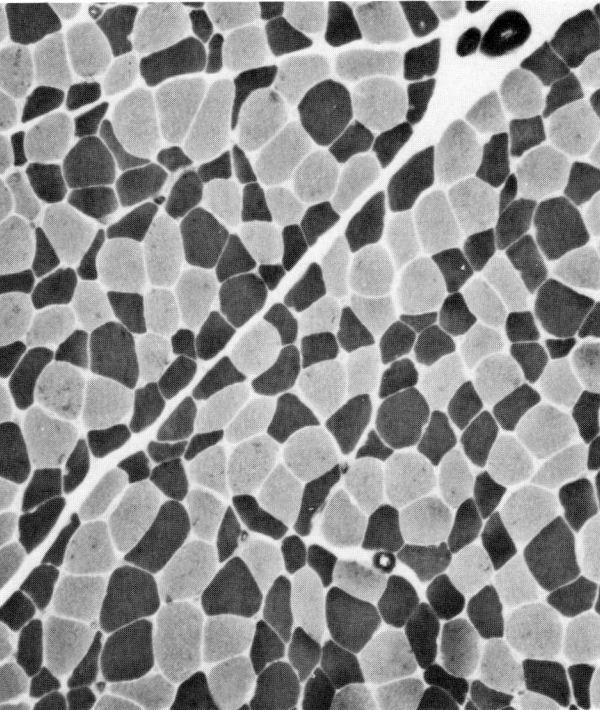

FIGURE 83.8   Type 2 fiber atrophy is a common change of uncertain significance. (Myosin adenosine triphosphatase stain.)

this texture also occurs in some congenital dystrophies. In polymyositis, there may be a loose edematous separation of fibers, but fibrosis is not usually characteristic of the active phase of the disease, except where associated with systemic sclerosis.

Changes in the intermyofibrillar network pattern are common in myopathic disorders. There is often a moth-eaten, whorled change to the intermyofibrillar network in LGMD and FSHD (Figure 83.7); the intermyofibrillar network loses its orderly arrangement and becomes swirled, resembling the current in an eddying stream. These changes may be seen in several diseases but tend to be much more common in the myopathies.

Other Changes

Selective changes in fiber types may be seen. Type 2 fiber atrophy is one of the most common abnormalities seen in muscle (Figure 83.8). This change, particularly if it is limited to type 2B fibers, is nonspecific and indicates a muscle that is subject to disuse. If a limb is casted and the muscle is examined some weeks later, selective atrophy of type 2 fibers is noted. Any chronic systemic illness tends to produce type 2 atrophy. It has been noted in rheumatoid arthritis, nonspecific collagen vascular diseases, cancer (hence the

name *cachectic atrophy*), mental retardation in children, and pyramidal tract disease. Therefore, type 2 fiber atrophy probably should be regarded as a nonspecific result of anything less than robust good health.

Type 1 fiber atrophy is more specific. It is seen in some of the congenital nonprogressive myopathies, such as nemaline myopathy and congenital fiber type disproportion, and is characteristic of myotonic dystrophy. Changes in the proportion of fibers in the biopsy are quite separate from changes in the fiber size. The name *fiber type predominance* has been given to a change in the relative numbers of a particular fiber type. Type 1 fiber predominance is a normal finding in the gastrocnemius and deltoid muscles. It is also the hallmark of congenital myopathies and many of the early dystrophies. Type 2 fiber predominance is seen in the lateral head of the quadriceps muscle. Type 2 predominance is seen occasionally in juvenile spinal muscular atrophy and motor neuron disease but is not firmly associated with any particular disease condition.

Some changes in muscle biopsies are pathognomonic of a particular disease. Thus, perifascicular atrophy, in which the atrophic fibers are more numerous around the edge of the muscle fascicles, is the hallmark of dermatomyositis. The presence of lipid vacuoles or abnormal pockets of glycogen characterizes the various metabolic myopathies. Enzyme defects, including phosphorylase deficiency, phosphofructokinase (PFK) deficiency, LDH deficiency, and adenylate deaminase deficiency, all can be detected with the appropriate histochemical stains. The interpretation of muscle biopsy usually includes the description of a constellation of changes and the subsequent association of these changes with a particular diagnosis. Illnesses that have characteristic biopsies include infantile spinal muscular atrophy, dermatomyositis, polymyositis, DMD, myotonic dystrophy, congenital muscular dystrophy (CMD), the congenital nonprogressive myopathies (including nemaline and central core disease), congenital fiber type disproportion, myotubular myopathy, lipid storage myopathies, acid maltase deficiency, phosphorylase deficiency, and FSHD. Although they are not disease specific, there are characteristic biopsy changes that indicate chronic denervation and acute simple denervation.

Immunocytochemical Studies

The use of biopsy material to identify missing proteins is increasing with the greater availability of commercial antibodies to the proteins of interest. If the DNA studies are unremarkable in a patient with DMD, as may be the case with a point deletion, the diagnosis rests on the demonstration of the absent or abnormal dystrophin in the tissue. All the sarcoglycans may be demonstrated using similar techniques. A deficiency of one of these proteins is increasingly recognized as a cause of muscular dystrophy. Because the sarcoglycans are part of a complex, when one is missing, all or some of the other sarcoglycans may be absent in the biopsy. α-Sarcoglycan is particularly prone to be lost, which makes it a suitable and economical screening tool. Absence of the laminin α_2 chain may be found in childhood muscular dystrophy. Histochemical studies may be used to look for various proteins, such as desmin, ubiquitin, and amyloid. In addition, biopsy material may give information about the type of inflammatory cell and the affinity for various markers, such as CD8 and CD4, which identify cells involved in cytotoxic mechanisms or in humoral mechanisms. Antibodies to the membrane attack complex may demonstrate the cells marked for destruction by the immune process, as in the vascular endothelium in dermatomyositis.

INHERITED MYOPATHIES

The muscular dystrophies are a group of primary muscle disorders that have a hereditary basis. They occur at all ages and with varying degrees of severity. Traditionally they are classified on clinical grounds and are recognized by their distinct clinical appearances. Increasing information about the molecular abnormalities in these illnesses has provided both reassurance and puzzlement to clinicians. The distinct clinical entities, such as BMD or DMD, are due to distinct molecular abnormalities; however, patients with similar molecular defects may show a wide variation in clinical severity that is not always easily explained.

For the most part, the known underlying molecular abnormalities in the dystrophies involve structural proteins, and it is useful to review these proteins as they occur in normal muscle (Brown 1997). The contractile proteins, actin and myosin, are arrayed with other proteins, such as troponin, to form the familiar thick and thin filaments. The reaction between actin and myosin results in realignment between the two molecules. In the sliding filament model, the thick and thin filaments form an array, which slides back and forth. The contractile proteins are connected to the "outside" of the cell by means of a complex of proteins that ultimately links up with the basal lamina. The first step in this connection is the protein dystrophin, which is located on the cytoplasmic face of the muscle membrane. This is a large protein (427 kD), which is coded by a gene on the short arm of the X chromosome. Dystrophin is related to spectrin and other structural proteins and consists of two ends separated by a long, flexible, rodlike region. The amino terminus binds to the actin molecule, and the carboxyl terminus, which is rich in cysteine, links dystrophin to a complex of glycoproteins in the sarcolemma. Two of these, the dystroglycans, form a direct link between dystrophin and part of the laminin molecule. α-Dystroglycan is a 156-kD protein located outside the membrane and linked to the laminin α_2 chain. It also connects with β dystroglycan, which is a 43-kD transmembrane component of the complex and is linked with dystrophin. The other glycoproteins are the sarcoglycans, of which there are four known at present, labeled alphabetically α (50 kD), β (43 kD), γ (35 kD), and δ sarcoglycans. All of them span the sarcolemmal membrane, but their relationship to the dystroglycans and their precise function is unclear. All are coded on different autosomal chromosomes and none on the X chromosome. The α_2 chain of laminin provides the anchor into the extracellular matrix because it is via the globular domain of this part of the molecule that α dystroglycan attaches to laminin. Another protein very closely related to dystrophin, with a molecular weight of 395 kD, is known as *utrophin*. This is not only similar in structure to dystrophin but seems to be able to replace some of the functions of dystrophin when the latter is deficient in experimental animals (Deconinck et al. 1997). It is also situated on the cytoplasmic face of the sarcolemma. Although it is present in the fetal and newborn animal, during development its territory is reduced until it is located only at the neuromuscular junctions. Significantly, in boys with dystrophin deficiency, utrophin may spread along the whole sarcolemmal membrane. Specific defects in this chain of proteins account for the occurrence of some but not all of the muscular dystrophies.

Dystrophin Deficiency (Duchenne's Muscular Dystrophy, Becker's Muscular Dystrophy, and Atypical Forms)

Pathophysiology

An absence or deficiency of dystrophin is implicated in two disorders that cause progressive destruction of muscle. The responsible gene is located on the short arm of the X chromosome at locus Xp21. It is an extremely large gene, comprising more than 2.5 million base pairs and 79 exons or coding regions. Approximately two-thirds of cases are associated with a detectable deletion or duplication of segments within the gene. The others are presumably due to point mutations too small to be detected using standard techniques. There are "hot spots" for these gene deletions, notably between exons 43 and 52 and particularly 44 and 49 (Nobile et al. 1997). Whether the deletion is in frame or out of frame (see Chapter 45) determines whether dystrophin is absent from the muscle or present in a reduced, altered form. This has clinical significance because the former is usually associated with the severe Duchenne's variety of the disease (DMD), whereas the latter situation may cause the milder Becker's variant (BMD) because the abnormal dystrophin preserves enough function to slow down the progress of the illness. The DNA code is read triplet by triplet. This *reading frame* must be maintained throughout the length of the gene for dystrophin to be produced. If a deletion removes a multiple of 3 base pairs, the reading frame may be intact upstream and downstream and may make limited sense, as if the sentence "You cannot eat the cat" were changed to "You not eat the cat," and some modified dystrophin may be formed. This is often the situation in the mild form of dystrophin deficiency. In the severe form, the reading frame is destroyed, as if a deletion resulted in the sentence "Yoc ann ote att hec at." There are exceptions to this rule, and frameshift deletions have been associated with the milder form of the disease, particularly at the 5' end of the gene in exons 3–7 (Muntoni et al. 1994).

The prevalence rate of DMD in the general population is approximately 3 per 100,000, and the incidence among liveborn males is 3 per 1,000. BMD is approximately one-tenth as common. Although the inheritance is clearly that of an X-linked recessive gene, almost one-third of cases are sporadic. Presumably this is due to a spontaneous mutation occurring either in the child or the parental germ cell.

It is not difficult to imagine that an absence of dystrophin would severely impair the integrity of the sarcolemmal membrane. Attention previously focused on this membrane because of electron microscopic evidence that it contains breaches associated with wedge-shaped areas of destruction in the adjacent muscle cell. It is assumed that the absence of a supporting protein renders the membrane susceptible to mechanical damage. This presumably means that molecules, such as calcium, would have unlimited access to the fiber and would initiate a whole chain of destructive processes, producing necrosis of the muscle fiber. The process would then involve continual degeneration, with repeated attempts at regeneration on the part of the surviving satellite cells. Eventually, however, this process leads to severe loss of muscle and replacement of the muscle fibers with fibrous tissue.

Several animals have been found to have dystrophin deficiency; the better known include the mdx mouse and the dog model. The situation in the mouse model is unusual. The animals appear to be relatively normal, except for a phase early in life during which pathological abnormalities in the muscle are noted. In the dogs, however, the dystrophin deficiency is associated with obvious weakness, and abnormal muscle is noted on microscopy, thus making this animal suitable for the evaluation of potential treatment.

Clinical Features

Severe Form (Duchenne's Muscular Dystrophy). Even in the severe variety, no abnormality is usually obvious at birth. Some time during the second year, when the boys begin walking, the early clumsiness seen in all toddlers persists. Soon the children have to place one hand on the knee to assume an upright position when rising from the floor (Gower's maneuver). It is often at this stage that the calf muscles are found to be rather firm and rubbery (pseudohypertrophy) (Figure 83.9). Within 2–3 years, parents notice that the child does not run properly and is never able to jump clear of the floor with both feet. In the absence of therapy, tightness is noted across several joints in the legs. The iliotibial bands and the heel cords are usually the first to become tight. This is particularly noticeable in boys who habitually walk on their toes.

By 5 or 6 years of age, stair climbing becomes labored, and the children use the railing to pull themselves upward. Some time between the ages of 2 and 6 years, there may be a period of apparent improvement, when the children gain motor skills. This is illusory because it simply represents the child's natural development, which has not yet been outpaced by the muscle weakness. At the age of 6 or 7 years, the boys often complain of sudden spontaneous falls. At first, these occur when the children are hurrying or are knocked off balance by their playmates. The fall is quite spectacular to the onlooker; the knees collapse abruptly and the child drops like a stone to the ground. At approximately 8–10 years of age, affected children cease to be able to climb stairs or stand up from the floor, and it is at approximately this time when they begin using a wheelchair for locomotion. Earlier studies suggested that these children began using a wheelchair and lost the ability to walk at approximately 9 years of age. In a population treated with bracing, reconstructive surgery, and physiotherapy, the average age of confinement to a wheelchair was 12.2 years. The true natural history of the disease is difficult to ascertain because many physicians and parents put considerable effort into keeping the children straight and the limbs supple.

Contractures of the hips, knees, and ankles become severe when the relatively untreated child spends much of the day in the wheelchair. The hips and knees are locked at 90 degrees, and the feet turn downward and inward in an exaggerated position of equinovarus. It is very difficult to get normal shoes to fit them, and it is impossible for them to sleep except in one position: usually with the knees propped up with pillows and slightly turned on one side. Handling

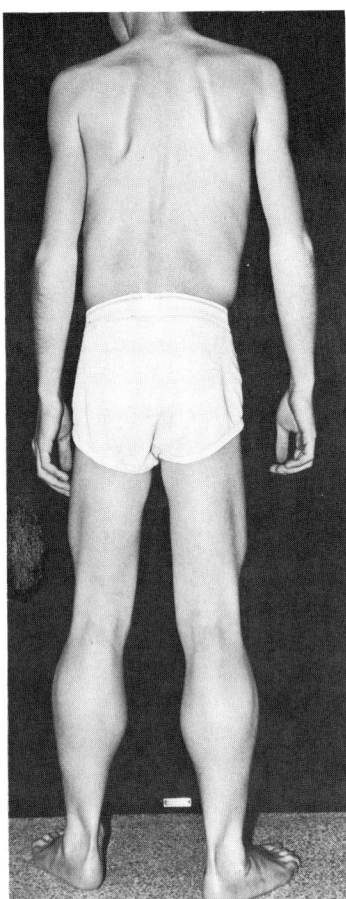

FIGURE 83.9   Duchenne's muscular dystrophy. Calf and thigh hypertrophy in an ambulatory 8-year-old patient.

the children at this stage becomes very difficult, and back pain and limb pain almost inevitably accompany this severe stage of muscular dystrophy. With the development of a severe scoliosis, respiratory function becomes compromised. The cardiac involvement is characterized by degeneration and fibrosis of the posterolateral wall of the left ventricle. Besides the abnormal electrocardiogram (ECG), valve motion, wall thickness, and wall motion are also abnormal. Affected children die from either respiratory failure or a cardiomyopathy that is relatively resistant to treatment.

Diagnosis. The least invasive test to confirm the diagnosis is to obtain DNA studies looking for a deletion in the dystrophin gene. In the 30% of patients in whom a deletion is not found, a muscle biopsy is necessary to establish the absence of dystrophin. Three antibodies are available against the ends (Dys-2 for the carboxyl terminal and Dys-3 for the amino terminal) and the rod region (Dys-1) of the molecule. Absence of the amino terminal, the end that binds with actin, appears to be associated with the more severe symptoms. In dystrophin deficiency, the protein is absent or the stain is irregular and fragmented. A few fibers

may demonstrate a rim of dystrophin. These are the revertant fibers, in which the gene has undergone a spontaneous change that allows it once again to code for dystrophin. Where there is doubt, immunoblotting may be used to show an absence of dystrophin in the tissue.

The serum concentration of creatine kinase (CK) is markedly elevated in this illness; levels greater than 10,000 mU/ml are common. Electromyography (EMG) shows myopathic changes (see Chapter 37B), and the muscle biopsy demonstrates variation in the size of fibers, fibrosis, groups of basophilic fibers, and opaque or hypercontracted fibers (hyaline fibers) (Figures 83.10–83.12).

Treatment

Physical Therapy. The primary aim of physical therapy is to keep the joints as loose as possible. Early on, the iliotibial bands and the heel cords give the greatest problems. Late in the course, elbow, wrist, and finger contractures add to the functional disability. Physical therapy generally is commenced at 3–4 years of age, when parents are taught to stretch the child's heel cords, hip flexors, and iliotibial bands. This program should be followed on a daily basis. Passive stretching of joints is directed not at increasing the range of motion but, rather, at preventing any further development of contractures. This should be explained carefully to the parents because they can be disheartened to see no improvement in the tightness, even after many months of therapy. A night splint, which is a plastic shell molded around the lower part of the leg to maintain the foot at right angles to the leg, is important at an early age. Ankle contractures are almost never seen in patients who use these splints conscientiously. Unfortunately, some patients, particularly those 6 or 7 years or older, cannot tolerate the splints. Parents often ask about an active exercise program. Such a program is largely unnecessary in a young child, who runs around to the best of his ability anyway. By the time a child is having difficulty walking or is in a wheelchair, muscle weakness is severe, and exercise is not known to increase muscle strength.

Bracing. The appropriate use of bracing may delay the child's progression to a wheelchair by approximately 2 years. A major factor responsible for the children's inability to stand or walk is weakness of the quadriceps. Such weakness causes the knee to collapse when it is even slightly flexed; the only stable position is in hyperextension. The boy is then reluctant to bend the knee in walking and may remain rooted to the ground, unable to move the feet. The addition of a long-leg brace (knee-foot orthosis) can help solve this problem. Such a device stabilizes the knee and prevents the knee from flexing. The children walk stiff-legged, but they do not have the same problem with falling that they had previously. Generally, children are ready for bracing when they have ceased to climb stairs, are having great difficulty arising from the floor, and are having frequent daily falls. On examination, a knee extensor muscle that is unable to straighten the knee against gravity is also

FIGURE 83.10 Duchenne's dystrophy: change in serum creatine kinase (CK) level with age. This is a scattergram of serum CK levels in individual patients. The lines represent the fifth, twenty-fifth, fiftieth, seventy-fifth, and ninety-fifth percentiles.

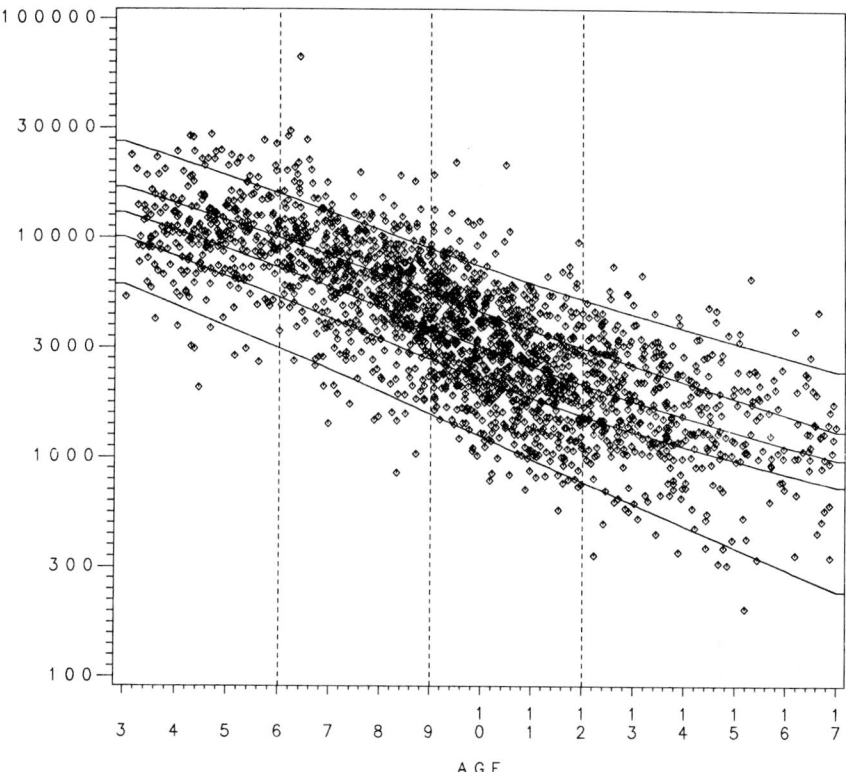

an indication for bracing. One often hears the comment that the weight of the brace makes it difficult for the child to walk. Because the brace basically functions as a pendulum, and slight elevation of the hip is sufficient to bring the leg forward, the weight of the brace is often not the problem it is believed to be. There may be some advantage to a lightweight, plastic knee-foot orthosis, but it should be remembered that it is difficult to keep the foot straight with such a device, whereas the high-top boot worn with the double-upright brace provides excellent stability. The choice between plastic and metal often comes down to personal preference of the patient or physician.

Surgery. Reconstructive surgery of the leg often accompanies bracing. Indeed, for most children, the two are performed during the same hospital admission. The purpose of leg surgery is to keep the leg extended and prevent contractures of the iliotibial bands and hip flexors. Shortening of the iliotibial bands is associated with a stance in which the boy's legs are widely abducted. As noted before, the long-leg brace is used like a pendulum. If the foot is widely abducted, the child cannot swing the leg forward. The only effect of lifting the hip in this case is that the leg tries to swing inward toward the midline. This is impossible because the abduction is due in the first place to the resistance of the iliotibial band contractures. A simple way to maintain function in the leg is to perform percutaneous tenotomies of the Achilles tendons, knee flexors, hip flexors, and iliotibial bands. This procedure often allows a

child who is becoming increasingly dependent on a wheelchair to resume walking.

The modern techniques of spinal stabilization are being used increasingly in the DMD population. Because of the extreme discomfort of a severe scoliosis and the respiratory problems associated with it, spinal surgery seems to have been well accepted by patients, and the management of the late stages of the disease has been remarkably changed.

Pharmacological Treatment. A large number of clinical trials have been carried out in DMD, most of them without the demonstration of any clear-cut improvement. Prednisone improves muscle strength and function. Although the duration of its effect is not certain, it seems to last for at least 3 years. The synthetic steroid deflazacort has a similar therapeutic effect and approximately half the side effects. It is available in Europe and Central and South America at the time of writing. The use of corticosteroids in DMD is not established but seems to be increasing, and there is some debate about the best time to use it. Corticosteroids may be viewed as agents that can "buy time" for the patient until some better treatment comes along. In this light, we usually delay treatment until 5 years of age, just before the expected decline in strength but at a stage where the muscles are relatively well preserved.

Gene Therapy. In theory, the treatment and cure of this illness would be a matter of replacing the defective gene. The illness is due to a negative effect, the lack of dystrophin, not to a positive effect due to the presence of a toxic gene prod-

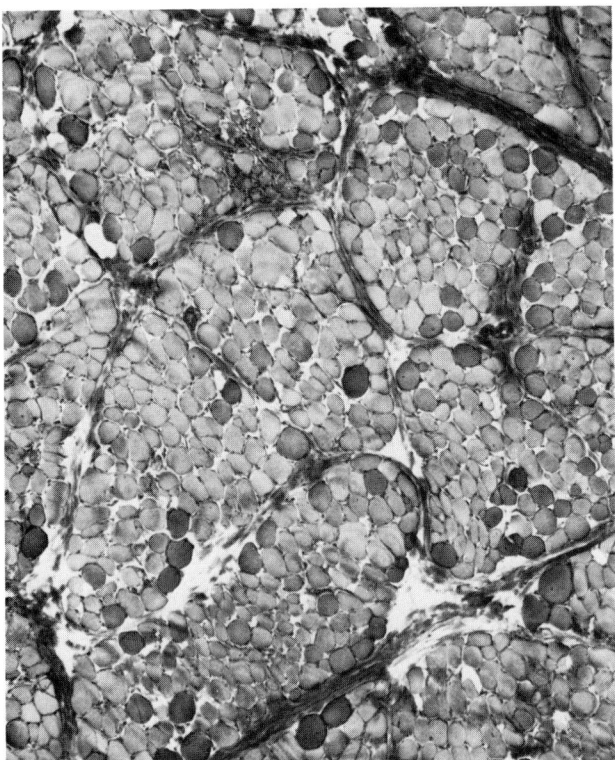

FIGURE 83.11 Duchenne's dystrophy: muscle biopsy. The fibers are of variable size and separated by connective tissue. Large, heavily stained opaque fibers are noted. (Verhoeff-Van Gieson stain.)

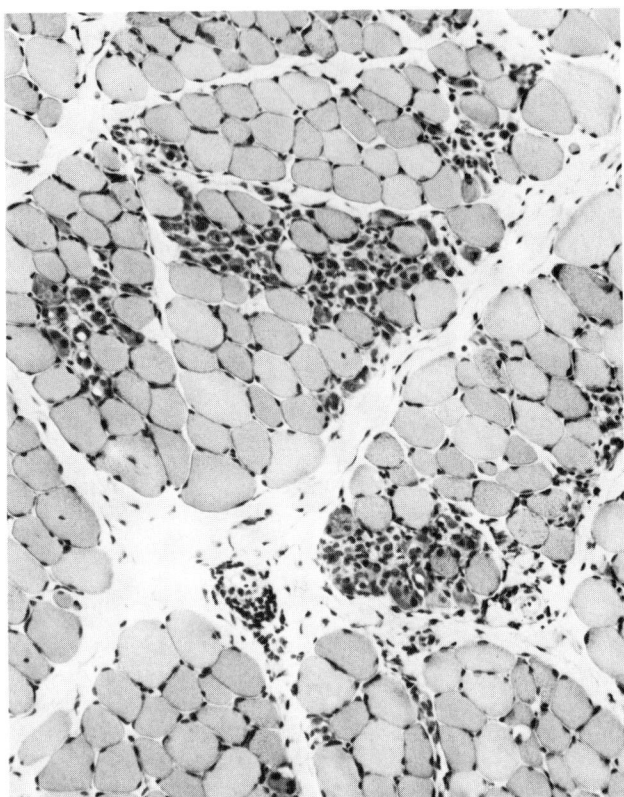

FIGURE 83.12 Duchenne's dystrophy. Groups of small, basophilic (darkly staining) fibers are scattered in the biopsy. (Hematoxylin-eosin stain.)

uct. The possibility of replacing old muscle with new is enticing and has occupied researchers for the last decade. The first attempt was to use normal myoblasts grown from unaffected muscle. These were then injected into the muscle with the hope that they would fuse with the dystrophic muscle and carry the normal gene with them. Although dystrophin was expressed in some of the muscle fibers, the percentage of fibers was so low that no clinical effect was detected. The reasons are many: The injected cells diffuse only a short distance, they are prone to rejection, and the surviving muscle proves resistant to fusion with these myoblasts. Attempts are ongoing to circumvent these drawbacks, but so far, myoblast transfer remains only a possibility for the future. More promising is the attempt to develop a vector into which the dystrophin gene can be inserted and which can carry the gene into the muscle. There are several problems to overcome. The large size of the gene makes it difficult to insert in the usual vectors. An abbreviated version of the full gene may be satisfactory, however. Certainly there are patients in whom such truncated genes occur naturally who are only mildly affected. The gene will have to work in conjunction with a promoter that allows dystrophin production to be limited to the muscle. The viral vector must also be proved safe. This can be accomplished by removal of some or all of the viral genes. At present, the adenovirus is the front runner from which a vector might be developed,

but other viruses, such as retroviruses, are also being considered. Initial animal experiments have given some encouragement to this approach, and human studies are planned.

Another possibility that is becoming increasingly popular is upregulating the dystrophinlike protein, utrophin. Animal studies have suggested that if the amount of utrophin can be increased in the dystrophin-deficient animal, there is both functional and pathological improvement. This finding is reinforced by the fact that utrophin is increased in patients with dystrophin deficiency. It is much easier to upregulate a gene that exists in the patient than it is to introduce a foreign gene to which the individual has had no prior exposure. It may also be possible to upregulate utrophin levels pharmacologically. Indeed, one of the effects of corticosteroids on cultured dystrophic cells is to increase utrophin levels.

Mild Form (Becker's Muscular Dystrophy). BMD shares all the characteristics of the severe form but has a milder course. The illness begins in the first decade, although the parents often notice the first signs of weakness later because of the mildness of the symptoms. Occasionally, the onset of symptoms is delayed until the fourth decade or later. The muscular hypertrophy, contractures, and pattern of weakness are similar to that seen in DMD. These boys, however, continue to walk independently past the age of 15 years and may not have to use a wheelchair until they are in their twenties or even later. A frequent complaint in teenagers with BMD is leg cramps and other muscle pains, which are often associated with exercise and are more severe than in DMD. A significant proportion of these patients has a cardiomyopathy that can be more disabling than the weakness. Cardiac transplantation has been very successful in some patients with this form of the illness. Diagnosis may require a quantitation of the dystrophin in the muscle because, in BMD, dystrophin may not be absent but may be reduced in amount or abnormal in size. Diagnosis requires immunoblotting studies.

Because the patients do not have much trouble in the first few years, aggressive physiotherapy, surgical reconstruction, and night splints are less often needed. Patients with BMD are less prone to develop kyphoscoliosis, perhaps because they are not confined to a wheelchair until after the spine has become fully mature. I have used corticosteroids only occasionally in patients with BMD. The stabilizing effect of steroids is less noticeable when the disease is already fairly stable. In every other respect, including bracing and genetic counseling, the disease can be treated identically to the severe form.

Other Phenotypes. With the development of genetic testing and dystrophin analysis, it is becoming clear that the concept that dystrophin deficiency is always associated with the BMD or DMD phenotype is false. There are notable exceptions, including one family in which males with dystrophin deficiency were asymptomatic (Morrone et al. 1997). In other examples, dystrophin deficiency has been associated with very mild late-onset weakness. Many patients have been described in whom the symptoms have been exercise intolerance, muscle pain, and myoglobinuria (Figarella-Branger et al. 1997). It appears that defects in the rod region of dystrophin may be more frequently associated with this mild phenotype. It is impractical to perform genetic testing on all patients with neuromuscular complaints, but the presence of muscle pain, mild weakness, an elevated serum CK, and large muscles warrants an analysis of dystrophin and its associated proteins. Attempts have been made to correlate the genetic abnormality with the clinical picture. Such correlations are inexact, but abnormalities in the amino terminal and at the carboxyl terminal domains of dystrophin are associated with the more severe form of disease. Alterations in the rod domain are more variable and may be associated with a mild phenotype. In-frame deletions and insertions are associated with a much more benign phenotype than out-of-frame alterations.

Genetic Counseling. Because DMD is an X-linked recessive disorder, the carrier state of all women related to an affected person by maternal linkage should be ascertained. Up to 30% of cases may be sporadic and due to new mutations or deletions. In the experience of many clinicians, an even higher percentage of new patients arriving in the clinic are sporadic cases, perhaps because genetic counseling is widely available and the women who carry the abnormal gene decide not to have children.

Genetic analysis of all potential carriers is advisable. In a family in which the disease is associated with a deletion, there is little problem in determining whether the woman is carrying the affected X chromosome using techniques that are presently available. Genetics laboratories now have the ability to identify the presence of a mutant gene over the background contributed by the normal allele. This involves an analysis of the gene "dosage," comparing two normal alleles that have a double dose against a deleted allele and a normal allele that have a single dose (Voskova-Goldman et al. 1997). Current diagnosis of carrier status when a deletion has been identified in a proband is based on an analysis of a gene dosage. Our diagnostic strategy uses fluorescence in situ hybridization to detect female carriers with major deletions in the dystrophin gene. Similarly, prenatal diagnosis using amniotic cells or chorionic villus biopsies can identify the affected fetus, and, more important, those who are unaffected. In families in whom the disease is associated with a point mutation too small to detect, carrier detection relies on the demonstration that the woman carries the same X chromosome as the affected individual. This necessitates linkage studies, which become reliable only if there are enough cases in the family and enough family members to provide reliable linkage.

Deficiencies of Specific Proteins and Limb-Girdle Dystrophies

The most dramatic developments in muscle disease over the last few years have related to a group of disorders that were clearly dystrophic but defied proper classification. The diagnosis of LGMD was traditionally used to cloak the clinician's uncertainty. In some patients, weakness was generally proximal but other characteristics were disparate. Some cases were dominantly inherited, others recessively. Some had more hip than shoulder weakness, others the reverse. The illness could be mild in late life, others severe and early. There was general recognition that the rubric contained a group of different illnesses. Beginning with the discovery that a defect in one of the sarcoglycans, probably γ, caused a severe form of dystrophy occurring in North Africa, a number of entities have been delineated that are characterized by defects in structural and other proteins. These include the sarcoglycans, the α_2 chain of laminin (merosin), calcium-activated protease, calpain3, and others. In addition, even when the precise molecular defect has not been identified, there are other forms of LGMD for which a gene locus has been assigned. The following sections outline the known protein abnormalities and then comment on the more amorphous forms of LGMD. The prevalence of these diseases as a group probably approaches 1 per 100,000 (van der Kooi et al. 1996).

Sarcoglycan Deficiencies

Four known sarcoglycans are expressed in muscle, and a possible fifth may exist, ε-sarcoglycan, with a wide distribution. The genes for the first four have been identified, and defects in each have been associated with a form of muscular dystrophy. The gene for α-sarcoglycan lies on chromosome 17, β on 4, γ on 13, and δ on 5. The numerologists among us may commit these to memory by recognizing that 17 minus 4 equals 13. (This begs the question of how to remember the last chromosome, unless you want to count the digits in the previous numbers.) The original cases of severe childhood muscular dystrophy, although described as α-sarcoglycan deficiency, were linked to chromosome 13, which is the locus of γ- rather than α-sarcoglycan. This illustrates one of the pitfalls in diagnostic testing for these illnesses. The sarcoglycans are a tightly knit family, and when one is absent, the others may also be missing. This is particularly true of α-sarcoglycan, making it both a useful screening tool and a misleading one on occasion. An absence of α-sarcoglycan is an indication to search for the abnormal gene, be it α, β, γ, or δ. These illnesses are not uncommon. Large population studies are not yet available, but surveys of muscle biopsies suggest that the sarcoglycanopathies may account for more than 10% of patients with a limb-girdle pattern and positive dystrophin (Duggan et al. 1997). It has been estimated that sarcoglycan deficiencies may account for up to 50% of patients with muscular dystrophy in North Africa.

There is not yet a wide enough experience to be able to separate the diseases clinically; all present with trunk and limb weakness and a serum CK concentration of 1,000 units and higher. Facial weakness is absent. Calf hypertrophy has been observed, but cardiac findings have not been prominent. A deficiency of γ-sarcoglycan seems to be mainly associated with severe weakness and mimics DMD in its progression and loss of ambulation. α-Sarcoglycan deficiencies are variable and may be severe or mild (Dincer et al. 1997). Some patients have been recorded in whom the onset of weakness was delayed until adult life and who continued to function without severe disability, despite proximal weakness. β-Sarcoglycan deficiency was described in the Amish community in southern Indiana. In these patients, the illness was milder than in a young girl with a Duchenne's muscular dystrophy–like picture who was also found to have a defect in β-sarcoglycan. The patients with δ-sarcoglycan deficiencies are not as frequently reported but also seem to have the severe phenotype. Intuitively, one might think that the severity of the disease in the sarcoglycanopathies, as in dystrophinopathy, depends on whether the protein is absent or reduced in amount and altered in structure but still retains some function. Although the diseases in many ways resemble dystrophin deficiency, information on response to treatment is inadequate. Physicians faced with a patient who has proximal weakness of early onset and a marked elevation of CK should obtain the appropriate studies for these diseases.

Calcium Activated Neutral Protease (Calpain3) Deficiency

A careful series of studies conducted over a decade by Fardeau's group documented the existence of a form of LGMD in an inbred population on Reunion Island in the Indian Ocean (Fardeau et al. 1996). The disease was localized to chromosome 15 and was associated with a mutation in the gene for muscle-specific calcium activated neutral protease (CANP-3, calpain3). It is presumably an autosomal recessively inherited illness. Since this description, cases have been described in the Amish in Northern Indiana, in Turkey, and in Brazil, which suggests that the illness is not limited by geography. The underlying pathophysiology of the illness is uncertain. CANP-3 is not a structural protein but an enzyme. It has been suggested that the enzyme has a regulatory role in the modulation and control of transcription factors and thus of gene expression.

The disease begins in childhood or in early adult life and is progressive. Most, but not all, cases have been mild to moderately progressive with loss of ambulation in adult life. Severe forms have been described. Weakness occurs in the hips first and then in the shoulders. There is no facial weakness, and the neck flexors and extensors are strong. Scapular winging, which is different from that seen in FSHD, is noted, with the whole of the medial scapular border jutting backward. The posterior thigh muscles are more severely affected than are the knee extensors, and the rectus abdominis muscles seem to be affected early. The concentration of serum CK is at first markedly elevated and then decreases and may become more normal later in the illness. Information on the effectiveness of treatment is not available, but it seems reasonable to apply the same principles to this disease as in the better-known illnesses, such as dystrophin deficiency.

Other Limb-Girdle Dystrophies and Classification

The ability to characterize and link this group of diseases with the location of their genes permits some clarification of this confusing group of syndromes. All are illnesses characterized by progressive symmetrical proximal weakness without facial weakness. The initial division is along the lines of dominant versus recessive inheritance. LGMD1 is dominant and LGMD2 recessive. The subsequent division depended on the ability to link the illness with a specific gene locus. The dominant group is divided into LGMD1A, which is linked to chromosome 5q and LGMD1B, which is not. A recent paper suggests that one form of LGMD, possibly 1B, is localized to chromosome 1q11-21 (van der Kooi et al. 1997). In this variety, there was a strong association with cardiac involvement. LGMD2A is calpain3 deficiency, and LGMD2B is an illness linked to chromosome 2p13.3. LGMD2C, LGMD2D, LGMD2E, and LGMD2F are γ-, α-, β-, and δ-sarcoglycan deficiencies, respectively. LGMD2G maps to chromosome 17q11-12 (α-sarcoglycan is at 17q21) and has some features (e.g., distal weakness and the presence of rimmed vacuoles on the biopsy) that may link it to the distal myopathy group (Moreira et al. 1997).

Emerin Deficiency (Emery-Dreifuss Dystrophy)

Pathophysiology

Emery-Dreifuss muscular dystrophy (EDMD) is an inherited, X-linked recessive disease. Similar phenotypes are reported in patients with diseases inherited as an autosomal dominant trait, but their emerin is normal. The gene for EDMD is located on the long arm of the X chromosome, close to the centromere (locus approximately Xq28). The gene codes for a unique protein, emerin, which has been localized to the inner nuclear membrane, from which it projects into the nucleoplasm (Manilal et al. 1996). Emerin may belong to a family of lamina-associated structural proteins. It is not immediately clear why a defect in this protein, which is ubiquitous, would cause a form of muscular dystrophy. Perhaps one clue is found in a report that describes its association with the intercalated discs of heart muscle as well as its nuclear location.

Clinical Features

EDMD is characterized by wasting and weakness of the upper arms, shoulders, and anterior compartment muscles in the legs. This weakness is associated with contractures, which occur early, particularly in the elbows, the posterior part of the neck, the paraspinal muscles, and the Achilles tendon. Elbow contractures are characteristic. They occur early and are severe. As the arm is extended, sudden resistance is met, which feels more like bone than the pressure of a tight tendon. The disorder is slowly progressive and often spreads to involve other muscle groups, such as those of the hip. Cardiac complications are frequent. Conduction block has been emphasized as a cause for the sometimes sudden, unexpected death of these patients. Atrial paralysis has been described in which the atria are electrically inexcitable and the heart responds only to ventricular pacing. There are also other cardiac problems, and ventricular myocardial disease with ventricular failure has been noted. Female carriers of the illness may develop the cardiac abnormalities at a later age; sudden death has been reported in such women. The severity of the cardiopathy in both men and women increases with age.

Diagnosis

The clinical picture of EDMD is distinctive. Confirmation of the diagnosis may be found in DNA studies showing a defect in the gene. Because emerin is present in many tissues, the diagnosis may also be made from a skin biopsy showing that the protein is absent from nuclei in the skin. The routine laboratory investigations simply confirm that the disease is myopathic. This is best demonstrated by muscle biopsy and EMG. The CK levels may be elevated. Every patient with the syndrome should have an ECG, which should be repeated at regular intervals. Other members of the family also should undertake regular ECGs because of the possibility of isolated cardiac involvement.

Treatment

Analysis and treatment of the cardiac problems are the most pertinent parts of therapy. Many patients with EDMD need a cardiac pacemaker; some may need treatment of congestive cardiac failure due to the ventricular failure. Because the atrial block may be sudden, unpredictable, and fatal, it may be wise to implant a pacemaker when the diagnosis is first made. It is important to realize that the pacemaker does not retard the development of a cardiomyopathy and only protects the patient against the complications of conduction block. Female carriers of the illness should be screened with ECG when they are older than 35 years.

Facioscapulohumeral Dystrophy

Pathophysiology

FSHD is inherited as an autosomal dominant trait. Its prevalence is around 1–2 per 100,000 population. The responsible gene has been localized to the end of the long arm of chromosome 4 (4q35) in many, but not all, families. The genetic abnormality is a deletion in a 3.3-kB repeating sequence. Digestion with the endonuclease *Eco*RI produces a fragment that is shorter than 34kB in most families with the illness compared with more than 40 kB for normal individuals. In the past, the results were clouded by the existence of an identical sequence, unrelated to the disease, on chromosome 10. The problem has since been solved, and DNA testing is reliable (Upadhyaya et al. 1997), although there are a few cases that show no abnormality in the chromosome 4 sequence. The severity of the illness bears a relationship to the size of the deletion: The smallest fragments tend to be associated with severe illness. Another phenomenon exhibited by these families is anticipation of the illness, where cases occur with more severity and at a younger age with successive generations. This suggests that the mutation is a dynamic one, which may become increasingly severe with each generation, as is the case with myotonic dystrophy. A puzzling feature of the abnormal region is that it does not seem to contain any actual genes. The suggestion has been made that the actual gene is slightly removed from the deleted area but that it is influenced by the changes in its neighboring environment (position effect variegation) (Fisher and Upadhyaya 1997).

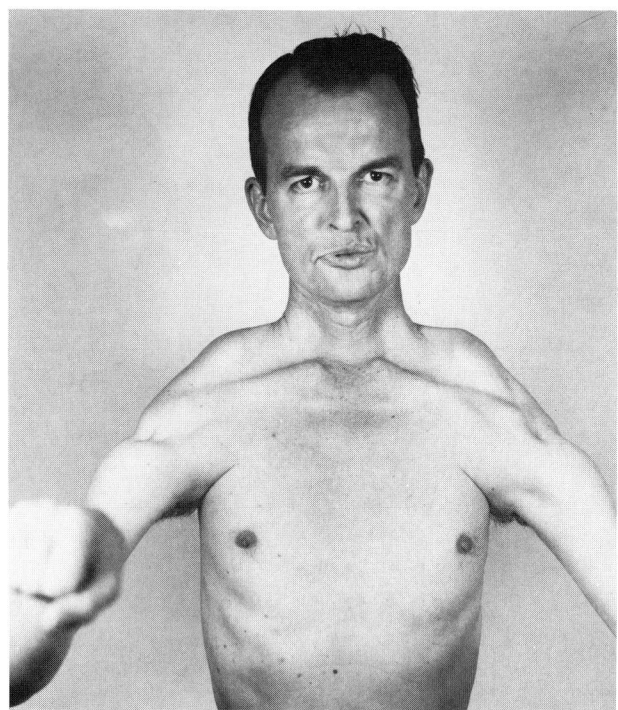

FIGURE 83.13 Facioscapulohumeral dystrophy. Notice the characteristic appearance of the shoulders, the downward-sloping clavicles, and the bulge in the region of the trapezius muscle, which is due to the scapula being displaced upward on attempted elevation of the arms. The patient also is attempting to purse his lips.

Clinical Features

FSHD varies in intensity even within the same family. Some patients may have mild facial weakness that can go unnoticed throughout life. Others may have total paralysis of the face and severe weakness of most other muscles in the body, and they may be confined to a wheelchair by the time they are 9 or 10 years old. In the typical variety, the disorder is first noted at the start of the teenage years. Facial weakness expresses itself as a difficulty in blowing up balloons or drinking through a straw. The child may be seen to sleep with the sclera of the eyes showing through partially opened lids. Facial expression is relatively preserved, but the smile is often flattened and transverse, as opposed to the upward curve of the usual smile. When the patient attempts to whistle, the lips move awkwardly and have a peculiar pucker (Figure 83.13). The mouth also may have a pouting quality, the so-called bouche de tapir.

Weakness of the shoulder muscles particularly affects the scapular fixators, and when the patient attempts to sustain the arms outstretched in front, the scapulae jut backward, with the inferomedial corner pointing backward. The deltoid muscle is usually quite bulky and its strength well preserved, provided the scapula is fixed, even late in the illness. The biceps and triceps muscles are often weak. The shoulders' unusual appearance is often noted in the locker room, and the child's "chicken wings" may be a source of embarrassment. The forearm muscles are less involved, although a discrepancy between the stronger wrist flexors and weaker wrist extensors often can be used to support the diagnosis. In spite of the lack of description of leg weakness in the name of this illness, the muscles of the legs are not spared in FSHD. Weakness of the hip flexor muscles and of the quadriceps is common, and the ankle dorsiflexors are weak, whereas strength is preserved in the plantar flexors. Often the ankle dorsiflexors are involved very early in the illness, and it is not unknown for a footdrop to be the presenting complaint, blending this illness with the scapuloperoneal syndromes. Asymmetry of the weakness is almost the rule, often leading the clinician to doubt the diagnosis of muscular dystrophy and to seek a superimposed peripheral nerve lesion where none exists. A severe form of FSHD may be noted in infancy. Unlike patients with the more typical, mildly disabling adult form, these babies have severe weakness. They may have no movement at all in the face, which remains passive and expressionless. Weakness of the limbs, although it conforms to the general pattern of FSHD, is so severe that these children may lose the ability to walk by 9 or 10 years of age. One striking feature of this illness is the extreme lumbosacral lordosis seen when the child walks or stands. This initially disappears on sitting, indicating that it is a compensatory mechanism the child uses to keep his or her balance. Deafness is frequent in these children. There is also an association with Coats' disease, an oxidative vascular degeneration of the retina.

Diagnosis

The diagnosis can be established reliably by DNA studies, EMG, muscle biopsy, and CK evaluations. The CK concentration usually is elevated severalfold above normal. The muscle biopsy may show general dystrophic features or more specific changes: tiny fibers scattered throughout the biopsy or scattered inflammatory cellular foci associated with muscle fibers and in the interstitial tissue in patients with more severe disease (Figures 84.14 and 84.15). EMG shows myopathic potentials (see Chapter 37B).

Treatment

The treatment of FSHD is supportive. There is no known way of reversing the illness. If the patient is unable to raise the arms above the head because of the lack of scapular fixation, surgical stabilization of the scapula may be beneficial (Twyman et al. 1996). This is particularly true in the majority of patients, in whom deltoid function is preserved. It is more usual for ambulatory patients to undertake this procedure. Wheelchair-confined patients, because of the severity of the general weakness, do not find the problems in shoulder movements to be out of proportion to the rest of the muscular weakness. Such patients find a forearm orthosis or ball-bearing feeder device to be more useful than undertaking rather lengthy surgery.

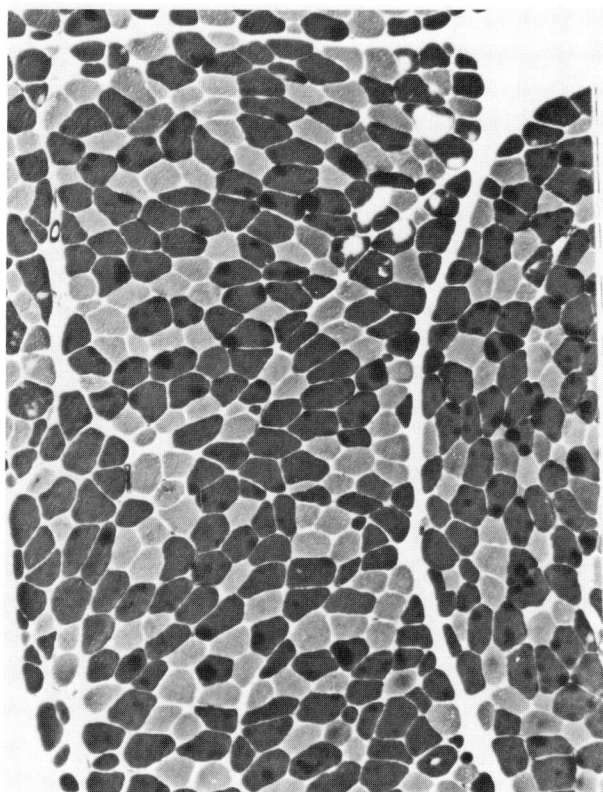

FIGURE 83.14 Facioscapulohumeral dystrophy. Note the variability in the size of fibers with scattered tiny fibers. (Myosin adenosine triphosphatase stain, pH 9.4.)

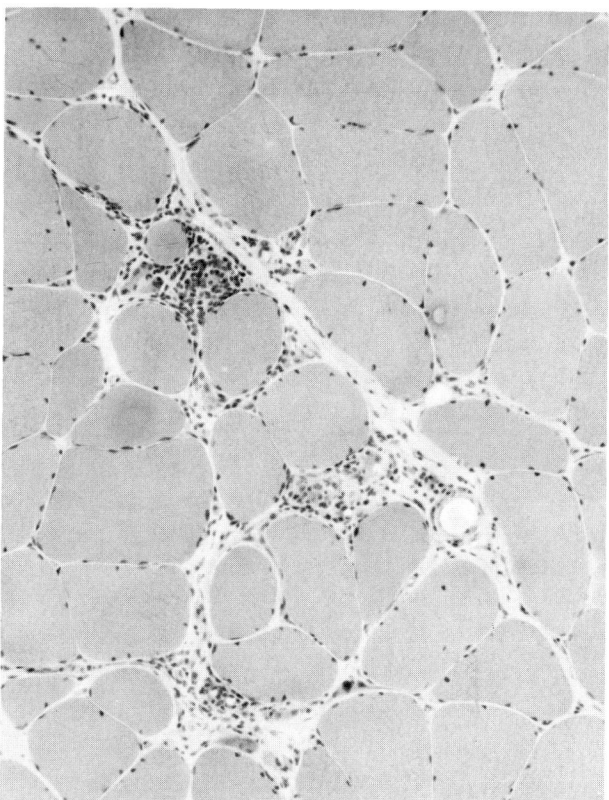

FIGURE 83.15 Facioscapulohumeral dystrophy. Cellular responses are noted in the biopsies from many patients with this illness. These are more often associated with necrotic fibers than with blood vessels. (Hematoxylin-eosin stain.)

An ankle-foot orthosis may be particularly beneficial for patients with a footdrop. Surgical transposition of the posterior tibial tendon to the dorsum of the foot is particularly useful in patients who have a marked intorsion of the foot when walking. The posterior tibial muscle remains relatively unaffected until very late in the illness. The posterior tibial tendon, in addition to its action of inversion, also dorsiflexes the foot. If patients have severe weakness of the anterior tibial group, overactivity of the posterior tibial muscle may be seen in an attempt to dorsiflex the foot and allow the toes to clear the ground. This results in marked inversion of the foot while walking and may lead to callus formation on the outer border of the foot. It also may make it impossible for the patient to use ankle-foot orthoses. Surgical transposition of the posterior tibial tendon to the dorsum of the foot can be a very effective reconstructive procedure, which may normalize the patient's walking. Prednisone has been tried in a small group of patients, but the results were not dramatic.

Scapuloperoneal Syndromes

There are a number of diseases in which weakness of the shoulder muscles and of the anterior compartment of the lower leg are the early symptoms. Some forms of scapuloperoneal dystrophy may be related to FSHD, but in others there was no linkage to the FSH site on 4q35. Further studies are needed in a larger population of patients with this symptom complex. In FSHD, there is a discrepancy between the strength of the ankle dorsiflexors, which are weak, and the plantar flexors, which are strong. The same is true of the scapuloperoneal syndrome, but facial weakness is only minor. Often, the patient presents with a footdrop, and shoulder weakness is found only on examination. The biopsy, EMG, and other laboratory tests are identical to those seen in FSH dystrophy in some cases but differ in others (Milanov and Ishpekova 1997). The disease may be inherited like an autosomal dominant trait, although an X-linked recessive pattern also has been described. The importance of differentiating this entity is simply that some patients with congenital nonprogressive diseases, such as nemaline myopathy, also may present with a scapuloperoneal distribution of weakness. It is therefore important to confirm the diagnosis with the appropriate tests in any patient with a scapuloperoneal syndrome. The only useful treatment is the application of ankle-foot orthoses, which may improve the patient's function by correcting the footdrop.

Distal Myopathies

Pathophysiology

There are several muscle diseases in which the pattern of weakness is distal, unlike the traditional proximal weakness that has come to be regarded as "myopathic." Classification of these illnesses is difficult. Some, such as Miyoshi's myopathy, are fairly clear-cut. Others seem to blend into each other and have features in common with the hereditary form of inclusion body myopathy, to which they may well be related. A proposal was made to classify the illnesses by their inheritance and whether they began late or early in life. Just when the picture seems clearer, another report appears of a patient with atypical features. The mechanism causing the weakness is not understood and awaits the discovery of the abnormal genes involved.

Miyoshi's Myopathy

Inherited as an autosomal recessive disease, Miyoshi's myopathy begins early, often in the teenage years (Bejaoui et al. 1995). The weakness is characteristically in the foot plantar flexors, with severe gastrocnemius atrophy. This causes a thin, tapering leg. Patients are unable to stand on their toes, and they walk up stairs in a clumsy, jerky fashion. The illness is progressive, although it remains confined to the legs. Ultimately, hip weakness develops and ambulation may become difficult in midlife. The serum CK concentration is extremely elevated, and levels of several thousand may be found even before the patient notices any symptoms. Originally described in the Japanese population, there are now several reports of this illness around the world. The illness has been linked to chromosome 2p12-14, which is the same location as one of the forms of LGMD. Families have been described in which some members exhibit a distal myopathy and others the more traditional proximal variety. The muscle biopsy shows dystrophic changes. In this variety there are no autophagic vacuoles.

Welander's Myopathy

Welander's myopathy was initially described in the Scandinavian population, where it is relatively common. Patients were affected for the first time between 40 and 60 years of age. The illness is inherited in an autosomal dominant fashion and begins in the hands, with later involvement of the legs and footdrop. The distal distribution may suggest a neuropathy, but the laboratory tests show little evidence of denervation and much evidence of a myopathy. Careful evaluation may show that there is, nevertheless, mild distal hypesthesia and temperature loss associated with some loss of small myelinated fibers, so that illness is not entirely restricted to the muscle. The muscle biopsy shows myopathic findings, superimposed on which are the rimmed vacuoles characteristic of several other distal myopathies. Serum CK concentration is normal or slightly elevated.

Other Distal Myopathies

Several other reports had initial findings of footdrop and anterior tibial weakness. Usually, the inheritance is autosomal dominant, and the illness begins in midlife or late adult life. Many patients do not notice their weakness, attributing it to the normal effects of aging. Muscle biopsy again shows the rimmed vacuoles. Another autosomal dominant distal disease has an earlier onset and is accompanied by neck flexor weakness, a feature that crops up in some other reports (Laing et al. 1995). A more severe variety of a distal myopathy is characterized by the storage of excess amounts of desmin (a protein associated with intermediate filaments in muscle), which appear as granulofilamentous material between the myofibrils and beneath the sarcolemma. In this family, the disease was autosomal dominant and began in the muscles of the lower leg. It spread rapidly, however, and involved arm, proximal trunk, respiratory, and bulbar muscles. Death occurred in the 40s and 50s from cardiorespiratory failure. A mother and daughter were reported with less severe disease (Ceuterick and Martin 1996). Cardiac abnormalities occur in many of the distal myopathies, although no systematic evaluation has been made. The clinician would be advised to be on the lookout for conduction abnormalities, and a periodic ECG may be helpful. Many of the illnesses described earlier in the chapter are on the borderland between the distal myopathies and the hereditary inclusion body myopathies; clarification of this issue awaits more certain knowledge of molecular pathogenetics. The recent finding that both the recessive form of distal myopathy and hereditary inclusion body myopathy link to the same locus reinforces this impression and leads to the suspicion that these diseases may be allelic.

Diagnosis

Myotonic dystrophy and the hereditary form of inclusion body myopathy also affect distal muscles more severely than proximal muscles. Hereditary neuropathies usually affect the peroneal muscles first and more severely, whereas in the distal myopathies with anterior compartment weakness, the anterior tibial tendon is most affected. The muscle biopsy may be fairly characteristic in some of these entities. CK is usually normal or shows mild-to-moderate elevation. In the Miyoshi form of disease, CK levels 10 times normal and higher are seen.

Treatment

Treatment of distal myopathy is largely symptomatic. In a patient with a severe wrist drop, a cock-up splint may be helpful to preserve hand function. Similarly, an ankle-foot orthosis may treat the footdrop.

Oculopharyngeal Dystrophy

Pathophysiology

Oculopharyngeal dystrophy is another illness with an uneven geographical distribution, although it is now being recognized worldwide. It is an inherited autosomal dominant disorder, with almost complete penetrance. Foci of the illness have been noted in Quebec; Montevideo, Uruguay; Germany; and the Spanish-American populations of Colorado, New Mexico, and Arizona. Isolated families have been described throughout the rest of the world. A hallmark of the illness is the presence of small intranuclear tubulofilaments. These occur as palisading filamentous inclusions. Nuclei may be packed with these small tubular filaments, which are approximately 8 nm in diameter. The filaments are unbranched and may be stacked side by side or may occur in tangles. Their origin is not known. A feature common to this illness, inclusion body myositis, and distal myopathy is the occurrence of rimmed autophagic vacuoles. Other features are also shared, such as the presence of amyloid, although this is a minor finding compared with its occurrence in inclusion body myopathy. Other reports suggest that there may be mitochondrial abnormalities in the illness. The disease has now been linked to chromosome 14q11.2-13 in several ethnically different families (Stajich et al. 1996), and the gene has recently been identified as producing poly A binding protein 2 (PAB2). It is localized to the nucleus and is involved in messenger RNA polyadenylation (Brais et al. 1998).

Clinical Features

Oculopharyngeal dystrophy begins at 30–40 years of age, with weakness of the eye muscles and mild ptosis. The ptosis may be quite asymmetrical initially, but eventually, as the muscles weaken, both lids become severely ptotic, and eye movements are diminished in all directions (Figure 83.16). There is considerable variation in the severity of the extraocular palsies, but ptosis is uniformly seen. Concomitant with or shortly after the development of ocular symptoms, patients notice difficulty with swallowing. Saliva pools in the pharynx, and at the extreme stages of the illness, it may be impossible for the patient to swallow anything. Muscle weakness is not limited to the eye. Facial weakness is seen in a number of patients, and hip and shoulder weakness is common in the late stages. Death occurs from emaciation and starvation. The terminal event is often pneumonia initiated by aspiration of secretions. Although the symptoms associated with the disease may be severe, patients' life spans may not be shortened, making the management of their nutritional status all the more important.

Diagnosis

Initially, laboratory tests should be used to differentiate oculopharyngeal dystrophy from other possible diagnoses.

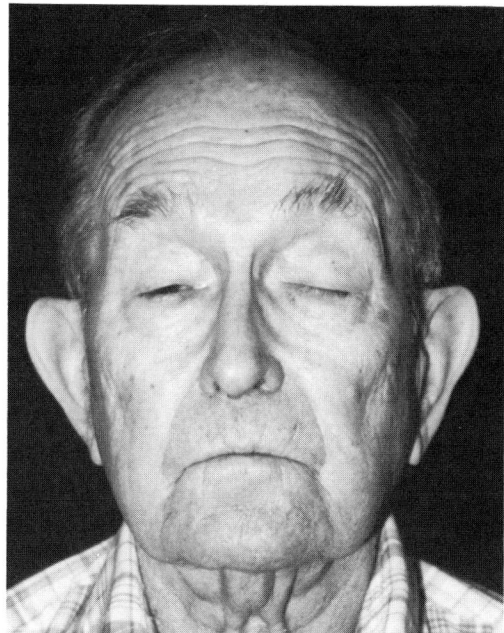

FIGURE 83.16   Oculopharyngeal dystrophy. The facial appearance of a patient who has ptosis and no eye movements.

Thus, repetitive nerve stimulation tests for abnormal fatigue of the evoked potential, as might be seen in myasthenia gravis, and the administration of edrophonium intravenously (Tensilon test) are important. The definitive tests are the demonstration of the genetic abnormality and the abnormal intranuclear filaments. Muscle biopsy shows the usual dystrophic findings, a random variation in the size of the fibers, necrotic fibers, some fibrosis, and occasional internal nuclei. In addition, autophagic vacuoles (rimmed vacuoles) are noted in the fibers (Figure 83.17), a feature common to this illness as well as to inclusion body myositis and hereditary distal myopathy.

Treatment

As in most of the muscular dystrophies, treatment of oculopharyngeal dystrophy is supportive. The swallowing difficulties may be treated first by a soft diet; pureed foods represent the next step in treatment. Feeding with a nasogastric tube may be a temporary solution, but a gastrostomy ultimately is needed. Surgery to correct the ptosis may be very successful, as opposed to the results seen in other causes of ptosis, such as myasthenia or Kearns-Sayre syndrome.

Congenital Muscular Dystrophies

CMD are a group of diseases that often appear at birth with hypotonia and severe trunk and limb weakness. Contractures of the joints are prominent, particularly at the ankles, knees, and hips. Mental retardation may be present, and magnetic resonance imaging (MRI) of the head shows a

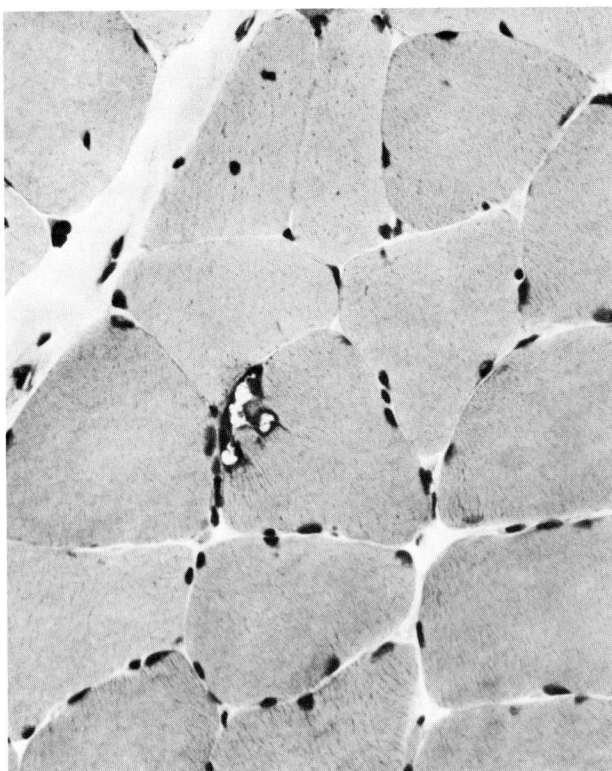

FIGURE 83.17 Oculopharyngeal dystrophy. Rimmed vacuoles are commonly seen in this illness. (Hematoxylin-eosin stain.)

striking increase in the signal from the white matter in many patients. Four groups of CMD are distinguished that are more or less clinically characterized, although the final sorting will have to wait for their genetic and molecular characterization. All are autosomal recessive in their inheritance, and all have a greater or lesser involvement of nervous tissue. The entities are merosin deficiency, Fukuyama type muscular dystrophy, Walker-Warburg disease, and muscle-eye-brain disease of Santavuori. There is an ongoing debate about how distinct these entities are, but, at least, Fukuyama type muscular dystrophy and merosin deficiency are distinct.

Laminin α₂ (Merosin) Deficiency

Laminin α_2, formerly known as merosin, is one of a large family of glycosylated proteins that is found in the basement membrane. It is made of three dissimilar chains: α_2, β_1, and γ_1. The amino termini separate to form a crosslike structure, and the other end of the molecule attaches to the dystroglycan complex. In the human, it is coded by a gene on chromosome 6. Laminin α_2 is found in muscle as well as skin and nerve. The fact that a deficiency of the laminin α_2 chain was found in the *dy/dy* mouse helped to explain a feature that had long puzzled researchers. This animal, a model for muscular dystrophy, had marked changes in both muscle and peripheral nerve. A report

describing laminin α_2 deficiency in children shifted the emphasis to a group of human muscle diseases that also have involvement of muscle and nervous tissue. CMDs have their onset in infancy. The hallmarks of the disease include severe weakness of trunk and limbs and hypotonia at birth. Extraocular muscles and face are usually spared. There are often prominent contractures of the feet and hips. Mental retardation may be found, and a striking MRI finding is increased signal from the white matter on T2-weighted images. Apart from occipital agyria, the structural defects characteristic of the other forms are not seen. For the most part, these children are severely disabled and many remain dependent on their caregivers for their whole lives. In 50% of cases, studies have shown an absence of laminin α_2 chain in the muscle. Laboratory studies reveal an elevated serum CK concentration, which is characteristic of any of the muscle diseases with membrane instability. EMG, in addition to demonstrating abnormalities in the muscle, also shows slowed nerve conduction velocities, as might be expected from the expression of laminin α_2 in the nerve tissue.

Milder forms of the illness are also noted with delayed onset and mild weakness (Tan et al. 1997). An absence of the protein is likely to cause marked destruction of muscle, but partial deficiencies have been found in which the symptoms are less severe. Again, this situation is akin to that seen in dystrophin deficiency. The diagnosis depends on the demonstration of an alteration of laminin α_2 in the muscle. Commercial antibodies are available for this purpose, but not all antibodies demonstrate the abnormality, particularly if part of the laminin α_2 chain is present. As in dystrophin deficiency, it may be advantageous to use at least two different antibodies. The diagnosis may be made from a skin biopsy rather than a muscle biopsy because laminin α_2 is expressed in the skin. Ultimately, the diagnosis rests on the demonstration of an abnormality in the gene on chromosome 6 because laminin α_2 may also be reduced as a secondary phenomenon in some of the other myopathies with membrane instability.

There are patients with identical symptoms who have neither an abnormality in the laminin α_2 gene nor any abnormality in the muscle protein. Many are without nervous system damage and have no clinical evidence of mental retardation or other central nervous system abnormalities (Figure 83.18). Lucencies may also be seen in these children on computed tomography (CT) scan of the head. Frequently, the muscle symptoms are milder, and, perhaps because there is no intellectual handicap, these children gain function as they grow older and may walk independently. The illness is either nonprogressive or slowly progressive. Parents are often mistakenly advised not to expect their child to survive beyond 10 years. Although survival may be compromised in these patients, many survive to adult life. The underlying cause of the abnormality in this group of children remains to be elucidated.

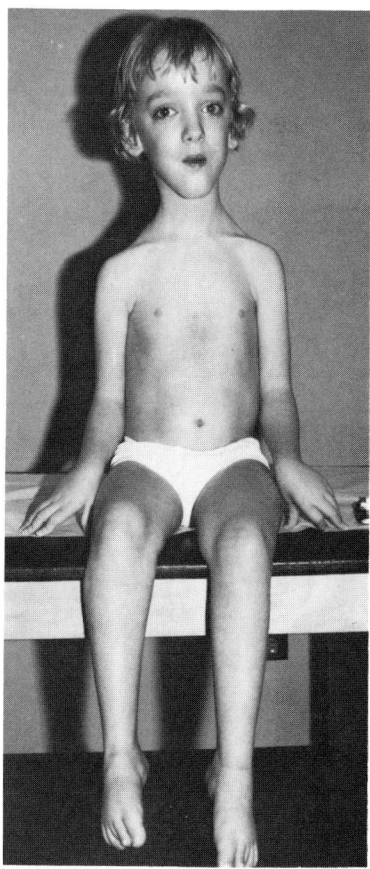

FIGURE 83.18   Congenital muscular dystrophy (non-Fukuyama type). This boy also had weakness and contractures of the limbs. His illness was relatively static. He had no mental retardation. Notice the similarity in facial appearance to the patient in Figure 83.19 even though these two children are unrelated.

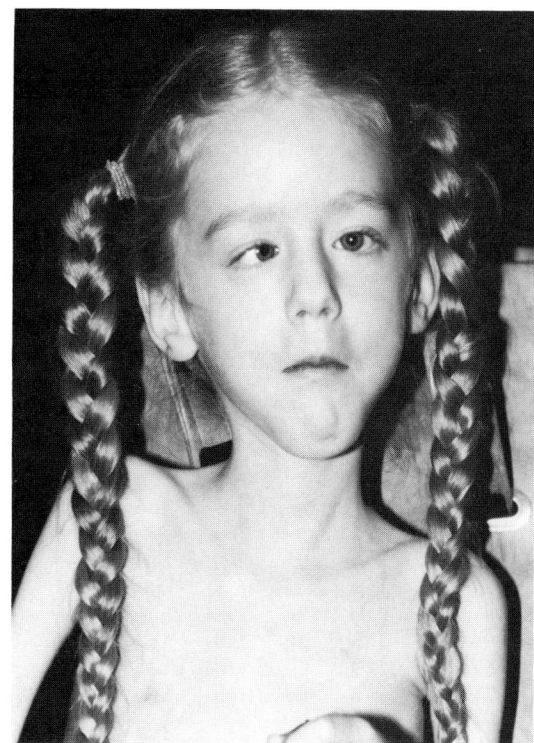

FIGURE 83.19   Congenital muscular dystrophy (Fukuyama type). This girl was severely retarded, had many seizures, and demonstrated marked contractures of the limbs. She was too weak to support her own weight. The disease was nonprogressive. Her two brothers also had the same illness.

Fukuyama Type Muscular Dystrophy, Walker-Warburg Disease, and Muscle-Eye-Brain Disease

Fukuyama type muscular dystrophy, Walker-Warburg disease, and muscle-eye-brain disease are confusing to the clinician because in many ways they seem to overlap, but increasing information about the genetics and the molecular abnormalities will, in time, reveal whether they are three distinct diseases or not (Leyten et al. 1996). All are characterized by a combination of muscle disease and central nervous system disease. The best known is the Fukuyama type.

Fukuyama Type Muscular Dystrophy.   Fukuyama type muscular dystrophy, like the other congenital dystrophies, is inherited as an autosomal recessive disease. The underlying mechanism of the illness is still uncertain, but the gene has been localized to chromosome 9q31-33. Laminin α_2 abnormalities have been described but cannot be the primary deficiency because the gene for that protein is on chromosome 6.

Clinical Features.   The children are usually normal at birth. Some are floppy, and joint contractures are present in 70% of the patients by the age of 3 months, with the hip, knee, and ankle commonly involved. The children often are severely mentally retarded, sometimes to the extent that speech is never developed and convulsions, either major motor seizures or petit mal, are common (Figure 83.19). Another curious finding is asymmetry of the skull, often noted on clinical examination. Testing these children for muscle strength is almost impossible, but weakness is diffuse and often disabling, so that the child never learns to walk. Weakness of the face and neck has been noted. Usually, these children are completely dependent on their parents and never attain any degree of unsupervised activity. The muscle disease is moderately or slowly progressive, and survival into early adult life is common.

Diagnosis.   Laboratory studies are helpful. The serum CK concentration usually is markedly elevated. The muscle biopsy shows dystrophic changes, with variability in the size of fibers and fibrosis. Internal nuclei are common, and the biopsy easily distinguishes this disorder from any of the congenital nonprogressive myopathies and from acquired illnesses, such as polymyositis. The Fukuyama variant does not resemble DMD, and the only real difficulty is in differentiating it from some of the other forms of congenital dystrophy. As in the other congenital dystrophies, muscle biopsy may be unusual and demonstrate changes that are

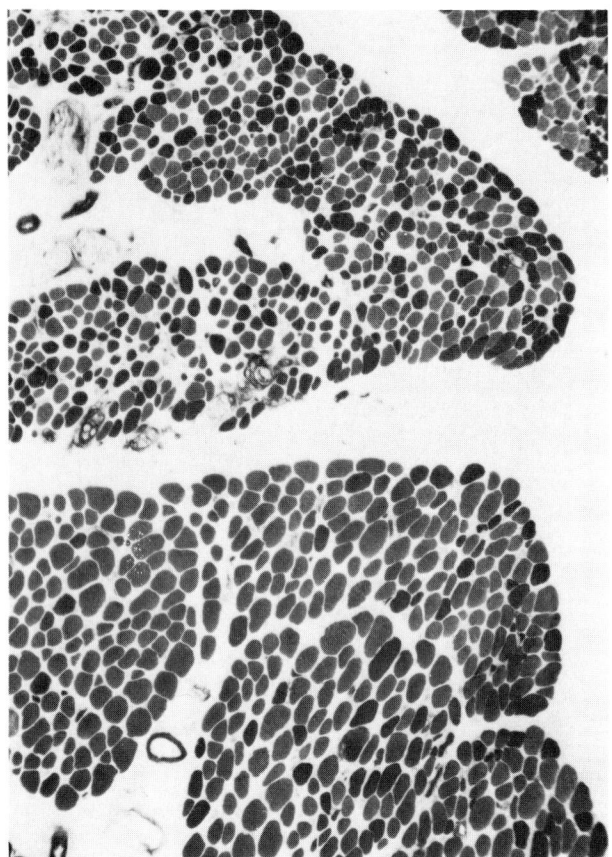

FIGURE 83.20   A biopsy from Fukuyama-type congenital muscular dystrophy. In addition to the variability in fiber size and the type 1 fiber predominance with fibrosis, notice the nonrandom distribution of atrophy. The fascicle in the lower part of the picture contains larger fibers than that in the upper part. (Myosin adenosine triphosphatase stain, pH 9.4.)

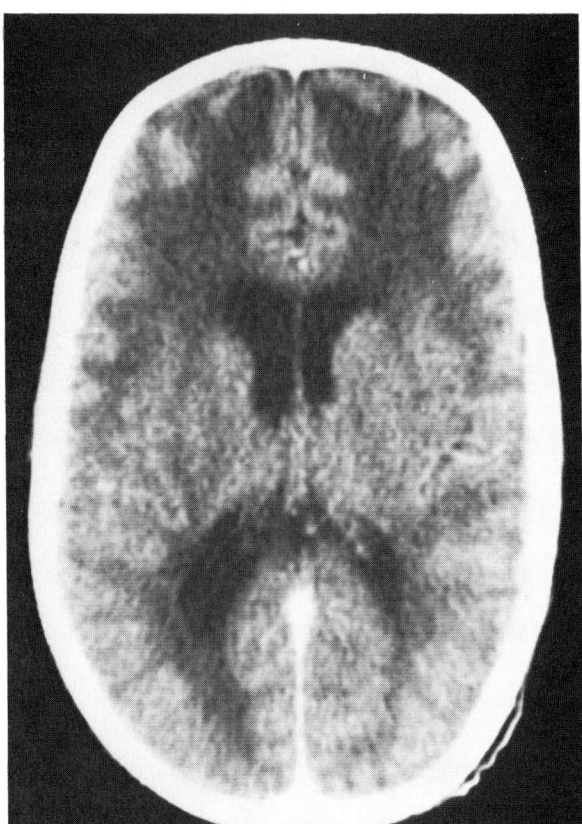

FIGURE 83.21   Computed tomographic scan of the head of a patient with Fukuyama muscular dystrophy demonstrating lucencies in the white matter, particularly toward the frontal poles.

interpreted as indicating an additional neurogenic component. The changes in fiber size may not be random, and some fascicles contain much smaller fibers than others do. This nonrandom change differs from denervation atrophy, in which there is a wide, random variability in the size of the fibers within the individual fascicles (Figure 83.20).

CT scans show a variety of abnormalities, but the most striking is the presence of lucencies, particularly in the frontal area (Figure 83.21). These changes seldom extend to the genu of the corpus callosum and spare the medial subependymal regions along the trigones and occipital horns. As the children grow older, these lucencies disappear in sequence from the occipital to the frontal region in a fashion resembling the progression of normal myelination. No explanation for the lucencies has been found. Occasionally, marked pallor of the myelin in the centrum semiovale has been noted, together with mild gliosis or edema. At autopsy, numerous brain malformations have been found, with agyria, pachygyria, and microgyria. There may be a cobblestone appearance to the cortex. There is an absence of lamination in the gray matter, with other abnormal cytoarchitecture. Heterotopias of the brainstem and basal meninges have been described, as has micropolygyria of the cerebellum. Ventricular dilatation, enlarged sulci, and aqueductal stenosis also have been noted. In short, there are marked abnormalities in the architecture of the brain.

Walker-Warburg Syndrome and Muscle-Eye-Brain Disease. The Walker-Warburg syndrome and the related muscle-eye-brain disease are characterized by the combination of muscular dystrophy, lissencephaly, cerebellar malformations, and severe retinal and eye malformations. Both are associated with more severe eye abnormalities than is Fukuyama type muscular dystrophy. Walker-Warburg is the more catastrophic disease, with death often occurring within the first 2 years. The eye changes are also more severe in Walker-Warburg, with microphthalmia, colobomas, congenital cataracts and glaucoma, corneal opacities, retinal dysplasia and nonattachment, hypoplastic vitreous, and optic atrophy. In muscle-eye-brain disease, a milder illness, high myopia is seen and possibly a preretinal membrane or gliosis, but the severe structural abnormalities of the eye are not present. The central nervous system findings are also different, and MRI may be a useful technique to separate the entities (van der Knaap et al. 1997). The changes in Walker-Warburg syndrome are more severe, with various combinations of hydrocephalus, aqueductal stenosis, cerebellar and pontine hypoplasia with a small posterior vermis, Dandy-Walker malformations, and an agyric or pachygyric cobblestone cortex. T1-weighted images show diffuse decreased white matter signal; T2-weighted images show an increased signal compatible with a defect in myelination. In muscle-eye-brain disease, white matter changes are more focal and the cortical changes milder. It is not yet certain how distinct the diseases are, but laminin α_2 was reported as preserved in muscle-eye-brain disease, which is distinct from both Walker-Warburg and Fukuyama type muscular dystrophy. Muscle-eye-brain disease is genetically distinct from Fukuyama type muscular dystrophy because linkage of the gene to chromosome 9 was excluded. One family had some members with the Fukuyama phenotype and some who appeared to have Walker-Warburg disease, with the disease localizing to chromosome 9q31-33. This suggests that the two entities were allelic, but further proof is needed.

Ocular Weakness and Dystrophies

Ocular dystrophies were described in older literature. Most patients who appear to have a form of dystrophy limited to the eye muscles are later found to have a more diffuse disease, such as oculopharyngeal dystrophy or Kearns-Sayre syndrome. The typical mitochondrial DNA deletion of Kearns-Sayre syndrome has been found in patients whose illness is limited to a chronic progressive external ophthalmoplegia. When an ocular dystrophy is suspected, it is important to rule out congenital myasthenic syndromes, hyperthyroid disease, and myasthenia gravis.

Kearns-Sayre Syndrome

Pathophysiology

A group of disorders known as the *mitochondrial myopathies* is caused by several different defects in respiratory chain function. The group includes Kearns-Sayre syndrome, other disorders of oxidative muscle metabolism with exercise intolerance, myoclonus epilepsy with ragged-red fibers, and mitochondrial encephalopathy associated with lactic acidosis and strokelike episodes. Most of these present with neurological complaints and are not discussed here. Kearns-Sayre syndrome is, however, likely to be seen first in the muscle clinic. Commonly, the illness is due to a large deletion in the mitochondrial DNA. Cells have many mitochondria, and not all the mitochondria are abnormal (heteroplasmy). The severity of the symptoms may depend as much on the ratio of mitochondria with deletions to wild-type (normal) mitochondria as it does on the number of abnormal mitochondria. Unlike some of the other mitochondrial diseases,

Kearns-Sayre syndrome is almost always a sporadic disease and not familial.

Clinical Features

Patients with Kearns-Sayre syndrome share common features but may differ widely in the severity of their symptoms and disability. The most striking feature is the development of a progressive external ophthalmoplegia. This may start in childhood or in adult life and progress to total immobility of the eyes. Associated with the ophthalmoplegia is retinitis pigmentosa, which may be difficult to see in the early stages because the pigment may be localized to the periphery of the retina and a mydriatic examination may be necessary for full visualization. The third feature is the presence of mitochondrial abnormalities in striated muscle and other tissues. Many patients have a moderate degree of weakness, and more patients complain of fatigue and sometimes pain with continued exertion. Other systems are also involved. Abnormalities in the nervous system may result in signs of spasticity with increased reflexes. Cerebellar incoordination is common, and nerve deafness may be noted. Endocrine abnormalities as diverse as hypoparathyroidism and dysmenorrhea have been reported. In children with the early and more severe form of the illness, mental retardation is associated with short stature. Cardiac conduction defects are common and may result in sudden death. For this reason, regular ECGs are recommended, and a pacemaker may be needed as the illness progresses.

Diagnosis

Laboratory studies are directed toward demonstrating widespread abnormalities. Muscle histochemistry is a useful screening tool. The presence of numerous ragged-red fibers in the trichrome stain against a background of relatively normal muscle is highly suggestive of the condition (Figure 83.22). It should be emphasized that ragged-red fibers also are seen in other diseases, although not in such quantities. Electron microscopic studies show bizarre distortions of the mitochondria. The biopsy may reveal scattered fibers that lack glycogen and cytochrome oxidase. Analysis of the mitochondrial DNA is important. Even though the typical clinical picture associated with ragged-red fibers in the biopsy makes the diagnosis apparent in many patients, there are some with few pathological changes and even normal biochemistry. Evidence of a defect in mitochondrial function may be found in high resting serum lactate levels. Cerebrospinal fluid protein is elevated, and plasma and cerebrospinal fluid folate levels have been reported as reduced.

In its fully developed form, the illness is unmistakable. When only some aspects of the illness are noted, they may be mistaken for other forms of chronic progressive external ophthalmoplegia. In Leigh disease, lactic acidosis is associated with a number of neurological problems, including deafness, blindness, ataxia, muscular weakness, and hypotonia.

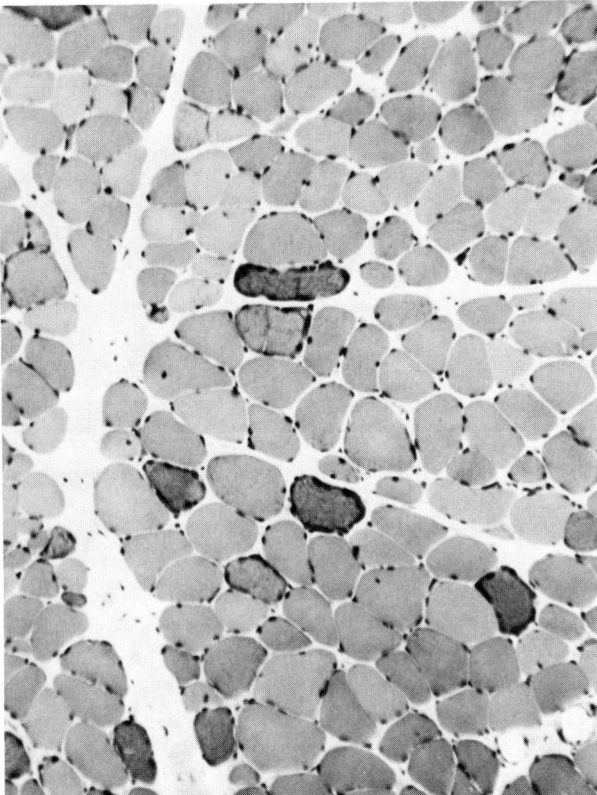

FIGURE 83.22   Kearns-Sayre syndrome. Typical appearance of the ragged-red fibers seen in the biopsy. Electron microscopy shows these fibers to be packed with abnormal mitochondria. (Modified Gomori trichrome stain.)

In Leigh disease, however, the ophthalmoplegia is unusual. Reye's syndrome (acute hepato-encephalopathy) is associated with elevations of blood ammonia and lactate. Kearns-Sayre syndrome sometimes may be associated with encephalopathic episodes, in which case it may be difficult to distinguish Kearns-Sayre from Reye's syndrome. Such episodes, however, are less common in Kearns-Sayre syndrome.

Treatment

Thiamine, folate, riboflavin, carnitine, ubiquinone, and the folate precursor methionine have been used but have not shown any uniform clinical benefit.

Other Muscular Dystrophies

Sometimes, very unusual forms of muscle disease are noted. They are mentioned here simply to allow the reader to share the general bewilderment as to their origin. Occasionally, a muscle disease that is clearly demonstrated to be myopathic by biopsy and EMG affects only one muscle or one limb. There are recurrent reports of such an illness affecting the quadriceps. Over a long period, other muscle

groups may become weak. This entity is best thought of as being a restricted variant of one of the other dystrophies or of inclusion body myositis; analysis of the biopsy for inclusions and muscle proteins or examination of other family members can clarify the situation. In branchial myopathy, there is enlargement of the masseter and temporalis muscles sufficient to make it difficult for the patient to wear glasses and causing a disfiguring lump over the angle of the jaw. This is not associated with any weakness. Treatment is difficult because simple resection of the muscle often is followed by recurrence of the muscle growth. Muscular hypertrophy also may be seen in other muscles. Sometimes, this occurs in response to denervation, but occasionally there is true hypertrophy of a single muscle, such as the gastrocnemius—a feature often noted in carriers of DMD.

Myotonic Dystrophy

Pathophysiology

Myotonic dystrophy is a muscle disorder characterized by muscle wasting and weakness associated with myotonia and a number of other systemic abnormalities. It is an inherited autosomal dominant disorder with an incidence of approximately 1 per 8,000 live births. It is one of the more common neuromuscular disorders. The gene is located on the chromosome 19q13.3. The genetic abnormality is unusual. A section of the gene in which there are repeating sequences of three nucleotides (CTG trinucleotide repeats) expands until the number of repeats exceeds the normal five to 30 to become hundreds or even thousands. The gene structure suggests that it encodes a serine threonine protein kinase. This would make sense because these kinases often play a role in the cell's signaling mechanisms, in the control of ion channels, and in the activation of second-messenger systems. The gene product is ubiquitously expressed in muscle and other tissues, such as the lens in the eye. Various studies have localized it to the neuromuscular junction and myotendinous junction, the sarcolemma, and the perinuclear region. In experimental animals, the myotonic dystrophy protein kinase gene (DMPK) does have an effect on the skeletal (but not cardiac) voltage-gated sodium channels. It decreases the peak sodium current. Other experiments indicate a higher intracellular calcium concentration in cells with an abnormality in the flux through the L-type calcium channel. However, the expansion is not in the coding region of the gene, and other experiments with knockout mice or mice that overexpress the protein show no marked abnormality in the muscle or other systems. This has led to the suggestion that the effect of the mutation is to alter the expression of one of the other adjacent genes. One candidate gene that flanks the DMPK gene is DMAHP. The expression of this gene is decreased in muscle, myoblasts, and heart when the DM expansion is introduced into the DNA (Thornton et al. 1997). The function of the *DMAHP* gene product is not yet clarified. In general, the size of the expansion is reflected in the severity of the illness. Children with severe congenital myotonic dystrophy may have very large expansions (>750 repeats). Mothers with more than 100 repeats are more at risk for having a child with the severe infantile form than are mothers with a smaller expansion. The phenomenon of anticipation, in which succeeding generations experience the illness earlier and more severely, is explained by the tendency of the expansion to grow with each meiosis. The reverse is true of some rare patients with paternally inherited myotonic dystrophy, in which the expansion is reduced, and the clinical state may return to normal or be very mild. The issue of relating the severity of the phenotype to the genetic defect is further complicated by the fact that the degree of the gene's expansion may vary among the different tissues in the body.

Clinical Features

Myotonia is demonstrated either by sharp percussion of the muscle with a reflex hammer or after firm voluntary contraction. Either maneuver elicits a sustained, involuntary contraction of the muscle, which fades slowly over a matter of seconds. Percussion of the thenar eminence, a popular way of eliciting myotonia, produces a sharp abduction of the thumb and a firm contraction of the thenar eminence, which gradually relaxes and allows the thumb to return to the resting position. It is often easier to demonstrate percussion myotonia if the posterior muscles of the forearm are percussed. The normal response to percussion of the forearm is also a brisk contraction of the finger extensors or the wrist extensors, but the wrist or fingers then fall into the resting position without delay. In the myotonic patient, there is a sharp extension of the fingers with a subsequent drift downward, toward the normal position, or even wrist extension that is maintained for some seconds. Patients seldom complain spontaneously about myotonia. When questioned, patients may confess to difficulty releasing a key after it has been firmly grasped or letting go of a hammer or vacuum cleaner, particularly in cold weather.

Few diseases are as easy to recognize as myotonic dystrophy once the diagnosis is considered. Conversely, the diagnosis frequently is missed because the presenting complaint may be apparently unrelated to the basic problem. Patients with myotonic dystrophy may be referred for evaluation of mental retardation, present themselves in the emergency room with fractures, or appear on the ward because they did not recuperate after cholecystectomy. The severity of myotonic dystrophy ranges from mild weakness in some adults to profound mental retardation and severe weakness in children.

The more typical picture is of an illness beginning in early teenage life, starting with noticeable weakness of the hands and often footdrop. Myotonic dystrophy is one of the rare forms of dystrophy that seems to affect the distal

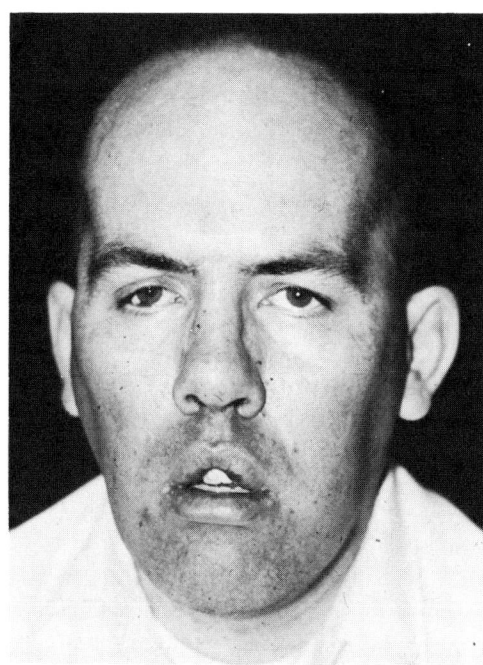

FIGURE 83.23 Myotonic dystrophy. The facial appearance includes ptosis, hollowing of the masseter and temples, and facial weakness.

muscles more severely. There is also a predilection for neck muscle involvement, and the sternocleidomastoid muscles are often atrophic and poorly defined. A rather long face with a mournful expression is accentuated by the hollowing of the temples associated with masseter and temporalis atrophy. In the fully developed disease, the eyes are hooded and the mouth slack and often tented (Figure 83.23). The muscular weakness is not limited to the distal muscles; shoulder, hip, and leg weakness may be quite prominent.

In middle age, repeated falls are common. As time goes by and the weakness of individual muscles becomes severe, the myotonia may be lost. It is not surprising to find a patient with advanced disease who has no myotonia of the small muscles of the hand, although there is pronounced myotonia of the deltoids or forearm muscles. The voice is also altered; it may be hollow and echoing, suggesting palatal weakness. The facial weakness makes it difficult to pronounce consonants. Difficulty in swallowing is common but usually a minor complaint. Recurrent dislocation of the jaw may be seen, particularly when the patient attempts to open the mouth wide, as in biting an apple.

Cardiac disease is a well-known complication of myotonic dystrophy, understanding of which has been increased by recent advances in both molecular techniques and cardiological investigations. Conduction disturbances and tachyarrhythmias occur commonly in myotonic dystrophy. These have been shown to have a broad correlation in severity with both neuromuscular disease and the extent of the molecular defect in some, but not all, studies. Clinical evidence of generalized cardiomyopathy is unusual. The rate of progression differs widely between individuals; sudden death may be caused by ventricular arrhythmias or by complete heart block, and this can occur at an early stage of disease. A familial tendency toward cardiac complications has been shown in some studies. The histopathology is of fibrosis (primarily in the conducting system and sinoatrial node), myocyte hypertrophy, and fatty infiltration. Electron microscopy shows prominent I-bands and myofibrillar degeneration. Myotonin protein kinase, the primary product of the myotonic dystrophy gene, may be located at the intercalated discs and have a different isoform in cardiac tissue. The role of other genes or the normal myotonic dystrophy allele in myotonic heart disease has yet to be determined. Finally, myotonic dystrophy should be considered in previously undiagnosed patients presenting to a cardiologist or general physician with suspected arrhythmia or conduction block.

Cardiac involvement is almost the rule in advanced myotonic dystrophy. There is often a conduction defect, and tachyarrhythmias are seen in more than one-half of patients. A more serious problem may be noted on radionuclide studies of cardiac function. After relatively mild exercise, the ventricular wall may balloon outward, and the ventricular ejection fraction decreases. This type of cardiomyopathy has been blamed for the frequent occurrence of sudden death in patients with myotonic dystrophy, although clinical symptoms of overt cardiomyopathy are uncommon, and sudden death is more likely to be due to ventricular arrhythmias. Postmortem studies show fibrosis, fatty infiltration, and myocyte hypertrophy (Phillips and Harper 1997). Suggestions for clinical management include a careful cardiac history and a 12-lead ECG at least every year, with a low threshold for use of 24-hour Holter monitoring. General anesthetic carries some risks, and the occurrence of complications, usually respiratory, was almost 10% in one series (Mathieu et al. 1997).

Somnolence is a common problem in the adult with myotonia. The uncontrollable urge to sleep may be mistaken for narcolepsy and is accompanied by a disturbance of the nighttime sleep pattern. Patients have been shown to have an abnormal central ventilatory response, with an absence of the usual hyperpnea, produced by an increasing carbon dioxide concentration. This is associated with an abnormal sensitivity to barbiturates, morphine, and other drugs that depress the ventilatory drive. Anesthesiologists should be made aware of the possibility of complications with these drugs.

A number of other organs are also commonly involved in the disease. Cataracts are almost universal, although slit-lamp examination may be needed to detect them. Commonly, multihued specks are found in the anterior and posterior subcapsular zones. Endocrine abnormalities include disturbances of the thyroid, pancreas, hypothalamus, and gonads. Testicular atrophy, with the disappearance of the seminiferous tubules, leads to infertility in the male. In the female, habitual abortion and menstrual irregularities are found. Although frank diabetes mellitus is probably no more common in the myotonic population than in any other population, a glucose tolerance test is often associated with abnormally high glucose levels, particularly late in the test. An overproduction of insulin has been associated with this finding and seems to be due to abnormal resistance of the insulin receptor. Smooth muscle involvement accounts for a number of problems. Cholecystitis and symptoms referable to gallbladder function are frequent. As noted, there is mild difficulty with swallowing, and peristalsis in the hypopharynx and the proximal esophagus is decreased. Patients often complain of constipation and urinary tract symptoms.

Diagnosis

DNA analysis is the definitive test for myotonic dystrophy and should be obtained from patients who have clinical evidence of the illness and from individuals at risk. Prenatal diagnosis is reliable and uses chorionic villus biopsies or cultured amniotic cells. The most helpful, simple laboratory study is the EMG. In addition to the presence of myopathic features, the characteristic myotonic discharges are seen (see Chapter 37B). On insertion of the needle, bursts of repetitive potentials are noted. These potentials wax and wane in both amplitude and frequency; when played over a loudspeaker, they resemble the sound of a diving airplane and therefore have been called "dive bomber" or "motorcycle" potentials. The muscle biopsy in the fully developed illness is markedly abnormal (Figures 83.24 and 83.25), demonstrating random variability in the size of fibers and fibrosis. In addition, multiple nuclei are peppered throughout the interior of the fibers. Ring fibers are numerous, in which small bundles of myofibrils are oriented at 90 degrees to the majority, rather like a thread wrapped around a stick. Other laboratory studies are less helpful. Serum muscle enzymes are often abnormal. Some patients demonstrate low levels of immunoglobulin G. Abnormalities seen on head MRI include cerebral atrophy, increased white matter signals on T2-weighted images, and thickening of the cranial vault (Miaux et al. 1997). These abnormalities seem to have little significance.

Treatment

Supportive treatment of myotonic dystrophy includes the use of ankle-foot orthoses to treat the footdrop. Wrist splints are less useful. In theory, they should give added function to the hand, but most myotonic patients prefer not to use them. Breathing exercises and postural drainage can be helpful in severe myotonia to ward off the frequent respiratory infections. Drugs such as quinine, phenytoin, procainamide, mexiletine, and acetazolamide have been used to treat the myotonia. Their lack of effect in a clinical situation is due mainly to the fact that the myotonic patient is not bothered by the myotonia but only by the weakness. Alleviating the myotonia does nothing to change this weakness. Mexiletine

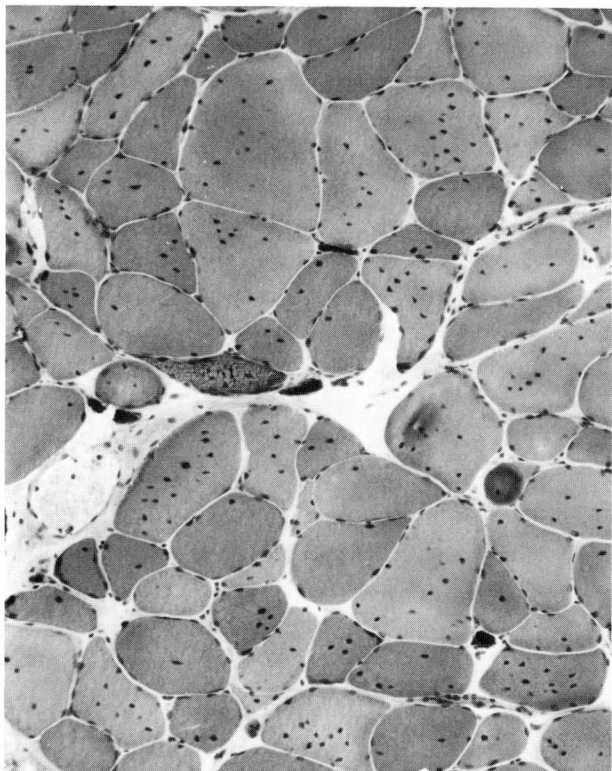

FIGURE 83.24   Myotonic dystrophy. There are numerous internal nuclei, some scattered pyknotic nuclear clumps, and marked variability in the size of fibers. One ring fiber can be identified by its circular, dark-staining appearance. (Hematoxylin-eosin stain.)

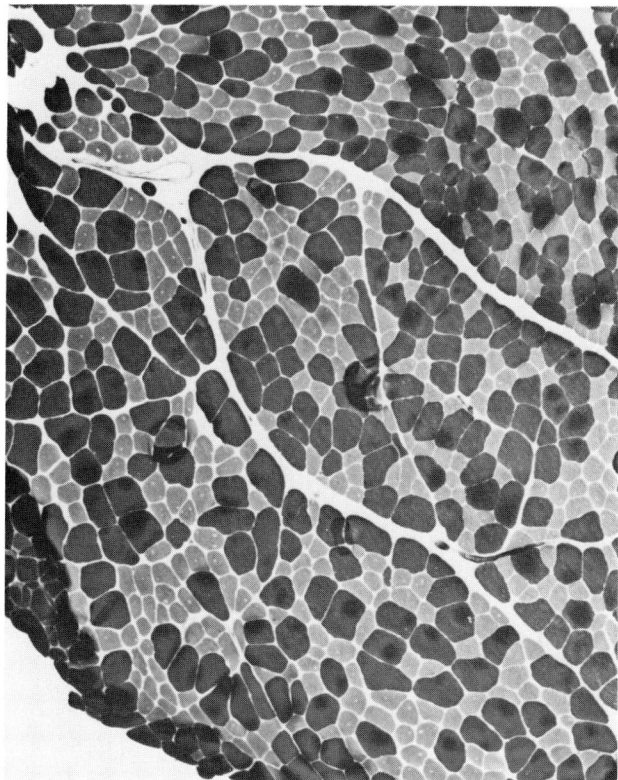

FIGURE 83.25   Myotonic dystrophy. This myosin adenosine triphosphatase stain at pH 9.4 demonstrates that the majority of type 1 fibers are small. Type 1 fiber atrophy is noted in early cases and is obscured as the disease becomes more severe.

has been tried in myotonic dystrophy but does not have the dramatic response seen in myotonia congenita.

Genetic Counseling

Once a patient has been identified as having myotonic dystrophy, it is important to examine all other members of the family and obtain DNA studies. The disorder is one of autosomal dominant inheritance with a strong penetrance. A curious problem makes genetic counseling less effective than it might be. Some people with quite marked disease can receive full genetic counseling but pay little attention to it. There is an element of denial of the illness that is distinctly different from that seen in other muscle diseases. Many affected family members do not seem to know they have the illness, including some family members who have been seen in the muscle clinic.

Congenital Myotonic Dystrophy

Congenital myotonic dystrophy may express itself in the newborn, almost always in infants of myotonic mothers. There may be extreme hypotonia and facial paralysis with failure to thrive and feeding difficulties. The children are prone to frequent respiratory infections, which may develop

into pneumonia. The upper lip forms an inverted V or "shark mouth" (Figure 83.26). Club feet are common, and the children are severely mentally retarded. The cause of the neonatal illness is the marked increase in the trinucleotide repeat region that seems to occur with maternal transmission, particularly if the mother has a sizable expansion herself.

Proximal Myotonic Myopathy

With the arrival of DNA testing it is now possible to say that there are forms of myotonic illness that, although bearing a superficial resemblance to myotonic dystrophy, are not that disease (Moxley 1996). Nor are they linked to any of the known channel defects. Whereas myotonic dystrophy's damage tends to be most severe in the distal muscles, patients with proximal myotonic myopathy experience stiffness, pain, and weakness more proximally. Like myotonic dystrophy, the illness is autosomal dominant, and cataracts are part of the illness. Gonadal atrophy and cardiac abnormalities have been described but not as frequently. One report has suggested that there may be neurological involvement with hyperintense areas on T2-weighted MRI images in the white matter. Progressive deafness has also been reported.

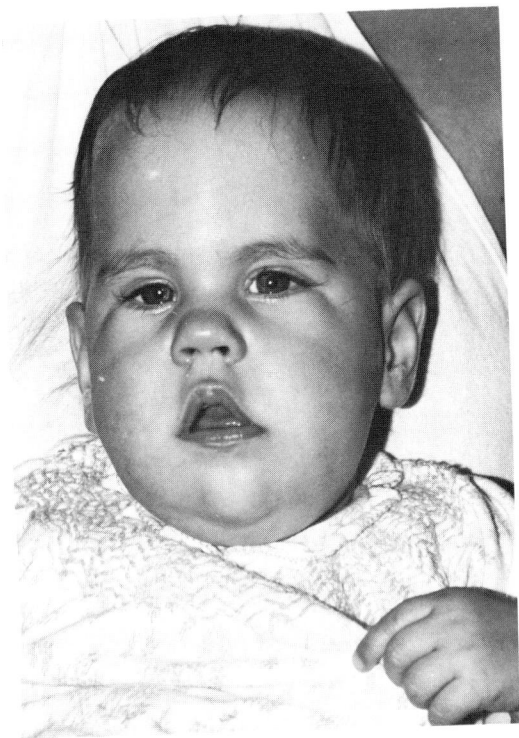

FIGURE 83.26 Infantile myotonic dystrophy. This child is severely retarded and has a marked inverted-V mouth.

The initial complaints are noted in adult life, rarely in childhood. The patient complains of a combination of muscle stiffness and an unusual muscle pain. Neither of these symptoms are identical to those of myotonic dystrophy; indeed, stiffness is seldom a complaint in the latter illness in spite of obvious clinical myotonia. The stiffness is a sense of a tight muscle, which produces a reluctance to move that impedes movement. It commonly affects the thighs and may be asymmetrical. Grip myotonia is noted, and the relaxation phase is jerky. The severity of the myotonia may vary from day to day, and a "warm-up" phenomenon is noted in which the stiffness disappears after repeated contraction and relaxation. The pain is a sense of discomfort and varies from sharp to a deep visceral ache. The prognosis in this illness is relatively good. The patient with proximal myotonic myopathy syndrome does not show the slow decline into helplessness and the early cardiorespiratory death so often noted in the myotonic dystrophy patient. Diagnostic testing includes the EMG, which shows myotonia, although this may happen only after a careful search in a number of muscles. Muscle biopsy shows nonspecific myopathic features. The CK may be elevated.

CHANNELOPATHIES

A group of illnesses ranging from myotonic syndromes to the periodic paralyses are recognized as abnormalities in ion channels (particularly sodium and chloride). The molec-ular basis for these illnesses is reorienting our classification as we discover it. The ion channels are fundamentally important in controlling the passage of ions across the cell membrane and in the shift of ions from one cell compartment to another. These proteins are associated with the cell membrane and are responsible for such phenomena as the muscle action potential. They may be influenced by the electrical potential across the cell membrane (voltage-gated) or by ligands, such as glutamate. Segments of these proteins have amino acid sequences that are remarkably similar across a wide range of species (conserved segments). It is logical that any change in the conserved segment of a protein might be expected to produce trouble for the organism. Some of these mutations are presumably lethal, affecting as they do such an important functional component of the cell. Other mutations may produce intermittent symptoms (e.g., the periodic paralyses).

Ion Channels

The calcium channel in muscle is made of five subunits: α-1, which is the most important and forms the ion pore across the membrane; α-2, β, γ, and δ. The type of α-1–subunit determines the sensitivity of the calcium channel. In muscle, this is sensitive to dihydropyridines, such as nifedipine. It is called an L-type channel because of its long-lasting effect (Greenberg 1997). The subunit is formed from four similar transmembrane regions (domains D1–4), each made of six membrane spanning proteins, S1–S6, all linked in series by "loops" that extend into the cytoplasm or extracellularly. S4 is highly charged, by virtue of the richness of positively charged amino acids, and may confer voltage sensitivity to the channel. Abnormalities in the calcium channel have been linked to several neurological conditions, including hypokalemic periodic paralysis (Hoffman et al. 1995).

The sodium channel is very similar in its makeup. The α-subunit, a 260-kD protein, confers the sodium channel activity with four domains made of six membrane-spanning proteins connected in similar fashion. Again the S4 segment is highly charged, which might make it suitable for responding to voltage changes. Mutations in a gene for the sodium channel have been found as a cause of hyperkalemic periodic paralysis and paramyotonia.

Defects in the chloride channel are seen in some patients with myotonia congenita, either autosomal dominant or recessive. The chloride channel has a different structure, being a homotetramer, in which each unit contains approximately a thousand amino acids.

The ryanodine receptor controls the flux of calcium from the sarcoplasmic reticulum into the cytoplasm. It plays an important part in the activation of the contractile mechanism, and in the condition termed malignant hyperthermia. Ryanodine receptors are made of four identical subunits, each of which is approximately 550 kD. The alkaloid ryanodine receptor interacts with the receptor, inhibiting at high concentrations and potentially activating at low concentrations. There are different types of receptor, and *RYR1* is found in muscle. The ryanodine receptor is associated with the L-type calcium channel with which it interacts.

Calcium-Channel Abnormalities (Familial Hypokalemic Periodic Paralysis)

Pathophysiology

Familial hypokalemic periodic paralysis is inherited as an autosomal dominant trait. The responsible gene has been tracked to chromosome 1q31-32 and is in fact the gene that encodes for the α-1–subunit of the dihydropyridine-sensitive calcium channel. The presumed voltage-sensitive S4 segment of domains 2 and 4 are affected. Two common mutations account for most patients. In both, there is a substitution of histidine for arginine. One is at position 528 and the other at 1239; the families are about evenly divided between the two. It appears that the Arg528His mutation is associated with incomplete penetrance of the disease in women, which accounts for the male preponderance of the illness. One report has also suggested that the same mutation may result in incomplete penetrance even in males (Sillen et al. 1997).

It is not easy to see why an abnormality of the calcium channel would cause periodic weakness, although the paralyzed muscle is inexcitable either by stimulation or by the application of calcium on isolated muscle strips. The sarcolemmal membrane of the muscle is unable to propagate an action potential. The response to calcium can be restored by stripping the muscle of its sarcolemmal membrane (with a local contraction of the underlying muscle). Studies on intact intercostal muscle fibers indicate that the resting membrane potential of the muscle fibers in patients with hypokalemic periodic paralysis is depolarized by approximately 5–15 mV compared with the normal value of –85 mV. Reducing the external potassium concentration in the medium further depolarizes the fibers to –50 mV and renders them inexcitable. The attacks of weakness are provoked by factors that lower the serum potassium. The serum potassium may fall as low as 1.5 mEq/liter during an attack, but weakness generally commences at much higher levels. An unexplained finding is the elevated intracellular sodium concentration in resting fibers. Also unexplained are the facts that membrane stability is restorable by removing sodium from the medium and that the sodium channel is not blocked by tetrodotoxin, as in normal muscle.

Clinical Features

Familial hypokalemic periodic paralysis may be noted at any age, but its onset is most common in the second decade. Age of onset may be earlier and the hypokalemia more pronounced in the Arg 1239His mutation (Fouad et al. 1997). The attack of weakness begins with a sensation of heaviness or aching in the legs or back. This sensation gradually increases and is associated with weakness of the proximal muscles. There also may be distal weakness as the attack develops. The paralysis may be severe enough that the patient cannot get up from bed or raise the head from the pillow. Respiratory muscles are not usually severely compromised, although a mild decrease in respiratory function may be seen. At the height of the weakness, the muscle is electrically and mechanically inexcitable, and reflexes are lost. The muscles feel swollen and may be firm to palpation. Usually an attack lasts for several hours, even up to a day, and the patient's strength returns as suddenly as it left. There is often a mild residual weakness that is slower to clear. Sometimes permanent weakness ensues. The attacks vary in both severity and frequency and may occur as often as several times a week but usually are isolated and separated by weeks to months. Because the disorder probably is associated with a shift in potassium, provocative factors include heavy exercise followed by a period of sleep or rest, a heavy carbohydrate load, or any other cause of increased insulin secretion. The attack commonly has its onset in the morning hours after waking, probably because sleep is associated with the movement of ions, such as potassium, across the muscle membrane. Epinephrine, norepinephrine, and corticosteroids may have a provocative effect on the illness. Attacks are most common in the third and fourth decades of life. There may be spontaneous improvement later in life.

Laboratory Studies

During an attack, there is usually, but not always, a fall in levels of serum potassium. The weakness may commence at levels that are at the low end of normal and may be quite profound by the time the serum potassium concentration reaches 2.0–2.5 mEq/liter. ECG changes also may be noted with bradycardia. Prolongation of the PR and QT intervals and T-wave flattening are associated with prominent U waves. If a spontaneous attack is not observed, provocative testing may be used. Because the common genetic defects cause a change in the size of the fragments after digestion with restriction endonucleases, genetic testing is not difficult and is probably the preferred test. Older provocative testing included the use of oral glucose, 2–5 g/kg to a maximum dose of 100 g to drive down the potassium and produce paralysis. If this is unsuccessful, the glucose load may be given with subcutaneous insulin 0.1 U/kg. More aggressive testing has been used in the past, with intravenous glucose, up to 3 g/kg over 60 minutes, accompanied by intravenous insulin, up to 0.1 U/kg 30 and 60 minutes into the glucose infusion. This aggressive testing usually is not necessary in patients with true periodic paralysis, however, and may cause a feeling of weakness in the normal individual. ECG monitoring should be carried out before and during this test. In the case of any pre-existing cardiac conduction abnormality, it may be wise to avoid the test. In other patients, potassium concentration should be measured every 15–30 minutes. The maximum change usually occurs within 3 hours, but the patient should be followed for at least 12 hours after the infusion. Muscle biopsy may be normal, although there are usually myopathic changes. A common feature of familial hypokalemic periodic paralysis is the presence of vacuoles within the fibers, particularly in association with permanent weakness. Tubular aggregates may also be noted, although they are more common in the hyperkalemic form of periodic paralysis.

Treatment

An attack of paralysis may be treated with 5–10 g of oral potassium. If this has no effect, the dose should be repeated in 1 hour. Renal function must be normal before potassium is administered to a patient with paralysis. Preventive treatment has focused on acetazolamide. This drug may produce a mild metabolic acidosis, which perhaps influences the potassium shifts that occur in the disease. Dichlorphenamide, another carbonic anhydrase inhibitor, also may be effective. Side effects of acetazolamide include tingling in the digits and a tendency for the formation of kidney stones. Hypersensitivity reactions also may be seen. Triamterene or spironolactone may be used as adjuncts, and the patient may need a low-sodium or low-carbohydrate diet for maximum effect.

Secondary Hypokalemic Paralysis

Periodic paralysis associated with thyrotoxicosis is well known, and the high incidence in Asian populations is well documented. This predisposition is inherited as an autosomal dominant trait, but the disease is sporadic and affects men more commonly than women. Kidney failure or adrenal failure may be associated with changes in potassium. A more common form of weakness with low potassium is noted in patients who are receiving potassium-depleting diuretics. Other compounds, such as licorice, have been implicated in attacks of weakness associated with potassium loss.

Sodium-Channel Abnormalities (Potassium-Sensitive Periodic Paralysis, Hyperkalemic Periodic Paralysis, Paramyotonia Congenita, and Myotonia Fluctuans)

Pathophysiology

The potassium-sensitive periodic paralysis and myotonias are associated with mutations in the α-subunit of the sodium channel; the gene is located on chromosome 17q. Even in the early descriptions of this group of illnesses, the association of decreased electrical activity, paralysis, and signs of hyperactivity (paramyotonia) was recognized. Molecular studies have helped to explain the reasons. The proper activity of the sodium channel depends on a complicated series of activation and deactivation processes that open the

pore to allow the passage of sodium but also protects the cell against inadvertent excess sodium flux. The channel may exist in a number of different states: closed, open, inactivated, and so forth. Physiological studies have suggested that the domain IV S3 segment has a dominant role in the recovery of inactivated channels, whereas the S4 segment is concerned with deactivation and inactivation of the open channel (Ji et al. 1996). Numerous mutations of the sodium channel have been described. Some of these impair fast inactivation of the sodium channel or shift the impulse to hyperpolarization. There is also evidence that two common mutations in hyperkalemic periodic paralysis in domain II, S5 and domain IV, S6 cause defective slow inactivation, adding to the problem and accentuating the weakness (Hayward et al. 1997). Mutations within the domain III–IV linker, which cause myotonia with or without weakness, do not impair slow inactivation.

Studies of muscle during a paralytic attack show that it is slightly depolarized. Decreased intracellular potassium levels have been noted, as well as an increase in sodium, water, and chloride content. Studies of intercostal muscle biopsies in vitro show a high level of spontaneous muscle activity, even in normal physiological saline. Increasing the external concentration of potassium gradually depolarizes the cells and is associated with an increase in sodium conductance. The sodium conductance increase was reversed by tetrodotoxin, implying that this part of the sodium channel function was not affected. Cultured myotubes from the muscle of a patient with this illness were used to examine the sodium currents. Raising the potassium concentration in the medium resulted in an increased open time or slowed inactivation of the sodium channel associated with sustained depolarization.

In patients with paramyotonia, when intact muscle fibers obtained from intercostal biopsy were cooled, this reduced the resting membrane potential from approximately –80 mV to –40 mV, at which point the fibers were inexcitable. As the muscle cools, it passes through a phase of hyperexcitability. Inexcitability is prevented by tetrodotoxin, which blocks the sodium channels. The physiological findings are reflected in the clinical features.

Clinical Features

Patients with hyperkalemic periodic paralysis have predominant symptoms of weakness that are provoked by exposure to potassium. There may be evidence of myotonia, and some patients complain of the symptom, but the predominant difficulty is recurrent bouts of paralysis. The allelic disease, paramyotonia congenita, causes different symptoms. In these patients, the predominant symptom is muscle stiffness, and bouts of weakness are mild, often provoked by exposure to cold. In some families, the distinction seems clear, but there are others with a somewhat mixed picture. The symptoms and signs of the two conditions are as follows.

Hyperkalemic Periodic Paralysis

As mentioned, potassium-sensitive periodic paralysis is inherited as an autosomal dominant trait, with strong penetrance and involvement of both sexes. Sometimes the illness is noted during infancy or early childhood. The infant's cry may become suddenly altered or unusual, or the child may be found lying quietly in the crib. Some parents notice an unusual stare these babies develop, particularly on exposure to cold. The first attack commonly occurs in the first few weeks of school because of the enforced sitting. By adolescence, the attacks are fairly well characterized. Often, rest after exercise provokes an attack, and the weakness develops quite rapidly, often within a matter of minutes. The weakness is milder than in the hypokalemic variety, and the attacks last for a shorter period. Patients may be able to walk off the symptoms if they undertake exercise early in the attack, but many prefer not to do so because an attack itself is mild and followed by a period of relative freedom from symptoms. In addition to rest after exercise, other provocative factors include exposure to cold, anesthesia, and sleep. Patients often avoid fruit juices (which contain much potassium), having noticed that they have a deleterious effect. Many patients talk about two kinds of attacks, light and heavy. During a light attack, there is a feeling of fatigue and mild weakness that usually disappears in less than an hour. A heavy attack, however, may be associated with more severe paralysis, even to the point where the patient is unable to arise from the chair or the bed. The frequency varies from two or three mild attacks a day to episodes months apart. Residual weakness may be noted into middle age and beyond.

Paramyotonia Congenita

In addition to the weakness, hyperkalemic periodic paralysis is associated with a form of myotonia that often involves the muscles of the face, eyes, tongue, and hands. Paramyotonia of the face may be noticed by stiffness of the expression, narrowing of the palpebral fissures, or dimpling of the chin due to contraction of the mentalis muscle. Unlike the myotonia in the common dystrophy, paramyotonia is accentuated by repeated exercise. Patients may complain of this as aching or stiffness. A clinical test is to have the patient forcibly close his or her eyes in a repetitive manner. After each repetition, the difficulty with relaxation may be accentuated until eventually the patient cannot open the eyes at all. Exposure to cold also has an unusual effect. It not only worsens the myotonia but may provoke muscle weakness, symptoms that the patients may notice themselves when swallowing ice cream or going out into the winter weather to shovel snow. A useful test for paramyotonia is to soak a small towel in ice water and lay it over the patient's eyes for 2 minutes. Eyelid myotonia is demonstrated by having the patient sustain an upward gaze for a few seconds and then look down. The eyelids remain up, baring the sclera above the iris. When muscle is sufficiently chilled, the paramyotonia disappears, and the muscle is flaccid and paralyzed. The weakness may far outlast the exposure to cold, and it is common for the muscle not to regain its full use for hours after returning to room temperature. Strong voluntary contraction also may be associated with a long-lasting decrease in strength, which is not clearly due to an increase in myotonia. Immersing the forearm in ice water may also produce obvious weakness, which may have been lacking on the initial examination.

Laboratory Studies

The diagnosis of these potassium-sensitive conditions relies on demonstration of the genetic defects, but the illness is suspected when high serum potassium levels coincide with bouts of weakness. In patients with paramyotonia, the EMG of the resting muscles at room temperature shows myotonia that is present on percussion or with movement of the needle. The most remarkable finding is the appearance of spontaneous activity on cooling the limb. Low-amplitude fibrillation activity appears as the muscle is cooled and is most intense when the muscle temperature is around 30°C. This spontaneous activity completely disappears as cooling continues. In contrast to myotonia, during the delayed muscle relaxation of paramyotonia, electrical activity of the muscle is not prominent. EMG studies may also be useful in demonstrating the worsening of the myotonic discharges with exposure to cold or to potassium. Because exercise may worsen symptoms, a brief exercise test has been proposed, searching for a decrease in the muscle compound action potential. This was seen in one mexiletine-responsive patient, even though symptoms of weakness were absent.

The ECG may show the changes of hyperkalemia, and the serum CK concentration may be elevated during or after an attack. Provocative testing, if considered, should be performed with care because the administration of potassium may be dangerous. If there is evidence of any cardiac abnormality, provocative testing is probably best avoided, and potassium should not be given intravenously as a provocative test. Oral potassium may be administered using approximately 1 mEq/kg. The maximum rise in potassium occurs 90–180 minutes after administration. If this dose of potassium does not provoke an attack and the index of suspicion is high, 2 mEq/kg orally may be used on a subsequent occasion.

Muscle biopsies frequently have been reported to show tubular aggregates in patients with paralysis, particularly in patients with fixed weakness. Marked myopathic changes have been noted, including internal nuclei, vacuoles, and fibrosis. The muscle biopsy may be abnormal in paramyotonia congenita and demonstrate variability in the size of fibers, with internal nuclei and occasional vacuoles.

Treatment

Acute attacks usually do not require treatment because they are mild and brief. Often, patients themselves learn to eat a candy bar or drink a sweet drink as a way of warding off an attack. If weakness is more severe, intravenous calcium gluconate has been recommended. Intravenous sodium chloride sometimes may abort an attack. Maintenance therapy with dichlorphenamide or acetazolamide can be helpful. The combination of hydrochlorothiazide with potassium may be effective, although the reason is not clear. Mexiletine, a drug related to lidocaine and tocainide, blocks the sodium channel. It may provide dramatic relief to patients with myotonia. It can be started at a dose of 200 mg tid. Most patients who derive benefit do so at relatively low doses.

Myotonia Fluctuans

Another dominantly inherited disorder of the sodium channel is characterized by muscle stiffness made worse by exercise or by potassium ingestion. The disease begins in adolescence and is characterized by bouts of stiffness. When the stiffness is present, it may affect extraocular, bulbar, or limb muscles. It is improved when the patient loosens up the limb, like the patient with myotonia congenita, but exercise is also associated with worsening of symptoms. Often, either following rest after 15–30 minutes of exercise or during exercise itself, the muscles become stiff and the patient incapacitated. Weakness of the muscles is not a part of this illness, unlike in paramyotonia congenita. The disorder has been associated with an abnormality in exon 22 and in exon 14 of the sodium channel gene. Treatment with mexiletine or with acetazolamide may be effective.

Secondary Hyperkalemic Periodic Paralysis

Weakness due to high levels of potassium may be seen in situations other than familial hyperkalemic periodic paralysis. The difference between secondary hyperkalemic periodic paralysis and the familial condition is that the levels of potassium are usually extremely high in secondary hyperkalemic periodic paralysis before weakness is noticed. Causes for secondary hyperkalemic periodic paralysis include renal failure or potassium administration associated with potassium-retaining diuretics.

Andersen's Syndrome

The occurrence of cardiac dysrhythmias with periodic weakness has been known for a considerable time, although it has not been accorded the importance it deserves. A series of reports emphasized the constellation of findings (periodic paralysis, cardiac dysrhythmias, and dysmorphic features) that have been termed *Andersen's syndrome* (Sansone et al. 1997). The disorder is inherited in an autosomal dominant fashion, but the known abnormalities in the sodium channel gene or the dihydropyridine calcium channel gene that characterize many of the other periodic paralyses are lacking. The known genetic abnormalities associated with the prolonged QT syndrome are also absent.

The bouts of paralysis may occur in early childhood but may also be delayed until later and may occur only rarely. Attacks have been recorded with both high and low potassium, in which regard it is different from the more standard hypokalemic variety, in which the potassium levels always veer to the lower values. Affected members of the family often show dysmorphic features, including wide-spaced eyes, low-set ears, a small chin, clinodactyly of the fifth finger, and syndactyly of the toes. Permanent muscle weakness has been found in several patients.

The importance of recognizing the syndrome lies in the frequent occurrence of cardiac involvement. This varies from a prolongation of the QT interval through ventricular tachycardia to fatal cardiac arrest. The risk of cardiac complication is high enough that provocative hypokalemic or hyperkalemic testing is not warranted. Several members of affected families have been described in whom only fragments of the syndrome exist (e.g., clinodactyly or an abnormal QT interval), so that a full evaluation of the pedigree is necessary.

Myotonia Congenita

Pathophysiology

There are two major forms of myotonia congenita: autosomal dominant and recessive. Both are associated with abnormalities in the chloride channel, the gene for which resides on chromosome 7q35. Introducing the mutant chloride channel into a cell system abolishes the chloride current and deranges the normal function of the chloride channel (Fahlke et al. 1997). Chloride conductance is also reduced in the patient's muscle, and the membrane resistance is greater than normal. The action potential in a normal muscle cell is associated with an outflow of potassium, which may accumulate in the transverse tubules simply because the physical structure of the tubule does not favor easy diffusion. Ordinarily, this does not present a problem because the chloride conductance is so large that the relatively free passage of chloride ions negates the effect of any small change in potassium. If chloride conductance is impeded, the increase in potassium concentration in the transverse tubules may lead to enough depolarization to activate the sodium channels again and hence lead to repetitive electrical discharge of the membrane, producing electrical and clinical myotonia.

Clinical Features

The dominant disease was originally described by Thomsen among members of his own family. It is usually milder than the recessive form described by Becker, in which myotonia may be associated with some weakness. It is sometimes difficult, when faced with a sporadic case, to decide on the pattern of inheritance. This is true because members of affected families who carry the abnormal mutation may be asymptomatic or only mildly involved. This necessitates a thorough evaluation of the family with the appropriate genetic testing.

On initial examination, especially if the patient has been sitting in the waiting room for some time, there may be apparent weakness because a muscle that is the site of severe myotonia cannot be used with full voluntary power. With repetitive activity, the muscle loosens up, and the strength usually returns to normal. This is particularly true of the proximal muscles of the limbs. The symptoms are described in a rather stereotyped way. After resting, the muscles are stiff and difficult to move. This is obvious when the patient arises from a chair. They move en bloc, with a stiff, wooden appearance, rather like the rusted Tin Man in the Wizard of Oz. As they continue, they then can walk freely and finally can run with ease. All the muscles of the body seem to share this abnormality, and, although it is most noticeable in the limbs, evidence of myotonia also can be found in the face and the tongue. In addition, particularly in the recessive form of the illness, muscular hypertrophy may be pronounced.

Diagnosis

In myotonia congenita, EMG shows well-marked myotonia with none of the associated dystrophic features. The muscle biopsy may demonstrate an absence of type 2B fibers. So far, no explanation for the finding has been noted. Muscle biopsy also may reveal some increase in the size of fibers and internal nuclei and other mild, nonspecific changes.

Treatment

Unlike patients with myotonic dystrophy, those with myotonia congenita may be quite disabled because of the myotonia. Treatment with mexiletine is worth trying and may provide dramatic relief in some patients. Older medicines include quinine, procainamide, and phenytoin.

METABOLIC DISEASES

Any disturbance in the biochemical pathways that support ATP levels in the muscle inevitably results in exercise intolerance. One common symptom is muscle fatigue, a sense that the muscle will no longer perform in a normal fashion. This is true fatigue and not simply a feeling of tiredness or weariness. It may be difficult for the patient to describe the fatigue in terms that the physician can understand because it has nothing to do with the sensations experienced by a healthy person after strenuous exercise. It has an unpleasant

quality, and patients describe it in terms of a barrier through which they cannot break. Other symptoms include muscle pain and sometimes muscle cramps. The normal fatigue of strenuous exercise is painless. Muscle pain after strenuous exercise (e.g., the next day) is almost universal in the untrained individual, but pain during exercise is more the hallmark of disturbed muscle function. Normally functioning muscle appears to have a series of safety mechanisms that prevent humans from exercising it to the point of destruction. In the metabolic muscle diseases, maintenance of ATP levels is impaired, and the protective mechanism that functions in the normal person is absent. If exercise is forced in a patient with a metabolic myopathy, muscle pain develops, and a muscle contracture subsequently may be found, in which state the muscle is hard, swollen, and tender. This reflects actual destruction of the muscle. It may be associated with the release of myoglobin into the blood and urine, sometimes noticed as a change in the color of the urine, which may resemble weak tea or cola. Fatigue, muscle pain, contractures, and myoglobinuria are increasingly severe effects of the biochemical defect. In the treatment of these illnesses, every effort should be made to prevent the development of myoglobinuria, which carries with it the potential complication of renal tubular necrosis. Although the final results are similar in many of the diseases, the illnesses can be grouped into three major categories: disorders of carbohydrate metabolism, disorders of lipid metabolism, and disorders of mitochondrial function. Finally, there are some conditions that, in theory, should disturb pathways for ATP maintenance but do not seem to cause any exercise intolerance. It should be noted that a tissue in which ATP levels are depleted is probably dead tissue. Even in the metabolic myopathies, the muscle seldom reaches this critical state. What does happen, however, is that most of the support pathways are overworked with the production of unwelcome by-products, which are probably responsible for the symptoms.

Disorders of Carbohydrate Metabolism

Myophosphorylase Deficiency

Pathophysiology. Intramuscular carbohydrate stores play an important part in the early stage of exercise, before the compensatory mechanisms of an increased supply of blood-borne metabolites and increased lipid metabolism supply the added demand. The first of the biochemical disorders to be recognized was a disorder of carbohydrate metabolism called *myophosphorylase deficiency* (McArdle's disease). In 1952, McArdle noted that a young man who presented with exercise intolerance experienced pain and tightness of his muscle on forced exercise. Ischemic forearm exercise caused a painful contracture of the muscle within a minute or so. Insertion of an EMG needle showed that there was no electrical activity, thereby differentiating this contracture from a muscle cramp. McArdle commented that the phenomenon resembled the reaction of a fish muscle poisoned by iodoacetate, a compound that blocks glycolysis. Subsequent studies showed the defect to be an absence of myophosphorylase activity, encoded by a gene on chromosome 11q13. There are two forms of phosphorylase: phosphorylase a, which is the active tetramer, and phosphorylase b, an inactive dimer. Conversion of the inactive form to the active form is catalyzed by phosphorylase b kinase, which itself is activated by a protein kinase under the control of cyclic adenosine monophosphate (AMP). Any abnormality of this cascade of reactions results in an absence of phosphorylase activity. Both phosphorylase a and phosphorylase b kinase deficiencies are known to cause exercise intolerance. The illnesses in both cases appear to be inherited as an autosomal recessive trait. Myophosphorylase deficiency is sometimes inherited as an autosomal dominant trait.

Clinical Features. The patient often notices symptoms during the first 10 years, but only in retrospect. As children, they may complain of being tired and unable to keep up with their playmates. The classic symptoms appear in teenage years. Fatigue and pain begin within the first few minutes of exercise, particularly if it is strenuous. There is a sensation of hitting a barrier, which causes the patient to slow down. If exercise is continued, pain develops within the muscle, which at first is deep and aching but gives way to the rapid development of a painful tightening of the muscle. When the muscle is examined, it is hard and contracted, and any attempt to straighten it results in great pain. The muscle contracture may last for several hours and can be differentiated from a muscle cramp on two counts: The EMG is electrically silent, and the duration of the contracture is far longer than that of a physiological cramp, which disappears after a few minutes at most. Another aspect of McArdle's disease is the development of the second-wind phenomenon. If, with the onset of fatigue, the patient slows down but does not stop, the abnormal sensation may disappear, and thereafter the muscle may function more normally. By gradually increasing the level of exercise again, the patient may be able to break through the barrier and, if so, may be able to exercise at an adequate level for long periods of time. This second-wind phenomenon, which is related to the phenomenon normally experienced by distance runners, may be marked in patients with phosphorylase deficiency. It probably is associated with a change in the blood supply in the muscle and with an intrinsic change in the muscle's metabolism. The second-wind phenomenon usually is associated with a rise in fatty acid use and may be blocked by nicotinic acid. Other unusual forms of phosphorylase deficiency have been described. One such patient was an infant girl who died of respiratory failure. Phosphorylase deficiency also has been noted in an occasional patient with proximal weakness who has neither cramps nor fatigue. On examination, the patients are superficially normal. There is neither wasting nor any detectable weakness, although the patient may be reluctant to exert full force during muscle strength testing because of the possibility of exacerbating muscle pain.

Diagnosis. A simple clinical test can be carried out using a hand dynamometer. A blood pressure cuff is inflated around the upper arm to occlude the blood supply. The patient is asked to grip the dynamometer, repetitively exercising the forearm. The patient should exert his or her maximum strength, and the rate should be approximately 20 times per minute. The importance of the dynamometer lies in the need to ensure that the patient is exerting maximum grip. The normal individual should be able to exercise in this fashion for a few minutes. If there is muscle fatigue, it occurs with the muscle in a relaxed position without an increase in muscle tone. The patient with phosphorylase deficiency often fatigues in less than 1 minute, and, concomitant with the fatigue, the muscles of the forearm shorten and the fist may remain clenched around the dynamometer. It should be emphasized that these tests are not benign because they undoubtedly result in muscle damage, and a negative test does not eliminate the possibility of a glycolytic defect. The usual laboratory tests (serum CK concentration, EMG, and muscle biopsy) may be unrevealing unless specific techniques for myophosphorylase and phosphorylase b kinase are included. The CK level is elevated if the patient has had a recent contracture or muscle fatigue, but it may be normal. The EMG is normal. Light microscopic examination of the muscle biopsy may show an increase in glycogen and the presence of subsarcolemmal blebs. Muscle necrosis also may be noted. Not infrequently, the routine stains are entirely normal. A useful screening test for this and other disorders of glycogen metabolism is the forearm exercise test. In normal exercise, lactate is produced as a result of anaerobic glycolysis. In phosphorylase deficiency and in other glycogenolytic defects, intracellular glycogen cannot be used, and therefore lactate production is either absent or less than normal. Peak lactate elevation of 3–4 times the resting level normally is noted within the first 3 minutes after exercise and is absent in patients with phosphorylase deficiency and other glycogenolytic defects. It is essential to do the test in a standardized fashion in a laboratory with established values for normal volunteers; otherwise, the results may be impossible to interpret.

Phosphofructokinase Deficiency

Pathophysiology. PFK is the enzyme that converts fructose 6-phosphate to fructose 1,6-diphosphate and is a step in the glycolytic chain downstream from that activated by phosphorylase. The reaction is rate limiting for glycolysis. PFK deficiency is inherited as an autosomal recessive trait, the gene is on chromosome 1, and heterozygotes have decreased but not absent levels of enzyme activity.

Clinical Features. PFK deficiency is almost identical clinically to phosphorylase deficiency, although it may be more severe. Most attacks are associated with nausea, vomiting, and muscle pain. There may also be mild hemolytic anemia, with increased levels of bilirubin and increased reticulocyte counts due to deficiency of red blood cell PFK. PFK, like phosphorylase, is a tetramer of different subunits, M and R. Muscle PFK is composed of identical M subunits, whereas the enzyme in the red blood cell comprises both M and R types. In PFK deficiency, the M subunit is missing, resulting in absence of muscle PFK and impairment of the PFK in the red blood cell because the R subunit is still preserved.

Phosphoglycerate Kinase Deficiency

Phosphoglycerate kinase is involved in another step in the glycolytic pathway. Its absence from muscle produces a predictable picture very similar to that of phosphorylase deficiency. There is no rise in venous lactate after exercise, as would be expected. The muscle biopsy, however, has been described as normal, with a normal glycogen concentration. Phosphoglycerate kinase is a single polypeptide, and many different point mutations of this enzyme have been described, most of which produce abnormalities in the red blood cell, with hemolytic anemia, mental retardation, and seizures. The gene for this disorder is on chromosome Xq13; hence, the inheritance is an X-linked recessive trait.

Phosphoglycerate Mutase Deficiency

Phosphoglycerate mutase exists as a dimer with M and B subunits. The predominant form in normal muscle is MM. A small amount of residual activity may be present in muscle as a result of the existence of the BB form. Patients with an absence of the enzyme have attacks of muscle pain and myoglobinuria and, in one case, typical attacks of gouty arthritis. The high uric acid level may be associated with an overactivity of the adenylate kinase-adenylate deaminase reaction, which is seen in many of the metabolic disorders and produces uric acid as its end product. Exercise testing shows some elevation of lactate, but not to the levels usually seen. Incremental bicycle ergometry in one patient was said to show a normal rise in lactate and a normal VO_{2max} and heart rate, which are difficult to explain. The gene for the illness is located at chromosome 7p12-13.

Lactate Dehydrogenase Deficiency

Exercise intolerance, fatigue, and myoglobinuria have been described in a young man due to LDH deficiency. There are some differences in the laboratory studies between this entity and the others discussed here. In most muscle diseases, muscle LDH and serum CK concentrations fluctuate together. In this illness, not surprisingly, there was a marked discrepancy between the high levels of CK and the low levels of LDH. Furthermore, because the action of LDH in exercise is to convert pyruvate to lactate, large amounts of pyruvate were produced even though no lactate was produced after ischemic forearm exercise. The gene is at chromosome 11p15.4.

Treatment of the Glycolytic Disorders

There are no effective forms of treatment for glycolytic disorders. The patient should be counseled to avoid situations that might precipitate myoglobinuria. Attempts have been made to bypass the metabolic block by using glucose or fructose. Sublingual administration of isoproterenol has been suggested, but patients generally obtain no benefit from this. Administration of branched-chain amino acids and a protein-enriched diet also has been suggested, but there is no evidence that these regimens are any more effective than a well-balanced diet. One maneuver that can be adopted is to develop the patient's awareness of the second-wind phenomenon. Graded exercise on a treadmill can be used to train the patient to recognize how to slow down with the first onset of symptoms and then resume exercise in small increments. The patient is best referred to an exercise physiology laboratory for this type of training.

Disorders of Lipid Metabolism

Carnitine Palmitoyl Transferase Deficiency

Pathophysiology. The synthesis of ATP that results from the oxidation of fatty acids is carried out by a system that is as complex as that seen in glycolysis. Although fatty acids are not used at the beginning of exercise, they become increasingly important after 20–30 minutes of endurance exercise, and after an hour, they represent the major energy supply. Consequently, defects in lipid metabolism give rise to symptoms after sustained activity. Carnitine palmitoyl transferase (CPT) is the enzyme that effects the linkage of carnitine to long-chain fatty acids, which is necessary to transport the fatty acid across the mitochondrial membrane from outside to inside (CPT-I). It is also responsible for unhooking carnitine when the complex reaches the inside (CPT-II). CPT-II deficiency is one of the more common biochemical abnormalities in muscle. The disorder is inherited as an autosomal recessive trait.

Clinical Features. Typically, the patient with CPT deficiency is a young adult male who experiences his first bout of weakness and myoglobinuria after strenuous exercise, such as mountain climbing or playing four sets of tennis. In retrospect, patients often experienced brief episodes of muscle pain as children, but these were shrugged off as growing pains or the more ordinary muscle cramps. Patients are particularly predisposed to these attacks if exercise is performed in the fasting state. This is not surprising because fasting throws the body into a dependency on fatty acids. Several patients with this illness have manifested the first symptoms during military training when they were required to undertake a forced march with a full backpack before breakfast. Attacks of myoglobinuria in CPT deficiency are often more severe, with a greater tendency to cause renal damage, than are those occurring in disorders of glycolysis. This may be due to the fact that the symptoms come on so rapidly in the glycolytic disorders that cessation of exercise immediately returns the muscle to its resting condition. In disorders of lipid metabolism, the patient is often far away from home and must out of necessity use muscles that have already been damaged. Second, even when the muscle stops working, it still depends on fatty acid metabolism. Frequently, respiratory paralysis accompanies severe attacks. Patients with CPT deficiency often notice that their stamina depends on their diet. Some carry a candy bar to be eaten during exercise. Others know that exercise in a fasting state is far more difficult for them. Despite these limitations, most patients with CPT deficiency are quite athletic. Usually, however, they are weight lifters or sprinters rather than marathon runners. Both activities draw on carbohydrate energy supplies and use glycolytic fibers, not the oxidative fibers. There is no abnormality on examination. Indeed, these patients are uniformly muscular, perhaps because their favorite exercise is weight lifting.

Diagnosis. In general, laboratory studies are unrevealing of CPT deficiency. The CK concentration may be normal unless the patient has had a recent attack of muscle damage. The muscle biopsy in CPT deficiency is normal, unless necrosis is associated with a recent bout of muscle damage. Biochemical analysis of the muscle biopsy reveals the deficiency of CPT, but the fact that one must suspect the diagnosis to ask for the assay makes it helpful only as a confirmatory test. One useful screening test is a respiratory exchange ratio (RER). The ratio of carbon dioxide produced to oxygen consumed gives an indication of the type of fuel being used by the patient. In a normal individual at rest, the RER is approximately 0.8 because fatty acids are the predominant source of fuel at rest. In CPT deficiency, the RER is seldom much below 1.0, even with the patient at complete rest. It may be worthwhile to obtain incremental bicycle ergometry results because, in addition to the RER, the VO_{2max} and $Work_{max}$ also can be determined. Both are likely to be decreased. The maximum heart rate is normal, indicating full effort. Forearm exercise testing is not of much value in CPT deficiency because the test stresses glycolytic pathways and hence is normal.

Treatment. Patients with CPT deficiency should be cautioned to avoid any situation that provokes muscle pain and puts them at risk for myoglobinuria. The physiological effect of fasting should be explained, and the patient should be warned not to attempt exercise under such conditions. The use of glucose tablets or candy bars during exercise may raise exercise tolerance slightly. If myoglobinuria is noted, the patient should be admitted to the hospital, and renal function should

be monitored. Forced alkaline diuresis may be helpful in some cases. All exercise should be discontinued and the patient put at bed rest until CK levels return to normal and renal function has been shown to be uncompromised.

Carnitine Deficiency Myopathy

Pathophysiology. Carnitine is an important compound in intermediary metabolism. It influences the balance between free coenzyme A (CoA) and acylated CoA in the mitochondria and is used to transfer long-chain fatty acids across the mitochondrial membrane under the action of the enzyme CPT. Carnitine supplied by the diet usually is supplemented by carnitine synthesized in the liver and kidney, which is transported to and then actively taken up by the muscle. Many metabolic processes produce acyl-CoA, which may then be employed in useful metabolic pathways, degraded by the liver, or excreted by the kidneys. The formation of acyl-carnitine is often a step in these processes, enabling the transport of fatty and organic acids across membranes, such as the mitochondrial membrane. A surplus of acyl-CoA may cause a wide variety of damage. It inhibits reactions as diverse as the oxidation of pyruvate, steps in the tricarboxylic acid cycle, and gluconeogenesis. Thus, an adequate amount of carnitine is necessary for normal function. The adequacy of the carnitine supply can be judged from its absolute value and the percentage of free (nonacylated) carnitine. If free carnitine is absent, carnitine deficiency exists, no matter how much total carnitine is present. Because 98% of the body carnitine is in muscle, it is not surprising that carnitine deficiency is associated with neuromuscular disease. In most patients with carnitine deficiency, the loss of free carnitine is due to a defect in some other enzyme system that results in an overproduction of organic acids or a defect in acyl-CoA disposal. Causes of secondary carnitine deficiency include multiple acyl-CoA dehydrogenase deficiencies, resulting in an overabundance of organic acids, which then bind the available carnitine; propionyl-CoA carboxylase deficiency; methylmalonyl-CoA mutase deficiency; and a number of mitochondrial disorders. Hemodialysis, cirrhosis, pregnancy, Reye's syndrome, valproate therapy, and renal Fanconi's syndrome also have been found to deplete carnitine stores. In muscle carnitine deficiency, serum levels of carnitine are often normal, but both total and free carnitine is reduced in the muscle. In systemic carnitine deficiency, muscle carnitine, liver carnitine, and serum carnitine are all decreased.

Clinical Features

Myopathic Carnitine Deficiency. The most common clinical picture in carnitine deficiency of the muscle is a slowly progressive weakness on which sudden exacerbations or a fluctuating course are superimposed. Fatigue and exercise-related pains have been described but usually do not constitute major complaints; myoglobinuria is almost always absent. The weakness is usually proximal, and the symptoms begin during childhood or early teenage life. In addition to the limb and some trunk weakness, facial and bulbar weakness have been described.

Systemic Carnitine Deficiency. Systemic carnitine deficiency also begins in infancy and childhood, but the muscular weakness occurs in association with encephalopathic crises resembling Reye's syndrome. The initial symptom of the encephalopathy usually is protracted vomiting, followed by changing levels of consciousness, culminating in coma. Hypoglycemia occurs in most patients, and there may be evidence of liver damage with an enlarged, tender liver or with increased serum levels of hepatic enzymes. Hypothrombinemia, hyperammonemia, and excess lipid in the liver are also common. Fasting, because it throws the body into a dependence on fatty acids, may exacerbate the symptoms of carnitine deficiency.

Diagnosis. The EMG frequently appears myopathic, but there are no specific findings that lead to the diagnosis of carnitine deficiency. The disorder may be suspected on muscle biopsy because of the accumulation of lipid droplets in muscle fibers (Figure 83.27), but the biochemical measurement of carnitine, both free and total, is necessary to establish the diagnosis. If abnormal, it will initiate the search for the underlying defect.

Treatment. The treatment of carnitine deficiency by replacing L-carnitine is not uniformly successful. Approximately 2–4 g per day have been given to adults in divided doses, with the equivalent of 100 mg/kg in infants and children. There have been no serious side effects, although patients may find L-carnitine unpleasant to take because of some accompanying nausea, and the "fishy odor" of the sweat. The results of such treatment vary. Some patients show dramatic improvement, whereas others feel no change at all. The effectiveness of other forms of treatment is equally variable. One patient responded to riboflavin in high doses and others to prednisone. Dietary manipulations, such as reducing the amount of long-chain fatty acids in the diet and supplying a medium-chain triglyceride diet, also are successful in some patients.

Other Disorders of Lipid Metabolism

There are other disorders involving lipid metabolism. The rest of the complicated chain of fatty acid metabolism probably does not always function normally. A number of patients with symptoms suggestive of CPT deficiency in fact prove to have normal amounts of the enzyme and must have some other abnormality, although what it may be has remained elusive.

Abnormalities of Mitochondrial Function

Pathophysiology

The final products of fatty acid metabolism and glycolysis are the two carbon fragments that enter the tricarboxylic

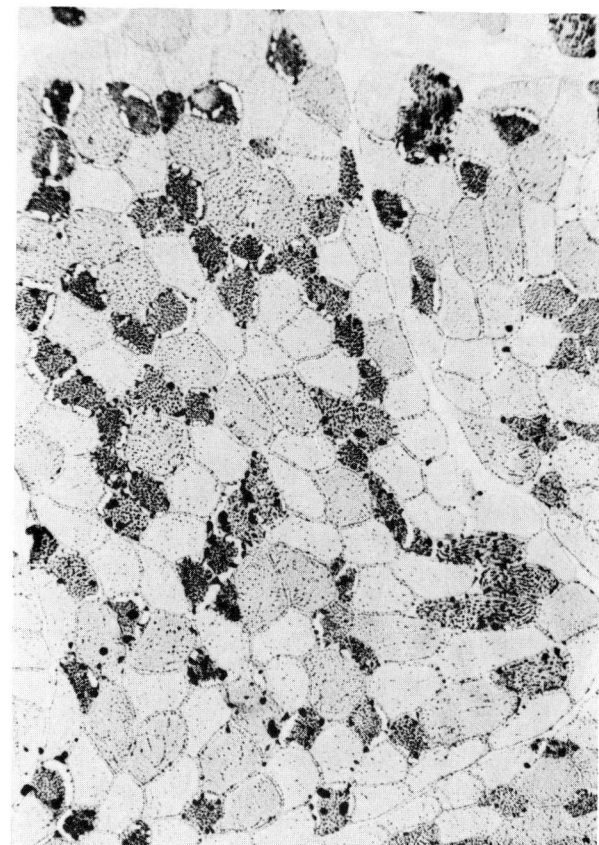

FIGURE 83.27   Carnitine deficiency. This lipid stain demonstrates deposition of fat in muscle fibers.

acid cycle. The final oxidative pathway involves the respiratory chain in mitochondria. Major disturbances in mitochondrial function produce severe neurological damage and abnormalities in the muscle. In a group of diseases known as the *mitochondrial myopathies*, the damage is less severe, and the symptoms are those of exercise intolerance. Under normal conditions, the rate of mitochondrial oxidation is coupled to the need for ATP. If ATP turnover is rapid, mitochondrial oxidation is turned on, with the resulting consumption of oxygen and other metabolites. When ATP turnover is minimal, mitochondrial oxidation is relatively quiescent. The body's response to the increased demands of exercise (and increased mitochondrial oxidation) is predictable. The higher oxygen consumption necessitates augmented delivery of oxygen to the muscle, evidenced by vasodilatation, tachycardia, increased cardiac output, and respiration. The heat generation that accompanies this oxidation results in sweating. Obviously, these are the normal accompaniments of vigorous exercise. When mitochondrial function is impaired, maintaining ATP levels at rest may be met only by mitochondrial oxidation that is fully turned on. In this situation, the patient at rest may experience all the symptoms that normally accompany vigorous exercise. In addition, because the oxidative mechanisms are insufficient to cope with the demand for ATP, anaerobic mechanisms come into play, which produce high lactate levels.

Clinical Features

The original description of a mitochondrial disorder was by Luft and colleagues in 1962, although the muscle symptoms were minor. Both patients were women who experienced sustained fever, profuse sweating, and heat intolerance. One preferred to spend her time in a room cooled to 4°C. Thirst and appetite were excessive, and polyuria was noted. General physical examination demonstrated a rapid heartbeat and respiration; profuse sweating; and warm, flushed skin. Blotchy erythematous changes of the skin over the legs were seen. Although some degree of muscle weakness was noted, it was mild and nonfocal. The muscle biopsy showed numerous ragged-red fibers, and electron microscopy revealed striking abnormalities in the mitochondria. Since then, other patients with more specific defects in the mitochondrial chain have been described. A number of patients had prominent muscle complaints. Symptoms often were noted in childhood, and exercise was associated with a heavy feeling in the limbs and muscle aches. After exercise, the patients often became tired, nauseated, and breathless. The illness progressed over the years until the patients were capable of only a limited amount of exercise. Acute attacks could be brought on by unaccustomed activity, fasting, or small quantities of alcohol. During one acute attack, a patient was noted to have bilateral ptosis, extraocular weakness, nystagmus, and profound generalized weakness of all the muscle groups. This was associated with a blood lactate level of 18 mEq/liter (normal resting level is less than 2 mEq/liter). Specific defects have been localized to complex 1, complex 3, and cytochrome oxidase.

Diagnosis

In their most severe forms, mitochondrial diseases can be detected at rest. As long as hyperthyroidism or intoxication with unusual compounds (e.g., dinitrophenol) that uncouple mitochondrial oxidation are ruled out, there are few explanations for patients at rest having high pulse and respiratory rates with a serum lactate level of more than 8 mEq/liter. In patients who are less severely affected, incremental bicycle ergometry is the most useful test. Increasing the workload even to low levels results in an excessive rise in pulse rate and oxygen consumption with a low Wmax. This discrepancy between normal VO_2max, normal heart rate, and a very low Wmax is characteristic of the illness. If bicycle ergometry is not available, incremental forearm exercise may demonstrate excessive lactate production for the levels of work used. If the disorder is suspected from the clinical history and the results of exercise testing, a mus-

cle biopsy should be carried out to confirm the diagnosis. Routine light microscopy of muscle may show ragged-red fibers or be relatively normal; abnormal mitochondria sometimes are seen on electron microscopy. Biochemical evaluation of the cytochrome chain is important to localize the defect. It must be realized that analysis of mitochondrial oxidation requires relatively large amounts of muscle. The introduction of noninvasive techniques to monitor muscle metabolism has had a major impact on the analysis of mitochondrial disorders, although it is perhaps less useful in the diagnosis of these conditions. Magnetic resonance spectroscopy of ^{31}P compounds permits the analysis of ATP, creatine phosphate, inorganic phosphate, and pH in muscle. In mitochondrial disorders, there is a rapid fall in levels of creatine phosphate and an abnormal accumulation of inorganic phosphates. Equally important, there is a delay in the recovery of phosphocreatine levels to normal after exercise. These techniques can be used to evaluate the effects of treatment in a way that invasive procedures, such as muscle biopsy, cannot.

Treatment

The treatment of most mitochondrial disorders is limited to the treatment of lactic acidosis when it occurs. Treatment with a "cocktail" of compounds, including riboflavin, ubiquinone, vitamin C, menadione, and niacin, has been popular.

Adenylate Deaminase Deficiency

Pathophysiology

Approximately 1–2% of the population has a deficiency of the enzyme myoadenylate deaminase (AMP deaminase, or AMPDA). The disorder is inherited as an autosomal recessive trait. The enzyme plays a role in supporting ATP levels by acting in conjunction with adenylate kinase. Adenylate kinase converts two molecules of adenosine diphosphate to one each of ATP and AMP. Adenylate deaminase then converts AMP to inosine monophosphate with production of ammonia. This reaction is called into play when the muscle is stressed.

Clinical Features

Early studies suggested that patients with AMPDA deficiency had various forms of myalgia. The problem is that many people with AMPDA deficiency have no symptoms of exercise intolerance. Indeed, we have seen it in perfectly normal individuals. A deficiency of the enzyme has been described in almost every condition from congenital hypotonia to amyotrophic lateral sclerosis. This and other evidence of poor correlation between the enzyme defect and the clinical symptoms make it difficult to know how to interpret the entity.

Diagnosis

There are no abnormalities on the muscle biopsy under light microscopy, although the histochemical reaction for AMPDA is absent. The forearm exercise test is, again, a useful screening test. Patients with AMPDA deficiency produce normal amounts of lactate but little or no ammonia and hypoxanthine, both of which are by-products of the AMPDA reaction.

INFLAMMATORY MYOPATHIES

Inflammatory cellular changes are seen in the muscle biopsies from a wide range of myopathies and dystrophies. In many of these instances, the changes are presumed to be secondary to some other underlying disorder. In the inflammatory myopathies, the basic disease is believed to be an abnormality of the immune system or a direct infection of the muscle itself. Polymyositis and dermatomyositis are examples of abnormalities of the immune system, whereas the various forms of viral, bacterial, and parasitic infection of the muscle represent infections of the muscle. Pathological involvement of the muscle also may be seen in other autoimmune diseases, such as rheumatoid arthritis. Such involvement often is overshadowed by the primary condition.

Polymyositis and Dermatomyositis

Polymyositis and dermatomyositis, together with inclusion body myositis, represent the three most common inflammatory diseases seen by the clinician. Dermatomyositis and polymyositis both have an autoimmune basis, but the basic mechanism is very different. In dermatomyositis, the illness is the result of a humoral attack on the muscle capillaries, whereas in polymyositis, the muscle fibers are under attack by cytotoxic T cells.

As in all autoimmune illnesses, the membrane-associated proteins, which are determined by the major histocompatibility complex (MHC), play an important role. These molecules may act as antigens if they find their way into an animal or human with a different characteristic type. In humans, the MHC system is equated with HLA typing. Class 1 antigens (HLA A, B, C) are present on the membranes of virtually all cells. Class 2 antigens (HLA DR) are not so widespread and are limited predominantly to the lymphoreticular system, vascular endothelium, and some epithelia. For a cell to be the target of an attack from a cytotoxic T cell, the two cells must share the HLA class 1 molecule. The reactions in which CD4 cells participate require class 2 molecules to be shared. There is a predominance of B8 and DR3 antigens in patients with myositis. Although muscle normally expresses class 1 HLA molecules, class 2 expression may be induced under the influ-

Table 83.1: Classification of polymyositis and dermatomyositis

Primary polymyositis (adult)
Dermatomyositis (adult)
Childhood dermatomyositis (or polymyositis) with vasculitis
Polymyositis associated with connective tissue disorders
   (overlap syndromes)
Polymyositis or dermatomyositis associated with neoplasia

ence of cytokines or other abnormal situations. T cells may be typed by means of a series of surface markers (CD markers) as to whether they are cytotoxic, helper, inducer, and so forth. Because CD8 cells are involved in cytotoxic mechanisms, analysis of the type of cell involved in the cellular response is one way to determine whether the primary process is due to cellular or humoral factors.

It is common to divide polymyositis and dermatomyositis into clinical groups, as shown in Table 83.1.

Dermatomyositis

Pathophysiology. Dermatomyositis affects the capillaries and small arterioles. The first evidence of the illness is deposition of the complement c5b-9 membrane attack complex, which is needed as part of the final stages of preparing the cell for destruction in antibody-mediated disease. Further evidence for humoral rather than cytotoxic factors is found in the relative preponderance of B and CD4 (helper) cells compared with CD8 (cytotoxic cells) in the inflammatory reaction associated with the blood vessels. With advancing disease, the capillaries are destroyed and the muscle undergoes changes that resemble micro-infarction. The fibers around the edge of the fascicles are particularly affected (perifascicular atrophy), but in advanced cases, necrotic and degenerating fibers are spread throughout the muscle.

Clinical Features. Dermatomyositis is an illness in which weakness is associated with a characteristic skin rash. It is the common form of myositis in childhood, but it also occurs in adults. Often, the first sign is a change in the child's behavior. The child becomes fretful and recalcitrant and may end up being a problem at home and at school. The rash usually occurs with onset of muscle weakness, although it may develop during the course of the disease. It is characteristically a purplish discoloration of the skin over the cheeks and eyelids. It often has a butterfly distribution and blanches on pressure. Another area that may be affected is a V-shaped distribution below the neck. The rash may spread widely over the body and be associated with edema of the skin, which frequently becomes scaly and weeping. The skin over the elbows, knees, and knuckles is particularly prone to develop a reddened, indurated appearance. Because the hallmark of the disease is the capillary abnormality, it may be helpful to use a hand lens to

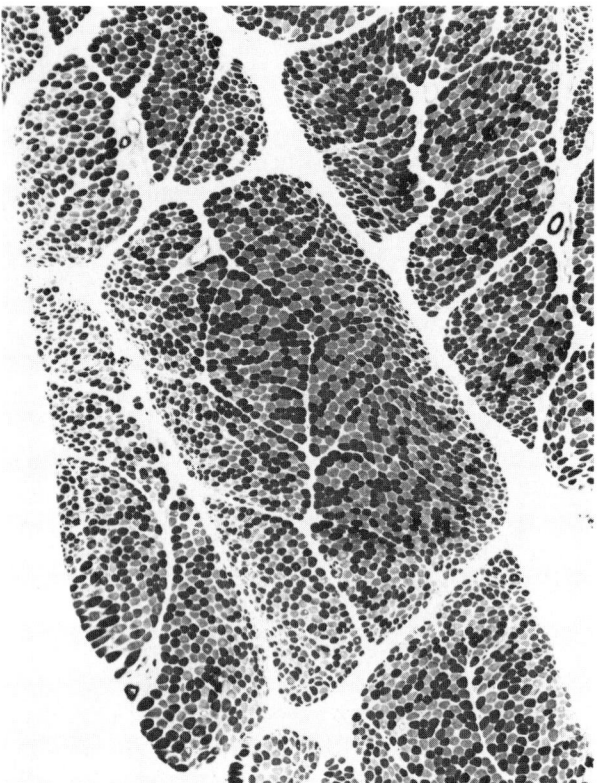

FIGURE 83.28 Dermatomyositis. Perifascicular atrophy. (Myosin adenosine triphosphatase stain, pH 9.4.)

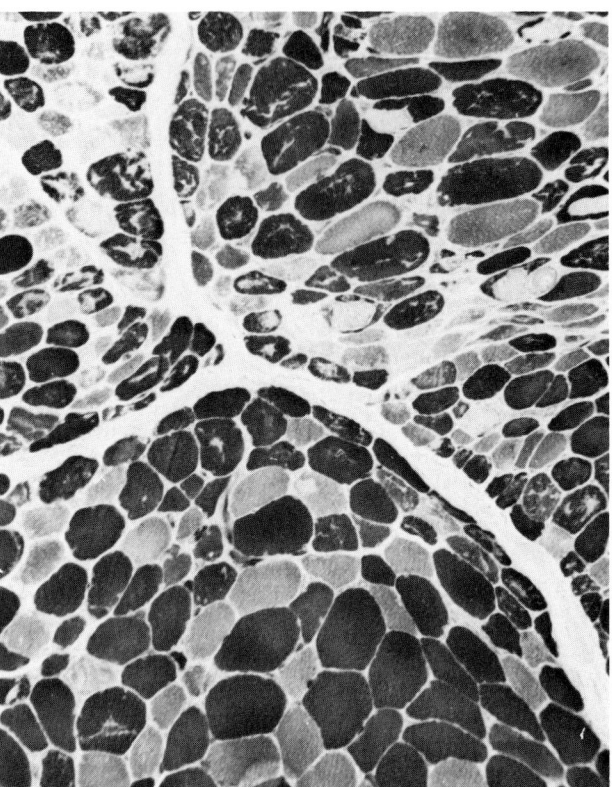

FIGURE 83.29 Polymyositis. Many of the fibers are undergoing a characteristic necrosis, indicated by pale areas in the center of the fiber. These areas spread until the entire fiber is a ghost fiber (upper left). (Myosin adenosine triphosphatase stain, pH 9.4.)

examine the skin around the nail beds. There, small hemorrhages and looped, dilatated, and sometimes thrombosed capillaries often may be combined with avascular areas. The cuticle is discolored. In chronic, long-standing dermatomyositis of childhood, the skin changes may be more disabling than the muscle weakness. In the terminal stage, the skin may be a shiny, fragile, shell-like covering that cracks at the slightest movement. Soft-tissue calcification also is seen in some patients as the disease progresses; it is usually late in the illness and is not necessarily an indication of active disease. The weakness itself is usually proximal more than distal and can be severe. Muscle pain is noted, but not in all patients. The illness often follows a relapsing-remitting course, although occasionally the illness is clearly monophasic even to the point of recovering spontaneously without treatment.

Tissues other than muscle may also be involved, as mentioned below in the section on polymyositis, with lung, heart, and gastrointestinal findings not uncommon.

Diagnosis. The serum CK concentrations are usually elevated in dermatomyositis but not universally. When abnormal, levels of several hundred to a thousand IU/ml are common. Even though the serum CK concentration is believed to reflect the activity of the disease, the correlation is imperfect. Thus, one can see a clinical exacerbation unac-

companied by marked changes in enzyme levels or patients whose illness appears quiescent who have moderately elevated levels of CK. The CK levels may rise several weeks before a clinical relapse occurs.

EMG demonstrates a combination of myopathic features together with indications of muscle hyperirritability. Thus, small polyphasic motor unit action potentials often are associated with increased insertional activity, fibrillations, and even positive sharp waves.

The muscle biopsy may be diagnostic because in no other disease is perifascicular atrophy noted (a crust of small fibers surrounding a core of more normal-sized fibers deeper in the fascicle) (Figure 83.28). MHC class 1 antibodies are also prominent in the perifascicular region. In addition, many fibers are undergoing changes of degeneration and necrosis that cause them to lose the staining characteristics with many of the enzyme reactions. Such fibers have been termed *ghost fibers* (Figure 83.29). When these changes are associated with collections of inflammatory cells around the blood vessels (Figure 83.30), the diagnosis is certain.

Unfortunately, many patients with dermatomyositis have less definite changes. Scattered fiber necrosis and phagocytosis, associated with some degree of perivascular cuffing, should always lead to the suspicion of dermatomyositis.

When the cellular responses are only associated with the muscle fibers themselves, the diagnosis is less secure because some forms of muscular dystrophy and other illnesses are associated with inflammatory responses around the muscle fibers.

Blood tests also provide evidence of an altered immune state with the development of unusual antibodies. These fall into different categories, depending on the type of antigen. One set is directed against the transfer RNA (tRNA) synthetases (antisynthetases), and of these, the Jo-1 antibody against histidyl tRNA synthetase seems to be particularly important. It is present in more than 20% of patients with polymyositis or dermatomyositis and is relatively specific to this disease group. A series of antibodies specific to myositis have also been found. Of these, anti Mi-2 seems to be specific to dermatomyositis, but the low frequency of its occurrence makes it only moderately useful as a diagnostic test. Antinuclear antibody and rheumatoid factors may be positive, particularly when evidence of other collagen vascular disease is noted.

Polymyositis

Pathophysiology. In polymyositis, the inflammatory reaction is associated more with the necrotic fibers than the blood vessels. Monoclonal antibodies demonstrate a high proportion of CD8 cells (cytotoxic cells) among the T cells around the necrotic fibers in the early phase of the disease. In one variety of polymyositis, T cells with unusual (γ/δ) receptor molecules have been found. The major unsolved question is how the immune system becomes activated. Viral mechanisms have long been suspected of playing a part in polymyositis and dermatomyositis. Coxsackie B virus has been implicated in both animals and humans as a cause of an acute myositis, and indirect evidence of Coxsackie B infection is found in a number of patients with polymyositis or dermatomyositis. Coxsackie B is of the same class of viruses as the encephalomyocarditis virus (EMCV), another virus causing myositis. These picornaviruses have a shell made up of several coat proteins. The sequence of amino acids in a region of one of these proteins is very similar to the sequence in an enzyme (histidyl tRNA synthetase, the antigen to the Jo-1 antibody) present in many patients with polymyositis and to sequences in the myosin light chain. The coat protein of EMCV demonstrates additional homology with the myosin heavy chain. The induction of polymyositis might be due to infection with one of the picornaviruses, such as Coxsackie B or EMCV, which might induce the formation of an antibody against these viruses. All this remains speculative, and supporting evidence is lacking at the present time. Other viruses, such as the human immunodeficiency virus, may infect the muscle tissue, directly damaging the vascular endothelium and releasing cytokines. Cytokines may then induce abnormal MHC expression and render the muscle tissue susceptible to destruction.

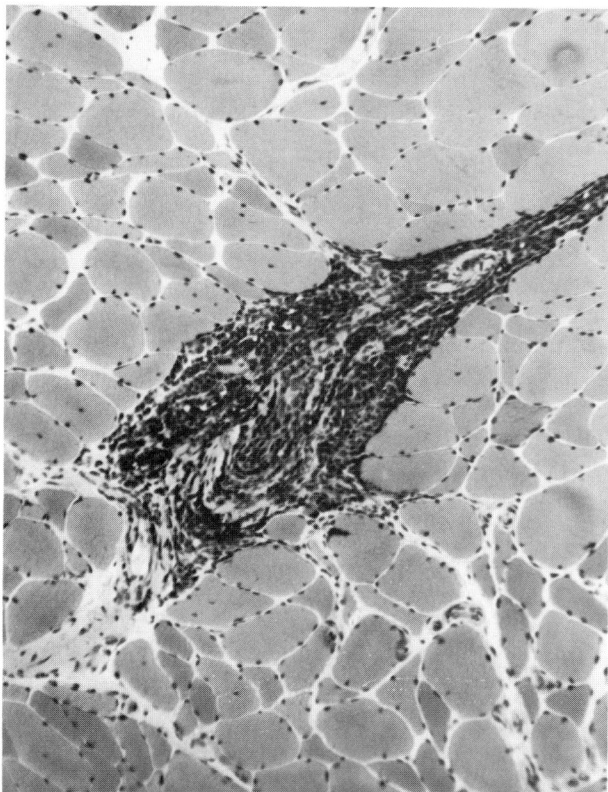

FIGURE 83.30 Polymyositis. A pronounced cellular response is associated with a blood vessel. In addition, there is abnormal variability in the size of fibers. (Hematoxylin-eosin stain.)

Clinical Features. Polymyositis is an acute or subacute illness that may occur at any age and produces widespread weakness, often more severe proximally than distally. It is not a common illness; the incidence is 5–10 per 1,000,000 population. It occurs at all ages but is most common in the 40- to 60-year-old population. It is slightly more frequent in women than in men, as are other autoimmune diseases. There is nothing very characteristic about the weakness. One would expect an inflammatory disorder of the muscle to cause severe pain, but such is not the case with polymyositis. Most patients with severe muscle pain have one of the varieties of ache, cramp, and pain disorders. Although there may be an aching, tender quality to the muscles in approximately one-half the patients with polymyositis, the more severe the pain, the less likely the diagnosis of polymyositis. The weakness may fluctuate from week to week or month to month, differentiating it from the steadily progressive dystrophies. There are often systemic symptoms at onset, such as malaise, fever, and anorexia. Sometimes, the illness is preceded by a viral prodrome, but such events are common enough in all our lives that their association with the onset of polymyositis may be no more than coincidental.

The neuromuscular examination reveals little that allows the clinician to make a specific diagnosis. The weakness may be similar in distribution to that seen in many other illnesses, such as LGMD or spinal muscular atrophy, although usually the distribution of weakness is diffusely proximal rather than the specific pattern of weakness seen in a muscular dystrophy. Eye muscles and bulbar muscles usually are not involved, but dysphagia associated with altered pharyngeal and esophageal motility may be seen, particularly in the overlap syndromes, where polymyositis is associated with other rheumatological diseases, such as scleroderma. Occasionally, the muscles may be sore to palpation and have a slightly nodular, grainy feel. This is more often discovered *after* the biopsy report has been seen than before. Tendon reflexes generally are decreased or absent in the established disease but may be increased early in the course of the condition.

Muscle is not the only tissue involved in inflammatory myopathies. There may be evidence of vascular abnormalities, such as Raynaud's phenomenon, especially in the overlap syndromes. Cardiac involvement ranges from conduction defects to congestive cardiac failure secondary to cardiomyopathy. Interstitial pneumonitis and fibrosis may cause a nonproductive cough and respiratory distress. Chest radiographs show changes in the majority of patients with patchy consolidation, particularly subpleural, and peribronchovascular thickening. The changes are reversible with treatment (Mino et al. 1997). Gastric and esophageal emptying also are delayed in the illness, indicating an abnormality in the smooth muscle of the upper gastrointestinal tract.

The natural history of polymyositis and dermatomyositis is not well defined. Attempts have been made to characterize the illness, but there has been no clear agreement on what diagnostic criteria can be used. The situation is complicated by the fact that most clinicians believe the illness should be treated with corticosteroids or immunosuppression; therefore, the course of the untreated illness will never be discovered. When the disease is relentlessly progressive, death usually occurs from inanition, intercurrent infection, or cardiac and respiratory failure, often complicated by the side effects of corticosteroid therapy. The course commonly relapses and remits, especially when the disease is treated with immunosuppression or corticosteroids. It is difficult to determine the mortality rate of the illness; some studies have placed this at 15–30%. A study of 69 patients put the 5-year survival rate at 66%, which is not very reassuring (Maugars et al. 1996). A substantial number of patients have profound disability even though the illness is burned out. The morbidity and mortality associated with high-dose immunosuppressive therapy, especially corticosteroids, has to be added to the prognosis of the disease.

Diagnosis. The diagnostic studies in polymyositis are similar to those in dermatomyositis, with serum CK concentrations, serum antibodies, EMG, and biopsy as the mainstay. CK levels may be quite markedly elevated during the course of the illness. Anti Jo-1 antibodies are found in one-fifth of the patients. Whereas the EMG is similar to that in dermatomyositis, the muscle biopsy is quite different. The perivascular inflammation seen in dermatomyositis is less prominent in polymyositis, and scattered fiber necrosis is seen associated with inflammatory reactions around and invading the fibers. Perifascicular atrophy is not seen.

Polymyositis Associated with Other Collagen Vascular Diseases (Overlap Syndromes)

Lupus erythematosus, systemic sclerosis, rheumatoid arthritis, and Sjögren's syndrome all may have weakness as a facet of the disease complex. The overlap syndromes are those in which features of at least two of these illnesses coexist. In one series, 15% of patients with polymyositis had associated collagen vascular disease. Predictably, the myositis may be seen in association with arthritis, features of scleroderma, nephritis, keratoconjunctivitis sicca, and Raynaud's phenomenon. The term *mixed connective tissue disorder* was used to indicate a combination in which polymyositis coexisted with Raynaud's phenomenon, sclerodactyly, arthritis, and pulmonary fibrosis. Mixed connective tissue disorder is characterized by a high titer of anti-μ1 ribonucleoprotein antibody.

Polymyositis or Dermatomyositis Associated with Neoplasia

A relationship between malignancy and polymyositis and, more particularly, dermatomyositis, has long been suspected. At one time, it was believed that the frequency of neoplasia in patients with dermatomyositis was approximately 50%, but subsequent studies showed that the incidence was much less, probably in the neighborhood of 10–20%. In elderly patients, particularly those with dermatomyositis, the frequency of an associated neoplasm is higher, reaching 100% in some series. The type of neoplasm is usually a carcinoma. The breast, lung, ovary, and stomach commonly have been implicated. The incidence of carcinoma may simply represent the normal incidence in the particular population of patients referred, but in some series, the frequency has exceeded that of the control population by many times. In practical terms, it is wise to carry out a rectal and vaginal examination and obtain a chest radiograph, hematological studies, and test for occult blood in the stools in any patient with adult-onset polymyositis or dermatomyositis.

Treatment of Polymyositis

There have been no good double-blinded trials of corticosteroid treatment in polymyositis. In the therapeutic trials that have been conducted, the criteria on which the diagnosis was made in the different studies were quite varied. Nevertheless, there is general agreement that polymyositis and dermatomyositis should be treated with corticosteroids or some other form of immunosuppression, or a combination of these (Mastaglia et al. 1997).

Daily prednisone may be used in the early stages of the disease in doses of up to 2 mg/kg or with a usual maximum of 100 mg. When significant improvement has occurred, the dose may be reduced to 60 mg daily, or conversion to an alternate-day dose may be considered after 2–3 months of prednisone therapy. It is difficult to know when to decrease the dosage further. As long as there is objective evidence that the patient is continuing to improve and the side effects of corticosteroids are not too severe, I usually maintain the high dose. When a plateau is reached, whether at normal strength or slightly below, the dose may be decreased slowly. The usual reduction is approximately 5 mg in the total daily dose each week until a level of 15 mg is reached; then the reduction continues in steps of 2.5 mg. If symptoms recur, it may be necessary to return to a higher level of prednisone. If there is no response after 8–10 weeks, the clinician should seriously consider some other form of treatment. The development of significant side effects may influence this regimen. Side effects may be minimized in some patients by careful attention to diet, salt restriction, high-potassium diet, H_2-receptor blockers, and the use of adjunctive calcium.

An increasingly popular alternative to corticosteroid therapy is treatment with azathioprine. It is tolerated easily by most patients in oral doses of 1.5–2.0 mg/kg per day. Before beginning treatment, a baseline complete blood count, platelet count, and liver function studies are obtained. Therapy often is initiated with a low dose (e.g., 50 mg/day in an adult). The dose then is increased gradually while monitoring the blood studies. With an effective dose (usually 2.0–3.0 mg/kg), the white blood cell count may be reduced to around 4,000, and the total lymphocytes to approximately 750 cells/ml. An abnormal decrease in platelets below 150,000/ml or a total neutrophil count of less than 1,000/ml is an indication for reducing the dosage or stopping the drug temporarily. Blood studies should be monitored twice a week at first. After a stable dose has been attained, blood studies can be monitored weekly and then monthly. Liver function tests are best monitored monthly at the beginning of treatment. An idiosyncratic response to azathioprine is seen in some patients. This consists of severe gastrointestinal distress, with nausea and vomiting associated with fever and some elevation of the liver function tests. The response disappears when the drug is withdrawn. If it is not certain that such an episode is due to azathioprine, a test dose of 25 mg can be given, which usually causes the symptoms to recur within an hour or so. There are advantages to combining prednisone and azathioprine therapy because a lower dose of both drugs may be used in combination than when each is used alone.

Cyclophosphamide, used in a similar way to that described for azathioprine, and methotrexate have been effective in some patients; methotrexate has been prominent in the rheumatology literature. Other recommended forms of treatment include low-dose total body or total lymphoid irradiation and plasmapheresis, but the response is often not very dramatic. Cyclosporine has been reported to show some benefit.

A recent development is the use of high-dose intravenous pooled human immunoglobulin (0.4 g/kg/day for 5 days). Initial trials suggested good benefit, but the cost is high (van der Meche and van Doorn 1997). A controlled, double-blind trial of intravenous immunoglobulin was carried out in patients with dermatomyositis and showed improvement in patients' functional ability and strength. Intravenous immunoglobulin was administered every month, with a total dose of 2 g/kg spread over a period of 2 days. The improvement was noted by the second or third treatment in most patients. Whether the improvement will be sustained over years is uncertain. The treatment itself poses some hazard. Thrombotic events may be seen in some patients. Common complications include vasomotor symptoms, headache, rash, leukopenia, and fever. Almost one-half of patients have some minor adverse event. In approximately 10% of patients in a recent series, the treatment had to be discontinued because of unacceptable side effects.

Inclusion Body Myositis and Myopathy

Pathophysiology

The muscle biopsy may demonstrate the presence of autophagic vacuoles in many diseases. Characteristic "rimmed" vacuoles may be profuse in an illness that has been termed *inclusion body myositis*. On light microscopy, the structures have a sharply demarcated central vacuole, around which is a rim of altered tissue that stains red with the trichrome stain. These are the inclusion bodies. Amyloid deposits are demonstrated in the muscle with Congo red and other stains. Electron microscopy demonstrates the presence of cytoplasmic tubulofilamentous structures. The filaments are paired and twisted together. They often are stacked in parallel arrays and are 15–21 nm in diameter, with an inner diameter of 3–6 nm. Filamentous bodies identical to those in the cytoplasm also are seen in the nucleus. There may also be other paired helical filaments 6–10 nm thick. The paired helical filaments may now be detected with light microscopy using a commercial antibody (Askanas et al. 1996).

There are also curious similarities to the changes seen in the brain in Alzheimer's disease. Investigating the muscle using antibodies or probes against several proteins (including β-amyloid, amyloid precursor protein, prion protein, ubiquitin, α-antichymotrypsin, neuronal microtubule-associated protein, and tau) has shown these all to be associated with the vacuoles. Ubiquitin and a hyperphosphorylated form of tau decorate the larger filaments, whereas β-amyloid is in the smaller paired helical filaments and associated with more amorphous structures. The possibility has been considered that inclusion body myositis is also a disease with an abnormality in protein processing. An interesting and unexplained finding is that there is a protein in the muscle that binds single-stranded DNA and localizes to the nucleus and the vacuoles.

An increased number of deletions of mitochondrial DNA have also been found in inclusion body myositis when compared with normal age-matched controls. This is probably reflected in the increased number of cytochrome oxidase–positive fibers and ragged-red fibers noted on the muscle biopsy. The findings do not cast any light on the etiology of the illness, which shares no clinical features with the mitochondrial disorders (Moslemi et al. 1997).

There are, in fact, two forms of inclusion body disease. The sporadic variety is associated with inflammatory changes in the muscle, and the hereditary variety, which lacks inflammatory changes. The two types of illness differ pathologically and in their clinical features.

Despite the fact that the histological hallmark of the disease is the inclusion body, the most abundant change in the biopsy from inclusion body myositis is the invasion of muscle fibers by CD8+ cytotoxic cells, suggesting a cell-mediated cytotoxicity with an immune basis. This is reinforced by the presence of the necessary MHC class I antigens on the invaded muscle fibers. On the other hand, a study of patients treated with prednisone showed that although the cellular reaction improved, the patient worsened along with the vacuolar changes, suggesting that the cellular response was secondary. Direct transfer of the β-amyloid protein precursor gene into cultured muscle cells reproduced some of the changes seen in inclusion body myositis.

Sporadic Inclusion Body Myositis

Clinical Features.   The illness is one of the most common to affect males older than 50 years; most patients are more than 30 years old. Although there is a male preponderance, women also are affected. The disease weakens the distal muscles of the arms and legs, but there is also early involvement of the quadriceps, which may be very weak. Finger flexors, especially of digits IV and V, are weak, and the wrist flexors are always more involved than the wrist extensors. The disease is sometimes asymmetrical. The progression is gradual but relentless, and disability may be severe. Facial weakness and dysphagia may be found in a number of the patients. Muscle pains are usually absent. Sometimes the sporadic form occurs in a familial setting (Sivakumar et al. 1997). It is nevertheless different from the hereditary form.

Diagnosis.   The diagnosis may be made from the muscle biopsy even if the clinical features are atypical. The required features are cellular invasion of non-necrotic fibers, rimmed vacuoles, and either amyloid deposition or filamentous deposits. If the muscle shows only cellular reaction, the diagnosis may be considered if the clinical picture is typical. The EMG may resemble that in polymyositis, but evidence of a peripheral neuropathy is noted on occasion. The CK concentration may be mildly elevated or high normal.

Treatment.   The disease generally has a chronic progressive course and is considered unresponsive to prednisone. Indeed, this is one of the criteria by which the diagnosis may be suspected. It is tempting to embark on a therapeutic trial when the inflammatory reaction is marked, but the side effects of corticosteroids in the elderly population are not to be taken lightly. A trial of high-dose intravenous immunoglobulin showed some improvement in leg function but did not show any effect in strength. Other reports have not shown any benefit (Griggs et al. 1995).

Hereditary Inclusion Body Myopathy

Some patients have biopsies that demonstrate the typical features of inclusion body myositis, but they have no cellular inflammatory component. These patients are separately classified on other counts: Their clinical picture is different from that of inclusion body myositis, the disease is often inherited, and the amount of amyloid in the biopsies is less. The pattern of inheritance may be either autosomal dominant or recessive. One type with a recessive inheritance was first reported in Iranian Jews but has now been described in Asians and Caucasians as well. Unlike those with sporadic inflammatory inclusion body myositis who have severe quadriceps weakness, these patients retained their quadriceps strength disproportionately, thereby leading to the term *quadriceps sparing*. The illness begins in early adult life and is progressive. Linkage studies have localized the gene for this type of inclusion body myopathy to chromosome 9 (Argov et al. 1997). Of major interest is that this is the same location as the gene for the autosomal recessive distal myopathy with rimmed vacuoles, a disease that appears very similar to hereditary inclusion body myopathy. This suggests that the two are the same disease or, less likely, are allelic. Autosomal dominant forms of hereditary inclusion body myopathy are also reported. They are clinically similar and begin earlier, often in the first two decades, with a slowly progressive course.

Polymyalgia Rheumatica

Clinical Features

Polymyalgia rheumatica is an illness characterized by severe muscle pain. The clinician should be cautious about the indiscriminate use of this diagnosis without full investigation because of two major implications: the high frequency of temporal arteritis and the effectiveness of corticosteroid therapy. The diagnosis should be limited to those with the typical picture, including increased erythrocyte sedimentation rate, and not used as an explanation for various aches, cramps, and pains. Women are affected more commonly than are men, and the disorder is rare under the age of 55 years. The patient develops muscle stiffness and pain and a feeling that the muscles have set. The arms are involved more commonly than the legs. Manipulation of the limb exacerbates the pain. The symptoms are particularly prominent in the morning when the patient arises and improve as the patient loosens up. These symptoms may be associated with chronic malaise, pyrexia, night sweats, and weight loss. On examination, there are no specific muscle abnormalities other than soreness. There may be tenderness over the temples, reflecting temporal arteritis. The frequency of this complication has been estimated at 20–30%.

Diagnosis

The erythrocyte sedimentation rate is elevated (often more than 70 mm/hour), and this should be considered an essential part of the diagnosis of polymyalgia rheumatica. There may be a mild hypochromic anemia. Otherwise, laboratory studies are generally normal. There is no elevation of the serum CK concentration, EMG may be normal, and muscle biopsy may show type 2 fiber atrophy, a nonspecific finding that is not helpful in the diagnosis.

Treatment

Polymyalgia rheumatica may be self-limiting but may take years to fade. For this reason, prednisone and the nonsteroidal anti-inflammatory drugs have been recommended as a treatment. The response to prednisone may be quite dramatic, with resolution of symptoms in hours to days. For the most part, the doses can be lower than those used in other inflammatory autoimmune diseases. It is possible to commence with 30–50 mg of prednisone daily in an adult and maintain this dose for 2 months before a gradual decrease. Maintenance on a low level of corticosteroids is often necessary for 2 years, and even then, only 24% of the patients were able to stop treatment in one prospective study.

Other Inflammatory Conditions

Muscle frequently shows subclinical involvement in chronic granulomatous diseases, such as sarcoidosis and tuberculosis. Bacterial infection (pyomyositis) is rare outside of tropical countries, although it has been recorded. The organism involved is often *Staphylococcus aureus*, and sometimes *Streptococcus*. Usually, the large muscle groups, such as those of the thigh, are the site of infection. The muscle is hot, painful, and swollen, and any movement exacerbates pain. Parasitic infections of muscles include those due to trichinosis, cysticercosis, and toxoplasmosis. In trichinosis, general symptoms of malaise and fever are associated with muscle pains and stiffness. There may be periorbital edema, and the jaw muscles commonly are involved. Laboratory studies include muscle biopsy, which may show evidence of hypersensitivity, such as eosinophilia and hypergammaglobulinemia. Treatment with thiabendazole has been recommended. Myopathies associated with the retroviruses,

such as human immunodeficiency virus, are discussed elsewhere (see Chapter 59).

CONGENITAL MYOPATHIES

Congenital Hypotonias

Hypotonic Children

Occasionally children exhibit a lack of tone at birth or shortly thereafter. In some, this hypotonia is accompanied by obvious weakness of the limbs, and the baby lies immobile in the crib. These children usually have one of the spinal muscular atrophies, a metabolic disorder (e.g., a mitochondrial myopathy), or, rarely, a toxic cause (e.g., botulism). Other babies move the limbs, if not normally, at least through their full range of movement, and do so spontaneously. Determining muscle strength in a baby is difficult; however, when no obvious weakness is discernible, the babies are classified in the category of congenital hypotonia. One of the most common causes of congenital hypotonia is secondary to damage to the central nervous system. Often, as such children grow older, the hypotonia is replaced by increased tone and an associated delay in intellectual development. This cerebral hypotonia is not due to any primary abnormality in the muscle but presumably accompanies a disturbance of reflex tone. Selective atrophy of type 2 muscle fibers may be noted on biopsy, changes that are not indicative of a primary disease of the muscle but are secondary to the neurological lesion. Babies with benign congenital hypotonia do not show any neurological abnormality other than hypotonia. Tendon reflexes are preserved or slightly diminished. Muscle biopsy and EMGs are normal, and serum CK levels are appropriate to the child's age. As time progresses, the children gain tone, and normal motor development ensues. In teenage life, these children may not gain the ranks of star high school athletes, but, nevertheless, for all intents and purposes, neuromuscular function is normal.

Congenital hypotonia with type 1 fiber predominance is a similar disorder (Figure 83.31). In these cases, the muscle biopsy shows a predominance of type 1 fibers that may be striking. Tendon reflexes may be absent, and the children often are less agile than the average student when they reach high school. Nevertheless, for all intents and purposes, they are perfectly capable of normal activity.

The only treatment necessary in all these conditions is to encourage the child to participate in play therapy, with the aim of increasing motor activity. A referral to an occupational therapist accomplishes this.

Prader-Willi Syndrome

Patients with Prader-Willi syndrome often present with congenital hypotonia and feeding difficulties. The diagnosis

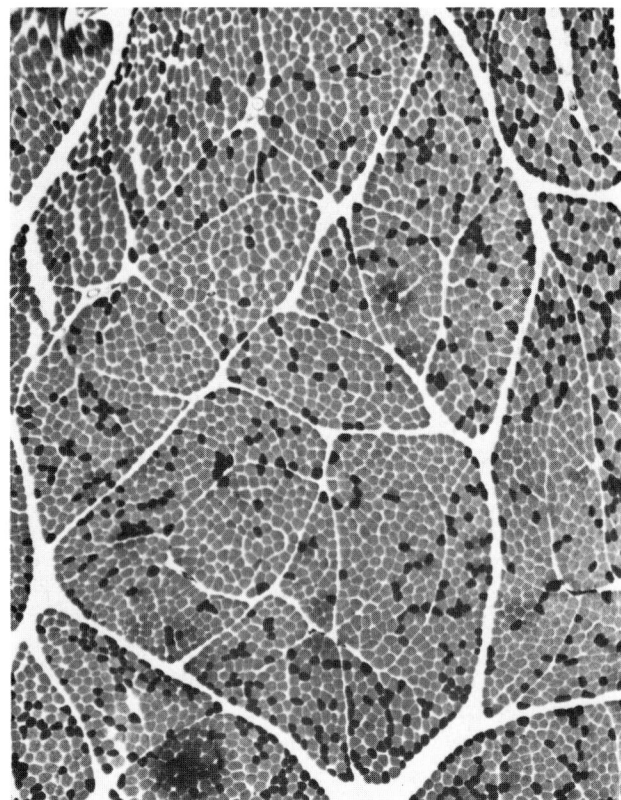

FIGURE 83.31 Congenital hypotonia with type 1 predominance. A biceps biopsy showing a change in the ratio of fiber types. In a normal child's muscle, the type 2 fibers are more numerous than the type 1. (Myosin adenosine triphosphatase stain, pH 9.4.)

sometimes is not revealed until the children start gaining weight, although, in retrospect, the characteristic features of almond eyes, disproportionately large head, large anterior fontanelle, mild micrognathia, gum anomalies, and genital hypoplasia have been present since birth. Mental retardation also is noted. As the children grow older, their hands and feet may be abnormally small, and the weight gain and excessive appetite characteristic of the illness is noted. There may be skin hypopigmentation, and the children often have unusually fair hair and sensitivity to sun exposure. Behavioral problems, such as theft of food, pica, and obsessive picking at the skin, as well as daytime somnolence and sleep apnea complicate the picture.

The prevalence of Prader-Willi syndrome is approximately 1 per 20,000, and it is caused by a deficient paternal gene on the long arm of chromosome 15 (15q11-13). The gene has been identified as encoding a polypeptide associated with a small nuclear ribonucleoprotein expressed in the brain. Studies of the homologous gene in the mouse have shown that it is subject to maternal imprinting, the phenomenon whereby alleles are processed slightly differently depending on whether they derive from the father or mother. Maternal imprinting is accomplished by methylation of some DNA loci in one parent but not the other and could account for the fact that the child must inherit the defective gene from the father.

Congenital Myopathies with Structural Changes in Muscle Fibers

Certain muscle illnesses manifest characteristic features that are visible on the muscle biopsy. These changes have been embodied in the names of the illnesses: central core disease, nemaline myopathy, myotubular myopathy, and fiber-type disproportion. Central core disease, nemaline myopathy, and fiber-type disproportion share many features in common, whereas myotubular myopathy seems to differ clinically from the others.

Central Core Disease

Pathophysiology. Central core disease was the first of the congenital nonprogressive myopathies to be described in the 1960s. The disease is inherited as an autosomal dominant trait, although sporadic cases are not uncommon. The faulty gene is on the long arm of chromosome 19 (19q13.1). The illness is associated with a mutation of the ryanodine receptor and is allelic to malignant hyperthermia. Malignant hyperthermia and central core disease certainly coexist in some families; however, the association is not always clear. Malignant hyperthermia does not always accompany central core disease, and in at least one family, the central core phenotype did not always accompany the gene defect.

The muscle shows a combination of type 1 fiber predominance with central cores, an area in the muscle fiber where the central myofibrils are in disarray. On cross-section of the muscle, many of the oxidative histochemical reactions and the periodic acid–Schiff stain demonstrate an unstained central core running through the center of the fibers (Figure 83.32).

Clinical Features. The patient with central core disease may be floppy shortly after birth, and, as in so many of these illnesses, congenital hip dislocation is common. As the child grows older, motor milestones are delayed, and, at an age when the child should be running easily, he or she is often ungainly and clumsy. The family recognizes before too long that the illness is not getting any worse. Strength, although below normal, usually is not impaired enough to be severely disabling. As in some of the other illnesses, the patients may be slender and short of stature. On examination, there is a diffuse weakness of the arms and legs. Mild facial and neck weakness also may be found. Deep tendon reflexes often are diminished, although, surprisingly, they are normal in some patients. Skeletal abnormalities, such as high-arched feet, a long face, and a high-arched palate, are not uncommon. In both central core disease and nemaline myopathy, a severe and disabling form of the illness

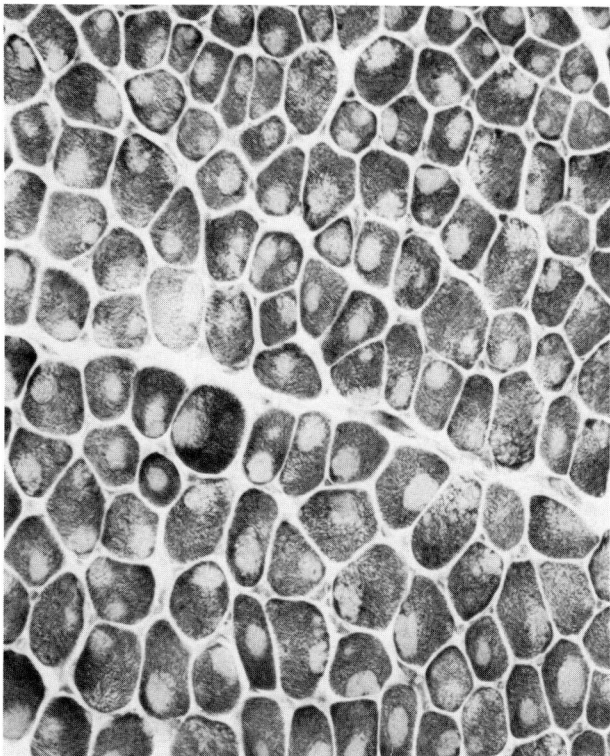

FIGURE 83.32 Central core disease. The unstained area in most of the fibers is characteristic of this illness. (Nicotinamide adenine dinucleotide dehydrogenase-tetrazolium reductase stain.)

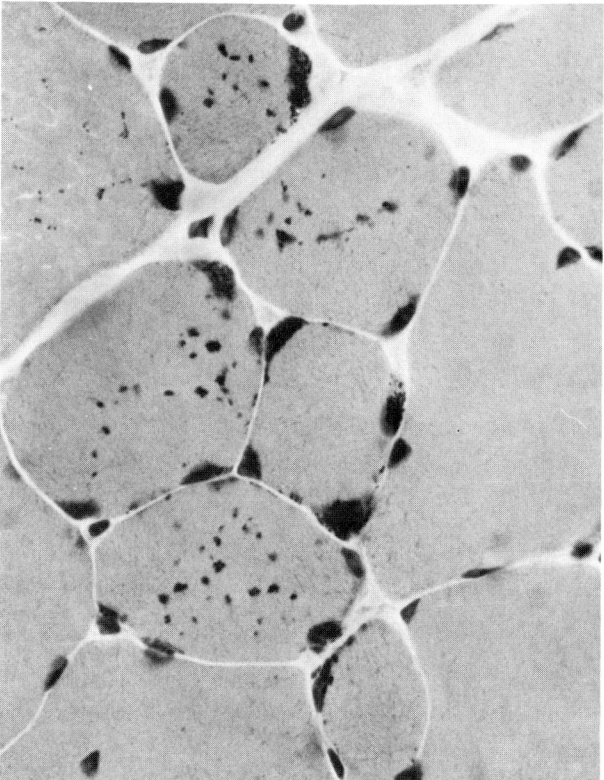

FIGURE 83.33 Nemaline myopathy. Although better demonstrated with the electron microscope, nemaline rods are also noted with histochemical reactions. The granular appearance of these fibers is due to the presence of many rods. (Modified Gomori trichrome stain.)

may be seen with respiratory failure. The muscle pathology does not appear to be any different, but the patient may be confined to a wheelchair, scarcely able to move arms or legs, and have a profound kyphoscoliosis. If this type of central core disease is noted, surgical stabilization of the back may be helpful, although the lack of respiratory reserve may prevent such an approach.

Diagnosis. The EMG shows nonspecific myopathic changes in central core disease. Serum CK level is usually normal, although mild elevation may be seen. The muscle biopsy is diagnostic.

Treatment. No specific treatment for central core disease is available, although bracing may be needed to correct a deformity, such as a footdrop. Any family in whom central core disease has been found should be advised about the possibility of malignant hyperthermia because this is a potentially fatal complication.

Nemaline Myopathy

Pathophysiology. This diagnosis of nemaline myopathy is based on the presence of small, rodlike particles in the muscle. They are usually found on the modified trichrome stain, but they are most accurately characterized on electron

microscopy (Figure 83.33). They originate in the Z disc and exhibit structural continuity with the thin filament. They have a regular structure, presenting as a tetragonal filamentous array when cut transversely and exhibiting periodic lines both perpendicular and parallel to the long axis. A major constituent of the rod structure is α-actinin, a protein normally present in the Z line. Desmin, which is a protein similar to α-actinin, and actin are also found in the rods. The disorder often is inherited as an autosomal dominant illness; however, autosomal recessive and sporadic cases are common. The gene for the dominant variety of the illness is localized tentatively to a region on the long arm of chromosome 1 (1q21-23). Although this is the same chromosome as the gene for α-actinin, linkage studies have excluded the possibility that this gene is the culprit. The gene for the recessive variety of nemaline myopathy is on 2q21.2-22. This raises the possibility that it involves one of the giant muscle proteins, nebulin or titin, the genes for which are in the same region (Pelin et al. 1997).

Clinical Features. The clinical picture of nemaline myopathy is heterogeneous. The most common is one in which hypotonia is noted early, succeeded by a diffuse weakness

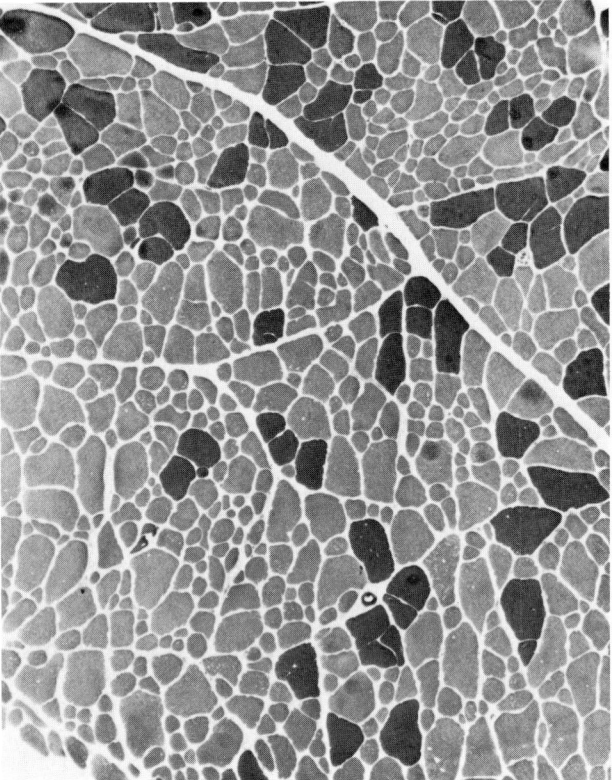

FIGURE 83.34 Nemaline myopathy. As in central core disease, nemaline myopathy shows predominance and atrophy of type 1 fibers. Note that the very smallest fibers in this biopsy are all type 1. (Myosin adenosine triphosphatase stain, pH 9.4.)

of the arms and legs, mild weakness of the face and other bulbar muscles, and a dysmorphic appearance. The face is long and narrow, with abnormalities of the jaw that may be either prognathous or abnormally short. The feet are often high-arched, and kyphoscoliosis is common as the children grow older. The disorder is considered nonprogressive, although some patients become weaker late in life. In some patients, respiratory failure out of proportion to the general weakness may ensue. Cardiomyopathy also has been noted. Another form may have its onset later in life and present with a mild proximal weakness. There is also a severe infantile variety that is fatal. These children have profound hypotonia and respiratory failure.

Diagnosis. In nemaline myopathy, EMG demonstrates the nonspecific myopathic changes. Serum CK levels may be normal or elevated. The muscle biopsy, in addition to demonstrating nemaline rods, often shows type 1 fiber predominance, selective atrophy of the type 1 fibers, and deficiency of type 2B fiber. Electron microscopic studies show the characteristic rods (Figure 83.34). These are most often in the cytoplasm, but intranuclear rods also have been noted and are equated with the severe infantile form (Goebel and Warlo 1997).

Treatment. No specific treatment for nemaline myopathy is available. Bracing and surgery may be recommended when necessary.

Centronuclear or Myotubular Myopathy

Pathophysiology. The term *centronuclear* or *myotubular myopathy* (MTM) was given to a group of diseases in which the pathological finding was the presence of fibers with internal nuclei, which were thought to resemble the myotube stage in the development of muscle fibers in culture. The best known form is a severe infantile illness that is often fatal, the hallmarks of which are extraocular, facial, and limb weakness, often with respiratory failure. The gene locus has been localized to the long arm of the X chromosome at Xq28. The gene has been identified and is known as the *MTM1* gene. It encodes for myotubularin, a protein with a tyrosine phosphatase domain (Laporte et al. 1997).

There appears to be another related gene on the X chromosome, *MTMR1*, and two other genes, *MTMR2* and *MTMR3*, on autosomal chromosomes. Perhaps changes in the last two account for the occurrence of the autosomally inherited variety of illness, some of which is dominant and some recessive. The relationship between the gene product and the disease has not yet been elucidated. Mild and intermediate forms do exist. Large deletions of the gene have not been described, but missense and nonsense mutations and point deletions have been found in a number of the X-linked families.

Clinical Features. The severe infantile variety of myotubular myopathy is inherited as an X-linked recessive disorder. It usually presents as severe hypotonia and respiratory distress. The disorder is usually fatal due to respiratory failure during the first few months. The weakness is severe and includes weakness of the facial and neck muscles as well as the extraocular muscles. Ptosis has not been as pronounced, but the eyes may appear puffy. The ribs are thin, and there are contractures at the hips and less often at the knees and ankles. Intermediate and milder forms of the illness are known. These vary between adults who have extraocular weakness, facial weakness, and mild difficulty with limb strength to adolescents who have more severe weakness and lose the ability to walk in early to middle adult life.

In the autosomal dominant form of myotubular myopathy, the illness is milder and occurs later in life. The illness is less common than the severe X-linked form. Ptosis, extraocular weakness, and facial weakness are noted, and a moderate limb weakness gives rise to some disability. Equinovarus deformity of the feet has been noted. The autosomal recessive variety, which is also less common, seems to be intermediate in severity between the other varieties. Reports of electrical or clinical seizures were prominent in the early literature but have not been emphasized recently.

Diagnosis. Laboratory studies show normal or slightly elevated serum CK level and a myopathic EMG. The muscle biopsy demonstrates characteristic features. With the routine hematoxylin-eosin or trichrome stains, there is quite marked variability in the size of fibers, most of which are small. In the center of many of these fibers is a large, plump nucleus, resembling the myotube stage of muscle development. With the oxidative enzyme reaction, many of the fibers have a darkly staining central spot. Almost all the fibers have a pale staining area, with the ATPase reaction that runs through the middle of the fiber. Although this looks superficially like a core, most central cores are not visible with an ATPase stain. When viewed in longitudinal section, the fiber has a long central area containing nuclei spaced at intervals. The biopsy shares features of the other congenital disorders, with type 1 fiber predominance and often type 1 fiber atrophy. The biopsy findings in the X-linked recessive illness appear similar. Although the muscle fibers superficially resemble myotubes, they are in fact quite different; hence, the preferred term *centronuclear myopathy*. The differentiation into well-marked histochemical fiber types and the cytoarchitecture of the fiber more resembles the adult fiber. Two fetal cytoskeletal proteins (vimentin and desmin), which are found in fetal myotubes, have been demonstrated in fibers from patients with myotubular myopathy by immunocytochemical studies. The electroencephalogram has been reported on occasions to show a paroxysmal disturbance.

Treatment. The treatment of the milder myotubular myopathy includes respiratory support where indicated, treatment of any concurrent seizure disorder, and general supportive measures. Treatment of the severe infantile form must be considered against the background of a very poor prognosis. The decision whether or not to provide life support for these children is a difficult one. Most die within the first 2 years.

Congenital Fiber-Type Disproportion

Pathophysiology. The biopsy in congenital fiber-type disproportion is characterized by a marked disproportion between the size of type 2 and type 1 fibers. The muscle biopsy shows the features of type 1 fiber atrophy and predominance. Originally, it was suggested that biopsies in which the mean diameter of the type 1 fibers was 15% smaller than that of the type 2 fibers were indicative of the illness. This assumption was a mistake, leading to the inclusion of patients with many different illnesses, such as CMD and FSHD. The diagnosis should only be made when the discrepancy between the type 1 and type 2 fibers is greater than 45% and when more than 75% of the fibers are type 1 (Figure 83.35). The reason for this discrepancy in fiber size is unknown. The illness is inherited as an autosomal dominant trait in approximately 40% of reported cases. There is considerable debate in the literature on the specificity of this illness, and many believe it to be a nonspecific biopsy finding. It is possible that this illness represents

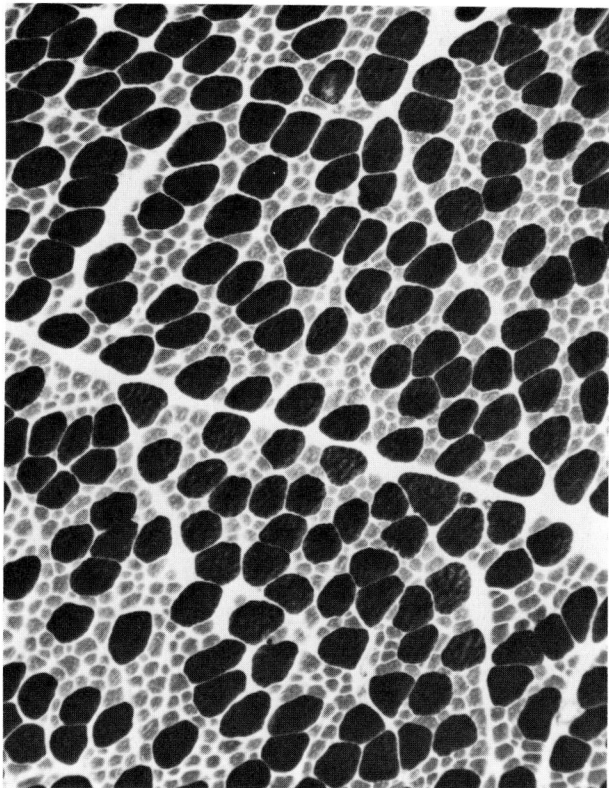

FIGURE 83.35 Congenital fiber-type disproportion. The diagnosis should not be made unless there is a clear discrepancy between hypertrophic type 2 fibers and atrophic type 1 fibers, as demonstrated in this picture. (Myosin adenosine triphosphatase stain, pH 9.4.)

nemaline myopathy without rods, a view that is strengthened by the fact that both rods and cores are inconsistently present in biopsies from patients with both of these illnesses. Only the appropriate DNA studies in the future will settle this question.

Clinical Features. The children are floppy at birth, with varying degrees of weakness. The weakness is diffuse, with frequent involvement of the face and neck. Sometimes in early childhood, there is improvement in strength, although whether this represents an improvement in the disease or the child's natural growth is not certain. Contractures, particularly of the Achilles tendons and congenital hip dislocation, commonly are seen. Respiratory complications are common during the first 2 years of life, when the disease can be quite severe. As the children grow older, they remain weak and are short, with low weight. Accompanying the illness are various deformities of the feet, high-arched palate, and kyphoscoliosis.

Diagnosis. In congenital fiber-type disproportion, EMG shows myopathic potentials, and the serum CK level may be normal to slightly elevated. The muscle biopsy is diagnostic.

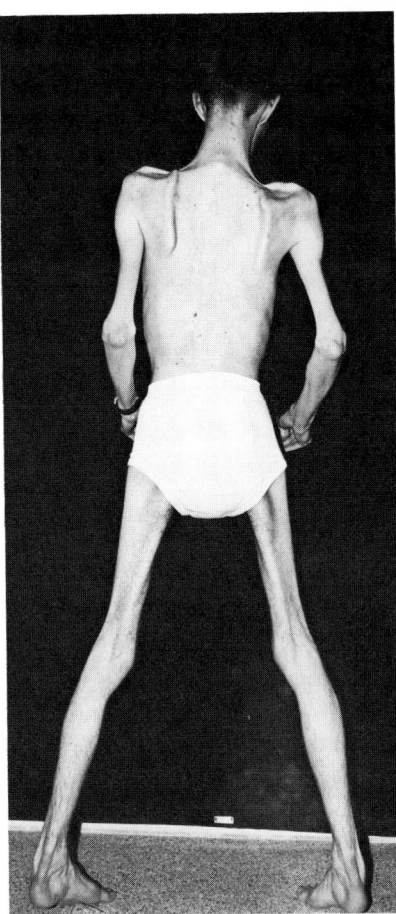

FIGURE 83.36 Congenital muscular dystrophy (stick man type). This boy has a nonprogressive weakness associated with limb contractures, which has been present from birth. There is no mental retardation. He is actually much stronger than his muscle bulk suggests.

Other Possible Clinical Entities

Clinical evaluation of patients with muscle disease now demands a proper analysis of the genetic and molecular mechanisms. It is an anachronism to try to describe muscle disease in the absence of this analysis. Nevertheless, one entity has always been puzzling: the child who has a static weakness, a skeletal appearance, and a biopsy that is dystrophic. I call this entity *stick man dystrophy*. Others have described similar cases as myosclerosis. It is uncertain whether this will turn out to be a distinct illness, although the patients are all remarkably similar. Often, this illness is called to the parents' attention when they see the child toe walking in early childhood. The muscles are extremely slender but generate a surprising amount of force for their mass, although strength is not normal (Figure 83.36). Contractures of the elbows, knees, and other joints are common. Kyphoscoliosis develops in early adult life. Treatment is limited to management of the contractures and kyphoscoliosis. If heel cord lengthening is attempted, it should be done cautiously because many of these children learn to walk and run with shortened heel cords. If these are lengthened, the children must relearn how to walk.

REFERENCES

Argov Z, Tiram E, Eisenberg I, et al. Various types of hereditary inclusion body myopathies map to chromosome 9p1-p1. Ann Neurol 1997;41:548–551.

Askanas V, Alvarez RB, Mirabella M, Engel WK. Use of anti-neurofilament antibody to identify paired-helical filaments in inclusion-body myositis. Ann Neurol 1996;39:389–391.

Bejaoui K, Hirabayashi K, Hentati F, et al. Linkage of Miyoshi myopathy (distal autosomal recessive muscular dystrophy) locus to chromosome 2p12-14. Neurology 1995;45:768–772.

Brown RH Jr. Dystrophin-associated proteins and the muscular dystrophies. Annu Rev Med 1997;48:457–466.

Ceuterick C, Martin JJ. Sporadic early adult-onset distal myopathy with rimmed vacuoles: immunohistochemistry and electron microscopy. J Neurol Sci 1996;139:190–196.

Deconinck N, Tinsley J, De Backer F, et al. Expression of truncated utrophin leads to major functional improvements in dystrophin-deficient muscles of mice. Nat Med 1997;3:1216–1221.

Dincer P, Leturcq F, Richard I, et al. A biochemical, genetic, and clinical survey of autosomal recessive limb girdle muscular dystrophies in Turkey. Ann Neurol 1997;42:222–229.

Duggan DJ, Gorospe JR, Fanin M, et al. Mutations in the sarcoglycan genes in patients with myopathy. N Engl J Med 1997;336:618–624.

Fahlke C, Beck CL, George AL Jr. A mutation in autosomal dominant myotonia congenita affects pore properties of the muscle chloride channel. Proc Natl Acad Sci U S A 1997;94:2729–2734.

Fardeau M, Hillaire D, Mignard C, et al. Juvenile limb-girdle muscular dystrophy. Clinical, histopathological and genetic data from a small community living in the Reunion Island. Brain 1996;119:295–308.

Figarella-Branger D, Baeta Machado AM, Putzu GA, et al. Exertional rhabdomyolysis and exercise intolerance revealing dystrophinopathies. Acta Neuropathol (Berl) 1997;94:48–53.

Fisher J, Upadhyaya M. Molecular genetics of facioscapulohumeral muscular dystrophy (FSHD). Neuromuscul Disord 1997;7:55–62.

Fouad G, Dalakas M, Servidei S, et al. Genotype-phenotype correlations of DHP receptor alpha1-subunit gene mutations causing hypokalemic periodic paralysis. Neuromuscul Disord 1997;7:33–38.

Goebel HH, Warlo I. Nemaline myopathy with intranuclear rods—intranuclear rod myopathy. Neuromuscul Disord 1997;7:13–19.

Greenberg DA. Calcium channels in neurological disease. Ann Neurol 1997;42:275–282.

Griggs RC, Askanas V, DiMauro S, et al. Inclusion body myositis and myopathies. Ann Neurol 1995;38:705–713.

Hayward LJ, Brown RH Jr, Cannon SC. Slow inactivation differs among mutant Na channels associated with myotonia and periodic paralysis. Biophys J 1997;72:1204–1219.

Hoffman EP, Lehmann-Horn F, Rudel R. Overexcited or inactive: ion channels in muscle disease. Cell 1995;80:681–686.

Ji S, George AL Jr, Horn R, Barchi RL. Paramyotonia congenita mutations reveal different roles for segments S3 and S4 of domain D4 in hSkM1 sodium channel gating. J Gen Physiol 1996;107:183–194.

Laing NG, Laing BA, Meredith C, et al. Autosomal dominant distal myopathy: linkage to chromosome 14. Am J Hum Genet 1995;56:422–427.

Laporte J, Guiraud-Chaumeil C, Vincent MC, et al. Mutations in the *MTM1* gene implicated in X-linked myotubular myopathy. ENMC International Consortium on Myotubular Myopathy. European Neuro-Muscular Center. Hum Mol Genet 1997;6:1505–1511.

Leyten QH, Gabreels FJ, Renier WO, ter Laak HJ. Congenital muscular dystrophy: a review of the literature. Clin Neurol Neurosurg 1996;98:267–280.

Manilal S, Nguyen TM, Sewry CA, Morris GE. The EDMD protein, emerin, is a nuclear membrane protein. Hum Mol Genet 1996;5:801–808.

Mastaglia FL, Phillips BA, Zilko P. Treatment of inflammatory myopathies. Muscle Nerve 1997;20:651–664.

Mathieu J, Allard P, Gobeil G, et al. Anesthetic and surgical complications in 219 cases of myotonic dystrophy. Neurology 1997;49:1646–1650.

Maugars YM, Berthelot JM, Abbas AA, et al. Long-term prognosis of 69 patients with dermatomyositis or polymyositis. Clin Exp Rheumatol 1996;14:263–274.

Miaux Y, Chiras J, Eymard B, et al. Cranial MRI findings in myotonic dystrophy. Neuroradiology 1997;39:166–170.

Milanov I, Ishpekova B. Differential diagnosis of scapuloperoneal syndrome. Electromyogr Clin Neurophysiol 1997;37:73–78.

Mino M, Noma S, Taguchi Y, et al. Pulmonary involvement in polymyositis and dermatomyositis: sequential evaluation with CT. AJR Am J Roentgenol 1997;169:83–87.

Moreira ES, Vainzof M, Marie SK, et al. The seventh form of autosomal recessive limb-girdle muscular dystrophy is mapped to 17q11-12. Am J Hum Genet 1997;61:151–159.

Morrone A, Zammarchi E, Scacheri PC, et al. Asymptomatic dystrophinopathy. Am J Med Genet 1997;69:261–267.

Moslemi AR, Lindberg C, Oldfors A. Analysis of multiple mitochondrial DNA deletions in inclusion body myositis. Hum Mutat 1997;10:381–386.

Moxley RT 3rd. Proximal myotonic myopathy: mini-review of a recently delineated clinical disorder. Neuromuscul Disord 1996;6:87–93.

Muntoni F, Gobbi P, Sewry C, et al. Deletions in the 5' region of dystrophin and resulting phenotypes. J Med Genet 1994;31:843–847.

Nobile C, Marchi J, Nigro V, et al. Exon-intron organization of the human dystrophin gene. Genomics 1997;45:421–424.

Pelin K, Ridanpaa M, Donner K, et al. Refined localisation of the genes for nebulin and titin on chromosome 2q allows the assignment of nebulin as a candidate gene for autosomal recessive nemaline myopathy. Eur J Hum Genet 1997;5:229–234.

Phillips MF, Harper PS. Cardiac disease in myotonic dystrophy. Cardiovasc Res 1997;33:13–22.

Sansone V, Griggs RC, Meola G, et al. Andersen's syndrome: a distinct periodic paralysis. Ann Neurol 1997;42:305–312.

Sillen A, Sorensen T, Kantola I, et al. Identification of mutations in the *CACNL1A3* gene in 13 families of Scandinavian origin having hypokalemic periodic paralysis and evidence of a founder effect in Danish families. Am J Med Genet 1997;69:102–106.

Sivakumar K, Semino-Mora C, Dalakas MC. An inflammatory, familial, inclusion body myositis with autoimmune features and a phenotype identical to sporadic inclusion body myositis. Studies in three families. Brain 1997;120:653–661.

Stajich JM, Gilchrist JM, Lennon F, et al. Confirmation of linkage of oculopharyngeal muscular dystrophy to chromosome 14q11.2-q13. Ann Neurol 1996;40:801–804.

Tan E, Topaloglu H, Sewry C, et al. Late onset muscular dystrophy with cerebral white matter changes due to partial merosin deficiency. Neuromuscul Disord 1997;7:85–89.

Thornton CA, Wymer JP, Simmons Z, et al. Expansion of the myotonic dystrophy CTG repeat reduces expression of the flanking *DMAHP* gene. Nat Genet 1997;16:407–409.

Twyman RS, Harper GD, Edgar MA. Thoracoscapular fusion in facioscapulohumeral dystrophy: clinical review of a new surgical method. J Shoulder Elbow Surg 1996;5:201–205.

Upadhyaya M, Maynard J, Rogers MT, et al. Improved molecular diagnosis of facioscapulohumeral muscular dystrophy (FSHD): validation of the differential double digestion for FSHD. J Med Genet 1997;34:476–479.

van der Knaap MS, Smit LM, Barth PG, et al. Magnetic resonance imaging in classification of congenital muscular dystrophies with brain abnormalities. Ann Neurol 1997;42:50–59.

van der Kooi AJ, Barth PG, Busch HF, et al. The clinical spectrum of limb girdle muscular dystrophy. A survey in The Netherlands. Brain 1996;119:1471–1480.

van der Kooi AJ, van Meegen M, Ledderhof TM, et al. Genetic localization of a newly recognized autosomal dominant limb-girdle muscular dystrophy with cardiac involvement (*LGMD1B*) to chromosome 1q11-21. Am J Hum Genet 1997;60:891–895.

van der Meche FG, van Doorn PA. The current place of high-dose immunoglobulins in the treatment of neuromuscular disorders. Muscle Nerve 1997;20:136–147.

Voskova-Goldman A, Peier A, Caskey CT, et al. DMD-specific FISH probes are diagnostically useful in the detection of female carriers of DMD gene deletions. Neurology 1997;48:1633–1638.

Chapter 84
Neurological Problems of the Newborn

Alan Hill and Joseph J. Volpe

Increased survival of premature newborns as a result of improved obstetrical care and especially of the treatment of neonatal respiratory disease has focused attention on the morbidity and mortality resulting from neurological complications. Rational management of newborn neurological problems must be based on sound principles of basic science, human and experimental pathology, and physiological and biochemical mechanisms.

Advances in fetal assessment, especially the use of real-time ultrasound (US) scanning, have increased awareness of the prenatal origin of many neurological abnormalities detected in the newborn. In many instances, methods of fetal assessment allow a limited neurological examination of the fetus. Intrauterine intervention for prevention of brain injury may be considered the primary objective for optimal management of neurological disorders that manifest in the newborn. Optimal management demands expertise from many disciplines, including obstetrics, neonatology, genetics, neurology, and neurosurgery. A cooperative team effort often is the most effective approach to neurological problems in neonates, especially when difficult ethical decisions are involved.

In this chapter, the practical aspects of diagnosis and management of relatively common neurological problems of the newborn encountered by practicing neurologists are reviewed.

GENERAL PRINCIPLES OF INVESTIGATION AND MANAGEMENT

The importance of a detailed history and neurological examination for the assessment of the newborn with neurological problems cannot be overemphasized. Although the general framework of the neurological examination used in older children is applicable to the newborn, observations must be interpreted on the basis of known maturational changes at different gestational ages. The examination should not be prolonged unnecessarily, especially in premature infants, because even routine handling may contribute to hypoxemia, hypertension, and hypotension.

Neurological examination is often limited by associated systemic illness and the use of complex life support systems, especially in premature infants. Therefore, considerable attention has been directed toward developing adjunctive noninvasive neurodiagnostic techniques for the assessment of neurological injury. The most important techniques and their principal applications are listed in Table 84.1.

Table 84.1: Diagnostic techniques for neurological assessment

Structural brain imaging
    Ultrasonography
    Computed tomography
    Magnetic resonance imaging
Neurophysiological studies
    Electroencephalography
    Brainstem auditory evoked responses
    Visual evoked responses
    Peripheral nerve conduction studies
Noninvasive techniques for continuous monitoring
    Intracranial pressure: anterior fontanelle monitors
    Cerebral blood flow velocity: Doppler ultrasound
Physiological brain imaging
    Nuclear magnetic resonance spectroscopy
    Positron emission tomography
    Near-infrared optical spectroscopy

NEONATAL SEIZURES

Seizures are the most common feature of significant neurological disease in the newborn. Prompt recognition and treatment are essential because seizures are often caused by serious underlying diseases that need to be identified and treated and because they may interfere with supportive care, such as ventilation and feeding. Experimental studies show a decrease in brain glucose concentration during prolonged seizures as well as excessive release of excitatory amino acids, which may interfere with DNA synthesis and subsequently with glial proliferation, differentiation, and myelination. Although the implications of these experiments for the human newborn are not clear, their relevance is suggested by in vivo studies with magnetic resonance (MR) spectroscopy, which have demonstrated an association between abnormally low phosphocreatine to inorganic phosphate ratios during seizures and long-term neurological sequelae (Shu et al. 1997).

Diagnosis

Table 84.2 summarizes the common types of neonatal seizures. These seizure types are not specific for cause, but some are seen more frequently with certain underlying conditions. Tonic seizures, which may represent decerebrate posturing, occur in up to 50% of premature newborns with severe intraventricular hemorrhage. Focal clonic seizures in the term newborn are most commonly associated with focal cerebral infarction or traumatic injury, such as cerebral contusion.

Differentiation of Seizures from Nonconvulsive Movements

Simultaneous monitoring with electroencephalography (EEG) and video display in newborns with movements suggestive of "subtle seizures" have not shown consistent electrographical discharges concomitant with the movement. This suggests that the abnormal movements may be nonictal brainstem release phenomena rather than seizures. Similarly, tonic extensor posturing in newborns with severe intraventricular hemorrhage is not usually accompanied by epileptiform discharges and responds poorly to anticonvulsant therapy (Sher 1997). Myoclonic seizures, which may evolve into infantile spasms, often have a dismal prognosis and must be distinguished from benign neonatal sleep myoclonus, which occurs in healthy newborns.

Jitteriness, an exaggerated startle response, is often confused with clonic seizures, especially because both jitteriness and clonic seizures occur in conditions such as hypoxic-ischemic or metabolic encephalopathies and in drug withdrawal. Jitteriness is distinguished clinically from seizures by the absence of associated ocular movements and the presence of stimulus sensitivity; the predominant movement is tremor that stops when the affected limb is passively flexed.

Table 84.2: Types of neonatal seizures

Neonatal seizure types	Clinical manifestations	Age distribution
Subtle	Eye deviation, blinking, fixed stare	Premature and term
	Repetitive mouth and tongue movements	
	Apnea	
	Pedaling, tonic posturing of limbs	
Tonic: focal or generalized	Tonic extension of limbs	Primarily premature
	Tonic flexion of upper limbs, extension of legs	
Clonic: multifocal or focal	Multifocal, clonic, synchronous, or asynchronous limb movements	Primarily term
	Nonordered progression	
	Localized clonic limb movements	
	Consciousness often preserved	
Myoclonic: focal, multifocal, or generalized	Single or several synchronous flexion jerks of upper more than lower limbs	Rare

Table 84.3: Major causes of neonatal seizures: clinical features and outcome

Cause	Most common age at onset	Relative frequency Premature	Full-term	Outcome (% of normal development)
Hypoxic-ischemic encephalopathy	<3 days	+++	+++	50
Intracranial hemorrhage				
Intraventricular hemorrhage	<3 days	++		<10
Primary subarachnoid hemorrhage	<1 day		++	90
Hypoglycemia	<2 days	+	+	50
Hypocalcemia				
Early-onset	2–3 days	+	+	50
Late-onset	>7 days		+	100
Intracranial infection				
Bacterial meningitis	>3 days	++	++	50
Intrauterine viral	>3 days	++	++	<10
Developmental defects	Variable	++	++	0
Drug withdrawal	<3 days	+	+	Unknown

+++ = most common; ++ = less common; + = least common.
Source: Reprinted with permission from JJ Volpe. Neurology of the Newborn (3rd ed). Philadelphia: Saunders, 1995.

Determination of the Underlying Cause

Diagnosis of the underlying cause allows specific treatment and a more precise prediction of outcome. Table 84.3 summarizes the major causes of neonatal seizures, their usual times of onset, and prognosis. Seizures are often caused by several factors (e.g., the combination of intracranial hemorrhage, metabolic derangement, and hypoxic-ischemic injury). Benign genetic epilepsies rarely have their onset in the neonatal period; the only example is benign familial neonatal epilepsy, an autosomal dominant trait for which a genetic locus has been identified on chromosome 20.

Electroencephalography

EEG, particularly continuous EEG monitoring (when available), is a valuable aid in the diagnosis of neonatal seizures, especially in newborns who are paralyzed, to assist ventilation, and in those with suspected subtle seizures. EEG correlates of neonatal seizures are focal or multifocal spikes or sharp waves and focal monorhythmic discharges. Sharp transients are normal in premature newborns and should not be confused with seizure activity. Similarly, the tracé alternant pattern of quiet sleep in normal term infants, in which normal low-amplitude reactivity is preserved between bursts, must be distinguished from the abnormal burst-suppression pattern, in which long periods of voltage suppression or absence of activity are recorded between bursts of high-voltage spikes and slow waves.

The interictal EEG may have prognostic value. Severe suppression of the background activity, whether or not interrupted by high-amplitude bursts, is associated with an abnormal outcome in more than 90% of cases. In contrast, normal background activity is associated with good outcome.

Management

Neonatal seizures require urgent treatment. Once adequate ventilation and perfusion are established, the blood glucose concentration is measured. If the glucose concentration is low, 10% dextrose should be administered in a dose of 2 ml/kg. In the absence of hypoglycemia, immediate treatment with anticonvulsant medications should be started, as outlined in Table 84.4. Studies for other underlying causes should proceed concurrently, and specific treatment should be initiated whenever possible.

Phenobarbital alone controls seizures in most newborns when adequate dosages are administered (up to 40 mg/kg loading dose). Phenytoin, 20 mg/kg, is given if seizures continue. Seizures usually respond to intravenous loading doses of phenobarbital and phenytoin. When these drugs fail, other anticonvulsants (diazepam, lorazepam, and primidone) may be effective, but they are not recommended as first-line drugs.

Phenobarbital may suppress seizures caused by hypocalcemia, and a favorable response does not exclude that diagnosis. Approximately 50% of newborns with hypocalcemia also have hypomagnesemia, which requires specific treatment.

Pyridoxine deficiency is a rare cause of neonatal seizures and should be considered whenever no other cause is determined. The diagnosis of pyridoxine deficiency cannot be excluded on the basis of lack of response to a single large dose of intravenous pyridoxine with concurrent EEG recording; rather, large doses (50–100 mg daily) should be given orally for several days.

Duration of Treatment and Outcome

The optimal duration of maintenance therapy for neonatal seizures has not been established. The duration of mainte-

Table 84.4:   Treatment of neonatal seizures

I. Ensure adequate ventilation and perfusion
II. Begin anticonvulsant therapy

	Acute therapy	Maintenance therapy (begin 12 hrs after loading dose)
Phenobarbital	20 mg/kg IV If necessary, additional 5–25 mg/kg IV in 5 mg/kg aliquots (Note: monitor blood pressure and respiration)	4–6 mg/kg/24 hrs IV/IM/PO
Phenytoin	2 doses of 10 mg/kg IV, diluted in normal saline (Note: monitor cardiac rate and rhythm)	5–10 mg/kg/24 hrs IV

III. Begin therapy for specific metabolic disturbances

	Acute therapy	Maintenance therapy
Hypoglycemia: glucose (10% solution)	2 ml/kg IV (0.2 g/kg)	Up to 8 mg/kg/min IV
Hypocalcemia: calcium gluconate (5% solution)	4 ml/kg IV (Note: monitor cardiac rhythm)	500 mg/kg/24 hrs PO
Hypomagnesemia: magnesium sulfate	0.2 ml/kg IM	0.2 ml/kg/24 hrs IM
Pyridoxine deficiency: pyridoxine	50–100 mg IV	100 mg PO daily for 2 wks

nance treatment for neonatal seizures depends on the risk of recurrence, the underlying cause (see Table 84.3), the neurological examination, and the EEG. Phenytoin is usually discontinued when intravenous therapy is stopped, because adequate serum levels are difficult to maintain with oral phenytoin in the newborn. If seizures have stopped and the neurological examination and EEG are normal, phenobarbital may be discontinued before discharge from the hospital. If phenobarbital is continued after discharge, discontinuation should be considered as early as 1 month later based on the neurological status and EEG. Phenobarbital may be discontinued in an infant whose examination is not normal if the EEG does not show epileptiform activity. Phenobarbital may have potential deleterious effects on brain development, and it is recommended that infants be maintained on phenobarbital for the briefest possible time (Holmes 1997).

HYPOXIC-ISCHEMIC BRAIN INJURY IN THE TERM NEWBORN

Hypoxic-ischemic encephalopathy results from reduced oxygen delivery to the brain and from the excessive accumulation of metabolites, such as lactate, free radicals, and excitotoxic amino acids. It is a major cause of morbidity and mortality in both premature and term infants. Hypoxic-ischemic cerebral injury in the premature newborn is discussed subsequently, together with intraventricular hemorrhage (see Hemorrhagic and Hypoxic-Ischemic Brain Injury in the Premature Newborn, later in this chapter). In this section, only hypoxic-ischemic injury in the term newborn is discussed. The pathophysiological and biochemical mechanisms that provide a rational approach to the diag-

nosis and management of neonatal hypoxic-ischemic encephalopathy are reviewed in detail elsewhere. Because most hypoxic-ischemic brain injury in term infants occurs antepartum and intrapartum, prevention depends principally on optimal obstetrical management. Advances in fetal heart rate monitoring, assessment of fetal movements, and the use of biophysical profile and scalp blood gases are aimed at reducing the frequency and severity of hypoxic-ischemic encephalopathy.

Diagnosis

Because asphyxia is mainly an intrauterine event, a history of maternal risk factors and abnormalities of labor and delivery must be documented carefully. An accurate history also may provide more precise information about the type of insult, which in turn may suggest a specific pattern of brain injury. The clinical features of hypoxic-ischemic encephalopathy are determined by the severity and timing of the insult. Acute total asphyxia may cause disproportionate injury to thalamus and brainstem nuclei, whereas prolonged partial asphyxia causes injury principally to cerebral cortex and subcortical white matter (Roland et al. 1998).

The initial features of severe asphyxia are depressed level of consciousness, periodic breathing (secondary to bilateral hemisphere dysfunction), hypotonia, and seizures. An apparent increase in alertness may occur between 12 and 24 hours, but seizures worsen and apnea may be noted. Between 24 and 72 hours of age, the level of consciousness deteriorates and brainstem abnormalities may become prominent. Specific patterns of weakness related to the distribution of neuronal injury may become evident (Table 84.5). After 72 hours, infants who survive show continued

Table 84.5: Neuropathological patterns of neonatal hypoxic-ischemic brain injury and clinical correlation

Pattern of injury	Neuropathological injury	Clinical features in neonatal period	Diagnostic technique	
			Computed tomographic scan	Ultrasound
Selective neuronal necrosis	Cerebral and cerebellar cortex, thalamus, brain-stem nuclei	Premature and term: coma, seizures, hypotonia, oculomotor abnormalities, abnormal sucking, swallowing	+ (late)	−
Status marmoratus	Thalamus, basal ganglia	Term > > premature: unknown	+	+
Parasagittal	Cerebral cortex, subcortical white matter in para-sagittal regions	Term: proximal limb weakness Upper > lower	+	−
Periventricular leukomalacia	Periventricular white matter	Premature: unknown (probably lower limb weakness)	± (early) + (late)	++
Focal/multifocal	Unilateral or bilateral cerebral cortex and subcortical white matter	Premature and term: variable hemiparesis/quadriparesis, stereotyped, nonhabituating reflex responses	++	+

− = not useful; ± = possibly useful; + = useful; ++ = very useful.

(although diminishing) stupor, abnormal tone, and brain-stem dysfunction with disturbances of sucking and swallowing. The temporal profile of clinical and EEG features of severe hypoxic-ischemic encephalopathy in the term newborn are summarized in Table 84.6.

The classification of hypoxic-ischemic encephalopathy into mild, moderate, and severe encephalopathy is useful for prediction of outcome. Mild encephalopathy is characterized by increased irritability, exaggerated Moro and tendon reflexes, and sympathetic overreactivity. Recovery is usually complete within 2 days, and no long-term sequelae exist. Moderate encephalopathy with lethargy, hypotonia, diminished reflexes, and seizures is associated with a 20–40% risk of abnormal outcome. Infants with severe encephalopathy, with coma, flaccid muscle tone, brainstem and autonomic dysfunction, seizures, and possible increased intracranial pressure, either die or survive with severe neurological abnormalities.

Severe hypoxic-ischemic encephalopathy causes widespread injury. The resulting clinical features are microcephaly, mental retardation, seizures, and spastic quadriparesis (see Chapter 67). Less severe encephalopathies mainly injure the parasagittal regions, causing shoulder weakness. Status marmoratus of the basal ganglia is the neuropathological finding associated with choreoathetosis and dystonic cerebral palsy. Unilateral focal lesions result in hemiplegia.

Electroencephalography and Cortical Evoked Responses

Hypoxic-ischemic encephalopathy is the single most important cause of seizures in term and premature newborns. Seizures associated with moderate or severe

encephalopathy begin during the first 24 hours after the original insult and are notoriously difficult to control. The pattern of background activity on EEG may have prognostic implications. Thus, infants with a normal EEG 1 week after the initial insult usually experience a favorable outcome.

The usefulness of the visual, auditory, and somatosensory evoked responses in the diagnosis and prognosis of hypoxic-ischemic encephalopathy is not definitely established (see Chapter 37A). Preliminary observations suggest a role for visual evoked responses in the diagnosis of periventricular leukomalacia (PVL) and for auditory evoked responses in the diagnosis of brainstem injury.

Metabolic Parameters

Hypoglycemia, hypocalcemia, hyponatremia (inappropriate antidiuretic hormone secretion), and acidosis may contribute to the neurological syndrome of hypoxic-ischemic encephalopathy. Metabolic derangements that are not corrected may worsen the cerebral injury.

Neuroimaging

Neuroimaging is useful for locating and quantitating cerebral injury. Abnormalities on delayed technetium brain scans performed in term newborns at 7 days of age correlate well with parasagittal focal and basal ganglia injury. Scanning with computed tomography (CT) in the term newborn (Figures 84.1 and 84.2) and US in the premature newborn are especially valuable. Decreased attenuation on CT performed

Table 84.6:   Clinical features of severe hypoxic-ischemic encephalopathy

	Time after insult			
Clinical features	*0–12 hrs*	*12–24 hrs*	*24–72 hrs*	*72 hrs*
Seizures	++	+++	++	±
Increased intracranial pressure (full-term)	–	±	+++	–
Stupor/coma	+++	++	+++	±
Apnea	+ (periodic breathing)	++	+++	±
Abnormal pupil/oculomotor responses	–	±	++	–
Hypotonia	+++	+++	+++	++
Limb weakness	++	+	+	++
Proximal, upper > lower (term)	±	±	±	±
Hemiparesis	±	±	±	±
Lower limbs (premature)	±	±	±	±
Electroencephalographical features	Amplitude (suppression) Frequency	Periodic pattern, ± multifocal sharp activity	Prominent periodic pattern + more voltage suppression, isoelectric pattern	

– = absent; ± = possibly present; + = present; ++ = more common; +++ = most common.

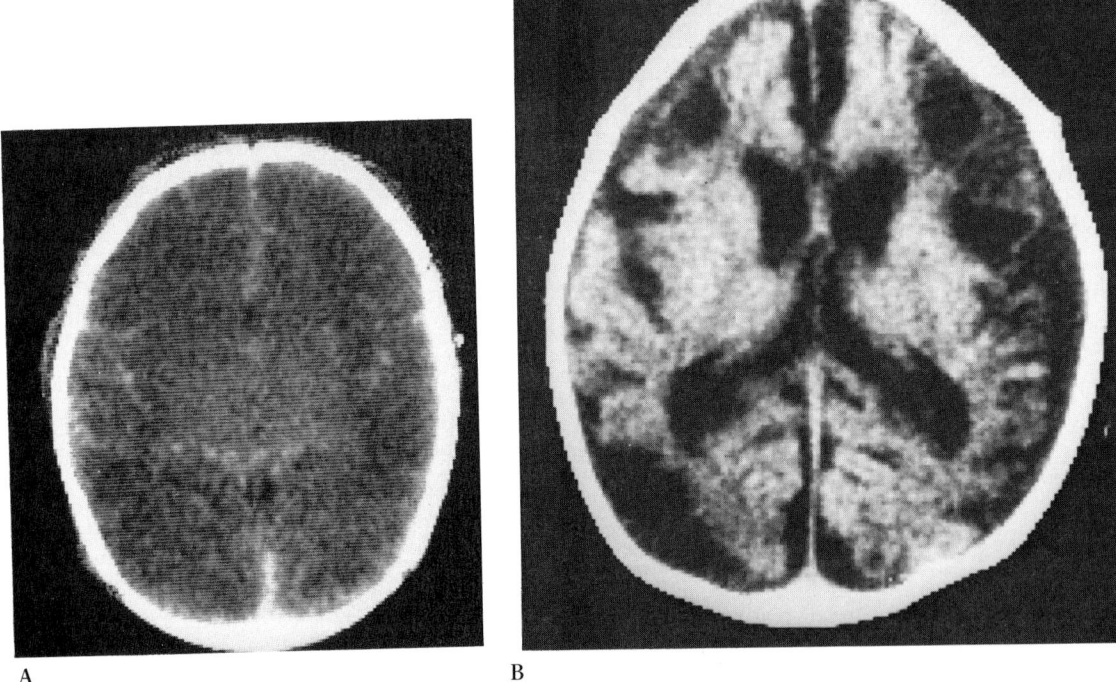

A   B

FIGURE 84.1   Computed tomographic scans of severely asphyxiated term newborn. **(A)** Scan at 3 days of age demonstrates diffuse low attenuation. **(B)** Scan at 5 months demonstrates wide sulci and enlarged ventricles consistent with severe generalized atrophy.

between 3 and 5 days of age shows the maximum severity of acute hypoxic-ischemic cerebral injury in the term newborn (see Figure 84.1). More precise anatomical delineation of mild brain injury or selective involvement of thalamus and basal ganglia or cerebellum may be assessed more accurately by magnetic resonance imaging (MRI) (Barkovich and Hallam 1997) after the hypoxic-ischemic episode.

Several newer techniques that provide insight into functional disturbances of newborn hypoxic-ischemic cerebral injury may have important implications for management. Positron emission tomography, single-photon emission CT, and near infrared spectroscopy show disturbances of cerebral blood flow. MR spectroscopy shows decreased brain levels of high-energy phosphates in asphyxiated infants (Wyatt 1997).

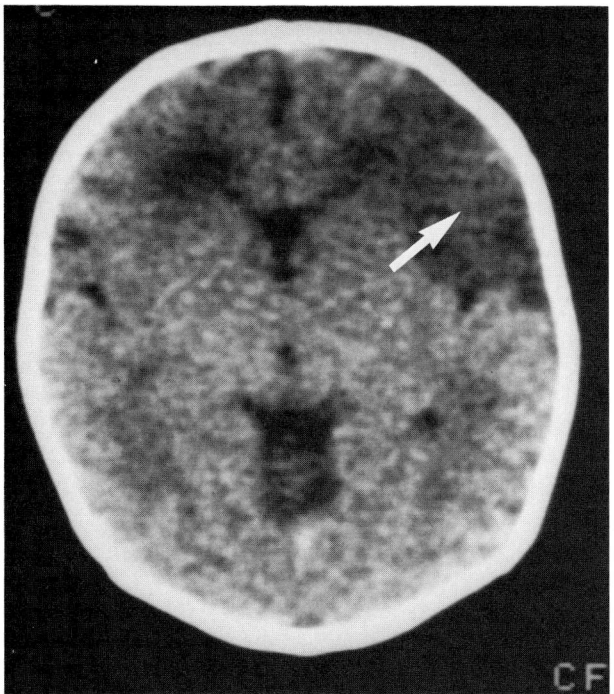
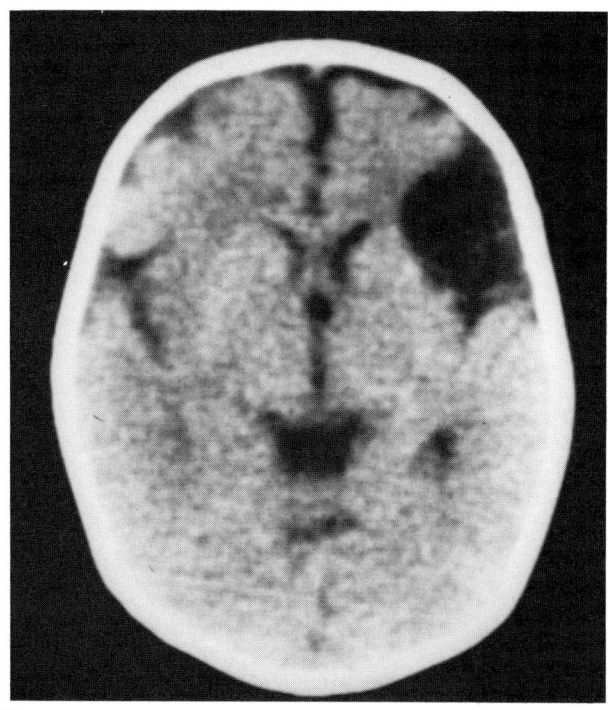

A   B

FIGURE 84.2 Computed tomographic scans demonstrate evolution of focal ischemic lesion in term infant who presented with focal seizures. (A) Scan at 3 days of age. Note low tissue attenuation in distribution of left middle cerebral artery (*arrow*). (B) Scan at 2 months of age. Note marked tissue loss in this region.

Management

Optimal management begins in utero by measures to prevent hypoxic-ischemic injury. Fetuses at risk must be identified early, monitored serially (discussed earlier), and considered for cesarean delivery when signs of fetal distress persist. An asphyxiated newborn requires immediate treatment to prevent additional hypoxic-ischemic cerebral injury. This includes close attention to ventilation, perfusion, blood glucose concentrations, control of seizures, and maintaining perfusion and function of other affected organs, including the heart, liver, kidneys, and gastrointestinal tract.

Maintenance of Adequate Ventilation

Maintaining adequate ventilation and avoidance of hypoxemia and hypercapnia are critical to outcome. Recognition of hypoxemia and hypercapnia has been facilitated by the availability of continuous transcutaneous oxygen and carbon dioxide monitoring. Significant hypoxemia may occur in the premature newborn during routine care, such as suctioning or venipuncture; minimal handling is recommended. Persistent postnatal hypoxemia is caused by the respiratory distress syndrome in premature newborns and by persistent fetal circulation and pulmonary hypertension in term newborns. Overcorrection of hypoxemia should be avoided because hyperoxemia may cause chronic lung injury and retrolental fibroplasia as well as pontosubicular necrosis, a specific pat-

tern of selective neuronal necrosis involving principally the hippocampal and pontine neurons. Hypercapnia is deleterious because it worsens intracellular acidosis, impairs cerebrovascular autoregulation, or both, with development of a pressure-passive cerebral circulation. The potential effects of hypocapnia on cerebral blood flow in the newborn have not been established. Experimental and human data do not support the use of hyperventilation in asphyxiated newborns, except perhaps in those with persistent fetal circulation.

Maintenance of Adequate Perfusion

The maintenance of adequate perfusion is critical to prevent further cerebral ischemia. Managing perfusion must be based on knowledge of normal systemic arterial blood pressure levels in the newborn at all gestational ages. Systemic hypotension must be avoided because cerebral blood flow is not autoregulated in asphyxiated newborns and reflects systemic blood pressure in a pressure-passive manner. Transient myocardial ischemia, a common cause of hypotension in asphyxiated newborns, may respond to inotropic agents such as dopamine. Other important causes of systemic hypotension that may cause decreased cerebral perfusion are patent ductus arteriosus and recurrent apneic spells with bradycardia. Because of the pressure-passive relationship between the systemic and cerebral circulations, systemic hypertension must be avoided also, especially in the premature infant, in whom the presence of vulnerable

Table 84.7: Prognostic factors in hypoxic-ischemic encephalopathy in term infants

Neonatal encephalopathy: severity and duration (>5–7 days)
Presence of seizures
Presence of brain swelling
Electroencephalography
Radiological investigations: computed tomography, ultrasound, magnetic resonance spectroscopy

germinal matrix capillaries predisposes to the development of intraventricular hemorrhage.

Hyperviscosity, secondary to polycythemia (venous hematocrit greater than 65%), may further impair cerebral perfusion in asphyxiated newborns, especially those who are small for gestational age. Jitteriness, apnea, poor feeding, and seizures are concomitant neurological features in approximately 40% of cases. Partial exchange transfusion with plasma is indicated in all symptomatic newborns with polycythemia and perhaps also in those who are asymptomatic.

Prevention of Metabolic Derangements

Fluid overload is an important consideration in the maintenance of metabolic homeostasis. Inappropriate antidiuretic hormone secretion is common during the first 3 days after a severe hypoxic-ischemic episode and may lead to hypo-osmolality and hyponatremia, which in turn increase brain water content (cerebral edema) and seizures. The role of glucose supplementation in the management of the asphyxiated newborn is unclear. We recommend maintaining blood glucose concentrations in the normal range.

Control of Brain Swelling

The contribution of brain swelling to neurological outcome in term newborns with hypoxic-ischemic encephalopathy is controversial. Experimental data from animals and human newborns suggest that brain swelling with increased intracranial pressure is a consequence rather than a cause of brain damage in severe hypoxic-ischemic encephalopathy. Clinical evidence of increased intracranial pressure, a bulging anterior fontanelle, is seen between 36 and 72 hours after the initial asphyxial episode. Mannitol reduces intracranial pressure in asphyxiated newborns, but its beneficial effect on outcome is uncertain. Surveillance of intracranial pressure by palpation of the anterior fontanelle or by noninvasive monitoring with the Ladd monitor may have prognostic value. Elevated intracranial pressures 36–72 hours after the asphyxial episode correlate with extensive low attenuation of tissue on CT and a poor outcome.

Prognosis

Selected aspects of the neurological syndrome and neurodiagnostic studies are helpful in determining outcome in

hypoxic-ischemic encephalopathy (Table 84.7). Because most instances of hypoxic-ischemic encephalopathy begin before birth, assessment of fetal well-being in utero is useful for prognosis. Apgar scores at 1 and 5 minutes are notoriously unreliable for prognosis because of interobserver variability, the effects of drugs given to the mother before delivery, and the stress of delivery, which may be reversible. Extended Apgar scores at 10, 15, and 20 minutes, however, are predictive of outcome.

The severity and duration of hypoxic-ischemic encephalopathy is the single most useful prognostic factor. Our experience since the 1970s indicates that newborns who have sustained intrapartum asphyxia but do not develop features of neonatal hypoxic-ischemic encephalopathy will not have subsequent neurological morbidity. The features of encephalopathy that are most predictive are its severity and duration and the occurrence of seizures. Neuroimaging (e.g., abnormalities on CT and MRI) also are predictive of poor outcome.

HEMORRHAGIC AND HYPOXIC-ISCHEMIC BRAIN INJURY IN THE PREMATURE NEWBORN

Periventricular-intraventricular hemorrhage (PIVH) is reported in approximately 20% of premature newborns of birth weight less than 1,500 g (Roland and Hill 1997). PIVH occurs on the first day in 50% of affected premature newborns and before the fourth day in 90%. PIVH originates from rupture of small vessels in the subependymal germinal matrix. Approximately 80% of germinal matrix hemorrhages extend into the ventricular system. Severe hemorrhages are accompanied by hemorrhagic lesions in the cerebral parenchyma. Parenchymal hemorrhages are usually unilateral and are probably hemorrhagic venous infarctions of the periventricular region (Volpe 1997).

Intraventricular hemorrhage rarely occurs in term newborns. In these infants, the initial site of hemorrhage is more variable and includes the choroid plexus, residual germinal matrix, vascular malformation, tumor, or hemorrhagic infarction of the thalamus.

Hypoxic-ischemic injury in the premature newborn affects predominantly the periventricular regions, resulting in PVL. This pattern of injury results in spastic diplegia, quadriplegia, or visual impairment because the corticospinal tracts and optic radiations are involved. More severe injury may affect the cerebral cortex, resulting in microcephaly and cognitive impairment.

Diagnosis

The high incidence of PIVH in premature infants has led to the use of routine US at 3–4 days in all newborns less than 32 weeks' gestation. Both CT and US scanning are informative, but US has replaced CT because it can be performed in the intensive care nursery and there is no ionizing radiation.

FIGURE 84.3   Cystic periventricular leukomalacia. Parasagittal ultrasound scan performed 5 weeks after intraventricular hemorrhage and hypoxic-ischemic insult. Note cystic lesion (*arrow*).

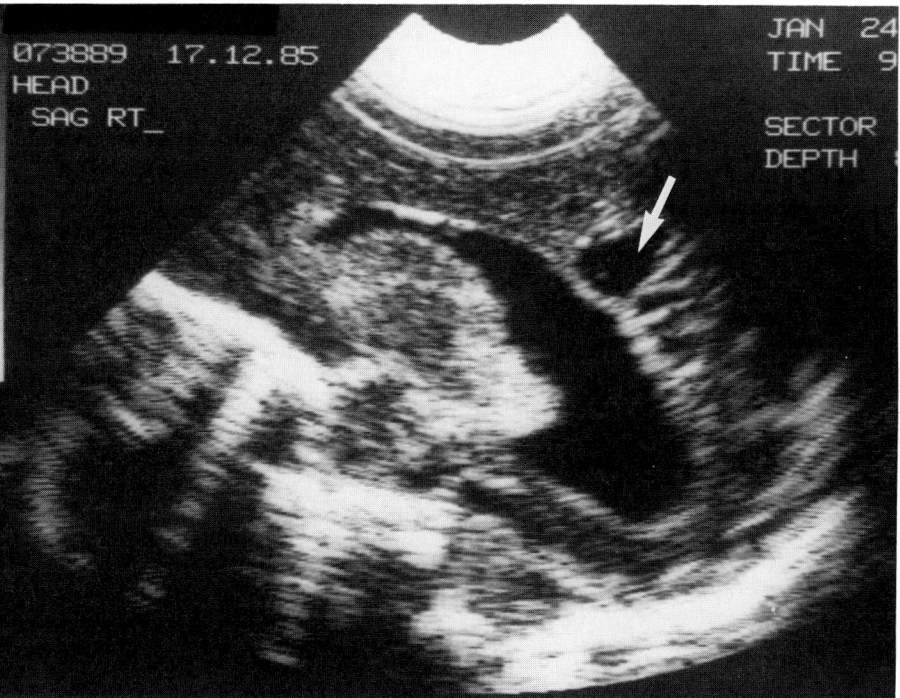

CT remains the technique of choice for demonstration of epidural, subdural, and subarachnoid hemorrhage, as well as most intracerebral and posterior fossa hemorrhages.

PIVH can be predicted on the basis of clinical features in 50% of cases. These usually are hemorrhages that have extended from the germinal matrix into the ventricular system. The spectrum of clinical features associated with PIVH ranges from an asymptomatic state, through stepwise neurological deterioration over several days, to rapid catastrophic deterioration characterized by coma, apnea, generalized tonic seizures, brainstem disturbances, and flaccid quadriparesis. Severe hemorrhage may be associated with the systemic abnormalities of metabolic acidosis, hypotension, bradycardia, and abnormal glucose and water homeostasis. Bloody or xanthochromic cerebrospinal fluid (CSF) at lumbar puncture suggests PIVH.

CT scans have limited value in assessing acute hypoxic-ischemic cerebral injury in premature newborns because the immature brain has a high water content and low attenuation is a normal feature. PVL may be suggested on routine US in premature newborns by increased echogenicity in the periventricular regions during the first days postpartum and subsequent cyst formation in the same areas during the following weeks (Figure 84.3). US is limited in its ability to distinguish between hemorrhagic and ischemic injury (Figure 84.4) and to reliably identify mild degrees of injury. After the neonatal period, PVL can be shown by CT or MRI.

Pathogenesis and Management

Table 84.8 summarizes the current concepts of pathogenesis and management of PIVH. Fluctuations of cerebral blood flow are a major factor in the pathogenesis of PIVH.

The primary management strategy for PIVH is prevention. Ideally, this is accomplished by preventing premature delivery. If premature delivery cannot be prevented, several strategies have been proposed, directed against the known intravascular, vascular, and extravascular mechanisms of hemorrhage. Muscle paralysis with pancuronium bromide in ventilated premature newborns has an established role in reducing the incidence and severity of PIVH by stabilizing fluctuations of cerebral blood flow velocity. The role of other agents is less well established. Phenobarbital may dampen fluctuations of systemic blood pressure and cerebral blood flow and have other cellular neuroprotective effects. However, one important study reported an increased incidence of PIVH in infants treated with phenobarbital. Indomethacin inhibits prostaglandin synthesis, thereby regulating cerebral blood flow. It prevents PIVH in animal models, but its efficacy in humans is inconclusive. Two other agents, vitamin E and ethamsylate, may hold promise for preventing PIVH, but the data are insufficient to recommend their routine use (see Table 84.8) (Roland and Hill 1997).

After PIVH has occurred, treatment is directed to prevent extension of hemorrhage, which occurs in 20–40% of cases, and to prevent further hypoxic-ischemic cerebral injury. Severe intraventricular hemorrhage may decrease circulating blood volume sufficiently to cause systemic hypotension that needs correction by blood transfusion.

Serial US and measurements of head circumference are needed in every newborn with PIVH for early diagnosis of the development of posthemorrhagic hydrocephalus (Figure 84.5). This complication is caused by arachnoiditis in the posterior

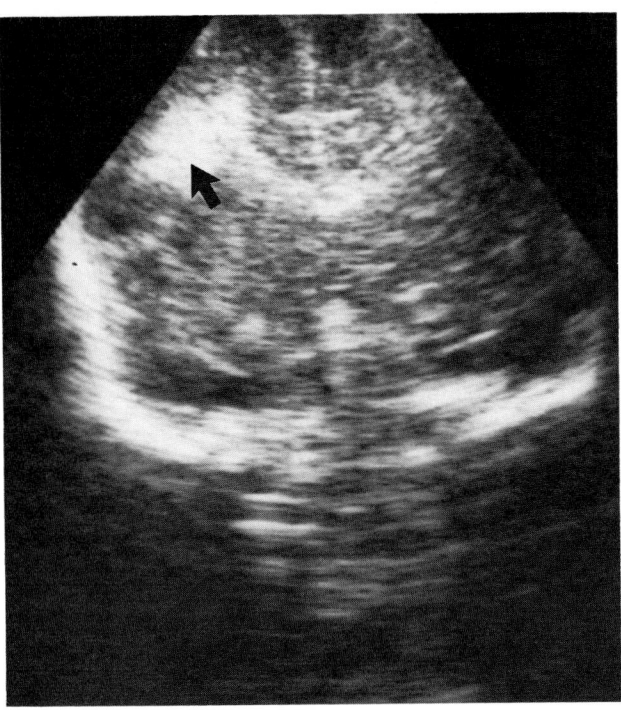

A

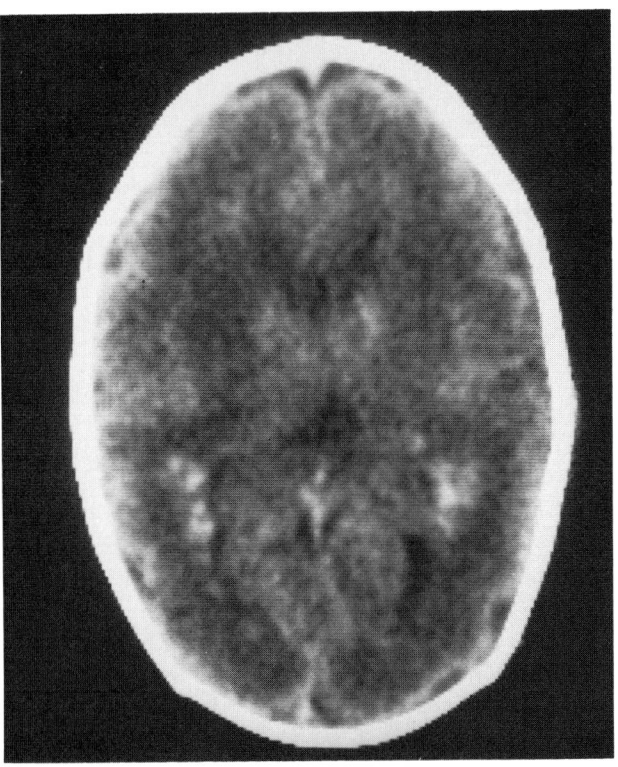

B

FIGURE 84.4 Hemorrhagic and nonhemorrhagic periventricular leukomalacia. (**A**) Ultrasound (US) scan demonstrates increased echoes in periventricular region (*arrow*). (**B**) In a computed tomographic scan performed at the same time, however, note the absence of hemorrhage in regions corresponding to increased echoes on US. This illustrates that echogenicity on US does not distinguish between ischemic and hemorrhagic injury.

fossa, by aqueductal obstruction, or both. Significant ventriculomegaly may precede measurable increases in head circumference. Factors that influence the management of posthemorrhagic hydrocephalus are the rate of progression, ventricular size, and intracranial pressure. In approximately 50% of premature newborns with posthemorrhagic hydrocephalus, ventriculomegaly arrests or resolves spontaneously without intervention, usually within 4 weeks (see Figure 84.5). In the other 50%, dilatation progresses beyond 4 weeks and requires intervention. However, rapid ventricular enlargement requires intervention in less than 4 weeks. The definitive treatment is placement of a ventriculoperitoneal shunt, but temporizing measures are often needed. These measures include CSF drainage by serial lumbar punctures, external ventriculostomy, ventricular catheter with subcutaneous reservoir or subgaleal shunt, and drugs that reduce CSF production, such as osmotic agents (isosorbide and glycerol) and carbonic anhydrase inhibitors and diuretics (acetazolamide and furosemide). In cases of rapidly progressive hydrocephalus, placement of a ventriculoperitoneal shunt is often indicated, despite the morbidity associated with shunt placement in small, premature infants.

Prognosis

The prognosis following PIVH relates to the severity of hemorrhage and to the concomitant hypoxic-ischemic cerebral injury. Germinal matrix hemorrhage alone is rarely a cause of significant neurological morbidity. Blood in the ventricles also has a relatively good prognosis unless ventricular dilatation occurs. Newborns with severe ventricular dilatation and intraparenchymal hemorrhage may die in the neonatal period, and most survivors develop posthemorrhagic hydrocephalus. Prognosis does not always correlate with the severity of PIVH and posthemorrhagic hydrocephalus; hypoxic-ischemic parenchymal injury, principally PVL, is the other important variable. However, PVL may be more difficult to document by ultrasonography. In severe cases, cystic lesions are observed after several weeks of age. At later ages, PVL may be documented by CT or MRI, especially T2-weighted images.

INFECTIONS OF THE CENTRAL NERVOUS SYSTEM

Bacterial infections of the central nervous system (CNS) in the newborn include bacterial meningitis, epidural and subdural empyema, and brain abscess.

Neonatal Meningitis

Bacterial meningitis occurs in approximately 1 per 2,000 term newborns and 3 per 1,000 premature newborns. The most common infecting organisms are *Escherichia coli* and group B hemolytic streptococcus, but several other nosocomial grampositive and gram-negative organisms must be considered.

Because as many as 20–30% of neonatal sepsis cases are complicated by meningitis and early diagnosis and treat-

Table 84.8:   Pathogenesis and management of periventricular-intraventricular hemorrhage

Pathogenesis	Management
Intravascular factors	
Fluctuating cerebral blood flow	Paralysis of ventilated preterm infants with pancuronium bromide
Increases in cerebral blood flow	Avoidance of systemic hypertension associated with routine handling and rapid volume expansion, exchange transfusions, colloid infusions, seizures, pneumothorax
	Indomethacin
	Decreases in cerebral blood flow
	Increases in cerebral venous pressure and flow
	Avoidance of systemic hypotension
	Avoidance of prolonged labor and difficult vaginal delivery
	Avoidance of pneumothorax, positive pressure ventilation, minimal handling
Platelet and coagulation disturbances	Avoidance of asphyxia
	Avoidance of maternal drug ingestion (such as aspirin)
	Prophylactic infusion of fresh, frozen plasma?
	Platelet infusion?
Vascular factors	
Venous vascular integrity	Ethamsylate, vitamin E?
Involuting vessels: subependymal germinal matrix	
Extravascular factors	
Poor vascular support: subependymal germinal matrix	
Direct external effects on vessels	

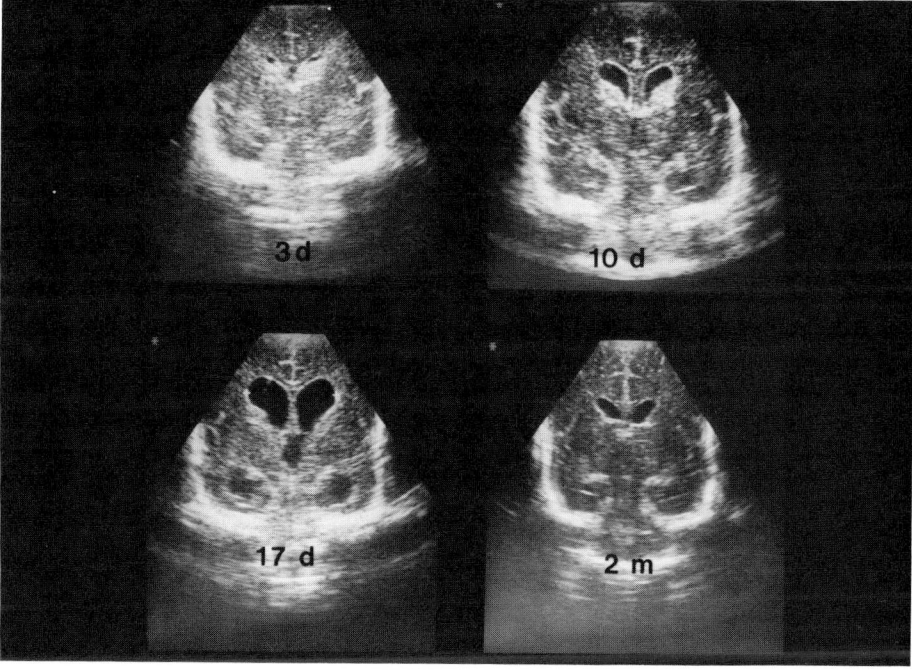

FIGURE 84.5 Composite of four ultrasound scans in coronal section demonstrating ventriculomegaly after intraventricular hemorrhage at 3 days of age, with spontaneous resolution by 2 months of age.

ment is critical to prevent morbidity and mortality, lumbar puncture must be performed as soon as a newborn seems sick; one cannot wait for the typical clinical features of meningitis, such as a bulging fontanelle, neck retraction, seizures, irritability, pallor, and poor feeding. The characteristic CSF profile is pleocytosis, increased protein concentration, decreased glucose concentration, and identification of the organism by Gram's stain and culture. Laboratory techniques that allow rapid detection of bacterial antigens also may be useful (e.g., immunoelectrophoresis, latex agglutination, and radioimmunoassays) (Trujillo and McCracken 1997).

Management

In an attempt to prevent neonatal meningitis, the American College of Obstetrics and Gynecology and the American Academy of Pediatrics recommend intravenous ampicillin during labor for mothers with positive rectal or genital cultures for group B streptococcus or other major risk factors

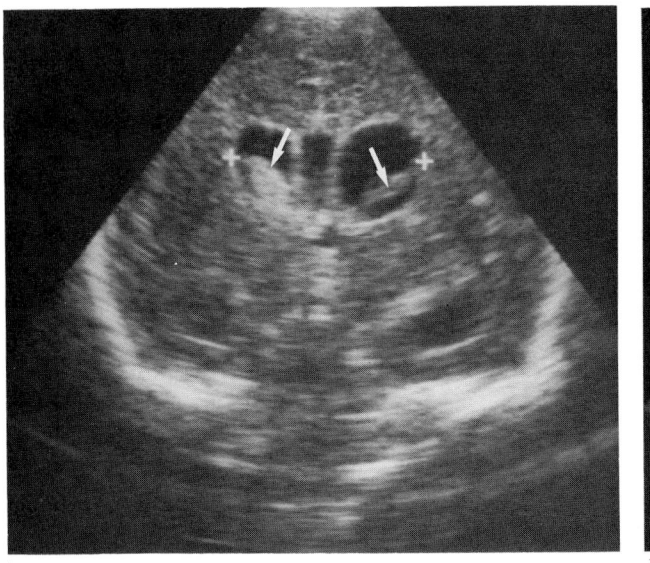 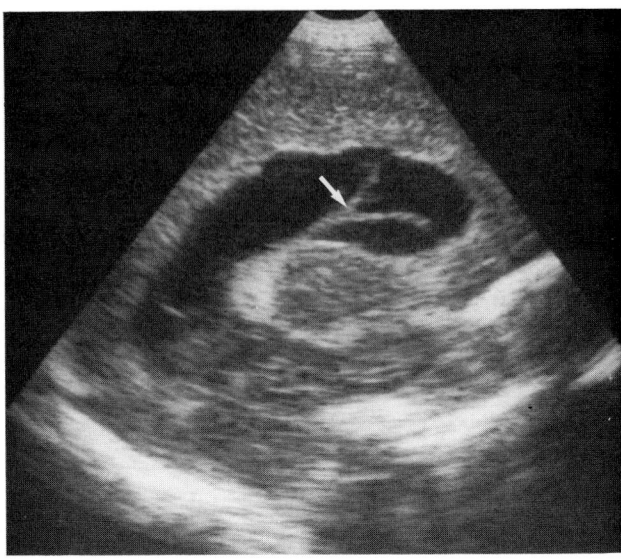

A   B

FIGURE 84.6   Ultrasound scans of newborn infant with bacterial meningitis and ventriculitis. Note intraventricular strands in both (**A**) coronal and (**B**) parasagittal images (*arrows*).

for neonatal sepsis. The initial empiric treatment of a neonate with bacterial meningitis of unknown cause is a combination of ampicillin, an aminoglycoside such as gentamicin, and possibly cefotaxime administered intravenously. The precise dosage varies according to the body weight and postnatal age of the affected infant. The optimal selection of antibiotics is determined by the resistances of the infecting organism. Parenteral antibiotic treatment should be maintained for at least 21 days.

In addition to antimicrobial therapy, supportive measures such as maintenance of fluid and electrolyte balance and control of blood pressure and blood gases are essential. Because the syndrome of inappropriate antidiuretic hormone secretion is common, fluids should be restricted to 30–40 ml/kg per day during the first few days of illness. Seizures are a common complication and should be treated with phenobarbital, phenytoin, or both (see Table 84.4). Serial measurements of head circumference and cranial US permit early diagnosis of the complications of ventriculitis, hydrocephalus, and subdural effusion.

Ventriculitis commonly causes hydrocephalus, either during the acute phase of the illness or subsequently (Figure 84.6). Treatment of meningitic hydrocephalus is external ventricular drainage, often with a reservoir for intermittent draining of CSF, instillation of antibiotics if active infection is present, or both. Most newborns require a permanent ventriculoperitoneal shunt after the infection is eradicated.

Cerebral abscess is a rare complication of neonatal meningitis. It occurs most frequently with *Citrobacter* infection and should be suspected when newborns with increased intracranial pressure respond poorly to treatment. Diagnosis is confirmed by US, CT, or both. The duration of antibiotic therapy is prolonged, and surgical exploration and drainage are sometimes needed. The mortality is 50%, and survivors often have neurological impairment.

Prognosis

The important variables that determine mortality are the type of infecting organism and the gestational age of the infant. Mortality is reportedly between 20–30% and is highest for gram-negative infections. Permanent neurological sequelae occur in 30–50% of survivors and include hydrocephalus, cerebral palsy, epilepsy, intellectual deficits, and deafness.

Viral and Parasitic Infections

Viral, protozoan (*Toxoplasma gondii*), and fungal infections occur in the newborn. The TORCH syndrome acronym is used as a reminder of the major nonbacterial neonatal infections: *t*oxoplasmosis, *o*thers (such as syphilis), *r*ubella, *c*ytomegalovirus (CMV), and *h*erpes simplex. All of the TORCH infections occur during pregnancy by transplacental inoculation, except for herpes simplex, which usually is contracted by passage of the fetus through an infected birth canal. Although most newborns with TORCH syndromes have clinical features of disease during the first month of life, symptoms can be delayed until later infancy and childhood (Bale 1997).

Congenital Rubella

The congenital rubella syndrome occurs when the fetus is infected before 20 weeks' gestation. The clinical features in the newborn are low birth weight, jaundice, hepatosplenomegaly, petechial rash, congenital heart disease, cataracts, sensorineural deafness, microcephaly, bone lesions, and thrombocytopenia. Less severely affected infants appear normal at birth and later show features of neurological and ocular defects, deafness, and congenital heart disease. Infected infants are highly infectious, may shed virus for several years, and must be considered a hazard to nonimmune women. Diagnosis is confirmed by virus culture (throat swab and urine) and demonstration of rubella-specific immunoglobulin M (IgM) in neonatal plasma. Neuroimaging may reveal periventricular calcifications, subependymal cysts, or PVL. The only effective management is prevention by universal immunization. Antiviral treatment is unavailable. Infants who survive may develop progressive sensorineural hearing loss, growth failure, or diabetes mellitus later in childhood.

Cytomegalovirus

CMV is the most common congenital viral infection and results either from primary maternal infection or from reactivation of virus in the mother. Almost all newborns with congenital CMV are asymptomatic. The fewer than 10% who are symptomatic have hepatosplenomegaly, jaundice, petechiae, microcephaly with periventricular calcifications, chorioretinitis, and blindness. In symptomatic cases, virus can be cultured from throat swabs or urine, and CMV-specific IgM is present in serum. Urine culture results are also positive in asymptomatic cases. Specific treatment is not available.

Most asymptomatic newborns with congenital CMV infection develop normally; only 10% develop deafness, microcephaly, or chorioretinitis. The mortality in symptomatic newborns is 20–30%, and most survivors have multiple, severe neurological sequelae.

Herpes Virus

Neonatal herpes infection may present as localized oral cutaneous or ophthalmic disease; localized disease of the CNS, such as meningitis; or disseminated disease with hepatosplenomegaly, severe disseminated intravascular coagulation, renal failure, and meningoencephalitis. Intranuclear inclusions may be detected in vesicular fluid, CSF, or conjunctival scrapings. A throat swab, as well as urine and stool samples, should be cultured. Negative culture results do not exclude the diagnosis. Studies of the CSF usually are consistent with viral meningoencephalitis, and diagnosis may be established quickly using polymerase chain reaction (see Chapter 59). A 14-day course of acyclovir (30 mg/kg per day given in evenly divided doses every 8 hours) should be started even before the results of cultures are known. Acyclovir may improve outcome but is not as effective as in postnatally acquired infection.

Toxoplasmosis

Toxoplasmosis is a parasitic infection that affects principally the CNS and the eye in the newborn. The result is extensive necrosis and calcification of the cerebral cortex and periventricular tissue. Cerebral injury in the periaque-

ductal region obstructs CSF flow and causes hydrocephalus. Cataracts and microphthalmia are the main eye abnormalities. Other organs that may be involved are the liver, bone marrow, lungs, muscles, and myocardium.

Antibody screening for neonatal infection may suggest congenital toxoplasmosis, but test results for toxoplasma-specific IgM often are negative. Examination of the CSF may show lymphocytosis, high protein content, and trophozoites. Diffuse intracerebral calcifications may be seen on skull radiography, CT, and US.

Spiramycin, pyrimethamine, and sulfadiazine are used to treat the infected mother and her infant during the first year. Approximately one-third of infected infants are symptomatic, and their mortality is 25%. Most survivors have significant neurological sequelae. In contrast, asymptomatic newborns have a good prognosis.

Human Immunodeficiency Virus

The number of newborns who are seropositive for human immunodeficiency virus is increasing. Transmission may occur in utero, during labor and delivery, or by breast-feeding. The vast majority of infected infants are asymptomatic during the newborn period but later develop evidence of opportunistic systemic infections (CMV, pneumocystis) and dementia caused by viral infection of the brain. Studies suggest that the risk of transmission may be reduced by a program of prenatal, perinatal, and postnatal therapy with zidovudine (Belman 1997).

MECHANICAL TRAUMA TO EXTRACRANIAL, CENTRAL, AND PERIPHERAL NERVOUS SYSTEM STRUCTURES

Traumatic injuries at birth have been greatly reduced by improvements in obstetrical management. This section discusses the diagnosis and management of traumatic injury according to its anatomical location.

Intracranial Hemorrhage

Other types of intracranial hemorrhage, such as primary subarachnoid, epidural, subdural, and intracerebellar hemorrhage, are usually associated with traumatic delivery or a bleeding diathesis and occur less commonly than PIVH (Figure 84.7). Subdural hemorrhage occurs in both premature and term newborns and results from laceration of major veins and sinuses. It is often related to excessive molding of the head. CT is the investigational technique of choice for diagnosis of subdural hemorrhage. Convexity subdural hematoma, especially if associated with midline shift, requires decompression by craniotomy or subdural tap. Subarachnoid hemorrhage is also of venous origin but is usually self-limited, originating from small vessels in the leptomeningeal plexus or

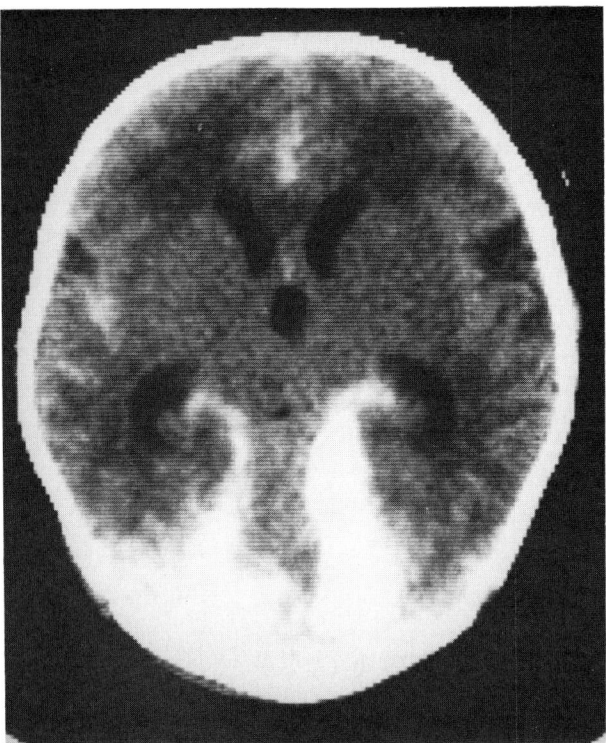

FIGURE 84.7 Computed tomographic scan of posterior fossa hemorrhage (intracerebellar and subdural).

bridging veins within the subarachnoid space. Infants may be asymptomatic with minor subarachnoid hemorrhage or present with seizures. Diagnosis may be suspected on the basis of uniformly bloodstained or xanthochromic CSF and confirmed by CT. In the absence of severe trauma or major hypoxic-ischemic injury, normal outcome is seen in 90% of cases. Table 84.9 summarizes the clinical features, management, and outcome of these types of intracranial hemorrhage.

Extracranial Hemorrhage

Extracranial hemorrhage is classified according to the tissue planes involved. Caput succedaneum is superficial bleeding between the skin and the epicranial aponeurosis; subgaleal hemorrhage is located between the aponeurosis and the periosteum of the skull; and cephalhematoma occurs in the deepest plane between the periosteum and cranial bones. The major clinical features and the usual outcome for extracranial hemorrhages are summarized in Table 84.10.

Extracranial hemorrhage rarely requires intervention, except for subgaleal hemorrhage, in which the amount of acute blood loss may cause shock. Urgent blood transfusion and surveillance for hyperbilirubinemia are sometimes needed. Cephalhematoma is often associated with skull fracture, but does not require treatment.

Skull Fractures

Skull fractures may be linear or depressed. Linear skull fractures usually are parietal in location. Bony continuity is lost without depression. Depressed skull fractures are called *ping-pong fractures* because the bone buckles inward without loss of continuity, like a depression in a ping-pong ball. Occipital diastasis is not an actual fracture but rather a traumatic separation of the squamous and lateral parts of the occipital bones that is usually associated with breech delivery.

Depressed skull fractures may be suspected clinically by palpation of the skull, but CT is needed to visualize the relation of the depressed bone to the cerebral surface. CT is useful also to show a linear fracture beneath a cephalhematoma. Occipital diastasis may be associated with posterior fossa subdural hemorrhage, cerebellar contusion, and brainstem compression without hemorrhage or contusion. The importance of recognizing fractures and diastases is to alert the physician to the possibility of a more serious intracranial disorder.

In the absence of intracranial lesions, treatment is required only when a depressed fracture impinges on the brain. Spontaneous elevation of the bone may occur with skull molding. Nonsurgical methods for elevation are digital pressure, a breast pump, or an obstetrical vacuum extractor. Surgical intervention usually is reserved for complicated fractures with extradural or subdural blood clot or bone fragments. A leptomeningeal cyst may develop at the site of a skull fracture. This unusual complication may be identified by transillumination of the region or radiographical evidence of a widening bony defect ("a growing fracture").

Spinal Cord Injury

Spinal cord injury is uncommon. It is caused by excessive torsion or traction. Injuries associated with breech delivery (75%) involve principally the lower cervical and upper thoracic regions, whereas injuries following vertex delivery more commonly involve the upper cervical and midcervical cord. Injuries of the lower thoracic and lumbar spinal cord are even less common and are usually related to vascular occlusion secondary to umbilical artery catheterization or air embolus from peripheral intravenous injection.

The neurological features reflect the segmental level of the lesion. Newborns with high cervical lesions are often stillborn or die quickly from respiratory failure in the absence of rapid ventilatory support. Lower cervical, upper thoracic lesions cause urinary retention, hypotonia, weakness, and areflexia of all limbs, evolving subsequently to spastic paraplegia or quadriplegia. Cord injuries are distinguished from neuromuscular disorders and brain injuries by the demonstration of a distinct sensory level of response to pinprick, urinary retention, and a patulous

Table 84.9:   Other types of intracranial hemorrhage

Type of hemorrhage	Clinical features	Diagnostic technique		Management	Prognosis
		Computed tomography	Ultrasound		
Epidural	Increased ICP ± unilateral fixed, dilated pupil Seizures (50%)	+	–	Immediate surgical evacuation	Poor
Subdural (convexity or infratentorial)	Variable: asymptomatic or increased ICP Brainstem disturbances Opisthotonus Seizures Coma	+	±	Close observation Surgery if deterioration or severe lesions	Hydrocephalus Focal abnormalities Major lesions: 100% mortality
Primary subarachnoid	Variable Minimal signs Seizures Well in interictal period	+	–	Seizure control Control of hydrocephalus	90% normal Hydrocephalus rare
Intracerebellar	Premature > term Brainstem dysfunction Increased ICP	+	+	Close observation Surgery if deterioration	Variable outcome

ICP = intracranial pressure.
+ = useful; – = not useful; ± = variable usefulness.

Table 84.10:   Clinical features and outcome of extracranial hemorrhage

	Most common location	Increases after birth	Crosses suture lines	Marked acute blood loss	Usual outcome
Caput succedaneum	Vertex	No	Yes	No	Resolves in first days of life
Subgaleal hemorrhage	Widespread—entire scalp	Yes	Yes	Yes	Resolves in 2–3 wks
Cephalhematoma	Unilateral—parietal	Yes	No	No	May calcify Resolves in weeks to months

anus. Autonomic dysfunction may cause wide fluctuations of body temperature.

Spinal cord injury in breech position can be minimized by cesarean delivery of all fetuses with a hyperextended head. Unfortunately, cesarean section does not entirely eliminate the risk because some fetuses sustain injuries in utero, perhaps caused by vertebral artery occlusion. Cord injury after vertex delivery may be a rare complication of forceps rotation. The diagnosis of spinal cord injury is made on the basis of the clinical features. Ultrasonography, radiography, and MRI of the spine are sometimes indicated to exclude surgically correctable lesions such as spinal dysraphism or extramedullary compression. Because the cord injury is a tear or intraparenchymal hemorrhage, surgical decompression and laminectomy generally are not helpful. Supportive management consists of adequate ventilation and prevention of urinary tract infection, decubitus ulcers, and contractures. High-dose corticosteroids have not been used in controlled trials in spinal cord injury in the newborn age group.

Traumatic Injury to the Peripheral Nervous System

Facial Paralysis

Facial paralysis occurs more commonly in utero by compression of the facial nerve against the bony sacral promontory than by the pressure of forceps blades during delivery. The clinical features are a unilateral widened palpebral fissure and flattened nasolabial fold with the infant at rest, and inability to close the eye completely or grimace when crying. Facial paralysis must be distinguished from *asymmetrical crying facies* resulting from congenital aplasia of the depressor angularis oris muscle.

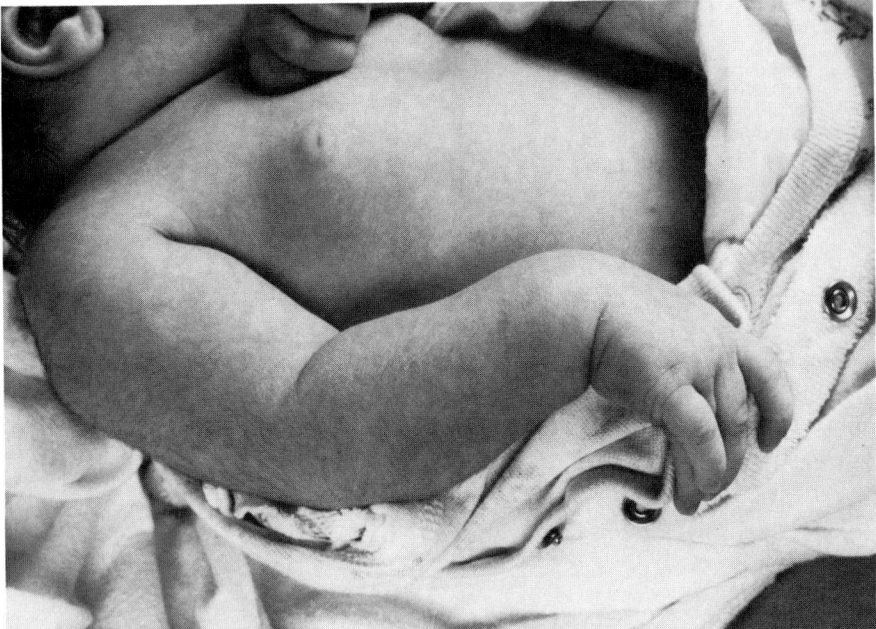

FIGURE 84.8   Brachial plexus injury in newborn. Upper extremity held adducted, internally rotated, and pronated. Note "waiter's tip" position of affected wrist and fingers.

Facial palsy is managed by the use of artificial tears and taping the affected eye closed at night to prevent corneal injury. Most cases recover within weeks or months.

Brachial Plexus Injury

Brachial plexus injury occurs in 0.5–2.6 per 1,000 live term births. The injury almost always occurs in large newborns who are difficult to deliver (Figure 84.8). The upper roots of the brachial plexus are involved most commonly (Erb's palsy). In other instances, lesions may involve the lower nerve roots down to the first thoracic root (Klumpke's palsy). Approximately 5% of cases are associated with diaphragmatic paralysis caused by injury of the third to fifth cervical roots. Such paralysis may result in tachypnea and hypoventilation, with consequent cyanosis and hypercapnia. Brachial plexus injury also may be associated with Horner's syndrome, fractured clavicle or humerus, subluxation of the shoulder or cervical spine, cervical cord injury, and facial palsy.

The neurological features of brachial plexus injury may be deduced from an understanding of the function of the involved cervical roots. Thus, involvement of the upper cervical roots results in loss of shoulder abduction and external rotation and of elbow flexion and supination, with variable impairment of wrist and finger extension (see Figure 84.8). Absence of the biceps reflex on the affected side and an impaired abduction phase of the Moro reflex are demonstrable. With involvement of the lower roots, paralysis extends to intrinsic hand muscles and includes an absent grasp reflex. Horner's syndrome occurs in one-third of such cases. Deficits of motor function and reflexes are usually more striking than are sensory deficits.

In the majority of cases, diagnosis is based primarily on careful neurological examination and may be confirmed if necessary by showing electromyographical evidence of denervation 2–3 weeks after the injury. Clinical suspicion of diaphragmatic paralysis should be confirmed by either fluoroscopy or US scanning. This complication necessitates careful surveillance of respiratory status and perhaps ventilatory support or surgical plication of the affected diaphragm. Other traumatic or bony lesions should be excluded by radiography of the cervical spine, clavicles, and humerus.

Management. The affected arm is usually painful and should be immobilized across the upper abdomen for 7–10 days. Passive range-of-motion exercises are then initiated to prevent contractures. Supportive wrist splints are important. The value of electrical stimulation techniques is controversial. Prognosis relates in large part to the severity of the injury and to the time of onset and rate of initial improvement. Evidence of improved arm function within 2 weeks is a favorable prognostic sign. As many as 88% recover by 4 months and 92% by 12 months. Surgical reconstruction of the plexus (e.g., nerve grafts, neuroma excision) should be considered in infants with no evidence of spontaneous recovery at 4 months (Laurent et al. 1993).

EFFECTS OF DRUGS AND TOXINS

Exposure of the fetus to medications and toxins may have profound adverse effects on the function of the newborn's central and peripheral nervous systems. These effects may be divided broadly into those that are teratogenic and those that cause passive addiction. It is often difficult to distin-

Table 84.11:   Major adverse effects of neuroactive drugs administered during pregnancy

Neuroactive drugs	Passive addiction	Known teratogenic	Neonatal seizures	Intrauterine growth retardation	Coagulation disorders (neonatal intracranial hemorrhage)
Alcohol	+	+	+	+	–
Heroin/methadone	+	–	+ (methadone)	+	–
Cocaine	+	+	?–	+	–
Benzodiazepines	+	–	–	–	–
Tricyclic antidepressants	+	–	+	–	–
Hydroxyzine (Atarax)	+	–	–	–	–
Ethchlorvynol (Placidyl)	+	–	–	–	–
Propoxyphene (Darvon)	+	–	+	–	–
Pentazocine (Talwin)	+	–	–	–	–
"Ts and blues" (pentazocine, tripelennamine)	+	–	+	–	–
Codeine	+	–	–	–	–
Hydantoins	–	+	–	–	+
Barbiturates	+	+	+ (short-acting)	–	+
Primidone	+	+	–	–	+
Valproate	–	+	–	±	–
Oxazolidine derivatives (trimethadione)	–	+	–	+	–

+ = present; – = not presetn ± = possible present.

guish between the adverse effects of a specific agent and those associated with confounding influences, such as intrauterine undernutrition, infection, genetic factors, and toxicity of other medications or exogenous substances.

Table 84.11 lists the major adverse effects of the most commonly used neuroactive agents taken during pregnancy. Prevention is the most important aspect of management, and women of childbearing age must be advised of the risks to the fetus of noxious agents before conception because the risk of malformations is greatest during the early weeks of gestation.

Teratogenic Effects and Intrauterine Growth Retardation

Congenital malformations and intrauterine growth retardation often are associated. In general, maternal alcohol abuse causes growth retardation and intellectual deficits, whereas anticonvulsant drugs cause congenital heart disease and cleft lip and palate. Exposure to valproate during the first weeks of gestation carries a 5% risk of neural tube defects. This risk may be diminished to some degree by preconceptional and periconceptional maternal folate supplementation. Because neural tube defects originate very early during pregnancy (5–6 weeks' gestation), folate administered after diagnosis of pregnancy is not helpful in this regard. Distinct syndromes of growth retardation, developmental delay, dysmorphism, and distal limb abnormalities are attributed to fetal exposure to phenytoin (Figure 84.9), barbiturates, alcohol, trimethadione, and valproate.

Microcephaly and mental retardation are the most disturbing teratogenic effects attributed to fetal exposure to

toxins. Microcephaly occurs in approximately 40% of infants who are passively addicted to heroin.

Risk of Intracranial Hemorrhage

A hemorrhagic diathesis may occur in newborns of mothers treated with phenytoin, barbiturates, and primidone caused by reduced vitamin K–dependent clotting factors (factors II, VII, IX, and X); either prothrombin or partial thromboplastin times are prolonged. Severe bleeding may take place in the skin and internal organs. All newborns exposed to anticonvulsant drugs during pregnancy should be treated with intravenous vitamin K immediately after delivery, and those with abnormal clotting factors should be given fresh frozen plasma. Exchange transfusion is indicated if the newborn has hemorrhagic disease.

Passive Addiction and Withdrawal Syndrome

Passive addiction occurs in 60–90% of newborns of mothers using neuroactive drugs (i.e., drugs that affect the CNS during pregnancy). The clinical features of addiction and withdrawal are similar for most drugs, but the time of withdrawal differs according to the half-life of elimination for the specific drug. Withdrawal symptoms usually start on the first day with heroin, alcohol, short-acting barbiturates, diazepam, tricyclic antidepressants, hydroxyzine, propoxyphene, and pentazocine; at 2–3 days of age with methadone and cocaine; as late as 7 days of age with longer-acting barbiturates; and at up to 21 days of age with chlordiazepoxide.

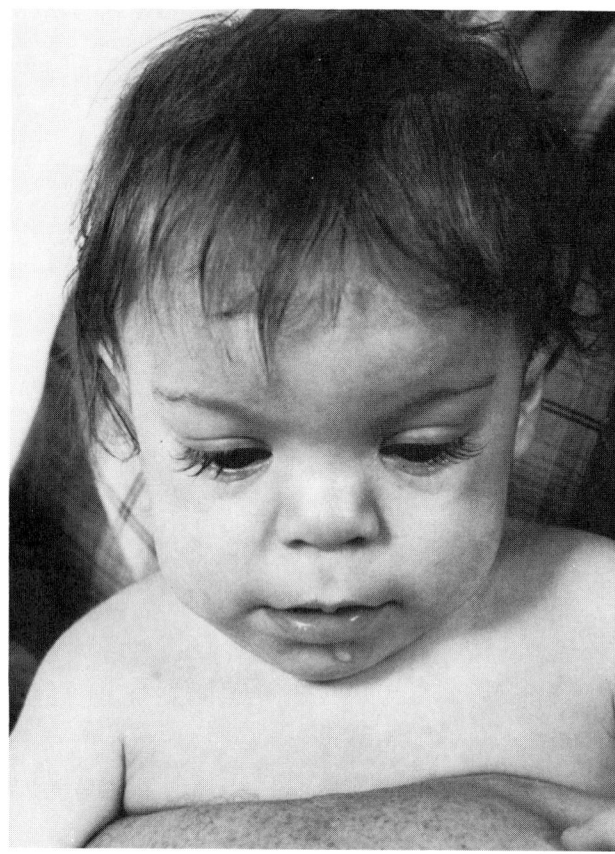

A

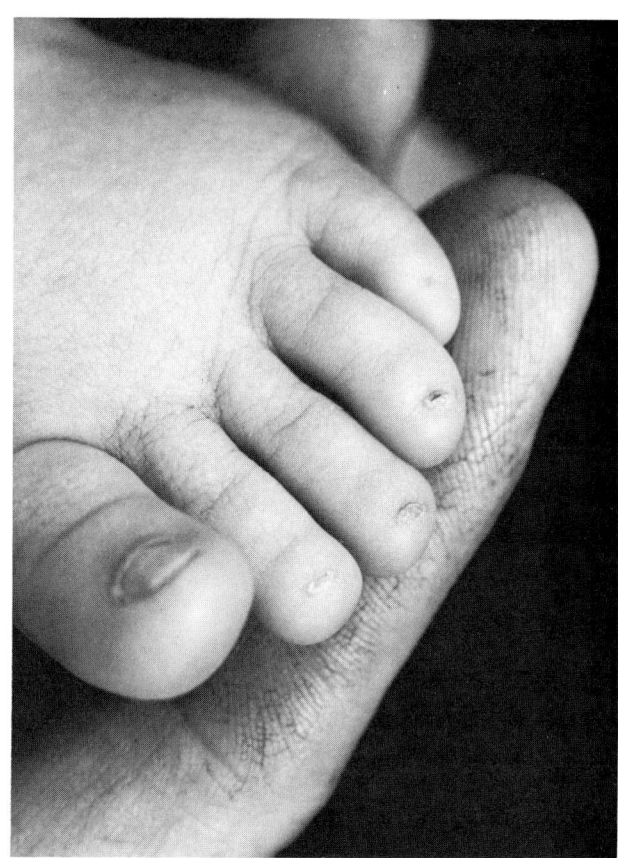

B

FIGURE 84.9   Infant with fetal hydantoin syndrome. (A) Typical facial appearance with broad, depressed nasal bridge and widely spaced eyes. (B) Hypoplasia of nails and distal phalanges.

The initial features of withdrawal reflect CNS overactivity: jitteriness, irritability, disturbed sleep-wake patterns, shrill cry, and frantic sucking. These may be accompanied by gastrointestinal disturbances, such as poor feeding, vomiting, and diarrhea, and less commonly by sneezing, tachypnea, and excessive sweating. Fever and seizures are uncommon manifestations of the neonatal withdrawal syndrome (see the exceptions listed in Table 84.11) and suggest the possibility of sepsis or other serious neonatal disorders.

The withdrawal syndrome associated with long-acting barbiturates and hydroxyzine may persist for several weeks. Newborns withdrawing from heroin often appear to recover initially, but later experience a significant worsening of symptoms that may persist for as long as 6 months.

Effective management requires early diagnosis. Attention is directed toward management of respiratory complications, infection, dehydration, and metabolic derangements. In addition, severe and persistent irritability, vomiting, and diarrhea may require treatment with paregoric, phenobarbital, chlorpromazine, or diazepam.

Oral paregoric (0.8–2.0 ml/kg/day, given in six to eight divided doses) and chlorpromazine (2–3 mg/kg/day given in four divided doses) are effective to control both the CNS and gastrointestinal symptoms. Paregoric is considered the preferred treatment because chlorpromazine may cause extrapyramidal disorders and a lowered seizure threshold. Treatment must be continued for several weeks and tapered gradually to avoid recurrence of symptoms.

Phenobarbital (loading dose of 20 mg/kg, followed by a maintenance dose of 5 mg/kg/day) or diazepam (0.5–1.0 mg intramuscularly every 8 hours) controls only the CNS abnormalities but does not relieve the gastrointestinal symptoms. They also cause sedation that may worsen feeding problems. Therefore, paregoric should be used first and phenobarbital added if CNS abnormalities are not controlled by paregoric alone.

REFERENCES

Bale JF. Perinatal Viral Infections. In K Roos (ed), Central Nervous System Infectious Diseases and Therapy. New York: Marcel Dekker, 1997;1–24.

Barkovich AJ, Hallam D. Neuroimaging in perinatal hypoxic-ischemic injury. Mental Retardation and Developmental Disabilities Research Reviews 1997;3:28–41.

Belman AL. Neurological Disorders Associated with Human Immunodeficiency Virus Infections in Children. In K Roos (ed),

Central Nervous System Infectious Diseases and Therapy. New York: Marcel Dekker, 1997;45–77.

Holmes GL. Epilepsy in the developing brain: lessons from the laboratory and clinic. Epilepsia 1997;38:12–30.

Roland EH, Hill A. Intraventricular hemorrhage and posthemorrhagic hydrocephalus. Clin Perinatol 1997;24:589–605.

Roland EH, Poskitt K, Rodriguez E, et al. Perinatal hypoxic-ischemic thalamic injury: clinical features and neuroimaging. Ann Neurol 1998;44:161–166.

Sher MS. Seizures in the newborn infant: diagnosis, treatment and outcome. Clin Perinatal 1997;24:735–772.

Shu SK, Ashwal S, Holshauser BA, et al. Prognostic value of H-MRS in perinatal CNS insults. Pediatr Neurol 1997;17:309–318.

Trujillo M, McCracken G. Neonatal Meningitis. In K Roos (ed), Central Nervous System Infectious Diseases and Therapy. New York: Marcel Dekker, 1997;25–44.

Volpe JJ. Brain injury in the premature infant—neuropathology, clinical aspects, pathogenesis and prevention. Clin Perinatol 1997;24:567–587.

Wyatt JS. Magnetic resonance spectroscopy and near-infrared spectroscopy in the assessment of the asphxiated term infant. Mental Retardation and Developmental Disabilities Research Reviews 1997;3:42–48.

Chapter 85
Neurological Problems of Pregnancy

D. Malcolm Shaner

Diseases of the nervous system develop and continue despite pregnancy. The good neurologist maintains a broad perspective, balancing the needs of the woman, her fetus, and her loved ones. Insofar as this audience creates an atmosphere for performance, the clinician may feel like a stage character prompted by cues from a scattered, incomplete, and occasionally contradictory literature. Still, neurologists who enjoy drama find gratification in caring for the pregnant woman with neurological disease.

NEUROLOGICAL COMPLICATIONS OF CONTRACEPTION

The neurologist can be helpful in planning pregnancy. The expected burden of the woman's neurological disease must be balanced against her perceived need for procreation. Asking her to consider the effect of a child on her life and how the child might be affected by her illness can be beneficial. Many women welcome the neurologist's uninvolved opinion.

The use of oral contraceptive agents containing more than 80 μg of estrogen is linked to increased incidence of stroke. Information on the use of agents containing less than 50 μg of estrogen in nondiabetic, nonhypertensive patients indicates that these agents pose no additional risk, or at most a true relative risk of ischemic stroke of no more than 2.5. Given the very low annual incidence of ischemic stroke in the normal population of women aged 15–44 of approximately 11.3 per 100,000, this small or nonexistent added risk can be considered safe. When women taking this dose smoke cigarettes, the risk of hemorrhagic stroke increases to an odds ratio of 3.64 with a 95% confidence interval of 0.95–13.87 (Petitti et al. 1998).

Some neurologists advise their female epileptic patients taking microsomal enzyme–inducing anticonvulsants to increase the dose of estrogen to at least 50 μg. Although this adjustment increases contraceptive effectiveness, the efficacy of the regimen is untested. The result is that barrier, spermicidal, or other contraceptive measures often are recommended for use simultaneously or exclusively. Valproic acid does not induce microsomal enzymes significantly, but there are no studies confirming lack of drug interaction with estrogen contraception.

Anticonvulsants do not affect efficacy or dose of medroxyprogesterone. Unwanted pregnancies with levonorgestrel use have occurred in women taking phenytoin and in women taking carbamazepine.

Some neurologists recommend against the use of hormonal contraceptives in women diagnosed with activated protein C resistance. Estrogen-containing oral contraceptive agents may worsen chronic inflammatory demyelinating polyneuropathy (CIDP), unmask systemic lupus erythematosus, worsen migraine, and produce chorea in patients with antiphospholipid antibody syndrome. The heightened risk of cerebral venous thrombosis (CVT) in women taking oral contraceptive agents increases with prothrombin or factor V gene mutations (Martinelli et al. 1998).

HEADACHE

Headache during pregnancy is common. Usually a patient visits the neurologist to receive reassurance that no serious medical problem is apparent. Of the headaches that occur during pregnancy, benign tension headaches are most frequent (see Chapter 73). There is no known association with hormones and, specifically, no association with the hormonal changes of pregnancy. Treatment for mild headaches often includes behavioral therapy and acetaminophen. For severe headaches, the use of a tricyclic antidepressant, such as amitriptyline or nortriptyline, may be helpful. Preschool children exposed in utero to tricyclic antidepressants have normal global IQ, language, and behavioral development. When treating significant comorbid depression, fluoxetine may be additionally helpful.

Approximately 80% of women with migraine clearly improve during pregnancy, but approximately 15% continue to have headaches. Prognosis is better for migraine without aura than migraine with aura. For women anticipating pregnancy, the physician may consider the discontinuation or reduction in dose of all migraine medications. Vigorous treatment with behavioral therapy, moist heat, and the judicious use of acetaminophen or opioid preparations can be considered. Migraine usually improves during the second and third trimesters. The diagnosis of complicated migraine, or de novo migraine with aura, should be made during pregnancy only after a thorough consideration of other diseases.

Pregnancy complicates usual migraine therapy. Ergotamine and dihydroergotamine are associated with high rates of fetal malformation and are contraindicated. For many other drugs, such as sumatriptan, data are incomplete, and their use cannot be advised. There are rare descriptions of fetal toxicity with propranolol, atenolol, and other beta blockers, with the exception of metoprolol. Although often safe during pregnancy, these drugs usually are discontinued or reduced to the lowest effective dose. Naproxen sodium is relatively safe throughout pregnancy but safest when used during the first two trimesters. Metoclopramide, acetaminophen, and meperidine do not increase fetal risk and may be of benefit. When physician and patient are convinced that prophylactic therapy is required, the benefit of metoprolol, propranolol, or verapamil may outweigh risks.

DISORDERS OF MUSCLE

Leg Muscle Cramps

Between 5% and 30% of pregnant women experience painful contraction of leg muscles. These contractions do not adversely affect the fetus or patient. The condition resolves rapidly postpartum. Typically, cramps occur in the morning or evening during the last trimester of pregnancy. Changes in the ionic concentration of potassium, magnesium, sodium, and calcium may be important in the pathogenesis. Magnesium lactate or magnesium citrate tablets (122 mg in the morning and 244 mg in the evening) relieves or considerably improves symptoms in approximately 80% of patients. Placebo is similarly effective in 40%. Some physicians report successful therapy using oral calcium carbonate or gluconate 500 mg three or four times daily. Passive stretch and massage are helpful for the acute cramp.

Restless Legs

Unpleasant paresthesias (described as creeping, crawling, aching, or fidgety) localized deep within both legs affect 10–27% of pregnant women. Usually they begin 30 minutes after lying down and are reported mainly in the last trimester. An irresistible desire to move the legs accompanies the discomfort.

In approximately 80% of patients complaining of restless legs, periodic movements of sleep occur (see Chapter 72). These are stereotyped flexion movements of the legs during non–rapid eye movement sleep, which may awaken the patient, leading to sleep loss and excessive daytime somnolence. Caffeine ingestion, uremia, alcohol use, iron deficiency, hypothyroidism, vitamin deficiency, rheumatoid arthritis, peripheral neuropathy, and medications are important, if only occasional, associated factors.

Folic acid, 500 mg daily, may be of benefit in treating restless legs during pregnancy. Anecdotal reports suggest a benefit from vitamin E, vitamin C, and magnesium supplements for restless legs that occur in nonpregnant patients. Electric vibrators, stretching, walking, decreased activity, and massage also may be helpful. For severe restless legs during pregnancy, L-dopa/carbidopa 25mg/100mg may be preferable to several other medications shown to be effective in nonpregnant patients. A single dose before bedtime, increasing to efficacy or using several doses through the night, has been helpful anecdotally. Advantages of L-dopa/carbidopa include its demonstrated clinical effectiveness for both restless legs and periodic movements of sleep and its low teratogenic potential.

Myasthenia Gravis

Fertility is unaffected by myasthenia gravis, and oral contraceptive agents do not weaken the myasthenic patient. No single study offers certainty with regard to the cumulative risk that pregnancy causes in the known myasthenic. Pregnancy did not worsen the long-term outcome of myasthenia gravis in one small prospective Italian study (Batocchi et al. 1999). Some of the best data indicate that approximately one-third of pregnant patients notice no clinical change, one-third experience an improvement at some time, and approximately two-thirds of known myasthenic patients weaken during pregnancy or puerperium. The puerperium and first trimester are times of greatest risk. The course of myasthenia for a future pregnancy cannot be predicted from the course of previous pregnancies.

The effect of thymectomy on myasthenia gravis usually is delayed. The potential mother can be advised that the procedure may be helpful for a pregnancy beginning approximately 1 year after surgery. Generally, the woman who may become pregnant is best served when the physician uses drugs other than azathioprine and cyclosporine. Azathioprine is teratogenic, and the safety of cyclosporine during gestation is uncertain.

Myasthenia gravis does not influence the contractile strength of the smooth muscle of the uterus, the frequency of postpartum hemorrhage, or the frequency of toxemia. Usually, the course of labor and delivery are unaffected. Premature labor may be more common in women with myasthenia but varies considerably among hospital studies.

The medical therapy of myasthenia gravis changes little with pregnancy. Anticholinesterase agents, including edrophonium (Tensilon), corticosteroids, and plasmapheresis, are relatively safe. Rapid drug metabolism during pregnancy may require increasing the frequency or dose of anticholinesterase drugs. Abortion is of no known benefit to myasthenia. Although human immunoglobulin has been used safely during pregnancy, the number of patients studied is small.

Regional anesthesia is preferred for cesarean section. When the patient is taking anticholinesterase agents, the metabolism of procaine is slowed and poorly predictable. In those patients, lidocaine is favored for local anesthesia. Neuromuscular blocking agents, such as curariform drugs, must be avoided. The use of magnesium sulfate as a tocolytic or as treatment for preeclampsia may precipitate myasthenic crisis and is contraindicated.

Perinatal mortality increases approximately five times that of the normal population to 6–8% for infants of myasthenic women. Approximately 2% of these are stillborn. Transient neonatal myasthenia affects 10–20% of infants born to women with myasthenia. Most infants who develop transient myasthenia do so within the first day, but weakness may begin up to 4 days after delivery and usually resolves within 3–6 weeks. Neonates must be observed carefully for at least 4 days. An imperfect correlation has been observed between maternal levels of antiacetylcholine receptor antibodies and the likelihood that the neonate will develop transient myasthenia.

Breast-feeding poses no significant difficulty. Cyclosporine and azathioprine are excreted in breast milk and carry immunosuppressive risks and tumorigenic potential and should be avoided. Corticosteroids also are secreted into breast milk but in small amounts. Large doses of anticholinesterase drugs taken by the mother may lead to gastrointestinal upset in the breast-fed newborn.

Myotonic Dystrophy

Pregnancy is uncommon in women who have advanced myotonic dystrophy. Physicians attribute this observation to ovarian failure. Before the development of advanced disease, there is no significant reduction in fertility. For women who are able to conceive, pregnancy can be hazardous for both mother and fetus. Myotonic weakness often worsens during the second half of pregnancy. Congestive heart failure is reported. Ineffective uterine contractions, premature labor, and breech presentation frequently complicate labor. Tocolysis may result in aggravation of myotonia. Oxytocin can stimulate the myotonic uterus to increased contraction. Myotonic dystrophy complicates obstetric anesthesia, and regional anesthesia is preferred. After delivery, hypotonic uterine dysfunction results in an increased risk of retained placenta and postpartum hemorrhage. One-half of the children born to women with myotonia inherit the disorder. Anticipation due to an increased number of triplet repeats (see Chapter 45) is responsible for the syndrome of congenital myotonic dystrophy (see Chapter 83). Many neonates are hypotonic, and high rates of morbidity are reported. Fetal myotonic dystrophy may affect fetal swallowing, causing polyhydramnios. Prenatal diagnostic testing with amniocentesis or chorionic villus biopsy is available.

Inflammatory Myopathy

Pregnancy worsens or activates polymyositis and dermatomyositis. Manifestations of collagen vascular disease commonly associated with myositis may complicate pregnancy. More than one-half of fetuses die, but surviving infants thrive. Immunosuppressive treatment usually is advised.

NEUROPATHY

Bell's Palsy

Facial nerve palsy is three to four times more common during pregnancy and the puerperium. Prognosis for recovery is unaltered by the pregnant state. Some researchers find an increased frequency of toxemia in patients with gestational facial palsy. Herpes simplex virus I is implicated in the cause of most facial palsies, and far less frequently, varicella zoster. Pharmacological therapy during pregnancy remains controversial. Prednisone, 1 mg/kg for 5 days, tapering rapidly over a total 10-day course when begun within 3 days of onset of facial weakness, appears to be effective in improving the prognosis in nongravid adults. Simultaneous acyclovir, 400 mg five times daily for 10 days is more effective than prednisone alone in a similar population (Adour et al. 1996). This combination of drugs has not been tested adequately during pregnancy, but individually, the drugs pose low risk. Patching of the eye and lubricating eye drops are helpful, particularly when the cornea is covered inadequately by the weak upper lid (see Chapter 74).

Carpal Tunnel Syndrome

Approximately one in five pregnant women report nocturnal hand paresthesias, primarily during the last trimester, often associated with peripheral edema. Excessive weight gain and fluid retention increase the frequency of these complaints. This irritation can be expected to disappear spontaneously within weeks after parturition. During pregnancy, conservative therapy is indicated. Splinting of the wrist in the neutral position at night is helpful. Additionally, some physicians inject corticosteroids into the carpal tunnel. When hand muscles supplied by the median nerve weaken, surgical decompression is indicated.

Meralgia Paresthetica

The expanding abdominal wall and the increased lordosis of pregnancy stretch the lateral femoral cutaneous nerve to the thigh as it penetrates the tensor fascia lata or at the inguinal ligament. This unilateral or bilateral affliction of late pregnancy resolves within 3 months postpartum.

Acute Polyradiculoneuropathy (Guillain-Barré Syndrome)

Pregnancy does not affect the frequency or course of acute polyradiculoneuropathy. Usually, infants of a mother without complications are born healthy. Some authors recommend fluid loading before plasmapheresis to prevent hypotension. Others suggest avoiding tocolytics in the presence of autonomic instability. Intravenous human immunoglobulin has been used safely during pregnancy, but the number of patients who received this therapy and were studied remains small.

Chronic Inflammatory Demyelinating Polyneuropathy

CIDP is three times more likely to relapse during the last trimester and puerperium than in the absence of pregnancy. Infants are unaffected. Corticosteroids, plasmapheresis, and intravenous immunoglobulin are used to treat exacerbations during pregnancy. Oral contraceptives can worsen CIDP.

Charcot-Marie-Tooth Disease Type 1

Small studies indicate that approximately one-half of women with Charcot-Marie-Tooth disease type 1 worsen during pregnancy (Rudnik-Schoneborn et al. 1993). The magnitude of the effect of pregnancy on this disease remains unclear. Risk is less when weakness begins in adulthood. After delivery, this deterioration improves in one-third and becomes persistently progressive in two-thirds. The course and outcome of pregnancy are unaffected. Epidural anesthesia for labor has been used safely.

Gestational Polyneuropathy

Distal symmetrical neuropathy affects malnourished women. Presumably, thiamine and possibly other nutrients are deficient in these patients. The acute presentation of symmetrical neuropathy and Wernicke's encephalopathy in the third and fourth months may be secondary to the thiamine deficiency associated with hyperemesis gravidarum.

Maternal Obstetric Palsy

Peripheral nerves are occasionally the objects of intrapartum compressive trauma by the fetal head, the application of forceps, and improperly positioned leg holders. Craniopelvic disproportion, dystocia, prolonged labor and primigravida status contribute to these injuries.

Unilateral lumbosacral (L4, L5, rarely S1) plexus injury is most common. The fetal brow strikes the nerves as they cross the posterior brim of the true pelvis. The sensory deficit associated usually involves more widespread sensory loss than that due to peroneal neuropathy. Peroneal nerve injuries often are caused when the nerve is compressed between a leg holder and the fibular head. Otherwise, the two neuropathies can be nearly identical in presentation. Less common obstetric palsies include those of the femoral and obturator nerves.

Most maternal obstetric palsies are neuropractic and recover within 6 weeks. In future pregnancies, women with recurrent craniopelvic disproportion, dystocia, or axonal degeneration with their initial neuropathy are candidates for cesarean delivery. Otherwise, a cautious trial of labor may be prudent.

WERNICKE'S ENCEPHALOPATHY

More than three-fourths of women experience nausea and vomiting during pregnancy, most commonly between 6 and 16 weeks of gestation. When vomiting becomes severe enough to result in weight loss or metabolic derangement requiring intravenous therapy, the term *hyperemesis gravidarum* is properly applied. Commonly, hyperemesis is isolated and idiopathic. Molar pregnancy, hyperthyroidism, and hepatitis are diagnostic considerations.

Apathy, drowsiness, memory loss, catatonia, ophthalmoplegia, nystagmus, ataxia, optic neuritis, and papilledema may result, typically between 14 and 20 weeks' gestation, and are described as features of Wernicke's encephalopathy. This condition is sometimes associated with gestational polyneuropathy and central pontine myelinolysis. Exacerbating factors include persistence of the hyperemesis over at least 3 weeks and the administration of intravenous glucose without other nutrients. Death and severe morbidity result when this condition is not treated. In a small study, only one-half of women with this condition delivered normal children.

The amount and duration of parenteral thiamine supplementation is unknown and must be titrated to the clinical state. Generally, parenteral therapy for at least 1 week is recommended or until a normal diet can be resumed. Despite therapy, some women continue to have ataxia and visual difficulties months to years afterward.

CHOREA GRAVIDARUM

Chorea of any cause beginning in pregnancy is chorea gravidarum. Historically, rheumatic heart disease (often fatal) was associated with most cases. Rheumatic heart disease has virtually disappeared. Today, the disease linked most strongly with this condition is the antiphospholipid antibody syndrome, with or without systemic lupus erythematosus. The physician may wish to consider additional etiologies, such as tardive dyskinesia due to neuroleptics, hyperthyroidism, Wilson's disease, vascular disease, other hypercoagulable states, and a variety of intoxications.

Chorea commonly presents during the second to fifth month of pregnancy and uncommonly may begin postpartum. Subtle, sometimes severe cognitive change may accompany the chorea. Usually, this condition resolves spontaneously within weeks to months, often shortly after delivery. Choice of therapy for this frequently benign condition depends on the severity of the disorder and other accompanying clinical manifestations. Expectant observation, the cautious use of haloperidol, and corticosteroids have been employed with success. Oral contraceptives also have been associated with the appearance of chorea. The mechanism by which pregnancy and oral contraceptives cause chorea is unknown (Cervera et al. 1997).

MULTIPLE SCLEROSIS

Uncomplicated multiple sclerosis has no apparent effect on fertility, pregnancy, labor, delivery, the rate of spontaneous abortions, congenital malformations, or stillbirths. The approximately 13% reduction in pregnancy rate among women with multiple sclerosis noted in one study may result from physical disability and from women deciding not to have children.

Despite several careful studies, the effect of pregnancy on the course of multiple sclerosis remains controversial. Small, prospective analyses challenge the long-held conclusion that multiple sclerosis worsens overall as a result of

pregnancy. Some authors suggest that pregnancy has either a beneficial effect or no significant effect on disease course (Runmarker and Andersen 1995; Stenager et al. 1994). Others believe that increased risk for relapse during the first 6 months postpartum is likely, but a full-term pregnancy may increase the overall interval to reach the point that a cane is needed (Damek and Shuster 1997).

Larger, retrospective studies describe a decrease in the exacerbation rate of multiple sclerosis during the last trimester and an increased rate during the 6 months after parturition. Studies that suggest an overall negative effect of pregnancy estimate an increase in relapse rate of 50–100%. Most commonly, women worsened during the first 3 months postpartum, and by 6 months, approximately 20–40% of women experienced disease aggravation. Medications have not prevented this postpartum exacerbation.

Glatiramer acetate, interferon-β-1a, and interferon-β-1b have not been studied adequately and currently are not indicated during pregnancy. Until information is available regarding safety, these medications should be discontinued before an anticipated pregnancy. Management strategies must cater to the individual patient. Anecdotal reports detail the success of plasmapheresis in a pregnant woman with rapidly progressive multiple sclerosis and in another woman with Devic's syndrome. Short-term courses of corticosteroids during pregnancy seem safe, but baclofen and tizanidine have not been well studied.

TUMORS

Primary Brain Neoplasms

Brain tumors of all types occur during pregnancy, but only at 38% of the rate expected in nonpregnant women of fertile age. Diminished fertility in women with these tumors probably explains this phenomenon. Studies show increased numbers of abortions before the appearance of tumor signs. We do not know if pregnancy worsens morbidity and mortality in women with brain tumors, but certain tumors grow during pregnancy. Meningiomas have estrogen receptors, which may explain their frequent enlargement during pregnancy. The frequency with which spinal hemangiomas rupture increases with gestation. Symptoms of meningioma, vascular tumors, and acoustic neuromas may remit postpartum.

The natural history of gestational brain tumors depends on anecdotal reports and literature reviews. These analyses suggest that gliomas usually present problems during the first trimester, meningiomas during and after the second trimester, and vascular tumors in the third trimester.

Malignant tumors, or tumors threatening compression of vital brain structures, commonly are operated on during pregnancy. Some benign tumors can wait several weeks postpartum to observe for spontaneous remission. Most women are delivered by cesarean section. Vaginal delivery is reserved for patients whose tumor would not pose a threat of herniation with the increased intracranial pressure associated with labor. Pregnancy interruption is considered when increased intracranial pressure, vision loss, or uncontrolled seizures develop.

Corticosteroids commonly relieve symptoms of brain tumors (see Chapter 58), but fetal hypoadrenalism may result from their use. Physicians usually defer potentially teratogenic chemotherapy until after delivery. Cranial radiation therapy during pregnancy may be helpful to the mother, but no dose of radiation can be considered completely safe for the fetus. The fetus usually is seriously affected when it receives doses greater than 0.1 Gy (10 rads), which may cause growth retardation, microcephaly, and eye malformations. The fetus may be affected by lower amounts of radiation, particularly early in gestation. Researchers estimate that in utero exposure to 0.01–0.02 Gy of radiation increases the frequency of leukemia by one case per 6,000 children treated. Estimates of the fetal dose during radiation for brain tumors range from 0.03–0.06 Gy (Sneed et al. 1995).

Pituitary Tumors

Bromocriptine reduces prolactinoma size usually within 6 weeks to 6 months. Although this drug has not demonstrated teratogenic potential, some authors recommend discontinuation of the medication unless it is clearly needed. Bromocriptine suppresses lactation. Puerperal maternal hypertension, seizures, stroke, and cerebral angiopathy have been reported anecdotally with its use. Data on other dopamine agonists during pregnancy are limited. Women with untreated hyperprolactinemia often are anovulatory and infertile. Treatment with dopamine agonists restores ovulation in 90% of patients. During pregnancy, medical therapy focuses on preventing complications of tumor growth.

The normal pituitary and usual pituitary tumor grow during pregnancy. The woman with a pituitary microadenoma (<10 mm) may be reassured that fewer than 5% of these tumors grow enough to become symptomatic. The risk for a macroadenoma becoming symptomatic ranges from 15.5% to 35.7% but is considerably less for patients who receive radiation or surgical therapy before pregnancy. Commonly, physicians advise women with macroadenomas to have transsphenoidal surgery before attempting pregnancy or to receive bromocriptine therapy during pregnancy. Visual fields and acuity can be checked monthly. Monitoring prolactin levels is not helpful. Magnetic resonance imaging (MRI) is indicated after delivery and should be performed for increasing symptoms. For the woman diagnosed during pregnancy with a symptomatic macroprolactinoma, therapeutic options include bromocriptine therapy, pregnancy termination, or surgery.

Usually, women with pituitary tumors deliver vaginally. Studies have not demonstrated tumor growth associated with breast-feeding. Pituitary apoplexy may occur. Uncommonly, a pituitary mass presenting in late pregnancy, or up to 1 year postpartum, may be lymphocytic hypophysitis.

Choriocarcinoma

Cerebral metastases are a common manifestation of this rare tumor of trophoblastic origin. The tumor metastasizes first to the lung and then from lung to brain. This often happens months after a molar pregnancy or abortion. Approximately 15% of tumors follow normal pregnancies. Women present with seizures, hemorrhage, infarction, or gradually progressive deficits. Tumor may invade the sacral plexus, cauda equina, or spinal canal. A ratio of serum to cerebrospinal fluid chorionic gonadotropin less than 60 suggests brain metastasis. Chemotherapy, radiation, and surgery have yielded successful results when the diagnosis is made early.

Idiopathic Intracranial Hypertension (Pseudotumor Cerebri)

Idiopathic intracranial hypertension (IIH) worsens with pregnancy. Some authors advise a delay in pregnancy until all signs and symptoms abate. Termination of pregnancy is of unknown value and is not indicated. Healthy babies usually result regardless of whether IIH begins before or during pregnancy.

Commonly, IIH develops during the fourteenth gestational week and disappears after 1–3 months, but it sometimes persists until the early puerperium. Typically, these women are obese and gain weight rapidly with pregnancy. Brain imaging is normal or may show slitlike ventricles. Protein levels may be slightly low in otherwise normal spinal fluid.

Frequent checks of optic fundi, visual acuity, and visual fields are recommended to monitor the condition and the results of treatment. Initial cerebrospinal fluid pressures that exceed 350 mm H_2O usually indicate more severe disease. Careful studies of the effectiveness of treatment are unavailable. Most physicians advise moderation in diet to produce a modest weight gain. Two-week courses of corticosteroids, most commonly dexamethasone or prednisone, may be added for vision loss. Four to six serial lumbar punctures can be performed, sometimes weekly, before considering optic nerve sheath fenestration or lumboperitoneal shunt.

The use of acetazolamide remains controversial; human studies are inadequate to determine its efficacy or teratogenic potential. Nevertheless, acetazolamide has been used to treat IIH during many pregnancies productive of healthy infants. Some physicians recommend restricting its use until after 20 weeks' gestation.

Headaches may be improved by acetaminophen with or without codeine. More aggressive therapy usually is reserved for vision loss. Adequate pain control during labor may decrease expected rises in intracranial pressure. Commonly, these patients are delivered vaginally with epidural analgesia. Recurrence in subsequent pregnancy is unusual.

EPILEPSY AND ITS TREATMENTS

Maternal Considerations

Women with epilepsy have approximately 15% fewer children than expected. Reasons offered for this decrease in fertility include menstrual irregularity, the effect of some antiepileptic medications on the ovaries, and an effect of seizures on reproductive hormones.

The effect of pregnancy on seizure frequency can be predicted from the control of epilepsy during the 9 months preceding gestation. The fewer seizures there are in the 9 months before conception, the lower the risk of worsening during the pregnancy. Women who have at least one seizure a month can be expected to have more seizures during pregnancy. Women who have fewer than one seizure in 9 months usually do not experience an increase in seizure frequency during pregnancy. Myriad studies have found the overall frequency of seizures to be increased at widely different rates. Most suggest that approximately one-fourth of women experience an increase in seizure frequency during gestation.

Elevated seizure frequency may result from lowered levels of circulating unbound antiepileptic drugs (AEDs). Pregnancy increases the drugs' volume of distribution and metabolism. However, even when blood levels are maintained adequately, approximately 10% of women can expect worsened seizure control. During labor, approximately 1–2% of epileptic women convulse, and another 1–2% have a seizure within 24 hours of delivery. Other factors that may contribute to increase in seizure frequency include hormonal changes, sleep deprivation, mild chronic respiratory alkalosis, the use of folic acid supplements, and emotional factors. Seizure type did not play a role in some studies, but in others, partial complex epilepsy worsened more often during gestation.

Convulsive seizures during pregnancy can result in blunt trauma to the mother. Trauma is the leading nonobstetric cause of maternal death in women with epilepsy, but the frequency is very low, and the relation to epilepsy remains obscure.

Controversy continues over whether seizures increase risks for developing eclampsia, preeclampsia, blood loss, placental abruption, and premature labor. For studies that claim increased risk, these risks are calculated to be approximately 1.5–3.0 times the risk of women without epilepsy. These reports have been based largely on retrospective and registry studies. The limited prospective data suggest that women with epilepsy have no or minimal additional risk for these complications.

Fetal Considerations

Nearly 90% of epileptic women deliver healthy, normal babies, but risks of miscarriage, stillbirth, prematurity, developmental delay, and major malformations are increased. Maternal seizures, AEDs, socioeconomic, genetic, and psychological aspects of epilepsy affect outcome.

Although AEDs may cause significant problems for the fetus, maternal seizures probably are more dangerous. Convulsive seizures cause fetal hypoxia and acidosis and carry the potential for blunt trauma to the fetus and placenta. Fetal heart rate slows during and for up to 20 minutes after a maternal convulsion, which suggests the presence of fetal asphyxia. The child of an epileptic mother experiencing convulsions during gestation is twice as likely to develop epilepsy as the child of a woman with epilepsy who does not convulse.

The rate of major birth defects in the general population has been estimated at approximately 2.0–4.8%, depending on the population studied and methodology employed. The risk of birth defects increases for infants of women with epilepsy to a rate of 3.5–6.0%, independent of the effect of medication. In general, use of a single AED increases the risk of congenital malformations to 4–8%. Researchers find a 5.5% frequency of malformations with two anticonvulsant drugs, 11% with three anticonvulsant drugs, and 23% with the use of four AEDs.

During the first 2.5 months of gestation, AEDs exert their most serious effects. Changes in medication must be made before or during the first trimester to be maximally useful. The neural tube closes between 3–4 weeks. Cleft lip and palate occur with exposure before 5 and 10 weeks, respectively, whereas congenital heart disease secondary to anticonvulsant exposure occurs before 6 weeks' gestation.

Phenytoin poses approximately a 10% risk of major congenital anomalies, and carbamazepine less than 10%. Studies disagree on whether these anomalies are dose dependent. Valproic acid increases the risk of neural tube defects and other malformations three- to 20-fold, to approximately 1–2%, and its teratogenic effects are dose related. Carbamazepine also is associated with neural tube defects, with a frequency of 0.5–1.0%. A syndrome described initially as *fetal hydantoin syndrome*—facial dimorphism, cleft lip and palate, cardiac defects, digital hypoplasia, and nail dysplasia—occurs with carbamazepine, primidone, and valproic acid and is more accurately called *fetal anticonvulsant syndrome*.

We lack adequate human studies of newer anticonvulsant drugs during pregnancy. The teratogenic potential of gabapentin, vigabatrin, tiagabine, zonisamide, lamotrigine, topiramate, clobazam, and oxcarbazepine is known incompletely. At this time, the physician may consider a re-evaluation of the need for these anticonvulsants and possible substitution with agents whose potential for risk is known. Trimethadione has such a high teratogenic potential that its use during pregnancy is contraindicated and should not be used in women who might become pregnant.

Common Advice and Management Strategy

The need for AED therapy should be re-evaluated before conception. Monotherapy at the lowest effective dose is preferred. Admonishing the patient against sleep deprivation and noncompliance with the drug regimen may be helpful when paired with a thorough description of the potential consequences of seizures and benefits of AEDs. AED levels can be monitored more frequently during gestation and the postpartum period and dosage adjusted as indicated. Women with a family history of neural tube defects probably should be weaned from valproic acid or carbamazepine, particularly if there is a suitable substitute.

Pregnant women with epilepsy who present to the neurologist already taking AEDs should be managed on an individual basis. During pregnancy, and particularly once the period of organogenesis has passed, changes in medications are likely to cause more harm than good.

Women who take folic acid supplements before and during pregnancy lower their risk of delivering a child with major malformations. The use of folic acid has become routine, but recommendations vary. The Department of Health in the United Kingdom and the Centers for Disease Control and Prevention in the United States have recommended, respectively, 5 mg and 4 mg of folic acid daily for women who have had a child with a neural tube defect and 0.4 mg for all other women planning pregnancy. Anticonvulsants inhibit the absorption of folic acid. Occasionally, folic acid lowers levels of anticonvulsants. Some authors suggest that 5 mg of folic acid be given daily to women treated with valproic acid or carbamazepine. Others recommend 2–4 mg daily for all women with epilepsy who are taking anticonvulsants, beginning as long as 3 months before conception until 12 weeks' gestation.

For patients taking AEDs during pregnancy, a second-trimester high-resolution ultrasound evaluation helps to exclude spina bifida aperta, cardiac anomalies, and limb defects. When the ultrasound is inconclusive, amniocentesis can be considered, and α-fetoprotein and acetylcholinesterase levels obtained.

A deficiency of vitamin K–dependent clotting factors occurs in some neonates born to women who take phenobarbital, primidone, carbamazepine, ethosuximide, or phenytoin. Infrequently reported, neonatal intracerebral hemorrhage may be attributed to this vitamin K deficiency. In an attempt to lower this risk, physicians prescribe oral vitamin K_1 10–20 mg daily beginning 2–4 weeks before expected delivery and until birth. Often, the neonate receives a single 1–2 mg intramuscular injection of vitamin K_1 immediately after delivery. When hemorrhage occurs, fresh frozen plasma acutely corrects the hemorrhagic state. When the expectant mother taking AEDs presents in labor without having received vitamin K_1 supplements, consider administering intravenous vitamin K_1 10 mg to the mother during labor, 2 mg to the neonate immediately postpartum, and fresh frozen plasma if needed on the basis of fetal cord coagulation studies.

Occasionally, seizures present for the first time during pregnancy. Pregnancy has little effect on the use of diagnostic examinations and treatment considerations. The most common causes of seizures during childbearing years include idiopathic epilepsy, trauma, congenital defects, neoplasms, meningitis, intracerebral hemorrhage, and drug or alcohol toxicity. In addition, pregnancy predisposes to certain conditions, such as eclampsia, water intoxication, thrombotic thrombocytopenic purpura, sinus or cortical venous thrombosis, and amniotic fluid embolus. Common iatrogenic causes include hyponatremia secondary to intravenous fluid infusion during the intrapartum period, and the use of epidural or parenteral anesthetics.

A single first-onset seizure resolving within minutes usually can be managed acutely without anticonvulsants. Once the physician determines the cause for the seizure and whether further seizures are likely, the need for anticonvulsant medication can be reviewed.

There are no special considerations during pregnancy when treating potentially fatal generalized convulsive status epilepticus. The choice of initial anticonvulsant regimen remains controversial. Physicians agree that familiarity with a specific treatment regimen and its prompt application generally has the best chance of success. Monotherapy with phenobarbital or lorazepam and combined therapies with phenytoin are effective.

Anticonvulsants are secreted in breast milk and ingested by the infant. Sedation and hyperirritability are reported. Infants may show withdrawal reactions from phenobarbital after lactational exposure. The World Health Organization Working Group on Human Lactation and the American Academy of Pediatrics disagree on the safety of breast milk containing ethosuximide, which may cause hyperexcitability and poor suckling. Known health benefits of breast milk probably outweigh potential subtle and theoretical effects of AEDs on the nervous system.

CEREBROVASCULAR DISEASE

Arteriovenous Malformations

The risk of repeat hemorrhage from a previously ruptured arteriovenous malformation (AVM) generally outweighs the risk from surgical excision or an obliterative procedure. Usually, surgical excision can be performed shortly after the diagnosis and before pregnancy is considered. When proton beam irradiation is performed, some authorities advise the woman to wait 2 years before conception. The decision about whether an unruptured AVM should be observed, excised, embolized, or irradiated remains controversial. No specific therapeutic course can be recommended for patients planning pregnancy.

The risk of hemorrhage from an AVM rises from a low point during childhood and teenage years to a higher risk during childbearing years. Whether pregnancy poses additional risk remains uncertain. The best retrospective review suggests that risk of hemorrhage during pregnancy resulting from an unruptured AVM may be as low as 3.5%. This is probably no different from the risk to non-pregnant women with unruptured AVMs. Multiple pregnancies do not increase the rate of hemorrhage. In the past, physicians routinely advised women with an AVM, previously ruptured or not, to avoid pregnancy. This conclusion might have been expected from information available from early retrospective studies that 87% of AVMs rupture during pregnancy and that 25–30% of initial ruptures are fatal. Subsequent analysis has contradicted these dismal estimates. Still, we have no prospective studies. The clinician must exercise caution in interpreting this information.

Women whose AVM is repaired surgically can undergo vaginal delivery. Physicians usually perform cesarean section for incompletely repaired or partially treated previously ruptured AVMs. Epidural anesthesia is preferred.

Intracranial Hemorrhage

Women presenting with pregnancy-associated stroke are as likely to have an infarct as an intracerebral hemorrhage. Intracerebral hemorrhage occurs 2.5 times more often during pregnancy, and almost 30 times more often during the 6 weeks postpartum. Up to 44% of these hemorrhages are associated with eclampsia and preeclampsia. In France, nearly one-half of women with intracerebral hemorrhage associated with eclampsia die (Sharshar et al. 1995). Additional diagnostic considerations include bleeding diatheses, cocaine toxicity, bacterial endocarditis, sickle cell disease, and metastatic choriocarcinoma. In approximately one-third of patients who have intracerebral hemorrhage, no specific cause is uncovered.

Subarachnoid hemorrhage is a common cause of nonobstetric maternal death. Hemorrhage from aneurysms and vascular malformations account for approximately one-fourth to just over one-third of intracranial hemorrhages. Management strategies are generally the same as those applied outside of pregnancy. Occasionally, definitive therapy for AVMs may be postponed until after delivery, whereas surgery or obliterative therapy for an aneurysm usually is urgent. The effects of some treatment agents, such as nimodipine, on the human fetus have not been studied well. However, the potentially fatal consequences of the vasospasm associated with subarachnoid hemorrhage make their use reasonable during pregnancy.

Anticonvulsants, specifically phenytoin, are unnecessary and ineffective in nongravid patients who have had an intracranial hemorrhage but not had a seizure. Data during pregnancy are unavailable. Anticonvulsants probably are best reserved for women who are in danger of herniating should intracranial pressure rise with a seizure or after the first convulsion.

Although many physicians recommend cesarean section for patients with gestational intracranial hemorrhage, mode of delivery does not affect outcome in the studies available (Sharma et al. 1995). Vaginal delivery can be performed with epidural anesthesia.

Ischemic Stroke

Most women who have a stroke before gestation complete uneventful pregnancies with excellent outcomes. Stroke during one pregnancy is not a risk factor for stroke in subsequent pregnancies, with the exception of women diagnosed with systemic lupus erythematosus or antiphospholipid antibody syndrome. Added risk is seen in women with conditions predisposing to stroke, such as embologenic cardiac disease and coagulopathies.

One woman has a stroke in every 10,000–20,000 deliveries. During pregnancy, risk of cerebral infarction does not exceed the risk in age-matched fertile controls. However, during the 6 weeks postpartum, the risk is approximately nine times that of the risk of nonpregnant women. Cesarean delivery and pregnancy-related hypertension are identified risk factors for stroke.

Eclampsia and preeclampsia are associated with approximately one-fourth of infarcts in the United States and approximately one-half of infarcts in France. In almost one-fourth to one-third of cases, the cause remains unclear. In the remainder, the stroke is symptomatic of a systemic illness, including premature atherosclerosis, hypertension, cardiac disease, hyperlipidemia, diabetes, arterial dissection, Takayasu's disease, vasculitis, antiphospholipid antibody syndrome, systemic lupus erythematosus, sickle cell disease, thrombotic thrombocytopenic purpura, CVT, coagulopathies, tobacco, cocaine, and other drug use. Stroke during labor or shortly after vaginal delivery may result from an amniotic fluid embolus.

When anticoagulation is indicated to lower the risk of gestational stroke, heparin is commonly the agent of choice. Heparin does not cross the placenta and is not associated with teratogenic effects. Warfarin is teratogenic, with highest risk during the period of 7–12 weeks gestation, with congenital malformations estimated at 28.5% and sometimes higher. Fetal wastage occurs in 18%. Some authors recommend that patients who require warfarin be counseled against pregnancy.

Prosthetic heart valves embolize at different rates, depending on whether they are aortic, mitral, bioprosthetic, or mechanical. Mechanical valves embolize and thrombose at the highest rate. Bioprosthetic valves are associated with better pregnancy outcomes, but some researchers postulate that gestation accelerates the natural rate of calcification and degeneration of these prostheses, ultimately leading to valve failure. We lack convincing studies that demonstrate an effect of pregnancy on these valves. Attempts to resolve the most pressing issue of anticoagulation in women with mechanical heart valves have been unsatisfactory.

The incidence of cerebral embolism associated with chronic atrial fibrillation during pregnancy is 2–10%. Anticoagulation for this condition is recommended throughout gestation usually, with high-dose subcutaneous heparin.

Women with circulating antiphospholipid antibodies and without a history of pregnancy loss do not require treatment to prevent stroke during pregnancy. Successful pregnancies without treatment are common. Women with very high antibody titers, habitual first-trimester abortion, a single miscarriage in the later trimesters, or antiphospholipid antibody syndrome, particularly with previous stroke, usually receive treatment. Various studies have examined the use of monotherapy or polytherapy in widely ranging doses and combinations of aspirin, prednisone, subcutaneous heparin, intravenous immunoglobulin and, occasionally, placebo. For women taking warfarin before pregnancy, subcutaneous high-dose heparin is substituted. Ideally, substitution is made just before conception and throughout gestation. Women with previous stroke and antiphospholipid antibody syndrome continue at high risk for additional thrombotic events during pregnancy. Stroke in these women may occur even at doses of heparin sufficient to produce therapeutic partial thromboplastin time. Some authors advise these women not to become pregnant (Petri 1997).

Like regular heparin, low-molecular-weight heparin does not cross the placenta and offers additional benefits, including reduced frequency of heparin-induced thrombocytopenia, osteoporosis, and bleeding complications. No blood test is required to monitor its safety. Data are unavailable on its use in patients with prosthetic valves. Relative safety has been demonstrated in small studies that include women with antiphospholipid antibody syndrome and active lupus disease, but clear indications for the use of this medication are still under investigation.

Aspirin at low dose (60–80 mg/day) has been used safely throughout pregnancy, but no longitudinal studies have confirmed the efficacy of aspirin in the prevention of stroke during pregnancy.

MRI can be used selectively to image the brain and venous and arterial circulation and is very useful during pregnancy. No study or clinical observations has detailed harmful effects of MRI on the mother or child, but detailed longitudinal studies on children with fetal exposure to MRI are lacking.

Two-dimensional echocardiography may be the test of greatest importance when evaluating a woman with gestational stroke. Computed tomography and selective angiography carry a small risk to the fetus and must be performed with adequate shielding. Angiography may help to diagnose the rare patient with postpartum benign angiopathy.

Cerebral Venous Thrombosis

Aseptic thrombosis of the cerebral venous system (CVT), in its most obvious clinical state, presents with puerperal headache worsening over several days, a change in behavior or personality, convulsive seizure, and weakness or numbness. The patient may be emotionally regressed, anxious, or lethargic, with mild to obvious neurological deficits, and, occasionally, papilledema. Initial symptoms generally begin 1 day to 4 weeks postpartum and peak in frequency 7–14 days postpartum.

CVT has been associated with hypercoagulable states, infection, sickle cell disease, dehydration, and ulcerative colitis in addition to gestation. Differential diagnoses include eclampsia, meningitis, and cerebral mass.

MRI is the initial imaging procedure of choice. Although it detects occlusion of major sinuses with high sensitivity, when smaller veins are involved, detection may be more difficult. Selective or digital subtraction angiography may be considered in some cases.

Geographic location influences the frequency of CVT. India reports a high frequency of puerperal CVT, estimated at 40–50 cases per 10,000 births. This high rate is attributed primarily to dehydration and has a predilection for women delivering at home. Incidence in the United States is comparatively low, approximately 9 per 100,000 deliveries.

CVT associated with pregnancy is relatively benign. Researchers in Mexico describe a mortality of approximately 10% for gestational CVT and 33% for CVT not associated with pregnancy. In the United States, estimates of the mortality of CVT from all causes suggest that approximately one in 10 patients die. However, death did not occur in a national survey of 4,454 cases of CVT in the United States. Cesarean section is a risk factor for CVT (Lanska and Kryscio 1997).

Researchers find diminished activity of protein S and antiphospholipid antibodies in women with gestational and puerperal CVT. Occasionally, multiple defects in coagulation are encountered in the same woman. Current theory suggests that proteins, such as C4b-binding protein, increase during pregnancy and the puerperium, creating a hypercoagulable state. Some women have conditions that predispose them to hypercoagulation during pregnancy, such as activated protein C resistance (factor V Leiden mutation), protein S deficiency, or antithrombin III antibodies. Homocystinuria (hyperhomocyst[e]inemia) may place patients at additional risk.

Heparin anticoagulation may be of benefit, particularly if the patient has concurrent thrombophlebitis in the pelvis and legs. Some observers recommend heparin therapy only when clinical indicators suggest that a poor prognosis is likely, particularly given the relatively benign CVT associated with pregnancy. Therapy with antifibrinolytic agents, such as urokinase, is controversial. Heparin and antifibrinolytic therapies are contraindicated when the patient has hemorrhaged intracranially. Long-term anticonvulsant therapy usually is unnecessary.

Eclamptic Encephalopathy

Preeclampsia (toxemia gravidarum) and eclampsia remain the principal causes of maternal perinatal morbidity and death. Edema, proteinuria, and hypertension after 20 weeks' gestation characterize the syndrome of preeclampsia. Epileptic seizures and this preeclamptic triad comprise the syndrome of eclampsia. Defining the terms *preeclampsia* and *eclampsia* in this way simplifies a complex disorder. Important and common manifestations, such as hepatic hemorrhage, disseminated intravascular coagulation, abruptio placentae, pulmonary edema, papilledema, oliguria, headache, hyperreflexia, hallucinations, and blindness seem relatively neglected in this definition. Occasionally, eclamptic seizures may precede the clinical triad of preeclampsia.

Preeclampsia develops in approximately 4–8% of the pregnancies in prospective studies. Eclampsia accounts for nearly one-half the intracranial hemorrhages and nearly one-half of cerebral infarcts in pregnancy and puerperium in French hospitals. In the United States, the figures are lower, 14% and 24%, respectively. Methodological problems plague these studies, and accurate estimates are difficult to obtain.

We lack a specific laboratory test for this disorder, and understanding of the pathogenesis remains incomplete. Geneticists have associated preeclampsia with a molecular variant of the angiotensinogen gene and suggest a possible genetic predisposition. Some authors postulate that damage to the fetal-placental vascular unit (such as defective placentation) may release products toxic to endothelium causing diffuse vasospasm and organ injury. None of these theories satisfactorily explain the tendency for preeclampsia or eclampsia to affect primarily young, primigravid women. Conditions considered to place women at added risk for preeclampsia include multifetal gestations, previous preeclampsia, insulin-treated diabetes mellitus, and chronic hypertension.

At autopsy, there is cerebral edema, hypertensive encephalopathy, subarachnoid, subcortical, and petechial hemorrhages, and infarction of multiple areas of the brain and brainstem. The occipital lobes, parietal lobes, and watershed areas injure most easily. Although any of these lesions may cause seizures, the patient may not convulse. This observation has led to criticism that the definition of eclampsia solely on the basis of a seizure is too restrictive.

Two theories compete to explain the genesis of cerebral disease. Elevated blood pressure may overcome protection that is usually provided by the precapillary arteriolar sphincter. Loss of autoregulation then leads to rupture of fragile capillaries, resulting in ring hemorrhages and thrombosis. Alternatively, diffuse cerebral endothelial dysfunction

may precipitate generalized cerebral vasospasm, producing the same pathology.

One review observed that many women diagnosed with preeclampsia or eclampsia had, in retrospect, clinical presentations most consistent with other diseases (Witlin et al. 1997). Most commonly, these included cerebral arterial infarction, hypertensive encephalopathy, and CVT. Eagerness to diagnose toxemia, possibly due to the frequency with which the condition naturally presents, may overestimate its incidence in epidemiological studies. The neurologist must consider alternative diagnoses carefully.

Severe preeclampsia is defined by the magnitude of blood pressure elevation and amount of proteinuria. Approximately 4–14% of preeclamptic pregnancies develop a syndrome called HELLP—an acronym for *h*emolysis, *e*levated *l*iver enzymes, and *l*ow *p*latelets. HELLP syndrome has been considered a form of severe preeclampsia with a high frequency of maternal and fetal injury. Patients complain of malaise, nausea, right upper quadrant pain, and vomiting. Occasionally, HELLP syndrome presents without the triad of preeclampsia and is considered a separable clinical entity.

Usual therapy for preeclampsia involves expectant management and antihypertensive medications. A systolic pressure greater than 169 mm Hg or a diastolic pressure greater than 109 mm Hg is considered severe. A review of the world literature on therapy found support for the treatment of severe hypertension with hydralazine, labetalol, or nifedipine. For milder hypertension (systolic pressure >140 mm Hg, or diastolic pressure of 90 mm Hg), methyldopa is considered first-line therapy, and labetalol, pindolol, oxprenolol, and nifedipine are second-line treatment.

Severe preeclampsia, eclampsia, or HELLP syndrome requires definitive therapy. All gestational products must be removed from the uterus by vaginal or cesarean delivery. Commonly, women are delivered within 24–48 hours of presentation.

Parenteral magnesium sulfate is used extensively to treat symptoms of severe preeclampsia while awaiting delivery. In a large clinical trial, women presenting for delivery with pregnancy-induced hypertension were given either phenytoin or magnesium sulfate. Among the women receiving magnesium, fewer developed seizures (Lucas et al. 1995). In a separate analysis of women with eclampsia, magnesium sulfate reduced recurrent convulsions better than regimens using either diazepam or phenytoin (Eclampsia Trial Collaborative Group 1995). The mechanism of action remains unclear. The most coherent theory suggests that magnesium sulfate affects the pathogenesis of cerebral disease, resulting in seizures, rather than functioning as an anticonvulsant itself. Usually, the drug is continued for a day after delivery. Antiepileptic agents commonly used to prevent and control eclamptic seizures include barbiturates, phenytoin, and benzodiazepines.

For some women, thrombocytopenic purpura and hemolytic uremic syndrome may overlap with or complicate toxemia and HELLP syndrome. Death and severe neurological disease is common. There may be improved survival with the use of plasma transfusion and plasmapheresis. Low-dose aspirin to prevent eclampsia was effective in small trials, but larger studies of women at high risk for preeclampsia showed no benefit of aspirin 60 mg taken daily (Caritis et al. 1998). Some researchers claim that the combination of aspirin with ketanserin, a selective serotonin-2 receptor blocker, may prevent preeclampsia in women with hypertension diagnosed before 20 weeks' gestation (Steyn and Odendaal 1997).

REFERENCES

Adour KK, Ruboyianes JM, Von Doersten PG, et al. Bell's palsy treatment with acyclovir and prednisone compared with prednisone alone: a double-blind, randomized, controlled trial. Ann Otol Rhinol Laryngol 1996;105:371–378.

Batocchi AP, Majolini L, Evoli A, et al. Course and treatment of myasthenia gravis during pregnancy. Neurology 1999;53:447–452.

Caritis S, Sibai B, Haurth J, et al. Low-dose aspirin to prevent preeclampsia in women at high risk. N Engl J Med 1998;338:701–705.

Cervera R, Asherson RA, Tikly M, et al. Chorea in the antiphospholipid syndrome. Clinical, radiologic, and immunologic characteristics of 50 patients from our clinics and the recent literature. Medicine 1997;76:203–212.

Damek DM, Shuster EA. Pregnancy and multiple sclerosis. Mayo Clin Proc 1997;72:977–989.

Eclampsia Trial Collaborative Group. Which anticonvulsant for women with eclampsia? Evidence from the Collaborative Eclampsia Trial. Lancet 1995;345:1455–1463.

Lanska DJ, Kryscio RJ. Peripartum stroke and intracranial venous thrombosis in the National Hospital Discharge Survey. Obstet Gynecol 1997;89:413–418.

Lucas MJ, Leveno KJ, Cunningham FG. A comparison of magnesium sulfate with phenytoin for the prevention of eclampsia. N Engl J Med 1995;333:201–205.

Martinelli I, Sacchi E, Landi G, et al. High risk of cerebral-vein thrombosis in carriers of a prothrombin-gene mutation and in users of oral contraceptives. N Engl J Med 1998;338:1793–1797.

Petitti DB, Sidney S, Quesenberry CP, Bernstein A. Ischemic stroke and use of estrogen and estrogen/progestogen as hormone replacement therapy. Stroke 1998;29:23–28.

Petri M. Pathogenesis and treatment of the antiphospholipid antibody syndrome. Med Clin North Am 1997;81:152–177.

Rudnik-Schoneborn S, Rohrig D, Nicholson G, Zerres K. Pregnancy and delivery in Charcot-Marie-Tooth disease type 1. Neurology 1993;43:2011–2016.

Runmarker B, Andersen O. Pregnancy is associated with a lower risk of onset and a better prognosis in multiple sclerosis. Brain 1995;118:253–261.

Sharma SK, Herrera ER, Sidawi JE, Leveno KJ. The pregnant patient with an intracranial arteriovenous malformation. Cesarean or vaginal delivery using regional or general anesthesia? Reg Anesth 1995;20:455–458.

Sharshar T, Lamy C, Mas JL for the Stroke in Pregnancy Study Group. Incidence and causes of strokes associated with pregnancy and puerperium. A study in public hospitals of Ile de France. Stroke 1995;26:930–936.

Sneed PK, Albright NW, Wara WM, et al. Fetal dose estimates for radiotherapy of brain tumors during pregnancy. Int J Radiat Oncol Biol Phys 1995;32:823–830.

Stenager E, Stenager EN, Jensen K. Effect of pregnancy on the prognosis for multiple sclerosis. A 5-year follow-up investigation. Acta Neurol Scand 1994;90:305–308.

Steyn DW, Odendaal HJ. Randomised controlled trial of ketanserin and aspirin in prevention of pre-eclampsia. Lancet 1997;350:1267–1271.

Witlin AG, Friedman SA, Egerman RS, et al. Cerebrovascular disorders complicating pregnancy—beyond eclampsia. Am J Obstet Gynecol 1997;176:1139–1148.

Chapter 86
Geriatric Neurology

Robert W. Hamill and David M. Pilgrim

The ideal end of life would require measurement by a photo finish, with all organ systems reaching the finish line simultaneously (i.e., the ultimate dead heat). Alternatively, we might accept that, like a great horse race, the brain—rhinencephalon in the lead—could win by a nose. Unfortunately, the aging brain is often the organ system that is too far in the lead. It begins to fail and does so over an extended period while the systemic organs, which have benefited from excellent preventative medicine and healthier lives, function well into the ninth decade and beyond. In fact, *successful aging* might be defined by the preservation until the end of our days of these most human functions and characteristics that are the brain's unique province. As the survival curves "rectangularize," (Mean life expectancy approaches maximum life span) we must enhance our understanding of the neurobiology of the aging brain to stave off age-related neurological disorders so that, at worst, there is a true compression of cumulative disability, including age-related neurological disease and dysfunction (Vita et al. 1998). Neurologists, as clinical neuroscientists, have the unique skills and knowledge base to lead investigations of the aging brain and to advance the care of disorders to which the brain exhibits unique vulnerability as it ages: the disorders of geriatric neurology.

The magnitude of the contribution of age-related neurological disease and dysfunction (ARNDD) to cumulative disability in the last quartile of life is substantial: 90% of individuals in long-term care facilities (nursing homes) and 50% of impaired elderly in the community have disabilities related to the nervous system. Demographics alone should signal neurologists that we have a critical role to play in understanding and remedying what will be the major medical and sociological tsunami of the next century: ARNDD.

The fundamental biological processes underlying the aging process remain unknown, but a number of theories exist: genetic, free radical, and protein oxidation theories have been reviewed by Masoro (1995). Regardless of the exact mechanisms determining life span and the resulting age-related changes in the biology of organisms, the price of long life for humans appears to be an increase in neurological disease. In addition, age-related alterations in the functional capabilities of the nervous system occur, simultaneously compromising normal physiology and underlying much of the dysfunction occurring in seniors. Because of their education and training in the basic and clinical neurosciences, neurologists are in a unique and critical position to evaluate and address the clinical dysfunctions that result in increased disabilities and dependence for older Americans. In fact, in one study, neurological consultation to a geriatrics unit provided 1.4 ± 1.1 new or revised neurological diagnoses in the 58 patients studied (Camicioli et al. 1998).

This chapter provides an overview of geriatric neurology. We present various aspects of the basic and clinical neurosciences related to the aging brain and review the clinical evaluation and treatment of the salient, and significant, clinical dysfunctions observed in geriatric age groups. Many of these disorders are covered in substantial detail in other chapters (e.g., those on dementia, depression, movement disorders, and autonomic dysfunction); this chapter addresses these clinical problems within the framework of geriatrics and gerontology. A number of monographs providing a more detailed review of geriatric neurology are available (Albert and Knoefel 1994; Barclay In press; Sage and Mark 1996).

DEMOGRAPHY, EPIDEMIOLOGY, AND ECONOMICS

Maximum life span (MLS), defined as the maximum observed life span of a species, is estimated to have increased only twofold over the last 3 million years of hominid evolution. The difference for today's society is that mean life expectancy (MLE) is estimated to have increased approximately 50%, or 25 years, during the twentieth century; thus, a large proportion of the population is now approaching the MLS. The oldest well-documented human, Jeanne Calment of France, died in 1998 at 122; this age represents an increase of approximately 10% in MLS in the twentieth century. The age of human MLS is compatible with the observation that the oldest age observed for most species is approximately 6 times the age of maturity, assuming that humans reach maturity at approximately 20 years of age (Rowe and Kahn 1998). Older individuals were initially termed the *young-old* (65–74) and the *old-old* (75+). The latter group was vulnerable to substantial frailty and disability. The old-old group was further subdivided to allow for the *oldest old*: those 85 and older. The old-old and oldest-old groups are rapidly growing. By the middle of the next century, the MLE will be approximately 83 years, and there will be approximately 25 million oldest-old and approximately one-half million seniors over the century mark.

Although data are accruing on brain biology in these age groups, we actually know very little about preventative strategies or supportive measures to protect against the onslaught of dysfunction and disability that currently occurs. Fewer than 100 brain autopsies have been performed in oldest-old individuals who were assessed cognitively before death (Kaye 1997). Thus, as MLE increases and more citizens have the potential to reach the century mark and become candidates to reach MLS, disease expression will likely increase as well. In fact, it is within this most senior population that the expression of disease mounts. The most common devastating clinical disorder in this population is Alzheimer's disease (AD), estimated to affect approximately 20% of subjects 75–85 years old and almost 50% of individuals older than 85. On the positive side, the obverse data are important to stress: 80% of individuals 75–85 years of age are functioning well cognitively, and at 90, 50% of seniors do not demonstrate functionally significant mental impairment. What is still unclear is whether, if we all live to our MLS, we will have the "invariable pathology of AD." We do know that not everyone with this pathological substrate exhibits dementia. Thus, compensatory mechanisms must exist to permit normal function despite altered brain substrate.

Essentially all studies of age-related disorders reveal substantial heterogeneity within both the control and diseased or dysfunctional groups. This heterogeneity suggests that within the normal aging control group, there are individuals who show very little decline in function with age, whereas others exhibit "age-related" decline. It may be that this heterogeneity reflects transition of function within individuals from normal to mildly abnormal to abnormal, a transition that reflects aging from successful to usual to diseased aging (to paraphrase Rowe and Kahn 1998). Thus, the "usual" may include disease but not altered physiology. As indicated below, it is critical to separate disease from aging, as well as usual from successful aging. Clinicians must resist the notion that dysfunction in seniors is secondary to age: Disease must be considered and excluded.

Remembering that major figures in government, the performing arts, and medicine have contributed substantially to society in their later years codifies the fact that aging is not necessarily associated with dysfunction. Benjamin Franklin was elected to a 3-year term as president of Pennsylvania in his eightieth year (before the establishment of the office of governor of Pennsylvania in 1790, the state executive was president of the Supreme Executive Council). This occurred after he had represented the United States in France from ages 76–79 and contributed to the Constitutional Convention at 81. Thomas Jefferson founded the University of Virginia at 76 and directed the plans for the school until his death at 83. Winston Churchill was Prime Minister of England for the second time at 77–81 and lived an active life until his death at 91. Goethe completed *Faust* at 82. George Burns was active in Hollywood until his death at age 100, and Bob Hope slowed down only in his mid-90s. In the medical field, Albert Schweitzer developed and directed his hospital in Africa well into his 80s, and Linus Pauling, winner of two Nobel prizes, died in 1994 at the age of 93. During the last 5 years of his life, Pauling wrote approximately five papers per year. Neurologists in their geriatric years have contributed substantially to our field. J. Purdon Martin, after his retirement at age 65, contributed original work on postencephalitic patients, and in his late 80s began work on a biography of Hughlings Jackson. He was still working on this effort when he died at age 92; MacDonald Critchley finished the Jackson biography in his ninety-seventh year, his last year of life. Thus, successful aging is not only possible but may be likely with improved preventative care, increased knowledge of the aging process, and therapies directed at age-related dysfunction.

The world's population is aging, and Western societies are leading the chronological curve. The proportion of the population older than 65 is expected to double before 2040, and the fastest-growing segment of older citizens is 85 and older; this group will increase by almost 50% by 2010. In 1990, there were 3.3 million people 85 and older in the United States, and an increase of more than sevenfold is expected by the year 2050. When the Baby Boomers reach 65, more than 20% of the population in the United States will be older than 65 years of age. Neurodegenerative dementias (AD, lobar atrophies); vascular dementias (multi-infarct dementia, Binswanger's disease); behavioral alterations, such as depression, Parkinson's disease, and other disorders of gait and balance, with their resultant falls; autonomic disorders; and stroke are all increased in senior citizens. Neurologists must be well versed in the geriatric principles of clinical care, and the role of neurology may expand to a more involved principal care provider model, probably as part of a multidisciplinary care team.

The cost of caring for senior citizens is staggering. In 1985, 12% of the American population (>65 years) accounted for 30% of the health care bills. By the year 2030, the 20% of the population that will be over age 65 will consume approximately 50% of the available health care dollars. A single illness—AD—cost more than $100 billion in 1999 alone. The amount of money directed at AD research represents less than 1% of the cost of caring for these individuals. Yet, investment in research is the most powerful way of saving some of the enormous health care costs consumed in life's last decade. For instance, if advances could stave off the major neurological disorders associated with age-related disease and dysfunction by only 5 years, the compression of disability and the reduction in health care costs would be substantial.

MULTIDISCIPLINARY ASSESSMENT

Multiple diseases are the rule in old patients. In addition, social problems are common. The patient's hearing aid may need adjustment, patients may need transportation to get to the doctor's office, and arrangements may be required to provide meals. These issues call for an approach very different from the usual neurological consultation. The clinician, patient, and family often feel overwhelmed.

Geriatricians approach this problem by forming multidisciplinary assessment teams. The team usually includes a nurse, social worker, and physician but also may include physician's assistants and nurse practitioners. Physical therapists, occupational therapists, psychiatrists, neurologists, physiatrists, optometrists, and audiologists commonly join the team for treating specific problems, bringing together the personnel and skills necessary to address the majority of clinical problems. It saves the patient multiple visits to different clinicians and sites. Also, teams may be formed to address specific diseases, such as stroke or dementia, or specific clinical problems, such as gait disorders, falls, or elder abuse. Although teams result in no additional cost to patients and lower costs by reducing hospitalizations and shortening lengths of stay (Inouye et al. 1993), the resources to maintain and manage these interdisciplinary efforts are increasingly difficult to muster in the current climate of care management.

ETHICS

One of the first principles of medical ethics is patient autonomy. This issue has special meaning in neurology because many neurological diseases cause difficulty with cognition, communication, integration of information, and executive function. Despite these difficulties, every effort must be made to discern the patient's wishes and to act accordingly. For instance, even patients with AD may be competent to make decisions about their care. That is, early in the disease course, the patient may experience substantial memory difficulties but still retain an understanding of issues and make proper judgments. These capabilities may be defined, and the patient's wishes may be presented and honored. Certain neuropsychological measures may be strongly associated with impaired competency, and clinical vignettes may serve as an adjunct tool for physicians making competency decisions. However, competency decisions are not easily arrived at. For instance, physicians involved in competency testing may reach consensus in controls (98%), but only 56% judgment agreement was achieved for patients with mild AD (Marson et al. 1997).

Advance Directives

Competency decisions involve assessing the patient's ability to comprehend issues, apply proper judgments, understand the implications of choices, and communicate decisions to the health care team. Questions may need to be direct and simple. The mental status assessment is critical to define the ability of patients to participate in decision making. For example, a patient with a large myocardial infarction and resultant embolic stroke with an aphasia and poor comprehension may need to make many decisions. Should cardiac catheterization be performed? Should the patient be resuscitated in the event of a cardiac arrest? Many patients with poor communication skills may be able to answer yes-or-no questions accurately. If this is the case, ask only very clear questions that require yes-or-no answers. Does the patient understand what the resuscitation effort means? Demonstrate with the paddles if necessary. Ask what the patient expects will happen if resuscitation is withheld. For example: Will you get better? Will you die? This approach requires time and the clear appreciation that the patient must comprehend each question asked. A family member or other health care provider should witness the interview to ensure agreement. This same approach may be used for any patient with neurological disorders that alter brain function (i.e., patients with dementia). Depression presents a special problem because the patient may refuse care because of the depression rather than because it is his or her preference.

If the patient is not competent, document the evidence of incompetency and obtain input from the family and other caregivers. Competency is also a legal concept, and statutes exist to protect patients; legal input should be obtained to ensure compliance. Advance directives, which provide written evidence of the patient's wishes, are very helpful in this circumstance. The more detailed the information, the better. Some physicians routinely record detailed discussions about these issues. Documentation of the patient's thoughts and wishes are then available if necessary. Even if written details are not available, many patients have clearly stated their wishes for care if they were to become incapacitated and unable to participate in decision making. Agreement among family members on the patient's wishes is critical. The physician must remain vigilant for potential ulterior motives and establish that uniform acceptance of the care decisions exists.

The clinical care issues that arise with progressive neurological disorders are substantial. Are complex but not immediately life-threatening illnesses treated? For instance, should we treat arrhythmias in end-stage AD or Huntington's disease? Are simple infections (urinary tract, pneumonia) treated or not? Do we continue to feed and hydrate people if they are no longer able to maintain nutritional support independently? If a patient has stated a preference that no heroic measures should be taken, what does that mean? Such a term does not cover food and water because such care is considered basic rather than heroic. Questions about feeding a patient with advanced disease may create great emotional difficulty for health professionals and caregivers. Evidence of hunger is the best indicator. If the patient does not appear hungry or pushes food away, pain or discomfort related to not eating seems unlikely. In this setting, forced feeding may produce emotional discomfort and stress for the patient. Thus, should there be an obligation to feed? Probably not. Patients with depression create a difficult problem, and such clinical dysfunction militates against using only the patient's indication of hunger to determine a course of action. Goldblatt (1997) addresses the decision-making processes on these ethical issues.

Alzheimer's Disease: Should the Patient Be Told the Diagnosis?

AD is a terrifying disease. The single concern of many patients who present to memory disorder centers is whether or not they have AD. Various strategies and rationales are presented to address the question of informing patients about this diagnosis. A reasonable strategy is that all patients should be informed, unless there is some likelihood that such information would lead to immediate adverse consequences (e.g., suicide). Patients must be informed so that they can make proper decisions about their care, finances, and relationships while they are still able. To restrict information also places enormous burdens on care providers, who then must continue to skirt these issues. It is often the family members who cannot deal with the diagnosis initially, and they may require special attention, including discussion sessions. The local Alzheimer's Association is an excellent resource for the patient and family, and families should contact the organization early in the disease.

Elder Abuse

AD, Parkinson's disease, and stroke are the only medical diagnoses shown to increase the risk of elder abuse and neglect. Neurologists may see more abused elders than other specialists and must remain vigilant for this possibility. Although physical injury may occur, it is rare. More commonly, the patient is neglected and presents with nonspecific signs, such as poor hygiene or nutrition or incorrect medicine use. Also, patients may be left alone for long periods and are at risk for injury. Occasionally, patients exist almost in isolation. These events may indicate caregiver burnout, and neurologists must know how to intercede in these events. Many communities have developed resources (e.g., public health or visiting nurses, home care teams) to investigate for these possibilities and to assist the caregiver and patient. Elder abuse will expand during the next century with the acceleration of ARNDD; heightened awareness of this issue by all care providers is critical (Lachs and Pillemer 1995).

Rationing

Rationing of care affects the elderly more than any other group. The age of the patient may be considered when applying any costly technology. Despite the clear evidence that aging is heterogeneous and that many seniors function well into their 80s, ageism exists. It must be challenged head-on, and decisions should be made individually, based on the expectation of remaining years with good function. This concept is sometimes referred to as *active life expectancy*. Health care rationing raises issues that span the domains of human and societal thought: Philosophical, religious, legal, societal commercial, societal responsibility, and professional views all abound. The idealists and the pragmatists frame the question of competing values of the individual and society. These issues are well reviewed (Buchanan 1997; Haber 1997; Rivlin 1997).

NEUROBIOLOGY OF AGING—RELATIONSHIP TO GERIATRIC NEUROLOGY

Anatomical and Neurochemical Changes with Age

During aging, neuronal cell loss occurs in specific regions in the central nervous system, but this change is not a generalized phenomenon. Within the brainstem, there is neuron loss in the locus ceruleus, substantia nigra, inferior olive, and probably the raphe. The cerebellum loses Purkinje's cells, and the large pyramidal neurons in the neocortex decrease. Earlier data on the hippocampus estimated neuronal losses at 25–40%, but later studies suggest that cell loss is restricted to the subiculum (40–50%) and hilus of the dentate gyrus (35–40%). This pattern of cell loss is clearly different from that observed in AD. Additionally, earlier data suggested that dendritic arbors are reduced with age, and fewer synapses are noted. However, other studies demonstrate that dendrites grow with age and may compensate for age-related neuronal loss. Thus, neuroplasticity exists in the aging brain. Connectivity between and among neurons is critical to maintain; thus, synapse counts in the aging brain may reflect the best index of functional capability. Although data are difficult to interpret because of technical issues, there is probably an approximately 20% reduction in synapse counts observed during aging, and these changes have regional specificity.

An increasingly interesting aspect of aging changes observed in the brain relate to white matter changes, particularly the increased signals seen in the periventricular area on T2-weighted magnetic resonance images (MRI). Although these changes occur with increasing frequency after the age of 65, they may not be apparent during gross examination of the brain at autopsy. Histologically, these white matter changes, termed *leukoaraiosis*, include loss of axons, myelin pallor, gliosis, loss of ependymal cells, and enlarged perivascular spaces. Small vessels in the white matter may exhibit thickened walls, and these changes, usually associated with the small vessel disease of hypertension and diabetes, may result in altered perfusion of the white matter and the resultant pathological changes. The relationship of these observed changes to the entity Binswanger's disease remains to be clarified. With the neuronal loss and white matter changes, brain weight and volume decrease, losing approximately 8–10% of their peak adult values over time. Generally, with age, these indices decrease, most noticeably after age 55.

Age-related changes in neurotransmitter systems remain to be fully clarified. For instance, reports vary depending on ages studied and brain regions sampled. Receptor systems are reported to be decreased or unchanged, depending on the site studied. Cholinergic, noradrenergic, serotoninergic, and dopaminergic neurotransmitters all appear to show some age-related decrements, but the inclusion of patients with subclinical diseases, specifically early AD or Parkinson's disease, may underlie some of the changes noted. Although there are studies that suggest declines in these systems with age, there is substantial heterogeneity, and the sample sizes for each decade studied remain small.

In the peripheral nervous system, changes are noted in the efferent target organ muscle, the motor and sensory components of the peripheral nerve, and the anterior horn cells (AHCs). For instance, there is muscle wasting, and isometric muscle strength declines gradually after the fifth decade. Morphological studies indicate that fiber atrophy and muscle fiber loss occur. Muscle endurance increases or remains stable. AHCs are reduced in aging, and estimates suggest that 350 nerve fibers per decade are lost in the lumbosacral roots (secondary to AHC loss). Myelin changes occur, and conduction is decreased. Changes in the sensory pathways are evident because vibratory sense decreases in the legs and, rarely, in the upper extremities. Touch is mildly reduced, and corneal sensitivity decreases. The pain threshold increases mildly, particularly to deep pain, but data conflict; thermal perception remains to be fully examined. Dorsal root ganglion cells demonstrate structural change and may decrease in number; sensory nerve fibers demonstrate progressive loss of myelinated fibers. Autonomic function is impaired in aging: Pupil reactivity decreases, autonomic control of heart and peripheral vasculature may be impaired (orthostatic hypotension [OH]), and temperature control mechanisms appear to be reduced, with hypothermia becoming a threat. Structural changes in peripheral ganglia and loss of intermediolateral column cells occur, but altered central integration may also exist because central monoaminergic pathways change with aging. Albert and Knoefel (1994) and Schochet (1998) reviewed the "normal" and pathological changes that occur with aging, and Drachman (1997) highlighted the investigative opportunities of the aging brain.

Higher Integrative and Intellectual Functions

The integrative functions of the brain are the most human features, which, when altered to pathological degrees, devolve to clinical dysfunction that may result in the loss of a sentient being. Clinically, we tend to focus on specific domains of cognition, such as attention and orientation, language, memory, visuospatial skills, conceptualization, and general intelligence, and specific alterations in various aspects of these cognitive skills may change in older persons (Albert 1994; Albert 1995). Aging and age-related neurological disorders alter brain function to varying degrees, from presumed "benign senescent forgetfulness" and "age-associated memory impairment" to pathological states of dementia and depression. This section addresses issues of neuropsychological assessment and integrative or intellectual functions in normal aging and the clinical dysfunction that results when these normal integrative functions are altered. We also consider three major clinical processes: dementia, depression, and delirium.

Neuropsychology of Aging

Most studies of higher cognitive functions in aging are cross-sectional in design (comparing young adults with older adults) and thus tend to highlight age-related change. Longitudinal studies (same individuals studied at different times from youth to aged) are most desirable, but such studies require half a century to complete and are extremely expensive. Nevertheless, a number of extant longitudinal studies will bring important and interesting data in the future (Albert 1995). Also, until quite recently, aging studies generally included subjects in the age groups 20–30 and 60–70. Because society's seniors are living well into their 80s, additional major efforts are needed to clarify whether the oldest old differ from younger seniors. Although previous ideas would have us all waiting for senile changes in brain function to occur after we begin receiving our Social Security checks, robust intellectual function continues in octogenarians and beyond. For instance, approximately 80–90% of subjects older than 65 and 75% of seniors older than 75 are not demented. A general overview would suggest that *crystallized intelligence* (learned information, vocabulary, skills, and overall judgment: in sum, wisdom) remains well preserved in old age, but *fluid intelligence* (interpretative problem solving, manipulation of data, discriminative functions, or dynamic processing of data: in sum, mental flexibility) demonstrates age-related decline. Crystallized intelligence and years of formal education showed little predictive power, whereas age and fluid intelligence were significant predictors of performance on "everyday memory" tests.

More recently, neuropsychological characterization of the oldest old reveal that the effects of aging were greatest in perceptual and constructional tasks and that memory function was quite well preserved (Howieson et al. 1993). Specifically, verbal measures of old learning and reasoning show relative sparing of age effects, whereas the single best predictor of age was altered perceptual reasoning, as demonstrated by visual perceptual tasks. Age also affected visuospatial memory more than verbal memory. Two other cognitive domains that appear to experience age-related effects include speed of information processing and explicit memory (Rowe and Kahn 1998). Fortunately, aging does not adversely affect working memory, a function on which the routines of daily life depend heavily. Thus, aging changes are not simply declines in fluid intelligence but undoubtedly reflect the perturbation of the integrative capacity of the brain, the basic substrate of which is still being defined. The main point for the neurological clinician is that it is important not to hold age hostage to any observed higher intellectual decline in senior citizens: Disease is the most likely cause, not age.

Assessment of Higher Cortical Functions

Clinical assessment of higher intellectual and integrative functions may be performed using streamlined bedside tests or more detailed neuropsychological testing (see Chapter 39). Although neuropsychological testing is needed to clarify difficult clinical pictures, bedside tests identify up to 85–90% of patients with altered mental status. Twenty-five years ago, Eric Pfeiffer developed the short portable mental status questionnaire (SPMSQ). Initial studies demonstrated 92% agreement between this test and the clinical diagnosis when the SPMSQ indicated definite impairment and 82% agreement when either no impairment or only mild impairment was present. This test examines orientation, previous memory and information, and attention with a simple subtraction test. Tests of recent memory (primary memory),

language, writing, calculations, visuospatial and constructional tasks, and comprehension are not included.

In the same year, the Mini-Mental State examination (MMSE) emerged and is currently one of the most frequently used tests. This test has a perfect score of 30; subjects with scores less than 27 are considered mildly impaired. Although these tests are useful, they are not very sensitive in identifying patients with early-onset dementia. Also, the MMSE is substantially influenced by education. The most valuable information is obtained from family members or close associates, who serve as collateral sources for reporting and substantiating loss of intellectual capabilities. Most clinicians arrive at a diagnosis of early dementia after the history and examination even when both of these short mental status examinations are normal. Patients with dementia performed significantly worse on tests of short-term memory, temporal orientation, visual perception, and language. In fact, three of these tests (visual retention, controlled oral word association, and temporal orientation) classified 89% of cases with a high degree of probability. Of note, an abnormal score in temporal orientation is clearly rare, occurring in only 4% of normal control cases. These three components of the examination may be administered in approximately 15 minutes. With the development of AD centers, the application of additional assessment tools (Consortium to Establish a Registry for Alzheimer's Disease [CERAD] protocols) have led to diagnostic accuracy approaching 100% without formal neuropsychological testing. The clinical assessment in these studies included the following brief cognitive scales: collateral source–derived Blessed Dementia Scale, Aphasia Battery, and the SPMSQ. A recently developed 7-minute neurocognitive screening battery appears to offer a highly sensitive screen for individuals with AD; it requires no clinical judgment and can be administered by nonphysician personnel (Solomon et al. 1998). Such a test may be highly useful in the current climate of increased time pressures on physicians.

The number of tools identified for assessing subjects in the geriatric age group is substantial; not surprisingly, each tool may be of unique value for a specific clinical syndrome but may have only weak appeal as a general assessment approach. Because older patients with cognitive changes often present with behavioral features such as depression, scales designed for multidimensional assessment may be considered. The frequently used scales include Sandoz Clinical Assessment-Geriatric, Brief Psychiatric Rating Scale (BPRS), Neurobehavioral Rating Scale (NRS), Global Assessment of Psychiatric Symptoms, Geriatric Rating Scale, Multidimensional Observation Scale for Elderly Subjects, and Geriatric Mental State. These approaches have all been constructed to assess various aspects of higher integrative and intellectual functions and behavioral change. Our suggestions are to choose one of these scales for an overall assessment of cognitive change and to recognize the need to expand the assessment to more psychiatric issues, if indicated (in this regard, choose the BPRS). The time required to complete these tests varies from 7 to 45 minutes, depending on the number of tests used. These psychometric studies may need to be completed during a second patient visit. No single test completely meets the clinician's needs, and full neuropsychological testing may be indicated in the small (<10%) number of patients who present difficulties in establishing the diagnoses with complete medical, neurological, and behavioral (psychiatric) evaluations.

Do patients who complain of memory loss progress to AD? This rather fundamental question is more apparent today because seniors are aware of AD and are terrified of its outcome. A basic axiom of memory, aging, and AD had been that patients with dementia generally do not complain of memory or intellectual failure. This is no longer the case since patients have become more aware of AD; it is estimated that approximately 60% of patients with AD complain of altered memory. Demographic studies also indicate that in an older population, 30–50% of subjects complain of memory loss. A component of memory loss in seniors may be age-associated memory impairment (also termed *benign senescent forgetfulness*). This interesting and partly understood clinical syndrome of memory impairment describes individuals with mild nonprogressive memory loss and cognitive impairment. However, the exact pathophysiology of this syndrome, its actual existence, and its relationship to the neurodegenerative dementias remain to be clarified; some have suggested a continuum between normal aging and senile dementia of the Alzheimer's type.

Nevertheless, many seniors state that their memory is "just not very good anymore," and they all do not progress to AD. Several studies have been designed to address these questions; clearly, longitudinal data are needed to construct the answer. Interesting points are emerging. Memory complaints do not correlate with memory performance on tests, and patients with tendencies toward somatization, anxiety, and negative views of their competence and capabilities were more likely to complain of memory loss (Hanninen et al. 1994). Also, depression and anxiety, reflecting the affective state of the informants, are major factors contributing to the complaint of cognitive decline in the elderly (Hanninen et al. 1994; Jorm et al. 1994). A comforting note is offered by Flicker and colleagues (1993), who determined that, in a relatively brief follow-up of 3–4 years, there was no evidence for progressive cognitive decline in patients who presented subjective perceptions of loss of cognitive skills. A caveat is the recognition that new memory complaints in individuals without previous concerns may indeed suggest the development of significant loss of memory or cognition (Schofield et al. 1997). Because there are age-related changes in neuropsychological function, the task now is to explain what this actually means both clinically and neuropathologically and whether or not these observed changes are harbingers of decline in higher integrative and intellectual functions. The answers are beginning to come.

CLINICAL EXAMINATION IN GERIATRIC NEUROLOGY

Functional Assessment

Functional impairment is a common problem of old age. Ninety-five percent of people aged 65–74 years are fully independent, but by age 85 years, only 60–65% of people are fully independent. Multiple diagnoses are common in old people, but function does not correlate with specific diseases or the number of diagnoses in a patient. As previously noted, variation is a rule of aging. The older the age, the larger the variation in function for virtually any variable measured. Accordingly, to establish a clear approach to the geriatric patient and arrive at an accurate diagnosis, the assessment must include a complete history, thorough examination, and functional assessment.

Physicians commonly underestimate functional impairment in older patients. To improve detection of impaired function, a number of instruments have been designed. The instruments are divided into tests of physical function, cognitive function, mood, and social support (Fleming et al. 1995). Many of these instruments were designed for primary care clinicians. The complete neurological examination, including functional testing, accomplishes many of the same goals. Such components of the neurological examination as behavioral and mental status testing, vision and hearing assessment, and motor control and balance testing are key elements of many geriatric assessment instruments.

Additional historic information relevant to the older patient, but not included as part of the usual neurological examination, include urinary incontinence (UI); assessing height, weight, and diet to determine nutritional status; and asking if the patient feels sad or depressed. One should also ask if the patient can get out of bed, prepare meals, and shop independently and about the presence of home environment and social supports. Does the patient need to climb stairs? Is the lighting adequate? Are there loose rugs or other obstacles that might cause a fall? How does the patient get in and out of the tub? Who is available to care for or help the patient in the event of an emergency?

Assessment scales generally describe physical and performance functions and cognitive and behavioral status. The scales listed below are in common use.

Physical Function Scales

The Katz activities of daily living (ADL) scale is the most commonly used. It measures self-care ability and can be administered by the patient. Barthel's index adds information about gait but requires administration by an interviewer. The Instrumental Activities of Daily Living scale measures the patient's ability to perform activities such as shopping, cooking, and housekeeping. The Framingham Disability scale includes questions about climbing stairs and lifting.

Cognitive Function Tests

The MMSE is a widely used and validated screening test for dementia, but its sensitivity is limited because it may not detect mild disease. The CERAD instruments are more sensitive to mild cognitive impairment but require some time to administer; the 7-Minute Screen may be a useful instrument for an office visit.

Mood Scales

A number of studies indicate that physicians overlook depression in patients in both the inpatient and outpatient settings. Scales to screen for the presence of depression should alert the physician to the possibility that depression is present, but they are not sufficiently accurate to establish the diagnosis. Examples of these scales include the BPRS, NRS, and the Hamilton Depression Scale.

Neurological Evaluation

Obtaining an accurate history from an old patient can be frustrating. Although such a statement may bias our view of the elderly population, neurologists are generally not asked to examine the "well elderly," and our sample of aging individuals is clearly skewed toward impaired seniors. Many changes occurring with aging and non-neurological dysfunction (hearing and visual impairments, slowed movements secondary to musculoskeletal changes), as well as alterations occurring in ARNDD (altered attention, memory, and communication), reduce the efficiency in performing clinical histories and neurological examinations. Also, seniors often have one or more other diagnoses and may be taking numerous medications. Both situations complicate the approach, and neurologists and patients may become frustrated, but assessments performed hastily may result in misleading data. The axiom, "If one has 30 minutes to spend with a patient, the first 25 should be spent on the history," clearly holds for geriatric neurology. In fact, the history obtained from a collateral source may be most critical for focusing the question at hand. Occasionally, with nonacute situations, a second visit is useful to focus the history and examination rather than initiating a series of unnecessary and poorly directed tests. Once the focus is developed, attending to the problem, rather than being misled by the large number of other diagnoses and symptoms, speeds the evaluation. Targeting the approach permits the experienced neurologist to emphasize certain parts of the examination. For example, developing experience with ARNDD allows the physician to direct the examination to identify such disorders as dementia, depression, encephalopathies related to medications, Parkinson's disease, gait disorders and falls, stroke, and cervical spondylosis.

Defining the neurological findings related to old age is difficult. Because the neurological examination requires skill and experience, neurologists would be required to examine many community-living elderly—a very time-consuming effort—to develop a good standard for what is normal. Our extant normative data are derived from subjects who tend to volunteer for studies at major centers and may not represent the norm but rather the "supernormal." These subjects, however, help us to accumulate knowledge on the best outcome for age, which is important to dispel the stereotype that "all is downhill." In either situation, a number of inclusion and exclusion criteria must be established to define what findings will be considered normal. Should one just describe the population? Should only disease-free individuals be included? Should people with relevant disease be excluded? For example, a patient with a history of lumbosacral radiculopathy would be excluded from the group used to describe ankle jerks, or cervical arthritis might exclude individuals because long-tract signs or segmental changes related to musculoskeletal disease would not necessarily be an age-related change within the nervous system. However, because the presence of degenerative bone disease of the vertebral bodies is exceedingly high in older citizens, an argument for including neurological changes secondary to other age-related conditions could be made. In assessing the literature on aging and neurological findings, these and any other variables must be identified. Although reports of neurological findings in aging continue to accumulate, Critchley's 1932 paper is the landmark. Two studies address specifically the oldest old and the "successfully aging" (Kaye et al. 1994; Odenheimer et al. 1994). We include here the findings considered common in most old people, but we emphasize that the cohorts of very old subjects are highly selected; many are remarkably well preserved and appear 10–20 years younger than their stated age.

Mental Status

Dementia is such a common problem in this age group that a careful mental status examination must be performed on all patients. Older patients are typically less educated than younger patients, and mental status tests should be designed to avoid poor performance resulting from poor education rather than cognitive impairment. Initially, attention and concentration require assessment because further aspects of the examination and the interpretation thereof depend on whether the patient is able to participate fully. Asking the patient to spell *world* forward and backward is an easy and commonly used test. Digit span forward and in reverse, days of the week or months of the year in reverse are other common tests of attention. Normal digit span is 7 forward and 5 in reverse, but this is often reduced to 6 forward and 3 in reverse in the elderly. If disordered attention is present (common in hospitalized patients in this age group), one must consider an encephalopathy (acute confusional state or delirium) before a diagnosis of dementia is entertained. Other tests of cognitive function have localizing value only if attention and concentration are normal or at least sufficiently preserved to permit examinations for aphasia, agnosia, and apraxia. At the bedside, there is no evidence that age alters the mental status examination, which remains normal in the absence of disease. It is useful to apply standardized tests to so that data collected on an individual may be viewed in a larger context and longitudinal characterization may be standardized. Also, these data may assist in discussing prognosis and used as an educational tool for the family.

Cranial Nerves

Visual acuity is often reduced as a result of one or more of the following: presbyopia, cataract, glaucoma, and senile macular degeneration. Upward gaze is commonly limited, pupils are smaller, accommodation is reduced, and pursuit eye movements are saccadic. Olfaction and hearing also decrease with age.

Motor

Tone may be altered in aging, the most common manifestation being mild rigidity or paratonia. Paratonia basically reflects failed relaxation and appears to indicate bihemispheric dysfunction or failed integration of cortical and striatal motor systems. Occasionally, paratonia is enhanced and moderate rigidity may exist in the lower extremities of a minority of old people, particularly those older than 85. Increased rigidity implies disordered striatal motor function, and the combination of spasticity and rigidity suggests bilateral white matter disease, most commonly the result of multiple small, deep infarcts (the lacunar state). Motor strength is generally preserved except for a mild reduction, especially proximally, with advancing age. However, because reduced activity, motor impersistence, or apraxia may adversely affect the examination, the examiner must be cognizant of other processes altering muscle strength.

Sensory

Vibratory and light touch sensation decrease with age, but position sense is generally well preserved. Ankle jerks are often absent, most likely secondary to age-related disorders of the afferent loop.

Gait

The gait may slow, and mild extrapyramidal signs, such as reduced arm swing and turning en bloc, may appear. Approximately 50% of people over the age of 85 years have mild extrapyramidal signs, stooped posture, reduced arm swing, and turning en bloc (Bennett et al. 1996). These changes may result from age-related loss of striatal dopamine. Shuffling is unusual, and although the marche à petits pas has been described as a "senile gait," this undoubtedly describes gaits secondary to disease, not age.

Neuroimaging Studies

Brain Magnetic Resonance Imaging and Computed Tomography

Brain images may show atrophy that increases with advancing age. The ventricles enlarge and the sulci widen. Ventricular enlargement is greater than sulcal widening. Atrophic changes are seen more frequently in the frontal lobes. Although the scans of patients with AD show more atrophy than the scans of control subjects, there is substantial overlap. Thus, generalized atrophy on a scan does not indicate AD or other degenerative brain disease. However, if patients are followed longitudinally with serial scans, there is an increased rate of ventricular enlargement, sulcal size, and total cerebrospinal fluid volumes in patients with AD, and control subjects show no increase in any of these measures. Accordingly, serial imaging may prove a useful test in evaluating patients with possible AD. However, clinical assessment alone generally provides the necessary diagnostic information. Frontal and temporal atrophy in the appropriate clinical setting may indicate the presence of Pick's disease. MRI is the preferred test in most clinical situations because of its greater sensitivity in detecting most disorders, its ability to demonstrate the gray-white matter junction and the lack of bone artifact. Also, MRI permits examining the volume of the hippocampus, amygdala, and entorhinal cortex; anatomical regions with substantial pathology; and architectural change with AD. These studies lend promise for an increased ability for structural imaging to enhance diagnostic accuracy. The only drawbacks of MRI are related to patient comfort and expense: Many older patients find the test difficult to tolerate. Although MRI is more sensitive than computed tomography (CT) in revealing white matter changes, it may be less specific: CT scans reveal more periventricular white matter lesions in patients who developed abnormal neurological signs subsequent to symptomatic cerebrovascular disease (Lopez et al. 1995).

Positron Emission Tomographic and Single-Photon Emission Computer Tomographic Scans

Positron emission tomography (PET) and single-photon emission CT are investigational techniques that show promise but are now only rarely useful in routine clinical settings. For most clinical situations, these studies reveal metabolic function (generally blood flow and oxygen use) in addition to structure. For instance, in early AD, there is reduced blood flow and oxygen use in the parietal cortices. Ligand studies using PET have demonstrated dopaminergic nerve terminals in the basal ganglia and striatal dopamine binding sites. These studies permit assessment of therapeutic interventions designed to enhance nerve terminal growth and neuronal survival (substantia nigra neurons) in Parkinson's disease. Studies overlapping MRI with PET have produced new data on functional brain anatomy, revealing information on the brain, behavior, and the ability of the brain to adapt to injury (neuroplasticity). MR spectroscopy offers the potential for a single technique with diagnostic discrimination of age-related neurodegenerative disorders: MR proton spectroscopy, specifically the myoinositol-to-creatinine ratio, distinguishes AD from other dementias and from normal seniors.

Normal-Pressure Hydrocephalus, Periventricular White Matter Changes, and Binswanger's Disease

Classically, patients with normal-pressure hydrocephalus (NPH) have a triad of gait disorder, incontinence, and dementia. The ventricles are enlarged, especially in the area of the frontal horns, and the periventricular white matter is altered. Shunting may ameliorate the symptoms, and the procedure is most beneficial to patients in whom the gait disorder is the most prominent complaint and dementia is of recent onset.

Because deep white matter infarcts typically occur in the frontal lobes around the ventricles, they may cause a syndrome similar to NPH. Classically, the infarct patient has stepwise deterioration, and the examination shows both spasticity and rigidity. The syndrome may be called *leukoariosis*, multiple lacunae, or Binswanger's disease, although the latter diagnosis still requires clarification. White matter abnormalities on MRI are common, occurring in 30–80% of elderly people in the absence of known neurological disease. Similar abnormalities are frequent in patients with NPH, and in turn, hydrocephalus is frequent in patients diagnosed as having deep hemisphere infarcts.

The frequent occurrence of white matter changes and ventricular dilatation result in frequent referrals to neurologists to rule out NPH, Binswanger's disease, or both. Many of these patients have no clinical evidence of neurological disease, and no further investigation is warranted. NPH is rare, and small vessel ischemic disease is common. Surgery can improve the symptoms and signs of NPH. However, we are not able to influence the course of the deficits caused by stroke. Therefore, every effort is made to avoid overlooking a case of NPH. In general, few patients present with NPH who have not had a previous head injury, meningitis, or another event, such as subarachnoid hemorrhage, which result in altered cerebrospinal fluid dynamics. Thus, historic data are critical to establish this diagnosis. Laboratory tests do not reliably predict who will respond to shunting. The lumbar puncture (LP) is simple and specific but insensitive (unless the patient improves after LP). If clinical symptoms improve after LP, the diagnosis of NPH is established. Sometimes the improvement is long lasting, and serial LPs can be used to treat the patient. However, the diagnosis of NPH remains problematic, especially if one uses response to treatment as an indication of its presence, because not all patients diagnosed as having NPH respond to treatment. If patients do not respond, does

that mean the diagnosis is incorrect? Are we overdiagnosing the illness? Do we really have a reliable way to diagnose the illness? The previous history of intracranial events predisposing to the development of NPH remains one of the best indicators of its presence and response to shunting. Because NPH is treatable, the overzealous search for the disorder unfortunately results in many diagnoses and subsequent shunts that do not help patients. Indeed, only 15% show substantial improvement.

Electrodiagnostic Studies

Electroencephalogram

On the electroencephalogram (EEG), the mean frequency of alpha waves decreases slightly with advancing age. The usual adult range is 8–12 Hz, with a mean of 10 Hz. At age 70 years, the mean is 9.5 Hz. After 80 years, the rate declines more rapidly, dropping to 8.5 Hz after age 90 and remaining at this level to at least age 100. The range of peak power frequency decreases with advancing age without much change in the average frequency (Figure 86.1), although the average frequency does drop after age 80.

Evoked Responses

Sensory evoked responses depend on normally functioning sensory receptors and peripheral nerves. Sensory receptor function and aspects of peripheral nerve conduction decrease with advancing age. Therefore, until we develop stimuli adequate to overcome the reduced sensitivity of the sensory receptors or establish means by which to interpret receptor and conduction changes, the interpretation of age-related evoked response changes must be viewed with caution. Despite these limitations, some observations appear to be reproducible: P3 latency increases with increasing age, and the latency of the P300 is prolonged in patients with dementia.

MAJOR DISORDERS IN GERIATRIC NEUROLOGY

Disorders of Higher Integrative Functions

Dementia

Dementia implies a reduction in cognitive capabilities from a normal premorbid level of intellectual and social functioning. The changes that emerge are multiple: memory, language, calculations, judgment, visuospatial skills, and behavior may all be altered. Frequently, a single deficit may be the lead abnormality, but other components of the dementia constellation must emerge for the clinical diagnosis to be established. The *Diagnostic and Statistical Manual of Mental Disorders* (4th ed.) (*DSM-IV*) defines *dementia* "as the development of multiple cognitive deficits that include memory impairment and at least one of the following: aphasia, apraxia, agnosia, or a disturbance in executive functioning. These deficits must be sufficiently severe to cause impairment in occupational or social functioning, and must represent a decline from a previously higher level of functioning." If other features of the dementing process do not emerge, a single deficit, such as memory or language, may be part of an amnestic or aphasic syndrome. Initially, these clinical abnormalities may be quite subtle, and even formal neuropsychological testing may not reveal a deficit substantial enough to render a diagnosis of dementia. There is considerable evidence that informant-based data may be more reliable than formal neuropsychological testing. An individual who knows the patient well can confirm that an individual has changed from premorbid levels. Clinical assessment, including formal neuropsychological tests, confirms the deficits. Subjects with dementia may also exhibit behavioral features at any time during the illness; depression and delusions may suggest a primary psychiatric illness, and supervening delirium should indicate an additional process, such as a systemic disorder or an adverse drug effect altering the presentation or course of dementia. *DSM-IV* also points out that historically, the term *dementia* tended to imply an irreversible process, although the course of dementia depends on its pathogenesis. Thus, dementia may remit, progress, or remain static.

The causes of dementia are many (Whitehouse 1993). Earlier and extant classification schemes for dementia have used the terms *cortical* and *subcortical dementia*, but this classification is problematic. Cortical dementia has been used to describe patients with memory disturbances and such neocortical dysfunction as aphasia, alexia, apraxia, agnosia, and acalculia ("the *A*s"). Patients with subcortical dementia usually demonstrate motor system alterations, including abnormal tone, posture, movements, and gait, as part of the initial presentation. Also, the subcortical memory disorder is characterized by a retrieval deficit, and overall cognition is slowed but without the prominent cortical dysfunction characterized by "the *A*s." However, because cortical processes (AD, Pick's disease, lobar atrophy) may have motor features, and because subcortical dementing processes (Huntington's disease, Parkinson's disease, progressive supranuclear palsy) may have apraxias, agnosias, and a degree of aphasia, the separation is somewhat artificial on clinical grounds. Also, some of the major pathology in AD, a "cortical dementia," is subcortical: Neuronal loss and transmitter change in the cholinergic basal forebrain and noradrenergic locus ceruleus occur in the diencephalon and brainstem. Thus, overlap clearly exists between the groups. Nevertheless, early in the course of a dementing illness, it is uncommon for a cortical process to produce substantial changes on the motor examination; that is, altered motor tone (rigidity), gait or balance disorders, and tremor are generally absent. Conversely, it is uncommon to see a prominent aphasia early in a dementing disorder due to disease in the diencephalon and midbrain, although language

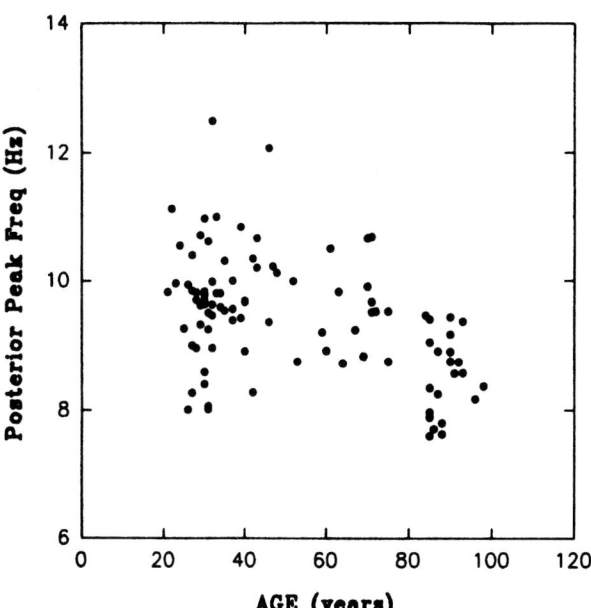

FIGURE 86.1   Scatterplot of the peak power frequency of the electroencephalogram and age in 97 subjects. Note five subjects older than age 84 with a peak frequency of less than 8 Hz.

output may be reduced or dysarthric. These general clinical axioms should assist the neurologist in targeting the primary locus of pathology and the diagnostic and treatment options. Reversible dementias are uncommon, accounting for approximately 15% of cases of dementia, and are generally restricted to depression, medications, and encephalopathies. Although metabolic disorders presenting as dementia are infrequent, occasionally hypothyroidism, vitamin B_{12} deficiency, hypercalcemia, and systemic organ failure (renal failure) may be discovered by laboratory tests.

In older citizens, a major cause of dementia is neurodegenerative disease. As indicated in Table 86.1, dementia of the Alzheimer's type is the leading etiology, with vascular disease second (if subjects with coexisting AD and vascular change are included, vascular diagnoses underlie dementia in approximately 12% of cases). AD reaches a prevalence of 25–45% between the ages of 75 and 90. Age is a leading factor in determining the expression of this illness: Prevalence at ages 60–65 is 1–3%; thereafter, the incidence increases for each decade, reaching an apparent plateau at 90 years of age, when prevalence approaches 50%. Most studies of dementing illnesses are drawn from neurological and psychiatric services, and primary brain diseases, such as AD, Huntington's disease, and Parkinson's disease, may be overrepresented compared with the general population of individuals who are demented. In particular, Huntington's and Parkinson's diseases generally represent a relatively small percentage of patients. Finally, as dementia patients have been studied in more detail, such clinical entities as frontal lobe dementia, lobar dementia, and Lewy

2280 NEUROLOGICAL DISEASES

Table 86.1: Disorders producing dementia: diagnoses in nine clinical series

Diagnosis	Number of patients	Percentage
Alzheimer's	499	
+ Parkinson's	10	
+ Vascular	8	
Total	517	65.9
Other progressive dementias		
Vascular multi-infarct dementia	85	
Parkinson's	10	
Huntington's	15	
Progressive supranuclear palsy	3	
Amyotrophic lateral sclerosis	1	
Kufs'	1	
Postanoxic	5	
Post-traumatic	8	
Postencephalitic	3	
Creutzfeldt-Jakob	3	
Total	134	17.1
Treatable dementias		
Neurosyphilis	2	
Fungal infections	2	
Tumor	22	
Alcohol	22	
Subdural hematoma	4	
Hydrocephalus	27	
Epilepsy	3	
Total	82	10.5
Reversible dementias		
Drug toxicity	21	
Metabolic	16	
Hepatic	1	
Hyponatremia	1	
Calcium (high or low)	4	
Vitamin B$_{12}$	2	
Thyroid	7	
Hypoglycemia	1	
Total	53	4.7
Cause uncertain	14	1.8
Grand total	800	100

Source: Reprinted with permission R Katzman, JW Rowe. Principles of Geriatric Neurology. Philadelphia: Davis, 1992.

Table 86.2: Illnesses causing dementia in 200 patients

	No. (%) of patients
Alzheimer's-type dementia	149 (74.5)*
Dementia due to drugs	19 (9.5)
Alcohol-related dementia	8 (4.0)
Hypothyroidism	6 (3.0)
Multi-infarct dementia	3 (1.5)
Other metabolic disease	
Hyperparathyroidism	2 (1.0)
Hyponatremia	2 (1.0)
Hypoglycemia	1 (0.5)
Other (cause known)	8 (4.0)
Other (cause unknown)	7 (3.5)
Benign senescent forgetfulness	3 (1.5)
Not demented	15 (7.5)

*Twelve of these patients also had Parkinson's disease.
Source: Reprinted with permission from EB Larson, BV Reifler, SM Sumi, et al. Diagnostic tests in the evaluation of dementia. Arch Intern Med 1986;146:1917–1922.

body dementia are occurring with more frequency; in some clinical pathological studies of dementia, Lewy body dementia represents 20% of the cases. In previous reviews, vascular dementia (multi-infarct dementia [MID]) usually ranked second or third in most studies (see Table 86.1), but recently the prevalence of vascular dementias appears to have decreased, possibly related to improved control of blood pressure (BP). However, the role of vascular disease and stroke in producing cognitive disorders appears to increase in the oldest old. In a series of 200 outpatients referred to a general medical and geriatric clinic for evaluation of cognitive decline, dementia related to medications, alcohol, and thyroid dysfunction was more frequent than vascular dementia; neurodegenerative dementia of the Alzheimer's type was the most frequent diagnosis (Table 86.2). Neuropathological studies suggest that MID may only account for 2.0–15.7% of patients with dementia, and patients with the combination of AD and MID may comprise 1.9–27.5% of the patients. However, haunting these studies is the realization that clear clinical and neuropathological criteria to establish a diagnosis of vascular dementia do not exist (Drachman 1993).

The evaluation of dementing illnesses requires careful history and examination and well-chosen laboratory and imaging studies. As indicated in Table 86.1, approximately 15% of dementias are either reversible or treatable. Consequently, it behooves the neurologist to ensure a complete assessment of all patients presenting with dementia. The National Institute on Aging's recommendation on diagnostic tests for dementia patients includes complete blood cell count (CBC), erythrocyte sedimentation rate, VDRL, serum folate, and cyanocobalamin. Also recommended are chemistry screen (electrolytes, glucose, liver function tests, renal function tests, calcium, albumin, total protein), serum phosphate, thyroid screen (thyroxin and triiodothyronine uptake) (thyrotropin, currently the best screening test for thyroid dysfunction, was not mentioned), urinalysis, electrocardiogram (ECG), chest radiograph, and CT scan of the brain. In 1986, Larson and co-workers evaluated the use of diagnostic tests in dementia and compared costs of tests to likelihood of revealing an unsuspected cause. For instance, the CBC was sufficiently sensitive to permit making the statement that "no more than 1.2% of persons who had a normal CBC would have abnormal cyanocobalamin levels." Additionally, the CT scan did not reveal any unsuspected pathology in their 200 patients, and the authors suggested that patients with chronic dementia probably do not need to be scanned unless the history and neurological examination suggest the possibility of structural disease. Patients who present subacutely or acutely with altered mentation, as well as those with

Table 86.3:   Genes associated with Alzheimer's disease

Chromosome	Gene	Type of genetic effect	Age at onset (range in yrs)	Other features
21	APP	Mutation	Sixth decade (41–67)	Familial; autosomal dominant
21	APP (?)	Trisomy 21	Fifth decade (>30)	Down syndrome; pathological features of Alzheimer's disease
14	S182/PS1 (presenilin 1)	Mutation	Fifth decade (29–62)	Familial; autosomal dominant; early aphasia, myoclonus, seizures, and extrapyramidal signs with rapid course
1	SPM2/PS2 (presenilin 2)	Mutation	Sixth decade (40–75)	Primarily Volga German families; autosomal dominant; incomplete penetrance demonstrated
19	Apolipoprotein E	Susceptibility	Adult life span	Modifier of age at onset; risk may be modified by ethnicity, family history, sex or age
6	HLA-A	Susceptibility	Adult life span	Modifier of age at onset; allele A2 earlier age at onset
Mitochondrial	Cytochrome-c oxidase I and II	Unknown	Unknown	Unknown

APP = amyloid precursor protein.

dementia who suddenly change, require scanning. As cost effectiveness begins to drive the health care system, the workup of patients with dementia will be influenced by approaches that provide the highest yield for the least cost. Larson's group demonstrated that focused assessment profiles would reduce costs by 68–79% per patient and might decrease costs on a national level from $2–3 billion to $450–630 million (in 1986 dollars).

The clinician must be sensitive to the expenses associated with evaluating dementia patients. Without a definitive diagnostic test for many of the neurodegenerative dementias, however, it is imperative to examine for all reasonable potential causes because once the diagnosis of dementia is rendered, further evaluations tend to cease unless the patient is enrolled in a research study. Over the last few years, investigations have raised the possibility that genetic markers of AD are identifiable. Six genes have been linked with clinical AD (Table 86.3). Familial AD is linked to chromosomes 1, 14, and 21. The presenilin mutations appear to alter the metabolism of amyloid and are associated with disease onset in the fifth and sixth decades of life. Mutation of the amyloid precursor protein (APP) gene on chromosome 21 results in familial AD with an early age of onset. The triplicate repeat of chromosome 21 in Down syndrome leads to AD in essentially all patients with trisomy 21 by the fifth decade (100% of these individuals whose brains have been studied at autopsy exhibit the classic neuropathological changes of AD). Two susceptibility genes have now been identified: the apolipoprotein E (ApoE) gene on chromosome 19 and the A2 allele of the HLA major histocompatibility complex on chromosome 6. Because individuals who are homozygous for these genes may not develop AD, they are not markers of AD. The ApoE-ε4 allele (ApoE-ε4) allele on chromosome 19 has been associated with an increased risk of developing AD in

adults between 60 and 80 years old, but in later years (the oldest old), the frequency of the ApoE-ε4 allele is the same in those who become demented and those who do not. However, ApoE-ε4 still carries an association with earlier-onset disease in this oldest-old group. In seniors, the frequency of the ApoE-ε2 allele appeared to be increased, raising the idea that ApoE-ε2 might be a longevity gene. This is probably not the case, although as more long-lived families are recognized and studied with the power of molecular genetics, such genes may become recognized. Similar to the observations with ApoE-ε4, individuals with the HLA-A2 allele have an earlier onset of dementia, and this observation is particularly interesting because it suggests that an inflammatory reaction is involved in the disease process. Furthermore, the observation that nonsteroidal anti-inflammatory drugs (NSAIDs) might delay the onset of AD is consonant with these data. Because aging has been associated with reduced immune surveillance, there might be a neuroimmune axis in the pathophysiology of AD. Despite these substantial advances in understanding the genetics of aging and AD, there is still no specific genetic marker for diagnosing dementing illnesses in the general population; the final diagnosis rests on examining the brain after death. Current criteria for establishing a definitive diagnosis of AD require correlative clinical and neuropathological data. A full discussion of dementia is available in Chapter 70.

The goals of evaluating dementia in elderly subjects are to identify reversible causes and initiate the appropriate treatment. Traditionally, the diagnosis of dementia of any cause casts a hopeless pall. However, there is now evidence that some therapeutic approaches to dementia are emerging. Medications that enhance central cholinergic activity show some promise in AD, and improved management of hypertension and stroke appears to be having a beneficial effect on patients with vascular dementias. The acetylcholinesterase inhibitor (AChE-I), tacrine hydrochloride, was the first medication approved for the treatment of AD by the U.S. Food and Drug Administration. The effectiveness in the initial study was minimal (treatment resulted in less decline in the assessment scale, but clinician assessment did not reveal a significant improvement with treatment). A further study suggests that some patients who can tolerate higher doses (160 mg/day) demonstrate improvement in function over 30 weeks compared with placebo-treated controls (Knapp et al. 1994). A problem exists with this study: 70% of the subjects had to withdraw because of abnormal liver function studies and gastrointestinal complaints. These adverse events reversed after discontinuing the medicine. A second AChE-I, donepezil, appears to have similar efficacy with fewer side effects and without the need to follow liver function tests. It is now the AChE-I of choice for the treatment of AD.

Ideally, medications that stop or retard the pathophysiological processes underlying AD would be the agents of choice. Research efforts are being directed at identifying agents that modify the metabolism of amyloid or alter the abnormal phosphorylation of microtubules and thus neurofilaments. Estrogen and NSAIDs delay the onset of AD, and vitamin E slows the progress of the disease. Additionally, agents that directly address the metabolism of microtubules and amyloid are being examined. For instance, the discovery of the connection between ApoE-ε4 and AD has opened new avenues for drug development. Different affinities exist between the microtubular-associated protein τ, the phosphorylated form of which may be the key molecule in developing neurofibrillary tangles (NFT), ApoE-ε4, and ApoE-ε3. ApoE-ε3 might assist in maintaining the structure of τ, and its absence (as in the ApoE-ε4 phenotype) may predispose to NFT development. A relationship between amyloid and ApoE-ε4 has also been suggested. Apparently, ApoE-ε4 binds with high affinity to amyloid, which becomes insoluble. This process may predispose to the development of plaques, and thus the ApoE-ε4 phenotype would also be a high risk for this neuropathological change. ApoE may be a pathological chaperon protein in patients with cerebral and systemic amyloid. Consonant with these hypotheses is the observation that ApoE-ε4 predisposes to more neuritic plaques and β-amyloid protein compared with AD brains lacking ApoE-ε4 (Gomez-Isla et al. 1996).

Another important aspect of therapy includes the recognition and treatment of affective disturbances. A substantial percentage of patients with dementia, secondary to many processes, are clinically depressed. Recognition of depression is critical. The antidepressants of choice are those with the least amount of anticholinergic activity. Newer-generation agents, such as the selective serotonin reuptake inhibitors, which have fewer side effects and do not impair cholinergic transmission, are the agents of choice. Treatment of the depression will not only improve the affective components of the illness but may also improve cognitive performance.

Two major events generally alter the ability to care for patients at home: behavioral changes and incontinence. Also, such care issues as maintaining general hygiene, nutrition, and normal sleep patterns are increasingly vexing to family members. The range of behavioral alterations is substantial. Agitation and restlessness, including wandering behavior and shadowing (following the care provider around like a shadow), are particularly troubling. The possible source of difficulties must be sought. Patients who are agitated may be depressed, be under some relatively sudden stress, have personal discomfort, or be bored. As mentioned above, depression occurs frequently and should be evaluated completely because antidepressant medication is very effective in these patients. Wanderers may feel lost and confused about where they are and require reassurance. Wandering and pacing may occur because of boredom and wanting to get around or in response to a normal bodily function (e.g., need to use the toilet, hunger, need for exercise, pain). The health care team and care providers must be sleuths with creative approaches to diagnose the possible causes of these behaviors.

UI is the second major event in the clinical course of patients with dementia that precipitates major care issues for the patient and family. A common cause may be urinary tract infection or other systemic process or medications such as diuretics. Patients develop apraxia and agnosias and may be unable to manage their clothing, find the bathroom, or distinguish a chair or a wastebasket from the toilet. Timing may be a key issue in that the urge to urinate cannot be resisted and mobility may be slowed such that the patient is unable to make it to the bathroom on time. Strategies include timed voiding and recognizing that advantage may be taken of the gastrocolic reflex: Patients are toileted after meals.

Patients who are unable to communicate effectively may become agitated and more confused, as well as acutely encephalopathic (delirious), from a host of systemic illnesses, metabolic changes, and pharmacological agents. Whenever a change in functional level or behavior occurs, such common etiologies as medication changes, urinary tract infection, and sources of pain must be examined. The critical issue is the diagnosis of the cause or causes of behavioral change. One of our patients had recurrent bouts of agitation, which went unrecognized until observation in the hospital revealed that these events were related to angina (as evidenced by his demeanor and ECG changes). His clinical picture improved and the symptoms fully resolved after treatment with nitroglycerin. Frequently, relatively banal events underlie the behavioral decompensation.

If there is no apparent cause for the behavioral change, a few guiding principles are helpful. First, medication is not always needed, and simple diversionary tactics, including change of activity, leaving the current environment, presenting ideas or stimuli (e.g., pictures, food such as ice cream) known to be positive for the patient, and reassurance and reorientation may be effective. Families are often particularly adept at identifying special tricks and should

FIGURE 86.2 Suicides by age, race, and sex, United States, 1988. (Reprinted with permission from National Institutes of Health. Diagnosis and treatment of depression in late life. In Consensus Development Conference, November 4–6, 1991 [review], Consensus Statement 1991;9:1–27.)

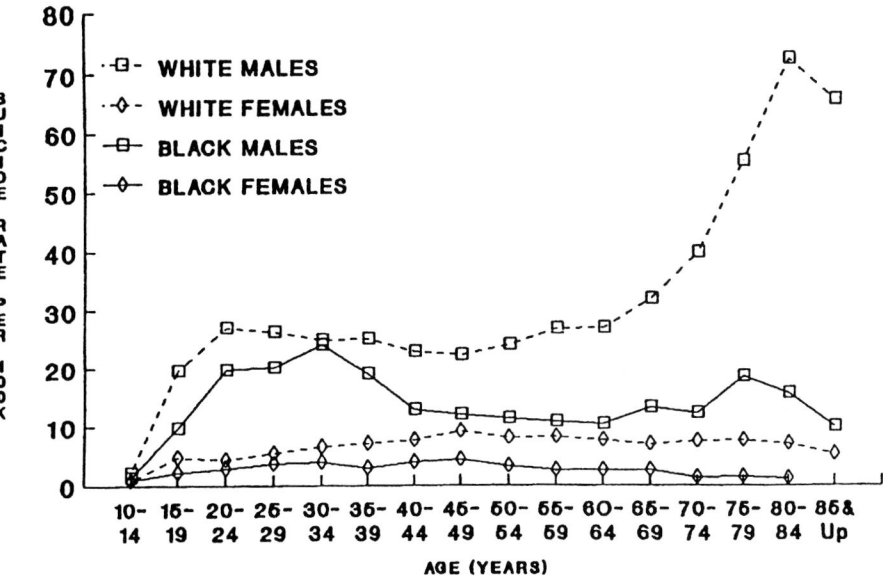

be encouraged to do so. Second, if medications are needed, the benzodiazepines should be avoided because they tend to be sedating and lead to more confusion, gait instability, and falls. Depending on the phenotype of the behavioral change, antidepressants or neuroleptics are probably the best choice, starting with a very low dose. As mentioned, depression may occur frequently and manifest as agitation with increased pacing, angry outbursts, and some affective display. In this situation, antidepressants might be tried initially. In other situations, neuroleptics may be needed to control abnormal behavior. The data supporting a very effective role for these agents are surprisingly limited, and other pharmacological approaches are needed. Two anticonvulsants, carbamazepine and valproic acid, have beneficial modifying effects on agitation and disruptive behavior. Trazodone, with its antidepressant effect and sedative qualities, appears to be particularly useful when administered before bed because it improves sleep and reduces the depression associated with dementia.

Depression

Depression symptoms listed in *DSM-IV* include depressed or irritable mood, loss of interest or pleasure in usual activities, changes in appetite and weight, disturbed sleep, motor agitation or retardation, fatigue and loss of energy, feelings of worthlessness, self-reproach, excessive guilt, suicidal thinking or attempts, and difficulty with thinking or concentration. There may be less specificity of clinical presentation in the elderly. Compared with depression in the young, late-life depression is more commonly associated with medical illness, such as diabetes mellitus, cardiovascular disease, or arthritis, and neurological disorders, such as dementia, Parkinson's disease, and stroke. Therefore, the clinician must differentiate somatic signs of depression from

signs of physical illness. An important issue in late-life depression is the high suicide rate of white men (Figure 86.2). The rate rises dramatically after age 64.

Depression is common, yet the diagnosis is frequently missed. The elderly may not reveal depressive symptoms, and furthermore, recognition of depression and anxiety in seniors may be hampered by complicating medical and neurological illnesses as well as by poor communication. Major depression was detected in 1% of community-dwelling elders, 5% of elders in primary care clinics, and 15–25% of nursing home residents. Each year, 13% of nursing home residents develop a new episode of major depression. An additional 18% develop new depressive symptoms. Depression is more common in women than in men, and there are no racial or ethnic differences. Depressive symptoms without major depression are present in 8–15% of community-dwelling elders. Bipolar disorder is present in 0.1% of community-dwelling elders and shows no racial or ethnic differences. Depression is a common accompaniment to Parkinson's disease, occurring in 20–30% of patients, and treatment may be difficult. Depression is also a frequent accompaniment of stroke, particularly with lesions in the left hemisphere.

Depression can present with cognitive impairment. The syndrome is called *pseudodementia* and is usually easily distinguished from dementia by the prominent affective disorder. Occasionally, neuropsychological testing suggests that depression may underlie the dementia observed in a patient. Patients with abulia from a frontal lesion can appear depressed. Causes of the frontal lesion include brain tumor, hydrocephalus, and rarely, multiple infarcts.

Antidepressants, electroconvulsive therapy, and psychotherapy are the mainstays of treatment. Many of the antidepressants have anticholinergic side effects, which are exaggerated in the elderly. Table 86.4 reviews the common

Table 86.4:   Antidepressants: pharmacology and adverse effects

Pharmacology	Adverse effects
Blockade of norepinephrine uptake at nerve endings	Tremors Tachycardia Erectile and ejaculatory dysfunction Blockade of the antihypertensive effects of guanethidine and guanadrel Augmentation of pressor effects of sympathomimetic amines
Blockade of serotonin uptake at nerve endings	Gastrointestinal disturbances Increase or decrease in anxiety (dose-dependent) Sexual dysfunction Extrapyramidal side effects Interactions with L-tryptophan, monoamine oxidase inhibitors, and fenfluramine
Blockade of dopamine uptake at nerve endings	Psychomotor activation Antiparkinsonian effect Aggravation of psychosis
Blockade of histamine H_1 receptors	Potentiation of central depressant drugs Sedation, drowsiness Weight gain Hypotension
Blockade of muscarinic receptors	Blurred vision Dry mouth Sinus tachycardia Constipation Urinary retention Memory dysfunction
Blockade of α_1-adrenergic receptors	Potentiation of the antihypertensive effect of prazosin, terazosin, doxazosin, and labetalol Postural hypotension, dizziness Reflex tachycardia
Blockade of dopamine D_2 receptors	Extrapyramidal movement disorders Endocrine changes Sexual dysfunction (men)

Source: Adapted with permission from E Richelson. Pharmacology of antidepressants—characteristics of the ideal drug. Mayo Clin Proc 1994;69:1071–1081.

clinical side effects of antidepressants (Richelson 1994). The antidepressant drugs with the fewest side effects include newer agents, such as the selective serotonin reuptake inhibitors and venlafaxine.

Delirium and Confusion

Delirium is a syndrome of rapid onset with fluctuating attention and distorted perception (see Chapter 4). It is frequently reversible. Onset occurs over hours to days. The three cardinal features are a disturbance of vigilance and heightened distractibility; the inability to maintain a coherent stream of thought; and the inability to carry out a sequence of goal-directed movements. Patients may be agitated or apathetic. Hallucinations are common. Other commonly used names to describe this clinical picture include *acute confusional state* and *toxic-metabolic encephalopathy*.

Patients with Wernicke's or other aphasias with fluent speech and paraphasic errors may at first appear confused. Frequent paraphasic errors, poor comprehension and processing of language, and the absence of distractibility usually indicate that aphasia is the main problem. Many demented patients are inattentive, but the history of disturbed memory as the main initial problem clarifies the diagnosis. Confusion related to urinary tract infection or pneumonia may be the initial sign of brain disease in a patient with dementia. After the confusion clears, memory returns to normal. Over the next year or two, persistent signs of disordered memory appear. Depression can be distinguished from delirium by the relative absence of fluctuation and the depressed affect.

Epidemiological studies reveal that delirium or encephalopathy is probably the most common nonspecific presentation of disease in older persons. The frequency ranges from 9–14% of patients after elective surgery to 20–50% of hospitalized medical patients. In two-thirds of patients, the diagnosis is overlooked or mistaken for another disorder. Difficulty in diagnosis is in part related to the frequent presence of inattention in demented patients and to not distinguishing between dementia and delirium. Old age and dementia are risk factors for the development of delirium. Recovery may be delayed. Although usually reversible, the disturbance may become permanent.

The etiology and pathogenesis of delirium vary because a number of events may produce the syndrome in older patients. Toxins and metabolic disorders are the most common causes of delirium, but structural brain lesions can produce a similar syndrome. The lesions may be multifocal or solitary. Single brain lesions that cause confusional states are usually located in the right hemisphere, especially the parietal lobe. A wide variety of brain insults result in the same syndrome. There may be a final common pathway, possibly related to cholinergic pathways.

The clinical assessment of the confused patient focuses heavily on the mental status examination, which shows abnormal attention. Useful tests include the digit span, months of the year in reverse, and spelling the word *world* in reverse. Confused patients have difficulty maintaining the task. The months in reverse might be reported as: December, November, October, August, September, October, November. The patient made two errors. First, the patient skipped a month, showing inattention to the task. Second, the patient was impersistent to the task, reverting to the months forward. Observation is very helpful. Patients often respond to stimuli normally ignored, such as a telephone in the hall or the public address system. They are usually disoriented about time and place and, rarely, to person. Because delirium may be an early presentation of events that lead to stupor and reduced level of consciousness, a careful systematic neurological examination indicates levels of the neuraxis that are dysfunctional. Also, an acute confusional state is often the first sign of any illness in an old person; thus, a full medical evaluation is indicated as well. In addition to the general neurological and medical evaluation, the neurological investigation should include a brain imaging study and often an LP. MRI is preferred, but a CT scan may be more appropriate in an agitated patient because it is faster and results in an image with less movement artifact. In delirium, the EEG pattern reveals diffuse background slowing and is classically reflective of a metabolic encephalopathy. A normal background should prompt a search for a cause of confusion other than a toxic-metabolic encephalopathy.

To initiate treatment, the pathophysiology of delirium must be fully understood. Treatment is then directed at the causative events. To manage the symptoms, antipsychotics and benzodiazepines may be helpful. High-potency antipsychotics, such as haloperidol, are widely used, but they are not very sedating and cause marked extrapyramidal side effects. Low-potency agents, such as chlorpromazine, are less likely to cause an extrapyramidal syndrome but may be too sedating. Midrange drugs, such as molindone or acetophenazine, offer a good compromise: Compared with haloperidol, the increased sedation is helpful in an agitated and confused patient. Additionally, these agents and the newer antipsychotics such as risperidone and olanzapine appear to have less affinity for dopamine (D_2) receptors and offer antipsychotic effects without causing an extrapyramidal syndrome.

Benzodiazepines are good sedatives, but they may worsen confusion. They may also compromise gait and cause a fall. They are particularly effective when sedation is the desired effect. Short-acting agents, like oxazepam or lorazepam, work well. Very-short-acting agents, such as triazolam, should not be used in the elderly because they cause an anxiety state as the effect wears off. The anxiety can be severe and lead to ischemic heart injury. Long-acting benzodiazepines (diazepam and chlordiazepoxide) are poor choices because their active metabolite (desmethyldiazepam) has a half-life of 50–100 hours, and gradual accumulation results in patients developing confusion and instability of gait and posture.

Disorders of Consciousness and Wakefulness

Syncope

Syncope, which may be defined as a transient loss of consciousness and unresponsiveness wherein the maintenance of motor tone is lost and patients sit or lie motionless and then recover spontaneously, is estimated to underlie more than 300,000 emergency room visits and account for up to 6% of medical admissions. Syncope is common; the incidence in an institutionalized population of seniors was 5–7%. Studies of institutionalized older citizens indicate that the annual incidence of syncope was 14%, and one-third of these patients had recurrent episodes. Observations in community-residing subjects are similar: The recurrence

rate is 13% for middle-aged people and 25% in older people. (See Chapter 2 for a full discussion of syncope.)

Determining the cause of syncope is not easy. Generally, approximately 40% of syncopal events remain undiagnosed, and the evaluation of elderly subjects with syncope is somewhat more problematic. Age-related physiological changes (decreased baroreceptor sensitivity, blunted heart rate responses, diminished renal conservation of sodium, reduced plasma renin and aldosterone responses), disease processes that increase with age (cerebrovascular, cardiovascular, diabetes mellitus), the presence of three or four chronic diseases, and the use of three times more medication in seniors all predispose elderly subjects to syncopal events and may preclude establishing a single etiological event (Kapoor 1994). Nevertheless, as indicated in Table 86.5, the initial history, physical examination, and ECG are still the most useful steps in establishing a diagnosis, yielding a diagnosis in 60–85% of diagnosable cases. The results of these initial studies and the neurological examination dictates the diagnostic studies (e.g., metabolic measures, image studies, EEG, more detailed cardiovascular studies) needed to fully explore potential causes. Clinical studies indicate that, unless the clinical picture suggests a focal neurological process or a seizure disorder, EEGs and CT scans are generally not useful in evaluating syncope.

Pathophysiological processes resulting in syncope alter central nervous function by changing the availability of two critical metabolic substrates, oxygen or glucose, or by altering electrical activity in the brain. In seniors, the presence of cardiac conduction abnormalities, cardiovascular disease, cerebrovascular disease, and medication is more likely to cause syncope, whereas noncardiovascular etiologies dominate in younger patients (Table 86.6).

Because a large percentage of patients with syncope remain undiagnosed with traditional tests, a number of new approaches have evolved. The postural (upright) tilt test has been espoused as a means to examine neurally mediated hypotension and bradycardia, a common cause of syncope. However, more studies are needed to clarify the role of the tilt test in older citizens.

A second evolving approach is intracardiac electrophysiological testing in patients with recurrent syncope. These studies offer promise because some reports indicate that a cause for syncope may be identifiable in approximately 70% of subjects and that 85% of patients did not experience syncope after the identified abnormality was treated. However, it is sometimes difficult to associate a specific finding with syncope. Thus, these studies generally produce inferences rather than proof. Nevertheless, when clinical characteristics are used as guidelines, these studies may be quite useful. A particularly useful test is loop ECG recordings that may be diagnostic in 25–35% of cases of syncope.

Treatment is directed at the underlying cause of syncope. In seniors, one must recognize that more than one event may compromise older patients and result in a syncopal event.

Table **86.5:** Diagnostic studies that established a cause of syncope

	Young (%)	Elderly (%)
History and physical examination	38	25
Electrocardiography	4	9
Electrocardiographic monitoring	8	17
Electroencephalography	0.5	0.5
Carotid massage	0	2
Electrophysiological studies	1	2
Cardiac catheterization	2	4
Cerebral angiography	0	1
Stress test	1	0

Source: Reprinted with permission from W Kapoor, D Snustad, J Peterson, et al. Syncope in the elderly. Am J Med 1986;80: 419–428.

Seizures

Neurological teaching has stressed that the onset of seizures during adult life generally heralds the presence of a structural lesion, such as tumor, abscess, or stroke (ischemic or hemorrhagic), and that the outcome is generally unfavorable. This notion is supported by some studies in the elderly reporting that tumors may account for 25–30% of seizures during adulthood. However, others have reported only a 2% occurrence of neoplastic processes among patients 69 years and older with the sudden onset of seizures. A summary of 18 clinical studies of seizures in the elderly is presented in Table 86.7. Of note are the high percentage of vascular etiologies (33%) and the wide range (0–36%) of tumor incidence. Also notable is the percentage of patients in whom the etiology of the seizure is unknown (7–68%), which suggests that, in fact, idiopathic epilepsy may occur throughout life. The exact profile of these unknown cases must be fully defined to determine whether subsequent events reveal a pathological substrate. This is especially so because these studies largely antedated the availability of MRI, which enhances lesion identification. Also, some of the reported series came from specialty units (neurology or neurosurgical services), and so the distribution of etiologies is biased toward structural disease, such as tumor. Surveys of general acute care outpatient and inpatient programs might reveal a broader range of etiologies, especially cardiovascular and metabolic (hypoglycemia). In summary, the general impression is that the leading processes underlying epilepsy in seniors may be cerebrovascular disease and idiopathic; after age 70, the likelihood of tumor being the cause is relatively small (see Chapter 71 for a full discussion).

Although seizure onset is frequent during the perinatal period and late childhood and adolescence, epidemiological studies also indicate that the incidence and prevalence of epilepsy increase with aging. In the Olmstead County, MN, registry, the incidence for seizures was 68.5 per 100,000 in subjects older than 60; this is almost twice the overall rate for the population. Other epidemiological and demographic studies of epilepsy in seniors report incidences of 100 per

Table **86.6:**   Causes of syncope

	Young (no. of patients)	Elderly (no. of patients)
Cardiovascular causes of syncope		
Ventricular tachycardia	13*	33
Sick sinus syndrome	3	12*
Carotid sinus syncope	0	5
Supraventricular tachycardia	5	0
Bradycardia	1	2
Second-degree atrioventricular block	1	1
Complete heart block	1	5
Pacemaker malfunction	2	1
Aortic stenosis	0	8
Myocardial infarction	1	4
Dissecting aortic aneurysm	1	0
Pulmonary embolus	2	0
Pulmonary hypertension	2	0
Total	32	71
Noncardiovascular causes of syncope		
Vasodepressor	29	3
Orthostatic hypotension	17	18
Situational	17	15
Drug-induced	2	7
Transient ischemic attack	1	7
Seizure	3*	3*
Subclavian steal	0	0
Trigeminal neuralgia	0	1
Psychiatric	3*	0
Total	72	54

*Diagnoses made on follow-up: ventricular tachycardia (one patient); sick sinus syndrome (one patient); seizure disorder (two young patients, three elderly patients); and conversion reaction (one patient).

Source: Reprinted with permission from W Kapoor, D Snustad, J Peterson, et al. Syncope in the elderly. Am J Med 1986;80:419–428.

100,000 (Hauser 1997; Scheuer and Cohen 1993). The striking point is the marked increase in epilepsy in seniors as they reach the eighth decade. Studies in long-term care facilities report an even higher incidence of new-onset seizures in the more frail elderly.

Approximately 65% of seizures in seniors are grand mal, 33% are partial seizures, and absence-type spells are rare. In a Mayo Clinic study of geriatric epilepsy, 80% of cases presented as partial seizures. The presence of a partial or focal ictal event often heralds the presence of focal disease, usually tumor or stroke. In contrast, metabolic, cardiovascular, or idiopathic etiologies usually result in generalized seizures. A surprising and important observation is that up to 30% of initial seizures in seniors may be severe and prolonged, qualifying for status epilepticus. Stroke patients are at a particularly high risk for seizures. The frequency with which seizures develop after a stroke varies (5–20%), but it may be as high as 50% in patients with involvement of the cortex in the area of the motor strip. Seizures in patients with subcortical lesions is quite uncommon, if not rare, in most series. A somewhat neglected observation is the

Table 86.7:   Etiology of seizures and epilepsy in the elderly

Etiology	Range (%)	Average (%)
Vascular	12–69	33
Tumor	0–36	13
Toxic or metabolic	0–18	8
Trauma	0–21	6
Miscellaneous	2–36	13
Idiopathic	7–68	27

Source: Compiled from 18 studies reported between 1953 and 1993; the latest, AB Ettinger, S Shinnar. New-onset seizures in an elderly hospitalized population. Neurology 1993;43:489–492, reporting 84% vascular and 8% idiopathic.

increased frequency of seizures in neurodegenerative disorders. There is a five- to 10-fold increase in risk of seizures in AD, and by year 10 of the illness, 15% of patients experience unprovoked seizures (Hesdorffer et al. 1996).

Except for the need to be cognizant of the increased susceptibility of seniors to the toxic side effects of anticonvulsants, which are probably related to altered metabolism and the presence of other medications, the treatment strategies for managing generalized and partial epilepsy in younger patients apply. Phenytoin or carbamazepine is generally used as the initial agent. Older individuals are particularly sensitive to carbamazepine; it must be started slowly, usually with 100-mg tablets, because the blood level may be adequate with quite low doses. Antiepileptic medications also have more side effects in seniors. For instance, cardiac conduction may be altered, and an increase in arrhythmias may occur with phenytoin and carbamazepine. Similarly, phenytoin, carbamazepine, or phenobarbital might aggravate osteoporosis in older women. Cognitive performance and gait and balance skills may also be impaired with a number of anticonvulsants. Consequently, anticonvulsants must be monitored closely, and if indicated, the free level of the agent examined because this level more accurately reflects the risk of drug toxicity. The newer pharmacological agents with reduced toxicity and drug interaction profiles may have a large role in treating seizures in the geriatric age group. We must point out that longitudinal studies have not been performed to determine if a single seizure in adults should be treated. Our policy has been to treat seizure patients with known structural disease (e.g., previous stroke, head trauma) because recurrent seizures occur more often in this setting. Also, patients who are particularly fragile and likely to not withstand a seizure should be treated. If a patient with a single seizure has no recurrence for 2 years and has a normal EEG, medications may be tapered and discontinued.

Sleep Disorders

Although human chronobiology predicts a 25-hour cycle of sleep and wakefulness, planetary events have given us the 24-hour clock. Societal structure and external events in daily living create further aberrations in the biological clock; the result is phase delays in our intrinsic sleep pattern. Although sleep has been extensively studied, we still have an incomplete understanding of the effect of aging on the incidence and prevalence of sleep-related disorders. The magnitude of sleep-disordered breathing among middle-aged adults has been highlighted (Young et al. 1993), and although in this study, aging appeared not to influence the prevalence of these disorders, the age group studied was 30–60 years old. In a review of the epidemiology of sleep disorders, the prevalence of sleep apnea in healthy elderly adults varied widely from zero to 75%. Most studies report values of 20–50%, suggesting that sleep apnea by itself is present in a high percentage of healthy seniors. Although respiratory disorders during sleep are a major category, sleep disorders cover a wide range of dysfunctions: central and obstructive sleep apneas, hypersomnias, insomnias, and associated neuromuscular and movement disorders (e.g., nocturnal cramps, periodic leg movements in sleep, and restless legs syndrome). Disordered sleep may result from age-related changes, but the clinician must first consider primary sleep disorders and sleep disorders secondary to medical, neurological, and psychiatric disturbances before attributing poor sleeping to the effects of age.

Various constellations of symptoms center on daytime sleepiness and fatigue or altered behavior. These complaints are not specific and may be attributed simply to aging. There is evidence that neuropsychological dysfunction may be adversely affected by oxygen desaturation during sleep disorders. The association of increased frequency of systolic hypertension, myocardial infarctions, and stroke with altered sleep may be a factor in these age-related sleep disorders. An interesting marker of the importance of sleep problems in seniors is the frequency with which disorders of sleep are mentioned as a reason for institutionalization of impaired family members. Seventy percent of caregivers cite nocturnal problems in their decision to place the patient in a long-term care facility. Surprisingly, sleep-related disturbances were rated higher than incontinence as a reason for placement. Only falls and dangerous behavior were listed more frequently. Significantly, the interrupted sleep patterns include those of the caregiver.

Age-related changes in the EEG during sleep remain to be fully characterized. Because changes during wakefulness may alter data collection and interpretations of EEG recordings during sleep, care must be taken to separate aging from disease in these baseline tracings. Age-related changes in the EEG characterization of sleep generally include an increase in stage I and decreases in stages III and IV, which supports an overall decline in slow-wave sleep. Rapid eye movement sleep remains unchanged into the fifth and sixth decade. Older individuals spend more time in bed but less time sleeping. They are also more easily aroused. Aging also tends to shift the sleep-wake cycle so that a phase advance occurs: Seniors tend to fall asleep and awaken earlier. There is a suggestion that the sleep cycle might be re-entrained with the use of bright light, and

Table 86.8: Causes of gait disorders in 50 patients in a neurological referral practice

Diagnosis	Frequency (%)
Myelopathy	16
Cervical spondylosis	
Vitamin B$_{12}$ deficiency	
Parkinsonism	10
Idiopathic Parkinson's disease	
Drug-induced parkinsonism	
Progressive supranuclear palsy	
Frontal gait disorder (gait apraxia)	20
Normal-pressure hydrocephalus	
Multiple strokes	
Binswanger's disease	
Cerebellar degeneration	8
Sensory imbalance	18
Neuropathy	
Multiple sensory deficits	
Toxic or metabolic encephalopathy	6
Other*	8
Undetermined	14
Total	**100**

*Causes include tumors, subdural hematoma, and depression.
Source: Reprinted with permission from L Sudarsky. Geriatrics: gait disorders in the elderly. N Engl J Med 1990;322:1441–1446.

patients with AD may benefit from this therapeutic approach as well.

Neurological clinicians must maintain vigilance about the presence of sleep-related disturbances in older citizens. The clinical picture may initially appear nonspecific: depressive symptoms, increased confusion or altered behavior, increased napping, easy fatigue, or nonspecific aches and pains may all be due to a sleep dysfunction. All too often, such symptoms may be explained away or attributed to aging or to an emotional or psychiatric problem. Seniors may be inappropriately evaluated because a bias of health care providers is that sleep-related disturbances are "part of normal aging." Further complicating the identification of sleep disturbances is that patients may not be aware of their nocturnal difficulties, and unless the spouse or companion is queried, critical historical data are not uncovered. If sleep dysfunction is suspected, nocturnal polysomnography and multiple sleep latency testing are required to establish a diagnosis. Abbreviated tests and home assessment systems provide inaccurate data that may overdiagnose or underdiagnose clinical syndromes.

The clinician reviews the clinical syndrome to diagnose primary disorders of sleep, such as sleep apnea syndromes, restless legs syndrome, and periodic leg movements (nocturnal myoclonus). He or she must also consider general medical illnesses, such as cardiopulmonary disease; pain syndromes, including arthritis; and psychiatric disorders, such as depression, which is often associated with poor sleeping. A number of neurological diseases that increase during aging may alter sleep. These include cerebrovascular disease, dementia (both AD and vascular dementias),

Parkinson's disease, and other neurodegenerative disorders, such as Shy-Drager syndrome and olivopontocerebellar atrophies. The importance of the neurological diseases is that some of them are associated with nocturnal respiratory failure and death. For a fuller discussion of sleep disorders, see Chapter 72.

Disorders of Movement

Strength and speed of movement decrease with increasing age. Many factors contribute to the decline. Alterations in the motor unit include reductions in the size and possibly the proportion of type II muscle fibers with advancing age. In addition, the oxidative capacity of exercising old muscle is less than that of young muscle. Finally, the number of alpha motor neurons in cervical and lumbar spinal cord decreases. Because both speed and strength require integration of central mechanisms, fewer cells in the motor cortex along with the decrease in the dendritic tree of pyramidal neurons and reduced synapses in the frontal cortex (layer III) probably contribute to the clinical picture. Also, the aforementioned changes in the substantia nigra and cerebellum contribute to the altered integration. Systemic changes, such as degenerative changes in the spine and joints, alter posture, cause pain, and, thus, slow movement.

Gait Disorders

No age-related neurological changes are as obvious as those related to gait and stance. Almost all people maintain a similar gait from early childhood to approximately 65–70 years. Older individuals tend to be slower and less steady. Minor obstacles that go unnoticed by young people may topple the senior. Approximately 50% of people older than 85 years have mild extrapyramidal signs, stooped posture, and reduced arm swing and turn en bloc.

Abnormal gaits observed in people younger than 65 years are well characterized: Hemiparesis, paraparesis, ataxia, extrapyramidal disorders, proprioceptive loss from peripheral nerve or spinal cord disease, and weakness from nerve or root lesions all produce fairly specific alterations of gait. The same syndromes that alter gait in the young account for most of the gait disorders of seniors (Table 86.8). (For a fuller discussion of gait disorders, see Chapter 26.)

Some gaits in seniors are well characterized, including those resulting from Parkinson's disease, spastic paraparesis from cervical spondylotic myelopathy, and cerebellar ataxia. Others are less well defined, including frontal gait disorder, marche à petits pas, gaits with associated nonparkinsonian extrapyramidal signs, and the fearful gait. Frontal gait disorder is a poorly characterized syndrome that appears to be common in the old and virtually nonexistent in the young. Nutt and colleagues. (1993) offered a framework to help clarify the difficult area of disordered gait in the elderly (Table 86.9).

There are two major components of walking: equilibrium and locomotion. Equilibrium consists of standing and maintaining balance on a narrow base. Locomotion consists of initiating and maintaining rhythmic stepping.

Equilibrium. Many responses and reflexes keep the body upright despite perturbations. Righting reflexes control the muscles responsible for moving the body from a lying or sitting to upright position. The systems responsible for this function receive input from vestibular, proprioceptive, visual, and touch receptors. Supporting reactions maintain the center of gravity over the feet. Anticipatory reflexes prepare the body posture for the next anticipated action. When the center of gravity deviates more than a certain distance beyond the center of the base formed by the feet, reactive responses are triggered. If the center of gravity is not brought back over the feet, rescue reactions begin. These involve the arms and legs: stepping or swinging the arms. If all these efforts fail, the person falls, and the protective reaction is to push out the arms to break the fall and limit the injury.

Locomotion. Locomotion is divided into two components: gait ignition and stepping. Gait ignition is the initiation of walking from standing still. To begin movement, the center of gravity first shifts onto one foot to allow the other to be raised. Then the center of gravity moves forward. Stepping is the rhythmic, alternating movement of the legs. All patients should be observed arising from a chair, standing, withstanding a push, initiating walking, during locomotion, and negotiating turns.

Most clinical studies of gaits have focused on static balance and posture or case reports of diseases that result in abnormal movement. The more difficult problem of the dynamics of walking is largely unstudied.

Falls

Falls are common, and the prevalence increases with advancing age. Some reports suggest that women have a higher frequency of falls than do men. Approximately 30% of people over the age of 65 years living in community fall, and more than 50% of nursing home residents fall. Falls are responsible for significant morbidity and mortality. They cause hip fracture and hospitalization. When patients fall, they reduce their activity because of fear of additional falls. The reduced activity leads to further disability. Falls may result from gait disorders, but most elders who fall do not have disorders of gait. Environmental factors are responsible for one-half of falls. These include surface abnormalities, such as slippery, sticky, or uneven floors; obstacles; poor lighting; and distractions. Seizures are a rare cause of falls and are usually readily identified by the clinical history. Transient ischemic attacks only rarely cause falls. Patients who fall as a result of transient ischemic attacks generally have additional symptoms of brainstem ischemia, such as dizziness, diplopia, ataxia, weakness, or sensory changes.

Table 86.9: Classification of gait syndromes

I. Lowest-level gait disorders
  A. Peripheral skeleto-motor problems
    1. Arthritic gait
    2. Myopathic gait
    3. Peripheral neuropathic gait
  B. Peripheral sensory problems
    1. Sensory ataxic gait
    2. Vestibular ataxic gait
    3. Visual ataxic gait
II. Middle-level gait disorders
  A. Hemiplegic gait
  B. Paraplegic gait
  C. Cerebellar ataxic gait
  D. Parkinsonian gait
  E. Choreic gait (and dystonic gait)
III. Highest-level gait disorders
  A. Cautious gait
  B. Subcortical dysequilibrium
  C. Frontal dysequilibrium
  D. Isolated gait ignition failure
  E. Frontal gait disorder
  F. Hysterical gait

Source: Reprinted with permission from JG Nutt, CD Marsden, PD Thompson. Human walking and higher-level gait disorders, particularly in the elderly. Neurology 1993;43:268–279.

Global reduction in brain perfusion may cause falling. These falls are associated with lightheadedness, vision loss, or loss of consciousness (see Syncope, earlier in this chapter). Common causes are cardiac disease, including arrhythmia and valvular heart disease, and OH. Drop attacks consist of sudden weakness of the postural muscles that cause a fall and, transiently, an inability to get up (see Chapter 3).

Disorders of Autonomic Control

Orthostatic Hypotension

Normally, assumption of the upright position is associated with maintenance of BP; not doing so results in OH. The definition of OH is surprisingly varied, although it is generally defined as a decrease of 20 mm Hg in systolic pressure and 10 mm Hg in diastolic pressure on standing. The frequency of this event in older citizens depends on the criteria used as well as the characteristics of the assessment. For instance, after standing, OH occurs in 10.4% of subjects examined at 1 minute, whereas 12% exhibit such change at 3 minutes. Pooling observations from these time points indicates that approximately 17% of subjects exhibit OH. OH occurs in approximately 20% of subjects older than 65 and in up to 30% of individuals older than 75. Despite many studies, it remains undecided whether OH in seniors is an age-related change or related to additional factors, such as disease, dehydration, and drugs. For instance, if patients with such covariates as hypertension, serious systemic disease, positive history of neurological or cardiac disease, abnormal chest radiograph or treadmill stress test, or multiple medications are excluded from studies, the change in arterial pressure after standing or tilt tests is not substantially different between younger and older individuals. Again we see the familiar theme of disease, other events, and other agents complicating the interpretation of what is an age-related alteration in clinical function. Disease, particularly hypertension, and medication (multiple agents exert a higher risk) are two of the major risk factors for OH in seniors rather than old age itself. Nevertheless, it is important to recognize OH in seniors because a number of adverse events occur in the setting of OH, including falls, fractures, poor overall function, increased morbidity, and mortality. Thus, the diagnosis and treatment of OH may preclude the development of more severe events.

A number of neurological disorders that occur in the elderly are associated with OH. Specifically, the neurodegenerative disorders (e.g., Parkinson's disease, olivopontocerebellar atrophy, and Shy-Drager syndrome), cerebrovascular disease, myelopathy, and peripheral neuropathies (primarily diabetes mellitus) are all associated with orthostasis. A careful history and physical and neurological examination generally indicates the presence of neurological disease as a cause of the OH.

An interesting association exists between meals and OH in older individuals. In young people, there is either no change or an increase in BP after meals, whereas in seniors there may be a decrease in BP. This decrease in BP appears to reach its maximum approximately 30 minutes after a meal, and BP may decline up to 25 mm Hg. This decrease occurs in seniors independent of any history of syncope or medications and is unrelated to specific diagnoses. Occasionally, postprandial syncope may be associated with the decrease in BP; studies of these patients indicate that there is no significant increase in heart rate and only an initial increase in plasma norepinephrine (NE) levels, which is not sustained. Subsequently, NE levels decline and are associated with decreasing BP. In contrast, nonsyncopal seniors exhibit a greater NE response to meals. Thus, symptomatic patients appear to have a failure in sympathetic neurohumoral responses (NE release) and compensatory cardiovascular reflexes (baroreflex-mediated cardioacceleration), which normally occurs after meals, as well as blood pooling in the splanchnic vascular bed. This phenomenon is not unusual, especially in frail elderly. In one study, up to 90% of nursing home residents showed a mean reduction of approximately 18 mm Hg in systolic BP after meals; a decrease of 20 mm Hg occurred in 36%, and 11% had a systolic BP of less than 100 mm Hg. Despite the magnitude of this disorder in these subjects, OH did not presage subsequent adverse effects in the follow-up period of 6 months. Nevertheless, being cognizant of this clinical syndrome should permit education of patients and staff and the institution of preventive measures to prevent falls and fractures, the risk of which may be increased with ambulation after meals.

Therapeutic approaches to OH in seniors should initially include identifying and altering the major determinants of OH (medications, fluid balance and nutrition, activity, and disease states). Because medications are a major etiological factor, all medication (prescription and over the counter) should be carefully reviewed, which may permit some to be discontinued and the regimens of some to be altered. After appropriate adjustments in medications or treatment for dehydration or changes related to disease, OH may improve and no further workup or treatment may be necessary. Enhanced physical activity, improved cardiovascular conditioning, and education about avoiding rapid changes in position also decreases the frequency and extent of BP changes. If OH persists and is associated with symptoms, it should be treated because it places the patient at an increased risk of adverse consequences (falls, fractures). Nonpharmacological approaches may be recommended. These include increasing fluid and salt intake (if congestive heart failure and hypertension are not present), exercise, support hose (especially elastic stockings that cover the thigh), and elevating the head of the bed (approximately 10–15 degrees) because the supine position predisposes to deconditioning of already dysfunctional orthostatic reflexes.

Pharmacological approaches include agents that alter prostaglandin synthesis and prostaglandin-mediated vasodilatation, the mineralocorticoid fludrocortisone, and sympathomimetic agents, such as α-receptor agonists. NSAIDs should be tried first because they have few side effects. Indomethacin at 100 mg twice daily may be effective. Newer NSAID agents have fewer gastrointestinal complications and are usually tried before indomethacin. Fludrocortisone is a popular choice if nonpharmacological means do not work. Adverse effects of this mineralocorticoid include supine hypertension, potassium loss, and fluid retention, resulting in congestive heart failure. Most patients respond to 0.1–0.6 mg daily, although a dose of 1.0–1.2 mg may be tried in refractory patients. Sympathomimetics, including α-receptor agonists, such as ergot alkaloids, phenylpropanolamine, midodrine, and caffeine, are suggested for postprandial hypotension (Low 1993).

Urinary Incontinence

The prevalence of UI in the elderly population is substantial: Estimates of UI in community-dwelling seniors are in the range of 5–34% (most authorities would accept a 10% prevalence in the well elderly), whereas in patients requiring institutional care, the prevalence may approach 50–60%. Incontinence may be transient, with 30–40% of patients recovering over a period of months to a year, depending on the etiology. The high rate in nursing homes relates to increased impairment of mobility and functional status, usually cognitive dysfunction, in these individuals. Nevertheless, UI may be the precipitating cause of admission to long-term care facilities in up to 89% of patients who have been receiving home care for chronic diseases. Patients with neurological diseases, such as AD, Parkinson's disease, or stroke, are often cared for at home until incontinence appears. At this point, the added burden may be more than the care provider is able to accept and results in institutionalization. The cost of UI is staggering: $3–5 billion are spent annually to manage the overall clinical and social costs of these patients. In addition, the psychosocial and hygienic issues related to an inability to control urine function may be devastating and result in increased isolation and depression for senior citizens.

Neurologists assess disorders of micturition in seniors to determine whether an alteration in neurological function may underlie the bladder dysfunction. The major causes of UI in seniors without known neurological disease are usually related to dysfunction of the lower urinary tract and include alterations in the musculature of the pelvic floor and structural changes in the bladder and its outflow tract. Nevertheless, because the nervous system integrates the neural and muscular structures that account for bladder function and because the dysfunction dictates different diagnostic and therapeutic choices, neurological assessment is critical in these patients. Bladder control depends on intact peripheral pathways, which provide sensory information about bladder fullness, and cortical control systems, which permit proper behavioral choices with voiding. It also depends on an integration system in the rostral pons (pontine micturition center), which receives sensory afferents and projects efferent reticulospinal pathways to the thoracolumbar and sacral autonomic areas affecting the detrusor reflex. Descending voluntary pathways from the mesial frontal cortex, which permits voluntary control over sacral motor neurons innervating the external sphincter, are also involved, as are peripheral efferents from the sacral autonomic and motor neurons, which project via the pelvic and pudendal nerves to innervate their appropriate targets. Thus, both peripheral and central lesions may interrupt the numerous circuits involved in bladder control and result in disorders of storage or release of urine. The clinical approach includes the neurological examination to assess for central and peripheral lesions, with particular attention paid to cognitive assessment and judgment, intraspinal pathways, and the sensory and motor pathways in the pelvis. Specifically, although such reflexes as the bulbocavernosus reflex may not correlate well with UI in the elderly, characterization of the sacral arcs involved in control of rectum and bladder and subserving sensory innervation of the perineum are important in evaluating incontinence.

The clinical picture of incontinence related to lesions at various levels of the neuraxis is discussed in Chapter 43. Clinical classifications of incontinence generally place neurological disorders in the *urge* and *overflow* categories. Urge incontinence is the result of not inhibiting the urge to void, and urine leakage occurs. These subjects perceive a full bladder but are unable to inhibit the micturition reflex long enough to get to a bathroom. Lesions interrupting frontal pathways, which inhibit the micturition reflex and excite pudendal motor neurons (both of which promote continence), result in urge incontinence and are usually the result of vascular disease. Neurodegenerative disorders, such as AD and Parkinson's disease, also interrupt the frontal control systems. Communicating hydrocephalus also compromises frontal fibers as they course along the lateral ventricles to brainstem and spinal sites. These lesions alter the ability to inhibit detrusor contractions. Spinal lesions above the level of the sacral cord may also produce this picture.

The International Continence Society terms the detrusor hyperactivity (DH) or motor instability resulting from neural dysfunction *detrusor hyperreflexia*. The more generic term, *DH*, is used to describe the same phenomenon when the etiology is unclear. Neurological disorders are not the only cause of urge incontinence because it occurs in association with urinary tract infection (cystitis and urethritis), bladder stones and diverticuli, and outflow obstruction, as in prostatic disease. DH due to such non-neurological disorders may also be termed *detrusor instability*. A subset of elderly patients with DH cannot empty their bladders. Normally, there is a relatively parallel change in bladder contraction and reflex integration, resulting in the bladder emptying more than 75% of its content. In approximately 33% of elderly institutionalized patients, bladder emptying was ineffective, and only 17% of the bladder volume was evacuated. This clinical picture is termed *DH with impaired contraction* (DHIC). The pathophysiology of this disorder remains to be fully clarified.

Patients with neurological disease are equally represented in subjects with DH and DHIC; therefore, clinically apparent neurological dysfunction does not appear to underlie DHIC. However, subtle changes in central integrating pathways, or changes in the peripheral autonomic neurons and neuromuscular synapses in the bladder and the sphincter muscles, would not be detected with current methods. Local changes in the bladder may eventually result in DHIC. It is important to consider DHIC because these patients may be at increased risk for urinary retention with therapeutic approaches to reduce the excitability of the detrusor.

The second type of incontinence that neural lesions may produce is overflow incontinence, the leakage of small amounts of urine from an overdistended bladder that is unable to empty properly. These patients may or may not feel the distended bladder and report the discomfort. The bladder may not contract secondary to lesions of the afferent or efferent peripheral nerves or the sacral autonomic centers controlling micturition. The bladder may contract but not fully empty, resulting in overflow. Supraspinal lesions (lesions rostral to the sacral cord) are the most common cause of this disorder, which is generally referred to as *detrusor-sphincter dyssynergy*. In seniors, vascular or compressive myelopathies, such as those due to cervical spondylosis, may be the most common cause of neurological overflow incontinence. Local changes in the pelvic anatomy that cause obstruction, such as prostate enlargement, urethral stricture, or a cystocele, may also cause overflow incontinence. In fact, these structural changes are more frequently the cause of this type of UI than are neural lesions in the older population.

The two other major categories of UI that relate to seniors are stress and functional incontinence. Stress incontinence is the involuntary loss of urine associated with increases in intra-abdominal pressure, usually occurring in the setting of exercise, lifting, laughing, or sneezing. Occasionally, the problem may be postural in character, with incontinence resulting on standing. The most frequent dysfunction resulting in this type of incontinence is weakness of the pelvic floor musculature and alterations in bladder outlet (sphincter) mechanisms. Functional incontinence results when subjects are unable to get to the toilet for proper voiding, usually secondary to altered mobility, or environmental factors, are cognitively impaired, and are either unable to find the bathroom or can no longer comprehend the functional needs. Elderly patients with Parkinson's disease may be unable to get to the toilet in time, and with an urge component also present, they are dually susceptible for UI. As patients with dementia progress, alterations in higher intellectual function may result in patients being unable to locate a bathroom or control urination. In severe dementia, patients may not be aware of their own incontinence.

More than one form of UI may occur in the same patient. In a review of 263 women and men older than 65 who were referred for evaluation, the symptoms of stress and urge incontinence occurred separately in 2–16%, whereas both symptom complexes were present in 68–82% of subjects. In another study of institutionalized patients, 35% of incontinent subjects exhibited more than one possible cause. Thus, assuming that the incontinence is related to the primary neurological disease is not tenable. Accordingly, careful assessment of patients is required, and even quite severely impaired AD patients are able to participate in these clinical evaluations.

The clinical approach to UI includes history and physical examination, with particular attention to the pelvic, rectal, and neurological examinations. Careful history taking should focus on characterizing the nature of the incontinence and determining whether a neurological disorder might be present and contributing to UI, as in urge and overflow incontinence. The rectal and pelvic examinations are important to evaluate local anatomical changes associated with UI, such as cystocele and rectocele. The neurological examination should focus on higher intellectual function and the motor system, including corticospinal and striatal motor system in patients with presumed functional incontinence. Motor and sensory system examinations, including the long tract signs and signs of myelopathy, indicate whether intraspinal or supraspinal lesions may be responsible. Both urge and overflow incontinence may result from such lesions. In addition to evaluating sphincter tone, the rectal examination should include a request for the patient to cough, to determine if there is reflex contraction of the rectum, and to voluntarily contract the rectum to examine for voluntary sphincter control. Last, the bulbocavernosus reflex may be examined because rectal sphincter contraction occurs after noxious stimulation of the penis or clitoris. If a catheter is in place, this reflex may be initiated by tugging the catheter. The anal reflex or wink (mediated by sacral roots S4-S5) may be examined, although its absence does not necessarily correlate with UI, and these reflexes may be absent in some normal elderly. Examination of perineal sensation also permits an assessment of sensory afferents. Because sacral roots S2-S4 innervate both the external urethral and anal sphincters, the integrity of sacral levels subserving bladder reflexes may be easily assessed on rectal examination. Examination of other peripheral nerves and reflexes indicates whether peripheral neuropathy may be contributing to the lack of urinary control.

Although urodynamic studies may eventually be needed, by careful collection of clinical data, a noninvasive approach may permit accurate diagnosis in a high percentage of patients. However, if the neurologist is not familiar with the more dynamic and functional aspects of assessing incontinence, referral to an incontinence clinic for urodynamic, gynecological, or urological examinations may be needed. Such studies have led to interesting observations. For instance, a substantial percentage of normal seniors have uninhibited detrusor contractions, particularly men. However, the mere presence of DH does not cause UI. Also, bladder capacity does not necessarily change with age unless uninhibited detrusor contractions are present. Last, postvoid residual volume does not correlate with UI, and surprisingly, the residual volume may be as high as 150 ml without associated UI.

The acronym DIAPPERS (delirium or confusional state, infection, atrophic urethritis or vaginitis, pharmaceuticals, psychological, endocrine, restricted mobility, stool impaction) summarizes the clinical approach to reversible factors or causes of UI. Table 86.10 summarizes the factors necessary for evaluating seniors with UI. These issues are important because they may either be the sole explanation for UI in the acute care setting or complicate bladder control in more chronic states. Stress incontinence is the most frequent cause of UI in women less than 75 years of age, whereas urge incontinence is more frequent in women older than 75 years. Overflow incontinence is present in probably less than 10% of seniors. Functional incontinence becomes a major diagnostic consideration in patients with neurological disorders that alter mental status and mobility.

Treatment of UI in seniors depends on determining the class of UI and the potential etiologies of the dysfunction. Primary neurological disorders require identification and treatment, and the management of UI may improve with enhanced functional ability of the patient. After treatment of the neurological illness, a number of additional

Table 86.10: Causes of transient incontinence

Delirium or confusional state
Infection—urinary (symptomatic)
Atrophic urethritis or vaginitis
Pharmaceuticals
Psychological, especially depression
Endocrine (hypercalcemia, hyperglycemia)
Restricted mobility
Stool impaction

Source: Reprinted with permission from NM Resnick. Noninvasive diagnosis of the patient with complex incontinence. Gerontology 1990; 36(Suppl. 2):8–18. With permission from S Karger AG, Basel.

Table 86.11: Primary treatments for different types of geriatric urinary incontinence

Type of incontinence	Primary treatments
Stress	Pelvic muscle (Kegel) exercises
	α-Adrenergic agonists
	Estrogen
	Biofeedback, behavioral training
	Surgical bladder neck suspension
Urge	Bladder relaxants
	Estrogen (if atrophic vaginitis)
	Training procedures (e.g., biofeedback, behavioral therapy)
	Surgical removal of obstructing or other irritating pathological lesions
Overflow	Surgical removal of obstruction
	Intermittent catheterization
	Indwelling catheterization
Functional	Behavioral therapies (e.g., prompted voiding, scheduled toileting)
	Environmental manipulations
	Incontinence undergarments and pads
	Bladder relaxants*
	External catheters
	Indwelling catheters*

*Selected patients.
Source: Reprinted with permission from JG Ouslander. Geriatric urinary incontinence. Dis Mon 1992;2:65–149.

approaches may be applied; the basic treatment approaches are outlined in Table 86.11. Pharmacological intervention may be beneficial. The range of agents and their selection depend on the presumed type of UI (Table 86.12). In brief, stress incontinence in men and women may be improved with exercise programs, estrogens in women to strengthen periurethral tissues, and α-agonists, which enhance internal sphincter strength. Urge incontinence may respond to anticholinergic medications, although the potential of retention should be recognized in those with DHIC. Because UI secondary to primary neurological events is usually associated with central lesions (e.g. stroke or system disorders, such as AD and Parkinson's disease) and causes DH with high-pressure uninhibited detrusor contractions, anticholinergic medications are the treatment of choice. The side effects of these medications must be monitored closely because in some situations they may exacerbate incontinence. Urge and overflow incontinence secondary to outlet obstruction may be managed with alpha-blocking agents, such as prazosin, or parasympathomimetics in situations wherein the contractile response is weak (detrusor hyporesponsiveness). Because up to 30% of subjects have mixed incontinence, a number of therapeutic interventions may have to be tried to effect a satisfactory response. Many pharmacological interventions may not produce substantial improvement and result in unacceptable side effects. In many situations, the use of intermittent catheterization in men and women or external clamps and collecting devices in men may be an acceptable alternative in managing UI.

Fecal Incontinence

Fecal incontinence (involuntary emptying of the rectum) implies dysfunction of the neural or muscular systems involved in normal bowel motility, control, and evacuation. Because areas of the neuraxis similar to those controlling bladder function are involved in the control of the rectum, fecal incontinence may accompany UI. The exact frequency of this association is not clear, but it probably approaches 25%. The neurological pathophysiology of fecal incontinence includes lesions of the mesial frontal lobes in the area

of the paracentral lobules, the descending tracts from these frontal control areas, and myelopathies, with interruption of control systems as they descend to the sacral area. Lesions of the sacral cord and peripheral neuropathies result in an inability to empty the rectum, with resultant leakage of liquid stool around impacted stool in the distended rectum.

As with UI, fecal incontinence in the geriatric age group more frequently results from non-neurological causes. For instance, chronic constipation with fecal impaction and secondary leakage of stool content is a common cause. Laxative abuse frequently underlies incontinence of stool. Previous surgeries for benign or malignant conditions, radiation therapy to the pelvis for malignancies, the presence of local disease involving the sacral outflow or muscular structures, and colorectal disorders may all result in primary fecal incontinence or constipation with secondary incontinence (Table 86.13). Disease processes interrupting supraspinal, spinal, and peripheral mechanisms controlling evacuation must be excluded.

Treatment of fecal incontinence rests with treating the underlying disorder. In patients with a combination of constipation and fecal incontinence, treatment is directed at constipation and may require strategic use of laxatives and enemas. Treatment may also include behavioral programs, including taking advantage of the gastrocolic reflex (the reflex activation of bowel evacuation after eating) by placing patients on the toilet shortly after eating. This reflex is active in children, but societal dictates result in control being exerted. Patients with diffuse brain disease, such as

Table 86.12: Examples of drugs used to treat urinary incontinence

Drug	Dosage	Mechanisms of action	Types of incontinence	Potential adverse effects
Anticholinergic and antispasmodic agents				
Tolterodine (Detrol)	1–2 mg bid	Increase bladder capacity	Urge with detrusor instability or hyper-reflexia	Dry mouth, blurry vision, elevated intraocular pressure, delirium, constipation
Oxybutynin (Ditropan)	2.5–5.0 mg tid	Increase bladder capacity	Urge with detrusor instability or hyperreflexia	Dry mouth, blurry vision, elevated intraocular pressure, delirium, constipation
Propantheline (Pro-Banthine)	15–30 mg tid	Increase bladder capacity	Urge with detrusor instability or hyperreflexia	Dry mouth, blurry vision, elevated intraocular pressure, delirium, constipation
Dicyclomine (Bentyl)	10–20 mg tid	Diminish involuntary bladder contractions	Urge with detrusor instability or hyperreflexia	Dry mouth, blurry vision, elevated intraocular pressure, delirium, constipation
Flavoxate (Urispas)	100–200 mg tid	Smooth muscle relaxation	Urge with detrusor instability or hyperreflexia	Dry mouth, blurry vision, elevated intraocular pressure, delirium, constipation
Imipramine (Tofranil)	25–50 mg tid	Increase bladder capacity	Stress or urgency	Dry mouth, blurry vision, elevated intraocular pressure, delirium, constipation, postural hypotension, cardiac conduction disturbances
α-Adrenergic agonists				
Pseudoephedrine	15–30 mg tid	Increase urethral smooth muscle contraction	Stress with sphincter weakness	Headache, tachycardia, elevation of blood pressure
Phenylpropanolamine	75 mg bid	Increase urethral smooth muscle contraction	Stress with sphincter weakness	Headache, tachycardia, elevation of blood pressure
Imipramine (Tofranil)	25–50 mg tid	Increase urethral smooth muscle contraction and bladder capacity	Stress with sphincter weakness	Headache, tachycardia, elevation of blood pressure
Conjugated estrogens[a]				
Oral (Premarin)	0.300–0.625 mg/day	Increase periurethral blood flow Strengthen periurethral tissues	Stress Urge associated with atrophic vaginitis	Endometrial cancer, elevated blood pressure, gallstones
Topical	0.5–1.0 g/application	Same as above	Same as above	None of significance
Cholinergic agonists				
Bethanechol[b]	10–30 mg tid	Stimulate bladder contraction	Overflow with acontractile bladder	Bradycardia, hypotension, bronchoconstriction, gastric acid secretion
α-Adrenergic antagonist				
Prazosin (Minipress)[c]	1–2 mg tid	Relax smooth muscle of urethra and prostatic capsule	Overflow or urge associated with prostatic enlargement	Postural hypotension

[a]With prolonged use, cyclical administration with a progestational agent should be considered in women with a uterus. Transdermal preparations are also available but have not been studied for treating incontinence.
[b]The efficacy of chronic bethanechol therapy is controversial.
[c]May provide some symptomatic relief in patients who are unwilling or unable to undergo prostatectomy.
Source: Reprinted with permission from JG Ouslander. Geriatric urinary incontinence. Dis Mon 1992;2:65–149.

Table 86.13: Etiologies of fecal incontinence

Neurological causes
   Stroke
   Neurodegenerative disorders
      Alzheimer's disease
      Frontal lobe dementias
      Parkinson's disease
   Myelopathy
      Extradural tumor
      Cervical spondylosis
      Lower motor neuron disorders
   Peripheral neuropathy
      Diabetes mellitus
      Infiltrative processes in sacral plexus
Medical causes
   Medication
   Laxatives
   Hyperosmotic feeding regimens
   Colorectal disorders
Structural causes
   Impaction
   Sphincter injury
   Pelvic surgery

AD, may no longer inhibit the reflex and have fecal incontinence after meals.

NEUROLOGISTS AS PRINCIPAL CARE PROVIDERS

Geriatric medicine appears to have confirmed the view proposed by Young in 1989, "There is no such thing as geriatric medicine, and it's here to stay." Will geriatric neurology follow the same course? It is difficult to say. Are neurologists consultants? Are neurologists currently serving as principal care providers for certain disorders (e.g., epilepsy, muscular dystrophy, multiple sclerosis, migraine, Parkinson's disease, AD)? If so, is neurology a principal care specialty? Because, as society successfully ages and more citizens reach the MLS, which approaches 80 years of age, many older citizens experience neurodegenerative disorders, such as AD and Parkinson's disease. The number of individuals with problems in the realm of geriatric neurology will continue to increase. Will neurologists see these patients for diagnostic reasons only? Will primary care providers manage therapy and seek input from neurologists only when situations become dire? In many ways, neurologists are better prepared for a role as a major care provider for older citizens than physicians considered primary care providers. This is true because the disorders are neurological, the fundamental knowledge base of clinical neuroscience is part of clinical training only in neurology. Other reasons are that the necessary clinical skills and assessment strategies require detailed knowledge and experience with the nervous system, and the evolving therapies are based on substantial knowledge of basic neuroscience and neuropharmacology.

As health care becomes more integrated, clinical care teams will develop, and neurologists will need to be part of the care teams for seniors. Conceivably, the primary care and preventive aspects of care for seniors may be delivered by generalists or nurse practitioners while the neurologist manages the care needs for the primary disorder, which for many seniors is a neurological dysfunction. Thus, training programs in neurology must ensure that neurologists have experience in caring for older citizens.

REFERENCES

Albert ML, Knoefel JE. Clinical Neurology of Aging. New York: Oxford University Press, 1994.

Albert MS. Age-Related Changes in Cognitive Function. In ML Albert, JE Knoefel (eds), Clinical Neurology of Aging. New York: Oxford University Press, 1994.

Albert MS. Predictors of cognitive change in older persons: MacArthur studies of successful aging. Psychol Aging 1995;10: 578–730.

Barclay L. Clinical Geriatric Neurology. Philadelphia: Lea & Febiger, In press.

Bennett DA, Beckett LA, Murray AM, et al. Prevalence of Parkinsonian signs and associated mortality in a community population of older people. N Engl J Med 1996;334:71–76.

Buchanan A. Philosophic perspectives on access to health care: distributive justice in health care. Mt Sinai J Med 1997;64:90–95.

Camicioli RM, Kaye JA, Brummel-Smith K. Recognition of neurologic diseases in geriatric inpatients. Acta Neurol Scand 1998; 97:265–270.

Diagnostic and Statistical Manual of Mental Disorders (4th ed). Washington, DC: American Psychiatric Association, 1994.

Drachman DA. New criteria for the diagnosis of vascular dementia: Do we know enough yet? Neurology 1993;43:243–245.

Drachman DA. Aging and the brain: a new frontier. Ann Neurol 1997;42:819–828.

Fleming KC, Evans JM, Weber DC, Chutka DS. Practical functional assessment of elderly persons: a primary care approach. Mayo Clin Proc 1995;70:890–910.

Flicker C, Ferris, SH, Reisberg B. A longitudinal study of cognitive function in elderly persons with subjective memory complaints. J Am Geriatr Soc 1993;41:1029–1032.

Goldblatt D. Advance directives. Semin Neurol 1997;17:287–289.

Gomez-Isla T, West HL, Reveck GW, et al. Clinical and pathological correlates of apolipoprotein E epsilon 4 in Alzheimer's disease. Ann Neurol 1996;39:62–70.

Haber JG. Philosophic perspectives on access to health care: putting the care into health care. Mt Sinai J Med 1997;64: 96–100.

Hanninen T, Reinikainen KJ, Helkala EL, et al. Subjective memory complaints and personality traits in normal elderly subjects. J Am Geriatr Soc 1994;42:1–4.

Hauser WA. Epidemiology of Seizures and Epilepsy in the Elderly. In AJ Rowan, RE Ramsay (eds), Seizures and Epilepsy in the Elderly. Boston: Butterworth–Heinemann, 1997;7–18.

Hesdorffer DC, Hauser WA, Annegers JF, et al. Dementia and adult onset unprovoked seizures. Neurology 1996;46:727–730.

Howieson DB, Holm LA, Kaye JA, et al. Neurologic function in the optimally healthy oldest old: neuropsychological evaluation. Neurology 1993;43:1882–1886.

Inouye SK, Wagner DR, Acampora D, et al. A controlled trial of a nursing-centered intervention in hospitalized elderly medical patients: the Yale Geriatric Care Program. J Am Geriatr Soc 1993;41:1353–1360.

Jorm AF, Christensen H, Henderson AS, et al. Complaints of cognitive decline in the elderly: a comparison of reports by subjects and informants in a community survey. Psychol Med 1994;24: 365–374.

Kapoor WN. Syncope in older persons. J Am Geriatr Soc 1994;42: 426–436.

Kaye JA. Oldest-old health brain function. Arch Neurol 1997;54: 1217–1221.

Kaye JA, Oken BS, Howieson DB, et al. Neurologic evaluation of the optimally healthy oldest old. Arch Neurol 1994;51: 1205–1211.

Knapp MJ, Knopman DS, Solomon PR, et al. A 30-week randomized controlled trial of high-dose tacrine in patients with Alzheimer's disease. JAMA 1994;271:985–991.

Lachs MS, Pillemer K. Abuse and neglect of elderly persons. N Engl J Med 1995;332:437–443.

Lopez OL, Becker JT, Jungreis CA, et al. Computed tomography—but not magnetic resonance imaging—identified periventricular white-matter lesions predict symptomatic cerebrovascular disease in probable Alzheimer's disease. Arch Neurol 1995;52:659–664.

Low PA. Neurogenic Orthostatic Hypotension. In RT Johnson, JW Griffin (eds), Current Therapy in Neurologic Disease. St. Louis: Mosby–Year Book, 1993;21–26.

Marson DC, McInturff B, Hawkins L, et al. Consistency of physician judgments of capacity to consent in mild Alzheimer's disease. J Am Geriatr Soc 1997;45:453–457.

Masoro E. Aging: Current Concepts. In E Masoro (ed), Handbook of Physiology Aging. New York: Oxford University Press, 1995.

Nutt JG, Marsden CD, Thompson PD. Human walking and higher-level gait disorders, particularly in the elderly. Neurology 1993;43:268–279.

Odenheimer G, Funkenstein HH, Beckett L, et al. Comparison of neurologic changes in "successfully aging" persons vs. the total aging population. Arch Neurol 1994;51:573–580.

Richelson E. Pharmacology of antidepressants—characteristics of the ideal drug. Mayo Clin Proc 1994;69:1071–1081.

Rivlin M. Can age-based rationing of health care be morally justified? Mt Sinai J Med 1997;64:113–119.

Rowe JW, Kahn RL. Successful Aging. New York: Pantheon, 1998.

Sage JI, Mark MH. Practical Neurology of the Elderly. New York: Dekker, 1996.

Scheuer ML, Cohen J. Seizures and Epilepsy in the Elderly. In O Devinsky (ed), Neurologic Clinics. Epilepsy I: Diagnosis and Treatment. Philadelphia: Saunders, 1993;787–804.

Schochet SS. Neuropathology of Aging. In J Riggs (ed), Neurologic Clinics. The Neurology of Aging. Philadelphia: Saunders, 1998;569–580.

Schofield PW, Jacobs D, Marder K, et al. The validity of new memory complaints in the elderly. Arch Neurol 1997;543:756–759.

Solomon PR, Hirschoff A, Kelly B, et al. A 7-minute neurocognitive screening battery highly sensitive to Alzheimer's disease. Arch Neurol 1998;53:349–355.

Vita AJ, Terry RB, Humbert HB, Fries JF. Aging, Health Risks, and Cumulative Disability. N Engl J Med 1998;338:1035–1041.

Whitehouse PJ. Dementia. Philadelphia: Davis, 1993.

Young T, Palta M, Dempsey J, et al. The occurrence of sleep-disordered breathing among middle-aged adults. N Engl J Med 1993;328:1230–1235.

INDEX

In this index, the letter "t" after a page number represents a table,
"f" represents a figure, and "cp" represents a color plate.

deep, 153
ideational, 694, 696f
lexical or surface, 153
motor, 695, 696f
in developmental disorders, 1591
phonological, 153, 687
Agyria, 1580
AIDS. *See* Human immunodeficiency virus
(HIV) infection and acquired
immunodeficiency syndrome (AIDS)
Air conduction in hearing, 737, 738
Air embolism, cerebral ischemia in, 1148
Airways
management of
in craniocerebral trauma, 1059–1060
in neurointensive care, 919–923
in spinal cord trauma, 1102
upper, resistance in, 1797, 1797f
Akathisia, 337
acute, 337
differential diagnosis in, 1800, 1801t
drug-induced, 1921t, 1922
tardive, 337, 1924
Akinesia, 117–119, 320
directional, 118, 119
endo-evoked and exo-evoked, 118, 119
eye movements in, 118–119
investigations in, 339t
limb, 118, 119, 121
and mutism, 38, 73, 121
pathophysiology of, 121–123
and rigidity
gait in, 343, 345, 347–348
in parkinsonism, 320–324,
1891–1905
spatial, 118
testing for, 118–119
types of, 118
Akinetopsia, cerebral, 693
β-Alaninemia, 1605t
Albendazole
in ascariasis, 1402
in cysticercosis, 1396
in echinococcosis, 1397
in gnathostomiasis, 1399
in strongyloidiasis, 1402
Albinism, 731
ocular, 731
oculocutaneous, 731
Albumin, cerebrospinal fluid levels in
multiple sclerosis, 1450, 1450t
Alcohol nerve block in trigeminal neuralgia,
1873–1874
Alcohol use and alcoholism, 1506t
amblyopia in, 1507
ataxia in, 316, 347, 1507, 1940
chronic progressive, 316
autonomic disorders in, 2139
blood levels of alcohol in, 53–54
cerebellar disorders in, 1940
degenerative, 316, 670, 1507–1508
and cluster headaches, 1864
cognitive function in, 1742
coma in, 53–54
craniocerebral trauma in, 1078
dementia in, 1742
folate deficiency in, 1499

glutamate and excitatory amino acids
in, 875t
hypothermia in, 1543
liver disease in, 1026f
Marchiafava-Bignami disease in, 1507
neuropathy in, 1506–1507, 2111–2112
nicotinic acid deficiency in, 1501
nutritional disorders in, 1505–1508,
2112
in pregnancy, 2253, 2253t
serotonin in, 887, 888t
sleep disorders in, 67, 68
thiamine deficiency in, 1940, 2112
in tremor, 1906, 1907
Wernicke-Korsakoff syndrome in, 1503,
1505, 1940
Aldosterone serum levels, 2150
in sleep cycle, 1784f
Alertness, 25, 37
in coma, 46
in delirium, 26, 27
Alexander's law, 246
Alexia, 151–152, 156, 686
acquired, 686
and agraphia, 151–153, 154t
in Broca's aphasia, 145, 151
central, 686
in cerebrovascular disorders, 151, 156,
1131
in posterior cerebral artery infarction,
1135
deep, 151–152, 686
developmental, 686, 1590–1591
diagnosis of, 1590, 1590t
features of, 154t
atypical, 1591, 1591t
letter-by-letter, 151
neglect, 686
peripheral, 686
phonological, 152, 686
primary, 686
pure, 134
surface, 151
treatment of, 1591
Alien hand syndrome, 73
Alkalosis, respiratory, with metabolic
acidosis, 1547, 1547f
Alleles, 778
Allesthesia, 120
Allochiria, motor, 120
Allodynia, 417, 2054, 2055
Allopurinol in Chagas' disease, 1393
Allyl chloride exposure, 1512
Alpers' disease, 1635
Alpha rhythm in electroencephalography,
474, 474f, 928f
in coma, 482, 483f, 1472
Alprostadil in erectile dysfunction, 756
Altitude changes
insomnia in, 1791
sickness in, 1020, 1467
Aluminum
in dialysis dementia, 1484, 1741
occupational exposure to, 1516
Alzheimer type II astrocytes
in hepatic encephalopathy, 1481
in Wilson's disease, 1925

Alzheimer's disease, 1703–1712, 1731
acetylcholine in, 879, 880t
biochemistry in, 1710
clinical features in, 1704–1705
cost of care in, 2271
course and prognosis in, 1712
diagnosis of
accuracy of, 1707
informing patient in, 2272
early-onset, 1706
electroencephalography in, 485,
1706–1707
epidemiology and etiology of, 1711–1712,
2279, 2280, 2280t
ethical issues in, 2271, 2272
familial, 1703–1704, 1706, 1710
genetic factors in, 1703–1704, 1706,
1706f, 1710
evaluation of, 2281, 2281t
heterogeneity of, 1706
historical aspects of, 1703–1704
incidence of, 2270
laboratory studies in, 1706–1707, 2280
language in, 153–154, 158, 1704–1705
late-onset, 1706
Lewy bodies in, 1706, 1713
memory in, 1704
and multi-infarct dementia, 2280
neurofibrillary tangles in, 1703, 1709,
1709f
neuroimaging in, 1707, 1708f
functional, 667, 1707
structural, 544, 1707
neuropsychiatric symptoms in, 1705
neuropsychological testing in, 2274, 2275
olfaction in, 265, 266
pathogenesis of, 1710
pathology in, 1707–1709, 1709f
cortical and subcortical, 2279
physical examination in, 1705
seizures in, 1705, 2287
serotonin in, 887, 888t
sleep disorders in, 66, 1807–1808
management of, 1825
polysomnography in, 1816
sundowning in, 1807, 1808
treatment of, 1712, 1715–1717
symptom management in, 862, 865
urinary continence in, 431, 2282
visuospatial skills in, 1705
Amantadine, 1356t
in influenza, 1371
mechanism of action, 882
in multiple sclerosis, 1454
in Parkinson's disease, 1896, 1898, 1898t
Amaurosis
fugax, 188, 1130
in giant cell arteritis, 1841, 1843
Leber's congenital, 730–731
Amblyopia
developmental, 203
nutritional, 191–192, 197, 1507
psychogenic, 729
tobacco-alcohol, 191, 197, 1507
toxic, 191
Ambu bag ventilation in neurointensive care,
919

Ambulation. *See* Gait; Walking
Amebic infections, 1389–1390
American Spinal Injury Association
    classification of spinal cord injury,
      1089, 1090–1092, 1091t, 1093f
Amino acids
  branched-chain, metabolism of, 1603f
    disorders in, 1602–1604, 1604t
  carrier molecules in cerebral capillaries,
    1547
  excitatory
    in amyotrophic lateral sclerosis, 2006
    clinical role of, 875, 875t
  in hepatic encephalopathy, 1480, 1482
  sulfur, metabolism of, 1601f
    disorders in, 1600–1602, 1601t
γ-Aminobutyric acid, 870–876
  chemistry and distribution of, 870
  in embryonic development, 1570, 1571
  in glutaric acidemia, 1602
  in hepatic encephalopathy, 1480
  receptors, 869f, 870
    clinical role of, 870, 871t
    subtypes of, 869f, 870
  in seizures, 870, 871t, 1766
γ-Aminobutyric acid transaminase, 870
trans-1–Aminocyclopentane-
    1,3–dicarboxylic acid, 872, 873
α-Amino-3–hydroxy-5–methylisoxazole-
    4–propionic acid receptors, 871,
    872
  clinical role of, 875
  pharmacology of, 873, 874f
Aminolevulinic acid in porphyria, 1620,
    1621, 2074
Aminolevulinic dehydratase deficiency, por-
    phyria in, 1621t, 2074, 2075, 2075t
Aminophylline, neurologic side effects in
    children, 1039–1040
Amiodarone, neuropathy from, 2117–2118,
    2117t
Amitriptyline
  in migraine, 1858
    menstrual, 1861t
  in multiple sclerosis, 1455
  in pain management, 2055
  in tension-type headache, 1870
  in vascular dementia and depression, 1728
Ammonia blood levels, 1614–1618
  elevated. *See* Hyperammonemia
  in hepatic encephalopathy, 1477,
    1479–1480, 1480f
    management of, 1481–1482
  in lysinuric protein intolerance, 1607
  in methylmalonic acidemia, 1611
Amnesia, 74–76, 679–681
  anterograde, 680
    assessment of, 681
    learning in, 680, 680f
  causes of, 680
  dissociative, 102
  in fugue states, 99–100, 102
  global, 679
    transient, in transient ischemic attack,
      1129–1130
  in hypoxia, 1467, 1469
  in Korsakoff's syndrome, 1505

neuroanatomy in, 74–75, 75f
neuropsychological assessment in, 681
post-traumatic, prognosis in, 1085
psychogenic, 102, 1743
  types of, 102t
rehabilitation in, 993, 994
retention-with-distraction tests in, 679, 680f
retrograde, 679–680
  assessment of, 681
semantic memory in, 679, 681
in shellfish poisoning, 1536t, 1538
transient, 76
  global, in transient ischemic attack,
    1129–1130
Amniotic fluid embolism, 1148
Amobarbital test of language laterality, 682,
    683t
Amoxicillin in Lyme disease, 1337
Amphetamines, 1524
  intracranial hemorrhage from, 1172, 1220
  neuropathy from, 2118
  raphe neuron injury from, 886
Amphotericin B, 1382–1383, 1382t
  in amebic meningoencephalitis, 1390
  in *Aspergillus* infection, 1381
  in blastomycosis, 1380
  in coccidioidomycosis, 1378–1379
  in cryptococcal infections, 1377
    in HIV infection and AIDS, 1418
  dosage of, 1382, 1382t
  in histoplasmosis, 1379–1380
  intrathecal administration of, 1383
  side effects of, 1382
Ampicillin in meningitis, 1319t, 1320, 1321t
Amplitude in nerve conduction studies, 498,
    499
Amputation after peripheral nerve trauma,
    1124
Amsler's grid chart in visual field
    measurement, 725, 726f
Amusia, auditory or sensory, 137
Amyloid deposits, 2096–2097
  in Alzheimer's disease, 1710
  in Down syndrome, 1713
  in peripheral nerves, 2072–2074
Amyloid precursor protein in Alzheimer's
    disease, 1704, 1706, 1706f,
    1707, 1710
  mutation of, 2281, 2281t
  processing of, 1710, 1711f
Amyloidosis, 1023
  amyloid light chain, 2096, 2097
  apolipoprotein A1, 2073
  autonomic nervous system in, 437, 1023,
    2139
  bladder function in, 437
  cerebral angiopathy in, 1148, 1171–1172,
    1173f
    intracranial hemorrhage in, 1172
    vasculitis in, 1233–1234
  familial, 1023
    DNA diagnosis of, 2074
    peripheral neuropathy in, 2072–2074
  gelsolin, 2073
  hypotension in, orthostatic, 2159, 2160
  polyneuropathy in, 1023, 2072–2074. *See
    also* Polyneuropathy, amyloid

primary systemic, 2096–2097
  clinical features in, 2096, 2096f
  laboratory features in, 2096–2097
  macroglossia in, 2096, 2096f
  sural nerve biopsy in, 2097, 2098f
  treatment of, 2097
sensory function in, 419, 424, 424f, 437,
    1023
sexual function in, 437
transthyretin, 2072–2073, 2074
Amyotrophic lateral sclerosis, 391,
    2005–2016
  classification of, 2005, 2006t
  clinical features in, 2007–2009, 2015–2016
  dementia in, 1720, 1733, 2014–2015
    and parkinsonism complex, 2016
  diagnosis of, 2009–2010
  differential diagnosis of, 1995, 1996,
    2002, 2003, 2010, 2091t
  dysarthria in, 175t, 2010
  etiology of, 2005–2007
  familial, 2004, 2005, 2015–2016
    autosomal dominant, 2015
    autosomal recessive juvenile, 2016
  genetic factors in, 2005
    and protein chemistry, 2015
    superoxide dismutase *(SOD1)* mutation
      in, 2005, 2009, 2015–2016
  glutamate excitotoxicity in, 2005–2006
  head drop or droop in, 2007, 2008f, 2013
  home and hospice care in, 2014
  laboratory studies in, 2009, 2010
  natural history of, 2009
  nutrition in, 2008, 2013–2014
  in paraneoplastic syndromes, 1306, 2016
  pathogenesis in, 2015
  prognosis in, 2009
  progressive muscle atrophy in, 1995,
    2002, 2004
  radiculopathies simulating, 2031
  respiratory system in, 2007, 2008, 2014
  sleep disturbances in, 1809
  speech and communication in, 2013
  sporadic, 2005
  treatment and management in, 2010–2014
    approach to patient in, 2010–2011
    of disability, 862–863
    drug therapy in, 2011, 2012t
    ethical and legal issues in, 2011–2012
    physical rehabilitation in, 2012–2013
    of symptoms, 861, 862–863, 2011,
      2012t
    team approach in, 2011
Amyotrophy
  benign focal, 1995–1996
  diabetic, 2026, 2101
  with disinhibition, dementia, and
    parkinsonism, 2017
  hypoglycemic, 2115
  monomelic, 365, 1996
  neuralgic, 444
Anal sphincter
  electromyography of, 748, 749f
  in fecal continence, 429–430, 757
Analgesics, 907–912
  adjuvant, 912
  nonopioid, 907–909, 908t

opioid, 909–912, 1521–1523. *See also*
    Opioids
rebound headache from, 906
Anancastic personality, 90
Anaplasia, 1241
    in astrocytoma, 1243, 1267–1270
    in ependymoma, 1245
    in meningioma, 1248–1249
Anarthria, pure, 684
Anatomical localization of lesion, 6–7
    false localizing signs in, 7
Ancrod in ischemic cerebrovascular disease,
    1159
Andersen's syndrome, 2216
Anemia, 1021–1022
    in folate deficiency, 1499
    in iron deficiency, 1021
        ischemic cerebrovascular disease in, 1153
    macrocytic, 1496–1497
    megaloblastic
        in folate deficiency, 1499
        in vitamin B_{12} deficiency, 1021–1022
    pernicious, 1497, 2112
    sickle cell, 1022
        cerebrovascular disorders in, 1154
        in children, 1041–1042
        ultrasonography in, 660
    in vitamin B_{12} deficiency, 1021–1022,
        1496–1497
Anencephaly, 1573, 1575
Anesthesia, 417
    dolorosa, 417, 1874
        symptom management in, 863
    hyperthermia in, malignant, 845
    in myasthenia gravis, 2180
        and pregnancy, 2259
    regional nerve blocks in, 913
Aneurysm
    aortic, 1014
        lumbosacral plexus disorders in,
            2041–2042
    intracranial, 640–641, 642, 1185–1198
        angiography in, 640–641, 936,
            1187–1188
            computed tomographic, 612–613,
                613f, 614f, 1185, 1187, 1187f
            magnetic resonance, 604–605, 606f,
                1185, 1187, 1188f
        in arteriovenous malformations, 1206,
            1211f
        causes of, 640
        classification of, 1188–1189, 1190t
        clinical signs in, 1185–1186
        in craniocerebral trauma, 1189
        dissecting, 1190
        in Ehlers-Danlos syndrome,
            1675–1676, 1676f
        in endocarditis, 1013–1014, 1013f, 1189
        epidemiology of, 1190–1191
        familial, 640, 1189, 1190–1191
        fusiform or dolichoectatic, 1190
        headache in, 1185, 1836–1837
        laboratory studies in, 1186–1188
        locations of, 640, 641f, 642f
        mycotic, 1189
            in endocarditis, 1013, 1013f, 1189
        oculomotor nerve palsy in, 1186, 1880

in Osler-Weber-Rendu syndrome, 1678
physical examination in, 1186
in pregnancy, 1197
prognosis in, 1191
rebleeding in, 1192–1194, 1193f
risk of hemorrhage in, 640
saccular or berry, 1189–1190
    in children, 1222
treatment of, 1191–1198
    balloon occlusion in, 1196, 1197f
    bypass graft in, 939, 939f
    coil occlusion in, 937–939, 938f,
        1196, 1198f
    comparison of methods in, 937–939
    in rebleeding, 1193–1194
    timing of surgery in, 936
in tumors, 1190
ultrasonography in, 660–662
unruptured, 1195–1196
vasospasm in, 640–641, 937, 1193
    and cerebral ischemia, 1193,
        1194–1195
    prevention of, 641, 937
Angelman's syndrome, 783
Angiitis
    allergic, 2106
    of central nervous system, isolated, 1231
    granulomatous, 1017, 1231
        intracranial hemorrhage in, 1172
Angina, nocturnal, 1810
Angioendotheliomatosis, neoplastic, 1147
Angiofibroma, facial, in tuberous sclerosis,
    1667, 1668f
Angiography, 617–643
    anatomy in, 619–633
    in aneurysms, intracranial, 640–641, 936,
        1187–1188
        computed tomographic technique,
            612–613, 613f, 614f, 1185, 1187,
            1187f
        magnetic resonance technique,
            604–605, 606f, 1185, 1187, 1188f
    of anterior cerebral artery
        anatomy in, 624–626, 625f
        in stenosis and occlusion, 634
    of aortic arch, 617
        anatomy in, 619, 619f, 620f
    in arteriovenous fistula
        cerebral, 637–639
        dural, 636–637
    in arteriovenous malformations, spinal, 1229
    in back and lower limb pain, 464
    in brain death, 56
    in carotid-cavernous fistula, direct, 635–636
    catheterization technique in, 619
    complications of, 617, 618–619, 1156
    computed tomography technique,
        609–613
        in aneurysms, intracranial, 612–613,
            613f, 614f, 1185, 1187, 1187f
        in stenosis of middle cerebral artery,
            611, 612f
    digital subtraction, 525, 618
    embolization in, 618, 642, 643
        nontarget, 618
    equipment in, 619
    of extracranial carotid arteries, 619–621

in fibromuscular dysplasia, 633, 633f, 634f
in headache, 290
    magnetic resonance technique, 290
    in migraine, 1850
in hypothalamic-pituitary disorders, 856
indications for, 525, 617, 618, 618t,
    1156–1157
of internal carotid artery
    anatomy in, 621–623
    in stenosis and occlusion, 633, 633f, 634f
interventional procedures in, 618, 642–643
intraoperative, 956
magnetic resonance technique, 525–526,
    595–609. *See also* Magnetic
    resonance angiography
of middle cerebral artery
    anatomy in, 626, 626f, 627f
    magnetic resonance technique, 603, 605f
    in stenosis and occlusion, 603, 605f,
        633–634
photographic subtraction, 617
of posterior cerebral artery
    anatomy in, 628–629, 629f
    in stenosis and occlusion, 634–635
principles of, 525
risk-benefit analysis of, 468–469
in sleep disorders, 1819
in stenosis and occlusion, intracranial,
    633–635
    computed tomography technique, 611,
        612f
    magnetic resonance technique, 603, 605f
    venous, 635
in subarachnoid hemorrhage, 936,
    1187–1188
in vasculitis, 1232
    in giant cell arteritis, 1842
venous, 629–632
    in stenosis and occlusion, intracranial,
        635
of vertebrobasilar circulation, 626–629
of Willis circle, 623–624, 624f
Angiokeratoma
    corporis diffusum, 1147, 1660, 1680
    in Fabry's disease, 1660, 1680, 2076,
        2077f
Angioma
    capillary, 1201
    cavernous, 564, 940–941, 1201
        clinical signs in, 1203–1204
        intracranial hemorrhage in, 1168
        magnetic resonance imaging in, 564,
            1168, 1168f, 1203, 1203f
        of pons, 940–941, 941f
    facial
        in Sturge-Weber syndrome, 1681, 1682f
        in Wyburn-Mason syndrome, 1696
    leptomeningeal, in Sturge-Weber
        syndrome, 1681, 1684f
    retinal, in von Hippel–Lindau disease,
        200, 200f
    spinal, 1228–1229
    venous, 564, 940, 940f, 1201
        magnetic resonance imaging in, 565f,
            1201, 1202f
        spinal, 1228
        treatment of, 940, 940f

Angiomatosis, cutaneomeningospinal,
1229
Angiomyolipoma, renal, in tuberous
sclerosis, 1671, 1671f, 1672
Angiopathy
cerebral, 1232
amyloid, 1148, 1171–1172, 1173f
intracranial hemorrhage in, 1172
vasculitis in, 1233–1234
autosomal dominant with subcortical
infarcts and leukoencephalopathy,
1146, 1850
in Susac's syndrome, 1147–1148
Angioplasty
in basilar artery stenosis, 619
complications of, 618–619, 1011
coronary, 1011
in subarachnoid hemorrhage and
vasospasm, 937, 937f, 1195,
1196f
Angiostrongyliasis, 1398–1399
Angiotensin, central nervous system function
of, 843t
Anhidrosis
in autonomic disorders, 2143, 2145
hyperpyrexia in, 2146
Animal models
of encephalomyelitis, experimental
allergic, 816, 817, 818, 1434
of multiple sclerosis, 817–818, 1458
of myasthenia gravis, 819, 2170
Animal neurotoxins, 1529–1531, 1530t
neuromuscular disorders from, 2185
Anismus, 433
Anisocoria, 48, 229–230
episodic, 230
examination in, 231–232, 231f, 724
investigations in, 232–233
simple, 230
Ankle-foot orthosis, 964, 964f, 987
Ankylosing spondylitis, 1979–1981. See also
Spondylitis, ankylosing
Annulus fibrosus, 441
Anomia, 135–136, 143, 683–684
and aphasia, 149, 150t, 683–684
bedside examination in, 144
Anorexia nervosa, 846
Anosmia, 264, 265
congenital, 266
Anosognosia, 694
in Alzheimer's disease, 1704
Anoxia, 1467–1474
in cardiopulmonary arrest, 1470–1471
coma in, 1468–1469
prognosis in, 1470–1471
in drug abuse, 1526
electroencephalography in, 483f, 484f
encephalopathy in, 1467–1474. See also
Encephalopathy, anoxic-ischemic
myoclonus in, 1919–1920
in neonate, 1573, 2240–2246
syncope in, 14, 1467
Anterior cord syndrome in spinal cord
trauma, 1097, 1097f
Anterior horn cells, 1990
age-related changes in, 2273
disorders of, 376

differential diagnosis of, 2040
and frontotemporal degeneration,
1715–1716
in paraneoplastic syndromes, 1306
Anthrax, 1346
Antibiotic therapy
in brain abscess, 1325–1326
in leptospirosis, 1338
in Lyme disease, 1337
in meningitis, 1319t, 1320,
1321t–1322t
in neonate, 2247–2248
in relapsing fever, 1338
in spinal epidural abscess, 1328
in syphilis, 1336
Anticholinergic drugs
delirium from, 32, 1525
in dizziness and vertigo, 740t, 741
overdose of, 1525
recreational use of, 1525
in urinary incontinence, 2294t
in detrusor hyperreflexia, 751–752
Anticholinergic serum activity assay in
delirium, 31
Anticoagulant drugs
in acute ischemic stroke, 1158–1159
in cardiogenic embolism, 1010,
1158–1159
intracranial hemorrhage from, 1170, 1181
in pregnancy, 2265, 2266–2267
in prevention of stroke, 1158
Anticodon, 786
Anticonvulsant drugs, 894, 895, 1769–1776,
1770t
in absence seizures, 1757
bioavailability of, 894
biotransformation of, 895
in breast-feeding, 2264
and calcium-channel activity, 891
in craniocerebral trauma, 1761–1762
discontinuation of, 1775–1776
distribution of, 895
in elderly, 2287
elimination of, 896
in febrile seizures, 1755–1756
interactions of, 896
with oral contraceptives, 2257
in Lennox-Gastaut syndrome, 1758
metabolism of, 895–896
genetic variations in, 895–896
physiological variations in, 896
monitoring of, 1775, 1775t
in myoclonic epilepsy
and encephalopathy, 1757
in infants, 1756
juvenile, 1756
in neonatal seizures, 2239–2240, 2240t
in nocturnal seizures, 1825
in pain management, 912, 2055
in pregnancy, 1763–1764, 2263–2264
fetal and neonatal effects of, 1764,
2253, 2254f, 2263–2264
guidelines on, 1764–1765, 1765t
selection of, 1774
and sodium-channel function, 890
spectrum of efficacy, 894
in status epilepticus, 1760–1761, 1760t,

1761t
titration rate of, 894–895
in West's syndrome, 1758
Antidepressant drugs
adverse effects of, 2284, 2284t
in depression, 109
in elderly, 2283–2284, 2284t
in migraine, 1858
in pain management, 912, 2055
pharmacology of, 2284t
Antidiuretic hormone, 853–854
central nervous system function of, 842t
deficiency of, 858
in diabetes insipidus, 854
inappropriate secretion of, 855–856,
1029, 1192
causes of, 855, 855t
in neonate, 2248
sodium serum levels in, 855–856, 1029,
1071, 1192, 1489
in multiple sclerosis, 1455
in nocturnal enuresis, 752
in orthostatic hypotension, 2160
Antiemetics in dizziness and vertigo, 740t,
741
Antigens
human leukocyte (HLA), 808. See also
HLA system
presentation of, 809
proliferation in central nervous system
tumors, 1240
receptor gene rearrangements, 807–808
superantigens, 816–817
Antihistamines in dizziness and vertigo,
740t, 741
Anti-Hu syndrome, 1303
Anti-inflammatory drugs, nonsteroidal
in Alzheimer's disease, 2281, 2282
in pain management, 907–909, 908t
Antimony in leishmaniasis, 1394
Antineuronal nuclear antibody type I, 2105
Antiphospholipid antibody syndromes,
1025–1026
cerebrovascular disease in, 1025, 1127,
1150
Antiretroviral drugs, 839
Antisense technology in gene therapy,
1259–1260
Antisocial personality, 90
Antithrombin III deficiency, 1149
Antitoxin
botulism, 1340, 2184
diphtheria, 1343, 2126
Antiviral drug therapy, 839
Anton's syndrome, 33, 190, 1135, 1722
Anus, sphincter of
electromyography of, 748, 749f
in fecal continence, 429–430, 757
Anxiety, 91, 96–98
γ-aminobutyric acid in, 871t
dizziness and vertigo in, 239, 240
generalized disorder, 96–97
pain complaints in, 905
panic disorder in, 97, 97t
and phobic depersonalization syndrome,
97
prevalence of, 996–997

in Charcot-Marie-Tooth disease, 2066,
2066f
complications in, 2062
in diabetes mellitus, 2099, 2099f
in floppy infant, 415
in hereditary neuropathy with pressure
palsies, 2068, 2069f
in hereditary sensory and autonomic
neuropathy, 2069, 2071f
indications for, 2053, 2053t
in inflammatory demyelinating
polyradiculoneuropathy, chronic,
2088
in leprosy, 2126f
in monoclonal gammopathy of
undetermined significance,
2092–2093
in Sjögren's syndrome, 2110, 2111f
of sural nerve. See Sural nerve,
biopsy of
in thiamine deficiency, 1503
in vasculitis, 2108, 2109f
skin, indications for, 2053
of temporal artery in giant cell arteritis,
291, 1842–1843
Biotin, 1609–1610
deficiency of, 1629
Biotinidase deficiency, 1609, 1629
Biotransformation of drugs, 895
Birth trauma, 2249–2252
brachial plexus injury in, 2252, 2252f
extracranial hemorrhage in, 2250, 2251t
facial paralysis in, 2251–2252
intracranial hemorrhage in, 2249–2250,
2250f, 2251t
skull fractures in, 2250
spinal cord injury in, 2250–2251
Birth weight in cerebral palsy, 1585
Birthmarks, 85
Bites
Bartonella infections in, 1345
Colorado tick fever in, 1366
ehrlichiosis in, 1344–1345
encephalitis in, 1364, 1365
hemorrhagic fever in, 1369
Lyme disease in, 1336–1337. *See also*
Lyme disease
malaria in, 1386–1389
plague in, 1346
rabies in, 1362–1363
rat-bite fever in, 1347
relapsing fever in, 1337–1338
Rocky Mountain spotted fever in, 1344
scorpion, 1530–1531, 1530t
snake, 1529–1530, 1530t
spider, 1530, 1530t
tick paralysis in, 1404, 1531
trypanosomiasis in, 1391
typhus in, 1343–1344
viral infections in, 830
Bithionol in fascioliasis, 1404
Bladder, 429–438, 751–755
in amyloid neuropathy and amyloidosis,
437
autonomic innervation of, 373, 429
clinical features of disorders, 2147
management of disorders, 2163–2164

tests and investigations in disorders,
2156
in brainstem disorders, 433–434
in cauda equina disorders, 436, 935
in cerebral cortex disorders, 431
cystometry of, 744, 745–747
in filling, 745–746, 747, 747f
decentralized or autonomous flaccid, 374
detrusor muscle of. *See* Detrusor muscle
of bladder
in diabetes mellitus, 436, 2100, 2103
drug therapy in disorders of, 981–982,
981t
in detrusor hyperreflexia, 751–752,
752t
in multiple sclerosis, 1454–1455
in elderly, 2291
in Guillain-Barré syndrome, 437
incomplete emptying of, 753–754
in elderly, 2291
postmicturition residual volume in, 744,
746f
in multiple sclerosis, 434–435, 1440
detrusor hyperreflexia of, 434, 435,
752, 753, 1454–1455
management of, 753, 754, 754f,
1454–1455
in multiple system atrophy, 432, 748, 2156
detrusor hyperreflexia of, 432, 748, 2156
management of disorders, 754,
2163–2164
in myotonic dystrophy, 437
in parkinsonism, 432–433
peripheral innervation of, 743, 744f
reflex, 373–374
rehabilitation in disorders of, 981–982
in spinal cord disorders, 373–374,
434–435, 752–755
clinical features in, 2147
detrusor hyperreflexia in, 752–753,
752f
management of, 752–753, 754, 755,
981–982
capsaicin in, 752–753, 752f
catheterization in, 754, 1109
in multiple sclerosis, 752, 753, 754,
754f
nerve and nerve root stimulators in,
755
surgery in, 755
in trauma, 981–982, 1109
retention of urine in, 754
in trauma, 373–374, 434, 752, 755,
1109, 2147
management of, 981–982, 1109
storage and voiding functions of, 429, 431
in stroke, 981
urodynamic studies of, 744–747, 981
catheterization in, 745–747
noninvasive, 744
Blaschko's lines in hypomelanosis of Ito,
1692
Blastomyces dermatitidis infection, 1380
treatment of, 1380, 1382t
Bleeding. *See* Hemorrhage
Bleeding disorders. *See* Hemorrhagic
disorders

Blepharospasm
benign essential, 235
central, 235
in dystonia, 332, 1909, 1910f
excessive eyelid closure in, 235, 235f
factitious or voluntary, 235
in Parkinson's disease, 235, 322
reflex, 235
Blinking, 236
rate of, 235, 236
reflex response, 273
in parkinsonism, 323
Blood
bacteria in, in craniocerebral trauma,
1074–1075
viruses in, 831–832
Blood-brain barrier, 1545–1547
in chemotherapy, 1235, 1312, 1547
drugs crossing, 1547
embryonic development of, 1546
in hepatic encephalopathy, 1479–1480
in multiple sclerosis, 1433, 1446
tight junctions in, 832, 1546t, 1547
transport mechanisms in, 1547
in traumatic brain injury, 1045, 1046,
1047f, 1051
in vasogenic cerebral edema,
1550, 1551
in viral infections, 832–833
Blood flow, cerebral. *See* Cerebral blood
flow
Blood-nerve barrier, 1114
Blood pressure
in autonomic disorders, 2140–2142
ambulatory monitoring of, 2149, 2152f
and carotid sinus massage, 2149–2150,
2153f
food ingestion affecting, 2149, 2150,
2151f
management of, 2158–2162
tests and investigations on, 2149–2154
and Valsalva's maneuver, 2149,
2153f
in coma, 41–42
in hypertension. *See* Hypertension
in hypotension. *See* Hypotension
in neonate, management of, 2243–2244
in vasovagal syncope, 2141, 2143f
Blood supply
of peripheral nerves, 1114
of pituitary, 848–849, 848f
of spinal cord, 375–376, 376f
anatomy of, 1225–1226, 1226f
disorders of, 1225–1230
magnetic resonance angiography of,
607–609
Blood volume, cerebral, 672
ratio to cerebral blood flow, 672, 673f,
674
Bobath approach in physical therapy, 961
Bobbing of eye, 49, 225, 225t
Body image in cenesthesic hallucinations,
111
Bombesin, central nervous system function
of, 842t
Bone
fractures of. *See* Fractures

ultrasonography in, 654, 656–657,
656f, 661f
ultrasonography of
in acute stroke, 654
in atherosclerosis, 661f
in recent transient ischemic attack or
stroke, 656–657, 656f
transcranial Doppler, 653, 656–657
in vasospasm, 662
posterior
anatomy in angiography, 628–629, 629f
branches of, 629, 629f
dementia in disorders of, 1722
fetal origin of, 628
infarction in territory of, 1132–1133,
1134–1135
stenosis and occlusion of, 634–635
clinical syndromes in, 1132–1133,
1134–1135
transcranial Doppler ultrasonography
of, 653
Cerebral blood flow, 672–673
autoregulation of, 672
in craniocerebral trauma, 1070
in subarachnoid hemorrhage, 1194
in brain death, 56, 929
in craniocerebral trauma
autoregulation of, 1070
as prognostic factor, 1083
disorders of. See Cerebrovascular
disorders
factors affecting, 928
and glucose metabolism, 1485
in hepatic encephalopathy, 1479
magnetic resonance imaging of, 673, 929
in migraine, 1851
monitoring in neurointensive care,
928–929
normal range in, 928
oxygen extraction fraction in, 672, 673,
673f, 674
prognostic patterns of, 674
in craniocerebral trauma, 1083
ratio to cerebral blood volume, 672, 673f,
674
in sleep, 1783, 1819
xenon 133 studies of, 928–929
in craniocerebral trauma, 1083
Cerebral blood volume, 672
ratio to cerebral blood flow, 672, 673f,
674
Cerebral capillaries, unique features of,
1547, 1547t
Cerebral palsy, 1585–1586
ataxia in, 1586, 1931
athetotic, 1911–1912
diagnosis of, 1585
floppy infant in, 411
gait in, 349–350
motor evoked potentials in, 495
prevention and treatment of, 1586
Cerebral perfusion pressure
in craniocerebral trauma, 926–927, 1068,
1069–1070
as prognostic factor, 1083–1084
monitoring in neurointensive care,
926–927, 1069–1070

Cerebral veins
anatomy in angiography, 629–632
deep, 630–632, 631f, 632f
superficial middle, 629–630, 630f
thrombosis of, 1163–1165, 1327–1328,
1468
infarction in, 1468
in oral contraceptive use, 2258
in pregnancy, 2266–2267
Cerebritis, 554, 554f
Cerebrocerebellum, 309
Cerebrospinal fluid, 1545
absorption of, 1548, 1549f
in Alzheimer's disease, 1706
in anoxic-ischemic encephalopathy, 1473
in coma, 40
in Creutzfeldt-Jakob disease, 1425
in delirium, 31
in encephalomyelitis, acute disseminated,
1461–1462
flow disorders of
headache in, 1832–1833
hydrocephalus in, 567–568
structural neuroimaging in, 559–562
in fungal infections, 1380
in coccidioidomycosis, 1378, 1379
cryptococcal, 1377, 1379f
in meningitis, 1375–1376
in Guillain-Barré syndrome, 2081
in headache, 290, 1832–1833, 1836
low pressure, 1832–1833, 1834f,
1835f, 1836f
in HIV infection and AIDS, 1417, 1418
in inflammatory demyelinating
polyradiculoneuropathy
acute, 2081
chronic, 2087
in leptomeningeal metastasis, 1286, 1286t
in Lyme disease, 1337
lymphocytosis of, 1836
in melanosis, neurocutaneous, 1693–1694
in meningitis
bacterial, 1318–1319, 1330
eosinophilic, 1386
fungal, 1375–1376
in HIV infection and AIDS, 1418
viral, 825, 1354
in multiple sclerosis, 1450–1451, 1450t,
1451f
pressure of, 1549
compared with rates of production and
absorption, 1548, 1549f
in headache, 1832–1833
low pressure in, 1832–1833, 1834f,
1835f, 1836f
measurement of, 1549
production of, 1548
compared with absorption, 1548, 1549f
serotonin in, 888t
sites in, 1548
in pseudotumor cerebri, 1553, 1833
in syphilis, 1335, 1336
in viral infections, 824t, 836, 837, 838
encephalitis, 1354–1355, 1358,
1364–1365
meningitis, 825, 1354
oligoclonal bands in, 837

poliovirus, 1992
polymerase chain reaction of, 837, 838
Cerebrovascular disorders, 1125–1224
alexia in, 151, 156, 1131
in posterior cerebral artery infarction,
1135
ambulation and walking after, 997–998
in amyloid angiopathy, 1148, 1171–1172,
1173f
intracranial hemorrhage in, 1172
vasculitis in, 1233–1234
aneurysms, 1185–1198. See also
Aneurysm, intracranial
angiography in. See Angiography
angioma
cavernous, 564, 940–941, 1168
venous, 564, 565f, 940
in antiphospholipid antibody syndromes,
1025, 1127, 1150
anxiety in, 996
in aortic disorders, 1014, 1127, 1148
aphasia in, 991, 1131
Broca's, 145
in children, 167–168
clinical tests in, 154–156
crossed, 153, 168
differential diagnosis in, 156
global, 148, 156
in middle cerebral artery territory
lesions, 1721
recovery and rehabilitation in, 158–159
transcortical, 150, 156
Wernicke's, 146–147, 156
arteriovenous fistulas, 637–639
arteriovenous malformations. See
Arteriovenous malformations,
intracranial
bladder dysfunction in, 981
brainstem syndromes in, 246, 299–307
capillary telangiectasia, 564, 940
in cardiac surgery, 1011–1012
in children, 1036, 1217
in cardiovascular disorders. See
Cardiovascular system, and
cerebrovascular disease
cerebellar, 1933–1934
in cerebral autosomal dominant
arteriopathy with subcortical
infarcts and leukoencephalopathy,
1146, 1850
cerebral blood flow monitoring in, 928–929
in cervical osteoarthritis, 1971
in children, 1215–1224. See also Children
and infants, cerebrovascular
disorders in
cognitive function in, 989, 994, 1721–1728
in children, 1223
in intracranial aneurysm and subarachnoid hemorrhage, 1186, 1191
in transient ischemic attack, 1129–1130
computed tomography in. See Computed
tomography, in cerebrovascular
disorders
in craniocerebral trauma, 1051, 1143
intracranial hemorrhage in. See
Craniocerebral trauma,
intracranial hemorrhage in

Coma, 25
  alpha, 38, 482, 483f, 1472
    electroencephalography in, 482, 483f
  in anoxic-ischemic encephalopathy,
      1468–1469
    cerebral edema in, 1469
    delayed deterioration in, 1469
    management of, 1473–1474
    persistent vegetative state in, 1469
    prognosis in, 1470–1471
  barbiturate induction of, 1072
  behavioral states confused with, 37–38,
      38t
  and brain death, 56, 1471–1472
  causes of, 38–40, 39t
  clinical approach to, 37–56
  common presentations in, 40–41
  in coronary artery bypass surgery, 1012,
      1012f
  in diabetes mellitus, nonketotic
      hyperosmolar, 1034, 1486, 1487
  differential diagnosis in, 52–55
  electroencephalography in, 55, 482, 483,
      483f
  Glasgow Coma Scale in. See Glasgow
      Coma Scale
  in hepatic encephalopathy, 1482
  history of patient in, 41
  in hyperthermia, 42, 1543
  initial examination and emergency
      therapy in, 40
  laboratory studies in, 53–54, 54t
  myoclonus in, 51, 53, 1919
  neurointensive care in, 918
  neurological examination in, 45–51
  physical examination in, 41–45
    prognostic indicators in, 1470, 1471t
  prognosis in, 55–56, 1085, 1470–1471
  pupillary light response in, 47–48, 52–53,
      1470, 1471t
  respirations in, 42, 46–47, 46f
  sleep compared with, 1786
  structural, 39t, 52–53
  toxic-metabolic, 39t, 52–53
  vigil, 38, 73
Communicating artery
  anterior, aneurysm of, 1186
  basilar, 299
    branches of, 300f
    posterior, 621, 622, 623f
    aneurysm of, 1187f
Communication. See also Speech and language
  adaptive aids in, 989, 991f
  in amyotrophic lateral sclerosis, 2013
Community setting, rehabilitation services
    in, 970
Compartment syndrome
  in electrical injuries, 1543
  tibial anterior, leg pain in, 459
Competency of patient in health care
    decisions, 2271–2272
Complement components in Guillain-Barré
    syndrome, 2083
Compliance measurements of tympanic
    membrane, 255–256, 257f
Compliance with therapy, acceptability of
    drugs affecting, 894

Comprehension
  auditory
    bedside examination of, 144
    in pure word deafness, 147–148
  in reading, 144, 686
  of sentences, 685
  of words, 682–683
Computed tomography, 521–594
  in adrenoleukodystrophy, 547–548, 1641f
  in affective disorders, 109
  in Alzheimer's disease, 1707
  in amyotrophic lateral sclerosis, 2009
  angiography in, 609–613
    applications of, 610–613
    in intracranial aneurysm, 612–613,
        613f, 614f, 1185, 1187, 1187f
    technique in, 609–610
  in aphasia, 156
    Broca's, 145
    and dementia, 153–154
  in back and lower limb pain, 463
  in basal ganglia disorders, 1912t, 1913
  in brachial plexus disorders, 2034
  in brain abscess, 1324, 1325, 1325f
  in central nervous system tumors, 1235
  in cerebrovascular disorders, 564, 929
    angiographic technique, 611–613
    in arteriovenous malformations, 1168,
        1205, 1206f
    and dementia, 1724f, 1726–1727
    dense middle cerebral artery sign in,
        1154, 1155f
    hemorrhage, 566, 566f, 1175
      in birth trauma, 2249, 2250, 2250f
      in head trauma, 550–551
      subarachnoid, 550–551, 936, 937,
          1187
      in tumors, 1169f, 1170
    infarction, 566–567, 566f, 567f, 1154,
        1155f
    transient ischemic attack or threatened
        stroke, 1154
  in cervical spondylosis
    and myelopathy, 1970, 1970f
    and radiculopathy, 2025
  in coma, 54–55
  in craniocerebral trauma, 548–552, 1064
    and coma, 55
    and headache, 1870
    indications for surgery in, 1067, 1068,
        1069
    prognostic information in, 1084, 1084t,
        1085
  in cysticercosis, 555f, 556, 1395, 1396
  in dementia
    in Alzheimer's disease, 1707
    and aphasia, 153–154
    in leukoaraiosis, 1725, 1726
    vascular, 1724f, 1726–1727
  in elderly, 2277
  of facial nerve, 275
  in Fukuyama type muscular dystrophy,
      2206, 2206f
  in headache, 289
    cluster, 1864
    in craniocerebral trauma, 1870
    in migraine, 1850

tension-type, 1869
  in hearing loss, 740
  in HIV infection and AIDS
    and lymphoma, 557, 557f, 558, 1413f
    and toxoplasmosis, 556, 556f,
        1410–1412, 1411f
  in holoprosencephaly, 559f, 1578f
  in hydrocephalus, 567, 1555, 1555f
    normal pressure, 1557
  in hypoglossal nerve disorders, 282
  in hypomelanosis of Ito, 1692
  in hypoxic-ischemic encephalopathy of
      neonate, 2241–2242, 2242f, 2243f
  in intervertebral disc herniation
    cervical, 1969f
    and radiculopathy, 2025
  in intracranial aneurysm, 1187, 1187f
    angiographic technique, 612–613, 613f,
        614f, 1185, 1187, 1187f
  in jugular foramen syndrome, 283
  in Krabbe's disease, 547
  in leukoaraiosis, 1725, 1726
  in longitudinal ligament ossification,
      posterior, 1966–1967, 1968f
  in lumbosacral plexus disorders, 2040
  in meningioma, 536, 573, 573f, 945, 1742f
  in meningitis, bacterial, 555f, 1318
    tuberculous, 555f
  in Menkes' syndrome, 1688
  in metachromatic leukodystrophy, 547
  in movement disorders, 339
  in multiple sclerosis, 1446, 1448f, 1450
  in orbital lesions, 572–574
  in Parkinson's disease, 1894
  in periventricular-intraventricular
      hemorrhage of premature infants,
      2244–2245
  in personality changes, 96
  in Pick's disease, 545
  principles of, 521–522
  in radiculopathy
    cervical, 1969f, 2025
    in disc degeneration and spondylosis,
        2025
    traumatic, 2022
  in real-time image-guided surgery, 957
  in schizophrenia, 114
  in seizures, 672, 1768
  single-photon emission. See Single-photon
      emission computed tomography
  in skull base lesions, 568–570
  in spinal cord trauma, 1092, 1100, 1104f,
      1105, 1106f
  spiral (helical or volume acquisition),
      521–522
  in Sturge-Weber syndrome, 1683, 1683f
  three-dimensional images in, 522, 522f
  in toxoplasmosis, 556, 556f, 1394f
    in HIV infection and AIDS, 556, 556f,
        1410–1412, 1411f
  in tuberous sclerosis, 1669, 1669f
COMT (catechol-O-methyl-transferase), 881
  inhibitors in Parkinson's disease, 1896,
      1898, 1898t
Concussion
  in craniocerebral trauma, 1045–1046
    acceleration, 1045–1046

neocortical, 38
rate of. *See* Mortality rate
Decarboxylase, 880, 885
Decisions on health care. *See* Health care
  decisions
Decompression
  posterior fossa, in trigeminal neuralgia,
    1874
  suboccipital, in cerebellar hemorrhage and
    infarction, 933
Decubitus ulcers, 979, 1103
Defecation, 429–430
  continence in. *See* Continence, fecal
  in Parkinson's disease, 433
  in spinal cord disorders, 435
  syncope in, 14
Degenerative disorders
  ataxia in. *See* Ataxia, in degenerative
    disorders
  axonal, 2046–2047, 2046f
    nerve conduction studies in, 503
  of cerebellum. *See* Cerebellum,
    degenerative disorders of
  in children, brain biopsy in, 955
  cortical-basal ganglia, 1720, 1904
    clinical features in, 1904
    course and treatment in, 1904
    functional neuroimaging in, 670, 1904
    pathology in, 1904
    positron-emission tomography in, 670,
      1904
    structural neuroimaging in, 545, 1904
  dementia in, 1703–1717, 1719–1720
    primary, 1703–1717
    progressive cortical syndromes,
      1731–1737
    and sleep disturbances, 1807–1808
  of frontal lobe, 1715, 1716
    diagnostic features in, 1736–1737
  frontotemporal, 1714–1715, 1731–1733
    diagnostic features in, 1736–1737
  glutamate and excitatory amino acids in,
    875, 875t
  hepatocerebral, 1482, 1741
    chronic, 1026
  hepatolenticular, 1622–1624, 1924–1925.
    See also Wilson's disease
  imaging techniques in, 544–545
  intracranial
    functional neuroimaging in, 667–668,
      669–670
    structural neuroimaging in, 544–545
  macular, in Kjellin's syndrome, 1950, 1950f
  neuronal, 2046
    of motor neurons, 1809
    of somatic neurons, 1807–1809
  peripheral nerve, 2046–2047, 2046f
  positron emission tomography in, cp38E.I
    in cortical-basal ganglia degeneration,
      670, 1904
  retinal, 191, 199
    in paraneoplastic syndromes, 1305–1306
  sleep disturbances in, 1807–1809
  of spinal cord, in vitamin B_{12} deficiency,
    1497, 1498f, 2112–2113
  of spine, 1967–1975. *See also* Spine,
    degenerative disorders of

spinocerebellar, neuropathy associated
    with, 2071–2072
striatonigral, 1809, 1900–1904
  in multiple system atrophy, 2134,
    2136f, 2137
  structural neuroimaging in, 545
of thalamus, 1717
wallerian, 1114, 2046, 2046f
  partial, 972
7–Dehydrocholesterol-delta-reductase
    deficiency, 1645
Dejerine-Klumpke palsy, 363, 2021, 2252
Dejerine-Roussy syndrome, 1135
Dejerine-Sottas disease, 2064, 2066, 2067
Delirium, 25–36, 37
  acute onset with fluctuating course, 26
  causes of, 32t
  clinical characteristics of, 26–28, 26t,
    2284
  compared with dementia, 34, 35t, 1701
  diagnosis of, 29–31, 2284
    scales and criteria in, 30
  differential diagnosis in, 31–34, 35t, 2284
  in elderly, 25, 2284–2285
    differential diagnosis in, 32, 2284
    drug-induced, 32–33
    epidemiology of, 2284
    prognosis in, 36
    risk factors for, 29, 30
  hallucinations in, 26–27, 36, 110, 111
  historical aspects of, 25
  in hypoxia, 1467
  management of, 34–36
    in elderly, 2285
  pathophysiology in, 28–29, 28f, 2285
  prognosis in, 36
  risk factors for, 29–30, 29t
  tremens, 33
Delta activity in electroencephalography,
    474
  focal, 479
  intermittent bursts, 479, 482f
Delusions, 110–114
  in Alzheimer's disease, 1705
  content of, 110
  in delirium, 27, 36
  diagnostic criteria on, 112, 113t
  differential diagnosis in, 111, 112t
  first-rank symptoms of Schneider in, 110,
    110t
Demeclocycline in inappropriate secretion of
    antidiuretic hormone , 856
Dementia, 1701–1702, 2278–2283
  alcoholic, 1742
  in Alzheimer's disease, 1703–1712, 1731.
    See also Alzheimer's disease
  in amyotrophic lateral sclerosis, 1720,
    1733, 2014–2015
    and parkinsonism complex, 2016
  and apraxia, progressive, 1735
  assessment procedures in, 1701–1702
  brain biopsy in, 955, 1702
  compared with delirium, 34, 35t, 1701
  cortical, 2279
    compared with subcortical dementia,
      1701, 1702t, 2279
    progressive focal syndromes, 1731–1737

in Creutzfeldt-Jakob disease, 1424, 1425
definitions of, 1701, 2278–2279
in degenerative disorders, 1703–1717,
    1719–1720
  corticobasal, 1720
  primary, 1703–1717
  progressive cortical, 1731–1737
  sleep disturbances in, 1807–1808
and depression, 107
  in Alzheimer's disease, 1705, 1712
  in elderly, 2282, 2283
  functional neuroimaging in, 668
  in vascular disorders, 1728
diagnostic criteria on, 1701, 1702t,
    2279–2280
in dialysis, 1028–1029, 1038, 1484, 1741
differential diagnosis of, 34, 35t
in Down syndrome, 1712–1713
drug-induced, 1742
in elderly. *See* Elderly, dementia in
electroencephalography in, 484–485, 1702
event-related evoked potentials in, 485
frequency of, 993
frontal, 1715, 1716
  diagnostic features in, 1736–1737
  familial, 1717
frontotemporal. *See* Frontotemporal
    dementia
functional neuroimaging in, 667–668,
    1702, 1725
in HIV infection and AIDS. *See* HIV
    infection and AIDS, dementia in
in Huntington's disease, 1719–1720,
    1914, 1916
in hydrocephalus, normal pressure,
    948–949, 1557, 1743
hysterical, 1743
in infections, 1739–1740
language in, 143, 153–154, 1733–1734,
    1735
  in frontotemporal dementia, 1732
  in progressive nonfluent aphasia,
    1733–1734
Lewy bodies in, 1713–1714, 1713f
  in Alzheimer's disease, 1706, 1713
  functional neuroimaging in, 668, 1713
  in Parkinson's disease, 1713, 1719,
    1894, cp75.II
in lipofuscinosis, neuronal ceroid, 1647,
    1647t, 1648, 1741
in metabolic disorders, 1740–1741
in multiple sclerosis, 1438, 1455,
    1742–1743
in neoplasms, 1741–1742
in parkinsonism. *See* Parkinsonism,
    dementia in
in Parkinson's disease, 1713, 1719, 1894
in Pick's disease, 1714–1715, 1737
in prion disease, 1720
and pseudodementia, 1743
pugilistica, 1742, 1905
semantic, 135, 681, 1734
  in Pick's disease, 1715
  reading in, 686
sleep disturbances in, 1807–1808
structural neuroimaging in, 544–545,
    545f, 1702

Dementia—*continued*
  subcortical, 1719, 2279
    compared with cortical dementia, 1701,
      1702t, 2279
    in supranuclear palsy, progressive, 1719,
      1900
  in thalamus disorders, 1717, 1722
  in toxic exposures, 1742
  in trauma, 1742, 1905
  treatment of, 948–949
    in elderly, 2281–2283
    in HIV infection and AIDS, 826–827,
      1416–1417
    symptom management in, 865
  urinary continence in, 431, 2282
    in elderly, 2282, 2292
  vascular, 1721–1728
    in anterior cerebral artery territory
      lesions, 1722
    computed tomography in, 1724f,
      1726–1727
    diagnostic criteria on, 1727–1728, 1728t
    functional neuroimaging in, 668, 1725
    incidence in stroke, 1722–1723
    ischemic score in, 1727, 1727t
    magnetic resonance imaging in, 545,
      545f, 1724f, 1726–1727
    in middle cerebral artery territory
      lesions, 1721–1722
    multi-infarct, 1723, 1724f, 1725
      structural neuroimaging in, 544–545,
        545f, 1724f
    pathogenesis of, 1724–1726, 1725t
    in posterior cerebral artery lesions,
      1722
    prevention and treatment of, 1728
    in single brain lesions, 1721
    in subcortical arteriosclerotic
      encephalopathy, 1723
    in subcortical infarctions, 1722
De Morsier's syndrome, 198, 730
Demyelination
  acute inflammatory, 819–820, 2030,
    2079–2086
    Guillain-Barré syndrome in. *See*
      Guillain-Barré syndrome
    in HIV infection and AIDS, 2121–2122
    in pregnancy, 2260
  in adrenoleukodystrophy, 548
    X-linked, 1640, 1641f
  in cancer therapy, 1312–1313
  in central pontine myelinolysis, 547
  in cerebellitis, 1464
  cerebral, 86
    hemiplegia in, 357
  chronic inflammatory, 819, 820, 1023,
    1995, 2030, 2086–2090
    in HIV infection and AIDS, 2121–2122
    polyradiculoneuropathy in. *See*
      Polyradiculoneuropathy, chronic
      inflammatory demyelinating
  combined central and peripheral disorder,
    1463
  in encephalomyelitis
    acute disseminated, 547, 1459–1463
    recurrent postinfectious and
      postvaccination, 1463

floppy infant in, 413
genetic factors in, 788
hemiplegia in, 357, 359
immune-mediated, 2047
in leukodystrophy
  globoid cell, 1660
  metachromatic, 1661
in leukoencephalitis, acute hemorrhagic,
  1463
in leukoencephalopathy, progressive
  multifocal, 1369–1370
in Marchiafava-Bignami disease, 1507
monoplegia in, 361
in multiple sclerosis, 546–547, 547f,
  1431–1459
in myelitis, transverse, 1463–1464
nerve conduction studies in, 503, 1432,
  1432f, 2048
onion bulb appearance in, 2047
in optic neuritis, 1464
in respiratory infections of children, 1039
segmental, 2047–2048, 2048f
of spinal cord
  bladder function in, 434–435
  hemiplegia in, 359
  monoplegia in, 361
  sexual function in, 436
structural neuroimaging in, 546–547, 547f
in viral infections, 829
Dendrites
  embryonic growth of, 1568–1569
    arborization and branching in, 1568,
      1569
    disorders of, 1568–1569
  injury in craniocerebral trauma, 1050
Denervation of muscles
  biopsy changes in, 2189, 2189f, 2190, 2190f
  in lower motor neuron disorders, 1991
  and reinnervation, 2189, 2190, 2190f
Dengue fever and hemorrhagic fever, 1369
Dens fracture, 582, 584f
Dentatorubropallidoluysian atrophy, 1948
Denver Developmental Screening Test, 81
Dependence on drugs, 1521
  opioid, 909, 1522, 1523
  stimulant, 1524
Depersonalization and phobic-anxiety
  syndrome, 97
Depression, 105–109, 995–996
  in aphasia, 108, 145
  in cerebrovascular disorders, 108, 996,
    997, 1163
  cognitive function in, 102
  and dementia
    in Alzheimer's disease, 1705, 1712
    in elderly, 2282, 2283
    functional neuroimaging in, 668
    vascular, 1728
  diagnostic criteria on, 106, 106t, 2283
  differentiated from dementia, 34, 35t
  dizziness and vertigo in, 240
  in elderly, 2275, 2276, 2283–2284
    and dementia, 2282, 2283
    and suicide rate, 2283, 2283f
  hallucinations in, 110
  in Huntington's disease, 108, 1914,
    1915–1916

in multiple sclerosis, 1438, 1455
in musculoskeletal pain, 398
in neurological disorders, 107–108, 108t
  treatment of, 109
norepinephrine and epinephrine in, 885,
  885t
pain complaints in, 905
in Parkinson's disease, 108, 321
prevalence of, 996–997
and pseudodementia, 1743
serotonin in, 887, 888t
sleep disorders in, 67, 107
  insomnia, 1790
in thyroid disorders, 1032
treatment of, 109, 997
  palliative, 865–866
Dermatan sulfate in mucopolysaccharidosis,
  1648, 1649, 1649t, 1650, 1651
Dermatochalasis, 234
Dermatomes, 369, 371f, 422, 423f
Dermatomyositis, 820, 2223–2225
  classification of, 2223, 2223t
  clinical features in, 2223–2224
  diagnosis of, 2224–2225, 2224f
  muscle biopsy in, 2191, 2224, 2224f
  in paraneoplastic syndromes, 1307, 2226
  pathophysiology in, 2223
  treatment of, 2226
Dermoid cyst
  orbital, structural neuroimaging in, 572
  pathology in, 1250–1251
  spinal, 1288
De Sanctis-Cacchione syndrome, 1620, 1697
Desipramine in pain management, 2055
Desmin, 2202, 2231, 2233
Desmoplasia, 1241
Desmopressin. *See* Antidiuretic hormone
Detrusor muscle of bladder
  areflexia of, 1455
  hyperreflexia of, 747, 751–753
    in elderly, 2291
    with impaired contraction, 2291
    in multiple sclerosis, 434, 435, 752,
      753, 1454–1455
    in multiple system atrophy, 432, 748,
      2156
  instability of, 746–747, 755
    in elderly, 2291
  in spinal cord trauma, 981
  and urethral sphincter dyssynergia, 748,
    981, 2291
Developmental disorders, 81–87, 1561–1582
  cerebral palsy, 1585–1586
  congenital malformations of brain in,
    1573–1582
    embryology of, 1561–1573
  delay, 81–85
    in cerebral malformations, 84
    in chromosomal disorders, 83–84, 84t
    diagnosis of, 81, 82t, 86–87
    global, 83, 86
    in intrauterine infections, 84–85
    parent response to, 86–87
  diagnosis of, 86–87
  dyslexia in, 1590–1591
  in intrauterine growth retardation, 2253
  learning disabilities in, 1587f, 1590–1594

nonverbal, 1592
mental retardation in, 1586
motor, 82–83, 1591
pervasive, 82, 1586–1590
  clinical features in, 1587–1589
  diagnosis of, 1586–1587, 1587t
  etiology of, 1589
  evaluation in, 1589
  treatment of, 1590
in pituitary disease
  in hyperfunction, 851, 852, 1030
  in hypofunction, 849–850
regression, 81, 85–86
  evaluation of, 86, 87t
  organs involved in, 85–86
  peripheral nerve disorders in, 86
sexual
  in delayed or absent puberty, 849–850
  in precocious puberty, 850
in speech and language, 81–82, 161–166.
    See also Speech and language,
    developmental disorders of
Devic's disease, 191, 359, 1435, 1452
Dexamethasone
  in cysticercosis, 1396
  in meningitis, 1320, 1323
    tuberculous, 1332
  in migraine, 1857, 1858
  in pituitary abscess, 934
  in spinal tumors, epidural metastatic, 1284
  suppression test
    in affective disorders, 109, 109t
    in Cushing's disease, 851, 852
Dextroamphetamine
  in narcolepsy, 1822, 1822t
  in rehabilitation, 976
Diabetes insipidus, 854–855, 1032
  central, 854, 1032
  nephrogenic, 854, 1032
Diabetes mellitus, 1033–1034
  arthropathy in, 2100
  bladder function in, 436, 2100, 2103
  cachexia in, 2026, 2102
  cardiac arrhythmias in, 2142–2143
  central nervous system in, 1034, 1037
  in children, 1037
  coma in, nonketotic hyperosmolar, 1034,
      1486, 1487
  dizziness and vertigo in, 247
  in Friedreich's ataxia, 1942, 1944
  gastrointestinal system in, 2100, 2103,
      2146, 2147
  hyperglycemia in, 1486–1488
    and neuropathy, 2097
  hypoglycemia in, 1485, 1486
    unawareness of, 2101
  hypotension in, orthostatic, 2100,
      2102–2103, 2140
  ischemic cerebrovascular disease in, 1126,
      1153
  ketoacidosis in, 1034, 1486–1488
    cerebral edema in, 1487–1488, 1552
    in children, 1037
  neuropathy in, 1033, 1037, 2097–2103
    asymmetrical, 2101–2102
    autonomic, 1033, 2100–2101,
        2102–2103, 2148

in children, 1037
  cranial nerve, 1033, 2098, 2101
  laboratory findings in, 2102
  large fiber, 2100
  mononeuropathy, 1033, 2098, 2101
  pain in, 2102
  pathology in, 2098–2100, 2099f
  pathophysiology of, 2097–2098
  patterns of, 2100–2102
  polyneuropathy, 1033, 2097, 2100–2101
  polyradiculoneuropathy, 1033,
      2026–2027, 2101
  small fiber, 2100
  somatic, 2148
  sural nerve biopsy in, 2099, 2099f
  symmetrical, 2100–2101
  treatment of, 2102–2103
  truncal, 2101
papillopathy in, 197, cp15.XVI
radiculopathy in, 423, 1033, 2026–2027,
    2101
  and lumbar radiculoplexopathy, 2099f,
      2101–2102
  and polyradiculoneuropathy, 1033,
      2026–2027, 2101
sexual function in, 436–437, 2100, 2103
sleep disturbances in, 1811
Diacylglycerol, 872, 879, 884
Diagnosis of neurological disorders, 3–8
  anatomic localization in, 6–7
  differential diagnosis in, 3, 7–8
  explained to patient and family, 865
    in Alzheimer's disease, 2272
  history-taking in, 3–5. *See also* History-
      taking
  inconclusive, 8
  laboratory tests in, 8. *See also* Laboratory
      tests
  neuroimaging in. *See* Neuroimaging
  neurological examination in, 3, 5–6. *See
      also* Neurological examination
  physical examination in, 6. *See also*
      Physical examination
Dialysis, 1028–1029, 1038, 1483–1484
  dementia in, 1028–1029, 1038, 1484,
      1741
  disequilibrium syndrome in, 1028,
      1483–1484
    and cerebral edema, 1484, 1552
  in hyperammonemia, 1617
  sleep disturbances in, 1811
  in uremic encephalopathy, 1483–1484
Diaminopeptide disorders, 1605, 1605t
3,4–Diaminopyridine
  in Lambert-Eaton syndrome, 2183
  in myasthenia gravis, 2178
Diarrhea in shellfish poisoning, 1536t, 1538
Diaschisis, 972, 1312
Diastematomyelia, 1962, 1962f
Diazepam
  in dizziness and vertigo, 740t, 741
  in pain management, 912
  in seizures, 1769
    febrile, 1755
    in status epilepticus, 1754, 1761,
        1761t
  in spasticity, 984t

in withdrawal symptoms of neonate, 2254
Dicyclomine in urinary incontinence, 2294t
Didanosine, neuropathy from, 1420, 2118
Dideoxycytidine, neuropathy from, 2117t,
    2118
Dideoxyinosine, neuropathy from, 2117t,
    2118
Dideoxynucleosides, neuropathy from,
    1420, 2117t, 2118
Diencephalic syndrome, 297
  in brain tumors of young children,
      1276
  growth hormone secretion in, 1037
  ischemic, 300t
    anatomy in, 300f, 301f
Diethylcarbamazine citrate
  in filariasis, lymphatic, 1400
  in loiasis, 1400
Diflunisal in pain management, 908t
Difluoromethylornithine in African
    trypanosomiasis, 1391–1392
Dihydroergotamine
  in cluster headache, 1866
  in migraine, 1855, 1855t, 1856t, 1857
    in children, 1876
    menstrual, 1860, 1860f, 1861, 1861t
Dihydrolipoyl dehydrogenase deficiency,
    1604, 1604t
Dihydropteridine reductase, 1598f
  deficiency of, 1599
Dihydroxyphenylalanine, 879. *See also* Dopa
L-Dihydroxyphenylserine in orthostatic
    hypotension, 2162
Diphenhydramine
  in dystonia, drug-induced, 1921
  in migraine, 1857
Diphtheria, 1342–1343
  antitoxin, 1342–1343, 2126
  faucial, 1342, 1343
  peripheral neuropathy in, 2125–2126
  vaccine, 1342–1343
Diphyllobothriasis, 1397
Diplophonia, 175
Diplopia, 203, 205–216
  in divergence disorders, 718
  fixation switch, 212–213
  in fovea displacement syndrome, 208
  guidelines in evaluation of, 205, 207t
  head posture in, 208–209, 209f
  history of, 208, 209t
  monocular, 207–208
    causes of, 208t
    pinhole test in, 207–208
  in muscle fatigue and weakness, 208, 214,
      382
  in oculomotor nerve palsy, 296
  in Parkinson's disease, 321
  physiological, 205, 207f
  signs associated with, 214–215
  spread of comitance in, 207
  treatment of, 215–216
  vertical, 205
    causes of, 208t
    three-step test in, 213–214, 213f
  visual confusion in, 205, 207f
Dipping in ocular bobbing, 225, 225t
Dipyridamole in stroke prevention, 1158

neurons in, 420, 2047
paraneoplastic disorders of, 2031
in sensory unit, 417, 418
ramus of, 2019
trauma of, 2021
Double crush syndrome, 2056
Doublecortin, 1580
Down syndrome, 1712–1713
atlantoaxial dislocation in, 1955
chromosome translocation in, 781, 782f
dementia in, 1712–1713
thyroid disorders in, 1038
Doxycycline
in brucellosis, 1345, 1346
in ehrlichiosis, 1345
in leptospirosis, 1338
in Lyme disease, 1337
in Rocky Mountain spotted fever, 1344
in syphilis, 1336
in typhus, 1343, 1344
Dracunculiasis, 1400–1401
Dreams, 62
and nightmares, 1813
in rapid eye movement sleep behavior
disorder, 1813
Drinking and thirst
compulsive, 855
in diabetes insipidus, 854, 855
hypothalamus center in, 854
in nocturnal drinking syndrome of
children, 1814
Drop attacks, 19–23, 1130
in atonic seizures, 1754–1755
causes of, 20t
Drug abuse, 1521–1527
botulism in, 1339
cerebrovascular disorders in, 1525–1526
in children, 1220
embolism, 1526
hemorrhage, 1172, 1174f, 1221, 1526
hypotension and anoxia, 1526
ischemia, 1144, 1145f, 1526
mechanisms of, 1525, 1525t
vasculitis, 1233, 1526
craniocerebral trauma in, 1078
dependence on drugs in, 1521
opioid, 909, 1522, 1523
stimulant, 1524
detection of, 1521, 1522t
neurological complications of, 1522t
overdose in, 1492
in pregnancy, fetal and neonatal effects of,
2253–2254
tolerance to drugs in, 1521
opioid, 909, 1522
withdrawal symptoms in. See Withdrawal
symptoms
Drug-induced disorders
in arrhythmias, 1012
in asthma, 1039–1040
ataxia in, 316, 1940
of autonomic nervous system, 2135t,
2139
cerebellar dysfunction in, 1940
chorea in, 329, 1921t
cognitive impairment in, 1742
coma in, 40, 41

differential diagnosis in, 53
delirium in, 32–33, 32t
dizziness and vertigo in, 244, 247
dyskinesia in, 1921–1924
in Parkinson's disease, 1808, 1825
epidural lipomatosis in, 1981
hemorrhagic disorders in, 1025
hyperprolactinemia in, 851
hypoglycemia in, 1486
intracranial hemorrhage in, 1170, 1172,
1181
in Lambert-Eaton syndrome, 2183–2184,
2184t
of liver
from acetaminophen, 907, 908t
from valproate, in children, 1040–1041
movement disorders in, 1921–1924,
1921t
muscle pain in, 400, 400t
myasthenia gravis in, 2181
mydriasis in, 230
neuroleptic malignant syndrome in, 845,
1922–1923
nightmares in, 1813
nystagmus in, gaze-paretic, 220
of olfaction, 267, 269t
optic neuropathy in, 192, 197
parkinsonism in, 1905, 1921t, 1922
in Parkinson's disease, 1896, 1897t
peripheral neuropathy in, 2117–2121,
2117t
porphyria in, acute intermittent, 1621
pseudotumor cerebri in, 1553, 1553t
research on, in approval process, 893–894
in rheumatoid arthritis, 1017
sexual behavior in, 100
of sleep, 67, 1789
insomnia in, 1789
in Parkinson's disease, 1808
tardive dyskinesia in, 328, 329–330,
1921t, 1923–1924
of taste sense, 268, 269t
tinnitus in, 260
vision loss in, gradual, 192
vitamin B_6 deficiency in, 1502
Drug therapy, 867–896
acceptability to patient, 894
in Alzheimer's disease, 1712, 2281–2283
in amyotrophic lateral sclerosis, 2011,
2012t
antiviral, 839
in aphasia, 158–159
in arrhythmias, neurological
complications of, 1012
in asthma, neurological complications of,
1039–1040
in attention-deficit hyperactivity disorder,
1593, 1594, 1594t
in autism, 1590, 1590t
in behavioral disorders, 996, 996t
bioavailability of drugs in, 894
biotransformation of drugs in, 895
in bladder disorders, 981–982, 981t
in detrusor hyperreflexia, 751–752,
752t
in multiple sclerosis, 1454–1455
compliance with, 894

in cramps, 399t
in delirium, 36
distribution of drugs in, 895
in Duchenne's muscular dystrophy, 2195
in dystonia, idiopathic torsion, 1908
ease of use in, 894
elimination of drugs in, 896
in erectile dysfunction, 756
in fungal infections, 1381–1383, 1382t
half-life of drugs in, 896
in headache. See Headache, drug therapy in
in HIV infection and AIDS. See HIV
infection and AIDS, drug therapy in
interactions of drugs in, 896
in children, 1039–1040
ion channels in, voltage-gated, 887–893
in ischemic cerebrovascular disease,
1157–1160
in leprosy, 1334
in malaria, 1388–1389
resistance to, 1388
in memory impairment, 994, 994t
metabolism of drugs in
genetic variations in, 895–896
physiological variations in, 896
in migraine. See Migraine, drug therapy in
in narcolepsy, 1822–1823, 1822t
neurotransmitters in, 867–887
in orthostatic hypotension, 2159–2162,
2160t
in elderly, 2290
in pain management, 863, 906–912,
2055–2056
in parasitic infections, 1385, 1386t
neurotoxicity of, 1385, 1386t
in Parkinson's disease, 1896–1898, 1898t
complications of, 1896, 1897t
placebo response in, 862
in pain management, 907
in rehabilitation, 976–977
research on, 893–894
in approval process, 893–894
design of studies in, 893
ethical issues in, 893
in restless legs syndrome, 1823–1824,
1823t
in rheumatoid arthritis, neurological side
effects of, 1017
in seizures, 1769–1776, 1770t. See also
Anticonvulsant drugs
in sleep apnea, 1821
in spasticity, 983–984, 984t
in spinal cord trauma, 1109
in subarachnoid hemorrhage and
vasospasm, 937, 1195
therapeutic index in, 894
titration rate in, 894–895
in Tourette's syndrome, 1918
in trigeminal neuralgia, 1873
in tuberculosis, 1331
in urinary incontinence of elderly, 2293,
2294t
in vestibular disorders, peripheral,
740–741, 740t
Drusen of optic nerve, 191, 193–194, cp15.II
pseudopapilledema in, 193
in retinitis pigmentosa, 194

congenital, 392, 393f, 414, 2203–2207
  myotonic, 2211, 2259
Duchenne's, 395, 2193–2196. *See also*
    Duchenne's muscular dystrophy
in dystrophin deficiency, 2192–2197
in emerin deficiency, 2199
Emery-Dreifuss, 394–395, 2199
facioscapulohumeral, 393–394, 394f,
    2199–2201
floppy infant in, 412, 414
Fukuyama type. *See* Fukuyama type
    muscular dystrophy
genetic factors in. *See* Genetics, in
    muscular dystrophy
immunocytochemical studies in, 2192
limb-girdle, 395, 2197–2199
  classification of, 2198–2199
  differential diagnosis in, 2001
in merosin deficiency, 2204
in muscle-eye-brain disease, 2204,
    2206–2207
muscle pain in, 399
myotonic, 394, 394f, 2202, 2208–2211
  bladder function in, 437
  bowel function in, 437
  cardiovascular disorders in, 2209–2210
  clinical features in, 2209–2210,
    2209f
  congenital, 2211, 2259
  diagnosis of, 2210
  facial appearance in, 2209, 2209f
  genetic counseling in, 2211
  muscle biopsy in, 2210, 2211f
  pathophysiology in, 2208–2209
  pregnancy in, 2259
  treatment of, 2210–2211
  trinucleotide repeat expansions in,
    789, 790f, 791f, 2208
ocular, 2207
oculopharyngeal, 393, 2203, 2203f,
    2204f
respiratory disorders in, 1804
scapuloperoneal, 394, 2201
sleep disorders in, 1804
  polysomnography in, 1818
stick-man, 392, 393f, 2234, 2234f
in Walker-Warburg syndrome, 2204,
    2206–2207
reflex sympathetic, 365, 426, 448, 904,
    2140
lower limb pain in, 460

Eales disease, 1148
Ear
  audiological testing of, 736–740
  congenital anomalies of, 1038–1039
  examination of, 736–740
    in hearing loss, 254, 255–256
  and hearing. *See* Hearing
  inner, microangiopathy in Susac's
      syndrome, 1147–1148
  middle, testing of, 738
  otoacoustic emissions of, 256
  and tinnitus, 260–261
Eating
  in anorexia nervosa, 846
  in bulimia nervosa, 846

nocturnal syndrome in children, 1814
Ebola virus, 1369
Echinococcosis, 1396–1397
  cerebral, seizures in, 1792
Echo sequences in magnetic resonance
    imaging, 523
Echocardiography in cardiogenic embolism,
    1010, 1156
Echolalia in parkinsonism, 322
Echoplanar imaging, 525
Echopraxia, 120
Echoviruses, 1364
Eclampsia
  encephalopathy in, 2267–2268
  ischemic stroke in, 2265
Economic factors. *See* Cost considerations
Ecstasy, 886, 1524
Ectoparasites, 1385, 1404
Ectopia. *See* Heterotopia
Edema
  cerebral, 1545, 1549–1552
    in anoxic-ischemic encephalopathy,
      1469, 1473
      in neonate, 2244
    cytotoxic, 1549, 1551–1552
    in diabetic ketoacidosis, 1487–1488,
      1552
    in dialysis disequilibrium syndrome,
      1484, 1552
    in hyperosmolality of serum,
      1490–1491, 1552
    in hypertensive encephalopathy, 1552
    inflammatory response in, 1549,
      1550–1551, 1550f
    in intracerebral hemorrhage, 1551
    in intracranial pressure increase, 1553
    in ischemic cerebrovascular disease,
      1162, 1550f, 1551
    in liver failure, 1026, 1026f,
      1551–1552
    in meningioma, 539
    molecular cascade in, 1549–1550
    posterior syndrome, 1552
    treatment of, 1552
      in neonate, 2244
    vasogenic, 1549, 1550–1551
  of optic disc, 193–197. *See also*
      Papilledema
  pulmonary
    neurogenic, 919, 920
    in subarachnoid hemorrhage, 1192
  of spinal cord, 582–583, 585f, 1107
    magnetic resonance imaging in,
      582–583, 585f, 1107
Edrophonium test
  in diplopia, 215
  in floppy infant, 415
  in myasthenia gravis, 2171–2172
Eflornithine in African trypanosomiasis,
    1391–1392
Ehlers-Danlos syndrome, 1147, 1675–1677
  arterial dissection in, 1676–1677
  carotid-cavernous fistula in, 1676
  hyperelasticity of skin in, 1675, 1675f
  intracranial aneurysm in, 1675–1676,
    1676f
  subtypes of, 1675

Ehrlichiosis, 1344–1345
Ejaculation, 430
  failure of, 756–757
  in spinal cord disorders, 435
  sympathetic thoracolumbar fibers in, 436
Elastance of brain in intracranial pressure
    increase, 1069
Elastase in cerebral edema, 1550, 1551
Elbow
  median nerve entrapment in, 447, 2057t,
    2059
  tennis injury of, 447
  ulnar nerve entrapment in, 447,
    2059–2060
Elderly, 2269–2295
  abuse of, 2272
  age-related neurological disease and
      dysfunction in, 2269, 2276
  Alzheimer's disease in, 2270. *See also*
      Alzheimer's disease
  anatomical and neurochemical changes in,
    2272–2273
  atrophic changes in, 544
    neuroimaging studies in, 2277
  autonomic nervous system in, 2273
    disorders of, 2138, 2289–2295
  cell loss in, 1254, 2272–2273
  clinical examination of, 2275–2278
  cognitive function in, 678, 2273–2275
    and competency in health care
        decisions, 2271–2272
    disorders of, 2278–2285
    testing of, 2276–2277
  cost of care for, 2271
  craniocerebral trauma in, 1078
  delirium in. *See* Delirium, in elderly
  dementia in, 2278–2283
    causes of, 2279–2280, 2280t
    and depression, 2282, 2283
    evaluation of, 2280–2281
    genetic markers in, 2281, 2281t
    reversible, 2279, 2280, 2280t
    treatment of, 2281–2283
  demographics of population, 2270
  depression in, 2275, 2276, 2283–2284
    and dementia, 2282, 2283
    and suicide rate, 2283, 2283f
  disequilibrium in, subcortical, 350–351,
    351t
  dizziness and vertigo in, 247, 248
  dorsal midbrain syndrome in, 294
  drug metabolism in, 896
  electroencephalography in, 484–485,
    2278, 2279f
  ethical issues in care of, 2271–2272
  evoked responses in, 2278
  falls and drop attacks in, 19, 22–23, 2289
    risk reduction in, 23
  fecal incontinence in, 2293–2295, 2295t
  functional assessment of, 2275–2276
  gait in, 346, 350–352
    assessment of, 2277
    disorders of, 2288–2289, 2288t, 2289t
    and falls, 22–23, 346
  headache in, 285, 286, 289
  hypotension in, orthostatic, 2289–2290
  mitochondrial disorders in, 1635–1636

Elderly—*continued*
  multidisciplinary assessment of, 2271
  nerve conduction studies in, 508, 509t
  neuroimaging studies in, 2277–2278
  neurological evaluation in, 2276–2277
  neurologists as principal care providers
      for, 2295
  neurotransmitters in, 2273
      acetylcholine, 879, 880t
  seizures in, 2286–2287, 2287t
  sleep patterns in, 60–61, 62f
      disorders of, 2287–2288
  successful aging in, 2257, 2270, 2276
  syncope in, 2285, 2286t
  urinary incontinence in, 2290–2293,
      2293t, 2294t
      in dementia, 2282, 2292
Electrical injuries, 1542–1543
Electrical polarity of cell membranes,
      embryonic development of, 1569
Electrical stimulation techniques
  functional, during exercise, 985
  in pain management, 907, 913, 950
  in spasticity, 983
Electrocardiography
  in coma, 54
  in Emery-Dreifuss muscular dystrophy,
      2199
  in Friedreich's ataxia, 1942, 1943, 1943f
  in ischemic cerebrovascular disease, 1162
  in periodic paralysis, hypokalemic, 2213
  in syncope, 14, 1036
Electrocerebral inactivity or silence in brain
      death, 56, 475, 484
Electrocochleography, 740
Electroconvulsive therapy
  in depression, 109
  language laterality in, 682, 683t
Electrocorticography, 473
Electrodes
  in electromyography, insertion of, 511
  in nerve conduction studies, 497–498
Electroencephalography, 473–486
  in affective disorders, 109
  age-related changes in, 484, 2278, 2279f
      in sleep, 2287
  alpha rhythm in, 474, 474f, 928f
      in coma, 482, 483f, 1472
  in Alzheimer's disease, 485, 1706–1707
  in anoxic-ischemic encephalopathy, 483f,
      484f, 1472
      in neonate, 2241
  in aphasia, 156
  in auditory agnosia, 163–164
  beta activity in, 474
  in brain death, 56, 475, 484, 1471
  burst suppression pattern in, 483, 483f,
      827
      in Creutzfeldt-Jakob disease, 1425,
          1426f
  clinical uses of, 475–485
  in coma, 55, 482, 483
      alpha, 482, 483f, 1472
  common abnormalities in, 474–475
  continuous monitoring, 927–928, 928f
      indications for, 927–928, 928t
  in corpus callosum agenesis, 1579

  in craniocerebral trauma, 480
      and prognosis, 1086
  in Creutzfeldt-Jakob disease, 485, 485f,
      1425, 1426f
  in delirium, 31, 31f
  delta activity in, 474
      focal, 479
      intermittent bursts, 479, 482f
  in dementia, 484–485, 1702
  digital systems in, 485–486
  in elderly, 484–485, 2278, 2279f
  electrocerebral inactivity or silence in, 56,
      475, 484
  in encephalitis, 1355
      herpes simplex, 483, 1358
  epileptiform discharges in, 475, 476
      lateralized, 477, 480f
  in focal cerebral lesions, 479–480, 481f,
      482f
  frequency domain topographical brain
      map obtained from, cp37A.I
  in headache, 290
      in migraine, 479, 1850
  in hepatic encephalopathy, 1477
  in holoprosencephaly, 1577
  in hypoxia, 482–483, 483f, 484f
  in infantile spasms, hypsarrhythmia in,
      477, 478f
  in infectious diseases, 483–484
  in intraoperative monitoring, 495, 956
  in Lennox-Gastaut syndrome, 477, 478f,
      1758
  light stimulation in, 475, 476f
  limitations of, 473–474
  in liver failure, 482, 483f
  magnetoencephalography compared with,
      486
  in measles and subacute sclerosing
      panencephalitis, 1367, 1367f
  in metabolic encephalopathy, 480–482,
      482f
  in movement disorders, 340
  in neurointensive care monitoring,
      927–928
      continuous, 927–928, 928f, 928t
  normal patterns in, 474, 474f
  periodic pattern in, 483, 484f
  in personality changes, 95–96
  physiological principles in, 473–474
  in premature infants, 1569
  in psychosis, 114
  recording techniques in, 475, 476f
  in schizophrenia, 114
  in seizures, 16–17, 476–477, 1767–1768
      absence, 1754
      anterior temporal spikes in, 477, 477f
      atonic, 1755
      centrotemporal spikes in, 1751
      epileptiform discharges in, 475, 476
          lateralized, 477, 480f
      intermittent delta waves in, 479, 482f
      intracranial monitoring in, 1767–1768
      in Lennox-Gastaut syndrome, 477,
          478f, 1758
      myoclonic
          with encephalopathy, 1757
          in infants, benign, 1756

      juvenile, 1756
      in neonate, 2239, 2241
      partial, 1748, 1751
      petit mal, 477, 478f
      prolonged recordings in, 1767
      psychogenic, 1763
      rolandic, 477, 479f, 1751
      and sleep, 1802, 1803, 1819
      spike-wave patterns in, 476, 477f
      tonic, 1754
      tonic-clonic, 476, 477f, 482f, 1753
      in West's syndrome, 1757–1758
  in sleep, 60, 61f, 474, 474f
      age-related changes in, 2287
      and seizures, 1802, 1803, 1819
  in syncope, 14
  theta activity in, 474
  voltage attenuation in, 475
  in West's syndrome, 1757–1758
Electrogustometry, 268
Electrolyte disorders, 1029–1039
Electromagnetic fields, exposure to, 1542
Electromyography, 509–518
  in amyotrophic lateral sclerosis, 2009,
      2010
  in amyotrophy, benign focal, 1996
  in back and lower limb pain, 463–464
  in botulism, 2184
  in brachial plexus disorders, 2033–2034
  complex repetitive discharges in, 512,
      513–514
  continuous muscle fiber activity in, 514
  corpus cavernosal, 751
  in cramps, 514
  in dermatomyositis, 2224
  discharge types in, 512
  in Duchenne's muscular dystrophy, 2194
  endplate activity in, 511, 511f
  in facial myokymia, 276
  fasciculation potentials in, 512, 513
  fibrillation potentials in, 511, 512
  in floppy infant, 414
  in Guillain-Barré syndrome, 2081
  in headache, tension-type, 1868
  insertional activity in, 509, 511
  interference pattern in, 510
  interpretation of, 516–518, 517f
  in Kennedy's disease, 2003
  in Lambert-Eaton syndrome, 2182
  in lumbosacral plexus disorders, 2039
  in motor neuron disorders, 516, 517,
      1991
      interpretation of, 517
      lower, 1991
      motor unit potentials in, 515
  motor unit potentials in, 509, 514–515
  in movement disorders, 340
  in multifocal motor neuropathy, 2090
  in multiple system atrophy, 748, 749f
  in muscle pain, 398
  in myasthenia gravis, 2172–2173, 2172f
  myokymic discharges in, 512, 513, 513f
  in myopathy, 516, 518
      motor unit potentials in, 515
  myotonic discharges in, 511
      in myotonic dystrophy, 2210
  in peripheral nerve trauma, 1118

Face—*continued*
  pain in, 285–291
    atypical, 1871
    differential diagnosis in, 289–291
    examination in, 288–289
    history of, 285–288
    location of, 287
    in temporomandibular joint disorders,
      287, 288, 290, 291, 1844–1845
    in trigeminal neuralgia, 1872–1874
    of unknown origin, 1871
  recognition of, 682, 688–691
    in prosopagnosia, 134, 690, 691–692
  reflexes of, 273
  spasm of, hemifacial, 235–236, 236f, 275,
    337, 1929
    botulinum toxin therapy in, 275, 951,
      1929
    neurosurgery in, 951, 1929
    and paretic contracture, 276
  vascular changes in autonomic disorders,
    2143
  weakness of, 273, 276, 382
    bilateral, 1884–1885
    disorders with, 393–394, 394f
    examination in, 383
    in motor neuron disorders, 273–274,
      273t
    speech in, 383
Facial artery, 620, 621f
Facial nerve, 271–276, 1884–1885
  acoustic reflex in disorders of, 256, 273
  anatomy of, 271–272, 272f, 1884
  branches of, 272, 1884
  clinical evaluation of, 273–274
  congenital disorders of, 1884
  in diabetes mellitus, 1033, 2101
  dysarthria in disorders of, 175t
  in facial movements, 272, 273, 273t, 1884
    overactivity of, 275–276
  herpes virus infection of, 274, 1885, 2259
  in leprosy, 1885, 2125
  in Lyme disease, 1885, 2126
  motor portion of, 271, 1884
    clinical features in disorders, 273–274,
      273t
  in multiple sclerosis, 1439
  paralysis of, 272, 273
    Bell's, 1885. *See also* Bell's palsy
    bilateral, 1884–1885
    diagnosis of, 274
    differential diagnosis of, 274
    neuroimaging in, 274–275
    in pregnancy, 2259–2260
    traumatic, 1884
      in birth injuries, 2251–2252
  in peripheral neuropathies, 2050, 2050t
  regeneration of, aberrant, 276, 1885
  sensory portion of (nervus intermedius),
    271, 272, 1884
    neuralgia of, 1874–1875
  in taste sense, 267, 271, 273, 1884
    disorders of, 268
  toxins affecting, 1884
  trauma of, 274, 275, 1884
    in birth injuries, 2251–2252
  tumors of, 274, 275, 1885

Facioscapulohumeral muscular dystrophy,
    393–394, 394f, 2199–2201
  clinical features in, 2200, 2200f
  diagnosis of, 2200
  pathophysiology in, 2199
  treatment of, 2200–2201
Factitious disorder, 103
Factor V Leiden mutation, 1042, 1127,
    1150
Failed back syndrome, 461, 914, 1975
Failure to thrive in Menkes' syndrome,
    1624, 1688
Fainting, 9, 13. *See also* Syncope
Fallot tetralogy, 1035, 1036
  syncope in, 12
Falls, 19–23
  in ataxia, 21, 343
  in cataplexy, 21–22, 67, 1792
  causes of, 20t
  in Duchenne's muscular dystrophy, 2193
  in elderly, 19, 22–23, 2289
  history of, 343
  in ischemic cerebrovascular disease, 19,
    20, 1130, 1163
  in narcolepsy, 21, 67, 1792
  in parkinsonism, 21, 321, 323
  in seizures, 20, 353
    atonic, 1754–1755
    in children, 353
    injuries related to, 1753
Falx
  cerebelli, 632
  cerebri, 632
Famciclovir, 1356t
  in herpes simplex virus infections, 2123
  mechanism of action, 839
  in varicella zoster virus infections, 1360,
    2124
Family
  history of, 5
    in brachial plexus disorders, 444
    in developmental regression, 85
    in floppy infant, 410–411, 410t
    genetic linkage analysis of, 794–797,
      795f
    in headaches, 288
    in intracranial aneurysm and
      subarachnoid hemorrhage, 1189,
      1190–1191
    in ischemic cerebrovascular disease,
      1125–1126
    in multiple sclerosis, 768
    in personality changes, 94
  impact of disease on, 865
    in dementia of elderly, 2282–2283
    informed about prognosis, 865
    and multiple sclerosis risk, 768,
      1437–1438, 1438t
    in rehabilitation process, 963
    in terminal illness, psychological support
      of, 866
Fanconi's syndrome, 1600
Farber's lipogranulomatosis, 1646
Faroe Islands, multiple sclerosis in, 768,
    769, 770f, 771f
Fas and Fas ligand, 814, 815f
Fascia iliaca, 2040, 2041

Fasciculation, 367–368, 384
  benign, 368, 384, 513
  electromyography potentials in, 512, 513
  in lower motor neuron disorders,
    1990–1991
Fasciculus, 1113, 1114
  medial longitudinal, 701, 702, 702f
    in vertical eye movements, 706–707,
      707f
    surgical repair of trauma, 1121–1122,
      1122f
    nerve grafts in, 1122, 1123f
Fascioliasis, 1404
Fast foot maneuver, 385
Fastigial nucleus in ocular motor system,
    706
Fat
  embolism, 1148
  malabsorption, 1500
  signal in magnetic resonance imaging, 523
Fatigue, 98–99
  chronic syndrome, 98, 99, 400, 1372
  differential diagnosis in, 59, 99
  exercise-induced, 390
  of eyelid, 208, 214
  in floppy infant, 409
  in metabolic muscle disorders, 2217
    in myophosphorylase deficiency, 2218
  in multiple sclerosis, 1441, 1454
  occupational therapy in, 962
  in postpolio syndrome, 1993
Fatty acid metabolism, 1630–1631, 2077,
    2219–2221
  beta-oxidation in, 1608f, 1630–1631
    disorders of, 1641
  carnitine in, 1607, 1608f, 1630,
    2220–2221
  carnitine palmitoyltransferase in,
    2219–2220
  in exercise, 390, 2219
  in hepatic encephalopathy, 1481
  in peroxisomes, 1636, 1637t
    disorders of, 1640, 1641
    pathways in, 1642f
Fazio-Londe disease, 2000
Felbamate in seizures, 1770t, 1771
Felbatol, 876
Femoral nerve
  at lumbosacral plexus
    anatomy of, 2038, 2039f
    hematoma affecting, 2040
    in pregnancy, 2042
  neuropathy of, 364t, 365, 459, 2057t,
    2062
    diabetic, 2026
    differential diagnosis in, 372t, 421–422
    lateral cutaneous, 421, 2057t, 2062
    pain in, 459
    sensory function in, 372t, 421–422
    site of compression in, 2057t
  stretch test of, 456
Fenamic acid in pain management, 908t
Fentanyl, transdermal, in pain management,
    910t, 911
Fernandez reaction in leprosy, 1333
Festination in parkinsonism, 321, 348
Fetal alcohol syndrome, 1569

Herniation—*continued*
  computed tomography in, 1969, 1969f
  lumbar. *See* Lumbar spine, disc
      herniation in
  magnetic resonance imaging in,
      575–577, 580f
    lumbar, 575, 580f, 1974, 1974f,
        1976f
    thoracic, 1971, 1972f
    in trauma, 588, 1107
  radiculoneuropathy in, 441, 1968,
      1969, 2022–2026
    cervical, 441, 1968, 1969,
        2022–2026
    lumbar, 1973, 1974, 1975,
        2022–2026
    thoracic, 1971, 1972f
  in trauma, 588
    magnetic resonance imaging in, 588,
        1107
Heroin, 1522
  neuropathy from, 2119
Herpes simplex virus, as vector in gene
    transfer therapy, 1260
Herpes simplex virus infections
  congenital, 1357, 2249
  encephalitis in, 825, 826, 829, 1358–1359
    aphasia in, 158
    computed tomography in, 554f
    and Cowdry type A inclusions, 1359,
        cp59B.I
    dementia in, 1739
    diagnosis of, 826, 836, 1358
    differential diagnosis of, 1359
    electroencephalography in, 483, 1358
    in HIV infection and AIDS, 829
    magnetic resonance imaging in, 552,
        1358, 1358f
    personality and behavior changes in,
        92–93, 1358
    structural neuroimaging in, 552, 554f
    treatment of, 826, 838, 839, 1359
  of facial nerve, 274, 1885, 2259
    Bell's palsy in, 2259
  meningitis in, 823, 825
  in neonate, 1357, 1359, 2249
  neural spread of, 833, 834
  treatment of, 1356t, 2123
    in encephalitis, 826, 838, 839, 1359
  trigeminal neuralgia in, 1883
  type 1, 2123
    encephalitis in, 1358–1359
  type 2, 2123
    encephalitis in, 1358
    in neonate, 1359
Herpes zoster virus infection, 1359–1360,
    2029–2030. *See also* Varicella
    zoster virus infections
Herpesviruses, 1357–1362
  cercopithecine herpesvirus type 1 (B
      virus), 1362
  cytomegalovirus. *See* Cytomegalovirus
      infections
  Epstein-Barr. *See* Epstein-Barr virus
      infections
  in facial nerve infection, 274, 1885, 2259
  herpes simplex

infection with. *See* Herpes simplex virus
    infections
  as vector in gene transfer therapy, 1260
  herpes zoster. *See* Varicella zoster virus
      infections
  human herpesvirus type 6 (HHV-6),
      1361–1362
    and HIV infection, 1361f
    and multiple sclerosis, 1361–1362,
        1435
Heschl's gyrus in language processes, 142
Hess screen test in diplopia, 210
Heterogeneity, genetic, 778, 788, 790f
  allelic, 778, 788
  linkage analysis of, 796
  nonallelic, 778, 788
Heterophoria, 204
Heterotopia, 1566, 1567, 1580–1581
  band, 562, 1580
  of brainstem nuclei, 1566
  bulk form, 562, 563f
  in encephalocele, 1575
  of gray matter, 562, 563f, 1580
  in holoprosencephaly, 1577
  of lens in homocystinuria, 1601, 1602t
  marginal glioneuronal, 1567–1568
  nodular, 562
    periventricular, 1580–1581
  subcortical laminar, 1580–1581
Heterotropia, 204. *See also* Strabismus
Heterozygote, 777
Heubner recurrent artery, 624, 624f
Hexacarbon solvent exposure, 1513–1514
n-Hexane, 1513, 1527
Hexosaminidase, 1655f
  deficiencies of, 1657, 1935, 1936f
    adult-onset, 2017
    ataxia in, 1935, 1936f
    differential diagnosis of, 2002, 2010
Hip
  osteoarthritis of, gait in, 353
  weakness of, 382, 395
Hippocampus
  in memory, 74–75, 75f, 76
  speech delay in disorders of, 81
  in traumatic brain injury, 1048–1049
Hippus, 229, 230–231
Hirschberg test in diplopia, 210–211, 212f
Hirschsprung's disease, 2139
Histamine, and cluster headaches,
    1864–1865, 1866
Histidine metabolism disorders, 1605, 1605t
Histidinemia, 1605
Histocompatibility complex, major,
    808–809. *See also* HLA system
Histogenesis disorders, structural
    neuroimaging in, 563–564
Histoplasmosis, 1379–1380, 1382t
Historical aspects
  of Alzheimer's disease, 1703–1704
  of delirium, 25
  of diagnostic techniques in viral
      infections, 836
  of migraine, 1845
  of myasthenia gravis, 2167–2168
  of neurointensive care, 917
  of vitamin B$_6$ deficiency, 1501

History-taking, 3–5
  chief complaint in, 4
  on family, 5
  in geriatric neurology, 2276
  in headache, 285–288
    in children, 1876
    cluster, 287, 288, 1863–1864
    in tension-type headache, 287, 288,
        1869
  in hypothalamic-pituitary disorders, 856
  in pain, 906
  in peripheral neuropathy, 2048–2049
  personal profile in, 4
  on present illness, 4
  on previous illness, 5
  in seizures, 4, 5, 15, 1767
  in sleep disorders, 68, 1787–1788
  systems review in, 4–5
HLA system, 806, 807, 808–809, 810f
  in autoimmune disorders, 816
  in central nervous system, 815
  and central tolerance, 813
  class I, 808, 808f, 809
  class II, 808, 809
  in myasthenia gravis, 2169, 2171
  in myopathy, inflammatory, 2223
  in narcolepsy, 1791, 1792, 1820
  in rheumatoid arthritis, 1978
  in spondyloarthropathy, inflammatory,
      1979
  and T cell activation, 809, 810
  and T cell receptors, 806f
Hoarseness, 173, 176
  and dysphagia, 181
Hodgkin's disease, 2005
  cerebellar degeneration in, 1933
  peripheral neuropathy in, 2106
Hoffmann's sign in cervical spine disorders,
    377–378
Hoffmann's syndrome in hypothyroidism,
    1032
Holmes-Adie syndrome, 229–230, 724,
    2139, 2145
  investigations in, 232–233
Holmes' tremor, 327, 1907
Holocarboxylase synthetase deficiency,
    1609, 1610, 1629
Holoprosencephaly, 1576–1577
  alobar, 559, 559f, 1577
  computed tomography in, 559f, 1578f
  lobar, 1577
  semilobar, 1577, 1578f
  structural neuroimaging in, 559, 559f
Homans' sign, 457
Home care
  in amyotrophic lateral sclerosis, 2014
  of elderly, 2282
Homeostasis
  glucose, 1484–1485
  lysine, 1606–1607
  osmotic, 1488–1489
  in sleep-wake cycle, 1787
  sodium, 854
  water, 854
Homer Wright rosette formations, 1241
  in medulloblastoma, 1241, 1247, 1248f
Homocarnosinase deficiency, 1605t

Hypertonia
    regional, and central hypotonia, 411
    spasticity in, 982–984
Hypertrichosis in ataxia-telangiectasia, 1685
Hypertropia, 204
    three-step test in, 213–214, 213f
Hyperuricemia in Lesch-Nyhan disease,
        1618, 1619
Hyperventilation
    in anxiety disorders, 97, 102
    central neurogenic, 46f, 47
    hypocapnia in, 1020
    syncope in, 14
    as therapy
        in craniocerebral trauma, 1072
        in intracerebral hemorrhage, 1181
        in intracranial pressure increase, 1072,
            1181
Hyperviscosity syndrome
    in leukemia, 1022
    in myeloma, 1023
Hypnotic drugs, 1523–1524
Hypoactivity in delirium, 27
Hypobetalipoproteinemia, 1622
    vitamin E deficiency in, 1939
Hypocalcemia, 1030, 1491
    cognitive function in, 1740
    neonatal seizure in, 2239, 2239t, 2240t
    in parathyroid disorders, 1030, 1033,
        1491
    symptoms in, 1491
    treatment of, 1491
Hypocapnia, 1020
Hypochondriasis, 101t
Hypogeusia, 267, 268
Hypoglossal nerve, 280–282, 1887–1888
    anatomy of, 280–281, 1887–1888
    clinical features in disorders, 281–282, 281f
    diagnosis of disorders, 282
    dysarthria in disorders, 175t, 281
    infections of, 282
    palsy of, 282, 1888
    trauma of, 1888
    tumors of, 282, 1888
Hypoglycemia, 1034, 1485–1486, 1486t
    acute, 1485
    amyotrophy in, 2115
    causes of, 1486, 1486t
    chronic, 1485
        cognitive function in, 1740
    in diabetes mellitus, 1485, 1486
        unawareness of, 2101
    encephalopathy in, 1034
    neonatal seizure in, 2239, 2239t, 2240t
    subacute, 1485
    syncope in, 13
Hypogonadism, 852
    and cerebellar ataxia, 1944–1945
Hypohidrosis in autonomic disorders, 2143,
        2145
Hypokalemia, 1029–1030
    paralysis in, 391
        periodic familial, 2213–2214
Hypokinesia, 117, 119, 320
    pathophysiology of, 121
    testing for, 119
Hypomagnesemia, 1030, 1491

Hypomania, 108
Hypomelanosis
    of Ito, 1691–1693
        swirling pigmentation in, cp69.I
    in tuberous sclerosis, 1666–1667, 1667f
Hypometria, 119
Hypomyelination, 86
Hyponasal speech, 173
Hyponatremia, 1029, 1071
    causes of, 1489, 1489t
    central pontine myelinolysis in, 1029,
        1489–1490
    in cerebral salt wasting, 856, 1071
    in inappropriate secretion of antidiuretic
        hormone, 855, 1029, 1071, 1192,
        1489
    osmolality of serum in, 1489
    in subarachnoid hemorrhage, 1192, 1489
    treatment of, 1489–1490
Hypo-osmolality of serum, 1489–1490
Hypoparathyroidism, 1033
    basal ganglia calcification in, 1927, 1928
    calcium serum levels in, 1030, 1033, 1491
Hypophonia, 321
Hypophosphatemia in epidermal nevus
        syndrome, 1691
Hypophyseal arteries and veins, 848, 848f
Hypophysectomy in pain management, 950
Hypophysitis, 853
    lymphocytic, 847, 853
Hypopigmentation
    in hypomelanosis of Ito, 1692
    in tuberous sclerosis, 1666–1667, 1667f
Hypopituitarism, 849–850, 849t, 1031–1032
    treatment of, 858
Hypoplasia
    cerebellar, 1562, 1581, 1582f, 1931
    cerebral, 1562, 1563f
    of optic nerve, 198, cp15.XVIII
        in children, 730
    pontocerebellar, 1563
Hypopnea, sleep-related, 1796
Hyporeflexia in lower motor neuron
        disorders, 1990
Hyposmia, 264, 265
Hypotension
    coma in, 41–42
    in craniocerebral trauma, 1051, 1060
        as prognostic factor, 1082
    dizziness and vertigo in, 247, 2140
    in neonate, 2243
    orthostatic, 2140–2142
        ambulatory monitoring of, 2149, 2152f
        in diabetes mellitus, 2100, 2102–2103,
            2140
        dizziness and vertigo in, 247, 2140
        drug-induced, 2140
        drug therapy in, 2159–2162, 2160t
            in elderly, 2290
        in elderly, 2289–2290
        factors influencing, 2140, 2140t
        food affecting, 2149, 2150, 2151f,
            2159
            in elderly, 2290
        heart rate in, 2141f, 2142f
        idiopathic, 2133
        management of, 2158–2162

non-neurogenic causes of, 2149, 2151t
        in spinal cord trauma, 2141
        symptoms in, 2140, 2140t
            and blood pressure changes,
                2140–2142, 2141f, 2142f
        syncope in, 13, 19
        tests and investigations in, 2149–2154
    spinal cord ischemia in, 1227
    syncope in, 10, 13, 2141–2142
        and falls, 19
Hypothalamus, 841–847
    in appetite, 845–846, 846f
    approach to disorders of, 856–858
    in circadian rhythms, 847, 1784
    drinking center of, 854
    embryonic development of, 847
    in emotions, 846
    in fever, 844–845
    glioma of, 540–542
    in libido, 846–847
    neuropeptides and hormones of, 841–843,
        842t–843t, 844t
        in pituitary regulation, 847, 847t, 849
    and pituitary function, 847, 847t, 849
        in hyperprolactinemia, 851
    in septo-optic dysplasia, 1578
    in sleep cycle, 1785, 1786
    in temperature regulation, 843–844, 845f,
        2146
Hypothermia, 1543–1544
    coma in, 42
    in hypothalamus disorders, 843, 2146
    management of, 2163
    in spinal cord trauma, 1109, 2146
    therapeutic, in craniocerebral trauma,
        1053–1054, 1073
Hypothyroidism, 1032
    in cancer therapy, 1311
    cerebellar dysfunction in, 1936
    in children, 1038, 1311
    cognitive function in, 1740
    dizziness and vertigo in, 247
    and myasthenia gravis, 2178
    peripheral neuropathy in, 2115
    thyroid-stimulating hormone levels in, 852
Hypotonia
    in cerebellar disorders, 311
    congenital, 2229–2230
        benign, 412
        with type 1 fiber predominance, 2229,
            2230f
    floppy infant in, 403–415
    in Krabbe's disease, 412, 1660
    in Menkes' syndrome, 1624, 1687–1688
    in Pompe's disease, 412, 1643, 1644
    with regional hypertonia, 411
Hypoventilation, 1797
    in obesity, 1798
    sleep-related, 1804, 1805
Hypovolemia
    shock in, compared with neurogenic
        shock, 1102, 1102t
    syncope in, 12
Hypoxanthine-guanine phosphoribosyl
        transferase, 1618f
    Lesch-Nyhan disease in deficiency of,
        1618–1619, 1680–1681

of spinal cord, 375–376, 1226, 1227
  in aortic surgery, 1015
Infections, 1315
  aphasia in, 158
  ataxia in, 1464, 1932–1933
    acute, 315, 1932
    chronic, 1932
  bacterial, 1317–1351. *See also* Bacterial
      infections
  brain biopsy in, 954–955, 1359
  of cerebellum, 1464, 1932–1933
  cerebral, structural neuroimaging in,
      552–556
  cerebrovascular disorders of children in,
      1219–1222
  congenital and perinatal, 1357
    cytomegalovirus, 84, 1357, 1360,
        1361
    developmental disorders in, 84–85
    rubella, 1357, 1368
    syphilis, 1335, 1336
    toxoplasmosis, 84–85, 1357, 1393,
        2248, 2249
      intracranial calcification and
          hydrocephalus in, 1393, 1394f
      seizures in, 1762
  in craniocerebral trauma, 1073–1075
  delirium in, 33–34
  dementia in, 1739–1740
  electroencephalography in, 483–484
  of facial nerve, 274, 1259, 1885
  fungal, 1375–1383. *See also* Fungal
      infections
  Guillain-Barré syndrome associated with,
      819, 829, 2079–2080, 2079t
    Campylobacter, 1346–1347,
        2079–2080, 2079t
  headache in, 1833–1836
  immune response to, 820–821
    in viral infections, 829, 832–833
  in intracranial pressure increase
      monitoring, 1073
  parasitic, 1385–1404. *See also* Parasitic
      infections
  peripheral neuropathy in, 2121–2127
  polarized, 831
  radiculopathy in, 828, 1355–1356,
      2028–2030
    in herpes zoster virus infection,
        2123–2124
    in HIV infection and AIDS, 828,
        1420–1421
  respiratory, 1039
    bacterial, 1348–1349
    in craniocerebral trauma, 1074
    viral, 830
  seizures in, 1762
  of spine, 589–594, 1975–1977. *See also*
      Spine, infections of
  viral, 823–839, 1353–1372. *See also* Viral
      infections
Inflammatory demyelinating
    polyradiculoneuropathy,
    2078–2090
  acute, 2030, 2079–2086
    Guillain-Barré syndrome in. *See*
        Guillain-Barré syndrome

  in pregnancy, 2260
  chronic. *See* Polyradiculoneuropathy,
      chronic inflammatory
      demyelinating
Inflammatory response
  in cerebral edema, 1549, 1550–1551,
      1550f
  in meningitis, bacterial, 1551
  systemic syndrome in, 1020
Influenza, 1371
Infundibulum of internal carotid artery, 640,
    641f
Inhalant abuse, 1513, 1525, 1527
Innominate artery
  anatomy in angiography of, 619
  occlusion of, subclavian steal syndrome
      in, 1129
Inositol triphosphate, 872, 878f, 879, 884
Inpatient rehabilitation services, 969–970
Insect bites. *See* Bites
Insecticide exposure, toxicity of, 1514–1515
Insomnia, 1788–1791
  in altitude changes, 1791
  causes of, 1789–1791, 1789t, 1790t
  chronic, 67, 1789–1791
  clinical manifestations in, 1789
  in delayed sleep-phase syndrome, 1802
  drug-induced, 1789
  drug therapy in, 1824t, 1825
  evaluation of, 1787
  fatal familial, 671, 1429, 1806, 2138
  idiopathic or primary, 1790–1791
  in medical disorders, 1809–1810
  in neurological disorders, 1790, 1790t
  prevalence of, 1789
  psychophysiological, 1791
  serotonin in, 888t
  short-term, 1789
  sleep restriction therapy in, 1824
  and sleep-state misperception, 1791
  stimulus-control therapy in, 1824
  transient, 1789
  treatment of, 1824–1825
Insula in speech and language, 151
Insulin
  central nervous system function of, 842t
  in glucose metabolism, 1484
  test of pituitary function, 857t
  therapy in diabetes mellitus, 2102
    hypoglycemia in, 1485
    and ketoacidosis, 1487
Insulinlike growth factors, 849
  in amyotrophic lateral sclerosis, 2011
Integrated care pathways in rehabilitation,
    968–969
Intellectual function, 71–78. *See also*
    Cognitive function
Intelligence quotient, 678
  in developmental language disorders, 166,
      167t
  in mental retardation, 1586
Intensive care, 917–930
  airway management and ventilatory
      support in, 919–923
  approach to patient in, 918–919
  in craniocerebral trauma, 1069–1073
    coagulopathy in, 1075

  gastrointestinal ulceration and
      hemorrhage in, 1077
  infections related to, 1074
  monitoring in, 1069–1071
  as prognostic factor, 1082
  examination in, 918, 919t
  historical aspects of, 917
  monitoring in, 918, 924–930
    in craniocerebral trauma, 1069–1071
    invasive, 924–927
    neuroelectrophysiological, 927–930
    parameters in, 925t
    with transcranial Doppler
        ultrasonography, 662, 929–930
  myopathy in, 924
  in neuromuscular weakness, 923–924
  neuropathy in, 924
    critical illness polyneuropathy,
        2115–2116
  observation skills in, 918
  psychosis in, 34
  scope of practice in, 917–918, 918t
  sleep disturbances in, 1811–1812
Intentional motor disorders, 117–123
  causes of, 123
  pathophysiology of, 121–123
Intercellular adhesion molecules,
    832, 833
Intercostobrachial nerve syndrome, 2061
Interferon, 1253
  α, 812, 812t
    in chronic inflammatory demyelinating
        polyradiculoneuropathy,
        2090
    in monoclonal gammopathy of
        undetermined significance, 2093
    as therapy in viral infections, 1356t
      in measles, 1367
  β, 812, 812t
    in multiple sclerosis therapy,
        1456–1457, 1458
  γ, 812, 812t
    in fever, 844
Interleukins (IL), 1253
  functions of, 811, 812, 812t
  IL-1, 812, 812t
    in fever, 844
  IL-2, 812, 812t
    in gene transfer therapy, 1260
    in T-cell regulation, 814
  IL-3, 812, 812t
  IL-4, 807, 812, 812t, 814
  IL-6, 812, 812t
    in fever, 844
  IL-10, 812, 812t, 814
  IL-12, 812t, 814
International Medical Society of
    Paraplegia classification of spinal
    cord injury, 1089, 1090–1092,
    1091t, 1093f
*International Statistical Classification of
    Diseases, Injuries, and Causes of
    Death,* 760
Interneurons, 1990
Interosseous nerve syndromes
  anterior, 447, 2059
  posterior, 447–448, 2060

Magnetic resonance imaging—*continued*
   plaque appearance in, 546–547, 1433, 1446
   spectroscopy technique, 1448–1450, 1449f
   in treatment monitoring, 1446, 1453, 1457
   in variants, 1451, 1452, 1453f
  in multiple system atrophy, 545, 546f, 1903, 1903f
  in neurofibroma, 576f, 1288f, 1295f, 1296
  in neurofibromatosis
   and schwannoma, 1295, 1295f, 1675f
   type 1, 563, 1673, 1674f
  in osteomyelitis, vertebral, 1975–1977, 1976f, 1977f
  in osteoporosis and vertebral fracture, 1964, 1964f
  in Parkinson's disease, 545, 1894
  in perineurial hypertrophic mononeuropathy, localized, 2063, 2064f
  in personality changes, 96
  in Pick's disease, 545, 1708f, 1715
  in pineal tumors, 535–536, 537f, 944
  principles of, 522–526
  in pseudotumor cerebri, 1553
  in radiculopathy
   cervical, 1969
   in disc degeneration and spondylosis, 2025
   traumatic, 2022
  in real-time image-guided surgery, 957
  relaxation processes in, 523
  repetition time in, 523
  in schizophrenia, 114
  in schwannoma, 542–543, 945, 1274, 1294–1295, 1295f
   of auditory canal, 1274f
   in neurofibromatosis, 1295, 1295f, 1675f
  in seizures, 16, 671, 672, 955, 1768
   in functional neuroimaging, 671, 1768
   spectroscopy technique, 1768
  spectroscopy technique. *See* Spectroscopy, magnetic resonance
  in spinal cord ischemia, 1227
  in spinal cord trauma, 582–585, 589, 1092, 1100, 1105–1108
   in central cord syndrome, 1095, 1096
   in cervical fracture, 1108f
   and edema, 582–583, 585f, 1107
   and epidural hematoma, 588–589, 592f, 1107
   and hemorrhage, 582–583, 586f, 1107
   in lumbar fracture, 1106f
  in spinal epidural abscess, 590–594, 1328, 1329f
  in spinal hemorrhage, 1230
  in spinal tumors
   ependymoma, 575, 577f, 578f, 1289, 1289f
   epidural metastatic, 1282, 1283f, 1294f
   extradural, 575, 579f
   extramedullary intradural, 575, 576f, 1288, 1288f
   intramedullary, 575, 577f, 578f

   leptomeningeal metastatic, 1286, 1286f
  in spondylitis, ankylosing, 1980, 1980f, 1981f
  in spondylosis, cervical, 443f
   and myelopathy, 1970, 1970f
   and radiculopathy, 2025
  in structural neuroimaging, 522–526
   in intracranial lesions, 526–568
   in orbital lesions, 572–574
   in skull base lesions, 568–570
   in spinal lesions, 574–594
  in Sturge-Weber syndrome, 1683, 1684f
  in toxoplasmosis, 556–557, 1410–1412, 1411f
  in tuberous sclerosis, 1667, 1669, 1669f, 1670f
  in venous thrombosis
   cerebral, 1165
   sinus, 605, 606f, 1165, 1328
  in von Hippel–Lindau disease, 1695
  in Walker-Warburg syndrome, 2207
  in Wilson's disease, 1623
Magnetic stimulation
  motor evoked potentials in, 494, 495
  nerve conduction studies in, 501–502
   in urogenital evaluation, 751
  transcranial, in upper motor neuron disorders, 1988
Magnetoencephalography, 486
  in seizures, 955, 1768
Maitotoxin, 1536
Malabsorption
  of fat, 1500
  neurological complications in, 1027, 2113–2114
  of vitamin B$_{12}$, 1496, 1498, 2112
  of vitamin E, 1499, 1500, 2113
Malaria, 1386–1389
  cerebellar signs in, 1933
  cerebral, 1386–1389
   seizures in, 1762
  multidrug resistance in, 1388
  postmalaria neurological syndromes in, 1389
Malignant syndrome, neuroleptic, 845, 1922–1923
Malingering, 103, 905
  consciousness impairment in, episodic, 18
  differentiated from stupor and coma, 53
  hemiplegia in, 360
  olfaction in, 263, 265
  pain in, 905
   in back and lower limb, 461–462
  vision loss in, transient, 189
Malnutrition, protein-calorie, 1509
Mandibular nerve, 1882
Manganese poisoning, 1492, 1518, 1742
Mania, 107
  diagnostic criteria on, 107, 107t
  norepinephrine and epinephrine in, 885, 885t
  secondary, 108, 108t
Mannitol
  in cerebral edema, 1552
  in ciguatera, 1536
  in craniocerebral trauma, 1068, 1072
  in intracerebral hemorrhage, 1181

Mannosidosis, 1653t
Manometry, esophageal, in dysphagia, 182, 183
Maple syrup urine disease, 1602–1604, 1604t
  differential diagnosis in, 1604, 1604t
Mapping studies, functional, 665–667
Marasmus, 1509
Marburg hemorrhagic fever, 1356, 1369
Marburg variant of multiple sclerosis, 1452
Marchiafava-Bignami disease, 1507
Marcus Gunn jaw-winking phenomenon, 234
Marcus Gunn pupil, 724
  in multiple sclerosis, 1439
Marfan's syndrome
  aortic aneurysm in, 1014
  ischemic cerebrovascular disease in, 1147
Marijuana, 1524
Marin-Amat syndrome, 1885
Marine toxins, 1535–1538, 1536t
Marinesco-Sjögren's syndrome, 1945
Markowsky prosencephalic vein, 639
Maroteaux-Lamy syndrome, 1649t, 1651
Masking of tinnitus, 261
Mastoiditis, headache in, 1834
Mathematical skills, 687–688, 1592
Matrix metalloproteinase, 810–811
Maturation, 1561
  neural, 1562–1573
Maxillary artery, internal, 620, 621f
Maxillary nerve, 1882
May-White syndrome, 1948
McArdle's disease, 2217–2218
McGregor's line in basilar impression, 1953, 1954f
McLeod's syndrome, 1929
McRae's line in basilar impression, 1953, 1954f
MDMA (ecstasy), 886, 1524
Measles, 1366–1368
  encephalomyelitis in, 1367
   acute disseminated, 1459, 1460, 1461t
   chronic or recurrent, 1459, 1460, 1461t
  immunotherapy in, 1357t
  inclusion body encephalitis in, 1367
  subacute sclerosing panencephalitis in, 827, 1367, 1368
   electroencephalography in, 1367, 1367f
  vaccine, 1368
  vitamin A in, 1356t, 1366–1367
Mebendazole
  in ascariasis, 1402
  in echinococcosis, 1397
  in larva migrans, neural, 1401
  in trichinosis, 1398
Meckel-Gruber syndrome, 1575f, 1580
Meclizine in dizziness and vertigo, 740t, 741
Median nerve
  conduction studies in carpal tunnel syndrome, 447, 499, 500f, 2058
   interpretation of, 504, 505f, 506f
  neuropathy of, 363–364, 364t, 2056–2059
   carpal tunnel syndrome in, 446–447, 2056–2059. *See also* Carpal tunnel syndrome
  in diabetes mellitus, 2101

Meningitis—*continued*
    corticosteroid therapy in, 1551
    diagnosis of, 1318–1320
    epidemiology in, 1318
    hydrocephalus in, 1554
    inflammatory response in, 1551
    in leptospirosis, 1338
    magnetic resonance imaging in, 554,
        1331f, 1332f
    in neonate, 2246–2248
        and ventriculitis, 2248, 2248f
    nosocomial, 1324
    in plague, 1346
    public health issues in, 1323–1324
    in syphilis, 1335
    tuberculous. *See* Tuberculosis,
        meningitis in
  chronic, 1981–1982
    adhesive, 1981–1982
  in craniocerebral trauma, 1073–1074
  electroencephalography in, 483
  eosinophilic, in parasitic infections, 1386
    in angiostrongyliasis, 1398
  fungal, 1375–1376, 1377
    in blastomycosis, 1380
    in candidiasis, 1380
    in coccidioidomycosis, 1378–1379, 1379f
    cryptococcal, 1376, 1377
        in HIV infection and AIDS, 557–558,
            1417–1418
    differential diagnosis in, 1376
    in histoplasmosis, 1379, 1380
    subacute or chronic, 1375–1376
  headache in, 1831, 1833–1836
  in HIV infection and AIDS, 823, 825,
    1417–1418, 1419
    cryptococcal, 557–558, 1417–1418
  Mollaret's, 1372, 1982
    headache in, 1834–1836
  neck pain and stiffness in, 448–449
  neoplastic
    headache in, 1831
    polyradiculoneuropathy in, 2027–2028,
        2027f
  recurrent, 1982
    aseptic, 825, 1372
  and uveitis, 1982, 1983t
  viral, 823–825, 1353–1354
    clinical features in, 825
    diagnosis of, 1354
    differential diagnosis in, 1354
    immune response in, 820–821
    in mumps, 1368
    in poliovirus infection, 1363
    recurrent, 1372
    treatment of, 825
Meningocele, spinal, 1961, 1961f
Meningococcal infection. *See Neisseria*
    meningitidis infection
Meningoencephalitis
  amebic, 1389–1390
  headache in, 1833
  in HIV infection and AIDS, 1419
  uveoretinal, 199–200, 200t
  viral, 823
Meningoencephalomyelitis, viral, 823
Meningohypophyseal trunk, 621, 622

Meningomyelocele, 1573, 1576
Meningoradiculitis, viral, 823
Menkes' syndrome, 1624, 1687–1689
  clinical features in, 1624, 1687–1688,
    1687t
  diagnosis of, 1624
  electron transport defects in, 1635
  genetic factors in, 1624, 1688–1689
  pathophysiology in, 1624
  treatment of, 1624, 1689
Menopause, migraine in, 1862–1863
Menstrual cycle
  hypersomnia in, 67
  migraine in, 1859–1862
    drug therapy in, 1860–1861, 1860f,
        1861t
Mental retardation, 1586
  dendrite differentiation and growth in, 1569
  diagnosis of, 1586
  etiology of, 1586
  in fragile X syndrome, 83, 782–783, 1586
  in hypomelanosis of Ito, 1692
  in muscular dystrophy, congenital, 2203,
    2204, 2205
    myotonic, 2211
  nonautistic, 1587f
  in thyroid disorders, 1038
  treatment of, 1586
  in tuberous sclerosis, 1667
Mental status. *See* Cognitive function
Meperidine
  in migraine, 1857
  in pain management, 909, 910t
Meptazinol in Lyme disease, 1337
Meralgia paresthetica, 459, 2062
  in pregnancy, 2260
Mercaptans in hepatic encephalopathy, 1481
Mercury poisoning, 1518, 1742
  cerebellar disorders in, 1940
Meretoja, 2073
Merosin deficiency, 2204
Mesencephalon. *See* Midbrain
Mesoneurium, 1113
Metabolism, 1484–1492, 1595–1662
  in acidemia, organic, 1607–1612
  of amino acids
    branched-chain, 1602–1604
    sulfur, 1600–1602
  of ammonia, 1614–1618
  ataxia in disorders of, 316–317,
    1934–1936
  of calcium, basal ganglia calcification in
    disorders in, 1927
  in Canavan's disease, 1606
  of carbohydrates, disorders of,
    2217–2219
  cerebellar dysfunction in disorders of,
    1934–1936
  cerebrovascular disease in disorders of
    in children, 1220–1221
    in homocystinuria, 1601, 1602
    ischemic, 1146–1147
  in cholesterol storage diseases, 1644–1645
  citric acid cycle in, 1863–1864
  coma in disorders of, 39t, 52–53
  consciousness impairment in disorders of,
    episodic

    in children, 18
    syncope in, 13–14
  of copper, 1622–1624
    in Menkes' syndrome, 1624, 1687–1689
    in Wilson's disease, 1622–1624,
        1924–1925
  delirium in disorders of, 29, 32, 32t
  dementia in disorders of, 1740–1741
  of drugs
    genetic variations in, 895–896
    physiological variations in, 896
  encephalopathy in disorders of,
    1484–1492, 1595–1662
    clinical manifestations in, 1475–1476,
        1596
    electroencephalography in, 480–482, 482f
  in Farber's lipogranulomatosis, 1646
  of fatty acids. *See* Fatty acid metabolism
  floppy infant in disorders of, 412
  of fructose, 1614, 2218
  of galactose, 1613
  of glucose. *See* Glucose, metabolism of
  of glycine, 1604–1605
  in glycogen storage disorders, 1643–1644
  of glycoproteins, 1652–1654
  headache in disorders of, 1868
  of histidine, 1605
  of homocystine, 1600–1602
  in hypoxic-ischemic encephalopathy of
    neonate, 2241, 2244
  inborn errors of, 1570, 1595–1662
    dementia in, 1741
    laboratory abnormalities in, 1596t
  in language disorders, developmental,
    165, 166t
  of lipids, disorders of, 2219–2221
  in lipoprotein deficiencies, 1621–1622
  in Lowe's oculocerebrorenal syndrome,
    1606
  of lysine, 1606–1607
  in lysosomal storage disorders, 1643
  mitochondrial, 391, 1624–1636. *See also*
    Mitochondria, metabolism disorders
  in mucolipidoses, 1652
  in mucopolysaccharidosis, 1648–1651
  myopathy in disorders of, 398–399, 2187,
    2217–2223
  in neuronal ceroid lipofuscinosis,
    1646–1648
  odors in disorders of, 1596, 1597t
    of branched-chain ketoacids, 1609, 1609t
    maple syrup urine disease, 1597t, 1602,
        1604
    in tyrosinemia, 1597t, 1600
  oxidative, 1624–1629
    encephalomyopathy in disorders of,
        1631–1636
    of fatty acids, 1630–1631
    and lactic acidosis, 1625–1627
    and Leigh disease, 1625, 1626f,
        1628–1629
    overview of, 1626f
  of oxygen, cerebral, in craniocerebral
    trauma, 1083
  peroxisomal disorders of, 1636–1643
  of phenylalanine, 1596–1599
  of porphyrins, 1620–1621

of purine, 1618–1619
of pyrimidine, 1620
seizures in disorders of, 1476, 1758–1759
in Smith-Lemli-Opitz syndrome,
1645–1646
in sphingolipidosis, 1654–1662
in sulfatase deficiency, multiple, 1652
of tryptophan, 1605–1606
of tyrosine, 1599–1600
Metabotropic receptors, 867
glutamate, 872–876
neuronal muscarinic, 879
Metachromasia, 1661
Metachromatic leukodystrophy. *See*
Leukodystrophy, metachromatic
Metal poisoning, 1516–1519
cerebellar disorders in, 1940
Metalloproteinase
in cerebral edema, 1550, 1551
matrix, 810–811
Metamorphopsia, 187
Metastases, 528–530, 1252, 1276–1279
brachial plexus disorders in, 362, 443,
1278, 1278f, 2035–2036
differentiated from radiation-induced
plexopathy, 2035, 2036–2037
to brain, 1252, 1252f, 1277–1278
neurosurgery in, 946
dural, 1277
lumbosacral plexus disorders in,
1278–1279, 1279f, 2042
of lymphoma, 528–530, 531f, 1024, 1250
leptomeningeal, 1285
peripheral neuropathy in, 2104
to pituitary, 853
to skull, 1277
spinal, 379f, 1252, 1281–1285
clinical features in, 1281–1282
compression of spinal cord in, 379–380
epidural, 379–380, 379f, 1281–1285
intramedullary, 1290–1291
leptomeningeal, 1285–1287
locations of primary tumors in, 1281,
1282, 1282t
neuroimaging in, 575, 579f,
1282–1283, 1283f
pain in, 460, 1281–1282
prognosis in, 1284
sensory function in, 420
treatment of, 1284–1285
Metatarsalgia, Morton's, 459
Methadone
in opioid withdrawal, 1523
in pain management, 910t, 911
Methamphetamine in narcolepsy, 1822,
1822t
Methaqualone overdose, 1524
Methionine malabsorption, 1601t
Methotrexate
in brain tumors, 1309, 1310
in multiple sclerosis, 1458
in spinal tumors, leptomeningeal
metastatic, 1287
N-Methyl-D-aspartate (NMDA) receptors,
871, 872, 873
antagonists in traumatic brain injury,
1052

clinical role of, 875–876
in hyperglycinemia, 1605
in migraine, 1851
pharmacology of, 873, 874f, 1052
in ischemic cerebrovascular disease,
1160
in seizures, 1766
Methyl bromide exposure, 1514
Methyl n-butyl ketone, 1513, 1527
Methylcobalamin, 1601f, 1601t, 1611
3–Methylcrotonyl–coenzyme A carboxylase,
1609t
3,4–Methylene deoxy-methamphetamine
(ecstasy), 886, 1524
Methylmalonic acidemia, 1611
Methylmalonyl–coenzyme A mutase, 1610f
deficiency of, 1611
Methylmalonyl–coenzyme A racemase,
1610f
Methylphenidate
in multiple sclerosis, 1454
in narcolepsy, 1822, 1822t
Methylprednisolone
in cluster headache, 1866
in migraine and pregnancy, 1862
in multiple sclerosis, 1456, 1458
in retrovirus infections, 1371
in spinal cord trauma, 1109
in vasculitis, 2108
Methysergide
in cluster headache, 1866
in migraine, 1858–1859
Metoclopramide in migraine, 1854, 1855,
1857
Metronidazole
in amebiasis, 1390
in brain abscess, 1325
in meningitis, 1322t
neuropathy from, 2117t, 2119
Metyrapone test of pituitary function, 857t
Mexiletine
in myotonia, 2216
in pain management, 2055–2056
Meyer's loop, 721
Miconazole in amebic meningoencephalitis,
1390
Microadenoma of pituitary, 539, 540, 541f
hyperprolactinemia in, 850, 851
in pregnancy, 2262
Microembolic signals in ultrasonography,
647, 657–658
Microflutter, ocular, 223–224
Microfold cells, 830
Microglial cells in immune response, 815
Micrographia in parkinsonism, 320, 323
Micropsia, 216
Microsurgery techniques, 956
in arteriovenous malformations, 1210,
1211, 1212, 1213t
Microtubule-associated protein 2 in
craniocerebral trauma, 1050
Micturition. *See* Urination
Midazolam in seizures, 1769
in status epilepticus, 1754–1755
Midbrain
dorsal syndrome of, 294, 294t, 706
differential diagnosis in, 294, 294t

eye movements in, 715, 717
hemiplegia and hemiparesis in disorders
of, 359t
hemorrhage from, 1198
clinical features in, 1176t, 1179–1180,
1179f
motor systems in, 342, 358f
oculomotor syndromes, 1879–1880,
1880t
reticular formation in, 702
in vertical eye movements, 706
stroke syndromes of, 299–300, 302t, 303f
anatomy in, 303f
ischemic, 300, 302t, 303f
symptoms in, 302t
in vergence eye movements, 706
in vertical eye movements, 714, 715
Migraine, 1845–1863
acephalic, 1848
γ-aminobutyric acid in, 871t
aura in, 287, 1847–1848
pathophysiology of, 1851
visual, 1849, 1850
basilar, 1848–1849
and cerebrovascular disease, 1146, 1849,
1862
cheiro-oral, 1848
in children, 1876–1877
classification of, 1845, 1846t
clinical features in, 1845–1849
compared with tension-type headache,
1868–1869
complicated, 357–358, 1849
facioplegic, 1849
confusional state in, 1848
definition of, 1845
differential diagnosis in, 289
dizziness and vertigo in, 248, 1847, 1848
drug therapy in, 1854–1859, 1854t,
1855t, 1856t
in children, 1876–1877
in menstrual migraine, 1860–1861,
1860f, 1861t
in pregnancy, 1862, 2258
prophylactic, 1858–1859, 1861, 1861t
symptomatic, 1854–1858
dysphrenic, 1848
electroencephalography in, 479, 1850
equivalent, 1848
evoked potentials in, visual, 1850
frequency of, 286, 1847
functional neuroimaging in, 674, 1851,
1852
genetic factors in, 1850
hemiplegia in, 357–358, 1849
genetic factors in, 1850
historical aspects of, 1845
hormonal factors in, 1859–1863
laboratory tests in, 1850
locations of pain in, 287, 1846
in neck, 449
management of, 1853–1859
in menopause, 1862–1863
menstrual, 1859–1862
management of, 1860–1862, 1860f,
1861t
true, 1859, 1861

Motor neuron disorders—*continued*
  neurodevelopmental approach to
    therapy in, 985
  primary lateral sclerosis, 1988
  pseudobulbar palsy, 1987
  signs and symptoms in, 1987, 1987t
  spasm and spasticity in. *See* Spasm and
    spasticity, in upper motor neuron
    disorders
  weakness in, 1987
    facial, 273–274, 273t
Motor neuropathy
  acute motor axonal neuropathy, 2079,
    2081, 2083
  acute motor sensory axonal neuropathy,
    2079, 2081, 2082, 2083
  hereditary, with sensory neuropathy,
    1942, 2063–2068
    Charcot-Marie-Tooth disease in. *See*
      Charcot-Marie-Tooth disease
  prednisone-responsive, 2087
  multifocal, 1994–1995, 2090–2091
    clinical features in, 2090
    with conduction block, 2090–2091
    differential diagnosis of, 1995, 1996,
      2091, 2091t
    laboratory studies in, 2090–2091
    treatment of, 2091
Motor unit, 367, 509
  embryonic development of, 1572
  muscle fiber-motor neuron ratio of, 509
  potentials in electromyography, 509,
    514–515
    amplitude of, 514
    discharge patterns in, 515
    duration of, 514
    phases of, 514–515
    profile of, 514
    quantitative measurement of, 510
    rise time of, 514
    stability of, 515
Mouth
  examination of
    in coma, 43
    in dysphagia, 181–182
  in oral apraxia, 177
  in oromandibular dystonia, 330, 330t,
    332, 1909, 1910f
  in swallowing process, 180, 181–182
  in taste sense, 267, 268
Movements, 1889–1930. *See also* Motor
    function
Moyamoya disease, 1143
  angiography in, 1143, 1143f
  in children, 1220
  in middle cerebral artery stenosis, 634,
    947, 948f, 1143
  neurosurgery in, 947, 948f
  transient ischemic attack in, 1143
Mucolipidoses, 1652
Mucopolysaccharidosis, 1648–1651
  clinical features in, 1648–1651, 1649t,
    1650f
  differential diagnosis in, 1651, 1651t
  genetic factors in, 1648, 1649t
Mucormycosis, 1378f, 1381
  in diabetes mellitus, 2101

Mulberry lesion in tuberous sclerosis, 1669,
    1670f
Multidisciplinary approach
  in amyotrophic lateral sclerosis clinic, 2011
  in craniocerebral trauma, 1082
  in geriatric neurology, 2271
  in rehabilitation, 960–964, 960t
    integrated care pathways in, 968
    local services in, 970–971
Multiple organ failure in burns, 1544
Multiple sclerosis, 546–547, 1431–1459
  acute tumorlike, 1452, 1453f
  age in, 1436, 1436f, 1438t
    in epidemics, 769, 770f
    and incidence rate, 768
    in migration studies, 768, 769
    and mortality rate, 766
    and prognosis, 1444–1445
  animal models of, 817–818, 1458
  and ankylosing spondylitis, 1980–1981
  annual cost of, 1431
  ataxia in, 316, 1440
  as autoimmune disease, 816, 817–818,
    1435, 1458
  autonomic disorders in, 2138
  benign, 1443, 1445
  bladder in, 434–435, 1440
    detrusor hyperreflexia of, 434, 435,
      752, 753, 1454–1455
    management of, 753, 754, 754f,
      1454–1455
    retention of urine in, 749, 754
  blood-brain barrier in, 1433, 1446
  bowel function in, 1440
  cerebellar pathway impairment in, 1440
  cerebrospinal fluid findings in,
    1450–1451, 1450t, 1451f
  clinical features in, 1438–1441, 1441t
  clinical neurological, 769
  cognitive impairment in, 1438,
    1742–1743
    management of, 1455
  computed tomography in, 1446, 1448f,
    1450
  course of, 1443–1444, 1443f
    exogenous factors affecting, 1444
  dementia in, 1438, 1455, 1742–1743
  depression in, 1438, 1455
  diagnostic criteria in, 1441, 1442t, 1446
  differential diagnosis in, 1441–1443,
    1442t, 2010
  disability and handicap in, 965t,
    1000–1001, 1000f
    progression of, 1444
    scales on, 1444, 1453
  environmental factors in, 768, 785, 817,
    1435
    migration studies of, 768–769
    viruses, 830, 1435
  epidemiology of. *See* Epidemiology, of
    multiple sclerosis
  etiology of, 1435
  evoked potentials in, 1451, 1451t
    brainstem auditory, 490–491, 1451,
      1451t
    somatosensory, 494, 1451, 1451t
    visual, 1451, 1451t

  facial myokymia in, 275, 276, 1439
  in Faroe Islands, 768, 769, 770f, 771f
  fatigue in, 1441, 1454
  gender differences in, 1436, 1444
  genetic factors in, 768, 785, 816, 817
    in epidemiology studies, 1437–1438
  geographic distribution of, 766–769,
    1436–1437, 1437f
  hemiplegia in, 357
  and herpesvirus type 6, 1361–1362, 1435
  immunology of, 817–818, 830, 1434, 1435
    measures of, 1453
  impulse conduction in, 1432, 1432f
  magnetic resonance imaging in. *See*
    Magnetic resonance imaging, in
    multiple sclerosis
  malignant, 1443, 1445
  monoplegia in, 361
  mortality rate in, 766, 1437
  motor function in, 1440, 1441, 1454
  multifactorial inheritance of, 785
  and myelopathy, 1445–1446
  oligodendrocytes in, 1433–1434
    in transplant grafts, 818
  and optic neuritis, 1438–1439, 1445, 1464
  pathology in, 1433–1435, 1433f, 1434f,
    1435f
  pathophysiology in, 1431–1432, 1432f
  plaque in, 1433–1434, 1433f, 1434f, 1435f
    magnetic resonance imaging of,
      546–547, 1433, 1446
  in pregnancy, 1444, 1445t, 1457, 2261
  primary affection, 769
  prognosis in, 1444–1445
  progressive, 1443, 1444
    and relapsing, 1443, 1444
    treatment of, 1458
  racial differences in, 1437
  rehabilitation in, 965, 965t, 999–1001
    in chronic and progressive disorders,
      971
    goals of, 969, 969f
    in inpatient unit, 970
    integrated care pathways in, 968–969,
      969f
    outcome measures in, 965, 965t,
      999–1001
      Barthel Index, 966, 968t
      Functional Independence Measure,
        966, 968t, 1000, 1001
    physical therapy in, 1000
    role of nurses in, 960–961
  relapsing, 1443, 1444
    and remitting, 1443, 1457
  remyelination in, 1434
  respiratory and sleep disorders in, 1807
  sensory function in, 1439, 1441
  sexual function in, 436, 756, 1440, 1455
  spasticity in, 1440, 1454
  structural neuroimaging in, 546–547, 547f
  treatment and management of,
    1452–1459
    in acute attacks, 1456
    disease-modifying, 1456–1458
    future trends in, 1458–1459
    immunosuppressive therapy in, 818, 1458
    in pregnancy, 1444, 1445t, 1457, 2261

in progressive disease, 1458
strategies in, 1456t
symptom management in, 861, 862, 1454–1455
tremor in, 1440, 1454
trigeminal neuralgia in, 1439, 1873
variants of, 1451–1452
pathology in, 1434–1435
viruses associated with, 830, 1435
Multiple system atrophy, 1807, 1808t, 1900–1904, 2133–2138
apnea in, 2148
ataxia in, 2148
autonomic nervous system in, 321, 1809, 1902–1903, 2133–2138, 2148
bladder dysfunction in, 432
detrusor hyperreflexia, 432, 748, 2156
management of, 754, 2163–2164
urinary incontinence in, 748, 2156
cerebellar or olivopontocerebellar atrophy in, 2134, 2136, 2136f, 2137, 2148
clinical and pathological features in, 1903–1904, 1903f, 2136
cognitive function in, 2148
compared with degenerative late-onset ataxia, 1949–1950
definition of, 2133
drug therapy in, 2164
dysphagia in, 2155, 2163
functional neuroimaging in, 669
magnetic resonance imaging in, 545, 546f, 1903, 1903f
norepinephrine and epinephrine in, 882–883, 884, 885t, 2150, 2154f
oligodendroglial inclusions in, 1903–1904, 2137, 2137f
parkinsonian, 2133–2134, 2136, 2136f, 2137, 2148
positron emission tomography in, 669
prognosis in, 2158
sexual function in, 321, 432
sleep disorders in, 1809
polysomnography in, 1816
sphincter electromyography in, 748, 749f, 2156
striatonigral degeneration in, 2134, 2136f, 2137
structural neuroimaging in, 545, 546f
sympathetic skin response in, 2155, 2157f
treatment and course of, 1904
Mumps, 1368
Munchausen syndrome, 103
by proxy, 103
Murmurs in coma, 43, 45
Murray Valley encephalitis, 1365
Muscarinic receptors, 877, 878f, 879
in various diseases, 880t
Muscle-eye-brain disease, 2204, 2206–2207
Muscles, 2187–2234
atrophy of
in amyotrophic lateral sclerosis, 2007f, 2008f
in amyotrophy, benign focal, 1996
biopsy in, 2189, 2190f
bulbospinal
trinucleotide repeat expansions in, 789, 791f, 2002, 2003

X-linked recessive, 2002–2004, 2003f
in floppy infant, 409, 412
in lower motor neuron disorders, 1990
in multifocal motor neuropathy, 1994, 1995
neurogenic, 367–368
in postpolio syndrome, 1992–1994
characteristic features in, 1993t
progressive, 2004
in amyotrophic lateral sclerosis, 1995, 2002, 2004
spinal. See Spinal muscular atrophy
type 1 fibers in, 2191, 2233, 2233f
type 2 fibers in, 2191, 2191f
biopsy of, 2188–2192. See also Biopsy, muscle
carnitine deficiency in, 1608, 1630
in channelopathies, 2212–2217
congenital disorders of, 2229–2234
dystrophy in, 2203–2207
continuous fiber activity of, 514
cramps of. See Cramps
denervation of
biopsy changes in, 2189, 2189f, 2190, 2190f
in lower motor neuron disorders, 1991
and reinnervation, 2189, 2190, 2190f
dystrophy of. See Dystrophy, muscular
electromyography of. See Electromyography
embryonic development of, 1572
in eye movements, 203, 204f, 204t, 205f
actions of, 203, 205f, 206f
balance assessment, 210–213
Hering's law of dual innervation, 203, 204, 206f
in monocular elevator deficiency or palsy, 715
in ophthalmoplegia. See Ophthalmoplegia
overaction of, 210
three-step test of, 213–214, 213f
weakness of, 382, 383, 393
in myasthenia gravis, 2168, 2169, 2178–2179
yoked arrangement of, 203, 204t, 701
fasciculation of. See Fasciculation
fiber types in, 2188, 2188f, 2189
disproportion or predominance of, 1572, 2191, 2233, 2233f
in congenital hypotonia, 2229, 2230f
in type 1 atrophy, 2191, 2233, 2233f
in type 2 atrophy, 2191, 2191f
fibrosis of, 2190–2191
functional evaluation of, 384–386
Hering's law of dual innervation, 203, 204, 206f
inflammatory disorders of, 820, 2223–2229
inherited disorders of, 2192–2212
ischemia of, 399
of lower limb, innervation of, 451, 453f
in metabolic disorders, 398–399, 2187, 2217–2223
motor endplate of, 509, 511, 511f
in motor unit, 509
ratio to motor neurons, 509
in myotonia. See Myotonia

in neck. See Neck, muscles in
nicotinic receptors in, 877–878
overuse syndromes of, 399–400
pain in, 397–401
in arm, 449–450
in back, 458
clinical features in, 397–398
drug-induced, 400, 400t
in encephalomyelitis, 98, 99
and eosinophilia from L-tryptophan, 2121
evaluation of, 398
mechanisms in, 397
in myopathies, 398–399, 398t
in myophosphorylase deficiency, 2218
in neck, 448–449
in overuse syndromes, 399–400
pathological conditions associated with, 397
in polymyalgia. See Polymyalgia
sleep disturbances in, 1811
trigger points in, 458, 1983, 1983f
in viral infections, 1356
palpation and percussion of, 386
range of motion, 386
in floppy infant, 405–407
reciprocal inhibition of, 203
segment-pointer, 367, 368t
strength of, 381–395
in back and lower limb pain, 456, 456t
evaluation of, 386
in floppy infant, 404–405
grading system on, 386, 386t, 456, 456t
measures in children and infants, 405, 408t
and weakness. See Weakness
tone of
age-related changes in, 407t
in cerebellar disorders, 311
in coma, 51, 53
in dystonia. See Dystonia
in elderly, assessment of, 2277
in floppy infant, 403–415
in gait and walking, 345
in hypertonia, 411, 982–984
in hypotonia. See Hypotonia
in motor neuron disorders, 1987, 1990
in radiculopathy, 368
resting, 403, 405f
in rigidity, 320
of upper limb, innervation of, 441, 442t
weakness of, 381–395. See also Weakness
Musculocutaneous nerve disorders
differential diagnosis of, 372t
entrapment neuropathy, 2060–2061
Mushroom poisoning, 1531, 1533, 1533t
Music, auditory agnosia for, 137
Mutations
heterogeneity in, 788, 790f
linkage analysis of, 794–797, 795f
in mitochondrial DNA, 784
new and sporadic, 780
rate of, 786
single base-pair, 787, 787f
of single genes, 777–780
single-nucleotide polymorphisms in, 786
two-hit phenomenon in, 781–782
types of, 787, 787f

in smell sense, 263–264
  clinical evaluation of, 264–265
Oligoclonal bands in cerebrospinal fluid, in
      multiple sclerosis, 1450, 1450t,
      1451f
Oligodendrocytes
  inclusions in multiple system atrophy,
      1903–1904, 2137, 2137f
  in multiple sclerosis, 1433–1434
  transplant grafts of, 818
Oligodendroglioma
  cognitive function in, 1742f
  neuroimaging in, 526, 527f, 1742f
  pathology in, 1244, 1245f
  treatment of, 1271
    surgery in, 934, 1271
Olivopontocerebellar atrophy, 1900–1903,
      2134
  ataxia in, 1944, 1945, 1949, 1950
  magnetic resonance imaging in, 545, 546f
  and multiple system atrophy, 1949–1950,
      2134, 2136f
  pathological findings in, 1949, 1949f
  structural neuroimaging in, 545, 546f
Onchocerciasis, 1399–1400
Oncogenes, 1254, 1256–1257
Ondansetron in multiple sclerosis, 1454
Ondine's curse, 1807
One-and-a-half syndrome, 1883
  eye movements in, 296, 714
    vertical, 715
  in pontine hemorrhage, 1179
Onion bulb appearance, 2047
  in Charcot-Marie-Tooth disease, 2066,
      2066f
  in chronic inflammatory demyelinating
      polyradiculoneuropathy, 2088
  in localized perineurial hypertrophic
      mononeuropathy, 2063, 2064f
Onuf's nucleus, 748, 2156
Oophorectomy in menstrual migraine,
      1861–1862
Opalski's cells in Wilson's disease, 1925
Ophthalmic artery, 621, 622
  transcranial Doppler ultrasonography of,
      653
Ophthalmic nerve, 1882
  herpes virus infections of, 1875, 1883
Ophthalmoplegia
  acute bilateral, 215, 215t
  chronic
    bilateral, 215, 216t
    progressive external, 234, 235, 237, 238
  combined vertical gaze, 293–294, 294t
    differential diagnosis in, 293–294, 294t
  in Graves disease, 1032
  internuclear, 49, 295, 713–714
    causes of, 714, 714t
    in cerebellar disorders, 313
    in multiple sclerosis, 1439
    nystagmus in, 295, 713, 714
  in Kearns-Sayre syndrome, 2207
  in migraine, 1849, 1850
  total, 296
    differential diagnosis in, 296, 296t
  in Wernicke's encephalopathy, 1503–1504
Opioids, 909–912, 1521–1523, 2056

abuse of, 1522
dependence on, 909, 1522, 1523
dosage of, 910t, 911
endogenous, 901, 902, 1522
epidural and intrathecal administration of,
    911–912
overdose of, 40, 1522–1523
pharmacology of, 1522
potency of, 909, 910t
receptors, 901, 902, 1522
selection of, 910–911
titration rate of, 911
tolerance to, 909, 1522
withdrawal from, 909, 910, 1523
Opium, 1521, 1522
Opsoclonus, 224, 314
  causes of, 224, 224t
  and myoclonus syndrome, paraneoplastic,
      1302–1303
  in neonates, 708
Optic chiasm
  axons in, 721
  compression in pituitary tumors,
      847–848, 850
  glioma of, 540–542. See also Glioma, of
      optic nerve and chiasm
  vision loss in disorders of, 187, 191
Optic nerve and disc, 193–198
  atrophy of, 197
    familial, 191
  coloboma of, 198
    disc in, cp15.XIX
  compression of, 191, 194
    unilateral disc edema in, 194, 195
  congenital anomalies of disc, 197–198
  cupping of disc, 197
  degenerative disorders of, 191
  demyelination of, 191
  in Devic's disease, 191, 359, 1435, 1452
  in diabetic papillopathy, 197, cp15.XVI
  double ring sign of, 198, 730
  drug-induced disorders of, 192, 197
  drusen of, 191, 193–194, cp15.II
    pseudopapilledema in, 193
    in retinitis pigmentosa, 194
  dysplasia of, 198
  edema of disc, 193–197. See also
      Papilledema
  glioma of, 540–542. See also Glioma, of
      optic nerve and chiasm
  hyperemia of disc, cp15.IX
    and edema, cp15.VII
  hypoplasia of, 198, cp15.XVIII
    in children, 730
  in hypothalamic-pituitary disorders, 856
  infarction of disc, 190
  ischemic neuropathy of
    anterior, 190, cp15.III
      unilateral disc edema in, 194–195
    posterior, 190
    retrobulbar, 197
    vision loss in, 190, 194
  Leber's hereditary neuropathy of, 196,
      1635, cp15.IX
    vision loss in, 190–191
  meningioma of, structural neuroimaging
      in, 573, 573f

morning glory appearance of disc, 198
in multiple sclerosis, 1439
neuritis of, 1464
  bilateral disc edema in, 197
  and multiple sclerosis, 1438–1439,
      1445, 1464
  retrobulbar, 197
  unilateral disc edema in, 194, 195–196
  vision loss in, 191, 194
  visual evoked potentials in, 488, 488f
normal appearance in optic neuropathy,
    197
nutritional neuropathy of, 1508
in pseudopapilledema, 193–194
radiation injury of, 196
recurrent neuropathy of, 1451–1452
retrobulbar neuropathy of, 197
in sarcoidosis, 191, 196, 1020, cp15.VIII
in septo-optic dysplasia, 559, 1577–1578
tilted disc, 197–198, cp15.XVII
in tobacco-alcohol amblyopia, 1507
toxic neuropathy of, 192, 197
traumatic neuropathy of, 190
in uremia, 1028
vision loss in disorders of, 187, 193–198,
    730
  gradual, 191, 192
  ischemic, 190
  sudden, 190–191
visual field in disorders of, 725, 728, 728f
Optokinetic system in eye movements, 701
Orbicularis oculi muscle
  in excessive eyelid closure, 235
  in insufficient eyelid closure, 235, 237
  myokymia of, 236
  reflexes of, 273
Orbicularis oris muscle reflex, 273
Orbital disorders
  in hyperthyroidism, 1032
  oculomotor nerve in, 1881
  structural neuroimaging in, 572–574
Orbitofrontal area
  functions of, 72, 73
  syndrome of, 92t
Orbivirus infections, 1366
Organic disorders
  behavioral, 89
  compared with functional disorders, 105,
      114–115
  personality change in, 91
Organochlorine pesticides, 1514
Organomegaly in POEMS syndrome, 1023,
    2094–2095
Organophosphate exposure, 1514–1515
Orgasm, 430
  in spinal cord disorders, 435–436
Oriental lung fluke, 1403–1404
Orientation
  bedside tests of, 77–78
  in delirium, 27
    assessment of, 30
  visual, 692, 693
    point localization in, 692–693
Ornithine, in lysinuric protein intolerance,
    1606–1607
Ornithine-ketoacid aminotransferase
    deficiency, 1616t

Peroxisomal assembly factor 1, 1638
Peroxisomes, 1636–1643
    ghost structures, 1637
    metabolic reactions in, 1636–1637, 1637t
        disorders of, 1637–1643
            classification of, 1637, 1637t
            diagnostic assays in, 1637, 1638t
            gene defects in, 1637, 1637t, 1638, 1638t
Perseveration, 695, 696, 696f
    cognitive, 121
    in language, 143
        speech therapy in, 992
    motor, 117, 121
        continuous, 121
        pathophysiology in, 121, 122
        recurrent, 121
Personality, 105
    changes in, 89–96
        computed tomography in, 96
        electroencephalography in, 95–96
        in frontal lobe disorders, 73, 91–92
        general and neurological examination in, 94–95
        history taking in, 94
        magnetic resonance imaging in, 96
        in temporal lobe syndromes, 92–94
        types of, 90–91
    multiple, 100
Personnel
    in multidisciplinary approach. See
        Multidisciplinary approach
    in rehabilitation services, 960–964, 960t
Pertussis, 1349
Pesticide exposure, 1492–1493, 1514–1515
Peyer's patches, 830
Peyote, 1531–1532, 1532t
pH of brain, 1547, 1547f
Phakomatosis
    Jadassohn's nevus, 1690
    retina in, 200
Phalen's test in carpal tunnel syndrome, 446, 2058
Pharmacogenetics, 895–896
Pharmacology, 867–896. See also Drug therapy
Pharyngeal artery, ascending, 620, 621f
Pharynx
    dystonia of, 1910
    in swallowing process, 180
        assessment of, 182
    in taste sense, 267
Phencyclidine, 873, 1525
Phenobarbital
    in seizures, 1770t, 1772
        in neonate, 2239, 2240, 2240t
        in status epilepticus, 1761, 1761t
    in spasticity, 984t
    in withdrawal symptoms of neonate, 2254
Phenotype, 777
    and genotype correlations in Friedreich's ataxia, 1943–1944
Phenylalanine
    metabolism of, 1597, 1598f
        disorders in, 1596–1599

serum levels of, 1596–1599
    differential diagnosis of disorders, 1597t
    in pregnancy, 1599
Phenylethanolamine-N-methyl transferase, 883
Phenylketonuria, 1596, 1597–1599, 1597t
    variants of, 1599
Phenylpropanolamine
    in diabetes mellitus, 2103
    intracranial hemorrhage from, 1172
    in urinary incontinence, 2294t
Phenytoin
    cerebellar dysfunction from, 1940
    fetal exposure to, 2253, 2254f, 2263
    genetic variations in metabolism of, 895–896
    neuropathy from, 2117t, 2120
    in seizures, 1770t, 1772–1773
        in craniocerebral trauma, 1076
        in elderly, 2287
        in neonate, 2239, 2240, 2240t
        in status epilepticus, 1761, 1761t
    in spasticity, 984t
    in uremic encephalopathy, 1483
Pheochromocytoma, 858–859, 1033
    cardiac arrhythmias in, 2142
    facial vascular changes in, 2143
    hypertension in, 858, 2142
        and norepinephrine plasma levels, 2151, 2155f
    in von Hippel–Lindau disease, 1694, 1694t, 1695
Phonagnosia, 137
Phonation, 141, 171, 684–685
    assessment of, 175–176, 177
    differential diagnosis of disorders, 175t
    in dysphonia, 141, 171, 172, 178
        spasmodic, 178, 326, 332, 1910
    familiar, recognition of, 137
    in phonological programming disorder, 162
    in phonological syntactic syndrome, 163
    substitution errors in, 143
Phonemes, 141
    errors in, 143, 684, 685
Phosphodiesterase activation, 872
Phosphoenolpyruvate carboxykinase, 1626f, 1629
Phosphofructokinase deficiency, 2218–2219
Phosphoglycerate kinase deficiency, 2219
Phosphoglycerate mutase deficiency, 2219
Phosphorylase deficiency, muscle, 2217–2218
Phosphorylation, 883–884
Photopsia, 187
Photosensitivity
    in porphyria, 1620, 1621
    in xeroderma pigmentosum, 1620, 1698
Phrenitis, 25
Physical examination, 6
    in Alzheimer's disease, 1705
    in giant cell arteritis, 289, 1841–1842
    in headache
        migraine, 1849–1850
        tension-type, 1869
    in hypothalamic-pituitary disorders, 856
    in intracranial aneurysm and subarachnoid hemorrhage, 1186

in intracranial arteriovenous malformations, 1204
    in myasthenia gravis, 2169
    in neurointensive care, 918, 919t
    in pain, 906
    in peripheral neuropathy, 2051–2052, 2051t
    in seizures, 15, 1767
    in sleep disorders, 68, 1788
        in apnea, 1799
    in urogenital disorders, 743
    in urinary incontinence, 2292
Physical therapy, 961–962, 984–989
    in amyotrophic lateral sclerosis, 2012–2013
    approaches in, 961–962, 985
    in Duchenne's muscular dystrophy, 2194
    gymnastic ball in, 961, 962f
    in multiple sclerosis, 1000
    in peripheral nerve trauma, 1124
    in postpolio syndrome, 1993
    proprioceptive neuromuscular facilitation in, 961
    in spasticity, 983
    in spinal muscular atrophy, 2000
Physicians
    in rehabilitation team, 960
    relationship with patient
        in Alzheimer's disease, 2272
        in amyotrophic lateral sclerosis, 2010–2011, 2012
        beneficial effects of, 862
        in cancer diagnosis and treatment, 1314
        discussion of prognosis in, 865
Physostigmine in anticholinergic overdose, 1525
Phytanic acid in Refsum's disease, 1641, 1642, 2077–2078
Pial cells, 1548
Pick bodies, 1714, 1715, 1716f, 1737
Pick cells, 1714
Pick's disease, 1714–1715
    clinical features in, 1714–1715
    diagnostic features in, 1737
    epidemiology and etiology of, 1715
    functional neuroimaging in, 667, 1715
    laboratory tests in, 1715
    language in, 158, 1714–1715
    pathology in, 1715, 1716f
    prognosis and management in, 1715
    structural neuroimaging in, 545, 1708f, 1715
Pickwickian syndrome, 1798
Pigmentation
    in hypomelanosis of Ito, 1692, cp69.I
    in tuberous sclerosis, 1666–1667, 1667f
Pili torti in Menkes' syndrome, 1624, 1687
Pilocarpine in pupil evaluation, 233
Pineal tumors, 944–945, 944f
    clinical features in, 1265
    cystic, 944
    germ cell, 535–536, 944, 945, 1250, 1274
    magnetic resonance imaging in, 535–536, 537f, 944
    pineal cell, 536, 537f
    treatment of, 1274
        radiation therapy in, 944, 945, 1274
Pinealoblastoma, 1274
    neuroimaging in, 536, 537f

Premotor areas, 1985
    apraxia in disorders of, 126
Preoptic area in sleep cycle, 1786
Presbyopia, 722
Presenilin genes in Alzheimer's disease, 1704,
        1706, 1710
Pressure sores, 979
    in spinal cord trauma, 1103
Presyncope, 247, 248
Pretectum of midbrain
    in vergence eye movements, 706
    in vertical eye movements, 714, 715
Priapism, 2147
Primidone
    in multiple sclerosis, 1454
    in seizures, 1770t, 1773
    in tremor, essential, 1906–1907
Priming of memory, 77, 993
Prion diseases, 1423
    dementia in, 1720
    insomnia in, fatal familial, 1806
Prisms in diplopia
    in assessment, 212, 212f
    in treatment, 216
Probenecid in syphilis, 1336
    in HIV infection and AIDS, 1418
Prochlorperazine
    in dizziness and vertigo, 740t, 741
    in migraine, 1855, 1857
        menstrual, 1860f
Progeria, 1678–1680, 1679f
Prolactin serum levels, 850–851, 850t,
        856–857
    in pituitary tumors, 850, 851, 856–857,
        1030
    in seizures, 17, 98, 850–851
        psychogenic, 1763
        tonic-clonic, 1752
    in sleep cycle, 1783, 1784f
Prolactinoma, 539, 850–851, 850t, 1030
    in pregnancy, 856, 2262
    treatment of, 856–857, 943, 1030
Prolidase deficiency, 1605t
Proliferating cell nuclear antigen, 1240
Proliferation, cellular, in tumors, 1253, 1254
    assessment of, 1239–1240
    endothelial cells in, 1242
Promethazine
    in dizziness and vertigo, 740t, 741
    in migraine, 1857
Pronator teres syndrome, 447, 2057t, 2059
Propantheline in urinary incontinence, 2294t
    in detrusor hyperreflexia, 752
    in multiple sclerosis, 1454
Propionic acid
    derivatives in pain management, 907–908,
        908t
    metabolism of, 1610f
    disorders in, 1610–1611
Propionic acidemia, 1610–1611
Propionyl–coenzyme A carboxylase, 1610f
    deficiency of, 1610
Propoxyphene in pain management, 910t
Propranolol
    in migraine, 1858
        in children, 1876
        menstrual, 1861t

in multiple sclerosis, 1454
in restless legs syndrome, 1824
in tremor, 1907, 1908
Proprioceptive neuromuscular facilitation,
        961
Propriospinal myoclonus, 336, 340, 1920
Proptosis, 208, 214
    examination in, 236
    eyelid retraction in, 235
    in Graves' disease, 1032
Prosencephalic vein of Markowsky, 639
Prosencephalon malformations, 1576
Prosody, 153
    acquired disorders of, 167
Prosopagnosia, 134, 690, 691–692, 1722
Prostaglandins in menstrual migraine, 1859
Prostate
    metastatic carcinoma of, 1277, 1281
        sensory loss in, 420
    urinary incontinence in enlargement of,
        2292
Prostatectomy, radical, pelvic nerve trauma
        in, 437
Prosthesis
    heart valve, embolism in, 2265–2266
    neural, 988
        in memory impairment, 994
Proteases
    calcium-activated neutral, deficiency of,
        2198
    in cerebral edema, 1550–1551, 1550f
    inhibitors in HIV infection and AIDS, 839
Protein
    dietary
        in hepatic encephalopathy, 1482
        in protein-calorie malnutrition, 1509
    glial fibrillary acid, 1565f
        in tumor diagnosis, 1239, 1239t
    myelin basic
        in encephalomyelitis, acute
            disseminated, 1462
        in multiple sclerosis, 1435
Protein C
    activated, resistance to, 1149, 1150
        in factor V Leiden mutation, 1042, 1150
    deficiency of, 1149
Protein-calorie malnutrition, 1509
Protein kinase C, activation by
        diacylglycerol, 872, 879, 884
Protein S deficiency, 1149–1150
Proto-oncogenes, 1254, 1256
Protozoal infections, 1385, 1386–1394. *See
        also specific infections*
    amebic, 1389–1390
    central nervous system disorders in, 1387t
    leishmaniasis in, 1394
    malaria in, 1386–1389
    sarcocystosis in, 1394
    toxoplasmosis in, 1393
    trypanosomiasis in, 1390–1393
PrP gene in transmissible spongiform
        encephalopathies, 1423, 1428t,
        1429
    in Creutzfeldt-Jakob disease, 1425, 1428
Pseudallescheria boydii infections, 1381,
        1382
Pseudobobbing of eye, 225, 225t

Pseudobulbar palsy, 299, 1987
Pseudoclaudication, 458, 462
Pseudocoma, 38, 38t
    differential diagnosis of, 53
Pseudodementia, 102, 108, 1743
    in elderly, 2283
Pseudodrusen, 194, cp15.XII
Pseudoephedrine in urinary incontinence,
        2294t
Pseudo-Foster Kennedy syndrome, 195, 195f
Pseudohallucinations, 110
Pseudo-Hurler's syndrome, 1652,
        1655–1656
Pseudomonas infection
    mallei, glanders in, 1346
    pseudomallei, melioidosis in, 1346–1347
Pseudonystagmus, pendular, 219–220
Pseudopalisading, 1241
    in glioblastoma multiforme, 1241, 1242,
        1242f
Pseudopapilledema, 193–194, cp15.I
    compared with papilledema, 194t
Pseudo-pseudoseizures, 101–102
Pseudoptosis of eyelid, 234
    in monocular elevator deficiency, 715
Pseudoseizures, 17, 101–102
    differential diagnosis of, 97–98
    management of, 104
    in sleep, 1803
Pseudotumor
    cerebri, 1552–1554
        clinical features in, 1552–1553
        drug-induced, 1553, 1553t
        drug therapy in, 1553
        false localizing sign in, 1553
        in Guillain-Barré syndrome, 2080
        headache in, 288, 289, 1552, 1833
            in pregnancy, 2262–2263
        in pregnancy, 2262–2263
        surgery in, 949, 1553–1554
        in vitamin A toxicity, 1508, 1553
    orbital, structural neuroimaging in,
        572–573
Pseudo–von Graefe's sign, 235, 1881
Pseudoxanthoma elasticum, 1147, 1677
Pseudo-Zellweger's syndrome, 1641
Psittacosis, 1348
Psoas muscle, 2038
    abscess of, 2041
    hemorrhage from, 2040
Psychiatric disorders
    in autonomic failure, 2148
    coma in, 41, 53
    differentiated from dementia, 34
    and hysteria, 102–103
    in lupus erythematosus, 1043
    pain complaints in, 905
    pseudoseizures in, 101
    sleep disorders in, 1812
        insomnia in, 1790
    speech in, 143
Psychogenic conditions
    amnesia in, 102, 102t, 1743
    asthenopia in, 216
    consciousness impairment in, episodic, 18
    movement disorders in, 1929–1930
    ocular deviation in, 711

Radiation therapy, 1235, 1541–1542
    in astrocytoma, 1266–1267, 1268
        of brainstem, 1270
        of cerebellum, 1269
        spinal, 1290
    brachial plexus disorders in, 1278, 1542,
        2036–2037
        differentiated from metastatic
            plexopathy, 443–444, 2035,
            2036–2037
        symptoms in, 363
    and cognitive function in brain tumors,
        1309, 1310, 1741
    in craniopharyngioma, 1275
    encephalopathy in, 1541
    in ependymoma, 1271, 1272
    in glioma, 943, 1268
        in optic pathway tumors, 1271
    gonadal dysfunction in, 1311
    growth hormone deficiency in,
        1310–1311
    ischemic cerebrovascular disease in, 1143
    lumbosacral plexus disorders in, 1279,
        1542, 2043
    in lymphoma of central nervous system,
        1274–1275
    in medulloblastoma, 1273, 1310
    in meningioma, 1273
    in metastatic tumors, 1277–1278
        spinal epidural, 1284
        spinal leptomeningeal, 1286–1287
    motor neuron disorders in, 2005, 2032
    in multiple sclerosis, 1458
    myelopathy in, 1227, 1541–1542
    necrosis in, 1312
        functional neuroimaging in, 675
        structural neuroimaging in, 548
    in oligodendroglioma, 1271
    oncogenetic potential of, 1311–1312
    optic neuropathy in, 196
    pathological findings in, 1312–1313
    in pineal tumors, 944, 945, 1274
    in pituitary tumors, 857–858, 943, 1030
    in pregnancy, 2262
    radiculoplexopathy in, 2043
    thyroid disorders in, 1311
    vision loss in, 192
    white matter disorders in, 548
Radicular arteries and veins, anatomy of,
        1225, 1226, 1226f
Radiculitis
    in HIV infection and AIDS, 828,
        1420–1421
    viral, 828, 1355–1356
Radiculoneuritis, viral, 1355–1356
Radiculoneuropathy in Lyme disease, 2029
Radiculopathy, 367–371, 2019–2032
    anatomy in, 2019–2020, 2020f
    cervical. See Cervical radiculopathy
    compared with peripheral neuropathy,
        370–371
    in diabetes mellitus, 423, 1033,
        2026–2027, 2101
        lumbar, 2099f, 2101–2102
        polyradiculoneuropathy in, 1033,
            2026–2027, 2101
        thoracic, 2026, 2101

differential diagnosis in, 369, 370–371,
        370t
    dorsal root ganglia disorders, acquired,
        2030–2031
    in Guillain-Barré syndrome, 2030,
        2079–2086
    hemiplegia in, 360
    in HIV infection and AIDS, 828,
        1420–1421, 2028, 2029f
        lumbosacral, 2028, 2123
    infectious, 828, 1355–1356, 2028–2030
        in herpes zoster virus infection,
            2123–2124
        in HIV infection and AIDS, 828,
            1420–1421
    in intervertebral disc herniation
        cervical, 441, 1968, 1969,
            2022–2026
        lumbar, 1973, 1974, 1975,
            2022–2026
    lumbar. See Lumbar radiculopathy
    lumbosacral. See Lumbosacral
        radiculopathy
    in Lyme disease, 2029, 2126
    monoplegia in, 361–362
    neurogenic muscle atrophy in, 367–368
    pain in, 368–369, 370t, 423
        cervical, 441–443, 443t, 1968–1969
        in disc degeneration and spondylosis,
            2022–2023, 2024f
        lumbar, 1973–1975
    and polyradiculoneuropathy. See
        Polyradiculoneuropathy
    in radiation therapy, 2043
    segment-pointer muscles in, 367, 368t
    sensory function in, 422–423
        in disc degeneration and spondylosis,
            2022–2023, 2024f
    simulating motor neuron disease,
        2031–2032
    thoracic. See Thoracic radiculopathy
    traumatic, 2021–2026
        avulsion injury in, 2021–2022
            reimplantation in, 1124
        cervical, 442, 2021–2022
        in disc degeneration and spondylosis,
            2022–2026
        reinnervation in, 2025, 2025f
        thoracic, 2021
Radiculoplexopathy
    in diabetes mellitus, 2099f, 2101–2102
    in radiation therapy, 2043
Radiography
    in back and lower limb pain, 463
    in brachial plexus disorders, 2034
    in craniocerebral trauma, 548–552,
        1064–1067
    in headache, 290
    in hyperostosis, diffuse idiopathic skeletal,
        1966, 1967f
    of lumbar spine, 1972, 1973f
        indications for, 1972, 1973t
    in osteopetrosis, 1965f
    in Paget's disease of bone, 1965, 1965f
    in spina bifida, 1960, 1960f
    in spinal cord trauma, 1100, 1100t,
        1103–1108

Radionuclide scans
    of cerebral blood flow, 928–929
    in headache, 290
Radiosurgery, 957
    in arteriovenous malformations, 941, 942,
        957
        intracranial, 942, 957, 1208,
            1211–1212, 1213t
        in Wyburn-Mason syndrome, 1697
    in astrocytoma, 1268
    in cluster headache, 1867
    in craniopharyngioma, 944
    in glioma, 943, 1268
    indications for, 957
    in metastatic tumors of brain, 957
    in pituitary tumors, 943
    in schwannoma, 945, 957
    in trigeminal neuralgia, 951, 957, 1874
Ragged-red fibers, 1632
    in Kearns-Sayre syndrome, 1633, 2207,
        2208f
    in myoclonic epilepsy, 1633t, 1634,
        1741
        inheritance in, 784, 784f
        structural neuroimaging in, 545, 546
Ramsay Hunt syndrome, 336, 828, 1359,
        1875, 1885
    ataxia in, 1936, 1945
    facial palsy in, 274, 275
    vertigo in, 242
Ramus of spinal nerves, 2019, 2020f
Random errors in outcome measures of
        rehabilitation, 967
Rankin Disability Scale, 967t
Raphe nucleus
    in nociception, 901
    serotonin receptors in, 886
ras proteins, 869
    in pituitary tumors, 853
Rash
    in coma, 44t
    in dermatomyositis, 2223
    in herpes zoster virus infection,
        2029–2030
    in Lyme disease, 1337, 2029
    in Rocky Mountain spotted fever, 1344
Rasmussen's encephalitis, 1372
    seizures in, 1372, 1752
Rat-bite fever, 1347
Raynaud's disease and phenomenon, 450
Reading, 686
    in alexia, 151–152, 1590–1591. See also
        Alexia
    in aphasia, 143
        and alexia, 151–152
        Broca's, 145, 151
        Wernicke's, 146, 151
    bedside assessment of, 144, 151
    in dementia, 154, 686
    in developmental language disorders, 166,
        167t
    neuroanatomical basis of, 142
    neuropsychological assessment of, 686, 687t
    phonological, 686
    processes in, 151, 155f
Rebound phenomenon in cerebellar
        disorders, 311

Receptors
  acetylcholine, 877–879. *See also*
      Acetylcholine, receptors
  γ-aminobutyric acid, 869f, 870, 871t
  dopamine, 881
  G protein-coupled, 867
  glutamate, 871–876. *See also* Glutamate,
      receptors
  growth factor, 1256–1257, 1261, 1269
    in glioma, 1269
  gustatory, 267
  in nociception, 418, 899–900, 2054
    activation of, 902
    muscle, 397
  olfactory, 263, 264, 264f
  opioid, 901, 902
  in sensory unit, 417, 418t
  serotonin, 886–887
    clinical role of, 887, 888t
  viral, 834–835, 834t
Recognition
  of faces, 682, 688–691
    in prosopagnosia, 134, 690, 691–692
  of familiar phonation, 137
  of objects. *See* Object recognition and use
Recruitment
  in electromyography, 515–516, 516f
  in sensorineural hearing loss, 258
Rectus muscles of eye, 203, 204f, 204t
  axis of rotation and muscle plane, 205f
  history in weakness of, 208
  palsy of, 206f
    clinical tests in, 211f
    head movements and posture in, 209,
        209f
Red glass test in diplopia, 210, 211f
Referred pain, 368–369, 418, 900
  to back and lower limb, 456, 461
  common syndromes in, 903t
  from muscles, 398
  nociceptive, 902
  patterns of, 369f
Reflex sympathetic dystrophy, 365, 426,
      448, 904, 2140
  lower limb pain in, 460
Reflexes
  acoustic. *See* Acoustic reflex
  autonomic, dysfunction of, 980–981
  in back and lower limb pain, 456–457,
      457t
  in brachial plexus disorders, 2032
  in brain death, 56
  bulbocavernous, 750
  in cerebellar disorders, 313, 313f, 1944
  in cervical spine disorders, 370, 377
  in coma, 51, 1470, 1471t
  facial, 273
  in floppy infant, 407–409
  gag, 173, 182, 278
  glabellar, 94, 273, 323
  in lower limb, 451, 452, 454t
    in coma, 51
  in lumbosacral plexus disorders, 2038–2039
  in motor neuron disorders, 1987, 1990
  in multiple sclerosis, 1440
  in myoclonus
    cortical, 1754

  reticular, 1754
  oculocephalic, 49–50, 50t
    in combined vertical gaze
        ophthalmoplegia, 293
    in parkinsonism, 323
  in personality changes, 94
  plantar, 51
  postural, 341, 342
    examination of, 344
    in floppy infant, 408
    rehabilitation of, 980–981
  pupillary light. *See* Pupils, light reaction of
  radial, inversion of, 370
  in radiculopathy, 441, 443t, 2023
  spinal cord function in, 369–370
    in coma, 51
    in spinal shock, 375, 407
  tonic neck, 407, 408–409
  vestibulo-ocular, 699, 700, 703
    in cerebellar disorders, 313, 313f
    in ocular motor apraxia, 708
Reflux, gastroesophageal. *See*
      Gastroesophageal reflux
Refractive errors, headache in, 1844
Refsum's disease, 1641–1642, 2077–2078
  infantile, 1638, 1638t
  peripheral neuropathy in, 2078
Regeneration of nerves, 421, 2046
  axons in, 976, 1116, 1118
  delayed or failed, 1118, 1124
  facial, aberrant, 276, 1885
  oculomotor, aberrant, 214, 1881
    eyelid retraction in, 235, 237, 1881
  time course of, 1116–1118
Regression, developmental, 81, 85–86, 87t
Rehabilitation, 862, 959–1001, 1163
  adaptive equipment in, 988–989
  in amyotrophic lateral sclerosis,
      2012–2013
  in aphasia, 158–159, 991–993. *See also*
      Aphasia, recovery and
      rehabilitation in
  assessment procedures in, 964, 965–968
    Barthel Index in, 965t, 966, 967t, 968t
    clinical usefulness of, 966–967
    floor and ceiling effects in, 967, 968t
    Functional Independence Measure in,
        965t, 966, 966t, 968t
    outcome measures in, 965–968,
        997–1001
    reliability and validity of, 967
    responsiveness of, 968
    scientific soundness of, 967–968
  in behavioral disorders, 995–996, 996t
  behavioral strategies in, 973
  biofeedback in, 986
  biological interventions in, 976, 976t
  in bladder dysfunction, 981–982, 981t
  in bowel dysfunction, 982
  in cerebral palsy, 1586
  in childhood cerebrovascular disorders,
      1223
  in chronic and progressive disorders, 971
  in cognitive impairment and disability,
      989–997
  common complications in, 977–997
  in community setting, 970

  in contractures, 980
  cortical and subcortical representational
      adaptations in, 974–976, 975f
  in craniocerebral trauma, 978, 978t
    functional outcome in, 998–999,
        999t
    prognostic factors in, 1077–1086
  definitions of, 959
  distributed network processing of signals
      in, 973–974, 973t
  drug therapy in, 976–977
  in dysautonomia, 980–981
  in dysphagia, 978–979, 979t
  functional outcomes in, 997–998
    in craniocerebral trauma, 998–999,
        999t
    in multiple sclerosis, 999–1001
    in Parkinson's disease, 999
    in spinal cord injury, 998, 999t
    in stroke, 997–998
  goals and aims of, 959–960
    categories of, 969, 969f
    determination of, 964
  in hemi-inattention, 995, 996t
  in inpatient unit, 969–970
  integrated care pathways in, 968–969
  local and regional services in, 970–971
  in memory disturbances, 993–995
  in multiple sclerosis. *See* Multiple
      sclerosis, rehabilitation in
  neural prostheses in, 988
  neuroscientific basis of interventions in,
      971–977
    potential mechanisms in, 971, 972t
  nursing care in, 960–961
  occupational therapy in, 962–963
  orthotic devices in, 963–964, 987–988
  outreach services in, 970
  pain management in, 982, 986
  in Parkinson's disease, 999
  in peripheral nerve trauma, 1124
  personnel in, 960–964, 960t
  physical therapy in, 961–962, 962f,
      984–989
  psychosocial aspects of, 963
  recovery of neuronal function in, 971–972
    in partially spared pathways, 972
  in right and left hemisphere dysfunction,
      comparison of, 121
  in seizures, 980
  skin care in, 979
  in sleep disorders, 982
  in spasticity, 982–984
  speech and language therapy in, 963,
      992–993
  in spinal cord ischemia, 1228
  in spinal cord trauma, 978, 978t, 980,
      1111
    functional outcome in, 998, 999t
    orthoses in, 987, 988
    skin care in, 979, 1103
  thromboembolism prevention in, 980
  treadmill training in, 986
Reiter's syndrome, 1979–1981
  neurological complications in, 1980,
      1981t
Relapsing fever, 1337–1338

in hemophilia, 1024
history-taking in, 4, 5, 15, 1767
in hyperglycinemia, 1605
in hyperprolactinemia, 850–851
in hypocalcemia, 1030
in hypomelanosis of Ito, 1692
hysterical, 101, 1762
idiopathic, 1745–1746
in infections, 1762
ion channels in, 1766
    calcium, 891, 1766
    sodium, 890, 1766
jack-knife, 1757
jacksonian, 1748
kindling in, 875t, 876, 887
in Lafora's disease, 1759
in Landau-Kleffner syndrome, 1758
language disorders in, 161
    aphasia, 158
    verbal auditory agnosia, 164
in Lennox-Gastaut syndrome. See
        Lennox-Gastaut syndrome
in lipofuscinosis, neuronal ceroid, 1647,
        1647t, 1648
in lupus erythematosus, 1018
magnetic resonance imaging in, 16, 671,
        672, 955, 1768
magnetoencephalography in, 955, 1768
membrane depolarizations in, 1569
in Menkes' syndrome, 1624, 1688
in metabolic disorders, 1476, 1758–1759
in migraine, 1848
in multiple sclerosis, 1438
in muscular dystrophy, Fukuyama type,
        2205
myoclonic, 336, 1754
    astasia in, 1758
    cortical reflex, 1754
    encephalopathy in, 1757
    epidemiology of, 765, 766f
    in infants, benign, 1756
    juvenile, 1746, 1756
        on awakening, 1803
    primary generalized, 1754
    progressive, 1758–1759
    with ragged-red fibers, 1633t, 1634,
            1741
        inheritance of, 784, 784f
        structural neuroimaging in, 545, 546
    reticular reflex, 1754
in neonate. See Neonates, seizures in
neuronal plasticity in, 1766
nocturnal, 1803
norepinephrine and epinephrine in, 885,
        885t
nystagmus in, 222–223
obsessive-compulsive behavior in, 99
occipital, 1749
    benign, 1751
with occipital paroxysms, 1751
olfaction in, 263, 267, 1749
paralysis after, transient, 356
parietal lobe, 1748–1749
partial, 1747–1752, 1747t
    clinical features in, 1748
    complex, 16, 1749–1751

compared with absence seizures, 16t,
        1750t
    epidemiology of, 765, 766f
drug therapy in, 1774
electroencephalography in, 1748, 1751
    motor, 1748
    sensory, 1748–1749
    simple, 1748–1749
pathophysiology in, 1765–1766
petit mal, 1714
    electroencephalography in, 477, 478f
    epidemiology of, 765, 766f
    functional neuroimaging in, 672
physical examination in, 15, 1767
in porphyria, 1621
positron emission tomography in, 671,
        672, 955, 1768, cp38E.II
in pregnancy. See Pregnancy, seizures in
prognosis in, 1746
prolactin serum levels in, 17, 98,
        850–851, 1752
    in psychogenic seizures, 1763
psychogenic, 17, 17t, 1762–1763
    compared with epileptic seizures, 17,
            17t, 1762–1763
    electroencephalography in, 1763
    prolactin serum levels in, 1763
    treatment of, 1763
psychomotor, benign, 1751
psychosis in, 111, 112, 114
in Rasmussen's encephalitis, 1372, 1752
recurrent, risk for, 1746
    in discontinuation of drug therapy,
            1775–1776
    in fever, 1755
rehabilitation in, 980
remote symptomatic, 1745
rolandic, 1751
    electroencephalography in, 477, 479f,
            1751
    in sleep, 1803
serotonin in, 887, 888t
sexual function in, 93, 100, 432
single or isolated, 766
single-photon emission computed
        tomography in, 671, 955,
        1768–1769, cp38E.II
and sleep, 1802–1804. See also Sleep, and
        seizures
startle, 1921
in status epilepticus, 1759–1761. See also
        Status epilepticus
in Sturge-Weber syndrome, 1682–1683,
        1684
surgery in, 955, 1776–1777
    indications for, 1776–1777
    procedures in, 1777
    results of, 1776, 1777t
syncope compared with, 9, 10t
temporal lobe, 93–94, 476
    complex partial, 1750
    electroencephalography in, 1751
    functional neuroimaging in, 671
    hallucinations in, 111, 1749, 1750
    mesial sclerosis in, 1765
    pathophysiology in, 1765
    sexual function in, 432

simple partial sensory, 1749
surgery in, 1777
in Todd's paralysis, 711
tonic, 1754
    in sleep, 1803
tonic-clonic, 15–16, 1752–1753
    on awakening, 1756
    clinical features in, 1752
    electroencephalography in, 476, 477f,
            482f, 1753
    epidemiology of, 765, 766f
    injuries in, 1752–1753
    phases in, 1752
in toxic encephalopathy, 1476
in tuberous sclerosis, 1667
in Unverricht-Lundborg disease, 1759
in uremic encephalopathy, 1483
violent behavior in, 1750–1751
vision loss in, transient, 189–190
in vitamin B_6 deficiency, 1501–1502
in West's syndrome, 1757–1758
Selegiline, 881
    in Parkinson's disease, 1896, 1898, 1898t
Self-care skills, 998–999
    in brain trauma, 998–999, 999t
    in spinal cord injury, 998, 999t
    in stroke, 998
Self-injury in Lesch-Nyhan disease, 1619,
        1619f, 1681, 1681f
Sella turcica, 847, 848f
    in empty sella syndrome, 847, 853
    tumors in region of, 853
Semantics, 141–142
    errors in, 143
    memory of, 135, 136, 681–682
        in amnesia, 679, 681
        in dementia, 135, 681, 686, 1715, 1734
        neuropsychological assessment of, 682
    in semantic pragmatic syndrome, 164–165
    and visual object recognition, 690–691
        for faces, 691–692
Semicircular canals, 700
    stimulation of, 702f
Senescence, cellular death in, 1254
Sensation, 417
Sensitivity and specificity of tests, 469
    limitations in, 471
Sensory function, 417–426
    age-related changes in, 2273
    in alcoholic neuropathy, 1506
    in amyloidosis, 419, 424, 424f, 437, 1023
    in ataxia, 310, 344, 345t, 347
        differential diagnosis in, 2050–2051,
                2051t
        and gait, 347
    in back and lower limb pain, 457
    in brachial plexus disorders, 2032, 2033
    brainstem in, 425
    case illustrations on disorders of,
            419–421, 423, 425
    chemosensory system in, 263
    dermatomes in, 369, 371f
    in diabetes mellitus, 1033
    distal symmetrical syndromes of, 423–424
    in dizziness and vertigo
        examination of, 249
        loss of, 247–248, 249

Spinal cord, 367–380
    anterior horn cells of. *See* Anterior horn
        cells
    arachnoiditis of, chronic adhesive,
        1981–1982
    autonomic dysfunction in disorders of,
        373–375, 2138
    bladder function in disorders of. *See*
        Bladder, in spinal cord disorders
    blood supply of, 375–376, 376f
        anatomy of, 1225–1226, 1226f
        disorders of, 1225–1230
        magnetic resonance angiography of,
            607–609
    cell counts in chronic primary autonomic
        failure, 2135–2136, 2137f
    central canal of, 1957, 1957f
    central cord syndrome of. *See* Central
        cord syndrome
    central pattern generators in, 342
    cervical. *See* Cervical spinal cord
    characteristics of lesions at different levels,
        376–378
        in trauma, 1092
    classification of disorders, 379–380, 379t
    clinical features in disorders of, 377–378
    compression of
        causes of, 935
        in epidural metastases, 379–380,
            1281–1285
        surgery in, 935, 1110, 1110t
    cysts of, 1288
        post-traumatic, 1101
            cervical, 583–584, 586f
            thoracic, 589
    degeneration in vitamin B$_{12}$ deficiency,
        1497, 1498f, 2112–2113
    demyelination of, 434–435, 436
        hemiplegia in, 359
        monoplegia in, 360
    in diastematomyelia, 1962, 1962f
    distributed network processing of signals
        in, 974
    edema of, 582–583, 585f, 1107
        magnetic resonance imaging in,
            582–583, 585f, 1107
    extramedullary disorders of
        differentiated from intramedullary
            disorders, 378–379
        intradural tumors, 574–575,
            1287–1288
    facial vascular changes in disorders of,
        2143
    falls in disease of, 21
    in fecal continence, 374, 757
    floppy infant in disorders of, 412
    gastrointestinal system in disorders of,
        374, 435, 982, 2147
        traumatic, 982, 1109
    hemisection syndrome of, 375, 1097,
        1098f
        hemiplegia in, 359, 360t
        monoplegia in, 361
        sensory signs in, 373
    hemorrhage, 1229–1230. *See also*
        Hemorrhage, spinal
    hypertension in disorders of, 2142

infarction of, 375–376, 1226, 1227
    in aortic surgery, 1015
intramedullary disorders of
    differentiated from extramedullary
        disorders, 378–379
    tumors, 575, 1288–1291
        syringomyelia in, 1958
ischemia of, 1226–1228
    in aortic disorders, 1014, 1227
    causes of, 1227–1228, 1227t
lateral and posterior column disease of,
    376
localization of lesions in transverse plane,
    371–375
lumbar, blood supply of, 1225
in motor function. *See* Motor function,
    spinal cord in
myelitis of. *See* Myelitis
in myelomeningocele, 1961, 1961f
myelopathy of. *See* Myelopathy
myoclonus in disorders of, 1920
nerve roots attached to, 2019–2020,
    2020f
pain in disorders of, 439, 440f
    in arm and neck, 439
    deep segmental, 439
    in ischemia, 1226
    post-traumatic, 1102
posterior and lateral column disease of,
    376
pyramidal tract disorders of, 376
in reflexes, 369–370
    in coma, 51
    in spinal shock, 375, 407
in respiratory function, 373
    sleep disturbances in disorders of, 1805
segmental innervation of, 367–371
in sensory function. *See* Sensory function,
    spinal cord in
in sexual function, 374–375, 435–436, 756
sleep disturbances in disorders of, 1805
spinal nerves corresponding to segments
    of, 423, 424f, 2020, 2021f
in syringomyelia, 1956–1959. *See also*
    Syringomyelia
tethered, 1961–1964, 1961t
    bladder function in, 435
    causes of, 1961, 1961t
    evoked potentials in, somatosensory,
        493, 493f
thoracic
    blood supply of, 1225
    clinical features in disorders of,
        377–378
    trauma of, 589, 1090, 1092
trauma of, 978, 978t, 1089–1111
    anterior cord syndrome in, 1097, 1097f
    in birth injuries, 2250–2251
    bladder function in, 373–374, 434, 752,
        755, 1109, 2147
        management of, 981–982, 1109
    bowel function in, 982, 1109
        management of, 1109
    Brown-Séquard syndrome in. *See*
        Brown-Séquard syndrome
    bulbar-cervical dissociation pattern in,
        1094

of cauda equina, 1098–1099, 1099f
causes of, 1090
central cord syndrome in, 375, 421,
    1094–1097, 1096f
cervical. *See* Cervical spinal cord,
    trauma of
cervicomedullary syndrome in, 1094,
    1095f
chronic syndromes in, 1101–1102,
    1101t
classification of, 1089, 1090–1092,
    1093f
clinical manifestations in, 1092–1102
complete, 1092, 1094t
complications in, 978, 978t
computed tomography in, 1092, 1100,
    1104f, 1105, 1106f
contractures in, 980
contusion and monoplegia in, 361
conus medullaris syndrome in,
    1097–1098, 1099f
coup and contrecoup, 378
cysts in, 583–584, 586f, 589, 1101
depression in, 996, 997
dis-complete syndrome in, 1092, 1102
distributed network processing of
    signals in, 974
drug therapy in, 1109
dysautonomia in, 980, 981
edema in, 582–583, 585f, 1107
in electrical injuries, 1542
epidemiology of, 1090
epidural hematoma in, 588–589, 592f,
    1107
functional outcome in, 998, 999t
hemorrhage in, 582–583, 586f, 1107
hyperhidrosis in, 2145
hypothermia in, 1109, 2146
immobilization in, 1102, 1109–1110
incomplete, 1092, 1094–1098, 1094t
level of, 1091–1092, 1091t
    and clinical manifestations, 1092
magnetic resonance imaging in. *See*
    Magnetic resonance imaging, in
    spinal cord trauma
management of, 1102–1111
    in field, 1102–1103
marshy cord syndrome in, 1101
monoplegia in, 361
multiple injuries in, 1091
myelography in, 1105
myelomalacia in. *See* Myelomalacia,
    post-traumatic
nerve root stimulators in, 755
neurological examination in, 1103
orthoses in, 987, 988
orthostatic hypotension in, 2141
pain in, 982, 1102
penetrating, 1101
posterior cord syndrome in, 1097,
    1098f
in pre-existing spinal disorders, 1091
radiography in, 1100, 1100t,
    1103–1108
rehabilitation in, 978, 978t, 980,
    1111
    functional outcome in, 998, 999t

Trauma—*continued*
  in noise exposure, 1542
  of oculomotor nerve, 1061, 1880
  of pelvic nerves, 437
  of peripheral nerves, 1113–1124. *See also*
      Peripheral nerves, trauma of
  personality changes in, 91, 94
  in radiation exposure, 1541–1542
  of sacral plexus, 363
  in seizures, 1752–1753
  seizures in, 980, 1076, 1761–1762
    prevention of, 1076, 1761–1762
  of spinal cord. *See* Spinal cord, trauma of
  of spine. *See* Spine, trauma of
  stress disorder in, 91, 97
    diagnostic criteria in, 98t
  taste sense in, 268
  of trigeminal nerve, 1883
  trochlear nerve palsy in, 1882
  in vibration exposure, 1543
Travel
  altitude changes in, 1020, 1467
    and insomnia, 1791
  interstate illusions or highway hallucinosis
      in, 216
  jet lag in, 67, 1784, 1789, 1802, 1823
Treadmill training in rehabilitation, 985, 986
Trematode infections, 1387t, 1402–1404
Tremor, 324–327, 1891t, 1905–1908
  action, 324
    of legs, 350
  in ataxia, 310, 312, 324, 347
  cerebellar, 347, 1907
  classification of, 325t
  cogwheel, 322
  compared with myoclonus, 336, 337
  differential diagnosis in, 325t
  in drug withdrawal, 1907–1908
  in dystonia, 331
  essential, 1905–1907
    alcohol response in, 1906, 1907
    clinical features in, 1905–1906, 1906f
    genetic factors in, 1906
    treatment of, 1906–1907
  examination in, 326–327, 327f
  of head, 310, 312, 324, 325, 1906
    in cerebellar ataxia, 347
    examination in, 326
  Holmes, 1907
  intention, 312, 324
  kinetic, 324
  of legs, 350
  in multiple sclerosis, 1440, 1454
  of palate, 173, 326
  parkinsonian, 322, 1892–1893, 1906
    examination in, 326
  peduncular, 312
  physiological, 1906, 1907
  postural, 324–325, 326, 1906
    drug-induced, 1921t
    orthostatic, 325, 326, 350, 1907
  resting, 324, 326
  rubral, 312, 327, 1907
  speech disorders in, 173, 326
  static, 324
  surgery in, 955, 1907
  terminal, 324, 326

  of vocal cords, 173, 176
  in Wilson's disease, 326, 329, 1924
  in writing, 325, 326, 327f, 1906, 1906f,
      1907
Treponema pallidum infection, 1334–1336.
    See also Syphilis
Triamcinolone in cluster headache, 1865
Triazolam in insomnia, 1824t, 1825
Triceps brachii reflex in cervical spine
    disorders, 370, 377
Trichinosis, 1398
Trichloroethylene, occupational exposure to,
    1516
Trichopoliodystrophy, 1624, 1687–1689.
    See also Menkes' syndrome
Trichorrhexis nodosa in Menkes' syndrome,
    1624, 1687
Trichothiodystrophy, 1697–1698, 1938
Triclabendazole in fascioliasis, 1404
Triethylene tetramine in Wilson's disease,
    1624, 1925
Trifluridine, 1356t
Trigeminal artery, persistent, 621, 621f, 622f
Trigeminal nerve, 1882–1883
  anatomy of, 1882
  dysarthria in disorders of, 175t
  herpes virus infections of, 1875, 1883, 2029
  mandibular division of, 1882
  maxillary division of, 1882
  motor portion of, 1882
  neuralgia of, 287, 1872–1874
    alcohol block in, 1873–1874
    clinical symptoms in, 1872
    course and prognosis in, 1873
    differential diagnosis in, 277
    drug therapy in, 1873
    epidemiology of, 1873
    etiology of, 1873
    laboratory tests in, 1873
    in multiple sclerosis, 1439, 1873
    pathology of, 1873
    physical examination in, 1872–1873
    postherpetic, 1875, 1883
    radiological findings in, 1873
    surgery in, 950–951, 1874
      radiosurgery technique, 951, 957, 1874
    thermocoagulation in, 1874
  numb chin and cheek syndromes in
      disorders of, 1882
  in olfaction, 263
    clinical evaluation of, 265
  ophthalmic division of, 1882
    herpes virus infections of, 1875, 1883
  sensory portion of, 1882
    neuropathy of, 1882, 2110–2111
    section procedure in neuralgia, 1874
    traumatic neuropathy of, 1883
    in trigeminal-levator synkinesis, 234, 235,
        237
Trigger points in fibromyalgia, 458, 1983,
    1983f
Triglycerides, medium chain, in nutritional
    management of seizures, 1776
Trihexyphenidyl in idiopathic torsion
    dystonia, 1908
Trimethoprim-sulfamethoxazole
  in melioidosis, 1347

  in meningitis, 1319t, 1322t
  in nocardiosis, 1350
  in shigellosis, 1347
  in Whipple's disease, 1348
Trisomy 21. *See* Down syndrome
Trochlear nerve, 1881–1882
  anatomy of, 1881–1882
  in diabetes mellitus, 1033, 2101
  eye movements in disorders of, 716
  palsy of, 1882
Trojan horse model of CNS viral infections,
    832
Trolard vein, 630, 630f
Tropical ataxic neuropathy, 2124
Tropical spastic paraparesis, 828, 1989,
    2124
Tropism, 834
Trypanosomiasis, 1390–1393
  African, 66, 1390–1392, 1812
    seizures in, 1762
  American, 1392–1393. *See also* Chagas'
      disease
Tryptophan, 885
  eosinophilia-myalgia syndrome from, 2121
  metabolism disorders, 1605–1606, 1606t
  neuropathy from, 2117t, 2121
Tuberculoma, 555, 1330
Tuberculosis, 1329–1332
  endarteritis and ischemic cerebrovascular
      disease in, 1144
  meningitis in, 555, 555f, 1330
    complications in, 1331–1332, 1331f,
        1332f
    computed tomography in, 555f
    magnetic resonance imaging in, 1331f,
        1332f
  prevention of, 1332
  psoas abscess in, 2041
  seizures in, 1762
  spinal, 1329, 1331, 1977, 1977f
    magnetic resonance imaging in, 1977,
        1977f
  spondylitis in, 589–590
Tuberin, 1666
Tuberous sclerosis, 1666–1672
  astrocytoma in
    retinal, 1670f
    subependymal giant cell, 534, 535f,
        563, 1244, 1669
  calcified nodules in, subependymal, 1669,
      1669f
  cardiac disorders in, 1671, 1671f
  cutaneous features in, 1666–1667, 1667f,
      1668f
  diagnostic criteria for, 1666, 1666t
  genetic factors in, 1666
  hamartoma in, 563
    astrocytic, cp15.XXIV
    retinal, 1669
  neurological features in, 1667–1669
  pulmonary disorders in, 1672
  renal disorders in, 1671–1672, 1671f
  retinal features in, 1669–1671, 1670f
Tularemia, 1346
Tullio's phenomenon, 717
Tumor necrosis factor, 1253
  α, 811, 812t

Van Allen amyloidosis, 2073
Vancomycin in meningitis, 1319t, 1320,
    1321t
Varicella zoster virus infections, 1359–1360,
    2029–2030
  congenital, 1357
  dorsal root ganglion in, 828, 2029
  of geniculate ganglion, 1875, 2123
  in HIV infection and AIDS, radiculitis in,
    2123
  myelitis in, 827
  ophthalmicus, 1359, 2029, 2030
  otic, 1359
    vertigo in, 242
  pain in, 420, 423, 442, 1359, 1360, 2030
    management of, 1875
  peripheral neuropathy in, 2123–2124
  reactivation of, 828, 829, 833, 1359
  spread of, 833, 834
  treatment of, 1356t, 1359, 1360, 2030
    immune globulin in, 1357t, 1359
    pain management in, 1875
  trigeminal neuralgia in, 1875, 1883, 2029
  vasculitis in, 1233, 1360, 2030
Vascular cell adhesion molecules, 810
  in viral infections of CNS, 832, 833
Vascular disorders, 1125–1234. *See also*
    specific disorders
  aneurysm, 1185–1198
  angiography in, 617–643
    computed tomographic, 609–613
    magnetic resonance, 595–609
  in cancer therapy, 1312
  cerebellar, 1933–1934
  cerebral, 1125–1224
    in children, 1215–1224
  in craniocerebral trauma, 550–552, 553f
    magnetic resonance angiography in,
    552, 553f
  dementia in, 1721–1728
  hemorrhage
    intracerebral, 1167–1183
    spinal, 1229–1230
    subarachnoid, 1185–1198
      spinal, 1229
  ischemia
    cerebral, 1125–1165
    spinal cord, 1226–1228
  malformations, 564–566, 940–942,
    1201–1213
    capillary telangiectasia, 564, 940
    cavernous angioma, 564, 940–941,
    941f
    intracranial, 564, 565f, 607,
    1201–1213
    magnetic resonance angiography in,
    607, 608
    spinal, 564–566, 608, 1228–1229
      neurosurgery in, 951–953
    venous angioma, 564, 940, 940f
  parkinsonism in, 1905
  of spinal cord, 1225–1230
    hemorrhage, 1229–1230
    ischemia, 1226–1228
    malformations, 564–566, 608,
    1228–1229
      neurosurgery in, 951–953

structural neuroimaging in, 564–567
  in craniocerebral trauma, 550–552, 553f
  vasculitis, 1015–1017, 1231–1234
Vasculitis, 1015–1017, 1231–1234,
    2106–2109. *See also* Arteritis
  brain biopsy in, 955
  of central nervous system, 1231–1234
  cerebrovascular disorders in
    in children, 1219
    hemorrhage, 1013, 1172, 1231
    ischemia, 1144–1146
  classification of, 2106, 2106t
  in drug abuse, 1233, 1526
  hypersensitivity, 2107
  lumbosacral plexus disorders in, 2043
  peripheral neuropathy in, 1015, 2105,
    2106–2109, 2106t
    clinical features in, 2107
    in giant cell arteritis, 1017, 1841, 1843,
    2107
    laboratory features in, 2107–2108
    pathogenesis in, 2107
    patterns of, 2107, 2108f
    in polyarteritis nodosa, 1015, 2106
    treatment of, 2108–2109
  retinal infarction in, 199
  in rheumatoid arthritis, 2109
  systemic necrotizing, 2106, 2106t, 2108
  in varicella zoster virus infections, 1233,
    1360
Vasoactive intestinal polypeptide, 842t
Vasoconstriction, reversible cerebral, 1232
  idiopathic segmental, 1148
Vasopressin. *See* Antidiuretic hormone
Vasospasm
  in drug abuse, 1526
  in subarachnoid hemorrhage, 640–641,
    660–662, 936
    angioplasty in, 937, 937f, 1195, 1196f
    cerebral ischemia in, 1193, 1194–1195
    drug therapy in, 937, 1195
    electroencephalography in, 928f
    neurointensive care monitoring in, 925t,
    928f, 930
    prevention of, 641, 937
    surgery in, 936, 937, 937f, 1193
    ultrasonography in, 661–662, 930
  syncope in, 13
Vasotonin, 885
VDRL test in syphilis, 1335, 1336
Vectors, 792
Vegetative state, persistent, 38, 38t, 1469
  ocular reflex in, 50
  outcomes in, 978, 978t
  prognosis in, 55–56
Velocity in nerve conduction studies, 498,
    499
  age affecting, 508, 508f, 509t
  in proximal and distal segments, 506–508
Venezuelan equine encephalitis, 1366
Venography, intracranial
  anatomy in, 629–633
  magnetic resonance technique, 605–607
Venom
  scorpion, 1530–1531, 1530t
  snake, 1529–1530, 1530t
  spider, 1530, 1530t

Ventilation. *See also* Respirations
  mechanical. *See* Ventilatory support
  minute, 920, 921
  spontaneous, 921
Ventilatory support, 919–923
  in amyotrophic lateral sclerosis, 2014
  assist/control, 920, 921–922
  in autonomic disorders, 2164
  bradycardia and cardiac arrest in, 2143,
    2145f
  bronchopulmonary dysplasia in, 1039
  continuous positive airway pressure in,
    920, 921
  in Guillain-Barré syndrome, 924, 2080,
    2083
  indications for, 919
  in myasthenia gravis, 923–924, 2180
  positive end-expiratory pressure in,
    920–921
  pressure control mode, 921, 922
  pressure support, 920, 922
    in myasthenia gravis, 923–924
  quality of life and ethical issues in,
    864–865
  in sleep apnea, 1821, 1822
  in spinal cord trauma, 1108
  synchronized intermittent mandatory,
    920, 921, 922
    in myasthenia gravis, 923–924
  weaning in, 922–923
  volume control mode, 921–922
  weaning from, 922–923
    in myasthenia gravis, 924
Ventral spinal nerve roots, 419f, 2019, 2020,
    2020f
  motor function in disorders of, 367–368
  ramus of, 2019
  trauma of, 2021
Ventricles, cerebral
  choroid plexus tumors of, 1246, 1246f
  in colpocephaly, 1579–1580
  in corpus callosum agenesis, 1579f, 1589
  ependymal cells of, 1548
  hemorrhage in, 1176t, 1180
  third, tumors of
    clinical features in, 1265
    colloid cyst, 1251, 1251f. *See also*
    Colloid cyst
    falls and drop attacks in, 20
Ventricular arrhythmias
  neurological complications in, 1011
  syncope in, 12, 19, 1011
Ventriculitis and bacterial meningitis in
    neonate, 2248, 2248f
Ventriculoatrial shunt in hydrocephalus, 1555
Ventriculoencephalitis, cytomegalovirus, in
    HIV infection and AIDS, 1417
Ventriculoperitoneal shunt in hydrocephalus,
    1555
Ventriculostomy, 931–932, 1070, 1072
  in cerebellar hemorrhage and infarction,
    932, 933
  in subarachnoid hemorrhage, 936
Verapamil
  in cluster headache, 1866
  in migraine, 1858
    menstrual, 1861t

Virchow-Robin spaces, 1548
Viremia, 831–832
    active, 831
    cell-associated, 831–832
    passive, 831
    primary, 831
    secondary, 831
    transit time in, 831
Viruses
    infection with. *See* Viral infections
    as vectors in gene transfer therapy, 1260
Vision, 187–192, 721–731
    acuity of, 721
        best corrected, 722
        examination of, 722
    and agnosia, 131–136, 688
        for faces, 134, 690, 691–692, 1722
        for objects, 690
    in amaurosis fugax, 188, 1130, 1841, 1843
    in ataxia, 311
        autosomal dominant, 1946, 1947
        optic, 692–693
    axis alignment in, 203, 204, 206f
        in diplopia, 205–216
        primary and secondary deviations in, 204, 206f
    causes of disorders in, 190t, 191t
    central, 721
        loss of, 187
    cerebral cortex areas in, 71–72, 721–722
    in cerebrovascular disorders, 1839
        in brainstem ischemic stroke syndromes, 299
    chiasmal loss of, 187, 191
    in children, 730–731, 730t
        transient loss of, 189–190
    color
        in achromatopsia, 689
        testing of, 723
    contrast sensitivity in, 722
    in convergence disorders, 717
    in diplopia, 205–216. *See also* Diplopia
    in divergence insufficiency, 718
    and evoked potentials, visual, 486–488
    examination of, 722–726
        in children, 730–731
        in dizziness and vertigo, 248
        in headache, 291
    eye movements in, 203, 205f, 206f
    false image in, 203, 206f
    in giant cell arteritis, 1841, 1843
    gradual loss of, 191–192
    and headache, 291, 1844
        in migraine, 188, 190, 1847–1848
    and hypernychthemeral syndrome, 1802
    in hypothalamic-pituitary disorders, 856
    in intracranial pressure increase, 1552, 1553
    in light stress, 188, 722–723
        testing of, 722–723
    in lipofuscinosis, neuronal ceroid, 1647, 1647t, 1648
    in multiple sclerosis, 1438–1439
    near
        measurement of, 722, 723f
        spasm of, 717–718, 718t

    in neuromyelitis optica, 191, 359
    and object recognition, 688–691
    in obscurations, transient, 188–189
    in onchocerciasis, 1399
    in parkinsonism, 321–322
    patterns of loss, 187, 189f
    peripheral, 187, 721
    prechiasmal loss of, 187, 191
    in pseudoxanthoma elasticum, 1677
    psychogenic disorders of, 729–730
    retrochiasmal loss of, 187
    and spatial skills. *See* Visual-spatial skills
    sudden loss of, 188–191
    transient loss of, 188–190, 188t
    type and severity of loss, 187
    in vitamin A deficiency, 1508
    in Wyburn-Mason syndrome, 1696
Visual evoked potentials. *See* Evoked potentials, visual
Visual fields, 726–729
    central
        loss of, 187
        measurement of, 725, 727f
    constricted, 725, 726f, 729–730
    nasal, 721
    patterns of disorders, 187, 189f
    peripheral, 187, 721–722
        measurement of, 725–726
    psychogenic disorders of, 726f, 729–730, 730f
    in Sturge-Weber syndrome, 1683
    temporal, 721, 722, 722f
    testing of, 724–726
        rules in interpretation of, 726–729, 726t
Visual grasp, 120
Visual-spatial skills, 692–694
    in Alzheimer's disease, 1705
    bedside tests of, 78, 78f
    central impairment of, 693–694
    in delirium, 27
    point localization in, 692–693
    primary impairment of, 692–693
Vitamin A
    deficiency of, 1508
    in measles, 1356t, 1366–1367
    toxicity of, 1508
        pseudotumor cerebri in, 1508, 1553
Vitamin B$_6$
    deficiency of, 1501–1502, 2112
        from isoniazid, 1502, 2112, 2119
        neonatal seizure in, 2239, 2240t
        peripheral neuropathy in, 2112
    in homocystinuria, 1601, 1602
    in multiple sclerosis and tremor, 1454
    neuropathy from, 2117t, 2120
        sensory, 1502
    in tuberculosis, 1331
    in Wilson's disease, 1624
Vitamin B$_{12}$
    deficiency of, 1021–1022, 1496–1499
        clinical features in, 1496
        cognitive function in, 1740
        diagnosis of, 1021, 1496–1497, 2113
            Schilling test in, 1021, 1497, 1498, 2113
        serum measurements in, 1497, 2113

    in gastric surgery, 1027, 1498
    in malabsorption, 1496, 1498, 2112
    from nitrous oxide, 1497, 1498, 2119
    peripheral neuropathy in, 2112–2113
    spinal cord degeneration in, 1497, 1498f, 2112–2113
    treatment of, 1021–1022, 1498–1499, 2113
    in methylmalonic acidemia, 1611
Vitamin D, 1508–1509
    deficiency of, 1508–1509
Vitamin E
    in Alzheimer's disease, 1712
    antioxidant functions of, 1500
    deficiency of, 1499–1501, 1938–1939, 2113
        ataxia in, 316, 1499, 1938–1939
        causes of, 1500, 1500t, 1939, 2113
        clinical features in, 1499–1500, 1938, 1939t
        diagnosis of, 1500, 2113
        in lipoprotein deficiency, 1621, 1622, 1939, 2078
        peripheral neuropathy in, 2113
        treatment of, 1500–1501, 1939, 2113
Vitamin K in pregnancy and seizures, 1764, 2253, 2264
Vocabulary. *See* Words
Vocal cords, 171
    abuse of, 173
    assessment of, 175–176, 177
    paralysis of, 174, 175–176, 176t
    tremor of, 173, 176
Vocalizations in coma, 45
Vogt-Koyanagi-Harada syndrome, 1979
Voice
    arrest of, 176
    in myasthenia gravis, 2169
Voltage-gated ion channels, 887–893. *See also* Ion channels
Vomiting. *See* Nausea and vomiting
Von Graefe's sign, 235
Von Hippel–Lindau disease, 1694–1696
    clinical features in, 1694–1695
    hemangioblastoma in, 575, 1249, 1694–1695, 1696
    molecular genetics in, 1695
    pheochromocytoma in, 1694, 1694t, 1695
    renal cell carcinoma in, 1694t, 1695
    retina in, 200, 200f, 1694, 1695, 1696
    systemic features in, 1695
    treatment of, 1696
Von Recklinghausen's disease, 563, 1672–1673. *See also* Neurofibromatosis, type 1
Vorbeireden, 102
Vowel sounds in speech, 171
    assessment of, 175–176, 177

Wakefulness, 25, 1782, 1782t
    ascending reticular activating system in, 1783
    behavioral and physiological criteria in, 59, 60t
    circadian rhythms in, 1784, 1786–1787
    disorders of. *See* Sleepiness
    maintenance test in sleep disorders, 1818
    neurobiology of, 1785–1786